Therapeutic Exercise

FOUNDATIONS AND TECHNIQUES

Seventh Edition

Therapeutic Exercise

FOUNDATIONS AND TECHNIQUES

Seventh Edition

Carolyn Kisner, PT, MS
Assistant Professor Emeritus
The Ohio State University
School of Health and Rehabilitation Sciences
Physical Therapy Division
Columbus, Ohio

Lynn Allen Colby, PT, MS
Assistant Professor Emeritus
The Ohio State University
School of Health and Rehabilitation Sciences
Physical Therapy Division
Columbus, Ohio

John Borstad, PT, PhD
Professor and Chair
College of St. Scholastica
School of Health Sciences
Department of Physical Therapy
Duluth, Minnesota

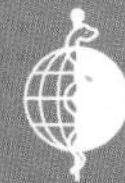

F.A. Davis Company • Philadelphia

F. A. Davis Company
1915 Arch Street
Philadelphia, PA 19103
www.fadavis.com

Printed in the United States of America

Last digit indicates print number: 10 9 8 7 6 5 4 3 2

Senior Acquisitions Editor: Melissa A. Duffield
Director of Content Development: George W. Lang
Senior Developmental Editor: Jennifer A. Pine
Art and Design Manager: Carolyn O'Brien

Library of Congress Cataloging-in-Publication Data

Names: Kisner, Carolyn, author. | Colby, Lynn Allen, author. | Borstad, John, author.
Title: Therapeutic exercise : foundations and techniques / Carolyn Kisner, Lynn Allen Colby, John Borstad.
Description: Seventh edition. | Philadelphia : F.A. Davis Company, [2018] | Includes bibliographical references and index.
Identifiers: LCCN 2017034666| ISBN 9780803658509 (alk. paper) | ISBN 0803658508 (alk. paper)
Subjects: | MESH: Exercise Therapy | Physical Therapy Modalities
Classification: LCC RM725 | NLM WB 541 | DDC 615.8/2—dc23 LC record available at https://lccn.loc.gov/2017034666

To Jerry, Craig and Kathleen, Jodi, and our grandchildren—as always, thank you for your love and support.
—CK

To Rick and my extended family—a source of constant support and joy.
—LC

To Alex and our children—for your support, inspiration, and hope.
—JB

To our parents—who were supportive throughout our lives.

To our students—who have taught us so much.

To our colleagues—who have been helpful and stimulating in our professional growth.
—LC, CK, and JB

Preface to the Seventh Edition

When Lynn Colby and I first began writing a book on therapeutic exercise over 30 years ago, it was simply an idea to fill a basic need in the education of physical therapists. Our first effort was a soft-cover product in outline form that was primarily marketed as a laboratory manual. The evolution of each succeeding edition came about from our creative insights and collaborative efforts to bring to the student and professional community the most up-to-date resource possible. Lynn has decided that this is the last edition with which she will be involved—I will miss her exceptional abilities, her collegiality, and the partnership that has grown over the years. I am at a loss to know how to thank her for her many years of love and dedication to this project and the friendship that has developed through our partnership. I simply say, thank you Lynn. Enjoy your well-deserved retirement.

For this edition we brought on a new co-author, John Borstad, PT, PhD. He was a contributor in our 6th edition and has been involved in other publications and research. You will see his name on many of the chapters in this edition as he has stepped into the roles of updating, revising, and editing. His biographical information follows in the About the Authors section. It is exciting to have him on board, and I look forward to our ongoing collaborative efforts.

The authors and contributors of this book have continually sought to incorporate current trends and research to support the foundational concepts of therapeutic exercise on which the student can learn and the practitioner can grow in their expertise of treating patients. In addition to the extensive and thorough revisions of content, the Focus on Evidence and Clinical Tips features, as well as links to video demonstrations of key interventions, are again highlighted in this edition. Whenever applicable, ***Clinical Practice Guidelines (CPGs)*** are included within the Focus on Evidence sections.

We have added a new chapter on Exercise in the Older Adult (Chapter 24). With this being such a critical area of practice in physical therapy, we anticipate that the content of the chapter will provide a foundation of information and suggested interventions that all practitioners will find useful when working with older individuals. There has also been important updating of information on use of the ICF language (International Classification of Functioning Disability and Health) in Chapter 1; an expansion of information on prevention, health, and wellness in Chapter 2; and incorporation of managing male incontinence in Chapter 25. With the expanding use of the Internet we decided to move some of our tables, boxes, and glossary online. When these resources are available, the reader will be referred to the F.A. Davis website associated with this edition for easy access to this feature.

As with previous editions, it is our hope that this updated text will provide a resource for learning and professional growth for the students and health-care practitioners who utilize therapeutic exercise.

Acknowledgments

We wish to acknowledge and express our sincere gratitude to the educators and clinicians who contributed their knowledge, insights, and professional perspectives to the revision of this edition.

A special thank you to Vicky Humphrey for editing the ancillary features for faculty that are associated with this edition and for her contributions to the pocket version ***Ther Ex Notes, ed. 2.***

A special thank you goes to Marsha Hall, Project Manager, Progressive Publishing Services, who spearheaded the copy-editing and production process. And once again, a special thank you to the F. A. Davis staff, particularly to our Senior Acquisitions Editor, Melissa Duffield, and to our Senior Developmental Editor, Jennifer Pine, both of who helped bring the 7th edition to fruition.

About the Authors

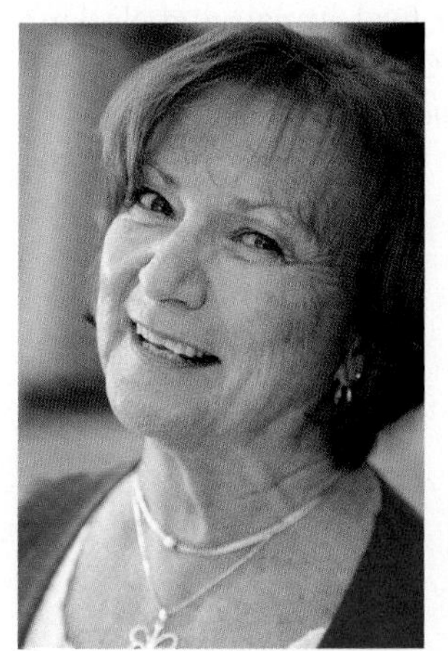

Carolyn Kisner, PT, MS

Carolyn was on the faculty at The Ohio State University for 27 years and was awarded Emeritus status after taking early retirement. During her tenure at OSU she received the Excellence in Teaching award from the School of Allied Medical Professions and was recognized as Outstanding Faculty by the Sphinx and Mortarboard Honor Societies. She organized and managed the honors and research program for the Physical Therapy Division, managed the Advanced Orthopedic track in the master's program, and advised numerous graduate students. Carolyn then taught at the College of Mount St. Joseph in Cincinnati for 7 years. During her tenure there she chaired the curriculum committee, which coordinated revision of the master's program and developed the entry-level Doctor of Physical Therapy program. She was awarded the Sister Adele Clifford Excellence in Teaching at the Mount and at the spring convocation in 2010 was awarded with the Lifetime Achievement in Physical Therapy.

Carolyn co-authored the textbook *Therapeutic Exercise: Foundations and Techniques* with Lynn Colby, PT, MS, first published in 1985. She and Lynn have always attempted to maintain current with the trends in physical therapy, which is reflected in each of the revisions of this book; they have also co-authored the pocket-sized flip book titled *Ther Ex Notes: Clinical Pocket Guide*. Her primary teaching experience includes medical kinesiology, orthopedic evaluation and intervention, therapeutic exercise, and manual therapy. She has presented numerous workshops on peripheral joint mobilization, spinal stabilization, kinesiology, gait, and functional exercise both nationally and internationally, including multiple visits to the Philippines, Brazil, Canada, and Mexico. Active clinical involvement throughout her career has primarily been in outpatient orthopedics and home health.

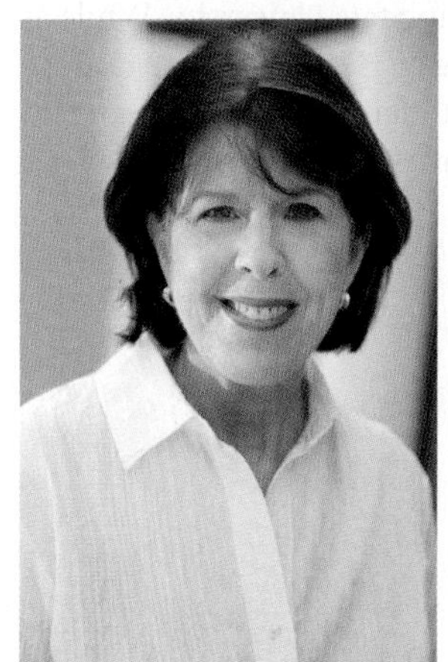

Lynn Allen Colby, PT, MS

Lynn Allen Colby is Assistant Professor Emeritus, The Ohio State University (OSU). She received her BS in physical therapy and MS in Allied Medicine from OSU, Columbus, Ohio. She is co-author of the textbook, *Therapeutic Exercise: Foundations and Techniques*, now in its 7th edition, and *Ther Ex Notes: Clinical Pocket Guide*.

Recently retired, she taught in the physical therapy program in the School of Allied Medical Professions at OSU for 35 years. As a faculty member, she also advised physical therapists enrolled in the postprofessional graduate program in Allied Medicine. Her primary teaching responsibilities in the physical therapy curriculum included therapeutic exercise interventions for musculoskeletal and neurological conditions and pediatric physical therapy. Experience in the clinical setting has included acute care in orthopedics, extended care in skilled nursing facilities, and inpatient and outpatient care in various pediatric settings.

During her long career in physical therapy, she was a recipient of the Excellence in Teaching Award from the School of Allied Medical Professions at OSU and was named the Ohio Physical Therapist of the Year in 2001 by the Ohio Physical Therapy Association. Most recently, she was honored by the OSU Alumni Association with the Ralph Davenport Mershon Award for Service and Leadership.

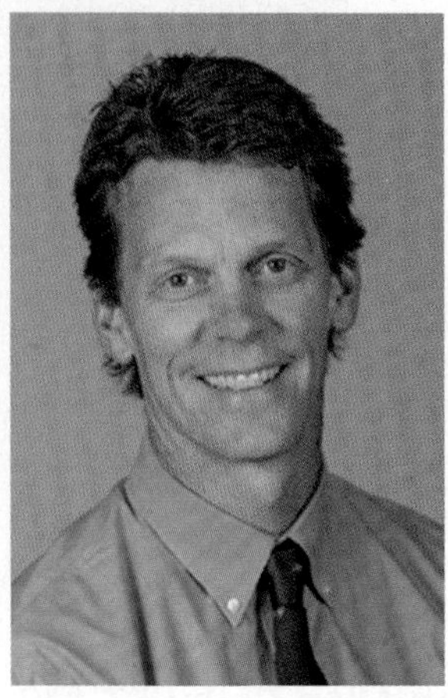

John Borstad, PT, PhD

John is professor and chair at the College of St. Scholastica in Duluth, Minnesota. After 7 years as a clinician, he began the academic phase of his career in 1999 at the University of Minnesota, earning a PhD in Rehabilitation Science in 2003. He spent the next 13 years on the faculty of the Physical Therapy Division in the School of Health and Rehabilitation Sciences at The Ohio State University. While at Ohio State, he was funded by the NIH, the Komen Foundation, and NHTSA to study shoulder biomechanics and to advise and train several MS and PhD students. John has presented his research at many national and international forums, including in Scotland, Japan, and Brazil. He was a co-author on the study that received the Rose Research Award for Excellence in Orthopaedic Physical Therapy Research in 2005 and received the School of Health and Rehabilitation Sciences Faculty Research Award in 2007. He moved back to his home state of Minnesota in 2016 to begin serving in academic leadership at St. Scholastica.

John has taught biomechanics, musculoskeletal science and application, evidence-based practice, and advanced therapeutic progressions during his academic career. In addition to being a contributor to the 6th edition of *Therapeutic Exercise: Foundations and Techniques*, he has co-authored textbook chapters related to the shoulder for Levangie and Norkin's *Joint Structure and Function: A Comprehensive Analysis* and for *Grieve's Musculoskeletal Physiotherapy*.

Contributors

Cynthia Johnson Armstrong, PT, DPT, CHT
Senior Instructor
Physical Therapy Program
University of Colorado
Aurora, Colorado

Susan Appling, PT, DPT, PhD, OCS, CMPT
Associate Professor, Clinical
Division of Physical Therapy Division
School of Health and Rehabilitation Sciences
The Ohio State University, Columbus, Ohio
Adjunct Associate Professor, Department of Physical Therapy
University of Tennessee Health Science Center
Memphis, Tennessee

Barbara Billek-Sawhney, PT, EdD, DPT, GCS
Professor Graduate School of Physical Therapy
Slippery Rock University
Slippery Rock, Pennsylvania

Elaine Bukowski, PT, DPT, MS, (D)ABDA
Professor Emerita of Physical Therapy
Stockton University
Galloway, New Jersey

Deborah Givens, PT, PhD, DPT,
Director, Division of Physical Therapy
University of North Carolina—Chapel Hill
Chapel Hill, North Carolina

Karen L Hock, PT, MS, CLT-LANA
Physical Therapist
The Ohio State University Comprehensive Cancer Center
Arthur G. James Cancer Hospital and Richard J. Solove Research Institute
The Stefanie Spielman Comprehensive Breast Center
Columbus, Ohio

Karen Holtgrefe, PT, DHSc, CWC
Physical Therapist and Certified Wellness Coach
Trihealth Outpatient Physical Therapy-Glenway
Cincinnati, Ohio

Barb Settles Huge, PT
Founder and Owner
BSH Wellness
President and Founder
Sisters Village, Inc 501c(3)
Fishers, Indiana

Vicky Humphrey, PT, MS
Lecturer, Physical Therapy Division
School of Health and Rehabilitation Sciences
The Ohio State University
Columbus, Ohio

Anne Kloos, PT, PhD, NCS
Professor Clinical Health, Physical Therapy Division
School of Health and Rehabilitation Sciences
The Ohio State University
Columbus, Ohio

Jonathan Rose, PT, SCS, MS, ATC
Assistant Professor
Department of Physical Therapy
College of Health Professions
Grand Valley State University
Grand Rapids, Michigan

Rajiv Sawhney, PT, DPT, MS, OCS
PIVOT Physical Therapy, Manager of Clinical Excellence
Adjunct Faculty
Chatham University
Pittsburgh, Pennsylvania

Jacob Thorp, PT, DHS, OCS, MTC
Associate Professor
East Carolina University
Greenville, North Carolina

Brief Contents

DavisPlus | **Chapters Available Online at DavisPlus:**

Contents

CHAPTER 1

Therapeutic Exercise: Foundational Concepts

VICKY N. HUMPHREY, PT, MS ■ LYNN ALLEN COLBY, PT, MS

Almost everyone, regardless of age, values the ability to function as independently as possible during activities of everyday life. Health-care consumers (patients and clients) typically seek out or are referred for physical therapy services because of physical impairments associated with disorders of the movement system caused by injury, disease, or health-related conditions that restrict their ability to participate in any number of activities that are necessary or important to them. Physical therapy services may also be sought by individuals who have no impairments or functional deficits but who wish to improve their overall level of fitness and quality of life or reduce the risk of injury or disease. An individually designed therapeutic exercise program is almost always a fundamental component of the physical therapy services provided. This stands to reason because the ultimate goal of a therapeutic exercise program is the achievement of an optimal level of symptom-free movement during basic to complex physical activities.

To develop and implement effective exercise interventions, a therapist must understand how the many forms of exercise affect tissues of the body and body systems and how those exercise-induced effects have an impact on key aspects of physical function as they relate to the human movement system. A therapist must also integrate and apply knowledge of anatomy, physiology, kinesiology, pathology, and the behavioral sciences across the continuum of patient/client management from the initial examination to discharge planning. To develop therapeutic exercise programs that culminate in positive and meaningful functional outcomes for patients and clients, a therapist must understand the relationships among physical functioning, health, and disability and apply these conceptual relationships to patient/client management to facilitate the provision of effective and efficient health-care services. Lastly, a therapist, as a patient/client educator, must know and apply principles of motor learning and motor skill acquisition to exercise instruction and functional training.

Therefore, the purpose of this chapter is to present an overview of the scope of therapeutic exercise interventions used in physical therapy practice. This chapter also discusses several models of health, functioning, and disability as well as patient/client management as they relate to therapeutic exercise and explores strategies for teaching and progressing exercises and functional motor skills based on principles of motor learning.

Therapeutic Exercise: Impact on Physical Function

Of the many procedures used by physical therapists in the continuum of care of patients and clients, therapeutic exercise takes its place as one of the key elements that lies at the center of programs designed to improve or restore an individual's function or to prevent dysfunction.[4]

Definition of Therapeutic Exercise

Therapeutic exercise[4,5] is the systematic, planned performance of physical movements, postures, or activities intended to provide a patient/client with the means to:

- Remediate or prevent impairments of body functions and structures.
- Improve, restore, or enhance activities and participation.
- Prevent or reduce health-related risk factors.
- Optimize overall health, fitness, or sense of well-being.

The beneficial effects of therapeutic exercise for individuals with a wide variety of health conditions and related physical impairments are documented extensively in the scientific literature[182] and are addressed in each of the chapters of this textbook.

Therapeutic exercise programs designed by physical therapists are *individualized* to the unique needs of each patient or client. A *patient* is an individual with impairments and functional deficits diagnosed by a physical therapist and is receiving physical therapy care to improve function and prevent disability.[4] A *client* is an individual without diagnosed movement dysfunction who engages in physical therapy services to promote health and wellness and to prevent dysfunction.[4] Because the focus of this textbook is on the management of individuals with body function and structure impairments, activity limitations, and participation restrictions, the authors have chosen to use the term "patient," rather than "client" or "patient/client," throughout this text. We believe that all individuals receiving physical therapy services must be active participants rather than passive recipients in the rehabilitation process to learn how to self-manage their health needs.

Components of Physical Function Related to Human Movement: Definition of Key Terms

The ability to function independently at home, in the workplace, within the community, or during leisure and recreational activities is contingent upon physical as well as psychological and social function. The multidimensional aspects of physical function encompass the diverse yet interrelated areas of movement performance that are depicted in Figure 1.1. These elements of function are characterized by the following definitions.

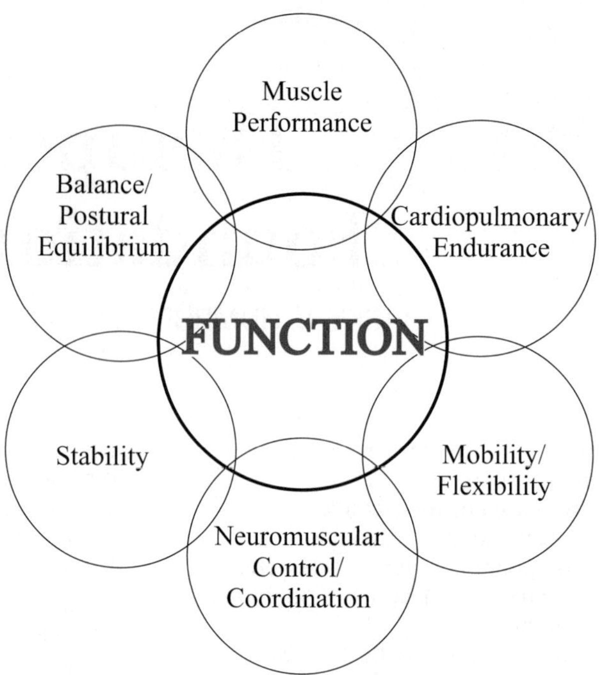

FIGURE 1.1 Interrelated components of physical function.

Balance. The ability to align body segments against gravity to maintain or move the body (center of mass) within the available base of support without falling; the ability to move the body in equilibrium with gravity via interaction of the sensory and motor systems.[4,94,107,125,166,169,170]

Cardiopulmonary endurance. The ability to perform moderate-intensity, repetitive, total body movements (walking, jogging, cycling, swimming, etc.) over an extended period of time.[2,115] A synonymous term is cardiopulmonary fitness.

Coordination. The correct timing and sequencing of muscle firing combined with the appropriate intensity of muscular contraction leading to the effective initiation, guiding, and grading of movement. Coordination is the basis of smooth, accurate, efficient movement and occurs at a conscious or automatic level.[139,142,165]

Flexibility. The ability to move freely, without restriction; used interchangeably with mobility.

Mobility. The ability of structures or segments of the body to move or be moved in order to allow the occurrence of range of motion (ROM) for functional activities (functional ROM).[4,177] Passive mobility is dependent on soft tissue (contractile and noncontractile) extensibility; in addition, active mobility requires neuromuscular activation.

Muscle performance. The capacity of muscle to produce tension and do physical work. Muscle performance encompasses strength, power, and muscular endurance.[4]

Neuromuscular control. Interaction of the sensory and motor systems that enables synergists, agonists, and antagonists, as well as stabilizers and neutralizers, to anticipate or respond to proprioceptive and kinesthetic information and, subsequently, to work in correct sequence to create coordinated movement.[102]

Postural control, postural stability, and equilibrium. Used interchangeably with static or dynamic balance.[73,166,169]

Stability. The ability of the neuromuscular system through synergistic muscle actions to hold a proximal or distal body segment in a stationary position or to control a stable base during superimposed movement.[73,169,177] Joint stability is the maintenance of proper alignment of bony partners of a joint by means of passive and dynamic components.[122]

The human movement system is the foundation for physical therapy and the focus for physical function.[160] The systems of the body that interact to control each of these elements of physical function react, adapt, and develop in response to forces and physical stresses (stress = force / area) placed upon tissues that make up the component parts of movement.[115,121,160] Gravity, for example, is a constant force that affects the musculoskeletal, neuromuscular, and circulatory systems. Additional forces, incurred during routine physical activities, help the body maintain a functional level of strength, cardiopulmonary fitness, and mobility. Imposed forces and physical stresses that are excessive can cause acute injuries, such as sprains and fractures, or chronic conditions, such as repetitive stress disorders.[121] The absence of typical forces on the body also can cause degeneration, degradation, or deformity. For example, the absence of normal weight bearing associated with prolonged bed rest or immobilization weakens muscle and bone.[2,3,17,121] Prolonged inactivity also leads to decreased efficiency of the circulatory and pulmonary systems.[2]

Impairment of any one or more of the body systems and subsequent impairment of any aspect of the human movement system, separately or jointly, can limit or restrict an individual's ability to carry out or participate in daily activities. Therapeutic exercise interventions involve the application of carefully graded physical stresses and forces that are imposed on the human movement system, specific tissues, or individual structures in a controlled, progressive, safely executed manner to enhance movement and improve the human experience.[5,160]

NOTE: In a recent article, Sahrmann[160]summarized the culmination of several decades of research by physical therapy leaders to more clearly define the role of physical therapy in health care. It has been proposed that physical therapy identify as a profession with a specific body system rather than with a type of intervention in order to gain professional recognition for content expertise. These proponents have defined the human movement system as a physiological system that represents the scope of practice and expertise of physical therapy. In this context, the human movement system is described as a separate physiological system comprised of interacting organs and systems including the nervous and musculoskeletal systems that produce movement and the pulmonary, cardiovascular, endocrine and integumentary systems that support movement.

Types of Therapeutic Exercise Interventions

Therapeutic exercise embodies a wide variety of activities, movements, and techniques. The individualized therapeutic exercise program is based on a therapist's determination of the underlying risk or cause of impairments in body function or structure, activity limitations, or participation restrictions as identified in the patient examination.[5] The types of therapeutic exercise interventions presented in this textbook are listed in Box 1.1.

NOTE: Although joint mobilization and manipulation procedures often are categorized as manual therapy techniques, not therapeutic exercise,[4] the authors of this textbook have chosen to include joint manipulative procedures under the broad definition of therapeutic exercise to address the full scope of soft tissue stretching techniques.

Exercise Safety

Regardless of the type of therapeutic exercise intervention, safety is a fundamental consideration whether the exercises are performed independently or under a therapist's direct supervision. Patient safety, of course, is paramount; nonetheless, the safety of the therapist also must be considered, particularly when the therapist is directly involved in the application of an exercise procedure or a manual technique.

Many factors can influence a patient's safety during exercise. Prior to engaging in exercise, a patient's health history and current health status must be explored. A patient unaccustomed to physical exertion may be at risk for the occurrence of an adverse effect from exercise associated with a known or an undiagnosed health condition. Medications can adversely affect a patient's balance and coordination during exercise or cardiopulmonary response to exercise. Therefore, risk factors must be identified and weighed carefully before an exercise program is initiated. Medical clearance from a patient's physician may be indicated before beginning an exercise program.

The environment in which exercises are performed also affects patient safety. Adequate space and a proper support surface for exercise are necessary prerequisites for patient safety. If exercise equipment is used in the clinical setting or at home, to ensure patient safety the equipment must be well maintained and in good working condition, must fit the patient, and must be applied and used properly.

Specific to each exercise in a program, the accuracy with which a patient performs an exercise affects safety, including proper posture or alignment of the body, execution of the correct movement patterns, and performance of each exercise

BOX 1.1 Therapeutic Exercise Interventions

- Aerobic conditioning and reconditioning
- Muscle performance exercises: strength, power, and endurance training
- Stretching techniques including muscle-lengthening procedures and joint mobilization/manipulation techniques
- Neuromuscular control, inhibition, and facilitation techniques and posture awareness training
- Postural control, body mechanics, and stabilization exercises
- Balance exercises and agility training
- Relaxation exercises
- Breathing exercises and ventilatory muscle training
- Task-specific functional training

with the appropriate intensity, speed, and duration. A patient must be informed of the signs of fatigue, the relationship of fatigue to the risk of injury, and the importance of rest for recovery during and after an exercise routine. When a patient is being directly supervised in a clinical or home setting while learning an exercise program, the therapist can control these variables. However, when a patient is carrying out an exercise program independently at home or at a community fitness facility, patient safety is enhanced and the risk of injury or re-injury is minimized by effective exercise instruction and patient education. Suggestions for effective exercise instruction and patient education are discussed in a later section of this chapter.

As mentioned, therapist safety also is a consideration to avoid work-related injury. For example, when a therapist is using manual resistance during an exercise designed to improve a patient's strength or is applying a stretch force manually to improve a patient's ROM, the therapist must incorporate principles of proper body mechanics and joint protection into these manual techniques to minimize his or her own risk of injury.

Throughout each of the chapters of this textbook, precautions, contraindications, and safety considerations are addressed for the management of specific health conditions, impairments, activity limitations, and participation restrictions and for the use and progression of specific therapeutic exercise interventions.

Classification of Health Status, Functioning, and Disability—Evolution of Models and Related Terminology

Background and Rationale for Classification Systems

Knowledge of the complex relationships among health status, functioning, and disability provides a foundation for the delivery of effective health-care services.[87,153,174] Without a common conceptual understanding and vocabulary, the ability to communicate and share information across disciplines and internationally is compromised for research, clinical practice, academia, policy making, and legislation.[153,176,199]

Disablement refers to the impact and functional consequence of acute or chronic conditions, such as disease, injury, and congenital or developmental abnormalities, that compromise basic human performance and an individual's ability to meet necessary, customary, expected, and desired societal functions and roles.[85,123,193] Disability is more than a consequence of a medical condition; rather, it is part of the human condition that is experienced by everyone either temporarily or permanently.[76,199] The disabling process depends on countless factors, such as access to quality care, severity and duration of the condition, motivation and attitude of the patient, and support from family and society. Depending on individual variables and social support, the disabling course is altered and levels of functioning vary among patients with the same medical diagnosis.[85,123,176,193] Defining a person's ability to function in the presence or absence of a health condition is a complex task that is better understood if practitioners, researchers, educators, policy makers, and legislators are using the same vocabulary and classification system.

Models of Functioning and Disability—Past and Present

Early Models

Several models that describe disability have been proposed worldwide over the past several decades. Two early theories were the Nagi model [123,124] and the International Classification of Impairments, Disabilities, and Handicaps (ICIDH) model for the World Health Organization (WHO).[67,75] The National Center for Medical Rehabilitation Research (NCMRR) created a third model that introduced individual risk factors for disability based on both physical and social risks.[126]

During the 1990s, physical therapists began to explore the potential use of disablement models and suggested that disablement schema and related terminology provided an appropriate framework for clinical decision-making in practice and research.[64,84,162] In addition, practitioners and researchers suggested that adoption of disablement-related language could be a mechanism to standardize terminology for documentation and communication in the clinical and research settings.[65] The American Physical Therapy Association (APTA) subsequently incorporated an extension of the Nagi disablement model and related terminology in its consensus document, the *Guide to Physical Therapist Practice* [4] (often called the *Guide*) in both its first edition in 1997 and second edition in 2001. Within the profession, this created a unifying force for documentation, communication, clinical practice, and research by designating a disablement framework for organizing and prioritizing clinical decisions made during the continuum of physical therapy care.

The conceptual frameworks of the Nagi, ICIDH, and NCMRR models, although applied widely in clinical practice and research, have been criticized internationally for their perceived focus on pathology.[41] These early models all describe a *unidirectional* path toward disability caused directly by the consequences of disease based on a medical-biological description without consideration of environmental or social influences.[41,176] In response to these criticisms, the WHO undertook a broad revision of its ICIDH model, and in 2001 the International Classification of Functioning, Disability, and Health (ICF) was introduced and characterized as a biopsychosocial model where environmental factors and personal factors are integrated into the concept of functioning and disability (Fig. 1.2).[76,77,173,174,175]

While the ICF is used to classify functioning and disability associated with health conditions, the WHO has a companion classification system to classify health conditions (diseases, disorders, and injuries) called the International Classification of Disease (ICD). Together, the use of these two classification systems provides a broader and more

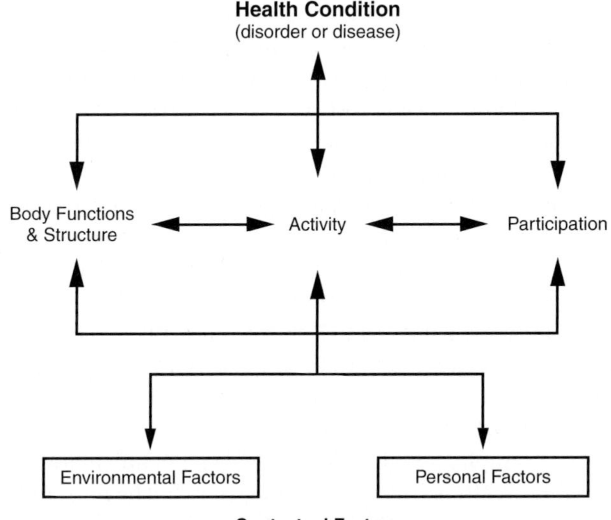

FIGURE 1.2 The ICF Framework.

meaningful picture of the health of both individuals and populations worldwide.[77]

The ICF—An Overview of the Model

Unlike previous models, the ICF does not focus on disability or on disease, but is intended to classify and code different health and health-related states experienced by everyone. The ICF takes a neutral approach to the human experience as it relates to components of health and functioning, experienced by all people, not just people with disabilities.[76,77,199] The ICF also includes both environmental and personal factors that influence how people with or without disability live and participate in society.[41,77,199]

As shown in Table 1.1, the ICF model organizes information about health into two basic parts. The first, labeled *Part 1: Functioning and Disability,* is subdivided into two components: (1) Body Functions and Structures and (2) Activities and Participation. The two *umbrella* terms, functioning and disability, are based on the classification of body functions and structures combined with activities and participation. *Functioning* is characterized by positive interactions that are defined by the integrity of body functions and structures and the ability to perform activities and participate in life situations. In contrast, *disability* is characterized by the negative interactions of health situations defined as impairments in body functions and structures, activity limitations, and participation restrictions.[76,77]

The second, labeled *Part 2: Contextual Factors,* also shown in Table 1.1, is subdivided into two components: (1) Environmental Factors and (2) Personal Factors. Contextual factors represent the complete background of an individual's life and living situation.[77] Environmental factors make up the physical, social, and attitudinal circumstances in which the individual lives either with or without a health problem.[77] These factors are external to the individual but have either facilitating or hindering influences on the individual's performance at the levels of body functions and structures, execution of activities, and participation in society. For this reason, Part 1 of the model is not classified separately from Part 2 as they are hierarchal in their coding to represent the biopsychosocial paradigm of a person's health condition.[1,77,144]

TABLE 1.1 An Overview of the International Classification of Functioning, Disability and Health (ICF)*

	Part 1: Functioning and Disability		**Part 2: Contextual Factors**	
Components	***Body Functions and Structures***	***Activities and Participation***	***Environmental Factors***	***Personal Factors***
Domains	Body functions Body structures	Life areas (tasks, actions)	External influences on functioning and disability	Internal influences on functioning and disability
Constructs	Changes in body functions (*physiological*) Changes in body structures (*anatomical*)	*Capacity*: Executing tasks in a standard environment *Performance:* Executing tasks in the current environment	Facilitating or hindering impact of features of the physical, social, and attitudinal world	Impact of attitudes of the person
Functioning				
Positive aspect	Functional and structural integrity	Activities Participation	Facilitators	Not applicable
Disability				
Negative aspect	Functional and/or structural Impairment	Activity limitation Participation restriction	Barriers Hindrances	Not applicable

*From *International Classification of Functioning, Disability and Health: ICF.* Geneva: World Health Organization, 2008, p 13, with permission.

Definitions of key terms are summarized in Box 1.2.[76,77,184] Numerous examples of these components are identified later in this chapter.

NOTE: The ICF classification and coding methodology is also unique from other models in its unit of measure. The *individual* is not placed in a classification, but rather the coding describes the *situation* of each person within an array of health and health-related domains. The coding used in ICF is complex and multifactorial, with inclusion of health, functioning, and environmental elements combined to describe the ability of an individual to perform activities and participate in society.[1,41,77,88,174,175]

Components of the ICF and Applications in Physical Therapy

Background

Traditionally, the physical therapy profession has been defined by a body of knowledge and clinical applications that are directed toward the elimination or remediation of disability.[150] However, as the physical therapy profession has evolved, the scope of practice has moved beyond solely the management and remediation of disability and now includes promoting the well-being of healthy individuals and preventing or reducing risk factors that may lead to disability while considering the external environmental and internal personal factors that influence each person's response to their health condition.[6]

BOX 1.2 Definition of Key Terms in the ICF

- **Impairments in body function:** Problems associated with the physiology of the body systems (including psychological functions).
- **Impairments in body structure:** Problems with the anatomical features of the body.
- **Activity limitations:** Difficulties an individual may have in executing actions, tasks, and activities.
- **Participation restrictions:** Problems an individual may experience with involvement in life situations, including difficulties participating in self-care; responsibilities in the home, workplace, or the community; and recreational, leisure and social activities.
- **Contextual factors:** The entire background of an individual's life and living situation composed of:
  - **Environmental factors:** Factors associated with the physical, social, and attitudinal environment in which people conduct their lives; factors may facilitate functioning (facilitators) or hinder functioning and contribute to disability (barriers).
  - **Personal factors:** Features of the individual that are not part of the health condition or health state; includes age, gender, race, lifestyle habits, coping skills, character, affect, cultural and social background, education, etc.

In 2008, the APTA officially endorsed the biopsychosocial framework, vocabulary, and classification system of the ICF. This began a continuing initiative over the past decade to integrate this framework and vocabulary into research, clinical documentation, education, policy making, and legislation.[5,77,141] To facilitate use of the ICF in clinical practice, several articles have been published to provide suggestions for integrating the ICF into specific components of physical therapy practice, ethics, and patient management.[1,48,49,144,153] In 2013, the third edition of the *Guide* was published and is available only in an electronic version in order to facilitate timely updates to reflect the rapid changes in physical therapy practice, including the integration of ICF as the adopted framework for defining the realm of functioning and disability.[5]

For example, use of ICF language for documentation in the clinical setting is being encouraged.[16,141] The most noteworthy application of the ICF can be found in a series of clinical practice guidelines developed and published by the specialty sections of the APTA. These guidelines use the ICF as the basis for describing and classifying care provided by physical therapists.[58,95] Information from the guidelines addressing the efficacy of therapeutic exercise interventions for health conditions and associated impairments commonly seen in orthopedic physical therapy practice is discussed in the regional chapters of this textbook.

Health Conditions

Health conditions, based on the terminology of the ICF framework, are acute or chronic diseases, disorders, or injuries or circumstances such as aging, pregnancy, or stress that have an impact on a person's level of function (see Fig. 1.2).[76,77] Health conditions are the basis of a medical diagnosis and are coded using the WHO's companion classification system, the International Classification of Disease (ICD).[77]

Physical therapists in all areas of practice treat patients with a multitude of health conditions. Knowledge of health conditions is important background information, but it does not tell the therapist how to assess impairments in body function or structure or how to assess when activities are limited or participation is restricted as a result of the health condition. Despite an accurate medical diagnosis and a therapist's thorough knowledge of specific health conditions, the experienced therapist knows that two patients with the same medical diagnosis, such as rheumatoid arthritis, and the same extent of joint destruction (confirmed radiologically) may have very different severities of impairment, activity limitation, and participation restriction. Consequently, they may have very different degrees of disability. This emphasizes the need for physical therapists to always assess the impact of a particular health condition on movement and function when designing meaningful management strategies to improve functional abilities.

Body Functions and Body Structures

As noted previously, the first component of classification in Part 1 of the ICF is body functions and structures (see Table 1.1). Body functions are the physiological functions of the body, whereas body structures describe the anatomical parts of the body. These domains of classification occur at the cellular, tissue, or body system level.

Types of Impairments

Impairments are defined by the loss of integrity of the physiological, anatomical, and/or psychological functions and structures of the body and are a partial reflection of a person's health status.

Some *impairments of body structure* are readily apparent during a physical therapy examination through visual inspection. Such impairments include joint swelling, scarring, presence of an open wound, lymphedema or amputation of a limb, or through palpation, such as adhesions, muscle spasm, and joint crepitus. Other structural impairments must be identified by a variety of imaging techniques, such as radiographic imaging to identify joint space narrowing associated with arthritis or magnetic resonance imaging (MRI) to identify a torn muscle or ligament.

Impairments of body function such as pain, reduced sensation, decreased ROM, deficits in muscle performance (strength, power, and endurance), impaired balance or coordination, abnormal reflexes, and reduced ventilation are those most commonly identified by physical therapists and managed with therapeutic exercise interventions. Some representative examples are noted in Box 1.3.

BOX 1.3 Common Body Function Impairments Managed With Therapeutic Exercise

Musculoskeletal
- Pain
- Muscle weakness/reduced torque production
- Decreased muscular endurance
- Limited range of motion due to:
  - Restriction of the joint capsule
  - Restriction of periarticular connective tissue
  - Decreased muscle length
  - Joint hypermobility
- Faulty posture
- Muscle length/strength imbalances

Neuromuscular
- Pain
- Impaired balance, postural stability, or control
- Incoordination, faulty timing
- Delayed motor development
- Abnormal tone (hypotonia, hypertonia, and dystonia)
- Ineffective/inefficient functional movement strategies

Cardiovascular/Pulmonary
- Decreased aerobic capacity (cardiopulmonary endurance)
- Impaired circulation (lymphatic, venous, and arterial)
- Pain with sustained physical activity (intermittent claudication)

Integumentary
- Skin hypomobility (e.g., immobile or adherent scarring)

Physical therapists typically provide care and services to patients with impairments associated with the musculoskeletal, neuromuscular, cardiovascular/pulmonary, and integumentary body systems when movement is compromised. In a biopsychosocial model, like the ICF, impairments are identified and documented as a first step to investigating the impact that a health condition has on activities and participation within the specific environment of the patient.

Primary and secondary impairments. Impairments may arise directly from the health condition (*direct/primary impairments*) or may be the result of preexisting impairments (*indirect/secondary impairments*). A patient, for example, who has been referred to physical therapy with a medical diagnosis of impingement syndrome or tendonitis of the rotator cuff (pathological condition), may exhibit primary impairments of body function, such as pain, limited ROM of the shoulder, and weakness of specific shoulder girdle and glenohumeral musculature during the physical therapy examination (Fig. 1.3 A and B). The patient may have developed

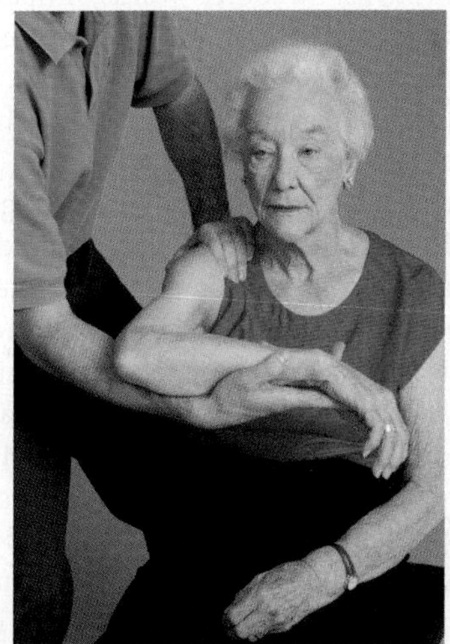
A

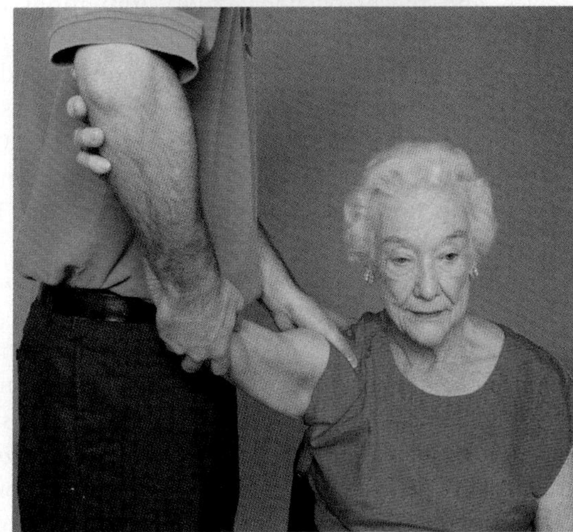
B

FIGURE 1.3 (A) Impingement syndrome of the shoulder and associated tendonitis of the rotator cuff (health condition/pathology) leading to **(B)** limited range of shoulder elevation (impairment of body function) are identified during the examination.

the shoulder pathology from a preexisting postural impairment (secondary impairment), which led to altered use of the upper extremity and impingement from faulty mechanics.

Composite impairments. When an impairment is the result of multiple underlying causes and arises from a combination of primary or secondary impairments, the term *composite impairment* is sometimes used. For example, a patient who sustained a severe inversion sprain of the ankle resulting in a tear of the talofibular ligament and whose ankle was immobilized for several weeks is likely to exhibit a balance impairment of the involved lower extremity after the immobilizer is removed. This composite impairment could be the result of chronic ligamentous laxity (body structure impairment) and impaired ankle proprioception from the injury or muscle weakness (body function impairments) due to immobilization and disuse.

Regardless of the types of physical impairment exhibited by a patient, a therapist must keep in mind that impairments manifest differently from one patient to another. An important key to effective patient management is to identify *functionally relevant impairments,* in other words, impairments that directly contribute to current or future activity limitations and participation restrictions in a patient's daily life. Impairments that can predispose a patient to secondary health conditions or impairments also must be identified.

Equally crucial for the effective management of a patient's condition is the need to analyze and determine, or at least infer and certainly not ignore, the *underlying causes* of the identified physical impairments of body function or body structure, particularly those related to impaired movement.[158,159,160] For example, are biomechanical abnormalities of soft tissues the source of restricted ROM? If so, which soft tissues are restricted, and why are they restricted? This information assists the therapist in the selection of appropriate, effective therapeutic interventions that target the *underlying causes* of the impairments, the impairments themselves, and the associated activity limitations and participation restrictions.

Although most physical therapy interventions, including therapeutic exercise, are designed to correct or reduce physical impairments of body function, such as decreased ROM or strength, poor balance, or limited cardiopulmonary endurance, the focus of treatment ultimately must be to improve performance of activities and participation in life events. From a patient's perspective, *successful outcomes* of treatment are determined by restoration of activities and participation levels.[144] A therapist cannot simply assume that intervening at the impairment level (e.g., with strengthening or stretching exercises) and subsequently reducing physical impairments (by increasing strength and ROM) generalize to improvement in a patient's level of activity and participation in work and social roles. Mechanisms for integrating task-specific training within the therapeutic exercise intervention are explored in a model of effective patient management presented in a later section of this chapter.

Activities and Participation

The second component of Part 1 of the ICF is Activities and Participation (see Table 1.1). *Activity* is defined as the execution of a task or action by an individual, whereas *participation* is the involvement of the individual in a life situation. The ICF structure of classification for this component is based on one single list of activities and life areas.[77] The therapist is encouraged to differentiate the components on a case by case basis depending on the patient's life situation. There has been extensive research to determine if these two components of functioning are distinct or interrelated.[1,26,89,144] Because of the varied environmental and personal influences (contextual factors), there is not a clear distinction between an individual's ability to perform a task and participation. Additional empirical research is recommended to provide a clearer operationalization of the two components to enhance data comparison between disciplines and countries.[77]

Activity Limitation and Participation Restriction

In the language of the ICF, *activity limitations* occur when a person has difficulty executing or is unable to perform tasks or actions of daily life (see Box 1.2).[41,76,77,173,174,175,184] For example, as shown in Figure 1.4, restricted ROM (impairment of body function) of the shoulder as the result of adhesive capsulitis (health condition) can limit a person's ability to reach overhead (activity limitation) while performing personal grooming or household tasks.

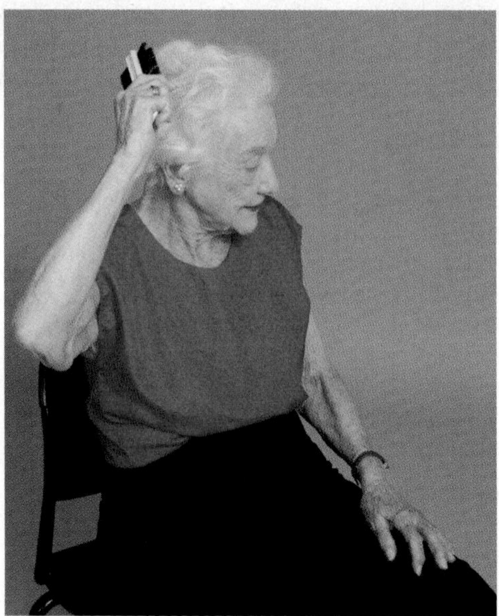

FIGURE 1.4 Limited ability to reach overhead (activity limitation) as the result of impaired shoulder mobility may lead to loss of independence in self-care and difficulty performing household tasks independently (participation restriction).

Many studies have linked body function impairments with activity limitations, particularly in older adults. Links have been identified between limited ROM of the shoulder and difficulty reaching behind the head or back while bathing and dressing,[185] between decreased isometric strength of lower extremity musculature and difficulty stooping and kneeling,[71] as well as a link between decreased lower extremity peak power and reduced walking speed and difficulty moving from sitting to standing.[140] However, it should also be noted that a single or even several mild impairments of body function or structure do not consistently result in activity limitations for all individuals. For example, results of a 2-year observational study of patients with symptomatic hip or knee osteoarthritis (OA) demonstrated that increased joint space narrowing (a body structure impairment that is considered an indicator of progression of the disease) confirmed radiologically was not associated with an increase in activity limitations as measured on a self-report assessment of physical functioning.[24] Furthermore, evidence from other studies suggests that the severity and complexity of impairments must reach a critical level, which is different for each person, before degradation of functioning begins to occur.[134,143] These examples reinforce the ICF construct that environmental and personal factors interact with all aspects of functioning and disability. Thus, each individual experiences a unique response to a health condition.

BOX 1.4 Common Tasks Related to Activity Limitations

Difficulties with or limitation of:

- Reaching and grasping
- Lifting, lowering, and carrying
- Pushing and pulling
- Bending and stooping
- Turning and twisting
- Throwing and catching
- Rolling
- Sitting or standing tolerance
- Squatting (crouching) and kneeling
- Standing up and sitting down (from and to a chair, the floor)
- Getting in and out of bed
- Moving around (crawling, walking, and running) in various environments
- Ascending and descending stairs
- Hopping and jumping
- Kicking or swinging an object

Activity limitation. Activities and participation require the performance of sensorimotor tasks—that is, total body actions that typically are *components or elements* of functional activities. Activity limitations involve technical and physiological problems that are task-specific and related to performance. Box 1.4 identifies a number of activity limitations that can arise from physical impairments in body function or structure, involve *whole-body movements or actions,* and are necessary component motions of simple to complex daily living tasks. Defining limitations in this way highlights the importance of identifying abnormal or absent component motions of motor skills through task analysis during the physical therapy examination and later integrating task-specific functional motions into a therapeutic exercise program.

When a person is unable or has only limited ability to perform any of the whole-body component motions identified in Box 1.4, activities may be limited and participation may be restricted. The following is an example of the interplay of activities and participation in everyday life. To perform a basic home maintenance task such as painting a room, a person must be able to grasp and hold a paintbrush or roller, climb a ladder, reach overhead, kneel, or stoop down to the floor. If any one of these component movements is limited, it may not be possible to perform the overall task of painting the room. If the individual views home maintenance as a personal or social role, the inability to perform the task of painting may result in participation restriction.

An essential element of a physical therapy examination and evaluation is the analysis of motor tasks to identify the component motions that are difficult for a patient to perform. This analysis helps the therapist determine why a patient is unable to perform specific daily living tasks. This information, coupled with identification and measurement of the impairments that are associated with the altered or absent component movement patterns, in turn, is used for treatment planning and selection of interventions to restore the ability to complete activities or to participate in personal, social, work, or life situations.

Participation restrictions. As identified in the ICF model (see Table 1.1), participation restrictions are defined as problems a person may experience in his or her involvement in life situations as measured against social standards (see Box 1.2).[76,77,173,174,175,184] More specifically, participation restriction is about not being able to take part in social practices in situations of significance or meaningfulness in the context of a person's attitudes and environment (contextual factors).[26,144]

Social expectations or roles that involve interactions with others and participation in activities are an important part of the individual. These roles are specific to age, gender, sex, and cultural background. Categories of activities or roles that, if limited, may contribute to participation restrictions are summarized in Box 1.5.

Contextual Factors

In the ICF, Part 2 consists of *contextual factors,* once again divided into two components: (1) *environmental factors* and (2) *personal factors.* These classifications represent the external and internal domains that influence functioning and disability, taking into consideration the complete

BOX 1.5 Areas of Functioning Associated With Participation Restrictions

- Self-care
- Mobility in the community
- Occupational tasks
- School-related tasks
- Home management (indoor and outdoor)
- Caring for dependents
- Recreational and leisure activities
- Socializing with friends/family
- Community responsibilities and service

background of an individual's life and living situation (see Table 1.1).

Environmental factors are outside of the individual, but every feature of the physical, social, and attitudinal world has either a facilitating or hindering impact on functioning and disability.[77]

Because disability is such a complex concept, the extent to which each aspect of functioning affects one's perceived level of disability is not clearly understood. An assumption is made that when impairments and activity limitations are so severe or of such long duration that they cannot be overcome to a degree acceptable to an individual, a family, or society, the perception of "being disabled" occurs.[143] The perception of disability is highly dependent on a person's or society's expectations of how or by whom certain roles or tasks *should* be performed.

Personal factors are unique to the individual and may include characteristics such as race, gender, family background, coping styles, education, fitness, and psychological assets.[77]

NOTE: Because personal factors are features of the individual, they are not part of the health condition, and they are not classified or coded in the ICF (see Table. 1.1). However, they must be considered in any provision of care because they will influence the outcome of the intervention.[77]

The Role of Prevention

Understanding the relationships among a health condition, impairments, activity limitations, participation restrictions, and the impact of environmental and personal factors on functioning is fundamental to the prevention or reduction of disability.[25,61,85] Disability is not caused by any one level of impairment or activity limitation or participation restriction; rather, the process is bidirectional and complex.

Take, for example, a relatively inactive person with long-standing osteoarthritis of the knees. The inability to get up from the floor or from a low seat (activity limitation) because of limited flexion of the knees and power deficits of the hip and knee extensors (impairments in body function) could indeed lead to restricted participation in life's activities and disability in several areas of everyday functioning. Disability could be expressed by problems in self-care (inability to get in and out of a tub or stand up from a standard height toilet seat), home management (inability to perform selected housekeeping, gardening, or yard maintenance tasks), or community mobility (inability to get into or out of a car or van independently).

The perception of disability possibly could be minimized if the patient's functional ROM and strength can be improved with an exercise program and the increased ROM and strength are incorporated into progressively more challenging functional activities or if the physical environment can be altered sufficiently with the use of adaptive equipment and assistive devices.

Adjusting expected roles or tasks within the family might also have a positive impact on the prevention or reduction of disability. Factors within the individual also can have an impact on the prevention, reduction, or progression of disability. Those factors include level of motivation or willingness to make lifestyle changes and accommodations as well as the ability to understand and cope with an adjusted lifestyle.[193] This example highlights that inherent in any discussion of disability is the assumption that it can be prevented or remediated.[25]

Categories of prevention. Prevention falls into three categories.[4]

- *Primary prevention:* Activities such as health promotion designed to prevent disease in an at-risk population.
- *Secondary prevention:* Early diagnosis and reduction of the severity or duration of existing disease and sequelae.
- *Tertiary prevention:* Use of rehabilitation to reduce the degree or limit the progression of existing disability and improve multiple aspects of function in persons with chronic, irreversible health conditions.

Therapeutic exercise, the most frequently implemented physical therapy intervention, has value at all three levels of prevention. Health and wellness have moved to the forefront of health care, and physical therapists are becoming involved in wellness screens, community health fairs, and annual check-ups as a form of primary prevention. The use of resistance exercises and aerobic conditioning exercises in weight-bearing postures is often advocated for the primary and secondary prevention of age-related osteoporosis.[40,70] In addition, therapists who work with patients with chronic musculoskeletal or neuromuscular diseases or disorders routinely are involved with tertiary prevention of disability.

Risk Factors

Modifying risk factors through an intervention, such as therapeutic exercise, is an important tool for preventing or reducing the impact of health conditions and subsequent impairments, activity limitations, and participation restrictions associated with disability. Risk factors are influences or characteristics that predispose a person to impaired functioning and potential disability. As such, they exist *prior to* the onset of a health condition and associated impairments, limitations, or restrictions.[25,85,193] Some factors that increase the risk of disabling conditions are biological characteristics, lifestyle behaviors, psychological characteristics, and the impact of the physical and social environments. Examples of each of these types of risk factor are summarized in Box 1.6.

Some of the risk factors, in particular lifestyle characteristics and behaviors and their impact on the potential for disease or injury, have become reasonably well known because of public service announcements and distribution of educational materials in conjunction with health promotion campaigns, such as *Healthy People 2010*[188] and *Healthy People 2020*.[189] Information on the adverse influences of health-related risk factors, such as a sedentary lifestyle, obesity, and smoking, has been widely disseminated by these public health initiatives. Although the benefits of a healthy lifestyle, which includes regular exercise and physical activity, are well founded and widely documented,[2,188,189] initial outcomes of a previous national campaign, *Healthy People 2000*,[191] suggest that an increased awareness of risk factors has not translated effectively into dramatic changes in lifestyle behaviors to reduce the risk of disease or injury.[50] This demonstrates that increased knowledge does not necessarily change behavior.

When a health condition exists, the reduction of risk factors by means of *buffers* (interventions aimed at reducing the progression of a pathological condition, impairments, limitations, restrictions, and potential disability) is appropriate.[85] This focus of intervention is categorized as secondary or tertiary prevention. Initiating a regular exercise program, increasing the level of physical activity on a daily basis, or altering the physical environment by removing architectural barriers or using assistive devices for a range of daily activities are examples of buffers that can reduce the risk of disability. (Refer to Chapter 2 of this textbook for additional information on prevention, reduction of health-related risk factors, and wellness.)

BOX 1.6 Risk Factors for Disability

Biological Factors
- Age, sex, and race
- Height/weight relationship
- Congenital abnormalities or disorders (e.g., skeletal deformities, neuromuscular disorders, cardiopulmonary diseases, or anomalies)
- Family history of disease; genetic predisposition

Behavioral/Psychological/Lifestyle Factors
- Sedentary lifestyle
- Cultural biases
- Use of tobacco, alcohol, and/or other drugs
- Poor nutrition
- Low level of motivation
- Inadequate coping skills
- Difficulty dealing with change or stress
- Negative affect

Physical Environment Characteristics
- Architectural barriers in the home, community, and workplace
- Ergonomic characteristics of the home, work, or school environments

Socioeconomic Factors
- Low economic status
- Low level of education
- Inadequate access to health care
- Limited family or social support

Summary

An understanding of the concepts of functioning and disability; of the relationships among the components of functioning, disability, and health; and of the various models and classification systems that have been developed over the past several decades provides a conceptual framework for practice and research. This knowledge also establishes a foundation for sound clinical decision-making and effective communication and sets the stage for delivery of effective, efficient, meaningful physical therapy care and services for patients.

Principles of Comprehensive Patient Management

An understanding of the concepts of functioning and disability, coupled with knowledge of the process of making informed clinical decisions based on evidence from the scientific literature, provides the foundation for comprehensive management of patients seeking and receiving physical therapy services. Provision of quality patient care involves the ability to make sound clinical judgments; solve problems that are important to a patient; and apply knowledge of the relationships among a patient's health condition(s), impairments, limitations in daily activities, and participation restrictions throughout each phase of management.

The primary purpose of this section of the chapter is to describe a model of patient management used in physical therapy practice. Inasmuch as clinical reasoning and evidence-based decision-making are embedded in each phase of patient management, a brief overview of the concepts and processes associated with clinical decision-making and evidence-based practice is presented before exploring a systematic process of patient management in physical therapy. Relevant examples of the clinical decisions a therapist must make are highlighted within the context of the patient management model.

Clinical Decision-Making

Clinical decision-making refers to a dynamic, complex process of reasoning and analytical (critical) thinking that involves making judgments and determinations in the context of patient care.[93] One of the many areas of clinical decision-making in which a therapist is involved is the selection, implementation, and modification of therapeutic exercise interventions based on the unique needs of each patient or client. To make effective decisions, merging clarification and understanding with critical and creative thinking is necessary.[101] A number of requisite attributes are necessary for making informed, responsible, efficient, and effective clinical decisions.[46,101,113,167] Those requirements are listed in Box 1.7.

There is a substantial body of knowledge in the literature that describes various strategies and models of clinical decision-making in the context of patient management by physical therapists.[43,46,65,79,80,92,93,148,151,152] One such model, the Hypothesis-Oriented Algorithm for Clinicians II (HOAC II), describes a series of steps involved in making informed clinical decisions.[152] The use of clinical decision-making in the diagnostic process also has generated extensive discussion in the literature.[19,22,42,46,59,62,83,84,149,158,183,187,201]

To assist in the decision-making process and ultimately improve patient care, tools known as *clinical prediction rules* (CPRs), first developed in medicine, also have been developed for use by physical therapists.[32,52] Some CPRs contain predictive factors that help a clinician establish specific diagnoses or improve the accuracy of prognoses, whereas others identify subgroupings of patients within large, heterogeneous groups who are most likely to benefit from a particular approach to treatment or specific therapeutic interventions. To date, some prediction tools in physical therapy have been developed to assist in the diagnosis of health conditions, including osteoarthritis in patients with hip pain[178] and deep vein thrombosis in patients with leg pain.[147] However, a greater number of CPRs in physical therapy have been established to predict likely responses of patients to treatment. As examples, CPRs have been developed to identify a subgrouping of patients with patellofemoral pain syndrome who are most likely to respond positively to lumbopelvic manipulation,[78] patients with low back pain most likely to respond to stabilization exercises,[72] and those with neck pain for whom thoracic spine manipulation is most likely to be effective.[35]

It is important to note, however, that little research, thus far, has focused on validation of published CPRs[15] or their impact on the effectiveness of patient care from specific therapeutic interventions. The results of two systematic reviews of the literature underscore these points. One review[15] concluded that there is considerable variation in the quality of studies used to validate CPRs developed for interventions used by physical therapists. The results of the other review of CPRs for musculoskeletal conditions[172] demonstrated that currently there is only limited evidence to support the use of these rules to predict the effectiveness of specific interventions or to optimize treatment. Additional information from studies directed toward clinical decision-making is integrated into the remainder of this section on patient management or is addressed in later chapters.

BOX 1.7 Requirements for Skilled Clinical Decision-Making During Patient Management

- Knowledge of pertinent information about the problem(s) based on the ability to collect relevant data by means of effective examination strategies
- Cognitive and psychomotor skills to obtain necessary knowledge of an unfamiliar problem
- Use of an efficient information-gathering and information-processing style
- Prior clinical experience with the same or similar problems
- Ability to recall relevant information
- Ability to integrate new and prior knowledge
- Ability to obtain, analyze, and apply high-quality evidence from the literature
- Ability to critically organize, categorize, prioritize, and synthesize information
- Ability to recognize clinical patterns
- Ability to form working hypotheses about presenting problems and how they might be solved
- Understanding of the patient's values and goals
- Ability to determine options and make strategic plans
- Application of reflective thinking and self-monitoring strategies to make necessary adjustments

Coordination, Communication, and Documentation

Health care continues to move in the direction of physical therapists being primary practitioners through whom consumers gain access to services without physician referral. As the coordinator of physical therapy care and services, the therapist has the responsibility to communicate verbally and through written documentation with all individuals involved in the care of a patient. The adoption of direct access has been scrutinized in regard to the ability of physical therapists to make sound clinical decisions and the potential for therapists to miss critical signs and symptoms (*red flags*) and neglect to refer patients when appropriate.[91] However, the literature shows several circumstances where therapists have shown evaluative and diagnostic skills resulting in appropriate decisions to involve other providers in the coordination of care of the patient.[23,68,91]

The following are descriptions of circumstances where it is appropriate for the physical therapist to communicate and coordinate care of the patient with another provider.[5]

- *Comanagement*: Sharing responsibility.
- *Consultation:* Providing or seeking professional expertise/judgement.

- *Supervision:* Delegation of some portion of treatment while remaining responsible for the care provided.
- *Referral:* Includes both referring to another provider and receiving referrals from another provider.

Even during the intervention or discharge phase of patient management, a therapist might make the clinical decision that referral to another practitioner is appropriate and complementary to the physical therapy services. This requires coordination and communication with other health-care practitioners. For example, a therapist might refer a patient who is generally deconditioned from a sedentary lifestyle and who is also obese to a nutritionist for dietary counseling to complement the physical therapy program designed to improve the patient's aerobic capacity (cardiopulmonary endurance) and general level of fitness.

Coordination, communication, and documentation are required of the physical therapist throughout the entire episode of patient management. This role encompasses many patient-related administrative tasks and professional responsibilities, such as writing reports (evaluations, plans of care, and discharge summaries); designing home exercise programs; contacting third-party payers, other health-care practitioners, or community-based resources; and participating in team conferences.

Evidence-Based Practice

Physical therapists who wish to provide high-quality patient care must make informed clinical decisions based on sound clinical reasoning and knowledge of the practice of physical therapy. An understanding and application of the principles of evidence-based practice provide a foundation to guide a clinician through the decision-making process during the course of patient care.

In recent years, evidence-based practice has been highlighted in the strategic plans of the APTA by establishing guidelines, setting goals for therapists to be engaged in applying and integrating research findings into everyday practice, and encouraging use of validated clinical practice guidelines.[8]

Definition and Description of the Process

Evidence-based practice is "the conscientious, explicit, and judicious use of current best evidence in making decisions about the care of an individual patient."[156] Evidence-based practice also involves combining knowledge of evidence from well-designed research studies with the expertise of the clinician and the values, goals, and circumstances of the patient.[157]

The process of evidence-based practice involves the following steps:[37,157]

1. Identify a patient problem and convert it into a specific question.
2. Search the literature and collect clinically relevant, scientific studies that contain evidence related to the question.
3. Critically analyze the pertinent evidence found during the literature search and make reflective judgments about the quality of the research and the applicability of the information to the identified patient problem.
4. Integrate the appraisal of the evidence with clinical expertise and experience and the patient's unique circumstances and values to make decisions.
5. Incorporate the findings and decisions into patient management.
6. Assess the outcomes of interventions and ask another question if necessary.

This process enables a practitioner to select and interpret the findings from the evaluation tools used during the examination of the patient and to implement effective treatment procedures that are rooted in sound theory and scientific evidence (rather than anecdotal evidence, opinion, or clinical tradition) to facilitate the best possible outcomes for a patient.

 **FOCUS ON EVIDENCE**

In a survey of physical therapists, all of whom were members of APTA, 488 respondents answered questions about their beliefs, attitudes, knowledge, and behavior about evidence-based practice.[90] Results of the survey indicated that the therapists believed that the use of evidence in practice was necessary and that the quality of care for their patients was better when evidence was used to support clinical decisions. However, most thought that carrying out the steps involved in evidence-based practice was time consuming and seemed incompatible with the demands placed on therapists in a busy clinical setting.

It is impractical to suggest that a clinician must search the literature for evidence to support each and every clinical decision that must be made. Despite time constraints in the clinical setting, when determining strategies to solve complex patient problems or when interacting with third-party payers to justify treatment, the "thinking therapist" has a professional responsibility to seek out evidence that supports the selection and use of specific evaluation and treatment procedures.[12]

Accessing Evidence

One method for staying abreast of evidence from the current literature is to read one's professional journals on a regular basis. It is also important to seek out relevant evidence from high-quality studies (randomized controlled trials, systematic reviews of the literature, etc.) from journals of other professions.[38] Journal articles that contain systematic reviews of the literature or summaries of multiple systematic reviews are an efficient means to access evidence because they provide a concise compilation and critical appraisal of a number of scientific studies on a topic of interest.

Evidence-based *clinical practice guidelines* for management of specific physical conditions or groupings of impairments also have been developed; they address the relative effectiveness of specific treatment strategies and procedures. These guidelines provide recommendations for management based on systematic reviews of current literature.[139,161] Initially, clinical practice guidelines that address four broadly defined musculoskeletal conditions commonly managed by physical therapists—specifically knee pain,[135] low back pain,[136] neck pain,[137] and shoulder pain[138]—were developed by the Philadelphia Panel, a panel of experts from physical therapy and medicine.

As mentioned previously in this chapter, a series of clinical practice guidelines has been created and published by several sections of the APTA. These guidelines provide evidence-based recommendations for physical therapy management (diagnosis, prognosis, selection of therapeutic interventions, and use of outcome measures) of a number of impairment/function-based groupings that are based on the ICF.[58] Some examples include clinical practice guidelines for management of neck pain,[33] knee pain and mobility impairments,[104] knee stability impairments,[105] hip pain and mobility deficits associated with osteoarthritis,[34] heel pain associated with plantar fasciitis,[117] and deficits associated with Achilles tendonitis.[29] All of the published clinical practice guidelines can be found at PTNow.org—a resource of the APTA.[7] More specific information from recently published guidelines is integrated into the regional chapters of this textbook.

If articles that contain systematic reviews of the literature on a specific topic have not been published, a therapist may find it necessary and valuable to perform an individual literature search to identify evidence applicable to a clinical question or patient problem. Journals exclusively devoted to evidence-based practice are another means to assist the practitioner who wants to identify well-designed research studies from a variety of professional publications without doing an individual search. These journals provide abstracts of research studies that have been critically analyzed and systematically reviewed.

Online bibliographic databases also facilitate access to evidence. Many databases provide systematic reviews of the literature relevant to a variety of health professions by compiling and critiquing several research studies on a specific patient problem or therapeutic intervention.[12,37,119] One example is the Cochrane Database of Systematic Reviews, which reports peer-reviewed summaries of randomized controlled trials and the evidence for and against the use of various interventions for patient care, including therapeutic exercise. Although a recent study [118] identified CENTRAL (Cochrane Central Registry of Controlled Trials), PEDro (Physiotherapy Evidence Database), PubMed, and EMBASE (Excerpta Medica Database) as the four most comprehensive databases indexing reports of randomized clinical trials of physical therapy interventions, only PEDro exclusively reports trials, reviews, and practice guidelines pertinent to physical therapy.[109] Easily accessed online databases such as these streamline the search process and provide a wealth of information from the literature in a concise format.

To further assist therapists in retrieving and applying evidence in physical therapist practice from the Cochrane online library, the *Physical Therapy* journal publishes a recurring feature called Linking Evidence and Practice (LEAP). This feature summarizes a Cochrane review and other scientific evidence on a single topic relevant to physical therapy patient care. In addition, LEAP presents case scenarios to illustrate how the results of the review of evidence can be applied to the decision-making process during patient management.

In support of evidence-based practice, relevant research studies are highlighted or referenced throughout each of the chapters of this text in relationship to the therapeutic exercise interventions, manual therapy techniques, and management guidelines presented and discussed. However, there is also an absence of research findings to support the use of some of the interventions presented. For such procedures, a therapist must rely on clinical expertise and judgment as well as each patient's response to treatment to determine the impact of these interventions on patient outcomes. Interventions without evidence to support efficacy should be used discriminately, and attempts to support and identify new research in those areas is a professional expectation. Examples of how to incorporate the ongoing process of clinical decision-making and application of evidence into each phase of patient management are presented in the following discussion of a model for patient management.

A Patient Management Model

The physical therapy profession has developed a comprehensive approach to patient management designed to guide a practitioner through a systematic series of steps and decisions for the purpose of helping a patient achieve the highest level of functioning possible.[6] This model is published online in the *Guide to Physical Therapist Practice* and is illustrated in Figure 1.5.

As described in the *Guide to Physical Therapist Practice,* the process of patient management has the following elements:[5,6,19,54]

1. A comprehensive *examination* including successive re-examination as indicated.
2. *Evaluation* of data collected.
3. Determination of a *diagnosis* based on impairments of body structure and function, activity limitations, and participation restrictions that result in movement dysfunction and/or are amenable to physical therapy intervention.
4. Establishment of a *prognosis* and plan of care based on patient-oriented goals.
5. Implementation of appropriate *intervention.*
6. Analysis and communication of *outcomes* resulting from interventions.

The ability to make timely decisions and appropriate judgments and to develop or adjust an ongoing series of working hypotheses makes transition from one phase of patient management to the next occur in an effective, efficient manner.

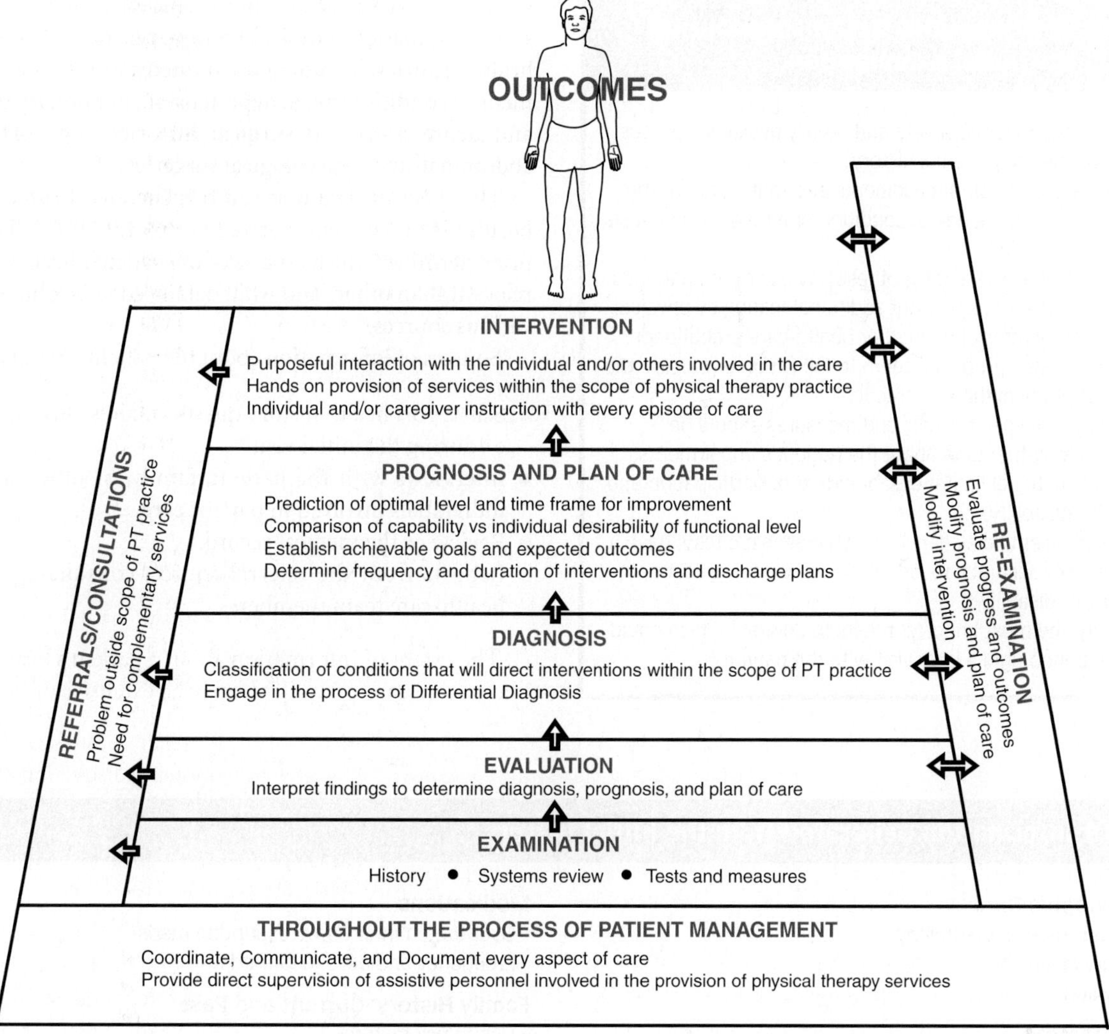

FIGURE 1.5 A comprehensive model of the patient management process.

Examination

The first component of the patient management model is a comprehensive examination of the patient. Examination is the systematic process by which a therapist obtains information about a patient's problem(s) and his or her reasons for seeking physical therapy services. During this initial data collection, the therapist acquires information from a variety of sources. The examination process involves both comprehensive screening and specific diagnostic testing. It is the means by which the therapist gathers sufficient information about the patient's existing or potential problems to ultimately formulate a diagnosis and determine whether these problems can be appropriately treated by physical therapy interventions. If treatment of the identified problems does not fall within the scope of physical therapy practice, referral to another health-care practitioner or resource is warranted. The examination is also the means by which baseline measurements of current impairments of body functions and structures, activity limitations, and participation restrictions are established as a reference point from which the results of therapeutic interventions can be measured and documented.

There are three distinct elements of a comprehensive examination:[5]

- The patient's health history
- A relevant systems review
- Specific tests and measures

Throughout the examination process, a therapist seeks answers to an array of questions and concurrently makes a series of clinical decisions that shape and guide the examination process. Examples of some questions to be asked and decisions to be made are noted in Box 1.8.

Health History

The health history is the mechanism by which a therapist obtains an *overview* of current and past information (both subjective and objective) about a patient's present condition(s), general health status (health risk factors and coexisting health problems), and why the patient has sought physical therapy

BOX 1.8 Key Questions to Consider During the Initial Examination

- What are the most complete and readily available sources for obtaining the patient's history?
- Is there a need to obtain additional information about the patient's presenting health condition or a medical diagnosis if one is available?
- Based on initial working hypotheses, which of the patient's signs and symptoms warrant additional testing by physical therapy or by referral to another health-care practitioner?
- Do the patient's problems seem to fall within or outside the scope of physical therapy practice?
- What types of specific tests and measures should be selected to gather data about the patient's impairments, activity/functional limitations, or extent of participation and resulting disability?
- Based on scientific evidence, which diagnostic tests have a high level of accuracy to identify impairments, functional deficits, or disability?
- What are the most important tests to do first? Which could be postponed until a later visit with the patient?

services. It has been shown in a multicenter study that patients seen in outpatient physical therapy practices have extensive health histories, including use of medications for a variety of medical conditions (e.g., hypertension, pulmonary disorders, and depression) and surgical histories (e.g., orthopedic, abdominal, and gynecological surgeries).[18]

The types of data that can be generated from a patient's health history are summarized in Box 1.9.[4,19,20,97] The therapist determines which aspects of the patient's history are more relevant than others and what data need to be obtained from various sources.

Sources of information about the patient's history include:

- Self-report health history questionnaires filled out prior to or during the initial visit.
- Interviews with the patient, family, or other significant individuals involved in patient care.
- Review of the medical record.
- Reports from the referral source, consultants, or other health-care team members.

The extent of information about a patient's health history that is necessary or available may be extensive or limited and

BOX 1.9 Information Generated from the Initial History

Demographic Data
- Age, sex, race, and ethnicity
- Primary language
- Education

Social History
- Family and caregiver resources
- Cultural background
- Social interactions/support systems

Occupation/Leisure
- Current and previous employment
- Job/school-related activities
- Recreational and community activities/tasks

Growth and Development
- Developmental history
- Hand and foot dominance

Living Environment
- Current living environment
- Expected destination after discharge
- Community accessibility

General Health Status and Lifestyle Habits and Behaviors: Past/Present (Based on Self or Family Report)
- Perception of health/disability
- Lifestyle health risks (smoking and/or substance abuse)
- Diet, exercise, and sleep habits

Medical/Surgical/Psychological History
- Previous inpatient or outpatient services

Medications
- Over-the-counter and prescription meds
- Frequency and dosage of meds

Family History: Current and Past
- Health risk factors
- Family illnesses

Cognitive/Social/Emotional Status
- Orientation and memory
- Communication
- Social/emotional interactions

Current Conditions/Chief Complaints or Concerns
- Conditions/reasons physical therapy services sought
- Patient's perceived level of daily functioning and disability
- Patient's needs and goals
- History, onset (date and course), mechanism of injury, and pattern and behavior of symptoms
- Family or caregiver needs, goals, and perception of patient's problems
- Current or past therapeutic interventions
- Previous outcome of chief complaint(s)

Functional Status and Activity Level
- Current/prior functional status: basic ADL and IADL related to self-care and home
- Current/prior functional status in work, school, and community-related IADL

Other Laboratory and Diagnostic Tests

Review of Systems: Any history of health conditions

may or may not be readily accessible prior to the first contact with the patient. Compare, for example, the information available to the therapist working in an acute care facility who has ready access to a patient's medical record versus the home health therapist who may have only a patient's medical diagnosis or brief surgical history. Regardless of the extent of written reports or medical/surgical history available, reviewing this information prior to the initial contact with the patient helps a therapist prioritize the questions asked and areas explored during the interview with the patient.

A general, verbal *review of systems* is conducted during the history-gathering phase to collect information about all major body systems relative to the patient's overall health condition.[5] The review of systems includes questions about past medical history, review of previous medical reports or lab work available, and other signs or symptoms experienced by the individual (see Table 1.2). This information is used to determine whether there are underlying conditions mimicking or masking musculoskeletal or neuromuscular symptoms or other signs indicative of complications that suggest the need for referral. This is especially important with the prevalence of patients being seen directly by the physical therapist through direct access.[5]

The interview is crucial for determining a patient's chief concerns and functional status—past, current, and desired. It also helps a therapist see a patient's problems from the patient's own perspective, specifically with regard to the perception of limitations in daily activities or participation restrictions in meaningful social or work roles. A patient almost always describes a current problem in terms of limited abilities or perceived quality of life, not the presenting impairment(s). For example, a patient might report, "My elbow really hurts when I pick up something heavy" or "I'm having trouble playing tennis (or bowling or unloading groceries from the car)." During the interview, questions that relate to symptoms (in this case, elbow pain) should identify

TABLE 1.2 Areas of Screening During the Patient Management Process

All Major Body Systems	*Review of Systems:* component of the Health History to determine need for referral for additional medical evaluation
Cardiovascular/pulmonary	Shortness of breath, pressure or pain in the chest, pulsating pain, history of heart or lung disease
Endocrine	History of thyroid or other hormonal conditions, medications
Eyes, Ears, Nose, and Throat	History of surgery or use of adaptive equipment
Gastrointestinal	Heartburn, reflux, diarrhea, constipation, vomiting, severe abdominal pain, swallowing problems
Genitourinary/reproductive	Bowel or bladder function, burning with urination, sexual function, unusual menstrual cycles, pregnancy
Hematological or lymphatic	Results of recent bloodwork or treatment, bleeding or lymphedema
Integumentary	History of skin cancer, dermatological conditions (eczema, psoriasis, etc.), lumps or growths
Neurological/musculoskeletal	History of CNS or peripheral nerve symptoms, muscular cramping, spasms, atrophy, weakness
Overall physical and emotional well-being	Persistent fatigue, malaise, fever, chills, sweats, unexplained weight change, depression, mood swings, suicidal thoughts
Human Movement System	***Systems Review:*** **component of the hands-on Examination specific to systems affecting movement**
Cardiovascular/pulmonary	Heart rate and rhythm, respiratory rate, blood pressure, and edema
Integumentary	Skin temperature, color, texture, integrity, scar formation, wound or incision healing
Musculoskeletal	Symmetry, gross ROM and strength, height and weight
Neuromuscular	General assessment of gross coordinated movement (e.g., balance, gait, locomotion, transfers, transitions) and motor function (motor control, motor learning)
Communication ability, affect, cognition, language, learning style	Ability to make needs known, consciousness, orientation (person, place, time), expected emotional/behavioral responses, learning preferences (e.g., learning barriers, educational needs)

location, intensity, description, and factors that provoke (aggravate) or alleviate symptoms in a 24-hour period.

Collecting health history data through a self-report questionnaire has been shown to be an accurate source of information from patients seen in an outpatient orthopedic physical therapy practice.[22] In addition, depending on a patient's condition and individual situation, the perceptions of family members, significant others, caregivers, or employers are often as important to the overall picture as the patient's own assessment of the current problems.

While taking a health history, it is useful to group the interview questions into categories to keep the information organized. Gathering and evaluating data simultaneously makes it easier to recognize and identify *patterns or clusters of signs and symptoms* and even to begin to formulate one or more initial "working" hypotheses about the patient's problem(s), which later will be supported or rejected as part of the diagnostic process. Making these judgments helps organize and structure the examination.[151,152,183] Experienced therapists tend to form working hypotheses quite early in the examination process, even while reviewing a patient's chart before the initial contact with the patient.[79,80,92,114,194] This enables a therapist to determine and prioritize which definitive tests and measures should be selected for the later portion of the examination.[80]

Systems Review

A brief but relevant screening of the body systems, known as a *systems review*,[4,5] is performed as a part of the hands on examination process after organizing and prioritizing data obtained from the health history. This baseline screening of the components of the movement system helps to determine which areas of tests and measures will be needed to determine specific diagnoses that impact function and the perception of disability. The systems typically screened by physical therapists are the cardiovascular and pulmonary, integumentary, musculoskeletal, and neuromuscular systems and a general overview of a patient's cognition, communication, and learning preferences (see Table 1.2).

Findings from the systems review, coupled with information about a patient's chief complaints and past history secured from the patient's health history, enable a therapist to begin to make decisions about the possible causes of a patient's impairments and functional deficits and to distinguish between problems that can and cannot be managed effectively by physical therapy interventions.[19] If a therapist determines that a patient has a condition or problem that falls outside the scope of physical therapy practice, then referral to or coordination with another health-care practitioner is appropriate.[4,19,21,59]

FOCUS ON EVIDENCE

In a case report,[68] a patient was referred to physical therapy 5 weeks after shoulder surgery. During the initial examination the physical therapist identified inconsistent signs and symptoms that were indicative of a possible infection or medical complication including bilateral diffuse multi-joint arthralgia, generalized fatigue, and other atypical signs. The therapist made the clinical decision to refer the patient back to the primary care physician where a secondary infection was confirmed. The result of this communication and coordination of care and services by the physical therapist was a positive outcome—the patient was able to fully participate in a rehabilitation program after the addition of antibiotic therapy to her medical care.

Specific Tests and Measures

Once it has been decided that a patient's problems/conditions are most likely amenable to physical therapy intervention, the next determination a therapist must make during the examination process is to decide which aspects of physical function require further investigation through the use of specific tests and measures.

Specific (definitive/diagnostic) tests and measures used by physical therapists provide in-depth information about body function and structure impairments, activity limitations, and participation restrictions.[4,53,57,97] The specificity of these tests enables a therapist to support or refute the working hypotheses formulated while taking the patient's health history and performing the systems review. These tests also give the therapist a clearer picture of a patient's current condition(s) and may reveal information about the patient not previously identified during the history and systems review. If treatment is initiated, the results of these specific tests and measures establish *objective baselines* from which changes in a patient's abilities as the result of interventions are measured.

Given the array of specific tests available to a therapist, the guidelines summarized in Box 1.10 should be considered when determining which definitive tests and measures need to be selected and administered.[4,53,54,146]

There are more than 20 general categories of specific tests and measures commonly performed by physical therapists.[4,180] Typically, testing involves multiple body systems to identify the scope of a patient's functioning or disability by targeting specific impairments, activity limitations, and participation restrictions. When examining a patient with chronic knee pain, for example, in addition to performing a thorough musculoskeletal examination, it also would be appropriate to administer tests that identify the impact of the patient's knee pain on the neuromuscular system (by assessing balance and proprioception) and the cardiopulmonary system (by assessing aerobic capacity).

Because many of the health-related conditions as the result of injury or disease discussed in this textbook involve the neuromusculoskeletal system, some examples of specific tests and measures that identify *musculoskeletal and neuromuscular impairments* are noted here. They include but are not limited to:

- Assessment of pain
- Goniometry and flexibility testing
- Joint mobility, stability, and integrity tests (including ligamentous testing)
- Tests of muscle performance (manual muscle testing and dynamometry)

BOX 1.10 Guidelines for Selection of Specific Tests and Measures

- Consider why particular tests are performed and how the interpretation of their results may influence the formulation of a diagnosis.
- Select tests and measures that provide accurate information and are valid and reliable and whose efficacy is supported by evidence generated from sound scientific studies.
- Administer tests that target multiple levels of functioning and disability: impairments, activity/functional limitations, and the patient's perceived level of participation restrictions.
- Prioritize tests and measures selected to gather in-depth information about key problems identified during the history and systems review.
- Decide whether to administer generic tests or tests that are specific to a particular region of the body.
- Choose tests that provide data specific enough to support or reject working hypotheses formulated during the history and systems review and to determine a diagnosis, prognosis, and plan of care when the data are evaluated.
- Select tests and measures that will help determine the types of intervention that most likely are appropriate and effective.
- To complete the examination in a timely manner, avoid collecting more information than is necessary to make informed decisions during the evaluation, diagnosis, and treatment planning phases of management.

- Posture analysis
- Assessment of balance, proprioception, and neuromuscular control
- Gait analysis
- Assessment of assistive, adaptive, or orthotic devices

Choice of specific tests and measures should be based on clinical decision-making used by the therapist to confirm or reject hypothesis about why the patient is experiencing less than optimal function and to provide data to support the diagnosis, prognosis, and plan of care.

Although specific testing of impairments is crucial, these tests do not tell the therapist how the impairments are affecting the patient's functional capabilities. Therefore, every examination should also include use of instruments that specifically measure extent of activity limitations and participation restrictions. These tools, often referred to as *functional outcome measures,* are designed to reflect the interaction of a patient's health condition and impairments in body function and structure with functional abilities and health-related quality of life.[11]

The Middle Class Tax Relief Act of 2012 mandated that functional outcomes be reported on the billing claims for Medicare and Medicaid patients receiving therapy services. As a result of this act, in 2013 requirements to report functional limitations and outcomes were established by the Centers for Medicare and Medicaid Services (CMS) for all outpatient therapy billing claims through the physician fee schedule final rule (77 Federal Regulation 68958). Functional Limitation Reporting, also referred to as "G-Code Reporting," uses a coding system based on the ICF classification of functioning, disability, and health to quantify the type and severity of functional limitation(s) identified through the use of tests and measures at the onset and throughout the "episode of care." The scope and specifics of this legislation and application of G-code reporting are beyond the scope of this textbook. Box 1.11 lists references and websites for those interested in learning more about this topic.

The format of functional testing procedures and instruments varies. The clinical decision-making skill of the therapist is paramount to the effective selection of the ideal test(s) to use to objectively describe the functional limits or abilities of patients based on the carefully synthesized results of examination and re-examination information. Some tests gather information by *self-report* (by the patient or family member);[96] others require *observation and rating of the patient's performance* by a therapist as various functional tasks are carried out.[11] Some instruments measure a patient's ease or difficulty of performing specific physical tasks. Other instruments incorporate temporal (time-based) or spatial (distance-based) criteria, such as measurement of walking speed or distance, in the format.[10] Test scores also can be based on the level of assistance needed (with assistive devices or by another person) to complete a variety of functional tasks.

Indices of disability measure a patient's perception of his or her degree of participation restriction. These self-report instruments usually focus on BADL and IADL, such as the ability or inability to care for one's own needs (physical, social, and emotional) or the level of participation in the community

BOX 1.11 Resources for Information on Functional Outcome Reporting (G-Codes)

- MLN Matters® Special Edition (SE) 1307: Outpatient Therapy Functional Reporting Requirements: http://www.cms.gov/outreach-and-education/medicare-learning-network-mln/mlnmattersarticles/downloads/se1307.pdf
- CMS Manual System Transmittal 165: Implementing the Claims-Based Data Collection Requirement for Outpatient Therapy Services — Section 3005(g) of the Middle Class Tax Relief and Jobs Creation Act (MCTRJCA) of 2012: https://www.cms.gov/Regulations-and-Guidance/Guidance/Transmittals/Downloads/R165BP.pdf
- CMS-1500 (02/12) Claim Form Example: Functional Limitation Reporting G-codes and Severity/Complexity Modifiers: https://medicare.fcso.com/Education_resources/0299021.pdf
- APTA Resources for Functional Limitation Reporting under Medicare: http://www.apta.org/Payment/Medicare/CodingBilling/FunctionalLimitation/

that is currently possible, desired, expected, or required. Information gathered with these instruments may indicate that the patient requires consultation and possible intervention by other health-care professionals to deal with some of the social or psychological aspects of disability.

Functional Limitation Reporting and G-code assignment do not require or limit specific tests to be used to define the functional limitation, its severity, or complexity when determining the G-code. It is the responsibility of the therapist to identify valid, objective tests to provide reliable results throughout the course of treatment from initial evaluation to discharge. Familiarity with evidence-based practice guidelines and use of resources for applying evidence as described earlier in this section will assist both the novice and veteran therapist to successfully accomplish this professional responsibility.

NOTE: It is well beyond the scope or purpose of this text to identify and describe the many tests and instruments that identify and measure impairments, activity limitations, and participation restrictions. The reader is referred to several resources in the literature that provide this information.[2,7,10,11,30,108]

Evaluation

Evaluation is a process characterized by the interpretation of collected data. The process involves analysis and integration of information to establish the diagnosis, prognosis, and plan of care using a series of sound clinical decisions.[4,5] Although evaluation is depicted as a distinct entity or phase of the patient management model (see Fig. 1.5), some degree of evaluation goes on at every phase of patient management, from examination through outcome. By pulling together and sorting out subjective and objective data from the examination, a therapist should be able to determine the following:

- A patient's general health status and its impact on current and potential function.
- The acuity or chronicity and severity of the current condition(s).
- The extent of structural and functional impairments of body systems and impact on functional abilities.
- Which impairments are related to which activity limitations.
- A patient's current, overall level of physical functioning (limitations *and* abilities) compared with the functional abilities needed, expected, or desired by the patient.
- The impact of physical dysfunction on social/emotional function.
- The impact of the physical environment on a patient's function.
- A patient's social support systems and their impact on current, desired, and potential function.

The decisions made during the evaluation process may also suggest that additional testing by the therapist or another practitioner is necessary before the therapist can determine a patient's diagnosis and prognosis for positive outcomes from physical therapy interventions. For example, a patient whose chief complaints are related to episodic shoulder pain but who also indicates during the health history that bouts of depression sometimes make it difficult to work or socialize should be referred for a psychological consultation and possible treatment.[19] Results of the psychological evaluation could be quite relevant to the success of the physical therapy intervention.

Addressing the questions posed in Box 1.12 during the evaluation of data derived from the examination enables a therapist to make pertinent clinical decisions that lead to the determination of a diagnosis and prognosis and the selection of potential intervention strategies for the plan of care.

During the evaluation, it is particularly useful to ascertain if and to what extent relationships exist among measurements of impairments, activity limitations, participation restrictions, and the patient's perceived level of disability. These relationships often are not straightforward as indicated in the following investigations.

FOCUS ON EVIDENCE

In a study of patients with cervical spine disorders,[70] investigators reported a strong correlation between measurements of impairments (pain, ROM, and cervical muscle strength) and functional limitations (functional axial rotation and lifting capacity) but a relatively weak statistical relationship between measurements of functional limitations and the patient's perceived level of disability, as determined by three self-report measures. In another study[185] that compared shoulder ROM with the ability of patients to perform basic self-care activities, a strong correlation was noted between the

BOX 1.12 Key Questions to Consider During the Evaluation and Diagnostic Processes

- What is the extent, degree, or severity of structural and functional impairments, activity/functional limitations, or participation restrictions/disability?
- What is the stability or progression of dysfunction?
- To what extent are any identified personal and environmental barriers to functioning modifiable?
- Is the current health condition(s) acute or chronic?
- What actions/events change (relieve or worsen) the patient's signs and symptoms?
- How do preexisting health conditions (comorbidities) affect the current condition?
- How does the information from the patient's medical/surgical history and tests and measures done by other health-care practitioners relate to the findings of the physical therapy examination?
- Have identifiable clusters of findings (i.e., patterns) emerged relevant to the patient's dysfunction?
- Is there an understandable relationship between the patient's extent of impairments and the degree of activity/functional limitation or participation restriction/disability?
- What are the causal factors that seem to be contributing to the patient's impairments, activity/functional limitations, or participation restriction/disability?

degree of difficulty of performing these tasks and the extent of shoulder motion limitation.

Although the results of these studies to some extent are related to the choice of measurement tools, these findings highlight the complexity of evaluating disability and suggest that identifying the strength or weakness of the links among the levels of functioning and disability may help a therapist predict more accurately a patient's prognosis. Evaluating these relationships and answering the other questions noted in Box 1.12 lay the foundation for determining a diagnosis and prognosis and developing an effective plan of care.

Diagnosis

The term *diagnosis* can be used in two ways—it refers to either a process or a category (label) within a classification system.[62,5] Both usages of the word are relevant to physical therapy practice. Physical therapists use a systematic process, sometimes referred to as differential diagnosis, to identify an appropriate diagnostic category amenable to physical therapy intervention.[5] The diagnosis is an essential and required element of patient management whose primary purpose is to guide the physical therapy prognosis, plan of care, and interventions.[4,53,97,129,158,183,202]

Diagnostic Process

The diagnostic process is a complex *sequence* of actions and decisions that includes (1) the collection of data (examination); (2) the analysis and interpretation of all relevant data collected, leading to the generation of working hypotheses (evaluation); and (3) organization of data, recognition of clustering of data (a pattern of findings), formation of a diagnostic hypothesis, and subsequent classification of data into categories.[4,43,59,149,159,183,202]

Through the diagnostic process a physical therapist identifies impairments of body structure and function that affect the human movement system, whereas a physician identifies disease.[59,84,97,129,149,187] For the physical therapist, the diagnostic process is a mechanism by which discrepancies and consistencies between a patient's current level of performance and desired level of function and his or her capacity to achieve that level of function are identified.[4]

Diagnostic Category

A diagnostic category (clinical classification) identifies and describes patterns or clusters of findings from the examination and conclusions from the evaluation. The purpose of this label is to guide the therapist in the development of a prognosis, plan of care, and interventions.[5]

A diagnostic category used in physical therapy should describe the impact of a health condition or disease on function of the human movement system at the level of the whole person.[4] This category, defined by the therapist, indicates the primary dysfunctions to be addressed in the selection of interventions and development of the plan of care.

The physical therapy profession has not officially adopted a specific classification system for diagnosis, although the ICF is recommended. The following are guidelines listed in the *Guide* for choosing a classification scheme that is relevant for the therapist to make a diagnosis:[5]

- The classification system must be within the legal boundaries placed on the profession and within societal approval.
- The health professional must use acceptable tests and measures to confirm the diagnostic decision.
- The diagnostic label must describe a condition or problem that is within the scope of intervention legally allowed by the clinician making the diagnosis.

As the profession of physical therapy has advanced to a doctoral level and the position as a primary care provider has evolved, the role of diagnostician has become the focus of both research and practice.[5,36,120,129,160] The exclusive use of ICD diagnostic categories does not always identify a problem within the scope of physical therapy intervention because this classification focuses primarily on the diagnosis of pathology. A diagnostic classification system developed by physical therapists is needed for delineating the knowledge base and scope of practice of physical therapy.[4,42,62,84,149,158,201] Because the diagnosis is intended to guide the treatment plan, a universally accepted diagnostic classification scheme would foster clarity of communication in practice and clinical research.[36,53,84,120]

Suffice it to say that it is well beyond the scope of this text to discuss the history and the future of the development of a classification system for accurately labeling diagnoses amenable to physical therapy intervention.

NOTE: The impairment/function-based diagnoses in the clinical practice guidelines developed by multiple practice sections of the APTA are based on the classification and coding system described in the ICF combined, as appropriate, with the ICD as recommended by the WHO. The diagnostic classifications in the approved clinical practice guidelines are linked to recommendations for physical therapy interventions based on "best evidence" from the scientific literature.[29,33,34,104,105,117] However, research shows that there continues to be a gap in the use of diagnostic classification systems and the selection of interventions that are directly related to the diagnostic label used by clinicians in practice.[120]

Prognosis and Plan of Care

After the initial examination has been completed, data have been evaluated, and a diagnosis has been established, a *prognosis* (see Fig. 1.5), including a plan of care, must be determined before initiating any interventions. A prognosis is a prediction of a patient's optimal level of function expected as the result of a plan for treatment during an episode of care and the anticipated length of time needed to reach specified functional outcomes.[4,97,141] Some factors that influence a patient's prognosis and functional outcomes are noted in Box 1.13.

Determining an accurate prognosis is, indeed, challenging even for experienced therapists. The more complex a patient's problems, the more difficult it is to project the patient's optimal level of function, particularly at the onset of treatment.

BOX 1.13 Factors That Influence a Patient's Prognosis/Expected Outcomes

- Complexity, severity, acuity, or chronicity and expected course of the patient's health condition(s) (pathology), impairments, and activity/functional limitations
- Patient's general health status and presence of comorbidities (e.g., hypertension, diabetes, and obesity) and risk factors
- The patient's previous level of functioning or disability
- The patient's living environment
- Patient's and/or family's goals
- Patient's motivation and adherence and responses to previous interventions
- Safety issues and concerns
- Extent of support (physical, emotional, and social)
- Health literacy of the patient

For example, if an otherwise healthy and fit 70-year-old patient who was just discharged from the hospital after a total knee arthroplasty is referred for home-based physical therapy services, it is relatively easy to predict the time frame that will be needed to prepare the patient to return to independence in the home and community. In contrast, it may be possible to predict only incremental levels of functional improvement at various stages of rehabilitation for a patient who has sustained multiple fractures and soft tissue injuries as the result of an automobile accident.

In these two examples of establishing prognoses for patients with musculoskeletal conditions, as with most other patient problems, the accuracy of the prognosis is affected in part by the therapist's clinical decision-making ability based on the following[4]:

- Familiarity with the patient's current health condition(s) and the surgical intervention(s) and previous history of diseases or disorders.
- Knowledge of the process and time frames of tissue healing.
- Experience managing patients with similar surgical procedures, pathological conditions, impairments, and functional deficits.
- Knowledge of the efficacy of tests and measures performed, accuracy of the findings, and effectiveness of the physical therapy interventions.

Plan of Care

The *plan of care,* an integral component of the prognosis, is established in coordination with the patient and, if indicated, others involved in the care of the patient. It should include the following components:[4]

- Patient goals that are functionally driven and time limited.
- Expected functional outcomes that are meaningful, utilitarian, sustainable, and measurable.
- Extent of improvement predicted and length of time necessary to reach that level.
- Specific interventions.
- Proposed frequency and duration of interventions.
- Specific discharge plans.

Setting Goals and Outcomes in the Plan of Care

Developing a plan of care involves *collaboration* and *negotiation* between the patient (and, when appropriate, the family) and the therapist.[4,84,97] The *anticipated goals* and *expected outcomes* documented in the plan of care must be patient centered—that is, the goals and outcomes must be meaningful to the patient.[141] These goals and outcomes also must be measurable and linked to each other. Goals describe the intended impact on functioning established with specific time limits.[4] Outcomes are the actual results of the episode of care measured with the specific tests and measures that were used to establish a baseline at the initial examination, and repeated periodically during the episode of care. Results are based on reduction of impairments, activity limitations, and participation restrictions coupled with achieving the optimal level possible of function, general health, and patient satisfaction.[4]

Establishing and prioritizing meaningful, functionally relevant goals and determining expected outcomes requires engaging the patient and/or family in the decision-making process from a therapist's first contact with a patient. Knowing what a patient wants to be able to accomplish as the result of treatment and ascertaining which accomplishments are the most important to the patient helps a therapist develop and prioritize intervention strategies that target the patient's functional limitations and associated impairments. This, in turn, increases the likelihood of successful outcomes from treatment.[132,141,142] Some key questions a therapist often asks a patient or the patient's extended support system that are critical for establishing anticipated goals and expected outcomes in the plan of care are listed in Box 1.14.[9,97,132,142]

An integral aspect of effective goal and outcome setting is explaining to a patient how the health condition and identified impairments are associated with the patient's activity limitations and participation restrictions and why specific interventions will be used. Discussing an expected time frame for achieving the negotiated goals and outcomes puts the treatment plan and the patient's expectation for progress in a realistic context. This type of information helps a patient and family members set goals that are not just meaningful, but also realistic and attainable. Setting up *short-term* and *long-term goals,* particularly for patients with severe or complex problems, is also a way to help a patient recognize incremental improvement and progress during treatment.

The plan of care also indicates the optimal level of improvement that will be reflected by the functional outcomes as well as how those outcomes will be measured. An outline of the specific interventions, their frequency and duration of use, and how the interventions are directly related to attaining the stated goals and outcomes also must appear in the plan. Finally, the plan of care concludes with the criteria for discharge. These criteria are addressed following a discussion of elements of intervention in the patient management process.

BOX 1.14 Key Questions to Establish and Prioritize Patient-Centered Goals and Outcomes in the Plan of Care

- What activities are most important to you at home, school, work, in the community, or during your leisure time?
- What activities do you currently need help with that you would like to be able to do independently?
- Of the activities you are finding difficult to do or cannot do at all at this time, and which ones would you like to be able to do better or do again?
- Of the problems you are having, which ones do you want to try to eliminate or minimize first?
- In what areas do you think you have the biggest problems during the activities you would like to do on your own?
- What are your goals for coming to physical therapy?
- What would you like to be able to accomplish through therapy?
- What would make you feel that you were making progress in achieving your goals?
- How soon do you want to reach your goals?

NOTE: Periodic re-examination of a patient and re-evaluation of a patient's response to treatment may necessitate modification of the initial prognosis and plan of care (see Fig. 1.5).

Intervention

Intervention, a component of patient management, is the purposeful interaction of the therapist with the patient and with other family members, caregivers, or providers as appropriate.[4,5] The therapist selects, prescribes, and implements interventions based on the examination, evaluation, diagnosis, prognosis, and goals established for the patient. Interventions are updated, progressed, or discontinued based on patient response, achievement of goals, or results of outcomes (see Fig. 1.5).

The *Guide* describes nine categories of intervention appropriate for use by physical therapists in the care of patients.[5] These categories are listed in Box 1.15. Clinical reasoning, decision-making, clinical practice guidelines, clinical prediction rules, and the use of evidence-based practice are tools that therapists use during the patient management process to assist in the selection of specific, individualized interventions.[37,38,91,95,120]

If interventions are to be considered effective, they must result in the reduction or elimination of body function or structure impairments, activity limitations, and/or participation restrictions and, whenever possible, reduce the risk of future dysfunction. Moreover, the efficacy of each intervention should be supported by sound evidence, preferably based on prospective, randomized, controlled research studies.

Although the intended outcome of therapeutic exercise programs has always been to enhance a patient's functional capabilities or prevent loss of function, until the past few decades the focus of exercise programs in physical therapy was on the resolution of impairments. Success was measured primarily by the reduction of the identified impairments or improvements in various aspects of physical performance, such as strength, mobility, or balance as depicted in Figure 1.6.

BOX 1.15 Categories of Intervention Used by Physical Therapists

- Patient or Client Instruction (universally used with all patients)
- Airway Clearance Techniques
- Assistive Technology: Prescription, Application, and as appropriate, Fabrication or Modification
- Biophysical Agents
- Functional Training in Self-Care and in Domestic, Education, Work, Community, Social, and Civic Life
- Integumentary Repair and Protection Techniques
- Manual Therapy Techniques
- Motor Function Training
- Therapeutic Exercise

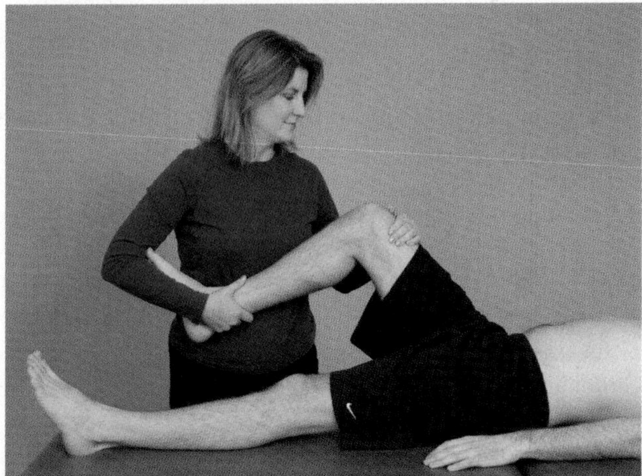

FIGURE 1.6 Manual resistance exercise, a procedural intervention, is a form of therapeutic exercise used during the early stage of rehabilitation if muscle strength or endurance is impaired.

In the past, it was assumed that if impairments were resolved, improvements in functional abilities would subsequently follow. Physical therapists now recognize that this assumption is not valid. To improve activity performance and participation in expected roles and to improve a patient's health-related quality of life, not only should therapeutic exercise interventions be implemented that correct functionally limiting impairments, but whenever possible, exercises should be task specific—that is, they should be performed using movement patterns that closely match a patient's intended or desired functional activities. In Figure 1.7, strengthening exercises are demonstrated using a task-specific lifting pattern.

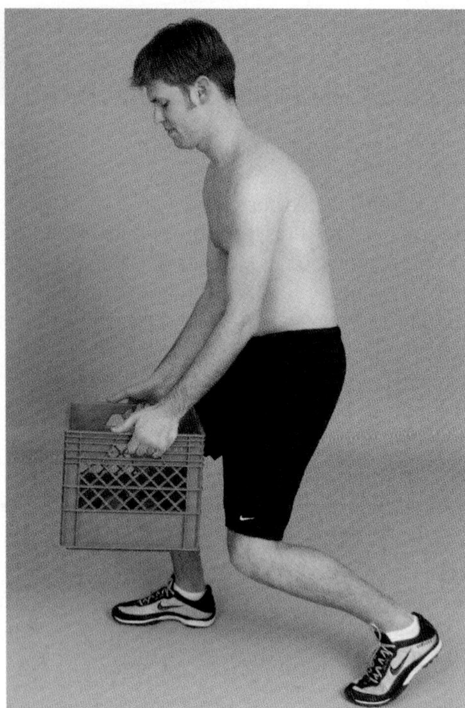

FIGURE 1.7 Task-specific strengthening exercises are carried out by lifting and lowering a weighted crate in preparation for functional tasks at home or work.

The importance of designing and implementing exercises that closely replicate the desired functional outcomes is demonstrated by the following study:

FOCUS ON EVIDENCE

Task-specific functional training was investigated in a study of the effects of a resistance exercise program on the stair-climbing ability of ambulatory older women.[39] Rather than having the subjects perform resisted hip and knee extension exercises in nonweight-bearing positions, they trained by ascending and descending stairs while wearing a weighted backpack. This activity not only improved muscle performance (strength and endurance), but also directly enhanced the subjects' efficiency in stair climbing during daily activities.

Another way to use therapeutic exercise interventions effectively to improve functional ability is to integrate safe but progressively more challenging functional activities that utilize incremental improvements in strength, endurance, and mobility into a patient's daily routine as early as possible in the treatment program. With this functionally oriented approach to exercise, the activities in the treatment program are specific to and directly support the expected functional outcomes. Selection and use of exercise procedures that target more than one goal or outcome are also appropriate and efficient ways to maximize improvements in a patient's function in the shortest time possible.

Effective use of any intervention must include determining the appropriate *intensity, frequency,* and *duration* of each intervention and periodic re-examination of a patient's responses to the interventions. While implementing therapeutic exercise interventions, a patient's response to exercise is continually monitored to decide when and to what extent to increase the difficulty of the exercise program or when to discontinue specific exercises. Each of the chapters of this textbook provides detailed information on factors that influence selection, application, and progression of therapeutic exercise interventions.

Patient or Client Instruction

Although patient instruction is one of the nine intervention categories, it is the only one that is specified to be used for every patient throughout the entire episode of care[5] (see Box 1.15). Because this intervention is universal for all patients, it is covered in more detail in this section. According to the revised third edition of the *Guide,* patient education is emphasized in the following way: *Patient or client instruction* is a type of intervention that physical therapists use with every individual they see. Education should include not only the patient, but also family members, caregivers, and other health professionals involved in the care of the patient.[5] There is no question that physical therapists perceive themselves as patient educators, facilitators of change, and motivators.[31,55,82,106,127] Patient education spans all three domains of learning: cognitive, affective, and psychomotor domains. Education ideally begins during a patient's initial contact with a therapist and involves the therapist *explaining* information, *asking* pertinent questions, and *listening* to the patient or a family member.

Patient-related instruction is the means by which a therapist helps a patient *learn* how to reduce his or her impairments and how to participate fully in the plan of care to achieve goals.[31] Patient-related instruction first may focus on providing a patient with background information, such as the interrelationship of the primary health condition and the associated impairments and limitations in activity or explaining the purpose of specific interventions in the plan of care. Instruction, such as physical therapist–directed exercise counseling,[181] may be implemented as an alternative to direct supervision of an exercise program and typically focuses on specific aspects of a treatment program, such as teaching a patient, family member, or caregiver a series of exercises to be carried out in a home program. Education may also help to prepare an individual for transition to a different role or setting or to understand risk factors for developing a problem and the need for health, wellness, or fitness programs. Therapists should also review health and wellness materials and clarify directions for safe use of equipment to be used at home.

A therapist must use multiple methods to convey information to a patient or family member, such as one-to-one, therapist-directed instruction; videotaped instruction; or written materials. Each has been shown to have a place in patient education as highlighted by the following studies.

FOCUS ON EVIDENCE

It has been shown that patients, who were taught exercises by a therapist, performed their exercises more accurately in a home program than patients whose sole source of information about their exercises was from reading a brochure.[51] In another study, the effectiveness of three modes of instruction in an exercise program were evaluated. The subjects who received in-person instruction by a therapist or two variations of videotaped instruction performed their exercise program more accurately than subjects who received only written instructions.[145]

However, written materials, particularly those with illustrations, can be taken home by a patient and used to reinforce verbal instructions from a therapist or videotaped instructions.

To be an effective patient educator, a therapist must possess an understanding of the process of learning, which most often is directed toward learning or modifying motor skills. As a patient educator, a therapist also must be able to recognize a patient's learning style, implement effective teaching strategies, and motivate a patient to *want* to learn new skills, adhere to an exercise program, or change health-related behaviors.

Outcomes

Simply stated, outcomes are results. Collection and analysis of outcome data related to health-care services are necessities, not options.[66] Measurement of outcomes is a means by which quality, efficacy, and cost-effectiveness of services can be assessed. Patient-related outcomes are monitored throughout an episode of physical therapy care—that is, intermittently during treatment and at the conclusion of treatment.[132] Evaluation of information generated from periodic re-examination and re-evaluation of a patient's response to treatment enables a therapist to ascertain if the anticipated goals and expected outcomes in the plan of care are being met and if the interventions that have been implemented are producing the intended results. It may well be that the goals and expected outcomes must be adjusted based on the extent of change or lack of change in a patient's function as determined by the level of the interim outcomes. This information also helps the therapist decide if, when, and to what extent to modify the goals, expected outcomes, and interventions in the patient's plan of care (see Fig. 1.5).

There are several broad areas of outcomes commonly assessed by physical therapists during the continuum of patient care. They are listed in Box 1.16.

BOX 1.16 Areas of Outcomes Assessed by Physical Therapists

- Level of a patient's physical functioning, including impairments, activity/functional limitations, participation restrictions, and perceived disability
- Extent of prevention or reduced risk of occurrence or recurrence of future dysfunction related to health conditions, associated impairments, activity/functional limitations, participation restrictions, or perceived disability
- Patient's general health status or level of well-being and fitness
- Degree of patient satisfaction
- Level of safety and patient/family understanding
- Adherence/compliance with home exercises or instructions

Functional Outcomes

The key to the justification of physical therapy services in today's cost-conscious health-care environment is the identification and documentation of successful patient-centered, functional outcomes that can be attributed to interventions.[4,10,30,63,179] As discussed previously (in the Tests and Measures section), functional limitation reporting became mandatory in 2013 for all outpatient therapy being billed to Medicare. G-code reporting is the methodology for providing a nonpayment code to track functional improvements for a patient over the course of the billing period.

Functional outcomes must be *meaningful*, *practical*, and *sustainable*.[179] Outcomes that have an impact on a patient's ability to function at work, in the home, or in the community in ways that have been identified as important by the patient, family, significant others, caregivers, or employers are considered *meaningful*. If the formulation of anticipated goals and expected outcome has been a collaborative effort between the patient and the therapist, the outcomes will be meaningful to the patient. The *practical* aspect of functional outcomes implies that improvements in function have been achieved in an efficient and cost-effective manner. Improvements in function that are maintained over time after discharge from treatment (to the extent possible given the nature of the health condition) are considered *sustainable*.

Measuring Outcomes

The expected outcomes identified in a physical therapy plan of care must be *measurable*. More specifically, changes in a patient's status over time must be *quantifiable*. As noted in the previous discussion of the examination component of the patient management model, many of the specific tests and measures used by physical therapists traditionally have focused on measurement of impairments (i.e., ROM, muscle performance, joint mobility/stability, and balance). The reduction of impairments may reflect the impact of interventions on the pathological condition but may or may not translate into improvements in a patient's health-related quality of life, such as safety and functional abilities. Hence, there is the need for measurement not only of impairments, but also of a patient's levels of physical functioning and perceived participation ability to accurately assess patient-related outcomes that include but are not limited to the effectiveness of physical therapy interventions, such as therapeutic exercise.

Impact of interventions on patient-related, functional outcomes. In response to the need to produce evidence that supports the effectiveness of physical therapy interventions for reducing movement dysfunction, a self-report instrument called OPTIMAL (Outpatient Physical Therapy Improvement in Movement Assessment Log) has been developed for measuring the impact of physical therapy interventions on function and has been tested for validity and reliability.[63] The instrument measures a patient's difficulty with or confidence in performing a series of 22 actions, most of which are related to functional mobility, including moving from lying to sitting and sitting to standing, kneeling, walking, running, climbing stairs, reaching, and lifting. In addition, to assist the therapist with setting goals for the plan of care, the patient is asked to identify three activities that he or she would like to be able to do without difficulty.

OPTIMAL also is considered to be a valid test for assisting in the assignment of G-codes for Functional Limitation Reporting. As such, in 2012 the APTA mapped each of the test activities in OPTIMAL to the Activity and Participation categories for G-code reporting to assist the clinician to use this tool more effectively. A number of studies that have investigated the benefits of exercise programs for individuals with impaired functional abilities[86,98,155] reflect the trend in research to include an assessment of changes in a patient's health-related quality of life as the result of interventions. Assessment of outcomes related to the reduction of risks of future injury or further impairment, prevention of further functional limitations or disability, adherence to a home program, or the use of knowledge that promotes optimal health and fitness may also help determine the effectiveness of the services provided. To substantiate that the use of physical therapy services for prevention is cost-effective, physical therapists are finding that it is important to collect follow-up data that demonstrate a reduced need for future physical therapy services as the result of interventions directed toward prevention and health promotion activities.

Patient satisfaction. Another area of outcomes assessment that has become increasingly important in physical therapy practice is that of *patient satisfaction*. An assessment of patient satisfaction during or at the conclusion of treatment can be used as an indicator of quality of care. Patient satisfaction surveys often seek to determine the impact of treatment based on the patient's own assessment of his or her status at the conclusion of treatment compared with that at the onset of treatment.[154] Instruments, such as the Physical Therapy Outpatient Satisfaction Survey (PTOPS)[154] or the MedRisk Instrument for Measuring Patient Satisfaction with physical therapy (MRPS),[13,14] also measure a patient's perception of many other areas of care. An important quality of patient satisfaction questionnaires is their ability to discriminate among the factors that influence satisfaction. Identification of factors that adversely influence satisfaction may enable the clinician to take steps to modify these factors to deliver an optimal level of services to patients.[14]

Factors that may influence the extent of patient satisfaction are noted in Box 1.17.[13,14,27,154]

BOX 1.17 Examples of Determinants of Patient Satisfaction*

- Interpersonal attributes of the therapist (communication skills, professionalism, helpfulness, and empathy) and the impact on the patient-therapist relationship
- Perception of a therapist's clinical skills
- Extent of functional improvement during the episode of care
- Extent of participation in goal setting in the plan of care
- The acuity of the patient's condition (higher satisfaction in acute conditions)
- Convenience of access to services
- Administrative issues, such as continuity of care, flexible hours for scheduling, waiting time at each visit, duration of treatments, and cost of care

*Determinants are not rank ordered.

FOCUS ON EVIDENCE

A recent systematic review of the literature addressed the degree of patient satisfaction with musculoskeletal physical therapy care and identified the factors that were associated with high patient satisfaction in outpatient settings across North America and Northern Europe.[74] The review included articles if they were a survey, clinical trial, qualitative study, or patient interview. Only 15 of several thousand articles met the inclusion criteria. A meta-analysis of pooled data from the included studies revealed that on a scale of 1 to 5 (5 being the highest level of satisfaction), the degree of patient satisfaction was 4.41 (95% confidence interval = 4.41–4.46), indicating that patients are highly satisfied with physical therapy care directed toward musculoskeletal conditions. One finding of interest in the studies reviewed is the quality of the patient-therapist relationship consistently ranked higher as an indicator of patient satisfaction than the extent of improvement in the patient's physical functioning as a result of the episode of care.

Discharge Planning

Planning for discharge begins early in the rehabilitation process. As previously noted, criteria for discharge are identified in a patient's plan of care. Ongoing assessment of outcomes is the mechanism by which a therapist determines when discharge from care is warranted. A patient is discharged from physical therapy services when the anticipated goals and expected outcomes have been attained.[4] The discharge plan often includes some type of home program, appropriate follow-up, possible referral to community resources, or re-initiation of physical therapy services (an additional episode of care) if the patient's needs change over time and if additional services are approved.

Discontinuation of services is differentiated from discharge.[4] *Discontinuation* refers to the ending of services prior to the achievement of anticipated goals and expected outcomes. Several factors may necessitate discontinuation of services, which may include a decision by a patient to stop services, a change in a patient's medical status such that progress is no longer possible, or the need for further services cannot be justified to the payer.

In conclusion, the patient management model discussed in this section establishes a comprehensive, systematic approach to the provision of effective and efficient physical therapy care and services to patients and clients. The model is a mechanism to demonstrate the interrelationships among the phases of the continuum of patient care set in a conceptual framework of functioning and disability; it is aimed at improving a patient's function and health-related quality of life. The management model also places an emphasis on reducing risk factors for disease, injury, impairments, or disability and promoting health and well-being in patients and clients seeking and receiving physical therapy services.

Strategies for Effective Exercise and Task-Specific Instruction

As discussed in the previous section of this chapter, patient-related instruction is an essential element of the intervention phase of patient management. As a patient educator, a therapist spends a substantial amount of time teaching patients, their families, or other caregivers how to perform exercises correctly and safely. An understanding of health literacy level and learning style, assessed during the examination screening, combined with the skill of the therapist to communicate in plain language with the patient or caregiver is critical to effective exercise instruction. Effective strategies founded on principles of motor learning that are designed to help patients initially learn an exercise program under therapist supervision and then carry it out on an independent basis over a necessary period of time contribute to successful outcomes for the patient.

Health Literacy

Health literacy is the degree to which individuals have the capacity to obtain, process, and understand basic health information and services needed to make appropriate health decisions[190] This definition was formulated by the National Library of Medicine and has been consistently incorporated into national initiatives to improve health-care access, quality, and outcomes and to teach healthy lifestyles.[189,190] Physical therapists have a professional and ethical responsibility to understand health literacy and to develop the teaching and communication skills required to provide quality patient instruction and education that fits the learning needs and literacy levels unique to each patient.[5,47,145] Communicating in plain language, including the use of easily understood handouts, brochures, videos, pictures, and feedback, closes the gap between what the professional knows and what the patient understands.[47,145,190] Teaching is an essential function in the practice of physical therapy; providing intervention without incorporating elements of health promotion and education can result in less than optimal outcomes for patients.

Preparation for Exercise Instruction

When preparing to teach a patient a series of exercises, a therapist should have a plan that will facilitate learning prior to and during exercise interventions. A positive relationship between the therapist and the patient is a fundamental aspect for creating a motivating environment that fosters learning. A collaborative relationship should be established when the goals for the plan of care are negotiated. This, of course, occurs before exercise instruction begins. Effective exercise instruction is also based on knowing a patient's learning style—that is, if he or she prefers to learn by watching, reading about, or doing an activity. This may not be known early in treatment, so several methods of instruction may be necessary.

Identifying a patient's attitudes toward exercise helps a therapist determine how receptive a patient is likely to be about learning and adhering to an exercise program. Answers to the following questions may help a therapist formulate a strategy for enhancing a patient's motivation to exercise:

- Does the patient believe exercise will lessen symptoms or improve function?
- Is the patient concerned that exercising will be uncomfortable?
- Is the patient accustomed to engaging in regular exercise?

One method for promoting motivation is to design the exercise program so the least complicated or stressful exercises are taught first, thus ensuring early success. Always ending an exercise session with a successful effort also helps maintain a patient's level of motivation. Additional suggestions to enhance motivation and promote adherence to an exercise program are discussed in this section following an overview of the concepts of motor learning and acquisition of simple to complex motor skills. Box 1.18 summarizes some practical suggestions for effective exercise instruction.

Concepts of Motor Learning: A Foundation for Exercise and Task-Specific Instruction

Integration of motor learning principles into exercise instruction optimizes learning an exercise or functional task. An exercise is simply a motor task (a psychomotor skill) that a therapist teaches and a patient is expected to learn.

Motor learning is a complex set of internal processes that involves the acquisition and *relatively permanent* retention of a skilled movement or task through practice.[130,163,164,192,196] In the motor learning literature a distinction is made between motor performance and motor learning. *Performance* involves acquisition of the ability to carry out a skill, whereas *learning* involves both acquisition and retention.[56,154,163] Therefore, a patient's ability to perform an exercise or any skilled movement early in the motor-learning process is not necessarily representative of having learned the new exercise or skill.

It is thought that motor learning probably modifies the way sensory information in the central nervous system is

BOX 1.18 Practical Suggestions for Effective Exercise Instruction

- Select a nondistracting environment for exercise instruction.
- Initially teach exercises that replicate movement patterns of *simple* functional tasks.
- Demonstrate proper performance of an exercise (safe vs. unsafe movements; correct vs. incorrect movements). Then have the patient model your movements.
- If appropriate or feasible, initially guide the patient through the desired movement.
- Use clear and concise verbal and written directions.
- Complement written instructions for a home exercise program with illustrations (sketches) of the exercise.
- Have the patient demonstrate an exercise to you as you supervise and provide feedback.
- Provide specific, action-related feedback rather than general, nondescriptive feedback. For example, explain *why* the exercise was performed correctly or incorrectly.
- Teach an entire exercise program in small increments to allow time for a patient to practice and learn components of the program over several visits.

organized and processed and affects how motor actions are produced. In addition, because motor learning is not directly observable, it must be measured by observation and analysis of how an individual performs a skill.

Types of Motor Tasks

There are three basic types of motor tasks: discrete, serial, and continuous.[163,164]

Discrete task. A discrete task involves an action or movement with a recognizable beginning and end. Isolating and contracting a specific muscle group (as in a quadriceps setting exercise), grasping an object, doing a push-up, locking a wheelchair, and kicking a ball are examples of discrete motor tasks. Almost all exercises, such as lifting and lowering a weight or performing a self-stretching maneuver, can be categorized as discrete motor tasks.

Serial task. A serial task is composed of a series of discrete movements that are combined in a particular sequence. For example, to eat with a fork, a person must be able to grasp the fork, hold it in the correct position, pierce or scoop up the food, and lift the fork to the mouth. Many functional tasks in the work setting, for instance, are serial tasks with simple as well as complex components. Some serial tasks require specific timing between each segment of the task or momentum during the task. Wheelchair transfers are serial tasks. A patient must learn how to position the chair, lock the chair, possibly remove an armrest, scoot forward in the chair, and then transfer from the chair to another surface. Some transfers require momentum, whereas others do not.

Continuous task. A continuous task involves repetitive, uninterrupted movements that have no distinct beginning and ending. Examples include walking, ascending and descending stairs, and cycling.

Recognizing the type of skilled movements a patient must learn to do helps a therapist decide which instructional strategies will be most beneficial for acquiring specific functional skills. Consider what must be learned in the following motor tasks of an exercise program. To self-stretch the hamstrings, a patient must learn how to position and align his or her body and how much stretch force to apply to perform the stretching maneuver correctly. As flexibility improves, the patient must then learn how to safely control active movements in the newly gained portion of the range during functional activities. This requires muscles to contract with correct intensity at an unaccustomed length. In another scenario, to prevent recurrence of a shoulder impingement syndrome or back pain, a patient may need to learn through posture training how to maintain correct alignment of the trunk during a variety of reaching or lifting tasks that place slightly different demands on the body.

In both of these situations, motor learning must occur for the exercise program and functional training to be effective. By viewing exercise interventions from this perspective, it becomes apparent why applications of strategies to promote motor learning are an integral component of effective exercise instruction.

Conditions and Progression of Motor Tasks

If an exercise program is to improve a patient's function, it must include performing and learning a variety of tasks. If a functional training program is to prepare a patient to meet necessary and desired functional goals, it must place demands on a patient under varying conditions. A taxonomy of motor tasks, proposed by Gentile,[56] is a system for analyzing functional activities and a framework for understanding the conditions under which simple to complex motor tasks can be performed. Figure 1.8 depicts these conditions and the dimensions of difficulty of motor tasks.

An understanding of the components of this taxonomy and the interrelationships among its components is a useful framework for a therapist to identify and increase the difficulty of functional activities systematically for a patient with impaired function.

There are four main task dimensions addressed in the taxonomy: (1) the environment in which the task is performed, (2) the intertrial variability of the environment that is imposed on a task, (3) the need for a person's body to remain stationary or to move during the task, and (4) the presence or absence of manipulation of objects during the task. Examples of simple to complex everyday activities characteristic of each of the 16 different but interrelated task conditions are shown in Figure 1.9.

Closed or open environment. Environmental conditions of a task address whether objects or people (around the patient) are stationary or moving during the task and if the surface on

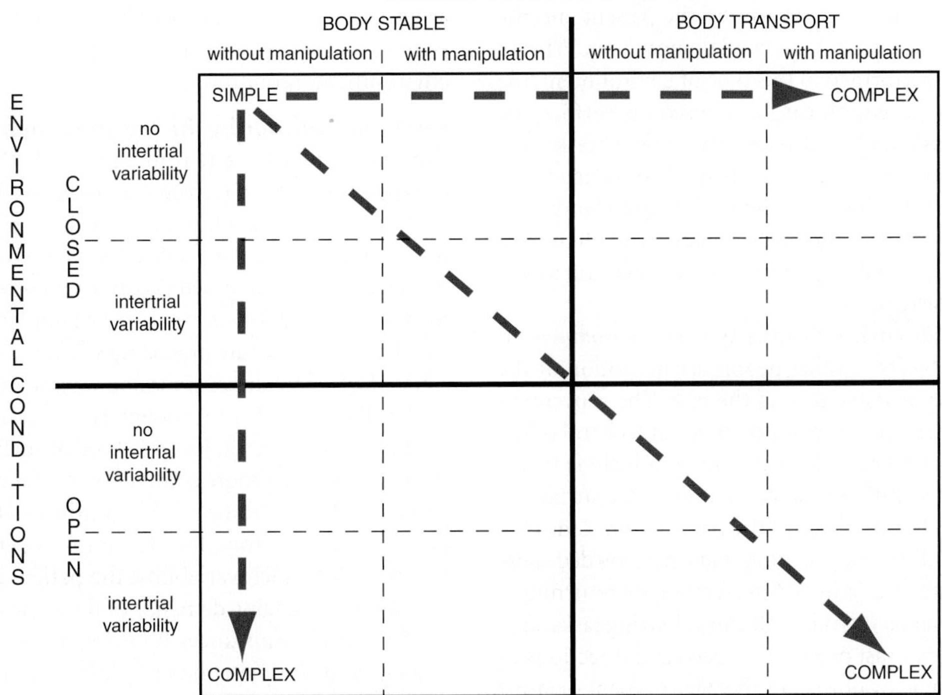

FIGURE 1.8 Taxonomy of motor tasks: dimensions of task difficulty. *(From Dennis, JK, and McKeough, DM: Mobility. In May, BJ [ed]:* Home Health and Rehabilitation—Concepts of Care. *Philadelphia: FA Davis, 1993, p 147, with permission.)*

		BODY STABLE		BODY TRANSPORT	
		without manipulation	with manipulation	without manipulation	with manipulation
CLOSED	without intertrial variability	Maintaining balance in sitting on bed while caregiver combs hair Maintaining balance in standing in hallway as caregiver buttons coat	Sitting at the table and eating a meal Sitting doing household accounts Sitting at desk to write a letter	Rolling over in bed Sit <=> stand from bed Tub transfers Bed <=> bathroom, using same route daily	Carrying a tray of food or drinks from the kitchen to the living room, using the same tray and same route each time
CLOSED	with intertrial variability	Maintaining sitting balance on different chairs in the room e.g., rocker, straight-backed chair, sofa. Maintaining standing balance on different surfaces: carpet, wood	Standing in the kitchen unloading a dish-washer Sitting on a low stool in the yard, bending over to weed the vegetable garden	Rolling over in a twin bed and a queen bed Sit <=> stand from different heights and surfaces Up and down curbs of different heights	Carrying a tray of food or drinks from the kitchen to the living room, using different trays and routes each time
OPEN	without intertrial variability	Maintaining balance in a moving elevator	Rearranging packages while standing in a moving elevator	Walking up or down a moving escalator or a moving sidewalk	Rearranging packages while walking up or down the moving escalator
OPEN	with intertrial variability	Maintaining sitting or standing balance in a moving bus	Drinking a cocktail on the deck of a cruise ship	Community ambulation Walking through a living room where children are playing	Shopping in the supermarket Walking a precocious pet on a leash

FIGURE 1.9 Activities of daily living in the context of the taxonomy of motor tasks. *(From Dennis, JK, and McKeough, DM: Mobility. In May, BJ [ed]:* Home Health and Rehabilitation—Concepts of Care, *ed. 2. Philadelphia: FA Davis, 1999, p 116, with permission.)*

which the task is performed is fixed or moving. A *closed environment* is one in which objects around the patient and the surface on which the task is performed do not move. When a functional task is performed in this type of environment, the patient's complete attention can be focused on performing the task and the task can be self-paced. Examples of tasks performed in a closed environment are drinking or eating while sitting in a chair and maintaining an erect trunk, standing at a sink and washing your hands or combing your hair, and walking in an empty hallway or in a room where furniture placement is consistent.

A more complex environment is an *open environment.* It is one in which objects or other people are in motion or the support surface is unstable during the task. The movement that occurs in the environment is not under the control of the patient. Tasks that occur in open environments include maintaining sitting or standing balance on a movable surface (a balance board or BOSU®; Fig. 1.10), standing on a moving train or bus, ascending or descending stairs in a crowded stairwell, crossing a street at a busy intersection, or returning a serve in a tennis match or volleyball game. During tasks such as these, the patient must predict the speed and directions of movement of people or objects in the environment or must anticipate the need to make postural or balance adjustments as the support surface moves. Consequently, the patient must pace the performance of the tasks to match the imposed environmental conditions.

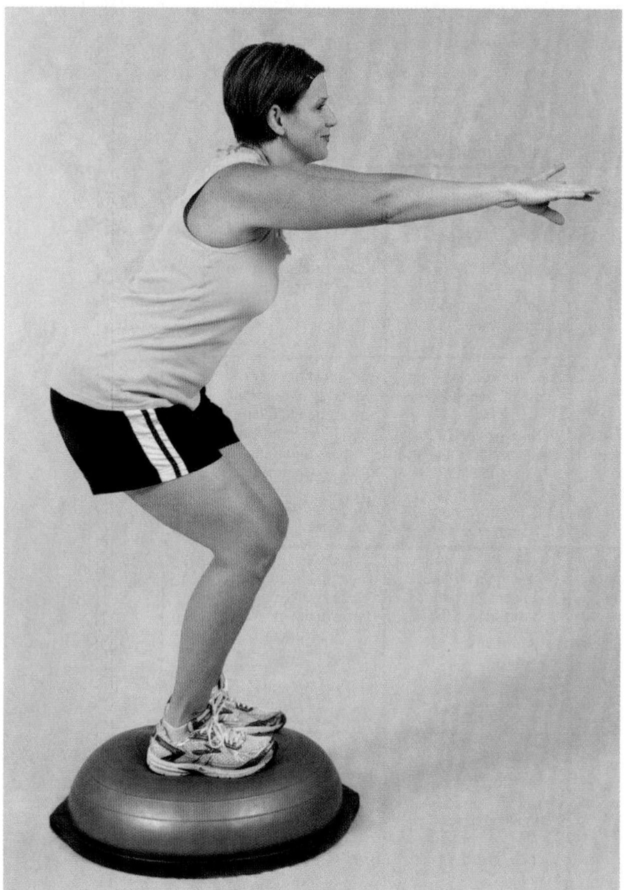

FIGURE 1.10 Learning to maintain standing balance on an unstable surface is an example of a motor skill that is performed in an open (moving) environment.

Intertrial variability in the environment—absent or present. When the environment in which a task occurs is constant (unchanging) from one performance of a task to the next, intertrial variability is absent. The environmental conditions for the task are predictable; therefore, little attention to the task is required, which often enables a patient to perform two tasks at one time. Some examples of tasks without intertrial variability are practicing safe lifting techniques using a box of the same dimensions and weight, practicing the tasks of standing up and sitting down from just one height or type of chair, or walking on just one type of surface.

A task becomes more complex when there is intertrial variability in the environmental conditions—that is, when the demands change from one attempt or repetition of a task to the next. With such variability, the patient must continually monitor the changing demands of the environment and adapt to the new circumstances by using a variety of movement strategies to complete the task. Lifting and carrying objects of different sizes and weight, climbing stairs of different heights, or walking over varying terrain are tasks with intertrial variability.

Body stable or body transport. In addition to environmental conditions, tasks are analyzed from the perspective of the person doing the task. Tasks that involve maintaining the body in a stable (stationary) position, such as maintaining an upright posture, are considered simple tasks, particularly when performed under closed environmental conditions. When the task requirements involve the patient moving from one place to another (body transport), such as performing a transfer, walking, jumping, or climbing, the task is more complex. When a body transport task is performed in an open environment with intertrial variability, such as walking in a crowded corridor or on different support surfaces, such as grass, gravel, and pavement, the task becomes even more complex and challenging.

Manipulation of objects—absent or present. Whether performing a task does or does not require upper extremity manipulation activities also affects the degree of difficulty of the task. When a task is performed without manipulating an object, it is considered less complex than if manipulation is a requirement of the task. Carrying a cup of coffee without spilling it while at home alone and walking from one room to another is a more complex task than walking with hands free. Doing the same task in a busy hallway further increases the complexity and difficulty of the task.

In summary, Gentile's taxonomy of motor tasks can be used to analyze the characteristics of functional tasks in the context of the task conditions. The taxonomy provides a framework to structure individual treatment sessions with a patient or to progress the level of difficulty of motor tasks throughout a functional training program.

Stages of Motor Learning

There are three stages of motor learning: cognitive, associative, and autonomous.[44,131,163,164] The characteristics of the learner are different at each stage of learning and consequently affect the type of instructional strategies selected by a therapist in an exercise and functional training program.

Cognitive Stage

When learning a skilled movement, a patient first must figure out *what* to do—that is, the patient must learn the goal or purpose and the requirements of the exercise or functional task. Then the patient must learn *how* to do the motor task safely and correctly. At this stage, the patient needs to think about each component or the sequencing of the skilled movement. The patient often focuses on how his or her body is aligned and how far and with what intensity or speed to move. In other words, the patient tries to get the "feel" of the exercise.

Because all of the patient's attention is often directed to the correct performance of the motor task, distractions in the environment, such as a busy, noisy exercise room (an open environment), may initially interfere with learning. During this stage of learning, errors in performance are common, but with practice that includes error correction, the patient gradually learns to differentiate correct from incorrect performance, initially with frequent feedback from a therapist and eventually by monitoring his or her own performance (self-evaluation).

Associative Stage

The patient makes infrequent errors and concentrates on fine-tuning the motor task during the associative stage of learning. Learning focuses on producing the most consistent and efficient movements. The timing of the movements and the distances moved also may be refined. The patient explores slight variations and modifications of movement strategies while doing the task under different environmental conditions (intertrial variability). The patient also uses problem-solving to self-correct errors when they do occur. At this stage, the patient requires infrequent feedback from the therapist and instead begins to anticipate necessary adjustments and make corrections even before errors occur.

Autonomous Stage

Movements are automatic in this final stage of learning. The patient does not have to pay attention to the movements in the task, thus making it possible to do other tasks simultaneously. Also, the patient easily adapts to variations in task demands and environmental conditions. Little, if any, instruction goes on in this phase of learning unless the patient encounters a recurrence of symptoms or other problems. In fact, most patients are discharged before reaching this stage of learning.

Variables That Influence Motor Learning—Considerations for Exercise Instruction and Functional Training

Motor learning is influenced by many variables, some of which can be manipulated by a therapist during exercise instruction or functional training to facilitate learning. Some of these variables include pre-practice considerations, physical or mental practice, and several forms of feedback. An understanding of these variables and their impact on motor learning is necessary to develop strategies for successful exercise instruction and functional training. A brief overview of these key variables that influence the acquisition and retention of skilled movements during each stage of motor learning is presented in this section. Because concepts and principles of motor learning encompass an extensive body of knowledge, the reader is referred to a number of in-depth resources for additional information.[45,56,111,128,130,131,163,164,192]

Pre-Practice Considerations

A number of variables can influence motor learning during an exercise session even before practice begins. A patient's *understanding* of the purpose of an exercise or task, as well as interest in the task, affects skill acquisition and retention. The more meaningful a task is to a patient, the more likely it is that learning will occur. Including tasks the patient identified as important during the initial examination promotes a patient's interest.

Attention to the task at hand also affects learning. The ability to focus on the skill to be learned without distracting influences in the environment promotes learning. Instructions given to a patient prior to practice about where his or her attention should be directed during practice also may affect learning. There is evidence in studies of nonimpaired individuals that learning is enhanced if a person attends to the outcomes of performing a task rather than to the details of the task itself.[116,200] This finding is addressed in more detail in a later discussion of feedback as it relates to motor learning.

Demonstration of a task prior to commencing practice also enhances learning. It is often helpful for a patient to observe another person, usually the therapist or possibly another patient, perform the exercise or functional task correctly and then model those actions. *Pre-practice verbal instructions* that describe the task also may facilitate skill acquisition, but they should be succinct. Extensive information about the task requirements early in the learning process may actually confuse a patient rather than enhance the learning process.

Practice

Motor learning occurs as the direct result of practice—that is, repeatedly performing a movement or series of movements in a task.[100,163,164] Practice is probably the single most important variable in learning a motor skill. The *amount*, *type*, and *variability* of practice directly affect the extent of skill acquisition and retention.[128,163,164] In general, the more a patient practices a motor task, the more readily it is learned. In today's health-care environment, most practice of exercises or functional tasks occurs at home independent of therapist supervision. A therapist often sets the practice conditions for a home program prior to a patient's discharge by providing guidelines on how to increase the difficulty of newly acquired motor skills during the later stages of learning.

The type of practice strategy selected also has a significant impact on how readily a motor task is learned.[45,100,111,128,131,163,164,196]

Common types of practice are defined in Box 1.19. The type of skill to be learned (discrete, serial, or continuous) and the patient's cognitive status and stage of motor learning determine which practice strategies are more appropriate than others.

Part versus whole practice. *Part practice* has been shown to be most effective in the early stage of learning for the acquisition of complex serial skills that have simple and difficult components. Depending on the patient's cognitive status, it is usually necessary to practice only the difficult dimensions of a task before practicing the task as a whole. *Whole practice* is more effective than part practice for acquiring continuous skills, such as walking and climbing stairs, or serial tasks in which momentum or timing of the components is the central focus of the learning process. Whole practice is also used for acquisition of discrete tasks, such as an exercise that involves repetitions of a single movement pattern.

Practice order—blocked, random, and random/blocked. During the initial phase of rehabilitation, practice usually is directed toward learning just a few exercises or functional motor tasks. During the initial (cognitive) stage of learning in which a new motor skill is acquired, *blocked-order practice* is the appropriate choice because it rapidly improves performance of skilled movements. A transition to *random-order* or *random/blocked-order practice* should be made as soon as possible to introduce variability into the learning process. *Variability of practice* refers to making slight adjustments (variations) in the conditions of a task—for example, by varying the support surface or the surroundings where a task is performed.[56,163,164]

Although blocked-order practice initially improves performance at a faster rate than random-order practice, random practice leads to better skill retention and generalizability of skills than blocked practice.[128] It is thought that varying tasks just slightly, as is done with random-order practice, requires more cognitive processing and problem-solving than blocked-order practice and, hence, culminates in greater retention of a newly acquired skill after practice has ceased. However, blocked-order practice may be preferable for patients with cognitive deficits because random-order practice may pose too great a challenge for the patient and subsequently interfere with the learning process.[103]

Random/blocked-order practice results in faster skill acquisition than random-order practice and better retention than blocked-order practice. Because random/blocked-order practice enables a patient to perform a task at least twice before changing to another variation of the task, this form of practice gives a patient the opportunity to identify and then immediately correct errors in a movement sequence before proceeding to the next variation of the task.[56,163]

Physical versus mental practice. Physical practice has long been a hallmark of exercise instruction and functional training in physical therapy, whereas mental practice (motor imagery practice) has its roots in sports psychology and sport-related training.[164,171] Over the past few decades, the applicability of mental practice as a treatment tool in the rehabilitation of patients with movement impairments has been investigated for its potential.[45,195] It is thought that mental rehearsal of a motor task reinforces the cognitive component of motor learning—that is, learning what to do when performing a task and refining how it is executed.

Most studies support the finding that physical practice of motor skills by overtly performing the task is superior to mental practice alone for learning motor tasks.[163,164] However, in sports training and rehabilitation, mental practice, when used in conjunction with physical practice, has been shown to enhance motor skill acquisition at a faster rate than use of physical practice alone.[111,112,128,133]

BOX 1.19 Types of Practice for Motor Learning

Part Versus Whole Practice

- *Part practice.* A task is broken down into separate dimensions. Individual and usually the more difficult components of the task are practiced. After mastery of the individual segments, they are combined in sequence so the whole task can be practiced.
- *Whole practice.* The entire task is performed from beginning to end and is not practiced in separate segments.

Blocked, Random, and Random/Blocked Practice Orders

- *Blocked-order practice.* The same task or series of exercises or tasks is performed repeatedly under the same conditions and in a predictable order; for example, the patient may consistently practice walking in the same environment, stepping to and from the same height platform, standing up from the same height chair, or lifting containers of equal size or weight; therefore, the task does not change from one repetition to the next.
- *Random-order practice.* Slight variations of the same task are carried out in an unpredictable order; for example, a patient could practice stepping to and from platforms of different heights or practice standing up from chairs of different heights or styles in a random order; therefore, the task changes with each repetition.
- *Random/blocked-order practice.* Variations of the same task are performed in random order, but each variation of the task is performed more than once; for example, the patient rises from a particular height or style chair and then repeats the same task a second time before moving on to a different height or style chair.

Physical Versus Mental Practice

- *Physical practice.* The movements of an exercise or functional task are actually performed.
- *Mental practice.* A cognitive rehearsal of how a motor task is to be performed occurs prior to actually executing the task; the terms *visualization* and *motor imagery practice* are used synonymously with mental practice.

Feedback

Second only to practicing a motor task, feedback is considered the next most important variable that influences motor learning.[128] *Feedback* is sensory information that is received and processed by the learner during or after performing or attempting to perform a motor skill.[56,128,130,163,164] There are a number of descriptive terms used to differentiate one type of feedback from another. The terms used to describe feedback are based on the source of feedback (*intrinsic* or *augmented/extrinsic*), the focus of feedback (*knowledge of performance* [KP] or *knowledge of results* [KR]), and the timing or frequency of feedback (the *feedback schedule*). Boxes 1.20 and 1.21 identify and define the various terms associated with the types and scheduling of feedback.

Several factors influence the types of feedback that can occur during exercise instruction or functional training and the effectiveness of feedback for skill acquisition (performance) and skill retention (learning). For example, a patient's physical and cognitive status and the stage of motor learning have a significant impact on the type of feedback that is most effective and the timing and frequency of augmented feedback implemented during practice sessions. It has also been suggested that a therapist should encourage a patient to provide input about his or her receptiveness to the type of feedback or feedback schedule used during practice, particularly once the patient has achieved a beginning level of skill acquisition. This active participation may promote a sense of self-control in the patient and is thought to have a positive impact on learning.[116]

BOX 1.20 Types of Feedback for Motor Learning

Knowledge of Performance (KP) Versus Knowledge of Results (KR)

- *KP.* Either intrinsic feedback sensed during a task or immediate, posttask, augmented feedback (usually verbal) about the *nature* or *quality* of the performance of a motor task.
- *KR.* Immediate, posttask, augmented feedback about the *outcome* of a motor task.

Intrinsic Feedback

- Sensory cues that are inherent in the execution of a motor task.
- Arises directly from performing or attempting to perform the task.
- May immediately follow completion of a task or may occur even before a task has been completed.
- Most often involves proprioceptive, kinesthetic, tactile, visual, or auditory cues.

Augmented (Extrinsic) Feedback

- Sensory cues from an external source that are supplemental to intrinsic feedback and that are not inherent in the execution of the task.
- May arise from a mechanical source or from another person.

BOX 1.21 Feedback Schedules

Concurrent Versus Postresponse Feedback

- *Concurrent.* Occurs during the performance of a task; also known as "real-time" feedback.
- *Postresponse (terminal).* Occurs after completing or attempting to complete a motor skill.

Immediate, Delayed, and Summary Postresponse Feedback

- *Immediate.* Information that is given directly after a task is completed.
- *Delayed.* Information that is given after a short interval of time has elapsed, allowing time for the learner to reflect on how well or poorly a task was executed.
- *Summary.* Information that is given about the average performance of several repetitions of a motor skill.

Variable Versus Constant Feedback

- *Variable (intermittent).* Occurs irregularly, randomly during practice of a motor task.
- *Constant.* Occurs on a regularly recurring, continuous basis during practice of a motor task.

In order to provide the most effective forms of feedback during exercise instruction and functional training, it is useful for a therapist to understand the benefits and limitations of several types and schedules of feedback for skill acquisition and skill retention.

Intrinsic feedback. Intrinsic feedback comes from all of the sensory systems of the learner, not from the therapist, and is derived from performing or attempting to perform any movement. Intrinsic feedback is inherent in the movement itself—that is, it occurs naturally during or after a task is performed.[56,128,163] It provides ongoing information about the quality of movement during a task and information about the outcomes (results) of a task, specifically if the goal of a task was achieved. In everyday life, intrinsic feedback is a continuous source of information that provides KP and KR as a person performs routine activities or tries to learn new motor skills.

Augmented feedback. Information about the performance or results of a task that is *supplemental* to intrinsic feedback is known as augmented feedback.[128,163,164,198] It is also referred to as *extrinsic feedback.*[56,131] Unlike intrinsic feedback, a therapist has control of the type, timing, and frequency of augmented feedback a patient receives during practice. Augmented/extrinsic feedback can be provided during or at the conclusion of a task to give information about the quality of the performance (KP) or the quality of the outcome of a task (KR).

NOTE: Although augmented feedback is a commonly used instructional tool to facilitate motor learning in healthy individuals, it is thought to be particularly necessary when teaching motor skills to patients who may receive inadequate or inaccurate intrinsic feedback as the result of impaired sensory systems from injury or disease.[56,128]

Therapists have many forms of augmented/extrinsic feedback from which to select for exercise instruction and functional training.[56,69,130,198] Some examples include *verbal* or *tactile* feedback directly from a therapist who is interacting with a patient during practice and *visual* or *auditory* feedback from a rehabilitative ultrasound imaging device (Fig. 1.11) or an electromyography (EMG) biofeedback unit. A videotaped replay of a previous performance is another source of augmented visual feedback.

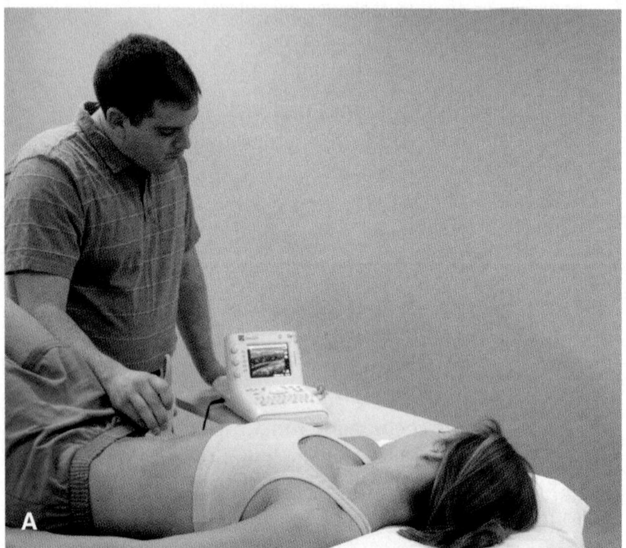

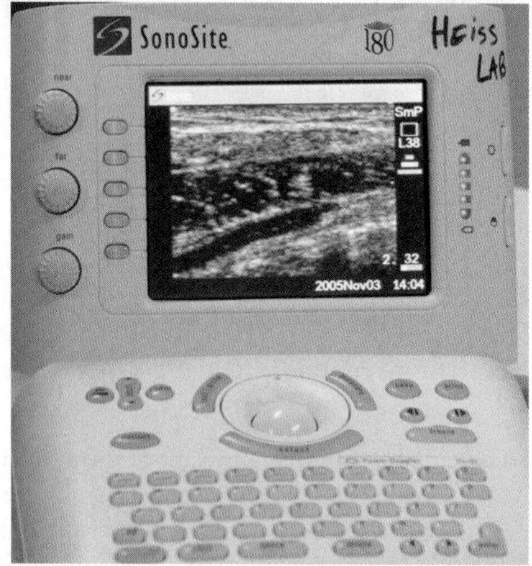

FIGURE 1.11 (A, B) Use of rehabilitative ultrasound imaging provides augmented (visual) feedback on the screen during exercise instruction to help the patient learn how to activate the transversus abdominis and internal oblique muscles.

KP versus KR. Over the past few decades, the selection and application of feedback have changed in the clinical setting. Traditionally, a therapist would have a patient focus on sensory information inherent in a motor task (intrinsic feedback) to "get the feel" of movements in the task, such as how it felt to weight shift from side to side while controlling the knees and maintaining standing balance. At the same time the therapist would provide ongoing feedback—usually verbal—about the quality of the patient's posture or knee control (KP) during the weight-shifting activity.

However, research, primarily with nonimpaired subjects, has shown that directing a person's attention to the outcomes of movements (KR) rather than to the details of the movements themselves enhances learning (retention of a motor skill) more effectively.[200] Consequently, therapists now tend to place greater emphasis on providing feedback about the outcomes (results) of performing a motor skill.[198]

Going back to the weight-shifting example—to employ KR during functional training, a therapist should have a patient perform weight shifts by reaching for objects placed in various positions just outside the patient's base of support. By giving the patient a target, the task becomes goal directed as the patient focuses on the intended results of the movement. The patient, therefore, learns to judge the effectiveness of his or her movements based on feedback received from external cues.[116,200]

The feedback schedule—timing and frequency of augmented feedback. The scheduling of feedback (see Box 1.21) during practice sessions involves the timing and frequency with which augmented/extrinsic feedback is provided. Feedback schedules affect motor skill acquisition and retention and should be adjusted during the learning process.

Concurrent feedback is a form of augmented feedback that occurs in "real time" as a patient is performing or attempting to perform a motor task. Visual feedback from a rehabilitative ultrasound-imaging unit (see Fig. 1.11) is an example of concurrent feedback and is useful when a patient is first learning how to perform an isometric contraction of the trunk stabilizing muscles because no observable movement of the body occurs.

Another form of concurrent feedback, the use of *manual guidance*, which provides tactile cues to the patient, may be necessary for patient safety and may help a patient understand the required movements of an exercise or functional task. However, excessive or long-term use of manual guidance may hamper motor learning in that it may not allow a patient to make "safe mistakes" while figuring out how to perform a movement. As mentioned in the discussion of the stages of motor learning, self-detection and self-correction of errors are absolutely necessary for learning to occur. The key is to use the least amount of concurrent feedback for the shortest time possible, so the patient does not become reliant on it to carry out a task.[56]

Immediate, postresponse feedback is another form of augmented/extrinsic feedback often used during the initial stage of learning. The therapist provides information, often verbally, about the outcome of the task (KR) immediately after each trial. Although immediate feedback after each trial may enhance early skill acquisition, it too does not allow time for problem-solving by the patient and detection of errors without input from the therapist. Consequently, although initial skill acquisition may occur rather quickly, learning, which includes retention, is delayed.[163]

As alternatives to immediate feedback, *delayed feedback* from the therapist after each repetition of a task or exercise or *summary feedback* after several trials have been completed gives the patient time for self-evaluation and problem-solving as to how the task was performed during practice, which in turn promotes retention and generalizability of the learned skills. Although use of delayed or summary schedules of feedback is associated with slower skill acquisition than concurrent or immediate feedback after every trial, it is thought that delaying the timing of feedback makes the patient pay attention to intrinsic feedback inherent in the task.[56,163,197]

FOCUS ON EVIDENCE

The impact of concurrent, immediate postresponse, and summary feedback schedules was investigated in a study of nonimpaired individuals.[197] When subjects practiced a partial weight-bearing activity, those who received concurrent visual feedback (by looking at a scale) achieved the skill more quickly than the subjects who received postresponse feedback (either immediate or summary). However, subjects who received concurrent feedback performed least well on a retention test 2 days after practice ended than the subjects in the two other groups who received postresponse feedback. In addition, summary feedback was found to enhance retention to a greater extent than immediate postresponse feedback.

The frequency with which a therapist provides augmented feedback also should be considered. A basic principle about augmented feedback is that "less is better." Although the greatest frequency of feedback is necessary during the cognitive (initial) stage of learning when a patient is first learning how to perform an exercise or a functional task, excessive or extended use of any form of augmented feedback can create dependence on the feedback and can be a deterrent to self-detection and correction of errors.[56,163,164] Excessive verbal feedback, for example, provided by a therapist after every trial also can be distracting and may interrupt a patient's attention to the task.

Rather than providing feedback after each repetition of an exercise, a therapist may want to consider varying the frequency of feedback (a variable feedback schedule) by giving the patient input following more than a single repetition and on a variable, less predictable basis. *Variable (intermittent)* feedback during practice has been shown to promote retention of a learned motor skill more effectively than *constant (continuous)* feedback given during or after each repetition.[69] A therapist must keep in mind, however, that constant (continuous) feedback improves skill acquisition (performance) more quickly during the initial stage of learning than variable (intermittent) feedback.[56]

It is also important to fade (decrease) the frequency of feedback over time to avoid the extended use of feedback. *Summary feedback,* particularly during the associative stage of learning, is an effective strategy to reduce the total amount of feedback given in a practice session. As augmented feedback is faded, a patient must explore slight modifications of a movement strategy and analyze the results. This promotes problem-solving, self-monitoring, and self-correction, all of which enable a patient to perform tasks independently and safely and to transfer learning to new task conditions.

Application of Motor-Learning Principles for Exercise Instruction Summarized

Box 1.22 summarizes the information discussed in this section with regard to qualities of the learner and effective strategies for exercise instruction and functional training founded on the principles and stages of motor learning.[44,130]

Adherence to Exercise

Effective patient-related instruction for a functionally oriented exercise program must include methods to foster *adherence.* This is particularly challenging when a patient is unaccustomed to regular exercise or when an exercise program must be carried out for an extended period of time. Positive outcomes from treatment are contingent not so much on designing the "ideal" exercise program for a patient, but rather on designing a program that a patient or family will actually follow.[81,82,186]

NOTE: Although the terms *adherence* and *compliance* are often used interchangeably by clinicians and in the literature, the term *adherence* has been selected for this discussion because it has a stronger connotation of active involvement of the patient and patient-therapist collaboration. In contrast, *compliance* tends to imply a more passive connotation with respect to a patient's behavior.

Factors that Influence Adherence to an Exercise Program

Many factors influence adherence to an exercise program.[28,60,64,81,82,110,116,127,168,186] These factors can be grouped into several categories: a patient's characteristics, factors related to a patient's health condition or impairments, and program-related variables.

Patient-Related Factors

The following patient-related factors can have a positive or negative impact on adherence: understanding the health condition, impairments, or exercise program; level of motivation, self-discipline, attentiveness, memory, and willingness and receptivity to change; degree of fatigue or stress; the availability of time to devote to an exercise program; the patient's self-perception of his or her compatibility with the therapist or the degree of control in the exercise program; socioeconomic and cultural background; the beliefs and attitudes about exercise and the value the patient places on the exercise program; and the patient's access to resources. The patient's age and sex also influence adherence to an exercise program, with men having higher adherence rates than women. The association between age and adherence is less clear.

BOX 1.22 Characteristics of the Learner and Instructional Strategies for the Three Stages of Motor Learning

COGNITIVE STAGE

Characteristics of the Learner

Must attend only to the task at hand; must think about each step or component; easily distractible; begins to understand the demands of the motor task; starts to get a "feel" for the exercise; makes errors and alters performance, particularly when given augmented feedback; and begins to differentiate correct versus incorrect and safe versus unsafe performance.

Instructional Strategies

- Initiate instruction in a nondistracting (closed) environment.
- Identify the purpose and functional relevance of the exercise or functional task.
- Demonstrate the ideal execution of the movements (modeling).
- Initially, guide or assist the patient through the movements. Reduce manual guidance feedback as soon as a patient can safely control movements.
- Point out the distance and speed of the movement (how far or fast to move).
- Emphasize the importance of controlled movements.
- Break complex movements into parts when appropriate.
- Have the patient verbally describe the sequence of component motions.
- Have the patient demonstrate each exercise or task but practice only a few motor tasks. Keep repetitions low and alternate tasks to ensure safety and avoid fatigue.
- Point out sensory cues (intrinsic feedback) to which the patient should attend.
- Provide frequent and explicit positive feedback related to KP and KR.
- Use a variety of forms of feedback (verbal, tactile, and visual) and vary.
- Initially use feedback after each repetition to improve performance (acquisition); gradually transition to variable and delayed feedback to enhance learning (retention).
- Introduce the concept of self-evaluation and self-correction of movements.
- Initially, use blocked-order practice; gradually introduce random-order practice.
- Allow trial and error to occur within safe limits.

ASSOCIATIVE STAGE

Characteristics of the Learner

Performs movements more consistently with fewer errors or extraneous movements; executes movements in a well-organized manner; refines the movements in the exercise or functional task; detects and self-corrects movement errors when they occur; is less dependent on augmented/extrinsic feedback from the therapist; and uses prospective cues and anticipates errors before they occur.

Instructional Strategies

- Emphasize practice of a greater number and variety of movements or tasks.
- Increase the complexity of the exercise or task.
- Vary the sequence of exercise or tasks practiced (random-order practice).
- Allow the patient to practice independently, emphasizing problem-solving and use of proprioceptive cues (intrinsic feedback) for error detection.
- Introduce simulation of functional tasks into the practice session.
- Continue to provide augmented feedback regarding KP and KR, but avoid the use of manual guidance.
- Delay feedback or use a variable feedback schedule to give the learner an opportunity to detect movement errors and self-correct them.
- Gradually fade feedback by decreasing the total amount of feedback but increase the specificity of feedback.
- Allow the learner to perform a full set of exercises or several repetitions of a functional task before providing feedback (summary feedback).
- Increase the level of distraction in the exercise environment.
- Prepare the patient to carry out the exercise program in the home or community setting.

AUTONOMOUS STAGE

Characteristics of the Learner

Performs the exercise program or functional tasks consistently and automatically and while doing other tasks; applies the learned movement strategies to increasingly more difficult tasks or new environmental situations; and, if appropriate, performs the task more quickly or for an extended period of time at a lower energy cost.

Instructional Strategies

- Set up a series of progressively more difficult activities the learner can do independently, such as increasing the speed, distance, and complexity of the exercises or task.
- Suggest ways the learner can vary the original exercise or task and use the task in more challenging situations encountered in everyday activities.
- If the patient is still in therapy, which at most is usually for just a recheck, incorporate little to no feedback unless a significant movement error is noted or a potentially unsafe situation arises.
- Provide assistance, as needed, to integrate the learned motor skills into fitness or sports activities.

Factors Related to the Health Condition or Impairments

The acuity, chronicity, severity, or stability of the primary health condition and related impairments and the presence of comorbidities all have an impact on adherence. Pain is obviously a deterrent to adherence and therefore must be minimized in an exercise program. When impairments are severe or long-standing, setting short-term goals that can be achieved regularly fosters adherence to an exercise program that must be followed over a long period of time.

Program-Related Variables

The complexity and necessary duration of an exercise program; the adequacy of instruction, supervision, and feedback from the therapist; whether the patient has had input into the plan of care; and the continuity of care from an inpatient to a home setting all can have an impact on adherence. Programs that address the interest level and motivational needs of a patient have higher adherence rates. In the outpatient setting, logistics, such as location and scheduling, the program's atmosphere created by the therapist/exercise instructor, and the availability of social support and individualized attention or counselling from personnel also are important factors that foster adherence.

Strategies to Foster Adherence

A therapist should expect that most patients will not dutifully adhere to any treatment program, particularly if regular exercise has not been a part of the patient's life prior to the occurrence of disease or injury. The most a therapist can hope to do is implement strategies that foster adherence. Some suggestions from a number of resources in the literature are noted in Box 1.23.[28,60,64,81,82,99,116,127,168,186]

BOX 1.23 Strategies to Foster Adherence to an Exercise Program

- Explore and try to appreciate the patient's beliefs about exercising or the value the patient places on exercising as a means to "get better."
- Help the patient identify personal benefits derived from adhering to the exercise program.
- Explain the rationale and importance of each exercise and functional activity.
- Identify how specific exercises are designed to meet specific patient-centered goals or functional outcomes.
- Allow and encourage the patient to have input into the nature and scope of the exercise program, the selection and scheduling of practice and feedback, and decisions of when and to what extent exercises are progressively made more difficult to enhance a patient's sense of self-control.
- Keep the exercise program as brief as possible.
- Identify practical and functionally oriented ways to do selected exercises during everyday tasks.
- Have the patient keep an exercise log.
- If possible, schedule follow-up visit(s) to review or modify exercises.
- Point out specific exercise-related progress.
- Identify barriers to adherence (not enough time in the day to do the exercises, discomfort during the exercises, and lack of necessary equipment); then suggest solutions or modify the exercise program.

Independent Learning Activities

Critical Thinking and Discussion

1. Critically analyze your own, an acquaintance's, or a family member's exercise history. Then identify how a regular regimen of exercise could improve your quality of life or theirs.
2. Research four health conditions (diseases, injuries, or disorders) that result in primary impairments of the (1) musculoskeletal, (2) neuromuscular, (3) cardiovascular/ pulmonary, and (4) integumentary systems. Identify characteristic impairments (signs and symptoms) associated with each health condition and hypothesize what activity limitations and participation restrictions are most likely to develop.
3. Why is it essential for a physical therapist to understand and be able to articulate (verbally or in written form) the interrelationships among impairments typically exhibited by patients with various health conditions, activity limitations, and participation restrictions?
4. Last month, you sprained your ankle (inversion sprain). You had to use crutches for several days, but since then you have been walking independently. Pain and swelling still return after vigorous activity, and your ankle feels unstable on uneven terrain. Using a model of functioning and disability as your frame of reference, identify specific activity limitations and at least one participation restriction that would most likely develop in your life as the result of your history and current problems.
5. Using your current knowledge of examination procedures, develop a list of specific tests and measures you would most likely choose to use when examining a patient whose primary impairments affect the (1) musculoskeletal, (2) neuromuscular, (3) cardiovascular and/or pulmonary, and (4) integumentary systems.

6. You have been asked to make recommendations for the adoption of one or more new measurement instruments to be used at your facility for data collection and analysis of patient-centered functional outcomes. Review the literature on musculoskeletal assessment and identify and summarize key features of five instruments that measure activity limitations associated with musculoskeletal impairments of the extremities, neck, or trunk. In addition, identify and summarize key features of five measurement instruments that assess a patient's restricted participation in societal, family, or work roles.
7. Three individuals just recently sustained similar fractures of the hip. All underwent an open reduction with internal fixation. The patients are an otherwise healthy 19-year-old college student who was in an automobile accident and wants to return to campus after discharge from the hospital; a 60-year-old person with a somewhat sedentary lifestyle who plans to return home after postoperative rehabilitation and wishes to return to work in an office as soon as possible; and an 85-year-old individual with severe age-related osteoporosis who has been residing in an assisted living facility for the past year. What issues must be considered when identifying anticipated goals and expected outcomes and determining appropriate interventions in the plans of care for these patients? In what ways would goals and expected outcomes differ for these patients?
8. Identify the key components of the patient management model described in this chapter and discuss how each of those components relates to the potential use of therapeutic exercise interventions.
9. Using the taxonomy of motor tasks discussed in this chapter, identify simple to complex activities that are necessary or important in your daily life. Identify at least 3 activities that fall within each of the 16 condition variables described in the taxonomy.
10. You are seeing a patient in the home setting for follow-up of a postoperative exercise program and progression of functional activities initiated in the hospital. The patient is a 55-year-old computer analyst who had a (L) total knee arthroplasty 10 days ago. You have completed your examination and evaluation. Other than a long-standing history of degenerative arthritis of the (L) knee, the patient has no other significant health-related problems. As you would expect, the patient has pain and limited ROM of the (L) knee and decreased strength of the (L) lower extremity. The patient is currently ambulating with axillary crutches, weight bearing as tolerated on the (L) lower extremity. As the patient recovers strength and ROM, design a series of progressively more challenging functional motor tasks the patient could practice with your supervision or independently at home based on the taxonomy of motor tasks described in this chapter.

REFERENCES

1. Allet, L, Burge, E, Monnin, D: ICF: clinical relevance for physiotherapy? A critical review. *Adv Physioth* 10:127–137, 2008.
2. American College of Sports Medicine: *ACSM's Guidelines for Exercise Testing and Prescription,* ed. 8. Philadelphia: Wolthers Kluwer/Lippincott Williams & Wilkins, 2010.
3. American College of Sports Medicine: Position stand: physical activity and bone health. *Med Sci Sports Exerc* 36:1985–1986, 2004.
4. American Physical Therapy Association: Guide to Physical Therapist Practice, ed. 2. *Phys Ther* 81:9–744, 2001, revised 2003.
5. American Physical Therapy Association: Guide to physical therapist practice, 3.0. Alexandria VA, 2014. Available at http://guidetoptpractice.org/. Accessed April 4, 2015.
6. American Physical Therapy Association: Today's physical therapist: a comprehensive review of a 21st century health care profession. Alexandria VA, 2011. Available at www.Moveforwardpt.com. Accessed March 31, 2015.
7. American Physical Therapy Association: PTNOW. Available at http://www.ptnow.org/ClinicalTools/Tests.aspx. Accessed June 26, 2015.
8. American Physical Therapy Association: APTA 2014 strategic plan. Alexandria VA, 2014. Available at www.apta.org/StrategicPlan. Accessed August 11, 2015.
9. Baker, SM, et al: Patient participation in physical therapy goal setting. *Phys Ther* 81:1118–1126, 2001.
10. Basmajian, J (ed): *Physical Rehabilitation Outcome Measures.* Toronto: Canadian Physiotherapy Association in cooperation with Health and Welfare Canada and Canada Communications Group, 1994.
11. Beaton, DE, and Schemitsch, E: Measures of health-related quality of life and physical function. *Clin Orthop* 413:90–105, 2003.
12. Beattie, P: Evidence-based practice in outpatient orthopedic physical therapy: using research findings to assist clinical decision-making. *Orthop Phys Ther Pract* 16:27–29, 2004.
13. Beattie, P, et al: Longitudinal continuity of care is associated with high patient satisfaction with physical therapy. *Phys Ther* 85(10):1046–1052, 2005.
14. Beattie, P, et al: MedRisk instrument for measuring patient satisfaction with physical therapy care: a psychometric analysis. *J Orthop Sports Phys Ther* 35:24–32, 2005.
15. Beneciuk, JM, Bishop, MD, and George, SZ: Clinical prediction rules for physical therapy interventions: a systematic review. *Phys Ther* 89(2): 114–124, 2009.
16. Bernsen, T: The future: documentation using the International Classification of Functioning, Disability and Health. In Kettenbach, G (ed): *Writing Patient/Client Notes: Ensuring Accuracy in Documentation.* Philadelphia: FA Davis, 2009, pp. 207–213.
17. Bloomfield, SA: Changes in musculoskeletal structure and function with prolonged bed rest. *Med Sci Sports Exerc* 29:197–206, 1997.
18. Boissonnault, WG: Prevalence of comorbid conditions, surgeries and medication use in a physical therapy outpatient population: a multi-centered study. *J Orthop Sports Phys Ther* 29:506–519, 1999.
19. Boissonnault, WG: Differential diagnosis: taking a step back before stepping forward. *PT Magazine Phys Ther* 8(11):46–54, 2000.
20. Boissonnault, WG: Patient health history including identification of health risk factors. In Boissonnault, WG (ed): *Primary Care for the Physical Therapist: Examination and Triage.* St. Louis: Elsevier Saunders, 2005, pp 55–65.
21. Boissonnault, WG: Review of systems. In Boissonnault, WG (ed): *Primary Care for the Physical Therapist: Examination and Triage.* St. Louis: Elsevier Saunders, 2005, pp 87–104.
22. Boissonnault, WG, and Badke, MB: Collecting health history information: the accuracy of a patient self-administered questionnaire in an orthopedic outpatient setting. *Phys Ther* 85:531–543, 2005.
23. Boissonnault, WG, Ross, MD: Physical therapists referring patients to physicians: a review of case reports and series. *J Orthop Sports Phys Ther* 42(5):446–454, 2012.

24. Botha-Scheepers, S, et al: Changes in outcome measures for impairment, activity limitation, and participation restriction over two years in osteoarthritis of the lower extremities. *Arthritis and Rheum* 59(12): 1750–1755, 2008.
25. Brandt, EN Jr, and Pope, AM (eds): *Enabling America: Assessing the Role of Rehabilitation Science and Engineering.* Washington, DC: Institute of Medicine, National Academies Press, 1997.
26. Buckhave, EB, LaCour, K, Huniche, L: The meaning of activity and participation in everyday life when living with hand osteoarthritis. *Scand J Occup Ther* 21:24–30, 2014.
27. Butler, RJ, and Johnson, WG: Satisfaction with low back pain care. *Spine J* 8:510–521, 2008.
28. Campbell, R, et al: Why don't patients do their exercises? Understanding non-compliance with physical therapy in patients with osteoarthritis of the knee. *J Epidemiol Community Health* 55:132–138, 2001.
29. Carcia, CR, et al: Achilles pain, stiffness, and muscle power deficits: Achille's tendinitis—clinical practice guidelines linked to the International Classification of Functioning, Disability and Health from the Orthopedic Section of the American Physical Therapy Association. *J Orthop Sports Phys Ther* 40(9):A1–A26, 2010.
30. Charness, AL: Outcomes measurement: intervention versus outcomes. *Orthop Phys Ther Clin North Am* 3:147, 1994.
31. Chase, L, et al: Perceptions of physical therapists toward patient education. In Shepard, KF, Jensen, GM (eds): *Handbook of Teaching for Physical Therapists.* Boston: Butterworth Heinemann, 1997, p 225.
32. Childs, JD, and Cleland, JA: Development and application of clinical prediction rules to improve decision making in physical therapist practice. *Phys Ther* 86(1):122–131, 2006.
33. Childs, JD, et al: Neck pain: clinical practice guidelines linked to the International Classification of Functioning, Disability and Health from the Orthopedic Section of the American Physical Therapy Association. *J Orthop Sports Phys Ther* 38(9):A1–A24, 2008.
34. Cibulka, TM, et al: Hip pain and mobility deficits: hip osteoarthritis—clinical practice guidelines linked to the International Classification of Functioning, Disability and Health from the Orthopedic Section of the American Physical Therapy Association. *J Orthop Sports Phys Ther* 39(4):A1–A25, 2009.
35. Cleland, JA, et al: Development of a clinical prediction rule for guiding treatment of a subgroup of patients with neck pain: use of thoracic spine manipulation, exercise, and patient education. *Phys Ther* 87(1):9–23, 2007.
36. Coffin-Zadai, CA: Disabling our diagnostic dilemmas. *Phys Ther* 87: 641–653, 2007.
37. Cormack, JC: Evidence-based practice: what it is and how to do it? *J Orthop Sports Phys Ther* 32:484–487, 2002.
38. Costa, LOP, et al: Core journals that publish clinical trials of physical therapy interventions. *Phys Ther* 90(11):1631–1640, 2010.
39. Cress, ME, et al: Functional training: muscle structure, function and performance in older women. *J Orthop Sports Phys Ther* 24:4–10, 1996.
40. Croakin, E: Osteopenia: implications for physical therapists managing patients of all ages. *PT Magazine Phys Ther* 9:80, 2001.
41. Dahl, TH: International Classification of Functioning, Disability and Health: an introduction and discussion of its potential impact on rehabilitation services and research. *J Rehabil Med* 34:201–204, 2002.
42. Dekker, J, et al: Diagnosis and treatment in physical therapy: an investigation of their relationship. *Phys Ther* 73:568–577, 1993.
43. DeLitto, A, and Snyder-Mackler, L: The diagnostic process: examples in orthopedic physical therapy. *Phys Ther* 75:203–211, 1995.
44. Dennis, JK, and McKeough, DM: Mobility. In May, BJ (ed): *Home Health and Rehabilitation: Concepts of Care*, ed. 2. Philadelphia: FA Davis, 1999, p 109.
45. Dickstein, R, and Deutsch, JE: Motor imagery in physical therapist practice. *Phys Ther* 87:942–953, 2007.
46. Edwards, I, et al: Clinical reasoning strategies in physical therapy. *Phys Ther* 84:312–330, 2004.
47. Ennis, K, Hawthorne, K, and Frownfelter, D: How physical therapists can strategically effect health outcomes for older adults with limited health literacy. *J Geriatr Phys Ther* 35:148–154, 2012
48. Escorpizo, R, et al: Creating an interface between the International Classification of Functioning, Disability and Health and physical therapist practice. *Phys Ther* 90(7):1053–1063, 2010.
49. Finger, ME, et al: Identification of intervention categories for physical therapy, based on the International Classification of Functioning, Disability and Health: a Delphi study. *Phys Ther* 86:1203–1220, 2006.
50. Francis, KT: Status of the year 2000 health goals for physical activity and fitness. *Phys Ther* 79:405–414, 1999.
51. Friedrich, M, Cernak, T, and Maderbacher, P: The effect of brochure use versus therapist teaching on patients' performing therapeutic exercise and on changes in impairment status. *Phys Ther* 76:1082–1088, 1996.
52. Fritz, JM: Clinical prediction rules in physical therapist practice: coming of age? *J Orthop Sports Phys Ther* 39(3):159–161, 2009.
53. Fritz, JM, and Wainner, RS: Examining diagnostic tests and evidence-based perspective. *Phys Ther* 81:1546–1564, 2001.
54. Fritz, JM: Evidence-based examination of diagnostic information. In Boissonnault, WG (ed): *Primary Care for the Physical Therapist: Examination and Triage.* St. Louis: Elsevier Saunders, 2005, pp 18–25.
55. Gahimer, JE, and Domboldt, E: Amount of patient education in physical therapy practice and perceived effects. *Phys Ther* 76:1089–1096, 1996.
56. Gentile, AM: Skill acquisition: action, movement, and neuromotor processes. In Carr, J, and Shepherd, R (eds): *Movement Science: Foundations for Physical Therapy in Rehabilitation.* Gaithersburg, MD: Aspen Publishers, 2000, pp 111–187.
57. Giallonardo, L: The guide to physical therapist practice: an overview for the orthopedic physical therapist. *Orthop Phys Ther Pract* 10:10, 1998.
58. Godges, JJ, and Irrgang, JJ: ICF-based practice guidelines for common musculoskeletal conditions. *J Orthop Sports Phys Ther* 38(4):167–168, 2008.
59. Goodman, CC, and Snyder, TEK: *Differential Diagnosis in Physical Therapy,* ed. 4. Philadelphia: Elsevier/Saunders, 2007.
60. Grindley, EJ, Zizzi, SS, and Nasypany, AM: Use of protection motivation theory, affect, and barriers to understand and predict adherence to outpatient rehabilitation. *Phys Ther* 88(12):1529–1540, 2008.
61. Guccione, A: Arthritis and the process of disablement. *Phys Ther* 74: 408–414, 1994.
62. Guccione, A: Physical therapy diagnosis and the relationship between impairment and function. *Phys Ther* 71:449–503, 1991.
63. Guccione, AA, et al: Development and testing of a self-report instrument to measure actions: Outpatient Physical Therapy Improvement in Movement Assessment Log (OPTIMAL). *Phys Ther* 85:515–530, 2005.
64. Hardman, AE: Physical activity and health: current issues and research needs. *Int J Epidemiol* 30(5):1193–1197, 2001.
65. Harris, BA: Building documentation using a clinical decision-making model. In Stewart, DL, and Abeln, SH (eds): *Documenting Functional Outcomes in Physical Therapy.* St. Louis: Mosby-Year Book, 1993, p 81.
66. Hart, DL, Geril, AC, and Pfohl, RL: Outcomes process in daily practice. *PT Magazine Phys Ther* 5:68, 1997.
67. Heerkens, YF, et al: Impairments and disabilities: the difference: proposal for the adjustment of the International Classification of Impairments, Disabilities and Handicaps. *Phys Ther* 74:430–442, 1994.
68. Heick, JD, and Boissonnault, WG: Physical therapist recognition of signs and symptoms of infection after shoulder reconstruction: a patient case report. *Physiother Theory Pract* Feb29(2):166–73,2013.
69. Herbert, WJ, Heiss, DG, and Basso, DM: Influence of feedback schedule in motor performance and learning of a lumbar multifidus muscle task using rehabilitative ultrasound imaging: a randomized clinical trial. *Phys Ther* 88(2):261–269, 2008.
70. Herman, KM, and Reese, CS: Relationship among selected measures of impairment, functional limitation, and disability in patients with cervical spine disorders. *Phys Ther* 81:903–914, 2001.
71. Hernandez, ME, Goldberg, A, and Alexander, NB: Decreased muscle strength relates to self-reported stooping, crouching, or kneeling difficulty in older adults. *Phys Ther* 90(1):67–74, 2010.
72. Hicks, GE, et al: Preliminary development of a clinical prediction rule for determining which patients with low back pain will respond to a stabilization exercise program. *Arch Phys Med Rehabil* 86:1753–1762, 2005.

73. Hodges, PW: Motor control. In Kolt, GS, and Snyder-Mackler, L (eds): *Physical Therapies in Sport and Exercise.* Edinburgh: Churchill Livingstone, 2003, pp 107–142.
74. Hush, JM, Cameron, K, and Mackey, M: Patient satisfaction with musculoskeletal physical therapy care: a systematic review. *Phys Ther* 91(1): 25–36, 2011.
75. ICIDH: *International Classification of Impairments, Disabilities and Handicaps: A Manual of Classification Relating to Consequences of Disease.* Geneva: World Health Organization, 1980.
76. ICF: *International Classification of Functioning, Disability and Health.* Geneva: World Health Organization, 2001.
77. ICF: *International Classification of Functioning, Disability and Health.* Geneva: World Health Organization, 2008.
78. Iverson, CA, Sutive, TG, and Crowell, MS: Lumbopelvic manipulation for the treatment of patients with patellofemoral pain syndrome: development of a clinical prediction rule. *J Orthop Sports Phys Ther* 38: 297–312, 2008.
79. Jensen, GM, Shepard, KF, and Hack, LM: The novice versus the experienced clinician: insights into the work of the physical therapist. *Phys Ther* 70:314–323, 1990.
80. Jensen, GM, et al: Attribute dimensions that distinguish master and novice physical therapy clinicians in orthopedic settings. *Phys Ther* 72:711–722, 1992.
81. Jensen, GM, and Lorish, C: Promoting patient cooperation with exercise programs: linking research, theory, and practice. *Arthritis Care Res* 7:181–189, 1994.
82. Jensen, GM, Lorish C, and Shepard, KF: Understanding patient receptivity to change: teaching for treatment adherence. In Shepard, KF, and Jensen, GM (eds): *Handbook of Teaching for Physical Therapists.* Boston: Butterworth-Heinemann, 1997, p 241.
83. Jensen, GM, et al: Expert practice in physical therapy. *Phys Ther* 80: 28–43, 2000.
84. Jette, AM: Diagnosis and classification by physical therapists: a special communication. *Phys Ther* 69:967–969, 1989.
85. Jette, AM: Physical disablement concepts for physical therapy research and practice. *Phys Ther* 74:380–386, 1994.
86. Jette, AM, et al: Exercise: It's never too late—the strong for life program. *Am J Public Health* 89:66–72, 1999.
87. Jette, AM: The changing language of disablement. *Phys Ther* 85:198–199, 2005.
88. Jette, AM: Toward a common language for function, disability, and health. *Phys Ther* 86:726–734, 2006.
89. Jette, AM, et al: Are the ICF activity and participation dimensions distinct? *J Rehabil Med* 35:145–149, 2003.
90. Jette, DU, et al: Evidence-based practice: beliefs, attitudes, knowledge, and behaviors of physical therapists. *Phys Ther* 83:786–805, 2003.
91. Jette, DU, et al: Decision-making ability of physical therapists: physical therapy intervention or medical referral. *Phys Ther* 86:1619–1629, 2006.
92. Jones, MA: Clinical reasoning in manual therapy. *Phys Ther* 72:875, 1992.
93. Jones, M, Jensen, G, and Rothstein, J: Clinical reasoning in physiotherapy. In Higgs, J, and Jones, M (eds): *Clinical Reasoning in the Health Professions.* Oxford: Butterworth-Heinemann, 1995, p 72.
94. Kauffman, TL, Nashner, LM, and Allison, LK: Balance is a critical parameter in orthopedic rehabilitation. *Orthop Phys Ther Clin N Am* 6:43–78, 1997.
95. Kelley, MJ, et al: Shoulder pain and mobility deficits: adhesive capsulitis. *J Orthop Sports Phys Ther* 43(5):A1–A31, 2013.
96. Kelo, MJ: Use of self-report disability measures in daily practice. *Orthop Phys Ther Pract* 11:22–27, 1999.
97. Kettenbach, G: *Writing Patient/Client Notes: Ensuring Accuracy in Documentation.* Philadelphia: FA Davis, 2009.
98. Krebs, DE, Jetle, AM, and Assmann, SF: Moderate exercise improves gait stability in disabled elders. *Arch Phys Med Rehabil* 79:1489–1495, 1998.
99. Lange, B, et al: Breathe: a game to motivate adherence of breathing exercises. *J Phys Ther Educ* 25(1):30–35, 2011.
100. Lee, T, and Swanson, L: What is repeated in a repetition: effects of practice conditions on motor skill acquisition. *Phys Ther* 71:150–156, 1991.
101. Leighton, RD, and Sheldon, MR: Model for teaching clinical decision making in a physical therapy professional curriculum. *J Phys Ther Educ* 11(Fall):23, 1997.
102. Lephart, S, Swanik, CB, and Fu, F: Reestablishing neuromuscular control. In Prentice, WE (ed): *Rehabilitation Techniques in Sports Medicine,* ed. 3. Boston: McGraw-Hill, 1999, p 88.
103. Lin, C-H, et al: Effect of task practice order in motor skill learning in adults with Parkinson's disease. *Phys Ther* 87(9):1120–113, 2007.
104. Logerstedt, DS, et al: Knee pain and mobility impairments: meniscal and articular cartilage lesions—clinical practice guidelines linked to the International Classification of Functioning, Disabilty and Health from the Orthopedic Section of the American Physical Therapy Association. *J Orthop Sports Phys Ther* 40(6):A1–A35, 2010.
105. Logerstedt, DS, et al: Knee stability and movement coordination impairments: knee ligament sprain—clinical practice guidelines linked to the International Classification of Functioning, Disability and Health from the Orthopedic Section of the American Physical Therapy Association. *J Orthop Sports Phys Ther* 40(4):A1–A37, 2010.
106. Lorish, C, and Gale, JR: Facilitating behavior change: strategies for education and practice. *J Phys Ther Educ* 13:31–37, 1999.
107. Lusardi, MM: Mobility and balance in later life. *Orthop Phys Ther Clin N Am* 6:305, 1997.
108. Magee, DJ: *Orthopedic Physical Assessment*, ed. 6. St. Louis: Elsevier/Saunders, 2013.
109. Maher, CG, et al: A description of the trials, reviews, and practice guidelines indexed in the PEDro database. *Phys Ther* 88(9):1068–1077, 2008.
110. Mahler, HI, Kulik, JA, and Tarazi, RY: Effects of videotape intervention at discharge on diet and exercise compliance after coronary bypass surgery. *J Cardiopulm Rehabil* 19(3):170–177, 1999.
111. Malouin, F, and Richards, CL: Mental practice for relearning locomotor skills. *Phys Ther* 90(2):240–251, 2010.
112. Maring, J: Effects of mental practice on rate of skill acquisition. *Phys Ther* 70:165–172, 1990.
113. May, BJ, and Dennis, JK: Clinical decision-making. In May, BJ (ed): *Home Health and Rehabilitation: Concepts of Care,* ed. 2. Philadelphia: FA Davis, 1999, p 21.
114. May, BJ, and Dennis, JK: Expert decision-making in physical therapy: a survey of practitioners. *Phys Ther* 71:190–202, 1991.
115. McArdle, WD, Katch, FI, and Katch, VL: *Nutrition, Energy, and Human Performance,* ed. 7. Philadelphia: Wolthers Kluwer/Lippincott Williams & Wilkins, 2009.
116. McNevin, NH, Wulf, G, and Carlson, C: Effects of attentional focus, self-control, and dyad training on motor learning: implications for physical rehabilitation. *Phys Ther* 80:373–385, 2000.
117. McPoil, TG, Martin, RL, and Cornwall, MW: Heel pain: Plantar fasciitis—clinical practice guidelines linked to the International Classification of Functioning, Disabilty, and Health from the Orthopedic Section of the American Physical Therapy Association. *The Journal of Orthop Sports Phys Ther* 38(4):A1–A18, 2008.
118. Michaleff, ZA, et al: CENTRAL, PEDro, PubMed, and EMBASE are the most comprehensive databases indexing randomized controlled trials of physical therapy interventions. *Phys Ther* 91(2):190–197, 2011.
119. Miller, PA, McKibbon, KA, and Haynes, RB: A quantitative analysis of research publications in physical therapy journals. *Phys Ther* 83: 123–131, 2003.
120. Miller-Spoto, M, and Gombatto, SP: Diagnostic labels assigned to patients with orthopedic conditions and the influence of the label on selection of interventions: a qualitative study of orthopaedic clinical specialists. *Phys Ther* 94:776–791, 2014.
121. Mueller, MJ, and Maluf, KS: Tissue adaptation to physical stress: a proposed "physical stress theory" to guide physical therapist practice, education, and research. *Phys Ther* 82:382–403, 2002.
122. Myers, JB, et al: Reflexive muscle activation alterations in shoulders with anterior glenohumeral instability. *Am J Sports Med* 32(4):1013–1021, 2004.

123. Nagi, S: Some conceptual issues in disability and rehabilitation. In Sussman MB (ed): *Sociology and Rehabilitation.* Washington, DC: American Sociological Association, 1965, pp 100–113.
124. Nagi, SZ: Disability concepts revisited: implications for prevention. In Pope, AM, and Tarlov, AR (eds): *Disability in America.* Washington, DC: National Academies Press, 1991.
125. Nashner, L: Sensory, neuromuscular and biomechanical contributions to human balance. In Duncan, P (ed): *Balance.* Alexandria, VA: American Physical Therapy Association, 1990, p 5.
126. National Advisory Board on Medical Rehabilitation Research, Draft V: *Report and Plan for Medical Rehabilitation Research.* Bethesda, MD: National Institutes of Health, 1992.
127. Nemshick, MT: Designing educational interventions for patients and families. In Shepard, KF, and Jensen, GM (eds): *Handbook of Teaching for Physical Therapists.* Boston: Butterworth-Heinemann, 1997, p 303.
128. Nicholson, DE: Teaching psychomotor skills. In Shepard, KF, and Jensen, GM (eds): *Handbook of Teaching for Physical Therapists.* Boston: Butterworth-Heinemann, 1997, p 271.
129. Norton, BJ: "Harnessing our collective professional power": diagnosis dialog. *Phys Ther* 87:635–638, 2007
130. O'Sullivan, SB, and Schmitz, TJ: *Improving Functional Outcomes.* Philadelphia: FA Davis, 2010.
131. O'Sullivan, SB, and Schmitz, TJ: *Physical Rehabilitation: Assessment and Treatment,* ed. 5. Philadelphia: FA Davis, 2007.
132. Ozer, MN, Payton, OD, and Nelson, CE: *Treatment Planning for Rehabilitation: A Patient-Centered Approach.* New York: McGraw-Hill, 2000.
133. Page, SJ, et al: Mental practice combined with physical practice for upper limb motor deficits in subacute stroke. *Phys Ther* 81:1455–1462, 2001.
134. Posner, JD, et al: Physical determinants in independence in mature women. *Arch Phys Med Rehabil* 76:373–380, 1995.
135. Philadelphia Panel: Evidence-based clinical practice guidelines on selected rehabilitation interventions for knee pain. *Phys Ther* 81: 1675–1700, 2001.
136. Philadelphia Panel: Evidence-based clinical practice guidelines on selected rehabilitation interventions for low back pain. *Phys Ther* 81: 1641–1674, 2001.
137. Philadelphia Panel: Evidence-based clinical practice guidelines on selected rehabilitation interventions for neck pain. *Phys Ther* 81: 1701–1717, 2001.
138. Philadelphia Panel: Evidence-based clinical practice guidelines on selected rehabilitation interventions for shoulder pain. *Phys Ther* 81: 1719–1730, 2001.
139. Philadelphia Panel: Evidence-based clinical practice guidelines on selected rehabilitation interventions: overview and methodology. *Phys Ther* 81:1629–1640, 2001.
140. Puthoff, ML, and Nielsen, DH: Relationships among impairments in lower extremity strength and power, functional limitations, and disability in older adults. *Phys Ther* 87(10):1334–1347, 2007.
141. Quinn, L, and Gordon, J: *Documentation for Rehabilitation: A Guide to Clinical Decision Making,* ed. 2, St. Louis: Saunders/Elsivier, 2010.
142. Randall, KE, and McEwen, IR: Writing patient-centered functional goals. *Phys Ther* 80(12):1197–1203, 2000.
143. Rantanen, T, et al: Disability, physical activity and muscle strength in older women: The Women's Health and Aging Study. *Arch Phys Med Rehabil* 80:130–135, 1999.
144. Rauch, A, et al: The utility of the ICF to identify and evaluate problems and needs in participation in spinal cord injury rehabilitation. *Top Spinal Cord Inj Rehabil* 15(4):72–86, 2010.
145. Reo, JA, and Mercer, VS: Effects of live, videotaped, or written instruction on learning an upper extremity exercise program. *Phys Ther* 84:622–633, 2004.
146. Riddle, DL, and Stratford, PW: Use of generic vs. region-specific functional status measures on patients with cervical spine disorders. *Phys Ther* 78:951–963, 1998.
147. Riddle, DL, et al: Preliminary validation of a clinical assessment for deep vein thrombosis in orthopedic outpatients. *Clin Orthop* 432:252–257, 2005.
148. Rivett, DA, and Higgs, J: Hypothesis generation in the clinical reasoning behavior of manual therapists. *J Phys Ther Educ* 11:40–49, 1997.
149. Rose, SJ: Physical therapy diagnosis: Role and function. *Phys Ther* 69:535–537, 1989.
150. Rothstein, JM: Disability and our identity. *Phys Ther* 74:375–378, 1994.
151. Rothstein, JM, and Echternach, JL: Hypothesis-oriented algorithm for clinicians: a method for evaluation and treatment planning. *Phys Ther* 66:1388–1394, 1986.
152. Rothstein, JM, Echternach, JL, and Riddle, DL: The Hypothesis-Oriented Algorithm for Clinicians II (HOAC II): A guide for patient management. *Phys Ther* 83:455–470, 2003.
153. Roush, SE, and Sharby, N: Disability reconsidered: the paradox of physical therapy. *Phys Ther* 91:1715–1727, 2011.
154. Roush, SE, and Sonstroen, RJ: Development of the Physical Therapy Outpatient Satisfaction Survey (PTOPS). *Phys Ther* 79:159–170, 1999.
155. Ruhland, JL, and Shields, RK: The effects of a home exercise program on impairment and health-related quality of life in persons with chronic peripheral neuropathies. *Phys Ther* 77:1026–1039, 1997.
156. Sackett, DL, et al: Evidence-based medicine: what it is and what it isn't. *BMJ* 312:71–72, 1996.
157. Sackett, DL, et al: *Evidence-Based Medicine: How to Practice and Teach EBM,* ed. 2. New York: Churchill Livingstone, 2000.
158. Sahrmann, SA: Diagnosis by physical therapists: a prerequisite for treatment. *Phys Ther* 68:1703–1706, 1988.
159. Sahrmann, S: Are physical therapists fulfilling their responsibilities as diagnosticians? *J Orthop Sports Phys Ther* 35:556–558, 2005.
160. Sahrmann, S: The human movement system: our professional identity. *Phys Ther* 94:1034–1042, 2014.
161. Scalzitti, DA: Evidence-based guidelines: application to clinical practice. *Phys Ther* 81:1622–1628, 2001.
162. Schenkman, M, and Butler, R: A model for multisystem evaluation, interpretation, and treatment of individuals with neurologic dysfunction. *Phys Ther* 69:538–547, 1989.
163. Schmidt, RA, and Lee, TD: *Motor Control and Learning: A Behavioral Emphasis,* ed. 4. Champaign, IL: Human Kinetics Publishers, 2005.
164. Schmidt, RA, and Wrisberg, CA: *Motor Learning and Performance: A Problem-Based Learning Approach,* ed. 3. Champaign, IL: Human Kinetics Publishers, 2004.
165. Schmitz, TJ: Coordination assessment. In O'Sullivan, SB, and Schmitz, TJ (eds): *Physical Rehabilitation: Assessment and Treatment,* ed. 4. Philadelphia: FA Davis, 2001, p 157.
166. Seyer, MA: Balance deficits: Examination, evaluation, and intervention. In Montgomery, PC, and Connolly, BH (eds): *Clinical Applications for Motor Control.* Thorofare, NJ: Slack, 2003, pp 271–306.
167. Seymour, CJ, and Dybel, GJ: Developing skillful clinical decision-making: evaluation of two classroom teaching strategies. *J Phys Ther Educ* 10:77–81, 1996.
168. Shuijs, EM, Kok, GJ, and van der Zee, J: Correlates of exercise compliance in physical therapy. *Phys Ther* 73:771–786, 1993.
169. Shumway-Cook, A, and Woollacott, MH: *Motor Control: Translating Research in Clinical Practice,* ed. 3. Philadelphia: Wolthers Kluwer/ Lippincott Williams & Wilkins, 2007.
170. Shumway-Cook, A, et al: The effect of multidimensional exercises on balance, mobility and fall risk in community-dwelling older adults. *Phys Ther* 77:46–57, 1997.
171. Sidaway, B, and Trzaska, A: Can mental practice increase ankle dorsiflexor torque? *Phys Ther* 85:1053–1060, 2005.
172. Stanton, TR, et al: Critical appraisal of clinical prediction rules that aim to optimize treatment selection for musculoskeletal conditions. *Phys Ther* 90(6):843–859, 2010.
173. Steiner, WA, et al: Use of the ICF model as a clinical problem-solving tool in physical therapy and rehabilitation medicine. *Phys Ther* 82:1098–1107, 2002.
174. Stucki, G, Ewert, T, and Cieza, A: Value and application of the ICF in rehabilitation medicine. *Disabil Rehabil* 24:932–938, 2002.

175. Stucki, G: International Classification of Functioning, Disability and Health (ICF): a promising framework and classification for rehabilitation medicine. *Am J Phys Med Rehabil* 84(10):733–740, 2005.
176. Stucki, G, Cieza, A, and Melvin, J: International Classification of Functioning, Disability and Health: a unifying model for the conceptual description of the rehabilitation strategy. *J Rehabil Med* 39:279–285, 2007.
177. Sullivan, PE, and Markos, PD: *Clinical Decision Making in Therapeutic Exercise.* Norwalk, CT: Appleton & Lange, 1995.
178. Sutive, TG, et al: Development of a clinical prediction rule for diagnosing hip osteoarthritis in individuals with unilateral hip pain. *J Orthop Sports Phys Ther* 38:542–550, 2008.
179. Swanson, G: Functional outcome report: The next generation in physical therapy reporting. In Stewart, DL, and Abeln, SH (eds): *Documenting Functional Outcomes in Physical Therapy.* St. Louis: Mosby-Year Book, 1993, p 101.
180. Task Force for Standards of Measurement in Physical Therapy: Standards for tests and measurements in physical therapy practice. *Phys Ther* 71:589–622, 1991.
181. Taylor, JD, Fletcher, JP, and Tiarks, J: Impact of physical therapist-directed exercise counseling combined with fitness center-based exercise training on muscular strength and exercise capacity in people with type 2 diabetes: a randomized clinical trial. *Phys Ther* 89(9):884–892, 2009.
182. Taylor, NF, et al: Therapeutic exercise in physiotherapy practice is beneficial: a summary of systematic reviews 2002–2005. *Aust J Physiother* 53(1):7–16, 2007.
183. Thoomes, EJ, and Schmit, MS: Practical use of the HOAC-II for clinical decision-making and subsequent therapeutic interventions in an elite athlete with low back pain. *J Orthop Sports Phys Ther* 41(2):108–117, 2011.
184. *Towards a Common Language for Functioning, Disability and Health.* Geneva: World Health Organization, 2001. Available at: http://www.who.int/classifications/icf/training/ icfbeginnersguide.pdf. Accessed July 8, 2011.
185. Triffitt, PD: The relationship between motion of the shoulder and the stated ability to perform activities of daily living. *J Bone Joint Surg Am* 80(1):41–46, 1998.
186. Turk, D: Correlates of exercise compliance in physical therapy. *Phys Ther* 73:783–786, 1993.
187. Umphried, D: Physical therapy differential diagnosis in the clinical setting. *J Phys Ther Educ* 9:39, 1995.
188. U.S. Department of Health and Human Services, Office of Disease Prevention and Health Promotion: *Healthy People 2010.* Washington, DC, 1998. Available at: http://www.healthypeople.gov/. Accessed August 2006.
189. U.S. Department of Health and Human Services, Office of Disease Prevention and Health Promotion: *Healthy People 2020.* Washington, DC: Available at: http://www.healthypeople.gov/. Accessed June 2011.
190. U.S. Department of Health and Human Services, Office of Disease Prevention and Health Promotion: *National Action Plan to Improve Health Literacy.* Washington, DC, 2010. Available at http://www.health.gov/communication/HLActionPlan/. Accessed June 2015.
191. U.S. Department of Health and Human Services, Public Health Service: *Healthy People 2000: National Health Promotion and Disease Prevention Objectives.* Washington, DC, 1991.
192. Van Sant, AE: Motor control, motor learning and motor development. In Montgomery, PC, Connolly, BH (eds): *Clinical Applications for Motor Control.* Thorofare, NJ: Slack, 2003, pp 25–52.
193. Verbrugge, L, and Jetle, A: The disablement process. *Soc Sci Med* 38:1, 1994.
194. Wainwright, SF, Shephard, K, and Harman, LB: Factors that influence the clinical decision making of novice and experienced physical therapists. *Phys Ther* 91(1):87–101, 2011.
195. Warner, L, and Mc Neill, ME: Mental imagery and its potential for physical therapy. *Phys Ther* 68:516–521, 1988.
196. Winstein, C, and Sullivan, K: Some distinctions on the motor learning/motor control distinction. *Neurol Rep* 21:42, 1997.
197. Winstein, C, et al: Learning a partial weight-bearing skill effectiveness of two forms of feedback. *Phys Ther* 76:985–993, 1996.
198. Winstein, C: Knowledge of results and motor learning: Implications for physical therapy. *Phys Ther* 71:140–149, 1991.
199. World Bank: World report on disability. Main report 2011. Washington, DC. Available at http://documents.worldbank.org/curated/en/2011/01/14440066/world-report-disability. Accessed June 30, 2015.
200. Wulf, G, Hob, M, and Prinz, W: Instructions for motor learning: differential effects of internal vs. external focus of attention. *J Motor Behav* 30: 169–179, 1998.
201. Zinny, NJ: Physical therapy management from physical therapy diagnosis: necessary but insufficient. *J Phys Ther Educ* 9:36, 1995.
202. Zinny, NJ: Diagnostic classification and orthopedic physical therapy practice: what we can learn from medicine. *J Orthop Sports Phys* Ther 34:105–109, 2004.

CHAPTER 2

Prevention, Health, and Wellness

SUSAN A. APPLING, PT, DPT, PHD, OCS, MTC
KAREN HOLTGREFE, PT, DHS, OCS

Transforming society by optimizing movement to improve the human experience.

APTA Vision Statement[8]

Physical therapists have long been advocates for prevention, health, and wellness. They not only work with patients in a rehabilitation environment, but they also have opportunity to work with clients to improve fitness, wellness, and overall health.[6,38] Their roles include education, direct intervention, research, advocacy, and collaborative consultation, as well as identification of risk factors and provision of services to mitigate those risks,[7] thus helping individuals bridge the gap between illness and wellness. Physical therapists and physical therapist assistants also work within their communities to influence and advocate for adapting environments to promote healthy lifestyles for all. In these ways, they can achieve the profession's vision of "transforming society by optimizing movement to improve the human experience."[8]

Key Terms and Concepts

Health. "A state of complete physical, mental, and social well-being and not merely the absence of disease or infirmity."[84] "A state of being associated with freedom from disease, injury, and illness that also includes a positive component (wellness) that is associated with a quality of life and positive well-being."[4]

Wellness. "A state of being that incorporates all facets and dimensions of human existence, including physical health, emotional health, spirituality, and social connectivity."[4] "An active process through which people become aware of, and make choices toward, a more successful existence."[48]

Health literacy. "The degree to which individuals have the capacity to obtain, process, and understand basic health information and services needed to make appropriate health decisions."[70]

Health promotion. "Any effort taken to allow an individual, group, or community to achieve awareness of—and empowerment to pursue—prevention and wellness."[4]

Public health. "The practice of preventing disease and promoting good health by providing the resources and creating environments that help people stay healthy."[9]

Health-related quality of life. "A broad multidimensional concept that usually includes self-reported measures of physical and mental health."[16]

Well-being. "A positive outcome that is meaningful for people and for many sectors of society, because it tells us that people perceive that their lives are going well."[19]

Fitness and physical activity. Refer to Chapter 7.

Chronic Disease, Prevention, and Health Care

Noncommunicable chronic diseases are primary causes of death and illness in the United States, with chronic diseases accounting for 7 of the top 10 causes of death.[34,83] The top four chronic conditions in terms of mortality include cardiovascular disease, cancers, chronic respiratory diseases, and diabetes. According to the Centers for Disease Control and Prevention (CDC), chronic diseases account for about two-thirds of deaths globally.[18]

Chronic Conditions Related to Behaviors

Chronic conditions are often attributable to behaviors. Some common risky behaviors include tobacco use and second-hand smoke exposure, physical inactivity and lack of regular exercise, poor diet and nutrition, and excessive alcohol use. These behaviors often lead to a cascade of health problems, including hypertension and stroke, obesity, and diabetes, among others. Approximately 78 million Americans are at increased risk for heart disease, diabetes, and cancer as a result of obesity alone.[69] In 2013, more than 76% of adults had at least one chronic condition, 19% had two to three chronic conditions, and 4% had more than four chronic conditions.[17] These conditions are common in the patients/clients with whom physical therapists intervene; therefore, risk factor assessment must be an integral part of physical therapist practice.

Health-Care Costs Due to Risky Behaviors

The risky life-style behaviors noted above result in increased costs for health care. In 2014, the US spent approximately $3.0 trillion dollars on health care, averaging about $9,523 per person, which was about 17.5% of the gross domestic product for that year.[20]According to the CDC, treating people with chronic disease accounts for about 86% of US health-care costs.[15] Although the health-care spending level is about twice as much as other industrialized nations, the US ranks 24th among those 30 nations in life expectancy.[9] Spending on prevention in the US is only about 3% of all health-care spending, while about 75% of health-care costs are related to treatment of largely preventable conditions.[37]

Investment in Prevention

To facilitate change and improve health behaviors, and thereby reduce health-care costs and spending, investment in prevention is critical. A 2009 report by the Trust for America's Health found that an investment of $10 per person per year on prevention and wellness programs could yield a net savings in health-care costs of more than $2.8 billion annually within 1 to 2 years and more than $16 billion annually within 5 years,[68] a significant return on investment. To that end, the Prevention and Public Health Fund (Prevention Fund) was created as a part of the Patient Protection and Affordable Care Act.[9] The purpose of the Prevention Fund is to provide money for investment in public health programs to improve the health of communities and the nation.[9] More than $4.7 billion has been allocated for prevention and public health programs since the inception of the Prevention Fund in 2012.[54] These activities and programs are typically community-based programs aimed to improve health, including those that reduce or prevent tobacco use, increase immunization rates, improve access to care, reduce transmission of HIV, and those that generally encourage healthy living.[9] Physical therapists have opportunity to facilitate behavior change to reduce risk factors in the individuals with whom they work, thereby reducing not only the economic burden of these conditions for the individual and society, but also improving the health of the individuals and the communities in which they live.

Wellness

There are varying definitions of wellness and models of the components of wellness, but there is general agreement on the multidimensional, interdependent nature of the concept of wellness.[2,13,24,48] The various components are summarized in Table 2.1. The National Wellness Institute utilizes The Six Dimensions of Health Model (SDH), which includes social, occupational, spiritual, physical, intellectual, and emotional dimensions.[48] Adams, Bezner, and Steinhardt describe six domains of wellness, including emotional, intellectual, physical, psychological, societal, and spiritual.[2] They developed the Perceived Wellness Survey (PWS) to assess wellness across and within those six domains of wellness. This tool is easy to administer and score, increasing its clinical utility for the physical therapist.[1] The Model for Healthy Living developed by the Church Health Center in Memphis, Tennessee, includes the domains of faith life, movement, medical, work, emotional, nutrition, and family and friends.[24] The Model of Healthy Living Assessment Wheel, shown in Figure 2.1, provides a description of each domain, as well as a rating system for self-assessment for individuals.[23] This tool is easily administered and has been used in community and faith-based settings.

Healthy People 2020

In 1979, following the Surgeon General's report on the health of the nation, the US government developed a national prevention agenda. Currently, the Office of Disease Prevention

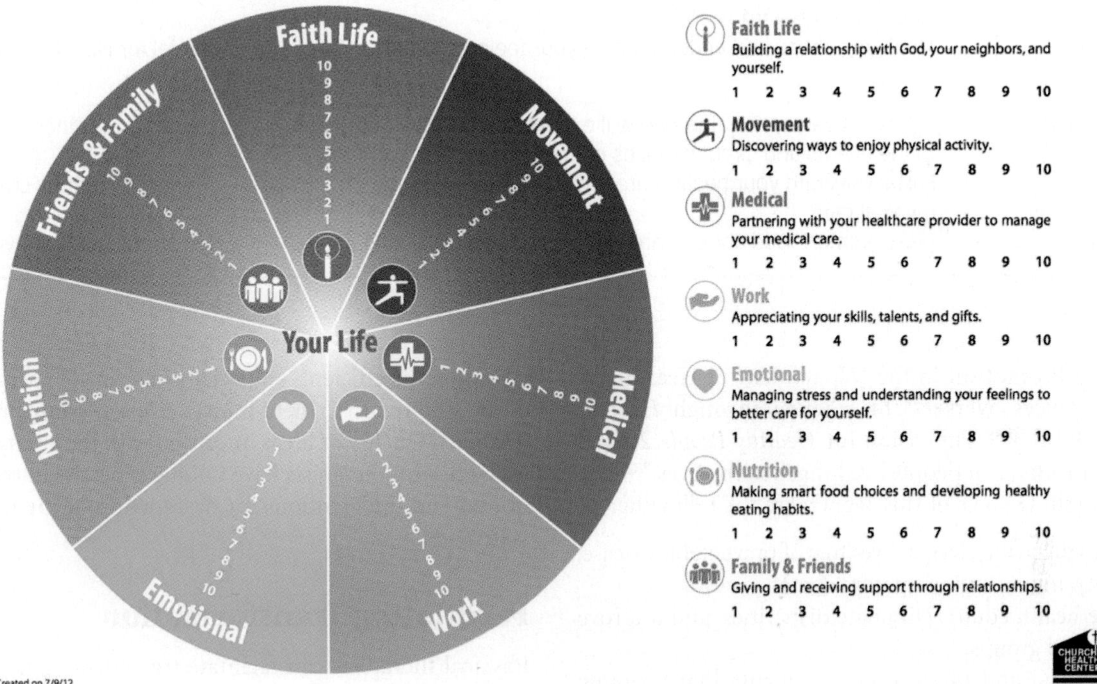

FIGURE 2.1 Model for Health Living Assessment Wheel. *(From* Church Health Reader, *Spring, 2013,*[24] *with permission. Available at http://chreader.org/wp-content/uploads/2014/12/Model-for-Healthy-Living-Assessment-Wheel.pdf)*

TABLE 2.1 Domains of Wellness by Model

Domain	Description	Model
Social	Interacting and contributing to one's community or environment; emphasizes interdependence of self with others	Six Dimensions of Health[48]
Social	The perception that salient others are available for support and that one provides support for others	Perceived Wellness Model[2,13]
Family & Friends	Giving and receiving support through relationships	Model for Healthy Living[24]
Occupational	Personal satisfaction and enrichment in one's life through work	Six Dimensions of Health[48]
Work	Appreciating your skills, talents, and gifts	Model for Healthy Living[24]
Spiritual	Finding and living a life that has meaning and purpose	Six Dimensions of Health[48]
Spiritual	A positive sense of meaning and purpose in life	Perceived Wellness Model[2,13]
Faith Life	Building a relationship with God, your neighbors, and yourself	Model for Healthy Living[24]
Physical	Making appropriate nutritional choices and participating in regular physical activity	Six Dimensions of Health[48]
Physical	Positive perceptions and expectancies of physical health	Perceived Wellness Model[2,13]
Movement	Discovering ways to enjoy physical activity	Model for Healthy Living[24]
Intellectual	Actively using your mind to develop new skills and learn new information	Six Dimensions of Health[48]
Intellectual	The perception that one is internally energized by the appropriate amount of intellectually stimulating activity	Perceived Wellness Model[2,13]

Continued

TABLE 2.1 Domains of Wellness by Model—cont'd

Domain	Description	Model
Emotional	Accepting and managing our feelings in all personal interactions	Six Dimensions of Health[48]
Emotional	The possession of a secure sense of self-identity and a positive sense of self-regard	Perceived Wellness Model[2,13]
Emotional	Managing stress and understanding your feelings to better care for yourself	Model for Healthy Living[24]
Psychological	A general perception that one will experience positive outcomes to the events and circumstances of life	Perceived Wellness Model[2,13]
Medical	Partnering with your health-care provider to manage your medical care	Model for Healthy Living[24]
Nutrition	Making smart food choices and developing healthy eating habits	Model for Healthy Living[24]

and Health Promotion in the Department of Health and Human Services oversees this agenda through *Healthy People 2020*.[1,23,50,68] The vision for *Healthy People 2020* is "a society in which all people live long, healthy lives."[72] The four overarching goals of this agenda are the following:

- Attain high-quality, longer lives free of preventable disease, disability, injury, and premature death.
- Achieve health equity, eliminate disparities, and improve health of all groups.
- Create social and physical environments that promote health for all.
- Promote quality of life, healthy development, and healthy behaviors across all life stages.

Leading health indicators. *Healthy People 2020* contains 42 topic areas and more than 1,200 objectives. Leading Health Indicators (LHI), a subset of *Healthy People 2020* objectives, have been identified since *Healthy People 2010*. LHIs were selected to communicate high-priority areas and actions to address the 26 identified objectives. The current LHI topic areas include access to care; clinical preventative services; environmental quality; injury and violence; maternal, infant, and child health; mental health; nutrition, physical activity, and obesity; oral health; reproductive and sexual health; social determinants of health; substance abuse; and tobacco use.[73] A progress update from March 2014 indicates that progress has been generally positive for the LHI, with 14 of the 26 indicators/objectives (53.9%) having either met their target or shown improvement.[74,75]

Role of Physical Therapists in Health Promotion and Wellness

Consider the American Physical Therapy Association (APTA) vision statement, "Transforming society by optimizing movement to improve the human experience".[8] Optimal movement is purposeful, efficient—especially in terms of energy expenditure, and reduces risk of injury or onset of impairments or disability. Quality of life is improved with the ability to move well. Physical therapists have unique expertise in the evaluation of and interventions for dysfunction of the movement system.

Facilitating Transformation

Physical therapists can facilitate transformation of society through the typical practice of working with patients in rehabilitation after onset of injury or illness or after surgery. Physical therapists can also facilitate this transformation by educating patients/clients to enhance health and wellness; identifying community resources available to the client to support a healthy lifestyle; advocating for community systems and resources to support health-enhancing behaviors and environments; influencing public policy at the local, state, and national levels; and advocating for reduction in health disparities. Through use of clinical reasoning, knowledge, and skills, and as experts in the human movement system, physical therapists can transform society by helping patients/clients optimize movement to promote health and wellness, prevent or reduce impairments, and reduce and/or prevent disability.

Promoting Health and Behavior Change

Due to the nature of physical therapist practice, with extended patient/client visits over a period of time, physical therapists are "uniquely qualified to lead the assault on lifestyle conditions."[32] Physical therapists have the opportunity to not only address patient/client specific impairments and functional limitations, but also to promote health and influence behavior change so that the outcome is improved individual health and function and improved health of the community. Through assessment of risk factors, education regarding impact of risk factors and behaviors, and interventions designed for the individual to address multiple components of wellness, the physical therapist can assist the patient/client in achieving better health and better health-related quality of life. Helpful resources for counseling patients and clients about nutrition and weight management can be found at myplate.gov and in the *2015-2020 Dietary Guidelines for Americans.*[71] Physical therapists can and should encourage their patients/clients to increase physical activity, eat a nutritious diet and manage weight, and have a positive outlook.

Assess State of Wellness

Physical therapists should take the opportunity to assess patient/client current state of wellness using an assessment tool, such as the Perceived Wellness Survey or the Model for Health Living Assessment Wheel (see Fig. 2.1).[1,23] These tools are easy to administer and provide insight in terms of perceived wellness in each category as well as across the domains. Balance across the domains is desired. Outcomes of interventions for these domains can be assessed with repeat administration. When obtaining the patient/client history, include questions about general health status and social and health habits, including current level of physical activity, tobacco use, nutrition and weight management, adequacy of sleep, and level of stress.[13] In addition to asking about these behaviors, discuss options for intervention with the patient/client, such as identifying smoking cessation or nutritional counseling and weight loss programs available in the area. Table 2.2 describes physical therapists' behaviors, knowledge, and skills needed for incorporating health and wellness into practice.[13]

TABLE 2.2 Health and Wellness Knowledge and Skills for Physical Therapists[13]

For all behaviors: normal and abnormal pathophysiology, epidemiology of injury and disease, risk factors, protective health behaviors, theories of health behavior change, ecological approaches to behavior change, counseling skills, local and community resources, history taking, rapport building, and ability to assess readiness to change

Behavior	Knowledge	Skill
Physical activity	▪ Age-and disease-specific exercise prescription for lifestyle-related conditions ▪ Physical activity guidelines	▪ Ability to ask the question "Are you physically active?" and provide guidance when the answer is "No" ▪ Personal experience with physical activity; role modelling ▪ Screening for physical activity ▪ Exercise prescription ▪ Counseling skills, including skill in motivational interviewing ▪ Time management (i.e., fitting regular physical activity into daily lifestyle)
Nutrition and weight management	▪ Population-based nutrition trends and data ▪ Overweight and obesity guidelines (e.g., BMI) ▪ Basic nutritional information and resources (e.g., ChooseMyPlate.gov)	▪ Ability to ask questions like "Do you eat five servings of fruits and vegetables per day?" and "Do you drink at least six to eight, 8-oz glasses of water per day?" and provide guidance when the answer is "No" ▪ Role modeling healthy eating habits ▪ Screening for malnutrition, undernutrition, and obesity ▪ Assessment of BMI ▪ Counseling skills, including skill in motivational interviewing ▪ Ability to recognize need to refer to a nutrition specialist
Smoking cessation	▪ Smoking information and resources ▪ 5 A's ▪ 5 R's	▪ Ability to ask the question "Do you smoke cigarettes?" and provide guidance when the answer is "Yes" ▪ Role modelling not smoking ▪ Screening for tobacco use and desire to quit ▪ Counseling skills, including skill in motivational interviewing ▪ Interprofessional collaboration ▪ Physical activity prescription to promote and support smoking cessation
Sleep	▪ Etiology, pathophysiology, diagnosis, treatment, prevention, and public health burden of sleep loss and disorders	▪ Ability to ask the questions "Do you get 7 to 8 hours of sleep each night?" "Are you tired in the morning?" "Do you fall asleep quickly?" "Are you sleepy during the day?" "Do you wake up at night?" and provide guidance if the answers indicate poor sleep hygiene

Continued

TABLE 2.2 Health and Wellness Knowledge, and Skills for Physical Therapists[13]—cont'd

Behavior	Knowledge	Skill
	▪ Recommend sleep habits and conditions conducive to sleep	▪ Role modeling healthy sleep habits ▪ Screening for sleep disorders ▪ Ability to provide instructions about optimal sleep habits ▪ Ability to recognize need to refer to another provider ▪ Physical activity prescription to enhance sleep
Stress management	▪ Difference between positive and negative stress ▪ Theory supporting relaxation techniques ▪ Role of physical activity in managing stress ▪ Resilience theory	▪ Ability to ask the question "Do you feel stressed?" and provide guidance when the answer is "Yes" ▪ Role modeling stress management ▪ Screening for stress ▪ Ability to instruct in relaxation techniques (e.g., deep breathing, PMR, visualization, meditation, autogenic training, biofeedback, massage) ▪ Physical activity prescription to manage stress, including tai chi and yoga ▪ Time management techniques ▪ Ability to recognize need to refer to another provider

*Taken from *Phys Ther* 95(10):1433–1444, 2014, with permission of the American Physical Therapy Association. © 2015 American Physical Therapy Association[13]

Function of the Physical Therapist

Roles of the physical therapist in prevention, health promotion, and wellness include:[4]

- *Identifying risk factors and interventions to reduce risk in individuals and communities.*
- *Preventing or slowing progression of functional decline and disability and enhancing activity in those with a diagnosed condition.*
- *Reducing disability by restoring skills and independence in those with chronic conditions.*
- *Screening:* Identifying individuals or groups who would benefit from education, intervention, or referral to an appropriate health-care provider.
- *Intervention:* Providing interventions as identified from screening sessions.
- *Consultation:* Providing expertise and knowledge.
- *Education:* Providing information on prevention, health, wellness, and fitness topics.
- *Critical Inquiry:* Obtaining, synthesizing, and utilizing current research; interpreting data; and/or participating in research.
- *Administration:* Planning, developing, and managing all aspects of a prevention or wellness project including budget, human resources, and space.

Prevention Activities

Examples for various prevention activities can be found in Table 2.3. When developing prevention activities, it is important to note that there are three types of prevention:[4]

- *Primary prevention:* Preventing a target problem or condition in an individual or in a community at risk; for example, developing fitness programs for children to prevent obesity or a back injury prevention program for warehouse workers.
- *Secondary prevention:* Decreasing the duration and severity of disease; for example, developing resistance programs for individuals with osteoporosis.
- *Tertiary prevention:* Decreasing the degree of disability and promoting rehabilitation for individuals with chronic or irreversible diseases; for example, developing fitness programs for individuals with spinal cord injury.

FOCUS ON EVIDENCE

Norman and her coauthors[50] assessed psychological well-being (Positive Affect Balance Scale), depression symptoms (Edinburgh Postnatal Depressions Scale), and physical activity (minutes per week) in postpartum women. The intervention group ($n = 62$) participated in an exercise and education program for 8 weeks led by a women's health physical therapist, while the control group ($n = 73$) was mailed the same educational material over the 8 weeks. The intervention group had a significant difference in well-being (improvement $p = 0.007$) and a reduced risk of developing postpartum depression ($P < 0.001$) compared with the control group but no difference in amount of physical activity.

Identifying Risk Factors

When developing specific programs related to health, wellness, and fitness, it is important to conduct risk assessments and preparticipation screenings. The reader is referred to the

TABLE 2.3 Prevention Activities

Screening Risk Assessment	Health Promotion, Wellness, and Fitness
Scoliosis	Education: Information flyer for parents on identification and treatment for idiopathic scoliosis.
Obesity	Intervention: Develop exercise/fitness program for overweight teens and adults. Include education on nutrition and weight management. Use myplate.gov for education and tracking tools.
Osteoporosis	Education: Develop community education programs related to osteoporosis (importance of exercise, reducing falls in the home). Administration: Develop a resistance and weight-bearing exercise class for individuals with osteoporosis. Screening: Perform Falls Risk Assessment at community health fair.
Falls	Critical Inquiry: Complete a literature review and identify the most appropriate measures of fall risk. Intervention: Develop exercise program to increase strength, balance, and coordination in older adults.
Work site assessment	Consultation: Work with human resource department of a company to identify ways to reduce workplace injuries. Educate: Educate employees and management on proper body mechanics, work station redesign, and ways to reduce injury risk.

American College of Sports Medicine (ACSM)[3] for several tools to assess these factors.

Preparticipation Screening

Prior to participation in moderate-intensity physical activity, the individual should be asked several questions as summarized in Box 2.1.[65] Individuals who answer yes to one or more questions should be evaluated further and may require consultation with their physician before starting some activities (see the appendix following Chapter 24). For higher-performing clients, the Functional Movement Screen (FMS) and the Selective Functional Movement Assessment (SFMA) can be used to assess movement patterns with seven activities.[25, 26] The FMS has been used to assess athletes, fireman, and military personnel. The SFMA is a similar assessment but is used with those with known musculoskeletal pain.[22,28,41,51]

BOX 2.1 Activity Prescreening Questions

1. Have you ever been diagnosed with a heart condition?
2. Have you ever been advised that you should only do physical activity under the direction of a physician?
3. Do you experience chest pain when you do physical activity?
4. Have you experienced chest pain during this past month when not physically active?
5. Have you been diagnosed with arthritis or osteoporosis, or have you experienced increased pain in your joints when physically active?
6. Are you currently taking prescription drugs for blood pressure or a heart condition?
7. Do you ever lose your balance or lose consciousness?
8. Are you aware of any condition that would prohibit you from doing physical activity?

Risk Assessment

The participant should be assessed for risk factors associated with specific conditions such as coronary artery disease (CAD) and osteoporosis, as shown in Box 2.2.[3, 47] Identification of risk factors guides the therapist when deciding how to proceed. If multiple risk factors, such as those associated with CAD, are identified, a participant may need to be referred to a physician prior to initiating a program. However, if the risk factors are minimal, the therapist should monitor and progress the chosen activities or exercises within established guidelines. (See Chapter 7 for guidelines related to aerobic exercise.)

An individual with identified risk factors for osteoporosis may require additional screening for balance and strength. The therapist can then develop an appropriate exercise program that reduces the risk of injury. (See Chapter 6 for precautions during resistance training and Chapter 8 for balance programs.)

Determining Readiness to Change

Once the preparticipation screenings and risk assessments are completed, but prior to individualized program development, it is important to know where the person is in terms of readiness for behavior change. There are multiple theories and models related to health promotion interventions that explain how behavior change occurs. Understanding several of these behavioral change theories can help guide the therapist and client toward the desired outcome.

BOX 2.2 Risk Factors for Coronary Artery Disease and Osteoporosis

Coronary Artery Disease Risk Factors
- Family history
- Cigarette smoking
- Hypertension
- Hypercholesterolemia
- Impaired fasting glucose level
- Obesity
- Sedentary lifestyle

Osteoporosis Risk Factors
- Bone mineral density score of −2.5 or less
- Postmenopausal
- Caucasian or Asian descent
- Family history of osteoporosis
- Low body weight
- Inactive lifestyle
- Insufficient calcium and vitamin E
- Insufficient fruits and vegetables in diet
- Smoking
- Excessive consumption of alcohol
- Prolonged bed rest
- Prolonged use of corticosteroids and other medications, including selective serotonin reuptake inhibitors, proton pump inhibitors, and some antacids

Behavioral Change Theories

Social cognitive theory. The underlying premise of the social cognitive theory is that learning occurs within a social context with a dynamic and reciprocal interaction between cognitive processes, environment, and behavior.[11,12] An individual must believe that he or she can change a particular behavior and that changing that behavior will lead to positive outcomes that outweigh possible negative outcomes one might experience.[27,33,42,44,67] For example, a patient/client may want to lose weight. In addition to the desire to change the behavior(s) causing the increased weight, the patient/client needs to believe that he or she is capable of succeeding (self-efficacy) and that the outcome will improve his or her health. If the patient/client decides to use exercise to lose weight, clear instructions on how to perform and progress the exercise program must be given. Feedback on performance must then occur to achieve the final outcome of weight reduction. Self-efficacy is one construct within this model. Many researchers have identified positive self-efficacy as the key to successful participation in physical activity.[56,64,80]

Health belief model. The health belief model (HBM), one of the most influential and widely used psychosocial approaches to explaining health-related behavior, was initially created to explain the failure of people to participate in programs to prevent or to detect disease.[27,59] The HBM has six constructs: perceived susceptibility, perceived severity, perceived benefits, perceived barriers, cues to action, and self-efficacy.[59] An individual must have sufficient concern about developing an illness (perceived threat, mediated by perceived susceptibility and perceived severity of disease). Next, the individual needs to believe that they can be successful following the health recommendations (self-efficacy) and that by doing so, it is possible to achieve the desired outcome (perceived benefit). The likelihood of taking the preventative action is mediated by the perceived benefits minus the perceived barriers of such action. Modifying factors to perceived threat include cues to action, such as a reminder card from the dentist, media campaigns, or illness of a loved one.[27] Using the example of losing weight, an individual would have to believe that being overweight puts him or herself at a greater risk for developing heart disease (perceived threat). This threat may be greater because of a family history. The individual may understand that modifying the diet can help with weight loss but is not sure of the best way to proceed or if they can even be successful with dieting. The person may consider joining a weight loss program but may not be sure he or she can afford the weekly fee (perceived barrier). If the perceived threat is sufficiently high, the individual may choose to join the weight loss program to obtain the desired benefit or may choose a different method of weight loss that does not have the same cost, such as using Internet resources, like myplate.gov.

Transtheoretical model. The transtheoretical model (TTM), also known as the stages of change model, was first described by Prochaska in 1979. The TTM "is an integrative framework for understanding how individuals and populations progress toward adopting and maintaining health behavior change for optimal health."[55]

The TTM has five stages of change:[27,44,55,59,67]

1. Precontemplation—no intention of making any changes within the next 6 months.
2. Contemplation—intend to make changes within the next 6 months.
3. Preparation—has begun to take steps toward making the desired change in behavior and plans to make the changes within the next 30 days.
4. Action—has changed the behavior for less than 6 months.
5. Maintenance—has changed the behavior for more than 6 months.

By knowing what stage an individual is in and knowing the beliefs they have regarding the need to change, the physical therapist can assist in planning the intervention, particularly if individuals are not ready to make any changes. It allows the therapist to give information needed at the appropriate time. Figure 2.2 depicts an algorithm for determining what stage of change an individual is in, using exercise as an example.

FOCUS ON EVIDENCE

Using the HBM, Chen[21] assessed older adults in a long-term care (LTC) facility about barriers to participating in physical activity. The residents interviewed identified five main barriers: (1) physical frailty and health problems, (2) fear of falling

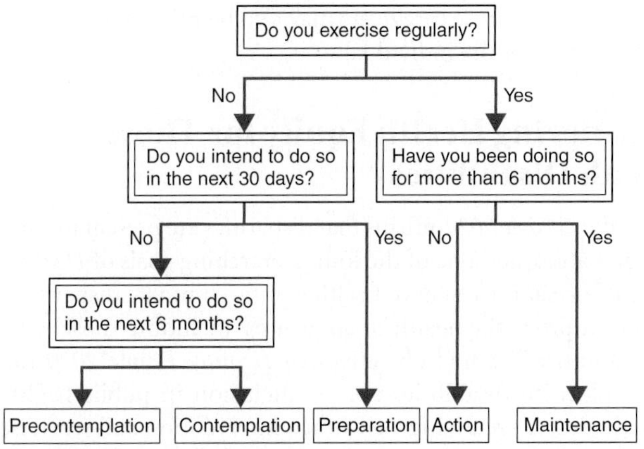

FIGURE 2.2 Transtheoretical Model Algorithm. *(Adapted from Reed et al: What makes a good staging algorithm: Examples from regular exercise.* Am J Health Promot *12(2):57-66, 1997)*[57]

and being injured, (3) past history of little to no physical activity, (4) limited knowledge about physical activity, and (5) restrictions within their environment. The author recommended addressing these modifiable barriers through careful planning, education, and interventions to increase physical activity in older adults living in LTC facilities to prevent further declines in function and mobility.

Motivation Affecting the Ability to Change

By definition, motivation is how we move ourselves or others to act.[64,67] When attempting to motivate an individual or group, several dimensions of motivation need to be considered. What is the *intrinsic* motivation? Is it the goal or expectation to do one's personal best? Is it the level of difficulty of the task and any potential incentives? Does the individual have the ability to learn and act on what they learn to be successful?

Next, what is the *performance* motivation? Positive and negative reinforcement or rewards can improve performance, as can success or failure. Generally, the best performance motivators are low failure and/or high successes.

Finally, what is the *task* motivation? This relates to knowledge and feedback on the performance and should include information on how to improve.

Physical Activity Guidelines

In October 2008, the US Department of Health and Human Services published *Physical Activity Guidelines for Americans,* which provides physical activity recommendations for persons 6 years and older and for specific subgroups.[78] This document is based on the findings of the Physical Activity Guidelines Advisory Committee, which conducted an extensive analysis of the scientific information on physical activity and health. Their findings suggest that some physical activity is better than none and that more activity is better than some. The guidelines include the minimal level of recommended physical activity to achieve most health benefits, although additional benefits occur with more activity. These health benefits include the reduction in risk for many chronic diseases. The Physical Activity Guidelines Advisory Committee also found that muscle strengthening and aerobic activities are beneficial and that the benefits of physical activity far outweigh the risks. A process is currently in place to update the guidelines.

Physical Activity Recommendations

In order to achieve the most health benefits, the following are identified for each age group.

Children and Adolescents

Children and adolescents (aged 6 years and older) should participate in at least 60 minutes of moderate to vigorous physical activity daily.

- At least 3 days a week, the activity level should be vigorous
- Both bone and muscle strengthening activities should be included in daily activity at least 3 days per week.
- Activities should be both age appropriate and fun.

Adults

Adults should participate in moderate intensity physical activity for a minimum of 150 minutes or vigorous intensity for 75 minutes per week.

- Episodes of at least 10 minutes count toward daily total.
- Muscles strengthening activities should be included at least 2 days per week.

Older Adults

Older adults (65 years and older) should follow adult guidelines as able.

- Participate in moderate intensity physical activity for a minimum of 150 minutes or vigorous intensity for 75 minutes per week.
- Include balance exercises to reduce risk of falls.
- Episodes of at least 10 minutes count toward daily total.
- Muscles strengthening activities should be included at least 2 days per week.

Adults With Disabilities

Adults with disabilities should follow adult guidelines as able. Those unable to meet the guidelines should:

- Engage in regular physical activity according to their abilities and should avoid inactivity.
- Consult with their health-care provider for an individualized program that is appropriate for their abilities.

Considerations for People With Disabilities

Individuals with disability encompass almost 19% of the US population.[14] The World Health Organization (WHO) defines disability as an "umbrella term, covering impairments, activity limitations, and participation restrictions. Disability is the interaction between individuals with a health condition (e.g., cerebral palsy, Down syndrome, and depression) and personal and environmental factors (e.g., negative attitudes, inaccessible transportation and public buildings, and limited social supports)."[82] In the WHO's ICF, disability and function are viewed as multifactorial and biopsychosocial phenomena, with both affected at the body, person, and society levels.[49]

Health Disparities and Risks

As a group, individuals with disability experience greater health disparities than those without disability.[60] Adults with disabilities and chronic conditions generally receive fewer preventive services and have poorer health status than those without disabilities with the same conditions.[58] These individuals are at higher risk of secondary conditions, including obesity, hypertension, cardiac disease, stroke, diabetes, arthritis, asthma, and depression, and are more likely to engage in unhealthy behaviors like smoking, poor diet, and inadequate physical activity.[58,60,61,79,82] According to the WHO, while people with disabilities have the same health-care needs as those without disabilities, those with disabilities are two times more likely to find health-care provider's with inadequate skill and facilities, 3 times more likely to be denied health care, and 4 times more likely to be treated poorly in the health-care system.[81]

People with disabilities, especially those with intellectual disabilities, have been described as having a "thinner margin of health,"[53] and therefore, physical activity is especially important. It is important to remember that individuals with disability are not "sick" but are more commonly in good health. However, their impairments of body functions and structures, activity limitations, and participation restrictions often put them at risk for and more vulnerable to health problems. Caretaker and family member attitudes of the individual's abilities and disability can contribute to learned helplessness, creating further barriers to physical activity. Additionally, individuals with disabilities typically have fewer opportunities to participate in health promoting behaviors, as facilities are often not designed to be inclusive or adaptive.

Children with disabilities often have individualized education plans and routinely work with physical therapists both within and outside of school systems. As these individuals become adults, access to physical therapy may be limited. Too often, health and fitness professionals lack adequate training and/or comfort level in working with persons with disabilities, especially intellectual disabilities. Often, attitudes of family and caregivers about their own levels of fitness can affect the attitude and fitness level of the person with disability, and education of those caregivers may also be necessary to facilitate fitness for the individual.

Achieving Health Equity for Those with Disabilities

Healthy People 2020 affirms that disparities are present for this population, and one of the four overarching goals of *Healthy People 2020* is to achieve health equity, eliminate disparities, and improve the health of all groups, including those with disabilities.[73] Some objectives in *Healthy People 2020* for people with disabilities are (1) inclusion in public health activities, (2) receiving well-timed intervention and services, (3) interaction with their environment without barriers, and (4) participation in everyday life activities. In order to meet these objectives, ways must be developed to include those with disabilities in public health programs.[79] Physical activity has a key role in increasing quality of years of healthy life and eliminating health disparities. As noted above in the *Physical Activity Guidelines for Americans,* those with disabilities should be physically active and avoid inactivity. Some objectives of a wellness program for people with disabilities are found in Box 2.3.

Resources. The National Center on Health, Physical Activity, and Disability (NCHPAD) is an excellent resource; it provides information on physical activity, health promotion, and disability, and it provides health promotion resources for professionals and for those with disabilities who want to achieve a healthy lifestyle.[46] The NCHPAD primarily serves persons with physical, sensory, and cognitive disabilities across the life span. Resources for professionals include tools for building inclusive communities, accessible fitness, inclusive fitness (i-Fit Tips), and a guidebook for healthy living with a spinal cord injury. There are also resources for individuals relating to living healthy with a variety of disabilities and ways to improve access in communities. The "Get the Facts" publication provides general exercise guidelines for individuals with disabilities, as well as a description of the NCHPAD's 14-week fitness program. Box 2.4 provides preliminary steps to exercise for persons with disabilities, taken from the NCHPAD.

BOX 2.3 Sample Objectives of a Wellness Program for Individuals With Disabilities

1. Reduce secondary conditions
2. Maintain functional independence throughout life span
3. Provide an opportunity for leisure and enjoyment
4. Enhance overall quality of life by reducing environmental barriers to good health

BOX 2.4 Preliminary Steps to Exercise (NCHPAD)[46]

1. Inform your physician, other health-care provider, or primary caregiver that you are considering starting an exercise program.
2. If possible, participate in a graded exercise test to determine your current level of fitness.
3. Find out the effects, if any, of your medication on exercise.
4. If possible, consult a trained exercise professional for an individualized exercise prescription.
5. Determine your goals and make sure they are S.M.A.R.T.**

**S.M.A.R.T. goals are Specific, Measurable, Attainable, Relevant, and Time Bound.

Role of physical therapist. Physical therapist interventions have a positive impact on overall health and wellness, primarily through patient/client education and movement. Physical therapists have opportunity to consult with individuals with disability and help them develop fitness programs to facilitate wellness. This is accomplished through interventions designed to improve muscle strength, flexibility, and endurance, as well as cardiovascular and pulmonary endurance. Major goals of fitness programs for individuals with developmental delay are provided in Box 2.5.[62]

Exercise adherence. Physical activity is important for all, especially so for those with disabilities, but adherence to a structured exercise program can be an issue. Some suggestions to improve exercise adherence in this population include using a buddy system to be physically active with a friend or caregiver, keeping an exercise log, and using a reward system (preferably not with food) when goals are achieved.[62] Remember, a "one size fits all" approach to physical activity does not work for individuals with disability. Consideration must be made for disability specific variability, an individual's comorbidities, and personal and environmental barriers to participation. By addressing these concerns with a fitness program and achieving improved physical activity and fitness levels, impairments of body functions and structures, activity limitations, and participation restrictions may be prevented, remediated, and improved.[5]

BOX 2.5 Major Goals of a Fitness Program for Individuals With Developmental Delay[62]

1. Aim to expend 200 to 400 calories a day. Fittest persons aim for 400 kcal/day while less fit aim for 200 kcal/day, working up to 300 kcal/day after 6 months of training.
2. Use the 3-2-1 principle when developing your fitness program:
   - 30 minutes of cardiovascular training (starting at 45%-55% max heart rate)
   - 20 minutes of strength training (may take longer to master; stress safety)
   - 10 minutes of flexibility exercises
3. Include a variety of activities; have one program for M/W/F, another for Tu/Th, and different activities for the weekend.
4. Aim for 30 to 60 minutes a day. This can be broken up into 4 sets of 15 minute bouts, 3 sets of 20 minute bouts, or 2 sets of 30 minute bouts. Do what works for the individual.
5. For a structured program, get physician clearance.

Mindfulness: Implications for Health and Wellness

Chronic or persistent pain, as well as chronic musculoskeletal conditions, have an effect on overall wellness. In the presence of chronic conditions, neurophysiological changes occur in the peripheral and central nervous systems. Integrating the principles of mindfulness with traditional exercise is an approach physical therapists can use to address these neuroplastic changes to help patients and clients with persistent symptoms deal with associated stress and anxiety.[45,52] Physical therapists routinely work on body and movement awareness, and the addition of mindful awareness may prove highly beneficial. Mindfulness can help a patient/client learn to separate the self from the illness and improve quality of life. Applications of mindful awareness include prevention of injury, rehabilitation, and increased tolerance of uncomfortable or painful medical treatments.

Mindfulness Defined

Mindfulness has been defined as "paying attention in a particular way: on purpose, in the present moment, and nonjudgementally."[39] Simply, it means paying full attention. Mindfulness has also been described as "…the non-judgmental observation of the ongoing stream of internal and external stimuli as they arise."[10] That is, recognizing that thoughts, perceptions, sensations, and emotions that enter one's awareness are observed, but are not judged in any way—not good or bad, not helpful or detrimental, and not important or unimportant. With distraction being a dominant condition of modern Western culture, mindfulness is a logical response. Mindfulness is one way to focus attention on the here and now, and this approach meets people where they are, viewing them as whole rather than broken. McManus describes seven qualities of mindful awareness based on the work of Kabat-Zinn.[40,45] These seven qualities include present moment awareness, fundamental kindness, nonjudging, acceptance, nonstriving, not knowing, and letting go. These are further described in Box 2.6.

BOX 2.6 Qualities of Mindful Awareness[45]

1. *Present Moment.* Mindfulness invites one to be in the moment and experience peace and well-being in the here and now.
2. *Fundamental Kindness.* Meeting oneself with kindness; being friendly toward ourselves.
3. *Nonjudging.* Judging experiences as good or bad results in triggers for automatic behaviors based on past experiences and can limit understanding of the self. Mindfulness allows one to be an impartial witness without those automatic behaviors.
4. *Acceptance.* Accepting one's thoughts, feelings, and actions just as they are.
5. *Nonstriving.* Efforts are directed at being fully aware of one's experience just as it is, without trying to force or change that experience.
6. *Not Knowing.* Mindfulness allows the temporary suspension of preconceived ideas, concepts, and expectations so that new learning can occur and life can be revealed rather than forced. It is meeting the world with a "beginner's mind."
7. *Letting Go.* Recognizing that life is change, mindfulness allows one to let go and be open to those changes.

Mindfulness Meditation

Mindfulness meditation is defined as "the deliberate training of the mind in present moment awareness" and generally results in increased compassion, understanding, inner peace, and well-being.[45] Mindfulness based stress reduction (MBSR) was first developed by Jon Kabat-Zinn in 1979 at the University of Massachusetts Medical Center and was originally housed in the Department of Physical Therapy there before moving to the College of Medicine.[45] The effects of MSBR and mindfulness meditation have been studied in persons with chronic pain, multiple sclerosis, depression and anxiety, cancer, and psoriasis and in high school, college, and elite athletes.

Research suggests that mindfulness meditation has a positive effect on attention regulation, body awareness, and emotional regulation.[36] MBSR programs promote acceptance without judgment to minimize anxiety and its effects on pain processing as well as encouraging movement and relaxation and translation of these skills to daily life.[35,52] Mindfulness meditation has been shown to have positive influence on immune response,[31] reduction in stress response,[30] reduction in serum cortisol levels, increased serum protein, and reduction in heart rate and blood pressure.[66] There is increasing evidence that mindfulness meditation can significantly attenuate the subjective experience of pain.[84] It has been suggested that mindfulness meditation–related pain relief may share a common final pathway with other cognitive techniques in pain modulation, with resultant reappraisal of faulty beliefs and restructuring of negative conditions.[84] MBSR has also been shown to decrease stress, anxiety, and depression associated with persistent pain, improve pain acceptance, and it shows promise in the treatment of central sensitization in those with chronic musculoskeletal disorders.[29,35,52,63]

Mindful Breathing

Mindful breathing is one method to integrate mindfulness in physical therapist interventions. Patients and clients often hold their breath when performing a painful movement or exercise that is very challenging. McManus advocates that every wellness program should include instruction in mindful breathing. She suggests that the practice of mindful breathing allows one to observe automatic mental, physical, and emotional reactions, which can play a role in symptom severity and distress.[45]

Mindful breathing involves observing the breath and breathing deeply during distress, and it can be taught as a part of mindfulness meditation (15 to 60 minutes) or as brief (5-minute) practices. One example of mindful breathing is found in Box 2.7. Further examples can be found in the McManus text,[45] or one can Google "mindful breathing exercises" for a host of examples. Other exercises in mindfulness meditation can be found by searching Google or YouTube. Numerous apps are also now available for use on mobile phones and tablets for the practice of mindfulness.

Mindful Eating

One often cited exercise to learn the skill of mindfulness, described by Kabat-Zinn, is the mindful eating exercise.[40] With this exercise, which lasts approximately 5 minutes or more, one practices mindful eating with a raisin. As with other mindfulness exercises, provide the instruction that when one finds the mind wandering from the task at hand, gently return one's attention to the raisin and what is being done with it. The raisin is first held in the hand and observed, examining the color and details of the raisin. One considers how the raisin came to be in one's hand, from its planting and growth, to its harvesting, and to its placement in the hand. It is moved in the hand, appreciating the texture, and it is smelled, noticing any response of the salivary glands or the stomach. It is placed in the mouth, with the sensation of that appreciated. It is then chewed, appreciating the sensation of that and both the texture and taste of the raisin and the body's response to it. Finally, the raisin is swallowed. The experience is then considered.

Developing and Implementing a Wellness Program

In general, there are several steps to follow when developing and implementing prevention, health, and wellness programs.[27,44] These steps are summarized in Box 2.8. The following case example illustrates the process.

BOX 2.7 Mindful Breathing Exercise (from McManus[45])

- Sit comfortably and avoid slouching. Sit so that your shoulders are aligned over your hips and both feet are on the floor. Close your eyes. Consider the quality of awareness you might bring to something in nature, such as how you might look at the ocean or mountains. This quality of awareness is open and nonjudging.
- Now bring this same quality of awareness to your inner landscape and observe your breathing. As you inhale, simply feel what part of your body moves. As you exhale, simply feel what part of your body moves as you exhale. Do not try to consciously change your breathing. Simply observe your breathing just as it is.
- You can experience the movement of your breathe in different places in your body. You might notice your belly move, your rib cage rising and falling, or your chest moving as you breathe. Each breath is unique. Simply experience the movement of your body as it occurs, moment to moment.

(Pause to allow participants to practice.)

- Now place one hand on your upper chest. Draw your stomach in slightly and breathe into your hand. Allow your breath to be of average size. You should feel your upper chest and rib cage rise and fall. Observe these sensations as they are. This is called upper chest or shallow breathing.

(Pause to allow for practice.)

- Observe how you feel.
- Now place your hand on your stomach at the level of your navel. As you inhale, imagine breathing into your hand. You should experience your stomach pushing forward into your hand as you breathe in. You may also feel your lower ribs flare out slightly. As you exhale, your stomach should gently fall. This is called diaphragmatic or abdominal breathing.

(Pause to allow for practice.)

- Observe how you feel.
- Now allow our breathing to return to whatever feels comfortable and natural for you. Simply observe your experience just as it is.

(Brief pause)

- Now, slightly round your shoulders and assume a slouched position. Notice how this affects your breathing.

(Pause to allow for practice.)

- Return to sitting upright and draw your shoulders blades back and down and your chest up slightly. This movement should be small and gentle. Notice how this movement affects your breathing.

(Pause to allow for practice.)

- Now, return to a comfortable position and breathing pattern that feels natural for you. Once again, observe your breath in and your breath out.

(Pause to allow for practice.)

- And now, gradually return your awareness to the room and let your eyes open.

BOX 2.8 Steps to Develop and Implement Prevention, Health, Wellness, and Fitness Programs

Step 1: Identify a Need

- Identify the intended audience
- Children
- Adults
- Older adults
- Industry/business
- School system
- Community
- Specific population (e.g., individuals with Parkinson's disease)

Step 2: Set Goals and Objectives

- Identify the purpose of the program
- Identify the goals to be achieved
  - Screening
  - Education
  - Exercise program
- Identify the objectives of the program

Step 3: Develop the Intervention

- Screenings: Identify valid and reliable right tools to use for the screening
- Education: Develop the program including handouts for participants
- Exercise: Develop the plan for each class
- Logistics
  - Secure a location for the program
  - Consider parking and access to the facility
  - Determine the time and length of the program
  - Determine the number of people who can attend based on the space
  - Identify who will do the program (self or with assistance)
  - Develop the presentation/program; include handouts for the participants
  - Develop a budget; determine costs and charge to the participants

Step 4: Implement the Intervention

- Recognize that even with the best of plans it is important to be adaptable and to be prepared for the unexpected

Step 5: Evaluate the Results

- For an educational session, ask the participants to evaluate the program; consider an additional follow-up assessment
- For an exercise class, record baseline data and assess progress during the program and at the end
- Ask participants to evaluate the exercise program
- Ask for feedback on what could be done to improve the program (e.g., different time, smaller class, longer sessions, etc.)

Case Example: Exercise and Osteoporosis

Step 1: Assessing the Need

- Gretchen, a physical therapist at ABC Hospital, completed an educational session for a local osteoporosis support group on the most recent research related to resistance training and weight-bearing exercise for increasing bone density.
- The women contacted Gretchen and asked her to develop a resistance training exercise class that included free weights and exercise equipment (as found in a fitness club).

NEED: An exercise class that educates women with osteoporosis about the safe way to perform resistance exercise.

Step 2: Set Goals and Objectives

Goal

Develop two education and exercise classes (level 1 and level 2) for women with osteoporosis that emphasize prevention of fractures and proper technique for resistance exercise and weight-bearing activities.

Objectives

1. Educate the participants on the effects of resistance training and weight-bearing exercise on bone health.
2. Educate the participants on the indications and contraindications of certain exercises for individuals with osteoporosis.
3. Educate the participants on the correct techniques for resistance exercise including free weights, resistance band and tubing, and exercise machines.
4. Have participants demonstrate the correct technique when performing resistance exercise.
5. Review implications related to posture and body mechanics during daily activities and during exercise.

Step 3: Develop the Intervention

Gretchen decided to develop two exercise classes: level 1 and level 2. To attend level 2 classes, participants had to complete the level 1 class. The level 1 exercise and education class consisted of four sessions as outlined in Table 2.4.

Gretchen decided to work collaboratively with the Occupational Therapy Department and together they conducted the final class, which emphasized the correct techniques for posture and body mechanics during daily activities. Once the number of classes and general content was decided, Gretchen started planning and developing the program.

- She reserved a medium-sized, open room in ABC hospital for 4 weeks and scheduled the class for Tuesday evenings from 6:00 p.m. to 8:30 p.m.
- She determined that the room be set up with tables and chairs in the front for lecture and discussion and with open space in the back for exercising. Classes would be limited to 20 people.
- She developed the content and objectives for each exercise/education session including handouts for participants. She put all developed material in a binder by week, including a presenter's checklist of what had to be brought to each class.
- She developed a brochure with times and location of the class and sent it to the osteoporosis support group. The cost of the level 1 exercise and education program was $25. Interested participants were to call and reserve a spot in the class.

TABLE 2.4 Sample: Level 1 Exercise and Educational Class Content for Osteoporosis

Session	Content/Plan
1	▪ Introduction ▪ Discussion about yearly height measurement ▪ Assessment of balance and flexibility of ankles, falls risk assessment ▪ Review and discussion of good posture ▪ Discussion on benefits of resistance training ▪ Perform exercises—shoulder blade retraction, chin tucks, sit to stand from a chair, pelvic tilt, heel/toe raises
2	▪ Brief review and questions related to material from first class ▪ Discussion on prevention of falls ▪ Discussion and demonstration of correct technique for performing strengthening exercises ▪ Perform exercises with resistance band: arms—bilateral horizontal abduction, rhomboids (band in doorway), leg press ▪ Perform exercises without band—standing hip abduction and step-ups
3	▪ Brief review and questions related to previous material ▪ Discussion of types of exercise to avoid (increase stress on vertebral bodies) ▪ Discussion and demonstration on how to lift weights correctly and how to determine starting weight ▪ Discussion on how to increase repetitions and weight during exercise ▪ Perform exercises with and without free weights—overhead press, seated fly, standing hip extension, prone bilateral scapular retraction, prone opposite arm and leg lift, lunges
4	▪ Review and questions over previous material ▪ Occupational therapy reviewed various adaptive equipment ▪ Demonstrated correct posture and body mechanics for brushing teeth, making bed, vacuuming ▪ Final questions ▪ Evaluation of program

Step 4: Implement the Program

The program had 10 participants and took place as scheduled for 4 weeks.

Step 5: Evaluate the Program

Participants were given a course evaluation sheet to complete regarding the location, time, content, and overall satisfaction with the program. In addition, Gretchen evaluated the participants' interest in the proposed level 2 class that would take place in a fitness center with equipment and consist of three sessions.

The overall evaluation of the program was positive, with a few individuals preferring a different day of the week or time of day for attendance. Altogether, 8 of the 10 participants were interested in participating in the level 2 class.

Additional Considerations for Developing Prevention, Health, and Wellness Programs

The following are additional points to consider:[43]

- The exercise or activity has to be specific to the goals of the individual. An individual training to run a marathon needs to run, not ride a bike. Specific principles and procedures for resistance training and aerobic exercise training can be found in Chapters 6 and 7, respectively.
- Consider asking the participants during the "assessing the need" component about what would motivate individuals to participate and then incorporate some of their suggestions.
- For children, the program should be fun and less structured but should take place for a specified period of time. The recommended amount of physical activity for children is 60 minutes (moderate and vigorous) every day.[76]
- For older adults, the program should start slowly to allow the participants to experience success. Consideration should be given to how the individuals can incorporate the various exercises or activities into their daily routines. The facility where the program is conducted should be well lit and easily accessible. The physical activity guidelines are the same for adults and older adults, 30 minutes a day of moderate intensity aerobic activity at least 5 days per week for a minimum of 10-minute bouts, unless they are unable because of chronic conditions. Older adults should also do exercises to maintain or improve balance to reduce fall risk.[77] Additional information on exercises in the older population in Chapter 24.
- If screenings are conducted, take-home materials with the results and with follow-up recommendations should be given to the participants.
- When making handouts for participants, keep in mind the audience. For children, make them colorful and fun. For older adults, make the print larger. Keep the language simple. Limit the amount of medical terminology used. Write information as clearly as possible.
- Include pictures of exercises whenever possible.
- Consider the time commitment for you and the participants and the cost involved.

Table 2.5 lists issues related to exercise adherence.

TABLE 2.5 Issues Affecting Exercise Adherence

Poor	Good
Poor or limited leadership	Effective leadership
Inconvenient class time or location	Part of regular routine or program
Injury	No injury
Boredom with exercise	Enjoyment—fun—variety
Poor individual commitment	Social support from group
Unaware of any progress being made	Regular updates on progress
Poor family support—disapproval	Family approval; positive reinforcement

Independent Learning Activities

Critical Thinking and Discussion

1. In the case example for developing an exercise program for women with osteoporosis, a second class (level 2) was proposed. Develop the level 2 class. Follow the steps outlined for developing and implementing this program including the content of each exercise session, use of fitness equipment for individuals with osteoporosis, and any handouts needed.
2. In this chapter, the differences in primary, secondary, and tertiary prevention were reviewed. For each of these categories, describe one screening program and one wellness program (exercise or education) that a physical therapist could provide.
3. One of the *Healthy People 2020* goals is to reduce the activity limitations (functional limitations) of individuals with chronic low back pain. Describe the limitations to

achieving this goal using one of the behavioral change theories. Identify strategies for obtaining this goal.

4. Using the five steps identified in this chapter, develop a prevention and wellness program for a group of fifth and sixth grade boys and girls (10 to 12 years of age) who have been identified as being at risk for type 2 diabetes because of obesity and sedentary lifestyle. Refer to Chapter 6 for special considerations when developing exercise programs for children.

REFERENCES

1. Adams, T, Bezner, J, and Steinhardt, M: Perceived wellness survey. Available at http://www.perceivedwellness.com/pws.pdf. Scoring instructions available at http://www.perceivedwellness.com/pws_scoring.htm. Accessed April 2016.
2. Adams, T, Bezner, J, and Steinhardt, M: The conceptualization and measurement of perceived wellness: integrating balance across and within dimensions. *Am J Health Promot* 11:208–218, 1997.
3. American College of Sports Medicine: *ACSM's Guidelines for Exercise Testing and Prescription*, ed. 8. Philadelphia: Lippincott Williams & Wilkins, 2010.
4. American Physical Therapy Association: *Guide to Physical Therapist Practice 3.0*. Available at http://guidetoptpractice.apta.org. Accessed March 2016.
5. American Physical Therapy Association: Physical fitness for special populations. Available at: http://www.apta.org/pfsp/. Accessed May 2016.
6. American Physical Therapy Association: Physical therapists' role in prevention, wellness, fitness, health promotion, and management of disease and disability. Available at http://www.apta.org/uploadedFiles/APTAorg/About_Us/Policies/Practice/ PTRoleAdvocacy.pdf#search=%22Role%20of%20Physical%20Therapists%20in%20Fitness%22. Accessed June 2016.
7. American Physical Therapy Association: Today's physical therapist: a comprehensive review of a 21st century health care profession. 2011. Available at http://www.apta.org/uploadedFiles/APTAorg/Practice_and_Patient_Care/PR_and_Marketing/Market_to_Professionals/TodaysPhysicalTherapist.pdf. Accessed May 2016.
8. American Physical Therapy Association: Vision statement for the physical therapy profession and guiding principles to achieve the vision. Available at http://www.apta.org/Vision/. Accessed March 2016.
9. American Public Health Association: Center for public policy issue brief. The prevention and public health fund: a critical investment in our nation's physical and fiscal health. Available at https://www.apha.org/~/media/files/pdf/topics/aca/apha_prevfundbrief_ june2012.ashx. Accessed March 2016.
10. Baer, RA: Mindfulness training as a clinical intervention: a conceptual and empirical review. *Clin Psychol Sci Prac* 10:125–143, 2003. Available at http://www.wisebrain.org/papers/MindfulnessPsyTx.pdf. Accessed May 2016.
11. Bandura, A: Self-efficacy: toward a unifying theory of behavioral change. *Psychol Rev* 84(2):191–215, 1977.
12. Bandura, A: *Social Foundations of Thought and Action*. Englewood Cliffs, NJ: Prentice Hall, 1986.
13. Bezner, JR: Promoting health and wellness: implications for physical therapist practice. *Phys Ther* 95(10):1433–1444, 2015. Available at http://dx.doi.org/ 10.2522/ptj.20140271. Accessed March 2016.
14. Brault, MW: Americans with disabilities: 2010 [brief]. Current populations report. Available at http://www.census.gov/prod/2012pubs/p70-131.pdf. Accessed May 2016.
15. Centers for Disease Control and Prevention: Chronic disease prevention and health promotion. Available at http://www.cdc.gov/chronicdisease/index.htm. Accessed June 2016.
16. Centers for Disease Control and Prevention: Health related quality of life. Available at http://www.cdc.gov/hrqol/index.htm. Accessed March 2016.
17. Centers for Disease Control and Prevention: Number of respondent-reported chronic conditions from 10 selected conditions among adults aged 18 and over, by selected characteristics: United States, selected years 2002–2013. Available at http://www.cdc.gov/nchs/hus/contents2014.htm#043. Accessed March 2016.
18. Centers for Disease Control and Prevention: Preventing chronic disease: eliminating the premature causes of death and disability in the US. Available at http://www.cdc.gov/chronicdisease/about/prevention.htm. Accessed March 2016.
19. Centers for Disease Control and Prevention: Well-being. Available at http://www.cdc.gov/hrqol/wellbeing.htm. Accessed March 2016.
20. Centers for Medicare and Medicaid Services: National health expenditures 2014 highlights. Available at https://www.cms.gov/Research-Statistics-Data-and-Systems/Statistics-Trends-and-Reports/NationalHealthExpendData/ Downloads/highlights.pdf. Accessed March 2016.
21. Chen, Y: Perceived barriers to physical activity among older adults residing in long-term care institutions. *J Clin Nurs* 19:432–439, 2010.
22. Chorba, RS, Chorba, DJ, Bouillon, LE, Overmyer, CA, Landis, JA: Use of a functional movement screening tool to determine injury risk in female collegiate athletes. *N Am J Sports Phys Ther* 5:47–54, 2010.
23. Church Health Center Wellness: The model for healthy living assessment wheel. Available at http://chreader.org/wp-content/uploads/2014/12/Model-for-Healthy-Living-Assessment-Wheel.pdf. Accessed April 2016.
24. Church Health Center Wellness: The model for healthy living. *Church Health Reader* Spring, 2013. Available at http://chreader.org/model-healthy-living/. Accessed April 2016.
25. Cook, G, Burton, L, and Hoogenboom, B: Pre-participation screening: the use of fundamental movements as an assessment of function - part 1. *N Am J Sports Phys Ther* 1:62–72, 2006.
26. Cook, G, Burton, L, and Hoogenboom, B: Pre-participation screening: the use of fundamental movements as an assessment of function - part 2. *N Am J Sports Phys Ther* 1:132–139, 2006.
27. Cottrell, RR, Girvan, JT, and McKenzie, JF. *Principles & Foundations of Health Promotion and Education*, ed. 5. Boston: Benjamin Cummings, 2012.
28. Cowen, VS: Functional fitness improvements after a worksite-based yoga initiative. *J Bodyw Mov Ther* 14:50–54, 2010. Available at http://dx.doi.org/10.1016/j.jbmt.2009.02.006.Accessed April 2016.
29. Cramer, H, Haller, H, Lauche, R, and Dobos, G: Mindfulness-based stress reduction for low back pain: a systematic review. *BMC Complement Altern Med.* 12:162, 2012.
30. Davidson, R, Abercrombie, J, Nitschke, JB, and Putnam, K: Regional brain function and disorders of emotion. *Curr Opin Neurobiol* 9(2): 228–234, 1999.
31. Davidson, RJ, et al: Alterations in brain and immune function produced by mindfulness meditations. *Psychosom Med* 65(4):564-570, 2003. doi: 10.1097/01.PSY.0000077505.67574.E3.
32. Dean, E: Physical therapy in the 21st century (part I): toward practice informed by epidemiology and the crisis of lifestyle conditions. *Physiother Theory Pract* 25:330–353, 2009.
33. Hays, L, et al: Exercise adoption among older, low-income women at risk for cardiovascular disease. *Public Health Nurs* 27:79–88, 2010.
34. Heron, M: Deaths: leading causes for 2013. *National Vital Statistics Reports* 65(2), 2008. Available at http://www.cdc.gov/nchs/data/nvsr/nvsr65/nvsr65_02.pdf. Accessed March 2016.
35. Hofmann, SG, Sawyer, AT, Witt, AA, and Oh, D: The effect of mindfulness-based therapy on anxiety and depression: a meta-analytic review. *J Consult Clin Psychol* 78:169, 2010.
36. Hozel, B, et al: How does mindfulness meditation work? Proposing mechanisms of action from a conceptual and neural perspective". *Perspect Psychol Sci*6(6): 537–559, 2011. doi: 10.1177/1745691611419671. PMID 26168376.
37. Institute of Medicine: For the public's health: investing in a healthier future. Available at http://www.nap.edu/download.php?record_id=13268#. Accessed March 2016.

38. Jewell, DV: The roles of fitness in physical therapy patient management: applications across the continuum of care. *Cardiopul Phys Ther J* 17: 47–62, 2006.
39. Kabat-Zinn, J: *Wherever You Go, There You Are: Mindfulness Meditation in Everyday Life.* New York: Hyperion, 1994.
40. Kabat-Zinn, J: *Full Catastrophe Living: Using the Wisdom of Your Body and Mind to Face Stress, Pain and Illness.* New York: Delacorte Press, 1990.
41. Kiesel, K, Plisky, P, and Butler, R: Functional movement test scores improve following a standardized off-season intervention program in professional football players. *Scand J Med Sci Sports* 21:287–292, 2011. doi: 10.1111/j.1600-0838.2009.01038.x.
42. Kosma, M, Cardinal, B, and Rintala, P: Motivating individuals with disabilities to be physically active. *Quest* 54:116–132, 2002.
43. McArdle, WD, Katch, FI, and Katch, VL: *Essentials of Exercise Physiology,* ed. 3. Philadelphia: Lippincott Williams & Wilkins, 2005.
44. McKenzie, J, Neiger, B, and Smelter, J: *Planning, Implementing, and Evaluating Health Promotion Programs,* ed. 4. San Francisco: Pearson Education, 2005.
45. McManus, CA: *Group Wellness Programs: For Chronic Pain and Disease Management.* Waltham, MA: Butterworth Heinmann, 2003.
46. National Center on Health, Physical Activity and Disability: Get the facts. Available at http://www.nchpad.org/Get~the~Facts/files/inc/b9f958ffcb.pdf. Accessed June 2016.
47. National Osteoporosis Foundation: Are you at risk? Available at http://nof.org/articles/2. Accessed April 2016.
48. National Wellness Institute: Six dimensions of wellness model. Available at http://c.ymcdn.com/sites/www.nationalwellness.org/resource/resmgr/docs/sixdimensionsfactsheet.pdf. Accessed April 2016.
49. National World Health Organization: International Classification of Functioning, Disability and Health (ICF). 2010. Available at http://www.who.int./classifications/icf/en/ index.html.Accessed June, 2016.
50. Norman, E, et al: An exercise and education group improves well-being of new mothers: a randomized controlled trial. *Phys Ther* 90:348–355, 2010.
51. O'Connor, FG, Deuster, PA, Davis, J, Pappas, CG, and Knapik JJ: Functional movement screening: predicting injuries in officer candidates. *Med Sci Sports Exerc* 43:2224–2230, 2011. doi: 10.1249/MSS.0b013e318223522d.
52. Pelletier, R, Higgins, J, and Bourbonnais, D: Addressing neuroplastic changes in distributed areas of the nervous system associated with chronic musculoskeletal disorders. *Phys Ther* 95(11):1582–1591, 2015. Available at http://dx.doi.org/10.2522/ptj.20140575. Accessed June 15, 2016.
53. Pope, A, and Tarlov, A (eds): *Institute of Medicine. Disability in America: Toward a National Agenda for Prevention.* Washington, DC: National Academy Press; 1991.
54. Prevention and Public Health Fund: Funding distributions. Available at http://www.hhs.gov/open/prevention/fy-2015-allocation-pphf-funds.html. Accessed April 2016.
55. Prochaska, JO, Johnson, S, and Lee P: The transtheoretical model of behavior change. In Shumaker, SA, Schron, EB, Ockene, JK, and McBee, WL (eds): *The Handbook of Health Behavior Change.* ed. 2. New York: Springer Publishing Company, 1998, pp 59–84.
56. Purdie, N, and McCrindle, A: Self-regulation, self-efficacy, and health behavior change in older adults. *Educ Gerontol* 28:379–400, 2002.
57. Reed, GR, Velicer, WF, Prochaska, JO, Rossi, JS, and Marcus, BH: What makes a good staging algorithm: Examples from regular exercise. *Am J Health Promot* 12(1):57–66, 1997.
58. Reichard, A, Stolzle, H, and Fox, MH: Health disparities among adults with physical disabilities or cognitive limitations compared to individuals with no disabilities in the United States. *Disabil Health J* April 4(2): 59–67, 2011. doi: 10.1016/j.dhjo.2010.05.003.
59. Rimer, BK, and Glanz, K: *Theory at a Glance: A Guide for Health Promotion Practice,* ed. 2 [NIH Pub. No. 05-3896]. Washington, DC: National Cancer Institute, 2005. Available at http://www.sneb.org/2014/Theory%20at%20a%20Glance.pdf. Accessed April 2016.
60. Rimmer, JH: Health promotion for people with disabilities: the emerging paradigm shifts from disability prevention to prevention of secondary conditions. *Phys Ther* 79:495–502, 1999.
61. Rimmer, JH, Chen, M-D, and Hsieh, K: A conceptual model for identifying, preventing, and managing secondary conditions in people with disabilities. *Phys Ther* 91:1728–1739, 2011.
62. Rimmer, JH: Developmental disability and fitness. National Center for Health, Physical Activity and Disability. Available at http://www.nchpad.org/104/800/Developmental~ Disability~and~Fitness. Accessed June 2016.
63. Santarnecchi, E, D'Arista, S, Egiziano, E, et al: Interaction between neuroanatomical and psychological changes after mindfulness-based training. *PloS One.* 9:e108359, 2014.
64. Self Determination Theory: An approach to human motivation and personality. Available at http://selfdeterminationtheory.org/about-the-theory/. Accessed April 2016.
65. Shephard, R: PAR-Q, Canadian home fitness test, and exercise screening alternatives. *Sports Med* 5:185–195, 1988.
66. Sudsuang, R, Chentanez V, and Veluvan, K: Effect of Buddhist meditation on serum cortisol and total protein level, blood pressure, pulse rate, lung volume and reaction time. *Physiol Behav* 50(3):543–548, 1991.
67. Thompson, C: *Prevention Practice and Health Promotion: A Health Care Professional's Guide to Health, Fitness, and Wellness,* ed. 2. Thorofare, NJ: Slack, Inc., 2015.
68. Trust for America's Health: Prevention for a healthier America: investments in disease prevention yield significant savings, stronger communities. Washington, DC. Available at http://healthyamericans.org/reports/prevention08/Prevention08.pdf. Accessed March 2016.
69. Trust for America's Health: The state of obesity 2015. Available at http://healthyamericans.org/reports/stateofobesity2015/. Accessed March 2016.
70. US Department of Health and Human Services: *Healthy People 2010.* Washington, DC: U.S. Government Printing Office, 2000. Originally developed for Ratzan, SC, and Parker, RM: Introduction. In Selden, CR, Zorn, M, Ratzan, SC, and Parker RM (eds): *National Library of Medicine Current Bibliographies in Medicine: Health Literacy.* NLM Pub. No. CBM 2000-1. Bethesda, MD: National Institutes of Health, US Department of Health and Human Services, 2000. Available at http://health.gov/communication/literacy/ quickguide/factsbasic.htm#one. Accessed February 2016.
71. US Department of Health and Human Services and US Department of Agriculture: *2015-2020 Dietary Guidelines for Americans,* ed. 8. 2015. Available at http://health.gov/dietaryguidelines/2015/guidelines/. Accessed June 2016.
72. US Department of Health and Human Services, Office of Disease Prevention and Health Promotion: History and development of healthy people. Available at https://www.healthypeople.gov/2020/about/History-and-Development-of-Healthy-People. Accessed April 2016.
73. US Department of Health and Human Services, Office of Disease Prevention and Health Promotion: Healthy People 2020 framework. Available at https://www.healthypeople.gov/sites/default/files/HP2020Framework.pdf. Accessed April 2016.
74. US Department of Health and Human Services, Office of Disease Prevention and Health Promotion: Healthy People 2020 leading health indicators. Available at https://www.healthypeople.gov/2020/Leading-Health-Indicators. Accessed April 2016.
75. US Department of Health and Human Services, Office of Disease Prevention and Health Promotion: *Healthy People 2020* leading health indicators: progress update. Available at https://www.healthypeople.gov/sites/default/files/LHI-ProgressReport-ExecSum_0.pdf. Accessed April 2016.
76. US Department of Health and Human Services, Office of Disease Prevention and Health Promotion: Physical activity guidelines. Available at http://health.gov/paguidelines/guidelines/chapter3.aspx. Accessed April 2016.
77. US Department of Health and Human Services, Office of Disease Prevention and Health Promotion: Physical activity guidelines. Available at http://health.gov/paguidelines/guidelines/older-adults.aspx. Accessed April 2016.
78. US Department of Health and Human Services, Office of Disease Prevention and Health Promotion: Physical activity guidelines. Available at http://health.gov/paguidelines/pdf/paguide.pdf. Accessed April 2016.

79. US Department of Health and Human Services, Office of Disease Prevention and Health Promotion: *Healthy People 2020*. Available at https://www.healthypeople.gov/2020/topics-objectives/topic/disability-and-health#4. Accessed June 2016.
80. Wilson, R, et al: Literacy, knowledge, self-efficacy, and health beliefs about exercise and obesity in urban low-income African American women. *JOCEPS* 53:7–13, 2008.
81. World Health Organization: Better health for people with disabilities infographic. Available at http://www.who.int/disabilities/facts/Infographic_en_pdf.pdf?ua=1. Accessed June 2016.
82. World Health Organization: Disability and health. Fact Sheet No. 352. Available at http://www.who.int/mediacentre/factsheets/fs352/en/. Accessed June 2016.
83. World Health Organization: Non-communicable diseases country profiles 2014. Available at http://apps.who.int/iris/bitstream/10665/128038/1/ 9789241507509_eng.pdf?ua=1. Accessed March 2016.
84. World Health Organization: Preamble to the constitution of the World Health Organization as adopted by the International Health Conference, New York, 19-22 June, 1946. Available at http://www.who.int/about/definition/en/print.html. Accessed February 2016.
85. Zeidan, F, Grant, JA, Brown, CA, McHaffie, JG, and Coghill, RC: Mindfulness meditation-related pain relief: evidence for unique brain mechanisms in the regulation of pain. *Neurosci Lett* 520:165–173, 2012.

CHAPTER 3

Range of Motion

CAROLYN KISNER, PT, MS

Range of motion is a basic technique used for the examination of movement and for initiating movement into a program of therapeutic intervention. Movement that is necessary to accomplish functional activities can be viewed, in its simplest form, as muscles or external forces moving bones in various patterns or ranges of motions. When a person moves, the intricate control of the muscle activity that causes or controls the motion comes from the central nervous system. Bones move with respect to each other at the connecting joints. The structure of the joints, as well as the integrity and flexibility of the soft tissues that pass over the joints, affects the amount of motion that can occur between any two bones. The full motion possible is called the **range of motion** (ROM). When moving a segment through its ROM, all structures in the region are affected: muscles, joint surfaces, synovial fluid, joint capsules, ligaments, fasciae, vessels, and nerves. ROM activities are most easily described in terms of joint range and muscle range. To describe joint range, terms such as flexion, extension, abduction, adduction, and rotation are used. Ranges of available joint motion are usually measured with a goniometer and recorded in degrees.[21] Muscle range is related to the functional excursion of muscles.

Functional excursion is the distance that a muscle is capable of shortening after it has been elongated to its maximum.[13] In some cases the functional excursion, or range of a muscle, is directly influenced by the joint it crosses. For example, the range for the brachialis muscle is limited by the range available at the elbow joint. This is true of one-joint muscles (muscles with their proximal and distal attachments on the bones on either side of one joint). For two-joint or multijoint muscles (those muscles that cross over two or more joints), their range goes beyond the limits of any one joint they cross. An example of a two-joint muscle functioning at the hip and knee is the hamstring muscle group. If it contracts and moves the knee into flexion while simultaneously moving the hip into extension, it shortens to a point known as *active insufficiency,* where it is too short to produce much tension. This is one end of its range. When it is fully lengthened and limits motion at one of the joints it crosses, it is known as *passive insufficiency.* This occurs in the hamstring muscle when the knee is extended and full range of hip flexion is limited (or conversely, when the hip is flexed full range and knee extension is limited). Two-joint or multijoint muscles normally function in the midportion of their functional excursion where ideal length-tension relations exist.[13]

To maintain normal ROM, the segments must be moved through their available ranges periodically, whether it is the available joint range or muscle range. It is recognized that many factors, such as systemic, joint, neurological, or muscular diseases; surgical or traumatic insults; or simply inactivity or immobilization for any reason, can lead to decreased ROM. Therapeutically, ROM activities are administered to maintain joint and soft tissue mobility to minimize loss of tissue flexibility and contracture formation.[7] Extensive research by Robert Salter has provided evidence of the benefits of movement on the healing of tissues in various pathological conditions in both the laboratory and clinical settings.[28-34]

The principles of ROM described in this chapter do not encompass stretching to increase range. Principles and techniques of stretching and joint manipulation for treating impaired mobility are described in Chapters 4 and 5.

Types of ROM Exercises

Passive ROM. Passive ROM (PROM) is movement of a segment within the unrestricted ROM that is produced entirely by an *external force;* there is little to no voluntary muscle contraction. The external force may be from gravity, a machine, another individual, or another part of the individual's own body.[9] PROM and passive stretching are not synonymous. (See Chapter 4 for definitions and descriptions of passive stretching.)

Active ROM. Active ROM (AROM) is movement of a segment within the unrestricted ROM that is produced by active contraction of the *muscles* crossing that joint.

Active-assistive ROM. Active-assistive ROM (A-AROM) is a type of AROM in which assistance is provided manually or mechanically by an outside force because the prime mover muscles need assistance to complete the motion.

Indications, Goals, and Limitations of ROM

Passive ROM

Indications for PROM

- In the region where there is acute, inflamed tissue, passive motion is beneficial; active motion would be detrimental to the healing process. Inflammation after injury or surgery usually lasts 2 to 6 days.
- When a patient is not able to or not supposed to actively move a segment(s) of the body, as when comatose, paralyzed, or on complete bed rest, movement is provided by an external source.
- PROM is indicated after surgical repair of contractile tissue when active motion would compromise the repaired muscle.

Goals for PROM

The primary goal for PROM is to decrease the complications that would occur with immobilization, such as cartilage degeneration, adhesion and contracture formation, and sluggish circulation.[9,27,33] Specifically, the goals are to:

- Maintain joint and connective tissue mobility.
- Minimize the effects of the formation of contractures.
- Maintain mechanical elasticity of muscle.
- Assist circulation and vascular dynamics.
- Enhance synovial movement for cartilage nutrition and diffusion of materials in the joint.
- Decrease or inhibit pain.
- Assist with the healing process after injury or surgery.
- Help maintain the patient's awareness of movement.

Other Uses for PROM

- When a therapist is examining inert structures, PROM is used to determine limitations of motion, joint stability, muscle flexibility, and other soft tissue elasticity.
- When a therapist is teaching an active exercise program, PROM is used to demonstrate the desired motion.
- When a therapist is preparing a patient for stretching, PROM is often used preceding the passive stretching techniques.

Limitations of Passive Motion

True passive, relaxed ROM may be difficult to obtain when muscle is innervated and the patient is conscious. Passive motion *does not:*

- Prevent muscle atrophy
- Increase strength or endurance
- Assist circulation to the extent that active, voluntary muscle contraction does

Active and Active-Assistive ROM

Indications for AROM

- When a patient is able to contract the muscles actively and move a segment with or without assistance, AROM is used.
- When a patient has weak musculature and is unable to move a joint through the desired range (usually against gravity), A-AROM is used to provide enough assistance to the muscles in a carefully controlled manner so the muscle can function at its maximum level and be progressively strengthened. Once patients gain control of their ROM, they are progressed to manual or mechanical resistance exercises to improve muscle performance for a return to functional activities (see Chapter 6).
- When a segment of the body is immobilized for a period of time, AROM is used on the regions above and below the immobilized segment to maintain the areas in as normal a condition as possible and to prepare for new activities such as walking with crutches.
- AROM can be used for aerobic conditioning programs (see Chapter 7) and is used to relieve stress from sustained postures (see Chapter 14).

Goals for AROM

If there is no inflammation or contraindication to active motion, the same goals of PROM can be met with AROM. In addition, there are physiological benefits that result from active muscle contraction and motor learning from voluntary muscle control. Specific goals are to:

- Maintain physiological elasticity and contractility of the participating muscles.
- Provide sensory feedback from the contracting muscles.
- Provide a stimulus for bone and joint tissue integrity.
- Increase circulation and prevent thrombus formation.
- Develop coordination and motor skills for functional activities.

Limitations of Active ROM

For strong muscles, AROM *does not* maintain or increase strength. It also *does not* develop skill or coordination except in the movement patterns used.

Precautions and Contraindications to ROM Exercises

Although both PROM and AROM are contraindicated under any circumstance when motion to a part is disruptive to the healing process (Box 3.1), complete immobility leads to adhesion and contracture formation, sluggish circulation, and a prolonged recovery time. In light of research by Salter[30] and others,[18] early, continuous PROM within a pain-free range has been shown to be beneficial to the healing and early recovery of many soft tissue and joint lesions (discussed later in the chapter). Historically, ROM has been contraindicated immediately after acute tears, fractures, and surgery, but because the benefits of controlled motion have demonstrated decreased pain and an increased rate of recovery, early controlled motion is used as long as the patient's tolerance is monitored.

It is imperative that the therapist recognizes the value as well as potential abuse of motion and stays within the range, speed, and tolerance of the patient during the acute recovery stage.[9] Additional trauma to the part is contraindicated. Signs of too much or the wrong motion include increased pain and increased inflammation (greater swelling, heat, and redness). See Chapter 10 for principles of when to use the various types of passive and active motion therapeutically.

Usually, AROM of the upper extremities and limited walking near the bed are tolerated as early exercises after myocardial infarction, coronary artery bypass surgery, and percutaneous transluminal coronary angioplasty. Careful monitoring of symptoms, perceived exertion, and blood pressure is necessary.[8,24] If the patient's response or the condition is life-threatening, PROM may be carefully initiated to the major joints along with some AROM to the ankles and feet to avoid venous stasis and thrombus formation. Individualized activities are initiated and progress gradually based on the patient's tolerance.[8,24]

Early mobility for patients on mechanical ventilation (initiated 1 to 2 days after intubation in one study[25] or less than 3 days in another study[35]) that includes sedative interruption followed by AROM, with progression to the activities of daily living (ADLs) of sitting, standing, and walking has been shown to improve patient status when compared with standard care as measured by duration of delirium, ventilator-free days, and functional outcome at hospital discharge.

BOX 3.1 Summary of Precautions and Contraindications to ROM Exercises

ROM should not be done when motion is disruptive to the healing process.

- Carefully controlled motion within the limits of pain-free motion during early phases of healing has been shown to benefit healing and early recovery.
- Signs of too much or the wrong motion include increased pain and inflammation.
- ROM should not be done when patient response or the condition is life-threatening.
- PROM may be carefully initiated to major joints and AROM to ankles and feet to minimize venous stasis and thrombus formation.
- After myocardial infarction, coronary artery bypass surgery, or percutaneous transluminal coronary angioplasty, AROM of upper extremities and limited walking are usually tolerated under careful monitoring of symptoms.
- Sedative interruption followed by AROM with progression to sitting, standing, and walking may be initiated early on mechanically ventilated patients

Note: ROM is not synonymous with stretching. For precautions and contraindications to passive and active stretching techniques, see Chapters 4 and 5.

Principles and Procedures for Applying ROM Techniques

Examination, Evaluation, and Treatment Planning

1. Examine and evaluate the patient's impairments and level of function, determine any precautions and their prognosis, and plan the intervention.
2. Determine the ability of the patient to participate in the ROM activity and whether PROM, A-AROM, or AROM can meet the immediate goals.
3. Determine the amount of motion that can be applied safely for the condition of the tissues and health of the individual.
4. Decide what patterns can best meet the goals. ROM techniques may be performed in the:
   a. *Anatomic planes of motion:* frontal, sagittal, and transverse
   b. *Muscle range of elongation:* antagonistic to the line of pull of the muscle
   c. *Combined patterns:* diagonal motions or movements that incorporate several planes of motion
   d. *Functional patterns:* motions used in ADLs
5. Monitor the patient's general condition and responses during and after the examination and intervention; note any change in vital signs; in the warmth and color of the segment; and in the ROM, pain, or quality of movement.
6. Document and communicate findings and intervention.
7. Re-evaluate and modify the intervention as necessary.

Patient Preparation

1. Communicate with the patient. Describe the plan and method of intervention to meet the goals.
2. Free the region from restrictive clothing, linen, splints, and dressings. Drape the patient as necessary.
3. Position the patient in a comfortable position with proper body alignment and stabilization but that also allows you to move the segment through the available ROM.
4. Position yourself so proper body mechanics can be used.

Application of Techniques

1. To control movement, grasp the extremity around the joints. If the joints are painful, modify the grip, still providing support necessary for control.
2. Support areas of poor structural integrity, such as a hypermobile joint, recent fracture site, or paralyzed limb segment.
3. Move the segment through its complete pain-free range to the point of tissue resistance. Do not force beyond the available range. If you force motion, it becomes a stretching technique.
4. Perform the motions smoothly and rhythmically, with 5 to 10 repetitions. The number of repetitions depends on the objectives of the program and the patient's condition and response to the treatment.

Application of PROM

1. During PROM, the force for movement is external; it is provided by a therapist or mechanical device. When appropriate, a patient may provide the force and be taught to move the part with a normal extremity.
2. No active resistance or assistance is given by the patient's muscles that cross the joint. If the muscles contract, it becomes an active exercise.
3. The motion is carried out within the free ROM—that is, the range that is available without forced motion or pain.

Application of AROM

1. Demonstrate the motion desired using PROM; then ask the patient to perform the motion. Have your hands in position to assist or guide the patient if needed.
2. Provide assistance only as needed for smooth motion. When there is weakness, assistance may be required only at the beginning or the end of the ROM or when the effect of gravity has the greatest moment arm (torque).
3. The motion is performed within the available ROM.

ROM Techniques VIDEO 3.1

The descriptions of positions and ROM techniques in this section may be used for PROM as well as A-AROM and AROM. When making the transition from PROM to AROM, gravity has a significant impact, especially in individuals with weak musculature. When the segment moves up against gravity, it may be necessary to provide assistance to the patient. However, when moving parallel to the ground (gravity eliminated or gravity neutral), the part may need only to be supported while the muscles take the part through the range. When the part moves downward, with gravity causing the motion, muscles antagonist to the motion become active and may need assistance in controlling the descent of the part. The therapist must be aware of these effects and modify the patient's position if needed to meet desired goals for A-AROM and AROM. Principles and techniques for progression to manual and mechanical resistance ROM to develop strength are described in Chapter 6.

CLINICAL TIP

- When transitioning from PROM to AROM, vary patient position to use gravity to either assist or resist the motion.
- Functional activities that are antigravity will require assistance when the muscle test grades are less than 3/5.

The following descriptions are, for the most part, with the patient in the supine position. Alternate positions for many motions are possible and, for some motions, necessary. For efficiency, perform all motions possible in one position; then change the patient's position and perform all appropriate motions in that position, progressing the treatment with minimal turning of the patient. Individual body types or environmental limitations might necessitate variations of the suggested hand placements. Use of good body mechanics by the therapist while applying proper stabilization and motion to the patient to accomplish the goals and avoid injury to weakened structures is the primary consideration.

NOTE: The term *upper hand,* or *top hand,* means the hand of the therapist that is toward the patient's head; the *bottom hand,* or *lower hand,* refers to the hand toward the patient's foot. Antagonistic ROMs are grouped together for ease of application.

Upper Extremity

Shoulder: Flexion and Extension (Fig. 3.1)

VIDEO 3.2

Hand Placement and Procedure

- Grasp the patient's arm under the elbow with your lower hand.
- With the top hand, cross over and grasp the wrist and palm of the patient's hand.
- Lift the arm through the available range and return.

NOTE: For normal motion, the scapula should be free to rotate upward as the shoulder flexes. If motion of only the glenohumeral joint is desired, the scapula is stabilized as described in the chapter on stretching (see Chapter 4).

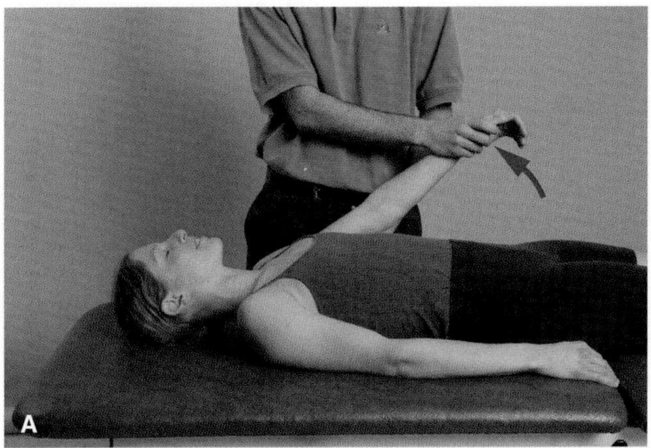

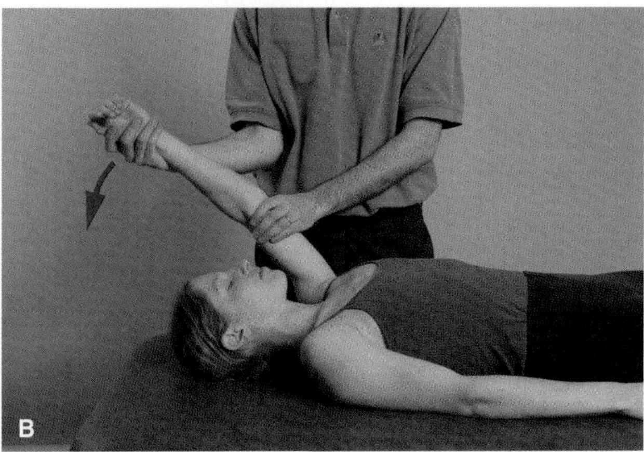

FIGURE 3.1 Hand placement and positions for **(A)** initiating and **(B)** completing shoulder flexion.

Shoulder: Extension (Hyperextension) (Fig. 3.2)

To obtain extension past zero, position the patient's shoulder at the edge of the bed when supine or position the patient side-lying, prone, or sitting.

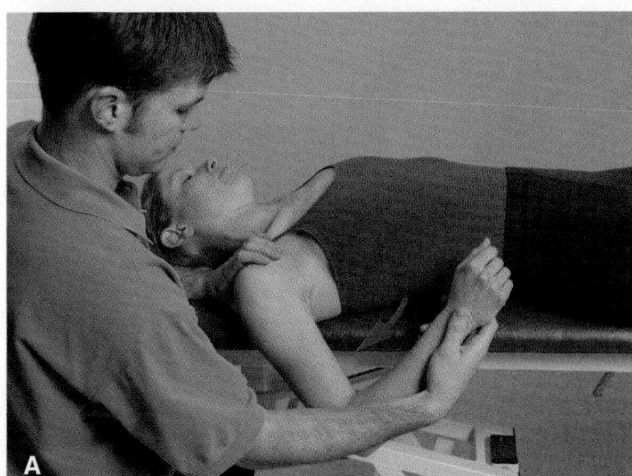

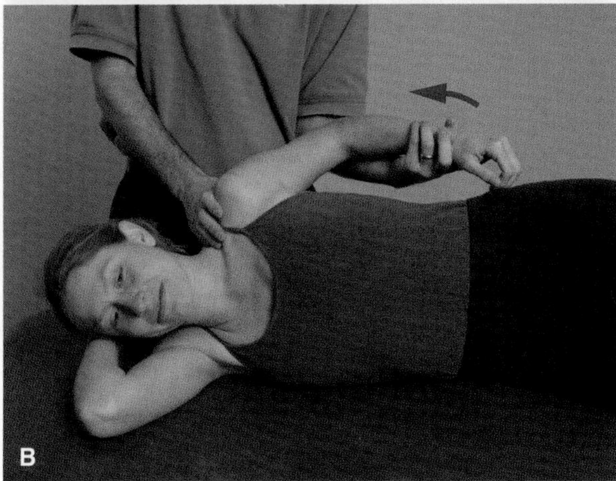

FIGURE 3.2 Hyperextension of the shoulder **(A)** with the patient at the edge of the bed and **(B)** with the patient side-lying.

Shoulder: Abduction and Adduction (Fig. 3.3)

Hand Placement and Procedure

Use the same hand placement as with flexion, but move the arm out to the side. The elbow may be flexed for ease in completing the arc of motion.

NOTE: To reach full range of abduction, there must be external rotation of the humerus and upward rotation of the scapula.

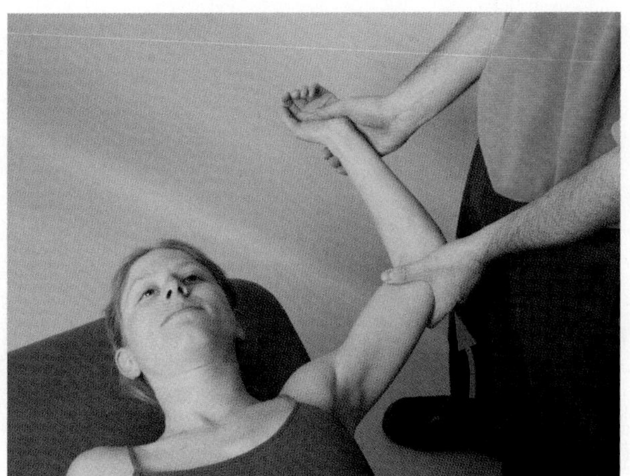

FIGURE 3.3 Abduction of the shoulder with the elbow flexed.

Shoulder: Internal (Medial) and External (Lateral) Rotation (Fig. 3.4)

If possible, the arm is abducted to 90°, the elbow is flexed to 90°, and the forearm is held in neutral position. Rotation may also be performed with the patient's arm at the side of the thorax, but full internal rotation is not possible in this position.

Hand Placement and Procedure

- Grasp the hand and the wrist with your index finger between the patient's thumb and index finger.
- Place your thumb and the rest of your fingers on either side of the patient's wrist, thereby stabilizing the wrist.

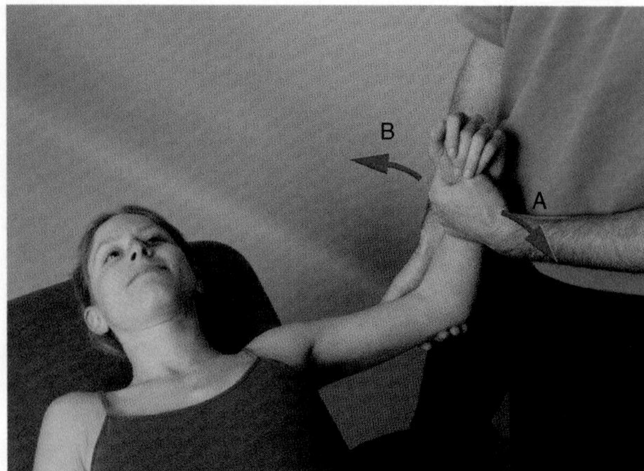

FIGURE 3.4 The 90/90 position for initiating **(A)** internal and **(B)** external rotation of the shoulder.

- With the other hand, stabilize the elbow.
- Rotate the humerus by moving the forearm like a spoke on a wheel.

Shoulder: Horizontal Abduction (Extension) and Adduction (Flexion) (Fig. 3.5)

To reach full horizontal abduction, position the patient's shoulder at the edge of the table. Begin with the arm either adducted or abducted 90°.

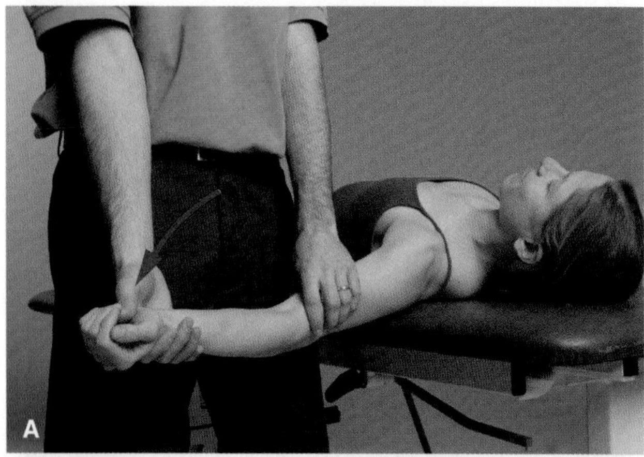

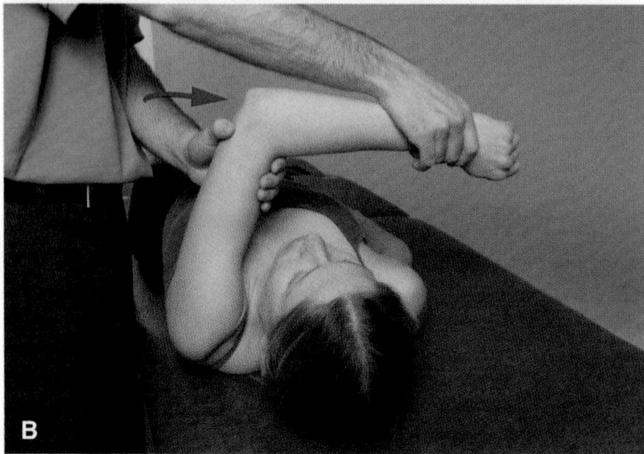

FIGURE 3.5 Horizontal **(A)** abduction and **(B)** adduction of the shoulder.

Hand Placement and Procedure

Hand placement is the same as with flexion, but turn your body and face the patient's head as you move the patient's arm out to the side and then across the body.

Scapula: Elevation/Depression, Protraction/Retraction, and Upward/Downward Rotation (Fig. 3.6)

Position the patient prone with his or her arm at the side (Fig. 3.6A) or side-lying facing toward you with the patient's arm draped over your bottom arm (Fig. 3.6B).

Hand Placement and Procedure

- Cup the top hand over the acromion process and place the other hand around the inferior angle of the scapula.
- For elevation, depression, protraction, and retraction, the clavicle also moves as the scapular motions are directed at the acromion process.
- For rotation, direct the scapular motions at the inferior angle of the scapula while simultaneously pushing the acromion in the opposite direction to create a force couple turning effect.

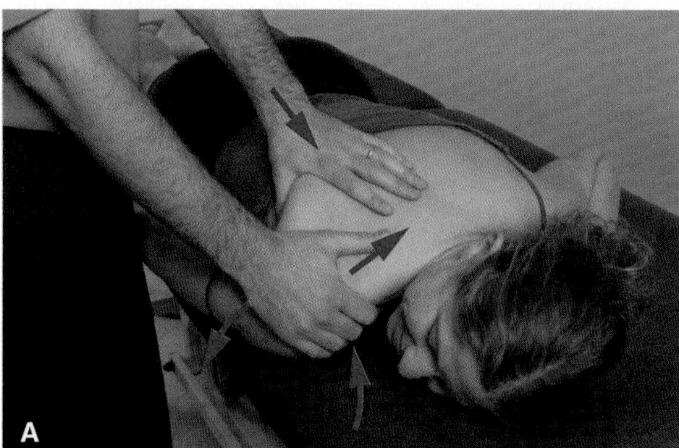

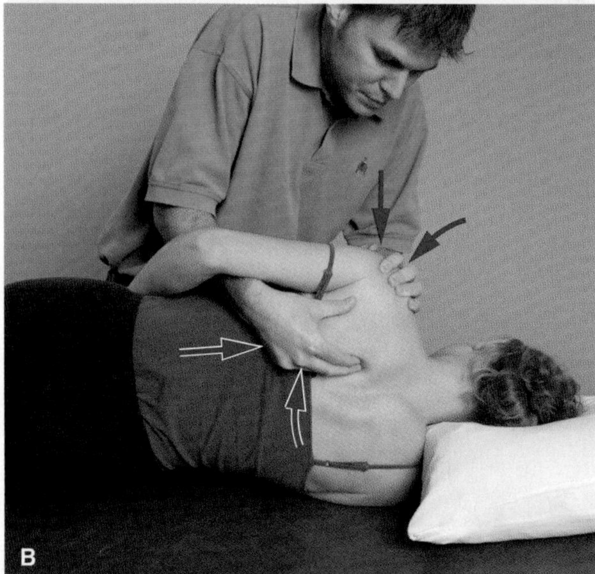

FIGURE 3.6 ROM of the scapula with the patient **(A)** prone and with the patient **(B)** side-lying.

Elbow: Flexion and Extension (Fig. 3.7)

VIDEO 3.3

Hand Placement and Procedure

- Grasp the distal forearm and support the wrist with one hand. This hand also controls forearm supination and pronation.
- With the other hand, support the elbow.
- Flex and extend the elbow with the forearm supinated and also with the forearm pronated.

NOTE: The scapula should not tip forward when the elbow extends, as it disguises the true range.

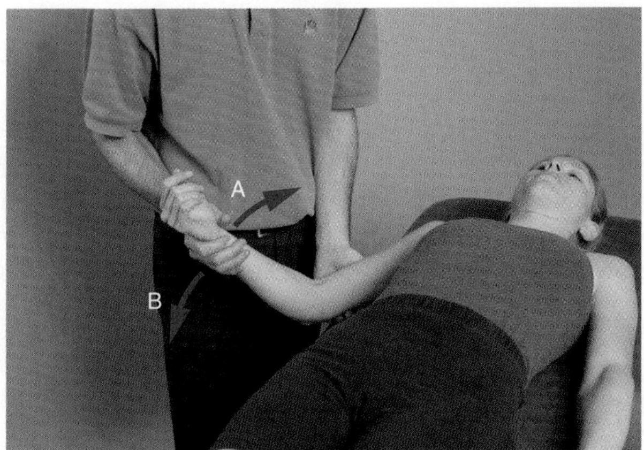

FIGURE 3.7 Elbow **(A)** flexion and **(B)** extension with the forearm supinated.

Elongation of Two-Joint Biceps Brachii Muscle

To extend the shoulder beyond zero, position the patient's shoulder at the edge of the table when supine or position the patient prone lying, sitting, or standing.

Hand Placement and Procedure

- First, pronate the patient's forearm by grasping the wrist and extend the elbow while supporting it.
- Then, extend (hyperextend) the shoulder to the point of tissue resistance in the anterior arm region. At this point, full available lengthening of the two-joint muscle is reached.

Elongation of Two-Joint Long Head of the Triceps Brachii Muscle (Fig. 3.8)

When the near-normal range of the triceps brachii muscle is available, the patient must be sitting or standing to reach the full ROM. With marked limitation in muscle range, ROM can be performed in the supine position.

Hand Placement and Procedure

- First, fully flex the patient's elbow with one hand on the distal forearm.
- Then, flex the shoulder by lifting up on the humerus with the other hand under the elbow.
- Full available range is reached when discomfort is experienced in the posterior arm region.

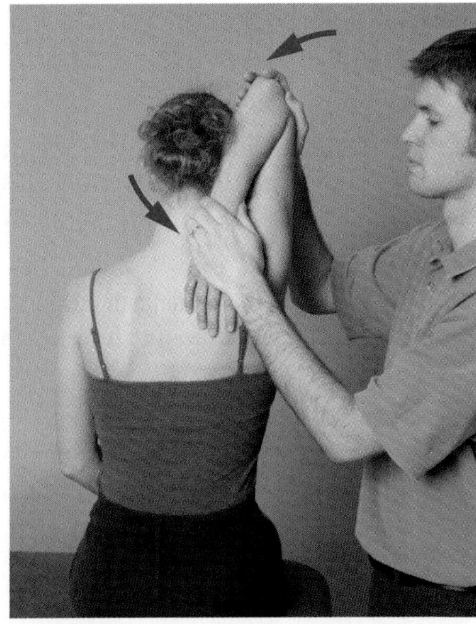

FIGURE 3.8 End ROM for the long head of the triceps brachii muscle.

Forearm: Pronation and Supination (Fig. 3.9)

Hand Placement and Procedure

Perform pronation and supination with the elbow flexed as well as extended. When the elbow is extended, prevent the shoulder from rotating by stabilizing the elbow.

- Grasp the patient's wrist, supporting the hand with the index finger and placing the thumb and the rest of the fingers on either side of the distal forearm.
- Stabilize the elbow with the other hand.
- The motion is a rolling of the radius around the ulna at the distal radius.

Alternate Hand Placement

Sandwich the patient's distal forearm between the palms of both hands.

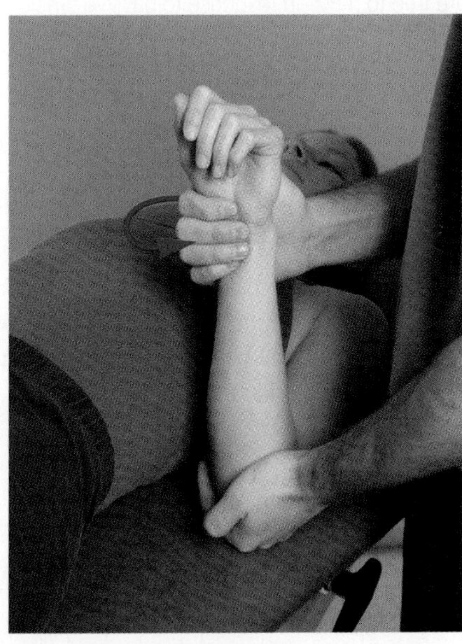

FIGURE 3.9 Pronation of the forearm.

PRECAUTION: Do not stress the wrist by twisting the hand; control the pronation and supination motion by moving the radius around the ulna.

Wrist: Flexion (Palmar Flexion) and Extension (Dorsiflexion); Radial (Abduction) and Ulnar (Adduction) Deviation (Fig. 3.10) VIDEO 3.4

Hand Placement and Procedure

For all wrist motions, grasp the patient's hand just distal to the joint with one hand and stabilize the forearm with your other hand.

NOTE: The range of the extrinsic muscles to the fingers affects the range at the wrist if tension is placed on the tendons as they cross into the fingers. To obtain full range of the wrist joint, allow the fingers to move freely as you move the wrist.

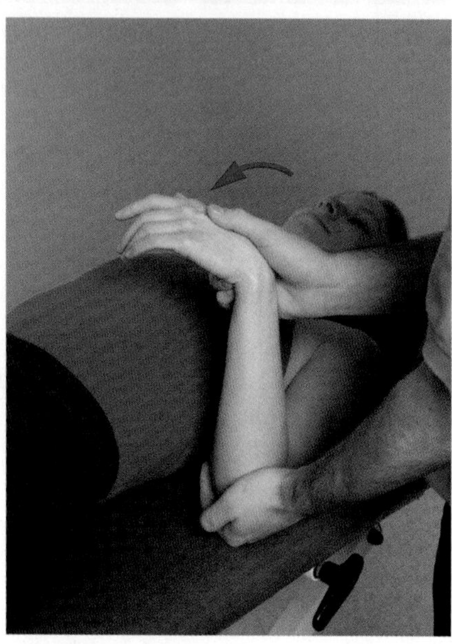

FIGURE 3.10 ROM at the wrist. Shown is wrist flexion; note that the fingers are free to move in response to passive tension in the extrinsic tendons.

Hand: Cupping and Flattening the Arch of the Hand at the Carpometacarpal and Intermetacarpal Joints (Fig. 3.11)

Hand Placement and Procedure

- Face the patient's hand; place the fingers of both of your hands in the palms of the patient's hand and your thenar eminences on the posterior aspect.
- Roll the metacarpals palmarward to increase the arch and dorsalward to flatten it.

Alternate Hand Placement

One hand is placed on the posterior aspect of the patient's hand with the fingers and thumb cupping the metacarpals.

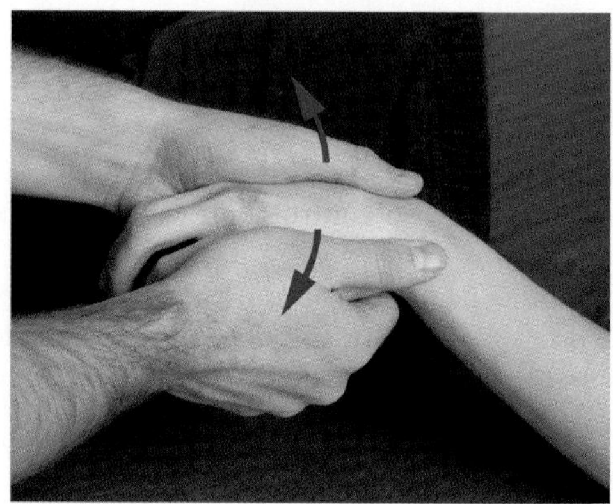

FIGURE 3.11 ROM to the arch of the hand.

NOTE: Extension and abduction of the thumb at the carpometacarpal joint are important for maintaining the web space for functional movement of the hand. Isolated flexion-extension and abduction-adduction ROM of this joint should be performed by moving the first metacarpal while stabilizing the trapezium.

Joints of the Thumb and Fingers: Flexion and Extension and Abduction and Adduction (Fig. 3.12) VIDEO 3.5

The joints of the thumbs and fingers include the metacarpophalangeal and interphalangeal joints.

Hand Placement and Procedure

- Depending on the position of the patient, stabilize the forearm and hand on the bed or table or against your body.

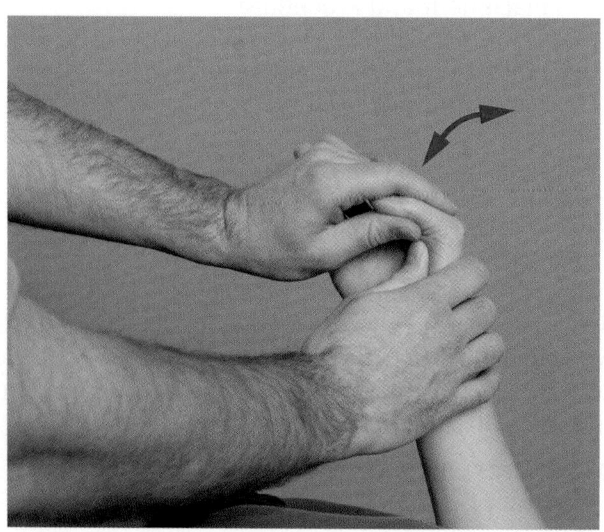

FIGURE 3.12 ROM to the metacarpophalangeal joint of the thumb.

- Move each joint of the patient's hand individually by stabilizing the proximal bone with the index finger and thumb of one hand and moving the distal bone with the index finger and thumb of the other hand.

Alternate Procedure

Several joints can be moved simultaneously if proper stabilization is provided. Example: To move all the metacarpophalangeal joints of digits 2 through 5, stabilize the metacarpals with one hand and move all the proximal phalanges with the other hand.

NOTE: To accomplish full joint ROM, do not place tension on the extrinsic muscles going to the fingers. Tension on the muscles can be relieved by altering the wrist position as the fingers are moved.

Elongation of Extrinsic Muscles of the Wrist and Hand: Flexor and Extensor Digitorum Muscles (Fig. 3.13)

General Technique

Hand Placement and Procedure

- First, move the distal interphalangeal joint and stabilize it; then move the proximal interphalangeal joint.
- Hold both these joints at the end of their range; then move the metacarpophalangeal joint to the end of the available range.
- Stabilize all the finger joints and begin to extend the wrist. When the patient feels discomfort in the forearm, the muscles are fully elongated.

NOTE: Motion is initiated in the distal-most joint of each digit to minimize compression of the small joints. Full joint ROM will not be possible when the extrinsic muscles are elongated.

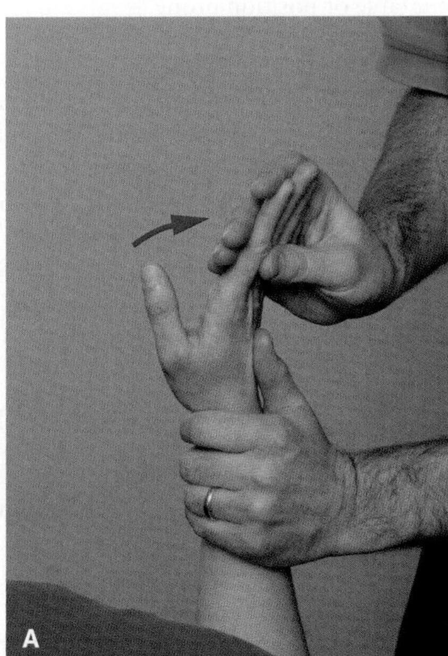

FIGURE 3.13 End of range for the extrinsic finger **(A)** flexors and

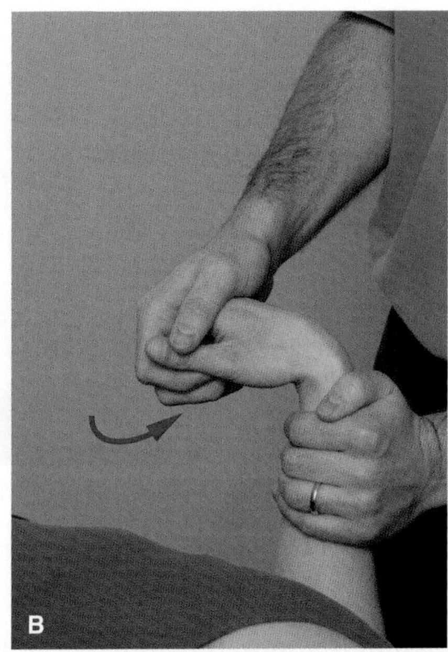

FIGURE 3.13 (B) extensors.

Lower Extremity

Combined Hip and Knee: Flexion and Extension (Fig. 3.14) VIDEO 3.6

To reach full range of hip flexion, the knee must also be flexed to release tension on the hamstring muscle group. To reach full range of knee flexion, the hip must be flexed to release tension on the rectus femoris muscle.

Hand Placement and Procedure

- Support and lift the patient's leg with the palm and fingers of the top hand under the patient's knee and the lower hand under the heel.
- As the knee flexes full range, swing the fingers to the side of the thigh.

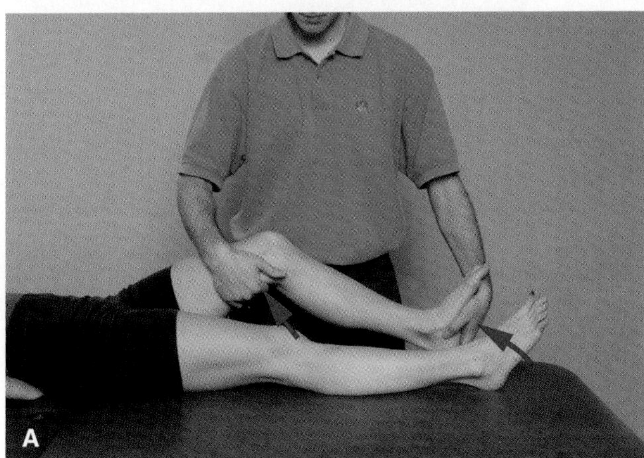

FIGURE 3.14 (A) Initiating and

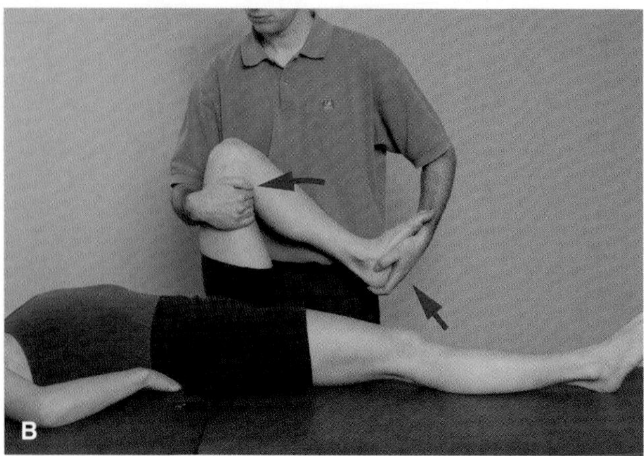

FIGURE 3.14—cont'd (B) completing combined hip and knee flexion.

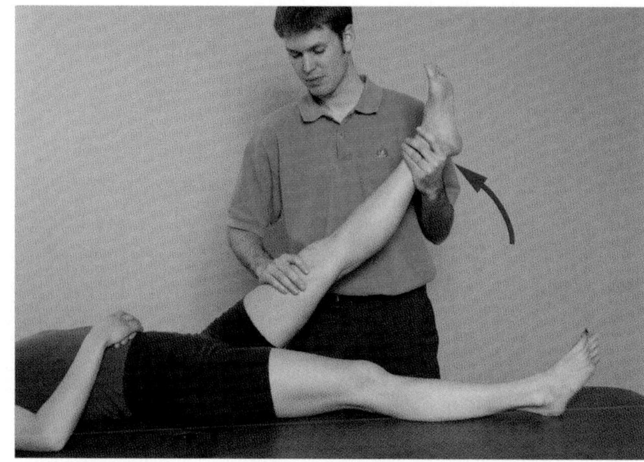

FIGURE 3.16 ROM to the hamstring muscle group.

Hip: Extension (Hyperextension) (Fig. 3.15)

Prone or side-lying must be used if the patient has near-normal or normal motion.

Hand Placement and Procedure

- If the patient is prone, lift the thigh with the bottom hand under the patient's knee; stabilize the pelvis with the top hand or arm.
- If the patient is side-lying, bring the bottom hand under the thigh and place the hand on the anterior surface; stabilize the pelvis with the top hand. For full range of hip extension, do not flex the knee full range, as the two-joint rectus femoris would then restrict the range.

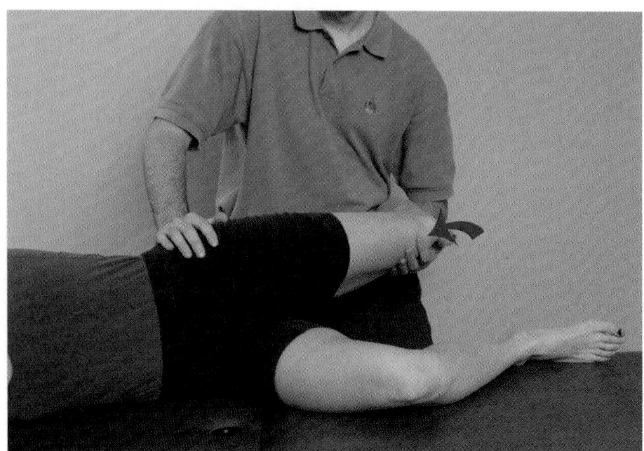

FIGURE 3.15 Hip extension with the patient side-lying.

Elongation of the Two-Joint Hamstring Muscle Group (Fig. 3.16)

Hand Placement and Procedure

- Place the lower hand under the patient's heel and the upper hand across the anterior aspect of the patient's knee.
- Keep the knee in extension as the hip is flexed.
- If the knee requires support, cradle the patient's leg in your lower arm with your elbow flexed under the calf and your hand across the anterior aspect of the patient's knee. The other hand provides support or stabilization where needed.

NOTE: If the hamstrings are so tight as to limit the knee from going into extension, the available range of the muscle is reached simply by extending the knee as far as the muscle allows and not moving the hip.

Elongation of the Two-Joint Rectus Femoris Muscle

Position the patient supine with knee flexed over the edge of the treatment table or position prone.

Hand Placement and Procedure

- When supine, stabilize the lumbar spine by flexing the hip and knee of the opposite lower extremity and placing the foot on the treatment table (hook-lying).
- When prone, stabilize the pelvis with the top hand (see Fig. 4.31).
- Flex the patient's knee until tissue resistance is felt in the anterior thigh, which means the full available range is reached.

Hip: Abduction and Adduction (Fig. 3.17)

Hand Placement and Procedure

- Support the patient's leg with the upper hand under the knee and the lower hand under the ankle.
- For full range of adduction, the opposite leg needs to be in a partially abducted position.
- Keep the patient's hip and knee in extension and neutral to rotation as abduction and adduction are performed.

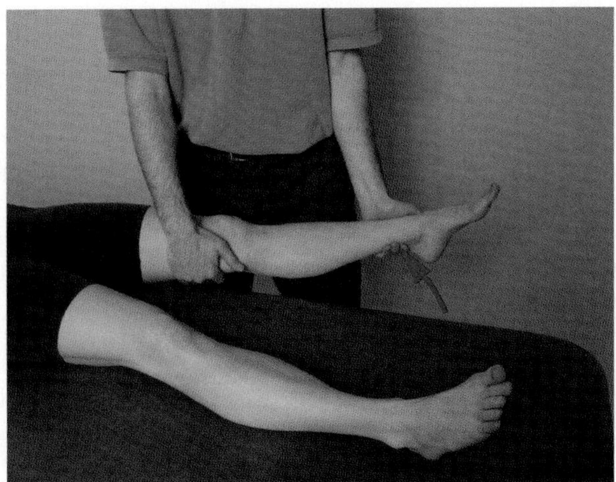

FIGURE 3.17 Abduction of the hip, maintaining the hip in extension and neutral to rotation.

Hip: Internal (Medial) and External (Lateral) Rotation

Hand Placement and Procedure With the Hip and Knee Extended

- Grasp just proximal to the patient's knee with the top hand and just proximal to the ankle with the bottom hand.
- Roll the thigh inward and outward.

Hand Placement and Procedure for Rotation With the Hip and Knee Flexed (Fig. 3.18)

- Flex the patient's hip and knee to 90°; support the knee with the top hand.
- If the knee is unstable, cradle the thigh and support the proximal calf and knee with the bottom hand.
- Rotate the femur by moving the leg like a pendulum.
- This hand placement provides some support to the knee but should be used with caution if there is knee instability.

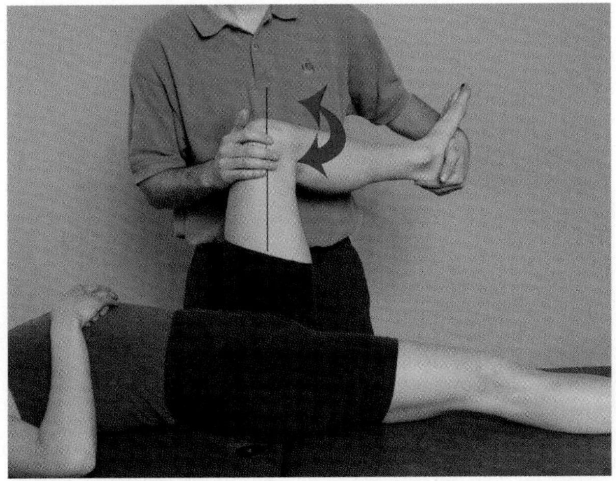

FIGURE 3.18 Rotation of the hip with the hip positioned in 90° of flexion.

Ankle: Dorsiflexion (Fig. 3.19) VIDEO 3.7

Hand Placement and Procedure

- Stabilize around the malleoli with the top hand.
- Cup the patient's heel with the bottom hand and place the forearm along the bottom of the foot.
- Pull the calcaneus distalward with the thumb and fingers while pushing upward with the forearm.

NOTE: If the knee is flexed, full range of the ankle joint can be obtained. If the knee is extended, the lengthened range of the two-joint gastrocnemius muscle can be obtained, but the gastrocnemius limits full range of dorsiflexion. Apply dorsiflexion in both positions of the knee to provide range to both the joint and the muscle.

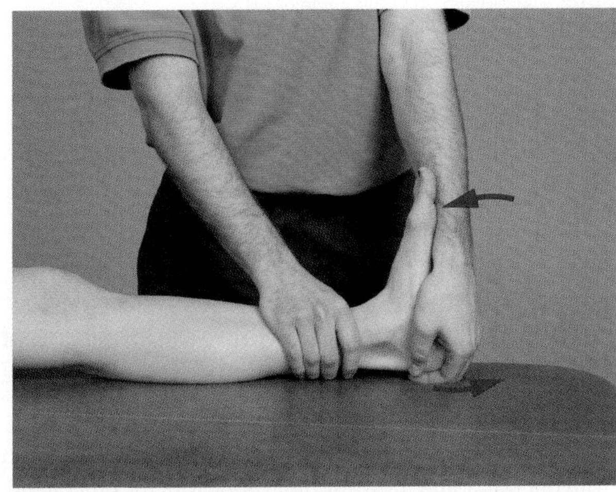

FIGURE 3.19 Dorsiflexion of the ankle.

Ankle: Plantarflexion

Hand Placement and Procedure

- Support the heel with the bottom hand.
- Place the top hand on the dorsum of the foot and push it into plantarflexion.

NOTE: In bed-bound patients, the ankle tends to assume a plantarflexed position from the weight of the blankets and the pull of gravity, so this motion may not need to be performed.

Subtalar (Lower Ankle) Joint: Inversion and Eversion (Fig. 3.20)

Hand Placement and Procedure

- Using the bottom hand, place the thumb medial and the fingers lateral to the joint on either side of the heel.
- Turn the heel inward and outward.

NOTE: Supination of the foot may be combined with inversion, and pronation may be combined with eversion.

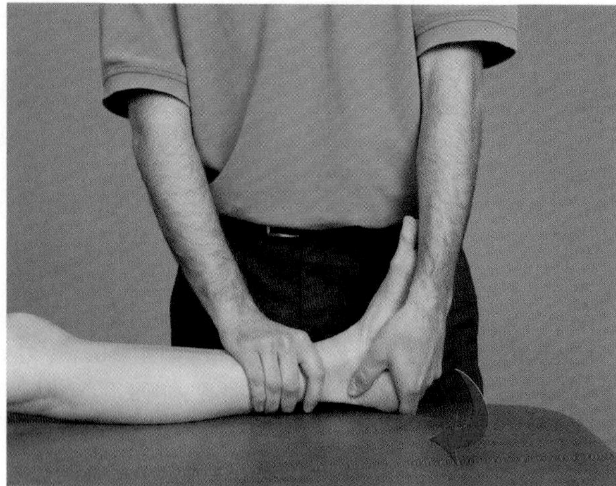

FIGURE 3.20 Inversion of the subtalar joint.

Transverse Tarsal Joint

Hand Placement and Procedure

- Stabilize the patient's talus and calcaneus with one hand.
- With the other hand, grasp around the navicular and cuboid.
- Gently rotate the midfoot by lifting and lowering the arch.

Joints of the Toes: Flexion and Extension and Abduction and Adduction (Metatarsophalangeal and Interphalangeal Joints) (Fig. 3.21)

Hand Placement and Procedure

- Stabilize the bone proximal to the joint that is to be moved with one hand, and move the distal bone with the other hand.
- The technique is the same as for ROM of the fingers.
- Several joints of the toes can be moved simultaneously if care is taken not to stress any structure.

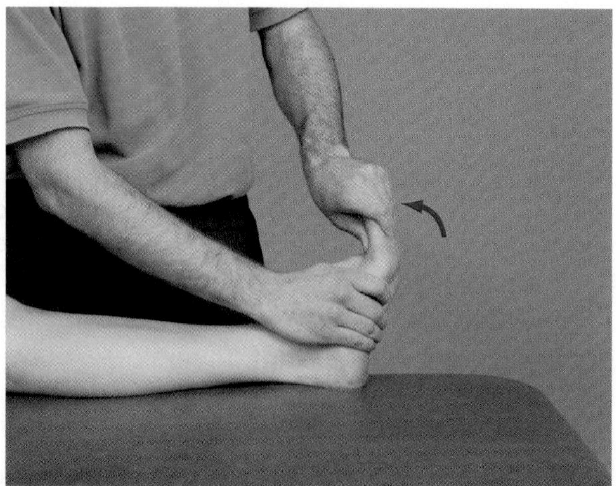

FIGURE 3.21 Extension of the metatarsophalangeal joint of the large toe.

Cervical Spine VIDEO 3.8

Stand at the end of the treatment table; securely grasp the patient's head by placing both hands under the occipital region.

Flexion (Forward Bending) (Fig. 3.22A)

Procedure

- Lift the head as though it were nodding (chin toward larynx) to flex the head on the neck.
- Once full nodding is complete, continue to flex the cervical spine and lift the head toward the sternum.

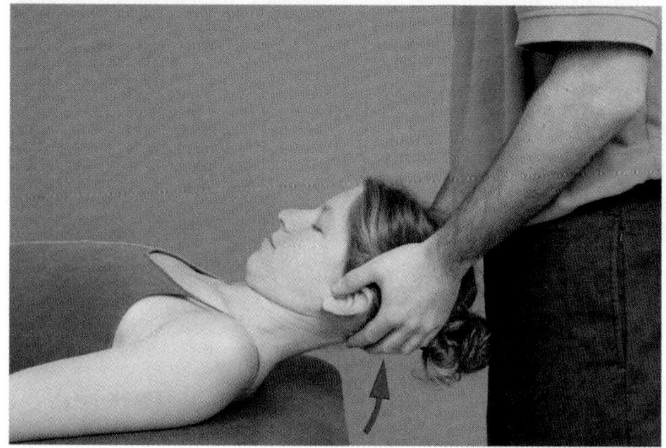

FIGURE 3.22 Cervical **(A)** flexion and

Extension (Backward Bending or Hyperextension)

Procedure

Tip the head backward.

NOTE: If the patient is supine, only the head and upper cervical spine can be extended; the head must clear the end of the table to extend the entire cervical spine. The patient may also be prone or sitting.

Lateral Flexion (Side Bending) and Rotation (Fig. 3.22B)

Procedure

Maintain the cervical spine neutral to flexion and extension as you direct the head and neck into side bending (approximate the ear toward the shoulder) and rotation (rotate from side to side).

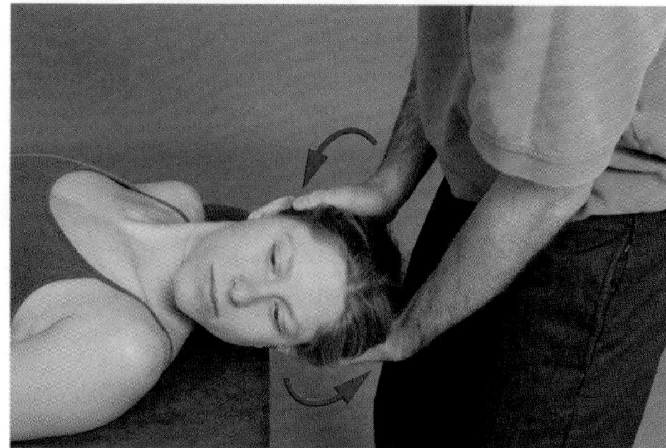

FIGURE 3.22 (B) rotation.

Lumbar Spine VIDEO 3.9

Flexion (Fig. 3.23)

Hand Placement and Procedure

- Bring both of the patient's knees to the chest by lifting under the knees (hip and knee flexion).
- Flexion of the spine occurs as the hips are flexed full range and the pelvis starts to rotate posteriorly.
- Greater range of flexion can be obtained by lifting under the patient's sacrum with the lower hand.

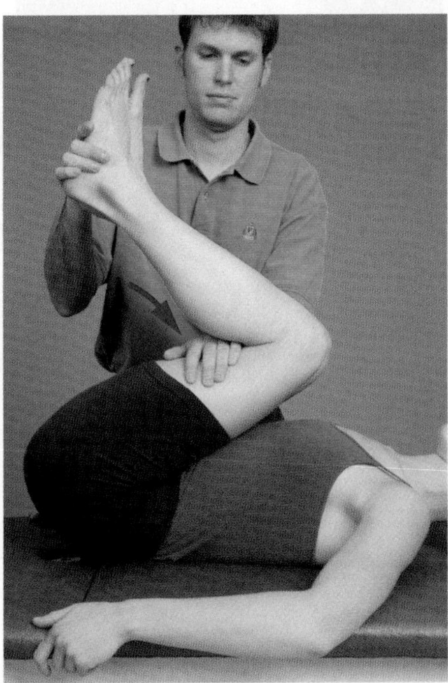

FIGURE 3.23 Lumbar flexion is achieved by bringing the patient's hips into flexion until the pelvis rotates posteriorly.

Extension

Position the patient prone for full extension (hyperextension).

Hand Placement and Procedure

With hands under the thighs, lift the thighs upward until the pelvis rotates anteriorly and the lumbar spine extends.

Rotation (Fig. 3.24)

Position the patient in the hook-lying position with hips and knees flexed and feet resting on the table.

Hand Placement and Procedure

- Push both of the patient's knees laterally in one direction until the pelvis on the opposite side comes up off the treatment table.
- Stabilize the patient's thorax with the top hand.
- Repeat in the opposite direction.

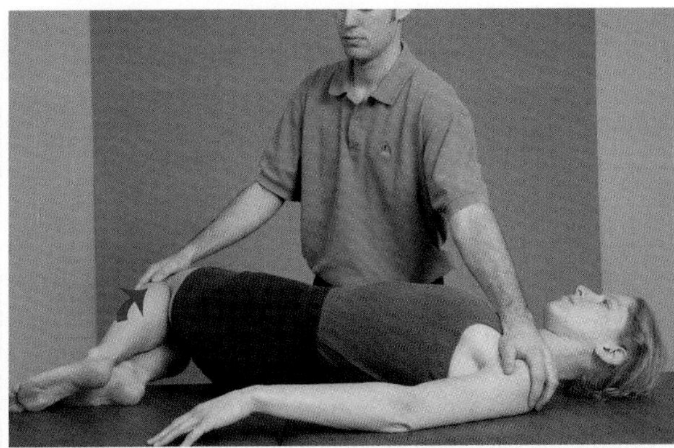

FIGURE 3.24 Rotation of the lumbar spine results when the thorax is stabilized and the pelvis lifts off the table as far as allowed.

CLINICAL TIP

Effective and efficient ROM can be administered by combining several joint motions that transect several planes resulting in oblique, functional, or diagonal patterns.

- For example, wrist flexion may be combined with ulnar deviation or shoulder flexion may be combined with abduction and lateral rotation.
- Use patterns that mimic functional activities such as moving hand behind head as in combing hair—add rotation of the neck. See also Box 3.3 at the end of the chapter.
- Proprioceptive neuromuscular facilitation (PNF) patterns of movement may be effectively used for PROM, AROM, or A-AROM techniques. See Chapter 6 for descriptions of these patterns.

Self-Assisted ROM

Patient involvement in self-care should begin as soon as the individual is able to understand and learn what to do. Even with weakness or paralysis, the patient can learn how to move the involved part and be instructed in the importance of movement within safe parameters. After surgery or traumatic injury, self-assisted ROM (S-AROM) is used to protect the healing tissues when more intensive muscle contraction is contraindicated. A variety of devices as well as use of a normal extremity may be used to meet the goals of PROM or A-AROM. Incorporation of S-AROM then becomes a part of the home exercise program (Box 3.2).

Manual Assistance

With cases of unilateral weakness or paralysis or during early stages of recovery after trauma or surgery, the patient can be taught to use the uninvolved extremity to move the involved

BOX 3.2 Self-assisted ROM Techniques

Forms of Self-assisted ROM
- Manual
- Equipment
  - Wand or T-bar
  - Finger ladder, wall climbing, ball rolling
  - Pulleys
  - Skate board/powder board
  - Reciprocal exercise devices

Guidelines for Teaching Self-assisted ROM
- Educate the patient on the value of the motion.
- Teach the patient correct body alignment and stabilization.
- Observe patient performance and correct any substitute or unsafe motions.
- If equipment is used, make sure all hazards are eliminated so application will be safe.
- Provide drawings and clear guidelines for number of repetitions and frequency.

Review the exercises at a follow-up session. Modify or progress the exercise program based on the patient response and treatment plan for meeting the outcome goals.

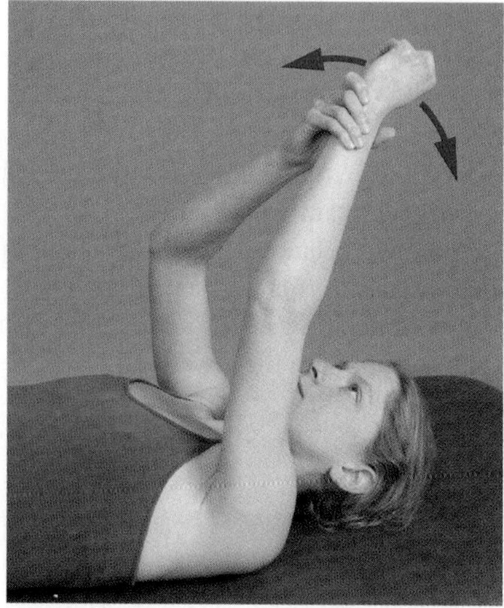

FIGURE 3.25 Patient giving self-assisted ROM to shoulder flexion and extension. Horizontal abduction and adduction can be applied with the same hand placement.

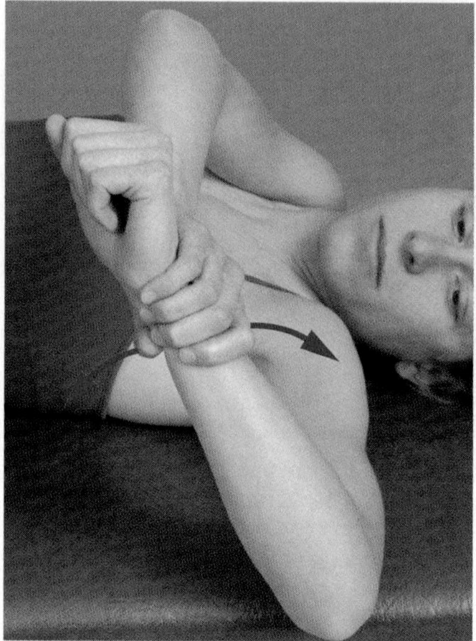

FIGURE 3.26 Arm position of patient for giving self-assisted ROM to internal and external rotation of shoulder.

extremity through ranges of motion. These exercises may be done supine, sitting, or standing. The effects of gravity change with patient positioning, so when lifting the part against gravity, gravity provides a resistive force against the prime motion and, therefore, the prime mover requires assistance. When the extremity moves downward, gravity causes the motion, and the antagonists need assistance to control the motion eccentrically.

Arm and Forearm

Instruct the patient to reach across the body with the uninvolved (or assisting) extremity and grasp the involved extremity around the wrist, supporting the wrist and hand.

- ***Shoulder flexion and extension.*** The patient lifts the involved extremity over the head and returns it to the side (Fig. 3.25).
- ***Shoulder horizontal abduction and adduction.*** Beginning with the arm abducted 90°, the patient pulls the extremity across the chest and returns it to the side.
- ***Shoulder rotation.*** Beginning with the arm at the patient's side in slight abduction and with the elbow resting on a small pillow to elevate it or abducted 90° and elbow flexed 90°, the patient moves the forearm "like a spoke on a wheel" with the uninvolved extremity (Fig. 3.26). It is important to emphasize rotating the humerus, not merely flexing and extending the elbow.
- ***Elbow flexion and extension.*** The patient bends the elbow until the hand is near the shoulder and then moves the hand down toward the side of the leg.
- ***Pronation and supination of the forearm.*** Beginning with the forearm resting across the body, the patient rotates the radius around the ulna. Emphasize to the patient not to twist the hand at the wrist joint.

Wrist and Hand

The patient moves the uninvolved fingers to the dorsum of the hand and the thumb into the palm of the hand.

- ***Wrist flexion and extension and radial and ulnar deviation.*** The patient moves the wrist in all directions, applying no pressure against the fingers (Fig. 3.27).

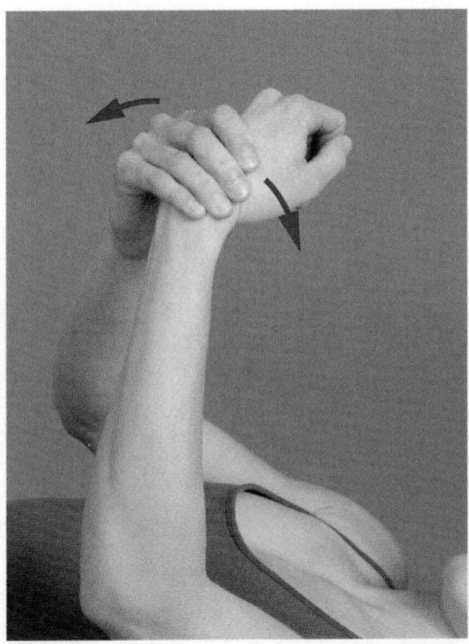

FIGURE 3.27 Patient applying self-assisted wrist flexion and extension with no pressure against the fingers.

- ***Finger flexion and extension.*** The patient uses the uninvolved thumb to extend the involved fingers and cups the normal fingers over the dorsum of the involved fingers to flex them (Fig. 3.28).

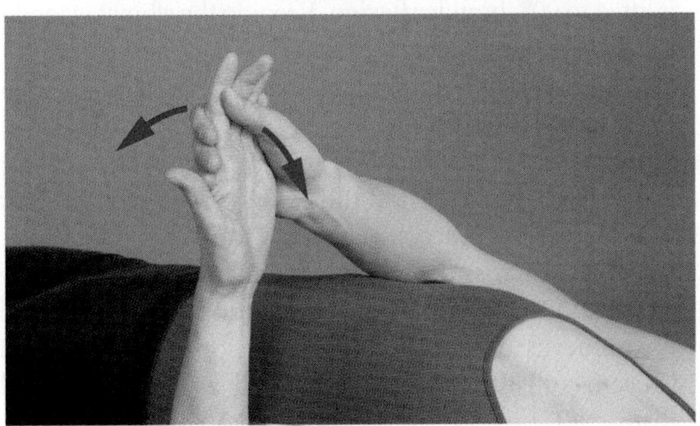

FIGURE 3.28 Patient applying self-assisted finger flexion and extension.

- ***Thumb flexion with opposition and extension with reposition.*** The patient cups the uninvolved fingers around the radial border of the thenar eminence of the involved thumb and places the uninvolved thumb along the palmar surface of the involved thumb to extend it (Fig. 3.29). To flex and oppose the thumb, the patient cups the normal hand around the dorsal surface of the involved hand and pushes the first metacarpal toward the little finger.

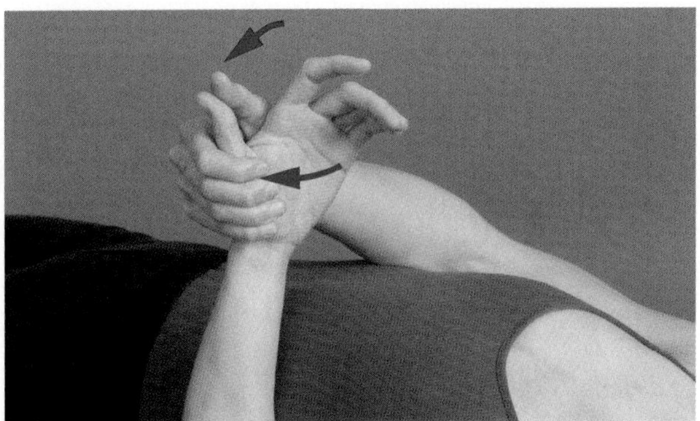

FIGURE 3.29 Patient applying self-assisted thumb extension.

Hip and Knee

- ***Hip and knee flexion.*** With the patient supine, instruct the patient to initiate the motion by lifting the involved knee by slipping his or her normal foot under the knee or with a strap or belt under the involved knee (Fig. 3.30). The patient can then grasp the knee with one or both hands to bring the knee up toward the chest to complete the range. With the patient sitting, he or she may lift the thigh with the hands and flex the knee to the end of its available range.

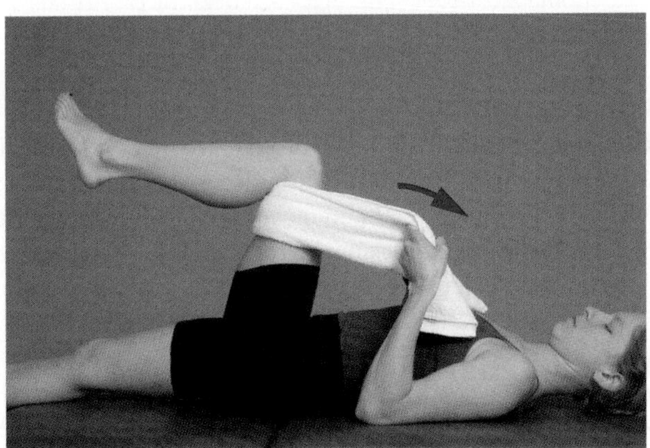

FIGURE 3.30 Self-assisted flexion of the hip.

- ***Hip abduction and adduction.*** It is difficult for the weak patient to assist the lower extremities into abduction and adduction when supine owing to the weight of the leg and the friction of the bed surface. It is necessary, though, for the individual to move a weak lower extremity from side to side for bed mobility. To practice this functional activity as an exercise, instruct the patient to slide the normal foot from the knee down to the ankle and then move the involved extremity from side-to-side. S-AROM can be performed sitting by using the hands to assist moving the thigh outward and inward.

- ***Combined hip abduction with external rotation.*** The patient sits on the floor or on a bed with the back supported, the involved hip and knee flexed, and the foot resting on the surface. The knee is moved outward (toward the table/bed) and back inward, with assistance from the upper extremities (Fig. 3.31).

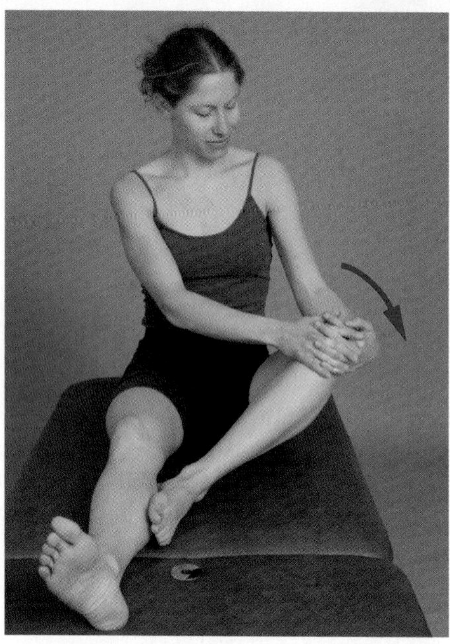

FIGURE 3.31 Self-assisted hip abduction and external rotation.

Ankle and Toes

- The patient sits with the involved extremity crossed over the uninvolved one so the distal leg rests on the normal knee. The uninvolved hand moves the involved ankle into dorsiflexion, plantarflexion, inversion, and eversion and toe flexion and extension (Fig. 3.32).

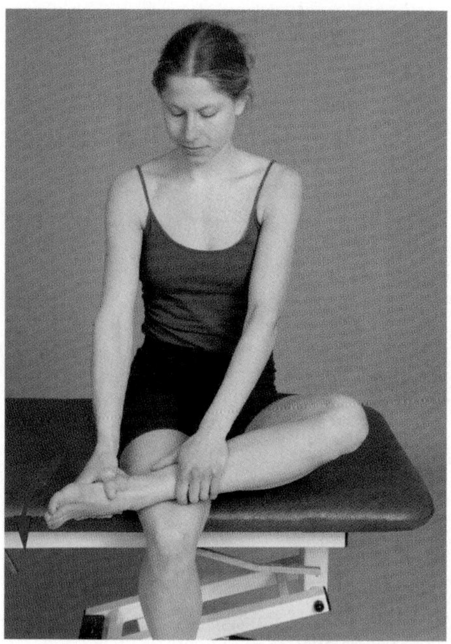

FIGURE 3.32 Position of patient and hand placement for self-assisted ankle and toe motions; shown is inversion and eversion.

Wand (T-Bar) Exercises

When a patient has voluntary muscle control in an involved upper extremity but needs guidance or motivation to complete the ROM in the shoulder or elbow, a wand (dowel rod, cane, wooden stick, T-bar, or similar object) can be used to provide assistance (Fig. 3.33).

The choice of position is based on the patient's level of function. Most of the techniques can be performed supine if maximum protection is needed. Sitting or standing requires greater control. Choice of position is also guided by the effects of gravity on the weak muscles. Initially, guide the patient through the proper motion for each activity to ensure that he or she does not use substitute motions. The patient grasps the wand with both hands, and the normal extremity guides and controls the motions.

- ***Shoulder flexion and return.*** The wand is grasped with the hands a shoulder width apart. The wand is lifted forward and upward through the available range, with the elbows kept in extension if possible (Fig. 3.33A). Scapulohumeral motion should be smooth; do not allow substitute motions such as scapular elevation or trunk movement.
- ***Shoulder horizontal abduction and adduction.*** The wand is lifted to 90° shoulder flexion. Keeping the elbows extended, the patient pushes and pulls the wand back and forth across the chest through the available range (Fig. 3.33B). Do not allow trunk rotation.
- ***Shoulder internal and external rotation.*** The patient's arms are at the sides, and the elbows are flexed 90°. Rotation of the arms is accomplished by moving the wand from side to side across the trunk while maintaining the elbows at the side (Fig. 3.33C). The rotation should occur in the humerus; do not allow elbow flexion and extension. To prevent substitute motions as well as provide a slight distraction force to the glenohumeral joint, a small towel roll may be placed in the axilla with instruction to the patient to "keep the roll in place."
- ***Shoulder internal and external rotation—alternate position.*** The patient's shoulders are abducted 90°, and the elbows are flexed 90°. For external rotation, the wand is moved toward the patient's head; for internal rotation, the wand is moved toward the waistline.
- ***Elbow flexion and extension.*** The patient's forearms may be pronated or supinated; the hands grasp the wand a shoulder -width apart. Instruct the patient to flex and extend the elbows.
- ***Shoulder hyperextension.*** The patient may be standing or prone. He or she places the wand behind the buttocks, grasps the wand with hands a shoulder width apart, and

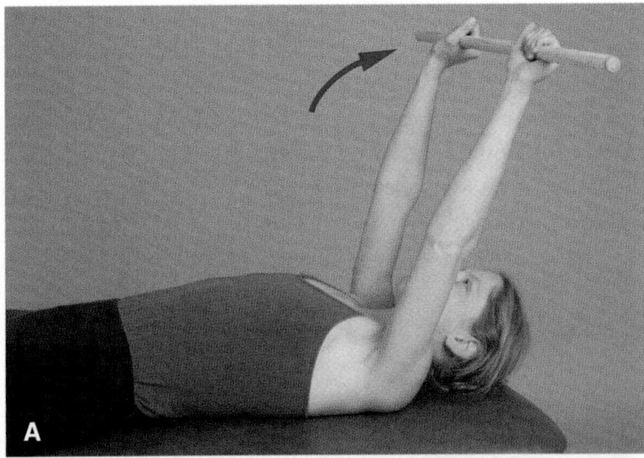

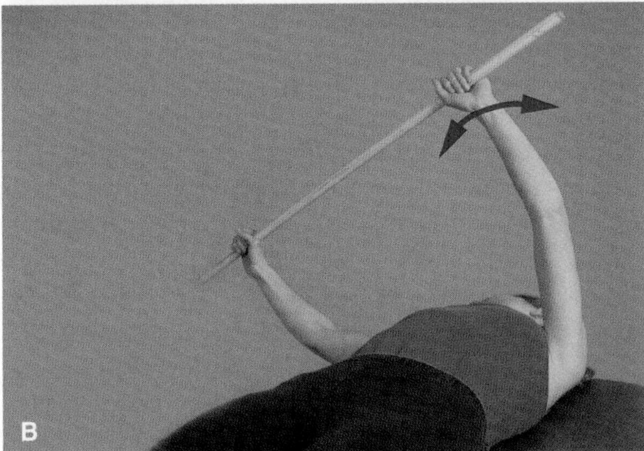

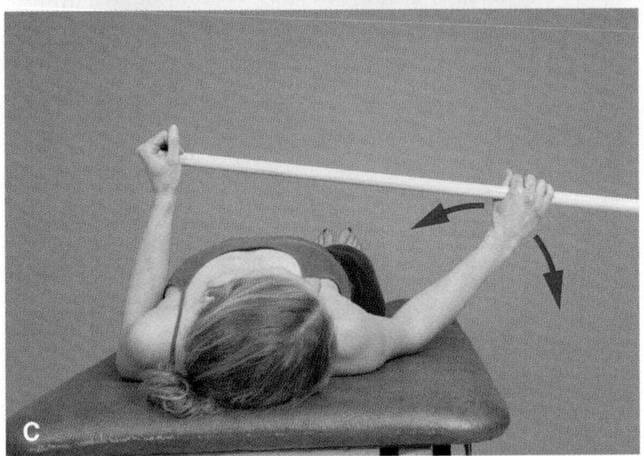

FIGURE 3.33 Patient using a wand for self-assisted shoulder **(A)** flexion, **(B)** horizontal abduction/adduction, and **(C)** rotation.

then lifts the wand backward away from the trunk. The patient should avoid trunk motion.

- ***Variations and combinations of movements.*** For example, the patient begins with the wand behind the buttocks and then moves the wand up the back to achieve scapular winging, shoulder internal rotation, and elbow flexion.

Wall Climbing

Wall climbing (or use of a device such as a finger ladder) can provide the patient with objective reinforcement and, therefore, motivation for performing shoulder ROM. Wall markings may also be used to provide visual feedback for the height reached. The arm may be moved into flexion or abduction (Fig. 3.34). The patient steps closer to the wall as the arm is elevated.

PRECAUTION: The patient must be taught the proper motions and not allowed to substitute with trunk side bending, toe raising, or shoulder shrugging.

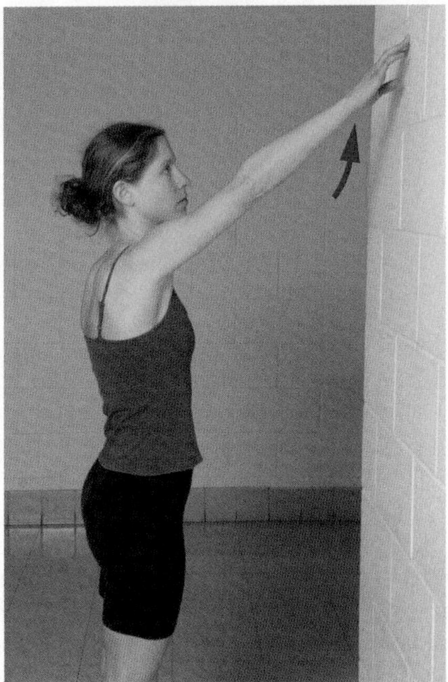

FIGURE 3.34 Wall climbing for shoulder elevation.

Overhead Pulleys

If properly taught, pulley systems can be effectively used to assist an involved extremity in performing ROM. The pulley has been demonstrated to utilize significantly more muscle activity than therapist-assisted ROM and continuous passive motion machines (described later in the chapter), so this form of assistance should be used only when muscle activity is desired.[6]

For home use, a single pulley may be attached to a strap that is held in place by closing the strap in a door. A pulley may also be attached to an overhead bar or affixed to the ceiling. The patient should be set up so the pulley is directly over the joint that is moving or so the line of pull is effectively moving the extremity and not just compressing the joint surfaces together. The patient may be sitting, standing, or supine.

Shoulder ROM (Fig. 3.35)

Instruct the patient to hold one handle in each hand, and with the normal hand, pull the rope and lift the involved extremity forward (flexion), out to the side (abduction), or in the plane of the scapula (scaption is 30° forward of the frontal plane). The patient should not shrug the shoulder (scapular elevation) or lean the trunk. Guide and instruct the patient so there is smooth motion.

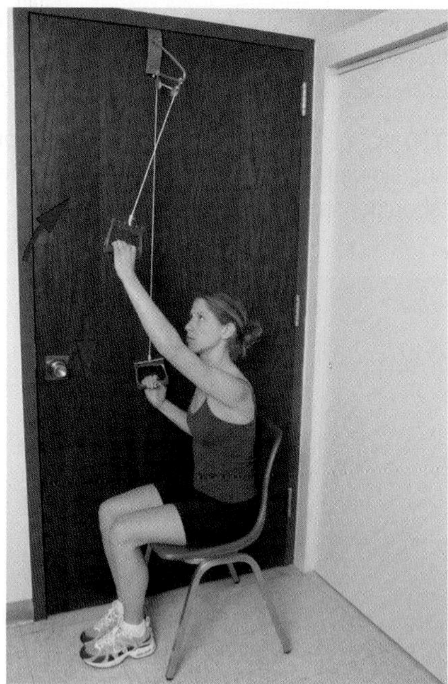

FIGURE 3.35 Use of overhead pulleys to assist shoulder elevation.

PRECAUTION: Assistive pulley activities for the shoulder are easily misused by the patient, resulting in compression of the humerus against the acromion process. Continual compression leads to pain and decreased function. Proper patient selection and appropriate instruction can avoid this problem. If a patient cannot learn to use the pulley with proper shoulder mechanics, these exercises should not be performed. Discontinue this activity if there is increased pain or decreased mobility.

Elbow Flexion

With the arm stabilized along the side of the trunk, the patient lifts the forearm and bends the elbow.

Skate Board/Powder Board

Use of a friction-free surface may encourage movement without the resistance of gravity or friction. If available, a skate with rollers may be used. Other methods include using powder on the surface or placing a towel under the extremity so it can slide along the smooth surface of the board. Any motion can be done, but most common are abduction/adduction of the hip while supine and horizontal abduction/adduction of the shoulder while sitting.

Reciprocal Exercise Unit

Several devices, such as a bicycle, upper body or lower body ergometer, or a reciprocal exercise unit, can be set up to provide some flexion and extension to an involved extremity using the strength of the normal extremity. Movable devices that can be attached to a patient's bed, wheelchair, or standard chair are available. The circumference of motion as well as excursion of the extremities can be adjusted. A reciprocal exercise unit has additional exercise benefits in that it can be used for reciprocal patterning, endurance training, and strengthening by changing the parameters of the exercise and monitoring the heart rate and fatigue. See Chapter 6 for principles of resistance exercise and Chapter 7 for principles of aerobic exercise.

Continuous Passive Motion

Continuous passive motion (CPM) refers to passive motion performed by a mechanical device that moves a joint slowly and continuously through a controlled ROM. The mechanical devices that exist for nearly every joint in the body (Fig. 3.36) were developed as a result of research by Robert Salter, who demonstrated that continual passive motion has beneficial healing effects on diseased or injured joint structures and soft tissues in animal and clinical studies.[28-34] Since the development of CPM, many studies have been done to determine the

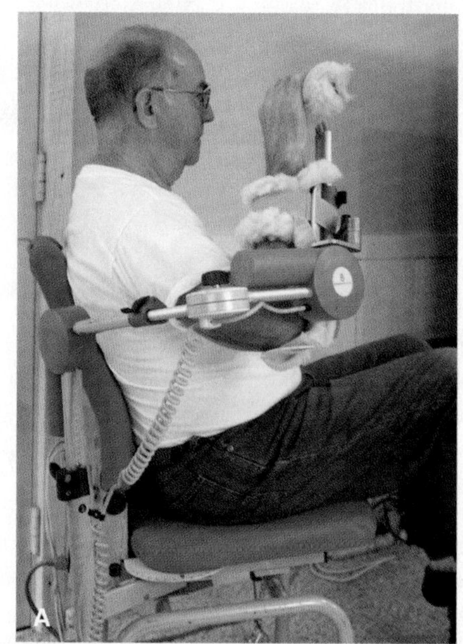

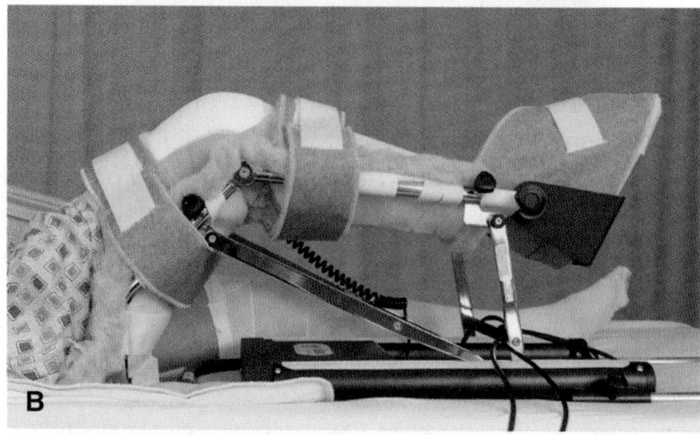

FIGURE 3.36 Continuous motion devices for **(A)** the shoulder and **(B)** the knee.

parameters of application, but because the devices are used for many conditions and studies have used various protocols with varying research designs, no definitive delineation has been established.[4,16,22]

Benefits of CPM

CPM has been reported to be effective in lessening the negative effects of joint immobilization in conditions such as arthritis, contractures, and intra-articular fractures[23]; some studies report improved recovery rate and ROM, particularly early in the recovery period after a variety of surgical procedures,[3,16,22,28-34,36] although other studies question the need for its use when long-term measures show little or no difference in outcomes compared with traditional therapy.[11,17,19] Suggested benefits of CPM include:

- Preventing development of adhesions and contractures and thus joint stiffness
- Providing a stimulating effect on the healing of tendons and ligaments
- Enhancing the healing of incisions over the moving joint
- Increasing synovial fluid lubrication of the joint and thus increasing the rate of intra-articular cartilage healing and regeneration
- Preventing the degrading effects of immobilization
- Providing a quicker return of ROM
- Decreasing postoperative pain

FOCUS ON EVIDENCE

Studies have compared short- and long-term outcomes of CPM use after various types of surgery using various parameters as well as CPM with other methods of early movement and positioning.[1,5,6,11,14,15,22,17,26,27,37,39] Some studies have shown no significant difference between patients undergoing CPM and those undergoing PROM or other forms of early motion.[5,14,15,27,38] Reports of the short-term benefits of CPM use after surgery were that patients gained ROM more quickly and therefore experienced earlier discharge from the hospital when CPM was used compared with other forms of intervention.[3] However, long-term functional gains are reported to be no different from those in patients who underwent other forms of early motion.[4,17,37,39]

The authors of an updated Cochrane Review of 24 randomized controlled trials in which CPM was used following total knee arthroplasty summarized that for patients who had CPM combined with physical therapy, the clinical effects on active knee flexion ROM, pain, function, and quality of life were not significant enough to justify its use as a routine intervention. There was no significant difference in passive knee flexion or passive or active knee extension.[11]

Another Cochrane Review looked at the use of CPM for the prevention of venous thromboembolism after total knee arthroplasty using 11 randomized controlled trials involving 808 patients. The authors concluded that there was insufficient evidence to state that CPM reduces thromboembolism after total knee arthroplasty.[12] They suggested that additional quality studies are needed.

Some studies have identified detrimental effects such as the need for greater analgesic intervention and increased postoperative blood drainage when using CPM[26,38] in contrast to claims that CPM decreases postoperative pain and complications.[29-33,36] The cost-effectiveness of the CPM equipment, patient compliance, utilization and supervision of equipment by trained personnel, length of hospital stay, speed of recovery, and determination of appropriate patient populations become issues to consider when making the choice of whether or not to utilize CPM devices.[15,20]

General Guidelines for CPM

General guidelines for CPM are as follows:[2,4,10,16,18,28,33]

1. The device may be applied to the involved extremity immediately after surgery while the patient is still under anesthesia or as soon as possible if bulky dressings prevent early motion.
2. The arc of motion for the joint is determined. A low arc of 20° to 30° is often used initially and progressed 10° to 15° per day as tolerated. The portion of the range used initially is based on the range available and patient tolerance. One study that looked at accelerating the range of knee flexion after total knee arthroplasty found that a greater range and earlier discharge were attained for that group of patients,[39] although there was no difference between the groups at 4 weeks.
3. The rate of motion is determined; usually 1 cycle/45 sec or 2 min is well tolerated.
4. The length of time on the CPM machine varies for different protocols—anywhere from continuous for 24 hours to continuous for 1 hour three times a day.[10,18,33] The longer periods of time per day reportedly result in a shorter hospital stay, fewer postoperative complications, and greater ROM at discharge,[10] although no significant difference was found in a study comparing CPM for 5 hr/day with CPM for 20 hr/day.[2] A study that compared short-duration CPM (3 to 5 hr/day) with long-duration CPM (10 to 12 hr/day) found that patient compliance and the most gained range occurred with a CPM duration of 4 to 8 hours.[4]
5. Physical therapy treatments are usually initiated during periods when the patient is not on CPM, including active-assistive and muscle-setting exercises. It is important that patients learn to use and develop motor control of the ROM as motion improves.
6. The duration minimum for CPM is usually less than 1 week or when a satisfactory range of motion is reached. Because CPM devices are portable, home use is possible in cases in which the therapist or physician deems that additional time would be beneficial. In these cases, the patient, a family member, or a caregiver is instructed in proper application.

7. CPM machines are designed to be adjustable, easily controlled, versatile, and portable. Some are battery operated (with rechargeable batteries) to allow the individual to wear the device for up to 8 hours while functioning with daily activities.

ROM Through Functional Patterns

To accomplish motion through functional patterns, first determine what pattern of movement is desired and then move the extremity through that pattern using manual assistance, mechanical assistance if it is appropriate, or self-assistance from the patient. Functional patterning can be beneficial in initiating the teaching of ADLs and instrumental activities of daily living (IADLs) as well as in instructing patients with visual impairments in functional activities. Utilizing functional patterns helps the patient recognize the purpose and value of ROM exercises and develop motor patterns that can be used in daily activities as strength and endurance improves. Box 3.3 identifies some examples and the basic motions that are utilized. When the patient no longer requires assistance to perform the pattern safely and correctly, the activity is incorporated into his or her daily activities so motor learning is reinforced and the motion becomes functional.

BOX 3.3 Functional ROM Activities

Early ROM training for functional upper extremity and neck patterns may include activities such as:

- Grasping an eating utensil: utilizing finger extension and flexion
- Eating (hand to mouth): utilizing elbow flexion and forearm supination and some shoulder flexion, abduction, and lateral rotation
- Reaching to various shelf heights: utilizing shoulder flexion and elbow extension
- Brushing or combing back of hair: utilizing shoulder abduction and lateral rotation, elbow flexion, and cervical rotation
- Holding a phone to the ear: utilizing shoulder lateral rotation, forearm supination, and cervical side bend
- Donning or doffing a shirt or jacket: utilizing shoulder extension, lateral rotation, and elbow flexion and extension
- Reaching out a car window to an ATM machine: utilizing shoulder abduction, lateral rotation, elbow extension, and some lateral bending of the trunk

Early ROM training for functional lower extremity and trunk patterns may include activities such as:

- Going from supine to sitting at the side of a bed: utilizing hip abduction and adduction followed by hip and knee flexion
- Standing up/sitting down and walking: utilizing hip and knee flexion and extension, ankle dorsi and plantarflexion, and some hip rotation
- Putting on socks and shoes: utilizing hip external rotation and abduction, knee flexion and ankle dorsi and plantarflexion, and trunk flexion

Independent Learning Activities

Critical Thinking and Discussion

1. Analyze a variety of functional activities, such as grooming, dressing, bathing, raising up from a chair, and getting in and out of a car; determine the functional ranges needed to perform each task.
2. Look at the effects of gravity or other forces on the ROM for each activity listed in #1. If you have a patient who is unable to do the activity because of an inability to control the range needed, determine how you would establish an exercise program to begin preparing the individual to develop the desired function.

Laboratory Practice

1. Perform PROM of the upper and lower extremities with your partner placed in a prone, side-lying, and sitting position.
   a. What are the advantages and disadvantages of each of the positions for some of the ranges, such as shoulder and hip extension, knee flexion with the hip extended, and rotation of the hip?
   b. Progress the PROM to A-AROM and AROM, and determine the effects of gravity and the effort required in these positions compared with that in the supine position.
2. Compare the ROMs of the hip, knee, and ankle when each of the two joint muscles is elongated over its respective joint versus when each of the muscles is slack.

REFERENCES

1. Alfredson, H, and Lorentzon, R: Superior results with continuous passive motion compared to active motion after periosteal transplantation: a retrospective study of human patella cartilage defect treatment. *Knee Surg Sports Traumatol Arthrosc* 7(4):232–238, 1999.
2. Basso, DM, and Knapp, L: Comparison of two continuous passive motion protocols for patients with total knee implants. *Phys Ther* 67:360–363, 1987.
3. Brosseau, L, et al: Efficacy of continuous passive motion following total knee arthroplasty: a metaanalysis. *J Rheumatol* 31(11): 2251–2264, 2004.
4. Chiarello, CM, Gunersen, L, and O'Halloran, T: The effect of continuous passive motion duration and increment on range of motion in total knee arthroplasty patients. *J Orthop Sports Phys Ther* 25(2):119–127, 1997.
5. Denis, M, et al: Effectiveness of continuous passive motion and conventional physical therapy after total knee arthroplasty: a randomized clinical trial. *Phys Ther* 86(2):174–185, 2006.
6. Dockery, ML, Wright, TW, and LaStayo, P: Electromyography of the shoulder: an analysis of passive modes of exercise. *Orthopedics* 11: 1181–1184, 1998.
7. Donatelli, R, and Owens-Burckhart, H: Effects of immobilization on the extensibility of periarticular connective tissue. *J Orthop Sports Phys Ther* 3: 67–72, 1981.
8. Fletcher, GF, et al: Exercise standards for testing and training: a scientific statement from the American Heart Association. *Circulation* 128: 873–934, 2013.
9. Frank, C, et al: Physiology and therapeutic value of passive joint motion. *Clin Orthop* 185:113–125, 1984.
10. Gose, J: Continuous passive motion in the postoperative treatment of patients with total knee replacement. *Phys Ther* 67:39–42, 1987.
11. Harvey, LA, Brosseau, L, and Herbert, R. Continuous passive motion following total knee arthroplasty in people with arthritis. *Cochrane Database of Systematic Reviews* 2: Art. No: CD004260, 2014.
12. He, ML, Xiao, ZM, Zeng, M, et al: Continuous passive motion for preventing venous thromboembolism after total knee arthroplasty. *Cochrane Database of Systematic Reviews* 7: Art. No: CD0008207, doi: 10.1002/14651858.pub3, 2014.
13. Houglum, PA and Bertoti, DB: *Brunnstrom's Clinical Kinesiology,* ed. 6. Philadelphia: FA Davis, 2012.
14. Kumar, PJ, et al: Rehabilitation after total knee arthroplasty: a comparison of 2 rehabilitation techniques. *Clin Orthop* 331:93–101, 1996.
15. LaStayo, PC, et al: Continuous passive motion after repair of the rotator cuff: a prospective outcome study. *J Bone Joint Surg Am* 80(7):1002–1011, 1998.
16. LaStayo, PC: Continuous passive motion for the upper extremity. In Hunter, JM, MacKin, EJ, and Callahan, AD (eds): *Rehabilitation of the Hand: Surgery and Therapy,* ed. 4. St. Louis: Mosby, 1995.
17. Lenssen A, et al: Effectiveness of prolonged use of continuous passive motin (CPM), as an adjunct to physiotherapy, after total knee arthroplasty. *BMC Musculoskeletal Disorders.* Available at http://www.medscape.com/viewarticle/574961_print. Accessed February 8, 2015.
18. McCarthy, MR, et al: The clinical use of continuous passive motion in physical therapy. *J Orthop Sports Phys Ther* 15:132–140, 1992.
19. Maniar, BN, Baviskar, JV, et al: To use or not to use continuous passive motion post-total knee arthroplasty. *J of Arthroplasty* 27(2):193–200, 2012.
20. Nadler, SF, Malanga, GA, and Jimmerman, JR: Continuous passive motion in the rehabilitation setting: a retrospective study. *Am J Phys Med Rehabil* 72(3):162–165, 1993.
21. Norkin, CC, and White, DJ: *Measurement of Joint Motion: A Guide to Goniometry,* ed. 4. Philadelphia: FA Davis, 2009.
22. O'Driscoll, SW, and Giori, NJ: Continuous passive motion (CPM) theory and principles of clinical application. *J Rehabil Res Dev* 37(2):179–188, 2000.
23. Onderko, LL and Rehman, S: Treatment of articular fractures with continuous passive motion. *Ortho Clin N Am* 44(3):345–356, 2013.
24. Pescatello, LS (ed): *ACSM's Guidelines for Exercise Testing and Prescription.* Philadelphia: Wolters Kluwert/Lippincott Williams & Wilkins Health, 2014.
25. Pohlman, MC, et al: Feasibility of physical and occupational therapy beginning from initiation of mechanical ventilation. *Crit Care Med* 38(11): 2089–2094, 2010.
26. Pope, RO, et al: Continuous passive motion after primary total knee arthroplasty: does it offer any benefits? *J Bone Joint Surg Br* 79(6): 914–917, 1997.
27. Rosen, MA, Jackson, DW, and Atwell, EA: The efficacy of continuous passive motion in the rehabilitation of anterior cruciate ligament reconstructions. *Am J Sports Med* 20(2):122–127, 1992.
28. Salter, RB: History of rest and motion and the scientific basis for early continuous passive motion. *Hand Clin* 12(1):1–11, 1996.
29. Salter, RB, Simmens, DF, and Malcolm, BW: The biological effects of continuous passive motion on the healing of full thickness defects in articular cartilage. *J Bone Joint Surg Am* 62:1232–1251, 1980.
30. Salter, RB: The prevention of arthritis through the preservation of cartilage. *J Can Assoc Radiol* 31:5–7, 1981.
31. Salter, RB, Bell, RS, and Keely, FW: The protective effect of continuous passive motion on living cartilage in acute septic arthritis. *Clin Orthop* 159:223–247, 1981.
32. Salter, RB: *Textbook of Disorders and Injuries of the Musculoskeletal System,* ed. 3. Baltimore: Williams & Wilkins, 1999.
33. Salter, RB, et al: Clinical application of basic research on continuous passive motion for disorders and injuries of synovial joints: a preliminary report of a feasibility study. *J Orthop Res* 1:325–342, 1984.
34. Salter, RB: Continuous passive motion: from origination to research to clinical applications. *J Rheumatol* 31:2104–2105, 2004.
35. Schweickert, WD, et al: Early physical and occupational therapy in mechanically ventilated, critically ill patients: a randomized controlled trial. *Lancet* 373(9678): 1874–1882, 2009.
36. Stap, LJ, and Woodfin, PM: Continuous passive motion in the treatment of knee flexion contractures: a case report. *Phys Ther* 66:1720–1722, 1986.
37. Wasilewski, SA, et al: Value of continuous passive motion in total knee arthroplasty. *Orthopedics* 13(3):291–295, 1990.
38. Witherow, GE, Bollen, SR, and Pinczewski, LA: The use of continuous passive motion after arthroscopically assisted anterior cruciate ligament reconstruction: help or hindrance? *Knee Surg Sports Traumatol Arthrosc* 1(2): 68–70, 1993.
39. Yashar, AA, et al: Continuous passive motion with accelerated flexion after total knee arthroplasty. *Clin Orthop* 345:38–43, 1997.

CHAPTER

4

Stretching for Improved Mobility

■ LYNN COLBY, PT, MS ■ JOHN BORSTAD, PT, PHD
■ CAROLYN KISNER, PT, MS

The term *mobility* is often defined as the ability of body structures or segments to move so that range of motion (ROM) for functional activities is allowed (*functional ROM*).[3] It can also be defined as the ability of an individual to initiate, control, or sustain active movements of the body to perform motor tasks (*functional mobility*).[41,116] Mobility, as it relates to functional ROM, is associated with both joint integrity and soft tissue *flexibility*. In this context, the soft tissues that cross or surround joints must have sufficient extensibility to allow an individual to perform their functional tasks and activities. Importantly, the ROM needed to perform functional activities does not necessarily mean full or "normal" ROM.

Sufficient soft tissue mobility and joint ROM must also be supported by a requisite level of muscle function, including strength, endurance, and neuromuscular control. Not only does adequate muscle function enable functional mobility, it also helps manage imposed physical loads and may help prevent musculoskeletal injury.[58,66,71,120,132,159]

Hypomobility, or reduced functional motion, is often caused by adaptive shortening or decreased extensibility in soft tissues. Potential factors leading to hypomobility include (1) prolonged immobilization of a body segment, (2) sedentary lifestyle, (3) postural malalignment with muscle length alterations, (4) impaired muscle performance (weakness) associated with musculoskeletal or neuromuscular disorders, (5) tissue trauma resulting in inflammation and pain, and (6) congenital or acquired deformities. Any factor that limits mobility by decreasing the extensibility of soft tissues may also lead to impaired muscular performance.[82] Hypomobility can contribute to activity limitations and participation restrictions in a person's life.[10,18]

Stretching interventions become an integral component of an individualized rehabilitation program when restricted mobility adversely affects function or increases the risk of injury. Stretching exercises also are considered an important element of fitness and sport-specific conditioning programs designed to promote wellness and reduce the risk of injury or re-injury.[58,120,132,159] *Stretching* is a general term used to describe any therapeutic maneuver designed to *increase* soft tissue extensibility with the intent of improving flexibility and ROM by elongating (lengthening) structures that have adaptively shortened and have become hypomobile.[70,155]

Only through a systematic examination, evaluation, and diagnosis of a patient's problems can a therapist determine what structures are restricting motion and if, when, and what types of stretching procedures are indicated. Early in the rehabilitation process, manual stretching and joint mobilization/manipulation, which involve direct, "hands-on" intervention by a practitioner, may be the most appropriate techniques. Later, self-stretching exercises performed independently by a patient after careful instruction and close supervision may be a more suitable intervention. In some situations the use of a mechanical stretching device is indicated, particularly when manual therapies have been ineffective. Regardless of the types of stretching used as an intervention, any gains in ROM should be used regularly during functional activities and strengthening exercises. The stretching interventions described in this chapter are designed to improve the extensibility of the contractile and noncontractile components of muscle-tendon units and periarticular structures. The efficacy of these interventions is explored throughout the chapter. In addition to the stretching procedures for the extremities illustrated in this chapter, self-stretching exercises for each region of the body are described and illustrated in Chapters 16 through 22. Joint mobilization/manipulation procedures for extremity joints are described and illustrated in Chapter 5 and for the temporomandibular joints, ribs, and sacrum in Chapter 15. Spinal manipulative techniques are presented in Chapter 16.

Definition of Terms Associated With Mobility and Stretching

Flexibility

Flexibility is the ability to rotate a single joint or series of joints smoothly and easily through an unrestricted, pain-free ROM.[82,100] Muscle length, joint integrity, and periarticular soft tissue extensibility all interact to determine flexibility.[3] Flexibility is maximized when the muscle-tendon units that cross a joint have adequate extensibility to deform and yield to a stretch force. In addition, the arthrokinematics of the moving joint (the ability of the joint surfaces to roll and slide) and the ability of periarticular connective tissues to deform also affect joint ROM and flexibility.

Dynamic and Passive Flexibility

Dynamic flexibility. This form of flexibility, also referred to as active mobility or active ROM, is the extent to which an active muscle contraction can rotate a joint through its available ROM. Dynamic flexibility depends on the ability of a muscle to contract through the ROM and on the degree and quality of tissue extensibility

Passive flexibility. This type of flexibility, also referred to as passive mobility or passive ROM, is the extent to which a joint can be passively rotated through its available ROM and depends on the extensibility of soft tissues that cross and surround a joint. Passive flexibility is a prerequisite for—but does not ensure—dynamic flexibility.

Hypomobility

Hypomobility refers to decreased mobility or restricted motion at a single joint or series of joints. Many pathological processes are associated with hypomobility, and there are many factors that may contribute to motion limitations. These factors are summarized in Table 4.1.

Contracture

Restricted motion can range from mild tightness to irreversible contractures. *Contracture* is defined as the adaptive shortening of the muscle-tendon unit and other soft tissues that cross or surround a joint, resulting in significant resistance to passive or active stretch and limited ROM.[12,33,51,82,104] The limitations associated with contractures can significantly compromise functional abilities.

There is no clear delineation of the extent of motion loss required due to decreased soft tissue extensibility to designate the limitation as a contracture. Contracture is most often defined as an almost complete loss of motion, whereas the term *shortness* is used to denote partial loss of motion.[82] *Tightness* is commonly used in the clinical and fitness settings to describe restricted motion due to adaptive shortening of soft tissue, in particular mild muscle shortening. *Muscle tightness* is also used to denote adaptive shortening of the contractile and noncontractile elements of muscle.[70]

Designation of Contractures by Location

Contractures are described as the side of the joint that has the tissue tightness. If the tightness is on the flexion side of the flexion/extension joint axis, it is called a flexion contracture. For the patient with shortened elbow flexors who cannot fully extend the elbow, they are said to have an elbow flexion contracture. The patient with tight hip adductors

TABLE 4.1 Factors Contributing to Restricted Motion

Contributing Factors	Examples
Prolonged immobilization: extrinsic factors ▪ Casts and orthotics ▪ Skeletal traction	Fractures, osteotomy, soft tissue trauma or repair
Prolonged immobilization: intrinsic factors	
▪ Pain	Microtrauma or macrotrauma; degenerative diseases
▪ Joint inflammation and effusion	Joint diseases or trauma
▪ Muscle, tendon, or fascial disorders	Myositis, tendonitis, fasciitis
▪ Skin disorders	Burns, skin grafts, scleroderma
▪ Bony block	Osteophytes, ankylosis, surgical fusion
▪ Vascular disorders	Peripheral lymphedema
Sedentary lifestyle and habitual faulty or asymmetrical postures	Confinement to bed or a wheelchair; prolonged positioning associated with occupation or work environment
Paralysis, tonal abnormalities, and muscle imbalances	Neuromuscular disorders and diseases: CNS or PNS dysfunction (spasticity, rigidity, flaccidity, weakness, muscle guarding, spasm)
Postural malalignment: congenital or acquired	Scoliosis, kyphosis

who cannot fully abduct the leg is said to have a hip adduction contracture.

Contracture Versus Contraction

The terms *contracture* and *contraction* (the process of active tension developing in a muscle during shortening or lengthening) are not synonymous and not to be used interchangeably.

Types of Contracture

One way to further define the term *contracture* is to describe contractures by the pathological changes in the different types of soft tissues involved.[32]

Myostatic contracture. In a myostatic (myogenic) contracture, although the musculotendinous unit has adaptively shortened and there is a significant loss of ROM, there is no specific muscle pathology present.[32] From a morphological perspective, although there may be a reduction in the number of sarcomere units in series, there is no decrease in individual sarcomere length. Myostatic contractures can be resolved in a relatively short time with stretching exercises.[32,51]

Pseudomyostatic contracture. Impaired mobility and limited ROM may also be the result of hypertonicity (i.e., spasticity or rigidity) associated with a central nervous system lesion, such as a cerebrovascular accident, a spinal cord injury, or traumatic brain injury.[32,51] Muscle spasm or guarding and pain may also cause a pseudomyostatic contracture. In both situations, the involved muscles appear to be in a constant state of contraction, giving rise to excessive resistance to passive stretch. Hence, the terms pseudomyostatic contracture or apparent contracture are used. If neuromuscular inhibition procedures to reduce muscle tension temporarily are applied, full, passive elongation of the apparently shortened muscle is then possible.

Arthrogenic and periarticular contracture. An arthrogenic contracture is the result of intra-articular pathology. These changes may include adhesions, synovial proliferation, joint effusion, irregularities in articular cartilage, or osteophyte formation.[51] A periarticular contracture develops when connective tissues that cross or attach to a joint or the joint capsule lose mobility, restricting normal arthrokinematic motion.

Fibrotic contracture and irreversible contracture. Fibrous changes in the connective tissue of muscle and periarticular structures can cause adherence of these tissues and subsequent development of a fibrotic contracture.[160] Although it is possible to stretch a fibrotic contracture and eventually increase ROM, it is often difficult to re-establish optimal tissue length.[33]

Permanent loss of soft tissue extensibility that cannot be reversed by nonsurgical intervention may occur when normal muscle and organized connective tissue are replaced with a large amount of relatively nonextensible fibrotic adhesions, scar tissue,[33] or heterotopic bone. These changes can occur after long periods of immobilization with tissues in a shortened position or after tissue trauma and the subsequent inflammatory response. The longer a fibrotic contracture exists or the more extensive the tissue replacement, the more difficult it becomes to regain optimal mobility and the more likely it is that the contracture will become irreversible.[33,145]

Selective Stretching

Selective stretching is a process whereby the overall function of a patient may be improved by applying stretching techniques to some muscles and joints while allowing motion limitations to develop in other muscles or joints. When determining which muscles to stretch and which to allow to become slightly shortened, the therapist must always keep in mind the functional needs of the patient and the importance of maintaining a balance between mobility and stability for maximum functional performance.

The decision to allow restrictions to develop in selected muscle-tendon units and joints typically is made in patients with permanent paralysis. For example:

- In a patient with spinal cord injury, stability of the trunk is necessary for independence in sitting. With thoracic and cervical lesions, the patient does not have active control of the back extensors. If the hamstrings are routinely stretched to improve or maintain their extensibility and moderate hypomobility is allowed to develop in the extensors of the low back, this enables a patient to lean into the slightly shortened structures and have some degree of trunk stability for long-term sitting. However, the patient must still have enough flexibility for independence in dressing and transfers. Too much limitation of motion in the low back can decrease function.
- Allowing slight hypomobility to develop in the long flexors of the fingers while maintaining mobility of the wrist extensors enables the patient with spinal cord injury, who lacks innervation of the intrinsic finger muscles, to regain the ability to grasp by using a tenodesis action.

Overstretching and Hypermobility

Overstretching is a stretch well beyond the normal length of muscle and ROM of a joint and the surrounding soft tissues,[82] resulting in *hypermobility* (excessive mobility).

- Creating selective hypermobility by overstretching may be necessary for certain healthy individuals with normal strength and stability who participate in sports that require extensive flexibility.
- Hypermobility can create detrimental joint *instability* if the static supporting structures and/or the dynamic muscular control of the joint are unable to maintain the joint in a stable, functional position during activities. Instability of a joint often causes pain and may predispose a person to musculoskeletal injury.

Overview of Interventions to Increase Mobility of Soft Tissues

Many therapeutic interventions are designed to improve the mobility of soft tissues to increase ROM and flexibility. Stretching and mobilization/manipulation are general terms that describe any therapeutic maneuver that increases the extensibility of restricted soft tissues.

The following terms describe techniques designed to increase soft tissue extensibility and joint mobility, some of which are addressed in depth later in this chapter.

Stretching: Manual or Mechanical/Passive or Assisted

An end-range stretch force will elongate shortened muscle-tendon units and/or periarticular connective tissues when a restricted joint is rotated just beyond its available ROM. The force can be applied by manual contact or a mechanical device and can be sustained or intermittent. When the patient is as relaxed as possible during the stretch, it is called *passive stretching*. If the patient assists in moving the joint through a greater range, it is called *assisted stretching*.

Self-Stretching

Any stretching exercise that is carried out independently by a patient after instruction and supervision by a therapist is referred to as *self-stretching*. In this case forces are applied by the patient at the end of available ROM for the purpose of elongating hypomobile soft tissues. Flexibility exercises are also performed independently, but this term usually indicates stretching that is part of a general conditioning and fitness program by individuals without mobility impairments.

Neuromuscular Facilitation and Inhibition Techniques

Neuromuscular facilitation and inhibition procedures are founded on the concept of reflexively decreasing tension in shortened muscles prior to or during the stretch. Because the use of inhibition or facilitation techniques to assist with muscle elongation is associated with an approach to exercise known as proprioceptive neuromuscular facilitation (PNF),[136,148] many clinicians and some authors refer to these procedures as PNF stretching,[29,36,131] active inhibition,[70] active stretching,[158] or facilitated stretching.[117] Stretching procedures based on principles of PNF are discussed in a later section of this chapter.

Muscle Energy Techniques

Muscle energy techniques are manipulative procedures that evolved out of osteopathic medicine designed to lengthen muscle and fascia and to mobilize joints.[21,26,157] The procedures employ voluntary muscle contractions by the patient in a precisely controlled direction and intensity against a counterforce applied by the practitioner (see additional information in Chapter 5 and a description of specific techniques for the sacroiliac (SI) joint in Chapter 15 and subcranial region in Chapter 16). Because principles of neuromuscular inhibition are incorporated into this approach, another term used to describe these techniques is *postisometric relaxation*.

Joint Mobilization/Manipulation

Joint manipulative techniques are skilled manual therapy interventions specifically applied to joint structures by the clinician to modulate pain and treat joint impairments that limit ROM.[64,78] Principles of use and basic techniques for the extremity joints are described and illustrated in detail in Chapter 5, and mobilization with movement techniques for the extremities are described and illustrated in the regional chapters (see Chapters 17 to 22). Techniques for the ribs, sacrum, and temporomandibular joints are presented in Chapter 15 and for the spinal joints in Chapter 16.

Soft Tissue Mobilization/Manipulation

Soft tissue manipulative techniques are designed to improve the extensibility of any soft tissue that limits mobility. These techniques involve the application of specific and progressive manual forces using sustained manual pressure or slow, deep stroking. Specially crafted instruments can also be used by clinicians to apply these forces. Many techniques, including friction massage,[70,138] myofascial release,[20,63,93,138] acupressure,[70,138,147] and trigger point therapy,[93,138,147] are designed to improve tissue mobility by manipulating connective tissue that binds soft tissues. Although they are useful adjuncts to manual stretching procedures, specific techniques are not described in this textbook.

Neural Tissue Mobilization (Neuromeningeal Mobilization)

Neural mobilization techniques are used to improve or restore nerve tissue mobility. Neural tissue mobility may become restricted by tissue adhesions or scar tissue following trauma or surgical procedures. Increased tension placed on nerve tissue by these adhesions during joint motion can lead to pain or neurological symptoms. After specific tests are conducted to determine neural tissue mobility, the neural pathway is mobilized through selective procedures.[19,70] These techniques are described in Chapter 13.

BOX 4.1 Indications for Stretching

- ROM is limited because soft tissues have lost their extensibility as the result of adhesions, contractures, and scar tissue formation, causing activity limitations or participation restrictions.
- Restricted motion may lead to structural deformities that are otherwise preventable.
- Muscle weakness and shortening of opposing tissue have led to limited ROM.
- May be a component of a total fitness or sport-specific conditioning program designed to prevent or reduce the risk of musculoskeletal injuries.
- May be used prior to and after vigorous exercise.

BOX 4.2 Contraindications to Stretching

- A bony block limits joint motion.
- There was a recent fracture, and bony union is incomplete.
- There is evidence of an acute inflammatory or infectious process (heat and swelling), or soft tissue healing could be disrupted in the restricted tissues and surrounding region.
- There is sharp, acute pain with joint movement or muscle elongation.
- A hematoma or other indication of tissue trauma is observed.
- Joint hypermobility already exists.
- Shortened soft tissues provide necessary joint stability in lieu of normal structural stability or neuromuscular control.
- Shortened soft tissues enable a patient with paralysis or severe muscle weakness to perform specific functional skills otherwise not possible.

Indications, Contraindications, and Potential Outcomes of Stretching Exercises

Indications and Contraindications for Stretching

There are situations in which stretching exercises are appropriate and safe; however, there are also instances when stretching should not be implemented. Boxes 4.1 and 4.2 list indications and contraindications for the use of stretching interventions.

Potential Benefits and Outcomes of Stretching

Increased Flexibility and ROM

The expected outcome of stretching exercises is to restore or increase muscle-tendon unit extensibility to regain or achieve the flexibility and ROM required for functional activities. As discussed throughout this chapter, a considerable body of evidence has shown that stretching, particularly static and PNF stretching procedures, improves flexibility and increases ROM. (The parameters of stretching exercises that determine effectiveness, such as intensity, duration, and frequency, are discussed later in this chapter.)

The underlying mechanisms for stretch-induced gains in ROM include biomechanical and neural changes in the contractile and noncontractile elements of the muscle-tendon unit and surrounding fascia. These changes are thought to be the result of increased muscle extensibility and length or decreased muscle stiffness (passive muscle-tendon tension).[56,97,99,105,125] (These underlying effects are discussed in the next section of this chapter.) Fascia may respond to the heat and mechanical stress generated during stretching by increasing its compliance.[128] There is also speculation that increased ROM following stretching may result from a change in an individual's perception or tolerance of the sensation associated with stretching.[87,152] This is supported by evidence showing that static stretching improves dorsiflexion ROM without changing the structure of the musculotendinous unit, a result attributed to improved tolerance to 6 weeks of stretching.[85]

General Fitness

In addition to improving flexibility and ROM, stretching exercises routinely are recommended for warm-up prior to or cool-down following strenuous physical activity. They are also considered to be an essential part of conditioning programs for general fitness, for recreational or workplace activities, and for training in preparation for competitive sports.

Other Potential Benefits

Potential benefits and outcomes traditionally attributed to stretching exercises include the prevention or reduced risk of soft tissue injuries, reduced post-exercise (delayed onset) muscle soreness, and enhanced physical performance.[47,66,71,132,] However, the evidence to support these potential benefits is inconclusive.

Injury prevention and reduced post-exercise muscle soreness. Although decreased flexibility has been associated with a greater risk of lower extremity musculotendinous injuries,[159] it is not likely that stretching exercises prevent or reduce injury risk. The vast majority of studies, analyzed in several critical reviews of the literature, indicate little, if any, link between an acute bout of stretching for warm-up prior to a strenuous event and the prevention or reduction in the likelihood of soft tissue injuries[67,120,125,140] or the severity or duration of post-exercise, delayed-onset muscle soreness.[67,68]

Enhanced performance. Another potential benefit attributed to stretching is enhanced physical performance—such as increased muscular strength, power, or endurance—or improvements in physical functioning such as walking or running speed and jumping abilities.

Consequently, it is common for an individual who is participating in a fitness or sport-related training program to perform stretching exercises prior to a strength training session. Stretching is also commonly performed just before participation in an athletic event requiring strength or power, such as sprinting or performing a vertical jump.

To effectively evaluate the impact of stretching on physical performance, a distinction must be made between a bout of stretching carried out just before a strenuous activity (*acute or pre-event stretching*) and a program of stretching exercises performed on a regular basis over a period of weeks (*chronic stretching*). A systematic review of the literature[124] and subsequent studies[30] indicate that acute static stretching either has no effect or decreases—rather than enhances—muscle performance (strength, power, or endurance) immediately following the stretching session. Acute stretching also provides no benefit or has a negative effect on the performance of activities that require strength, such as sprinting or jumping.[9,56,109,124,133] These performance decrements are greatest when static stretches are held for longer than 90 seconds. To the contrary, acute *dynamic* stretching appears to lead to enhanced performance, especially with longer duration stretches (>90 seconds).[9] *Dynamic stretching* is defined as a controlled movement through the active ROM for each joint.[54] Similarly, performing stretching exercises as part of a comprehensive conditioning program on a regular basis over a period of weeks (*chronic stretching*) not only increases flexibility, but also appears to have beneficial effects on physical performance. This approach to stretching has been found to improve strength or power,[59,84,124,133] perhaps because of an alteration in the length-tension relationships of the stretched muscles. Participating in a stretching program on a regular basis also has been shown to improve gait economy[59] and enhance the performance of physical activities, such as sprinting and jumping abilities.[124,133]

Properties of Soft Tissue: Response to Immobilization and Stretch

The ability of the body to move without restriction during functional activities depends on active neuromuscular control and the passive extensibility of soft tissues. As noted above, the soft tissues that can become restricted and impair mobility include muscles with their contractile and noncontractile elements and various types of connective tissue (tendons, ligaments, joint capsules, fascia, and skin). In most instances, decreased extensibility of connective tissue is the primary cause of restricted mobility in both healthy individuals and patients after injury, disease, or surgery.

A period of immobilization is often used to protect joints or tissues after injury or surgery, which may result in soft tissue morphological adaptations. Each type of soft tissue has unique properties that affect its response to immobilization and its ability to regain extensibility after immobilization. When stretching procedures are applied to these soft tissues, the direction, velocity, intensity (magnitude), duration, and frequency of the stretch force, as well as tissue temperature, tension, and stiffness, all interact to affect the unique soft tissue responses and outcomes. Specifically, mechanical characteristics of contractile and noncontractile soft tissue and the neurophysiological properties of contractile tissue will affect tissue lengthening. In addition, increased extensibility of the muscle-tendon unit following stretching may result from a modification of the stretch sensation, such as the onset of end-range discomfort, perceived by an individual.[99,152]

Most of the information on the biomechanical, biochemical, and neurophysiological responses of soft tissues to immobilization and remobilization is derived from animal studies; as such, the exact physiological mechanism by which stretching increases the extensibility of human tissues is still unclear. However, studies using ultrasound imaging on musculotendinous tissue in humans have provided confirmation of previous experiments on tendon adaptability to stress using isolated material.[86,96] Specifically, decreased muscle stiffness, quantified as a decrease in shear elastic modulus using ultrasound elastography, has been identified as the likely mechanism for increased extensibility.[1,108] An understanding of the properties of these tissues and their responses to immobilization and stretch is the basis for selecting and applying the safest, most effective stretching procedures for patients with impaired mobility.[59]

When soft tissue is stretched, elastic, viscoelastic, or plastic changes occur. Both contractile and noncontractile tissues have elastic and plastic qualities, while only noncontractile connective tissues have viscoelastic properties.

- A stretched soft tissue is *elastic* if it returns to its prestretch resting length directly after a short-duration stretch force is removed.[24,39,90,91,111]
- *Viscoelasticity,* or viscoelastic deformation, is a time-dependent property of soft tissue. A viscoelastic tissue initially resists deformation, such as a change in length, when a stretch force is applied but will slowly lengthen if the force is sustained. The viscoelastic tissue will gradually return to its prestretch configuration after the stretch force is removed.[90,97,98,111,152]
- *Plasticity,* or plastic deformation, is the tendency of soft tissue to assume a new and greater length after a stretch force is removed.[90,145,152]

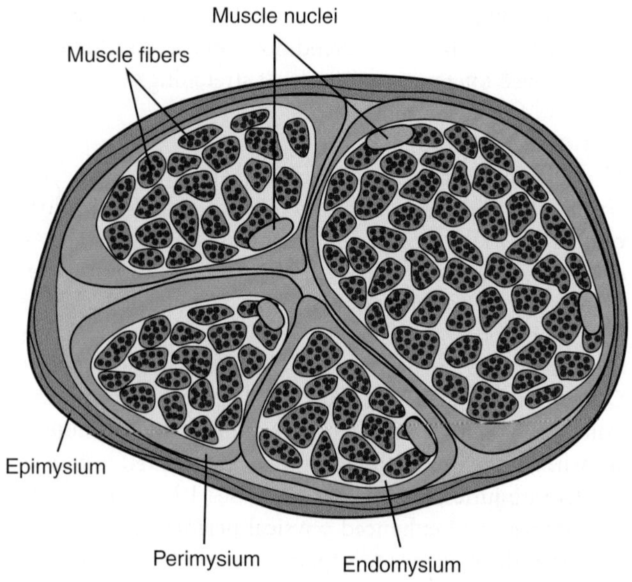

Muscle nuclei
Muscle fibers
Epimysium
Perimysium
Endomysium

FIGURE 4.1 Muscular connective tissue. Cross-sectional view of the connective tissue in a muscle shows how the perimysium is continuous with the outer layer of epimysium. *(From Chleboun, G: Muscle structure and function. In Levangie, PK, and Norkin, CC [eds]:* Joint Structure and Function: A Comprehensive Analysis, *ed. 5. Philadelphia: FA Davis, 2011, p 117, with permission.)*

Mechanical Properties of Noncontractile Soft Tissue

Noncontractile soft tissue permeates the entire body and is organized into various types of connective tissue to support the structures of the body. Ligaments, tendons, joint capsules, fascia, noncontractile tissue in muscles (Fig. 4.1), and skin all possess connective tissue characteristics that can lead to the development of adhesions and contractures. Any of these tissues can lose extensibility and contribute to reduced mobility. When these tissues restrict joint ROM and require stretching, it is important to understand how they respond to the intensity and duration of stretch forces and to recognize that the only way to increase the extensibility of connective tissue is to remodel its basic architecture.[33]

Composition of Connective Tissue

Connective tissue is composed of three types of fiber: collagen, elastin and reticulin, and nonfibrous ground substance consisting of proteoglycans and glycoproteins.[34,145]

Collagen fibers. Collagen fibers are responsible for the strength and stiffness of tissue and resist tensile deformation. Tropocollagen crystals form the building blocks of collagen microfibrils. Each additional level of composition of the fibers is arranged in an organized relationship and dimension (Fig. 4.2). There are six classes with 19 types[29] of collagen. As collagen fibers develop and mature, they bind together, initially with unstable hydrogen bonding, then convert to stable covalent bonding. The stronger these bonds, the greater the mechanical stability of the tissue. Tissue with a larger proportion of collagen provides greater stability.

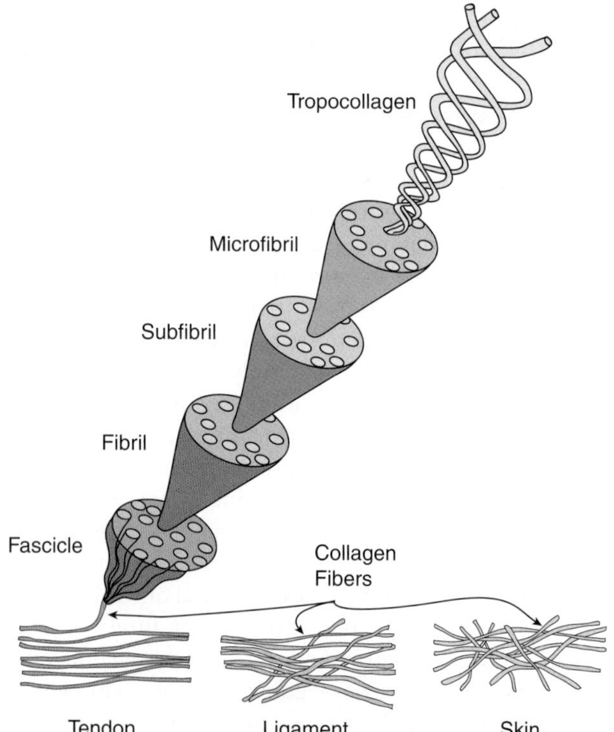

FIGURE 4.2 Composition of collagen fibers showing the aggregation of tropocollagen crystals as the building blocks of collagen. Organization of the fibers in connective tissue is related to the function of the tissue. Tissues with parallel fiber orientation, such as tendons, are able to withstand greater tensile loads than tissue, such as skin, in which the fiber orientation appears more random.

Elastin fibers. Elastin fibers provide extensibility. They show a great deal of elongation with small loads and fail abruptly without deformation at higher loads. Tissues with higher amounts of elastin have greater flexibility.

Reticulin fibers. Reticulin fibers provide tissue with bulk.

Ground substance. Ground substance is an organic gel containing water and is made up of proteoglycans (PGs) and glycoproteins. The PGs function to hydrate the matrix, stabilize the collagen networks, and resist compressive forces—especially important in cartilage and intervertebral discs. The type and amount of PGs are proportional to the types of compressive and tensile stress that the tissue is functionally subjected to.[34] Glycoproteins provide linkage between the main tissue matrix components and between the cells and the matrix opponents. The ground substance functions to reduce friction between fibers, transport nutrients and metabolites within the tissue, and maintain space between fibers to help prevent excessive cross-linking between them.[44,145]

Mechanical Behavior of Noncontractile Tissue

The mechanical behavior of the various noncontractile tissues is determined by the proportion of collagen and elastin fibers, the proportion of PGs, and by the structural orientation of the fibers. Those tissues that withstand high tensile loads are high in collagen fibers; those that withstand greater compressive loads have greater concentrations of PGs. The composition of the tissue changes when the loading environment changes.[34]

Collagen is the structural element that absorbs most of the tensile stress. Its mechanical behavior is explained with reference to the stress-strain curve described in the following paragraphs. With an externally applied load, collagen fibers elongate quickly as wavy fibers align and straighten. With increased loading, tension increases and the fibers stiffen. Continued loading will progressively increase fiber strain until a point where bonds between collagen fibers begin to break. When a substantial number of bonds are broken, the fibers themselves will ultimately fail. Failure of collagen due to tensile loading occurs at less than 10% increase in fiber length, whereas elastin may lengthen 150% without failure. However, collagen is five times as strong as elastin. The alignment and orientation of collagen fibers in a particular tissue reflects the typical tensile loading pattern acting on that tissue (see Fig. 4.2):

- In tendons, collagen fibers are parallel and can resist the greatest tensile load. Their fiber alignment is in series with muscle fibers to transmit muscle forces to the bone.
- In skin, collagen fibers have a random orientation and so are limited in resisting higher levels of tension.
- In ligaments, joint capsules, and fascia, collagen fiber alignment varies so that they can resist multidirectional forces. Ligaments that resist major joint stresses have a more parallel orientation of collagen fibers and a larger cross-sectional area.[113]

Interpreting Mechanical Behavior of Connective Tissue: The Stress-Strain Curve

The stress-strain curve illustrates the mechanical strength of structures (Fig. 4.3) and is used to interpret what is happening to connective tissue under stress from an externally applied load.[34,143,145] When a tensile load is applied to a structure, it produces elongation; the stress-strain curve illustrates the strength properties, stiffness, and amount of energy the material can store before failure of the structure.

- *Stress* is force (or load) per unit area. Mechanical stress is the internal reaction or resistance to an externally applied load.
- *Strain* is the amount of deformation or lengthening that occurs when an external load (such as a stretch force) is applied to a structure.

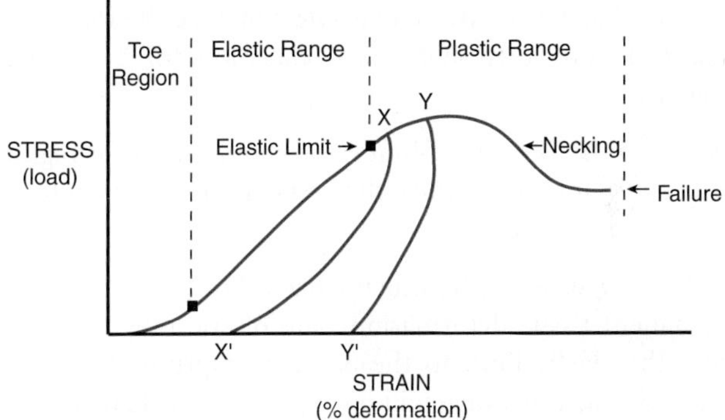

FIGURE 4.3 Stress-strain curve. When stressed, the wavy collagen fibers straighten (toe region). With additional stress, recoverable deformation occurs in the elastic range. Once the elastic limit is reached, sequential failure of the collagen fibers and tissue occurs in the plastic range, resulting in release of heat and new length when the stress is released. The length from the stress point (X) results in a new length when released (X′); the heat released is represented by the area under the curve between these two points. Y to Y′ represents additional length from additional stress into the plastic region with more heat released. Necking is the region in which there is considerable weakening of the tissue, and less force is needed for deformation. Total failure quickly follows even under small loads.

Types of Stress

There are three kinds of stress that develop in a structure in response to an applied load:

- *Tension*—the resistance to a force applied in a manner that will lengthen the tissue. A stretching force results in tension stress.
- *Compression*—resistance to a force applied in a manner that approximates tissue. Weight bearing through a joint will produce compression stresses.
- *Shear*—resistance to two or more forces that are applied in opposing directions.

Regions of the Stress-Strain Curve

Toe region. Because collagen fibers are wavy and within a three-dimensional matrix at rest, their first response to loading is to straighten and align. This response occurs with minimally applied force and results in small increases in tissue stress. The toe region of the stress-strain curve represents this behavior and is the range in which most functional activity normally occurs.

Elastic range/linear phase. Adjacent to the toe region, stress and strain have a direct relationship such that a change in stress results in a proportional change in strain. This is called the linear region, and its slope depends on the specific tissues response to loading. A tissue that responds to loading with a rapid rise in strain, such as bone, will have a steep slope and higher stiffness than a tissue that responds with a smaller rise in strain. With respect to stretching, tissue stress beyond the toe region aligns collagen fibers in the direction of applied force. As strain increases, some microfailure between the collagen bonds begins and water may be displaced from the ground substance. If strain does not increase beyond the linear region or is not maintained, the tissue returns to its original size and shape when the load is released. (See the following discussion on creep and stress-relaxation for prolonged stretch.)

Elastic limit The elastic limit is the end of the linear region and the point beyond which the tissue does not return to its original shape and size.

Plastic range. Strain beyond the elastic limit begins to cause permanent tissue deformation. The plastic range extends from the elastic limit to the point of rupture and tissue strained into this range will have permanent deformation after the external load is released. Plastic deformation results from sequential failure (microfailure) of the bonds between collagen fibrils and eventually of collagen fibers. Because collagen is crystalline, individual fibers rupture rather than stretch, a process that may result in increased length from stretching.

Ultimate strength. The maximum strain the tissue can sustain is its ultimate strength. Once this point is reached, further increase in strain does not result in increased stress due to tissue macrofailure. The region of necking is reached in which there is considerable weakening of the tissue, and it rapidly fails. Experimentally, maximum tensile deformation (strain) of isolated collagen fibers prior to failure is 7% to 8%, while whole ligaments may withstand strains of 20% to 40% before failing.[113]

Failure. Failure is reached when the tissue ruptures and loses its integrity.

Structural stiffness. The slope of the linear portion of the curve (elastic range) is known as Young's modulus or the modulus of elasticity and represents the stiffness of the tissue.[34] Tissues with greater stiffness have a steeper slope in the elastic region, with less elastic deformation as stress increases. Contractures and scar tissue have greater stiffness, probably because of a greater degree of bonding between collagen fibers and their surrounding matrix. Tissues with less stiffness will demonstrate greater elongation than those with greater stiffness under similar external loads.[34]

CLINICAL TIP

The grades of ligament injuries (strains) are related to the stress-strain curve.

- **Grade I**—Microfailure: rupture of some fibers after deformation into the early part of the plastic range.
- **Grade II**—Macrofailure: rupture of an increased number of fibers and partial failure after deformation into the later part of the plastic range.
- **Grade III**—Complete rupture or tissue failure after deformation beyond the plastic range.

Time and Rate Influences on Tissue Deformation

Because connective tissue has viscoelastic properties, the amount of time and the rate at which an external load is applied to tissue will affect its response.

Rate dependence. When a load is rapidly applied to a viscoelastic tissue, the slope of the stress-strain curve will be steeper than if the load is applied slowly. In essence, the tissue becomes stiffer when the load is applied at a high rate. This increased stress response protects the tissue by keeping deformation below the plastic range and minimizing the potential for failure. Viscoelasticity is an extremely valuable tissue property because it allows the body to tolerate high loads applied over short durations—a combination often encountered during high velocity events or activities. A tissue load that is applied gradually during a stretch will minimize this rate-dependent response.

Creep. When a gradually increasing external load is applied to a viscoelastic tissue and then sustained, the tissue will continue to slowly elongate during the maintained stretch (Fig. 4.4A). This slow adaptation to sustained loading is a time-dependent property of a viscoelastic tissue. The amount of tissue deformation depends on the amount of force and the rate at which the force is applied. Low-magnitude loads reaching the elastic range and applied for long periods of time increase connective tissue deformation and allow gradual rearrangement of collagen fiber bonds (remodeling) and redistribution of water to surrounding tissues.[33,91,143] Increasing the temperature of the tissue enhances creep and the extensibility of the tissue.[150,154] Complete recovery from creep may occur over time, but not as rapidly as recovery from a short duration load. Long-duration stretches applied to chronic contractures take advantage of this tissue property.

Stress-relaxation. When a sub-failure load is applied to a viscoelastic tissue and kept constant, there is a gradual decrease in the force required to maintain the amount of deformation[33] (Fig. 4.4B). This response is also a function of the viscoelastic qualities of the connective tissue and redistribution of water content. Stress-relaxation is the underlying principle used in prolonged stretching procedures in which the stretch position is maintained for several hours or days. Recovery versus permanent changes in length is dependent on both the amount of deformation and the length of time the deformation is maintained.[33]

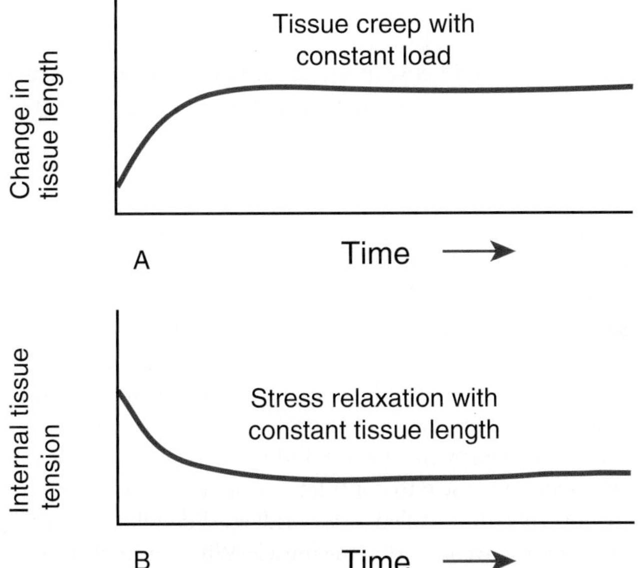

FIGURE 4.4 Tissue responses to prolonged stretch forces as a result of viscoelastic properties. **(A)** Effects of creep. A constant load, applied over time, results in increased tissue length until equilibrium is reached. **(B)** Effects of stress-relaxation. A load applied with the tissue kept at a constant length results in decreased internal tension in the tissue until equilibrium is reached.

Cyclic loading and connective tissue fatigue. Repetitive loading of tissue within a short time duration increases heat production and may cause failure at strain levels lower than what is needed for a single load. Similarly, the greater these repetitive loads, the fewer number of cycles needed to reach failure. This phenomenon is referred to as connective tissue fatigue. Examples of connective tissue fatigue from cyclic loading are stress fractures and overuse syndromes. These represent situations where the load intensity and number of repetitions exceed the endurance limit, below which an apparently infinite number of cycles of low loading will not cause failure. Animal studies confirm that cyclic loading will result in decreased ligament stiffness, indicative of tissue damage, sooner than will static loading.[142]

Summary of Mechanical Principles for Stretching Connective Tissue

- Connective tissue deformation (stretch) varies depending on the magnitude of loading and the rate of load application. Permanent changes in tissue length or flexibility requires breaking of collagen bonds and realignment of the fibers. Tissue failure begins as microfailure of fibrils and fibers before complete failure occurs. Complete tissue failure can occur as a single maximal event or from repetitive submaximal stress. Microfailure that induces permanent lengthening can occur through creep, stress-relaxation, and controlled cyclic loading.
- Healing and adaptive remodeling capabilities allow the tissue to respond to repetitive and sustained loads if time is allowed between bouts. This is important for increasing both flexibility and tensile strength of the tissue. If healing and remodeling time is not allowed, a breakdown of tissue (failure) occurs as in overuse syndromes and stress fractures. Intensive stretching is usually not done every day in order to allow time for healing. If the inflammation from the microruptures is excessive, additional scar tissue, which could become more restrictive, is laid down.[33]
- It is imperative that the individual use any newly gained range to allow the remodeling of tissue and to train the muscle to control the new range. Without functional use of the newly gained range, the tissue may gradually return to its shortened length.

Changes in Collagen Affecting the Stress-Strain Response

Effects of Immobilization

Immobilization causes collagen turnover and weak bonding between the new, nonstressed fibers, resulting in decreased stiffness. There is also greater cross-linking between disorganized collagen fibers and decreased effectiveness of the ground substance in maintaining space and lubrication between the fibers, resulting in adhesion formation.[44,143] The rate of return to normal tensile strength for immobilized tissue is slow. For example, after 8 weeks of immobilization, the anterior cruciate ligament in monkeys failed at 61% of maximum load; after 5 months of reconditioning, it failed at 79%; and after 12 months of reconditioning, it failed at 91%.[112,114] There was also a reduction in energy absorbed and a decrease in stiffness prior to failure following immobilization.[112]

Effects of Inactivity (Decrease of Normal Activity)

Inactivity decreases the size and amount of collagen fibers, resulting in weakening of the tissue.[34] With collagen decrease there is a proportional increase in the predominance of elastin fibers, resulting in increased tissue compliance. Recovery from these changes takes about 5 months of regular cyclic loading. Physical activity has a beneficial effect on the strength of connective tissue.

Effects of Age

Aging decreases maximum tensile strength and stiffness of tissue, and the rate of adaptation to loading is slower. There is an increased tendency for overuse syndromes, fatigue failures, and tears with stretching.[113]

Effects of Corticosteroids

Corticosteroid use has a long-lasting deleterious effect on the mechanical properties of collagen with a subsequent decrease in tensile strength.[34] Adverse effects from corticosteroid injections include decreased collagen synthesis and organization, necrosis, and an increased ratio of type III to type I collagen.[37] There is fibrocyte death next to the injection site with delay in reappearance up to 15 weeks.[113]

Effects of Injury

Damaged tissue follows a predictable healing pattern (see Chapter 10), with newly synthesized type III collagen bridging the injury site. This collagen is structurally weaker than mature type I collagen. As remodeling progresses, the collagen eventually matures to type I. Remodeling usually begins about 3 weeks post-injury and continues for several months to a year, depending on the size of the connective tissue structure and the magnitude of the rupture.

Other Conditions Affecting Collagen

Nutritional deficiencies, hormonal imbalances, and dialysis may predispose connective tissue to injury at lower levels of loading than normal.[34]

Mechanical and Physiological Properties of Muscle Tissue

Muscle is composed of both contractile and noncontractile connective tissues. The contractile elements of muscle (Fig. 4.5) give it the characteristics of contractility and irritability.

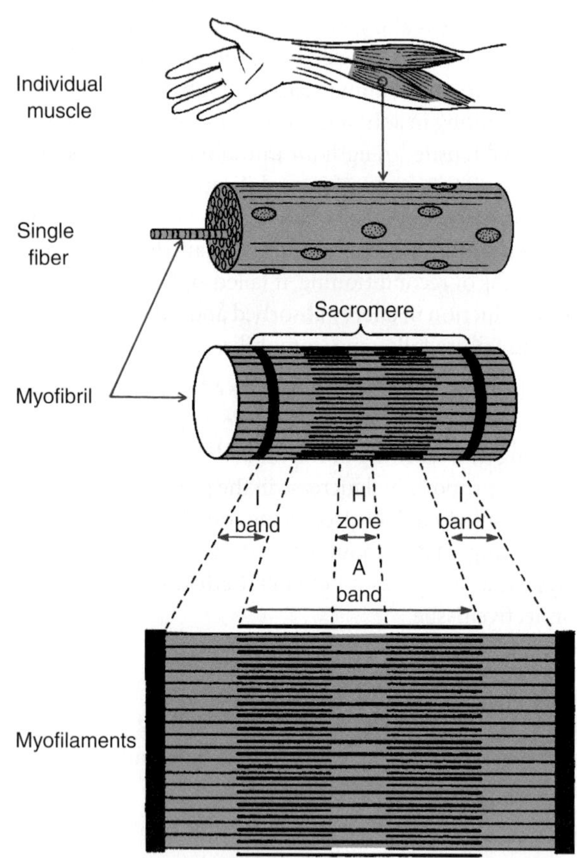

FIGURE 4.5 Structure of skeletal muscle.

The noncontractile connective tissues in and around muscle (see Fig. 4.1) have the same properties as all connective tissue, including the ability to resist deforming forces.[24,97,98] The noncontractile connective tissue structures of muscle are the *endomysium,* which is the innermost layer that separates individual muscle fibers and myofibrils; the *perimysium,* which encases fiber bundles; and the *epimysium,* which is the fascial sheath enveloping the entire muscle. It is this connective tissue framework of muscle that is the primary source of a muscle's resistance to passive elongation.[24,33,111] Tissue adhesions within and between the collagen fibers of these structural tissues can resist and restrict movement and result in joint contracture.[33]

Contractile Elements of Muscle

Individual muscles are composed of many muscle fibers that lie in parallel with one another. A single muscle fiber is made up of many myofibrils. Each myofibril is composed of even smaller structures called sarcomeres, which lie in series (end-to-end) within a myofibril. The sarcomere is the contractile unit of the myofibril and is composed of overlapping myofilaments of actin and myosin proteins. The sarcomeres give muscle the ability to contract and relax. When a motor unit stimulates a muscle to contract, the actin-myosin filaments form connections called cross-bridges, slide relative to each other, and actively shorten the muscle. When a muscle relaxes, the myofilaments slide apart slightly, and the muscle returns to its resting length (Fig. 4.6).

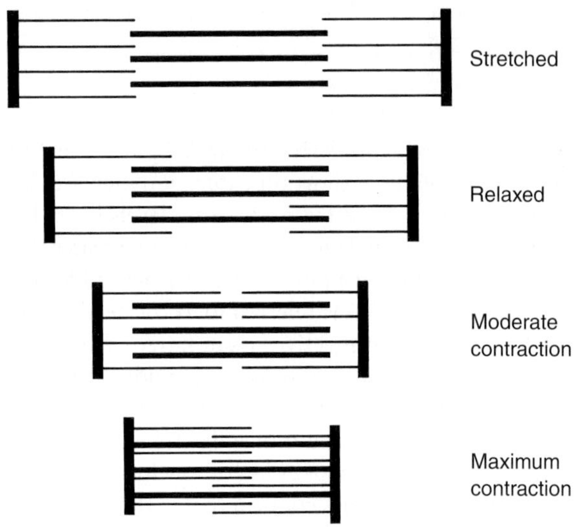

FIGURE 4.6 A model of myofilament sliding. Elongation and shortening of the sarcomere, the contractile unit of muscle.

Mechanical Response of the Contractile Unit to Stretch and Immobilization

There are a number of changes in the anatomical structure and physiological function of the sarcomeres that can occur over time. These changes can result from a stretch during an exercise or from extended periods of immobilization followed by remobilization. The noncontractile structures in and around muscle also affect a muscle's response to stretch and immobilization.[31,90]

Response to Stretch

When a muscle is stretched and elongates, the stretch force is transmitted to the muscle fibers through the endomysium and perimysium. It is hypothesized that molecular interactions link these noncontractile elements to the sarcomere and enable this force transduction.[39]

During a passive stretch, both longitudinal (in series) and lateral (in parallel) force transduction occurs in muscle.[39] During initial lengthening, tension rises sharply in the series elastic component. With continued lengthening there is mechanical disruption of the cross-bridges as the myofilaments slide apart, leading to abrupt lengthening of the sarcomeres,[39,55,90,91] sometimes referred to as *sarcomere give.*[55] When the stretch force is released, the individual sarcomeres return to their resting length[39,90,91] (see Fig. 4.6). As noted previously, the property of muscle promoting return to its resting length after short-term stretch is called elasticity. For longer lasting or more permanent (viscoelastic or plastic) length increases to occur the stretch force must be maintained over an extended period of time.[39,90,152]

Response to Immobilization and Remobilization

Morphological changes. If a muscle is subjected to prolonged immobilization, it is not used during functional activities and the physical stresses placed on it are substantially diminished. This results in decay of contractile protein in the immobilized muscle, as well as decreases in muscle fiber diameter, the number of myofibrils, and intramuscular capillary density. The outcome of this process is muscle *atrophy* and *weakness.*[13,17,60,77,80,90,106,141] As the immobilized muscle atrophies, an increase in fibrous and fatty tissue in muscle also occurs.[106]

The composition of muscle affects its response to immobilization, with atrophy occurring more quickly and more extensively in tonic (slow-twitch) postural muscle fibers than in phasic (fast-twitch) fibers.[90,91] The duration and position of immobilization also affect the extent of atrophy and weakness, with longer duration leading to greater atrophy and loss of functional strength. Atrophy can begin within as little as a few days to a week.[79,80,141] Accompanying the decrease in cross-sectional size of muscle fibers with atrophy, an even more significant deterioration in motor unit recruitment occurs as reflected by electromyographic (EMG) activity.[90,91] Both of these factors compromise the force-producing capabilities of the muscle.

Immobilization in a shortened position. In studies using animals, when a muscle is immobilized in a shortened position for several weeks there is a reduction in muscle length, the number of muscle fibers, and the number of sarcomeres in series within myofibrils as the result of *sarcomere absorption.*[77,90,137] This absorption occurs at a faster rate than the muscle's ability to regenerate sarcomeres in an attempt to restore itself. This decrease in the overall muscle length and the number of sarcomeres results in muscle atrophy and weakness. It has also been suggested that a muscle immobilized in a shortened position atrophies and weakens at a faster rate than a muscle immobilized in a lengthened state.[17]

With muscle shortening due to immobilization, there is a shift to the left in its length-tension curve, decreasing its capacity to produce maximum tension as it contracts at its normal resting length.[24] The decrease in muscle length also results in an earlier onset of passive tension as the muscle is stretched. This mechanical alteration is related to the new muscle length and to the increased proportion of connective tissue to muscle tissue that results from immobilization. Importantly, the increase in connective tissue and early onset of passive tension also serves to protect the shorter and weaker muscle when it is elongated.[33,60]

Immobilization in a lengthened position. Sometimes a muscle is immobilized in a lengthened position for a prolonged period of time. This occurs with some surgical procedures, such as a limb lengthening,[14] the application of a series of positional casts (serial casts),[72] or the use of a dynamic orthosis to stretch a long-standing contracture and increase ROM.[12,101] There is some evidence from animal studies,[137] but very limited evidence from studies involving human skeletal muscle,[14] to suggest that a muscle held in a lengthened position for an extended time adapts by increasing the number of sarcomeres in series, sometimes referred to as *myofibrillogenesis.*[39] It is theorized that sarcomere addition maintains the optimal functional overlap of actin and myosin filaments in the muscle[90] and may be relatively permanent if the newly gained length is used on a regular basis in functional activities.

The minimum time necessary for an elongated muscle (fiber) to become a longer muscle (fiber) by adding sarcomeres in series is not known. In animal studies, increased muscle length as the result of sarcomere number addition required continuous immobilization in a lengthened position for several weeks.[90] It is speculated that this same process contributes to gains in muscle length (indirectly quantified by increases in joint ROM) following the use of serial casts,[72] dynamic orthoses,[101] and perhaps as the result of stretching exercises.[39] Interestingly, direct evidence of sarcomere adaptation in human skeletal muscle was recently reported following long-term, continuous limb distraction used to lengthen a patient's femur.[14]

Adaptation. The adaptation of the contractile units of muscle (an increase or decrease in the number of sarcomeres) to prolonged positioning in either lengthened or shortened positions is transient, lasting only 3 to 5 weeks if the muscle resumes its pre-immobilization use and degree of lengthening for functional activities.[80,90] In clinical practice, this underscores the need for patients to use full-range motions during a variety of functional activities to maintain the stretch-induced gains in muscle extensibility and joint ROM.

Neurophysiological Properties of Skeletal Muscle

The neurophysiological properties of the muscle-tendon unit will also influence a muscle's response to stretch and the effectiveness of stretching interventions. In particular, two sensory organs of muscle-tendon units, the *muscle spindle* and the *Golgi tendon organ* (GTO), are mechanoreceptors that convey information to the central nervous system about the physical environment within the muscle-tendon unit. This information often results in muscle responses that may impact the effectiveness of a stretch.

Muscle Spindle

The muscle spindle is the major sensory organ of muscle and is sensitive to quick and sustained (tonic) stretch (Fig. 4.7). The main function of muscle spindles is to detect and convey information about muscle length changes and the velocity of those changes.

Muscle spindles are small, encapsulated receptors composed of afferent sensory fiber endings, efferent motor fiber endings, and specialized muscle fibers called *intrafusal fibers.* Intrafusal muscle fibers are bundled together and lie between and parallel to the extrafusal muscle fibers that make up the main body of a skeletal muscle.[60,73,94,119] Intrafusal muscle fibers connect at their ends to extrafusal muscle fibers, so when a muscle is stretched, intrafusal fibers are also stretched. Intrafusal muscle fibers can also contract, but only their ends (polar regions), not their central portion (equatorial region), are contractile. Consequently, when an intrafusal muscle fiber is stimulated and contracts, it lengthens the central portion and activates the sensory receptors in the nuclear bag and chain. Small-diameter motor neurons, known as *gamma* motor neurons, innervate the contractile polar regions of intrafusal muscle fibers and adjust the sensitivity of muscle spindles to detect length changes. Large-diameter *alpha* motor neurons innervate extrafusal fibers.

There are two general types of intrafusal muscle fibers: *nuclear bag fibers* and *nuclear chain fibers,* named based on the arrangement of their nuclei in the equatorial region. Primary (type Ia) afferent endings, which arise from nuclear bag fibers, sense and cause muscle to respond to both quick and sustained stretch. However, secondary (type II) afferents from the nuclear chain fibers are sensitive only to sustained stretch.

The primary and secondary afferents synapse on alpha or gamma motoneurons, which, when stimulated, cause excitation of their own extrafusal or intrafusal muscle fibers, respectively. There are essentially two ways to stimulate these sensory afferents by means of stretch—one is by overall lengthening of the muscle and the other is by contraction of the intrafusal muscle fibers via the gamma efferent neural pathways.

Golgi Tendon Organ

The GTO is a sensory organ located near the musculotendinous junctions of extrafusal muscle fibers. The function of a GTO is to monitor changes in tension of muscle-tendon units. These encapsulated nerve endings are woven among collagen strands of a tendon and transmit sensory information via Ib fibers. These sensory organs are sensitive to even slight changes of tension on a muscle-tendon unit brought on by passive stretch or active muscle contractions during normal movement.

When muscle tension develops, GTO activation signals to the spinal cord inhibit alpha motoneuron activity and decrease tension in the muscle-tendon unit.[22,60,73,119] With respect to the neuromuscular system, *inhibition* is a state of decreased neuronal activity and altered synaptic potential, which diminishes the capacity of a muscle to contract.[71,73,94]

Originally, the GTO was thought to respond only to high levels of muscle tension as a protective mechanism for muscle. However, the GTO has since been shown to have a low threshold for firing, functioning to continuously monitor and adjust the force of active muscle contractions during movement or the tension in muscle during passive stretch.[57,119]

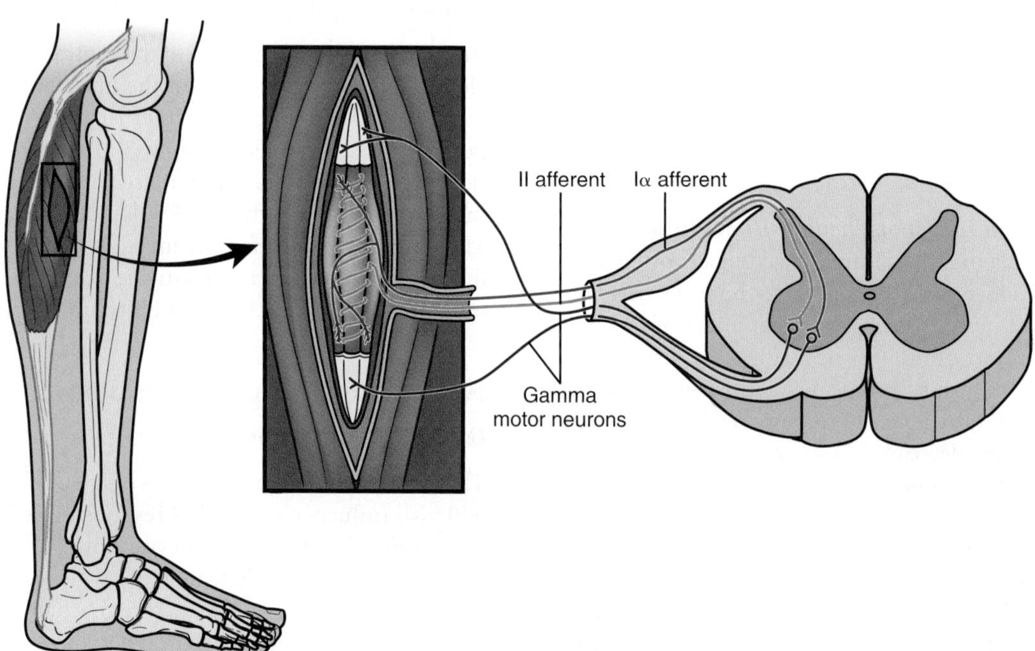

FIGURE 4.7 Muscle spindle showing intrafusal and extrafusal muscle fibers, stretch receptors, afferent and efferent nerve fibers, and spinal cord processes.

Neurophysiological Response of Muscle to Stretch

Stretch reflex. When a quick or sustained stretch force is applied to a muscle-tendon unit, the primary and secondary afferents of intrafusal muscle fibers sense these length changes. These afferent signals synapse with alpha motor neurons in the spinal cord to activate extrafusal muscle fibers. This motor response is known as the stretch reflex, defined as an increase or facilitation of active tension in the muscle being stretched. This increased tension resists lengthening and is thought to compromise the effectiveness of the stretching procedure.[8,43] When the stretch reflex is activated in a muscle being lengthened, decreased activity (inhibition) in the muscle(s) on the opposite side of the joint also may occur.[94,148] This is referred to as *reciprocal inhibition* but to date has only been documented in studies using animal models.[22,131,152] To minimize activation of the stretch reflex and the subsequent increase in muscle tension, a slowly applied, low-intensity, prolonged stretch is considered preferable to a quickly applied, short-duration stretch.

Autogenic inhibition. In contrast, the GTO has an inhibitory effect on the level of muscle tension in the muscle-tendon unit in which it lies, particularly if the stretch force is prolonged. This effect is called *autogenic inhibition*.[60,94,119] Inhibition of the contractile components of muscle by the GTO is thought to contribute to reflexive muscle relaxation during a stretching maneuver, enabling a muscle to be elongated against less muscle tension. Consequently, if a low-intensity, slow stretch force is applied to muscle, the stretch reflex is less likely to be activated as the GTO fires and inhibits tension in the muscle, allowing the parallel elastic component (the sarcomeres) of the muscle to remain relaxed and to lengthen.

In summary, current evidence suggests that improvement in muscle extensibility attributed to stretching procedures is more likely due to tensile stresses placed on the viscoelastic, noncontractile connective tissue in and around muscle than to inhibition (reflexive relaxation) of the contractile elements of muscle.[22,97,98,99,131]

Determinants and Types of Stretching Exercises

There are a number of essential elements that determine the effectiveness and outcomes of stretching interventions. The determinants (parameters) of stretching, all of which are interrelated, include *alignment* and *stabilization* of the body or body segment during stretching; the *intensity, duration, speed, frequency*, and *mode* of stretch; and the integration of neuromuscular factors and functional activities into stretching programs. By manipulating the determinants of stretching interventions, which are defined in Box 4.3, a therapist has many options from which to choose when designing stretching programs that are safe and effective and meet the needs, functional goals, and capabilities of many patients. Each of these determinants is discussed in this section of the chapter.

BOX 4.3 Determinants of Stretching Interventions

- *Alignment:* Positioning a limb or the body such that the stretch force is directed to the appropriate muscle group.
- *Stabilization:* Fixation of a bony segment that has an attachment of the muscle to be stretched.
- *Intensity of stretch:* Magnitude of the stretch force applied.
- *Duration of stretch:* Length of time the stretch force is applied during a stretch cycle.
- *Speed of stretch:* Rate of initial application of the stretch force.
- *Frequency of stretch*: Number of stretching sessions per day or per week.
- *Mode of stretch:* Form or manner in which the stretch force is applied (static, ballistic, or cyclic), degree of patient participation (passive, assisted, or active), or the source of the stretch force (manual, mechanical, or self).

Most investigations comparing the type, intensity, duration, and frequency of effective stretching have been carried out with healthy, young adults as subjects. The findings and recommendations of these studies are difficult to generalize and apply to patients with long-standing contractures or other forms of tissue restriction. Therefore, many decisions, particularly those related to the type, intensity, duration, and frequency of stretching, must continue to be based on a balance of scientific evidence and sound clinical judgments by the therapist.

There are four broad categories of stretching exercises: static stretching, cyclic (intermittent) stretching, ballistic stretching, and stretching techniques based on the principles of PNF.[38,47,69,163] Each of these forms of stretching are effective in elongating tissue and increasing ROM. Each can be accomplished in various ways—manually or mechanically, passively or actively, and by a therapist or independently by a patient—giving rise to many terms that are used in the literature to describe stretching interventions. The stretching interventions listed in Box 4.4 are defined and discussed in this section.

Alignment and Stabilization

Just as appropriate alignment and effective stabilization are fundamental components of muscle testing, goniometry, and all therapeutic exercises, they are also essential elements of effective stretching.

Alignment

Proper alignment or positioning of the patient and the specific muscles and joints to be stretched is necessary for patient comfort and stability during stretching. Alignment influences the baseline amount of tension present in soft tissue and

BOX 4.4 Types of Stretching

- Static stretching
- Cyclic/intermittent stretching
- Ballistic stretching
- Proprioceptive neuromuscular facilitation stretching procedures (PNF stretching)
- Manual stretching
- Mechanical stretching
- Self-stretching
- Passive stretching
- Active stretching

consequently affects the available joint ROM. In addition to the alignment of the muscles and joint to be stretched, the alignment of the trunk and adjacent joints must also be considered. For example, to effectively stretch the rectus femoris, a muscle that crosses two joints, the lumbar spine and pelvis, should be maintained in a neutral position as the knee is flexed and the hip extended. Because effective stretching requires maximizing the distance between origin and insertion, alignment that compromises this requirement—such as pelvis anterior tilt or hip flexion or abduction in our example—must be avoided (Fig. 4.8 A and B). Similarly, when a patient is self-stretching to increase shoulder flexion, the trunk should be erect, not slumped (Fig. 4.9 A and B).

NOTE: Throughout this and later chapters, recommendations for appropriate alignment and positioning during stretching procedures are identified. If it is not possible for a patient to attain the recommended postures because of discomfort, restrictions of motion of adjacent joints, inadequate neuromuscular control, or insufficient cardiopulmonary capacity, the therapist must critically analyze the situation to determine an alternative position.

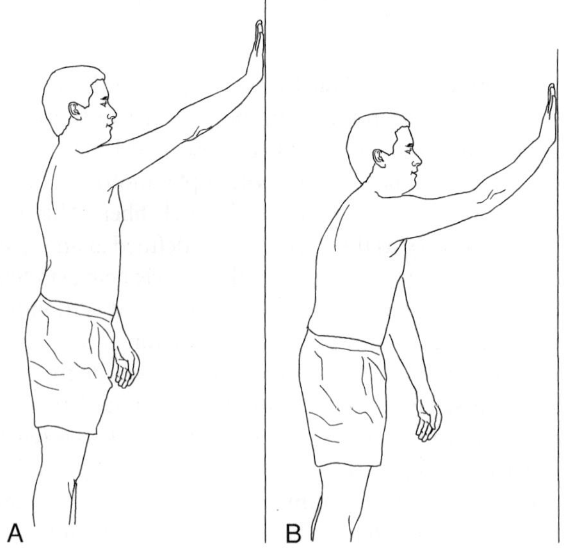

FIGURE 4.9 (A) Correct alignment when stretching to increase shoulder flexion: Note that the cervical and thoracic spine is erect. **(B)** Incorrect alignment: Note the forward head and rounded spine.

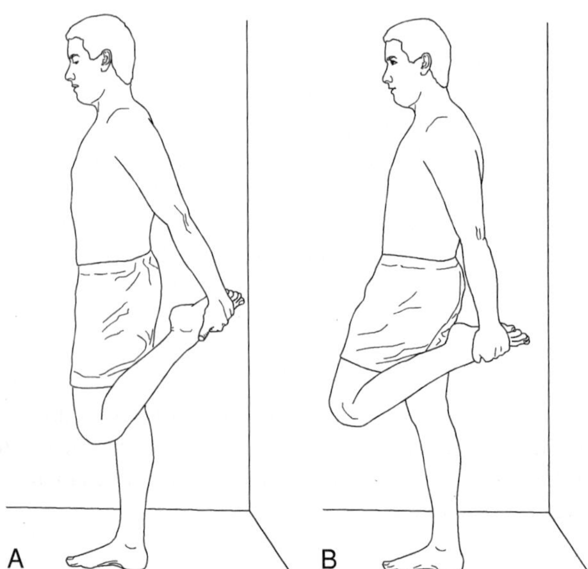

FIGURE 4.8 (A) Correct alignment when stretching the rectus femoris: The lumbar spine, pelvis, and hip are held in a neutral position as the knee is flexed. **(B)** Incorrect position of the hip in flexion. In addition, avoid anterior pelvic tilt, hyperextension of the lumbar spine, and abduction of the hip.

Stabilization

To achieve an effective stretch of a specific muscle or muscle group and associated periarticular structures, it is imperative to stabilize (fixate) either the proximal or distal attachment site of the muscle-tendon unit being elongated. Without stabilization, the attachment sites are free to move with the tissue, reducing the ability to effectively maximize the origin-insertion distance. Either site may be stabilized, but for manual stretching, it is common for a therapist to stabilize the proximal attachment and move the distal segment, as shown in Figure 4.10 A.

For self-stretching procedures, a stationary object, such as a chair or a doorframe, or active muscle contractions by the patient may provide stabilization of one segment as the other segment moves. During self-stretching, it is often the distal attachment that is stabilized as the proximal segment moves (Fig. 4.10 B).

Stabilization of multiple body segments also helps maintain the proper alignment necessary for an effective stretch. For example, when stretching the iliopsoas, the pelvis and lumbar spine must maintain a neutral position as the hip is extended to avoid stress to the low back region (see Fig. 4.26). Sources of stabilization include manual contacts; straps or belts; body weight; or a firm surface, such as a table, wall, or floor.

Intensity of Stretch

The intensity of a stretch is determined by the tensile load placed on soft tissue to elongate it. There is general agreement among clinicians and researchers that stretching should be

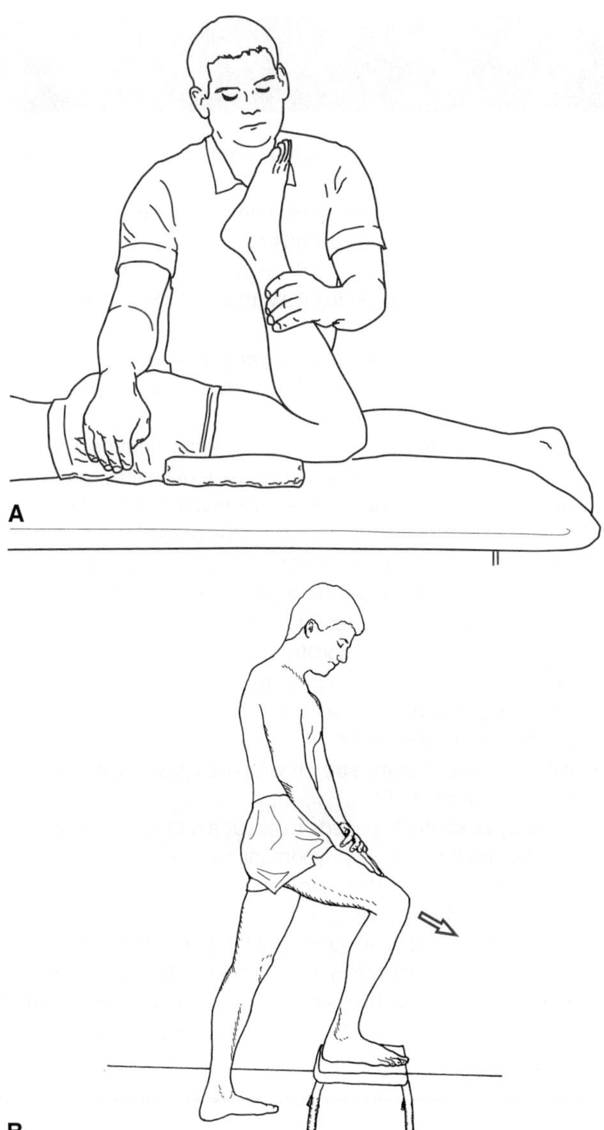

FIGURE 4.10 (A) The proximal attachment (femur and pelvis) of the muscle being stretched (the quadriceps) is stabilized as the distal segment is moved to increase knee flexion. (B) During this self-stretch of the quadriceps, the distal segment (tibia) is stabilized through the foot as the patient moves the proximal segment (femur) by lunging forward.

applied at a *low intensity* by means of a *low load*.[2,12,14,28,47,69,92] Low-intensity stretching in comparison to high-intensity stretching is more comfortable for the patient and minimizes voluntary or involuntary muscle guarding, enabling the patient to remain relaxed or assist with the stretching maneuver.

Low-intensity stretching results in optimal rates of improvement in ROM without exposing tissues, possibly weakened by immobilization, to excessive loads and potential injury.[92] Low-intensity stretching has also been shown to elongate dense connective tissue, a significant component of chronic contractures, more effectively and with less soft tissue damage and post-exercise soreness than a high-intensity stretch.[4]

Duration of Stretch

One of the most important decisions a therapist makes when selecting and implementing a stretching intervention is the duration of stretch that is expected to be safe, effective, practical, and efficient for each situation. The duration of stretch refers to the period of time a stretch force is applied and tissues are held in a lengthened position. Duration most often refers to how long a *single cycle* of stretch is applied. If more than one repetition of stretch (*stretch cycle*) is carried out during a treatment session, the cumulative time of all the stretch cycles reflects the total duration of stretch, also referred to as the *total elongation time*. In general, the shorter the duration of a single stretch cycle, the greater the number of repetitions needed during a stretching session. Many combinations of duration and cycle have been studied to determine optimal effectiveness.

FOCUS ON EVIDENCE

In a study by Cipriani and associates,[25] two repetitions of 30-second hamstring stretches were found to be equally effective as six repetitions of 10-second stretches. Similarly, Johnson et al reported that three 30-second stretches were equally effective as nine 10-second stretches for increasing hamstring length,[76] while Sainz de Baranda and associates showed that 180 seconds of daily stretch was also effective to increase hamstring length regardless of whether the individual stretch repetitions were of 15, 30, or 45 seconds.[127] In contrast, Roberts and Wilson[122] found that over the course of a 5-week period and equal total duration times, three 15-second hamstring stretches each day yielded significantly greater stretch-induced gains in ROM than nine daily 5-second stretches.

Despite many studies over several decades, there is lack of agreement on the ideal combination of single stretch duration and number of stretch repetitions that leads to the greatest and most sustained stretch-induced gains in ROM or reduction of muscle stiffness. Ultimately, the duration of stretch must be applied in context with the other stretching parameters of intensity, frequency, and mode. Key findings from a number of studies are summarized in Box 4.5.

Several descriptors are used to differentiate between a long-duration versus a short-duration stretch. Terms such as *static, sustained, maintained,* and *prolonged* are used to describe a long-duration stretch, whereas terms such as *cyclic, intermittent,* or *ballistic* are used to characterize a short-duration stretch. There is no specific time period assigned to any of these descriptors, nor is there a time frame that distinguishes a long-duration from a short-duration stretch.

Static Stretching

Static stretching* is a commonly used method of stretching in which soft tissues are elongated just beyond the point of

*2,7,8,25,38,42,43,52,87,107,110,122,151,161

BOX 4.5 Intensity, Duration, Frequency, and Mode of Stretch—Evidence-Based Interrelationships and Impact on Stretching Outcomes

- There is an inverse relationship between intensity and duration as well as between intensity and frequency of stretch.
  - The lower the intensity of stretch, the longer the time the patient will tolerate stretching and the soft tissues can be held in a lengthened position.
  - The higher the intensity, the less frequently the stretching intervention can be applied to allow time for tissue healing and resolution of residual muscle soreness.
- A low-load, long-duration stretch is considered the safest form of stretch and yields the most significant, elastic deformation and long-term, plastic changes in soft tissues.
- Manual stretching and self-stretching in hypomobile but healthy subjects[7-9,25,52] and prolonged mechanical stretching in patients with chronic contractures[72,75,92,102] yield significant stretch-induced gains in ROM.
- In the well elderly, stretch cycles of 15, 30, and 60 seconds applied to the hamstrings for four repetitions have all been shown to produce significant gains in ROM with the greatest and longest-lasting improvements occurring with the use of repeated 60-second stretch cycles.[52]
- In healthy young and/or middle-age adults:
  - Stretch durations of 15, 30, 45, 60, or 120 seconds to lower extremity musculature produced significant gains in ROM.[7,25,43,156]
  - Stretch cycles of 30- and 60-second durations applied to the hamstrings for one repetition daily are both more effective for increasing ROM than one repetition daily of a 15-second stretch cycle but are equally effective when compared with each other.[7,9]
  - Two repetitions daily of a 30-second static stretch of the hamstrings yield significant gains in hamstring flexibility similar to those seen with six repetitions of 10-second static stretches daily.[25]
  - There seems to be no additional benefit to holding each stretch cycle beyond 60 seconds.[7,83]
  - Three cycles of 30-second and 1-minute stretches are no more effective for improving ROM than one cycle of each duration of stretch.[7]
- Longer total durations of passive stretch yield longer-lasting decreases in muscle-tendon stiffness than short-duration stretches.[56,97,125]
  - A 2-minute passive stretch yields only a transient decrease in stiffness of the gastrocnemius muscle of healthy, young adults, whereas 4-minute and 8-minute stretches reduce stiffness for up to 20 minutes after stretching.[125]
- When the total duration of stretch (total elongation time) is equal, cyclic stretching is equally effective and possibly more comfortable than static stretching.[135]
- For patients with chronic, fibrotic contractures:
  - Common durations of manual stretching or self-stretching (several repetitions of 15-second or 30-second stretches) may not be effective.[92,107]
  - Use of prolonged static stretch with orthotics or casts is more effective.[75,92,102]
- Frequency of stretching needs to occur a minimum of two times per week for healthy hypomobile individuals, but more frequent stretching is necessary for patients with soft tissue pathology to achieve gains in ROM.[9]
- Although stretch-induced gains in ROM often persist for several weeks to a month in healthy adults after cessation of a stretching program, permanent improvement in mobility can be achieved only by use of the newly gained ROM in functional activities and/or with a maintenance stretching program.[156]

tissue resistance and then held in the lengthened position with a sustained stretch force over a period of time. The duration of static stretch can be predetermined prior to stretching or be based on the patient's tolerance and response during the stretch.

There is considerable variability in defining the duration of a static stretch. The term has been used to describe a single stretch cycle ranging from as short as 5 seconds to as long as 5 minutes per repetition when either a manual stretch or self-stretch is employed.[†] If a mechanical device provides the static stretch, the time frame can range from almost an hour to several days or weeks.[15,72,75,92,101] (See additional information on mechanical stretching later in this section.)

FOCUS ON EVIDENCE

In a systematic review of the effectiveness of hamstring stretching,[38] a 30-second manual or self-stretch performed for one or more repetitions was the most frequently used duration per repetition of static stretch. A median duration of 30-seconds per repetition has also been reported in a review on calf muscle stretching effectiveness.[161]

Static stretching is well accepted as an effective method to increase flexibility and ROM[2,38,69,70,87,110,125,152] and is considered safer than ballistic stretching.[42] Early research established that tension created in muscle during static stretching is approximately half that created during ballistic stretching.[149] This is consistent with our current understanding of the viscoelastic properties of connective tissue, which lies in and around muscles, and of the neurophysiological properties of the contractile elements of muscle.

As described earlier in this chapter, noncontractile soft tissues are known to yield to a low-intensity, continuously applied stretch force, as used in static stretching. Furthermore, a low-intensity, slowly applied, continuous, end-range static stretch does not appear to cause significant neuromuscular activation of the stretched muscle.[22,99] However, the assertion

†7,8,14,25,52,87,92,110,122,151,161

that static stretching contributes to neuromuscular relaxation (inhibition) of the stretched muscle through activation of the GTO is not supported by experimental evidence in human research studies.[22,131]

Static Progressive Stretching

Static progressive stretching is a term that characterizes how static stretching is applied for maximum effectiveness. The shortened soft tissues are held in a comfortably lengthened position until a degree of relaxation is felt by the patient or therapist. Then the shortened tissues are incrementally lengthened even further and again held in the new end-range position for an additional duration of time.[15,75] This approach involves periodically adjusting joint or segment alignment to increase the stretch force and capitalize on the stress-relaxation properties of soft tissue[102] (see Fig. 4.4B).

Most studies that have explored the merits of static *progressive* stretching have examined the effectiveness of a dynamic orthosis (see Fig. 4.13), which allows the patient to control the degree of joint angular displacement.[15,75] Manual stretching and self-stretching are also routinely applied in this manner.

Cyclic (Intermittent) Stretching

A relatively short-duration stretch force that is repeatedly but gradually applied, released, and then reapplied multiple times during a single treatment session is described as a cyclic (intermittent) stretch.[50,103,135] With cyclic stretching, the end-range stretch force is applied at a slow velocity, in a controlled manner, and at relatively low intensity. For these reasons, cyclic stretching is not synonymous with ballistic stretching, which is characterized by high-velocity movements.

There is no clear differentiation between cyclic stretching and static stretching that is repeated several times during a treatment session. According to some authors, in cyclic stretching, each cycle of stretch is held between 5 and 10 seconds.[50,135] However, others refer to stretches of 5- and 10-second duration as static.[25,122] There is also no consensus on the minimum number of repetitions during a treatment session needed to differentiate cyclic stretching from static stretching. In practice, this determination is often based on the patient's response to stretching.

Although the evidence is limited, cyclic loading has been shown to increase flexibility as effectively or more effectively than static stretching.[103,135]

FOCUS ON EVIDENCE

In a study of nonimpaired young adults, 60 seconds of cyclic stretching of calf muscles caused tissues to yield at slightly lower loads than one 60-second, two 30-second, or four 15-second static stretches, possibly due to decreased muscle stiffness.[103] In another study that compared cyclic to static stretching,[135] the authors speculated that heat production might occur because of the movement inherent in cyclic stretching and cause soft tissues to yield more readily to stretch. The authors of the latter study also concluded that cyclic stretching was more comfortable than a prolonged static stretch.

Speed of Stretch

Importance of a Slowly Applied Stretch

To minimize muscle activation during stretching and reduce the risk of injury to tissues and poststretch muscle soreness, a stretch force should be applied and released at a slow rate. A slowly applied stretch is less likely to increase tensile stresses on connective tissues[97,98] or to activate the stretch reflex. A slowly applied stretch also moderates the viscoelastic effects of connective tissue, making them more compliant. In addition, a stretch force applied at a low velocity is easier for the therapist or patient to control making it safer than a high-velocity stretch.

Ballistic Stretching

A rapid, forceful intermittent stretch—that is, a high-velocity and high-intensity stretch—is commonly called ballistic stretching.[2,7,8,47,163] It is characterized by fast joint movement that quickly elongates the targeted soft tissues. For example, a rapidly produced straight leg raise can be used to ballistically stretch the hamstrings. Although both static and ballistic stretching have been shown to improve flexibility equally, ballistic stretching is thought to cause greater trauma to stretched tissues and greater residual muscle soreness than static stretching.[153]

Dynamic stretching, noted earlier as a stretch shown to enhance performance, uses controlled movement to stretch muscle groups.[54] Dynamic stretching is similar to ballistic stretching in that it moves the joint through its ROM, yet differs by doing so at low velocities and intensities. As dynamic stretching is emerging as a viable replacement for static stretching prior to athletic activities,[9] it may also have the potential to be appropriate for general fitness or rehabilitation programs.

Although ballistic stretching safely increases ROM in young, healthy subjects participating in a conditioning program,[65] it is, for the most part, not recommended for elderly or sedentary individuals or patients with musculoskeletal pathology or chronic contractures. The rationale for this recommendation is based on the following:[33]

- Tissues weakened by immobilization or disuse are easily injured.
- Dense connective tissue found in chronic contractures does not yield easily with high-intensity, short-duration stretch; rather, it becomes more brittle and tears more readily.

High-Velocity Stretching in Conditioning Programs and Advanced-Phase Rehabilitation

Although controversial, there are situations in which high-velocity stretching is appropriate for certain individuals. For example, a highly trained athlete involved in a sport, such as gymnastics, that requires significant dynamic flexibility may need to incorporate high-velocity stretching in a conditioning program. Also, a young, active patient in the final phase of rehabilitation who wishes to return to high-demand recreational or sport activities after a musculoskeletal injury may need to perform carefully progressed, high-velocity stretching activities prior to beginning plyometric training or simulated, sport-specific exercises or drills.

When high-velocity stretching is deemed appropriate, low-intensity stretches are recommended while paying close attention to effective stabilization. The following self-stretching progression is designed to improve dynamic flexibility using a transition from static stretching to dynamic stretching and then to ballistic stretching.[163]

- Static stretching → Slow, short end-range stretching → Slow, full-range stretching → Fast, short end-range stretching → Fast, full-range stretching.
- The stretch force is initiated by having the individual actively contract the muscle group opposite the muscle and connective tissues to be stretched.

Frequency of Stretch

Frequency of stretching refers to the number of individual sessions per day or per week that a patient carries out the planned intervention. The optimal frequency of stretching is based on factors such as the underlying cause of impaired mobility, the quality and level of tissue healing, and the chronicity and severity of a contracture, as well as a patient's age, use of corticosteroids, and previous response to stretching. Because few studies have attempted to determine the optimal frequency of stretching within a day or a week, decisions on treatment frequency often depend on experience and best judgment. Frequency typically ranges from two to five sessions per week with time between sessions as needed for tissue healing and to minimize post-exercise soreness. Ultimately, the decision is based on the clinical discretion of the therapist and the response and needs of the patient.

A therapist must be aware of signs of tissue damage that may result from repetitive stretching. The correct balance between collagen tissue microfailure and subsequent repair is needed to allow an increase in soft tissue lengthening. With excessive loading frequency, tissue breakdown may exceed repair and tissue macrofailure becomes possible. In addition, if there is progressive loss of ROM over time rather than a gain in range, continued low-grade inflammation from repetitive stress may be causing excessive collagen formation and hypertrophic scarring.

Mode of Stretch

Stretching exercises can be executed in a variety of ways. The mode of stretch refers to how the stretch force is applied and who is actively participating in the process. Categories include, but are not limited to, *manual* and *mechanical stretching* or *self-stretching*, as well as *passive, assisted,* or *active stretching.* Regardless of the mode of stretching selected and implemented, it is imperative that the shortened muscle remains relaxed and that the restricted connective tissues yield as easily as possible to the stretch. To facilitate this, stretching should be preceded by either low-intensity active exercise or therapeutic heat to warm the tissues that are to be lengthened.

There is no best form or type of stretching. What is important is that the therapist and patient have many modes of stretching from which to choose. Box 4.6 lists some questions a therapist needs to answer to determine which forms of stretching are most appropriate and likely to be most effective for each patient at different stages of a rehabilitation program.

Manual Stretching

Characteristics. During manual stretching, the clinician or caregiver applies an external force that lengthens the targeted tissue beyond the point of tissue resistance. The therapist manually controls the site of stabilization and the direction, rate of application, intensity, and duration of stretch. Manual stretching can be performed passively, with assistance from the patient, or even independently by the patient.

Manual stretching typically employs a controlled, static stretch applied at an intensity consistent with the patient's comfort level. It is held for 15 to 60 seconds and repeated for at least several repetitions. The intensity is often increased as tolerated for subsequent repetitions in an effort to achieve progressive lengthening.

CLINICAL TIP

Remember—stretching and ROM exercises are not synonymous terms. Stretching takes soft tissue structures *beyond* their available length to *increase* ROM. ROM exercises stay within the limits of available tissue length to *maintain* mobility.

BOX 4.6 Considerations for Selecting Methods of Stretching

- Based on the results of your examination, what tissues are involved and impairing mobility?
- Is there evidence of pain or inflammation?
- How long has the hypomobility existed?
- What is the stage of healing of restricted tissues?
- What form(s) of stretching have been implemented previously? How did the patient respond?
- Are there any underlying diseases, disorders, or deformities that might affect the choice of stretching procedures?
- Does the patient have the ability to actively participate in, assist with, or independently perform the exercises? Consider the patient's physical capabilities, age, ability to cooperate, or ability to follow and remember instructions.
- Is assistance from a therapist or caregiver necessary to execute the stretching procedures and appropriate stabilization? If so, what is the size and strength of the therapist or the caregiver who is assisting the patient with a stretching program?

Effectiveness. Despite widespread use of manual stretching by clinicians, its effectiveness for increasing tissue extensibility is debatable. Although some investigators[43] report that manual stretching increases muscle length and ROM in nonimpaired subjects, other investigators have reported a negligible effect from manual stretching,[61] especially in the presence of long-standing contractures associated with tissue pathology.[92] The short duration of typical manual stretching may be responsible for these disparate outcomes.

Application. The following are points to consider about the use of manual stretching:

- Manual stretching may be most appropriate in the early stages of a stretching program when a therapist wants to determine how a patient responds to varying intensities or durations of stretch and when optimal stabilization is most critical.
- Passive manual stretching by the therapist or caregiver is appropriate if a patient lacks neuromuscular control of the body segment to be stretched and cannot perform a self-stretch.
- When the patient has adequate neuromuscular control of the body segment to be stretched, it is often helpful to ask them to assist the therapist with the stretch, particularly if the patient is apprehensive about moving or having difficulty relaxing. When the patient concentrically contracts the muscle opposite the target muscle to assist with joint movement, the target muscle tends to relax reflexively and allow elongation. This is one of several stretching procedures based on PNF techniques that are discussed later in this chapter.
- Using procedures and hand placements similar to those described for self-ROM exercises (see Chapter 3), the patient can also independently lengthen target muscles and periarticular tissues with manual stretching. This is usually described as *self-stretching* and is discussed in more detail as the next topic in this section.

NOTE: Specific guidelines for the application of manual stretching, as well as descriptions and illustrations of manual stretching techniques for the extremities (Figs. 4.16 through 4.34), are presented in later sections of this chapter.

Self-Stretching

Characteristics. Self-stretching (also referred to as flexibility exercises or active stretching) is a type of stretching procedure done independently by the patient after careful instruction and supervised practice. Self-stretching enables the patient to maintain or increase the extensibility gained as the result of direct intervention by a therapist. This form of stretching is often an integral component of a home exercise program and is necessary for long-term self-management of many musculoskeletal and neuromuscular disorders.

Effectiveness. To facilitate effectiveness, the patient must be taught to perform self-stretching procedures *correctly* and *safely.* Factors identified earlier in the chapter such as alignment, stabilization, intensity, dose, and mode must all be addressed with the patient to prevent re-injury and maintain function.

Application. The guidelines for the intensity, speed, duration, and frequency that apply to manual stretching are also appropriate for self-stretching. Static stretching for a 30- to 60-second duration per repetition is considered the safest type of self-stretching.

Self-stretching can be carried out in several ways:

- Using positions for self-ROM exercises described in Chapter 3, a patient can passively move the distal segment of a restricted joint with one or both hands to elongate a shortened muscle while stabilizing the proximal segment (Fig. 4.11 A).

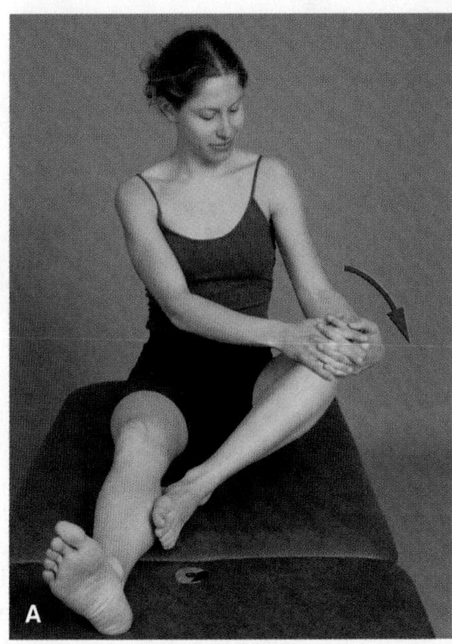

FIGURE 4.11 (A) When manually self-stretching the adductors and internal rotators of the hip, the patient moves the distal segment (femur) while stabilizing the proximal segment (pelvis) with body weight.

- If the distal attachment of a shortened muscle is stabilized on a support surface, body weight can be used as the source of the stretch force to elongate the shortened muscle-tendon unit (Fig. 4.11 B).
- Neuromuscular inhibition, using PNF stretching techniques, can be integrated into self-stretching procedures to promote relaxation in the muscle that is being elongated.
- Low-intensity active stretching (referred to by some as *dynamic ROM*[8]), using repeated, short-duration, end-range active muscle contractions of the muscle opposite the target muscle is another form of self-stretching exercise.[8,151,158]

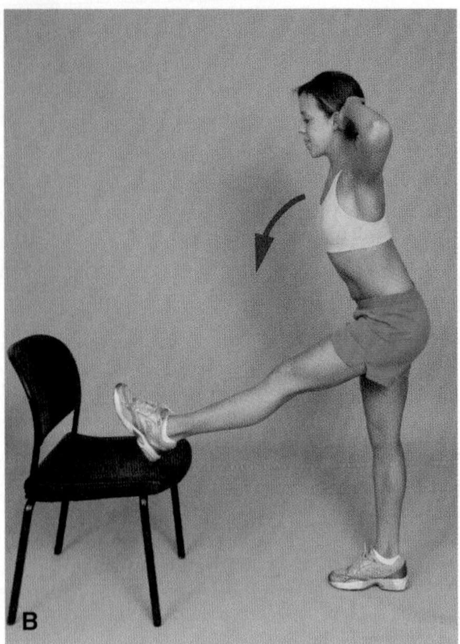

FIGURE 4.11—cont'd (B) When self-stretching the hamstrings, the distal segment (tibia) is stabilized through the foot on the surface of a chair as the patient bends forward and moves the proximal segment. The weight of the upper body is the source of the stretch force.

Mechanical Stretching

Characteristics. Mechanical stretching devices apply a very low-intensity stretch force over a prolonged period of time to create relatively permanent lengthening of soft tissues, presumably due to plastic deformation.

There are many ways to use equipment to stretch shortened tissues and increase ROM. The equipment can be as simple as a cuff weight or weight-pulley system or as sophisticated as some adjustable orthotic devices or automated stretching machines.[12,15,75,89,92,101,135] These mechanical stretching devices provide either a constant load with variable displacement or constant displacement with variable loads.

Effectiveness. Studies[15,75] about the efficacy of the two categories of mechanical loading devices base their effectiveness on the short-term soft tissue properties of either creep or stress-relaxation and on the long-term effects of plastic deformation.

Be cautious when interpreting studies or product information reporting "permanent" lengthening through the use of mechanical stretching devices. The term permanent may mean that length increases were maintained for as little as a few days or a week after discontinuing use of a stretching device, while long-term follow-up may indicate that tissues have returned to their shortened state.

Application. It is often the responsibility of a therapist to recommend the type of stretching device that is most suitable to the patient and to teach them how to safely use and monitor the equipment in the home setting. A therapist may also be involved in the fabrication of serial casts or orthoses used for mechanical stretching.

Each form of mechanical stretching listed below has been shown to be effective, particularly in reducing long-standing contractures:

- Stretch force applied with a cuff weight (Fig. 4.12) as low as a few pounds.[92]

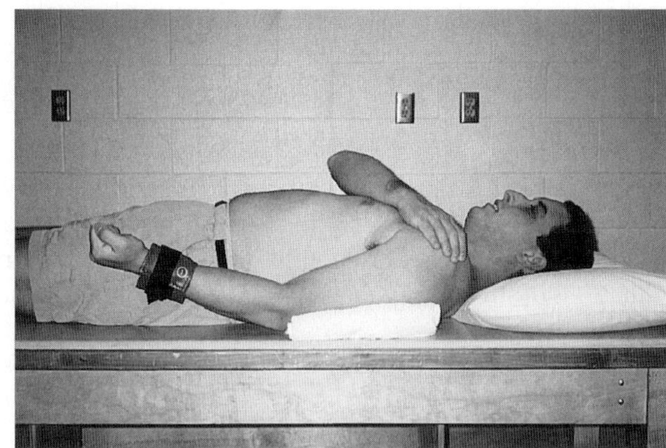

FIGURE 4.12 Low-load mechanical stretch with a cuff weight and self-stabilization of the proximal humerus to stretch the elbow flexors and increase end-range elbow extension.

- Devices such as the Joint Active Systems™ adjustable orthosis (Fig. 4.13) allow a patient to control and adjust the stretch force during a session.[15,75]

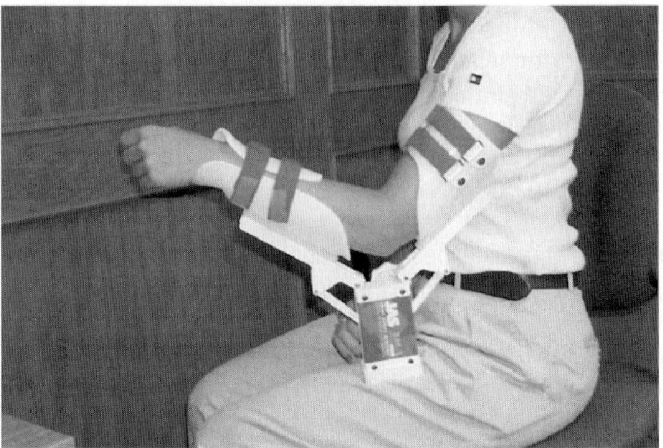

FIGURE 4.13 JAS orthosis is a patient-directed device that applies a static progressive stretch. *(Courtesy of Joint Active Systems, Effingham, IL.)*

- Orthotics with a preset load that remains constant while the orthotic is in place.

Duration of Mechanical Stretch

Mechanical stretching involves a substantially longer overall duration of stretch than is practical with manual stretching or self-stretching exercises. Mechanical stretch durations reported in the literature range from 15 to 30 minutes to as long as 8 to 10 hours per session[15,56,75] or continuous throughout the day except for time out of the device for hygiene and exercise.[12]

Serial casts are worn for days or weeks before being removed and then reapplied.[72] The duration is dependent on the type of device; patient tolerance; and the cause, severity, and chronicity of impairment. Longer duration stretches are typically required for patients with chronic contractures stemming from neurological or musculoskeletal disorders rather than healthy subjects with mild hypomobility.[15,72,75,92,102,107]

FOCUS ON EVIDENCE

Light and colleagues[92] compared the effects of mechanical and manual stretching on nonambulatory elderly nursing home residents with long-standing bilateral knee flexion contractures. Both types of stretches were applied twice a day, 5 days per week, for a 4-week period. Low-intensity, prolonged mechanical stretching (a 5- to 12-lb stretch force applied by a weight-pulley system for 1 hour) was applied to one knee, and manual passive stretching was applied to the other knee by a therapist (three repetitions of 1-minute static stretches). At the conclusion of the study, the mechanical stretching procedure was found to be considerably more effective than the manual stretching procedure for reducing knee flexion contractures. The subjects also reported that the prolonged mechanical stretch was more comfortable than the manual stretching procedure. The investigators recognized that the total duration of mechanical stretch (40 hours) was substantially longer over the course of the study than the total duration of manual stretch (2 hours) but believed that the manual stretching procedures were practical and typical of the clinical setting.

Proprioceptive Neuromuscular Facilitation Stretching Techniques

PNF stretching techniques,[22,69,99,115,131] sometimes referred to as *active stretching*[158] or *facilitative stretching*,[117] integrate active muscle contractions into stretching. These techniques are used to inhibit or facilitate muscle activation and to increase the likelihood that the muscle to be lengthened remains as relaxed as possible as it is stretched.

The traditional explanation of the underlying mechanisms of PNF stretching is that reflexive muscle relaxation occurs during the stretch as the result of autogenic or reciprocal inhibition. This inhibition leads to decreased tension in muscle fibers and decreased resistance to elongation by the contractile elements of the target muscle. However, this explanation has come into question in recent years.

Current thinking suggests that gains in ROM during or following PNF stretching techniques cannot be attributed solely to autogenic or reciprocal inhibition, which involves the spinal processing of proprioceptive information. Rather, increased ROM is the result of more complex mechanisms of sensorimotor processing, most likely combined with viscoelastic adaptation of the muscle-tendon unit and increases in the patient's tolerance to stretching.[22,99,131] Regardless of these competing explanations, numerous studies have demonstrated that the various PNF stretching techniques can increase flexibility and ROM.[8,36,50,115,158] However, the degree of neuromuscular relaxation associated with the PNF stretching maneuvers investigated was not determined in these studies. There is also some evidence[99] that PNF stretching yields greater gains in ROM than static stretching, but there is no consensus on whether one PNF technique is significantly superior to another.

Types of PNF Stretching VIDEO 4.1

There are several types of PNF stretching procedures, all of which have been shown to improve ROM. They include:

- Hold-relax (HR) or contract-relax (CR)
- Agonist contraction (AC)
- Hold-relax with agonist contraction (HR-AC)

With classic PNF, these techniques are always performed with combined muscle groups acting in diagonal patterns.[117,118,148] Over time the techniques have been modified by clinicians and others to include stretching in a single plane or opposite the line of pull of a specific muscle group.[8,27,63,71,99,115,158] (For a description of the PNF diagonal patterns, refer to Chapter 6.)

CLINICAL TIP

PNF stretching techniques require that a patient has normal innervation and voluntary control of either the range-limiting target muscle or the muscle on the opposite side of the joint. As such, these techniques cannot be used effectively for patients with paralysis or spasticity resulting from neuromuscular diseases or injury. Furthermore, because PNF stretching procedures are designed to affect the contractile elements of muscle, as opposed to noncontractile connective tissues, they are more appropriate to use when muscle spasm limits motion and less appropriate for long-standing fibrotic contractures.

Hold-Relax and Contract-Relax

With the HR and CR procedures,[27,71,99,115,117,118] the range-limiting target muscle is first lengthened to the point of tissue resistance or to the extent that is comfortable for the patient. The patient then actively performs a *prestretch, end-range, isometric contraction* of the range-limiting target muscle against manual resistance applied by the clinician. This contraction is held for about 5 seconds and followed by *voluntary* relaxation of the target muscle. The limb is then passively moved by the clinician into the new range as the range-limiting muscle is elongated. Clinicians with experience using PNF report that the HR and CR techniques appear to make passive elongation of muscles more comfortable for a patient than manual passive stretching.[71] A sequence for using the HR and CR technique to stretch shortened pectoralis major muscles bilaterally and increase horizontal abduction of the shoulders is illustrated in Figure 4.14.

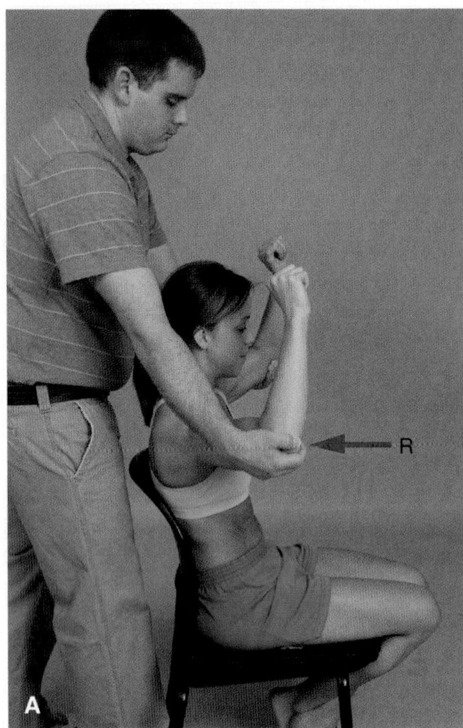

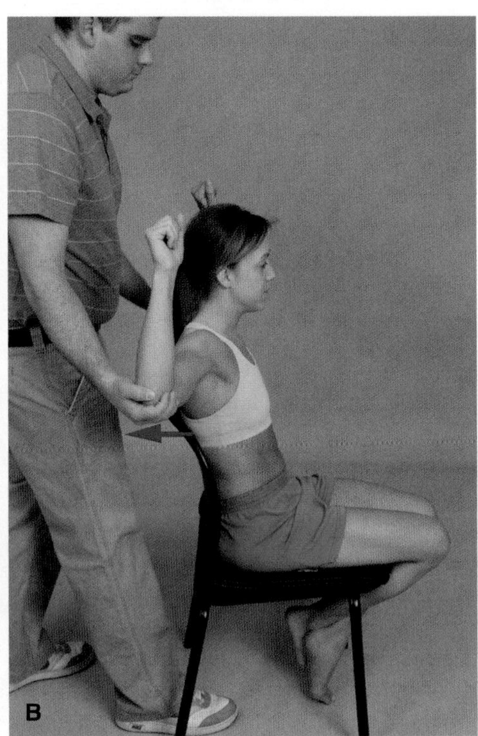

FIGURE 4.14 Hold-relax (HR) procedure to stretch the pectoralis major muscles bilaterally. **(A)** The therapist horizontally abducts the shoulders bilaterally to a comfortable position. The patient isometrically contracts the pectoralis major muscles against the therapist's resistance for about 5 to 10 seconds. **(B)** The patient relaxes voluntarily, and the therapist passively lengthens the pectoralis major muscles by horizontally abducting the shoulders into the newly gained range. After a 10-second rest with the muscles maintained in a comfortably lengthened position, the entire sequence is repeated several times.

NOTE: Although the terms *CR* and *HR* often are used interchangeably, in classic PNF the technique descriptions are not identical. Both techniques are performed in diagonal patterns, but in the CR technique, the axial rotators of the limb are allowed to contract concentrically in the prestretch phase, while all other muscle groups of the diagonal pattern contract isometrically. In contrast, the prestretch isometric contraction occurs in all muscles of the diagonal pattern during the HR technique.[118,148]

As noted earlier, the traditional explanation for PNF effectiveness is that neuromuscular relaxation results from autogenic inhibition following the prestretch isometric contraction of the target muscle.[95,117,118] Some investigators[99] have challenged this assumption, attributing the gains in flexibility to the viscoelastic properties of the muscle-tendon unit. These studies report a postcontraction sensory discharge (increased EMG activity) in the range-limiting muscle after the prestretch contraction, suggesting that the muscle was not reflexively relaxed prior to stretch. However, the results of another study[28] indicated no evidence of a postcontraction elevation in EMG activity with the HR or CR techniques.

In light of the mixed evidence about the extent of neuromuscular relaxation achieved after the prestretch contraction, practitioners must determine the effectiveness of the HR or CR techniques based on the responses of their patients.

PRECAUTION: Multiple repetitions of maximal prestretch isometric contractions have been shown to result in an acute increase in arterial blood pressure, most notably after the third repetition.[29]

CLINICAL TIP

It is not necessary for the patient to perform a maximal isometric contraction of the range-limiting target muscle prior to stretch. To minimize the adverse effects of the Valsalva maneuver (elevation in blood pressure associated with a high-intensity effort), have the patient breathe regularly while performing *submaximal* (low-intensity) isometric contractions held for about 5 seconds with each repetition of the HR or CR procedure. From a practical perspective, a submaximal contraction is also easier for the therapist to control if the patient is strong.

Agonist Contraction

Another PNF stretching technique is the *agonist contraction* (AC), a term that may be misleading.[28,71,115] The "agonist" in this case refers to the muscle *opposite* the range-limiting target muscle, while the "antagonist" refers to the range-limiting muscle. It may help to frame this paradigm as the short muscle (the antagonist) preventing the prime mover (the agonist) from actively achieving full movement. *Dynamic ROM* (DROM)[8] and *active stretching*[158] are other terms that have been used to describe the AC procedure.

With the AC procedure, the patient *concentrically contracts (shortens) the muscle opposite the range-limiting muscle* and then holds the end-range position for at least several seconds.[22,28,71,115] The movement of the limb is controlled independently by the patient and is deliberate and slow, not ballistic. In most instances, the shortening contraction is performed without the addition of resistance. For example, if the hip flexors are the range-limiting target muscle group, the patient performs end-range prone leg lifts by contracting the hip extensors concentrically and holding at the end range for several seconds. After a brief rest period, the patient repeats the procedure.

Increased muscle length and joint ROM using the AC procedure have been reported. However, when the effectiveness of the AC technique has been compared with that of static stretching, the evidence is mixed.

FOCUS ON EVIDENCE

Two studies have compared the effect of the AC procedure, referred to as DROM, to static stretching of the hamstrings of healthy subjects over a 6-week period. One study[151] demonstrated that DROM is as effective as static stretching, but the other study[8] showed that one daily session of a 30-second static stretch was almost three times as effective in increasing hamstring flexibility as was six repetitions of a 5-second end-range DROM hold performed daily.

In a study of young adults with hypomobile hip flexors and periodic lumbar or lower-quarter pain, investigators compared active stretching with the AC procedure to static passive stretching.[158] Both techniques resulted in increased hip extension with no significant difference between the AC and passive stretching groups.

In addition to the evidence related to the AC stretching procedure, clinicians have observed the following:

- The AC technique seems to be especially effective when significant antagonist muscle guarding restricts muscle lengthening and joint movement but is less effective in reducing chronic contractures.
- AC is also useful when the patient cannot generate a strong, pain-free contraction of the range-limiting muscle, which is needed for the HR and CR procedures.
- AC is also useful for initiating neuromuscular control in newly gained joint ROM to re-establish dynamic flexibility.
- The AC technique is least effective if a patient has close to normal flexibility.

PRECAUTION: Avoid full-range, ballistic movements when performing concentric contractions of the agonist muscle group.

CLINICAL TIP

If, while performing an AC technique, the agonist is contracting in a very shortened position, have the patient rest after each repetition to avoid muscle cramping.

Classic PNF theory suggests that when the agonist is activated and contracts concentrically, the antagonist (the range-limiting muscle) is reciprocally inhibited, allowing it to relax and lengthen more readily.[117,122] However, the theoretical mechanism of reciprocal inhibition has been substantiated only in animal studies.[119] Evidence of reciprocal inhibition during the AC procedure has not been demonstrated in human subjects.[22,119,131] In fact, increased EMG activity, not reciprocal inhibition, has been identified in the range-limiting muscle during the AC stretching procedure.[28,115]

Hold-Relax With Agonist Contraction

The HR-AC stretching technique combines the HR and AC procedures. The HR-AC technique is also referred to as the CR-AC procedure[22] or the slow reversal hold-relax technique.[148] To perform the HR-AC procedure, move the limb to the point that tissue resistance is felt in the range-limiting target muscle; then have the patient perform a resisted, prestretch isometric contraction of the range-limiting muscle, *followed* by voluntary relaxation of that muscle and an immediate concentric contraction of the muscle *opposite* the range-limiting muscle.[28,117,148]

For example, to stretch knee flexors, extend the patient's knee to a comfortable end-range position and then have the patient perform an isometric contraction of the knee flexors against resistance for about 5 seconds. Tell the patient to voluntarily relax and then actively extend the knee as far as possible, holding any newly gained range for several seconds.

FOCUS ON EVIDENCE

Studies comparing two PNF stretching procedures have produced differing results. In one study,[50] the HR-AC technique produced a greater increase in ankle dorsiflexion range than the HR technique alone, while both HR-AC and HR alone produced a greater increase than manual passive stretching. However, another study[71] reported no significant difference in ROM between the use of the HR and HR-AC techniques.

PRECAUTIONS: Recognize the same precautions as described for both the HR and AC procedures and follow the CLINICAL TIPS to minimize complications and discomfort.

Integration of Function Into Stretching

Importance of Strength and Muscle Endurance

As previously discussed, the strength of soft tissue is altered when it is immobilized for a period of time.[23,106] The magnitude of peak tension produced by muscle decreases, and the tensile strength of noncontractile tissues decreases. A muscle group that has been elongated while its opposing muscle group has been in a shortened state for an extended period of time also becomes weak.[82,90,91] Therefore, it is critical to include low-load resistance exercises to improve muscle performance (strength and endurance) as early as possible in a stretching program.

Initially, emphasis should be on developing neuromuscular control and strength of the agonist, the muscle group opposite the range-limiting target muscle. For example, if the elbow flexors are the range-limiting muscle group, emphasize contraction of the elbow extensors in the newly gained range. Early use of the agonist enables the patient to elongate the hypomobile structures actively and use the recently gained ROM.

As ROM approaches a "normal" or functional level, the muscles that were range limiting and then stretched must also be strengthened to maintain an appropriate balance of strength between agonists and antagonists throughout the ROM. Manual and mechanical resistance exercises are effective ways to load and strengthen muscles, but functional weight-bearing activities, such as those mentioned below, will specifically strengthen antigravity muscle groups.

Use of Increased Mobility for Functional Activities

As mentioned previously, gains in flexibility and ROM achieved as the result of a stretching program are transient, lasting only about 4 weeks after the cessation of stretching.[156] The most effective means of achieving permanent increases in ROM and reducing functional limitations is to integrate functional activities that use the newly gained range on a regular basis into the stretching program. Use of functional activities to maintain mobility also lends diversity and interest to a stretching program, which may benefit patient compliance.

Active movements should be performed within the pain-free ROM. As soon as even small increases in tissue extensibility and ROM have been achieved, have the patient use the gained range by performing motions that *simulate* functional activities. Have the patient transition to using all of the available ROM while doing specific functional tasks when they are ready.

Functional movements that are practiced should complement the stretching program. For example, if a patient has been performing stretching exercises to increase shoulder mobility, have the patient fully use the available ROM by reaching as far as possible behind the back and overhead when grooming or dressing or by reaching for or placing objects on a high shelf (Fig. 4.15). Gradually increase the weight of objects placed on or removed from a shelf to strengthen shoulder musculature simultaneously.

If the focus of a stretching program has been to increase knee flexion after removal of a long-leg cast, emphasize flexing both knees before standing up from a chair or when stooping to pick up an object from the floor. These weight-bearing activities also strengthen the quadriceps that were held in a shortened position and likely became weak while the leg was immobilized.

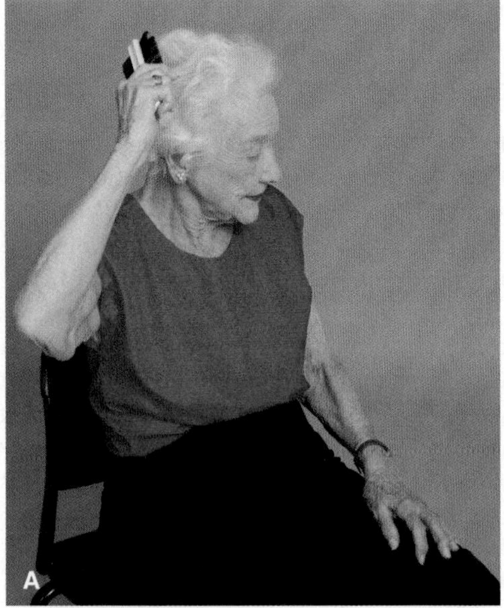

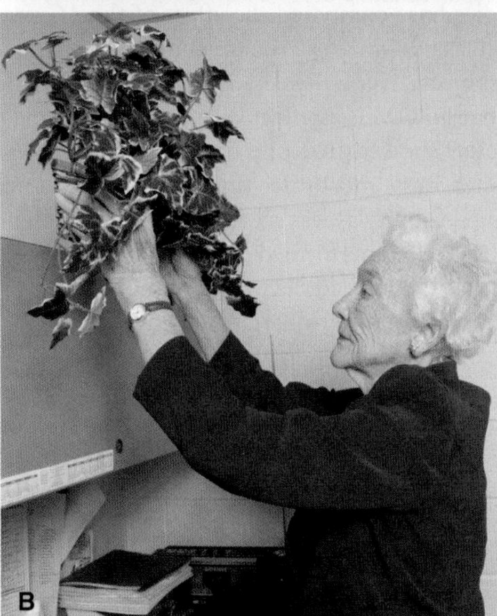

FIGURE 4.15 (A, B) Stretching-induced gains in ROM are used during daily activities.

Procedural Guidelines for Application of Stretching Interventions

The following guidelines are central to the development and implementation of stretching interventions. The results of an examination and evaluation of a patient's status determine the need for and types of stretching procedures that will be most effective in the patient's plan of care. This section identifies general guidelines to be addressed before, during, and after stretching procedures, as well as specific guidelines for the application of manual stretching. Special considerations for teaching self-stretching exercises to the patient and the use of mechanical stretching devices are listed in Boxes 4.7 and 4.8.

BOX 4.7 Special Considerations for Teaching Self-Stretching Exercises

- Be sure to carefully teach the patient all elements of self-stretching procedures, including appropriate alignment and stabilization, intensity, duration, and frequency. Because many self-stretching exercises are performed using a portion of the body weight as the stretch force (by moving the body over a fixed distal segment), emphasize the importance of performing a slow, sustained stretch, not a ballistic stretch that creates momentum and may lengthen but can potentially injure hypomobile soft tissues.
- Make sure the patient is taught to carry out stretching exercises on a firm, stable, comfortable surface to maintain proper alignment.
- Supervise the patient and make suggestions or corrections to be certain the patient performs each exercise using safe biomechanics that protect joints and ligaments, especially at the end of the ROM. Pay particular attention to maintaining postural alignment and effective stabilization.
- Emphasize the importance of warming up the tissues prior to stretching with low-intensity, rhythmic activities such as cycling. Stretching should not be the first activity in an exercise routine because cold tissue may be easier to injure.
- If appropriate and possible, teach the patient how to independently incorporate neuromuscular inhibition techniques, such as the hold-relax procedure, into selected stretching exercises.
- Provide written instructions with illustrations to which the patient can refer when independently performing the self-stretching exercises.
- Demonstrate how items commonly found around the house, such as a towel, belt, broomstick, or homemade weight, can be used to assist with stretching activities.
- Emphasize the importance of using the gained ROM during appropriately progressed functional activities.

BOX 4.8 Special Considerations for Use of Mechanical Stretching Devices

- Become thoroughly familiar with the manufacturer's product information.
- Become familiar with stretching protocols recommended by the manufacturer; seek out research studies that provide evidence of the efficacy of the equipment or protocols.
- Determine if modifying a suggested protocol is warranted to meet your patient's needs. For example, should the suggested intensity of stretch or recommended wearing time (duration and frequency) be modified?
- Check the fit of a device before sending it home with a patient. Teach the patient how to apply and safely adjust the device and how to maintain it in good working order. Be sure that the patient knows who to contact if the equipment appears to be defective.
- Teach the patient where and how to inspect the skin to detect areas of excessive pressure from the stretching device and potential skin irritation.
- If the mechanical stretching device is "homemade," such as a cuff weight, check to see if the equipment is safe and effective.
- Have the patient keep a daily record of using the stretching device.
- Re-examine and re-evaluate the patient and equipment periodically to determine the effectiveness of the mechanical stretching program and to modify and progress the program as necessary.
- Be sure the patient complements the use of mechanical stretching with active exercises.

Examination and Evaluation of the Patient

- Carefully review the patient's history and perform a comprehensive systems review.
- Select and perform appropriate tests and measurements. Determine the ROM available in involved and adjacent joints and assess if active and/or passive mobility is impaired.
- Determine if hypomobility is related to other impairments of body structure or function and if it is causing activity limitations or participation restrictions.
- Determine if soft tissues are the source of the impaired mobility. If so, differentiate between joint capsule, periarticular structures, noncontractile tissue, and muscle length restrictions as the cause of limited ROM. Be sure to assess joint play and fascial mobility.
- Evaluate the irritability of the involved tissues and estimate their stage of healing. When moving the patient's extremities or spine, pay close attention to the patient's reaction to movements. This not only helps identify the stage of healing of involved tissues; it also helps determine the probable dosage (such as intensity and duration) of stretch that stays within the patient's comfort range.
- Assess the strength of muscles in which there is motion limitation and realistically consider the value of stretching the range-limiting structures. Ideally, an individual should have the capability of developing adequate strength to control and use any newly gained ROM safely.
- Consider the outcome goals (i.e., functional improvements) that the patient hopes to achieve as the result of the intervention program and determine if those goals are realistic.
- Analyze the impact of any factors that could adversely affect the projected outcomes of the stretching program.

Preparation for Stretching

- Review the goals and desired outcomes of the stretching program with the patient. Obtain the patient's consent to initiate treatment.
- Select the stretching techniques that will be most effective and efficient.

- Warm up the soft tissues to be stretched by the application of local heat or by active, low-intensity exercises. Warming up tight structures may increase their extensibility and decrease the risk of injury from stretching.
- Have the patient assume a comfortable, stable position that allows the correct plane of motion for the stretching procedure. *The direction of stretch is exactly opposite the direction of the joint or muscle restriction.*
- Explain the procedure to the patient and be certain he or she understands.
- Free the area to be stretched of any restrictive clothing, bandages, or orthotics.
- Explain to the patient that it is important to be as relaxed as possible and that the stretching procedures are meant to remain within his or her tolerance level.

Application of Manual Stretching Procedures

- Move the extremity slowly through the free range to the point of tissue restriction.
- Grasp the areas proximal and distal to the joint in which motion is to occur. The grasp should be firm but not uncomfortable for the patient. Use padding, if necessary, in areas with minimal subcutaneous tissue, reduced sensation, or over a bony surface. Use the broad surfaces of your hands to spread forces over a larger surface area.
- Firmly stabilize the proximal segment (manually or with equipment) and move the distal segment.
- To stretch a multijoint muscle, stabilize either the proximal or distal segment to which the range-limiting muscle attaches. Stretch the muscle over one joint at a time and then over all joints simultaneously until the optimal length of soft tissues is achieved. To minimize compressive forces in small joints, stretch the distal joints first and proceed proximally.
- Consider incorporating a prestretch, isometric contraction of the range-limiting muscle (the HR procedure).
- To minimize joint compression during the stretch, a gentle (grade I) distraction to the moving joint can be applied.
- Apply the stretch using a slow, sustained rate. Remember, the direction of the stretching movement is directly *opposite* the line of pull of the range-limiting muscle. Ask the patient to assist you with the stretch or apply a passive stretch to lengthen the tissues. Take the hypomobile soft tissues to the point of firm tissue resistance and then move just beyond that point. The force must be enough to place tension on soft tissue structures but not so great as to cause pain or injure the structures. The patient should experience a *pulling sensation*, but not pain, *in the structures being stretched*. When stretching adhesions of a tendon within its sheath, the patient may describe a "stinging" sensation as adhesions are mobilized.
- Maintain the stretch position for 30 seconds or longer. During this time, the tension in the tissues should slowly decrease. When tension decreases, move the extremity or joint a little farther to progressively lengthen the hypomobile tissues.
- Gradually release the stretch force and allow the patient and therapist to rest momentarily while maintaining the range-limiting tissues in a comfortably elongated position. Then repeat the sequence several times.
- If the patient does not seem to tolerate a sustained stretch, use several very slow, gentle, intermittent stretches with the muscle in a lengthened position.
- If deemed appropriate, apply selected soft tissue mobilization procedures, such as fascial massage or cross-fiber friction massage, at or near the sites of adhesion during the stretching maneuver.

CLINICAL TIP

Do not attempt to gain the full range in one or two treatment sessions. Resolving mobility impairment is a slow, gradual process. It may take several weeks of stretching to see significant results. Between stretching sessions, it is important to use the newly increased range to maintain what has been gained.

After Stretching

- Apply cold to the soft tissues that have been stretched and allow these structures to cool in a lengthened position. Cold may minimize poststretch muscle soreness that can occur as the result of microtrauma during stretching. When soft tissues are cooled in a lengthened position, increases in ROM are more readily maintained.[73,102]
- Have the patient perform active ROM and strengthening exercises through the gained range immediately after stretching. With your supervision and feedback, have the patient use the gained range by performing simulated functional movement patterns that are part of daily living, occupational, or recreational tasks.
- Strengthen the antagonistic muscles in the newly gained range to ensure adequate neuromuscular control and stability as flexibility increases.

Precautions for Stretching

There are a number of general precautions that apply to all forms of stretching interventions. In addition, some special precautions must be taken when advising patients about stretching exercises that are part of community-based fitness programs or commercially available exercise products marketed to the general public.

General Precautions

- Do not passively force a joint beyond its normal ROM. Remember, normal (typical) ROM varies among individuals. In adults, flexibility is greater in women than in men.[162] When treating older adults, be aware of age-related changes in flexibility.

FOCUS ON EVIDENCE

Some studies suggest that flexibility decreases with age, particularly when coupled with decreased activity levels.[4,5] However, a study of more than 200 adults ages 20 to 79 who regularly exercised demonstrated that hamstring length did not significantly decrease with age.[162]

- Use extra caution in patients with known or suspected osteoporosis due to disease, prolonged bed rest, age, or prolonged use of steroids.
- Protect newly united fractures; be certain there is appropriate stabilization between the fracture site and the joint in which the motion takes place.
- Remember that a longer lever arm creates greater torque at a joint. Always be aware that the point of force application on each of the segments will influence the tensile load on the target tissue.
- Avoid vigorous stretching of muscles and connective tissues that have been immobilized for an extended period of time. Connective tissues, such as tendons and ligaments, lose their tensile strength after prolonged immobilization.[90] High-intensity, short-duration stretching procedures tend to cause more trauma and resulting weakness of soft tissues than low-intensity, long-duration stretch.
- Progress the dosage (intensity, duration, and frequency) gradually to minimize soft tissue trauma and postexercise muscle soreness. If a patient experiences joint pain or muscle soreness lasting more than 24 hours after stretching, it is likely that too much stretch force caused an inflammatory response. This, in turn, can result in increased scar tissue formation. Patients should experience no more residual discomfort than a transitory feeling of tenderness.
- Avoid stretching edematous tissue, as it is more susceptible to injury than normal tissue and continued irritation usually causes increased pain and edema.
- Avoid overstretching weak muscles, particularly those that support body structures in relation to gravity.

Special Precautions for Mass-Market Flexibility Programs

To develop and maintain a desired level of fitness, many people participate in physical conditioning programs at home or in the community. Self-stretching exercises are often an integral component of these programs. As a result, individuals frequently learn self-stretching procedures in fitness classes or from popular videos or television programs. Although much of the information in these resources is usually safe and accurate, there may also be errors or potential problems in flexibility programs designed for the mass market. These problems are possible any time the assessment of an individual's specific limitations is not obtained by a trained professional and a "one-size-fits-all" approach is used.

Common Errors and Potential Problems

Nonselective or poorly balanced stretching activities. General flexibility programs may advise stretching body regions that are already mobile or even hypermobile, while neglecting regions that are tight from faulty posture or inactivity. For example, in the sedentary population, some degree of hypomobility tends to develop in the hip flexors, trunk flexors, shoulder extensors and internal rotators, and scapular protractors from sitting in a slumped posture. Yet, if the commercially available flexibility routines overemphasize exercises that stretch posterior muscle groups and fail to include exercises to stretch the tight anterior structures, faulty postures may worsen rather than improve.

Insufficient warm-up. Individuals involved in flexibility programs may fail to warm up prior to stretching.

Ineffective stabilization. Programs often lack effective methods of self-stabilization. Therefore, an exercise may fail to stretch the intended tight structures and may transfer the stretch force to structures that are already mobile or even hypermobile.

Use of ballistic stretching. Although a less common problem than in the past, some exercise routines still recommend ballistic stretching. Because this form of stretching is not well controlled, it increases the likelihood of post-exercise muscle soreness and significant injury to soft tissues.

Excessive intensity. The phrase "no pain, no gain" is often used inappropriately as the guideline for intensity of stretch. An effective flexibility routine should be progressed gradually by remaining within each individual's pain tolerance levels.

Abnormal biomechanics. Some popular stretching exercises do not respect the biomechanics of the region. For example, the "hurdler's" stretch is designed to simultaneously stretch the hamstrings of one lower extremity and the quadriceps of the opposite extremity but may impose detrimental strain on the medial capsule and ligaments of the flexed knee.

Insufficient information about age-related differences. A single flexibility program does not fit all age groups. As a result of the normal aging process, mobility of connective tissues diminishes.[4,5,77] Consequently, elderly individuals typically exhibit less flexibility than young adults. Even an adolescent after a growth spurt temporarily exhibits restricted flexibility, particularly in two-joint muscle groups. Flexibility programs marketed to the general public may not be sensitive to these normal, age-related differences in flexibility.

Strategies for Risk Reduction

- Whenever possible, assess the appropriateness and safety of exercises in a "prepackaged" flexibility program.
- If a patient you are treating is participating in a community-based fitness class, review the exercises in the program

and determine their appropriateness and safety for your patient.

- Stay up to date on current exercise programs, products, and trends by reviewing the content and safety of your patient's home exercise videos.
- Determine whether a class or video is intended for individuals of the same age or with similar physical conditions.
- Eliminate or modify those exercises that are inconsistent with the intervention plan you have developed for your patient.
- See that the flexibility program maintains a balance of mobility between antagonistic muscle groups and emphasizes stretching those muscle groups that often become shortened with age, faulty posture, or a sedentary lifestyle.
- Teach your patient the basic principles of self-stretching and to evaluate fitness materials that they are using. Encourage them to select only safe and appropriate stretching exercises while avoiding those that perpetuate impairments or have no value.
- Make sure your patient understands the importance of warming up prior to stretching. Give suggestions on how to warm up before stretching.
- Be certain that the patient knows how to provide effective self-stabilization and isolate a stretch to specific muscle groups.
- Teach your patient how to determine the appropriate intensity of stretch; be sure your patient knows that, at most, postexercise muscle soreness should be mild and last no more than 24 hours.

Adjuncts to Stretching Interventions

Practitioners managing patients with structural or functional impairments, including chronic pain, muscle guarding or imbalances, and restricted mobility, may find it useful to integrate complementary therapies that address the body, mind, and spirit, such as relaxation training, Pilates, yoga, or tai chi into a patient's plan of care to improve function and quality of life. Other interventions that are useful adjuncts to a stretching program include superficial or deep heat, cold, massage, biofeedback, and joint traction.

Complementary Approaches

Relaxation Training

Relaxation training has been used for many years by a variety of practitioners[49,53,74,129,146] to help patients learn to relieve or reduce pain; muscle tension; anxiety or stress; and associated physical impairments or medical conditions, including tension headaches, high blood pressure, and respiratory distress. Some of the many approaches used to achieve beneficial relaxation include progressive relaxation, biofeedback, stress and anxiety management, and imagery. A brief overview of techniques is presented in this section.

There are a number of physiological, behavioral, cognitive, and emotional responses that occur during total body relaxation.[146] These key indicators are decreased muscle tension, lowered blood pressure, lowered heart and respiratory rates, increased skin temperature in the extremities, constricted pupils, little to no body movement, eyes closed and flat facial expression, jaw and hands relaxed, and decreased distractibility.

Common Elements of Relaxation Training

The purpose of relaxation training is to reduce muscle tension in the entire body or the painful or restricted region by using conscious effort and thought. Training typically occurs in a quiet environment with low lighting and soothing music or an auditory cue on which the patient may focus. The patient performs deep breathing exercises or visualizes a peaceful scene. When giving instructions, the therapist uses a calm and soft tone of voice.

Examples of Approaches to Relaxation Training

Autogenic training. This approach, advocated by Schultz and Luthe[129] and Engle,[49] involves conscious relaxation through autosuggestion and a progression of exercises as well as meditation.

Progressive relaxation. This technique, pioneered by Jacobson,[74] uses systematic, distal-to-proximal progression of voluntary contraction and relaxation of muscles. It is sometimes incorporated into childbirth education.

Awareness through movement. The system of therapy developed by Feldenkrais[53] combines sensory awareness, movements of the limbs and trunk, deep breathing, conscious relaxation procedures, and self-massage to remediate muscle tension and pain by altering muscle imbalances and abnormal postural alignment.

Sequence for Progressive Relaxation Techniques

- Place the patient in a quiet area and in a comfortable position and be sure that restrictive clothing is loosened.
- Have the patient breathe in a deep, relaxed manner.
- Ask the patient to contract the distal musculature in the hands or feet voluntarily for several (5 to 7) seconds and then consciously relax those muscles for 20 to 30 seconds.
- Suggest that the patient try to feel a sense of heaviness in the hands or feet and a sense of warmth in the muscles just relaxed.
- Progress to a more proximal area of the body and have the patient actively contract and actively relax the more proximal musculature. Eventually have the patient isometrically contract and consciously relax the entire extremity.
- Suggest to the patient that he or she should feel a sense of relaxation and warmth throughout the entire limb and eventually throughout the whole body.

Pilates

Pilates is an approach to exercise that combines Western theories of biomechanics, core stability, and motor control with Eastern theories of the interaction of body, mind, and spirit.[6] Components of a Pilates exercise session typically include deep breathing and core stabilization exercises, focus on activation and relaxation of specific muscle groups, posture control and awareness training, strength training (primarily using body weight as resistance), balance exercises, and flexibility exercises.[134]

Although Pilates training may be part of community-based fitness programs for healthy adults, therapists may also incorporate elements of Pilates into individualized intervention programs for patients with a variety of diagnoses. Despite limited research, Pilates exercises appear to have a positive benefit on function (including improved flexibility, strength, and pain control) and quality of life in healthy individuals[130] and those with impairments.[81,126]

Heat

Warming up prior to stretching is an important element of rehabilitation and fitness programs. It is well documented in human and animal studies that as intramuscular temperature increases, the extensibility of contractile and noncontractile soft tissues likewise increases. In addition, as the temperature of muscle increases, the amount of force required and the time the stretch force must be applied decrease.[88,89,123,154] There is also a decrease in the rate of firing of the type II efferents from the muscle spindles and an increase in the sensitivity of the GTO, which makes it more likely to fire.[57] It is also believed that when tissues relax and more easily lengthen, stretching is associated with less muscle guarding and is more comfortable for the patient.[88,89]

CLINICAL TIP

Although stretching is often thought of as a warm-up activity performed prior to vigorous exercise,[132] an appropriate warm-up, typically through low-intensity active exercise, must be carried out *in preparation* for stretching.

Methods of Warm-Up

Superficial heat (hot packs or paraffin) or deep-heating modalities (ultrasound or shortwave diathermy) provide different mechanisms to heat tissues.[104,121] These thermal agents are used primarily to heat small areas such as individual joints, muscle groups, or tendons and may be applied prior to or during the stretching procedure.[46,83,123] There is no consensus as to whether heating modalities should be applied prior to or during the stretching procedure.

Low-intensity, active exercises, which generally increase circulation and core body temperature, also can be used as a mechanism to warm up large muscle groups prior to stretching.[43,83] Some common warm-up exercises are a brief walk, nonfatiguing cycling on a stationary bicycle, use of a stair-stepping machine, active heel raises, or a few minutes of active arm exercises.

Effectiveness of Warm-Up Methods

Thermal agents or warm-up exercises used alone without stretching have either little or no effect on improving muscle flexibility.[16,43,65,135] While some evidence indicates that heat combined with stretching produces greater long-term gains in tissue length than stretching alone,[45,46] other studies have not shown differences in ROM gain between these two methods.[43,65,83,139]

Cold

The application of cold prior to stretching (cryostretching) compared with heat has been studied,[139] and advocates suggest it decreases muscle tone and makes the muscle less sensitive during stretch in healthy subjects[62] and in patients with spasticity or rigidity secondary to upper motor neuron lesions.[148] While the use of cold immediately after soft tissue injury effectively decreases pain and muscle spasm, once healing and scar formation begin, cold makes healing tissues less extensible and more susceptible to microtrauma during stretching.[33,88] Cooling soft tissues in a lengthened position *after* stretching has been shown to promote more lasting increases in soft tissue length and to minimize poststretch muscle soreness.[89]

CLINICAL TIP

The authors of this text recommend that cold be applied to injured soft tissues during the first 24 to 48 hours after injury to minimize swelling, muscle spasm, and pain. Remember, stretching is contraindicated in the presence of inflammation that occurs during the acute phase of tissue healing (see Chapter 10). When inflammation subsides and stretching is indicated, the authors advocate warming soft tissues prior to or during a stretching maneuver. After stretching, cold should be applied to soft tissues held in a lengthened position to minimize poststretch muscle soreness and to promote longer-lasting gains in ROM.

Massage

Massage for Relaxation

Local muscle relaxation can be enhanced by massage, particularly with light or deep stroking techniques.[40,138] Self-massage with light stroking techniques is used to enhance relaxation in some approaches to pain or stress and anxiety management.[53] In sports and conditioning programs,[11,138] massage is used for general relaxation purposes or to enhance recovery after strenuous physical activity, although the efficacy of the latter is not well founded.[144] Because massage has been shown to increase circulation to muscles and decrease muscle spasm, it can be a useful adjunct to stretching exercises.

Soft Tissue Mobilization/Manipulation Techniques

Another broad category of massage is soft tissue mobilization/manipulation. Although these techniques involve various forms of deep massage, the primary purpose is not relaxation but to increase the mobility of adherent or shortened connective tissues including fascia, tendons, and ligaments.[20]

There are several soft tissue mobilization/manipulation techniques that are used clinically to improve soft tissue mobility. These techniques are often specific to a tissue or specific adhesion, and the rationale for their use is based primarily on the mechanical effects of stress and strain. Stresses during the technique are applied for a long enough duration for creep and stress-relaxation of tissues to occur. With *myofascial massage*,[20,93] stretch forces are applied across fascial planes or between muscle and septae. With *friction massage*,[35,70,138] deep circular or cross-fiber (perpendicular to tissue fiber orientation) massage is applied to break up adhesions or minimize rough surfaces between tendons and their synovial sheaths. *Instrument-assisted soft tissue mobilization* uses specially crafted tools to release fascial restrictions and scar tissue. Friction massage is also used to increase the mobility of scar tissue in muscle as it heals. Theoretically, stresses applied to maturing scar tissue align the collagen fibers along the lines of stress to encourage normal mobility. These forms of connective tissue massage, as well as many other approaches and techniques of soft tissue mobilization, are useful interventions for patients with restricted mobility.

Biofeedback

Biofeedback is another tool that can help a patient learn and practice the process of relaxation. A patient, with proper instruction, can monitor and learn to reduce the amount of muscle tension through biofeedback instrumentation.[49,146] Through the visual or auditory feedback provided by the instrumentation, the patient can begin to sense or feel the relaxed muscle. By voluntarily reducing muscle tension, pain can be decreased and flexibility increased. Biofeedback can also be used to help a patient increase voluntary muscle activation, such as when learning how to perform quadriceps setting exercises after knee surgery.

Joint Traction or Oscillation

Slight manual distraction of joint surfaces prior to stretching a muscle-tendon unit can be used to inhibit joint pain and muscle spasm around a joint (see Chapter 5).[35,70,78] Pendular motions of a joint use the weight of the limb to distract the joint surfaces and simultaneously oscillate and relax the limb. The joint may be further distracted by adding a 1- or 2-lb weight to the extremity, which causes a stretch force on joint tissues.

Manual Stretching Techniques in Anatomical Planes of Motion

As with the ROM exercises described in Chapter 3, the manual stretching techniques in this section are described with the patient in a *supine* position. Alternative patient positions, such as prone or sitting, are indicated for some motions and are noted when necessary. Manual stretching procedures in an aquatic environment are described in Chapter 9.

Effective manual stretching techniques require adequate stabilization of the patient and sufficient strength and good body mechanics of the therapist. Depending on the size (height and weight) of the therapist and the patient, modifications in the patient's position and suggested hand placements for stretching or stabilization may have to be made by the therapist.

Each description of a stretching technique is identified by the anatomical plane of motion that is to be increased followed by a notation of the muscle group being stretched. Limitations in functional ROM usually are caused by shortening of multiple muscle groups and periarticular structures, and they affect movement in combined (as well as anatomical) planes of motion. In this situation, however, stretching multiple muscle groups simultaneously using diagonal patterns (i.e., D_1 and D_2 flexion and extension of the upper or lower extremities as described in Chapter 6) is *not* recommended and therefore is not described in this chapter. The authors believe that combined, diagonal patterns are appropriate for maintaining available ROM with passive and active exercises and increasing strength in multiple muscle groups but are ineffective for *isolating* a stretch force to specific muscles or muscle groups of the extremities that are shortened and restricting ROM. Special considerations for each region being stretched are also noted in this section.

Prolonged passive stretching techniques using mechanical equipment are applied using the same points of stabilization as manual stretching. The forces used in mechanical stretching are applied at a lower intensity and over a much longer period than with manual stretching. The stretch force is provided by weights or orthotics rather than the strength or endurance of a therapist. The patient is stabilized with belts, straps, or counterweights.

NOTE: Manual stretching procedures for the musculature of the cervical, thoracic, and lumbar spine may be found in Chapter 16.

Selected self-stretching techniques of the spine and extremities that a patient can do without assistance from a therapist can be found in Chapters 16 through 22.

Upper Extremity Stretching

The Shoulder: Special Considerations

Many muscles that move the arm attach to the scapula rather than the thorax. Therefore, when muscles of the shoulder girdle are stretched, it is imperative to stabilize the scapula. Without scapular stabilization some of the stretch force will be transmitted to the scapulothoracic muscles. This subjects these muscles to possible overstretching, limits the effectiveness of the applied stretch, and disguises the actual ROM of the glenohumeral (GH) joint. Remember:

- When the scapula is stabilized and not allowed to abduct or upwardly rotate, only 120° of shoulder flexion and abduction can occur at the GH joint.
- The humerus must be externally rotated to gain full ROM of abduction.
- Muscles most apt to become shortened are those that *prevent* full shoulder flexion, abduction, and external rotation. It is rare to find restrictions in structures that prevent shoulder adduction and extension to neutral.

Shoulder Flexion VIDEO 4.2

To increase flexion of the shoulder, stretch the shoulder extensors (Fig. 4.16).

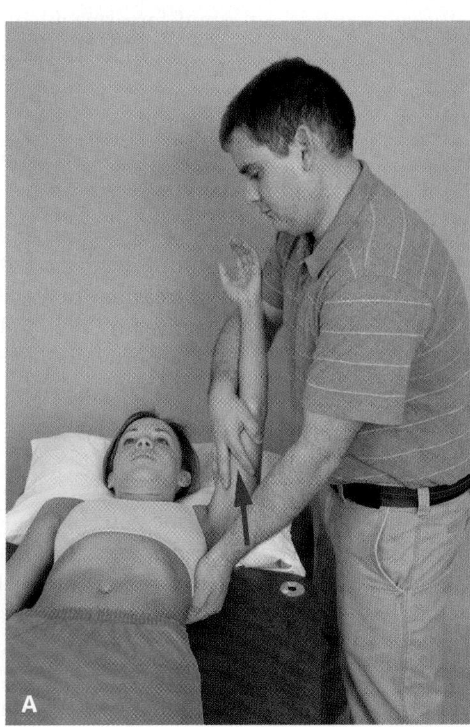

FIGURE 4.16 (A) Hand placement and stabilization of the scapula to stretch the teres major and increase shoulder flexion.

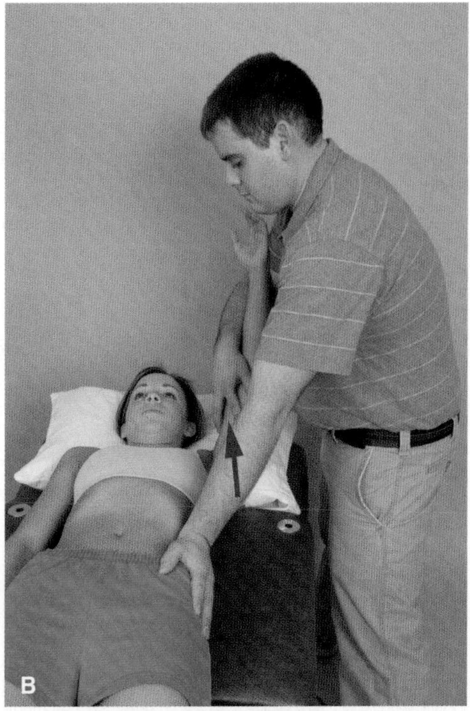

FIGURE 4.16 (B) Hand placement and stabilization of the pelvis to stretch the latissimus dorsi and increase shoulder flexion.

Hand Placement and Procedure

- Grasp the posterior aspect of the distal humerus just above the elbow.
- Stabilize the axillary border of the scapula to stretch the teres major or stabilize the lateral aspect of the thorax and superior aspect of the pelvis to stretch the latissimus dorsi.
- Move the patient's arm into full shoulder flexion to elongate the shoulder extensors.

Shoulder Hyperextension VIDEO 4.3

To increase hyperextension of the shoulder, stretch the shoulder flexors (Fig. 4.17).

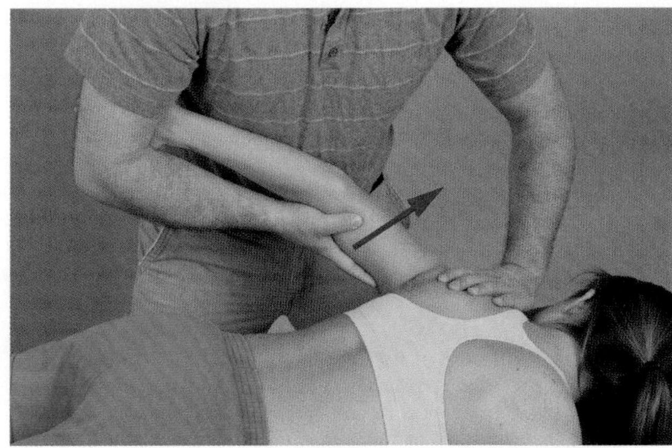

FIGURE 4.17 Hand placement and stabilization of the scapula to increase extension of the shoulder beyond neutral.

Patient Position

Place the patient in a prone position.

Hand Placement and Procedure

- Support the forearm and grasp the distal humerus.
- Stabilize the posterior aspect of the scapula to prevent substitute movements.
- Move the patient's arm into full hyperextension of the shoulder to elongate the shoulder flexors.

Shoulder Abduction

To increase abduction of the shoulder, stretch the adductors (Fig. 4.18).

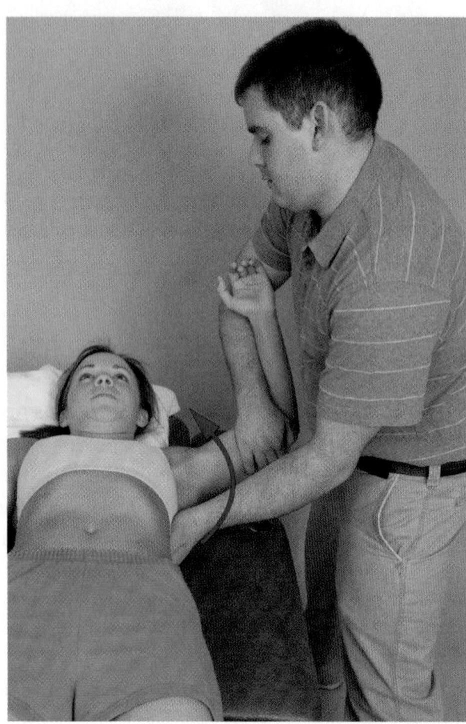

FIGURE 4.18 Hand placement and stabilization of the scapula for the stretching procedure to increase shoulder abduction.

Hand Placement and Procedure

- With the elbow flexed to 90°, grasp the distal humerus.
- Stabilize the axillary border of the scapula.
- Move the patient into full shoulder abduction to lengthen the adductors of the shoulder.

Shoulder Adduction

To increase adduction of the shoulder, stretch the abductors. It is rare when a patient is unable to adduct the shoulder fully to 0° (so the upper arm is at the patient's side). Even if a patient has worn an abduction orthotic after a soft tissue or joint injury of the shoulder, when he or she is upright the constant pull of gravity elongates the shoulder abductors so the patient can adduct to a neutral position.

Shoulder External Rotation VIDEO 4.4

To increase external rotation of the shoulder, stretch the internal rotators (Fig. 4.19).

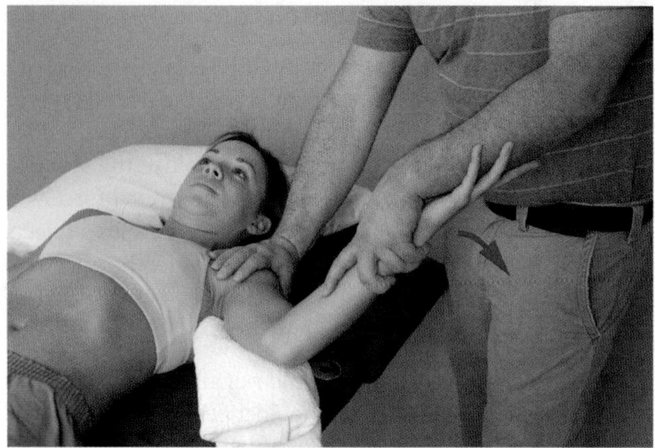

FIGURE 4.19 Shoulder position (slightly abducted and flexed) and hand placement at the mid to proximal forearm to increase external rotation of the shoulder. A folded towel is placed under the distal humerus to maintain the shoulder in slight flexion. The table stabilizes the scapula.

Hand Placement and Procedure

- Abduct the shoulder to a comfortable position—initially 30° or 45° and later to 90° if the GH joint is stable—or place the arm at the patient's side.
- Flex the elbow to 90° so the forearm can be used as a lever.
- Grasp the volar surface of the mid-forearm with one hand.
- Stabilization of the scapula is provided by the table on which the patient is lying.
- Externally rotate the patient's shoulder by moving the patient's forearm closer to the table. This fully lengthens the internal rotators.

PRECAUTION: Because it is necessary to apply the stretch forces across the intermediate elbow joint when elongating the internal and external rotators of the shoulder, be sure the elbow joint is stable and pain-free. In addition, keep the intensity of the stretch force very low, particularly in patients with osteoporosis.

Shoulder Internal Rotation

To increase internal rotation of the shoulder, stretch the external rotators (Fig. 4.20).

Hand Placement and Procedure

- Abduct the shoulder to a comfortable position that allows internal rotation to occur without the thorax blocking the motion (initially to 45° and eventually to 90°).
- Flex the elbow to 90° so the forearm can be used as a lever.
- Grasp the dorsal surface of the midforearm with one hand, stabilize the anterior aspect of the shoulder, and support the elbow with your other forearm and hand.
- Move the patient's arm into an internal rotation to lengthen the external rotators of the shoulder.

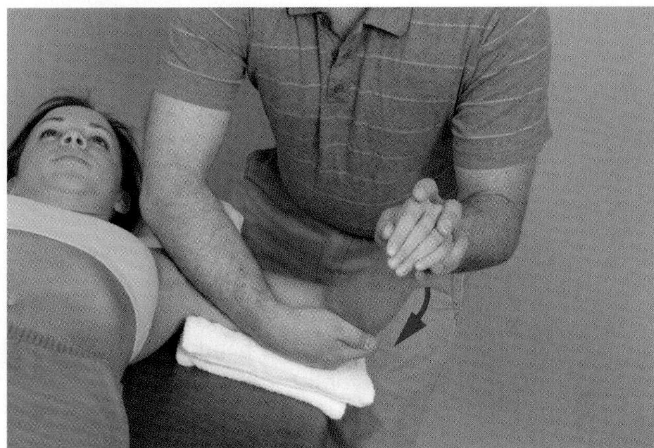

FIGURE 4.20 Hand placement and stabilization of the shoulder to increase internal rotation of the shoulder.

Shoulder Horizontal Abduction

To increase horizontal abduction of the shoulder, stretch the pectoralis muscles (Fig. 4.21).

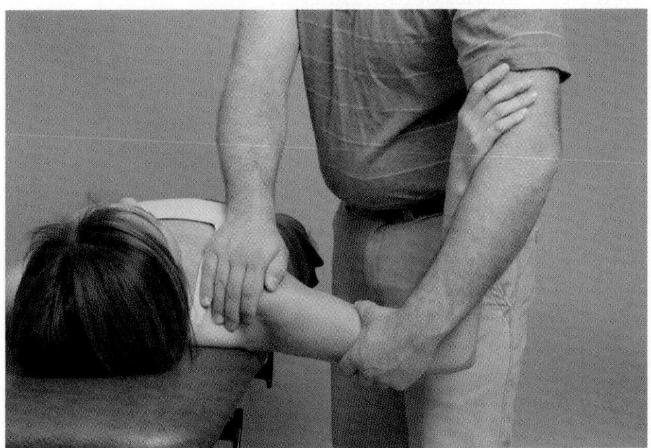

FIGURE 4.21 Hand placement and stabilization of the anterior aspect of the shoulder and chest to increase horizontal abduction of the shoulder past neutral (to stretch the pectoralis major).

Patient Position

To reach full horizontal abduction in the supine position, the patient's shoulder must be at the edge of the table. Begin with the shoulder in 60° to 90° of abduction. The patient's elbow may also be flexed.

Hand Placement and Procedure

- Grasp the anterior aspect of the distal humerus.
- Stabilize the anterior aspect of the shoulder.
- Move the patient's arm below the edge of the table into full horizontal abduction to stretch the horizontal adductors.

NOTE: The horizontal adductors are usually tight bilaterally. Stretching techniques can be applied bilaterally by the therapist, or a bilateral self-stretch can be done by the patient by using a corner or wand (see Figs. 17.30 through 17.32).

Scapular Mobility

To have full shoulder motion, a patient must have normal scapular mobility. (See the scapular mobilization/manipulation techniques in Chapter 5.)

The Elbow and Forearm: Special Considerations

Several muscles that cross the elbow, such as the biceps brachii and brachioradialis, also influence supination and pronation of the forearm. Therefore, when stretching the elbow flexors and extensors, the techniques should be performed with the forearm pronated as well as supinated.

Elbow Flexion

To increase elbow flexion, stretch the one-joint elbow extensors.

Hand Placement and Procedure

- Grasp the distal forearm just proximal to the wrist.
- With the arm at the patient's side supported on the table, stabilize the proximal humerus.
- Flex the patient's elbow just past the point of tissue resistance to lengthen the elbow extensors.

To increase elbow flexion with the shoulder flexed, stretch the long head of the triceps (Fig. 4.22).

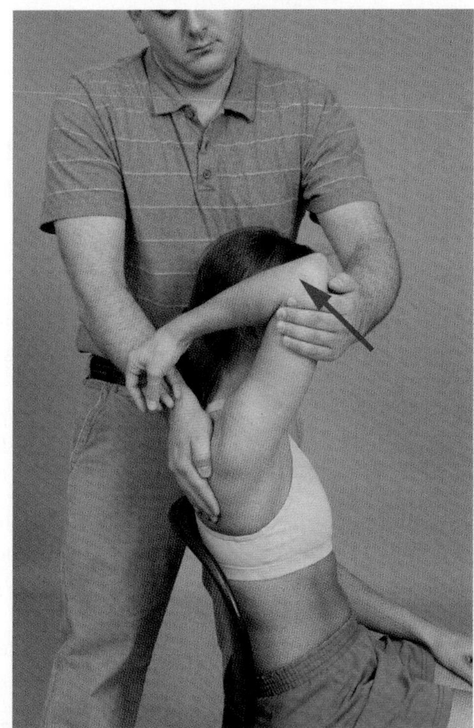

FIGURE 4.22 Hand placement and stabilization to increase elbow flexion with shoulder flexion (to stretch the long head of the triceps brachii).

Patient Position, Hand Placement, and Procedure

- With the patient sitting or lying supine with the arm at the edge of the table, flex the patient's shoulder as far as possible.

- While maintaining shoulder flexion, grasp the distal forearm and flex the elbow just past the point of resistance to lengthen the long head of the triceps.

Elbow Extension VIDEO 4.5

To increase elbow extension, stretch the elbow flexors (Fig. 4.23).

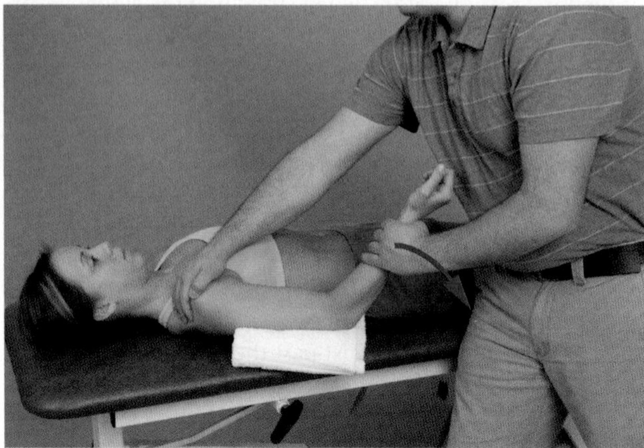

FIGURE 4.23 Hand placement and stabilization of the scapula and proximal humerus for stretching procedures to increase elbow extension.

Hand Placement and Procedure

- Grasp the distal forearm.
- With the upper arm at the patient's side supported on the table, stabilize the scapula and anterior aspect of the proximal humerus.
- Extend the elbow just past the point of tissue resistance to lengthen the elbow flexors.

NOTE: Be sure to do this with the forearm in supination, pronation, and neutral position to stretch each of the elbow flexors.

To increase elbow extension with the shoulder extended, stretch the long head of the biceps.

Patient Position, Hand Placement, and Procedure

- With the patient lying supine close to the side of the table, stabilize the anterior aspect of the shoulder, or with the patient lying prone, stabilize the scapula.
- Pronate the forearm, extend the elbow, and then extend the shoulder.

PRECAUTION: It has been reported that heterotopic ossification (the appearance of ectopic bone in the soft tissues around a joint) can develop around the elbow after traumatic or burn injuries.[48] It is believed that *vigorous, forcible* passive stretching of the elbow flexors may increase the risk of this condition developing. Passive or assisted stretching should therefore be applied very gently and gradually in the elbow region. Use of active stretching techniques, such as agonist contraction, might also be considered.

Forearm Supination or Pronation

To increase supination or pronation of the forearm.

Hand Placement and Procedure

- With the patient's humerus supported on the table and the elbow flexed to 90°, grasp the distal forearm.
- Stabilize the humerus.
- Supinate or pronate the forearm just beyond the point of tissue resistance.
- Be sure the stretch force is applied to the radius rotating around the ulna. Do not twist the hand, thereby avoiding stress to the wrist articulations.
- Repeat the procedure with the elbow extended. Be sure to stabilize the humerus to prevent internal or external rotation of the shoulder.

The Wrist and Hand: Special Considerations

VIDEO 4.6

The extrinsic muscles of the fingers cross the wrist joint and therefore may influence the ROM of the wrist. Wrist motion may also be influenced by the position of the elbow and forearm because the wrist flexors and extensors attach proximally on the epicondyles of the humerus.

When stretching the musculature of the wrist, the stretch force should be applied proximal to the metacarpophalangeal (MCP) joints, and the fingers should be relaxed.

Patient Position

When stretching the muscles of the wrist and hand, have the patient sit in a chair adjacent to you with the forearm supported on a table to stabilize the forearm effectively.

Wrist Flexion

To increase wrist flexion.

Hand Placement and Procedure

- The forearm may be supinated, in midposition, or pronated.
- Stabilize the forearm against the table and grasp the dorsal aspect of the patient's hand.
- To elongate the wrist extensors, flex the patient's wrist and allow the fingers to extend passively.
- To further elongate the wrist extensors, extend the patient's elbow.

Wrist Extension

To increase wrist extension (Fig. 4.24).

Hand Placement and Procedure

- Pronate the forearm or place it in midposition and grasp the patient at the palmar aspect of the hand. If there is a severe wrist flexion contracture, it may be necessary to place the patient's hand over the edge of the treatment table.
- Stabilize the forearm against the table.
- To lengthen the wrist flexors, extend the patient's wrist, allowing the fingers to flex passively.

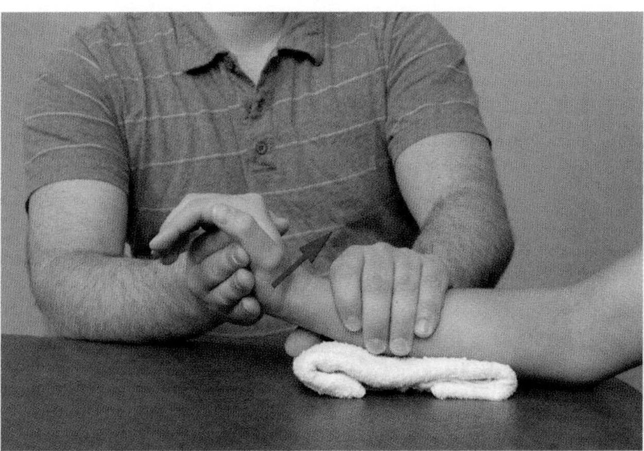

FIGURE 4.24 Hand placement and stabilization of the forearm for stretching procedure to increase extension of the wrist.

Radial Deviation

To increase radial deviation.

Hand Placement and Procedure

- Grasp the ulnar aspect of the hand along the fifth metacarpal.
- Hold the wrist in midposition.
- Stabilize the forearm.
- Radially deviate the wrist to lengthen the ulnar deviators of the wrist.

Ulnar Deviation

To increase ulnar deviation.

Hand Placement and Procedure

- Grasp the radial aspect of the hand along the second metacarpal, not the thumb.
- Stabilize the forearm.
- Ulnarly deviate the wrist to lengthen the radial deviators.

The Digits: Special Considerations VIDEO 4.7

The complexity of the relationships among the joint structures and the intrinsic and multijoint extrinsic muscles of the digits requires careful examination and evaluation of the factors that contribute to loss of function in the hand because of motion limitations. The therapist must determine if a limitation is from joint restrictions, decreased muscle-tendon unit extensibility, or adhesions of tendons or ligaments. The digits should always be stretched individually, not simultaneously. If an extrinsic muscle limits motion, lengthen it over one joint while stabilizing the other joints. Then, hold the lengthened position and stretch it over the second joint, and so forth, until normal length is obtained. Begin the motion with the most distal joint to minimize shearing and compressive stresses to the surfaces of the small joints of the digits. Specific interventions to manage adhesions of tendons are described in Chapter 19.

CMC Joint of the Thumb

To increase flexion, extension, abduction, or adduction of the carpometacarpal (CMC) joint of the thumb.

Hand Placement and Procedure

- Stabilize the trapezium with your thumb and index finger.
- Grasp the first metacarpal (not the first phalanx) with your other thumb and index finger.
- Move the first metacarpal in the desired direction to increase CMC flexion, extension, abduction, and adduction.

MCP Joints of the Digits

To increase flexion, extension, abduction, or adduction of the MCP joints of the digits.

Hand Placement and Procedure

- Stabilize the metacarpal with your thumb and index finger.
- Grasp the proximal phalanx with your other thumb and index finger.
- Keep the wrist in midposition.
- Move the MCP joint in the desired direction for stretch.
- Allow the interphalangeal (IP) joints to flex or extend passively.

PIP and DIP Joints

To increase flexion or extension of the proximal and distal interphalangeal (PIP and DIP) joints.

Hand Placement and Procedure

- Grasp the middle or distal phalanx with your thumb and finger.
- Stabilize the proximal or middle phalanx with your other thumb and finger.
- Move the PIP or DIP joint in the desired direction for stretch.

Stretching Specific Extrinsic and Intrinsic Muscles of the Fingers

Elongation of extrinsic and intrinsic muscles of the hand is described in Chapter 3. To stretch these muscles beyond their available range, the same hand placement and stabilization are used as with passive ROM. The only difference in technique is that the therapist moves each segment into the stretch range.

Lower Extremity Stretching

The Hip: Special Considerations VIDEO 4.8

Because muscles of the hip attach to the pelvis or lumbar spine, the pelvis must always be stabilized when lengthening muscles about the hip. If the pelvis is not stabilized, the stretch force is transferred to the lumbar spine and unwanted compensatory motion results.

Hip Flexion

To increase flexion of the hip with the knee flexed, stretch the gluteus maximus.

Hand Placement and Procedure

- Flex the hip and knee simultaneously.
- Stabilize the opposite femur in extension to prevent posterior tilt of the pelvis.

- Move the patient's hip and knee into full flexion to lengthen the one-joint hip extensor.

Hip Flexion With Knee Extension

To increase flexion of the hip with the knee extended, stretch the hamstrings (Fig. 4.25 A and B).

Hand Placement and Procedure

- With the patient's knee fully extended, support the patient's lower leg with your arm or shoulder.
- Stabilize the opposite extremity along the anterior aspect of the thigh with your other hand or a belt or with the assistance of another person.

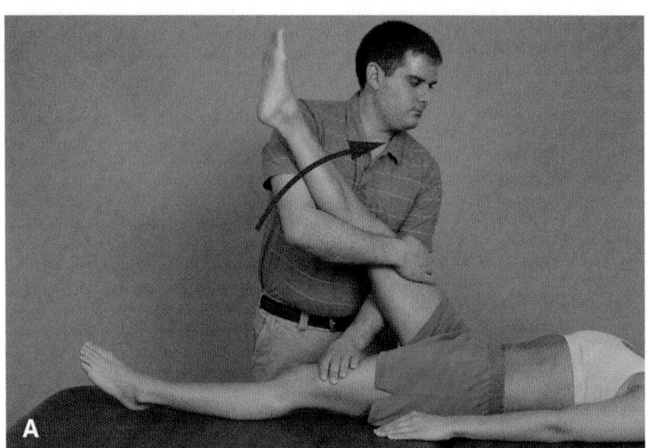

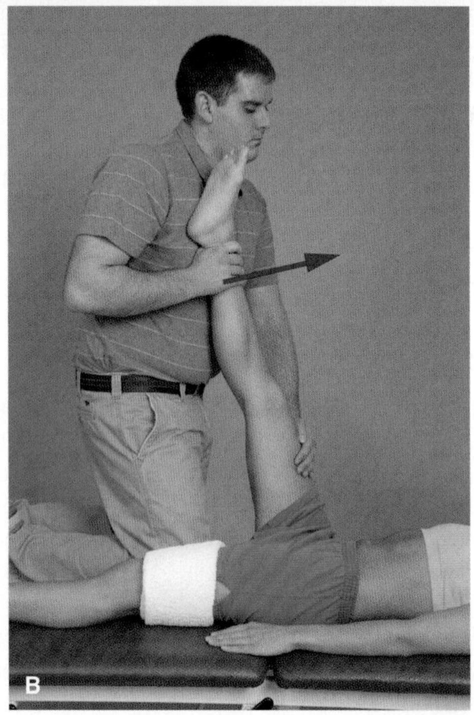

FIGURE 4.25 Hand placement and stabilization of the opposite femur to stabilize the pelvis and low back for stretching procedures to increase hip flexion with knee extension (stretch the hamstrings) with the therapist **(A)** standing by the side of the table or **(B)** kneeling on the table.

- With the knee at 0° extension and the hip in neutral rotation, flex the hip as far as possible.

NOTE: Externally rotate the hip prior to hip flexion to isolate the stretch force to the medial hamstrings and internally rotate the hip to isolate the stretch force to the lateral hamstrings.

Alternative Therapist Position

Kneel on the mat and place the patient's heel or distal tibia against your shoulder (see Fig. 4.25 B). Place both of your hands along the anterior aspect of the distal thigh to keep the knee extended. The opposite extremity is stabilized in extension by a belt or towel around the distal thigh and held in place by the therapist's knee.

Hip Extension VIDEO 4.9

To increase hip extension, stretch the iliopsoas (Fig. 4.26).

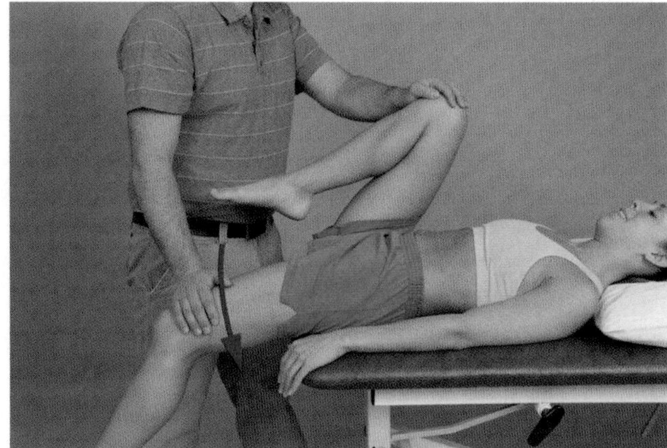

FIGURE 4.26 Hand placement and stabilization of the pelvis to increase extension of the hip (stretch the iliopsoas) with the patient lying supine. Flexing the knee when in this position also elongates the rectus femoris.

Patient Position

Have the patient positioned close to the edge of the treatment table so the hip being stretched can be extended beyond neutral. The opposite hip and knee are flexed toward the patient's chest to stabilize the pelvis and spine.

Hand Placement and Procedure

- Stabilize the opposite leg against the patient's chest with one hand or, if possible, have the patient assist by grasping around the thigh and holding it to the chest to prevent an anterior tilt of the pelvis during stretching.
- Move the hip to be stretched into extension or hyperextension by placing downward pressure on the anterior aspect of the distal thigh with your other hand. Allow the knee to extend so the two-joint rectus femoris does not restrict the range.

Alternate Position

Have the patient assume the prone-lying position (Fig. 4.27).

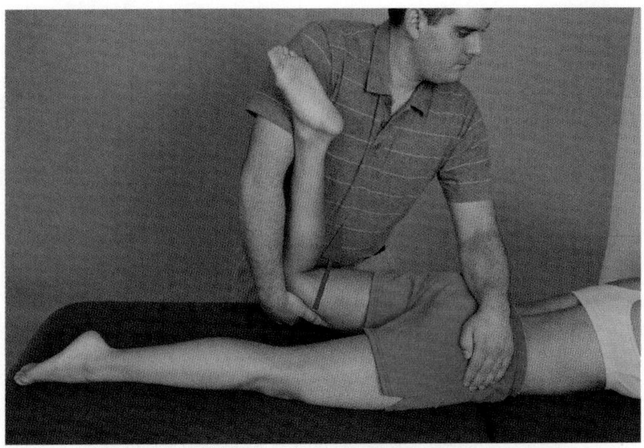

FIGURE 4.27 Hand placement and stabilization to increase hyperextension of the hip with the patient lying prone.

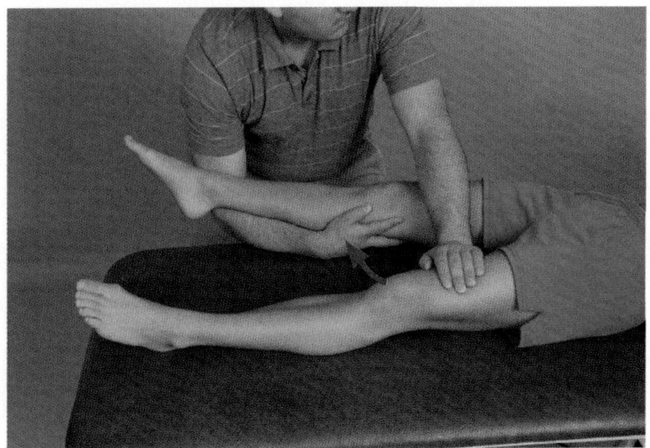

FIGURE 4.28 Hand placement and stabilization of the opposite extremity (or pelvis) for the stretching procedure to increase abduction of the hip.

Hand Placement and Procedure

- Support and grasp the anterior aspect of the patient's distal femur.
- Stabilize the patient's pelvis with a downward force on their buttocks.
- Extend the patient's hip by lifting the femur off the table.

Hip Extension With Knee Flexion

To increase hip extension and knee flexion simultaneously, stretch the rectus femoris.

Patient Position

Use either of the positions previously described for increasing hip extension in the supine or prone positions (see Figs. 4.26 and 4.27).

Hand Placement and Procedure

- With the hip held in full extension on the side to be stretched, move your hand to the distal tibia and gently flex the knee of that extremity as far as possible.
- Do not allow the hip to abduct or rotate.

Hip Abduction VIDEO 4.10

To increase abduction of the hip, stretch the adductors (Fig. 4.28).

Hand Placement and Procedure

- Support the distal thigh with your arm and forearm.
- Stabilize the pelvis by placing pressure on the opposite anterior iliac crest or by maintaining the opposite lower extremity in slight abduction.
- Abduct the hip as far as possible to stretch the adductors.

NOTE: You may apply your stretch force cautiously at the medial malleolus only if the knee is stable and pain-free. An abduction force applied at this location creates a great deal of stress to the medial supporting structures of the knee and is generally not recommended by the authors.

Hip Adduction VIDEO 4.11

To increase adduction of the hip, stretch the tensor fasciae latae and iliotibial (IT) band (Fig. 4.29).

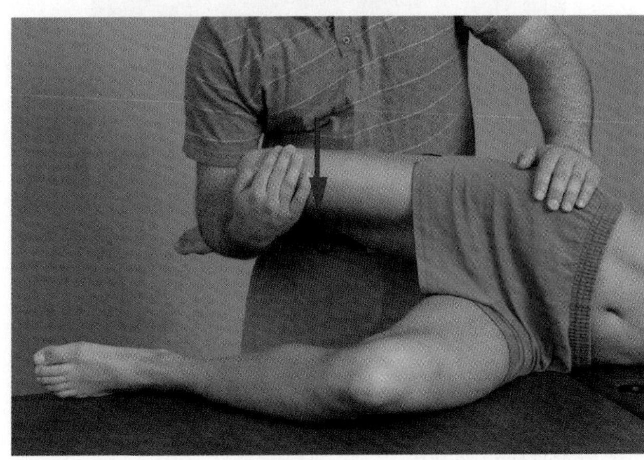

FIGURE 4.29 Patient positioned side-lying. Hand placement and procedure to stretch the tensor fasciae latae and IT band.

Patient Position

Place the patient in a side-lying position with the hip to be stretched uppermost. Flex the bottom hip and knee to stabilize the patient.

Hand Placement and Procedure

- Stabilize the pelvis at the iliac crest with your proximal hand.
- With the knee flexed, extend the patient's hip to neutral or into slight hyperextension, if possible. Moving the hip into a small amount of flexion and abduction prior to extending it may help orient the IT band for the stretch.
- Let the patient's hip adduct with gravity and apply an additional stretch force with your other hand to the lateral aspect of the distal femur to further adduct the hip.

NOTE: If the patient's hip cannot be extended to neutral, the hip flexors must be stretched before the tensor fasciae latae can be stretched.

Hip External Rotation

To increase external rotation of the hip, stretch the internal rotators (Fig. 4.30 A).

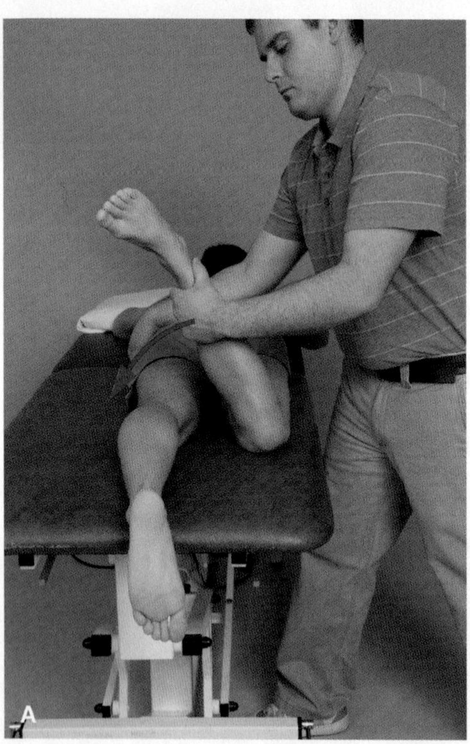

FIGURE 4.30 (A) Hand placement and stabilization of the pelvis to increase external rotation of the hip.

Patient Position

Place the patient in a prone position with the hips extended and knee flexed to 90°.

Hand Placement and Procedure

- Grasp the distal tibia of the extremity to be stretched.
- Stabilize the pelvis by applying pressure with your other hand across the buttocks.
- Apply pressure to the lateral malleolus or lateral aspect of the tibia and externally rotate the hip as far as possible.

Alternate Position and Procedure

Sitting at the edge of a table with hips and knees flexed to 90°:

- Stabilize the pelvis by applying pressure to the iliac crest with one hand.
- Apply the stretch force to the lateral malleolus or lateral aspect of the lower leg and externally rotate the hip.

NOTE: When you apply the stretch force against the lower leg in this manner, thus crossing the knee joint, the knee must be stable and pain-free. If the knee is not stable, it is possible to apply the stretch force by grasping the distal thigh, but the leverage is poor and there is a tendency to twist the skin.

Hip Internal Rotation

To increase internal rotation of the hip, stretch the external rotators (Fig. 4.30 B).

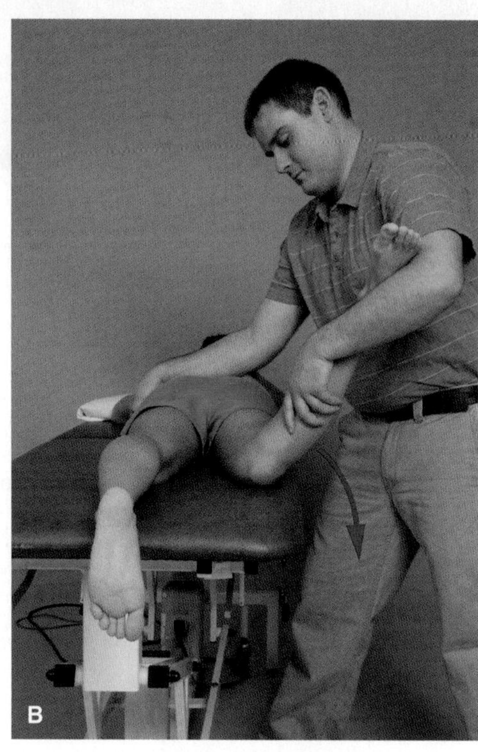

FIGURE 4.30 (B) Hand placement and stabilization of the pelvis to increase internal rotation of the hip with the patient prone.

Patient Position and Stabilization

Position the patient the same as when increasing external rotation, described previously.

Hand Placement and Procedure

Apply pressure to the medial malleolus or medial aspect of the tibia and internally rotate the hip as far as possible.

The Knee: Special Considerations

VIDEO 4.12

The position of the hip during stretching influences the flexibility of the flexors and extensors of the knee. The flexibility of the hamstrings and the rectus femoris must be examined and evaluated separately from the one-joint muscles that affect knee motion.

Knee Flexion

To increase knee flexion, stretch the knee extensors (Fig. 4.31).

Patient Position

Have the patient assume a prone position.

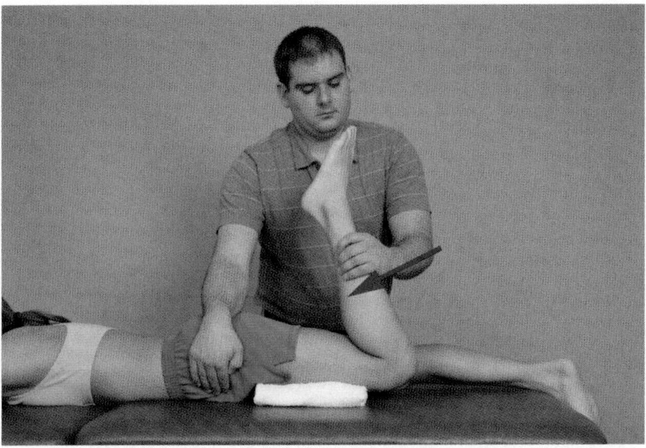

FIGURE 4.31 Hand placement and stabilization to increase knee flexion (stretch the rectus femoris and quadriceps) with the patient lying prone.

Hand Placement and Procedure

- Stabilize the pelvis by applying downward pressure across the buttocks.
- Grasp the anterior aspect of the distal tibia and flex the patient's knee.

PRECAUTION: Place a rolled towel under the thigh just above the knee to prevent compression of the patella against the table during the stretch. Stretching the knee extensors too vigorously in the prone position can traumatize the knee joint and cause swelling.

Alternate Position and Procedure

- Have the patient sit with the thigh supported on the treatment table and leg flexed over the edge as far as possible.
- Stabilize the anterior aspect of the proximal femur with one hand.
- Apply the stretch force to the anterior aspect of the distal tibia and flex the patient's knee just past the point of tissue resistance.

NOTE: This position is useful when working in the 0° to 100° range of knee flexion. The prone position is best for increasing knee flexion from 90° to 135°.

Knee Extension

To increase knee extension in the midrange, stretch the knee flexors (Fig. 4.32).

Patient Position

Place the patient in a prone position and put a small, rolled towel under the patient's distal femur, just above the patella.

Hand Placement and Procedure

- Grasp the distal tibia with one hand and stabilize the buttocks to prevent hip flexion with the other hand.
- Slowly extend the knee to stretch the knee flexors.

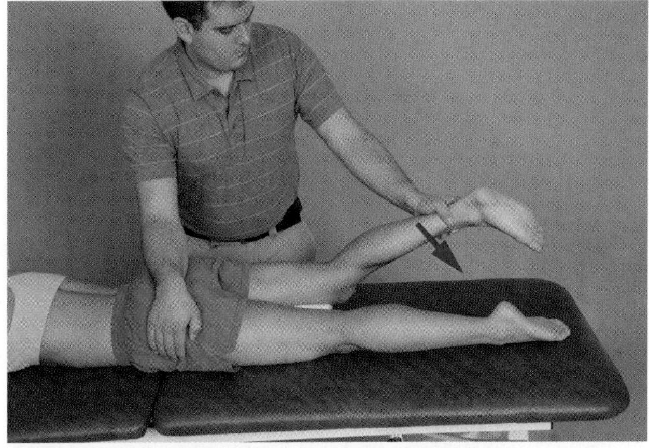

FIGURE 4.32 Hand placement and stabilization to increase midrange knee extension with the patient lying prone.

End-Range Knee Extension VIDEO 4.13

To increase end-range knee extension (Fig. 4.33).

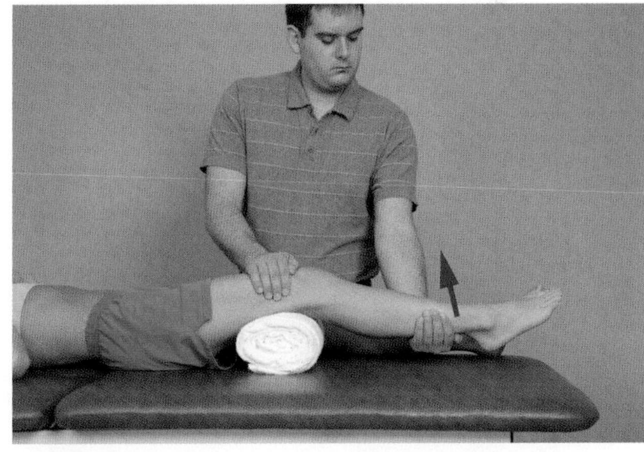

FIGURE 4.33 Hand placement and stabilization to increase terminal knee extension.

Patient Position

Patient assumes a supine position.

Hand Placement and Procedure

- Grasp the distal tibia of the knee to be stretched.
- Stabilize the hip by placing your hand or forearm across the anterior thigh. This prevents hip flexion during stretching.
- Apply the stretch force to the posterior aspect of the distal tibia and extend the patient's knee.

The Ankle and Foot: Special Considerations VIDEO 4.14

The ankle and foot are composed of multiple joints. Consider the mobility of these joints (see Chapter 5) as well as the multijoint muscles that cross these joints when increasing ankle and foot ROM.

Ankle Dorsiflexion

To increase dorsiflexion of the ankle with the knee extended, stretch the gastrocnemius muscle (Fig. 4.34).

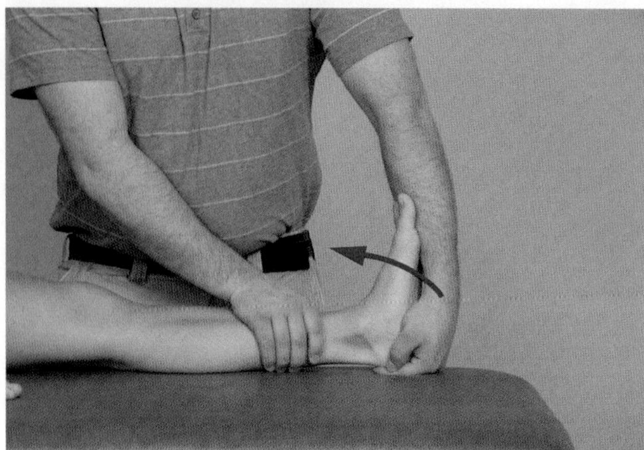

FIGURE 4.34 Hand placement and procedure to increase dorsiflexion of the ankle with the knee extended (stretching the gastrocnemius).

Hand Placement and Procedure

- Grasp the patient's heel (calcaneus) with one hand, maintain the subtalar joint in a neutral position, and place your forearm along the plantar surface of the foot.
- Stabilize the anterior aspect of the tibia with your other hand.
- Dorsiflex the talocrural joint of the ankle by pulling the calcaneus in an inferior direction with your thumb and fingers while gently applying pressure in a superior direction just proximal to the heads of the metatarsals with your forearm.

To increase dorsiflexion of the ankle with the knee flexed, stretch the soleus muscle. The knee must be flexed to eliminate the effect of the two-joint gastrocnemius muscle. Hand placement, stabilization, and stretch force are the same as when stretching the gastrocnemius.

PRECAUTION: When stretching the gastrocnemius or soleus muscles, avoid placing too much pressure against the heads of the metatarsals and stretching the long arch of the foot. Overstretching the long arch of the foot can cause a flat foot or a rocker-bottom foot.

Ankle Plantarflexion

To increase plantarflexion of the ankle.

Hand Placement and Procedure

- Support the posterior aspect of the distal tibia with one hand.
- Grasp the foot along the tarsal and metatarsal areas.
- Apply the stretch force to the anterior aspect of the foot and plantarflex the foot.

Ankle Inversion and Eversion

To increase inversion and eversion of the ankle. Inversion and eversion of the ankle occur at the subtalar joint as a component of pronation and supination. Mobility of the subtalar joint (with appropriate strength) is particularly important for walking on uneven surfaces.

Hand Placement and Procedure

- Stabilize the talus by grasping just distal to the malleoli with one hand.
- Grasp the calcaneus with your other hand and move it medially and laterally at the subtalar joint.

Stretching Specific Muscles of the Ankle and Foot

Hand Placement and Procedure

- Stabilize the distal tibia with your proximal hand.
- Grasp around the foot with your other hand and align the motion and force opposite the line of pull of the tendons. Apply the stretch force against the bone to which the muscle attaches distally.
  - *To stretch the tibialis anterior (which inverts and dorsiflexes the ankle),* grasp the dorsal aspect of the foot across the tarsals and metatarsals and plantarflex and abduct the foot.
  - *To stretch the tibialis posterior (which plantarflexes and inverts the foot),* grasp the plantar surface of the foot around the tarsals and metatarsals and dorsiflex and abduct the foot.
  - *To stretch the peroneals (which evert the foot),* grasp the lateral aspect of the foot at the tarsals and metatarsals and invert the foot.

Toe Flexion and Extension

To increase flexion and extension of the toes. It is best to stretch any musculature that limits motion in the toes individually. With one hand, stabilize the bone proximal to the restricted joint, and with the other hand, move the phalanx in the desired direction.

Neck and Trunk

Stretching techniques to increase mobility in the cervical, thoracic, and lumbar spine may be found in Chapter 16.

Self-Stretching Techniques

Examples of self-stretching techniques, performed independently by the patient after appropriate instruction, may be found in Chapters 17 through 22 (upper and lower extremities) and Chapter 16 (neck and trunk).

Independent Learning Activities

Critical Thinking and Discussion

1. What physical findings from the patient examination would lead you to decide that stretching exercises were an appropriate intervention?
2. Discuss the advantages and disadvantages of various stretching exercises, specifically manual stretching, self-stretching, and mechanical stretching. Under what circumstances would one form be a more appropriate choice than another?
3. Discuss how the effectiveness of a stretching program is influenced by the responses of contractile and noncontractile soft tissues to stretch.
4. Explain how factors such as intensity, rate, duration, and frequency of stretch can be used to maximize stretching effectiveness.
5. Discuss how your approach to and application of stretching would differ when developing stretching exercises for a healthy young adult with limited mobility in the (a) shoulder, (b) knee, or (c) ankle in contrast to an elderly individual with osteoporosis and limited motion in the same regions.
6. Explain the procedures for and rationale behind each of the following types of neuromuscular inhibition: HR, HR-AC, CR, and AC. Under what circumstances would you choose one technique over another?
7. Select a popular exercise video. Review and critique the flexibility exercises on the video. Were the flexibility exercises appropriately distributed across body regions and joints? Were the exercises executed safely and correctly? Were the exercises appropriate for the target population?
8. Your patient has been attending a Pilates class over the past few months but is now receiving your therapy services for management of a chronic hamstring strain. How could you integrate your patient's participation in these classes with your plan of care?

Laboratory Practice

1. Manually stretch as many major muscle groups of the upper and lower extremities as is *safe* and *practical* with the patient in supine, prone, side-lying, and/or seated.
2. While considering individual muscle actions and lines of pull, demonstrate how to specifically and fully elongate the following muscles: pectoralis major, biceps brachii, brachioradialis, brachialis, triceps, extensor or flexor carpi ulnaris or radialis, flexor digitorum superficialis or profundus, rectus femoris versus the iliopsoas, gastrocnemius versus soleus, and the tibialis anterior and posterior.
3. Teach your partner how to stretch major muscle groups of the upper and lower extremities using either body weight or a cuff weight as the stretch force. Be sure to include effective stabilization procedures for these stretching techniques whenever possible.
4. Using either the hold-relax or contract-relax and the hold-relax agonist contraction PNF stretching techniques, stretch at least two muscle groups at the shoulder, elbow, wrist, hip, knee, and ankle. Be sure to position, align, and stabilize your partner properly.
5. Design an effective and efficient series of self-stretches that a person who works at a desk most of the day could incorporate into a daily home exercise routine. Demonstrate and teach each self-stretching exercise to your laboratory partner.
6. Identify a recreational/sport activity that your partner enjoys and design and demonstrate a program of self-stretching exercises to prepare your partner for the activity.
7. Design a program of progressive relaxation exercises for total body relaxation. Then, implement the relaxation training sequence with your partner.

REFERENCES

1. Akagi, R, and Takahashi, H: Effect of a 5-week static stretching program on hardness of the gastrocnemius muscle. *Scand J Med Sci Sports* 24: 950–957, 2014.
2. American College of Sports Medicine: *ACSM's Resource Manual for Guidelines for Exercise Testing and Prescription,* ed. 6. Baltimore: Wolters Kluwer/Lippincott Williams & Wilkins, 2010.
3. American Physical Therapy Association: *Guide to Physical Therapist Practice,* 3.0. Available at: http://guidetoptpractice.apta.org. Accessed March 2015.
4. Amundsen, LR: The effect of aging and exercise on joint mobility. *Orthop Phys Ther Clin North Am* 2:241, 1993.
5. Amundsen, LR: Effects of age on joints and ligaments. In Kauffman, TL (ed): *Geriatric Rehabilitation Manual.* New York: Churchill Livingstone, 1999, pp 14–16.
6. Anderson, BD, and Spector, A: Introduction to Pilates-based rehabilitation. *Orthop Phys Ther Clin North Am* 9:395–411, 2000.
7. Bandy, W, Irion, J, and Briggler, M: The effect of time and frequency of static stretch on flexibility of the hamstring muscle. *Phys Ther* 77: 1090–1096, 1997.
8. Bandy, W, Irion, J, and Briggler, M: The effect of static stretch and dynamic range of motion training on the flexibility of the hamstring muscles. *J Orthop Sports Phys Ther* 27(4):295–300, 1998.
9. Behm, DG, and Chaouachi, A: A review of the acute effects of static and dynamic stretching on performance. *Eur J Appl Physiol* 111: 2633–2651, 2011.
10. Beissner, KL, Collins JE, and Holmes, H: Muscle force and range of motion as predictors of function in older adults. *Phys Ther* 80:556–563, 2000.
11. Benjamin, PJ, and Lamp, SP: *Understanding Sports Massage.* Champaign, IL: Human Kinetics, 1996.
12. Blanton, S, Grissom, SP, and Riolo, L: Use of a static adjustable ankle-foot orthosis following tibial nerve block to reduce plantar-flexion contracture in an individual with brain injury. *Phys Ther* 82(11):1087–1097, 2002.
13. Bloomfield, SA: Changes in musculoskeletal structure and function with prolonged bed rest. *Med Sci Sports Exerc* 29:197–206, 1997.

14. Boakes, JL, et al: Muscle adaptation by serial sarcomere addition 1 year after femoral lengthening. *Clin Orthop Rel Res* 456:250–253, 2007.
15. Bonutti, PM, et al: Static progressive stretch to re-establish elbow range of motion. *Clin Orthop* 303:128–134, 1994.
16. Boone, L, Ingersoll, CD, and Cordova, ML: Passive hip flexion does not increase during or following ultrasound treatment of the hamstring muscle. *Sports Med Training Rehabil* 9(3):189–198, 2000.
17. Booth, FW: Physiologic and biochemical effects of immobilization on muscle. *Clin Orthop* 219:15–20. 1994.
18. Brach, J, and Van Swearingen, JM: Physical impairment and disability: relationship to performance of activities of daily living in community-dwelling older men. *Phys Ther* 82:752–761, 2002.
19. Butler, DS: *The Sensitive Nervous System.* Adelaide, Australia: Noigroup Publications, 2000.
20. Cantu, RI, and Grodin, AJ: *Myofascial Manipulation: Theory and Clinical Application,* ed. 2. Gaithersburg, MD: Aspen, 2001.
21. Chaitow, L: *Muscle Energy Techniques,* ed. 3. St. Louis: Elsevier, 2007.
22. Chalmers, G: Re-examination of the possible role of the Golgi tendon organ and muscle spindle reflexes in proprioceptive neuromuscular facilitation muscle stretching. *Sports Biomech* 3:159–183, 2004.
23. Chandler, JM: Understanding the relationship between strength and mobility in frail elder persons: A review of the literature. *Top Geriatr Rehabil* 11:20–37, 1996.
24. Chleboun, G: Muscle structure and function. In Levangie, PK, and Norkin, CC (eds): *Joint Structure and Function: A Comprehensive Analysis,* ed. 5. Philadelphia: FA Davis, 2011, pp 108–137.
25. Cipriani, D, Abel, B, and Purrwitz, D: A comparison of two stretching protocols on hip range of motion: implications for total daily stretch duration. *J Strength Cond Res* 17:274–278, 2003.
26. Clark, MA: Muscle energy techniques in rehabilitation. In Prentice, WE, and Voight, ML (eds): *Techniques in Musculoskeletal Rehabilitation.* New York: McGraw-Hill, 2001, pp 215–223.
27. Clark, S, et al: Effects of ipsilateral anterior thigh soft tissue stretching on passive unilateral straight leg raise. *J Orthop Sports Phys Ther* 29(1): 4–9, 1999.
28. Condon, SN, and Hutton, RS: Soleus muscle electromyographic activity and ankle dorsiflexion range of motion during four stretching procedures. *Phys Ther* 67:24–30, 1987.
29. Cornelius, WL, Jensen, RL, and Odell, ME: Effects of PNF stretching phases on acute arterial blood pressure. *J Appl Physiol* 20:222–229, 1995.
30. Cramer, JT, et al: An acute bout of static stretching does not affect maximal eccentric isokinetic peak torque, the joint angle at peak torque, mean power, electromyography, or mechanomyography. *J Orthop Sports Phys Ther* 37(3):130–139, 2007.
31. Culav, EM, Clark, CH, and Merrilees, MJ: Connective tissue matrix composition and its relevance to physical therapy. *J Orthop Sports Phys Ther* 79:308–319, 1999.
32. Cummings, GS, Crutchfeld, CA, and Barnes, MR: *Soft Tissue Changes in Contractures,* vol 1. Atlanta: Stokesville, 1983.
33. Cummings, GS, and Tillman, LJ: Remodeling of dense connective tissue in normal adult tissues. In Currier, DP, and Nelson, RM (eds): *Dynamics of Human Biologic Tissues.* Philadelphia: FA Davis, 1992, pp 45–73.
34. Curwin, S: Joint structure and function. In Levangie, PK, and Norkin, CC (eds): *Joint Structure & Function: A Comprehensive Analysis,* ed. 5. Philadelphia: FA Davis, 2011, pp 64–107.
35. Cyriax, J: *Textbook of Orthopedic Medicine: Treatment by Manipulation,* ed. 11. Philadelphia: WB Saunders, 1984.
36. Davis, DS, et al: The effectiveness of 3 proprioceptive neuromuscular facilitation stretching techniques on the flexibility of the hamstring muscle group. *J Orthop Sports Phys Ther* 34(1):33A–34A, 2004.
37. Dean, BJF, et al: The risks and benefits of glucocorticoid treatment for tendinopathy: a systematic review of the effects of local glucocorticoid on tendon. *Sem Arthritis Rheum* 43:570–576, 2014.
38. Decoster, LC, et al: The effect of hamstring stretching on range of motion: a systematic literature review. *J Orthop Sports Phys Ther* 35: 377–387, 2005.
39. DeDeyne, PG: Application of passive stretch and its implications for muscle fibers. *Phys Ther* 81(2):819–827, 2001.
40. DeDomenico, G, and Wood, EC: *Beard's Massage,* ed. 4. Philadelphia: WB Saunders, 1997.
41. Dennis, JK, and McKeough, DM: Mobility. In May, BJ (ed): *Home Health and Rehabilitation: Concepts of Care.* Philadelphia: FA Davis, 1999, pp 109–143.
42. de Vries, HA: Evaluation of static stretching procedures for improvement of flexibility. *Res Q* 33:222–229, 1962.
43. de Weijer, VC, Gorniak, GC, and Shamus, E: The effect of static stretch and warm-up exercise on hamstring length over the course of 24 hours. *J Orthop Sports Phys Ther* 33(12):727–732, 2003.
44. Donatelli, R, and Owens-Burkhart, H: Effects of immobilization on the extensibility of periarticular connective tissue. *J Orthop Sports Phys Ther* 3:67–72, 1981.
45. Draper, DO, and Richard, MD: Rate of temperature decay in human muscle following 3 MHz ultrasound: the stretching window revealed. *J Athletic Training* 30:304–307, 1996.
46. Draper, DO, et al: Shortwave diathermy and prolonged stretching increase hamstring flexibility more than prolonged stretching alone. *J Orthop Sports Phys Ther* 34(1):13–20, 2004.
47. Dutton, M: *Orthopedic Examination, Evaluation, and Intervention,* ed. 4. New York: McGraw-Hill, 2004, pp 521-556.
48. Ellerin, BE, et al: Current therapy in the management of heterotopic ossification of the elbow: a review with case studies. *Am J Phys Med Rehabil* 78(3):259–271, 1999.
49. Engel, JM: Relaxation and related techniques. In Hertling, D, and Kessler, RM (eds): *Management of Common Musculoskeletal Disorders,* ed. 4. Philadelphia: Lippincott Williams and Wilkins, 2006, pp 261–266.
50. Etnyre, BR, and Abraham, LD: Gains in range of ankle dorsiflexion using three popular stretching techniques. *Am J Phys Med* 65:189–196, 1986.
51. Euhardy, R: Contracture. In Kauffman, TL (ed): *Geriatric Rehabilitation Manual.* New York: Churchill-Livingstone, 1999, pp 77–80.
52. Feland, JB, et al: The effect of duration of stretching of the hamstring muscle group for increasing range of motion in people aged 65 years or older. *Phys Ther* 81(5):1110–1117, 2001.
53. Feldenkrais, M: *Awareness Through Movement.* New York: Harper & Row, 1985.
54. Fletcher, IM: The effect of different dynamic stretch velocities on jump performance. *Eur J Appl Physiol* 109:491–498, 2010.
55. Flitney, FW, and Hirst, DG: Cross-bridge detachment and sarcomere "give" during stretch of active frog's muscle. *J Physiol* 276:449–465, 1978.
56. Fowles, JR, Sale, DG, and MacDougall, JD: Reduced strength after passive stretch of the human plantarflexors. *J Appl Physiol* 89:1179–1188, 2000.
57. Fukami, Y, and Wilkinson, RS: Responses of isolated Golgi tendon organs of the cat. *J Physiol* 265:673–689, 1977.
58. Gilchrist, J, et al: A randomized controlled trial to prevent noncontact anterior cruciate ligament injury in female college soccer players. *Am J Sports Med* 36(8):1476–1483, 2008.
59. Godges, JJ, MacRae, PG, and Engelke, KA: Effects of exercise on hip range of motion, trunk muscle performance, and gait economy. *Phys Ther* 73: 468–477, 1993.
60. Guyton, AC, and Hall, JE: *Textbook of Medical Physiology,* ed. 13. Philadelphia: WB Saunders, 2016, pp 75-93.
61. Halbertsma, JPK, et al: Repeated passive stretching: acute effect on the passive muscle moment and extensibility of short hamstrings. *Arch Phys Med Rehabil* 80:407–414, 1999.
62. Halkovich, LR, et al: Effect of Fluori-Methane® spray on passive hip flexion. *Phys Ther* 61:185–189, 1981.
63. Hanten, WP, and Chandler, SD: The effect of myofascial release leg pull and sagittal plane isometric contract-relax technique on passive straight-leg raise angle. *J Orthop Sports Phys Ther* 20:138–144, 1994.
64. Hengeveld, E, and Banks, K: *Maitland's Peripheral Manipulation,* ed. 5. Oxford, UK: Butterworth Heinemann, 2014, pp 1-87.
65. Henricson, AS, et al: The effect of heat and stretching on range of hip motion. *J Orthop Sports Phys Ther* 6(2):110–115, 1984.

66. Herbert, LA: Preventative stretching exercises for the workplace. *Orthop Phys Ther Pract* 11:11, 1999.
67. Herbert, RD, Gabriel, M: Effects of stretching before and after exercising on muscle soreness and risk of injury: Systematic review. *BMJ* 325:468–472, 2002.
68. Herbert, RD, de Noronha, M, and Kamper, SJ: Stretching to prevent or reduce muscle soreness after exercise. *Cochrane Database of Systematic Reviews* 7:1–48, 2011.
69. Hertling, D: Soft tissue manipulations. In Hertling, D, and Kessler, RM (eds): *Management of Common Musculoskeletal Disorders,* ed. 4. Philadelphia: Lippincott Williams & Wilkins, 2006, pp 179–259.
70. Hertling, D, and Kessler, RM: Introduction to manual therapy. In Hertling, D, and Kessler, RM (eds): *Management of Common Musculoskeletal Disorders,* ed. 4. Philadelphia: Lippincott Williams & Wilkins, 2006, pp 112–132.
71. Hulton, RS: Neuromuscular basis of stretching exercise. In Komi, PV (ed): *Strength and Power in Sports.* Boston: Blackwell Scientific, 1992, pp 29–38.
72. Ito, CS: Conservative management of joint deformities and dynamic posturing. *Orthop Phys Ther Clin N Am* 2(1):25–38, 1993.
73. Iyer, MB, Mitz, AR, and Winstein, C: Motor 1: lower centers. In Cohen, H (ed): *Neuroscience for Rehabilitation.* Philadelphia: Lippincott Williams & Wilkins, 1999, pp 209–242.
74. Jacobson, E: *Progressive Relaxation.* Chicago: University of Chicago Press, 1929.
75. Jansen, CM, et al: Treatment of a knee contracture using a knee orthosis incorporating stress-relaxation techniques. *Phys Ther* 76(2):182–186, 1996.
76. Johnson, AW, et al: Hamstring flexibility increases the same with 3 or 9 repetitions of stretching held for a total time of 90 s. *Phys Ther Sport* 15:101–105, 2014.
77. Jokl, P, and Konstadt, S: The effect of limb immobilization on muscle function and protein composition. *Clin Orthop* 174:222–229, 1983.
78. Kaltenborn, FM: *The Kaltenborn Method of Examination and Treatment, Vol 1: The Extremities,* ed. 5. Oslo: Olaf Norlis Bokhandel, 1999.
79. Kannus, P, et al: The effects of training, immobilization and remobilization on musculoskeletal tissue. I. Training and immobilization. *Scand J Med Sci Sports* 2:100–118, 1992.
80. Kannus, P, et al: The effects of training, immobilization and remobilization on musculoskeletal tissue. II. Remobilization and prevention of immobilization atrophy. *Scand J Med Sci Sports* 2:164–176, 1992.
81. Keays, KS, et al: Effects of Pilates exercises on shoulder range of motion, pain, mood, and upper extremity function in women living with breast cancer: A pilot study. *Phys Ther* 88:494–510, 2008.
82. Kendall, F, et al: *Muscles, Testing and Function: With Posture and Pain,* ed. 5. Philadelphia: Lippincott Williams & Wilkins, 2005.
83. Knight, CA, et al: Effect of superficial heat, deep heat, and active exercise warm-up on the extensibility of the plantar flexors. *Phys Ther* 81(6): 1206–1214, 2001.
84. Kokkonen, J, et al: Chronic static stretching improves exercise performance. *Med Sci Sports Exerc* 39(10):1825–1831, 2007.
85. Konrad, A, and Tilp, M: Increased range of motion after static stretching is not due to changes in muscle and tendon structures. *Clin Biomech* 29: 636–642, 2014.
86. Kubo, K, et al: Measurement of viscoelastic properties of tendon structures in vivo. *Scand J Med Sci Sports* 12(1):3–8, 2002.
87. Law, RYW, et al: Stretch exercises increase tolerance to stretch in patients with chronic musculoskeletal pain: A randomized, controlled trial. *Phys Ther* 89(10):1016–1026, 2009.
88. Lehmann, JF, and DeLateur, BJ: Therapeutic heat. In Lehmann, JF (ed): *Therapeutic Heat and Cold,* ed. 4. Baltimore: Williams & Wilkins, 1990.
89. Lentell, G, et al: The use of thermal agents to influence the effectiveness of a low-load prolonged stretch. *J Orthop Sports Phys Ther* 16(5): 200–207, 1992.
90. Lieber, RL: *Skeletal Muscle Structure, Function, and Plasticity: The Physiological Basis of Rehabilitation,* ed. 3. Philadelphia: Wolters Kluwer/Lippincott Williams & Wilkins, 2010.
91. Lieber, RL, and Boodine-Fowler, SC: Skeletal muscle mechanisms: implications for rehabilitation. *Phys Ther* 73:844–856, 1993.
92. Light, KE, et al: Low-load prolonged stretch vs. high-load brief stretch in treating knee contractures. *Phys Ther* 64(3):330–333, 1984.
93. Liston, C: Specialized systems of massage. In De Domenico, G, and Wood, EC (eds): *Beard's Massage,* ed. 4. Philadelphia: WB Saunders, 1997, pp 163–171.
94. Lundy-Ekman, L: *Neuroscience: Fundamentals for Rehabilitation,* ed. 2. Philadelphia: WB Saunders, 2002.
95. Macefield, G, et al: Decline in spindle support to alpha motoneurons during sustained voluntary contractions. *J Physiol* 440:497–512, 1991.
96. Maganaris, CN: Tensile properties of in vivo human tendinous tissue. *J Biomech* 35(8):1019–1027, 2002.
97. Magnusson, SP, et al: Biomechanical responses to repeated stretches in human hamstring muscle in vivo. *Am J Sports Med* 24:622–628, 1996.
98. Magnusson, SP, et al: A mechanism for altered flexibility in human skeletal muscle. *J Physicol* 497:291–298, 1996.
99. Magnusson, SP, et al: Mechanical and physical responses to stretching with and without pre-isometric contraction in human skeletal muscle. *Arch Phys Med Rehabil* 77:373–378, 1996.
100. McClure, M: Exercise and training for spinal patients. Part B. Flexibility training. In Basmajian, JV, and Nyberg, R (eds): *Rational Manual Therapies.* Baltimore: Williams & Wilkins, 1993, p 359.
101. McClure, PW, Blackburn, LG, and Dusold, C: The use of splints in the treatment of stiffness: biologic rationale and an algorithm for making clinical decisions. *Phys Ther* 74:1101–1107, 1994.
102. McHugh, MP, et al: Viscoelastic stress relaxation in human skeletal muscle. *Med Sci Sports Exerc* 24:1375–1381, 1992.
103. McNair, PJ, et al: Stretching at the ankle joint: viscoelastic responses to hold and continuous passive motion. *Med Sci Sports Exerc* 33: 354–358, 2001.
104. Monroe, LG: Motion restrictions. In Cameron, MH (ed): *Physical Agents in Rehabilitation,* ed. 2. Philadelphia: WB Saunders, 2003, pp 111–128.
105. Morse, CI, et al: The acute effects of stretching on the passive stiffness of the human gastrocnemius muscle-tendon unit. *J Physiol* 586:97–106, 2008.
106. Mueller, MJ, and Maluf, KS: Tissue adaptation to physical stress: A proposed "physical stress theory" to guide physical therapist practice, education, and research. *Phys Ther* 82(4):383–403, 2002.
107. Muir, IW, Chesworth, BM, and Vandervoort, AA: Effect of a static calf-stretching exercise on resistive torque during passive ankle dorsiflexion in healthy subjects. *J Orthop Sports Phys Ther* 29:107–113, 1999.
108. Nakamura, M, et al: Acute effects of static stretching on muscle hardness of the medial gastrocnemius muscle belly in humans: An ultrasonic shear-wave elastography study. *Ultrasound Med Biol* 40(9):1991–1997, 2014.
109. Nelson, AG, et al: Acute effects of passive muscle stretching on sprint performance. *J Sports Sci* 23:449–454, 2005.
110. Nelson, RT, and Bandy, WD: Eccentric training and static stretching improve hamstring flexibility of high school males. *J Ath Training* 39: 31–35, 2004.
111. Neuman, DA: *Kinesiology of the Musculoskeletal System: Foundations for Rehabilitation,* ed. 2. St. Louis: Mosby, 2010.
112. Noyes, FR: Functional properties of knee ligaments and alterations induced by immobilization. *Clin Orthop* 123:210–242, 1977.
113. Noyes, FR, et al: Advances in understanding of knee ligament injury, repair, and rehabilitation. *Med Sci Sports Exerc* 16:427–443, 1984.
114. Noyes, FR, et al: Biomechanics of ligament failure. *J Bone Joint Surg Am* 56:1406–1418, 1974.
115. Ostering, LR, et al: Differential response to proprioceptive neuromuscular facilitation (PNF) stretch technique. *Med Sci Sports Exerc* 22: 106–111, 1990.
116. O'Sullivan, SB: Assessment of motor function. In O'Sullivan, SB, and Schmitz, TJ (eds): *Physical Rehabilitation: Assessment and Treatment,* ed. 4. Philadelphia: FA Davis, 2001, pp 177–212.
117. O'Sullivan, SB: Strategies to improve motor control and motor learning. In O'Sullivan, SB, and Schmitz, TJ (eds): *Physical Rehabilitation: Assessment and Treatment,* ed. 4. Philadelphia: FA Davis, 2001, pp 363–411.

118. O'Sullivan, SB: Interventions to improve motor control and motor learning. In O'Sullivan, SB, and Schmitz, TJ (eds): *Improving Functional Outcomes in Physical Rehabilitation.* Philadelphia: FA Davis, 2010, pp 12–41.
119. Pearson, K, and Gordon, J: Spinal reflexes. In Kandel, ER, Schwartz, JH, and Jessell, TM (eds): *Principles of Neural Science,* ed. 4. New York: McGraw-Hill, 2000, pp 713–736.
120. Pope, RP, et al: A randomized trial of pre-exercise stretching for prevention of lower limb injury. *Med Sci Sports Exerc* 32:271–277, 2000.
121. Rennie, S, and Michlovitz, SL: Biophysical effects of temperature elevation. In Bellew, JW, Michlovitz, SL, and Nolan, TP (eds): *Modalities for Therapeutic Intervention,* ed. 6. Philadelphia: FA Davis, 2016, pp 62–68.
122. Roberts, JM, and Wilson, K: Effect of stretching duration on active and passive range of motion in the lower extremity. *Br J Sports Med* 33: 259–263, 1999.
123. Rose, S, et al: The stretching window, part two: rate of thermal decay in deep muscle following 1 MHz ultrasound. *J Athletic Training* 31: 139–143, 1996.
124. Rubini, EC, Costa, ALL, and Gomes, PSC: The effects of stretching on strength performance. *Sports Med* 37(3):213–224, 2007.
125. Ryan, ED, et al: The time course of musculotendinous stiffness responses following different durations of passive stretching. *J Orthop Sports Phys Ther* 38(10):632–639, 2008.
126. Rydeard, R, Leger, A, and Smith, D: Pilates-based therapeutic exercise: effects on subjects with nonspecific, chronic low back pain and functional disability—a randomized controlled trial. *J Orthop Sports Phys Ther* 36(7):472–484, 2006.
127. Sainz de Baranda, P, and Ayala, F: Chronic flexibility improvement after 12 week of stretching program utilizing the ACSM recommendations: Hamstring flexibility. *Int J Sports Med* 31:389–396, 2010.
128. Schleip, R: Fascial plasticity—a new neurobiological explanation: part 1. *J Bodywork Movement Ther* 7(1):11–19, 2003.
129. Schultz, JH, and Luthe, W: *Autogenic Training: A Psychophysiologic Approach in Psychotherapy.* New York: Grune & Stratton, 1959.
130. Segal, NA, Hein, J, and Basford, JR: The effects of Pilates training on flexibility and body composition: an observational study. *Arch Phys Med Rehabil* 85:1977–1981, 2004.
131. Sharman, MJ, Creswell, AG, and Riek, S: Proprioceptive neuromuscular facilitation stretching: mechanisms and clinical implications. *Sports Med* 36:929–939, 2006.
132. Shehab, R, et al: Pre-exercise stretching and sports-related injuries: Knowledge, attitudes, and practices. *Clin J Sports Med* 16:228–231, 2006.
133. Shrier, I: Does stretching improve performance? A systematic and critical review of the literature. *Clin J Sport Med* 14:267–273, 2004.
134. Smith, E, and Smith, K: *Pilates for Rehab: A Guidebook for Integrating Pilates in Patient Care.* Minneapolis, MN: OPTP, 2005.
135. Starring, DT, et al: Comparison of cyclic and sustained passive stretching using a mechanical device to increase resting length of hamstring muscles. *Phys Ther* 68:314–320, 1988.
136. Sullivan, PE, and Markos, PD: *Clinical Decision Making in Therapeutic Exercise.* Norwalk, CT: Appleton & Lange, 1995.
137. Tabary, JC, et al: Physiological and structural changes in the cat soleus muscle due to immobilization at different lengths by plaster casts. *J Physiol (Lond)* 224:231–244, 1972.
138. Tappan, FM, and Benjamin, PJ: *Tappan's Handbook of Healing Massage Techniques.* Stamford, CT: Appleton & Lange, 1998.
139. Taylor, BF, Waring, CA, and Brashear, TA: The effects of therapeutic heat or cold followed by static stretch on hamstring muscle length. *J Orthop Sports Phys Ther* 21:283–286, 1995.
140. Thacker, SB, et al: The impact of stretching on sports injury risk: A systematic review of the literature. *Med Sci Sports Exerc* 36:371–378, 2004.
141. Thompson, LV: Skeletal muscle adaptations with age, inactivity, and therapeutic exercise. *J Orthop Sports Phys Ther* 32(2):33–57, 2002.
142. Thornton, GM, Schwab, TD, and Oxland, TR: Fatigue is more damaging than creep in ligament revealed by modulus reduction and residual strength. *Ann Biomed End* 35(10):1713–1721, 2007.
143. Threlkeld, AJ: The effects of manual therapy on connective tissue. *Phys Ther* 72:893–902, 1992.
144. Tiidus, PM: Manual massage and recovery of muscle function following exercise: A literature review. *J Orthop Sports Phys Ther* 25:107–112, 1997.
145. Tillman, LJ, and Cummings, GS: Biologic mechanisms of connective tissue mutability. In Currier, DP, Nelson, RM (eds): *Dynamics of Human Biologic Tissues.* Philadelphia: FA Davis, 1992, p 1–44.
146. Townsend, MC: *Psychiatric Mental Health Nursing: Concepts of Care,* ed. 3. Philadelphia: FA Davis, 2000.
147. Travell, JG, and Simons, DG: *Myofascial Pain and Dysfunction Trigger Point Manuals,* vol 2. Baltimore: Williams & Wilkins, 1992.
148. Voss, DE, Ionla, MK, and Myers, BJ: *Proprioceptive Neuromuscular Facilitation,* ed. 3. Philadelphia: Harper & Row, 1985.
149. Walker, SM: Delay of twitch relaxation induced by stress and stress relaxation. *J Appl Physiol* 16:801–806, 1961.
150. Warren, CG, Lehmann, JF, and Koblanski, JN: Elongation of rat tail tendon: effect of load and temperature. *Arch Phys Med Rehabil* 52: 465–474, 1971.
151. Webright, WG, Randolph, BJ, and Perin, DH: Comparison of nonballistic active knee extension in neural slump position and static stretch techniques on hamstring flexibility. *J Orthop Sports Phys Ther* 26: 7–13, 1997.
152. Weppler, CH, and Magnuson, SP: Increasing muscle extensibility: a matter of increasing length or modifying sensation. *Phys Ther* 90(3): 438–449, 2010.
153. Wessel, J, and Wan, A: Effect of stretching on intensity of delayed-onset muscle soreness. *J Sports Med* 2:83–87, 1994.
154. Wessling, KC, Derane, DA, and Hylton, CR: Effect of static stretch vs. static stretch and ultrasound combined on triceps surae muscle extensibility in healthy women. *Phys Ther* 67:674–679, 1987.
155. Wilkinson, A: Stretching the truth: A review of the literature on muscle stretching. *Aust J Physiother* 38:283–287, 1992.
156. Willy, RW, et al: Effect of cessation and resumption of static hamstring muscle stretching on joint range of motion. *J Orthop Sports Phys Ther* 31:138–144, 2001.
157. Wilson, E, et al: Muscle energy techniques in patients with acute low back pain: a pilot clinical trial. *J Orthop Sports Phys Ther* 33(9): 502–512, 2003.
158. Winters, MV, et al: Passive versus active stretching of hip flexor muscles in subjects with limited hip extension: a randomized clinical trial. *Phys Ther* 84(9):800–807, 2004.
159. Witvrouw, E, et al: Muscle flexibility as a risk factor for developing muscle injuries in male professional soccer players: a prospective study. *Am J Sports Med* 31:41–46, 2003.
160. Wong, K, Trudel, G, and Laneuville, O: Noninflammatory joint contractures arising from immobility: animal models to future treatments. *BioMed Res Int,* 2015, Article ID 848290, 6 pages, http://dx.doi.org/10.1155/2015/848290.
161. Youdas, JW, et al: The effect of static stretching of the calf muscle-tendon unit on active ankle dorsiflexion range of motion. *J Orthop Sports Phys Ther* 33(7):408–417, 2003.
162. Youdas, JW, et al: The influence of gender and age on hamstring muscle length in healthy adults. *J Orthop Sports Phys Ther* 35(4): 246–252, 2005.
163. Zachazewski, JE: Flexibility in sports. In Sanders, B (ed): *Sports Physical Therapy.* Norwalk, CT, Appleton & Lange, 1990, pp 201–229.

CHAPTER

5

Peripheral Joint Mobilization/Manipulation

CAROLYN KISNER, PT, MS

Joint mobilization, also known as manipulation, refers to manual therapy techniques that are used to modulate pain and treat joint impairments that limit range of motion (ROM) by specifically addressing the altered mechanics of the joint. The altered joint mechanics may be due to pain and muscle guarding, joint effusion, contractures or adhesions in the joint capsules or supporting ligaments, or aberrant joint motion. Joint mobilization stretching techniques differ from other forms of passive or self-stretching (described in Chapter 4) in that they specifically address restricted capsular tissue by replicating normal joint mechanics while minimizing abnormal compressive stresses on the articular cartilage in the joint.[17]

Historically, mobilization has been the preferred term to use as therapists began using the passive, skilled joint techniques because mobilization had a less aggressive connotation than manipulation. High-velocity thrust (HVT) techniques, typically called manipulation, were not universally taught or used by most practitioners. However, with the increased level of education[3,5] and current practice of physical therapy,[2] both non-thrust and thrust manipulation techniques are skills that therapists are learning and safely using in many practice settings. The *Manipulation Education Manual for Physical Therapist Professional Degree Programs*[2] as well as the *Guide to Physical Therapist Practice*[8] couple the terms "mobilization" and "manipulation" in order to demonstrate their common usage.

An editorial[25] described problems with using the terms interchangeably without clear definitions. The authors cited confusion in interpreting research and describing outcomes when the techniques used are not specifically described. They also indicated possible confusion in communicating with patients and with referral sources. It is therefore critical that the practitioner clearly understands and defines the characteristics of the techniques used when referring to manipulative techniques.

In this text, the terms "mobilization" and "manipulation" will be used interchangeably, with the distinction made between non-thrust and thrust techniques. The procedures section in this chapter describes documentation and the importance of identifying rate, range, and direction of force application, as well as target, relative structural movement, and patient position whenever referring to mobilization/manipulation intervention techniques.[24] This information should be used in all documentation and communication in order to minimize discrepancies in interpretation of outcomes.

To use joint mobilization/manipulation techniques for effective treatment, the practitioner must know and be able to examine the anatomy, arthrokinematics, and pathology of the neuromusculoskeletal system and to recognize when the techniques are indicated or when other techniques would be more effective for regaining lost motion. Indiscriminate use of joint techniques, when not indicated, could lead to potential harm to the patient's joints. We assume that, prior to learning the techniques presented in this text, the student or therapist has had (or will be concurrently learning) orthopedic examination and evaluation and therefore will be able to choose appropriate, safe techniques for treating the patient's impairments. The reader is referred to several resources for additional study of examination and evaluation procedures.[6,12,17,20] When indicated, joint manipulative techniques are safe, effective means of restoring or maintaining joint play and can also be used for treating pain.[12,17]

Principles of Joint Mobilization/Manipulation

Definitions of Terms

Mobilization/Manipulation

As noted in the introductory paragraphs, mobilization and manipulation are two terms that have come to have the same meaning[3,21] and are therefore interchangeable. In general, they are passive, skilled manual therapy techniques applied to joints and related soft tissues at varying speeds and amplitudes using physiological or accessory motions for therapeutic purposes. The varying speeds and amplitudes can range from a small-amplitude force applied at fast velocity to a large-amplitude force applied at slow velocity—that is, there is a continuum of intensities and speeds at which the technique could be applied.[12,17]

Thrust manipulation/HVT. Thrust refers to high-velocity, short-amplitude techniques.[12,30] The thrust is performed at the end of the pathological limit of the joint and is intended to alter positional relationships, snap adhesions, or stimulate joint receptors.[30] Pathological limit means the end of the available ROM when there is restriction.

NOTE: The terms thrust and manipulation are often used interchangeably,[4] but with the trend to use manipulation to include all manipulative techniques, including non-thrust techniques, this text will not use these two terms interchangeably.

Self-Mobilization (Auto-Mobilization)

Self-mobilization refers to self-stretching techniques that specifically use joint traction or glides that direct the stretch force to the joint capsule. When indicated, these techniques are described in the chapters on specific regions of the body.

Mobilization With Movement

Mobilization with movement (MWM) is the concurrent application of sustained accessory mobilization applied by a therapist and an active physiological movement to end-range applied by the patient. Passive end-of-range overpressure, or stretching, is then delivered without pain as a barrier. The techniques are always applied in a pain-free direction and are described as correcting joint tracking from a positional fault.[23,26] Brian Mulligan of New Zealand originally described these techniques.[26] MWM techniques related to specific peripheral joint regions are described in Chapters 17 through 22.

Physiological Movements

Physiological movements are movements the patient can do voluntarily (e.g., the classic or traditional movements, such as flexion, abduction, and rotation). The term *osteokinematics* is used when these motions of the bones are described.[13]

Accessory Movements

Accessory movements are movements in the joint and surrounding tissues that are necessary for normal ROM but that cannot be actively performed by the patient.[30] Terms that relate to accessory movements are *component motions* and *joint play*.

Component motions. These are motions that accompany active motion but are not under voluntary control. The term is often used synonymously with accessory movement. For example, motions such as upward rotation of the scapula and rotation of the clavicle, which occur with shoulder flexion, and rotation of the fibula, which occurs with ankle motions, are component motions.

Joint play. Joint play describes the motions that occur between the joint surfaces and also the distensibility or "give" in the joint capsule, which allows the bones to move. The movements are necessary for normal joint functioning through the ROM and can be demonstrated passively, but they cannot be performed actively by the patient.[30] The movements include distraction, sliding, compression, rolling, and spinning of the joint surfaces. The term *arthrokinematics* is used when these motions of the bone surfaces within the joint are described.[13]

NOTE: Procedures to distract or slide the joint surfaces to decrease pain or restore joint play are the fundamental joint mobilization techniques described in this text.

Resting Position

The *resting position, open-pack position,* and *loose-pack position* are terms that describe the position of the joint where the greatest mobility is possible; that is, where the least amount of tension is placed on the joint capsule and supporting ligaments. This position is typically used for testing joint play and for applying the initial mobilization treatment.

Manipulation Under Anesthesia

Manipulation under anesthesia is a procedure used to restore full ROM by breaking adhesions around a joint while the patient is anesthetized. The technique may be a rapid thrust or a passive stretch using physiological or accessory movements. Therapists may assist surgeons in the application of these skilled techniques in the operating room and continue with follow-up care.

Muscle Energy

Muscle energy techniques use active contraction of deep muscles that attach near the joint and whose line of pull can cause the desired accessory motion. The technique requires the therapist to provide stabilization to the segment on which the distal aspect of the muscle attaches. A command for an isometric contraction of the muscle is given that causes accessory movement of the joint. Several specific muscle energy techniques are described for the sacroiliac joint in Chapter 15 and for the subcranial region of the cervical spine in Chapter 16.

Basic Concepts of Joint Motion: Arthrokinematics

Joint Shapes

The type of motion occurring between bony partners in a synovial joint is influenced by the shape of the joint surfaces. The shape may be described as *ovoid* or *sellar.*[13,17,19,33]

- In ovoid joints, one surface is convex and the other is concave (Fig. 5.1 A).
- In sellar (saddle) joints, one surface is concave in one direction and convex in the other, with the opposing surface convex and concave, respectively—similar to a horseback rider being in complementary opposition to the shape of a saddle (Fig. 5.1 B).

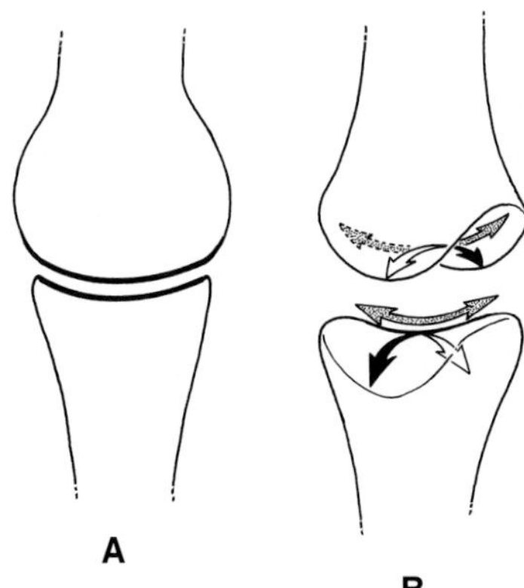

FIGURE 5.1 (A) With ovoid joints, one surface is convex and the other is concave. **(B)** With saddle (sellar) joints, one surface is concave in one direction and convex in the other, with the opposing surface convex and concave, respectively.

Types of Motion

As a bony lever moves about an axis of motion, there is also movement of the bone surface on the opposing bone surface in the joint.

- The movement of the bony lever is called *swing* and is classically described as flexion, extension, abduction, adduction, and rotation. The amount of movement can be measured in degrees with a goniometer and is called ROM.
- Motion of the bone surfaces in the joint is a variable combination of *rolling* and *sliding*, or *spinning.*[13,17,19,33] These accessory motions allow greater angulation of the bone as it swings. For the rolling, sliding, or spinning to occur, there must be adequate capsule laxity or joint play.

Roll

Characteristics of one bone rolling on another (Fig. 5.2) are as follows:

- The surfaces are incongruent.
- New points on one surface meet new points on the opposing surface.
- Rolling results in angular motion of the bone (swing).
- Rolling is always in the same direction as the swinging bone motion whether the surface is convex (Fig. 5.3 A) or concave (Fig. 5.3 B).
- Rolling, if it occurs alone, causes compression of the surfaces on the side to which the bone is swinging and separation on the other side. Passive stretching using bone angulation alone may cause stressful compressive forces to portions of the joint surface, potentially leading to joint damage.

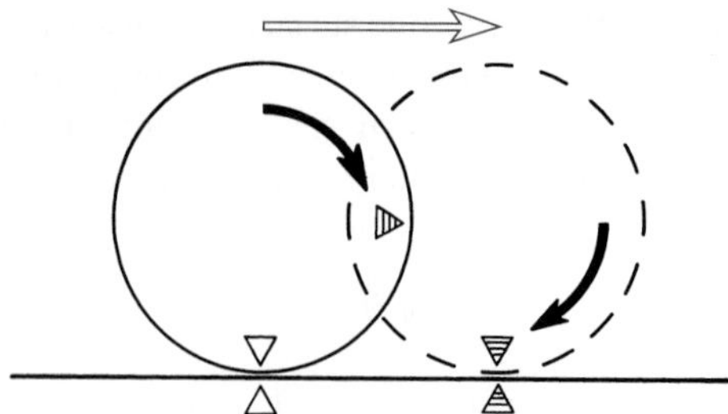

FIGURE 5.2 Representation of one surface rolling on another. New points on one surface meet new points on the opposing surface.

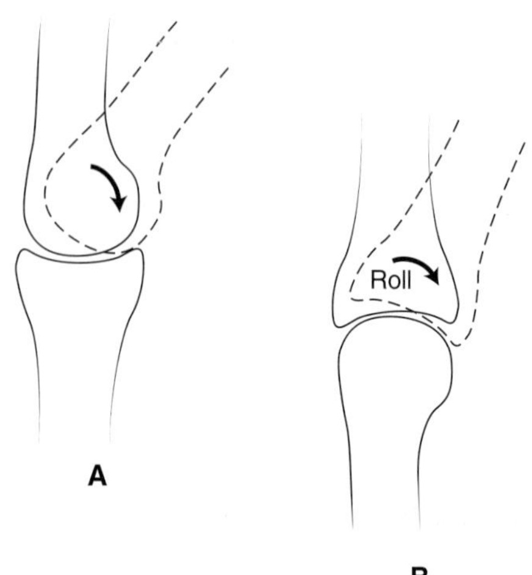

FIGURE 5.3 Rolling is always in the same direction as bone motion, whether the moving bone is **(A)** convex or **(B)** concave.

- In normally functioning joints, pure rolling does not occur alone but in combination with joint sliding and spinning.

Slide/Translation

Characteristics of one bone sliding (translating) across another include the following:

- For a pure slide, the surfaces must be congruent, either flat (Fig. 5.4 A) or curved (Fig. 5.4 B).
- The same point on one surface comes into contact with the new points on the opposing surface.

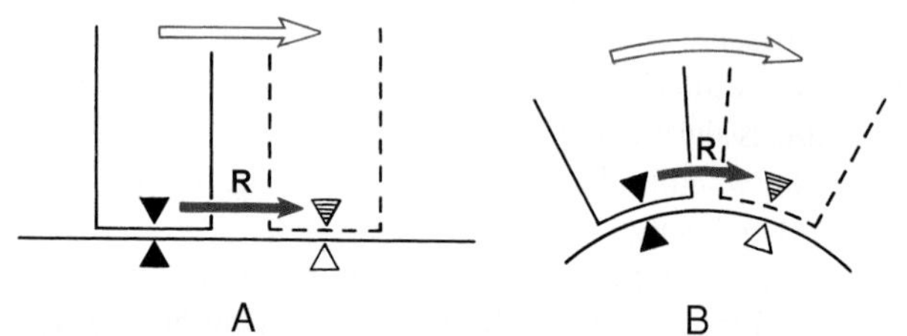

FIGURE 5.4 Representation of one surface sliding on another, whether **(A)** flat or **(B)** curved. The same point on one surface comes into contact with new points on the opposing surface.

- Pure sliding does not occur in joints because the surfaces are not completely congruent.
- The direction in which sliding occurs depends on whether the moving surface is concave or convex. Sliding is in the opposite direction of the angular movement of the bone if the moving joint surface is convex (Fig. 5.5 A). Sliding is in the same direction as the angular movement of the bone if the moving surface is concave (Fig. 5.5 B).

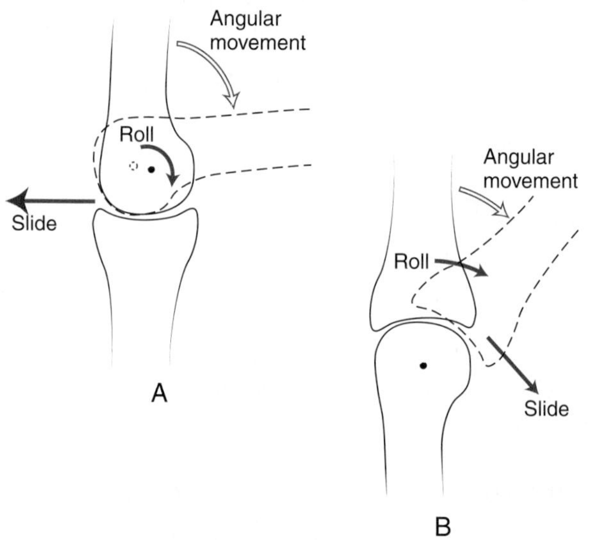

FIGURE 5.5 Representation of the concave-convex rule. **(A)** If the surface of the moving bone is convex, sliding is in the direction opposite to that of the angular movement of the bone. **(B)** If the surface of the moving bone is concave, sliding is in the same direction as the angular movement of the bone.

NOTE: This mechanical relationship is known as the *convex-concave rule* and is the theoretical basis for determining the direction of the mobilizing force when joint gliding techniques are used.[15]

FOCUS ON EVIDENCE

Several studies[11,14,16] have examined the translational movement of the humeral head with shoulder motions and have documented translations opposite to what is predicted by the convex-concave rule. Hsu and associates[15] proposed that this apparent contradiction to the convex-concave rule is the result of asymmetrical tightening of the shoulder joint capsule during movement resulting in translation of the moving bone opposite to the direction of capsular tightening. They documented that stretching the tight capsule with translations that affect the restricting tissues leads to greater ROM in cadaver shoulder joints. This apparent contradiction is further discussed in an editorial that points out the potential misinterpretation of the results of studies that appear to negate the convex-concave arthrokinematic descriptors; that it is important to recognize the size of the joint surfaces, starting position/

relationship of the joint surface, not just the end position, as well as effect of capsule tightness .[28]

Combined Roll-Sliding in a Joint

- The more congruent the joint surfaces are, the more sliding there is of one bony partner on the other with movement.
- The more incongruent the joint surfaces are, the more rolling there is of one bony partner on the other with movement.
- When muscles actively contract to move a bone, some of the muscles may cause or control the sliding movement of the joint surfaces. For example, the caudal sliding motion of the humeral head during shoulder abduction is caused by the rotator cuff muscles, and the posterior sliding of the tibia during knee flexion is caused by the hamstring muscles. If this function is lost, the resulting abnormal joint mechanics may cause microtrauma and joint dysfunction.
- The joint mobilization techniques described in this chapter use the sliding component of joint motion to restore joint play and reverse joint hypomobility. Rolling (passive angular stretching) is not used to stretch tight joint capsules because it causes joint compression.

CLINICAL TIP

When the therapist applies a passive accessory motion to the articulating surface using the slide component of joint motion, the technique is called translatoric glide, translation, or simply glide.[17] It is used to control pain when applied gently or to stretch the capsule when applied with a stretch force.

Spin

Characteristics of one bone spinning on another include the following:

- There is rotation of a segment about a stationary mechanical axis (Fig. 5.6).

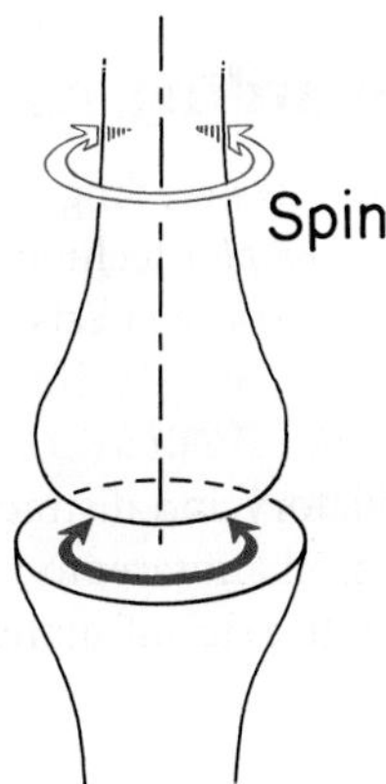

FIGURE 5.6 Representation of spinning. There is rotation of a segment about a stationary mechanical axis.

- The same point on the moving surface creates an arc of a circle as the bone spins.
- Spinning rarely occurs alone in joints but in combination with rolling and sliding.
- Three examples of spin occurring in joints of the body are the shoulder with flexion/extension, the hip with flexion/extension, and the radiohumeral joint with pronation/supination (Fig. 5.7).

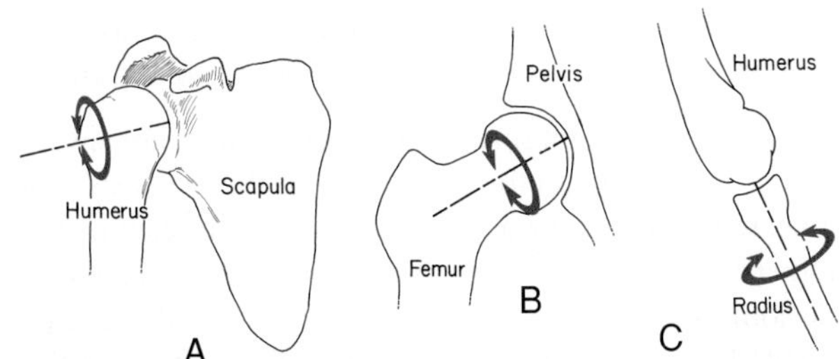

FIGURE 5.7 Examples of joint spin locations in the body. **(A)** Humerus with flexion/extension; **(B)** Femur with flexion/extension; **(C)** Head of the radius with pronation/supination.

Passive-Angular Stretching Versus Joint-Glide Stretching

- Passive-angular stretching procedures, as when the bony lever is used to stretch a tight joint capsule, may cause increased pain or joint trauma because:
  - The use of a lever magnifies the force at the joint.
  - The force causes compression of the joint surfaces in the direction of the rolling bone (see Fig. 5.3).
  - The roll without a slide does not replicate normal joint mechanics.
- Joint glide stretching procedures, as when the translatoric slide component of the joint function is used to stretch a tight capsule, are safer and more selective because:
  - The force is applied close to the joint surface and controlled at an intensity compatible with the pathology.
  - The direction of the force replicates the sliding component of the joint mechanics and does not compress the cartilage.
  - The amplitude of the motion is small yet specific to the restricted or adherent portion of the capsule or ligaments. Thus, the forces are selectively applied to the desired tissue.

Other Accessory Motions That Affect the Joint

Compression

Compression is the decrease in the joint space between bony partners.

- Compression normally occurs in the extremity and spinal joints when weight bearing.

- Some compression occurs as muscles contract, which provides stability to the joints.
- As one bone rolls on the other (see Fig. 5.3), some compression also occurs on the side to which the bone is angulating.
- Normal intermittent compressive loads help move synovial fluid and thus help maintain cartilage health.
- Abnormally high compression loads may lead to articular cartilage changes and deterioration.[19]

Traction/Distraction VIDEO 5.1

Traction and distraction are not synonymous. Traction is a longitudinal pull. Distraction is a separation, or pulling apart.

- Separation of the joint surfaces (distraction) does not always occur when a traction force is applied to the long axis of a bone. For example, if traction is applied to the shaft of the humerus when the arm is at the side, it results in a glide of the joint surface (Fig. 5.8 A). Distraction of the glenohumeral joint requires a force to be applied at right angles to the glenoid fossa (Fig. 5.8 B).

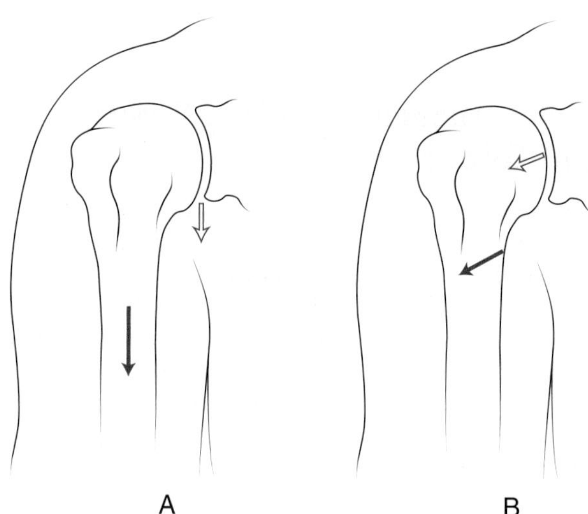

FIGURE 5.8 (A) Traction applied to the shaft of the humerus results in caudal gliding of the joint surface; **(B)** Distraction of the glenohumeral joint requires separation at right angles to the glenoid fossa.

- For clarity in this textbook, whenever there is to be a pulling force applied to the long axis of a bone, the term *long-axis traction* is used. Whenever the surfaces are to be separated, the term *distraction, joint traction,* or *joint separation* is used.

CLINICAL TIP

For joint mobilization/manipulation techniques, distraction is used to control or relieve pain when applied gently or to stretch the capsule when applied with a stretch force. For patient comfort a slight distraction force is used when applying stretch gliding techniques.

Effects of Joint Motion

Joint motion stimulates biological activity by moving synovial fluid, which brings nutrients to the avascular articular cartilage of the joint surfaces and intra-articular fibrocartilage of the menisci.[19] Atrophy of the articular cartilage begins soon after immobilization is imposed on joints.[1,8,9]

Extensibility and tensile strength of the articular and periarticular tissues are maintained with joint motion. With immobilization there is fibrofatty proliferation, which causes intra-articular adhesions as well as biochemical changes in tendon, ligament, and joint capsule tissue, which in turn causes joint contractures and ligamentous weakening.[1]

Afferent nerve impulses from joint receptors transmit information to the central nervous system and therefore provide awareness of position and motion. With injury, swelling within the joint, or joint degeneration, there is a potential decrease in an important source of proprioceptive feedback that may affect an individual's balance response.[13,34] Joint motion provides sensory input relative to:[36,37]

- Static position and sense of speed of movement (type I receptors found in the superficial joint capsule)
- Change of speed of movement (type II receptors found in deep layers of the joint capsule and articular fat pads)
- Sense of direction of movement (type I and III receptors; type III found in joint ligaments).
- Regulation of muscle tone (type I, II, and III receptors)
- Nociceptive stimuli (type IV receptors found in the fibrous capsule, ligaments, articular fat pads, periosteum, and walls of blood vessels)

Indications and Limitations for Use of Joint Mobilization/Manipulation

Gentle mobilizations may be used to treat pain and muscle guarding, whereas stretching techniques are used to treat restricted movement in order to improve the functional mobility.

Pain, Muscle Guarding, and Spasm

Painful joints, reflex muscle guarding, and muscle spasm can be treated with *gentle joint-play* techniques to stimulate neurophysiological and mechanical effects.[12]

Neurophysiological Effects

Small-amplitude oscillatory and distraction movements are used to stimulate the mechanoreceptors that may inhibit the transmission of nociceptive stimuli at the spinal cord or brain stem levels.[30,33]

Mechanical Effects

Small-amplitude distraction or gliding movements of the joint are used to cause synovial fluid motion, which is the vehicle for bringing nutrients to the avascular portions of the articular cartilage (and intra-articular fibrocartilage when present). Gentle joint-play techniques help maintain nutrient exchange and thus prevent the painful and degenerating effects of stasis when a joint is swollen or painful and cannot move through the ROM. When applied to treat pain, muscle guarding, or muscle spasm, these techniques should not place stretch on the reactive tissues (see section on Contraindications and Precautions).

Reversible Joint Hypomobility

Reversible joint hypomobility can be treated with *progressively vigorous joint-play stretching* techniques to elongate hypomobile capsular and ligamentous connective tissue. Sustained or oscillatory stretch forces are used to distend the shortened tissue mechanically.[12,17]

Positional Faults/Subluxations

A faulty position of one bony partner with respect to its opposing surface may result in limited motion or pain. This can occur with a traumatic injury, after periods of immobility, or with muscle imbalances. The faulty positioning may be perpetuated with maladapted neuromuscular control across the joint, so whenever attempting active ROM, there is faulty tracking of the joint surfaces resulting in pain or limited motion. MWM techniques attempt to realign the bony partners while the person actively moves the joint through its ROM.[26] Thrust techniques are used to reposition an obvious subluxation, such as a pulled elbow or capitate-lunate subluxation.

Progressive Limitation

Diseases that progressively limit movement can be treated with joint-play techniques to maintain available motion or retard progressive mechanical restrictions. The dosage of distraction or glide is dictated by the patient's response to treatment and the state of the disease.

Functional Immobility

When a patient cannot functionally move a joint for a period of time, the joint can be treated with nonstretch gliding or distraction techniques to maintain available joint play and prevent the degenerating and restricting effects of immobility.

FOCUS ON EVIDENCE

DiFabio[7] summarized evidence on the effectiveness of manual therapy (primarily mobilization/manipulation) for patients with somatic pain syndromes in the low back region and concluded that there was significantly greater improvement in patients receiving manual therapy than in controls. Boissonnault and associates[5] cited several studies that demonstrated the effectiveness of manual therapy interventions (defined as "a continuum of skilled passive movements to the joints and/or related soft tissues that are applied at varying speeds and amplitudes") in patients with low back pain as well as shoulder impingement, knee osteoarthritis, and cervical pain. However, there is a lack of randomized, controlled studies on the effects of mobilization for all the peripheral joints. Case studies that describe patient selection and/or interventions using joint mobilization/manipulation techniques are identified in various chapters in this text (see Chapters 15 and 17 to 22).

Limitations of Joint Mobilization/ Manipulation Techniques

Joint techniques cannot change the disease process of disorders such as rheumatoid arthritis or the inflammatory process of injury. In these cases, treatment is directed toward minimizing pain, maintaining available joint play, and reducing the effects of any mechanical limitations (see Chapter 11).

The skill of the therapist affects the outcome. The techniques described in this text are relatively safe if directions are followed and precautions are heeded. However, if these techniques are used indiscriminately on patients not properly examined and screened for such maneuvers or if they are applied too vigorously for the condition, joint trauma or hypermobility may result.

Contraindications and Precautions

The only true contraindications to mobilization/manipulation stretching techniques are hypermobility, joint effusion, and inflammation.

Hypermobility

- The joints of patients with potential necrosis of the ligaments or capsule should not be mobilized with stretching techniques.
- Patients with painful hypermobile joints may benefit from gentle joint-play techniques if kept within the limits of motion. Stretching is not done.

Joint Effusion

There may be joint swelling (effusion) due to trauma or disease. Rapid swelling of a joint usually indicates bleeding in the joint and may occur with trauma or diseases such as hemophilia. Medical intervention is required for aspiration of the blood to minimize its necrotizing effect on the articular cartilage. Slow swelling (more than 4 hours) usually indicates serous effusion (a build-up of excess synovial fluid) or edema in the joint due to mild trauma, irritation, or a disease such as arthritis.

- Do not stretch a swollen joint with mobilization or passive stretching techniques. The capsule is already on a stretch by being distended to accommodate the extra fluid. The limited motion is from the extra fluid and muscle response to pain, not from shortened fibers.
- Gentle oscillating motions that do not stress or stretch the capsule may help block the transmission of a pain stimulus so it is not perceived and also may help improve fluid flow while maintaining available joint play.
- If the patient's response to gentle techniques results in increased pain or joint irritability, the techniques were applied too vigorously or should not have been done with the current state of pathology.

Inflammation

Whenever inflammation is present, stretching increases pain and muscle guarding and results in greater tissue damage. Gentle oscillating or distraction motions may temporarily inhibit the pain response. See Chapter 10 for an appropriate approach to treatment when inflammation is present.

Conditions Requiring Special Precautions for Stretching

In most cases, joint mobilization/manipulation techniques are safer than passive angular stretching, in which the bony lever is used to stretch tight tissue and joint compression results. Mobilization may be used with *extreme care* in the following conditions if the signs and the patient's response are favorable.

- Malignancy
- Bone disease detectable on radiographs
- Unhealed fracture (The site of the fracture and the stabilization provided will dictate whether or not manipulative techniques can be safely applied.)
- Excessive pain (Determine the cause of pain and modify treatment accordingly.)
- Hypermobility in associated joints (Associated joints must be properly stabilized so the mobilization force is not transmitted to them.)
- Total joint replacements (The mechanism of the replacement is self-limiting, and therefore the mobilization techniques may be inappropriate.)
- Newly formed or weakened connective tissue such as immediately after injury, surgery, or disuse or when the patient is taking certain medications such as corticosteroids (Gentle progressive techniques within the tolerance of the tissue help align the developing fibrils, but forceful techniques are destructive.)
- Systemic connective tissue diseases such as rheumatoid arthritis, in which the disease weakens the connective tissue (Gentle techniques may benefit restricted tissue, but forceful techniques may rupture tissue and result in instabilities.)
- Elderly individuals with weakened connective tissue and diminished circulation (Gentle techniques within the tolerance of the tissue may be beneficial to increase mobility.)

Procedures for Applying Passive Joint Techniques

Examination and Evaluation

If the patient has limited or painful motion, examine and decide which tissues are limiting function and the state of pathology. Determine whether treatment should be directed primarily toward relieving pain or stretching a joint or soft tissue limitation.[5,12]

Quality of Pain

The quality of pain when testing the ROM helps determine the stage of recovery and the dosage of techniques used for treatment (see Fig. 10.2).

- If pain is experienced *before* tissue limitation—such as the pain that occurs with muscle guarding after an acute injury or during the active stage of a disease—gentle pain-inhibiting joint techniques may be used. The same techniques also can help maintain joint play (see the next section on Grades or Dosages of Movement). Stretching under these circumstances is contraindicated.
- If pain is experienced *concurrently* with tissue limitation—such as the pain and limitation that occur when damaged tissue begins to heal—the limitation is treated cautiously. Gentle stretching techniques specific to the tight structure are used to improve movement gradually yet not exacerbate the pain by reinjuring the tissue.
- If pain is experienced *after* tissue limitation is met because of stretching of tight capsular or periarticular tissue, the stiff joint can be aggressively stretched with joint-play techniques and the periarticular tissue with the stretching techniques described in Chapter 4.

Capsular Restriction

The joint capsule is limiting motion and should respond to mobilization techniques if some or all of the following signs are present.

- The passive ROM for that joint is limited in a capsular pattern. (These patterns are described for each peripheral joint under the respective sections on joint problems in Chapters 17 through 22).
- There is a firm capsular end-feel when overpressure is applied to the tissues limiting the range.
- There is decreased joint-play movement when mobility tests (articulations) are performed.
- An adhered or contracted ligament is limiting motion if there is decreased joint play and pain when the fibers of the ligament are stressed; ligaments often respond to joint mobilization techniques if applied specific to their line of stress.

Subluxation or Dislocation

Subluxation or dislocation of one bony part on another and loose intra-articular structures that block normal motion may respond to thrust techniques. Some of the simpler thrust techniques for extremity joints are described in the respective chapters in this text; thrust techniques for the spine are described in Chapter 16.

Documentation

Use of standardized terminology for communication is recommended in order to facilitate research on effective outcomes using mobilization/manipulation. A task force formed by the American Academy of Orthopaedic Manual Physical Therapists published recommendations regarding the characteristics to use in the description of manipulative techniques.[24] These are listed in Box 5.1.

The principles describing the *rate of application of the force, location in range of available movement,* and *direction and target of force* that the therapist applies are described in this section. The actual *target of force, structural movement,* and *patient position* are specific to each joint technique; these are described in the section on peripheral joint mobilization techniques in this chapter, for the temporomandibular joint in Chapter 15, and for the spine in Chapter 16.

Grades or Dosages of Movement for Non-Thrust and Thrust Techniques

Two systems of grading dosages (or rate of application) and their application in the range of available motion have been popularized.[12,17]

Non-Thrust Oscillation Techniques (Fig. 5.9)

The oscillations may be performed using physiological (osteokinematic) motions or joint-play (arthrokinematic) techniques.

Dosage and Rate of Application

Grade I. Small-amplitude rhythmic oscillations are performed at the beginning of the range. They are usually rapid oscillations, like manual vibrations.

BOX 5.1 Characteristics to Describe Mobilization and Manipulation Techniques for Documentation[24]

1. *Rate of application of the force*
2. *Location in range of available movement*
3. *Direction of force as applied by the therapist*
4. *Target of force* (The specific structure to which the force is applied is described identifying palpable anatomical structures.)
5. *Relative structural movement* (The structure that is to move is identified first, followed by the structure that is kept stable.)
6. *Patient position*

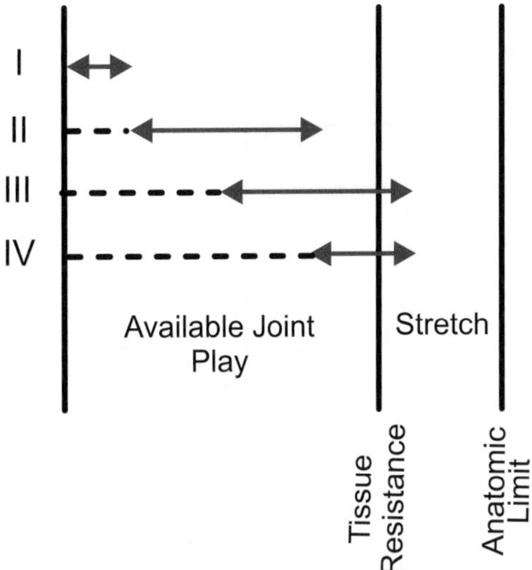

FIGURE 5.9 Representation of oscillation techniques. *(Adapted from Hengeveld, E, and Banks, K: Maitland's Peripheral Manipulation, ed. 4. Oxford: Butterworth Heinemann, 2005.[12])*

Grade II. Large-amplitude rhythmic oscillations are performed within the range, not reaching the limit. They are usually performed at two or three per second for 1 to 2 minutes.

Grade III. Large-amplitude rhythmic oscillations are performed up to the limit of the available motion and are stressed into the tissue resistance. They are usually performed at two or three per second for 1 to 2 minutes.

Grade IV. Small-amplitude rhythmic oscillations are performed at the limit of the available motion and stressed into the tissue resistance. They are usually rapid oscillations, like manual vibrations.

Indications

- Grades I and II are primarily used for treating joints limited by pain or muscle guarding. The oscillations may have an inhibitory effect on the perception of painful stimuli by repetitively stimulating mechanoreceptors that block nociceptive pathways at the spinal cord or brain stem levels.[30,38] These nonstretch motions help move synovial fluid to improve nutrition to the cartilage.
- Grades III and IV are primarily used as stretching maneuvers.
- Vary the speed of oscillations for different effects, such as low amplitude and high speed, to inhibit pain or slow speed to relax muscle guarding.

Non-Thrust Sustained Joint-Play Techniques (Fig. 5.10)

This grading system describes only joint-play techniques that separate (distract) or glide/translate (slide) the joint surfaces.

Dosages and Rate of Application

As indicated by the name, rate of application is slow and sustained for several seconds followed by partial relaxation and then repeated depending on the indications.

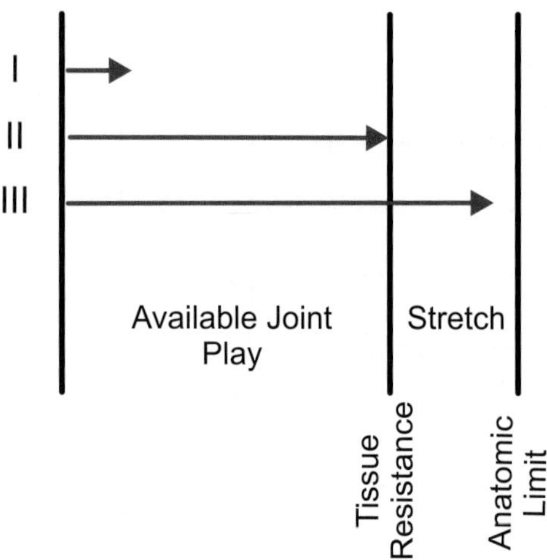

FIGURE 5.10 Representation of sustained joint-play techniques. *(Adapted from Kaltenborn, FM, et al:* Manual Mobilization of the Joints: Joint Examination and Basic Treatment, Vol I: The Extremities, *ed. 8. Oslo, Norway: Norli, 2014.*[17]*)*

Grade I (loosen). Small-amplitude distraction is applied when no stress is placed on the capsule. It equalizes cohesive forces, muscle tension, and atmospheric pressure acting on the joint.

Grade II (tighten). Enough distraction or glide is applied to tighten the tissues around the joint. Kaltenborn[15] called this "taking up the slack."

Grade III (stretch). A distraction or glide is applied with an amplitude large enough to place stretch on the joint capsule and surrounding periarticular structures.

Indications

- Grade I distraction is used with all gliding motions and may be used for relief of pain. Apply intermittent distraction for 7 to 10 seconds with a few seconds of rest in between for several cycles. Note the response and either repeat or discontinue.
- Grade II distraction is used for the initial treatment to determine the sensitivity of the joint. Once the joint reaction is known, the treatment dosage is increased or decreased accordingly.
- Gentle grade II distraction applied intermittently may be used to inhibit pain. Grade II glides may be used to maintain joint play when ROM is not allowed.
- Grade III distractions or glides are used to stretch the joint structures and thus increase joint play. For restricted joints, apply a minimum of a 6-second stretch force followed by partial release (to grade I or II), then repeat with slow, intermittent stretches at 3- to 4-second intervals.

Comparison of Oscillation and Sustained Techniques

When using either grading system, dosages I and II are low intensity and so do not cause a stretch force on the joint capsule or surrounding tissue, although by definition, sustained grade II techniques take up the slack of the tissues, whereas grade II oscillation techniques stay within the slack. Grades III and IV oscillations and grade III sustained stretch techniques are similar in intensity in that they all are applied with a stretch force at the limit of motion. The differences are related to the rhythm or speed of repetition of the stretch force.

- For clarity and consistency, when referring to dosages in this text, the notation *graded oscillations* means to use the dosages as described in the section on oscillation techniques. The notation *sustained grade* means to use the dosages as described in the section on sustained joint-play techniques.
- The choice of using oscillating or sustained techniques depends on the patient's response.
  - When dealing with managing pain, either grade I or II oscillation techniques or slow intermittent grade I or II sustained joint distraction techniques are recommended; the patient's response dictates the intensity and frequency of the joint-play technique.
  - When dealing with loss of joint play and thus decreased functional range, sustained techniques applied in a cyclic manner are recommended; the longer the stretch force can be maintained, the greater the creep and plastic deformation of the connective tissue.
  - When attempting to maintain available range by using joint-play techniques, either grade II oscillating or sustained grade II techniques can be used.

Thrust Manipulation/High Velocity Thrust

HVT is a small-amplitude, high-velocity technique.

Application

- Prior to application, the joint is moved to the limit of the motion so that all slack is taken out of the tissue, then a quick thrust is applied to the restricting tissue. It is important to keep the amplitude of the thrust small so as not to damage unrelated tissues or lose control of the maneuver.
- HVT is applied with one repetition only.

Indications

HVT is used to snap adhesions or is applied to a dislocated structure to reposition the joint surfaces.

Positioning and Stabilization

- The patient and the extremity to be treated should be positioned so the patient can relax. To relax the muscles crossing the joint, techniques of inhibition (see Chapter 4) may be used prior to or between mobilization techniques.
- Examination of joint play (passive accessory motion) and the first treatment are initially performed in the loose pack or the resting position for that joint so that the greatest capsule laxity is possible. In some cases, the position to use is the one in which the joint is least painful.
- With progression of treatment, the joint is positioned at or near the end of the available range prior to application of the mobilization force. This places the restricting tissue in

its most lengthened position where the stretch force can be more specific and effective.[17]

- Firmly and comfortably stabilize one joint partner, usually the proximal bone. A belt, one of the therapist's hands, or an assistant holding the part may provide stabilization. Appropriate stabilization prevents unwanted stress to surrounding tissues and joints and makes the stretch force more specific and effective.

Direction and Target of Treatment Force

- The treatment force (either gentle or strong) is applied as close to the opposing joint surface as possible. It is imperative that the therapist be able to identify anatomical landmarks and use these as guides for accurate hand placement and force application. The larger the contact surface, the more comfortable the patient will be with the procedure. For example, instead of forcing with your thumb, use the flat surface of your hand.
- The direction of movement during treatment is either parallel or perpendicular to the treatment plane. *Treatment plane* was described by Kaltenborn[17] as a plane perpendicular to a line running from the axis of rotation to the middle of the concave articular surface. The plane is in the concave partner, so its position is determined by the position of the concave bone (Fig. 5.11).

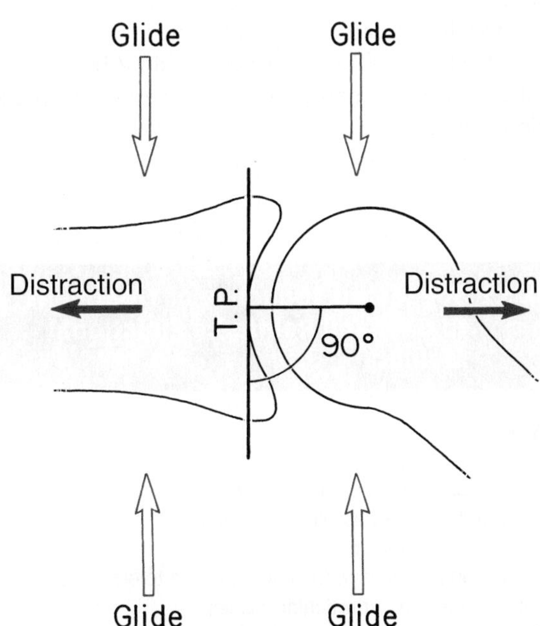

FIGURE 5.11 Treatment plane (T.P.) is at right angles to a line drawn from the axis of rotation to the center of the concave articulating surface and lies in the concave surface. Joint traction (distraction) is applied perpendicular to and glides parallel to the T.P.

- Distraction techniques are applied perpendicular to the treatment plane. The entire bone is moved so the joint surfaces are separated.
- *Gliding techniques are applied parallel to the treatment plane.* The direction of gliding may be determined by using the convex-concave rule (described earlier in the chapter). If the surface of the moving bony partner is convex, the treatment glide should be opposite to the direction in which the bone swings. If the surface of the moving bony partner is concave, the treatment glide should be in the same direction (see Fig. 5.5). Or, if a restricted feel is identified during the examination, the glide is performed in the direction that stretches the restriction.
- The entire bone is moved so there is gliding of one joint surface on the other. The bone should not be used as a lever; it should have no arcing motion (swing), which would cause rolling and thus compression of the joint surfaces.

Initiation and Progression of Treatment (Fig. 5.12)

1. The initial treatment is the same whether treating to decrease pain or increase joint play. The purpose is to determine joint reactivity before proceeding. Use a sustained grade II distraction of the joint surfaces with the joint held in resting position or the position where the greatest mobility is detected.[17] Note the immediate joint response relative to irritability and range.
2. The next day, evaluate the joint response or have the patient report the response at the next visit.
   - If there is increased pain and sensitivity, reduce the amplitude of treatment to grade I oscillations.
   - If the joint is the same or better, perform either of the following: Repeat the same maneuver if the goal of treatment is to maintain joint play, or progress the maneuver to stretching techniques if the goal of treatment is to increase joint play.
3. To maintain joint play by using gliding techniques when ROM techniques are contraindicated or not possible for a period of time, use sustained grade II or grade II oscillation techniques.
4. To progress the stretch technique, move the bone to the end of the available ROM[17] and then apply a sustained grade III distraction or glide technique. Progressions include prepositioning the bone at the end of the available range and rotating it prior to applying grade III distraction or glide techniques. The direction of the glide and rotation is dictated by the joint mechanics. For example, laterally rotate the humerus as shoulder abduction is progressed; medially rotate the tibia as knee flexion is progressed.

CLINICAL TIP

For effective mobilization:

- Warm the tissue around the joint prior to stretching. Modalities, massage, or gentle muscle contractions increase the circulation and warm the tissues.

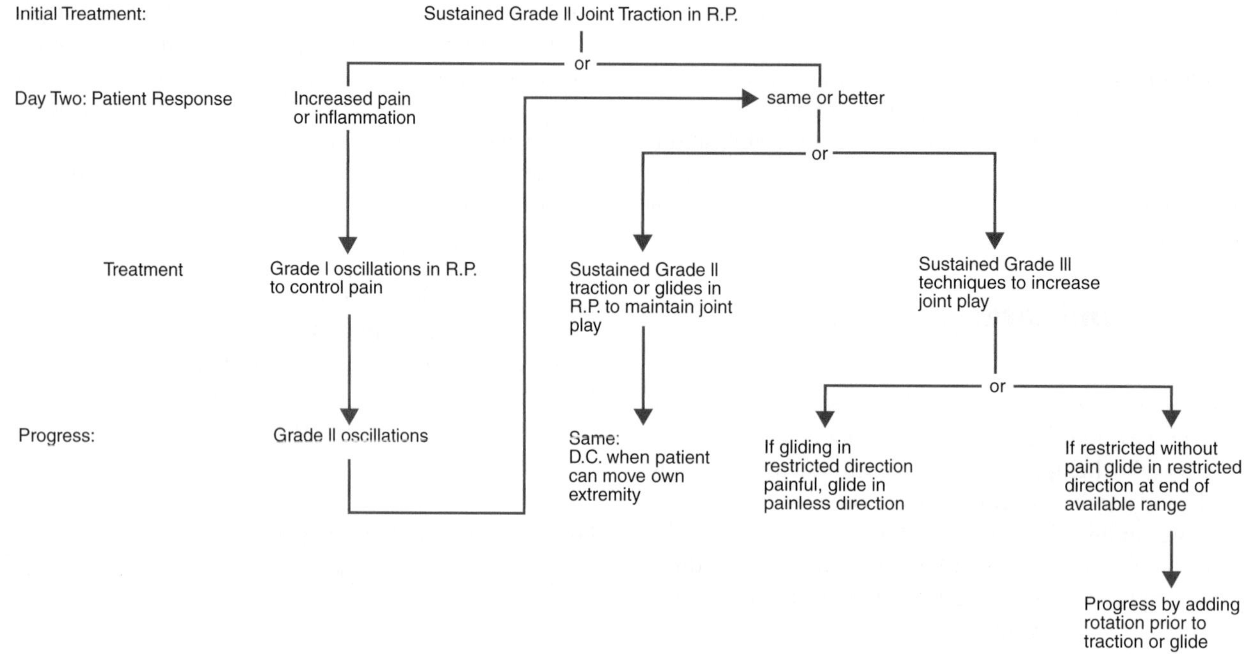

FIGURE 5.12 Initiation and progression of treatment.

- Muscle relaxation techniques and grade I and II oscillation techniques may inhibit muscle guarding and should be alternated with sustained stretching techniques, if necessary.
- When using grade III gliding techniques, a grade I distraction should be used with it. A grade II or III distraction should not be used with a grade III glide to avoid excessive trauma to the joint.
- If gliding in the restricted direction is too painful, begin gliding mobilizations in the painless direction. Progress to gliding in the restricted direction when mobility improves and pain decreases.
- When stretching to increase joint play, move the bony partner through the available range of joint play first—that is, "take up the slack." When tissue resistance is felt, apply the stretch force against the restriction.
- Incorporate MWM techniques (described in the following section) as part of the total approach to treatment.

Patient Response

- Stretching maneuvers usually cause soreness. Perform the maneuvers on alternate days to allow the soreness to decrease and tissue healing to occur between stretching sessions. The patient should perform ROM into any newly gained range during this time.
- If there is increased pain lasting longer than 24 hours after stretching, the dosage (amplitude) or duration of treatment was too vigorous. Decrease the dosage or duration until the pain is under control.
- The patient's joint and ROM should be reassessed after treatment and again before the next treatment. Alterations in treatment are dictated by the joint response.

Total Program

Mobilization techniques are one part of a total treatment program when there is decreased function. If muscles or connective tissues are also limiting motion, PNF stretching and passive stretching techniques are alternated with joint mobilization during the same treatment session. Interventions should also include appropriate ROM, strengthening, and functional exercises, so the patient learns effective control and use of the gained mobility (Box 5.2).

BOX 5.2 Suggested Sequence of Treatment to Gain and Reinforce Functional Mobility

1. Warm the tissues
2. Relax the muscles
   - Hold-relax inhibition technique
   - Grade I or II joint oscillation techniques
3. Joint mobilization stretches
   - Position and dosage for level of tissue tolerance
5. Passive stretch periarticular tissues
6. Patient actively uses new range
   - Reciprocal inhibition
   - Active ROM
   - Functional activities
7. Maintain new range; patient instruction
   - Self-stretching
   - Auto-mobilization
   - Active, resistive ROM
   - Functional activities using the new range

Mobilization With Movement: Principles of Application

Brian Mulligan's concept of MWM is the natural continuance of progression in the development of manual therapy from active self-stretching exercises, to therapist-applied passive physiological movement, to passive accessory mobilization techniques.[23] MWM is the concurrent application of pain-free accessory mobilization with active and/or passive physiological movement.[26] Passive end-range overpressure or stretching is then applied without pain as a barrier. These techniques are applicable when:

- No contraindication for manual therapy exists (described earlier in the chapter).
- A full orthopedic examination has been completed, and evaluation of the results indicates local musculoskeletal pathology.
- A specific biomechanical analysis reveals localized loss of movement and/or pain associated with function.
- No pain is produced during or immediately after application of the technique.[22]

Principles and Application of MWM in Clinical Practice

Comparable sign. One or more comparable signs are identified during the examination.[12] A comparable sign is a positive test sign that can be repeated after a therapeutic maneuver to determine the effectiveness of the maneuver. For example, a comparable sign may include loss of joint play movement, loss of ROM, or pain associated with movement during specific functional activities, such as lateral elbow pain with resisted wrist extension, painful restriction of ankle dorsiflexion, or pain with overhead reaching.

Passive techniques. A passive joint mobilization is applied using the principles described in the previous section following the principles of Kaltenborn.[17] Utilizing knowledge of joint anatomy and mechanics, a sense of tissue tension, and sound clinical reasoning, the therapist investigates various combinations of parallel or perpendicular accessory glides to find the pain-free direction and grade of accessory movement. This may be a glide, spin, distraction, or combination of movements. This accessory motion must be pain-free.[26]

Accessory glide with active comparable sign. While the therapist sustains the pain-free accessory force, the patient is requested to perform the comparable sign. The comparable sign should now be significantly improved—that is, there should be increased ROM, and the motion should *be free of the original pain.*[26]

No pain. The therapist must continuously monitor the patient's reaction to ensure no pain is produced. Failure to improve the comparable sign would indicate that the therapist has not found the correct direction of accessory movement, the grade of movement, or that the technique is not indicated.

Repetitions. The previously restricted and/or painful motion or activity is repeated 6 to 10 times by the patient while the therapist continues to maintain the appropriate accessory mobilization. Further gains are expected with repetition during a treatment session, particularly when *pain-free* passive overpressure is applied to achieve end-range loading.

Description of techniques. Techniques applicable to the extremity joints are described throughout this text in the treatment sections for various conditions (see Chapters 17 through 22).

Patient Response and Progression

Pain as a guide. Successful MWM techniques should render the comparable sign painless while significantly improving function during the application of the technique.

Self-treatment. Once patient response is determined, self-treatment is often possible using MWM principles with sports-type adhesive tape and/or the patient providing the mobilization component of the MWM concurrent with the active physiological movement.[10]

Total program. Having restored articular function with MWMs, the patient is progressed through the ensuing rehabilitation sequences of the recovery of muscular power, endurance, and neural control. Sustained improvements are necessary to justify ongoing intervention.

Theoretical Framework

Mulligan postulated a positional fault model to explain the results gained through his concept. Alternatively, inappropriate joint tracking mechanisms due to an altered instantaneous axis of rotation and neurophysiological response models have also been considered.[10,22,23,27] For further details of the application of the Mulligan concept as it applies to the spine and extremities, refer to *Manual Therapy, "NAGS," "SNAGS," "MWMS," etc.*[26]

FOCUS ON EVIDENCE

Early research on the MWM approach confirms its benefits; however, the mechanism by which it affects the musculoskeletal system, whether mechanical or physiological, has yet to be fully determined.[4,18,29,31,32,35] A study by Paungmali and associates[31] measured a significant reduction in pain, increased grip strength, and increased sympathetic nervous system response immediately following MWM for chronic lateral epicondylalgia compared with a placebo intervention, results that were similar to those in studies of spinal manipulation. They interpreted this to imply that there is a multisystem response to manipulation whether the spine or the elbow is manipulated.

Peripheral Joint Mobilization Techniques

The following are suggested joint distraction and gliding techniques for use by entry-level therapists and those attempting to gain a foundation in joint mobilization of extremity joints. A variety of adaptations can be made from these techniques. Some adaptations are described in the respective chapters in which specific impairments and interventions are discussed (see Chapters 17 through 22). The distraction and glide techniques should be applied with respect to the dosage, frequency, progression, precautions, and procedures as described earlier in this chapter. Manipulation and HVT techniques for the spine are described in Chapter 16.

NOTE: Terms, such as proximal hand, distal hand, lateral hand, or other descriptive terms, indicate that the therapist should use the hand that is more proximal, distal, or lateral to the patient or the patient's extremity.

Shoulder Girdle Complex

Joints of the shoulder girdle consist of three synovial articulations—sternoclavicular, acromioclavicular, and glenohumeral—and the functional articulation of the scapula gliding on the thorax (Fig. 5.13). To gain full elevation of the humerus, the accessory and component motions of clavicular elevation and rotation, scapular rotation, and external rotation of the humerus, as well as adequate joint play, are necessary. The clavicular and scapular techniques are described following the glenohumeral joint techniques. For a review of the mechanics of the shoulder complex, see Chapter 17.

Glenohumeral Joint

The concave glenoid fossa receives the convex humeral head.

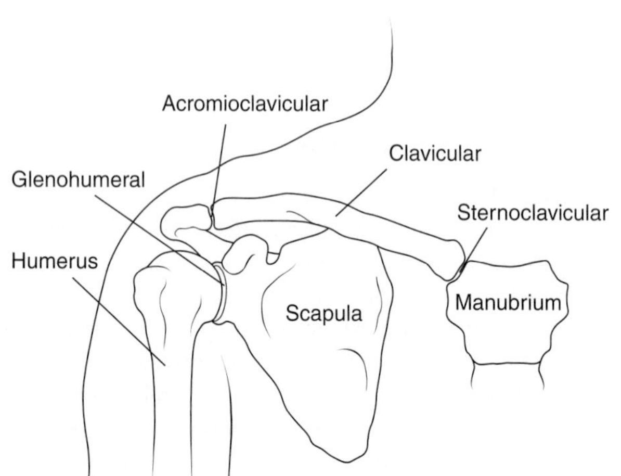

FIGURE 5.13 Bones and joints of the shoulder girdle complex.

Resting position. The shoulder is abducted 55°, horizontally adducted 30°, and rotated so the forearm is in the horizontal plane with respect to the body (called plane of the scapula).

Treatment plane. The treatment plane is in the glenoid fossa and moves with the scapula as it rotates.

Stabilization. Fixate the scapula with a belt or have an assistant help.

Glenohumeral Distraction (Fig. 5.14)

VIDEO 5.1

Indications

Testing; initial treatment (sustained grade II); pain control (grade I or II oscillations); general mobility (sustained grade III).

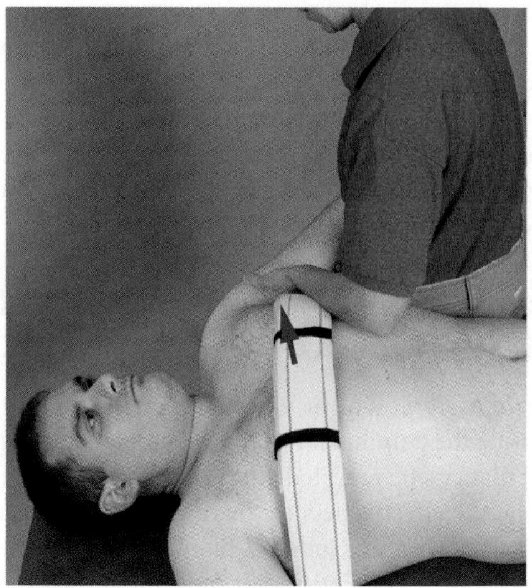

FIGURE 5.14 Glenohumeral joint: distraction in resting position. Note that the force is perpendicular to the T.P. in the glenoid fossa.

Patient Position

Supine, with arm in the resting position.

Therapist Position and Hand Placement

- Stand at the patient's side, facing toward his or her head.
- Use the hand nearer the part being treated (e.g., left hand if treating the patient's left shoulder) and place it in the patient's axilla with your thumb just distal to the joint margin anteriorly and fingers posteriorly. Support the forearm between your trunk and elbow.
- Your other hand supports the humerus from the lateral surface.

Mobilizing Force

With the hand in the axilla, move the humerus laterally.

NOTE: The entire arm moves in a translatoric motion away from the plane of the glenoid fossa. Distractions may be performed with the humerus in any position (see Figs. 5.17, 5.19, and 17.20). You must be aware of the amount of scapular rotation and adjust the distraction force against the humerus, so it is perpendicular to the plane of the glenoid fossa.

Glenohumeral Caudal Glide in Resting Position (Fig. 5.15) VIDEO 5.2

Indications

To increase abduction (sustained grade III); to reposition the humeral head if superiorly positioned.

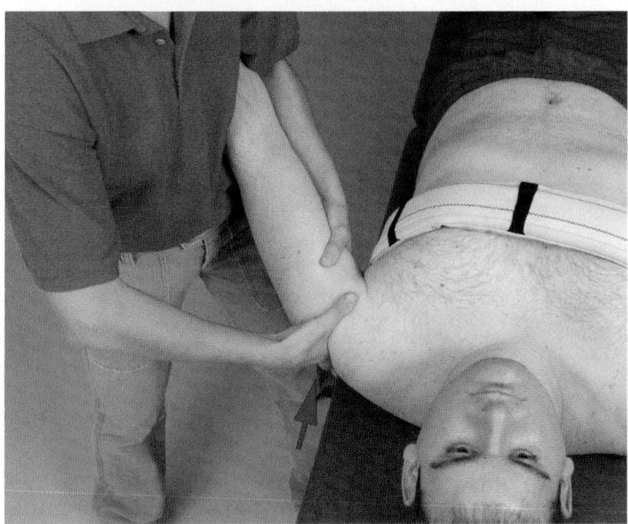

FIGURE 5.15 Glenohumeral joint: caudal glide in the resting position. Note that the distraction force is applied by the hand in the axilla, and the caudal glide force is from the hand superior to the humeral head.

Patient Position

Supine, with arm in the resting position.

Therapist Position and Hand Placement

- Stand lateral to the patient's arm being treated and support the forearm between your trunk and elbow. Place one hand in the patient's axilla to provide a grade I distraction.
- The web space of your other hand is placed just distal to the acromion process.

Mobilizing Force

With the superiorly placed hand, glide the humerus in an inferior direction.

Glenohumeral Caudal Glide (Long Axis Traction)

Patient Position

Supine, with arm in the resting position.

Hand Placement and Mobilizing Force

Support the patient's forearm between your trunk and elbow. Grasp around the distal arm with both hands and apply the force in a caudal direction as you shift your body weight toward the patient's feet.

Glenohumeral Caudal Glide Progression (Fig. 5.16)

Indication

To increase abduction.

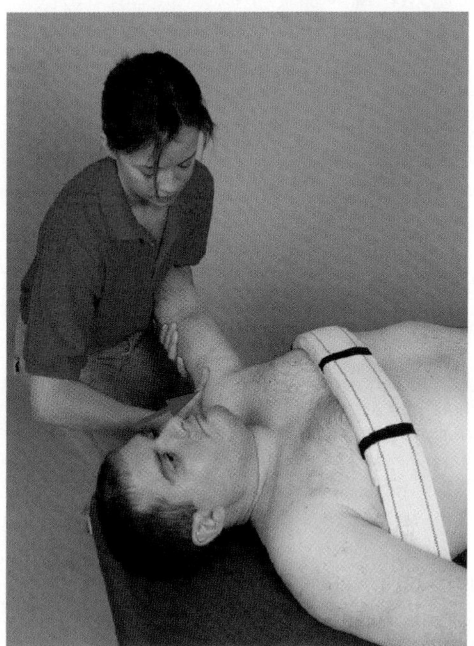

FIGURE 5.16 Glenohumeral joint: caudal glide with the shoulder near 90°.

Patient Position

- Supine or sitting, with the arm abducted to the end of its available range.
- External rotation of the humerus should be added to the end-range position as the arm approaches and goes beyond 90°.

Therapist Position and Hand Placement

- With the patient *supine,* stand facing the patient's feet and stabilize the patient's arm against your trunk with the hand farthest from the patient. Slight lateral motion of your trunk provides grade I distraction via a long-axis traction.
- With the patient *sitting,* stand behind the patient and cradle the distal humerus with the hand farthest from the patient; this hand provides a grade I distraction via a long-axis traction.
- Place the web space of your other hand just distal to the acromion process on the proximal humerus.

Mobilizing Force

With the hand on the proximal humerus, glide the humerus in an inferior direction with respect to the glenoid fossa of the scapula.

Glenohumeral Elevation Progression (Fig. 5.17)

Indication

To increase elevation beyond 90° of abduction.

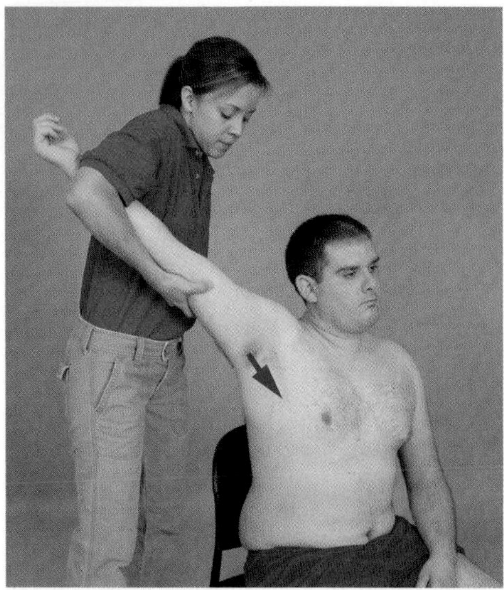

FIGURE 5.17 Glenohumeral joint: elevation progression in the sitting position. This is used when the range is greater than 90°. Note the externally rotated position of the humerus; pressure against the head of the humerus is toward the axilla.

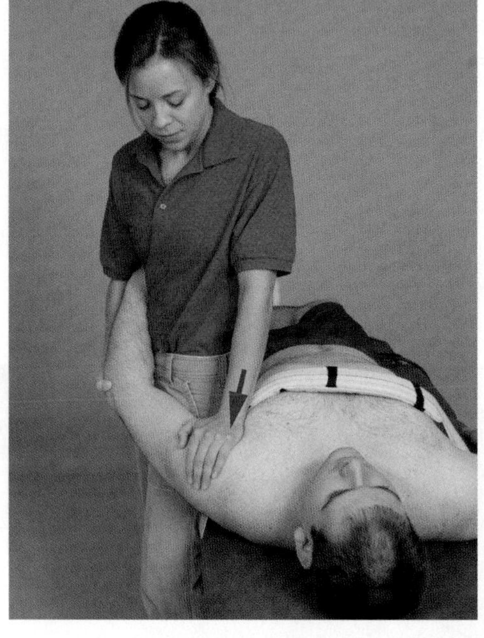

FIGURE 5.18 Glenohumeral joint: posterior glide in the resting position.

Patient Position

Supine or sitting, with the arm abducted and externally rotated to the end of its available range.

Therapist Position and Hand Placement

- Hand placement is the same as for caudal glide progression.
- Adjust your body position so the hand applying the mobilizing force is aligned with the treatment plane in the glenoid fossa.
- With the hand grasping the elbow, apply a grade I distraction force (this is a long axis traction as pictured in Fig. 5.17).

Mobilizing Force

- With the hand on the proximal humerus, glide the humerus in a progressively anterior direction against the inferior folds of the capsule in the axilla.
- The direction of force with respect to the patient's body depends on the amount of upward rotation and protraction of the scapula.

Glenohumeral Posterior Glide, Resting Position (Fig. 5.18) VIDEO 5.3

Indications

To increase flexion; to increase internal rotation.

Patient Position

Supine, with the arm in resting position.

Therapist Position and Hand Placement

- Stand with your back to the patient between the patient's trunk and arm.
- Support the arm against your trunk, grasping the distal humerus with your lateral hand. This position provides grade I distraction to the joint.
- Place the lateral border of your top hand just distal to the anterior margin of the joint, with your fingers pointing superiorly. This hand gives the mobilizing force.

Mobilizing Force

Glide the humeral head posteriorly by moving the entire arm as you bend your knees.

Glenohumeral Posterior Glide Progression (Fig. 5.19)

Indications

To increase posterior gliding when flexion approaches 90°; to increase horizontal adduction.

Patient Position

Supine, with the arm flexed to 90° and internally rotated and with the elbow flexed. The arm may also be placed in horizontal adduction.

Hand Placement

- Place padding under the scapula for stabilization.
- Place one hand across the proximal surface of the humerus to apply a grade I distraction.
- Place your other hand over the patient's elbow.
- A belt placed around your pelvis and the proximal aspect of the patient's humerus may be used to apply the distraction force.

Mobilizing Force

Glide the humerus posteriorly by pushing down at the elbow through the long axis of the humerus.

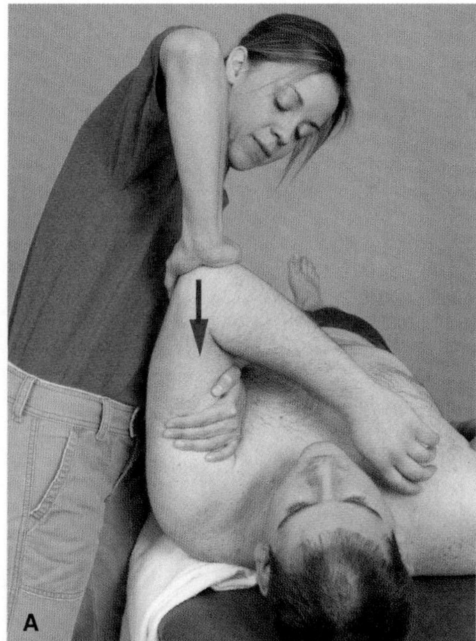

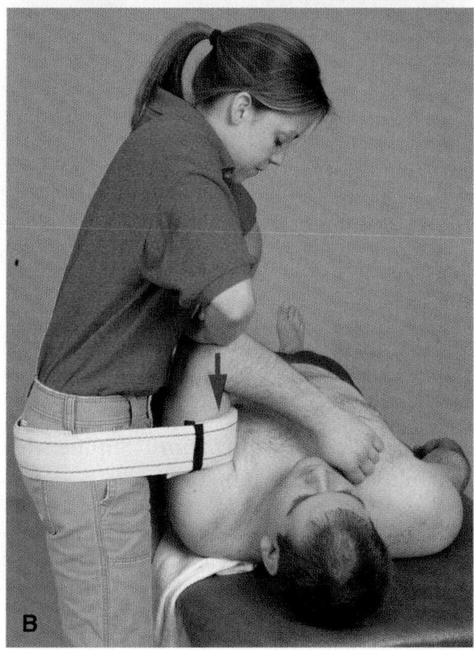

FIGURE 5.19 Glenohumeral joint: posterior glide progression. **(A)** One hand or **(B)** a belt is used to exert a grade I distraction force.

Glenohumeral Anterior Glide, Resting Position (Fig. 5.20) VIDEO 5.4

Indications

To increase extension; to increase external rotation.

Patient Position

Prone, with the arm in resting position over the edge of the treatment table, supported on your thigh. Stabilize the acromion with padding. The supine position may also be used.

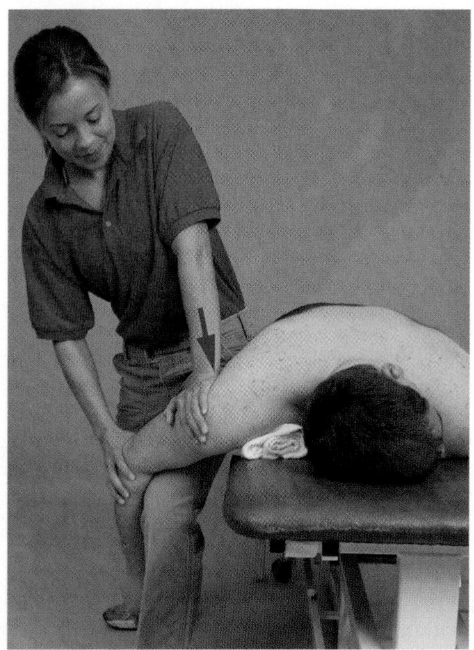

FIGURE 5.20 Glenohumeral joint: anterior glide in the resting position.

Therapist Position and Hand Placement

- Stand facing the top of the table with the leg closer to the table in a forward stride position.
- Support the patient's arm against your thigh with your outside hand; the arm positioned on your thigh provides a grade I distraction.
- Place the ulnar border of your other hand just distal to the posterior angle of the acromion process, with your fingers pointing superiorly; this hand gives the mobilizing force.

Mobilizing Force

Glide the humeral head in an anterior and slightly medial direction. Bend both knees so the entire arm moves anteriorly.

PRECAUTION: Do not lift the arm at the elbow and thereby cause angulation of the humerus. Such angulation could lead to anterior subluxation or dislocation of the humeral head. Do not use this position to progress external rotation. Placing the shoulder in 90° abduction with external rotation and applying an anterior glide may cause anterior subluxation of the humeral head.

Glenohumeral External Rotation Progressions (Fig. 5.21) VIDEO 5.5

Indication

To increase external rotation.

Techniques

Because of the danger of subluxation when applying an anterior glide with the humerus externally rotated, use a distraction progression or elevation progression to gain range.

- *Distraction progression*: Begin with the shoulder in resting position, externally rotate the humerus to end-range, and

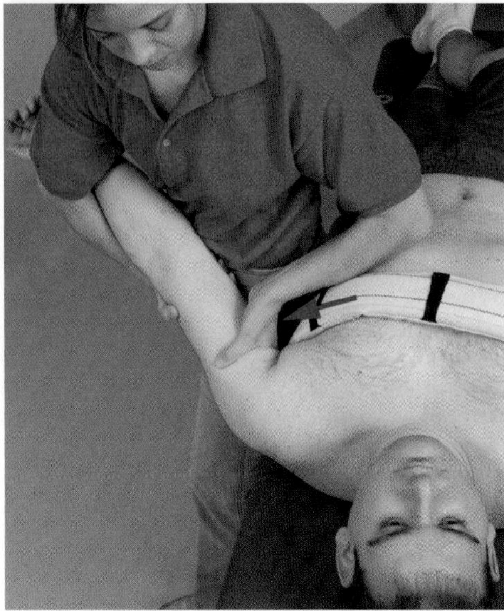

FIGURE 5.21 Glenohumeral joint: distraction for external rotation progression. Note that the humerus is positioned in the resting position with maximum external rotation prior to the application of distraction stretch force.

then apply a grade III distraction perpendicular to the treatment plane in the glenoid fossa.

- *Elevation progression* (see Fig. 5.17): This technique incorporates end-range external rotation.
- Several research studies have documented increased external rotation by using a posterior glide. This is particularly beneficial when the humeral head is anteriorly displaced in the glenoid fossa and the posterior capsule is tight.[11,14,15,16]

Acromioclavicular Joint

Indication. To increase mobility of the joint.

Stabilization. Fixate the scapula with your more lateral hand around the acromion process.

Anterior Glide of Clavicle on Acromion (Fig. 5.22)

Patient Position

Sitting or prone.

Hand Placement

- With the patient sitting, stand behind the patient and stabilize the acromion process with the fingers of your lateral hand.
- The thumb of your other hand pushes downward through the upper trapezius and is placed posteriorly on the clavicle, just medial to the joint space.
- With the patient prone, stabilize the acromion with a towel roll under the shoulder.

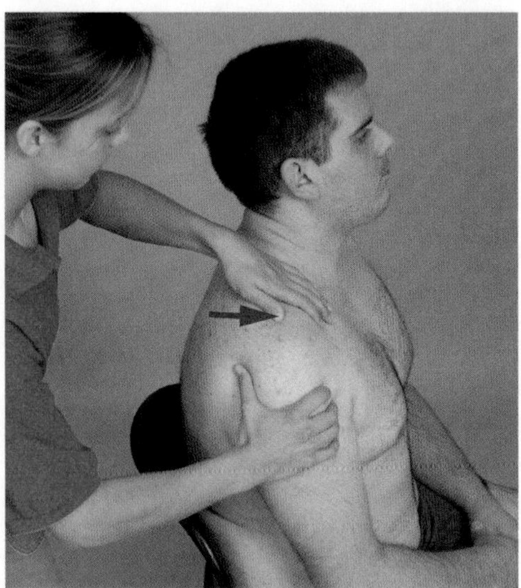

FIGURE 5.22 Acromioclavicular joint: anterior glide.

Mobilizing Force

Push the clavicle anteriorly with your thumb.

Sternoclavicular Joint

Joint surfaces. The proximal articulating surface of the clavicle is convex superiorly/inferiorly and concave anteriorly/posteriorly with an articular disk between it and the manubrium of the sternum.

Treatment plane. For protraction/retraction, the treatment plane is in the clavicle. For elevation/depression, the treatment plane is in the manubrium.

Patient position and stabilization. Supine; the thorax provides stability to the sternum.

Sternoclavicular Posterior Glide and Superior Glide (Fig. 5.23)

Indications

Posterior glide to increase retraction; superior glide to increase depression of the clavicle.

Hand Placement

- Place your thumb on the anterior surface of the proximal end of the clavicle.
- Flex your index finger and place the middle phalanx along the caudal surface of the clavicle to support the thumb.

Mobilizing Force

- *Posterior glide*: Push with your thumb in a posterior direction.
- *Superior glide*: Push with your index finger in a superior direction.

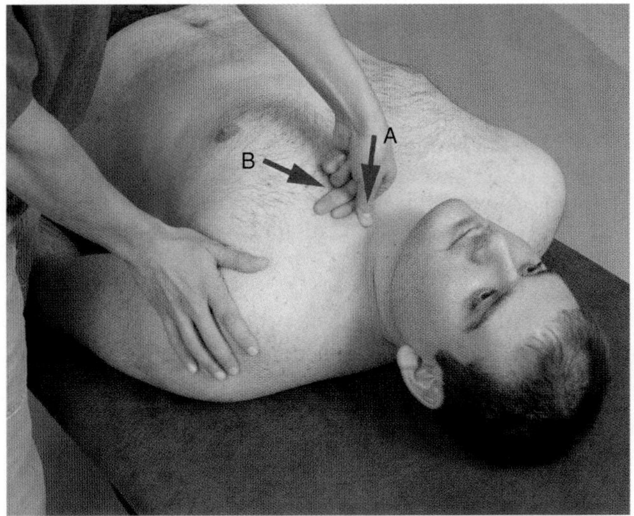

FIGURE 5.23 Sternoclavicular joint: posterior and superior glides. **(A)** Press down with the thumb for posterior glide; **(B)** Press upward with the index finger for superior glide.

Sternoclavicular Anterior Glide and Caudal (Inferior) Glide (Fig. 5.24)

Indications

Anterior glide to increase protraction; caudal glide to increase elevation of the clavicle.

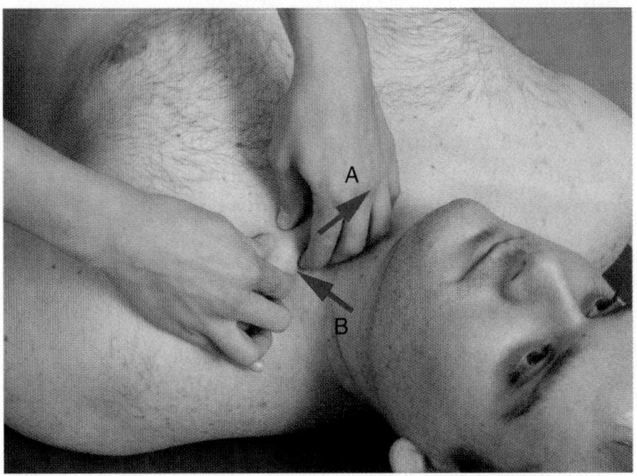

FIGURE 5.24 Sternoclavicular joint: anterior and inferior glides. **(A)** Pull the clavicle upward for an anterior glide; **(B)** Press caudalward with the curled fingers for an inferior glide.

Hand Placement

Your fingers are placed superiorly and thumb inferiorly around the clavicle.

Mobilizing Force

- *Anterior glide*: lift the clavicle anteriorly with your fingers and thumb.
- *Caudal glide*: press the clavicle inferiorly with your fingers.

Scapulothoracic Soft-Tissue Mobilization (Fig. 5.25) VIDEO 5.6

The scapulothoracic articulation is not a true joint, but the soft tissue and muscles supporting the articulation are mobilized to obtain scapular motions of elevation, depression, protraction, retraction, upward and downward rotation, and winging for normal shoulder girdle mobility.

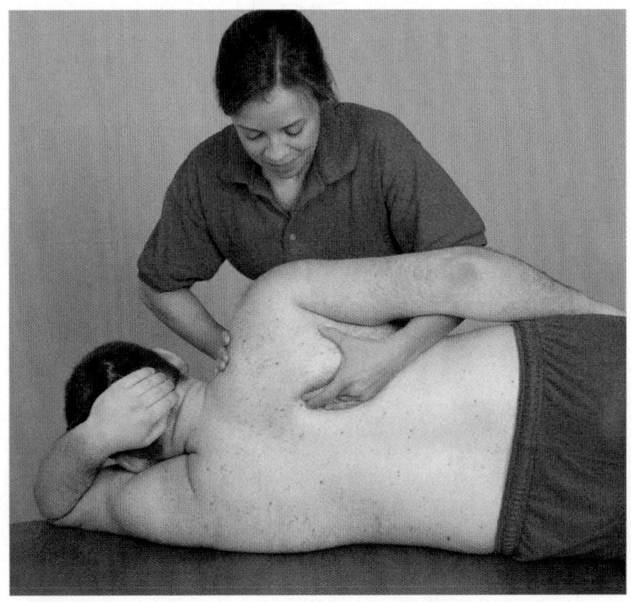

FIGURE 5.25 Scapulothoracic articulation: elevation, depression, protraction, retraction, upward and downward rotations, and winging.

Patient position. If there is considerable restriction in mobility, begin prone and progress to side-lying, with the patient facing you. Support the weight of the patient's arm by draping it over your inferior arm and allowing it to hang so the scapular muscles are relaxed.

Hand placement. Place your superior hand across the acromion process to control the direction of motion. With the fingers of your inferior hand, scoop under the medial border and under the inferior angle of the scapula.

Mobilizing force. Move the scapula in the desired direction by lifting from the inferior angle or by pushing on the acromion process.

Elbow and Forearm Complex

The elbow and forearm complex consists of four joints: humeroulnar, humeroradial, proximal radioulnar, and distal radioulnar (Fig. 5.26). For full elbow flexion and extension, accessory motions of varus and valgus (with radial and ulnar glides) are necessary. The techniques for each of the joints as well as accessory motions are described in this section. For a review of the joint mechanics, see Chapter 18.

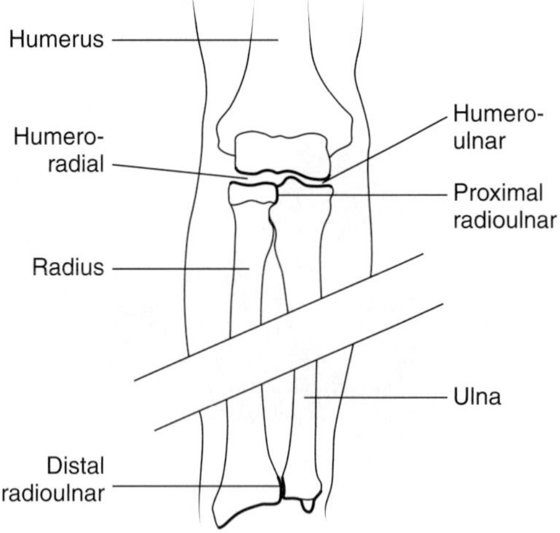

FIGURE 5.26 Bones and joints of the elbow complex.

Humeroulnar Articulation

The convex trochlea articulates with the concave olecranon fossa.

Resting position. Elbow is flexed 70°, and forearm is supinated 10°.

Treatment plane. The treatment plane is in the olecranon fossa, angled approximately 45° from the long axis of the ulna (Fig. 5.27).

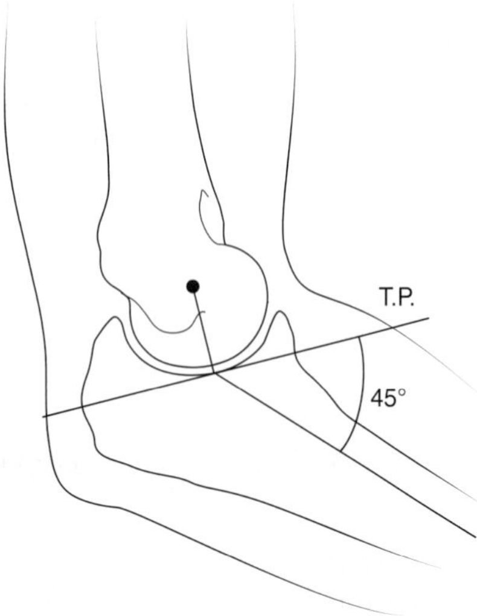

FIGURE 5.27 Lateral view of the humeroulnar joint, depicting the treatment plane (T.P.).

Stabilization. Fixate the humerus against the treatment table with a belt or use an assistant to hold it. The patient may roll onto his or her side and fixate the humerus with the contralateral hand if muscle relaxation can be maintained around the elbow joint being mobilized.

Humeroulnar Distraction and Progression (Fig. 5.28 A) VIDEO 5.7

Indications

Testing; initial treatment (sustained grade II); pain control (grade I or II oscillation); to increase flexion or extension (grade III or IV).

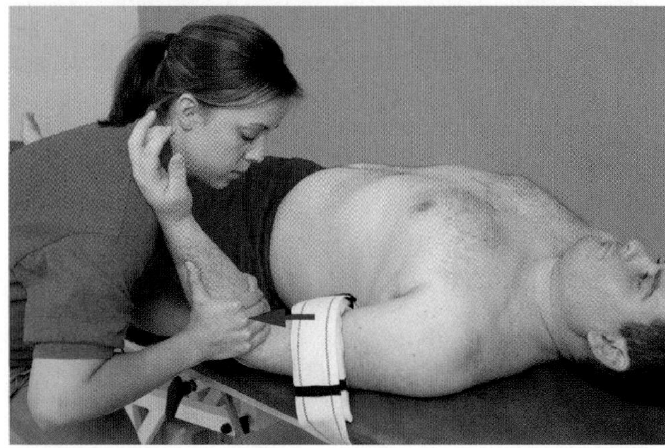

FIGURE 5.28 Humeroulnar joint: **(A)** Distraction;

Patient Position

Supine, with the elbow over the edge of the treatment table or supported with padding just proximal to the olecranon process. Rest the patient's wrist against your shoulder, allowing the elbow to be in resting position for the initial treatment. To stretch into either flexion or extension, position the joint at the end of its available range.

Hand Placement

- When in the resting position or at end-range flexion, place the fingers of your medial hand over the proximal ulna on the volar surface; reinforce it with your other hand.
- To isolate the mobilization force to the humeroulnar articulation, be sure that your hand is not in contact with the proximal radius.
- When at end-range extension, stand and place the base of your proximal hand over the proximal portion of the ulna and support the distal forearm with your other hand.

Mobilizing Force

Apply force against the proximal ulna at a 45° angle to the shaft of the bone.

Humeroulnar Distal Glide (Fig. 5.28 B)

Indication

To increase flexion.

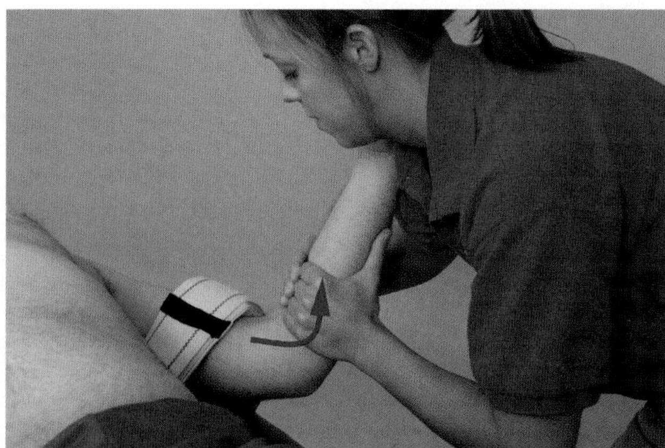

FIGURE 5.28—cont'd (B) Humeroulnar distraction with distal glide (scoop motion).

Patient Position and Hand Placement

- Supine, with the elbow over the edge of the treatment table.
- Begin with the elbow in resting position. Progress by positioning it at the end-range of flexion.
- Place the fingers of your medial hand over the proximal ulna on the volar surface; reinforce it with your other hand. To isolate the mobilization force to the humeroulnar articulation, be sure that your hand is not in contact with the proximal radius.

Mobilizing Force

First apply a distraction force to the joint at a 45° angle to the ulna, then while maintaining the distraction, direct the force in a distal direction along the long axis of the ulna using a scooping motion.

Humeroulnar Radial Glide

Indication

To increase varus. This is an accessory motion of the joint that accompanies elbow flexion and is therefore used to progress flexion.

Patient Position

- Side-lying on the arm to be mobilized, with the shoulder laterally rotated and the humerus supported on the table.
- Begin with the elbow in resting position; progress to end-range flexion.

Hand Placement

Place the base of your proximal hand just distal to the elbow; support the distal forearm with your other hand.

Mobilizing Force

Apply force against the ulna in a radial direction.

Humeroulnar Ulnar Glide

Indication

To increase valgus. This is an accessory motion of the joint that accompanies elbow extension and is therefore used to progress extension.

Patient Position

- Same as for radial glide except a block or wedge is placed under the proximal forearm for stabilization (using distal stabilization).
- Initially, the elbow is placed in resting position and is progressed to end-range extension.

Mobilizing Force

Apply force against the distal humerus in a radial direction, causing the ulna to glide ulnarly.

Humeroradial Articulation VIDEO 5. 8

The convex capitulum articulates with the concave radial head (see Fig. 5.26).

Resting position. Elbow is extended and forearm is supinated to the end of the available range.

Treatment plane. The treatment plane is in the concave radial head perpendicular to the long axis of the radius.

Stabilization. Fixate the humerus with one of your hands.

Humeroradial Distraction (Fig. 5.29)

Indications

To increase mobility of the humeroradial joint; to manipulate a pushed elbow (proximal displacement of the radius).

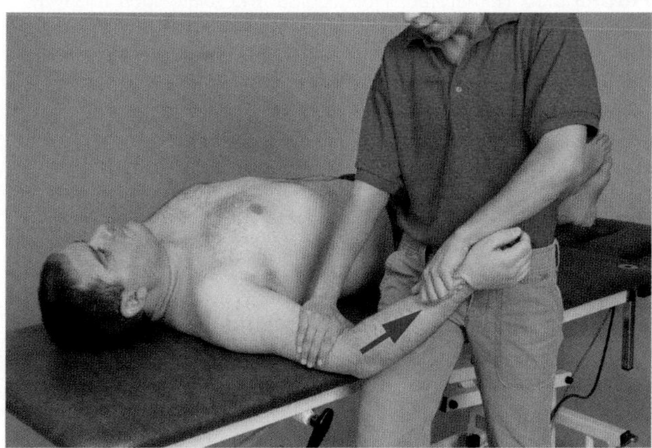

FIGURE 5.29 Humeroradial joint: distraction.

Patient Position

Supine or sitting, with the arm resting on the treatment table.

Therapist Position and Hand Placement

- Position yourself on the ulnar side of the patient's forearm so you are between the patient's hip and upper extremity.
- Stabilize the patient's humerus with your superior hand.
- Grasp around the distal radius with the fingers and thenar eminence of your inferior hand. Be sure you are not grasping around the distal ulna.

Mobilizing Force

Pull the radius distally (long-axis traction causes joint traction).

Humeroradial Dorsal/Volar Glides (Fig. 5.30)

Indications

Dorsal glide head of the radius to increase elbow extension; volar glide to increase flexion.

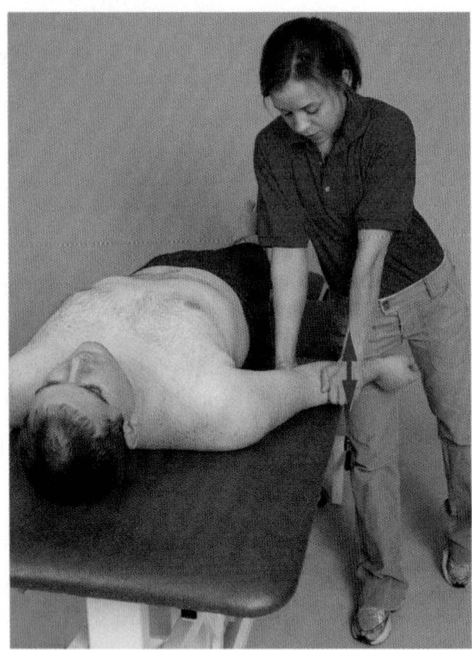

FIGURE 5.30 Humeroradial joint: dorsal and volar glides. This may also be done sitting, as in Figure 5.32, with the elbow positioned in extension and the humerus stabilized by the proximal hand (rather than the ulna).

Patient Position

Supine or sitting with the elbow extended and supinated to the end of the available range.

Hand Placement

- Stabilize the humerus with your hand that is on the medial side of the patient's arm.
- Place the palmar surface of your lateral hand on the volar aspect and your fingers on the dorsal aspect of the radial head.

Mobilizing Force

- Move the radial head dorsally with the palm of your hand or volarly with your fingers.
- If a stronger force is needed for the volar glide, realign your body and push with the base of your hand against the dorsal surface in a volar direction.

Humeroradial Compression (Fig. 5.31)

Indication

To reduce a pulled elbow subluxation.

Patient Position

Sitting or supine.

Hand Placement

- Approach the patient right hand to right hand or left hand to left hand. Stabilize the elbow posteriorly with the other hand. If supine, the stabilizing hand is under the elbow supported on the treatment table.
- Place your thenar eminence against the patient's thenar eminence (locking thumbs).

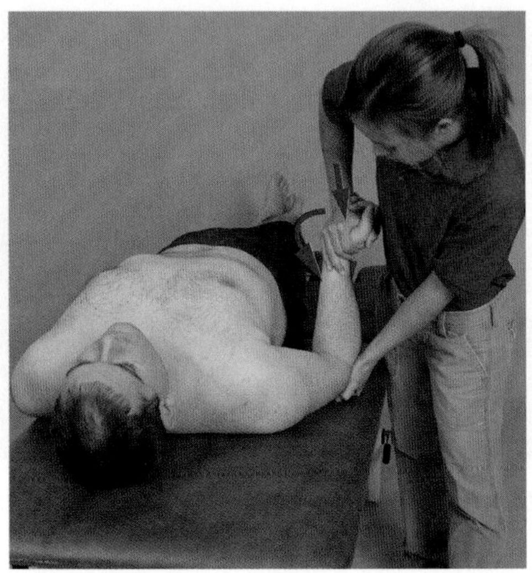

FIGURE 5.31 Humeroradial joint: compression mobilization. This is a quick thrust with simultaneous supination and compression of the radius.

Mobilizing Force

Simultaneously, extend the patient's wrist, push against the thenar eminence, and compress the long axis of the radius while supinating the forearm.

NOTE: To replace an acute subluxation, an HVT is used.

Proximal Radioulnar Joint

The convex rim of the radial head articulates with the concave radial notch on the ulna (see Fig. 5.26).

Resting position. The elbow is flexed 70°, and the forearm is supinated 35°.

Treatment plane. The treatment plane is in the radial notch of the ulna, parallel to the long axis of the ulna.

Stabilization. Proximal ulna is stabilized.

Proximal Radioulnar Dorsal/Volar Glides (Fig. 5.32) VIDEO 5.8

Indications

Dorsal glide to increase pronation; volar glide to increase supination.

Patient Position

- Sitting or supine, begin with the elbow flexed 70° and the forearm supinated 35°.
- Progress by placing the forearm at the limit of the range of pronation or supination prior to administering the respective glide.

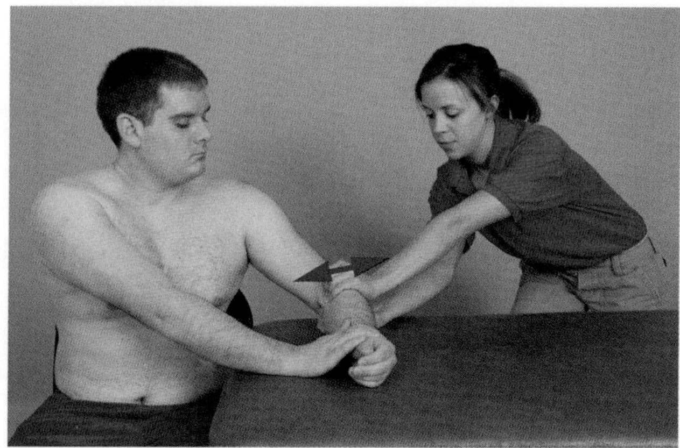

FIGURE 5.32 Proximal radioulnar joint: dorsal and volar glides.

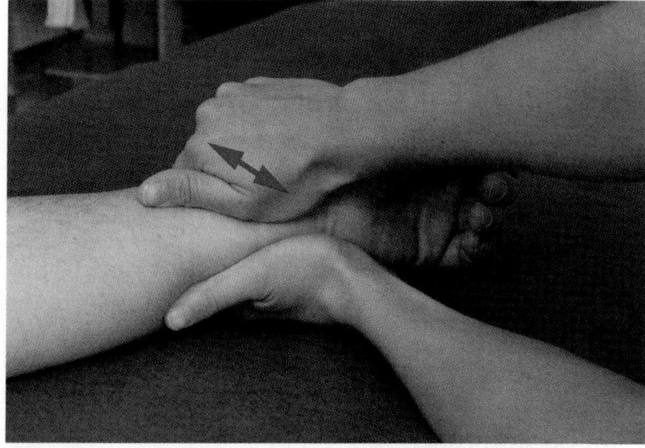

FIGURE 5.33 Distal radioulnar joint: dorsal and volar glides.

Hand Placement

- Approach the patient from the dorsal or volar aspect of the forearm. Fixate the ulna with your medial hand around the medial aspect of the forearm.
- With your other hand, grasp the head of the radius between your flexed fingers and palm of your hand.

Mobilizing Force

- Force the radial head volarly or dorsally by pushing with your palm or pulling with your fingers.
- If a stronger force is needed, rather than pulling with your fingers, move to the other side of the patient, switch hands, and apply the force with the palm of your hand.

Distal Radioulnar Joint

The concave ulnar notch of the radius articulates with the convex head of the ulna.

Resting position. The resting position is with the forearm supinated 10°.

Treatment plane. The treatment plane is the articulating surface of the radius, parallel to the long axis of the radius.

Stabilization. Distal ulna.

Distal Radioulnar Dorsal/Volar Glides (Fig. 5.33)

Indications

Dorsal glide to increase supination; volar glide to increase pronation.

Patient Position

Sitting, with the forearm on the treatment table. Begin in the resting position and progress to end-range pronation or supination.

Hand Placement

Stabilize the distal ulna by placing the fingers of one hand on the dorsal surface and the thenar eminence and thumb on the volar surface. Place your other hand in the same manner around the distal radius.

Mobilizing Force

Glide the distal radius dorsally to increase supination or volarly to increase pronation parallel to the ulna.

Wrist and Hand Complex

When mobilizing the wrist, begin with general distractions and glides that include the proximal row and distal row of carpals as a group. For full ROM, individual carpal mobilizations/manipulations may be necessary. They are described following the general mobilizations. For a review of the mechanics of the wrist complex, see Chapter 19 (Fig. 5.34).

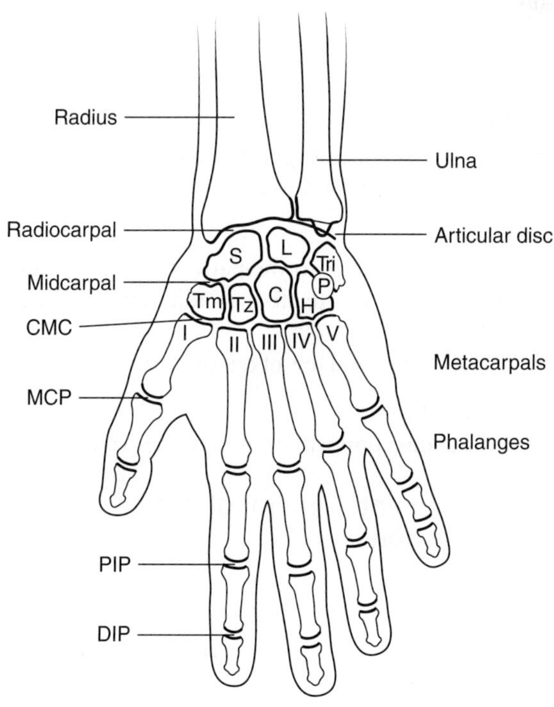

FIGURE 5.34 Bones and joints of the wrist and hand.

Radiocarpal Joint

The concave distal radius articulates with the convex proximal row of carpals, which is composed of the scaphoid, lunate, and triquetrum.

Resting position. The resting position is a straight line through the radius and third metacarpal with slight ulnar deviation.

Treatment plane. The treatment plane is in the articulating surface of the radius perpendicular to the long axis of the radius.

Stabilization. Distal radius and ulna.

Radiocarpal Distraction (Fig. 5.35)

Indications

Testing; initial treatment; pain control; general mobility of the wrist.

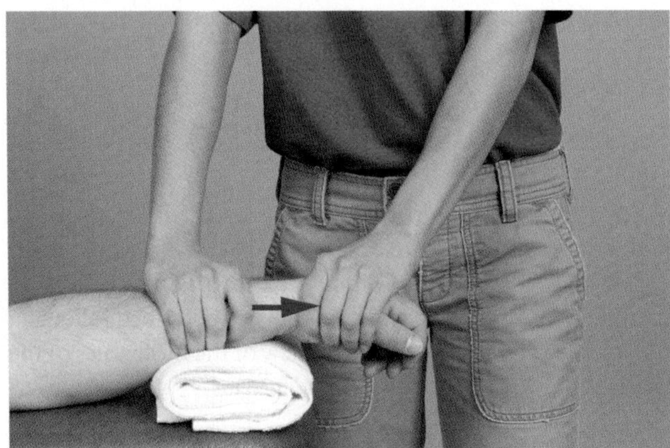

FIGURE 5.35 Wrist joint: general distraction.

Patient Position

Sitting, with the forearm supported on the treatment table and wrist over the edge of the table.

Hand Placement

- With the hand closest to the patient, grasp around the styloid processes and fixate the radius and ulna against the table.
- Grasp around the distal row of carpals with your other hand.

Mobilizing Force

Pull in a distal direction with respect to the arm.

Radiocarpal Joint: General Glides and Progression

Indications

Dorsal glide to increase flexion (Fig. 5.36 A); volar glide to increase extension (Fig. 5.36 B); radial glide to increase ulnar deviation; ulnar glide to increase radial deviation (Fig. 5.37).

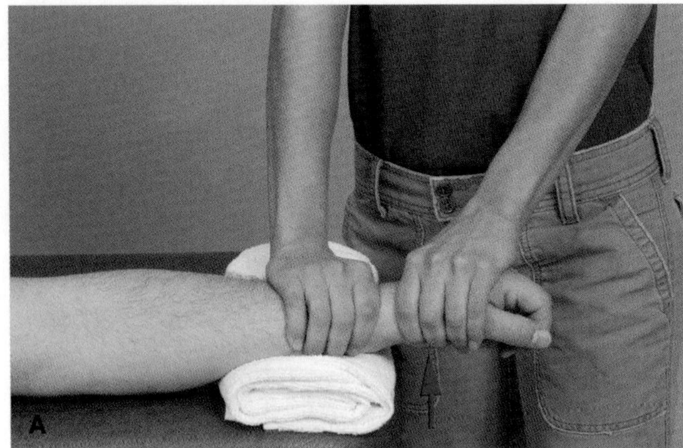

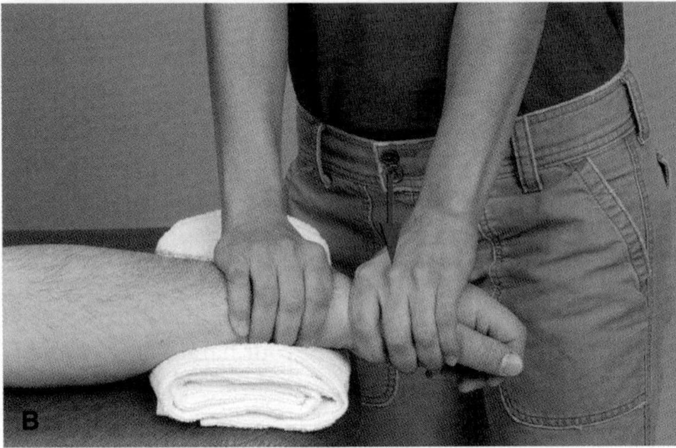

FIGURE 5.36 Wrist joint: general mobilization. **(A)** Dorsal glide; **(B)** Volar glide.

Patient Position and Hand Placement

- Sitting with forearm resting on the table in pronation for the dorsal and volar techniques and in midrange position for the radial and ulnar techniques.

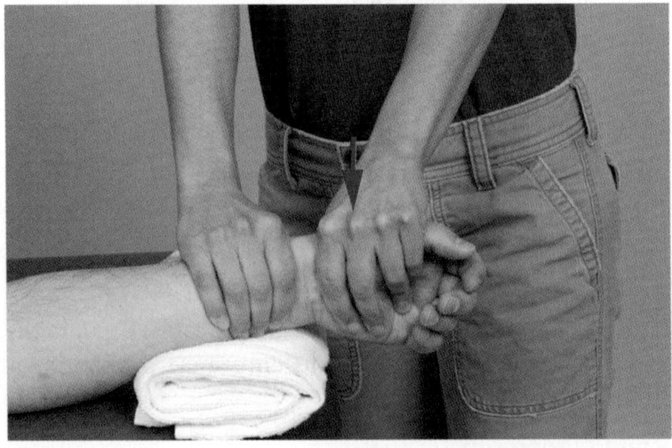

FIGURE 5.37 Wrist joint: general mobilization—ulnar glide.

- Progress by moving the wrist to the end of the available range and gliding in the defined direction.
- Specific carpal gliding techniques described in the next sections are used to increase mobility at isolated articulations.

Mobilizing Force

The force comes from the hand around the distal row of carpals.

Specific Carpal Mobilizations (Figs. 5.38 and 5.39)

Specific techniques to mobilize individual carpal bones may be necessary to gain full ROM of the wrist. Specific biomechanics of the radiocarpal and intercarpal joints are described in Chapter 19. To glide one carpal on another or on the radius, utilize the following guidelines.

Patient and Therapist Positions

- The patient sits.
- Stand and grasp the patient's hand so the elbow hangs unsupported.
- The weight of the arm provides slight distraction to the joints, so you then need only to apply the glides.

Hand Placement and Indications

Identify the specific articulation to be mobilized and place your index fingers on the volar surface of the bone to be stabilized. Place the overlapping thumbs on the dorsal surface of the bone to be manipulated. The rest of your fingers hold the patient's hand so it is relaxed.

To increase flexion. Place the stabilizing index fingers under the bone that is *convex* (on the volar surface) and the mobilizing thumbs overlapped on the dorsal surface of the bone that is *concave*.

- Thumbs on the dorsum of the concave radius, index fingers stabilize scaphoid.
- Thumbs on the dorsum of the concave radius, index fingers stabilize lunate (see Fig. 5.38).

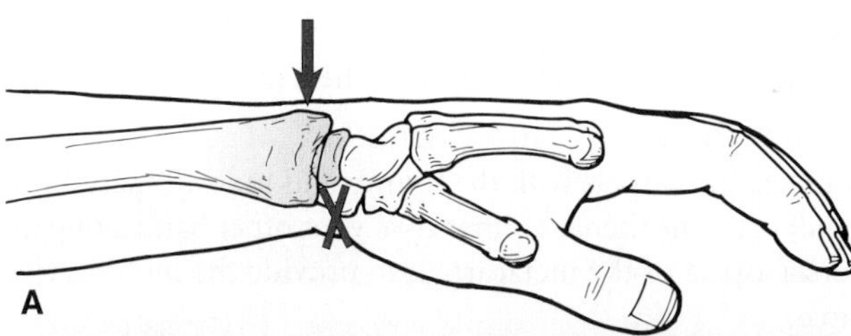

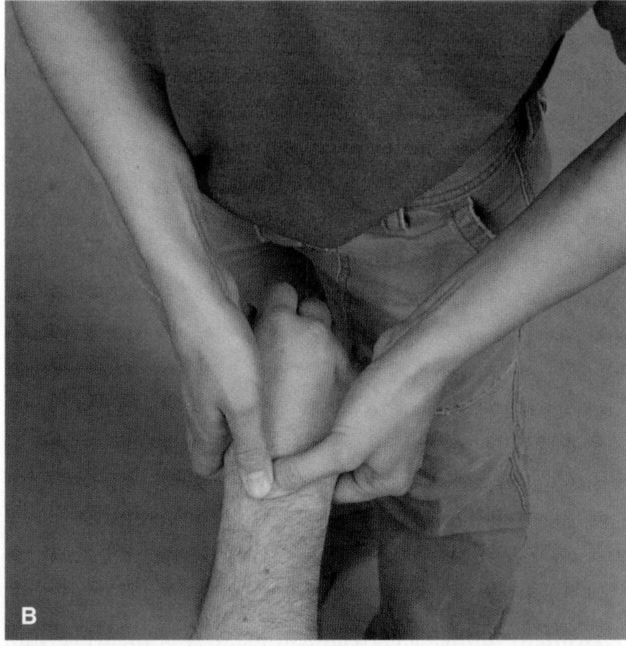

FIGURE 5.38 Specific carpal mobilizations: stabilization of the distal bone and volar glide of the proximal bone. Shown is stabilization of the scaphoid and lunate with the index fingers and a volar glide to the radius with the thumbs to increase wrist flexion: **(A)** Drawing of the side view, with the arrow depicting placement of thumbs on the radius and the "x" depicting placement of stabilizing index fingers; **(B)** Illustrates superior view of overlapping thumbs on the radius.

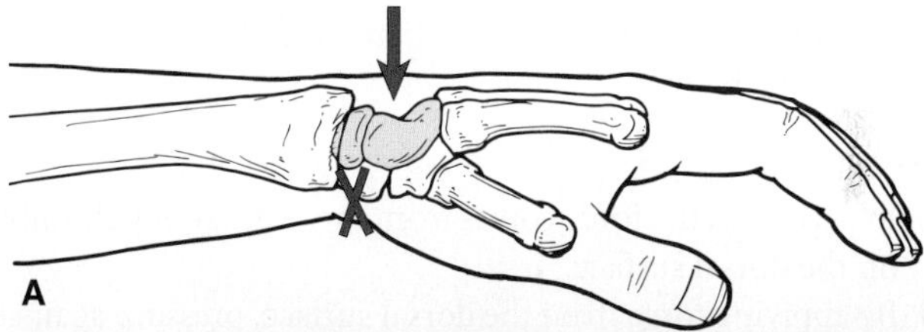

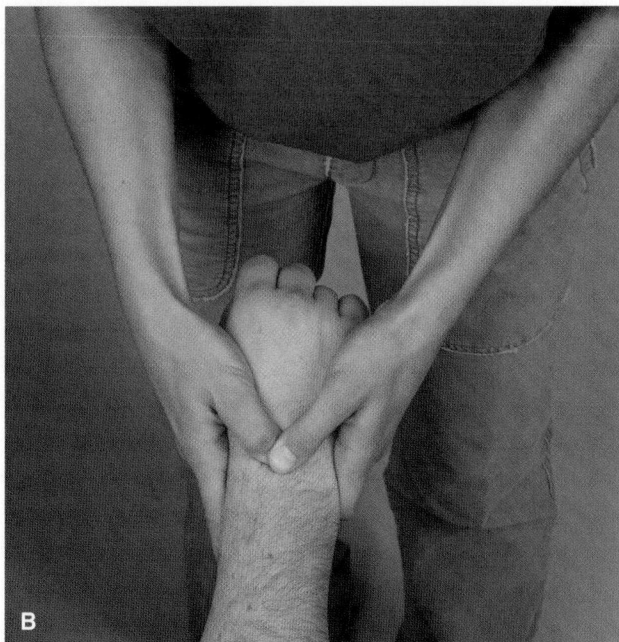

FIGURE 5.39 Specific carpal mobilizations: stabilization of the proximal bone and volar guide of the distal bone. Shown is stabilization of the lunate with the index fingers and volar glide to the capitate with the thumbs to increase extension: **(A)** Drawing of the side view, with the arrow depicting placement of thumbs on the capitate and the "x" depicting placement of stabilizing index fingers; **(B)** Illustrates superior view of overlapping thumbs on the capitate.

- Thumbs on dorsum of trapezium-trapezoid unit, index fingers stabilize scaphoid.
- Thumbs on dorsum of concave lunate, index fingers stabilize capitate.
- Thumbs on dorsum of concave triquetrum, index fingers stabilize hamate.

To increase extension. Place the stabilizing index fingers under the bone that is *concave* (on the volar surface). Overlap the thumbs and place on the dorsal surface of the bone that is *convex*. The thumbs provide the manipulating force.

- Thumbs on dorsum of convex scaphoid, index fingers stabilize radius.
- Thumbs on dorsum of convex lunate, index fingers stabilize radius.
- Thumbs on dorsum of convex scaphoid, index fingers stabilize trapezium-trapezoid unit.
- Thumbs on dorsum of convex capitate, index fingers stabilize lunate (see Fig. 5.39).
- Thumbs on dorsum of convex hamate, index fingers stabilize triquetrum.

Mobilizing Force

- In each case, the force comes from the overlapping thumbs on the dorsal surface.
- By applying force from the dorsal surface, pressure against the nerves, blood vessels, and tendons in the carpal tunnel and Guyon's canal is minimized, and a stronger mobilization force can be used without pain.
- An HVT technique can be used by providing a quick downward and upward flick of your wrists and hands while pressing against the respective carpals.

Ulnar-Meniscal-Triquetral Articulation

To unlock the articular disk, which may block motions of the wrist or forearm, apply a glide of the ulna volarly on a fixed triquetrum.

Carpometacarpal and Intermetacarpal Joints of Digits II to V

Opening and closing of the hand and maintenance of the arches in the hand requires general mobility between the carpals and metacarpals.

Carpometacarpal Distraction (Fig. 5.40)

Stabilization and Hand Placement

Stabilize the respective carpal with thumb and index finger of one hand. With your other hand, grasp around the proximal portion of a metacarpal.

Mobilizing Force

Apply long-axis traction to the metacarpal.

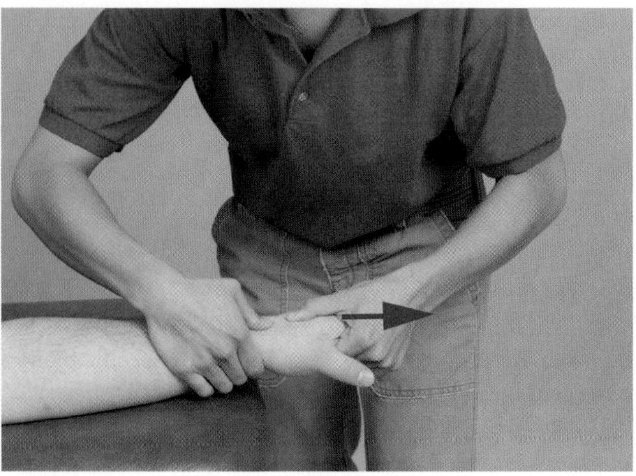

FIGURE 5.40 Carpometacarpal joint: distraction.

Carpometacarpal and Intermetacarpal: Volar Glide

Indication

To increase mobility of the arch of the hand.

Stabilization and Hand Placement

Stabilize the carpals with the thumb and index finger of one hand; place the thenar eminence of your other hand along the dorsal aspect of the metacarpals to provide the mobilization force.

Mobilizing Force

Glide the proximal portion of the metacarpal volar ward. See also the stretching technique for cupping and flattening the arch of the hand described in Chapter 4.

Carpometacarpal Joint of the Thumb

The CMC of the thumb is a saddle joint. The trapezium is concave, and the proximal metacarpal is convex for palmar abduction/adduction (metacarpal moving perpendicular away from and toward the palm of the hand). The trapezium is convex, and the proximal metacarpal is concave for radial abduction/adduction (metacarpal moving in the plane of the hand away and toward the radius; previously called flexion/extension).

Resting position. The resting position is midway between radial abduction/adduction and between palmar abduction/adduction.

Stabilization. Fixate the trapezium with the hand that is closer to the patient.

Treatment plane. The treatment plane is in the trapezium for abduction-adduction and in the proximal metacarpal for flexion-extension.

Carpometacarpal Distraction (Thumb)

Indications

Testing; initial treatment; pain control; general mobility.

Patient Position

The patient is positioned with forearm and hand resting on the treatment table.

Hand Placement

- Fixate the trapezium with the hand that is closer to the patient.
- Grasp the patient's metacarpal by wrapping your fingers around it (see Fig. 5.41 A).

Mobilizing Force

Apply long-axis traction to separate the joint surfaces.

Carpometacarpal Glides (Thumb) (Fig. 5.41)

Indications

- Ulnar glide to increase radial adduction.
- Radial glide to increase radial abduction.
- Dorsal glide to increase palmar abduction.
- Volar glide to increase palmar adduction.

Patient Position and Hand Placement

- Stabilize the trapezium by grasping it directly or by wrapping your fingers around the distal row of carpals.
- Place the thenar eminence of your other hand against the base of the patient's first metacarpal on the side opposite the desired glide. For example, as pictured in Figure 5.41 A, the surface of the thenar eminence is on the radial side of the metacarpal to cause an ulnar glide.

Mobilizing Force

Apply the force with your thenar eminence against the base of the metacarpal. Adjust your body position to line up the force as illustrated in Figure 5.41 A through D.

Metacarpophalangeal and Interphalangeal Joints of the Fingers

In all cases, the distal end of the proximal articulating surface is convex and the proximal end of the distal articulating surface is concave.

NOTE: Because all the articulating surfaces are the same for the digits, all techniques are applied in the same manner to each joint.

Resting position. The resting position is in light flexion for all joints.

Treatment plane. The treatment plane is in the distal articulating surface.

Stabilization. Rest the forearm and hand on the treatment table; fixate the proximal articulating surface with the fingers of one hand.

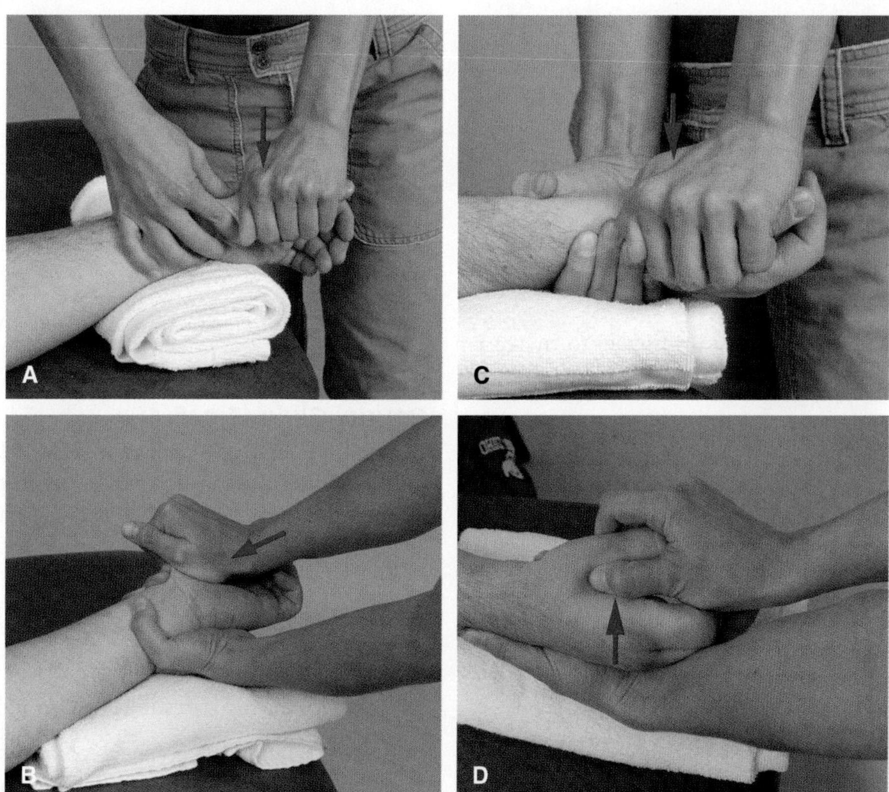

FIGURE 5.41 Carpometacarpal joint of the thumb. **(A)** Ulnar glide to increase radial adduction; **(B)** Radial glide to increase radial abduction; **(C)** Dorsal glide to increase palmar abduction; **(D)** Volar glide to increase palmar adduction. Note that the thumb of the therapist is placed in the web space between the index and thumb of the patient's hand to apply a volar glide.

Metacarpophalangeal and Interphalangeal Distraction (Fig. 5.42)

Indications

Testing; initial treatment; pain control; general mobility.

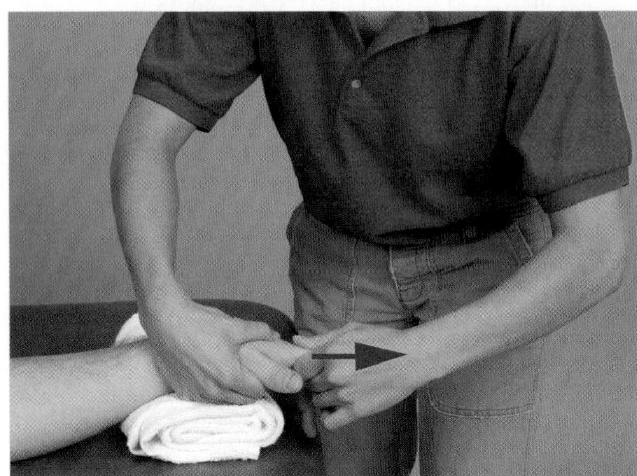

FIGURE 5.42 Metacarpophalangeal joint: distraction.

Hand Placement

Use your proximal hand to stabilize the proximal bone; wrap the fingers and thumb of your other hand around the distal bone close to the joint.

Mobilizing Force

Apply long-axis traction to separate the joint surface.

Metacarpophalangeal and Interphalangeal Glides and Progression

Indications

- Volar glide to increase flexion (Fig. 5.43).
- Dorsal glide to increase extension.
- Radial or ulnar glide (depending on finger) to increase abduction or adduction.

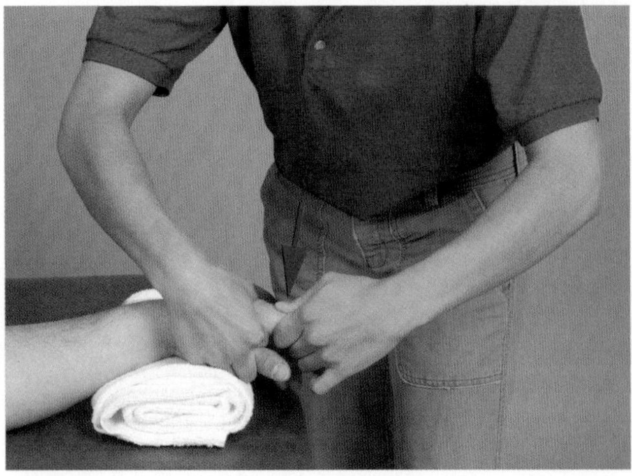

FIGURE 5.43 Metacarpophalangeal joint: volar glide.

Mobilizing Force

The glide force is applied by the thumb or thenar eminence against the proximal end of the bone to be moved. Progress by taking the joint to the end of its available range and applying slight distraction and the glide force. Rotation may be added prior to applying the gliding force.

Hip Joint

The concave acetabulum receives the convex femoral head (Fig. 5.44). Biomechanics of the hip joint are reviewed in Chapter 20.

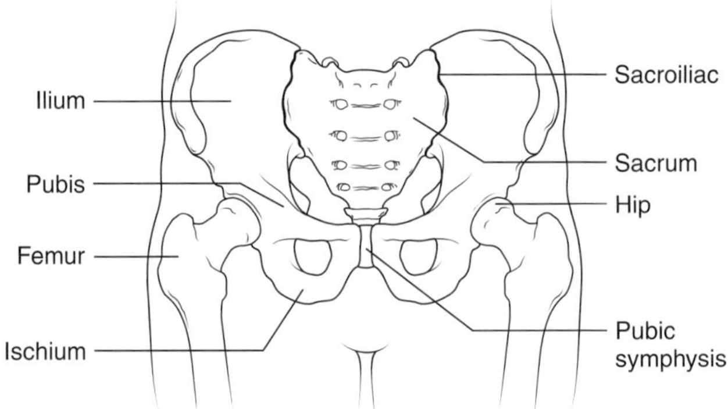

FIGURE 5.44 Bones and joints of the pelvis and hip.

Resting position. The resting position is hip flexion 30°, abduction 30°, and slight external rotation.

Stabilization. Fixate the pelvis to the treatment table with belts.

Treatment plane. The treatment is in the acetabulum.

Hip Distraction of the Weight-Bearing Surface, Caudal Glide (Fig. 5.45)

Because of the deep configuration of this joint, traction applied perpendicular to the treatment plane causes lateral glide of the superior, weight-bearing surface. To obtain separation of the weight-bearing surface, a caudal glide is used.

Indications

Testing; initial treatment; pain control; general mobility.

Patient Position

Supine, with the hip in resting position and the knee extended.

PRECAUTION: In the presence of knee dysfunction, this position should not be used; see alternate position following.

Therapist Position and Hand Placement

Stand at the end of the treatment table; place a belt around your trunk and then cross the belt over the patient's foot and around the ankle. Place your hands proximal to the malleoli,

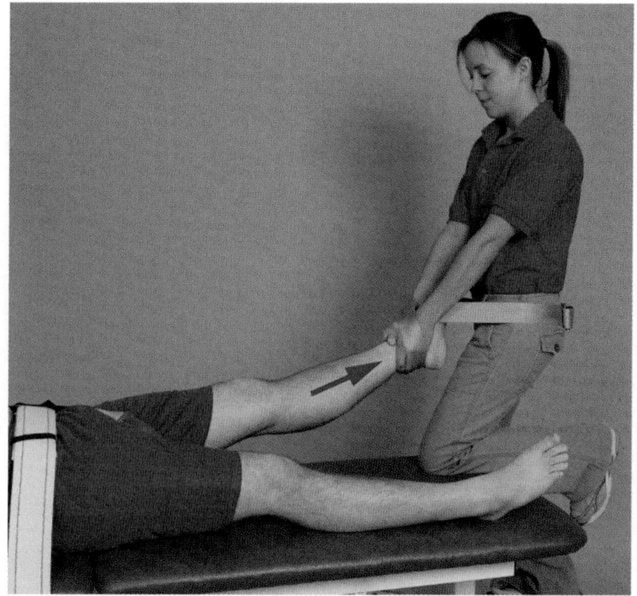

FIGURE 5.45 Hip joint: distraction of the weight-bearing surface.

under the belt. The belt allows you to use your body weight to apply the mobilizing force.

Mobilizing Force

Apply a long-axis traction by pulling on the leg as you lean backward.

Alternate Position and Technique for Hip Caudal Glide

- Patient supine with hip and knee flexed and foot resting on table.
- Wrap your hands around the epicondyles of the femur and distal thigh. Do not compress the patella.
- The force comes from your hands and is applied in a caudal direction as you lean backward.

Hip Posterior Glide (Fig. 5.46) VIDEO 5.9

Indications

To increase flexion; to increase internal rotation.

Patient Position

- Supine, with hips at the end of the table.
- The patient helps stabilize the pelvis and lumbar spine by flexing the opposite hip and holding the thigh against the chest with the hands.
- Initially, the hip to be mobilized is in resting position; progress to the end of the range.

Therapist Position and Hand Placement

- Stand on the medial side of the patient's thigh.
- Place a belt around your shoulder and under the patient's thigh to help hold the weight of the lower extremity.
- Place your distal hand under the belt and distal thigh. Place your proximal hand on the anterior surface of the proximal thigh.

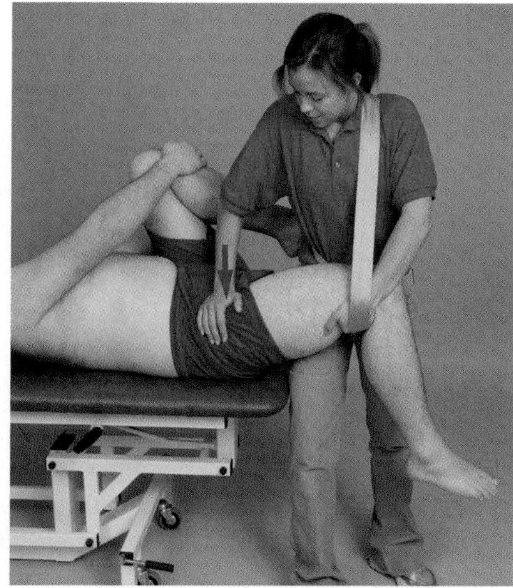

FIGURE 5.46 Hip joint: posterior glide.

Mobilizing Force

Keep your elbows extended and flex your knees; apply the force through your proximal hand in a posterior direction.

Hip Anterior Glide (Fig. 5.47) VIDEO 5.10

Indications

To increase extension; to increase external rotation.

Patient Position

Prone, with the trunk resting on the table and hips over the edge. The opposite foot is on the floor.

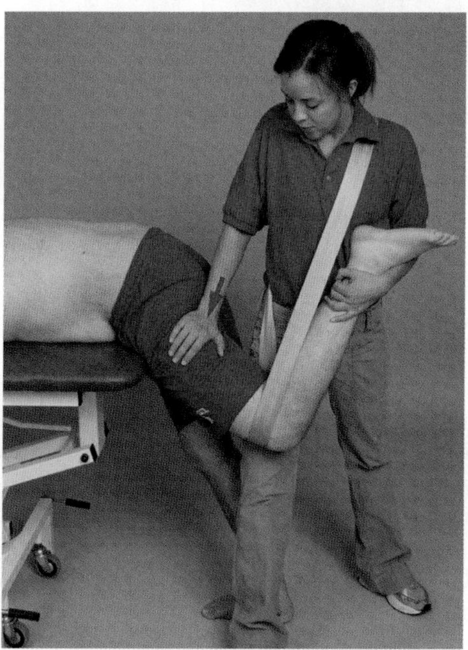

FIGURE 5.47 Hip joint: anterior glide. **(A)** Prone;

Therapist Position and Hand Placement

- Stand on the medial side of the patient's thigh.
- Place a belt around your shoulder and the patient's thigh to help support the weight of the leg.
- With your distal hand, hold the patient's leg.
- Place your proximal hand posteriorly on the proximal thigh just below the buttock.

Mobilizing Force

Keep your elbow extended and flex your knees; apply the force through your proximal hand in an anterior direction.

Alternate Position

- Position the patient side-lying with the thigh comfortably flexed and supported by pillows.
- Stand posterior to the patient and stabilize the pelvis across the anterior superior iliac spine with your cranial hand.
- Push against the posterior aspect of the greater trochanter in an anterior direction with your caudal hand.

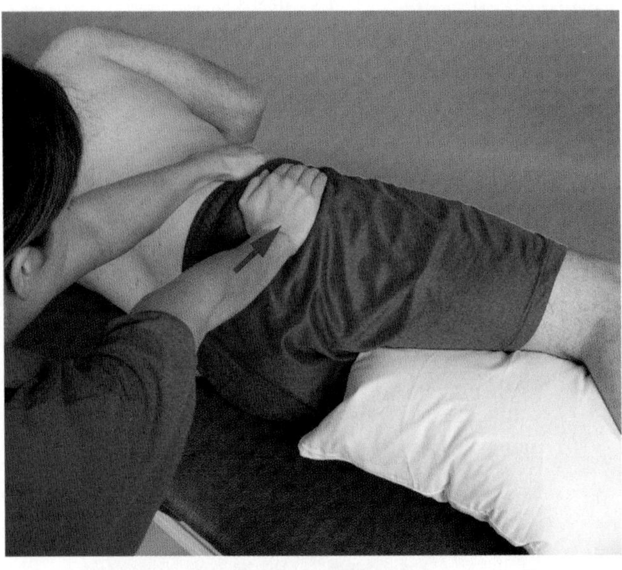

FIGURE 5.47—cont'd (B) Side-lying.

Knee Joint Complex

The knee joint consists of two articulating surfaces between the femoral condyles and tibial plateaus with a fibrocartilaginous disc between each articulation, as well as the articulation of the patella with the femoral groove (Fig. 5.48). As the knee flexes, medial rotation of the tibia occurs, and as it extends, lateral rotation of the tibia occurs. In addition, the patella must glide caudally against the femur during flexion and glide cranially during extension for normal knee mobility. These mechanics are described in Chapter 21.

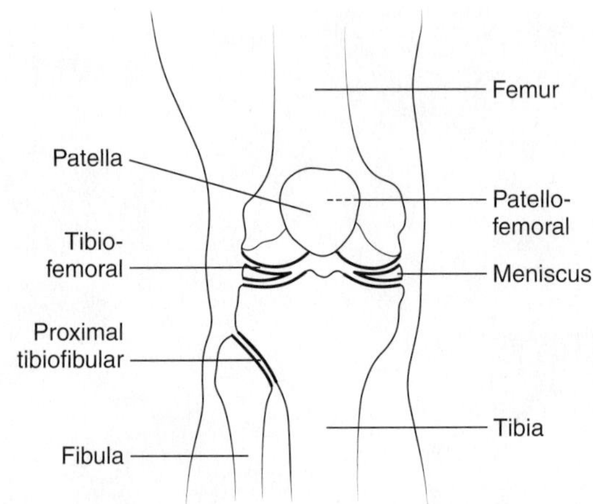

FIGURE 5.48 Bones and joints of the knee and leg.

Tibiofemoral Articulations

The concave tibial plateaus articulate on the convex femoral condyles. Biomechanics of the knee joint are described in Chapter 21.

Resting position. The resting position is 25° flexion.

Treatment plane. The treatment plane is along the surface of the tibial plateaus; therefore, it moves with the tibia as the knee angle changes.

Stabilization. In most cases, the femur is stabilized with a belt or by the table.

Tibiofemoral Distraction: Long-Axis Traction (Fig. 5.49)

Indications

Testing; initial treatment; pain control; general mobility.

Patient Position

- Sitting, supine, or prone, beginning with the knee in the resting position.
- Progress to positioning the knee at the limit of the range of flexion or extension.
- Rotation of the tibia may be added prior to applying the traction force. Use internal rotation at end-range flexion and external rotation at end-range extension.

Hand Placement

Grasp around the distal leg, proximal to the malleoli with both hands.

Mobilizing Force

Pull on the long axis of the tibia to separate the joint surfaces.

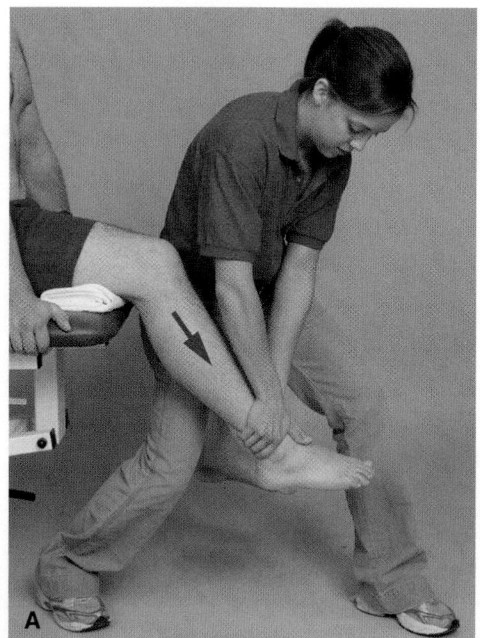

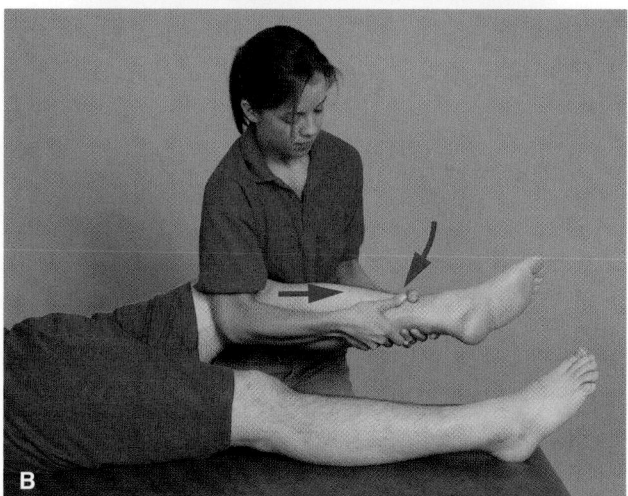

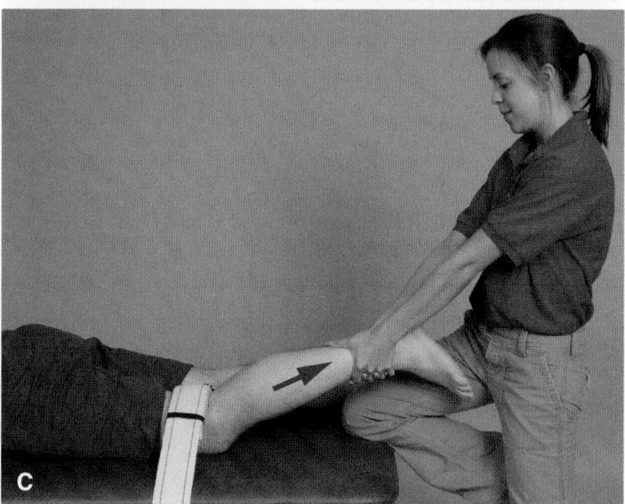

FIGURE 5.49 Tibiofemoral joint: distraction. **(A)** Sitting; **(B)** Supine; **(C)** Prone.

Tibiofemoral Posterior Glide (Fig. 5.50)

Indications

Testing; to increase flexion.

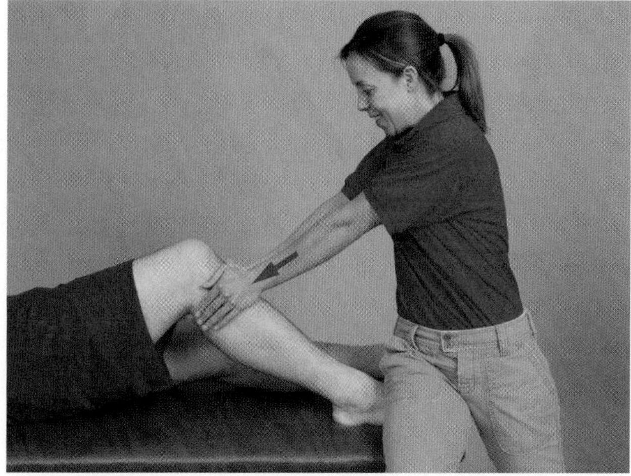

FIGURE 5.50 Tibiofemoral joint: posterior glide (drawer).

Patient Position

Supine, with the foot resting on the table. The position for the drawer test can be used to mobilize the tibia either anteriorly or posteriorly, although no grade I distraction can be applied with the glides in this position.

Therapist Position and Hand Placement

Sit on the table with your thigh fixating the patient's foot. With both hands, grasp around the tibia, fingers pointing posteriorly and thumbs anteriorly.

Mobilizing Force

Extend your elbows and lean your body weight forward; push the tibia posteriorly with your thumbs.

Tibiofemoral Posterior Glide: Alternate Positions and Progression (Fig. 5.51)

Patient Position

- Sitting, with the knee flexed over the edge of the treatment table, beginning in the resting position (Fig. 5.51). Progress to near 90° flexion with the tibia positioned in internal rotation.
- When the knee flexes past 90°, position the patient prone; place a small rolled towel proximal to the patella to minimize compression forces against the patella during the mobilization.

Therapist Position and Hand Placement

- When in the resting position, stand on the medial side of the patient's leg. Hold the distal leg with your distal hand and place the palm of your proximal hand along the anterior border of the tibial plateaus.

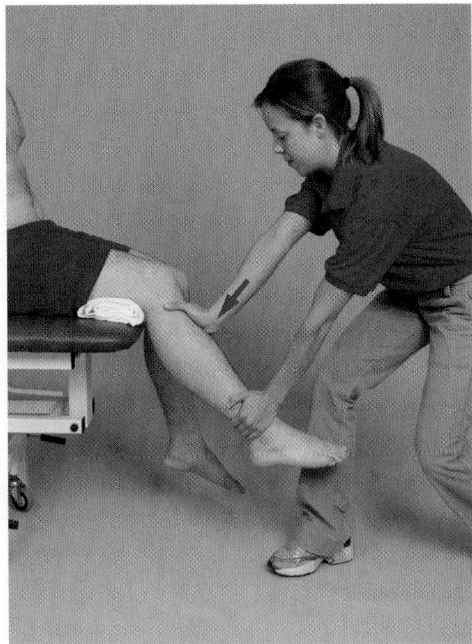

FIGURE 5.51 Tibiofemoral joint: posterior glide, sitting.

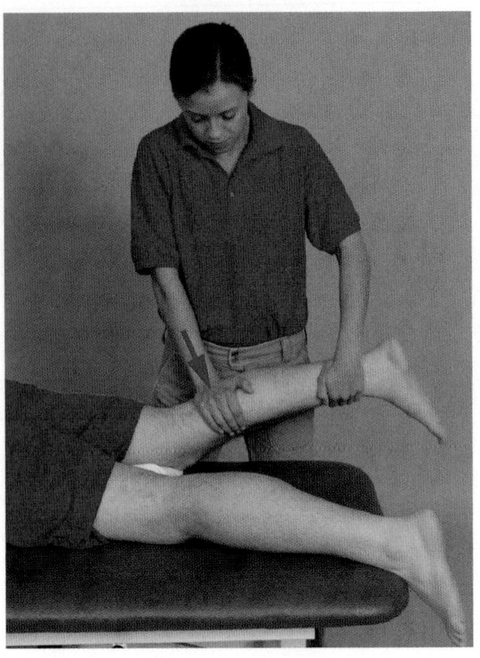

FIGURE 5.52 Tibiofemoral joint: anterior glide.

- When near 90°, sit on a low stool; stabilize the leg between your knees and place one hand on the anterior border of the tibial plateaus.
- When prone, stabilize the femur with one hand and place the other hand along the border of the tibial plateaus.

Mobilizing Force

- Extend your elbow and lean your body weight onto the tibia, gliding it posteriorly.
- When progressing with medial rotation of the tibia at the end of the range of flexion, the force is applied in a posterior direction against the medial side of the tibia.

Tibiofemoral Anterior Glide (Fig. 5.52)

VIDEO 5.11

Indication

To increase extension.

Patient Position

- Prone, beginning with the knee in resting position; progress to the end of the available range. Place a small pad under the distal femur to prevent patellar compression.
- The drawer test position can also be used. The mobilizing force comes from the fingers on the posterior tibia as you lean backward (see Fig. 5.50).

Hand Placement

Grasp the distal tibia with the hand that is closer to it and place the palm of the proximal hand on the posterior aspect of the proximal tibia.

Mobilizing Force

Apply force with the hand on the proximal tibia in an anterior direction. The force may be directed to the lateral or medial tibial plateau to isolate one side of the joint.

Alternate Position and Technique

- If the patient cannot be positioned prone, position him or her supine with a fixation pad under the tibia.
- The mobilizing force is placed against the femur in a posterior direction.

Patellofemoral Joint

The patella must have mobility to glide distally on the femur for normal knee flexion, and glide proximally for normal knee extension.

Patellofemoral Joint, Distal Glide (Fig. 5.53)

Patient Position

Supine, with knee extended; progress to positioning the knee at the end of the available range in flexion.

Hand Placement

Stand next to the patient's thigh, facing the patient's feet. Place the web space of the hand that is closer to the thigh around the superior border of the patella. Use the other hand for reinforcement.

Mobilizing Force

Glide the patella in a caudal direction, parallel to the femur.

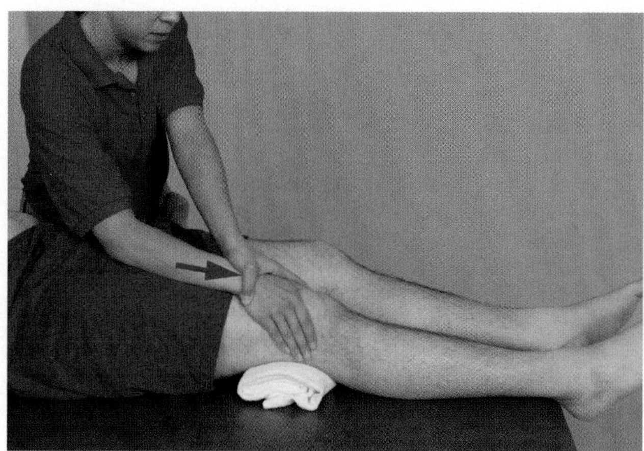

FIGURE 5.53 Patellofemoral joint: distal glide.

PRECAUTION: Do not compress the patella into the femoral condyles while performing this technique.

Patellofemoral Medial or Lateral Glide (Fig. 5.54)

Indication

To increase patellar mobility.

Patient Position

Supine with the knee extended. Side-lying may be used to apply a medial glide (see Fig. 21.10).

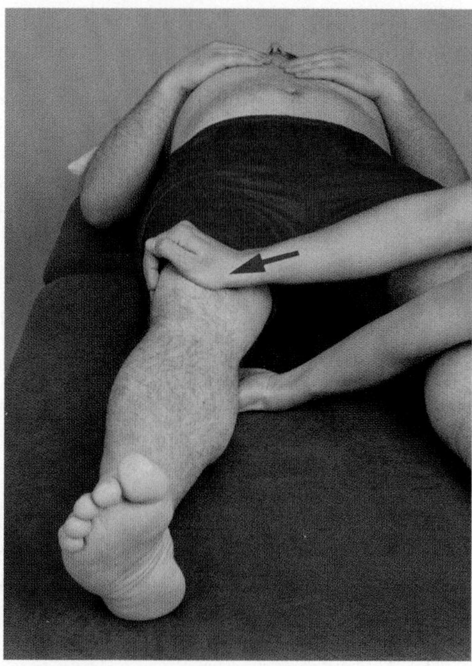

FIGURE 5.54 Patellofemoral joint: lateral glide.

Hand Placement

Place the heel of your hand along either the medial or lateral aspect of the patella. Stand on the opposite side of the table to position your hand along the medial border and on the same side of the table to position your hand along the lateral border. Place the other hand under the femur to stabilize it.

Mobilizing Force

Glide the patella in a medial or lateral direction, against the restriction.

Leg and Ankle Joints

The joints of the leg consist of the proximal and distal tibiofibular joints; accessory motions at these joints occur during all ankle and subtalar joint motions (see Fig. 5.48 and Fig. 5.57 A). The complex mechanics of the leg, foot, and ankle in weight-bearing and nonweight-bearing conditions are described in Chapter 22.

Tibiofibular Joints

Proximal Tibiofibular Articulation: Anterior (Ventral) Glide (Fig. 5.55)

Indications

To increase movement of the fibular head; to reposition a posteriorly subluxed head.

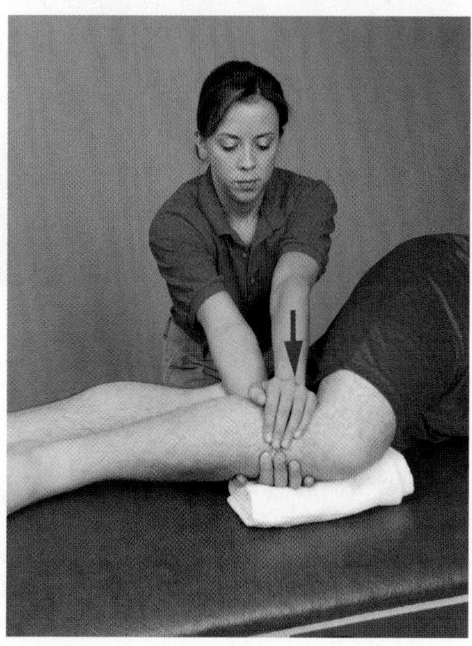

FIGURE 5.55 Proximal tibiofibular joint: anterior glide.

Patient Position

- Side-lying, with the trunk and hips rotated partially toward prone.
- The top leg is flexed forward so the knee and lower leg are resting on the table or supported on a pillow.

Therapist Position and Hand Placement

- Stand behind the patient, placing one of your hands under the tibia to stabilize it.
- Place the base of your other hand posterior to the head of the fibula, wrapping your fingers anteriorly.

Mobilizing Force

Apply the force through the heel of your hand against the posterior aspect of the fibular head, in an anterior-lateral direction.

Distal Tibiofibular Articulation: Anterior (Ventral) or Posterior (Dorsal) Glide (Fig. 5.56)

Indication

To increase mobility of the mortise when it is restricting ankle dorsiflexion.

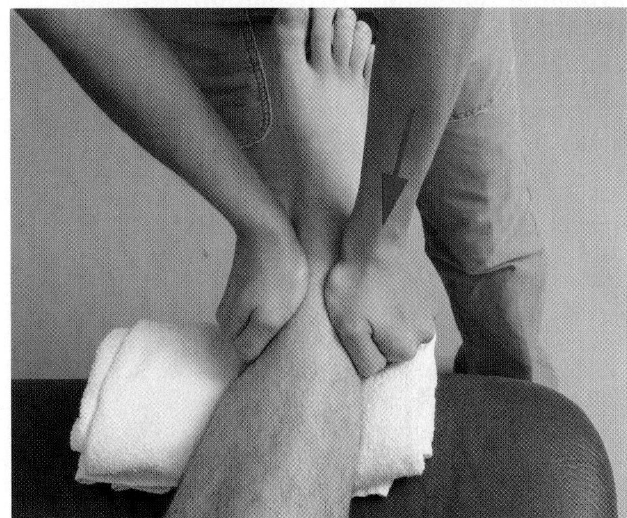

FIGURE 5.56 Distal tibiofibular articulation: posterior glide.

Patient Position

Supine or prone.

Hand Placement

Working from the end of the table, place the fingers of the more medial hand under the tibia and the thumb over the tibia to stabilize it. Place the base of your other hand over the lateral malleolus, with the fingers underneath.

Mobilizing Force

Press against the fibula in an anterior direction when prone and in a posterior direction when supine.

Talocrural Joint (Upper Ankle Joint) (Fig. 5.57)

The convex talus articulates with the concave mortise made up of the tibia and fibula.

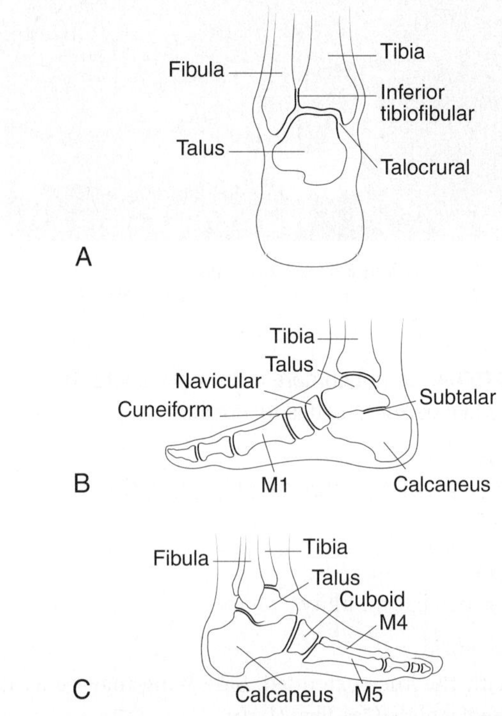

FIGURE 5.57 **(A)** Anterior view of the bones and joints of the lower leg and ankle; **(B)** Medial view; **(C)** Lateral view of the bones and joint relationships of the ankle and foot.

Resting position. The resting position is 10° plantarflexion.

Treatment plane. The treatment plane is in the mortise, in an anterior-posterior direction with respect to the leg.

Stabilization. The tibia is strapped or held against the table.

Talocrural Distraction (Fig. 5.58) VIDEO 5.12

Indications

Testing; initial treatment; pain control; general mobility.

Patient Position

Supine, with the lower extremity extended. Begin with the ankle in resting position. Progress to the end of the available range of dorsiflexion or plantarflexion.

Therapist Position and Hand Placement

- Stand at the end of the table; wrap the fingers of both hands over the dorsum of the patient's foot, just distal to the mortise.
- Place your thumbs on the plantar surface of the foot to hold it in resting position.

Mobilizing Force

Pull the foot along the long axis of the leg in a distal direction by leaning backward.

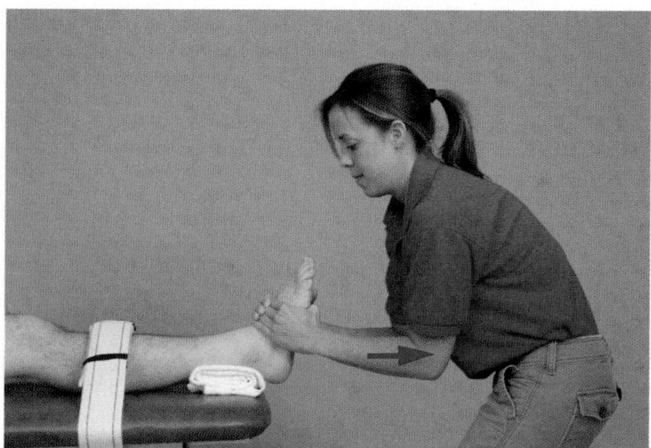

FIGURE 5.58 Talocrural joint: distraction.

Talocrural Dorsal (Posterior) Glide (Fig. 5.59)

Indication

To increase dorsiflexion.

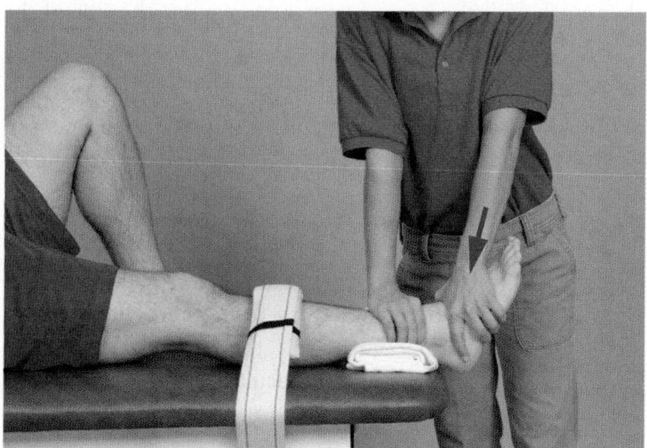

FIGURE 5.59 Talocrural joint: posterior glide.

Patient Position

Supine, with the leg supported on the table and the heel over the edge.

Therapist Position and Hand Placement

- Stand to the side of the patient.
- Stabilize the leg with your cranial hand or use a belt to secure the leg to the table.
- Place the palmar aspect of the web space of your other hand over the talus just distal to the mortise.
- Wrap your fingers and thumb around the foot to maintain the ankle in resting position. Grade I distraction force is applied in a caudal direction.

Mobilizing Force

Glide the talus posteriorly with respect to the tibia by pushing against the talus.

Talocrural Ventral (Anterior) Glide (Fig. 5.60)

Indication

To increase plantarflexion.

Patient Position

Prone, with the foot over the edge of the table.

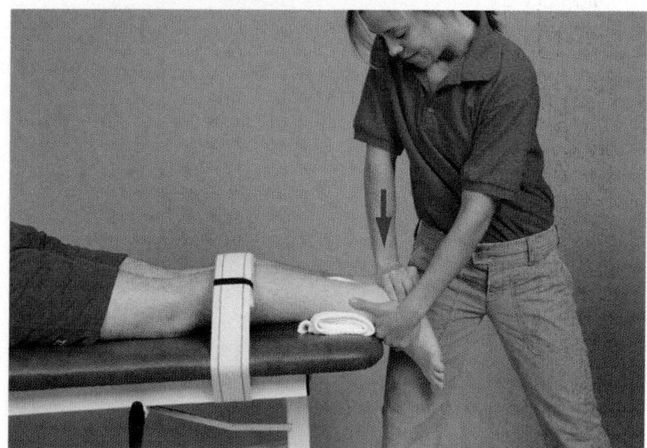

FIGURE 5.60 Talocrural joint: anterior glide.

Therapist Position and Hand Placement

- Working from the end of the table, place your lateral hand across the dorsum of the foot to apply a grade I distraction.
- Place the web space of your other hand just distal to the mortise on the posterior aspect of the talus and calcaneus.

Mobilizing Force

Push against the calcaneus in an anterior direction (with respect to the tibia); this glides the talus anteriorly.

Alternate Position

- Patient is supine. Stabilize the distal leg anterior to the mortise with your proximal hand.
- The distal hand cups under the calcaneus.
- When you pull against the calcaneus in an anterior direction, the talus glides anteriorly.

Subtalar Joint (Talocalcaneal), Posterior Compartment

The articulations between the calcaneus and talus are divided by the tarsal canal. The complex mechanics of these separate articulations are described in Chapter 22. Only mobilization of the posterior compartment is described here. The calcaneus is convex, articulating with a concave talus in the posterior compartment.

Resting position. The resting position is midway between inversion and eversion.

Treatment plane. The treatment plane is in the talus, parallel to the sole of the foot.

Stabilization. Dorsiflexion of the ankle stabilizes the talus. Alternatively, the talus is stabilized with one of your hands.

Subtalar Distraction (Fig. 5.61) VIDEO 5.13

Indications

Testing; initial treatment; pain control; general mobility for inversion/eversion.

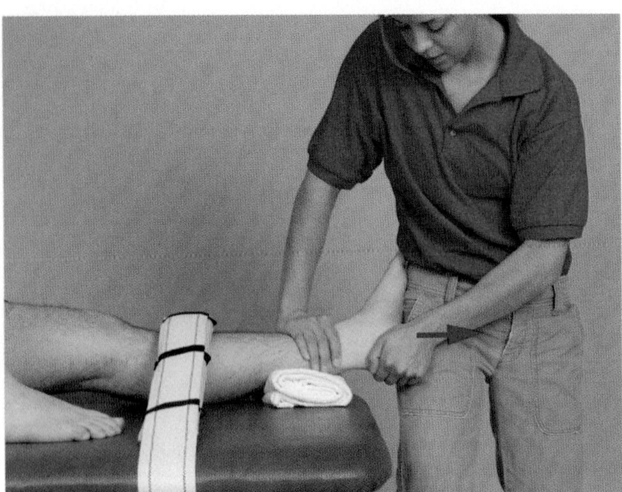

FIGURE 5.61 Subtalar (talocalcaneal) joint: distraction.

Patient and Therapist Positions and Hand Placement

- Supine, with the leg supported on the table and heel over the edge.
- Externally rotate the patient's hip so the talocrural joint can be stabilized in dorsiflexion with pressure from your thigh against the plantar surface of the patient's forefoot.
- The distal hand grasps around the calcaneus from the posterior aspect of the foot. The other hand fixes the talus and malleoli against the table.

Mobilizing Force

Pull the calcaneus distally with respect to the long axis of the leg.

Subtalar Medial Glide or Lateral Glide (Fig. 5.62)

Indications

Medial glide to increase eversion; lateral glide to increase inversion.

Patient Position

Side-lying or prone, with the leg supported on the table.

Therapist Position and Hand Placement

- Align your shoulder and arm parallel to the bottom of the foot.
- Stabilize the talus with your proximal hand.
- Place the base of the distal hand on the side of the calcaneus medially to cause a lateral glide and laterally to cause a medial glide.
- Wrap the fingers around the plantar surface.

Mobilizing Force

Apply a grade I distraction force in a caudal direction and then push with the base of your hand against the side of the calcaneus parallel to the plantar surface of the heel.

Alternate Position

Same as the position for distraction, moving the calcaneus in the medial or a lateral direction with the base of the hand.

Intertarsal and Tarsometatarsal Joints

When moving in a dorsal-plantar direction with respect to the foot, all of the articulating surfaces are concave and convex in the same direction. For example, the proximal articulating surface is convex, and the distal articulating surface is concave.

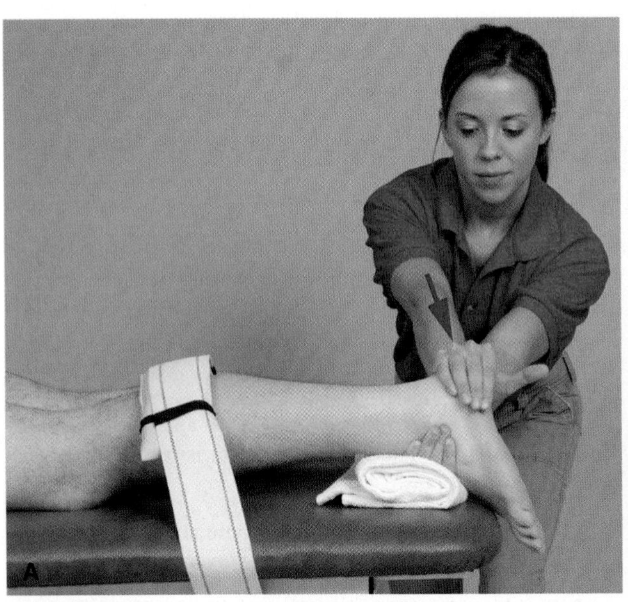

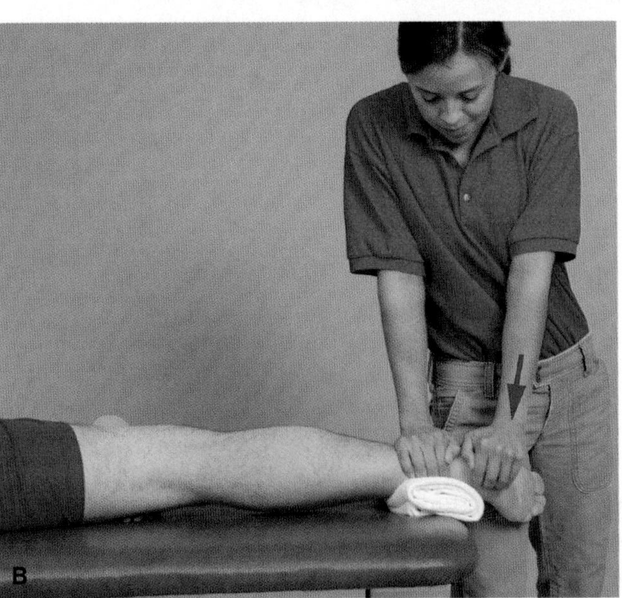

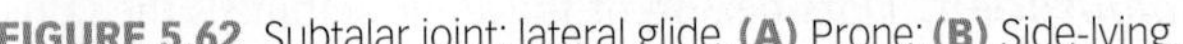

FIGURE 5.62 Subtalar joint: lateral glide. (A) Prone; (B) Side-lying.

The technique for mobilizing each joint is the same. The hand placement is adjusted to stabilize the proximal bone partner so the distal bone partner can be moved.

Intertarsal and Tarsometatarsal Plantar Glide (Fig. 5.63)

Indication

To increase plantarflexion accessory motions (necessary for supination).

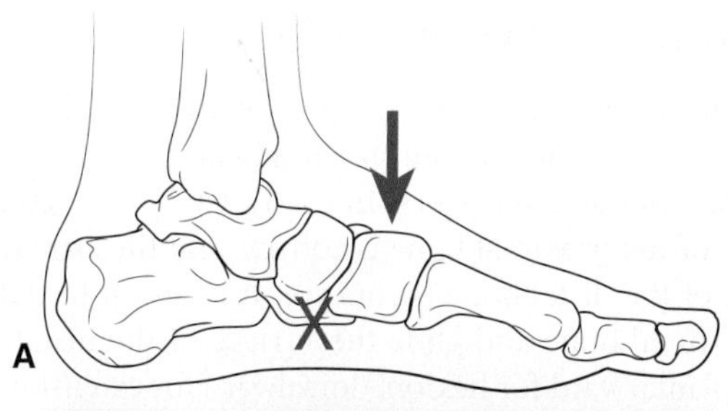

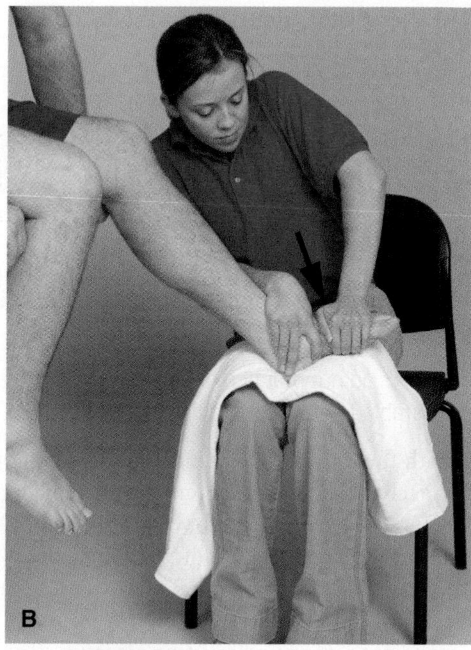

FIGURE 5.63 Plantar glide of a distal tarsal bone on a stabilized proximal bone. Shown is stabilization of the navicular with the therapist's index finger and plantar glide of the cuneiform to increase the arch of the foot: **(A)** Drawing of the medial side of the foot, with the "x" depicting placement of the stabilizing index finger and the arrow depicting the downward force from the thenar eminence of the therapist's hand; **(B)** Illustrates application of the technique.

Patient Position

Supine, with hip and knee flexed, or sitting, with knee flexed over the edge of the table and heel resting on your lap.

Stabilization and Hand Placement

- Fixate the more proximal bone with your index finger on the plantar surface of the bone.
- To mobilize the tarsal joints along the medial aspect of the foot, position yourself on the lateral side of the foot. Place the proximal hand on the dorsum of the foot with the fingers pointing medially, so the index finger can be wrapped around and placed under the bone to be stabilized.
- Place your thenar eminence of the distal hand over the dorsal surface of the bone to be moved and wrap the fingers around the plantar surface.
- To mobilize the lateral tarsal joints, position yourself on the medial side of the foot, point your fingers laterally, and position your hands around the bones as just described.

Mobilizing Force

Push the distal bone in a plantar direction from the dorsum of the foot.

Intertarsal and Tarsometatarsal Dorsal Glide (Fig. 5.64)

Indication

To increase the dorsal gliding accessory motion (necessary for pronation).

Patient Position

Prone, with knee flexed.

Stabilization and Hand Placement

- Fixate the more proximal bone.
- To mobilize the lateral tarsal joints (e.g., cuboid on calcaneus), position yourself on the medial side of the patient's leg and wrap your fingers around the lateral side of the foot (as in Fig. 5.64).
- To mobilize the medial bones (e.g., navicular on talus), position yourself on the lateral side of the patient's leg and wrap your fingers around the medial aspect of the foot.

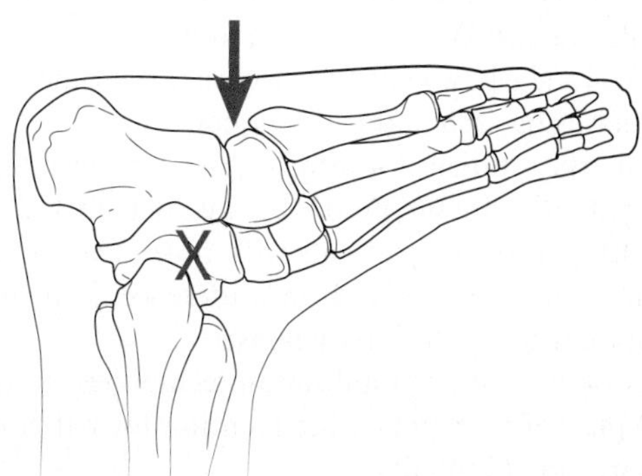

FIGURE 5.64 Dorsal gliding of a distal tarsal on a proximal tarsal. Shown is stabilization of the calcaneus with compression through the talus, and dorsal glide of the cuboid: **(A)** Drawing of the lateral side of the foot, with "x" depicting the stabilization and the arrow depicting the downward (dorsal) force from the base of the therapist's hand;

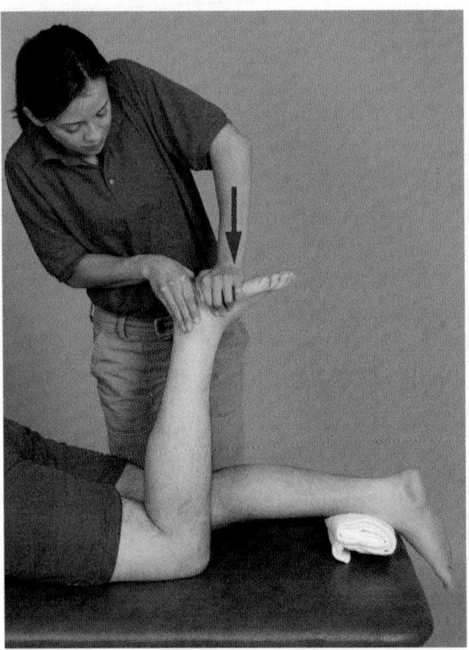

FIGURE 5.64—cont'd (B) Illustrates application of the technique.

- Place your second metacarpophalangeal joint against the bone to be moved.

Mobilizing Force

Push from the plantar surface in a dorsal direction.

Alternate Technique

Same position and hand placements as for plantar glides, except the distal bone is stabilized and the proximal bone is forced in a plantar direction. This is a relative motion of the distal bone moving in a dorsal direction.

Intermetatarsal, Metatarsophalangeal, and Interphalangeal Joints

The intermetatarsal, metatarsophalangeal, and interphalangeal joints of the toes are stabilized and mobilized in the same manner as the fingers. In each case, the articulating surface of the proximal bone is convex, and the articulating surface of the distal bone is concave. It is easiest to stabilize the proximal bone and glide the surface of the distal bone either plantarward for flexion, dorsalward for extension, and medially or laterally for adduction and abduction.

Independent Learning Activities

Critical Thinking and Discussion

1. An individual is immobilized in a cast for 4 to 6 weeks following a fracture. In general, what structures lose their elasticity, and what restrictions do you feel when testing range of motion, joint play, and flexibility?
2. Describe the normal arthrokinematic relationships for the extremity joints and define the location of the treatment plane for each joint.
3. Using the information from Activity 1, define a specific fracture, such as a Colle's fracture of the distal forearm. Identify what techniques are necessary to gain joint mobility and ROM in the related joints such as the wrist, forearm, and elbow joints, connective tissues, and muscles. Practice using each of the techniques.
4. Explain the rationale for using passive joint techniques to treat patients with limitations because of pain and muscle guarding or to treat patients with restricted capsular or ligamentous tissue. What is the difference in the way the techniques are applied in each case?
5. Describe how joint mobilization techniques fit into the total plan of therapeutic intervention for patients with impaired joint mobility.
6. Explain the difference between passive joint mobilization techniques and MWM techniques.

Laboratory Practice

With a partner, practice mobilizing each joint in the upper and lower extremities.

PRECAUTION: Do not practice on an individual with a hypermobile or unstable joint.

1. Begin with the joint in its resting position and apply distraction techniques at each intensity (sustained grades I, II, and III) to develop a feel for "very gentle," "taking up the slack," and "stretch." Do not apply a vigorous stretch to someone with a normal joint. Be sure to use appropriate stabilization.
2. With the joint in its resting position, practice all appropriate glides for that joint. Be sure to use a grade I distraction with each gliding technique. Vary the techniques between sustained and oscillation.
3. Practice progressing each technique by taking the joint to a point that you determine to be the "end of the range" and:
   - Apply a distraction technique with the extremity in that position.
   - Apply the appropriate glide at that range (be sure to apply a grade I distraction with each glide).
   - Add rotation (e.g., external rotation for shoulder abduction) and then apply the appropriate glide.

REFERENCES

1. Akeson, WH, et al: Effects of immobilization on joints. *Clin Orthop* 219:28–37, 1987.
2. American Physical Therapy Association: *Guide to Physical Therapist Practice 3.0*, Available at http://guidetoptpractice.apta.org/. Accessed March 26, 2015.
3. American Physical Therapy Association Manipulation Task Force Manipulation Education Committee: *Manipulation Education Manual for Physical Therapist Professional Degree Programs.* Alexandria, VA: American Physical Therapy Association, 2004.
4. Backstrom, KM: Mobilization with movement as an adjunct intervention in a patient with complicated De Quervain's tenosynovitis: a case report. *J Orthop Sports Phys Ther* 32(3):86–97, 2002.
5. Boissonnault, W, Bryan, JM, and Fox, KJ: Joint manipulation curricula in physical therapist professional degree programs. *J Orthop Sports Phys Ther* 34(4):171–181, 2004.
6. Cyriax, J: *Textbook of Orthopaedic Medicine, Vol I: The Diagnosis of Soft Tissue Lesions,* ed. 8. London: Bailliere & Tindall, 1982.
7. DiFabio, RP: Efficacy of manual therapy. *Phys Ther* 72:853–864, 1992.
8. Donatelli, R, and Owens-Burkhart, H: Effects of immobilization on the extensibility of periarticular connective tissue. *J Orthop Sports Phys Ther* 3: 67–72, 1981.
9. Enneking, WF, and Horowitz, M: The intra-articular effects of immobilization on the human knee. *J Bone Joint Surg Am* 54:973–985, 1972.
10. Exelby, L: Mobilizations with movement: a personal view. *Physiotherapy* 81(12):724–729, 1995.
11. Harryman, DT, et al: Translation of the humeral head on the glenoid with passive glenohumeral motion. *J Bone Joint Surg Am* 72: 1334–1343, 1990.
12. Hengeveld, E, and Banks, K: *Maitland's Peripheral Manipulation,* ed. 4. Oxford: Butterworth Heinemann, 2005.
13. Houglum, PA and Bertoti, DB: *Brunnstrom's Clinical Kinesiology*, ed. 6. Philadelphia: FA Davis, 2012.
14. Howell, SM, et al: Normal and abnormal mechanics of the glenohumeral joint in the horizontal plane. *J Bone Joint Surg Am* 70:227–232, 1988.
15. Hsu, AT, et al: Changes in abduction and rotation range of motion in response to simulated dorsal and ventral translational mobilization of the glenohumeral joint. *Phys Ther* 82(6):544–556, 2002.
16. Itoi, E, et al: Contribution of axial arm rotation to the humeral head translation. *Am J Sports Med* 22:499–503, 1994.
17. Kaltenborn, FM, Evjenth, O, Kaltenborn, TB, et al: *Manual Mobilization of the Joints: Joint Examination and Basic Treatment, Vol I: The Extremities,* ed. 8. Oslo, Norway: Norli, 2014.
18. Kavanagh, J: Is there a positional fault at the inferior tibiofibular joint in patients with acute or chronic ankle sprains compared to normals? *Manual Ther* 4(1):19–24, 1999.
19. Levangie, PK, and Norkin, CC: *Joint Structure and Function: A Comprehensive Analysis,* ed. 5. Philadelphia: FA Davis, 2011.
20. Magee, DJ: *Orthopedic Physical Assessment,* ed. 6. St. Louis: Saunders, 2014.
21. McDavitt, S: Practice affairs corner—a revision for the Guide to Physical Therapist Practice: mobilization or manipulation? Yes! That is my final answer! *Orthop Phys Ther Pract* 12(4):15, 2000.
22. Meadows, J: *Orthopedic Differential Diagnosis in Physical Therapy: A Case Study Approach.* Toronto: McGraw-Hill, 1999.
23. Miller, J: The Mulligan concept—the next step in the evolution of manual therapy. *Orthop Division Rev* 2:9–13, 1999.
24. Mintken, PE, et al: A model for standardizing manipulation terminology in physical therapy practice. *J Orthop Sports Phys Ther* 38:A1, 2008.
25. Mintken, PE, et al: Moving past sleight of hand. *J Orthop Sports Phys Ther* 40(8):536–537, 2010.
26. Mulligan, BR: *Manual Therapy: "NAGS," "SNAGS," "MWMS", etc.,* ed. 6. Wellington: Plane View Press, 2010.
27. Mulligan, BR: Mobilizations with movement (MWMs). *J Manual Manipulative Ther* 1(4):154–156, 1993.
28. Neumann, DA: The convex-concave rules of arthrokinematics: flawed or perhaps just misinterpreted? *J Ortho Sports Phys Ther* 42(2):53–55, 2012.
29. O'Brien, T, and Vincenzino, B: A study of the effects of Mulligan's mobilization with movement of lateral ankle pain using a case study design. *Manual Ther* 3(2):78–84, 1998.
30. Paris, SV: Mobilization of the spine. *Phys Ther* 59(8):988–995, 1979.
31. Paungmali, A, et al: Hypoalgesic and sympathoexcitatory effects of mobilization with movement for lateral epicondylalgia. *Phys Ther* 83(4): 374–383, 2003.
32. Vincenzino, B, and Wright, A: Effects of a novel manipulative physiotherapy technique on tennis elbow: a single case study. *Manual Ther* 1(1):30–35, 1995.
33. Warwick, R, and Williams, S (eds): Arthrology. In *Gray's Anatomy,* British ed. 35. Philadelphia: WB Saunders, 1973.
34. Wegener, L, Kisner, C, and Nichols, D: Static and dynamic balance responses in persons with bilateral knee osteoarthritis. *J Orthop Sports Phys Ther* 25(1): 13–18, 1997.
35. Wilson, E. Mobilizations with movement and adverse neutral tension: an exploration of possible links. *Manipulative Phys Ther* 27(1):40, 1995.
36. Wyke, B: The neurology of joints. *Ann R Coll Surg* 41:25–50, 1967.
37. Wyke, B: Articular neurology: a review. *Physiotherapy* 58(3):94–99, 1972.
38. Wyke, B: *Neurological aspects of pain for the physical therapy clinician.* Columbus, OH: Physical Therapy Forum, 1982.

CHAPTER 6

Resistance Exercise for Impaired Muscle Performance

LYNN COLBY, PT, MS ■ JOHN BORSTAD, PT, PHD

Muscle performance is the capacity of a muscle to do work (force × distance).[9] Despite the simplicity of the definition, muscle performance is a complex component of functional movement and is influenced by all of the body systems. Factors that affect muscle performance include the morphological qualities of muscle; neurological, biochemical, and biomechanical influences; and metabolic, cardiovascular, respiratory, cognitive, and emotional function. A healthy and fully functioning muscular system is critical for not only meeting the physical demands imposed on the body, but for allowing individuals to be mobile, recreate, work, and pursue meaningful experiences.

The key elements of muscle performance are *strength*, *power*, and *endurance*.[9] If any one or more of these elements is impaired, activity limitations and participation restriction or increased risk of dysfunction may ensue. Factors such as injury, disease, immobilization, disuse, and inactivity may impair muscle performance, leading to weakness and muscle atrophy. When deficits in muscle performance are present, resistance exercises are an appropriate therapeutic intervention to select.

Resistance exercise is an activity in which dynamic or static muscle contraction is resisted by an outside force applied manually or mechanically.[95,236] Resistance exercise, also referred to as *resistance training*,[6,7,161] is an essential element of rehabilitation programs for persons with impaired function. In addition, resistance exercise is an integral component of conditioning programs for those who wish to promote or maintain health and physical well-being, enhance performance of motor skills, and reduce the risk of injury and disease.[6,7,231]

A comprehensive examination and evaluation of the patient or client are the foundations on which a therapist determines whether a program of resistance exercise is warranted and likely to be effective. Many factors will influence this determination and decisions about how the exercises are designed, implemented, and progressed. Factors such as the underlying pathology; the extent and severity of muscle performance impairments; the presence of other deficits; the stage of tissue healing after injury or surgery; and the patient's or client's age, overall level of fitness, and ability to cooperate and learn must all be considered. Once a resistance exercise program is developed and prescribed, the therapist should initially implement the program directly or teach and supervise the exercises to ensure a smooth transition to an independent, home-based program.

This chapter provides a foundation of information on resistance exercise, identifies the determinants of resistance training programs, summarizes the principles and guidelines for application of manual and mechanical resistance exercise, and explores a variety of regimens for resistance training. It also addresses the available scientific evidence on the relationship between improvements in muscle performance and enhanced functional abilities. The specific techniques described and illustrated in this chapter focus on manual resistance exercise for the extremities, primarily used during the early phase of rehabilitation. Additional exercises performed independently by the patient or client using resistance equipment are described and illustrated in Chapters 16 through 23.

Muscle Performance and Resistance Exercise: Definitions and Guiding Principles

The three elements of muscle performance[9]—strength, power, and endurance—can all be enhanced by resistance exercise. To what extent each of these elements is altered by exercise depends on how the principles of resistance training are applied and how factors such as the intensity, frequency, and duration of exercise are manipulated. Because the physical demands of work, recreation, and everyday living usually involve all three aspects of muscle performance, most resistance training programs should address the optimum proportion of strength, power, and muscular endurance that will meet an individual's needs and goals. In addition to positively impacting muscle performance, resistance training can produce many other benefits.[6,7,8] These potential benefits are listed in Box 6.1. After a brief description of the three elements of muscle performance, the guiding principles of exercise prescription and training are discussed in this section.

Strength, Power, and Endurance

Strength

Muscle strength is a broad term that refers to the extent that the contractile elements of muscle produce force. Implicit in this definition is the idea that with adequate strength, the contractile tissue generates enough force to meet the physical and functional demands placed on the system.[175,184,202] In practice, muscle strength is the greatest measurable force that is exerted by a muscle or muscle group to overcome resistance during a *single* maximum effort.[9] *Functional strength* relates to the ability of the neuromuscular system to produce the appropriate amount of force, during functional activities in a smooth and coordinated manner.[41,211] Insufficient muscular strength can contribute to major functional losses of even the most basic activities of daily living.

Strength training. The development of muscle strength is an integral component of most rehabilitation or conditioning programs for individuals of all ages and abilities.[6,8,83,162,213] *Strength training (strengthening exercise)* is the systematic practice of using muscle force to raise, lower, or control heavy external loads for a relatively low number of repetitions or over a short period of time.[7,32,95] The most common adaptation to strength training is an increase in the maximum force-producing capacity of muscle, primarily the result of neural adaptations and increased muscle fiber size.[7,8,184]

BOX 6.1 Benefits of Resistance Exercise

- Enhanced muscle performance through restoration, improvement or maintenance of muscle strength, power, and endurance
- Increased strength of connective tissues: tendons, ligaments, and intramuscular connective tissue
- Increased bone mineral density and/or less bone demineralization
- Decreased joint stress during physical activity
- Reduced risk of soft tissue injury during physical activity
- Improved capacity for repair and healing of damaged soft tissues and for tissue remodeling
- Improved balance
- Enhanced physical performance during daily living, occupational, and recreational activities
- Positive changes in body composition: ↑ lean muscle mass or ↓ body fat
- Enhanced feeling of physical well-being
- Positive perception of disability and quality of life

Power

Muscle power is related to the strength and speed of movement and is defined as the work (force × distance) produced by a muscle per unit of time (force × distance/time).[175,184,202] In other words, power is the *rate* of performing work. The rate at which a muscle produces a force and the relationship between force and velocity are key factors that affect muscle power.[32,202] Because work can be produced over a very brief or a very long period of time, power can represent a single burst of high-intensity activity (such as lifting a heavy piece of luggage onto an overhead rack or performing a high jump) or repeated bursts of less intense activity (such as climbing a flight of stairs). The terms *anaerobic power* and *aerobic power*, respectively, are sometimes used to differentiate these two aspects of power.[184]

Power training. Many motor tasks are somewhat ballistic movements that involve both strength and speed. Therefore, re-establishing muscle power may be an important priority in a rehabilitation program. Muscle strength is a necessary foundation for developing muscle power. Power can be gained by either increasing the work a muscle must perform during a specified period of time or reducing the amount of time required to produce the work. The greater the intensity (force and/or distance) of the exercise and the shorter the time period taken to generate force, the greater is the muscle power. For power training regimens, such as *plyometric training* or *stretch-shortening drills*, the time of movement is the variable that is most often manipulated[277] (see Chapter 23).

Endurance

Endurance is a broad term that refers to the ability to perform repetitive or sustained activities over a prolonged period of time. *Cardiopulmonary endurance* (*total body endurance*) is associated with repetitive, dynamic motor activities, such as walking, cycling, swimming, or upper extremity ergometry, which involve use of the large muscles of the body.[6,7] This aspect of endurance is explored in Chapter 7.

Muscle endurance (sometimes referred to as *local endurance*) is the ability of a muscle to contract repeatedly against an external load, generate and sustain tension, and resist fatigue over an extended period of time.[6,7,224] The term *aerobic power* sometimes is used interchangeably with muscle endurance. Maintenance of balance and proper alignment of the body segments requires endurance of the postural muscles. In fact, almost all daily living tasks require some degree of both muscle and cardiopulmonary endurance.

Although muscle strength and endurance are associated, they do not always correlate well with each other. Just because a muscle group is strong, it is still possible for muscular endurance to be impaired. For example, a worker may have the strength to lift a 10-lb object several times, but they may not have sufficient endurance of the upper extremity or trunk muscles to lift 10-lb objects several hundred times during the course of a day's work without excessive fatigue or potential injury.

Endurance training. *Endurance training* (*endurance exercise*) is the systematic practice of using muscle force to raise, lower, or control a light external load for many repetitions over an extended period of time.[7,8,184,202,248] The key parameters of endurance training are low-intensity muscle contractions, a high number of repetitions, and a prolonged time period. Unlike strength training, muscles adapt to endurance training by increases in their oxidative and metabolic capacities, which allows better delivery and use of oxygen. For many patients with impaired muscle performance, endurance training has a more positive impact on improving function than strength training. In addition, using lower levels of resistance in an exercise program minimizes potentially harmful joint reaction forces, produces less irritation to soft tissues, and is more comfortable for the patient than heavy resistance exercise.

Overload Principle

Description

The overload principle is a foundational element that guides the use of resistance exercise in improving muscle performance. The overload principle states that if muscle performance is to improve, a resistance load that exceeds the metabolic capacity of the muscle must be applied—that is, the muscle must be challenged to perform at a level greater than that to which it is accustomed.[7,8,123,162,184,198] If the external demands remain constant after the muscle has adapted to exercise, the level of muscle performance can be maintained but not increased.

Application of the Overload Principle

The overload principle focuses on progressively loading muscle by manipulating factors such as the intensity or volume of exercise. The *intensity* of resistance exercise refers to how much external resistance is imposed on the muscle, whereas the *volume* of exercise includes variables such as repetitions, sets, or frequency, any combination of which can be adjusted to progressively increase the demands on the muscle.

- In a strength training program, the amount of external resistance applied to the muscle is incrementally and progressively increased.
- For endurance training, emphasis is placed on increasing the *time* a muscle contraction is sustained or the *number of repetitions* performed rather than the amount of external resistance.

PRECAUTION: To ensure safety, the application of the overload principle must always be done in the context of the underlying pathology, age of the patient, stage of tissue healing, the patient response, and the overall abilities and goals of the patient. The muscle and related body systems must be given time to *adapt* to the demands of increased intensity or volume before subsequent increases.

Specific Adaptation to Imposed Demands (SAID) Principle

The SAID principle[7,184] is another foundational element applied to a muscle performance program. This principle refers to the concept that to improve a specific muscle performance element, the resistance program should be matched to that elements constructs. For example, to increase muscle power the exercise program should consist of interventions that increase work demands while decreasing the time that work is accomplished. This principle applies to all body systems and is an extension of Wolff's law (i.e., body systems adapt over time to the stresses placed on them). The SAID principle guides therapists to determine the exercise parameters that will create specific training effects to best meet the patient's functional needs and goals.

Specificity of Training

Specificity of training, also referred to as specificity of exercise, is a widely accepted concept suggesting that the adaptive effects of training, such as improvement of strength, power, and endurance, are highly specific to the training method employed.[7,176] Whenever possible, exercises incorporated in a program should mimic the anticipated function. For example, if the desired functional activity requires greater muscular endurance than strength, lower intensity exercises performed over a longer time should be emphasized.

Specificity of training must also incorporate the optimal mode (type) and velocity of exercise,[24,74,197,217] the patient or joint position,[155,156,270] and the movement patterns used during exercise. For example, if the desired functional outcome is the ability to ascend and descend stairs, exercise should be performed eccentrically and concentrically in a weight-bearing pattern and progressed to the desired speed. Regardless of the simplicity or complexity of the motor task performed, task-specific practice always must be emphasized. It has been suggested that the basis of specificity of training is related to morphological and metabolic changes in muscle as well as neural adaptations to the training stimulus associated with motor learning.[210]

Transfer of Training

In contrast to the SAID principle, carryover of training effects from one variation of exercise or task to another also has been reported. This phenomenon is called transfer of training, overflow, or a cross-training effect. Transfer of training has been reported to occur on a very limited basis with respect to the velocity of training[137,260] and the type or mode of exercise.[74] Furthermore, it has been suggested that a cross-training effect can occur from an exercised limb to a nonexercised, contralateral limb in a resistance training program.[268,269]

A muscle strengthening program has been shown to have a transfer effect by moderately improving muscular endurance.[17] In contrast, endurance training has little to no cross-training effect on muscle strength.[7,16,95] In fact, when endurance training and strength training are combined, there appears to be a detrimental effect on the ability to improve strength.[102,146] Strength training at one speed of exercise has been shown to provide some improvement in strength at higher or lower speeds of exercise.[137,260] However, the overflow effects are substantially less than the effects that result from using specificity of training principles.

Despite the evidence that a small degree of transfer of training occurs from a resistance exercise program, most studies support the importance of designing an exercise program that most closely replicates the desired functional activities.

Reversibility Principle

Adaptive changes in the body's systems in response to a resistance exercise program are transient unless training-induced improvements are regularly used for functional activities or unless an individual participates in a maintenance program of resistance exercises.[6,7,45,82,184]

Detraining, reflected by reductions in muscle performance, begins a week or two after the cessation of resistance exercises and continues until training effects are lost.[7,82,161,199] For this reason, it is imperative that gains in strength and endurance are incorporated into daily activities as early as possible in a rehabilitation program. It is also advisable for patients to participate in a maintenance program of resistance exercises as an integral component of a lifelong fitness program.

Skeletal Muscle Function and Adaptation to Resistance Exercise

Knowing the factors that influence the force-producing capacity of normal muscle during an active contraction is fundamental to understanding how the neuromuscular system adapts to resistance training. This knowledge, in turn, provides a basis on which a therapist is able to make sound clinical decisions when designing resistance exercise programs for patients with weakness and functional limitations or to reduce injury risk in healthy individuals.

Factors That Influence Tension Generation in Normal Skeletal Muscle

NOTE: For a brief review of the structure of skeletal muscle, refer to Chapter 4 of this textbook. For in-depth information on muscle structure and function, numerous resources are available.[175,176,184,202]

Morphological, biomechanical, neurological, metabolic, and biochemical factors all affect the tension-generating capacity of *normal* skeletal muscle. Each of these factors contributes to the *magnitude, duration,* and *speed* of force production and the muscles' susceptibility to fatigue. Properties of muscle and key neural factors and their impact on tension generation during an active muscle contraction are summarized in Table 6.1.[7,175,176,184,202]

Additional factors—such as the energy stores available to muscle; the influence of fatigue and recovery from exercise; and a person's age, gender, and psychological/cognitive status—affect a muscle's ability to develop and sustain tension. A therapist must recognize that these factors affect both a patient's performance during exercise and the potential outcomes of the exercise program.

Energy Stores and Blood Supply

Muscle needs adequate sources of energy to contract, generate tension, and resist fatigue. Muscle also requires an adequate blood supply to provide the tissue with oxygen and nutrients and to transport waste products from muscle to other organs. The degree of vascularization is related to the predominant fiber type that constitutes the tissue, which directly affects the fatigue profile of the muscle. The three main energy systems (the ATP-PC system, the anaerobic/glycolytic/lactic acid system, and the aerobic system) are reviewed in Chapter 7.

Fatigue

Fatigue is a complex phenomenon that affects muscle performance and must be considered in a resistance exercise

TABLE 6.1 Determinants and Correlates That Affect Tension Generation of Skeletal Muscle

Factor	Influence
Cross-section and size of the muscle (includes muscle fiber number and size)	The larger the muscle diameter, the greater its tension-producing capacity
Muscle architecture—fiber arrangement and fiber length (also relates to cross-sectional diameter of the muscle)	Short fibers with pennate and multipennate design are typical in high force-producing muscles (ex. quadriceps, gastrocnemius, deltoid, biceps brachii)
	Long fibers with parallel design are typical in muscles with fast shortening rates but lower force production (ex. sartorius, lumbricals)
Fiber-type distribution of muscle—type I (tonic, slow-twitch) and type IIA & IIB (phasic, fast-twitch)	High percentage of type I fibers favors low force production, slow rate of maximum force development, resistance to fatigue
	High percentage of type IIA and IIB fibers favors rapid high force production and rapid fatigue
Length-tension relationship of muscle at time of contraction	Muscle produces greatest tension when it is near or at the physiological resting length at the time of contraction
Moment arm between muscle force vector and axis of joint rotation	Greater tension is produced with longer moment arm
Recruitment of motor units	The greater the number and synchronization of motor units firing, the greater the force production
Rate of motor unit firing	The higher the firing frequency, the greater the tension
Type of muscle contraction	Force output from greatest to least—eccentric, isometric, concentric muscle contraction
Speed of muscle contraction (force-velocity relationship)	Concentric contraction: $\uparrow$ speed $\rightarrow$ $\downarrow$ tension. Eccentric contraction: $\uparrow$ speed $\rightarrow$ $\uparrow$ tension

program. There are several types of fatigue, each with its own definition.

Muscle (local) fatigue. Most relevant to resistance exercise is the phenomenon of skeletal muscle fatigue. Muscle fatigue—the diminished response of muscle to a repeated stimulus—is reflected in a progressive decrement in the amplitude of motor unit potentials.[176,184] This occurs during exercise when a muscle repeatedly contracts statically or dynamically against an imposed load.

Muscle fatigue is an acute physiological response to exercise that is normal and reversible. It is characterized by a gradual decline in the force-producing capacity of the neuromuscular system. This is a temporary decline that leads to a decrease in muscle strength.[23,52,176,241]

The diminished contractile response of the muscle is caused by a complex combination of factors, which include disturbances in the contractile mechanism of the muscle itself (associated with a decrease in energy stores, insufficient oxygen, reduced sensitivity and availability of intracellular calcium, and a build-up of H^+) and perhaps reduced excitability at the neuromuscular junction or inhibitory (protective) influences from the central nervous system (CNS).[176,184,202]

The fiber-type distribution of a muscle, which can be divided into two broad categories (type I and type II), affects its resistance to fatigue.[176,184,202] Type II (phasic, fast-twitch) muscle fibers are further divided into two additional classifications (types IIA and IIB) based on contractile and fatigue characteristics. In general, type II fibers generate a great amount of tension within a short period of time, with type IIB being geared toward anaerobic metabolic activity and having a tendency to fatigue more quickly than type IIA fibers. Type I (tonic, slow-twitch) muscle fibers generate a low level of muscle tension but can sustain the contraction for a long time. These fibers are geared toward aerobic metabolism, as are type IIA fibers. However, type I fibers are more resistant to fatigue than type IIA. Table 6.2 compares the characteristics of muscle fiber types.[7,175,176,202]

Because muscles are composed of varying proportions of tonic and phasic fibers, their function becomes specialized. For example, a heavy distribution of type I (slow twitch, tonic) fibers is found in postural muscles, allowing them to sustain a low level of tension for extended periods of time. Functionally, postural muscles are suited to hold the body erect against gravity or stabilize against repetitive loads. On the other end of the fatigue spectrum, muscles with a large distribution of type IIB (fast twitch, phasic) fibers can produce high increases of tension over a relatively short time. These muscles function to move heavy loads but are susceptible to fatigue.

Clinical signs of muscular fatigue during exercise are summarized in Box 6.2.[184,202] When these signs and symptoms develop during resistance exercise, the therapist should decrease the load on the exercising muscle or stop the exercise and shift to another muscle group to allow time for the fatigued muscle to rest and recover. When resistance exercises are part of a home program, the therapist should teach the patient to recognize signs of fatigue and the strategies to minimize its effects.

Cardiopulmonary (general) fatigue. This type of fatigue is the systemic diminished response of an individual to a stimulus as the result of prolonged physical activity such as walking, jogging, cycling, or repetitive work. Cardiopulmonary fatigue is related to the body's ability to use oxygen efficiently. Cardiopulmonary fatigue associated with endurance training is probably caused by a combination of the following factors:[23,108]

- Decreased blood sugar (glucose) levels
- Decreased glycogen stores in muscle and liver
- Depletion of potassium, especially in the elderly patient

Threshold for fatigue. The threshold for fatigue is the level of exercise that cannot be sustained indefinitely.[23] A patient's threshold for fatigue could be noted as the length of time a contraction is maintained or the number of repetitions of an exercise that initially can be performed. This sets a baseline

TABLE 6.2 Muscle Fiber Types and Resistance to Fatigue

Characteristics	Type I	Type IIA	Type IIB
Resistance to fatigue	High	Intermediate	Low
Capillary density	High	High	Low
Energy system	Aerobic	Aerobic	Anaerobic
Diameter	Small	Intermediate	Large
Twitch rate	Slow	Fast	Fast
Maximum muscle-shortening velocity	Slow	Fast	Fast

BOX 6.2 Signs and Symptoms of Muscle Fatigue

- An uncomfortable sensation in the muscle, with pain and cramping possible
- Shaking or trembling of the contracting muscle
- An unintentional slowing of contraction velocity with successive repetitions of an exercise
- Active movements are jerky or inconsistent
- Inability to complete the movement pattern through the full range of available motion during dynamic exercise against the same level of resistance
- Use of substitute motions—that is, incorrect movement patterns—to complete the activity
- Inability to continue low-intensity physical activity
- Decline in peak torque during isokinetic testing

from which adaptive changes in physical performance can be measured.

Factors that influence fatigue. A patient's health status, diet, or lifestyle (sedentary or active) all influence fatigue thresholds. In patients with neuromuscular, cardiopulmonary, inflammatory, cancer-related, or psychological disorders, the onset of fatigue is often irregular.[3,52,90] For instance, it may occur abruptly, more rapidly, or at predictable intervals.

It is advisable for a therapist to become familiar with the patterns of fatigue associated with different diseases and medications. In multiple sclerosis, for example, the patient usually awakens rested and functions well during the early morning. By mid-afternoon, however, the patient reaches a fatigue threshold and becomes notably weak. By early evening, fatigue often diminishes and strength returns. Patients with cardiac, peripheral vascular, and pulmonary diseases, as well as patients with cancer undergoing chemotherapy or radiation therapy, all have deficits that compromise the oxygen transport system. Therefore, these patients fatigue more readily and require a longer recovery period from exercise.[3,90]

Environmental factors, such as outside or room temperature, air quality, and altitude, also influence how quickly the onset of fatigue occurs and how much time is required for recovery from exercise.[163,184]

Recovery From Exercise

Adequate time for recovery from fatiguing exercise must be built into every resistance exercise program. This applies to both intrasession and intersession recovery. After vigorous exercise, the body must be given time to restore itself to a state that existed prior to the exercise. Recovery from acute exercise, in which the force-producing capacity of muscle returns to 90% to 95% of the pre-exercise capacity, usually takes 3 to 4 minutes, with the greatest proportion of recovery occurring in the first minute.[49,233]

Oxygen and energy stores replenish quickly in muscle recovery. Lactic acid is removed from skeletal muscle and blood within approximately 1 hour after exercise, and glycogen stores are replaced over several days.

FOCUS ON EVIDENCE

Studies over several decades have demonstrated that if light exercise is performed during the recovery period (*active recovery*), recovery from exercise occurs more rapidly than with total rest (*passive recovery*).[28,49,107,233] Faster recovery with light exercise is probably the result of neural as well as circulatory influences.[49,233]

CLINICAL TIP

Muscle performance (strength, power, or endurance) only improves over time if a patient is allowed adequate time to recover from fatigue after each exercise session.[28,107] With insufficient rest intervals during a resistance exercise program, a patient's performance plateaus or deteriorates. Evidence of overtraining or overwork weakness may become apparent (see additional discussion in the Overtraining and Overwork section of this chapter). It has also been shown that fatigued muscles are more susceptible to acute strains.[182]

Age

Muscle performance capability will change across the life span. Whether the goal of a resistance training program is to remediate impairments and activity limitations or enhance fitness and performance, an understanding of "typical" changes in muscle performance and response to exercise during each phase of life is necessary to prescribe effective, safe resistance exercises for individuals of all ages. Key aspects of how muscle performance changes throughout life are discussed in this section and summarized in Box 6.3.

Early Childhood and Preadolescence

In absolute terms, muscle strength increases *linearly* with chronological age in both boys and girls from birth through puberty.[183,249,274] Muscle endurance also increases linearly during the childhood years.[274] Much of these linear increases are attributed to the development of muscle mass. Muscle fiber number is essentially determined prior to or shortly after birth,[231] although there is speculation that fiber number may continue to increase into early childhood.[274] The rate of fiber growth (increase in cross-sectional area) is relatively consistent from birth to puberty. Change in fiber type distribution is relatively complete by the age of 1, shifting from a predominance of type II fibers to a more balanced distribution of type I and type II fibers.[274]

Throughout childhood, boys have slightly greater absolute and relative muscle mass (kilograms of muscle per kilogram of body weight) than girls, with boys approximately 10% stronger than girls from early childhood to puberty.[183] This difference may be associated with differences in relative muscle mass, although social expectations may also contribute to the observed difference in muscle strength.

It is well established that an appropriately designed resistance exercise program can improve muscle strength in children above and beyond gains attributable to typical growth and development. These training-induced strength gains in prepubescent children occur primarily as the result of neuromuscular adaptation—that is, without a significant increase in muscle mass.[22,84] Reviews of the literature[83,85] have cited many studies that support these findings. However, there is concern that children who participate in resistance training may be at risk for injuries, such as an epiphyseal or avulsion fractures, because the musculoskeletal system is immature.[22,27,95,253]

The American Academy of Pediatrics,[5] the American College of Sports Medicine (ACSM),[6] and the Centers for Disease Control and Prevention (CDC)[36] support youth participation in resistance training programs if they are designed appropriately, initiated at a reasonable age, and carefully supervised (Fig. 6.1). With this in mind, two important questions need

BOX 6.3 Summary of Age-Related Changes in Muscle and Muscle Performance Through the Life Span

Infancy, Early Childhood, and Preadolescence

- At birth, muscle accounts for about 25% of body weight.
- Total number of muscle fibers is established prior to birth or early in infancy.
- Postnatal changes in distribution of type I and type II fibers in muscle are relatively complete by the end of the first year of life.
- Muscle fiber size and muscle mass increase linearly from infancy to puberty.
- Muscle strength and muscle endurance increase linearly with chronological age in boys and girls throughout childhood until puberty.
- Muscle mass (absolute and relative) and muscle strength is approximately 10% greater in boys than girls from early childhood to puberty.
- Training-induced strength gains occur equally in both sexes during childhood *without* evidence of hypertrophy until puberty.

Adolescence

- Rapid acceleration in muscle fiber size and muscle mass, especially in boys. During puberty, muscle mass increases more than 30% per year.
- Rapid increase in muscle strength in both sexes.
- Marked difference in strength levels develops between boys and girls.
- In boys, muscle mass and body height and weight peak before muscle strength peaks; in girls, strength peaks before body weight peaks.
- Relative strength gains through resistance training are comparable between the sexes, with significantly greater muscle hypertrophy in boys.

Young and Middle Adulthood

- Muscle mass peaks in women between 16 and 20 years of age; muscle mass in men peaks between 18 and 25 years of age.
- Muscle mass constitutes approximately 40% of total body weight during early adulthood, with men having slightly more muscle mass than women.
- Muscle continues to develop into the second decade, especially in men.
- Muscle strength and endurance reach a peak during the second decade, earlier for women than men.
- Decreases in muscle mass begin to occur as early as 25 years of age.
- Starting in the third decade, strength declines between 8% and 10% per decade through the fifth or sixth decade.
- Strength and muscle endurance decline less rapidly in physically active adults.
- Improvements in strength and endurance are possible with only modest increases in physical activity.

Late Adulthood

- Muscle strength declines at a rate of 15% to 20% per decade during the sixth and seventh decades and declines at a rate of 30% per decade thereafter.
- By the eighth decade, skeletal muscle mass will have decreased by 50% compared to peak muscle mass.
- Muscle fiber size (cross-sectional area), type I and type II fiber quantity, and the number of alpha motoneurons all decrease.
- Preferential atrophy of type II muscle fibers occurs.
- Muscle contraction speed and peak power production both decrease.
- Endurance and maximum oxygen uptake gradually but progressively decrease.
- The force-producing capacity of muscle is reduced.
- Performance of functional skills begins to decline during the sixth decade.
- Significant deterioration in functional abilities by the eighth decade is associated with a decline in muscular endurance.
- With a resistance training program, significant improvements in muscle strength, power, and endurance is possible during late adulthood.

to be addressed: At what point during childhood is a resistance training program appropriate? And, what constitutes a safe training program?

There is general consensus that during the toddler, preschool, and even the early elementary school years, free play and organized but age-appropriate physical activities are effective methods to promote fitness and improve muscle performance rather than structured resistance training programs. The emphasis throughout most or all of the first decade of life should be on recreation and learning motor skills.[264]

There is lack of agreement, however, on when and under what circumstances resistance training is an appropriate form of exercise for prepubescent children. Although age-appropriate physical activity on a regular basis has been recommended for children for some time,[5,6,36] it has become popular for older (preadolescent) boys and girls to participate in sport-specific training programs (including resistance exercises) before, during, and even after the season. In theory, these training programs enhance athletic performance and reduce the risk of sport-related injury. Rehabilitation programs for prepubescent children who sustain injuries during everyday activities also may include resistance exercises. Consequently, an understanding of the effects of exercise in this age group must be the basis for establishing a safe program with realistic goals.

FOCUS ON EVIDENCE

In the preadolescent age group, many studies have shown that improvements in strength and muscular endurance are similar to training-induced gains in young adults.[27,85,86,141] As with adults, when training stops strength levels gradually return to a pretraining level.[82] This suggests that some

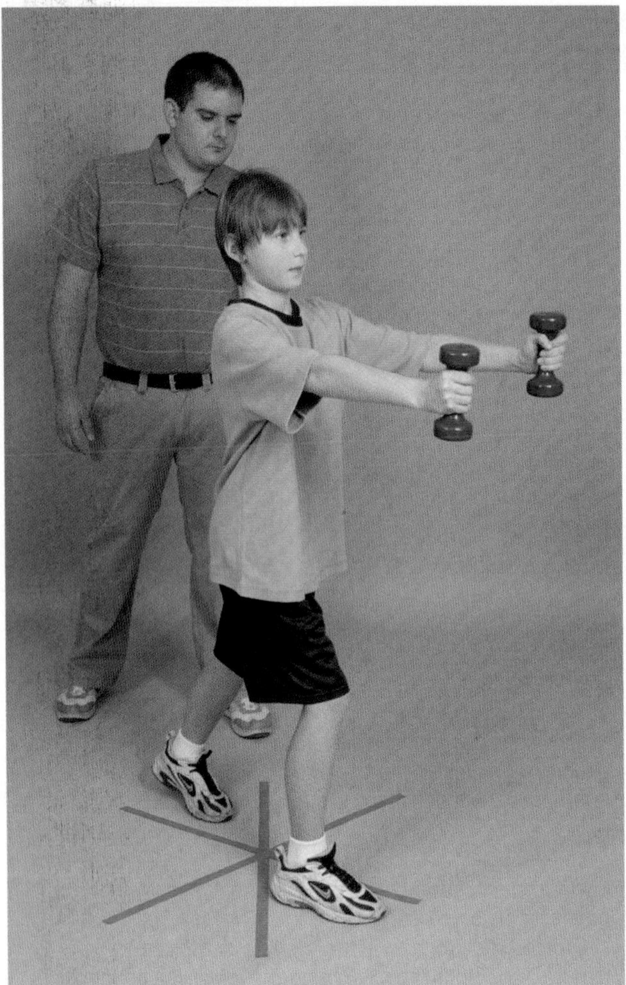

FIGURE 6.1 Resistance training, if initiated during the preadolescent years, should be performed using body weight or light weights and carefully supervised.

maintenance level of training could be useful in children as with adults.[83]

Although training-induced gains in strength and muscular endurance are well documented, there is insufficient evidence to suggest that a structured resistance training program for children, when coupled with a general sports conditioning program, reduces injuries or enhances sports performance.[5] However, other health-related benefits of a balanced exercise program have been noted, including increased cardiopulmonary fitness, decreased blood lipids levels, and improved psychological well-being.[22,27,82,141] These findings suggest that participation in a resistance training program during preadolescence may be of value if the program is performed at an appropriate level (low loads and repetitions), incorporates sufficient rest periods, and is closely supervised.[5,22,83,253]

Adolescence

As hormonal levels change at puberty, there is rapid acceleration in the development of muscle strength, especially in boys. During this phase of development, typical strength levels become markedly different in boys and girls, due in part to hormonal differences between the sexes. Strength in adolescent boys increases about 30% per year between ages 10 and 16, with muscle mass peaking before muscle strength.[34,183] In adolescent girls, peak strength develops before peak mass.[88] Overall, muscle mass increases more than 5-fold in boys and approximately 3.5-fold in girls during the adolescent years.[34,183] Although most longitudinal studies of growth stop at age 18, strength continues to develop, particularly in males, well into the second and even into the third decade of life.[183]

As with prepubescent children, resistance training during puberty also results in significant strength gains. During puberty, these gains average 30% to 40% above that which is expected as the result of normal growth and maturation.[83] A balanced training program for the adolescent involved in a sport often includes off-season and preseason aerobic conditioning and low-intensity resistance training, followed by more vigorous, sport-specific training during the season.[22] The benefits of strength training noted during puberty are similar to those that occur in prepubescent children.[82,86]

Young and Middle Adulthood

Although data on typical strength and endurance levels during the second through the fifth decades of life are more often from studies of men than women, a few generalizations can be made that seem to apply to both sexes.[178] Strength peaks earlier in women than men, with women reaching a peak during the second decade and most men peaking by age 30. After these peaks, strength then declines approximately 1% per year,[274] or 8% per decade.[100] This decline in strength appears to be minor until about age 50[264] and tends to occur at a later age or slower rate in active adults versus those who are sedentary.[104,274] The potential for improving muscle performance with a resistance training program (Fig. 6.2 A and B) or by participation in even moderately demanding activities several times a week is high during this phase of life. Guidelines for young and middle-aged adults participating in resistance training as part of an overall fitness program have been published by the ACSM[8] and the CDC.[35]

Late Adulthood

In most cases, the rate of decline in the tension-generating capacity of muscle accelerates to approximately 15% to 20% per decade for men and women in their sixties and seventies, and it increases to 30% per decade thereafter.[104,178] However, the rate of decline may be significantly less (only 0.3% decrease per year) in elderly men and women who maintain a high level of physical activity.[113] These findings suggest that loss of muscle strength during the advanced years may be due, in part, to progressively greater inactivity and disuse.[39] Loss of muscle in the lower extremity and trunk strength and stability during late adulthood—most notably during the seventies, eighties, and beyond—is associated with a gradual deterioration of functional abilities and an increase in the frequency of falling.[39,125]

The decline in muscle strength and endurance in the elderly is associated with many factors in addition to progressive

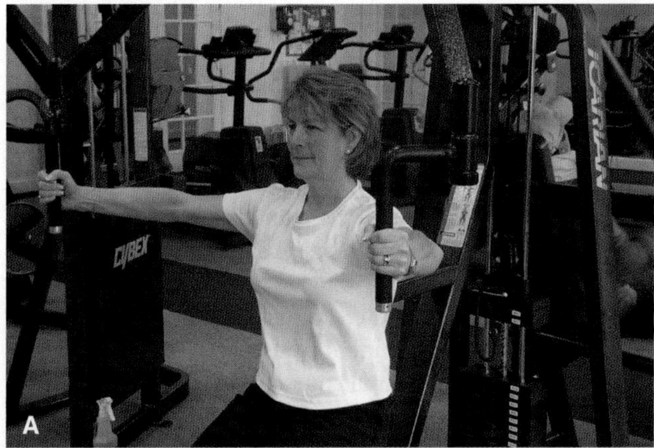

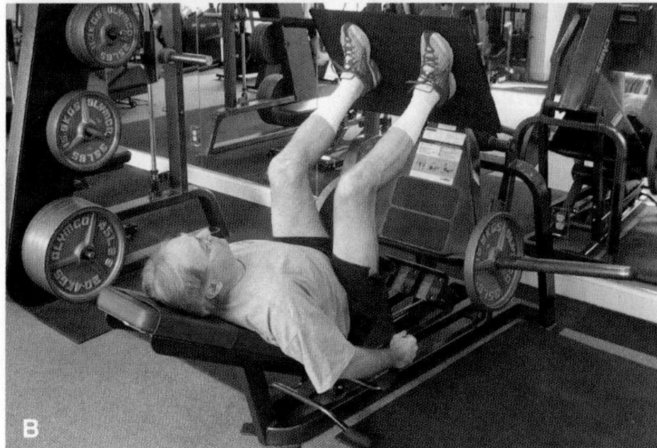

FIGURE 6.2 Conditioning and fitness programs for active young and middle-aged adults include resistance training with a balance of (A) upper extremity and (B) lower extremity strengthening exercises.

disuse and inactivity. It is difficult to determine if these factors are causes or effects of an age-related decrease in strength. Neuromuscular factors include decreased muscle mass (atrophy), decreased number of type I and II muscle fibers with a corresponding increase in connective tissue in muscle, decreased cross-sectional size of muscle, selective atrophy of type II fibers, and change in the length-tension relationship of muscle associated more with loss of flexibility than with deficits in motor unit activation and firing rate.[35,100,136,229,258,264,279] The number of motor units also appears to decline after age 60.[136]

In addition to decreases in muscle strength, declines in the speed of muscle contraction, muscle endurance, and the ability to recover from muscular fatigue occur with advanced age.[136,258] The time needed to produce the same absolute and relative levels of torque output is longer in the elderly compared with younger adults, as is the time necessary to achieve relaxation after a voluntary contraction.[100] Consequently, as the rate of movement declines, so does the ability to generate muscle power during activities that require quick responses, such as rising from a low chair or making balance adjustments to prevent a fall. Deterioration of muscle power with age has a stronger relationship to functional limitations and disability than does muscle strength.[220]

Information on changes in muscle endurance with aging is limited. There is some evidence to suggest that the ability to sustain low-intensity muscular effort also declines with age, a change attributed to reduced blood supply and capillary density in muscle, decreased mitochondrial density, changes in enzymatic activity level, and decreased glucose transport.[100] As a result, muscle fatigue may tend to occur more readily in the elderly. In the healthy and active elderly population, the decline in muscle endurance appears to be minimal well into the seventies.[136]

During the past few decades, as the health-care community and the public have become more aware of the benefits of resistance training during late adulthood, a greater number of older adults are participating in fitness programs that include resistance exercises. ACSM and the CDC have published guidelines for resistance training for healthy adults over 60 to 65 years of age.[6,37] (For additional information on exercise in the older population, see Chapter 24.)

Psychological and Cognitive Factors

An array of psychological factors can influence muscle performance and how easily, vigorously, or cautiously a person moves. Just as injury and disease adversely affect muscle performance, so can a person's mental status. For example, fear of pain, injury, or re-injury; depression related to physical illness; or impaired attention or memory as the result of age, head injury, or the side effects of medication can all adversely affect motor ability. In contrast, psychological factors can also positively influence physical performance.

The principles and methods employed to maximize motor performance and learning as functions of effective patient education are discussed in Chapter 1. These principles and methods should be applied in a resistance training program to develop a requisite level of muscle strength, power, and endurance for functional activities. The following interrelated psychological factors, as well as other aspects of motor learning, may influence muscle performance and the effectiveness of a resistance training program.

Attention

A patient must be able to focus on a given task to learn how to perform it correctly. Attention involves the ability to process relevant data while screening out irrelevant information from the environment and to respond to internal cues from the body. Both are necessary when first learning an exercise and later when carrying out an exercise program independently. Attention to form and technique during resistance training is necessary for patient safety and optimal long-term training effects.

Motivation and Feedback

If a resistance exercise program is to be effective, a patient must be willing to put forth and maintain sufficient effort and adhere to the program over time. Using meaningful activities that are perceived as having potential usefulness or periodically modifying an exercise routine help maintain a patient's interest in resistance training. Charting or graphing a patient's strength gains, for example, also helps sustain motivation. Incorporating gains in muscle performance into functional activities as early as possible puts improvements in strength to practical use, thereby making those improvements meaningful.

The importance of feedback for learning an exercise or motor skill is discussed in Chapter 1. In addition, feedback can have a positive impact on a patient's motivation and subsequent adherence to an exercise program. For example, some computerized equipment, such as isokinetic dynamometers, provide visual or auditory signals that let the patient know if each muscle contraction during a particular exercise is within a specific range of intensity or work that is likely to cause a training effect. Documenting improvements over time, such as the amount of external resistance used during various exercises or walking distance or speed, also provides positive feedback to sustain a patient's motivation in a resistance exercise program.

Physiological Adaptations to Resistance Exercise

The use of resistance exercise in rehabilitation and conditioning programs has a substantial impact on all systems of the body. Resistance training is equally important for patients with impaired muscle performance and individuals who wish to improve or maintain their level of fitness, enhance performance, or reduce their injury risk. When body systems are exposed to a greater than usual, but appropriate level of resistance exercises, they initially react with a number of *acute* physiological responses before adapting—that is, body systems accommodate over time to the newly imposed physical demands.[6,7,184] Training-induced adaptations to resistance exercise, known as *chronic* physiological responses, are summarized in Table 6.3 and discussed in this section. Key differences in adaptations from strength training versus endurance training are noted.

Adaptations to overload create changes in muscle performance and, in part, determine the effectiveness of a resistance training program. The time course for these adaptations to occur varies from one individual to another depending on a person's health status and previous level of participation in a resistance exercise program.[8]

Neural Adaptations

It is well accepted that the initial, rapid gain in the tension-generating capacity of skeletal muscle from a resistance training program is attributed largely to neural responses, not adaptive changes in muscle itself.[103,176,195,225] This is reflected by an increase in electromyographic (EMG) activity during the first 4 to 8 weeks of training, with little to no evidence of muscle fiber hypertrophy. It is also possible that increased neural activity is the source of additional gains in strength late in a resistance training program after muscle hypertrophy has plateaued.[162,184]

TABLE 6.3 Physiological Adaptations to Resistance Exercise

Variable	Strength Training Adaptations	Endurance Training Adaptations
Skeletal muscle structure	Muscle fibers hypertrophy: greatest in type IIB fibers Possible hyperplasia of muscle fibers Fiber type composition: remodeling of type IIB to type IIA; no change in type I to type II distribution (i.e., no conversion) ↓ or no change in capillary bed density: ↓ in mitochondrial density and volume	Minimal or no muscle fiber hypertrophy ↑ in capillary bed density ↑ in mitochondrial density and volume (↑ number and size)
Neural system	Motor unit recruitment (↑ # of motor units firing) ↑ rate of firing (↓ twitch contraction time) ↑ synchronization of firing	No changes
Metabolic system and enzymatic activity	↑ ATP and PC storage ↑ myoglobin storage Triglycerides storage: change not known ↑ creatine phosphokinase ↑ myokinase	↑ ATP and PC storage: ↑ myoglobin storage ↑ of stored triglycerides ↑ creatine phosphokinase ↑ myokinase
Body composition	↑ lean (fat-free) body mass; ↓ % body fat	No change in lean body mass; ↓ % body fat
Connective tissue	↑ tensile strength of tendons, ligaments, and connective tissue in muscle ↑ bone mineral density; no change or possible ↑ in bone mass	↑ tensile strength of tendons, ligaments, and connective tissue in muscle ↑ in bone mineralization with land-based, weight-bearing activities

The initial neural responses to resistance exercise are attributed to motor learning and improved coordination[103,161,163,184] through *increased recruitment* in the number of motor units firing and an *increased rate and synchronization* of motor unit firing.[103,161,217,225] It is speculated that these changes are the result of decreased inhibition of the CNS, decreased sensitivity of the Golgi tendon organ, or changes at the myoneural junction of the motor unit.[103,225]

Skeletal Muscle Adaptations

Hypertrophy

As noted previously, the tension-producing capacity of muscle is directly related to the physiological cross-sectional area of the individual muscle fibers. *Hypertrophy* is an increase in the size of an individual muscle fiber caused by increased myofibrillar volume.[198,258] After an extended period of moderate- to high-intensity resistance training, usually by 4 to 8 weeks,[1,271] but possibly as early as 2 to 3 weeks with very high-intensity resistance training,[243] hypertrophy becomes an increasingly important adaptation that accounts for muscle strength gains.

Although the mechanism of hypertrophy is complex and the stimulus for growth is not clearly understood, hypertrophy of skeletal muscle appears to be the result of increased protein (actin and myosin) synthesis and decreased protein degradation. Hypertrophy is also associated with biochemical changes that stimulate uptake of amino acids.[161,184,198,258]

The greatest increases in protein synthesis and hypertrophy are associated with high-volume, moderate-resistance exercise performed eccentrically.[161,223] Furthermore, it is the type IIB muscle fibers that appear to increase in size most readily with resistance training.[184,202]

Hyperplasia

Although the topic has been debated for many years and evidence of the phenomenon is sparse, there is some thought that a portion of the increase in muscle size that occurs with heavy resistance training is caused by *hyperplasia*, an increased *number* of muscle fibers. It has been suggested that this increase in fiber number, observed in laboratory animals,[111,112] is the result of longitudinal splitting of fibers.[13,134,191] It has been postulated that fiber splitting occurs when individual muscle fibers increase in size to a point at which they are inefficient and then subsequently split to form two distinct fibers.[111]

Critics of the concept of hyperplasia suggest that evidence of fiber splitting actually may be caused by inappropriate tissue preparation in the laboratory.[109] The general opinion in the literature is that hyperplasia either does not occur, or if it does occur to a slight degree, its impact is insignificant.[96,176,181]

Muscle Fiber Type Adaptation

As previously mentioned, type IIB (phasic) muscle fibers preferentially hypertrophy with heavy resistance training. In addition, a substantial degree of plasticity exists in muscle fibers with respect to contractile and metabolic properties.[229] Transformation of type IIB to type IIA is common with endurance training,[229] as well as during the early weeks of heavy resistance training,[243] making the type II fibers more resistant to fatigue. There is some evidence of type I to type II fiber type conversion in the denervated limbs of laboratory animals,[208,286] in humans with spinal cord injury, and after an extended period of weightlessness associated with space flight.[229] However, there is little to no evidence of type II to type I conversion under training conditions in rehabilitation or fitness programs.[184,229]

Vascular and Metabolic Adaptations

Adaptations of the cardiovascular and respiratory systems as the result of low-intensity, high-volume resistance training are discussed in Chapter 7. Opposite to what occurs with endurance training, with muscle hypertrophy from high-intensity, low-volume training, capillary bed density actually decreases because of the increased number of myofilaments per fiber.[7] Athletes who participate in heavy resistance training actually have fewer capillaries per muscle fiber than endurance athletes and even untrained individuals.[148,256] Other changes associated with metabolism, such as a decrease in mitochondrial density, also occur with high-intensity resistance training.[7,161] This change is associated with reduced oxidative capacity of muscle.

Adaptations of Connective Tissues

Although the evidence is limited, it appears that resistance training for muscle strength increases the tensile strength of tendons, ligaments, and bone.[47,247,287]

Tendons, Ligaments, and Connective Tissue in Muscle

Increased tendon strength probably occurs at the musculotendinous junction, whereas increased ligament strength may occur at the ligament-bone interface. It is believed that tensile strength increases in these tissues from resistance training function to support the adaptive strength and size changes of muscle.[287] Consequently, the stronger ligaments and tendons may be less prone to injury. The connective tissue in muscle also thickens, giving more support to the enlarged fibers.[184] It is also thought that noncontractile soft tissue strength may develop more rapidly with eccentric resistance training than with other types of resistance exercises.[246,247]

Bone

Numerous sources indicate that bone mineral density is highly correlated with muscle strength and the level of physical activity across the life span.[228] Consequently, physical activities and exercises, particularly those performed in weight-bearing positions, are typically recommended to minimize or prevent age-related bone loss[218] and to reduce the risk of fractures or improve bone density when osteopenia or osteoporosis is already present.[51,228]

FOCUS ON EVIDENCE

Although the evidence from prospective studies is limited and mixed, resistance exercises performed with adequate intensity and with site-specific loading through weight bearing have been shown to increase or maintain bone mineral density.[150,154,168,190,201] In contrast, a number of studies in young, healthy women[222] and postmenopausal women[219,234] have reported that there was no significant increase in bone mineral density with resistance training. However, the resistance exercises in these studies were not combined with site-specific weight bearing. In addition, the intensity of the weight training programs may not have been high enough to have an impact on bone density.[168,228] The time course of the exercise program also may not have been long enough. It has been suggested that it may take as long as 9 to 12 months of exercise for detectable and significant increases in bone mass to occur.[8] In the spine, although studies to date have not shown that resistance training prevents spinal fractures, there is some evidence to suggest that the strength of the back extensors closely correlates with vertebral bone mineral density.[234]

Research continues to determine the most effective forms of exercise to enhance bone density and prevent age-related bone loss and fractures. For additional information on prevention and management of osteoporosis, refer to Chapters 11 and 24.

BOX 6.4 Determinants of a Resistance Exercise Program

- *Alignment* of body segments during each unique exercise
- *Stabilization* of proximal or distal joints to prevent substitute motions
- *Intensity:* the exercise load or level of resistance
- *Volume:* the total number of repetitions and sets in an exercise session
- *Exercise order:* the sequence in which muscle groups are exercised during a session
- *Frequency:* the number of exercise sessions per day or per week
- *Rest interval:* the time allotted for recuperation between exercise sets and sessions
- *Duration:* total time committed to a resistance training program
- *Mode*: the type of muscle contraction, type of resistance, arc of movement used, and primary energy system utilized during exercise
- *Velocity:* the rate at which each exercise is performed
- *Periodization:* the variation of intensity and volume during specific periods of resistance training
- *Integration of exercises into functional activities:* exercises that approximate or replicate functional demands

Determinants of Resistance Exercise

Many interrelated factors determine whether a resistance exercise program is appropriate, effective, and safe. This holds true when resistance training is a part of a rehabilitation program for individuals with known or potential impairments in muscle performance, when it is incorporated into a general conditioning program to improve the fitness level of healthy individuals, or as part of a comprehensive exercise program intended to increase performance and reduce injury risk.

Each factor discussed in this section and noted in Box 6.4 should be considered when designing a resistance program to improve one or more aspects of muscle performance and achieve desired functional outcomes. Appropriate *alignment* and *stabilization* are two constant factors for any exercise designed to improve muscle performance. A suitable *dosage* of exercise must also be determined. In resistance training, dosage includes *intensity, volume, frequency,* and *duration* of exercise. Each separate dosage factor is a mechanism by which the muscle can be progressively overloaded to improve muscle performance. The *velocity* of exercise and the *mode (type)* of exercise must also be considered. Finally, the appropriate *rest interval* between sessions must be determined. ACSM denotes the key determinants of a resistance training program by the acronym FITT, which represents frequency, intensity, time, and type of exercise.[6]

Consistent with the SAID principle discussed in the first section of this chapter, the determinants of resistance exercise must be specific to the patient's desired functional goals. Additional factors, such as the underlying cause of the muscle performance deficits; the extent of impairment; and the patient's age, medical history, mental status, and social situation, may also affect the design and implementation of a resistance exercise program.

Alignment and Stabilization

Just as correct alignment and effective stabilization are basic elements of manual muscle testing and dynamometry, they are also crucial in resistance exercise. To strengthen a specific muscle or muscle group effectively and avoid substitute motions, appropriate positioning of the body and alignment of a limb or body segment are essential. *Substitute motions* are compensatory movement patterns caused by muscle action of a stronger adjacent agonist or a muscle group that normally serves as a stabilizer.[152] Substitute motions must be avoided if the resistance exercises are to optimally benefit the target muscle or muscle group. If the principles of alignment and stabilization for manual muscle testing[132,152] are applied whenever possible during resistance exercise substitute motions can usually be avoided.

Alignment

Alignment and muscle action. Proper alignment is determined by considering the fiber orientation, the line of pull, and the specific action desired of the muscle to be strengthened. The patient or body segment must be positioned so the direction of movement of a limb or segment of the body replicates the action of the muscle or muscle groups to be strengthened. For example, to strengthen the gluteus medius, the hip must remain slightly extended and the pelvis must be shifted slightly forward as the patient abducts the lower extremity against the applied resistance. If the hip is flexed as the leg abducts, the adjacent tensor fasciae latae becomes the prime mover and detracts from the beneficial effect to the gluteus medius (Fig. 6.3).

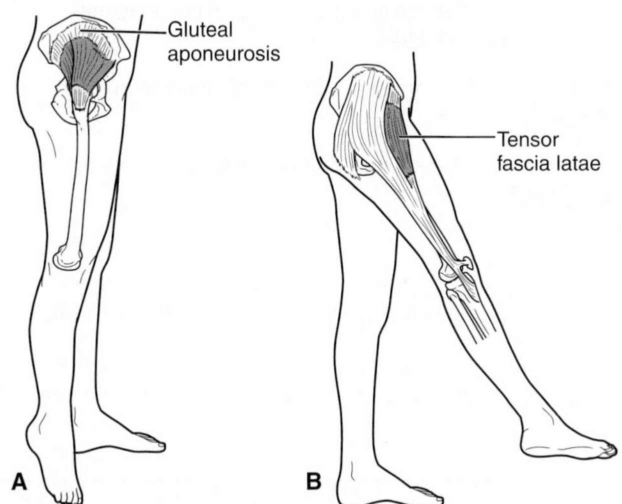

FIGURE 6.3 When performing hip abduction, emphasize maintaining the hip in extension and slight external rotation to **(A)** strengthen the gluteus medius. Allowing the hip to flex while attempting abduction **(B)** puts the TFL in in line to abduct the hip and minimizes benefit to the gluteus medius.

Alignment and gravity. The alignment or position of the patient or limb with respect to gravity will also be important during some forms of resistance exercise, particularly if body weight or free weights (dumbbells, barbells, and cuff weights) are the source of resistance. The patient or limb should be positioned in a way that considers how both gravity and a weight provide external resistance to the muscle being strengthened.

Staying with the example of strengthening the gluteus medius, if a cuff weight is placed around the lower leg, the patient must be positioned in side-lying so that the muscle contraction overcomes the external resistance applied by both gravity and the cuff weight. However, if the patient were positioned in supine, the cuff weight and gravity's resistance force become oriented to optimally resist hip flexion rather than abduction.

Stabilization

Stabilization refers to holding down a body segment or holding the body steady.[152] Effective stabilization is imperative during resistance exercise to maintain appropriate alignment, ensure the correct muscle action and movement pattern, and avoid unwanted substitute motions. Exercising on a stable surface, such as a firm treatment table, helps achieve stabilization. Body weight also provides a source of stability during exercise. It is most common to stabilize the body segment that has the proximal attachment of the muscle being strengthened, but sometimes the distal segment is stabilized. For example, when strengthening the plantarflexors against the resistance of an elastic band in a long-sitting position, the proximal muscle attachment on the leg must be stabilized. However, if strengthening against the resistance of body weight and gravity while standing, the distal segment foot is now stabilized by contact with the ground.

Stabilization for resistance exercise can be achieved through external or internal means.

- *External stabilization* can be applied manually by the therapist or the patient with equipment such as belts and straps or by using gravity to hold the body against a firm support surface such as the back of a chair or the surface of a treatment table.
- *Internal stabilization* is achieved by an isometric contraction of an adjacent muscle group that does not impact the desired movement pattern but holds the proximal body segment of the muscle being strengthened firmly in place. For example, when performing a bilateral straight leg raise while positioned in supine, the abdominals contract to stabilize the pelvis and lumbar spine as the hip flexors raise the legs. This form of stabilization is effective only if the fixating muscle group is strong enough or not fatigued.

Exercise Intensity

The *intensity* of exercise in a resistance training program is the amount of external resistance imposed on the contracting muscle during each repetition of an exercise. The amount of resistance is also referred to as the *exercise load* or *training load*—that is, the extent to which the muscle is loaded or how much weight is raised, lowered, or held.

Remember, consistent with the overload principle, muscle performance improves only if the muscle is subjected to an exercise load that is greater than what is usually experienced. One way to progressively overload a muscle is to gradually increase the amount of resistance used in the exercise program.[6,8,95,162,163]

Submaximal Versus Maximal Exercise Loads

Many factors determine whether resistance exercise is carried out against submaximal or maximal muscle loading. These factors include the goals and expected functional outcomes of the exercise program; the cause and extent of muscle performance deficits; the stage of healing of injured tissues; and the patient's age, general health, and fitness level. In general, the level of resistance is lower in rehabilitation programs for persons with impairments than in conditioning programs for healthy individuals.

Indications for submaximal loading for moderate to low-intensity exercise versus near-maximal or maximal loading for high-intensity exercise are summarized in Table 6.4.

PRECAUTION: Resistance exercises that cause pain indicate that the intensity level is too great. Also, there is a direct

TABLE 6.4 Indications for Low-Intensity Versus High-Intensity Exercise

Low Intensity	High Intensity
In the early stages of soft tissue healing when injured tissues must be protected	When the goal of exercise is to increase muscle strength and power and possibly increase muscle size
After prolonged immobilization when the articular cartilage is not able to withstand large compressive forces or when bone demineralization may have occurred, increasing the risk of pathological fracture	For otherwise healthy adults in the advanced phase of a rehabilitation program after a musculoskeletal injury in preparation for returning to high-demand occupational or recreational activities
To evaluate the patient's response to resistance exercise, especially after an extended period of inactivity	In a conditioning program for individuals with no known pathology
When initially learning an exercise to emphasize the correct form	For individuals training for competitive weight lifting or body building
For most children or older adults	
When the goal of exercise is to improve muscle endurance	
To warm-up and cool-down prior to and after a session of exercise	
During slow-velocity isokinetic training to minimize compressive forces on joints	

relationship between increasing exercise intensity requiring maximal effort and cardiovascular risks. Patients need continual reminders to incorporate rhythmic breathing into each repetition of an exercise to minimize these risks.

Initial Exercise Load (Amount of Resistance) and Documentation of Training Effects

It is always challenging to estimate how much external resistance to apply during resistance exercises, particularly at the beginning of a strengthening program. When applying manual resistance, the decision is entirely subjective, based on the therapist's judgment about the patients' effort, performance, and response during exercise. In an exercise program using mechanical resistance, the determination can be made quantitatively.

Repetition Maximum

One method of calculating an appropriate exercise load for training is to determine a repetition maximum. This term was first reported decades ago by DeLorme in his investigations of an approach to resistance training called progressive resistive exercise (PRE).[60,61] A *repetition maximum* (RM) is defined as the greatest amount of weight or load that can be moved with control through the full, available range of motion (ROM) a specific number of times before fatiguing.

Use of a RM. There are two main reasons for determining a RM: (1) to identify an initial exercise load (amount of weight) to be used during exercise for a specified number of repetitions and (2) to document a baseline measurement of the dynamic strength of a muscle or muscle group against which exercise-induced improvements in strength can be compared. DeLorme reported use of a 1-RM (the greatest amount of weight a subject can move through the available ROM just one time) as the baseline measurement of a subject's maximum effort but used a multiple RM, specifically a 10-RM, (the amount of weight that could be lifted and lowered 10 times through the ROM) during training.[61]

Despite criticism that establishing a 1-RM involves some trial and error, it is a frequently used method for measuring muscle strength in research studies and has been shown to be a safe and reliable measurement tool prior to beginning conditioning programs with healthy young adults and athletes[95,163] as well as active older adults.[194,252,262]

PRECAUTION: Use of a 1-RM as a baseline measurement of dynamic strength is inappropriate for some patient populations because one maximum effort may require an unsafe amount of exertion. For example, it is not safe for patients with joint impairments, patients who are recovering from or who are at risk for soft tissue injury, or patients with known or at risk for osteoporosis or cardiovascular pathology.

CLINICAL TIP

To avoid the trial and error associated with establishing a 1-RM or to eliminate the need for an at-risk patient to exert a single maximum effort, formulas have been developed and tables have been published[16,135] that enable a therapist to calculate a 1-RM for each muscle group to be strengthened based on the patient performing a greater number of repetitions against a reduced load.

Another practical, time-saving way to establish a baseline RM is for a therapist to select a specific amount of resistance (weight) and document how many repetitions can be completed through the full range before the muscle begins to fatigue. If six repetitions, for example, were completed, the baseline resistance would be based on a 6-RM. Remember, a sign of fatigue is the inability to complete the full, available ROM against the applied resistance.

Alternative Methods of Determining Baseline Strength or an Initial Exercise Load

Cable tensiometry[184] and isokinetic or handheld dynamometry[53] are alternatives to a RM for establishing a baseline measurement of dynamic or static strength. A percentage of body weight has also been proposed to estimate the amount of external resistance to be used in a strength training program.[226] Some examples for several exercises are noted in Box 6.5. The percentages indicated are meant as guidelines for the advanced stage of rehabilitation and are based on 10 repetitions of each exercise at the beginning of an exercise program. Percentages vary for different muscle groups.

When a maximum effort is inappropriate, the level of perceived loading, as measured by the Borg CR10 scale,[29] is also a useful tool in estimating an appropriate level of resistance and sufficient exercise intensity for muscle strengthening.[8] Box 6.6 provides the category scale used with the Borg CR10.[29]

Training Zone

After establishing the baseline RM, the amount of external resistance to be used at the initiation of resistance training is often calculated as a *percentage* of a 1-RM for a particular muscle group. At the beginning of an exercise program the percentage necessary to achieve training-induced adaptations in strength ranges from low (30% to 40%) for sedentary, untrained individuals to very high (>80%) for highly trained individuals. For healthy but untrained adults, a typical training zone usually falls between 40% and 70% of the baseline 1-RM.[6,8,13] The lower percentage of this range is safer at the beginning of a program to enable an individual to focus on learning correct exercise form and technique before progressing to higher loads.

Exercising at a low to moderate percentage of the established RM is recommended for children and the elderly.[6,8] For patients with significant deficits in muscle strength or to train for muscular endurance, using a low load—possibly at the 30% to 50% level—is safe yet challenging.

BOX 6.5 Percentage of Body Weight as an Initial Exercise Load for Selected Exercises

- Universal bench press: 30% body weight
- Universal leg extension: 20% body weight
- Universal leg curl: 10% to 15% body weight
- Universal leg press: 50% body weight

BOX 6.6 Borg CR10 Scale for Estimating Perceived Exertion[29]

0	Nothing at all	
0.3		
0.5	Extremely weak	Just noticeable
0.7		
1	Very weak	
1.5		
2	Weak	Light
2.5		
3	Moderate	
4		
5	Strong	Heavy
6		
7	Very strong	
8		
9		
10	Extremely strong	"Maximal"
11		
•	Absolute maximum	Highest possible

Exercise Volume

In resistance training, the *volume* of exercise is the summation of the total number of repetitions and sets of a particular exercise during a single exercise session multiplied by the intensity of the exercise.[6,8,162] The same combination of repetitions and sets is not and should not be used for all muscle groups.

There is an inverse relationship between the sets and repetitions of an exercise and the intensity of the resistance. The higher the intensity or external resistance, the lower the number of repetitions and sets are possible. Conversely, the lower the external resistance, the greater the number of repetitions and sets are possible. Therefore, the external resistance directly dictates how many repetitions and sets are possible.

Repetitions. The number of repetitions in an exercise program refers to the number of times a particular movement is performed consecutively. More specifically, it is the number of muscle contractions performed to move the limb through a series of continuous and complete excursions against a specific exercise load.

If the RM designation is used, the number of repetitions at a specific exercise load is reflected in the designation. For example, 10 repetitions with a 20-lb load is designated as a 10-RM. If a 1-RM has been established as a baseline level of dynamic strength, the percentage of the 1-RM that is used as the exercise load will directly influence the number of repetitions a patient is able to perform before fatiguing. The "average," untrained adult, when exercising with a load that is equivalent to 75% of the 1-RM, is able to complete approximately 10 repetitions before needing to rest.[16,184] At 60% intensity, about 15 repetitions are possible, and at 90%, intensity only 4 or 5 repetitions are usually possible.

For practical reasons, after a beginning exercise load is selected, the target number of repetitions performed for each exercise before a brief rest is often within a range rather than an exact number of repetitions. For example, a patient might be able to complete between 8 and 10 repetitions against a specified load before resting. This is sometimes referred to as a *RM zone*[184] and gives the patient flexibility in their exercise program.

The target number of repetitions selected depends on the patient's status and whether the goal of the exercise is to improve muscle strength or endurance. No optimal number of repetitions for strength training or endurance training has been identified, although greater strength has been reported for exercise programs using from a 2- to 3-RM to a 15-RM.[16,164]

Sets. A predetermined number of consecutive repetitions grouped together is known as a *set* or *bout* of exercise. After each set of a specified number of repetitions, there is a brief interval of rest. For example, during a single exercise session to strengthen a particular muscle group, a patient might be directed to lift an exercise load 8 to 10 times, rest, and then lift the load another 8 to 10 times. This sequence describes two sets of an 8- to 10-RM.

As with repetitions, there is no optimal number of sets per exercise session, but two to four sets are a common recommendation for adults.[6] As few as one set and as many as six sets have yielded positive training effects.[8,162] Single-set exercises at low intensities are most common in the very early phases of a resistance exercise program or in a maintenance program. Multiple-set exercises are used to progress the program and have been shown to be superior to single-set regimens in advanced training.[164]

Training to Improve Strength, Power, or Endurance: Impact of Exercise Load and Repetitions

Because many variations of intensity and volume cause positive training-induced adaptations in muscle performance, there is a substantial amount of latitude for selecting an exercise load/repetition and set scheme for each exercise. Clinicians can improve their ability to select appropriate exercise volume parameters for their patients and clients by determining if their goal is to improve muscle strength, power, or endurance.

To Improve Muscle Strength

In DeLorme's early studies,[60,61] three sets of a 10-RM performed for 10 repetitions over the training period led to strength gains. Current recommendations for strength training vary somewhat. One resource[15] suggests that a threshold of 40% to 60% of maximum effort is necessary for adaptive strength gains to occur in a healthy but untrained individual. However, other resources recommend using a moderate exercise load (60% to 80% of a 1-RM) that causes fatigue after 8 to 12 repetitions for 2 or 3 sets.[6,162] When fatigue no longer occurs after the target number of repetitions has been completed, the level of resistance is increased to overload the muscle once again.

To Improve Muscle Power

Power can be developed and improved by modifying the intensity and speed of training. The recommended intensity for power training ranges for 20% to 70% of 1-RM, while the rate of exercises should be explosive or ballistic. The mean training combination from over 350 studies showing an overall small increase in power was 3.8 sets of 6.4 repetitions of an exercise performed rapidly at 81% of the 1-RM.[188] Not surprisingly, there is a linear relationship between increased training variables, especially resistance load, and improved power. Three to four sessions per week is recommended to increase power of both the upper and lower extremities.[188] Chapter 23 provides additional detail on strategies to improve power.

To Improve Muscle Endurance

Training to improve muscle endurance involves performing many repetitions of an exercise against a submaximal load.[7,162,248] For example, as many as 3 to 5 sets of 40 to 50 repetitions against a low amount of external resistance or a light grade of elastic resistance might be used. When increasing the number of repetitions or sets becomes inefficient, the load can be increased slightly.

Endurance training also can be accomplished by maintaining an isometric muscle contraction for incrementally longer periods of time. Because endurance training is performed against very low levels of resistance, it can be initiated very early in a rehabilitation program without risk of injury to healing tissues.

CLINICAL TIP

When injured muscles are immobilized, type I (slow twitch) muscle fibers atrophy at a faster rate than type II (fast twitch) fibers.[198] There is also a slow to fast muscle fiber type conversion with disuse. These changes give rise to a much faster rate of atrophy of antigravity muscles compared with their antagonists,[176] underscoring the need for early initiation of endurance training following injury or surgery.

Exercise Order

The sequence in which resistance exercises are performed during an exercise session has an impact on muscle fatigue and adaptive training effects. When several muscle groups are exercised in a single session, as is the case in most rehabilitation or conditioning programs, large muscle groups should be exercised before small muscle groups and multijoint exercises should be performed before single-joint exercises.[8,95,161,162]

In addition, after an appropriate warm-up, higher intensity exercises should be performed before lower intensity exercises.[8]

Exercise Frequency

Frequency in a resistance exercise program refers to the number of exercise sessions per day or per week.[6,8] Frequency also may refer to the number of times per week specific muscle groups are exercised or certain exercises are performed.[6,162] As with other aspects of dosage, frequency is dependent on other determinants, such as intensity and volume, as well as the patient's goals, general health status, previous participation in a resistance exercise program, and response to training. The greater the intensity and volume of exercise, the more time is needed between exercise sessions to recover from the temporary fatigue effects. A common cause of a decline in performance from overtraining (see discussion later in the chapter) is excessive frequency, inadequate rest intervals, and progressive fatigue.

Some forms of exercise should be performed less frequently than others because they require greater recovery time. It has been known for some time that high-intensity *eccentric* exercise, for example, is associated with greater microtrauma to soft tissues and a higher incidence of delayed-onset muscle soreness than concentric exercise.[14,99,204] Therefore, rest intervals between exercise sessions are longer and the frequency of exercise is less for eccentric exercises than with other forms.

Although an optimal frequency per week has not been determined, a few generalizations can be made. Initially in an exercise program, short sessions of exercises sometimes can be performed on a daily basis several times per day as long as the intensity of exercise and number of repetitions are low. This frequency is often indicated for early postsurgical patients when the operated limb is immobilized and the extent of exercise is limited to nonresisted isometric (setting) exercises meant to minimize the risk of muscle atrophy. As the intensity and volume of exercise increases, a frequency of two to three times per week, every other day, or up to five exercise sessions per week is common.[6,8,95,161] A rest interval of 48 hours when training major muscle groups can be achieved by alternating sessions by exercising the upper extremities one day and the lower extremities the next day.

Frequency can be reduced for a maintenance program, usually to two times per week. With prepubescent children and the very elderly, frequency typically is limited to no more than two to three sessions per week.[6,8,36,37] Highly trained athletes involved in body building, power lifting, and weight lifting, who know their own response to exercise, often train at a high intensity and volume up to 6 days per week.[8,162,164]

Exercise Duration

Exercise *duration* is the total number of weeks or months during which a resistance exercise program is carried out. Depending on the cause of impaired muscle performance, some patients require only a month or two of training to return to the desired level of function or activity, whereas others need to continue the exercise program for a lifetime to maintain optimal function.

As noted earlier in the chapter, strength gains observed early in a resistance training program (after 2 to 3 weeks) are primarily the result of neural adaptation. For significant changes to occur in muscle, such as hypertrophy or increased vascularization, at least 6 to 12 weeks of resistance training is required.[1,6,184]

Rest Interval (Recovery Period)

Purpose of rest intervals. Rest is a critical element of a resistance training program and is necessary to allow time for the body to recuperate from muscle fatigue or to offset adverse responses such as exercise-induced, delayed-onset muscle soreness. Only with an appropriate balance of progressive loading and adequate rest intervals can muscle performance improve. Therefore, rest between sets of exercise and between exercise sessions must be carefully implemented.

Integration of rest into exercise. Rest intervals for each exercising muscle group are dependent on the intensity and volume of exercise. In general, with a higher exercise intensity a longer rest interval is needed. For moderate-intensity resistance training, a 2- to 3-minute rest period after each set is recommended. A shorter rest interval is adequate after low-intensity exercise. Longer rest intervals (>3 minutes) are appropriate with high-intensity resistance training, particularly when exercising large, multijoint muscles.[6,8] While the muscle group that was just exercised is resting, resistance exercises can be performed by another muscle group in the same extremity or by the same muscle group in the opposite extremity.

Patients with pathological conditions that make them more susceptible to fatigue, as well as children and the elderly, should rest at least 3 minutes between sets by performing a nonresisted exercise, such as low-intensity cycling, or performing the same exercise with the opposite extremity. Remember, active recovery is more efficient for neutralizing the effects of muscle fatigue than passive recovery.

Rest between exercise sessions must also be considered. When strength training is initiated at moderate intensities (typically in the intermediate phase of a rehabilitation program after soft tissue injury), a 48-hour rest interval between exercise sessions—that is, training every other day—allows the patient adequate time for recovery.

Mode of Exercise

The *mode* of exercise in a resistance exercise program refers to the form of exercise, the type of muscle contraction that occurs, and the manner in which the exercise is carried out. For example, a patient may perform an exercise dynamically or statically or in a weight-bearing or nonweight-bearing position. Mode of exercise also encompasses the form of resistance—that is, how the exercise load is applied. External resistance can be applied manually or mechanically.

As with other determinants of resistance training, the modes of exercise selected are based on a multitude of factors already highlighted throughout this section. A brief overview of the various modes of exercise is presented in this section. An in-depth explanation and analysis of each of these types of exercise can be found in the next section of this chapter and in Chapter 7.

Type of Muscle Contraction

Figure 6.4 depicts the types of muscle contraction that may be performed in a resistance exercise program, with their relationships to each other and to muscle performance noted.[175,202,236]

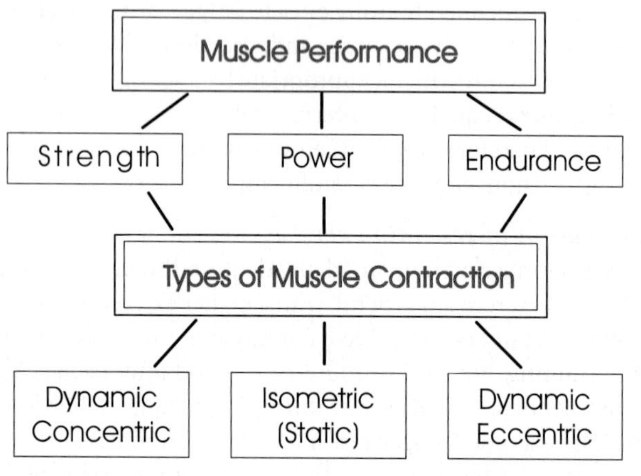

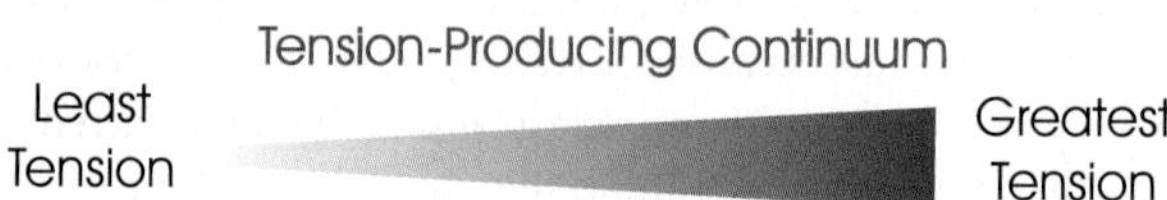

FIGURE 6.4 Types of muscle contractions: their relationships to muscle performance and their tension-generating capacities.

- Static or dynamic muscle contractions are two broad categories of exercise.
- Static contractions can refer to isometric contractions done internally—often called muscle setting—or against an unmovable external resistance.
- Dynamic resistance exercises can be performed using *concentric* (muscle shortening) or *eccentric* (muscle lengthening) contractions, or both.
- When the velocity of limb movement is held consistent by a rate-controlling device, the term *isokinetic* contraction is sometimes used.[236] An alternative perspective is that this is simply a dynamic (shortening or lengthening) contraction that occurs under controlled conditions.[175]

Position for Exercise: Weight Bearing or Nonweight Bearing

The patient's body or extremity position relative to a weight-bearing surface also alters the mode of exercise. When a nonweight-bearing position is assumed and the distal segment (foot or hand) moves freely during exercise, the term *open-chain exercise* is most often used. When a weight-bearing position is assumed and the body moves over a fixed distal segment, the term *closed-chain exercise* is commonly used.[175,202,236] Concepts and issues associated with the use of this terminology are addressed later in this chapter.

Forms of Resistance

- *Manual* resistance and *mechanical* resistance are the two broad methods by which external resistance can be applied.
- A *constant* or *variable* load can be imposed through mechanical resistance such as free weights or weight machines.
- *Accommodating* resistance[133] can be implemented by use of an isokinetic dynamometer that controls the velocity by adjusting the external resistance to meet the internal effort during exercise.
- *Body weight* or partial body weight is also a source of resistance if the exercise occurs in an antigravity position. Although an exercise performed against only the resistance of the weight of a body segment (and no additional external resistance) is defined as an active rather than an active-resistive exercise, a substantial amount of resistance from the weight of the body can be imposed by altering a patient's position. For example, progressive loads can be placed on upper extremity musculature during push-ups by starting with wall push-ups while standing, progressing to push-ups while leaning against a countertop, push-ups in a horizontal position (Fig. 6.5), and finally push-ups with the feet elevated above the hands.

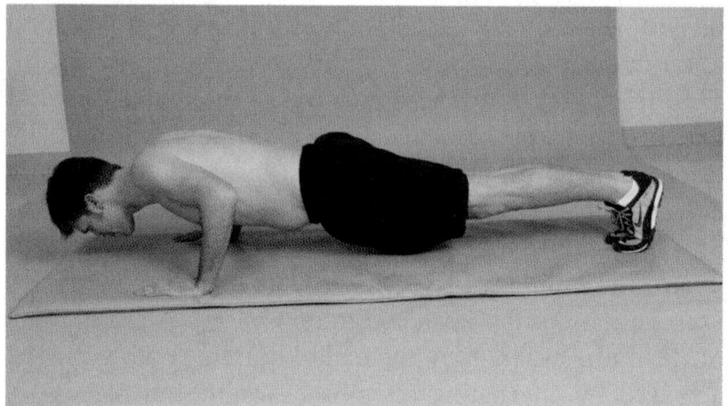

FIGURE 6.5 Body weight serves as the source of resistance during a push-up.

Energy Systems

Modes of exercise can also be classified by the energy systems used during the exercise. Anaerobic exercise involves high-intensity effort carried out over a low number of repetitions because muscles rapidly fatigue at near-maximal intensity. Strengthening exercises are categorized as anaerobic. Aerobic exercise is associated with low-intensity, high-repetition effort over an extended period of time. This mode of exercise primarily increases muscular and cardiopulmonary endurance. (Refer to Chapter 7 for an in-depth explanation.)

Range of Movement: Short-Arc or Full-Arc Exercise

External resistance through the full joint range of movement (full-arc exercise) is necessary to develop strength over the entire ROM. However, sometimes resistance exercises are executed through only a portion of the available range, which is referred to as short-arc exercise. Short-arc exercise is used when a painful or unstable arc of motion must be avoided or to protect healing tissues after injury or surgery.

Mode of Exercise and Application to Function

Mode-specific training is essential if a resistance training program is to have a positive impact on function. When tissue healing allows, the type of muscle contractions performed or the position in which an exercise is carried out should mimic the desired functional activity as closely as possible.[197]

Velocity of Exercise

The velocity at which a muscle contracts significantly affects the tension that the muscle produces and subsequently affects muscular strength and power.[209] Exercise velocity is frequently manipulated in a resistance training program to prepare the patient for the variety of functional activities that occur across the wide spectrum of movement velocities.

Force-Velocity Relationship

The force-velocity relationship is different during concentric and eccentric muscle contractions, as depicted in Figure 6.6.

Concentric Muscle Contraction

During a maximum effort concentric muscle contraction, as muscle shortening velocity increases, the force the muscle can generate *decreases*. EMG activity and torque also decrease as a muscle shortens at faster contractile velocities, possibly because the muscle may not have sufficient time to develop peak tension.[50,175,202,236,278]

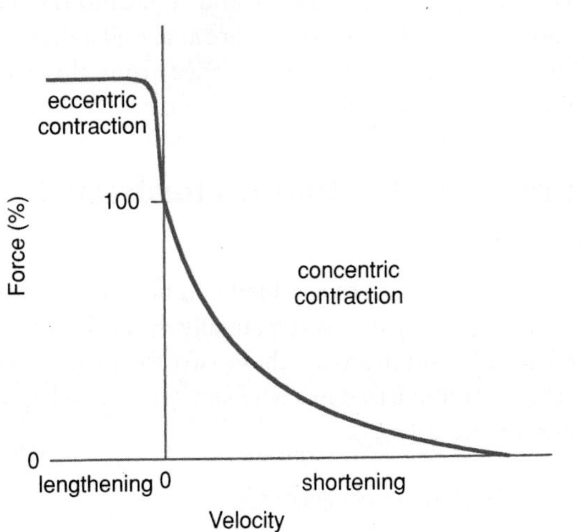

FIGURE 6.6 Force-velocity curve for concentric and eccentric exercise. *(From Levangie, PK, and Norkin, CC:* Joint Structure and Function—A Comprehensive Analysis, *ed. 5. Philadelphia: FA Davis, 2011, p. 121, with permission.)*

Eccentric Muscle Contraction

During a maximum effort eccentric contraction, as the velocity of active muscle lengthening increases, force production in the muscle initially *increases* to a point but then *quickly levels off*.[38,59,175,202,236] The initial increase in force production may be a protective response of the muscle when it is first overloaded. It is thought that this increase may be important for shock absorption or rapid deceleration of a limb during quick changes of direction.[72,236] The force increase may also be caused by passive tension of the noncontractile tissue in muscle.[59] In contrast, other research indicates that eccentric force production is essentially unaffected by velocity and remains constant at slow and fast velocities.[50,115]

Application to Resistance Training

A range of slow to fast exercise velocities should be integrated into an exercise program. Resistance training with free weights is safe and effective only at slow to medium velocities of limb movement so the patient can maintain control of the moving weight. Because many functional activities require higher velocities of limb movement, training at only slow velocities is inadequate. The development of the isokinetic dynamometer during the late 1960s[133,192] gave clinicians a tool to implement resistance training at fast as well as slow velocities. In recent years, some variable resistance exercise units (pneumatic and hydraulic) and elastic resistance products have provided additional options for safely training at fast velocities.

Velocity-specific training is fundamental to a successful rehabilitation program. Study results have shown that training-induced strength gains from a resistance exercise program primarily occur at the training velocities,[24,74,142] with limited transfer of training effects above and below the training velocities.[137,260] Accordingly, training velocities for resistance exercises should be chosen to match or approach the demands of the desired functional activities.[53,142]

Isokinetic training, using *velocity spectrum rehabilitation* regimens, and *plyometric training,* also known as *stretch-shortening drills,* often emphasize high-speed training. These approaches to exercise are discussed later in this chapter and in Chapter 23, respectively.

Periodization and Variation of Training

Periodization, also known as *periodized training,* is an approach to resistance training that partitions a training program into specific time intervals and establishes *systematic variation* in exercise intensity and repetitions, sets, or frequency.[94,162] This approach to training was developed for highly trained athletes preparing for weight lifting or power lifting competition. The intention of periodization is to optimally progress training programs, prevent overtraining and psychological staleness prior to competition, and optimize performance during competition.

Periodization breaks the training calendar into cycles, or phases, that sometimes extend over an entire year. The goal is to prepare for a "peak" performance at the time of competition. Different types of exercises at varying intensities, volume, frequency, and rest intervals are performed over each of the cycles. Although periodization is commonly implemented prior to a competitive event, evidence to support its efficacy is limited.[94,164,184] Periodized training concepts are introduced here because certain applications may be appropriate in the clinical setting for injured athletes during the advanced stage of rehabilitation.[89]

Integration of Function

Balance of Stability and Active Mobility

Functional movements and tasks require a balance of active movement superimposed on a stable background of neuromuscular control. Stability is also necessary to control quick changes of direction during functional movements. Stability is achieved through proper agonist and antagonist muscle activation at individual joints, while mobility requires the correct activation sequencing and intensity across multiple muscle groups. For example, a person must be able to hold the trunk erect and stabilize the spine to grasp, lift, and transport a heavy object. Because of this interaction among stability and active movement, a resistance exercise program must address both the static and dynamic strength of the trunk and extremities.

Balance of Strength, Power, and Endurance

Functional tasks encompass many combinations of muscle strength, power, and endurance, requiring motor capabilities that produce slow and controlled movements, rapid movements, repeated movements, and long-term positioning. Analysis of the tasks a patient would like to be able to do provides the framework for a task-specific resistance exercise program.

Task-Specific Movement Patterns With Resistance Exercise

To prepare the patient for the demands of their regular functional activities, resistance should be incorporated into task-specific movement patterns. Applying resistance during exercise in anatomical planes, diagonal patterns, and combined task-specific movement patterns is an important strategy in a carefully progressed resistance exercise program. Use of simulated functional movements under controlled, supervised conditions is a means to return a patient safely to independent functional activities.[197]

Pushing, pulling, lifting, and holding activities can initially be done against a low level of resistance for a low number of repetitions. Over time, the intensity and dose of the resistance is progressed until the patient returns to using the same movements during functional activities in an unsupervised work or home setting. The key to successful self-management is to teach a patient how to judge the speed, level, and duration of muscle force in combination with the appropriate timing necessary to perform a motor task safely and efficiently.

Types of Resistance Exercise

The types of resistance exercise selected for a rehabilitation or training program are contingent on many factors, including the cause and extent of primary and secondary impairments. Deficits in muscle performance; the stage of tissue healing; the tolerance of joints to compression and movement; the general abilities (physical and cognitive) of the patient; the availability of equipment; and, of course, the patient's goals and the intended functional outcomes of the program must all be considered. A therapist has a large spectrum of exercises from which to choose for a resistance exercise program that will meet the individual needs of each patient. There is no one best form or type of resistance training. Prior to selecting specific types of resistance exercise for a patient's rehabilitation program, a therapist should consider the questions listed in Box 6.7.

Application of the SAID principle is key to making sound exercise decisions. In addition to selecting the appropriate types of exercise, a therapist must also make informed decisions about the intensity, volume, order, frequency, rest interval, and other factors discussed in the previous section of this chapter for effective progression of resistance training. Table 6.5 summarizes general guidelines for progression of exercise.

The types of exercise presented in this section are static and dynamic, concentric and eccentric, isokinetic, and open-chain and closed-chain. In addition, manual and mechanical, and constant and variable resistance exercise will also be discussed. The benefits, limitations, and applications of each of these forms of resistance exercise are analyzed and discussed. When available, supporting evidence from the scientific literature is summarized.

Manual and Mechanical Resistance Exercise

From a broad perspective, a load can be applied to a contracting muscle in two ways: manually or mechanically. The benefits and limitations of these two forms of resistance training are summarized in a later section of this chapter (see Boxes 6.15 and 6.16).

Manual Resistance Exercise

Manual resistance exercise is a type of active-resistive exercise in which external resistance is provided by a therapist or other health professional. A patient can also be taught to apply

BOX 6.7 Selecting Types of Resistance Exercise: Questions to Consider

- Based on the results of your examination and evaluation, what are the type and extent of muscle performance deficits you will need to address?
- Based on the underlying pathology causing the deficits in muscle performance or on the stage of tissue healing, what types of resistance exercise would be most appropriate?
- What are the goals and anticipated functional outcomes of the resistance training program?
- Will dynamic strength or static strength be more effective to achieve the desired outcomes?
- Which types of resistance exercise are most compatible with the desired goals?
- Are there restrictions or limitations to the patients' positioning during resistance exercise?
  - Is weight bearing contraindicated, restricted, or fully permissible?
  - Is there hypomobility of affected or adjacent joints (due to pain or contracture) that may affect how the patient is positioned?
  - Is there a portion of the ROM in which the patient cannot safely or comfortably perform resistance exercises due to hypermobility?
  - Are there cardiovascular or respiratory impairments that may affect positioning?
- Will the patient be expected to perform the exercises independently using mechanical resistance, or will manual resistance applied by the therapist be most appropriate?
- What types of equipment will be available or needed for exercises?
- What types of exercises will replicate or approximate the functional activities required by the patient?

TABLE 6.5 Progression of a Resistance Training Program: Factors to Consider

Factors	Progression
Intensity (exercise load)	Submaximal → maximal (or near-maximal) Low load → high load
Body position (nonweight bearing or weight bearing)	Variable: depending on pathology and impairments, weight-bearing restrictions (pain, swelling, instability) and goals of the rehabilitation program
Repetitions and sets	Low volume → high volume
Frequency	Variable: depends on intensity and volume of exercise
Type of muscle contraction	Static → dynamic Concentric and eccentric: variable progression
Range of motion	Short arc → full arc Stable portion of range → unstable portion of range
Plane of movement	Uniplanar → multiplanar
Velocity of movement	Slow → fast velocities
Neuromuscular control	Proximal → distal control
Functional movement patterns	Simple → complex Single joint → multijoint Proximal control → distal control

self-generated manual resistance to certain muscle groups. Although the amount of resistance cannot be measured quantitatively, this technique is useful in the early stages of an exercise program when the muscle to be strengthened is weak and can overcome only minimal to moderate resistance. It is also useful when the range of joint movements needs to be carefully controlled. The amount of external resistance provided is limited only by the strength of the therapist.

NOTE: Techniques for application of manual resistance exercises in anatomical planes and diagonal patterns are presented in later sections of this chapter.

Mechanical Resistance Exercise

Mechanical resistance exercise is a form of active-resistive exercise in which external resistance is applied through the use of equipment or mechanical apparatus. The amount of resistance can often be measured quantitatively and incrementally progressed over time. Mechanical resistance is useful when the amount of external resistance necessary is greater than what the therapist can apply manually.

NOTE: Systems and regimens of resistance training that involve the use of mechanical resistance, such as PRE, circuit weight training, and velocity spectrum rehabilitation, and the advantages and disadvantages of various types of resistance equipment are addressed later in this chapter.

Isometric Exercise (Static Exercise)

Isometric exercise is a static form of exercise in which a muscle contracts and produces force without an appreciable change in the length of the muscle and without visible joint motion.[175,202] Although there is no mechanical work accomplished (force × distance), a measurable amount of tension and force output are produced by the muscle. Sources of external resistance for isometric exercise include a manually applied force, a weight held in a static joint position, body weight, or an immovable object.

Repetitive isometric contractions, for example a set of 20 per day, held for 6 seconds each against near-maximal resistance, has been shown to be an effective method to improve isometric strength. A *cross-exercise effect* (a limited increase in strength of the contralateral, unexercised muscle group), as the result of transfer of training, also has been observed with maximum isometric training.[63]

Rationale for Use of Isometric Exercise

The need for static strength and endurance is apparent in almost all aspects of body control during functional activities. Recall that most functional activities require a combination of static control at one body region and dynamic activity at another. Loss of static muscle strength occurs rapidly with immobilization and disuse, with estimates from 8% per week[180] to as much as 5% per day.[200]

Functional demands often involve the need to hold a position against either a high level of resistance for a short period of time or a low level of resistance over a prolonged period of time. Of these two aspects of static muscle performance, it is suggested that muscular endurance plays a more important role than muscle strength in maintaining sufficient postural stability and preventing injury during daily living tasks.[184] For example, the postural muscles of the trunk and lower extremities contract isometrically to maintain the body's upright position against gravity and provide stability for balance and functional movements. Dynamic stability of joints during functional activities is achieved by activating and maintaining a low level of co-contraction—that is, concurrent isometric contractions of antagonist muscles that surround joints.[186] The importance of isometric strength and endurance in the elbow, wrist, and finger musculature, for example, is apparent when a person holds and carries a heavy object for an extended period of time.

With these examples in mind, there can be no doubt that isometric exercises are an important part of a rehabilitation program designed to improve functional abilities. The rationale and indications for isometric exercise in rehabilitation are summarized in Box 6.8.

Types of Isometric Exercise

Several forms of isometric exercise can be used to serve different therapeutic purposes during successive phases of rehabilitation. All but one type—muscle setting—incorporate some form of significant resistance and therefore are used to improve static strength or develop sustained muscular control. Because no appreciable resistance is applied during muscle setting, this type of isometric contraction is technically not a form of resistance exercise. However, it is included in this discussion to show a continuum of isometric exercise that can be used for multifaceted goals in a rehabilitation program.

Muscle-setting exercises. Setting exercises involve low-intensity isometric contractions performed against little to no resistance. They are used to decrease muscle pain and spasm and to promote relaxation and circulation during the *acute* stage of healing after soft tissue injury. A common example of muscle setting is the activation of the quadriceps muscles after a knee injury or surgery.

Because muscle setting is performed against no appreciable resistance, it does not improve muscle strength except in very weak muscles. However, setting exercises can slow muscle atrophy and maintain mobility between muscle fibers when a joint is immobilized to protect healing tissues during the very early phase of rehabilitation.

Stabilization exercises. This form of isometric exercise is used to develop a submaximal but sustained level of co-contraction to improve postural stability or dynamic joint stability. Stabilization exercises typically consist of isometric contractions against resistance in antigravity or weight-bearing positions if weight bearing is permissible.[186] External resistance is usually provided by body weight or applied manually.

BOX 6.8 Isometric Exercise: Summary of Rationale and Indications

- To minimize muscle atrophy when joint movement is restricted by external immobilization (casts, orthotics, or skeletal traction)
- To begin re-establishing neuromuscular control of healing tissues when joint movement is not advisable after soft tissue injury or surgery
- To develop postural or joint stability
- To improve muscle strength when use of dynamic resistance exercise could compromise joint integrity or cause joint pain
- To develop static muscle strength at particular points in the ROM consistent with specific task-related needs

Several terms are used to describe specific types of stabilization exercises. They include *rhythmic stabilization* and *alternating isometrics,* two techniques associated with proprioceptive neuromuscular facilitation (PNF) described later in the chapter.[212,272] Stabilization exercises that focus on trunk/postural control are often referred to as *dynamic, core,* and *segmental* stabilization exercises. Applications of these exercises are addressed in Chapter 16. Equipment, such as the BodyBlade® (see Fig. 6.50) and stability balls, are designed for dynamic stabilization exercises.

Multiple-angle isometrics. This term refers to a system of isometric exercise in which resistance is applied at multiple joint positions within the available ROM.[53] This approach is used when the goal of exercise is to improve strength throughout the ROM when joint motion is permissible but dynamic resistance exercise is painful or inadvisable.

Characteristics and Effects of Isometric Training

Effective use of isometric exercise in a resistance training program depends on an understanding of its characteristics, potential benefits, and limitations.

Intensity of muscle contraction. The amount of tension that can be generated during an isometric muscle contraction depends in part on joint position and the subsequent length of the muscle at the time of contraction.[270] The greatest amount of isometric force will be generated at the joint angle at which there is maximum actin and myosin protein overlap and the best potential for cross-bridge formation. Isometric force potential decreases as the joint angle moves progressively further away from this optimal angle. An exercise intensity of at least 60% of a muscle's maximum voluntary contraction is sufficient to improve strength.[156,270] The amount of external resistance against which the muscle is able to hold varies by joint angle and needs to be adjusted at different points in the range. As strength increases from isometric exercise, the external resistance must be progressively increased to continue to overload the muscle.

CLINICAL TIP

When performing isometric exercises, to avoid potential injury to the contracting muscle, apply and release the resistance gradually. This helps to grade the muscle tension and ensures that the muscle contraction is pain-free. This technique also minimizes the risk of uncontrolled joint movement at the onset or completion of the exercise.

Duration of muscle activation. To achieve adaptive changes in static muscle performance, an isometric contraction should be held for 6 seconds and no more than 10 seconds because muscle fatigue develops rapidly. This duration allows sufficient time for peak tension to develop and for metabolic changes to occur in the muscle.[128,184] A 10-second contraction allows a 2-second rise time, a 6-second hold time, and a 2-second fall time.[53]

Repetitive contractions. Sets of repetitive contractions, held for 6 to 10 seconds each, decreases muscle cramping and increases the effectiveness of the isometric regimen.

Joint angle and mode specificity. Gains in muscle strength occur only at or closely adjacent to the joint angle at which resistance is applied—known as the training angle.[155,156,270] Physiological overflow is minimal, occurring no more than 10° in either direction from the training angle.[156] Therefore, when performing multiple-angle isometrics, resistance at four to six different angles in the joint ROM is recommended. Additionally, isometric resistance training is mode specific, causing increases in static strength with little to no impact on dynamic strength.

Sources of resistance. It is possible to perform a variety of isometric exercises with or without equipment. For example, multiple-angle isometrics can be carried out against manual resistance or by simply having the patient push against an immovable object, such as a doorframe or a wall.

Equipment designed for dynamic exercise can be adapted for isometric exercise. A weight-pulley system that provides resistance greater than the force-generating capacity of a muscle leads to a resisted isometric exercise. Most isokinetic devices can be set up with the velocity set at 0° per second at multiple joint angles for isometric resistance at multiple points in the ROM.

PRECAUTION: Patients will often hold their breath during isometric exercise, particularly when performed against substantial external resistance. This is likely to cause a pressor response as the result of the Valsalva maneuver, causing a rapid increase in blood pressure.[87] Rhythmic breathing, emphasizing exhalation during the contraction, should always be performed by the patient during isometric exercise to minimize this response.

CONTRAINDICATION: High-intensity isometric exercises are contraindicated for patients with a history of cardiac or vascular disorders.

Dynamic Exercise: Concentric and Eccentric

A muscle causes joint movement and excursion of a body segment through two unique contraction types—concentric or eccentric. As represented in Figure 6.7, the term *concentric exercise* refers to a form of dynamic muscle activation in which tension develops and physical shortening of the muscle occurs as an external resistance is overcome by internal force, as when lifting a weight. In contrast, *eccentric exercise* involves dynamic muscle activation and tension production that is below the level of external resistance so that physical lengthening of the muscle occurs as it controls the load, as when lowering a weight.

During concentric and eccentric exercise, resistance can be applied in several ways: (1) constant resistance, such as body

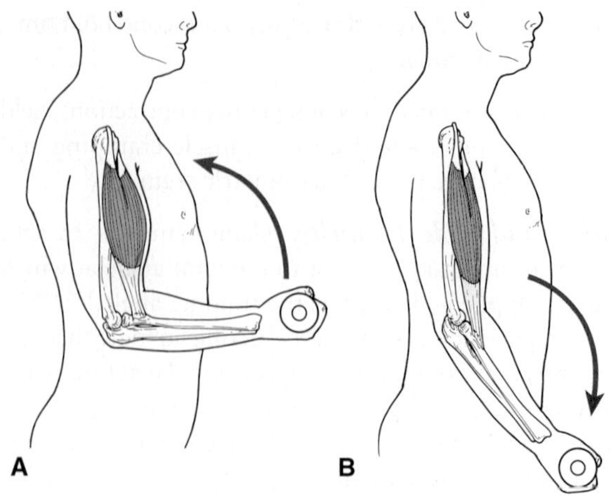

FIGURE 6.7 **(A)** Concentric and **(B)** eccentric strengthening of the elbow flexors occurs as a weight is lifted and lowered.

weight, a free weight, or a simple weight-pulley system; (2) a weight machine or elastic bands that provide variable resistance; or (3) an isokinetic device that maintains the velocity of limb movement.

NOTE: Although the term *isotonic* (meaning equal tension) has been used frequently to describe a resisted, dynamic muscle contraction, application of this terminology is incorrect. In fact, when a body segment moves through its available range, the tension that the muscle is capable of generating *varies* through the range as the muscle shortens or lengthens. This is due to the changing length-tension relationship of the muscle and the changing torque of the external load.[175,202,236] Therefore, in this textbook "isotonic" is not used to describe dynamic resistance exercise.

Rationale for Use of Concentric and Eccentric Exercise

Both concentric and eccentric exercises have distinct value in rehabilitation and conditioning programs. Concentric muscle contractions accelerate body segments, whereas eccentric contractions decelerate body segments. Eccentric contractions also act as a source of energy absorption during high-impact activities.[59,169]

A combination of concentric and eccentric muscle action is used in many daily activities, such as walking up and down inclines, ascending and descending stairs, rising from a chair and sitting back down, or picking up or setting down an object. It is therefore advisable to incorporate a variety of concentric and eccentric resistance exercises in a rehabilitation progression for patients with impaired muscle performance.

Special Considerations for Eccentric Training

Eccentric training is considered an essential component of rehabilitation programs. Eccentric exercises are appropriate following musculoskeletal injury or surgery and in conditioning programs to reduce the risk of injury or re-injury associated with activities that involve high-intensity deceleration, quick changes of direction, or repetitive eccentric muscle contractions.[10,169,205,242] Eccentric training also is thought to improve sport-related physical performance.[8,169]

Traditionally, training that emphasizes high-intensity eccentric loading, such as eccentric isokinetic training or *plyometric training* (see Chapter 23), has been initiated during the advanced phase of rehabilitation to prepare a patient for high-demand sports or work-related activities.[169] Recently, however, progressive eccentric training early in the rehabilitation process has been advocated to more effectively reduce the deficits in strength and physical performance that often persist following a musculoskeletal injury or surgery. However, the safety of early implementation of eccentric resistance exercise is still being evaluated in controlled studies.

FOCUS ON EVIDENCE

Gerber and colleagues[105] conducted a randomized, prospective clinical trial to evaluate a gradually progressed, eccentric exercise program initiated during the *early* phase of rehabilitation (approximately 2 to 3 weeks postoperatively) following arthroscopically assisted anterior cruciate ligament (ACL) reconstruction. All study participants began a 15-week traditional, but "accelerated" (early weight-bearing and ROM) exercise program immediately after surgery. After the first 2 to 3 postoperative weeks, half of the participants (experimental group) performed 12 weeks of gradually progressed, lower extremity training on a motorized eccentric ergometer. A control group followed the same 12 week graduated program on a standard exercise cycle that provided only concentric resistance.

Knee effusion and stability and knee and thigh pain were measured preoperatively and at 15 and 26 weeks postoperatively. Quadriceps strength and single-leg long jump distance were measured prior to surgery and at 26 weeks postoperatively. Results of the study indicated that there were no significant differences in knee or thigh pain and knee effusion and stability between groups at any point during the investigation. Importantly, quadriceps strength and physical performance improved significantly in the eccentric training group but not in the control group. This study demonstrated that the addition of progressively graduated eccentric resistance training during early rehabilitation following ACL reconstruction was safe and effective in reducing strength deficits and improving physical performance.

A 1-year follow-up study by Gerber and colleagues[106] involving 80% of the original study participants demonstrated that quadriceps strength and physical performance continued to be superior in the eccentric training group.

Characteristics and Effects of Concentric and Eccentric Exercise

A summary of the characteristics and effects of eccentric versus concentric resistance exercise is noted in Box 6.9.

BOX 6.9 Eccentric Versus Concentric Exercise: Summary of Characteristics

- Greater external loads can be controlled with eccentric exercise.
- Training-induced gains in muscle strength and mass are greater with maximum-effort eccentric training than with maximum-effort concentric training.
- Adaptations associated with eccentric training are more mode and velocity specific than are adaptations from concentric training.
- Eccentric muscle contractions are more efficient metabolically and generate less fatigue than concentric contractions.
- Following *unaccustomed,* high-intensity eccentric exercise, there is greater incidence and severity of delayed-onset muscle soreness than there is after concentric exercise.

Exercise load and strength gains. A maximum concentric contraction produces less force than a maximum eccentric contraction under the same conditions (see Fig. 6.6). In other words, greater loads can be lowered than lifted. This difference in the magnitude of loads that can be controlled by concentric versus eccentric muscle contractions may be associated with the contributions of the contractile and noncontractile components of muscle. When a load is lowered during an eccentric exercise, the force exerted by the load is controlled not only by the active, contractile components of muscle, but also by the noncontractile connective tissue in and around the muscle. In contrast, when a weight is lifted during concentric exercise, only the contractile components of the muscle contribute to lifting the load.[59]

With a concentric contraction, greater numbers of motor units must be recruited to control the same load compared with an eccentric contraction, suggesting that concentric exercise has less mechanical efficiency than eccentric exercise.[59,72] Consequently, it requires more effort by a patient to control the same load during concentric exercise than during eccentric exercise. As a result, when a weight is lifted and lowered, maximum resistance during the concentric phase of an exercise does not provide a maximum load during the eccentric phase.

If a resistance exercise program involves maximum effort during eccentric and concentric exercise and if the exercise load is increased gradually, eccentric training increases eccentric strength over the duration of a program to a greater degree than concentric training increases concentric strength. This may occur because greater loads can be used for eccentric than concentric training.[223]

CLINICAL TIP

Given that eccentric exercise requires recruitment of fewer motor units to control a load than does concentric exercise, when a muscle is very weak—less than a fair (3/5) muscle grade—active eccentric muscle contractions against no external resistance (other than gravity) can be used to generate active muscle contractions and develop a beginning level of strength and neuromuscular control. In other words, in the presence of substantial muscle weakness, it may be easier to lower the limb against gravity than to raise the limb.

PRECAUTION: There is greater stress on the cardiovascular system (i.e., increased heart rate and arterial blood pressure) during eccentric exercise than during concentric exercise,[59] possibly because greater loads can be used for eccentric training. This underscores the need for rhythmic breathing during high-intensity exercise. (Refer to the Contraindications to Resistance Exercise section of this chapter for additional information on cardiovascular precautions.)

Velocity of exercise. The velocity at which dynamic exercises are performed directly affects the force-generating capacity of the neuromuscular unit.[50,72] Consider that a certain amount of external resistance will result in a contraction of zero velocity (isometric) for a muscle group. If that amount of external resistance is decreased slightly, a concentric contraction will now be able to raise the load, but only with a slow-velocity, high-tension contraction. As the external resistance decreases further, a concentric contraction requires still lower levels of tension to overcome the load and can do so with greater shortening velocity. In contrast, if the amount of external resistance that generates the isometric contraction is increased slightly, an eccentric contraction can lower the external load with high tension at a slow velocity. Progressive increases in the external load will demand increasingly greater eccentric tension at increased velocity until force generating capacity plateaus (see Fig. 6.6).

CLINICAL TIP

A common misconception regarding high-intensity resistance training is that if a weight is lifted quickly (concentric contraction) and lowered slowly (eccentric contraction), the slow eccentric contraction will increase strength because it generates greater tension. In fact, if the load is constant, less tension is generated during the eccentric than the concentric phase. The only way to develop greater tension is to increase the weight of the applied load during the eccentric phase of each exercise cycle. This usually requires assistance from an exercise partner to help lift the load during each concentric contraction. This is a highly intense form of exercise and should be undertaken only by healthy individuals training for high-demand sports or weight lifting competition. This technique is not appropriate for individuals recovering from musculoskeletal injuries.

Energy expenditure. Compared across similar exercise loads, eccentric exercise is more efficient at a metabolic level than concentric exercise[223]—that is, eccentric muscle contractions consume less oxygen and energy stores than concentric contractions.[40] Therefore, the use of eccentric activities such as downhill running may improve muscular endurance more efficiently than similar concentric activities because muscle fatigue occurs less quickly with eccentric exercise.[59,223]

Specificity of training. It is not yet known if the training effects of exercises using concentric or eccentric contractions are mode specific. Although there is substantial evidence to support specificity of training,[25,74,197,230,261] there is also some evidence to suggest that training using one mode leads to strength gains in the other mode.[78] For the most part, however, eccentric training is more mode specific than concentric training.[223] Eccentric exercise also appears to be more velocity specific than concentric exercise.[223] Therefore, because transfer of training in general is quite limited, selection of exercises that simulate the functional movements needed by the patient is always a prudent choice.

Cross-training effect. Both concentric[268] and eccentric[269] training have a cross-training effect—that is, a slight increase in strength occurs over time in the same muscle group of the contralateral, unexercised extremity. This effect also occurs with high-intensity exercise using a combination of concentric and eccentric contractions (lifting and lowering a weight).

The cross-training effect may be caused by repeated contractions of the unexercised extremity in an attempt to stabilize the body during high-effort exercise. Although cross-training is an interesting phenomenon, there is no evidence to suggest that it has a positive impact on a patient's functional capabilities.

Exercise-induced muscle soreness. Repeated and rapidly progressed, high-intensity eccentric muscle contractions are associated with a significantly higher incidence and severity of delayed-onset muscle soreness (DOMS) than occurs with high-intensity concentric exercise.[14,42,99,204] Why DOMS occurs more readily with eccentric exercise is speculative, but it may be the result of greater damage to muscle and connective tissue when heavy loads are controlled and lowered.[14,42] It also has been suggested that the higher incidence of DOMS may adversely affect the training-induced gains in muscle strength.[59,74,99]

It should be noted that there is at least limited evidence to suggest that if the intensity and volume of concentric and eccentric exercise are equal, there is no significant difference in the degree of DOMS after exercise.[92] Further, if the intensity and volume of eccentric exercise is progressed gradually, DOMS does not occur.[105]

Dynamic Exercise: Constant and Variable Resistance

The most common system of dynamic resistance training is *progressive resistance exercise* (PRE). A later section of this chapter, which covers systems of training using mechanical resistance, addresses PRE.

Dynamic Exercise: Constant External Resistance

Dynamic exercise against constant external resistance (DCER) is a form of resistance training in which a limb moves through a ROM against a constant external load,[162] provided by free weights such as a handheld or cuff weight, weight machines, or weight-pulley systems.

This terminology—DCER exercise—is used in place of the term "isotonic (equal tension)" exercise because although the external load does not change, the torque imposed by the weight and the tension generated by the muscle both change throughout the range of movement.[175,236] If the imposed load is less than the torque generated by the muscle, the muscle contracts concentrically and accelerates the load; if the load exceeds the muscle's torque production, the muscle contracts eccentrically to decelerate the load (see Fig. 6.7).

DCER exercise has an inherent limitation. When lifting or lowering a constant load, the contracting muscle is challenged maximally at only the one point in the ROM in which the maximum torque of the resistance matches the maximum torque output of the muscle. A therapist needs to be aware of the changing external torque of the exercise and the changing length-tension relationship of the muscle and modify body position and external resistance accordingly to match where in the range the maximum load needs to be applied (see Figs. 6.46 and 6.47). Despite this limitation, DCER exercise has been and continues to be a mainstay of rehabilitation and fitness programs for effective muscle loading and subsequent training-induced improvements in muscle performance.

Variable Resistance Exercise

Variable resistance exercise, a form of dynamic exercise, addresses the primary limitation of dynamic exercise against a constant external load. Specially designed resistance equipment imposes varying levels of resistance to the contracting muscles to load the muscles more effectively at multiple points in the ROM. The resistance is altered throughout the range by means of a weight-cable system that moves over an asymmetrically shaped cam, by a lever arm system (Fig. 6.8), or by hydraulic or pneumatic mechanisms.[237] How effectively this equipment varies the resistance to match muscle torque curves is questionable.

Dynamic exercise with elastic resistance products (bands and tubing) can also be thought of as variable resistance exercise because of the inherent properties of the elastic material and its response to stretch.[139,145,232] In addition to the progressive resistance increases inherent to elastic bands or tubing, the change in the orientation that the force is applied to the body will also contribute to the variable resistance profile of these products. (Refer to the final section of this chapter for additional information on exercise with elastic resistance devices.)

NOTE: When dynamic exercise is performed against manual resistance, a skilled therapist can vary the load applied to

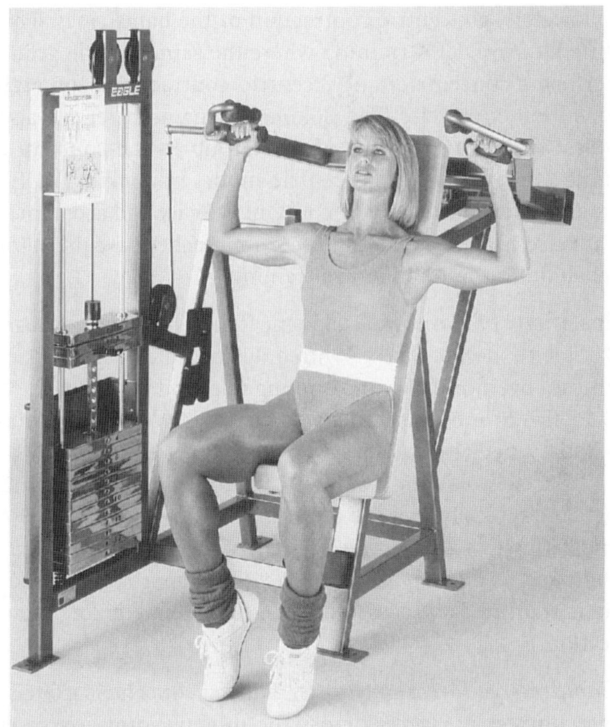

FIGURE 6.8 Cybex/Eagle Fitness Systems shoulder press provides variable resistance throughout the range of motion. *(Courtesy of Cybex, Division of Lumex, Ronkonkoma, NY.)*

the contracting muscle throughout the ROM. The therapist adjusts the resistance based on the patient's effort and response so the muscle is appropriately loaded throughout the ROM.

Special Considerations for DCER and Variable Resistance Exercise

Excursion of limb movement. During either DCER or variable resistance exercise, the excursion of limb movement is controlled exclusively by the patient (with the exception of exercising on resistance equipment that has a range-limiting device). When free weights, weight-pulley systems, and elastic devices are used, additional muscles may be recruited to control the arc and direction of limb movement.

Velocity of exercise. Although most daily living, occupational, and sport activities occur at medium to fast velocities of limb movement, dynamic exercises are most often performed at a relatively slow velocity to avoid momentum and uncontrolled movements, which could jeopardize the safety of the patient. (As a point of reference, dynamic exercise with a free weight typically is performed at about 60° per second.[53]) Consequently, the training-induced improvements in muscle strength that occur only at slow velocities may not prepare the patient for activities that require rapid bursts of strength or quick changes of direction.

CLINICAL TIP

Hydraulic and pneumatic variable resistance equipment and elastic resistance products allow safe, moderate- to high-velocity resistance training.

Isokinetic Exercise

Isokinetic exercise is a form of dynamic exercise in which the velocity of the joint angular velocity is predetermined and held constant by a rate-limiting device known as an isokinetic dynamometer (Fig. 6.9).[53,76,133,192] The term *isokinetic* refers to movement that occurs at a constant velocity. Unlike DCER exercise in which a specific amount of resistance is selected and superimposed on the contracting muscle, in isokinetic exercise the *velocity* of limb movement—not the load—is maintained during the effort. The external resistance force encountered by the muscle will vary according to the amount of force applied to the equipment.[4,133]

Because the external resistance adjusts to the effort applied to the equipment, isokinetic exercise is also called *accommodating resistance exercise.*[133] If an individual gives maximum effort during exercise, the torque they produce will vary across the range of joint motion due to changes in muscle length and internal moment arms. An isokinetic dynamometer quantifies this variable torque and accommodates or adjusts the external resistance so that velocity is held constant. When the movement being performed is in the vertical plane, the dynamometer will adjust to the combination of gravity and muscle force. Although early advocates of isokinetic training suggested it was superior to resistance training with free weights or weight-pulley systems, this claim has not been well supported by evidence. Today, isokinetic training is regarded as one of many tools that can be integrated into the later stages of rehabilitation.[5]

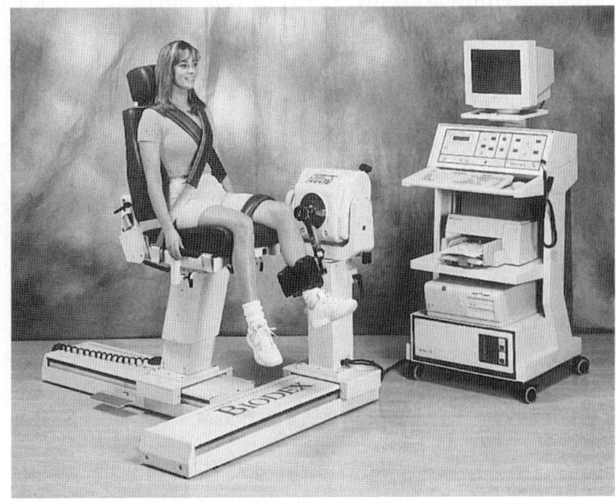

FIGURE 6.9 Biodex isokinetic dynamometer is used for testing and training. *(Courtesy of Biodex Medical Systems, Inc., Shirley, NY.)*

Characteristics of Isokinetic Training

A brief overview of the key characteristics of isokinetic exercise is provided in this section. For more detailed information on isokinetic testing and training, a number of resources are available.[4,53,75,76,116]

Constant velocity. Fundamental to the concept of isokinetic exercise is that joint angular velocity is preset and controlled by the unit and remains relatively constant throughout the ROM. Due to limb inertia, there is usually a short period at the start and end ranges of exercise motion where angular velocity is not constant.

Range and selection of training velocities. Isokinetic dynamometry affords a wide range of exercise velocities. Current dynamometers can adjust the velocity of limb movement from 0° per second (isometric mode) up to 500° per second. As shown in Table 6.6, training velocities are classified as slow, medium, and fast. This range provides a mechanism by which a patient can prepare for the demands of functional activities that occur across a range of movement velocities.

Training velocities should be matched as specifically as possible to the demands of the anticipated functional tasks. The faster training velocities are similar to the velocities of limb movements inherent in some functional motor skills such as walking or lifting.[4,283] For example, the average angular velocity of the lower extremity during walking has been calculated at 230° to 240° per second.[5,53,283] Despite this example, the velocity of limb movements during many functional activities far exceeds the fastest training velocities available with dynamometry.

The training velocities selected may also be based on the mode of exercise (concentric or eccentric) to be performed. As noted in Table 6.6, the range of training velocities recommended for concentric exercise is greater than the range of velocities for eccentric training.[4,76,116]

Reciprocal versus isolated muscle training. One advantage of isokinetic dynamometry is the ability to provide resistance to opposing muscle groups at a joint, referred to as reciprocal training. For example, the training parameter can be set so the patient performs concentric contraction of the quadriceps followed by concentric contraction of the hamstrings. This differs from DCER training where the same muscle group performs concentric and eccentric contractions for each repetition of exercise. The isokinetic dynamometer can also be set to target the same muscle group in the concentric mode, followed by the eccentric mode, mimicking DCER training with the benefit of constant velocity and accommodating resistance.[282] Both of these approaches have merit for rehabilitation and functional training.

TABLE 6.6 Classification of Velocity of Training in Concentric Isokinetic Exercises*

Classification	Angular Velocity
Isometric	0°/sec
Slow	30°–60°/sec
Medium	60°–180°or 240°/sec
Fast	180 or°240°–360°/sec or greater

*Training velocities tend to be substantially slower for eccentric training, ranging from 30° to 120°/sec with most eccentric training initiated between 60° and 120°/sec.

Specificity of training. Isokinetic training for the most part is velocity specific [23,116,142] with only limited evidence of significant overflow from one training velocity to another.[137,260] Evidence of mode specificity (concentric versus eccentric) with isokinetic exercise is less clear.[10,76,115,197,230]

Because isokinetic exercise tends to be velocity specific, patients typically exercise at several velocities (between 90° and 360° per second) using a system of training known as *velocity spectrum rehabilitation.*[4,53,76] (This approach to isokinetic training is discussed later in the Isokinetic Regimens section.)

Compressive forces on joints. During concentric exercise the compressive forces across the moving joint are lower at faster angular velocities than they are at slower velocities.[4,53,75,76] This effect is consistent with the constructs that muscle force decreases as movement velocity increases during concentric contractions and that lower muscle forces minimize joint reaction forces.

Accommodation to fatigue. Because the external resistance encountered is directly proportional to the force applied to the resistance arm of the isokinetic unit, lower muscle force output does not necessarily result in cessation of motion. This means that as the contracting muscle fatigues, the patient is still able to perform additional repetitions at the constant velocity even though the force output of the muscle is diminishing.

Accommodation to a painful arc. If a patient experiences transient pain at some portion of the arc of motion during exercise and uses less force to move through that arc, isokinetic training accommodates by reducing the external resistance applied to the limb. If the patient stops a resisted motion because of the sudden onset of pain, the external resistance is eliminated as soon as the patient stops pushing against the torque arm of the dynamometer.

Training Effects and Carryover to Function

Numerous studies have shown that isokinetic training is effective for improving one or more of the muscle performance parameters (strength, power, and endurance).[10,24,76,137,185,197] In contrast, only a limited number of studies have investigated the relationship between isokinetic training and improvement in the performance of functional skills. Two such studies indicated that high-velocity concentric and eccentric isokinetic training was associated with increased velocity of a tennis serve and throwing a ball.[78,193]

Limitations in carryover. Several factors inherent in the design of most types of isokinetic equipment may limit the extent to which isokinetic training carries over to improvements in functional performance. Although isokinetic training affords a spectrum of velocities for training, the velocity of limb movement during many daily living and sport-related activities far exceeds the maximum velocity settings available on isokinetic equipment. In addition, limb movements during most functional tasks occur at multiple velocities, not at a constant velocity, depending on the conditions of the task.

Furthermore, isokinetic exercise usually isolates a single muscle or opposing muscle groups, involves movement of a single joint, is uniplanar, and does not involve weight bearing. Although isolation of a single muscle can be beneficial in remediating strength deficits, most functional activities require contraction of multiple muscle groups and movement spanning multiple joints in several planes of motion. It is important to note, however, that some of these limitations can be addressed by adapting the setup of the equipment to allow multi-axis movements in diagonal planes, multijoint resisted movements, or closed-chain training.

Special Considerations for Isokinetic Training

Availability of Equipment

From a pragmatic perspective, one limitation of isokinetic exercise is that a patient can incorporate this form of exercise into a rehabilitation program only by going to a facility where the equipment is available. In addition, the patient will require assistance to set up the equipment and may need supervision during exercise. These availability considerations contribute to the high costs associated with a rehabilitation program using isokinetic dynamometry.

Appropriate Setup

The positioning recommended by the product manufacturers may need to be altered to ensure that the exercise is safe for a particular joint. For example, although the 90°/90° position of the shoulder and elbow is recommended for strengthening the shoulder rotators, it may be safer to exercise the patient in the resting position or with the arm at the side.

Initiation and Progression of Isokinetic Training During Rehabilitation

Isokinetic training typically is begun in the later stages of rehabilitation, when active motion through the full or available ROM is pain-free. Suggested guidelines for implementation and progression are summarized in Box 6.10.[4,53,76,116]

BOX 6.10 Progression of Isokinetic Training for Rehabilitation

- Initially, to keep resistance low, submaximal isokinetic exercise is implemented before maximal effort isokinetic exercise.
- When avoiding an unstable or painful portion of the ROM is necessary, short-arc movements are used before full-arc motions.
- Slow to medium training velocities (60°–180°/sec) are used before progressing to faster velocities.
- Maximal concentric contractions at multiple velocities are performed before introducing eccentric isokinetic exercises for the following reasons:
  - Concentric isokinetic exercise is easier to learn and is fully under the control of the patient.
  - The velocity of movement of the resistance arm is not controlled by the patient during eccentric isokinetic exercise but is robotically controlled by the dynamometer.

Open Kinetic Chain and Closed Kinetic Chain Exercise

Background

In clinical practice and the rehabilitation literature, functional activities and exercises are often categorized as having weight-bearing or nonweight-bearing characteristics. The descriptors closed kinetic chain and open kinetic chain are commonly used and are similar in meaning to weight bearing and nonweight bearing, respectively. These concepts, extended to the analysis of human movement during the 1950s by Steindler,[244] were proposed to provide a system for classifying two unique approaches to function and exercise.

Steindler[244] described the open kinetic chain as the combination of sequentially arranged joints in which the terminal segment is free to move. He proposed that the term applies to completely unrestricted movement in space of a peripheral segment of the body, as in waving the hand or swinging the leg. Open-chain exercises typically focus on motion at a single joint. In contrast, closed kinetic chain exercises are those in which the terminal segment meets considerable external resistance such that distal movement is restrained. This implies that with the terminal segment fixed, external resistance moves proximal segments and joints over the stationary distal segment. Closed kinetic chain exercises are said to emphasize joint compression and are considered more functional in nature than open kinetic chain exercises. Both Steindler and Brunnstrom noted that the action of a muscle changes when the terminal segment is free to move versus when it is fixed in place. For example, in an open kinetic chain the tibialis posterior muscle functions to invert and plantarflex the foot and ankle. In contrast, during the stance phase of gait, the tibialis posterior functions to first decelerate pronation of the subtalar joint and then supinate the same joint to improve foot rigidity for terminal push-off.

Controversy and Inconsistency in Use of Open-Chain and Closed-Chain Terminology

Although this terminology to describe exercises is prevalent in clinical practice and the rehabilitation literature, there is lack of consensus about how—or even if—it should be used and about what constitutes an open kinetic chain versus a closed kinetic chain exercise.[25,67,68,118,239,275]

One source of inconsistency is whether or not weight bearing is an inherent component of closed kinetic chain activities. Steindler[244] did not specify that weight bearing must occur for a motion to be categorized as closed kinetic chain, but many of his examples, particularly in the lower extremities, involved weight bearing. In the rehabilitation literature, closed kinetic chain exercises both do[57,93] and do not[122,239] include weight bearing as a necessary element. One resource suggests that all weight-bearing exercises involve some elements of closed kinetic chain activity, but not all closed kinetic chain exercises are performed in weight-bearing positions.[239] For example, squat exercises are considered a weight-bearing and closed kinetic chain activity, while leg press exercises are not weight bearing yet may be considered closed kinetic chain.

Another point of ambiguity is whether or not the terminal segment must be absolutely fixed in place on a surface to be classified as a closed kinetic chain motion. Although Steindler[244] described this as one condition of a closed kinetic chain motion, another condition allows that if the "considerable external resistance" is overcome, there can be movement of the terminal segment. These two concepts can appear to be at odds with each other, creating uncertainty regarding the correct use of this terminology.

Lifting a handheld weight or pushing against the force arm of an isokinetic dynamometer are consistently cited in the literature as examples of open kinetic chain exercises.* Although there is no axial loading in these exercises, if the terminal segment is overcoming considerable external resistance an argument could be made for calling these closed kinetic chain exercises.[*56,57,79,93,122,221,245,275,280]

Given the complexity of human movement, it is not surprising that a single classification system using two descriptors cannot adequately classify the multitude of movements found in functional activities and therapeutic exercise interventions.

Alternatives to Open Kinetic Chain and Closed Kinetic Chain Terminology

To address the unresolved issues associated with this terminology, several authors have offered alternative or additional terms to classify activities and exercises. One suggestion is to use the terms, *distally fixated* and *nondistally fixated* instead of closed kinetic chain and open kinetic chain.[196] The terms *distal segment fixed* and *distal segment free* are also commonly used substitutes. Another suggestion is to add a third descriptor dubbed *partial kinetic chain*[275] to describe exercises in which the distal segment (hand or foot) meets resistance but is not absolutely stationary, such as using a leg press machine, stepping machine, or slide board. The term *closed kinetic chain* is then reserved for instances when the terminal segment does not move.

Another classification system categorizes exercises as either *joint isolation exercises* (movement of only one joint segment) or *kinetic chain exercises* (simultaneous movement of multiple segments linked by more than one joint).[153,213] Boundaries of movement of the distal segment (movable or stationary) or loading conditions (weight bearing or nonweight bearing) are not parameters of this terminology. However, other, more complex classification systems do take these conditions into account.[68,174]

An additional option is to describe the specific conditions of exercises, where most open kinetic chain exercises are described as single-joint nonweight-bearing exercises and most closed kinetic chain exercises are identified as multiple-joint weight-bearing exercises.[126]

Despite the suggested alternatives, open and closed kinetic chain terminology continues to be widely used in clinical practice and the literature.† Therefore, recognizing the inconsistencies and limitations of the terminology and that many exercises and functional activities involve a combination of "open" and "closed" conditions, the authors of this textbook will continue to use open and closed kinetic chain terminology to describe exercises. The commonly used shortened versions (open-chain and closed-chain) will also be used throughout the text.[†26,32,56,57,70,76,77,118,122,143,189,250,280]

Characteristics of Open Kinetic Chain and Closed Kinetic Chain Exercises

The following operational definitions and characteristics of open- and closed-chain exercises are presented for clarity and as the basis for the discussion of exercises described throughout this textbook. The parameters of the definitions are those most frequently noted in the current literature. Common characteristics of open- and closed-chain exercises are compared in Table 6.7.

Open-Chain Exercises

Open-chain exercises involve motions in which the distal segment (hand or foot) is free to move in space, without necessarily causing simultaneous motions at adjacent joints.[56,77,79,93,153] Limb movement only occurs *distal* to the moving joint, and muscle activation occurs in the muscles that cross the moving joint. For example, during knee flexion in an open-chain exercise (Fig. 6.10), the action of the hamstrings is independent of recruitment of other hip or ankle musculature. Open-chain exercises also are typically performed in nonweight-bearing positions.[57,93,189,285] During resistance training, the external load is applied to the moving distal segment.[56,77,79,93,122,153,189,239,275]

Closed-Chain Exercises

Closed-chain exercises involve motions in which the body or proximal segments move on a distal segment that is fixed or stabilized on a support surface. Movement at one joint causes simultaneous motions at distal and proximal joints in a relatively predictable manner. For example, when performing a bilateral short-arc squatting motion (mini-squat) (Fig. 6.11) and then returning to an erect position, as the knees flex and extend, the hips and ankles move in predictable patterns.

TABLE 6.7 Characteristics of Open-Chain and Closed-Chain Exercises

Open-Chain Exercises	Closed-Chain Exercises
Distal segment moves in space	Distal segment remains fixed or in contact with support surface
Independent joint movement; no predictable joint motion in adjacent joints	Interdependent joint movements; relatively predictable movement patterns in adjacent joints
Movement of body segments distal to the moving joint only	Movement of body segments may occur distal and/or proximal to the moving joint
Muscle activation occurs predominantly in the prime mover and is isolated to muscles crossing the moving joint	Muscle activation occurs in multiple muscle groups, both distal and proximal to the moving joint
Typically performed in nonweight-bearing positions	Typically but not always performed in weight-bearing positions
Resistance is applied to the moving distal segment	Resistance is applied simultaneously to multiple moving segments
External rotary loading of joints is typical	Axial loading of joints through body-weight is typical
External stabilization (manually or with equipment) often required	Internal stabilization by means of muscle action, joint compression and congruency, and postural control

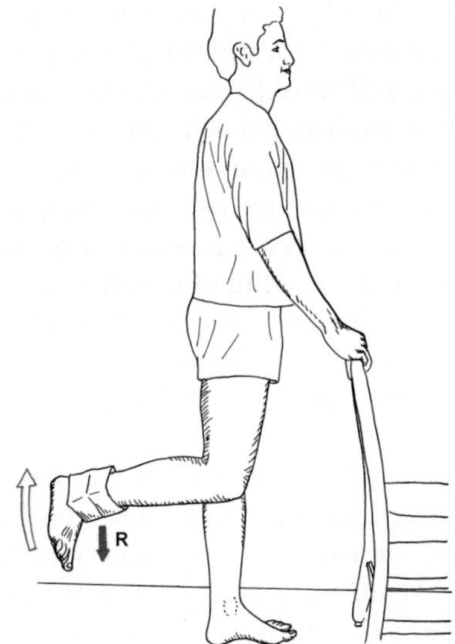

FIGURE 6.10 Open-chain resisted knee flexion.

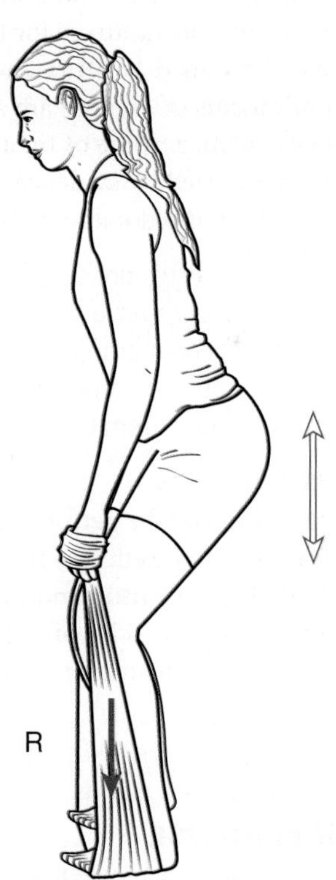

FIGURE 6.11 Bilateral closed-chain resisted hip and knee flexion/extension.

Closed-chain exercises are typically performed in weight-bearing positions.[56,78,93,122,189,285] Examples in the upper extremities include balance activities in quadruped, press-ups from a chair, wall push-offs, or prone push-ups; examples in the lower extremities include lunges, squats, step-up or step-down exercises, or heel rises.

NOTE: In this textbook, the scope of closed-chain exercises includes weight-bearing activities in which the distal segment *moves but remains in contact with the support surface,* as when using a bicycle, cross-country ski machine, or stair-stepping machine. In the upper extremities, chin-ups at an overhead bar qualify as a nonweight-bearing closed-chain activity.

Rationale for Use of Open-Chain and Closed-Chain Exercises

The rationale for selecting open- or closed-chain exercises is based on the goals of an individualized rehabilitation program and a critical analysis of the potential benefits and limitations inherent in either form of exercise. Because functional activities involve many combinations of both open- and closed-chain motions, it is appropriate to include task-specific open- and closed-chain exercises into rehabilitation and conditioning programs. Both types can be successfully integrated into treatment sessions and home programs to add training variation and appropriately challenge the patient.

 **FOCUS ON EVIDENCE**

There is no evidence to support the global assumption that closed-chain exercises are "more functional" than open-chain exercises. A review of the literature by Davies[54] indicated there is a substantial body of evidence that both open- and closed-chain exercises are effective for reducing upper and lower extremity muscle performance deficits. However, of these studies, very few randomized, controlled trials demonstrated that the muscle performance improvements were associated with a reduced functional limitation or improved physical performance.

A summary of the benefits and limitations of open- and closed-chain exercises and the rationale for their use follows. Whenever possible, presumed benefits and limitations or comparisons of both forms of exercise are analyzed in light of existing scientific evidence. Some of the reported benefits and limitations are supported by evidence, while others are often based on opinion or anecdotal reports.

NOTE: Most reports and investigations comparing or analyzing open- or closed-chain exercises have focused on the knee, in particular the ACL or patellofemoral joint. Far fewer articles have addressed the application or impact of open- and closed-chain exercises on the upper extremities.

Isolation of Muscle Groups

Open-chain exercises improve the performance of individual muscles or muscle groups more effectively than closed-chain exercises. The potential for substitute motions that compensate for and mask strength deficits of individual muscles is likely greater with closed-chain exercise than open-chain exercise.

 **FOCUS ON EVIDENCE**

In a study of the effectiveness of a closed-chain-*only* resistance training program after ACL reconstruction, residual muscle weakness of the quadriceps femoris was identified.[238] The investigators suggested that this residual strength deficit might have been avoided with the inclusion of open-chain quadriceps training in the postoperative rehabilitation program.

Control of Movements

During open-chain resisted exercises, a greater level of motion control is possible with a *single* moving joint than with multiple moving joints, as occurs during closed-chain training. With open-chain exercises, stabilization is usually applied externally by a therapist's manual contacts or with belts or straps. In contrast, during closed-chain exercises the patient most often uses muscular stabilization to control joints or structures proximal and distal to the targeted joint. This improved ability to isolate motion to the target joint during open-chain training is particularly advantageous during the early phases of rehabilitation.

Joint Approximation

Almost all muscle contractions include a compressive component that approximates the joint surfaces and provides stability to the joint in both open- or closed-chain situations.[175,202,236] Additional joint approximation occurs during weight bearing and is associated with lower levels of shear forces at a moving joint. This has been demonstrated at the knee, with decreased anterior or posterior tibiofemoral translation during weight-bearing activities.[284,285] The joint approximation that occurs with the axial loading and weight bearing during closed-chain exercises is thought to cause an increase in joint congruency, which in turn contributes to stability during the exercise.[56,77]

Co-activation and Dynamic Stabilization

Because most closed-chain exercises are performed in weight-bearing positions, it is widely assumed that they stimulate joint and muscle mechanoreceptors, facilitate co-activation of agonists and antagonists (co-contraction), and consequently promote dynamic stability.[212,251,265] During a standing squat, for example, the quadriceps and hamstrings contract concurrently to control knee and hip motion, respectively, making this exercise an appropriate choice for improving knee stability. In studies of muscle activation during lower extremity closed-chain exercises, these assumptions have been both supported[31,48,276] and refuted.[80]

Upper extremity closed-chain exercises are also thought to promote co-activation of the scapular and glenohumeral stabilizers and improve dynamic stability of the shoulder complex.[77,275] While plausible, evidence of shoulder girdle muscle co-contraction during weight-bearing exercises, such as a prone push-up or a press-up from a chair, is limited.[170] Some open-chain exercises are also thought to encourage muscle co-contraction. Exercises such as alternating isometrics associated with PNF,[212.251,265] stretch-shortening drills performed in nonweight-bearing positions,[277] use of a Body-Blade® (see Fig. 6.50), and high-velocity isokinetic training may all stimulate co-activation of muscle groups and promote dynamic stability. Evidence of a co-contraction effect using these open-chain approaches is currently limited.

In studies of high-velocity, concentric isokinetic training of knee musculature,[71,117] co-activation of agonist and antagonist muscle groups was noted briefly at the end the range of knee extension. Investigators speculated that the knee flexors contracted eccentrically to decelerate the limb just before contact was made with the extension ROM stop. In contrast, there was no evidence of co-activation of knee musculature during maximum effort, slow-velocity (60° per second) isokinetic training.[167] It is possible that only high-velocity isokinetic exercise elicits this co-contraction effect.

PRECAUTION: High-load, open-chain exercise may have an adverse effect on unstable, injured, or recently repaired joints, as demonstrated in the ACL-deficient knee.[80,143,276,284]

Proprioception, Kinesthesia, Neuromuscular Control, and Balance

Conscious awareness of joint position and movement is one of the foundations of motor learning during the early phase of training for neuromuscular control of functional movements. After soft tissue or joint injury, proprioception and kinesthesia may be disrupted and alter neuromuscular control. Re-establishing the use of sensory information from the injured region to effectively initiate and control movement is a high priority in rehabilitation.[173] Studies have shown that proprioception and kinesthesia improve after rehabilitation of the ACL-reconstructed knee.[17,171]

It is thought that closed-chain training elicits greater proprioceptive and kinesthetic feedback than open-chain training. Theoretically, because multiple muscle groups are activated across several moving joints, closed-chain exercises trigger sensory receptors in a greater number of muscles and intra-articular and extra-articular structures. The weight-bearing element of closed-chain exercises, which increases joint approximation, is believed to stimulate the mechanoreceptors and enhance sensory input for the control of movement.[122,171-174,221,251,276]

FOCUS ON EVIDENCE

Despite the assumption that proprioception and kinesthesia are enhanced to a greater extent under closed-chain than open-chain conditions, the evidence is mixed. One study[172] demonstrated that kinesthesia in patients with unstable shoulders improved to a greater extent with a program of closed-chain *and* open-chain exercises compared with a program of open-chain exercises only. In contrast, subjects evaluated for their ability to detect knee position showed no significant differences during closed- versus open-chain conditions.[255]

Lastly, closed-chain training is the obvious choice to improve upright balance and postural control. Balance training is an essential element of rehabilitation for patients after musculoskeletal injuries or surgery to restore functional abilities and reduce the risk of re-injury.[149] Activities and parameters to challenge the body's balance mechanisms are discussed in Chapter 8.

Carryover to Function and Injury Prevention

There is ample evidence to demonstrate that both open- and closed-chain exercises effectively improve muscle strength, power, and endurance.[54,56,57] Evidence also suggests that if there is a comparable level of external loading applied to a muscle group, EMG activity is similar regardless of whether open-chain or closed-chain exercises are performed.[25,68]

That being said, and consistent with the principles of motor learning and task-specific training, if exercises are to have a beneficial effect on functional outcomes, they should be selected based on their ability to simulate the patients' functional requirements and goals.[56,118,239,275]

FOCUS ON EVIDENCE

In a study of 24 healthy subjects, closed-chain barbell squats and open-chain isokinetic knee extension were compared for their effects on a vertical jump test. Subjects were randomized into two groups and trained twice each week for 6 weeks, progressively increasing the amount of external resistance used for exercise. The close chain group improved 10% in their vertical jump performance, while the open-chain group did not improve relative to their baseline performance.[15] Closed-chain training, specifically a program of jumping activities, has also been shown to decrease landing forces through the knees and reduce the risk of knee injuries in female athletes.[129]

Implementation and Progression of Open-Chain and Closed-Chain Exercises

Principles and general guidelines for the implementation and progression of open-chain and closed-chain exercises are similar with respect to variables such as intensity, volume, frequency, and rest intervals. These variables were discussed earlier in the chapter. Relevant features of closed-chain exercises and guidelines for progression are summarized in Table 6.8.

Introduction of Open-Chain Training

Because open-chain training typically is performed in non-weight-bearing postures, it may be the only option when weight bearing is contraindicated or must be significantly restricted. Soft tissue pain and swelling or restricted motion of any segment of the chain may also necessitate the use of open-chain exercises at adjacent joints. For example, after a tibia fracture the lower extremity is usually immobilized in a long leg cast and weight bearing is restricted for at least a few weeks. During this period, open-chain hip strengthening exercises can still be initiated and gradually progressed until partial weight-bearing and closed-chain activities are permissible.

Any activity that involves open-chain motions can be easily replicated with open-chain exercises, first by developing isolated control and strength of the weak musculature and then by combining motions to simulate functional patterns.

Closed-Chain Exercises and Weight-Bearing Restrictions: Use of Unloading

If weight bearing must be restricted, a safe alternative to open-chain exercises may be to perform closed-chain exercises while partial weight bearing on the involved extremity. This is simple to achieve in the upper extremity; but in the lower extremity, because the patient is in an upright position during

TABLE 6.8 Parameters and Progression of Closed-Chain Exercises

Parameters	Progression
% Body weight	Partial → full weight-bearing (LE: aquatic exercise, parallel bars, overhead harnessing; UE: wall push-up → modified prone push-up → prone push-up) Full weight bearing + additional weight (weighted vest or belt, handheld or cuff weights, elastic resistance)
Base of support	Wide → narrow Bilateral → unilateral Fixed on support surface → sliding on support surface
Support surface	Stable → unstable/moving (LE: floor → rocker board, wobble board, sideboard, treadmill) (UE: floor, table or wall → rocker or side board, ball) Rigid → soft (floor, table → carpet, foam) Height: ground level → increasing height (low step → high step)
Balance	With external support → no external support Eyes open → eyes closed
Excursion of limb movement	Small → large ranges Short arc → full arc (if appropriate)
Plane or direction of movement	Uniplanar → multiplanar Anterior → posterior → diagonal (forward walking → retrowalking; forward step-up → backward step-up) Sagittal → frontal or transverse (forward-backward sliding → side to side sliding; forward or backward step-up → lateral step-up)
Speed of movement or directional changes	Slow → fast

closed-chain exercises, axial loading in one or both lower extremities must be reduced.

Two methods for reducing lower extremity weight bearing during closed-chain exercise are aquatic therapy, as described in Chapter 9, or using parallel bars to unload the limb during standing. The buoyancy of water assists with lower extremity unloading, but the resistance of the water can limit movement velocity and pools are not always accessible. A limitation of using parallel bars is the difficulty in controlling the amount of weight bearing during exercises. An alternative strategy, if available, is the use of a bodyweight-supported treadmill training system to unload the lower extremities.[151] These systems enable the patient to perform a variety of closed-chain exercises and to begin ambulation at functional speeds early in rehabilitation.

Progression of Closed-Chain Exercises

The parameters and suggestions for progression of closed-chain activities noted in Table 6.8 are not all inclusive and are flexible. As a rehabilitation program progresses, more advanced forms of closed-chain training, such as plyometric training and agility drills (discussed in Chapter 23), can be introduced.[58,79] The selection and progression of activities is always based on the discretion of the therapist as they consider the patient's response to the current exercises and their functional needs.

General Principles of Resistance Training

The principles of resistance training presented in this section apply to both manual and mechanical resistance exercises for persons of all ages, but they are not hard and fast rules. There are many instances when these principles may need to be modified based on therapist judgment. Additional guidelines specific to the application of manual resistance exercise, PNF, and mechanical resistance exercise are addressed in later sections of this chapter.

Examination and Evaluation

As with all forms of therapeutic exercise, a comprehensive examination and evaluation is the cornerstone of an individualized resistance training program. Therefore, prior to initiating any form of resistance exercise:

- Perform a thorough examination of the patient, including a health history, systems review, and selected tests and measurements.
  - Determine qualitative and quantitative baselines of strength, muscular endurance, ROM, and overall level of functional performance against which progress can be measured.
  - Administer a standardized outcome measure that is valid and reliable for the patient's condition.
- Evaluate the findings to determine if the use of resistance exercise is appropriate or inappropriate at this time. Some questions that may help with this interpretation are noted in Box 6.11. Be sure to identify the most functionally relevant impairments, the goals the patient is seeking to achieve, and the expected functional outcomes of the exercise program.
- Establish how resistance training will be integrated into the plan of care with other therapeutic exercise interventions,

BOX 6.11 Is Resistance Training Appropriate? Questions to Consider

- Were deficits in muscle performance identified? If so, do these deficits appear to be contributing to limitations of functional abilities that you have observed or that the patient or family has reported?
- Could identified muscle performance deficits cause future functional limitations?
- What is the irritability and current stage of healing of involved tissues?
- Is there evidence of tissue swelling?
- Is there pain? If so, is pain present at rest or with movement, noted at a specific portion of the ROM, or located in specific tissues?
- Are there other deficits such as impaired mobility, balance, sensation, coordination, or cognition that are adversely affecting muscle performance?
- What are the patient's goals or desired functional outcomes? Are they realistic in light of the identified muscle performance deficits?
- Given the patient's current status, are resistance exercises indicated? Contraindicated?
- Will the identified muscle performance deficits be eliminated or minimized with resistance exercises?
- Should one type of muscle performance be emphasized over another?
- Will the patient require supervision or assistance over the course of the exercise program or can the program be carried out independently?
- What is the expected frequency and duration of the resistance training program? Will a maintenance program be necessary?
- Are there any precautions specific to the patient's physical status, general health, or age that may warrant special consideration?

such as stretching, joint mobilization techniques, balance training, and cardiopulmonary conditioning exercises.

- Re-evaluate periodically to document progress and determine if and how the dosage of exercises (intensity, volume, frequency, and rest) and the types of resistance exercise should be adjusted to continue to challenge the patient.

Preparation for Resistance Exercises

- Select and prescribe the forms of resistance exercise that are appropriate and expected to be effective, such as choosing manual or mechanical resistance exercises, or both.
- If implementing mechanical resistance exercise, determine what equipment is needed and available.
- Review the anticipated goals and expected functional outcomes with the patient.
- Explain the exercise plan and procedures. Be sure that the patient and/or family understands and gives consent.
- Have the patient wear nonrestrictive clothing and supportive shoes appropriate for exercise.
- If possible, select a firm but comfortable support surface for exercise.
- Demonstrate each exercise and the desired movement pattern.

Implementation of Resistance Exercises

NOTE: These general guidelines apply to the use of *dynamic* exercises against manual *or* mechanical resistance. In addition to these guidelines, refer to special considerations and guidelines unique to the application of manual and mechanical resistance exercises in the chapter sections that follow.

Warm-Up

Warm-up prior to resistance exercises using light, repetitive, dynamic, site-specific movements without applying resistance. For example, prior to lower extremity resistance exercises, have the patient walk on a treadmill for 5 to 10 minutes followed by flexibility exercises for the trunk and lower extremities.

Placement of Resistance

- Resistance is most often applied to the distal end of the segment on which the muscle to be strengthened attaches. For example, to strengthen the anterior deltoid, resistance is applied to the distal humerus as the patient flexes the shoulder (Fig. 6.12). Distal placement of resistance generates the greatest amount of external torque with the least amount of manual or mechanical resistance.
- Resistance may be applied across an intermediate joint if that joint is stable and pain-free and if there is adequate muscle strength supporting the joint. For example, to strengthen the anterior deltoid using mechanical resistance, a handheld weight is a common source of resistance.

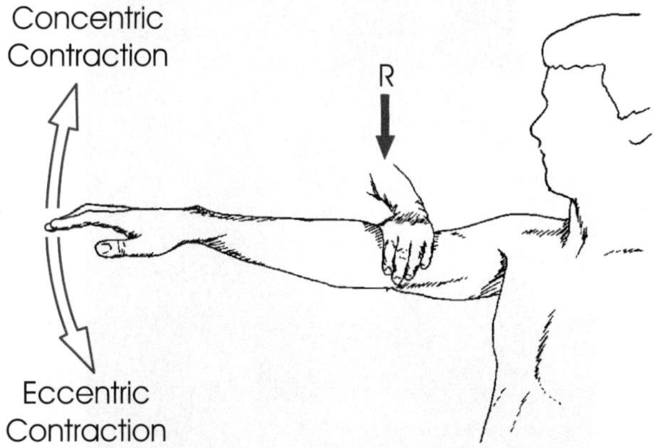

FIGURE 6.12 Resistance (R) is applied to the distal end of the segment being strengthened. Resistance is applied in the *direction opposite* to that of limb movement to resist a concentric muscle contraction and in the *same direction* as limb movement to resist an eccentric contraction.

- If pressure from the external load is uncomfortable for the patient, the therapist can either change the location of resistance or enlarge the area over which the resistance is applied.

Direction of Resistance

During concentric exercise resistance is applied in the direction directly opposite to the desired motion, whereas during eccentric exercise resistance is applied in the same direction as the desired motion (see Fig. 6.12). When using manual resistance, the force will be most mechanically effective if applied perpendicular to the segment through the entire arc of motion.

Stabilization

Stabilization is necessary to avoid unwanted, substitute motions.

- For nonweight-bearing resisted exercises, external stabilization is applied to the proximal segment on which the muscle to be strengthened attaches. For example, with biceps brachii muscle strengthening, stabilization should occur at the anterior shoulder as elbow flexion is resisted (Fig. 6.13). When appropriate, belts or straps can be effective sources of external stabilization.
- During multijoint resisted exercises in weight bearing, the patient must use muscle activation and control to stabilize nonmoving segments.

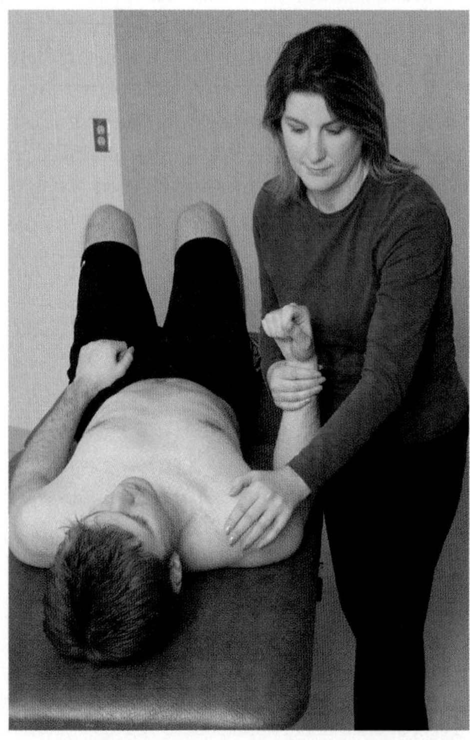

FIGURE 6.13 Stabilization is applied at the proximal attachment of the muscle being strengthened. In this figure, the proximal humerus and scapula are stabilized as elbow flexion is resisted.

Intensity of Exercise/Amount of Resistance

NOTE: The intensity of the exercise must be consistent with the intended goals of resistance training and the type of muscle contraction as well as other aspects of dosage.

- Initially, have the patient practice the movement pattern against a minimal load to learn the correct exercise technique.
- Have the patient exert a forceful but controlled and pain-free effort. The level of resistance should be such that movement performance is smooth and nonballistic.
- Adjust the alignment, stabilization, or the amount of resistance if the patient is unable to complete the available ROM, muscular tremor develops, or substitute motions occur.

Number of Repetitions, Sets, and Rest Intervals

- In general, for most adults, use 8 to 12 repetitions of a specific motion against a moderate exercise load. This quantity typically induces the expected acute and chronic responses of muscular fatigue and adaptive gains in muscular strength.
- Decrease the amount of resistance if the patient cannot complete the minimum target number of 8 repetitions.
- After a brief rest, perform additional repetitions—a second set of 8 to 12 repetitions, if possible.
- For progressive overloading, initially increase the number of repetitions or sets; at a later point in the exercise program, gradually increase the resistance.

Verbal or Written Instructions

When teaching an exercise using mechanical resistance or when applying manual resistance, use simple instructions that are easily understood. Do not use medical terminology or jargon. For example, tell the patient to "Bend and straighten your elbow" rather than "Flex and extend your elbow." Be sure that descriptions of resistance exercises to be performed as part of a home program are written and clearly illustrated.

Monitoring the Patient

Observe the patient execute the exercises and modify any ineffective or incorrectly performed techniques (position, stabilization, speed, and fatigue). Assess the patient's responses before, during, and after exercise using combinations of subjective and objective information. Regularly monitor the patient's vital signs to evaluate the physiological responses to exercise relative to subjective and objective information. Adhere to relevant precautions discussed in the next section of the chapter.

Cool-Down

Cool-down after a series of resistance exercises using rhythmic, unresisted movements such as arm swinging, walking, or stationary cycling. Gentle stretching is also appropriate after resistance exercise.

Precautions for Resistance Exercise

Regardless of the goals of a resistance exercise program and the types of exercises prescribed and implemented, the exercises must not only be effective but *safe*. The therapist's interpretation of the examination's findings will help determine effectiveness, while awareness of precautions maximizes patient safety. General precautions for resistance training are summarized in Box 6.12. Additional information about several of these precautions is presented in the following section.

Valsalva Maneuver

The Valsalva maneuver or phenomenon, defined as an expiratory effort against a closed glottis, must be avoided during resistance exercise. The Valsalva maneuver is characterized by the following sequence. A deep inspiration is followed by closure of the glottis and contraction of the abdominal muscles. This increases intra-abdominal and intrathoracic pressures, which in turn forces blood from the heart, causing an abrupt, temporary increase in arterial blood pressure.[144]

During exercise the Valsalva phenomenon occurs most often with *high-effort* isometric[87] and dynamic[179] muscle contractions. It has been shown that the rise in blood pressure induced by an isometric muscle contraction is proportional to the percentage of maximum voluntary force exerted.[179] A Valsalva maneuver superimposed on a maximum effort contraction will increase the risk of cardiovascular injury. Although the Valsalva phenomenon is thought to occur most often with isometric[87,144] and eccentric[59] resistance exercise, a recent study[179] indicated that the rise in blood pressure appears to be based more on extent of effort—not strictly on the type (mode) of muscle contraction.

At-Risk Patients

The risk of complications from a rapid rise in blood pressure is particularly high in patients with a history of coronary artery disease, myocardial infarction, cerebrovascular disorders, or hypertension. Also at risk are patients who have undergone neurosurgery or eye surgery or who have intervertebral disk pathology. The breathing of high-risk patients must be monitored closely during exercise.

BOX 6.12 General Precautions During Resistance Training

- Keep the ambient temperature of the exercise setting comfortable for vigorous exercise.
- Select clothing for exercise that facilitates heat dissipation and sweat evaporation.
- Caution the patient that pain should *not* occur *during* exercise.
- Do not initiate resistance training at a maximal level of resistance, particularly with eccentric exercise to minimize delayed-onset muscle soreness (DOMS). Use light to moderate exercise during the recovery period.
- Avoid use of heavy resistance during exercise for children, older adults, and patients with osteoporosis.
- Do not apply resistance across an unstable joint or distal to a fracture site that is not completely healed.
- Have the patient avoid breath-holding during resisted exercises to prevent the Valsalva maneuver; emphasize exhalation during exertion.
- Avoid uncontrolled, ballistic movements as they compromise safety and effectiveness.
- Prevent incorrect or substitute motions by adequate stabilization and an appropriate level of resistance.
- Avoid exercises that place excessive, unintended secondary stress on the back.
- Be aware of medications a patient is using that can alter acute and chronic responses to exercise.
- Avoid cumulative fatigue due to excessive frequency of exercise and the effects of overtraining or overwork. Incorporate adequate rest intervals between exercise sessions to allow adequate time for recovery.
- Discontinue exercises if the patient experiences pain, dizziness, or unusual or precipitous shortness of breath.

CLINICAL TIP

Although resistance training is often recommended for individuals at risk for or a history of cardiovascular disorders, it is important to determine those individuals for whom resistance training is safe and appropriate. In addition to knowledge of screening guidelines for resistance training,[6] close communication with a patient's physician is essential. After clearance for exercise, low-intensity resistance training (30% to 40% intensity for upper body exercises and 50% to 60% intensity for lower body exercises) is recommended.[6]

Risk Prevention During Resistance Exercise

- Caution the patient about breath-holding.
- Ask the patient to breathe rhythmically, count, or talk during exercise.
- Have the patient exhale when lifting and inhale when lowering an exercise load.[8]
- Restrict high-risk patients from doing high-intensity resistance exercises.

Substitute Motions

When the external resistance is too great for the target muscle to manage during exercise, substitute motions can occur. Similarly, when muscle performance declines during exercise because of fatigue or pain, a patient may recruit other muscles or use alternate movements to compensate.[152] For example, if the deltoid or supraspinatus muscles are weak or abduction of the arm is painful, a patient may elevate the scapula and laterally flex the trunk to the opposite side to elevate the arm. To avoid substitute motions during exercise, the appropriate amount of resistance must be applied and correct stabilization must be used.

Overtraining and Overwork

Exercise programs, in which heavy resistance is applied or exhaustive training is performed repeatedly, must be progressed cautiously to avoid a problem known as overtraining or overwork. These terms refer to deterioration in muscle performance and physical capabilities (either temporary or permanent) that can occur in healthy individuals or in patients with certain neuromuscular disorders.

In most instances, the uncomfortable sensation associated with acute muscle fatigue induces an individual to cease exercising. This is not necessarily the case in highly motivated athletes who are said to be *overreaching* in their training program[101] or in patients who may not adequately sense fatigue because of impaired sensation associated with a neuromuscular disorder.[211]

Overtraining

The term *overtraining* is commonly used to describe a decline in physical performance in healthy individuals participating in high-intensity, high-volume strength and endurance training programs.[101,166] The terms *chronic fatigue*, *staleness*, and *burnout* are also used to describe this phenomenon. When overtraining occurs, the individual progressively fatigues more quickly and requires more time to recover from strenuous exercise because of physiological and psychological factors.

Overtraining is brought on by inadequate rest intervals between exercise sessions, too rapid progression of exercises, and inadequate diet and fluid intake. Fortunately, in healthy individuals, overtraining is a preventable, reversible phenomenon that can be resolved by periodically decreasing the volume and frequency of exercise.[101,161,164,166]

Overwork

The term *overwork*, sometimes called *overwork weakness*, refers to progressive deterioration of strength in muscles already weakened by nonprogressive neuromuscular disease.[211] This phenomenon was first observed more than 50 years ago in patients recovering from polio who were actively involved in rehabilitation.[21] In many instances the decrement in strength that was noted was permanent or prolonged. More recently, overwork weakness has been reported in patients with other nonprogressive neuromuscular diseases, such as Guillain-Barré syndrome.[52] Postpolio syndrome is also thought to be related to long-term overuse of weak muscles.[90]

Overwork weakness has been experimentally produced in laboratory animals,[124] providing some insight into its cause. When strenuous exercise was initiated soon after a peripheral nerve lesion, the return of functional motor strength was slowed, suggesting excessive protein breakdown in the denervated muscle.

Prevention is the key to dealing with overwork weakness. Patients in resistance exercise programs who have impaired neuromuscular function or a systemic, metabolic, or inflammatory disease that increases susceptibility to muscle fatigue must be monitored closely, progressed slowly and cautiously, and re-evaluated frequently to determine their response to resistance training. These patients should not exercise to exhaustion and should be given longer and more frequent rest intervals during and between exercise sessions.[3,52]

Exercise-Induced Muscle Soreness

Almost every individual who begins a resistance training program experiences muscle soreness. This effect is especially common in those who are unaccustomed to exercise and if the program includes eccentric exercise. Exercise-induced muscle soreness falls into two categories: acute and delayed onset.

Acute Muscle Soreness

Acute muscle soreness develops during or directly after strenuous exercise performed to the point of muscle exhaustion.[43] This response occurs from the inadequate blood flow and oxygenation, combined with a temporary build-up of metabolites such as lactic acid and potassium in the exercised muscle.[7,43] The sensation is characterized as a feeling of burning or aching in the muscle. It is thought that the noxious metabolic waste products stimulate free nerve endings and cause pain. This soreness experienced during intense exercise is transient and subsides quickly after stopping the exercise when adequate blood flow and oxygen are restored to the muscle. An appropriate cool-down period of low-intensity exercise (active recovery) can facilitate this process.[49]

Delayed-Onset Muscle Soreness

With vigorous and unaccustomed resistance training or any form of muscular overexertion, DOMS, which is noticeable in the muscle belly or at the myotendinous junction,[66,97,138] develops approximately 12 to 24 hours after the exercise session. As was already pointed out in the discussion of concentric and eccentric exercise in this chapter, high-intensity eccentric muscle contractions consistently cause the most severe DOMS symptoms.[14,59,72,92,97,207] Box 6.13 lists the signs and symptoms over the time course of DOMS. Although the time course varies, the signs and symptoms, which can last up to 10 to 14 days, gradually dissipate.[14,72,92]

Etiology of DOMS. Despite years of research dating back to the early 1900s, the underlying mechanisms (mechanical, neural, or/or cellular) of tissue damage associated with DOMS is still unclear.[42,187] Several theories have been proposed, with some subsequently refuted. Early investigators proposed the *metabolic waste accumulation theory,* which suggested that both acute and delayed-onset muscle soreness

BOX 6.13 Delayed-Onset Muscle Soreness: Clinical Signs and Symptoms

- Muscle soreness and aching beginning 12 to 24 hours after exercise, peaking at 48 to 72 hours, and subsiding 2 to 3 days later
- Tenderness with palpation throughout the involved muscle belly or at the myotendinous junction
- Increased soreness with passive lengthening or active contraction of the involved muscle
- Local edema and warmth
- Muscle stiffness reflected by spontaneous muscle shortening[62] before the onset of pain
- Decreased ROM during the time course of muscle soreness
- Decreased muscle strength prior to onset of muscle soreness that persists for up to 1 to 2 weeks after soreness has remitted[39]

was caused by a build-up of lactic acid in muscle after exercise. Although this is a source of muscle pain with acute exercise, this theory has been disproved as a cause of DOMS.[266] Multiple studies have shown that it requires only about 1 hour of recovery after exercise to exhaustion to remove almost all lactic acid from skeletal muscle and blood.[97]

The *muscle spasm theory* was also proposed as the cause of DOMS, suggesting that a feedback cycle of pain caused by ischemia and a build-up of metabolic waste products during exercise led to muscle spasm.[65] This build-up, it was hypothesized, caused the DOMS sensation and an ongoing reflex pain-spasm cycle that lasted for several days after exercise. The muscle spasm theory has been discounted in subsequent research that showed no increase in EMG activity and, therefore, no evidence of spasm in muscles with delayed soreness.[2]

Although studies on the specific etiology of DOMS continue, current research seems to suggest that DOMS is linked to some form of contraction-induced, mechanical disruption or microtrauma of muscle fibers and/or connective tissue in and around muscle that results in tissue degeneration.[42,99] Evidence of tissue damage such as elevated blood serum levels of creatine kinase is present for several days after exercise and is accompanied by inflammation and edema.[2,98,99]

The temporary loss of strength and the perception of soreness associated with DOMS appear to occur independently and follow different time courses. Strength deficits develop prior to the onset of soreness and persist after soreness has remitted.[62,204] Thus, force production deficits appear to be the result of muscle damage, possibly myofibrillar damage at the Z bands,[42,203] which directly affects the structural integrity of the contractile units of muscle, rather than neuromuscular inhibition as the result of pain.[203,204]

Prevention and treatment of DOMS. Prevention and treatment of DOMS at the initiation of an exercise program have been either ineffective or, at best, marginally successful. It is a commonly held opinion in clinical and fitness settings that the initial onset of DOMS can be prevented or at least kept to a minimum by progressing the intensity and volume of exercise *gradually*,[46,72] by performing low-intensity warm-up and cool-down activities,[64,72,235] or by gently stretching the exercised muscles before and after strenuous exercise.[64,235] Although these techniques are regularly advocated and employed, little to no evidence in the literature supports their efficacy in the prevention of DOMS.

There is some evidence to suggest that the use of repetitive concentric exercise prior to DOMS-inducing eccentric exercise does not entirely prevent but does reduce the severity of muscle soreness and other markers of muscle damage.[206] Paradoxically, a regular routine of eccentric exercise performed prior to the onset of DOMS or after an initial episode of DOMS has developed can minimize its effects.[7,42,43,46] This response is often referred to as the "repeated-bout effect," whereby a bout of eccentric exercise protects the muscle from damage from subsequent bouts of eccentric exercise.[187] It may well be that with repeated bouts of the same level of eccentric exercise or activity that caused the initial episode of DOMS, the muscle adapts to the physical stress and prevents additional episodes of DOMS.[7,42,169,187]

To date, the efficacy of DOMS treatment has been mixed. Evidence shows that continuation of a training program that has induced DOMS does not worsen the muscle damage or slow the recovery process.[42,207] Light, high-speed isokinetic, concentric exercise has been reported to reduce muscle soreness and hasten the remediation of strength deficits associated with DOMS,[120] but other reports suggest no significant improvement in strength or relief of muscle soreness with light exercise.[69,267]

The effectiveness of therapeutic modalities and massage techniques is also questionable. Electrical stimulation to reduce soreness has been reported to be effective[62,147] and ineffective.[267] Although cryotherapy, specifically cold water immersion, after vigorous eccentric exercise reduces signs of muscle damage, little to no effect on the perpetuation of muscle tenderness or strength deficit is reported.[81] Also, there is no significant evidence that post-exercise massage, despite its widespread use in sports settings, reduces the signs and symptoms of DOMS.[147,259,267] Other treatments, such as hyperbaric oxygen therapy and nutritional supplements, also have limited benefits.[46] However, use of compression sleeves[160,165] and topical salicylate creams, which provide an analgesic effect, may reduce the severity of and hasten the recovery from DOMS-related symptoms.

FOCUS ON EVIDENCE

In a prospective study[160,165] of DOMS that was induced by maximal eccentric exercise, the use of a compression sleeve over the exercised muscle group resulted in no increase in circumferential measurements of the upper arm, suggesting the prevention of soft tissue swelling. In participants wearing a sleeve, there was also a more rapid reduction in the perception of muscle soreness and a more rapid amelioration of deficits in peak torque than in those who did not wear the compression sleeve.

In summary, although some interventions for the treatment of DOMS appear to have potential, a definitive treatment has yet to be determined.

Pathological Fracture

When an individual has or is at high risk for osteoporosis or osteopenia, the risk of pathological fracture from participating in a resistance exercise program must be considered. *Osteoporosis,* which is discussed in greater detail in Chapter 11 and in Chapter 24, is a systemic skeletal disease characterized by reduced mineralized bone mass that is associated with an imbalance between bone resorption and bone formation, leading to fragility of bones. In addition to the loss of bone mass, there also is narrowing of the bone shaft and widening of the medullary canal.[7,30,168]

The changes associated with osteoporosis make the bone less able to withstand physical stress making them highly susceptible to pathological fracture. A *pathological fracture,* or fragility fracture, is the failure of bone already weakened by disease that results from minor stress to the skeletal system.[30,110,201] Pathological fractures most commonly occur in the vertebrae, femurs, wrists, and ribs.[110,168] Therefore, to design and implement a safe exercise program, a therapist needs to know if a patient has a history of osteoporosis and, as such, an increased risk of pathological fracture. If there is no known history of osteoporosis, the therapist must be able to recognize those factors that place a patient at risk for osteoporosis.[30,51,168] As noted in Chapter 11, postmenopausal women, for example, are at high risk for primary (type I) osteoporosis. Secondary (type II) osteoporosis is associated with prolonged immobilization or disuse, restricted weight bearing, or extended use of certain medications, such as systemic corticosteroids or immunosuppressants.

Prevention of Pathological Fracture

Numerous studies have demonstrated that physical activity that includes resistance training has positive osteogenic effects. Consequently, in addition to aerobic exercises that involve weight-bearing, resistance exercises have become an essential element of rehabilitation and conditioning programs for individuals with or at risk for osteoporosis.[6,7,218,228] Therefore, individuals who are at risk for pathological fracture often engage in resistance training with a goal of increasing bone density.

Successful, safe resistance training must impose a great enough load to satisfy the overload principle and achieve the goals of the exercise program but not so heavy a load as to cause a pathological fracture. Guidelines and precautions during resistance training to reduce the risk of pathological fracture for individuals with or at risk for osteoporosis are summarized in Box 6.14.[201,218,228]

BOX 6.14 Resistance Training Guidelines and Precautions to Reduce the Risk of Pathological Fracture

- *Intensity of exercise.* Avoid high-intensity, high-volume weight training. Depending on the severity of osteoporosis, begin weight training at a minimal intensity (40% to 60% of 1-RM) and progress to moderate-intensity (60% to <80% of 1-RM) only if indicated.
- *Repetitions and sets.* Initially, perform only one set of several exercises, using 8 to 12 repetitions of each exercise for the first 6 to 8 weeks.
  - Progress intensity and volume (repetitions) gradually; eventually work up to three or four sets of each exercise at moderate levels of intensity.
- *Frequency.* Perform resistance exercises two to three times per week.
- *Type of exercise.* Integrate weight-bearing activities into resistance training, but use the following precautions:
  - Avoid high-impact activities such as jumping or hopping. Perform most strengthening exercises in weight-bearing postures that involve low impact, such as lunges or step-ups/step-downs against additional resistance (handheld weights, a weighted vest, or elastic resistance).
  - Avoid high-velocity movements.
  - Avoid trunk flexion with rotation and end-range resisted flexion of the spine. Such combinations can place excessive loading on the anterior portion of the vertebrae, potentially resulting in anterior compression fracture, wedging of the vertebral body, and loss of height.
  - Avoid lower extremity weight-bearing activities that involve torsional movements of the hips, particularly if there is evidence of osteoporosis of the proximal femur.
  - To avoid loss of balance during lower extremity exercises while standing, have the patient hold onto a stable surface such as a countertop. If the patient is at high risk for falling or has a history of falls, perform exercises in a chair to provide weight bearing through the spine.
  - In group exercise classes, keep participant-instructor ratios low; for patients at high risk for falling or with a history of previous fracture, consider direct supervision on a one-to-one basis from another trained person.

Contraindications to Resistance Exercise

There are only a few instances when resistance exercises are contraindicated. Resistance training is most often contraindicated during periods of acute inflammation and with some acute diseases and disorders. By carefully selecting the appropriate type (mode) of exercise (static versus dynamic; weight bearing versus nonweight bearing) and keeping the initial intensity of the exercise at a low to moderate level, adverse effects from resistance training can almost always be avoided.

Pain

If a patient experiences severe joint or muscle pain during active movements against no external load, dynamic resistance exercises should not be initiated. During testing, if a patient experiences acute muscle pain during a resisted isometric contraction, resistance exercises should not be initiated. Lastly, if a patient experiences pain that cannot be eliminated by reducing the external resistance, the exercise should be stopped.

Inflammation

Dynamic and static resistance training is absolutely contraindicated in the presence of inflammatory neuromuscular disease. For example, in patients with acute anterior horn cell disease (Guillain-Barré) or inflammatory muscle disease (polymyositis, dermatomyositis) resistance exercises may actually cause irreversible deterioration of strength through damage to muscle. *Dynamic* resistance exercises are contraindicated in the presence of acute inflammation of a joint. The use of dynamic resisted exercise can irritate the joint and cause more inflammation. Gentle setting exercises against negligible resistance are appropriate.

Severe Cardiopulmonary Disease

Severe cardiac or respiratory diseases or disorders associated with acute symptoms contraindicate resistance training. For example, patients with severe coronary artery disease, carditis, cardiac myopathy, congestive heart failure, or uncontrolled hypertension or dysrhythmias should not participate in vigorous physical activities, including a resistance training program.[6]

After myocardial infarction or coronary artery bypass graft surgery, resistance training should be postponed for at least 5 weeks (that includes participation in 4 weeks of supervised cardiac rehabilitation endurance training) and until clearance from the patient's physician has been received.[6]

Manual Resistance Exercise

Definition and Use

Manual resistance exercise is a form of active resistive exercise in which the resistance force is applied to either a dynamic or a static muscular contraction by the therapist.

- When joint motion is permissible, resistance is usually applied throughout the available ROM.
- Resistance is applied during exercise carried out in anatomical planes of motion, in diagonal patterns associated with PNF techniques,[159,265] or in combined patterns of movement that simulate functional activities.
- A specific muscle may also be strengthened by resisting the action of that muscle, as described in manual muscle-testing procedures.[132,152]
- In rehabilitation programs, manual resistance exercise, which may be preceded by active-assisted and active exercise, is part of the continuum of active exercises available to a therapist to improve or restore muscular performance.

There are many advantages to the use of manual resistance exercises, but there also are disadvantages and limitations to this form of resistance exercises. These issues are summarized in Box 6.15.

Guidelines and Special Considerations

The general principles for the application of resistance exercises discussed in the preceding section of this chapter also apply to manual resistance exercise. In addition, there are some special considerations unique to manual resistance exercises that should be followed. The following guidelines apply to manual resistance exercise carried out in anatomical planes of motion and in diagonal patterns association with PNF.

BOX 6.15 Manual Resistance Exercise: Advantages and Disadvantages

Advantages
- Most effective during the early stages of rehabilitation when muscles are weak (MMT of 4/5 or less).
- Effective form of exercise for transition from assisted to mechanically resisted movements.
- More finely graded resistance than mechanical resistance.
- Resistance is adjusted throughout the ROM as the therapist responds to the patient's efforts or a painful arc.
- Muscle works maximally at all portions of the ROM.
- The range of joint movement can be carefully controlled by the therapist to protect healing tissues or to prevent movement into an unstable portion of the range.
- Useful for dynamic or static strengthening.
- Direct manual stabilization prevents substitute motions.
- Can be performed in a variety of patient positions.
- Placement of resistance is easily adjusted.
- Gives the therapist an opportunity for direct interaction and continuous monitoring of the patient's performance.

Disadvantages
- Exercise load (amount of resistance) is subjective; it cannot be measured or quantitatively documented for purposes of establishing a baseline or exercise-induced improvements in muscle performance.
- Amount of resistance is limited to the strength of the therapist; therefore, resistance imposed is not adequate to strengthen already strong muscle groups.
- Speed of movement is slow to moderate, which may not carry over to most functional activities.
- Cannot be performed independently by the patient for most muscle groups.
- Not useful in home program unless caregiver assistance is available.
- Labor and time intensive for the therapist.
- Impractical for improving muscular endurance; too time-consuming.

Body Mechanics of the Therapist

- Select a treatment table on which to position the patient that is a suitable height or adjust the height of the patient's bed, if possible, to enhance use of proper body mechanics.
- Assume a position close to the patient to avoid stresses on your low back and to maximize control of the patient's upper or lower extremity.
- Use a wide base of support to maintain stability while applying resistance; shift your weight to move as the patient moves his or her limb.

Application of Manual Resistance and Stabilization

- Review the principles and guidelines for placement and direction of resistance and stabilization (see Figs. 6.12 and 6.13). Stabilize the proximal attachment of the contracting muscle with one hand, when necessary, while applying resistance distally to the moving segment. Use appropriate hand placements (manual contacts) to provide tactile and proprioceptive cues to help the patient better understand in which direction to move.[251]
- Grade and vary the amount of resistance to equal the abilities of the muscle throughout the available ROM.

CLINICAL TIP

When applying manual resistance, the therapist must possess well-developed skills in order to provide enough resistance to challenge but not overpower the patient's efforts, especially when the patient has significant weakness.

- Gradually apply and release the resistance so movements are smooth, not unexpected or uncontrolled.
- Hold the patient's extremity close to your body so some of the force applied is from the weight of your body not just the strength of your upper extremities. This enables you to apply a greater amount of resistance, particularly as the patient's strength increases.
- When applying manual resistance to alternating isometric contractions of agonist and antagonist muscles to develop joint stability, maintain manual contacts at all times as the isometric contractions are repeated. As a transition is made from one muscle contraction to another, no abrupt relaxation phase or joint movements should occur between the opposing contractions.

Verbal Commands

- Coordinate the timing of the verbal commands with the application of resistance to maintain control when the patient initiates a movement.
- Use simple, direct verbal commands.
- Use different verbal commands to facilitate isometric, concentric, or eccentric contractions. To resist an *isometric* contraction, tell the patient to "Hold," "Don't let me move you," or "Match my resistance." To resist a *concentric* contraction, tell the patient to "Push" or "Pull." To resist an *eccentric* contraction, tell the patient to "Slowly let go as I push or pull you."

Number of Repetitions and Sets/Rest Intervals

- As with all forms of resistance exercise, the number of repetitions is dependent on the response of the patient.
- For manual resistance exercise, the number of repetitions also is contingent on the strength and endurance of the therapist.
- Build in adequate rest intervals for the patient *and* the therapist; after 8 to 12 repetitions, both the patient and the therapist typically begin to experience some degree of muscular fatigue.

Techniques: General Background

The manual resistance exercise techniques described in this section are for the upper and lower extremities, performed concentrically in anatomical planes of motion. The direction of limb movement would be the opposite if manual resistance were applied to an eccentric contraction. The exercises described are performed in nonweight-bearing positions and involve movements to isolate individual muscles or muscle groups.

Consistent with Chapter 3, most of the exercises described and illustrated in this section are performed with the patient in a *supine position.* Variations in the therapist's position and hand placements may be necessary, depending on the size and strength of the therapist and the patient. Alternative patient positions, such as prone or sitting, are described when appropriate or necessary. Ultimately, a therapist must be versatile and able to apply manual resistance with the patient in all positions to meet the needs of many patients with significant differences in abilities, limitations, and pathologies.

NOTE: In all illustrations in this section, the direction in which resistance (R) is applied is indicated with a solid arrow.

Reciprocal motions, such as flexion/extension and abduction/adduction, are often alternately resisted in an exercise program in which strength and balanced neuromuscular control in both agonists and antagonists are desired. Resistance to reciprocal movement patterns also enhances a patient's ability to reverse the direction of movement smoothly and quickly, a neuromuscular skill that is necessary in many functional activities. Reversal of direction requires muscular control of both prime movers and stabilizers and combines concentric and eccentric contractions to decrease momentum and make a controlled transition from one direction to the opposite direction of movement.

Manual resistance in diagonal patterns associated with PNF are described and illustrated in the next section of this chapter. Additional resistance exercises to increase strength, power, endurance, and neuromuscular control in the extremities can be found in Chapters 17 through 23. In these chapters many examples and illustrations of resisted eccentric exercises, exercises in weight-bearing positions, and exercises in functional movement patterns are featured. Resistance exercises for the cervical, thoracic, and lumbar spine are described and illustrated in Chapter 16.

Upper Extremity

Shoulder Flexion VIDEO 6.1

Hand Placement and Procedure

- Apply resistance to the anterior aspect of the distal arm or to the distal portion of the forearm if the elbow is stable and pain-free (Fig. 6.14).
- Stabilization of the scapula and trunk is provided by the treatment table.

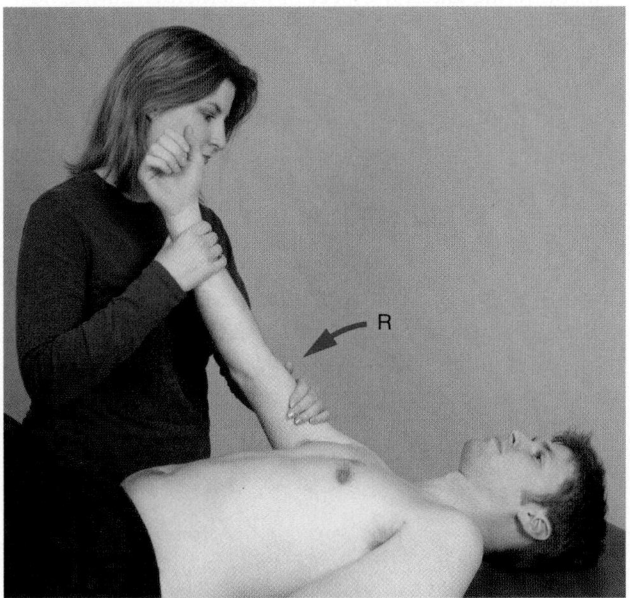

FIGURE 6.14 Resisted shoulder flexion.

Shoulder Extension

Hand Placement and Procedure

- Apply resistance to the posterior aspect of the distal arm or the distal portion of the forearm.
- Stabilization of the scapula is provided by the table.

Shoulder Hyperextension

The patient assumes the supine position, close to the edge of the table, side-lying, or prone so hyperextension can occur.

Hand Placement and Procedure

- Apply resistance in the same manner as for extension of the shoulder.
- Stabilize the anterior aspect of the shoulder if the patient is supine.
- If the patient is side-lying, adequate stabilization must be given to the trunk and scapula. This usually can be done if the patient is positioned close to the edge of the table and the therapist uses their trunk to stabilize.
- If the patient is lying prone, manually stabilize the scapula.

Shoulder Abduction and Adduction

Hand Placement and Procedure

- Apply resistance to the distal arm with the patient's elbow flexed to 90°. To resist abduction (Fig. 6.15), apply resistance to the lateral aspect of the arm. To resist adduction, apply resistance to the medial aspect of the arm.

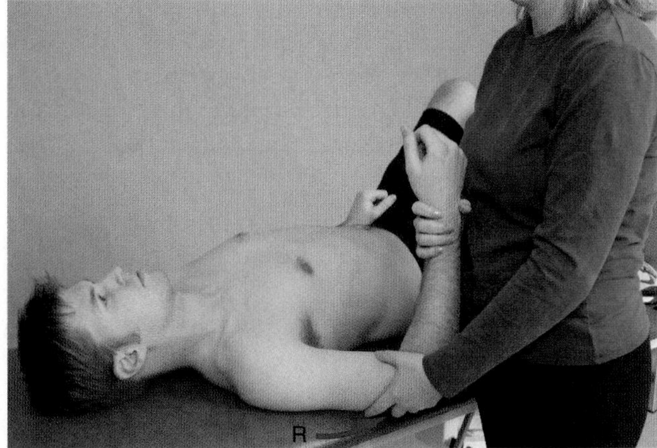

FIGURE 6.15 Resisted shoulder abduction.

- Stabilization (although not pictured in Fig. 6.15) is applied to the superior aspect of the shoulder, if necessary, to prevent the patient from *initiating* abduction by shrugging the shoulder (elevation of the scapula).

PRECAUTION: Allow the glenohumeral joint to externally rotate when resisting abduction above 90° to avoid impingement.

Elevation of the Arm in the Plane of the Scapula

Hand Placement and Procedure

- Same as previously described for shoulder flexion.
- Apply resistance as the patient elevates the arm in the plane of the scapula (30° to 40° anterior to the frontal plane of the body).[175,211]

CLINICAL TIP

Although scapular plane elevation is not a motion of the shoulder that occurs in one of the anatomical planes of the body, resistance in the scapular plane is thought to have its merits. The evidence is inconclusive[227,273] as to whether the torque-producing capabilities of the key muscle groups of the glenohumeral joint are greater when the arm elevates in the plane of the scapula versus the frontal or sagittal planes. However, the glenohumeral joint is considered to be more stable with less risk of soft tissue impingement when strength training is performed in the scapular plane.[183,211] (See additional discussion in Chapter 17.)

Shoulder Internal and External Rotation

Hand Placement and Procedure

- Flex the elbow to 90° and position the shoulder midway between full adduction and 90° abduction. A towel can be placed under the distal arm to approach the plane of the scapula.

- Apply resistance to the distal forearm during internal rotation and external rotation (Fig. 6.16A).
- Stabilize at the level of the clavicle during internal rotation; the back and scapula are stabilized by the table during external rotation.

Alternate Procedure

Alternate alignment of the humerus (Fig. 6.16 B). If the mobility and stability of the glenohumeral joint permit, the shoulder can be positioned in 90° of abduction during resisted rotation.

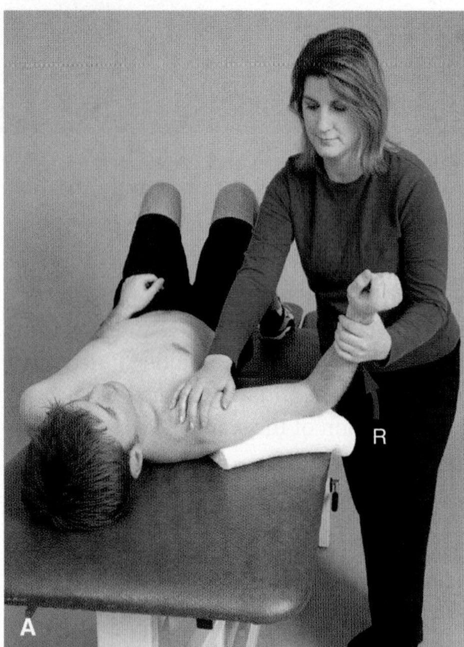

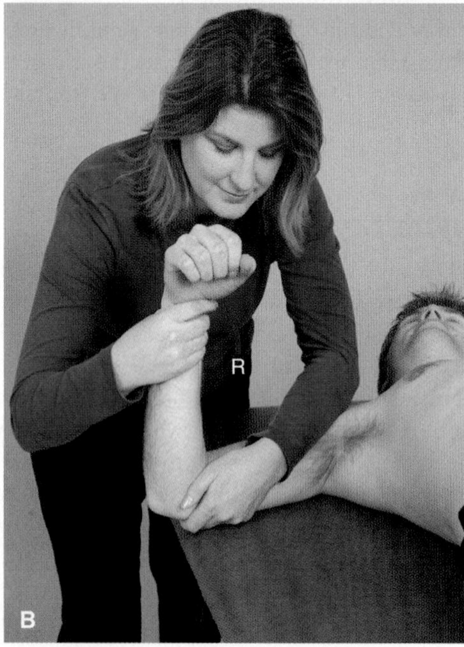

FIGURE 6.16 (A) Resisted external rotation of the shoulder with the shoulder positioned in flexion and abduction (approaching the plane of the scapula). **(B)** Resisted internal rotation of the shoulder with the shoulder in 90° of abduction.

Shoulder Horizontal Abduction and Adduction

Hand Placement and Procedure

- Flex the shoulder and elbow to 90° and place the shoulder in neutral rotation.
- Apply resistance to the distal arm just above the elbow during horizontal adduction and abduction.
- Stabilize the anterior aspect of the shoulder during horizontal adduction. The table stabilizes the scapula and trunk during horizontal abduction.
- To resist horizontal abduction from 0° to 45°, the patient must be close to the edge of the table while supine or be placed side-lying or prone.

Elevation and Depression of the Scapula Video 6.2

Hand Placement and Procedure

- Have the patient assume a supine, side-lying, or sitting position.
- Apply resistance along the superior aspect of the shoulder girdle just above the clavicle during scapular elevation (Fig. 6.17).

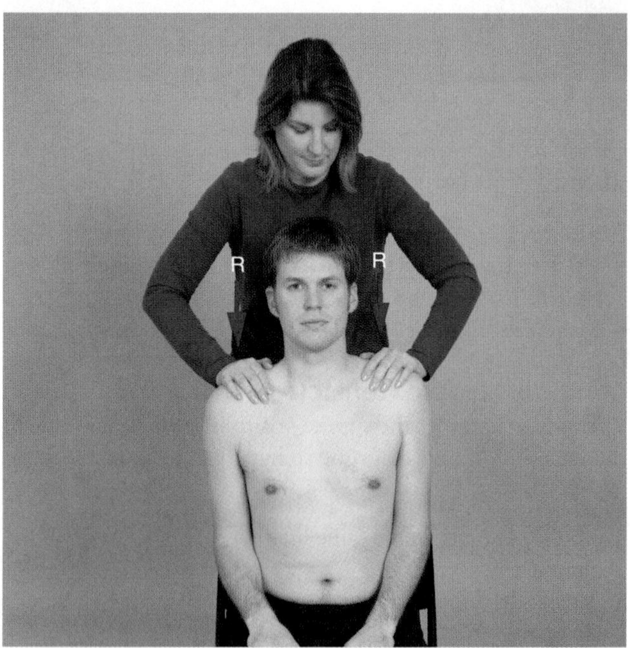

FIGURE 6.17 Elevation of the shoulders (scapulae), resisted bilaterally.

Alternate Procedures: Scapular Depression

To resist unilateral scapular depression in the supine position, have the patient attempt to reach down toward the foot and push the hand into the therapist's hand. When the patient has adequate strength, the exercise can be performed to include weight bearing through the upper extremity by having the patient sit on the edge of a low table and lift the body weight with both hands.

Protraction and Retraction of the Scapula

Hand Placement and Procedure

- Apply resistance to the anterior portion of the shoulder at the head of the humerus to resist protraction and to the posterior aspect of the shoulder to resist retraction.
- Resistance may also be applied directly to the scapula if the patient sits or lies on the side, facing the therapist.
- Stabilize the trunk to prevent trunk rotation.

Elbow Flexion and Extension VIDEO 6.3

Hand Placement and Procedure

- To strengthen the elbow flexors, apply resistance to the anterior aspect of the distal forearm (Fig. 6.18).
- The forearm may be positioned in supination, pronation, and neutral to resist individual flexor muscles of the elbow.
- To strengthen the elbow extensors, place the patient prone (Fig. 6.19) or supine and apply resistance to the distal forearm.
- Stabilize the upper portion of the humerus during both motions.

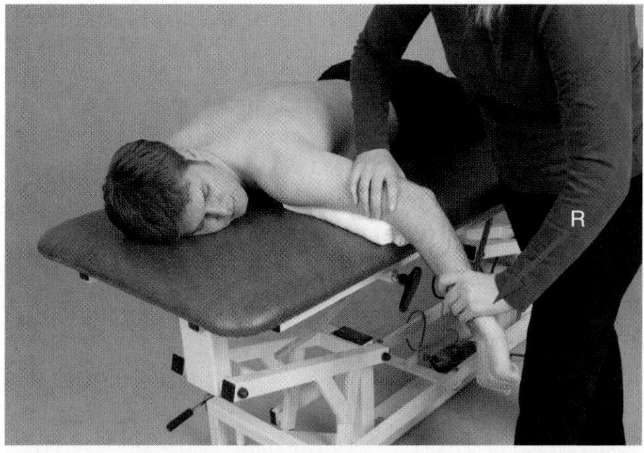

FIGURE 6.19 Resisted elbow extension.

Forearm Pronation and Supination VIDEO 6.4

Hand Placement and Procedure

- Apply resistance to the radius of the distal forearm with the patient's elbow flexed to 90° (Fig. 6.20) to prevent rotation of the humerus.

PRECAUTION: Do not apply resistance to the hand to avoid twisting forces at the wrist.

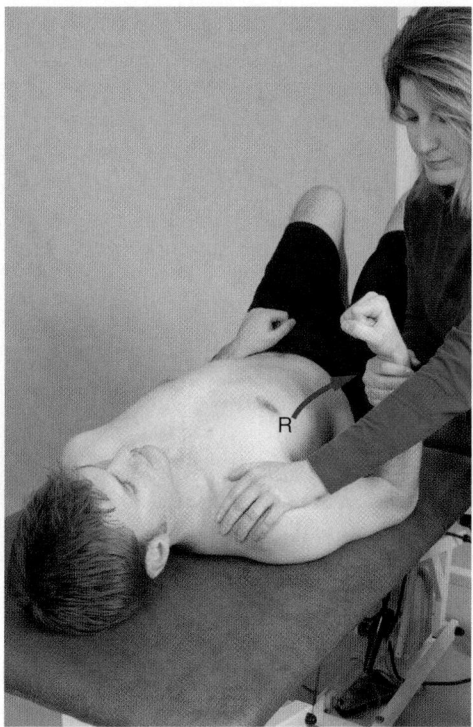

FIGURE 6.18 Resisted elbow flexion with proximal stabilization.

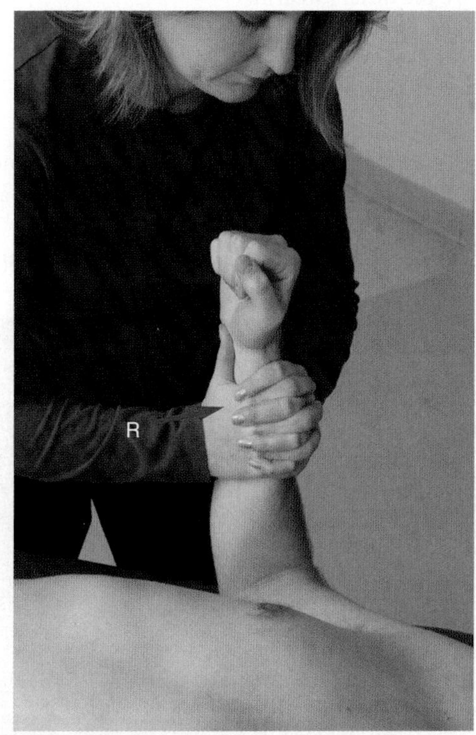

FIGURE 6.20 Resisted pronation of the forearm.

Wrist Flexion and Extension VIDEO 6.5

Hand Placement and Procedure

- Apply resistance to the volar and dorsal aspects of the hand at the level of the metacarpals to resist flexion and extension, respectively (Fig. 6.21).
- Stabilize the volar or dorsal aspect of the distal forearm.

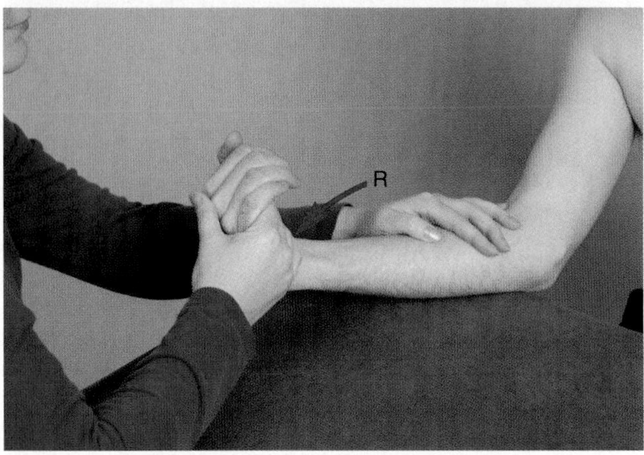

FIGURE 6.21 Resisted wrist flexion and stabilization of the forearm.

Wrist Radial and Ulnar Deviation

Hand Placement and Procedure

- Apply resistance to the second and fifth metacarpals alternately to resist radial and ulnar deviation.
- Stabilize the distal forearm.

Motions of the Fingers and Thumb VIDEO 6.6

Hand Placement and Procedure

- Apply resistance just distal to the joint that is moving. Resistance is applied to one joint motion at a time (Figs. 6.22 and 6.23).
- Stabilize the joints proximal and distal to the moving joint.

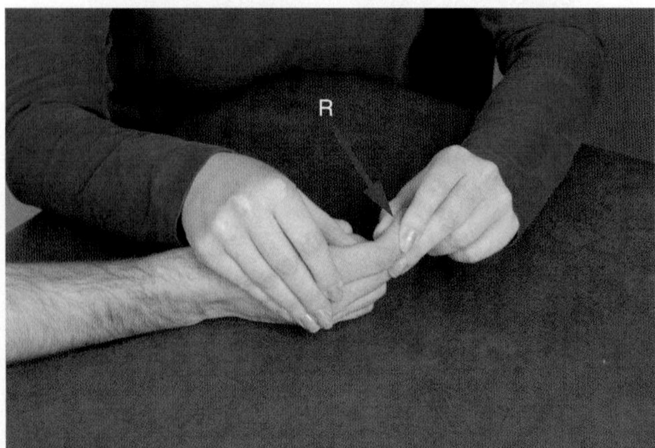

FIGURE 6.22 Resisted flexion of the proximal interphalangeal (PIP) joint of the index finger with stabilization of the metacarpophalangeal (MCP) and distal interphalangeal (DIP) joints.

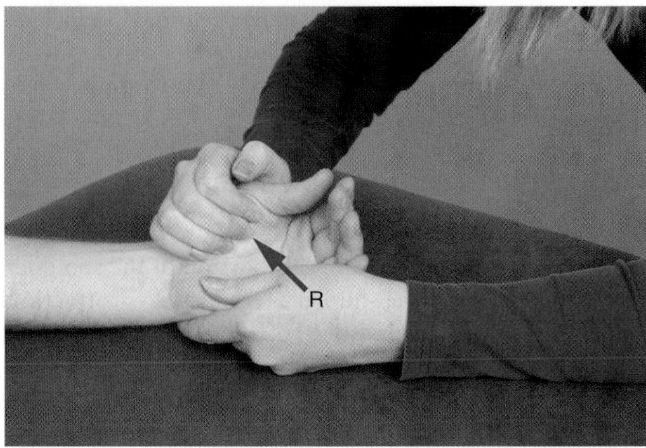

FIGURE 6.23 Resisted opposition of the thumb.

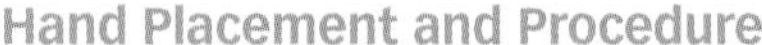

Lower Extremity

Hip Flexion With Knee Flexion VIDEO 6.7

Hand Placement and Procedure

- Apply resistance to the anterior portion of the distal thigh (Fig. 6.24). Simultaneous resistance to knee flexion may be applied at the distal and posterior aspect of the lower leg, just above the ankle.
- Stabilization of the pelvis and lumbar spine is provided by adequate strength of the abdominal muscles.

PRECAUTION: If the pelvis rotates anteriorly and lumbar spine lordosis increases during resisted hip flexion, the patient can flex the contralateral hip and knee and plant the foot on the table to stabilize the pelvis and protect the low back region.

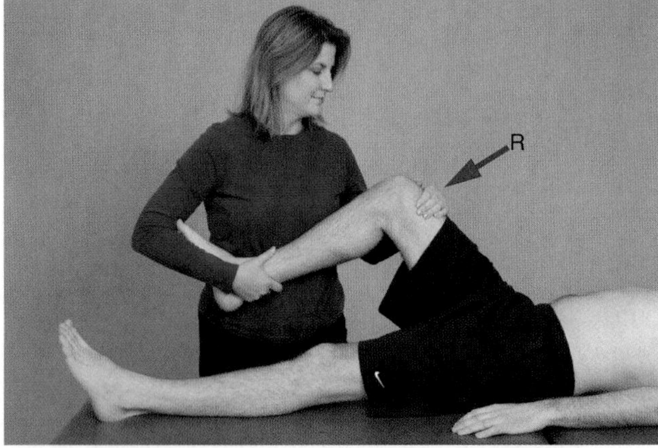

FIGURE 6.24 Resisted flexion of the hip with the knee flexed.

Hip Extension

Hand Placement and Procedure

- Apply resistance to the posterior aspect of the distal thigh with one hand and to the inferior and distal aspect of the heel with the other hand (Fig. 6.25).
- Stabilization of the pelvis and lumbar spine is provided by the table.

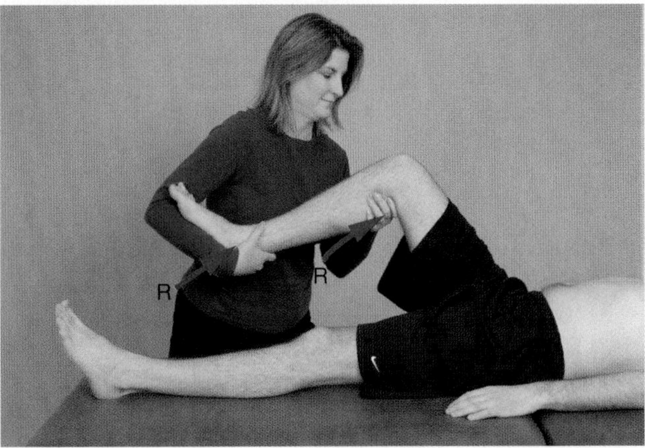

FIGURE 6.25 Resisted hip and knee extension with the hand placed at the popliteal space to prevent hyperextension of the knee.

Hip Hyperextension

Patient position: prone.

Hand Placement and Procedure

- With the patient in a prone position, apply resistance to the posterior aspect of the distal thigh (Fig. 6.26).
- Stabilize the posterior aspect of the pelvis to avoid motion of the lumbar spine.

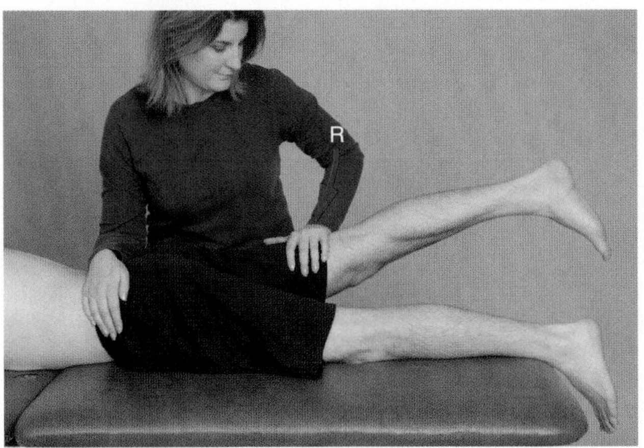

FIGURE 6.26 Resisted end-range hip extension with stabilization of the pelvis.

Hip Abduction and Adduction

Hand Placement and Procedure

- Apply resistance to the lateral and the medial aspects of the distal thigh to resist abduction (Fig. 6.27) and adduction, respectively, or to the lateral and medial aspects of the distal leg just above the malleoli if the knee is stable and pain-free.
- Stabilization is applied to the pelvis to avoid hip-hiking from substitute action of the quadratus lumborum and to keep the thigh in neutral position to prevent external rotation of the femur and subsequent substitution by the iliopsoas.

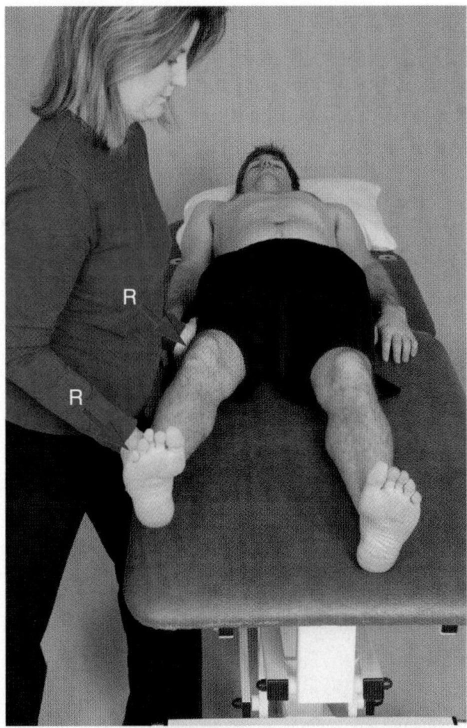

FIGURE 6.27 Resisted hip abduction.

Hip Internal and External Rotation

Patient position: supine with the hip and knee extended.

Hand Placement and Procedure

- Apply resistance to the lateral aspect of the distal thigh to resist external rotation and to the medial aspect of the thigh to resist internal rotation.
- Stabilize the pelvis.

Patient position: supine with the hip and knee flexed (Fig. 6.28).

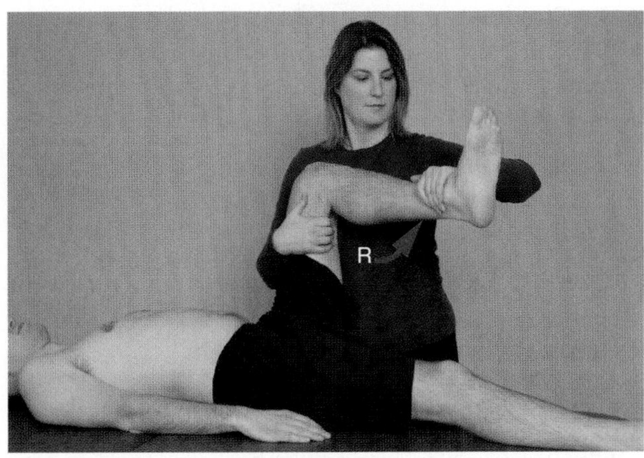

FIGURE 6.28 Resisted external rotation of the hip with the patient lying supine.

Hand Placement and Procedure

- Apply resistance to the medial aspect of the lower leg just above the malleolus during external rotation and to the lateral aspect of the lower leg during internal rotation.
- Stabilize the anterior aspect of the pelvis as the thigh is supported to keep the hip in 90° of flexion.

Patient position: prone, with the hip extended and the knee flexed (Fig. 6.29).

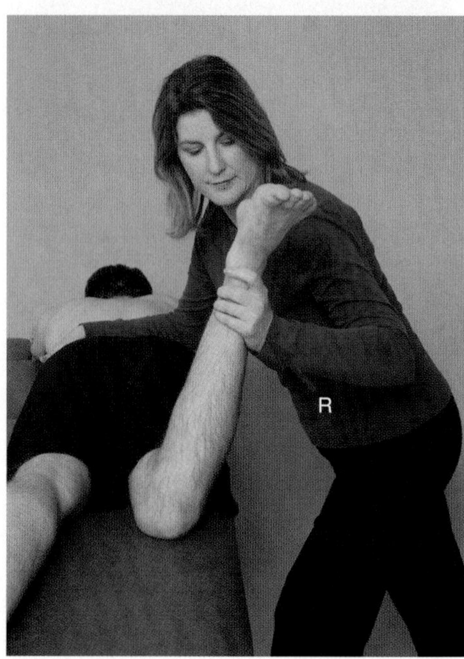

FIGURE 6.29 Resisted internal rotation of the hip with the patient lying prone.

Hand Placement and Procedure

- Apply resistance to the medial and lateral aspects of the lower leg.
- Stabilize the pelvis by applying pressure across the buttocks.

Knee Flexion VIDEO 6.8

- Resistance to knee flexion may be combined with resistance to hip flexion, as described earlier with the patient supine.

Alternate patient position: prone with the hips extended (Fig. 6.30).

Hand Placement and Procedure

- Apply resistance to the posterior aspect of the lower leg just above the heel.
- Stabilize the posterior pelvis across the buttocks.

Additional patient position: sitting at the edge of a table with the hips and knees flexed and the back supported and stabilized.

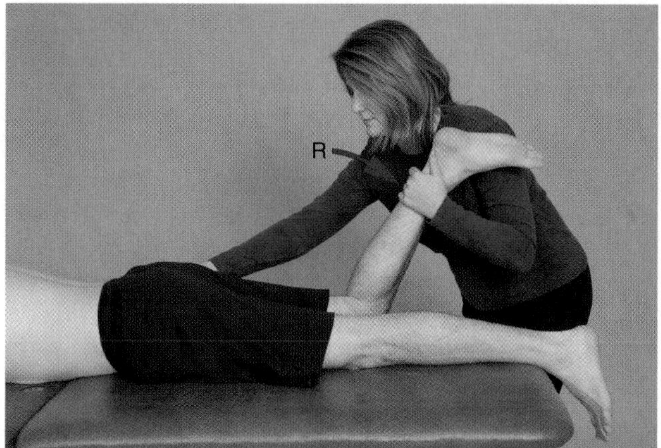

FIGURE 6.30 Resisted knee flexion with stabilization of the hip.

Knee Extension

Alternate Patient Positions

- If the patient is lying supine on a table, the hip must be abducted and the knee flexed so the lower leg is over the side of the table. This position should not be used if the rectus femoris or iliopsoas is tight because it causes an anterior tilt of the pelvis and places stress on the low back.
- If the patient is prone, place a rolled towel under the anterior aspect of the distal thigh; this allows the patella to glide normally during knee extension.
- If the patient is sitting, place a rolled towel under the posterior aspect of the distal thigh (Fig. 6.31).

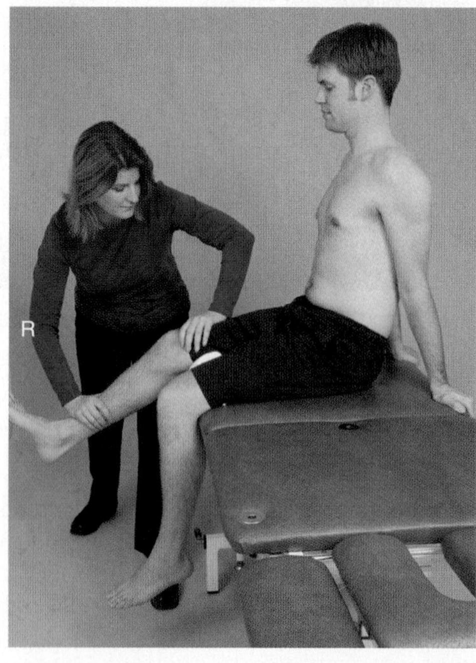

FIGURE 6.31 Resisted knee extension with the patient sitting and stabilizing the trunk with the upper extremities and the therapist stabilizing the thigh.

Hand Placement and Procedure

- Apply resistance to the anterior aspect of the lower leg.
- Stabilize the femur, pelvis, or trunk as necessary.

Ankle Dorsiflexion and Plantarflexion VIDEO 6.9

Hand Placement and Procedure

- Apply resistance to the dorsum of the foot just above the toes to resist dorsiflexion (Fig. 6.32 A) and to the plantar surface of the foot at the metatarsals to resist plantarflexion (Fig. 6.32 B).
- Stabilize the lower leg.

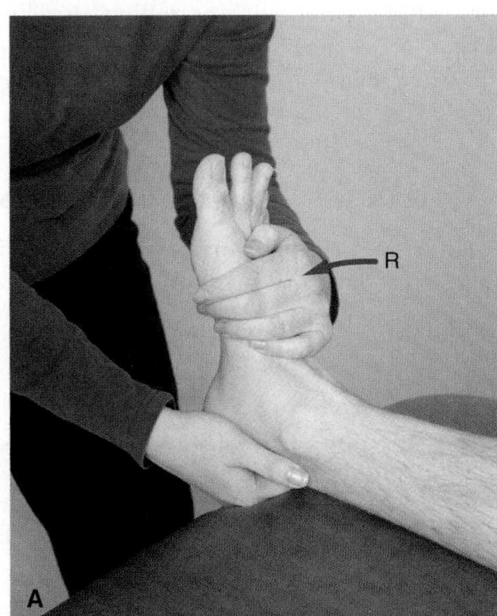

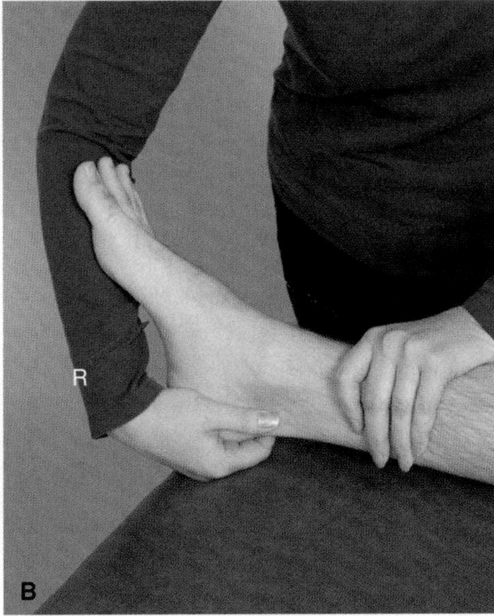

FIGURE 6.32 (A) Resisted dorsiflexion. **(B)** Resisted plantarflexion of the ankle.

Ankle Inversion and Eversion

Hand Placement and Procedure

- Apply resistance to the medial aspect of the first metatarsal to resist inversion and to the lateral aspect of the fifth metatarsal to resist eversion.
- Stabilize the lower leg.

Flexion and Extension of the Toes

Hand Placement and Procedure

- Apply resistance to the plantar and dorsal surfaces of the toes as the patient flexes and extends the toes.
- Stabilize the joints above and below the joint that is moving.

Proprioceptive Neuromuscular Facilitation: Principles and Techniques

PNF is an approach to therapeutic exercise that combines functionally based diagonal patterns of movement with techniques of neuromuscular facilitation to evoke motor responses and improve neuromuscular control and function. This widely used approach to exercise was developed during the 1940s and 1950s by the pioneering work of Kabat, Knott, and Voss.[159] Their work integrated the analysis of movement during functional activities with then current theories of motor development, control, and learning and principles of neurophysiology as the foundations of their approach to exercise and rehabilitation. Long associated with neurorehabilitation, PNF techniques also have widespread application for rehabilitation of patients with musculoskeletal conditions that result in altered neuromuscular control of the extremities, neck, and trunk.[127,251,263]

PNF techniques can be used to develop muscular strength and endurance; to facilitate stability, mobility, neuromuscular control, and coordinated movements; and to lay a foundation for the restoration of function. PNF techniques are useful throughout the continuum of rehabilitation from the early phase of tissue healing when isometric techniques are appropriate to the final phase of rehabilitation when high-velocity, diagonal movements can be performed against maximum resistance.

Hallmarks of this approach to therapeutic exercise are the use of diagonal patterns and the application of sensory cues—specifically proprioceptive, cutaneous, visual, and auditory stimuli—to elicit or augment motor responses. Embedded in this philosophy and approach to exercise is that the stronger muscle groups of a diagonal pattern facilitate the responsiveness of the weaker muscle groups. The focus of discussion of PNF in this chapter deals with the use of PNF patterns and techniques as an important form of resistance exercise for the development of strength, muscular endurance, and dynamic stability.

Although PNF patterns for the extremities can be performed unilaterally or bilaterally and in a variety of weight-bearing and nonweight-bearing positions, only unilateral patterns with the patient in a supine position are described and illustrated. In Chapter 4 of this text the use of several PNF stretching techniques are described. As noted in Chapter 3, diagonal patterns can also be used for passive and active ROM. Additional application of diagonal patterns for the extremities and trunk, some using resistance equipment, are described in the regional chapters later in this text.

Diagonal Patterns

PNF patterns are composed of *multijoint, multiplanar, diagonal,* and *rotational* movements of the extremities, trunk, and neck. Multiple muscle groups contract simultaneously during the execution of these patterned motions. There are two pairs of diagonal patterns that can be used for the upper and lower extremities: diagonal 1 (D_1) and diagonal 2 (D_2). Each diagonal pattern can be performed when moving in either a flexion or extension direction. Hence, the terminology used is D_1Flexion or D_1Extension and D_2Flexion or D_2Extension of the upper or lower extremities. The patterns encompass motion at each joint of the extremity but are identified by the motions that occur at the most proximal joints—the shoulder or the hip. In other words, a pattern is named by *the position of the shoulder or hip when the diagonal pattern has been completed.* Within each pattern, flexion or extension is coupled with abduction or adduction as well as external or internal rotation. Table 6.9 summarizes the component motions of each of the diagonal patterns.

As mentioned, the diagonal patterns can be carried out unilaterally or bilaterally. Bilateral patterns can be done *symmetrically* (e.g., D_1Flexion of both extremities), *asymmetrically* (D_1Flexion of one extremity coupled with D_2Flexion of the other extremity), or *reciprocally* (D_1Flexion of one extremity and D_1 Extension of the opposite extremity). Furthermore, there are patterns specifically for the scapula or pelvis and techniques that integrate diagonal movements into functional activities, such as rolling, crawling, and walking. There are several in-depth resources that describe and illustrate the many variations and applications of PNF techniques.[212,251,265]

Basic Procedures With PNF Patterns

A number of basic procedures that involve the application of multiple types of sensory cues are superimposed on the diagonal patterns to elicit the best possible neuromuscular responses.[212,251,265] Although the diagonal patterns can be

TABLE 6.9 Component Motions of PNF Patterns: Upper and Lower Extremities

Joints or Segments	Diagonal 1: Flexion (D_1Flx)	Diagonal 1: Extension (D_1Ext)	Diagonal 2: Flexion (D_2Flx)	Diagonal 2: Extension (D_2Ext)
Upper Extremity Component Motions				
Shoulder	Flexion-adduction-external rotation	Extension-abduction-internal rotation	Flexion-abduction-external rotation	Extension-adduction-internal rotation
Scapula	Elevation, abduction, upward rotation	Depression, adduction, downward rotation	Elevation, abduction, upward rotation	Depression, adduction, downward rotation
Elbow	Flexion or extension	Flexion or extension	Flexion or extension	Flexion or extension
Forearm	Supination	Pronation	Supination	Pronation
Wrist	Flexion, radial deviation	Extension, ulnar deviation	Extension, radial deviation	Flexion, ulnar deviation
Fingers and thumb	Flexion, adduction	Extension, abduction	Extension, abduction	Flexion, adduction
Lower Extremity Component Motions				
Hip	Flexion-adduction-external rotation	Extension-abduction-internal rotation	Flexion-abduction-internal rotation	Extension-adduction-external rotation
Knee	Flexion or extension	Flexion or extension	Flexion or extension	Flexion or extension
Ankle	Dorsiflexion, inversion	Plantarflexion, eversion	Dorsiflexion, eversion	Plantarflexion, inversion
Toes	Extension	Flexion	Extension	Flexion

used with various forms of mechanical resistance (e.g., free weights, simple weight-pulley systems, elastic resistance, or even an isokinetic unit), the interaction between the patient and therapist, a prominent feature of PNF, provides the greatest amount and variety of sensory input, particularly in the early phases of re-establishing neuromuscular control.

Manual Contacts

The term *manual contact* refers to how and where the therapist's hands are placed on the patient. Whenever possible, manual contacts are placed over the agonist muscle groups or their tendinous insertions. These contacts allow the therapist to apply resistance to the appropriate muscle groups and cue the patient as to the desired direction of movement. For example, if wrist and finger extension is to be resisted, manual contact is on the dorsal surface of the hand and wrist. In the extremity patterns, one manual contact is placed distally and the other manual contact can be placed more proximally. Placement of manual contacts is adjusted based on the patient's response and their skill at performing and controlling the pattern.

Maximal Resistance

The amount of resistance applied during dynamic concentric muscle contractions is the greatest amount possible that still allows the patient to move smoothly and without pain through the available ROM. Resistance should be adjusted throughout the pattern to accommodate strong and weak components of the pattern.

Position and Movement of the Therapist

The therapist remains positioned and aligned along the diagonal planes of movement with shoulders and trunk facing in the direction of the moving limb. Use of effective body mechanics is essential. Resistance should be applied through body weight, not only through the upper extremities. The therapist must use a wide base of support, move with the patient, and pivot over the base of support to allow rotation to occur in the diagonal pattern.

Stretch

Stretch stimulus. The stretch stimulus is the act of physically placing the patient's body segments in positions that lengthen the muscles that will contract during the diagonal movement pattern. For example, prior to initiating D_1Flexion of the lower extremity, the lower limb is placed in D_1Extension to lengthen the flexors.

Considerable importance is placed on rotation during the stretch stimulus. It is believed that the rotational component elongates the muscle fibers and spindles of the agonist muscles for a given pattern, increasing the excitability and responsiveness of those muscles. The stretch stimulus is sometimes described as "winding up the part" or "taking up the slack."

Stretch reflex. The stretch reflex is facilitated by a rapid stretch or overpressure just past the point of tension to an agonist muscle that is positioned for a stretch stimulus. The stretch reflex is usually directed to a distal muscle group to elicit a phasic muscle contraction that initiates a given diagonal movement pattern. The quick stretch is followed by sustained manual resistance to the agonist muscles to maintain their tension. For example, to initiate D_1Flexion of the upper extremity, a quick stretch is applied to the already elongated wrist and finger flexors followed by application of resistance. A quick stretch also can be applied to any agonist muscle group at any point during the execution of a diagonal pattern to further stimulate an agonist muscle contraction or direct a patient's attention to a weak component of a pattern. (See additional discussion of the use of *repeated contractions* in the next section, which describes special PNF techniques.)

PRECAUTION: Use of a stretch reflex, even prior to resisted isometric muscle contractions, is not advisable during the early stages of soft tissue healing after injury or surgery. It is also inappropriate with acute or active arthritic conditions.

Normal Timing

A sequence of distal to proximal coordinated muscle contractions and joint motions occurs during the diagonal patterns. The distal component motions of the pattern should be completed halfway through the full pattern. Correct sequencing of movements promotes neuromuscular control and coordinated movement.

Traction

Traction is the slight separation of joint surfaces, theoretically, to inhibit pain and facilitate movement during execution of the movement patterns.[212,251,265] Traction is most often applied manually during flexion patterns.

Approximation

The gentle compression of joint surfaces by means of manual compression or weight bearing during the movement patterns stimulates co-contraction of agonists and antagonists to enhance dynamic stability and postural control via joint and muscle mechanoreceptors.[212,251,265]

Verbal Commands

Auditory commands and cues are given to enhance motor output. The tone and volume of the verbal commands are varied to help maintain the patient's attention. A sharp verbal command is given simultaneously with the application of the stretch reflex to synchronize the phasic, reflexive motor response with a sustained volitional effort by the patient. Verbal cues then direct the patient throughout the movement patterns. As the patient learns the sequence of movements, verbal cues can be more succinct.

Visual Cues

The patient is asked to follow the movement of a limb with both head and eye motion to further enhance correct movement throughout the full ROM.

Upper Extremity Diagonal Patterns

NOTE: All descriptions for manual contacts are for the patient's right (R) upper extremity. During each pattern tell the patient to watch their moving hand. Be sure that rotation shifts *gradually* from full internal to full external rotation (or vice versa) throughout the ROM. By midrange, the arm should be in neutral rotation. Manual contacts may be altered from the suggested placements as long as contact remains on the appropriate surfaces. The therapist should manually resist all patterns through the full, available ROM.

D_1Flexion VIDEO 6.10

Starting Position (Fig. 6.33 A)

Position the upper extremity in shoulder extension, abduction, and internal rotation; elbow extension; forearm pronation; and wrist and finger extension with the hand about 8 to 12 inches from the hip.

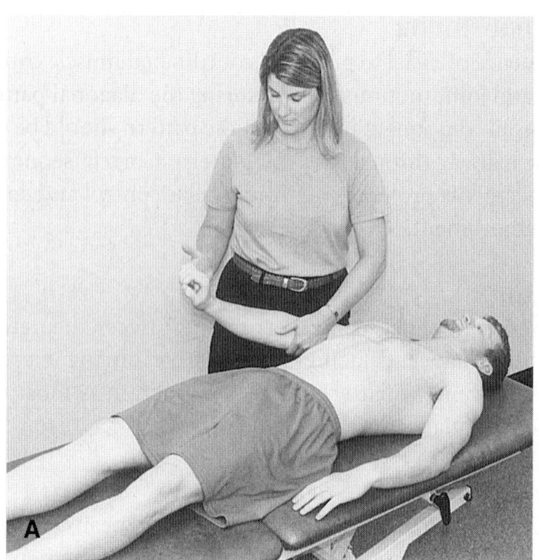

FIGURE 6.33 (A) Starting position and

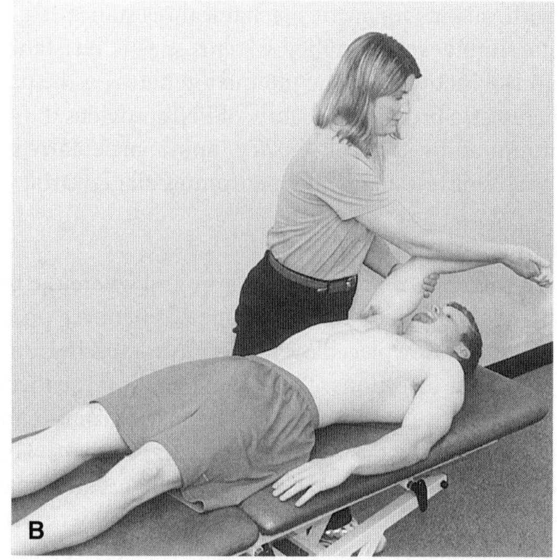

FIGURE 6.33 (B) ending position for D_1 flexion of the upper extremity.

Hand Placement

Place the index and middle fingers of your (R) hand in the palm of the patient's hand and your left (L) hand on the volar surface of the distal forearm or at the cubital fossa of the elbow.

Verbal Commands

Apply a quick stretch to the wrist and finger flexors and tell the patient to "Squeeze my fingers; turn your palm up; pull your arm up and across your face," as you resist the pattern.

Ending Position (Fig. 6.33 B)

Complete the pattern with the arm across the face in shoulder flexion, adduction, external rotation; partial elbow flexion; forearm supination; and wrist and finger flexion.

D_1Extension

Starting Position (Fig. 6.34 A)

Begin as described for completion of D_1Flexion.

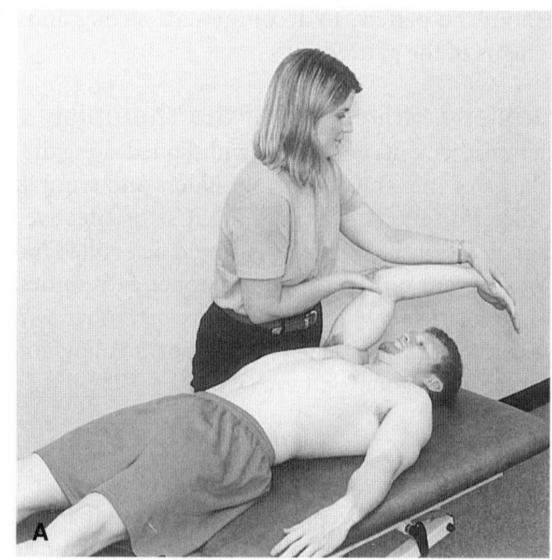

FIGURE 6.34 (A) Starting position and

Hand Placements

Grasp the dorsal surface of the patient's hand and fingers with your (R) hand using a *lumbrical grip.* Place your (L) hand on the extensor surface of the arm just proximal to the elbow.

Verbal Commands

As you apply a quick stretch to the wrist and finger extensors, tell the patient, "Open your hand" (or "Wrist and fingers up"); then "Push your arm down and out."

Ending Position (Fig. 6.34 B)

Finish the pattern in shoulder extension, abduction, internal rotation; elbow extension; forearm pronation; and wrist and finger extension.

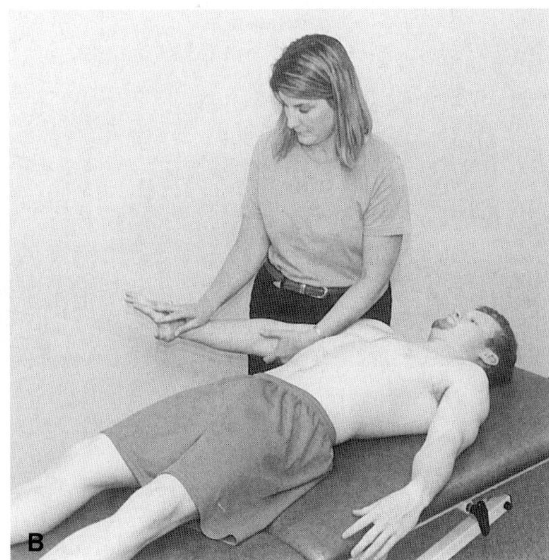

FIGURE 6.34—cont'd (B) ending position for D_1 extension of the upper extremity.

D_2Flexion VIDEO 6.11

Starting Position (Fig. 6.35 A)

Position the upper extremity in shoulder extension, adduction, and internal rotation; elbow extension; forearm pronation; and wrist and finger flexion. The forearm should lie across the umbilicus.

Hand Placement

Grasp the dorsum of the patient's hand with your (L) hand using a lumbrical grip. Grasp the dorsal surface of the patient's forearm close to the elbow with your (R) hand.

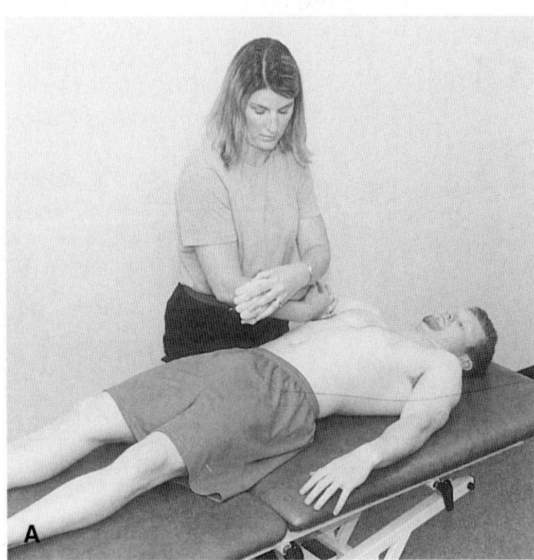

FIGURE 6.35 (A) Starting position and

Verbal Commands

As you apply a quick stretch to the wrist and finger extensors, tell the patient, "Open your hand and turn it to your face;" "Lift your arm up and out;" "Point your thumb out."

Ending Position (Fig. 6.35 B)

Finish the pattern in shoulder flexion, abduction, and external rotation; elbow extension; forearm supination; and wrist and finger extension. The arm should be 8 to 10 inches from the ear; the thumb should be pointing to the floor.

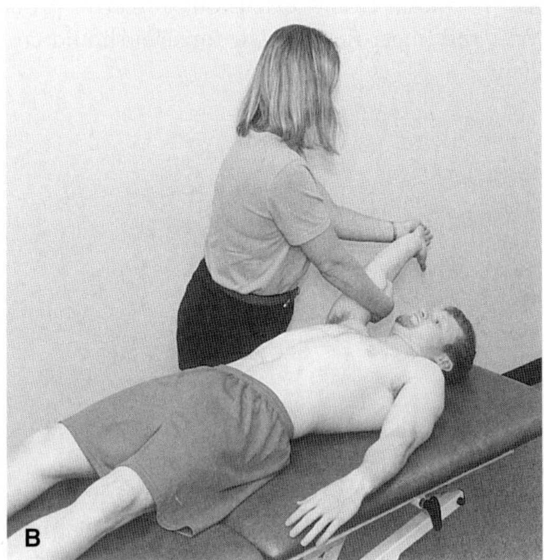

FIGURE 6.35 (B) ending position for D_2 flexion of the upper extremity.

D_2Extension

Starting Position (Fig. 6.36 A)

Begin as described for completion of D_2Flexion.

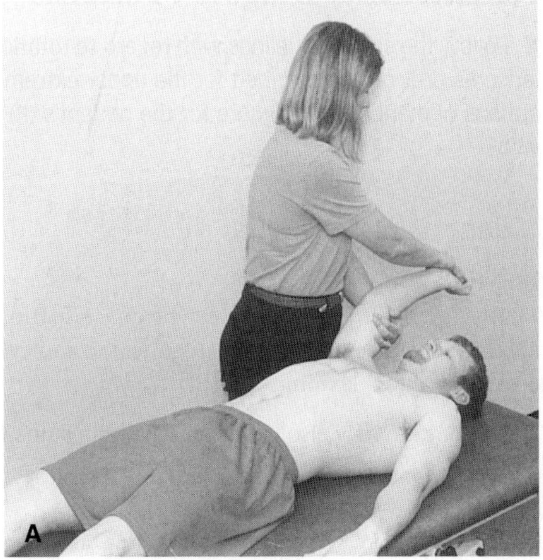

FIGURE 6.36 (A) Starting position and

Hand Placement
Place the index and middle fingers of your (R) hand in the palm of the patient's hand and your (L) hand on the volar surface of the forearm or distal humerus.

Verbal Commands
As you apply a quick stretch to the wrist and finger flexors, tell the patient, "Squeeze my fingers and pull down and across your chest."

Ending Position (Fig. 6.36 B)
Complete the pattern in shoulder extension, adduction, and internal rotation; elbow extension; forearm pronation; and wrist and finger flexion. The forearm should cross the umbilicus.

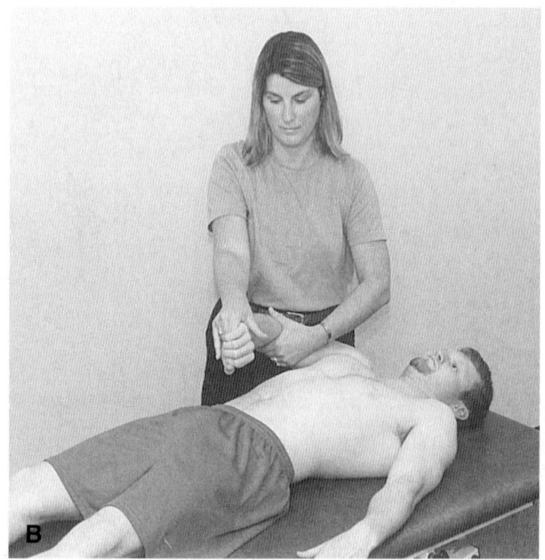

FIGURE 6.36—cont'd (B) ending position for D_2 extension of the upper extremity.

Lower Extremity Diagonal Patterns

NOTE: Follow the same guidelines with regard to rotation and resistance as previously described for the upper extremity. All descriptions of manual contacts are for the patient's (R) lower extremity.

D_1Flexion VIDEO 6.12

Starting Position (Fig. 6.37 A)
Position the lower extremity in hip extension, abduction, and internal rotation; knee extension; plantar flexion and eversion of the ankle; and toe flexion.

NOTE: This pattern may also be initiated with the knee flexed and the lower leg over the edge of the table.

Hand Placement
Place your (R) hand on the dorsal and medial surface of the foot and toes and your (L) hand on the anteromedial aspect of the thigh just proximal to the knee.

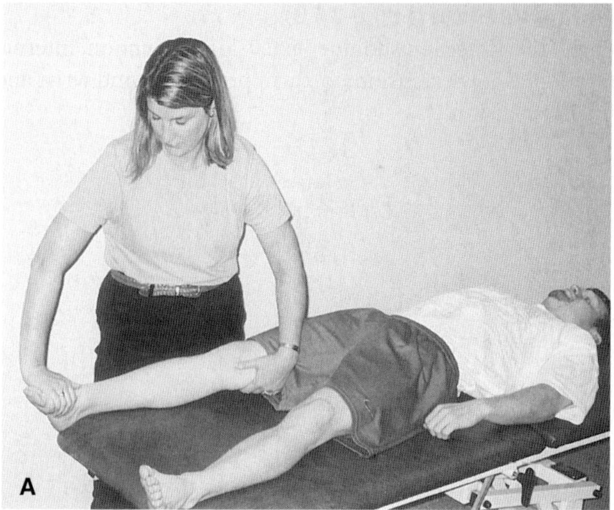

FIGURE 6.37 (A) Starting position and

Verbal Commands
As you apply a quick stretch to the ankle dorsiflexors and invertors and toe extensors, tell the patient, "Foot and toes up and in; bend your knee; pull your leg over and across."

Ending Position (Fig. 6.37 b)
Complete the pattern in hip flexion, adduction, and external rotation; knee flexion (or extension); ankle dorsiflexion and inversion; toe extension. The hip should be adducted across the midline, creating lower trunk rotation to the patient's (L) side.

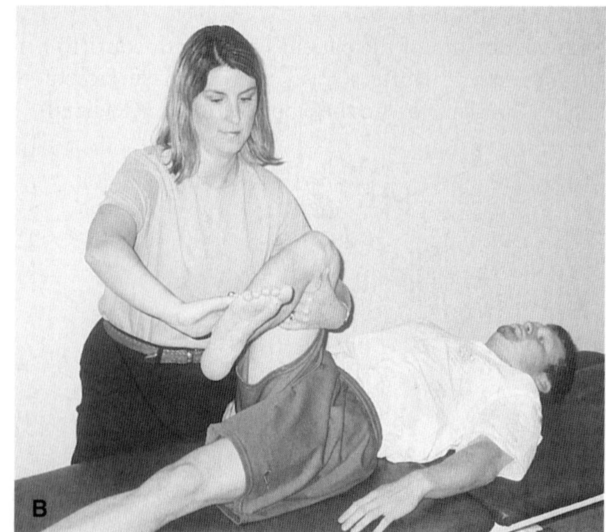

FIGURE 6.37 (B) ending position for D_1 flexion of the lower extremity.

D_1Extension

Starting Position (Fig. 6.38 A)
Begin as described for completion of D_1Flexion.

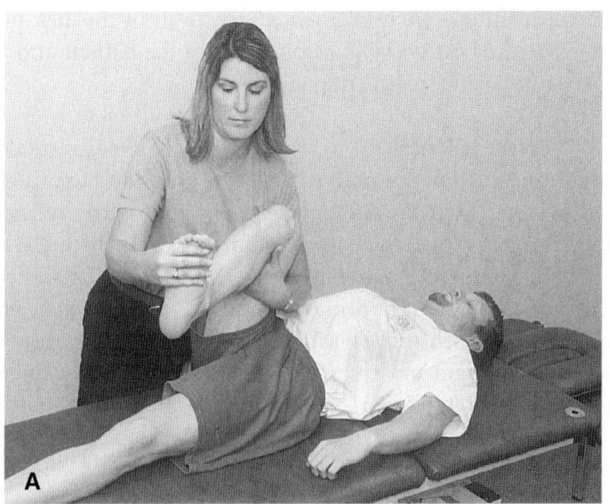

FIGURE 6.38 (A) Starting position and

Hand Placement

Place your (R) hand on the plantar and lateral surface of the foot at the base of the toes. Place your (L) hand (palm up) at the posterior aspect of the knee at the popliteal fossa.

Verbal Commands

As you apply a quick stretch to the plantarflexors of the ankle and toes, tell the patient, "Curl (point) your toes; push down and out."

Ending Position (Fig. 6.38 B)

Finish the pattern in hip extension, abduction, and internal rotation; knee extension or flexion; ankle plantarflexion and eversion; and toe flexion.

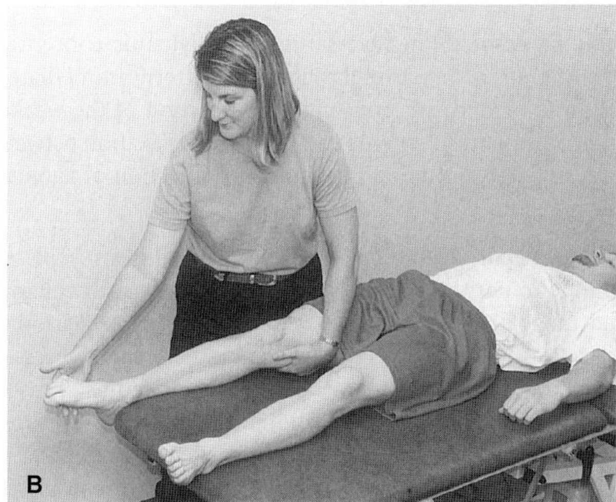

FIGURE 6.38 (B) ending position for D_1 extension of the lower extremity.

D_2Flexion VIDEO 6.13

Starting Position (Fig. 6.39 A)

Place the lower extremity in hip extension, adduction, and external rotation; knee extension; ankle plantarflexion and inversion; and toe flexion.

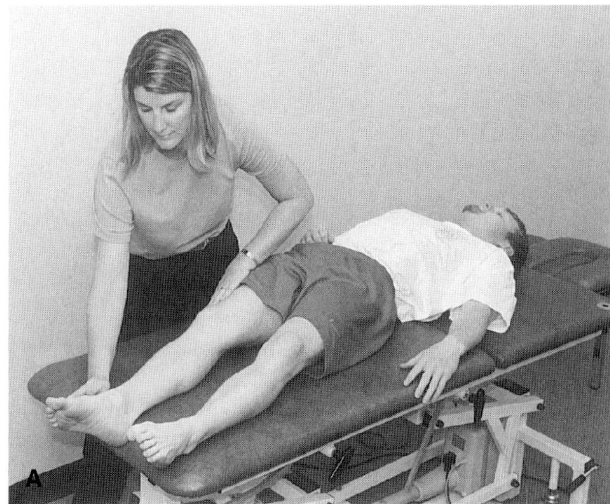

FIGURE 6.39 (A) Starting position and

Hand Placement

Place your (R) hand along the dorsal and lateral surfaces of the foot and your (L) hand on the anterolateral aspect of the thigh just proximal to the knee. The fingers of your (L) hand should point distally.

Verbal Commands

As you apply a quick stretch to the ankle dorsiflexors and evertors and toe extensors, tell the patient, "Foot and toes up and out; lift your leg up and out."

Ending Position (Fig. 6.39 B)

Complete the pattern in hip flexion, abduction, and internal rotation; knee flexion (or extension); ankle dorsiflexion and eversion; and toe extension.

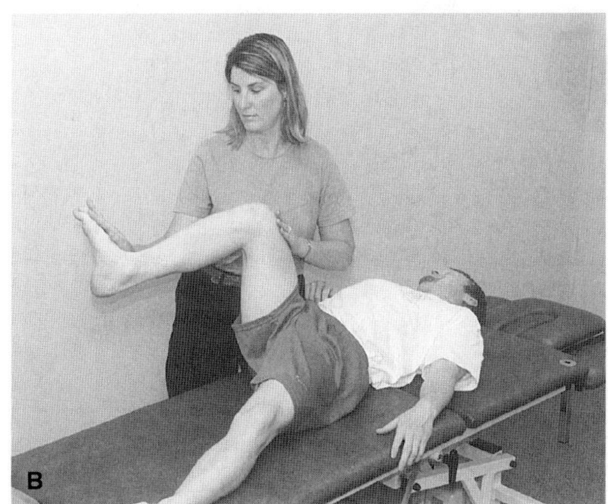

FIGURE 6.39 (B) ending position for D_2 flexion of the lower extremity.

D_2Extension

Starting Position (Fig. 6.40 A)

Begin as described for the completion of D_2Flexion.

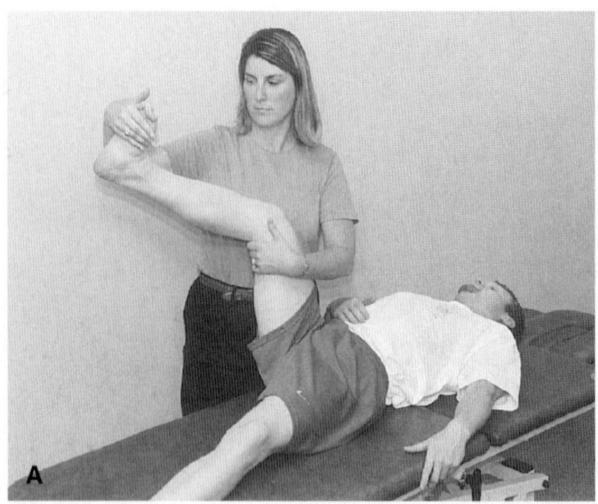

FIGURE 6.40 (A) Starting position and

Hand Placement

Place your (R) hand on the plantar and medial surface of the foot at the base of the toes and your (L) hand at the posteromedial aspect of the thigh, just proximal to the knee.

Verbal Commands

As you apply a quick stretch to the plantarflexors and invertors of the ankle and toe flexors, tell the patient, "Curl (point) your toes down and in; push your leg down and in."

Ending Position (Fig. 6.40 B)

Complete the pattern in hip extension, adduction, and external rotation; knee extension; ankle plantarflexion and inversion; and toe flexion.

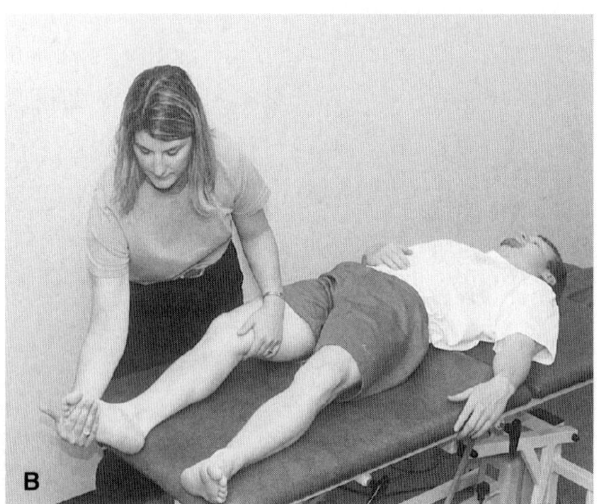

FIGURE 6.40 (B) ending position for D_2 extension of the lower extremity.

Specific Techniques With PNF

There are a number of specific additional techniques that may be used during the execution of a PNF pattern to further stimulate weak muscles and enhance movement or stability. These techniques are implemented selectively by the therapist to evoke the best possible response from the patient and to focus on specific treatment goals.

Rhythmic Initiation

Rhythmic initiation is used to promote the ability to initiate a movement pattern. After the patient voluntarily relaxes, the therapist moves the patient's limb passively through the available range of the desired movement pattern several times so the patient becomes familiar with the sequence of movements within the pattern. Rhythmic initiation also helps the patient understand the rate at which movement is to occur. Practicing assisted or active movements (without resistance) also helps the patient learn a movement pattern.

Repeated Contractions

Repeated, dynamic contractions, initiated with repeated quick stretches followed by resistance, are applied at any point in the ROM to strengthen a weak agonist component of a diagonal pattern.

Reversal of Antagonists

Many functional activities involve quick reversals of the direction of movement. This is evident in diverse activities such as sawing or chopping wood, dancing, playing tennis, or grasping and releasing objects. The reversal of antagonists technique involves stimulation of a weak agonist pattern by first resisting static or dynamic contractions of the antagonist pattern. The reversals of a movement pattern are instituted just before the previous pattern has been fully completed.

There are two categories of reversal techniques available to strengthen weak muscle groups.

Slow reversal. Slow reversal involves dynamic concentric contraction of a stronger agonist pattern immediately followed by dynamic concentric contraction of the weaker antagonist pattern. There is no voluntary relaxation between patterns. This promotes rapid, reciprocal action of agonists and antagonists.

Slow reversal hold. *Slow* reversal hold adds an *isometric* contraction at the end of the range of a pattern to enhance end-range holding of a weakened muscle. With no period of relaxation, the direction of movement is then rapidly reversed by means of *dynamic* contraction of the agonist muscle groups quickly followed by isometric contraction of those same muscles. This is one of several techniques used to enhance dynamic stability, particularly in proximal muscle groups.

Alternating Isometrics VIDEO 6.14

Another technique to improve isometric strength and stability of the postural muscles of the trunk or proximal stabilizing muscles of the shoulder girdle or hip is alternating isometrics. Manual resistance is applied in a single plane on one side of a body segment and then on the other. The patient is instructed to "hold" his or her position as resistance is alternated from one direction to the opposite direction. No joint movement should occur. This procedure isometrically strengthens agonists and antagonists, and it can be applied to one extremity, to both extremities simultaneously, or to the trunk. Alternating isometrics can be applied with the extremities in weight-bearing or nonweight-bearing positions.

For example, if a patient assumes a side-lying position, manual contacts are alternately placed on the anterior aspect of the trunk and then on the posterior aspect of the trunk. The patient is told to maintain (hold) the side-lying position as the therapist first attempts to push the trunk in a posterior and then anterior direction (Fig. 6.41 A). Manual contacts are maintained on the patient as the therapist's hands are moved alternately from the anterior to posterior surfaces. Resistance is gradually applied and released. The same can be done unilaterally or bilaterally in the extremities (Fig. 6.41 B).

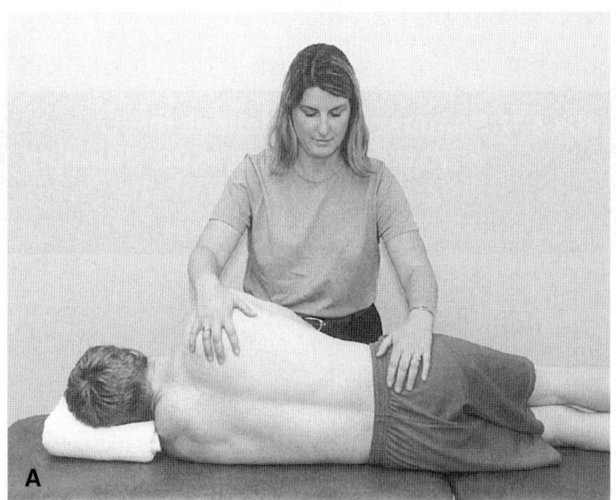

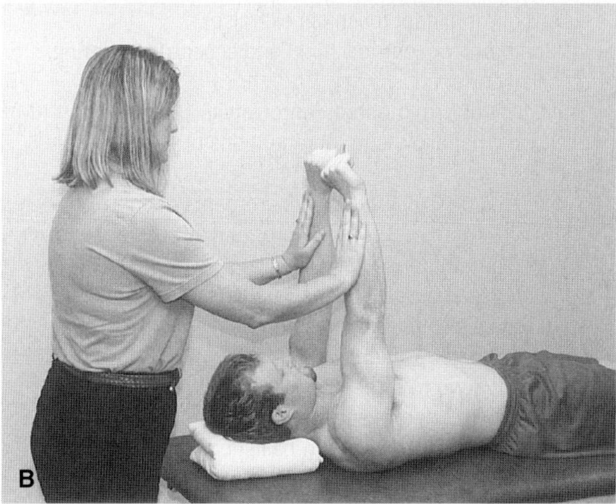

FIGURE 6.41 (A) Use of alternating isometrics to improve static strength of the proximal musculature by alternately placing both hands and applying resistance to the anterior aspect of the body and then to the posterior aspect of the body. **(B)** Use of alternating isometrics in the upper extremities.

Rhythmic Stabilization

Rhythmic stabilization is used as a progression of alternating isometrics and is designed to promote stability through co-contraction of the proximal stabilizing musculature of the trunk as well as the shoulder and pelvic girdle regions of the body. Rhythmic stabilization typically is performed in weight-bearing positions to incorporate joint approximation into the procedure, hence further facilitating co-contraction. The therapist applies multidirectional, rather than unidirectional, resistance by placing manual contacts on opposite sides of the body and applying resistance simultaneously in opposite directions as the patient holds the selected position. Multiple muscle groups around joints—most importantly the rotators—must contract to hold the position.

For example, the patient is told to hold the exercise position as the therapist pushes against the posterior aspect of the body with one hand and simultaneously pushes against the anterior aspect of the body with the other hand (Fig. 6.42). Manual contacts are then shifted to the opposite surfaces and isometric holding against resistance is repeated. There is no voluntary relaxation between contractions.

Use of these special techniques, as well as others associated with PNF, gives the therapist a significant variety of methods for increasing muscle strength and promoting dynamic stability and controlled mobility.

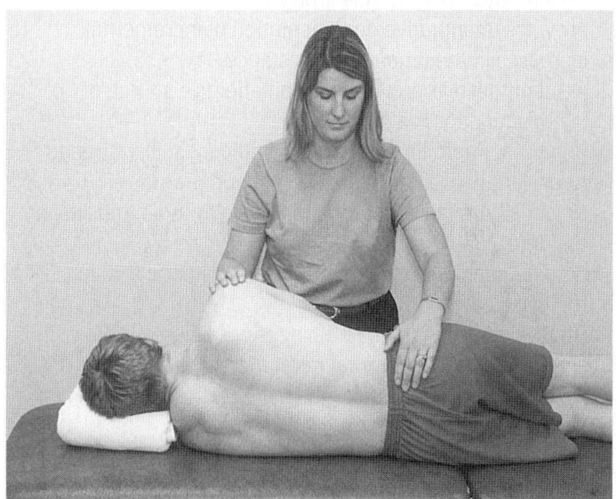

FIGURE 6.42 Use of rhythmic stabilization to improve stability of the trunk by simultaneously applying resistance in opposite directions to the anterior and posterior surfaces of the trunk, emphasizing isometric contractions of the trunk rotators.

Mechanical Resistance Exercise

Mechanical resistance exercise is any form of exercise in which external resistance is applied by means of some type of exercise equipment. Frequently used terms that denote the use of mechanical resistance are *resistance training, weight training,* and *strength training.*[5-8,16,35]

Mechanical resistance exercise is an integral component of rehabilitation and fitness/conditioning programs for individuals of all ages. The advantages and disadvantages of using mechanical resistance in an exercise program are noted in Box 6.16.

Application in Rehabilitation Programs

Mechanical resistance exercise is commonly implemented in rehabilitation programs to eliminate or reduce deficits in muscular performance caused by an array of pathological conditions and to restore or improve functional abilities. Guidelines for integration of mechanical resistance exercises into an individualized rehabilitation program for patients with specific conditions are detailed in Chapters 16 through 23.

BOX 6.16 Mechanical Resistance Exercise: Advantages and Disadvantages

Advantages

- Establishes a quantitative baseline measurement of muscle performance against which improvement can be judged.
- Most appropriate during intermediate and advanced phases of rehabilitation when muscle strength is 4/5 or greater or when the strength of the patient exceeds the therapist's strength.
- Provides exercise loads far beyond that which can be applied manually by a therapist to induce a training effect for already strong muscle groups.
- Provides quantitative documentation of incremental increases in the amount of resistance.
  - Quantitative improvement is an effective source of motivation for the patient.
- Useful for improving dynamic or static muscular strength.
- Adds variety to a resistance training program.
- Practical for high-repetition training to improve muscular endurance.
- Some equipment provides variable resistance through the ROM.
- High-velocity resistance training is possible and safe with some forms of mechanical resistance (hydraulic and pneumatic variable resistance machines, isokinetic units, and elastic resistance).
  - Potentially better carryover to functional activities than relatively slow-velocity manual resistance exercises.
  - Appropriate for independent exercise in a home program after careful patient education and a period of supervision.

Disadvantages

- Not appropriate when muscles are very weak or soft tissues are in the very early stages of healing, with the exception of some equipment that provides assistance, support, or control against gravity.
- Equipment that provides constant external resistance maximally loads the muscle at only one point in the ROM.
- No accommodation for a painful arc (except with hydraulic, pneumatic, or isokinetic equipment).
- Expense for purchase and maintenance of equipment.
- With free weights and weight machines, gradation in resistance is dependent on the manufacturer's increments of resistance.

Application in Fitness and Conditioning Programs

There is general consensus that training with weights or other forms of mechanical resistance is an important component of comprehensive health and fitness programs. As in rehabilitation programs, resistance training complements aerobic training and flexibility exercises in conditioning and fitness programs. Guidelines for a balanced resistance training program for the healthy but untrained adult (less than 50 to 60 years of age) recommended by the ACSM[6,8] and the CDC[35] are summarized in Box 6.17.

NOTE: Special considerations for resistance exercises in the older adult population are presented in Chapter 24.

BOX 6.17 Summary of Guidelines for Resistance Training in Conditioning Programs for Healthy Adults (<50–60 years old)

- Prior to resistance training, perform warm-up activities followed by flexibility exercises.
- Perform dynamic exercises through the full, available, and pain-free ROM and target the major muscle groups of the body (approximately 8–10 muscle groups of the upper and lower extremities and trunk) for total body muscular fitness.
- Balance flexion-dominant (pulling) exercises with extension-dominant (pushing) exercises.
- Include both concentric (lifting) and eccentric (lowering) muscle contractions.
- *Intensity:* Perform moderate-intensity (60% to 80% of 1-RM) exercises that allow 8 to 12 repetitions of each exercise per set.
  - Increase intensity gradually (increments of approximately 5% of 1-RM) to progress the program as strength and muscular endurance improve.
- *Sets:* Two sets, progressing to four sets of each exercise.
- *Rest intervals:* 2 to 3 minutes between sets. While resting one muscle group, exercise a different muscle group.
- *Frequency:* Two to three times per week.
- Use slow to moderate speeds of movement.
- Use rhythmic, controlled, non-ballistic movements.
- Exercises should not interfere with normal breathing.
- Whenever possible, train with a partner for feedback and assistance.
- Cool-down after completion of exercises.
- Reduce the resistance and volume when reinitiating weight training after a layoff of more than 1 to 2 weeks.

Special Considerations for Children and Adolescents

Resistance Training

There is growing evidence that children and adolescents can achieve health-related benefits from resistance training and can safely engage in weight-training programs if designed appropriately and closely supervised.[6,36,114,119,253] Use of body weight as a source of resistance and equipment specifically designed to fit children and adolescents will contribute to program safety (Fig. 6.43).

Training-induced strength, power, and performance gains in children and adolescents have been documented,[83,85,119,281] but sport-related injury prevention remains questionable.[83,281] As with adults, information on the impact of strength training on the enhancement of functional motor skills is limited.

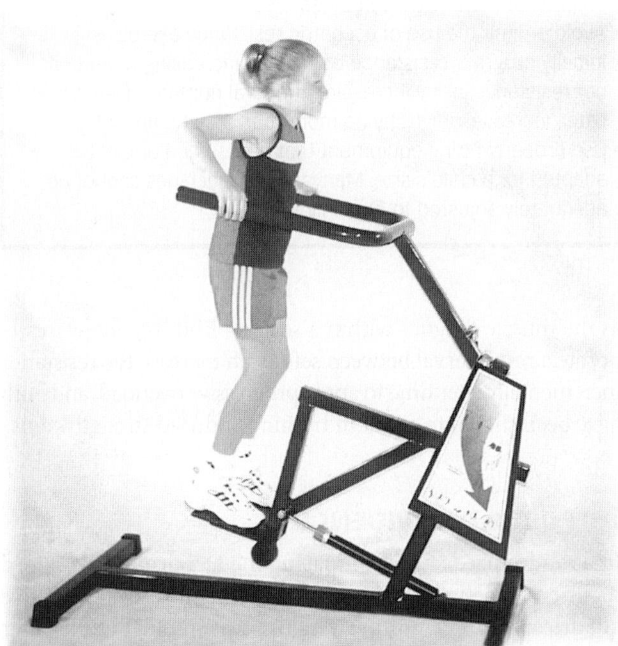

FIGURE 6.43 Youth resistance training on Kids-N-Motion® equipment (Triceps-Dip), specifically designed and sized for a child's use. *(Courtesy of Youth Fitness International, Moncks Corner, SC; www.youthfit.com/.)*

FOCUS ON EVIDENCE

Research has shown that some acute and chronic responses to exercise in children are similar to those of adults, while other responses are quite different. For example, because of an immature thermo-regulation system, children dissipate body heat less easily, fatigue more quickly, and therefore need longer rest periods than young adults to recover from exercise.[73,281] Such differences in response to resistance exercise must be considered when designing and implementing strength training programs for children.

The American Academy of Pediatrics,[5] ACSM,[6] the Canadian Society for Exercise Physiology,[20] and the CDC[36] support youth involvement in resistance training—but only if a number of special guidelines and precautions are consistently followed. Although the risk of injury from resistance training is quite low if performed at an appropriate intensity and volume,[86,253] exercise-induced soft tissue or growth plate injuries have been noted if guidelines and precautions are not followed. Guidelines and special considerations for resistance training in children as a component of regular physical activity are summarized in Box 6.18.[5,6,36,83,84,114,253] Consistent with adult guidelines, a balanced program of dynamic exercise for major muscle groups includes warm-up and cool-down periods.

Specific Resistance Training Regimens

As resistance training gained acceptance, many specific systems of exercise were developed to improve muscle strength, power, and endurance. All of these systems are based on the overload principle, and most use some form of mechanical resistance to load the muscle. The driving force behind the development of these regimens seems to be to design the "optimal"—that is, the most effective and efficient—method to improve muscular performance and functional abilities.

Several frequently used regimens of resistance training for rehabilitation and for fitness and conditioning programs—PRE, circuit weight training, and velocity spectrum isokinetic training—are presented in this section. Some approaches to advanced training, such as plyometric exercises (stretch-shortening drills) to develop muscle power, are presented in Chapter 23.

Progressive Resistance Exercise

PRE is a system of dynamic resistance training in which a constant external load is applied to the contracting muscle by some mechanical means and incrementally increased. The RM is used as the basis for determining and progressing the amount of resistance used during training.

FOCUS ON EVIDENCE

The results of countless studies have demonstrated that PRE improves the force-generating capacity of muscle and may improve physical performance. It is important to note that the participants in many of these studies were young, healthy adults rather than patients with impairments associated with injury and disease.

However, a systematic literature review[254] indicated that PRE was also beneficial for patients with a variety of pathological

BOX 6.18 Resistance Training for Children: Guidelines and Special Considerations

- No formal resistance training for children younger than 6 to 7 years of age; age-appropriate physical activity through organized and free play is recommended.
- At age 6 to 7, introduce the *concept* of an exercise session; encourage 60 or more minutes of moderate-intensity physical activity daily;[36] focus on aerobic activities (active exercises without weights).
  - Include weight-bearing exercises, such as push-ups and jumping activities for bone strengthening 3 days per week.
  - Emphasize a variety of short-duration, play-oriented exercises to prevent boredom, overheating, and muscle fatigue.
  - As a small portion of daily physical activity, perform muscle-strengthening exercises against the resistance of body weight (sit-ups, chin-ups). Postpone including exercises with light weights added for several years.
- When introducing weight-training in the prepubescent years:
  - Maintain *close* and *continuous supervision* by trained personnel or a parent who has received instruction.
  - Always perform warm-up activities for at least 5 to 10 minutes before initiating resistance exercises.
  - Focus on proper form, exercise technique, and safety (alignment, stabilization, and controlled/nonballistic movements).
  - Emphasize low-intensity exercise throughout childhood to avoid potential injury to a child's growing skeletal system and to joints and supportive soft tissues.
  - Emphasize adequate hydration.
- *Intensity:* Select low exercise loads that allow 8 to 15[7,83] repetitions.
  - Progress gradually to moderate-intensity (60% to 80% of an estimated 1-RM) exercise loads.
  - Do not use near-maximal or maximal exercise loads or participate in power lifting or body building until physical and skeletal maturity has been reached.
- *Sets and rest intervals:* Initially perform only one set, progressing to two to three sets of each exercise; rest at least 3 minutes between sets of exercises.
- *Frequency:* Limit the frequency of resistance training to no more than two sessions per week.
- Emphasize multi-joint, combined movements.
- Avoid or limit the use of eccentric resistance exercises.
- Initially progress resistance training by increasing repetitions, not resistance, or by increasing the total number of exercises. Later, increase weight by no more than 5% at a time.[6,83]
- Use properly fitting equipment that is designed or can be adapted for a child's size. Many weight machines cannot be adequately adjusted to fit a child's stature.

conditions including musculoskeletal injuries, osteoarthritis, osteoporosis, hypertension, adult-onset (type II) diabetes, and chronic obstructive pulmonary disease. Specific findings of some of the studies identified in this systematic review are presented in later chapters of this textbook.

Delorme and Oxford Regimens

The concept of PRE was introduced by DeLorme,[60,61] who originally used the term *heavy resistance training*[60] and later *load-resisting exercise*[61] to describe a new system of strength training. DeLorme proposed and studied the use of three sets of resistance training with progressive loading during each set, using a percentage of a 10-RM. Other investigators[288] developed a modified regimen, the Oxford technique, with regressive loading in each set (Table 6.10).

The DeLorme technique builds a warm-up period into the protocol, whereas the Oxford technique decreases the resistance as the muscle fatigues within a session. Both regimens incorporate a rest interval between sets, both increase the resistance incrementally over time to apply progressive overload, and both have been shown to result in training-induced strength gains.

TABLE 6.10 Comparison of Two PRE Regimens

DeLorme Regimen	Oxford Regimen
Determination of a 10-RM	Determination of a 10
10 reps @ 50% of the 10-RM	10 reps @ 100% of the 10
10 reps @ 75% of the 10-RM	10 reps @ 75% of the 10
10 reps @ 100% of the 10-RM	10 reps @ 50% of the 10

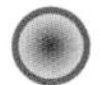 **FOCUS ON EVIDENCE**

In a randomized study comparing the DeLorme and Oxford regimens, no significant difference was found in adaptive quadriceps muscle group strength gains in older adults after a 9-week exercise program.[91]

Many variations of PRE protocols have been proposed and studied since the DeLorme and Oxford systems were introduced, most aiming to determine the optimal intensity, number of repetitions and sets, frequency, and progression of loading. In reality, an ideal combination of these variables does not exist. Extensive research has shown that many combinations of exercise load, repetitions and sets, frequency, and rest intervals significantly improve strength.[16,95,163] The typical PRE program produces training-induced strength gains using 2 to 3 sets of 6 to 12 repetitions of a 6- to 12-RM.[8,16,95,162,163] This gives a therapist wide latitude when designing an effective resistance training program.

DAPRE Regimen

Knowing when and by how much to increase the resistance in a PRE program is often imprecise and arbitrary. A common guideline is to increase the weight by 5% to 10% when all prescribed repetitions and sets can be completed easily without significant fatigue. The Daily Adjustable Progressive Resistive Exercise (DAPRE) technique[157,158] is a more systematic and objective system that takes into account the different rates at which individuals progress during rehabilitation or conditioning programs. The system is based on a 6-RM working weight (Table 6.11). The adjusted working weight, which is based on the maximum number of repetitions possible using the working weight in Set #3 of the regimen, determines the working weight for the next exercise session (Table 6.12).

NOTE: It should be pointed out that the recommended increases or decrease in the adjusted working weight are based on progressive loading of the quadriceps muscle group.

Circuit Weight Training

Another system of mechanical resistance training that has been developed is *circuit weight training*.[19,32,163] A preestablished sequence or circuit of exercises targeting major muscle groups is performed in succession at individual exercise stations. Typically, minimal rest is provided between the 8 to 12 individual circuit stations, which add cardiovascular system conditioning to the strengthening program. An example of a circuit weight training sequence is shown in Box 6.19.

TABLE 6.11 DAPRE Technique

Sets	Repetitions	Amount of Resistance
1	10	50% 6-RM*
2	6	75% 6-RM
3	Maximum possible	100% 6-RM
4	Maximum possible	100% adjusted working weight**

*6-RM = working weight
**See Table 6.13 for calculation of the adjusted working weight.

TABLE 6.12 Calculation of the Adjusted Working Weight for the DAPRE Regimen

Adjustment of Working Weight		
Repetitions in Set 3	Set 4	Next exercise session 3
0–2	↓ 5–10 lb	↓ 5–10 lb
3–4	↓ 0–5 lb	Same weight
5–6	Keep same weight	↑ 5–10 lb
7–10	↑ 5–10 lb	↑ 5–15 lb
11 or more	↑ 10–15 lb	↑ 10–20 lb

BOX 6.19 Example of a Resistance Training Circuit

Station #1: Bench press → #2: Leg press or squats → #3: Sit-ups → #4: Upright rowing → #5: Hamstring curls → #6: Prone trunk extension → #7: Shoulder press → #8: Heel raises → #9: Push-ups → #10: Leg lifts or lowering

Each resistance exercise is performed at an exercise station for a specified number of repetitions and sets. Typically, intensity (resistance) is lower and repetitions are higher than in other forms of weight training. For example, two to three sets of 8 to 12 repetitions at 90% to 100% 10-RM or 10 to 20 repetitions at 40% to 50% 1-RM are performed,[9,184] with a minimum amount of rest (15 to 20 seconds) between sets and stations. The program is progressed by increasing the number of sets or repetitions, the resistance, the number of exercise stations, and the number of circuit revolutions.

Exercise order is an important consideration when setting up a weight training circuit.[15,32,162] Exercises with free weights or weight machines should alternate among upper extremity, lower extremity, and trunk musculature and between muscle groups involved in pushing or pulling actions. This enables one muscle group to rest and recover from exercise while exercising another group so that muscle fatigue is minimized. Ideally, larger muscle groups should be exercised before smaller muscle groups. Multijoint exercises that recruit multiple muscle groups should be performed before exercises that recruit an isolated muscle group to minimize the risk of injury from fatigue.

Isokinetic Regimens

It is well established that isokinetic training improves muscle performance, but its effectiveness in carryover to functional tasks is less clear. Studies support[78,193] and refute[121,221] that isokinetic training improves function. Ideally, when isokinetic training is implemented in a rehabilitation program, it should be performed at velocities that closely match or at least approach the expected velocities of movement of specific functional tasks to have the most positive impact on function. Because many functional movements occur at a variety of medium to fast speeds, isokinetic training typically is performed at medium and fast velocities.[4,53,58,76]

Current isokinetic technology makes it possible to align training speeds to the movement velocities of some lower extremity functions such as walking.[53,283] This is less possible in the upper extremities where some functional movements occur at velocities that far exceed the capabilities of isokinetic dynamometers.[76] For example, overhead throwing velocities are well beyond 1000° per second.

It is also widely accepted that isokinetic training is relatively speed specific, with only limited transfer of training.[142,260]

Therefore, *speed-specific isokinetic training* matched to the velocity of a specific functional task is advocated.[4,55,76]

Velocity Spectrum Rehabilitation

To deal with the problem of limited physiological overflow of training effects from one training velocity to another, a regimen called *velocity spectrum rehabilitation* (VSR) has been advocated.[53,76,95] With this system of training, isokinetic exercises are performed across a range of angular velocities.[240]

NOTE: The guidelines for VSR that follow are for *concentric* isokinetic training. General guidelines for eccentric isokinetics are identified at the conclusion of this section.

Selection of training velocities. Typically, medium (60° or 90° to 180° per second) and fast (180° to 360° per second) angular velocities are selected for VSR. Although isokinetic units are designed for velocities faster than 360° per second, they are not used for VSR training because the limb must accelerate to the preset speed before encountering resistance from the torque arm of the dynamometer. At very high speeds, this acceleration phase consumes most of the arc of motion so that resistance is met in only a small portion of the ROM, limiting the potential for benefit.

It is proposed that the effects of isokinetic training only carry over to movements that are within 15° to 30° per second of the training velocity.[53,142] Therefore, some protocols use 30° per second increments for VSR training. Of course, if a patient trains at medium and fast velocities (from 60° or 90° to 360° per second) in one exercise session, this strategy necessitates nine different training velocities for one agonist/antagonist muscle pair, giving rise to a time-consuming exercise session. For this reason, a more common protocol is to use as few as three training velocities.[4,76,240]

Repetitions, sets, and rest. A typical VSR protocol might have the patient perform 1 or 2 sets of 8 to 10 repetitions of agonist/antagonist muscle groups (reciprocal training) at multiple velocities.[4,53,76] For example, at medium velocities training could occur at 90°, 120°, 150°, and 180° per second. A second series would then be performed at decreasing velocities—180°, 150°, 120°, and 90° per second. Because many combinations of repetitions, sets, and different training velocities lead to improvement in muscle performance, the therapist has many options when designing a VSR program. A 15- to 20-second rest between sets and a 60-second rest between exercise velocities is recommended.[245] The suggested frequency for VSR is a maximum of three times per week.[4]

Intensity. Submaximal effort exercise on the dynamometer can be used for a brief warm-up period. However, this is not a replacement for a more general form of upper or lower body warm-up exercises, such as cycling or upper-extremity ergometry. When training to improve endurance, exercises are carried out at a submaximal intensity (effort) but to improve strength or power, maximal intensity exercise is used.

During the early stages of isokinetic training, it is useful to begin with submaximal intensity exercise at medium and slow velocities so the patient gets the "feel" of the device while protecting the muscle. As the training program progresses, it is usually safe for the patient to exert maximum effort at medium speeds. Slow-velocity training is eliminated when the patient begins to exert maximum effort. During the advanced phase of rehabilitation, training with maximum-effort at fast velocities is emphasized as long as exercises are pain-free.[58] Additional aspects to a progression of isokinetic training regimens include short-arc to full-arc exercises and concentric to eccentric movements.[58]

PRECAUTION: Training with maximum effort at slow velocities is rarely indicated because of the excessive shear forces produced across joint surfaces.[53,76]

Eccentric Isokinetic Training: Special Considerations

Because eccentric isokinetic training became available more gradually as technology evolved, there is less guidance on exercise parameters and minimal evidence supporting its efficacy. Most current guidelines are based on clinical opinion or anecdotal evidence. Key differences in eccentric versus concentric isokinetic guidelines are listed in Box 6.20. Several resources describe pathology-specific guidelines for eccentric isokinetic training based on clinical experience.[4,53,76,115,116]

PRECAUTION: Eccentric isokinetic training is appropriate only during the final phase of a rehabilitation program, when additional challenge to individual muscle groups is needed due to persistent strength and power deficits. Because eccentric isokinetic training may not accurately match the functional

BOX 6.20 Key Differences in Eccentric Versus Concentric Isokinetic Training

Eccentric isokinetic exercise is:

- Introduced only *after maximal* effort concentric isokinetic exercise can be performed without pain at several velocities
- Implemented only after functional ROM has been restored
- Performed at slower velocities across a narrower velocity spectrum than concentric isokinetic exercise—usually between 60° and 120°/sec per second for the general population and up to 180°/sec for athletes
- Carried out at submaximal levels for a longer time frame to avoid extensive torque production and lessen the risk of DOMS
- Most commonly performed in a continuous concentric-eccentric pattern for a muscle group during training, whereas concentric isokinetics involves reciprocal training of agonist/antagonist muscle groups

way in which eccentric contractions occur, medium training velocities are considered safer than fast velocities. Sudden, rapid, motor-driven movements of the dynamometer's torque arm against a limb could injure healing tissue.

Equipment for Resistance Training

There is a large variety of resistance training exercise equipment available on the market. The equipment ranges from simple to complex, compact to space-consuming, and inexpensive to expensive. An assortment of simple but versatile handheld and cuff weights or elastic resistance products is useful in clinical and home settings, whereas multiple pieces of variable resistance equipment may be useful for advanced-level resistance training. The literature distributed by manufacturers, product demonstrations at professional meetings, and studies of these products reported in the research literature are the main sources of information about new products on the market.

Although most equipment is *load resisting* (augments the resistance of gravity), a few pieces of equipment can be adapted to be *load assisting* (eliminates or diminishes the resistance of gravity) to improve the strength of weak muscles. Equipment can be used for static or dynamic, concentric or eccentric, and open-chain or closed-chain exercises to improve muscular strength, power, or endurance, neuromuscular stability or control, as well as cardiopulmonary fitness.

Ultimately, the right equipment choice depends on the needs, abilities, and goals of the person using the equipment. Other factors that influence equipment choice are the *availability*, the *cost* of purchase and/or maintenance, the *ease of use*, the *versatility*, and the *space requirements*. Once the appropriate equipment has been selected, its safe and effective use is the highest priority. General principles for equipment use are listed in Box 6.21.

Free Weights and Simple Weight-Pulley Systems

Types of Free Weights

Free weights are incremental weights that are held in the hand or secured to an extremity or the trunk. They include commercially available dumbbells, barbells, weighted balls (Fig. 6.44), cuff weights, weighted vests, and even sandbags. Free weights can even be fashioned from readily available materials and objects for use in a home exercise program.

BOX 6.21 General Principles for the Selection and Use of Equipment

- Base the selection of equipment on a comprehensive examination and evaluation of the patient.
- Determine when in the exercise program the use of equipment should be introduced and when it should be altered or discontinued.
- Determine if the equipment can or should be set up and used independently by a patient.
- Teach appropriate exercise form and technique with the equipment before adding resistance.
- Teach and supervise the application and use of the equipment before allowing a patient to use the equipment independently.
- Adhere to all safety precautions when applying and using equipment.
  - Be sure all attachments, cuffs, collars, and straps are secured and that the equipment is appropriately adjusted to the individual patient prior to the exercise.
  - Apply padding for comfort, if necessary, especially over bony prominences. Stabilize or support appropriate structures to prevent unwanted movement and undue stress on body parts.
  - If exercise machines are used independently, be certain that set-up and safety instructions are clearly illustrated and affixed directly to the equipment.
- Use available range-limiting attachments when ROM must be restricted to protect healing tissues or unstable structures.
- Give explicit instructions on how, when, and to what extent to change or adapt the equipment to provide a progressive overload when the patient is using the equipment in a home program.
- When transitioning from one type of resistance equipment to another, be certain that the newly selected equipment and method of set-up provides a similar level of torque production to the prior equipment to avoid insufficient or excessive loads.
- When the exercise has been completed:
  - Disengage the equipment and leave it in proper condition for future use.
  - Never leave broken or potentially hazardous equipment available for future use.
- Set up a regular routine of maintenance, replacement, or safety checks for all equipment.

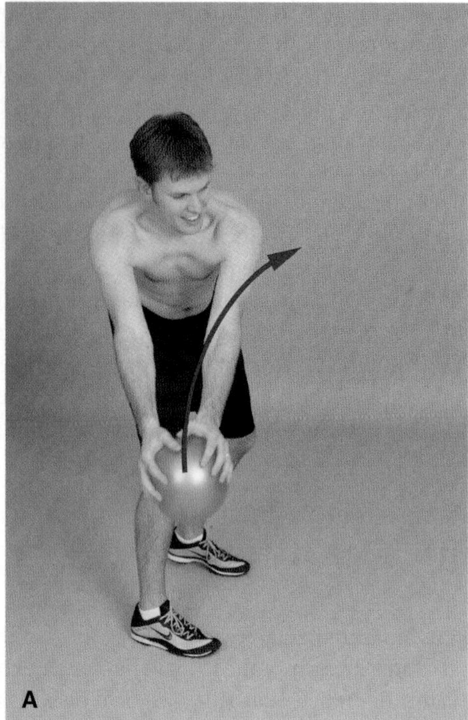

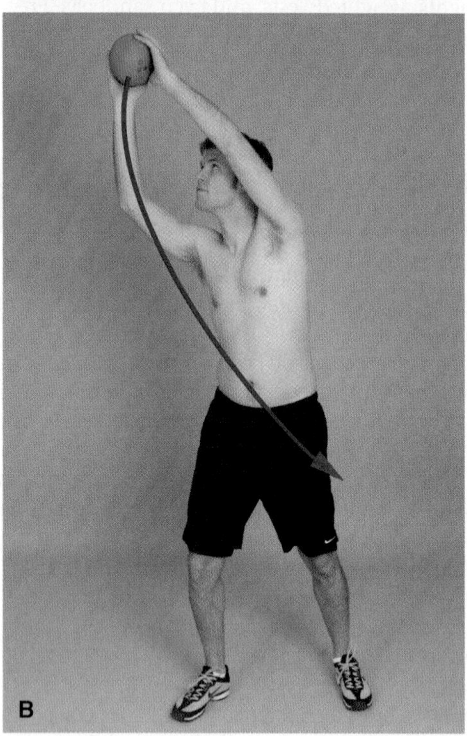

FIGURE 6.44 (A & B) Holding a weighted ball while performing combined patterns of movement provides resistance to upper extremity and trunk muscles and augments the resistance of body weight to lower extremity muscle groups during weight-bearing activities.

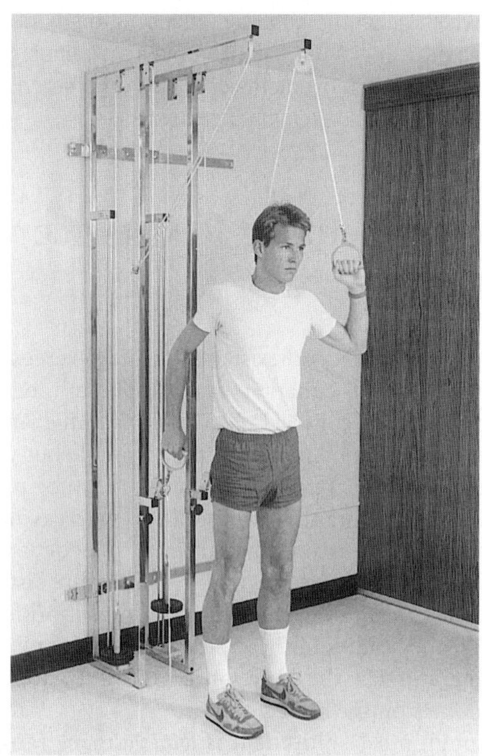

FIGURE 6.45 Multi-Exercise Pulley Unit can be used to strengthen a variety of muscle groups. *(Courtesy of N–K Products Company, Inc., Soquel, CA.)*

Simple Weight-Pulley Systems

Free-standing or wall-mounted simple weight-pulley systems are commonly used for resisted upper and lower extremity or trunk exercises (Fig. 6.45). Permanent or interchangeable weights are available. Permanent systems typically have stacks of individual weight plates in 5- to 10-lb increments. The amount of resistance used for exercise can be easily adjusted by selecting a certain number of stacked plates with the placement of a single weight key or pin.

NOTE: The simple weight-pulley systems described here are those that impose a relatively constant (fixed) load. Variable resistance weight machines, some of which incorporate pulleys into their designs, are discussed later in this section.

Characteristics of Free Weights and Simple Weight-Pulley Systems

Free weights and weight-pulley systems impose a constant load. In these systems the external resistance maximally challenges the contacting muscle at only one portion of the ROM, which depends on the patient's positioning. The weight that is selected for exercise cannot be greater than what the muscle can control at this particular point in the ROM. In addition, there is no accommodation for a painful arc if the patient needs to reduce their internal effort at some point in the ROM.

When using free weights, it is possible to vary the point in the ROM at which the maximum exercise load is experienced by changing the patient's position with respect to gravity or the direction of the resistance load. For example, shoulder flexion may be resisted with the patient standing or supine and holding a weight in the hand.

- *Patient position:* standing (Fig. 6.46)—Maximum resistance is experienced and maximum external torque is produced

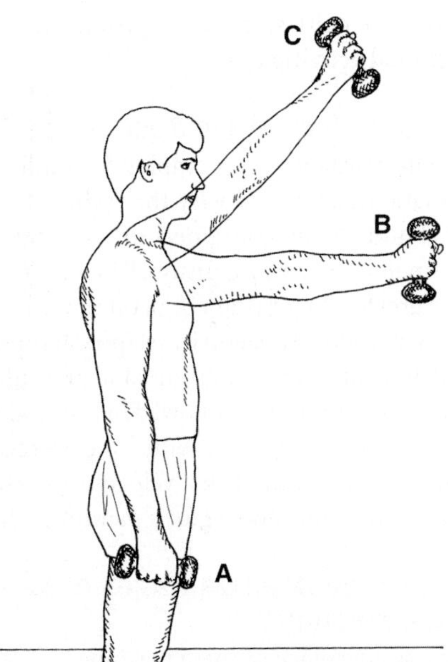

FIGURE 6.46 When the patient is standing and lifting a weight: **(A)** Zero torque is produced in the shoulder flexors when the shoulder is at 0° of flexion; **(B)** maximum torque is produced when the shoulder is at 90° of flexion; and **(C)** torque again decreases as the arm moves from 90° to 180° of shoulder flexion.

when the shoulder is at 90° of flexion. No torque is produced by the weight when the shoulder is at 0° of flexion. External torque progressively decreases as the patient lifts the weight from 90° to 180° of flexion. In addition, when the weight is at the side (in the 0° position of the shoulder), it causes traction force on the extremity; when overhead, it causes compression force through the upper extremity joints.

- *Patient position:* supine (Fig. 6.47)—Maximum resistance is experienced and maximum external torque is produced when the shoulder is at 0° of flexion. No torque is produced

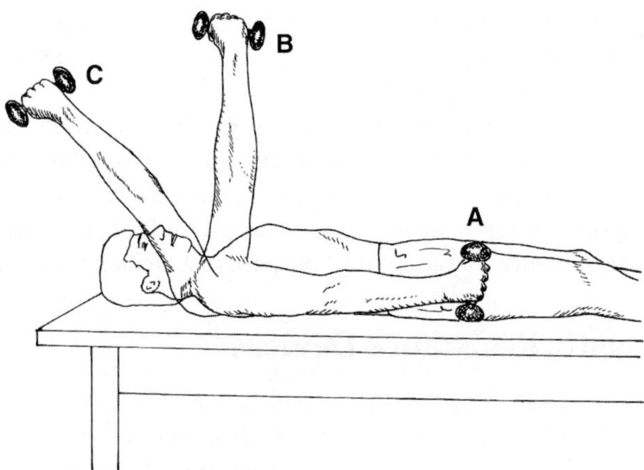

FIGURE 6.47 When the patient is supine and lifting a weight: **(A)** Maximum torque is produced at 0° of shoulder flexion; **(B)** zero torque is produced at 90° of shoulder flexion; and **(C)** the shoulder extensors are active and contract eccentrically against resistance from 90° to 180° of shoulder flexion.

by the weight at 90° of shoulder flexion. In this position the load creates a compression force on the extremity. The shoulder flexors are not active between 90° and 180° of shoulder flexion. Instead, the shoulder extensors contract eccentrically to control the descent of the arm and weight.

The therapist must determine at which portion of the patient's ROM maximum strength is needed and then choose the optimum position in which the exercise should be performed to gain maximum benefit from the exercise.

Simple weight-pulley systems provide maximum resistance when the angle of the pulley is at right angles to the moving bone. As the angle of the pulley becomes more acute, the load creates more compression through the moving bones and joints and offers less effective resistance.

Unlike many weight machines, neither free weights nor pulleys provide external stabilization. When a patient lifts or lowers a weight to and from an overhead position, muscles of the scapula and shoulder abductors, adductors, and rotators must synergistically contract to stabilize the arm and keep it aligned in the correct plane of motion. The need for concurrent contraction of adjacent stabilizing muscle groups can be viewed as an advantage or a disadvantage. Because muscular stabilization is necessary to control the plane or pattern of movement, less external resistance can be controlled with free weights than can be managed with a weight machine that offers stabilization.

Advantages and Disadvantages of Free Weights and Simple Weight-Pulley Systems

- Exercises can be performed in many positions, including supine, side-lying, prone, sitting, or standing. Many muscle groups in the extremities and trunk can be strengthened by simply repositioning the patient.
- Free weights and simple weight-pulley systems are typically used for dynamic, nonweight-bearing exercises but also can be set up for isometric exercise and resisted weight-bearing activities.
- Stabilizing muscle groups are recruited; however, because there is no external source of stabilization and movements must be controlled entirely by the patient, it may take more time for the patient to learn correct alignment and movement patterns.
- Many movement patterns are possible, incorporating single plane or multiplanar motions. An exercise can be highly specific to one muscle or generalized to several muscle groups. Movement patterns that replicate functional activities can be resisted.
- If a large enough assortment of graduated free weights is available, resistance can be increased by very small increments. The weight plates of pulley systems have larger increments of resistance, usually a minimum of 5 pounds per plate.
- Most exercises with free weights and weight-pulley systems must be performed slowly to minimize acceleration and momentum and prevent uncontrolled, end-range movements that could compromise patient safety. It is thought

that exclusively performing slow movements during strengthening activities has less carryover to many daily living activities compared with incorporating both slow- and fast-velocity exercises.

- Dumbbells and barbells that allow adjustable resistance through interchangeable plates are versatile and can be used for patients with many different levels of strength, but they require patient or personnel time for proper assembly.
- Bilateral lifting exercises with barbell weights often require the assistance of a spotter to ensure patient safety, thus increasing personnel time.

Variable Resistance Units

Variable resistance exercise equipment falls into two broad categories: specially designed weight-cable (weight-pulley) machines and hydraulic and pneumatic units. Both categories of equipment impose a variable load on the contracting muscles consistent with the changing torque-producing capabilities of the muscles throughout the available ROM.

Variable Resistance Weight-Cable Systems

Variable resistance weight-cable machines (Fig. 6.48) use a cam (an elliptical or kidney-shaped disk) in their design. The cam is designed to vary the load (torque) applied to the contracting muscle even though the weight remains constant. In theory, the cam is configured to match the torque output of the contracting muscle. This system varies the external load imposed on the contracting muscle based on the physical dimensions of the "average" individual. How effectively this design provides truly accommodating resistance throughout the full ROM is debatable.

During each repetition of an exercise, the same muscle group contracts both concentrically and eccentrically to manage the external resistance. As with simple weight-pulley systems and free weights, exercises must be performed at relatively slow velocities, thus compromising carryover to many functional activities.

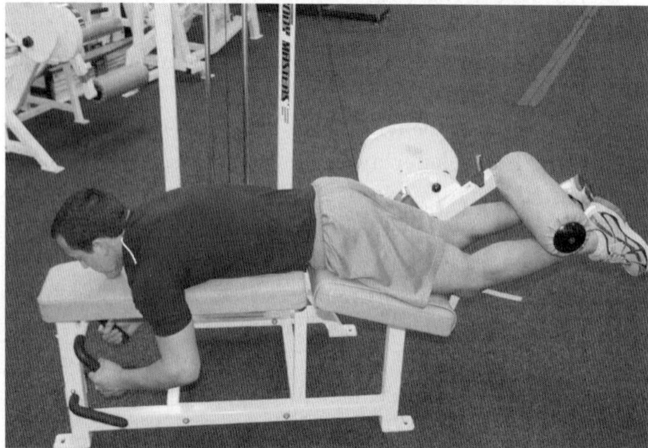

FIGURE 6.48 Variable resistance by means of a cam mechanism in the weight-pulley system is applied to concentric and eccentric contractions of the hamstrings as the knees flex and extend.

Hydraulic and Pneumatic Resistance Devices

Other variable resistance units employ hydraulic or pressurized pneumatic resistance to vary the resistance throughout the ROM. Fluid or air contained in a cylinder is forced through a small opening by a piston. The faster the piston is pushed, the greater the resistance encountered.

These devices allow concentric, reciprocal muscle work to agonist and antagonist muscle groups and, in some machines, provide concentric resistance followed by controlled eccentric return through the ROM. Patients can exercise safely at medium and, to some extent, fast velocities. These units also allow a patient to accommodate for a painful arc in the ROM.

Advantages and Disadvantages of Variable Resistance Machines

- The obvious advantage of these machines is that the resistance is adjusted in an attempt to match a muscle's torque-generating capabilities throughout the ROM. The contracting muscle is subjected to near maximal loads at multiple points in the ROM rather than just through one small portion of the range.
- Most pieces of equipment are designed to isolate and exercise specific muscle groups. For example, resisted squats are performed on one machine and hamstring curls on another. Consequently, numerous units are needed to exercise all major muscles groups.
- Unlike functional movement, most machines allow only single-plane movements, although some newer units now offer a dual-axis design allowing multiplanar motions that strengthen multiple muscle groups and more closely resemble functional movement patterns.
- The equipment is adjustable to allow individuals of varying heights to perform each exercise in a well-aligned position.
- Each unit provides substantial external stabilization to guide or limit movements. This makes it easier for the patient to learn how to perform the exercise correctly and safely and helps maintain appropriate alignment without assistance or supervision.
- One of the main disadvantages of weight machines is the initial expense and ongoing maintenance costs. Multiple machines, usually 8 to 10 or more, must be purchased to target multiple major muscle groups. Multiple machines also require a large amount of space in a facility.

Elastic Resistance Devices

Elastic resistance products are widely used in rehabilitation and have been shown to be an effective method of providing sufficient resistance to improve muscle strength.[139] Resistance training with elastic products is also a feasible alternative to training with weight machines[44] and free weights,[11] generating comparably high levels of muscle activation during exercises.

Quantitative analysis of the resistance supplied by elastic products or the level of muscle activation during their use suggests that their effectiveness requires not only the application of biomechanical principles, but also an understanding of the physical properties of elastic resistance material.[130,131,140,145,214,216,232,257]

Types of Elastic Resistance

Elastic resistance products, specifically designed for use during exercise, fall into two broad categories: elastic bands and elastic tubing. Elastic bands and tubing are produced by several manufacturers under different product names, the most familiar of which is Thera-Band® Elastic Resistance Bands and Tubing (Hygenic Corp., Akron, OH). Both types of products are available in an assortment of thicknesses or diameters that provide progressive levels of resistance. Color-coding denotes the thickness of the product and grades of resistance.

Properties of Elastic Resistance: Implications for Exercise

A number of studies describing the physical characteristics of elastic resistance have provided quantitative information about its material properties. Knowledge of this information enables a therapist to use elastic resistance more effectively for therapeutic exercise programs.

Effect of elongation of elastic material. Elastic resistance provides a form of variable resistance because the force generated changes as the material is elongated. Specifically, as it is stretched, the amount of resistance (force) produced by an elastic band or tubing increases depending on the *relative change* in the length of the material *(percentage of elongation/deformation)* from the start to the end of elongation. There is a relatively predictable and *linear* relationship between the percentage of elongation and the tensile force of the material.[131,140,145,216,232]

To determine the percentage of elongation, the stretched length must be compared with the resting length of the elastic material. The *resting length* of a band or tubing is its length when it is laid out flat and there is no stretch applied. The actual length of the material before it is stretched has no effect on the force imparted. Rather, it is the percentage of elongation that affects the tensile forces.[216]

The formula for calculating the percentage of elongation/deformation is:[139,232]

$$\text{Percent of elongation} = (\text{stretched length} - \text{resting length}) \div \text{resting length} \times 100$$

Using this formula, if a 2-ft length of red tubing, for example, is stretched to 4 feet, the percentage of elongation is 100%. With this in mind, it is understandable why a 1-ft length stretched to 2 feet (100% elongation) generates the same force as a 2-ft length of the same color tubing stretched to 4 feet.[214,215]

Furthermore, the *rate* at which elastic material is stretched does not seem to have a significant effect on the amount of resistance encountered.[216] Consequently, when a patient is performing a particular exercise, so long as the percentage of elongation of the tubing or band is the same from one repetition to the next, the resistance encountered is the same regardless of whether the exercise is performed at slow or fast velocity.

Determination and quantification of resistance. To help clinicians make decisions about the grade (color) of elastic material to select for a patient's exercise program, a number of studies have quantified the resistance imparted by elastic bands or tubing.[131,140,145,216,232,257] These studies measured and compared the tensile forces generated by various grades of elastic bands or tubing in relation to the percentage of elongation of the material. The forces expected at specific percentages of elongation of each grade of bands or tubing can be calculated by means of linear regression equations. Detailed specifications about the material properties of one brand of elastic resistance products, Thera-Band®, are available at www.thera-bandacademy.com/.

During exercise, the percentage of deformation and resulting resistance (force) from the material is not the only factor that must be considered. The amount of torque (force × distance) imposed by the elastic material on the bony lever is also an important consideration. Just because the tension produced by an elastic band or tubing increases as it is stretched, it does not mean that the imposed torque necessarily increases from the beginning to the end of an exercise. In addition to the resistance (force) imposed by the elastic material as it is stretched, the length of the external moment arm will change as the angle of the elastic resistance vector with respect to the moving limb will modify the torque generated by the elastic material.[140] Studies have indicated that bell-shaped torque curves occur during exercises with elastic material, with the peak torque near midrange.[140,215] As in all forms of dynamic resistance exercise, the length-tension relationship of the contracting muscle also affects its ability to respond to the changing external load.

Fatigue characteristics. Elastic resistance products tend to fatigue over time, which causes the material to lose some of its force-generating property.[139] The extent of this *material fatigue* is dependent on the number of times the elastic band or tubing has been stretched (number of stretch cycles) and the percentage of deformation with each stretch.[232]

Studies have shown that the decrease in tensile force is significant but small, with much of the decrease occurring within the first 20[216] or 50[139] stretch cycles. However, in the former study, investigators found that after this small, initial decrease in tensile force occurred, there was no appreciable decrease in the force-generating potential of the tubing after more than 5,000 cycles of stretch. This translates to performing 10 repetitions each of 4 different exercises, 3 times a day, every day for 6 weeks with the same piece of tubing before it needs replacing.

Elastic materials also display a property called *viscoelastic creep.* If a constant load is placed on elastic material, in time it becomes brittle and eventually ruptures. Environmental conditions, such as heat and humidity, also affect the force-generating potential of elastic bands and tubing.[139]

Application of Elastic Resistance

Selecting the appropriate grade of material. The thickness (stiffness) of the material affects the level of resistance. Heavier grades of elastic generate greater tension when stretched and, therefore, impart greater levels of resistance.[131,139,232] As already noted, corresponding levels of resistance have been published for the different grades of bands and tubing. Therapists and patients should be aware that color-coding schemes and their corresponding levels of resistance might not be consistent across manufacturers.

FOCUS ON EVIDENCE

In a study[257] comparing similar colors and lengths of Thera-Band® and Cando tubing (Cando Fabrication Enterprises, White Plains, NY), investigators measured (by means of a strain gauge) the forces generated under similar conditions. They found no appreciable differences between the two products except for the thinnest (yellow) and thickest (silver/grey) grades. In those two grades the Cando tubing produced approximately 30% to 35% higher levels of force than the Thera-Band® product. Despite these small differences, investigators suggested that it is prudent to use the same product with the same patient.

Selecting the appropriate length. Elastic bands or tubing come in large rolls and can be cut to length for the specific exercise to be performed and the height of a patient or the length of the extremities. The length of the elastic material should be sufficient to attach it *securely* at both ends. It should be taut but not stretched (*resting length*) at the beginning position of an exercise.

Because the percentage of elongation of the material affects the tension produced, it is essential that the same length of elastic material is used each time a particular exercise is performed. Otherwise, the imposed load may vary between exercise sessions even though the same grade of elastic is used.

Securing bands or tubing. One end of the material is often tied or attached to a fixed object such as a doorknob, table leg, or D-ring or can be secured by having the patient stand on it. The other end is then grasped or fastened to a nylon loop, which is then placed around a limb segment. The elastic material can also be secured to a harness on a patient's trunk for resisted walking activities. The material can also be held in both hands or looped under both feet for bilateral exercise. Figure 6.49 A, B, and C depicts upper or lower extremity and trunk strengthening activities using elastic resistance.

Setting up an exercise. With elastic resistance, the maximum external resistance torque occurs when the material is on a stretch and angled 90° to the lever arm (moving bone). The therapist should determine the limb position at which maximum resistance is desired during the exercise and then

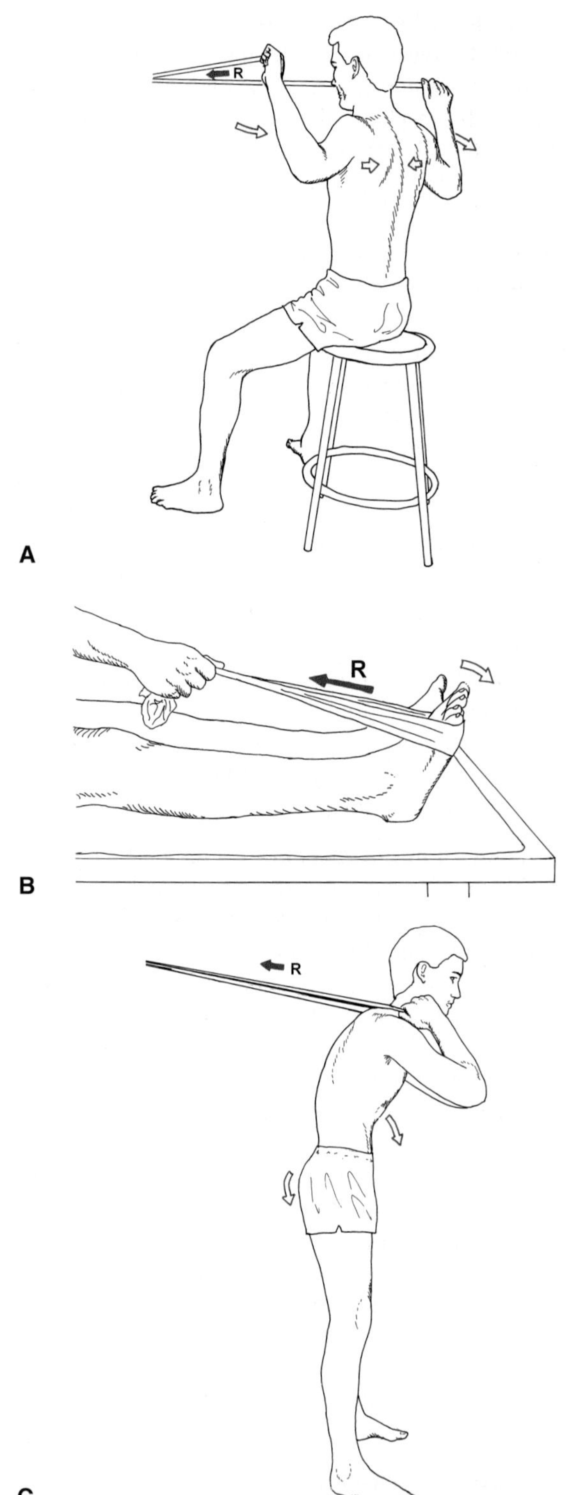

FIGURE 6.49 Use of elastic resistance to strengthen **(A)** upper or **(B)** lower extremity or **(C)** trunk musculature.

secure the elastic material so that a right angle is formed between the material and limb at that position. When the material is at an acute angle to the moving bone, there is less resistance but greater joint compressive force.

It is important to position the patient and elastic material in the same manner from one exercise session to the next. Each time a patient performs a specific exercise, in addition to using the same length of elastic material, the relationship between the patient and the attachment site of the material should be consistent. A resource by Page and Ellenbecker[214] describes setups for numerous exercises using elastic resistance.

Progressing exercises. Exercises can be progressed by increasing the number of repetitions performed with the same grade of resistance or by using the next higher grade of elastic band or tubing.

Advantages and Disadvantages of Exercise With Elastic Resistance

Advantages

- Elastic resistance products are portable and relatively inexpensive, making them an ideal choice for home exercise programs.
- Because elastic resistance is not significantly gravity dependent, elastic bands and tubing are extremely *versatile*, allowing many combinations of limb and trunk movement patterns and patient positions.[139,140,215]
- It is safe to exercise at moderate to fast velocities with elastic resistance because the patient does not have to overcome the inertia of a rapidly moving weight. As such, it is appropriate for plyometric training (see Chapter 23).

Disadvantages

- One of the most significant drawbacks to the use of elastic resistance is the need to refer to a table of figures for quantitative information about the level of resistance for each color-coded grade of material. This makes it difficult to know which grade to select initially and to what extent changing the grade of the band or tubing changes the level of resistance.
- As with free weights, there is no source of stabilization or control of extraneous movements when an elastic band or tubing is used for resistance. The patient must use muscular stabilization to ensure that the correct movement pattern occurs.
- Although the effects of material fatigue are small with typical clinical use, elastic bands and tubing should be replaced on a routine basis to ensure patient safety.[139,232] When many individuals use the same precut lengths of bands or tubing, it may be difficult to determine how much use has occurred and when replacement is necessary.
- Some elastic products contain latex, which is a fairly common allergen, thus eliminating use by some individuals. However, there are latex-free products on the market at a relatively comparable cost.

Equipment for Dynamic Stabilization Training

BodyBlade®

The BodyBlade® (Fig. 6.50) is a dynamic, reactive device that produces oscillatory resistance proportional to an oscillatory force generated by the patient.[33,177] During exercise, agonist and antagonist muscle groups rapidly contract in an attempt to control the instability created by oscillations of the blade. The greater the amplitude or flex of the blade, the greater the resistance. This provides progressive resistance that the patient controls.

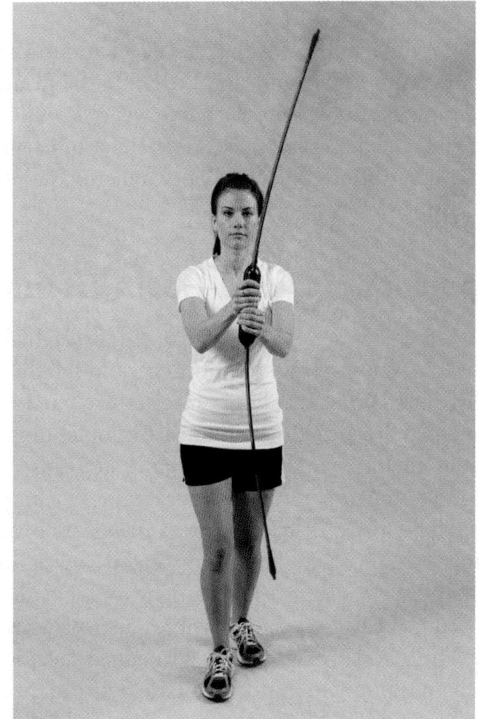

FIGURE 6.50 Dynamic stabilization exercises of the upper extremity and trunk using the BodyBlade®.

Initially, the oscillating blade is maintained in single positions in space, particularly those positions in which dynamic stability is required for functional activities. The patient can progress the exercises by moving the upper extremity through various planes of motion (from sagittal to frontal and ultimately to transverse) while maintaining oscillations of the blade. The goal of this type of resistance is to develop proximal joint stability as a foundation of controlled mobility.

FOCUS ON EVIDENCE

Lister and colleagues[177] conducted a within-subject trial to determine the extent of activation of the scapula stabilizing muscles during upper extremity exercise with three forms of resistance (a cuff weight, elastic resistance, and a BodyBlade®). Healthy college athletes ($n = 30$) performed shoulder flexion and abduction with each type of equipment as activity in the upper trapezius, lower trapezius, and serratus anterior muscles was quantified with EMG. The study demonstrated that significantly greater muscle activity occurred in each of the three scapular stabilizers during exercises with the blade than with either the cuff weight or elastic resistance. The investigators recommended use of a blade in shoulder rehabilitation to develop scapular stability during arm movements.

Swiss Balls (Stability Balls)

Heavy-duty vinyl balls, usually 20 to 30 inches in diameter, are used for a variety of trunk and extremity stabilization exercises. Using elastic resistance or free weights while on the ball increases the difficulty of exercises. Refer to Chapters 16 and 23 for descriptions of a number of dynamic stabilization exercises using stability balls.

Equipment for Closed-Chain Training

Many closed-chain exercises are performed in weight-bearing positions to develop strength, endurance, and stability across multiple joints. Typically, these exercises use partial or full body weight as the source of resistance. Examples in the lower extremities include squats, lunges, and step-ups or step-downs, and in the upper extremities examples include push-ups, press-ups, and pull-ups. These exercises are progressed by adding resistance with handheld weights, a weighted belt or vest, or elastic resistance. Changing from bilateral to unilateral weight bearing (when feasible) also progresses the exercise. The following equipment is designed specifically for closed-chain training to improve muscle performance across multiple joints.

Body Weight Resistance: Multipurpose Exercise Systems

The Total Gym® system uses a glide board, which can be set at 10 incline angles, enabling a patient to perform bilateral or unilateral closed-chain strengthening and endurance exercises in positions that range from partially reclining to standing (Fig. 6.51 A and B). The level of resistance on the Total Gym apparatus is increased or decreased by adjusting the angle of the glide board on the incline.

Performing squatting exercises in a semi-reclining position allows the patient to begin closed-chain training in a partially loaded (partial weight-bearing) condition early in the rehabilitation program. Later, the patient can progress to forward lunges (where the foot slides forward on the glide board) while in a standing position.

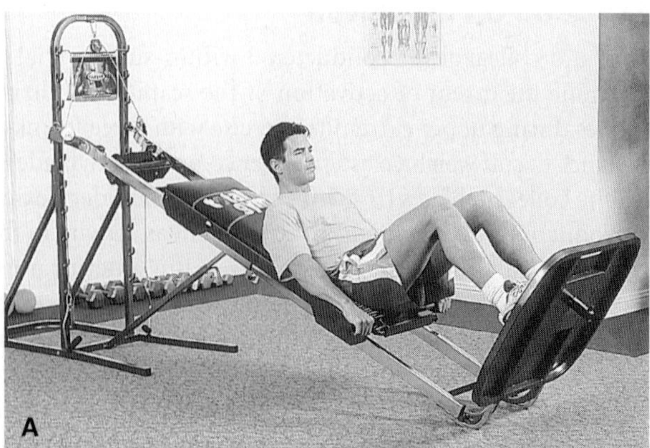

FIGURE 6.51 Closed-chain training in the **(A)** semi-reclining position and

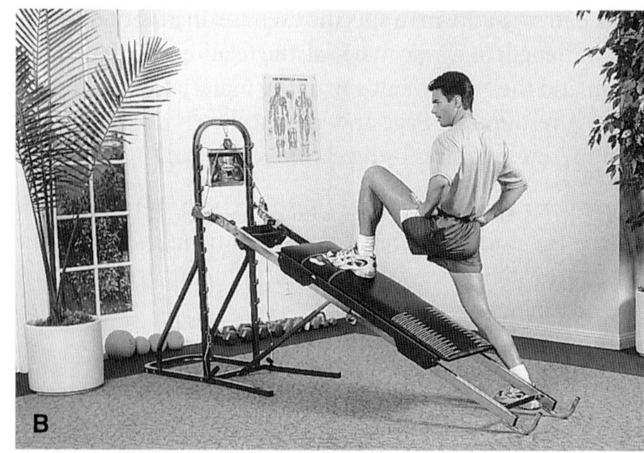

FIGURE 6.51 (B) standing position using the Total Gym® system. *(Courtesy of Total Gym®, San Diego, CA.)*

CLINICAL TIP

The Total Gym® system also can be set up for trunk exercises and open-chain exercises for the upper or lower extremities.

Slide Boards

The ProFitter® (Fig. 6.52) consists of a moving platform that slides side to side across an elliptical surface against adjustable resistance. While it is most often used with the patient standing for lower extremity rehabilitation, it can also be used for

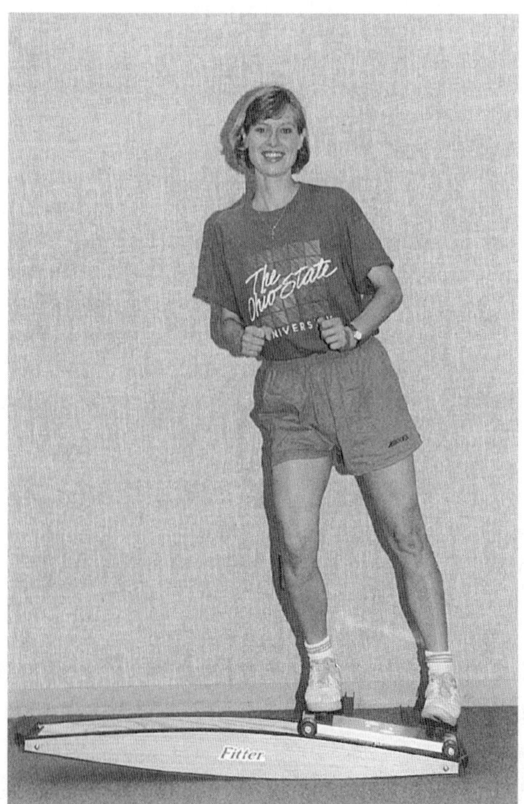

FIGURE 6.52 Pro Fitter provides closed-chain resistance to lower extremity musculature in preparation for functional activities.

upper extremity and trunk stability exercises. Medial-lateral or anterior-posterior movements are possible.

Balance Equipment

A balance board (wobble board) or BOSU® (in the shape of a half sphere with a flat and round side) is used primarily for stabilization, proprioceptive, and perturbation training. Bilateral or unilateral weight bearing through the upper or lower extremities can be performed on this equipment to develop strength and stability. Some balance boards, such as the BAPS (Biomechanical Ankle Platform System) board, have interchangeable half spheres in several sizes that progressively increase the difficulty of the balance activity. Refer to Chapters 8 and 23 for examples of balance activities using various types of equipment.

Mini-Trampolines (Rebounders)

Mini-trampolines enable the patient to begin gentle, bilateral or unilateral bouncing activities on a resilient surface to decrease the impact on joints. A patient can jog, jump, or hop in place. "Mini-tramps" that have a waist-height bar attached to their frame for the patient to hold onto during exercise provide additional safety.

Reciprocal Exercise Equipment

Similar to other types of equipment that can be used for closed-chain training, reciprocal exercise devices strengthen multiple muscle groups across multiple joints. They also are appropriate for low-intensity, high-repetition resistance training to improve muscular endurance, reciprocal coordination of the upper or lower extremities, and cardiopulmonary fitness. They are often used for warm-up or cool-down exercises prior to or following more intense resistance training. Resistance is imparted by an adjustable friction device or by a hydraulic or pneumatic mechanism.

Stationary Exercise Cycles

Upright or recumbent stationary exercise cycles are used to increase lower extremity strength and endurance. An upright cycle requires greater patient trunk control and balance than does a recumbent cycle. A few exercise cycles provide resistance to the upper extremities as well. Resistance can be graded to progressively challenge the patient. Distance, speed, or duration of exercise can be monitored.

Exercise cycles provide resistance to muscles during repetitive, nonimpact, and reciprocal extremity movements. Passive cycles resist only concentric muscle activity as the patient performs pushing or pulling movements. Motor-driven exercise cycles can be adjusted to provide eccentric as well as concentric resistance. Adjusting the seat placement alters the ROM that occurs in the lower extremity joints.

Portable Resistive Reciprocal Exercise Units

A number of portable resistive exercisers are effective alternatives to an exercise cycle for repetitive, reciprocal exercise. One such product, the Chattanooga Group Exerciser® (Fig. 6.53), can be used for lower extremity exercise by placing the unit on the floor in front of a chair or wheelchair. This is particularly appropriate for a patient who is unable to get on and off an exercise cycle. In addition, it can be placed on a table for upper extremity exercise. Resistance can be adjusted to meet the abilities of individual patients and to progress the exercise when appropriate.

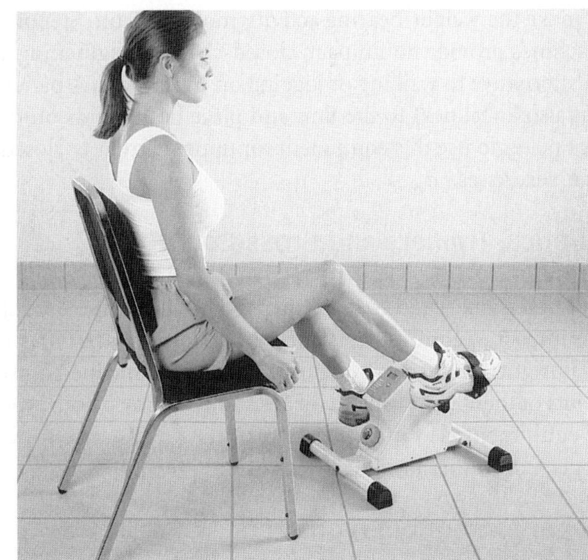

FIGURE 6.53 Resisted reciprocal exercise using the Chattanooga Exerciser.® *(Courtesy of Chattanooga Group, Inc., Hixon, TN.)*

Stair-Stepping Machines

The StairMaster® (Fig. 6.54) and the Climb Max 2000® are examples of stepping machines that allow the patient to perform reciprocal pushing movements against adjustable resistance

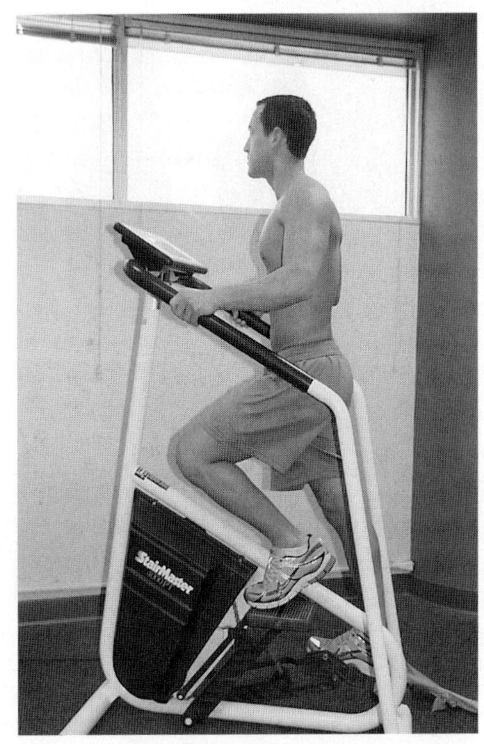

FIGURE 6.54 A stepping machine provides resistance during alternating lower extremity-pushing movements that simulate stair-climbing.

to make the weight-bearing activity more difficult. Stepping machines provide nonimpact, closed-chain strengthening as an alternative to walking or jogging on a treadmill. A patient can also kneel next to the unit and place both hands on the foot plates to use this equipment for upper extremity closed-chain exercises.

Elliptical Trainers and Cross-Country Ski Machines

Elliptical trainers and cross-country ski machines also provide nonimpact, reciprocal resistance to the lower extremities in an upright, weight-bearing position. Variable incline adjustments of these units expand the resistance options. Both types of equipment also incorporate reciprocal resistance to the upper extremities into their designs.

Upper Extremity Ergometers

Upper extremity ergometers provide resistance primarily to the upper extremities to increase strength and muscular endurance (Fig. 6.55). Forward and reverse cycling at varying speeds is possible. As with stationary cycles, upper extremity ergometers also are used to improve cardiopulmonary fitness. Typically the patient is seated, but some ergometers can be used in a standing position to minimize the arm elevation necessary with each revolution. This is particularly helpful for patients with impingement syndromes of the shoulder.

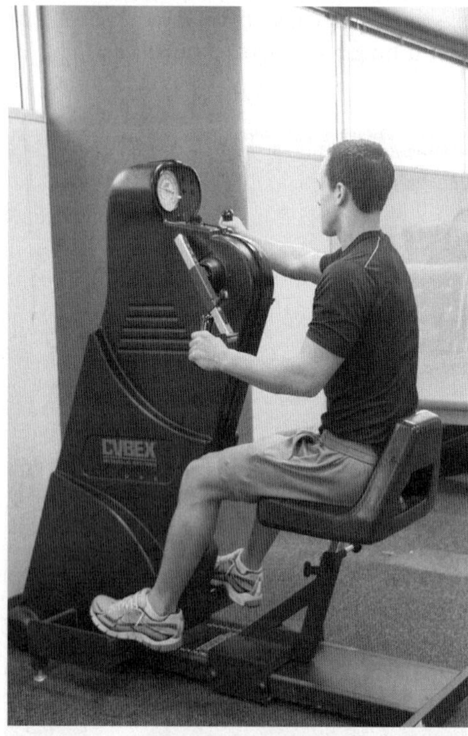

FIGURE 6.55 An upper extremity ergometer is used for upper body strength and endurance training and cardiopulmonary fitness.

Isokinetic Testing and Training Equipment

Isokinetic dynamometers (rate-limiting devices that control the velocity of motion) provide accommodating resistance during dynamic exercises of the extremities or trunk (see Fig. 6.9). The equipment supplies resistance proportional to the force generated by the person using the machine. The preset rate of movement (degrees per second) cannot be exceeded no matter how vigorously the person pushes against the force arm. Therefore, the muscle contracts to its fullest capacity at all points in the ROM.

Features of Isokinetic Dynamometers

Features include computerized testing capabilities; passive and active modes that permit open-chain, concentric and eccentric testing and training; and velocity settings from 0° per second for isometric exercise, up to 500° per second for the concentric mode, and up to 250° per second for the eccentric mode. Computer programming can limit limb movement to a specified range. Single-joint, uniplanar, open-chain movements are most common, but adaptations are available that permit a limited number of multiplanar movement patterns and multijoint, closed-chain exercises. Reciprocal training of agonist and antagonist and concentric/eccentric training of the same muscle group are possible.

Advantages and Disadvantages of Isokinetic Equipment

The characteristics of isokinetic exercise and equipment have already been presented in an earlier section of this chapter. The advantages and disadvantages of isokinetic dynamometers include the following.

Advantages

- If the patient puts forth a maximum effort, isokinetic equipment provides maximum resistance through the entire ROM.
- Both high- and low-velocity training can be done safely and effectively.
- The equipment accommodates for a painful arc of motion.
- As a patient fatigues, exercise can still continue.
- Isolated strengthening of muscle groups is possible to correct strength deficits in specific muscle groups.
- External stabilization keeps the patient and moving segment well aligned.
- Concentric and eccentric contractions of the same muscle group can be performed repeatedly, or reciprocal exercise of opposite muscle groups can be performed, allowing one muscle group to rest while its antagonist contracts; the latter method minimizes muscle ischemia.
- Computer-based visual or auditory cues provide feedback to the patient so submaximal to maximal work can be carried out more consistently.

Disadvantages

- The equipment is large and expensive to purchase and maintain.
- Setup time and assistance from personnel are necessary if a patient is to exercise multiple muscle groups.
- Most units allow only open-chain (nonweight-bearing) movement patterns, which do not translate to many lower extremity and some upper extremity functions.
- Although functional movements typically occur in combined patterns and at varying velocities, most exercises are performed in a single plane and at a constant velocity.
- Although the range of concentric training velocities (up to 500° per second) is comparable to some lower extremity limb speeds during functional activities, even the upper limits of this range of velocities cannot begin to approximate the rapid limb speeds that are necessary during many sports-related motions, such as throwing. In addition, the eccentric velocities available, at best, only begin to approach medium-range speeds, far slower than the velocity of movement associated with quick changes of direction and deceleration. Both of these limitations in the range of training velocities compromise carryover to functional goals.

Independent Learning Activities

Critical Thinking and Discussion

1. What physical findings from an examination and evaluation of a patient would lead you to determine that resistance exercises were an appropriate intervention?
2. What are the benefits and limitations of isometric, dynamic, and isokinetic exercises?
3. Compare and contrast constant resistance and variable resistance.
4. What are the key changes that occur in muscle strength and endurance throughout the life span?
5. You have been asked to design a resistance exercise program as part of a total fitness program for a group of 7- to 9-year-old soccer players (boys and girls).
   a. Indicate the exercises you would include, the equipment you need, and the guidelines for intensity, volume, frequency, and rest.
   b. What special precautions during resistance training should be taken with children and why?
6. Analyze five daily living tasks or recreational activities that you currently perform or would like to be able to perform effectively and efficiently. Identify the aspects of muscle performance (strength, power, and endurance) that are involved in each task. Propose two exercises for each task that would help to improve the muscle performance aspects you identified.
7. Develop an instructional presentation that deals with the appropriate and effective use of elastic resistance products.
8. You have been asked to help design a circuit weight training sequence at a soon-to-open fitness facility at the outpatient treatment center where you work. Select equipment to meet the needs of beginning and advanced individuals. Establish general guidelines for intensity, repetitions and sets, order of exercise, rest intervals, and frequency.

Laboratory Practice

1. Perform manual resistance exercise to all muscle groups of the upper and lower extremities in the following positions: supine, prone, side-lying, and sitting. What are the major limitations to effective, full-range strengthening in each of these positions?
2. Apply manual resistance exercises to each of the muscles of the wrist, fingers, and thumb.
3. Practice upper extremity and lower extremity D_1 and D_2 PNF exercises on your laboratory partner's right *and* left extremities.
4. Determine a 1-RM and 10-RM for the following muscle groups: shoulder flexors, shoulder abductors, shoulder external rotators, elbow flexors and extensors, hip abductors, hip flexors, knee flexors, and extensors. Select one upper and one lower extremity muscle group. Determine a 1-RM or 10-RM with free weights in two positions. Determine where in the ROM maximum resistance is encountered. Then determine a 1-RM or 10-RM with a pulley system. Compare your results.
5. Set up and safely apply exercises with elastic bands or tubing to strengthen the major muscle groups of the upper and lower extremities. Identify the point in each exercise where the external resistance is greatest and consider how this will impact effectiveness. Include a dynamic open-chain, a dynamic closed-chain, and an isometric exercise for each muscle group.
6. Demonstrate a series of simulated functional activities that could be used in the final stages of rehabilitation to continue to improve muscle performance as a transition into independent functional activities for a mail carrier, a nurse's aide who works in a skilled nursing facility, a ski instructor, a package delivery truck driver, and a day-care worker.

REFERENCES

1. Abe, T, et al: Time course for strength and muscle thickness changes following upper and lower body resistance training in men and women. *Eur J Appl Physiol* 81:174–180, 2000.
2. Abraham, WM: Factors in delayed muscle soreness. *Med Sci Sports Exerc* 9:11–20, 1977.
3. Aitkens, S, et al: Moderate resistance exercise program: its effects in slowly progressive neuromuscular disease. *Arch Phys Med Rehabil* 74:711–715, 1993.
4. Albert, MS, and Wooden, MJ: Isokinetic evaluation and treatment. In Donatelli, RA (ed): *Physical Therapy of the Shoulder,* ed. 3. New York: Churchill Livingstone, 1997, p 401.
5. American Academy of Pediatrics: Strength training by children and adolescents: policy statement. *Pediatr* 121(4):835–840, 2008.
6. American College of Sports Medicine: *ACSM's Guidelines for Exercise Testing and Prescription,* ed. 9. Philadelphia: Lippincott Williams & Wilkins, 2014.
7. American College of Sports Medicine: *ACSM's Resource Manual for Guidelines for Exercise Testing and Prescription,* ed. 7. Philadelphia: Lippincott Williams & Wilkins, 2012.
8. American College of Sports Medicine: Position stand: progression models in resistance training for healthy adults. *Med Sci Sports Exerc* 41:687–708, 2009.
9. American Physical Therapy Association: *Guide to Physical Therapist Practice 3.0.* Available at http://guidetoptpractice.apta.org/. Accessed March 2015.
10. Amiridis, IG, et al: Concentric and/or eccentric training-induced alterations in shoulder flexor and extensor strength. *J Orthop Sports Phys Ther* 25:26–33, 1997.
11. Andersen, LL, et al: Muscle activation and perceived loading during rehabilitation exercises: comparison of dumbbells and elastic resistance. *Phys Ther* 90:538–549, 2010.
12. Andersen, LL, et al: Neuromuscular activation in conventional therapeutic exercises and heavy resistance exercises: implications for rehabilitation. *Phys Ther* 86:683–697, 2006.
13. Antonio, J, and Gonyea, WJ: Skeletal muscle fiber hyperplasia. *Med Sci Sports Exerc* 25:1333–1345, 1993.
14. Armstrong, RB: Mechanisms of exercise-induced delayed onset muscular soreness: a brief review. *Med Sci Sports Exerc* 15:529–538, 1984.
15. Augustsson, J, et al: Weight training of the thigh muscles using closed vs. open kinetic chain exercises: a comparison of performance enhancement. *J Orthop Sports Phys Ther* 27:3–8, 1998.
16. Baechle, TR, Earle, RW, and Wathen, D: Resistance training. In Baechle, TR, and Earle, RW (eds): *Essentials of Strength Training and Conditioning,* ed. 3. Champaign, IL: Human Kinetics, 2008.
17. Barrett, DS: Proprioception and function after anterior cruciate ligament reconstruction. *J Bone Joint Surg* 73:833–837, 1991.
18. Beattie, K, et al: The effect of strength training on performance in endurance athletes. *Sports Med* 44:845–865, 2014.
19. Beckham, SG, and Earnest, CP: Metabolic cost of free weight circuit training. *J Sports Med Physical Fitness* 40(2):118–125, 2000.
20. Behm, DG, et al: Canadian Society for Exercise Physiology position paper: resistance training in children and adolescents. *Appl Physiol Nutr Metab* 33:547–561, 2008.
21. Bennett, R, and Knowlton, G: Overwork weakness in partially denervated skeletal muscle. *Clin Orthop* 12:22–29, 1958.
22. Bernhardt, DT, et al: Strength training by children and adolescents. *Pediatr* 107:1470–1472, 2001.
23. Bigland-Richie, B, and Woods, J: Changes in muscle contractile properties and neural control during human muscle fatigue. *Muscle Nerve* 7:691–699, 1984.
24. Bishop, KN, et al: The effect of eccentric strength training at various speeds on concentric strength of the quadriceps and hamstring muscles. *J Orthop Sports Phys Ther* 13:226–229, 1991.
25. Blackard, DO, Jensen, RL, and Ebben, WP: Use of EMG analysis in challenging kinetic chain terminology. *Med Sci Sports Exerc* 31:443–448, 1999.
26. Blackburn, JR, and Morrissey, MC: The relationship between open and closed kinetic chain strength of the lower limb and jumping performance. *J Orthop Sports Phys Ther* 27:430–435, 1998.
27. Blimkie, C: Benefits and risks of resistance training in youth. In Cahill, B, and Pearl, A (eds): *Intensive Participation in Children's Sports.* Champaign, IL: Human Kinetics, 1993, p 133.
28. Bonen, A, and Belcastro, AN: Comparison of self-directed recovery methods on lactic acid removal rates. *Med Sci Sports Exerc* 8: 176–178, 1976.
29. Borg, E, Kaijser, L: A comparison between three rating scales for perceived exertion and two different work tests. *Scand J Med Sci Sports* 16:57–69, 2006.
30. Bottomley, JM: Age-related bone health and pathophysiology of osteoporosis. *Orthop Phys Ther Clin North Am* 7:117–132, 1998.
31. Brask, B, Lueke, R, and Sodeberg, G: Electromyographic analysis of selected muscles during the lateral step-up exercise. *Phys Ther* 64: 324–329, 1984.
32. Brosky, JA, and Wright, GA: Training for muscular strength, power and endurance and hypertrophy. In Nyland, J (ed): *Clinical Decisions in Therapeutic Exercise: Planning and Implementation.* Upper Saddle River, NJ: Pearson Education, 2005, pp 171–230.
33. Buteau, JL, Eriksrud, O, and Hasson, SM: Rehabilitation of a glenohumeral instability utilizing the BodyBlade. *Physiother Theory Pract* 23(6):333–349, 2007.
34. Carron, AV, and Bailey, DA: Strength development in boys from 10–16 years. *Monogr Soc Res Child Dev* 39:1–37, 1974.
35. Centers for Disease Control and Prevention: How much physical activity do adults need? Available at http://www.cdc.gov/physicalactivity/everyone/guidelines/adults.html. Accessed March 18, 2016.
36. Centers for Disease Control and Prevention: How much physical activity do children need? Available at http://www.cdc.gov/physicalactivity/everyone/guidelines/children.html. Accessed March 18, 2016.
37. Centers for Disease Control and Prevention: How much physical activity do older adults need? Available at http://www.cdc.gov/physicalactivity/everyone/guidelines/ olderadults.html. Accessed March 18, 2016.
38. Chandler, JM, and Duncan, PW: Eccentric versus concentric force-velocity relationships of the quadriceps femoris muscle. *Phys Ther* 68:800, 1988.
39. Chandler, JM: Understanding the relationship between strength and mobility in frail older persons: a review of the literature. *Top Geriatr Rehabil* 11:20, 1996.
40. Chung, F, Dean, E, and Ross, J: Cardiopulmonary responses of middle-aged men without cardiopulmonary disease to steady-rate positive and negative work performed on a cycle ergometer. *Phys Ther* 79:476–487, 1999.
41. Clark, MA, Foster, D, and Reuteman, P: Core (trunk) stabilization and its importance for closed kinetic chain performance. *Orthop Phys Ther Clin North Am* 9:119–135, 2000.
42. Clarkson, PM, and Hubal, MJ: Exercise-induced muscle damage in humans. *Am J Phys Med Rehabil* 81(11 Suppl):S52–S69, 2002.
43. Clarkson, PM, and Tremblay, I: Exercise induced muscle damage, repair, and adaptation in humans. *J Appl Physiol* 65:1–6, 1988.
44. Colado, JC, and Triplett, NT: Effects of a short-term resistance program using elastic bands and weight machines for sedentary middle-aged women. *J Strength Cond Res* 22:1441–1448, 2008.
45. Connelly, DM, and Vandervoort, AA: Effects of detraining on knee extensor strength and functional mobility in a group of elderly women. *J Orthop Sports Phys Ther* 26:340–346, 1997.
46. Connolly, DA, Sayers, SP, and McHugh, MP: Treatment and prevention of delayed onset muscle soreness. *J Strength Cond Res* 17:197–208, 2003.
47. Conroy, BP, and Earle, RW: Bone, muscle, and connective tissue adaptations to physical activity. In Beachle, TR, and Earle, RW (eds): *Essentials of Strength Training and Conditioning,* ed. 3. Champaign, IL: Human Kinetics, 2008, 93–118.
48. Cook, TM, et al: EMG comparison of lateral step-up and stepping machine exercise. *J Orthop Sports Phys Ther* 16:108–113, 1992.

49. Corder, KP, et al: Effects of active and passive recovery conditions on blood lactate, rating of perceived exertion, and performance during resistance exercise. *J Strength Conditioning Res* 14:151–156, 2000.
50. Cress, NM, Peters, KS, and Chandler, JM: Eccentric and concentric force-velocity relationships of the quadriceps femoris muscle. *J Orthop Sports Phys Ther* 16:82–86, 1992.
51. Croarkin, E: Osteopenia in the patient with cancer. *Phys Ther* 79: 196–201, 1999.
52. Curtis, C, and Weir, J: Overview of exercise responses in healthy and impaired states. *Neurol Rep* 20:13, 1996.
53. Davies, GJ: *A Compendium of Isokinetics in Clinical Usage and Rehabilitation Techniques,* ed. 4. Onalaska, WI: S & S Publishing, 1992.
54. Davies, GJ: The need for critical thinking in rehabilitation. *J Sports Rehabil* 4:1–22, 1995.
55. Davies, GJ, and Ellenbecker, TS: Application of isokinetics in testing and rehabilitation. In Andrews, JR, Harrelson, GL, and Wilk, KE (eds): *Physical Rehabilitation of the Injured Athlete,* ed. 4. Philadelphia: WB Saunders, 2012, pp 548–570.
56. Davies, GJ, et al: The scientific and clinical rationale for the integrated approach to open and closed kinetic chain rehabilitation. *Orthop Phys Ther Clin North Am* 9:247–267, 2000.
57. Davies, GJ, Heiderscheit, BC, and Clark, M: Open and closed kinetic chain rehabilitation. In Ellenbecker, TS (ed): *Knee Ligament Rehabilitation.* New York: Churchill Livingstone, 2000, p 219.
58. Davies, GJ, and Zillmer, DA: Functional progression of a patient through a rehabilitation program. *Orthop Phys Ther Clin North Am* 9:103–118, 2000.
59. Dean, E: Physiology and therapeutic implications of negative work: a review. *Phys Ther* 68:233–237, 1988.
60. DeLorme, TL: Heavy resistance exercise. *Arch Phys Med Rehabil* 27: 607–630, 1946.
61. DeLorme, T, and Watkins, A: Techniques of progressive resistance exercise. *Arch Phys Med Rehabil* 29:263–273, 1948.
62. Denegar, CR, et al: Influence of transcutaneous electrical nerve stimulation on pain, range of motion, and serum cortisol concentration in females experiencing delayed onset muscle soreness. *J Orthop Sports Phys Ther* 11:100–103, 1989.
63. DeVine, K: EMG activity recorded from an unexercised muscle during maximum isometric exercise of contralateral agonists and antagonists. *Phys Ther* 61:898–903, 1981.
64. DeVries, HA: Electromyographic observations on the effects static stretching has on muscular distress. *Res Q* 32:468–479, 1961.
65. DeVries, HA: Quantitative electromyographic investigation of the spasm theory of muscle pain. *Am J Phys Med Rehabil* 45:119–134, 1966.
66. Dierking, JK, et al: Validity of diagnostic ultrasound as a measure of delayed onset muscle soreness. *J Orthop Sports Phys Ther* 30:116–122, 2000.
67. DiFabio, RP: Editorial: Making jargon from kinetic and kinematic chains. *J Orthop Sports Phys Ther* 29:142–143, 1999.
68. Dillman CJ, Murray, TA, and Hintermeister, RA: Biomechanical differences of open- and closed-chain exercises with respect to the shoulder. *J Sport Rehabil* 3:228–238, 1994.
69. Donnelly, AE, Clarkson, PM, and Maughan, RJ: Exercise-induced damage: effects of light exercise on damaged muscle. *Eur J Appl Physiol* 64:350–353, 1992.
70. Doucette, SA, and Child, DD: The effect of open and closed chain exercise and knee joint position on patellar tracking in lateral patellar compression syndrome. *J Orthop Sports Phys Ther* 23:104–110, 1996.
71. Draganich, LF, Jaeger, RJ, and Kraji, AR: Coactivation of the hamstrings and quadriceps during extension of the knee. *J Bone Joint Surg Am* 71:1075–1081, 1989.
72. Drury, DG: The role of eccentric exercise in strengthening muscle. *Orthop Phys Ther Clin North Am* 9:515–527, 2000.
73. Duarte, JA, et al: Exercise-induced signs of muscle overuse in children. *Int J Sports Med* 20:103–108, 1999.
74. Duncan, PW, et al: Mode and speed specificity of eccentric and concentric exercise training. *J Orthop Sports Phys Ther* 11:70–75, 1989.
75. Dvir, Z: *Isokinetics: Muscle Testing, Interpretation, and Clinical Application.* Edinburgh: Churchill Livingstone, 2004.
76. Ellenbecker, TS: Isokinetics in rehabilitation. In Ellenbecker, TS (ed): *Knee Ligament Rehabilitation.* New York: Churchill Livingstone, 2000, p 277.
77. Ellenbecker, TS, and Cappel, K: Clinical application of closed kinetic chain exercises in the upper extremities. *Orthop Phys Ther Clin North Am* 9:231–245, 2000.
78. Ellenbecker, TS, Davies, GJ, and Rowinski, MJ: Concentric versus eccentric isokinetic strengthening of the rotator cuff. *Am J Sports Med* 16: 64–69, 1988.
79. Ellenbecker, TS, and Davies, GJ: *Closed Kinetic Chain Exercise: A Comprehensive Guide to Multiple-Joint Exercises.* Champaign, IL: Human Kinetics, 2001.
80. Escamilla, RF, et al: Biomechanics of the knee during closed kinetic chain and open kinetic chain exercises. *Med Sci Sports Exerc* 30: 556–569, 1998.
81. Eston, R, and Peters, D: Effects of cold water immersion symptoms of exercise-induced muscle damage. *J Sports Sci* 17:231–238, 1999.
82. Faigenbaum, A, et al: The effects of strength training and detraining on children. *J Strength Conditioning Res* 10:109–114, 1996.
83. Faigenbaum, AD, and Bradley, DF: Strength training for the young athlete. *Orthop Phys Ther Clin North Am* 7:67–90, 1998.
84. Faigenbaum, AD, et al: Effects of different resistance training protocols on upper body strength and endurance development in children. *J Strength Cond Res* 15:459–465, 2001.
85. Faigenbaum, AD, et al: The effects of different resistance training protocols on muscular strength and endurance development in children. *Pediatr* 104(1):e5, 1999.
86. Falk, B, and Tenenbaum, G: The effectiveness of resistance training in children: a meta-analysis. *Sports Med* 22:176–186, 1996.
87. Fardy, P: Isometric exercise and the cardiovascular system. *Phys Sports Med* 9:43–53, 1981.
88. Faust, MS: Somatic development of adolescent girls. *Soc Res Child Dev* 42:1–90, 1977.
89. Fees, M, et al: Upper extremity weight training modifications for the injured athlete: a clinical perspective. *Am J Sports Med* 26:732–742, 1998.
90. Fillyaw, M, et al: The effects of long-term nonfatiguing resistance exercise in subjects with post-polio syndrome. *Orthopedics* 14:1252–1256, 1991.
91. Fish, DE, et al: Optimal resistance training: comparison of DeLorme with Oxford techniques. *Am J Phys Med and Rehabil* 92:903–909, 2003.
92. Fitzgerald, GK, et al: Exercise-induced muscle soreness after concentric and eccentric isokinetic contractions. *Phys Ther* 7:505–513, 1991.
93. Fitzgerald, GK: Open versus closed kinetic chain exercise: issues in rehabilitation after anterior cruciate ligament surgery. *Phys Ther* 77: 1747–1754, 1997.
94. Fleck, SJ: Periodized strength training: a critical review. *J Strength Condition Res* 13:82–89, 1999.
95. Fleck, SJ, and Kraemer, WJ: *Designing Resistance Training Programs,* ed. 4. Champaign, IL: Human Kinetics, 2014.
96. Folland, JP, and Williams, AG: The adaptations to strength training. Morphological and neurological contributions to increased strength. *Sports Med* 37:145–168, 2007.
97. Francis, KT: Delayed muscle soreness: a review. *J Orthop Sports Phys Ther* 5:10, 1983.
98. Franklin, ME, et al: Effect of isokinetic soreness-inducing exercise on blood levels of creatine protein and creatine kinase. *J Orthop Sports Phys Ther* 16:208–214, 1992.
99. Friden, J, Sjostrom, M, and Ekblom, B: Myofibrillar damage following intense eccentric exercise in man. *Int J Sports Med* 4:170, 1983.
100. Frontera, WR, and Larsson, L: Skeletal muscle function in older people. In Kauffman, TL, Barr, JO, Moran, M (eds): *Geriatric Rehabilitation Manual,* ed. 2. New York: Churchill Livingstone, 2007, pp 9–11.
101. Fry, AC: The role of training intensity in resistance exercise, overtraining, and overreaching. In Kreider, R, Fry, A, and O'Toole, M (eds): *Overtraining in Sport.* Champaign, IL: Human Kinetics, 1998, p 107.

102. Fyfe, JJ, Bishop, DJ, and Stepto, NK: Interference between concurrent resistance and endurance exercise: molecular bases and the role of individual training variables. *Sports Med* 44:743–762, 2014.
103. Gabriel, DA, Kamen, G, and Frost, G: Neural adaptations to resistive exercise: mechanisms and recommendations for training practices. *Sports Med* 36:133–149, 2006.
104. Gajdosik, RL, Vander Linden, DW, and Williams, AK: Concentric isokinetic torque characteristics of the calf muscles of active women aged 20 to 84 years. *J Orthop Sports Phys Ther* 29:181–190, 1999.
105. Gerber, JP, et al: Safety, feasibility, and efficacy of negative work exercise via eccentric muscle activity following anterior cruciate ligament reconstruction. *J Orthop Sports Phys Ther* 37(1):10–25, 2007.
106. Gerber, JP, et al: Effects of early progressive eccentric exercise on muscle size and function after anterior cruciate ligament reconstruction: a 1-year follow-up study of a randomized clinical trial. *Phys Ther* 89(1):51–59, 2009.
107. Gisolti, C, Robinson, S, and Turrell, ES: Effects of aerobic work performed during recovery from exhausting work. *J Appl Physiol* 21:1767–1772, 1966.
108. Gollnick, P, et al: Glycogen depletion patterns in human skeletal muscle fibers during prolonged work. *J Appl Physiol* 34:45–57, 1973.
109. Gollnick, PD, et al: Muscular enlargement and number of fibers in skeletal muscle of rats. *J Appl Physiol* 50:936–943, 1981.
110. Golob, AL, and Laya, MB: Osteoporosis. Screening, prevention, and management. *Med Clin N Am* 99:587–606, 2015.
111. Gonyea, WJ: Role of exercise in inducing increases in skeletal muscle fiber number. *J Appl Physiol* 48:421–426, 1980.
112. Gonyea, WJ, Ericson, GC, and Bonde-Petersen, F: Skeletal muscle fiber splitting induced by weightlifting in cats. *Acta Physiol Scand* 99: 105–109, 1977.
113. Greig, CA, Botella, J, and Young, A: The quadriceps strength of healthy elderly people remeasured after 8 years. *Muscle Nerve* 16: 6–10, 1993.
114. Griesemer, B, and Ided, B: Strength training by children and adolescents. *Pediatrics* 107(6):1470–1472, 2001.
115. Hageman, PA, Gillaspie, D, and Hall, LD: Effects of speed and limb dominance on eccentric and concentric isokinetic testing of the knee. *J Orthop Sports Phys Ther* 10:59–65, 1988.
116. Hageman, PA, and Sorensen, TA: Eccentric isokinetics. In Albert, M (ed): *Eccentric Muscle Training in Sports and Orthopedics,* ed. 2. New York: Churchill Livingstone, 1995, p 115.
117. Hagood, S, et al: The effect of joint velocity on the contribution of the antagonist musculature to knee stiffness and laxity. *Am J Sports Med* 18:182–187, 1990.
118. Harbst, KB, and Wilder, PA: Neurophysiologic, motor control, and motor learning basis of closed kinetic chain exercises. *Orthop Phys Ther Clin North Am* 9:137–149, 2000.
119. Harries, SK, Lubans, DR, and Callister, R: Resistance training to improve power and sports performance in adolescent athletes: A systematic review and meta-analysis. *J Sci Med Sport* 15:532–540, 2012.
120. Hasson, S, et al: Therapeutic effect of high speed voluntary muscle contractions on muscle soreness and muscle performance. *J Orthop Sports Phys Ther* 10:499–507, 1989.
121. Heiderscheit, BC, McLean, KP, and Davies, GJ: The effects of isokinetic vs. plyometric training on the shoulder internal rotators. *J Orthop Sports Phys Ther* 23:125–133, 1996.
122. Heiderscheit, BC, and Rucinski, TJ: Biomechanical and physiologic basis of closed kinetic chain exercises in the upper extremities. *Orthop Phys Ther Clin North Am* 9:209–218, 2000.
123. Hellebrandt, FA, and Houtz, SJ: Mechanisms of muscle training in man: experimental demonstration of the overload principle. *Phys Ther Rev* 36:371–383, 1956.
124. Herbison, GJ, et al: Effect of overwork during reinnervation of rat muscle. *Exp Neurol* 41:1–14, 1973.
125. Hernandez, ME, Goldberg, A, and Alexander, NB: Decreased muscle strength relates to self-reported stooping, crouching, or kneeling difficulty in older adults. *Phys Ther* 90(1):67–74, 2010.
126. Herrington, L, and Al-Sherhi, A: A controlled trial of weight-bearing versus nonweight-bearing exercises for patellofemoral pain. *J Orthop Sports Phys Ther* 37(4):155–159, 2007.
127. Hertling, D, and Kessler, RM: *Management of Common Musculoskeletal Disorders: Physical Therapy Principles and Methods,* ed. 4. Philadelphia: Lippincott Williams & Wilkins, 2006.
128. Hettinger, T, and Muller, EA: Muscle strength and muscle training. *Arbeitsphysiol* 15:111–126, 1953.
129. Hewett, TE: The effect of neuromuscular training on the incidence of knee injury in female athletes: a prospective study. *Am J Sports Med* 27(6):699–706, 1999.
130. Hintermeister, RA, et al: Electromyographic activity and applied load during shoulder rehabilitation exercises using elastic resistance. *Am J Sports Med* 26:210–220, 1998.
131. Hintermeister, RA, et al: Quantification of elastic resistance knee rehabilitation exercises. *J Orthop Sports Phys Ther* 28:40–50, 1998.
132. Hislop, HJ, and Montgomery, J: *Daniels and Worthingham's Muscle Testing: Techniques of Manual Examination,* ed. 7. Philadelphia: WB Saunders, 2002.
133. Hislop, HJ, and Perrine, J: The isokinetic concept of exercise. *Phys Ther* 41:114–117, 1967.
134. Ho, K, et al: Muscle fiber splitting with weight lifting exercise. *Med Sci Sports Exerc* 9:65, 1977.
135. Hoffman, J: Resistance training. In Hoffman, J (ed): *Physiological Aspects of Sport Training and Performance.* Champaign, IL: Human Kinetics, 2002, pp 77–92.
136. Hopp, JF: Effects of age and resistance training on skeletal muscle: a review. *Phys Ther* 73:361–373, 1993.
137. Housh, D, and Housh T: The effects of unilateral velocity-specific concentric strength training. *J Orthop Sports Phys Ther* 17:252–256, 1993.
138. Howell, JN, Chleboun, G, and Conaster, R: Muscle stiffness, strength loss, swelling, and soreness following exercise-induced injury in humans. *J Physiol* 464:183–196, 1993.
139. Hughes, C, and Maurice, D: Elastic exercise training. *Orthop Phys Ther Clin North Am* 9:581–595, 2000.
140. Hughes, CJ, et al: Resistance properties of Thera-Band® tubing during shoulder abduction exercise. *J Orthop Sports Phys Ther* 29: 413–420, 1999.
141. Isaacs, L, Pohlman, R, and Craig, B: Effects of resistance training on strength development in prepubescent females. *Med Sci Sports Exerc* 265(Suppl):S210, 1994.
142. Jenkins, WL, Thackaberry, M, and Killan, C: Speed-specific isokinetic training. *J Orthop Sports Phys Ther* 6:181–183, 1984.
143. Jenkins, WL, et al: A measurement of anterior tibial displacement in the closed and open kinetic chain. *J Orthop Sports Phys Ther* 25: 49–56, 1997.
144. Jones, H: The Valsalva procedure: its clinical importance to the physical therapist. *Phys Ther* 45:570–572, 1965.
145. Jones, KW, et al: Predicting forces applied by Thera-Band® tubing during resistive exercises [abstract]. *J Orthop Sports Phys Ther* 27:65, 1998.
146. Jones, TW, et al: Performance and neuromuscular adaptations following different ratios of concurrent strength and endurance training. *J Strength Cond Res* 27:3342–3351, 2013.
147. Jonhagen, S, et al: Sports massage after eccentric exercise. *Am J Sports Med* 32(6):1499–1503, 2004.
148. Kadi, F, et al: Cellular adaptation of the trapezius muscle in strength-trained athletes. *Histochem Cell Biol* 111:189–195, 1999.
149. Kauffman, TL, Nashner, LM, and Allison, LK: Balance is a critical parameter in orthopedic rehabilitation. *Orthop Phys Ther Clin North Am* 6:43–79, 1997.
150. Kelley, GA, Kelley, KS, and Tran, ZV: Resistance training and bone mineral density in women: a meta-analysis of controlled trials. *Am J Phys Med Rehabil* 80:65–77, 2001.
151. Kelsey, DD, and Tyson, E: A new method of training for the lower extremity using unloading. *J Orthop Sports Phys Ther* 19:218–223, 1994.
152. Kendall, FP, et al: *Muscles: Testing and Function with Posture and Pain,* ed. 5. Philadelphia: Lippincott Williams & Wilkins, 2005.

153. Kernozck, TW, McLean, KP, and McLean, DP: Biomechanical and physiologic factors of kinetic chain exercise in the lower extremity. *Orthop Phys Ther Clin North Am* 9:151, 2000.
154. Kerr, D, et al: Resistance training over 2 years increases bone mass in calcium-replete postmenopausal women. *J Bone Miner Res* 16(1): 175–181, 2001.
155. Kitai, TA, and Sale, DG: Specificity of joint angle in isometric training. *Eur J Appl Physiol* 58:744–748, 1989.
156. Knapik, JJ, Mawadsley, RH, and Ramos, MU: Angular specificity and test mode specificity of isometric and isokinetic strength training. *J Orthop Sports Phys Ther* 5:58–65, 1983.
157. Knight, KL: Knee rehabilitation by the daily adjustable progressive resistive exercise technique. *Am J Sports Med* 7:336–337, 1979.
158. Knight, KL: Quadriceps strengthening with DAPRE technique: case studies with neurological implications. *Med Sci Sports Exerc* 17: 646–650, 1985.
159. Knott, M, and Voss, DE: *Proprioceptive Neuromuscular Facilitation, Patterns, and Techniques,* ed. 2. Philadelphia: Harper & Row, 1968.
160. Kraemer, WJ, et al: Continuous compression as an effective therapeutic intervention in treating eccentric-exercise-induced muscle soreness. *J Sport Rehabilitation* 10:11–23, 2001.
161. Kraemer, WJ, and Ratamess, NA: Physiology of resistance training: current issues. *Orthop Phys Ther Clin North Am* 9:467–513, 2000.
162. Kraemer, WJ, and Ratamess, NA: Fundamentals of resistance training: progression and exercise prescription. *Med Sci Sports Exerc* 36: 674–688, 2004.
163. Kraemer, WJ, Duncan, ND, and Volek, JS: Resistance training and elite athletes: adaptations and program considerations. *J Orthop Sports Phys Ther* 28:110–119, 1998.
164. Kraemer, WJ, et al: Influence of resistance training volume and periodization on physiological and performance adaptations in collegiate women tennis players. *Am J Sports Med* 28:626–633, 2000.
165. Kraemer, W, et al: Influence of compression therapy on symptoms following soft tissue injury from maximal eccentric exercise. *J Orthop Sports Phys Ther* 31:282–290, 2001.
166. Kuipers, H: Training and overtraining: an introduction. *Med Sci Sports Exerc* 30:1137–1139, 1998.
167. Kvist, J, et al: Anterior tibial translation during different isokinetic quadriceps torque in anterior cruciate ligament deficient and nonimpaired individuals. *J Orthop Sports Phys Ther* 31:4–15, 2001.
168. Lane, JN, Riley, EH, and Wirganowicz, PZ: Osteoporosis: diagnosis and treatment. *J Bone Joint Surg Am* 78(4):618–632, 1996.
169. LaStayo, PC, et al: Eccentric muscle contractions: their contributions to injury, prevention, rehabilitation, and sport. *J Orthop Sports Phys Ther* 33(10):557–571, 2003.
170. Lear, LJ, and Gross, MT: An electromyographical analysis of the scapular stabilizing synergists during a push-up progression. *J Orthop Sports Phys Ther* 28:146–157, 1998.
171. Lephart, SM, et al: Proprioception following ACL reconstruction. *J Sports Rehabil* 1:188–196, 1992.
172. Lephart, SM, et al: The effects of neuromuscular control exercises on functional stability in the unstable shoulder. *J Athletic Training* 33S: 15, 1998.
173. Lephart SM, et al: The role of proprioception in rehabilitation of athletic injuries. *Am J Sports Med* 25:130–137, 1997.
174. Lephart, SM, and Henry, TJ: The physiological basis for open and closed kinetic chain rehabilitation for the upper extremity. *J Sport Rehabil* 5:71–87, 1996.
175. Levangie, PK, and Norkin, CC: *Joint Structure and Function: A Comprehensive Analysis,* ed. 5. Philadelphia: FA Davis, 2011.
176. Lieber, RL: *Skeletal Muscle Structure, Function, and Plasticity: The Physiological Basis of Rehabilitation Techniques,* ed. 3. Philadelphia: Lippincott Williams & Wilkins, 2010.
177. Lister, JL, et al: Scapular stabilizer activity during BodyBlade, cuff weights, and Thera-Band use. *J Sport Rehabil* 16:50–67, 2007.
178. Lindle, RS, et al: Age and gender comparisons of muscle strength of 654 women and men aged 20–93 yr. *J Appl Physiol* 83:1581–1587, 1997.
179. MacDougal, JD, et al: Arterial pressure responses to heavy resistance exercise. *J Appl Physiol* 58(3):785–790, 1985.
180. MacDougall, JD, et al: Effect of training and immobilization on human muscle fibers. *Eur J Appl Physiol* 43:25–34, 1980.
181. MacDougall, JD: Hypertrophy or hyperplasia. In Komi, PV (ed): *Strength and Power in Sport,* ed. 2. Oxford: Blackwell Science, 2003, pp 252–264.
182. Mair, SD, et al: The role of fatigue in susceptibility to acute muscle strain injury. *Am J Sports Med* 24:137–143, 1996.
183. Malina, RM, Bouchard, C, and Bar-Or, O (eds): *Growth, Maturation, and Physical Activity,* ed 2. Champaign, IL: Human Kinetics, 2004.
184. McArdle, WD, Katch, FL, and Katch, VL (eds): *Exercise Physiology: Nutrition, Energy, and Human Performance,* ed. 8. Philadelphia: Wolters Kluwer/Lippincott Williams & Wilkins, 2015.
185. McCarrick, MS, and Kemp, JG: The effect of strength training and reduced training on rotator cuff musculature. *Clin Biomech* 15(1 Suppl): S42–S45, 2000.
186. McGill, SM, and Cholewicki, J: Biomechanical basis of stability: an explanation to enhance clinical utility. *J Orthop Sports Phys Ther* 31: 96–99, 2001.
187. McHugh, MP: Recent advances in the understanding of the repeated bout effect: the protective effect against muscle damage from a single bout of eccentric exercise. *Scand J Med Sci Sports* 13(2):88–97, 2003.
188. McMaster, DT, et al: The development, retention and decay rates of strength and power in elite rugby union, rugby league and American football. *Sports Med* 43:367–384, 2013.
189. Mellor, R, and Hodges, PW: Motor unit synchronization of the vasti muscles in closed and open chain tasks. *Arch Phys Med Rehabil* 86: 716–721, 2005.
190. Menkes, A, et al: Strength training increases regional bone mineral density and bone remodeling in middle-aged and older men. *J Appl Physiol* 74:2478–2484, 1993.
191. Mikesky, AE, et al: Changes in muscle fiber size and composition in response to heavy resistance exercise. *Med Sci Sports Exerc* 23: 1042–1049, 1991.
192. Moffroid, M, et al: A study of isokinetic exercise. *Phys Ther* 49:735–747, 1969.
193. Mont, MA, et al: Isokinetic concentric versus eccentric training of shoulder rotators with functional evaluation of performance enhancement in elite tennis players. *Am J Sports Med* 22:513–517, 1994.
194. Morganti, CM, et al: Strength improvements with 1 yr of progressive resistance training in older women. *Med Sci Sport Exerc* 27:906–912, 1995.
195. Moritani, T, and deVries, HA: Neural factors vs. hypertrophy in the time course of muscle strength gain. *Am J Phys Med Rehabil* 58: 115–130, 1979.
196. Morrissey, MC, et al: Effects of distally fixated leg extensor resistance training on knee pain in the early period after anterior cruciate ligament reconstruction. *Phys Ther* 82:35–42, 2002.
197. Morrissey, MC, Harman, EA, and Johnson, MJ: Resistance training modes: Specificity and effectiveness. *Med Sci Sport Exerc* 27:648–660, 1995.
198. Mueller, MJ, and Maluf, KS: Tissue adaptation to physical stress: a proposed "physical stress theory" to guide physical therapist practice, education, and research. *Phys Ther* 82(4):383–403, 2002.
199. Mujika, I, and Padilla, S: Muscular characteristics of detraining in humans. *Med Sci Sports Exerc* 33:1297–1303, 2001.
200. Müller, EA: Influence of training and inactivity on muscle strength. *Arch Phys Med Rehabil* 51(8):449–462, 1970.
201. Nelson, ME, et al: Effects of high-intensity strength training on multiple risk factors for osteoporotic fractures. *JAMA* 272(24):1909–1914, 1994.
202. Neumann, DA: *Kinesiology of the Musculoskeletal System—Foundations for Rehabilitation,* ed. 2. St. Louis: Mosby/Elsevier, 2010.
203. Newman, D: The consequences of eccentric contractions and their relationship to delayed onset muscle pain. *Eur J Appl Physiol* 57: 353–359, 1988.
204. Newman, D, Jones, D, and Clarkson, P: Repeated high force eccentric exercise effects on muscle pain and damage. *J Appl Physiol* 63: 1381–1386, 1987.

205. Niederbracht, Y, et al: Effects of a shoulder injury prevention strength training program on eccentric external rotation muscle strength and glenohumeral joint imbalance in female overhead activity athletes. *J Strength Cond Res* 22:140–145, 2008.
206. Nosaka, K, and Clarkson, PM: Influence of previous concentric exercise on eccentric exercise-induced damage. *J Sports Sci* 15:477–483, 1997.
207. Nosaka, K, and Clarkson, PM: Muscle damage following repeated bouts of high force eccentric exercise. *Med Sci Sports Exerc* 27(9): 1263–1269, 1995.
208. Oakley, CR, and Gollnick, PD: Conversion of rat muscle fiber type: a time course study. *Histochemistry* 83(6):555–560, 1985.
209. Osternig, LR, et al: Influence of torque and limb speed on power production in isokinetic exercise. *Am J Phys Med Rehabil* 62: 163–171, 1983.
210. O'Sullivan, SB: Strategies to improve motor function. In O'Sullivan, SB, Schmitz, TJ, and Fulk, GD (eds): *Physical Rehabilitation: Assessment and Treatment,* ed. 6. Philadelphia: FA Davis, 2014, 393–443.
211. O'Sullivan, SB, and Portney, LG: Examination of motor function: motor control and motor learning. In O'Sullivan, SB, Schmitz, TJ, and Fulk, GD (eds): *Physical Rehabilitation: Assessment and Treatment,* ed. 6. Philadelphia: FA Davis, 2014, 161–205.
212. O'Sullivan, SB, and Schmitz, TJ: *Improving Functional Outcomes in Physical Rehabilitation.* Philadelphia: FA Davis, 2010.
213. Palmitier, RA, et al: Kinetic chain exercise in knee rehabilitation. *Sports Med* 11:402–413, 1991.
214. Page, P, and Ellenbecker, TS (eds): *The Science and Clinical Application of Elastic Resistance.* Champaign, IL: Human Kinetics, 2003.
215. Page, P, McNeil, M, and Labbe, A: Torque characteristics of two types of resistive exercise [abstract]. *Phys Ther* 80:S69, 2000.
216. Patterson, RM, et al: Material properties of Thera-Band® tubing. *Phys Ther* 81(8):1437–1445, 2001.
217. Petersen, SR, et al: The effects of concentric resistance training and eccentric peak torque and muscle cross-sectional area. *J Orthop Sports Phys Ther* 13:132–137, 1991.
218. Pomerantz, EM: Osteoporosis and the female patient. *Orthop Phys Ther Clin North Am* 3:71–84, 1996.
219. Pruitt, LA, et al: Weight-training effects on bone mineral density in early postmenopausal women. *J Bone Miner Res* 7(2):179–185, 1992.
220. Puthoff, ML, and Nielsen, DH: Relationships among impairments in lower extremity strength and power, functional limitations, and disability in older adults. *Phys Ther* 87:1334–1347, 2007.
221. Rivera, JE: Open versus closed kinetic rehabilitation of the lower extremity: a functional and biomechanical analysis. *J Sports Rehabil* 3:154–167, 1994.
222. Rockwell, JC, et al: Weight training decreases vertebral bone density in premenopausal women: a prospective study. *J Clin Endocrinol Metab* 71(4):988–983, 1990.
223. Roig, M, et al: The effects of eccentric versus concentric resistance training on muscle strength and mass: a systematic review with meta-analysis. *Br J Sports Med* 43:556–568, 2009.
224. Rothstein, JM: Muscle biology. Clinical considerations. *Phys Ther* 62(12):1823–1830, 1982.
225. Sale, DG: Neural adaptation to resistance training. *Med Sci Sports Exerc* 20(5 Suppl):S135–S145, 1988.
226. Sanders, MT: Weight training and conditioning. In Sanders, B (ed): *Sports Physical Therapy.* Norwalk, CT: Appleton & Lange, 1990, 1–535.
227. Sapega, AA, and Kelley, MJ: Strength testing about the shoulder. *J Shoulder Elbow Surg* 3:327–345, 1994.
228. Schueman, SE: The physical therapist's role in the management of osteoporosis. *Orthop Phys Ther Clin North Am* 7:199, 1998.
229. Scott, W, Stevens, J, and Binder-Macleod, SA: Human skeletal muscle fiber type classifications. *Phys Ther* 81(11):1810–1816, 2001.
230. Seger, JY, and Thorstensson, A: Effects of eccentric versus concentric training on thigh muscle strength and EMG. *Int J Sports Med* 26: 45–52, 2005.
231. Servedio, FJ: Normal growth and development: physiologic factors associated with exercise and training in children. *Orthop Phys Ther Clin North Am* 6:417, 1997.
232. Simoneau, GG, et al: Biomechanics of elastic resistance in therapeutic exercise programs. *J Orthop Sports Phys Ther* 31:16–24, 2001.
233. Sinacore, DR, Bander, BL, and Delitto, A: Recovery from a 1-minute bout of fatiguing exercise: characteristics, reliability and responsiveness. *Phys Ther* 74:234–241, 1994.
234. Sinaki, M, et al: Can strong back extensors prevent vertebral fractures in women with osteoporosis? *Mayo Clin Proc* 71(10):951–956, 1996.
235. Smith, CA: The warm-up procedure: To stretch or not to stretch. A brief review. *J Orthop Sports Phys Ther* 19(1):12–17, 1994.
236. Smith, LK, Weiss, EL, and Lehmkuhl, LD: *Brunnstrom's Clinical Kinesiology,* ed. 5. Philadelphia: FA Davis, 1996.
237. Smith, MJ, and Melton, P: Isokinetic vs. isotonic variable-resistance training. *Am J Sports Med* 9:275–279, 1981.
238. Snyder-Mackler, L, et al: Strength of the quadriceps femoris muscle and functional recovery after reconstruction of the anterior cruciate ligament. *J Bone Joint Surg Am* 77(8):1166–1173, 1995.
239. Snyder-Mackler, L: Scientific rationale and physiological basis for the use of closed kinetic chain exercise in the lower extremity. *J Sport Rehabil* 5:2, 1996.
240. Soderberg, GJ, and Blaschak, MJ: Shoulder internal and external rotation peak torque through a velocity spectrum in differing positions. *J Orthop Sports Phys Ther* 8(11):518–524, 1987.
241. Stackhouse, SK, Reisman, DS, and Binder-Macleod, SA: Challenging the role of pH skeletal muscle fatigue. *Phys Ther* 81(12):1897–1903, 2001.
242. Stanton, P, and Purdam, C: Hamstring injuries in sprinting: the role of eccentric exercise. *J Orthop Sports Phys Ther* 10(9):343–349, 1989.
243. Staron, RS, et al: Skeletal muscle adaptations during the early phase of heavy-resistance training in men and women. *J Appl Physiol* 76: 1247–1255, 1994.
244. Steindler, A: *Kinesiology of the Human Body under Normal and Pathological Conditions,* ed. 2. Springfield, IL: Charles C Thomas, 1977.
245. Stiene, HA, et al: A comparison of closed kinetic chain and isokinetic joint isolation exercise in patients with patellofemoral dysfunction. *J Orthop Sports Phys Ther* 24(3):136–141, 1996.
246. Stone, MH, and Karatzaferi, C: Connective tissue and bone responses to strength training. In Komi, PV (ed): *Strength and Power in Sport,* ed. 2. Oxford: Blackwell Science, 2003, pp 343–360.
247. Stone, MH: Implications for connective tissue and bone alterations resulting from resistance exercise training. *Med Sci Sports Exerc* 20 (5 Suppl):S162–S168, 1988.
248. Stone, WJ, and Coulter, SP: Strength/endurance effects from three resistance training protocols with women. *J Strength Conditioning Res* 8(4):231–234, 1994.
249. Stout, JL: Physical fitness during childhood and adolescence. In Campbell, SK, Palisano, RJ, and Orlin, MN (eds): *Physical Therapy for Children,* ed. 4. Philadelphia: WB Saunders, 2012, 205–238.
250. Straker, JS, and Stuhr, PJ: Clinical application of closed kinetic chain exercises in the lower extremity. *Orthop Phys Ther Clin North Am* 9: 185–207, 2000.
251. Sullivan, PE, and Markos, PD: *Clinical Decision Making in Therapeutic Exercise.* Norwalk, CT: Appleton & Lange, 1995.
252. Taaffe, DR, et al: Once-weekly resistance exercise improves muscle strength and neuromuscular performance in older adults. *J Am Geriatr Soc* 47(10):1208–1214, 1999.
253. Tanner, SM: Weighing the risks: strength training for children and adolescents. *Phys Sports Med* 21:104–116, 1993.
254. Taylor, NF, Dodd, KJ, and Damiano, DL: Progressive resistance exercise in physical therapy: a summary of systemic reviews. *Phys Ther* 85: 1208–1223, 2005.
255. Taylor, RA, et al: Knee position error detection in closed and open kinetic chain tasks during concurrent cognitive distraction. *J Orthop Sports Phys Ther* 28(2):81–87, 1998.
256. Tesch, PA, Thurstensson, A, and Kaiser, P: Muscle capillary supply and fiber type characteristics in weight and power lifters. *J Appl Physiol* 56(1):35–38, 1984.
257. Thomas, M, Müller, T, and Busse, MW: Comparison of tension in Thera-Band® and Cando tubing. *J Orthop Sports Phys Ther* 32(11): 576–578, 2002.

258. Thompson, LV: Skeletal muscle adaptations with age, inactivity, and therapeutic exercise. *J Orthop Sports Phys Ther* 32(2):44–57, 2002.
259. Tiidus, PM: Manual massage and recovery of muscle function following exercise: a literature review. *J Orthop Sports Phys Ther* 25(2): 107–112, 1997.
260. Timm, KE: Investigation of the physiological overflow effect from speed-specific isokinetic activity. *J Orthop Sports Phys Ther* 9(3): 106–110, 1987.
261. Tomberlin, JP, et al: Comparative study of isokinetic eccentric and concentric quadriceps training. *J Orthop Sports Phys Ther* 14:31–36, 1991.
262. Tracy, BL, et al: Muscle quality. II. Effects of strength training in 65- to 75-year old men and women. *J Appl Physiol* 86(1):195–201, 1999.
263. Tyler, TF, and Mullaney, M: Training for joint stability. In Nyland, J (ed): *Clinical Decisions in Therapeutic Exercise: Planning and Implementation.* Upper Saddle River, NJ: Pearson Education, 2006, 248–254.
264. Vandervoort, AA: Resistance exercise throughout life. *Orthop Phys Ther Clin North Am* 10(2):227–240, 2001.
265. Voss, DE, Ionta, MK, and Myers, BJ: *Proprioceptive Neuromuscular Facilitation,* ed. 3. New York: Harper & Row, 1985.
266. Waltrous, B, Armstrong, R, and Schwane, J: The role of lactic acid in delayed onset muscular soreness. *Med Sci Sports Exerc* 13:80, 1981.
267. Weber, MD, Servedio, F, and Woodall, WR: The effect of three modalities on delayed onset muscle soreness. *J Orthop Sports Phys Ther* 20: 236–242, 1994.
268. Weir, JP, et al: The effect of unilateral concentric weight training and detraining on joint angle specificity, cross-training and the bilateral deficit. *J Orthop Sports Phys Ther* 25(4):264–270, 1995.
269. Weir, JP, et al: The effect of unilateral eccentric weight training and detraining on joint angle specificity, cross-training and the bilateral deficit. *J Orthop Sports Phys Ther* 22(5):207–215, 1995.
270. Weir, JP, Housh, TJ, and Wagner, LI: Electromyographic evaluation of joint angle specificity and cross-training following isometric training. *J Appl Physiol* 77:197, 1994.
271. Weiss, LW, Coney, HD, and Clark, FC: Gross measures of exercise-induced muscular hypertrophy. *J Orthop Sports Phys Ther* 30(3):143–148, 2000.
272. Westcott, WL, and Baechle TR: *Strength Training Past 50,* ed 2. Champaign, IL: Human Kinetics, 2007.
273. Whitcomb, LJ, Kelley, MJ, and Leiper, CI: A comparison of torque production during dynamic strength testing of shoulder abduction in the coronal plane and the plane of the scapula. *J Orthop Sports Phys Ther* 21(4):227–232, 1995.
274. Wilder, PA: Muscle development and function. In Cech, DJ, and Martin, S (eds): *Functional Movement Development Across the Life Span.* Philadelphia: WB Saunders, 1995, p 13.
275. Wilk, K, Arrigo, C, and Andrews, J: Closed and open kinetic chain exercise for the upper extremity. *J Sports Rehabil* 5:88–102, 1995.
276. Wilk, KE, et al: A comparison of tibiofemoral joint forces and electromyography during open and closed kinetic chain exercises. *Am J Sports Med* 24(4):518–527, 1996.
277. Wilk, KE, et al: Stretch-shortening drills for the upper extremities: theory and clinical application. *J Orthop Sports Phys Ther* 17: 225–239, 1993.
278. Wilke, DV: The relationship between force and velocity in human muscle. *J Physiol* 110:249–280, 1950.
279. Williams, GN, Higgins, MJ, and Lewek, MD: Aging skeletal muscle: physiologic changes and effects of training. *Phys Ther* 82(1): 62–68, 2002.
280. Witvrouw, E, et al: Open versus closed kinetic chain exercises in patellofemoral pain: a 5-year prospective, randomized study. *Am J Sports Med* 32(5):1122–1130, 2004.
281. Woodall, WR, and Weber, MD: Exercise response and thermoregulation. *Orthop Phys Ther Clin North Am* 7:1, 1998.
282. Wu, Y, et al: Relationship between isokinetic concentric and eccentric contraction modes in the knee flexor and extensor muscle groups. *J Orthop Sports Phys Ther* 26(3):143–149, 1997.
283. Wyatt, MP, and Edwards, AM: Comparison of quadriceps and hamstrings torque values during isokinetic exercise. *J Orthop Sports Phys Ther* 3(2):48–56, 1981.
284. Yack, HJ, Colins, CE, and Whieldon, T: Comparison of closed and open kinetic chain exercise in the anterior cruciate ligament deficient knee. *Am J Sports Med* 21(1):49–54, 1993.
285. Yack, HJ, Riley, LM, and Whieldon, T: Anterior tibial translation during progressive loading the ACL-deficient knee during weight-bearing and nonweight-bearing isometric exercise. *J Orthop Sports Phys Ther* 20(5): 247–253, 1994.
286. Yarasheski, KE, Lemon, PW, and Gilloteaux, J: Effect of heavy resistance exercise training on muscle fiber composition in young rats. *J Appl Physiol* 69(2):434–437, 1990.
287. Zernicke, RF, and Loitz-Ramage, B: Exercise-related adaptations in connective tissue. In Komi, PV (ed): *Strength and Power in Sport,* ed. 2. Oxford: Blackwell Science, 2003, 96–113.
288. Zinowieff, AN: Heavy resistance exercise: the Oxford technique. *Br J Phys Med* 14(6):129–132, 1951.

CHAPTER

7

Principles of Aerobic Exercise

KAREN HOLTGREFE, PT, DHSC

There are numerous sources from which to obtain information on training for endurance in athletes and healthy young people and for individuals with chronic diseases such as coronary heart disease, diabetes, and others.[2-4] Using the most recent research, the American College of Sports Medicine (ACSM) published basic guidelines for many of the more common chronic conditions.[2-4] This chapter uses information from these well-known sources to demonstrate that the physical therapist can use aerobic-type activity when working with either healthy individuals or patients with a variety of conditions. In addition, some fundamental information about cardiovascular and respiratory parameters in children and the elderly, as well as the young or middle-aged adult, is presented so the physical therapist can be prepared to treat individuals of all ages.

Key Terms and Concepts

Physical Activity

Physical activity as defined by ACSM[2] and the Centers for Disease Control and Prevention (CDC)[6] is "any bodily movement produced by the contraction of skeletal muscles that result in a substantial increase over resting energy expenditure."

Exercise

Exercise is any planned and structured physical activity designed to improve or maintain physical fitness.

Physical Fitness

Fitness is a general term used to describe the ability to perform physical work. Performing physical work requires cardiorespiratory functioning, muscular strength and endurance, and musculoskeletal flexibility. Optimum body composition is also included when describing fitness.

To become physically fit, individuals must participate regularly in some form of physical activity that uses large muscle groups and challenges the cardiorespiratory system. Individuals of all ages can improve their general fitness status by participating in activities that include walking, biking, running, swimming, stair climbing, cross-country skiing, and/or training with weights.

Fitness levels can be described on a continuum from poor to superior based on energy expenditure during a bout of physical work.[11,12] These ratings are often based on direct or indirect measurement of the body's maximum oxygen consumption. Oxygen consumption is influenced by age, gender, heredity, inactivity, and disease.

Maximum Oxygen Consumption

Maximum oxygen consumption ($VO_{2\ max}$) is a measure of the body's capacity to use oxygen.[2,4,11,12] It is usually measured when performing an exercise that uses many large muscle groups such as swimming, walking, and running. It is the maximum amount of oxygen consumed per minute when the individual has reached maximum effort. It is usually expressed relative to body weight, as milliliters of oxygen per kilogram of body weight per minute (mL/kg per minute). It is dependent on the transport of oxygen, the oxygen-binding capacity of the blood, cardiac function, oxygen extraction capabilities, and muscular oxidative potential.

Endurance

Endurance (a measure of fitness) is the ability to work for prolonged periods of time and the ability to resist fatigue.[11,12] It includes muscular endurance and cardiovascular endurance. Muscular endurance refers to the ability of an isolated muscle group to perform repeated contractions over a period of time, whereas cardiovascular endurance refers to the ability to perform large muscle dynamic exercise, such as walking, swimming, and/or biking for long periods of time.

Aerobic Exercise Training (Cardiorespiratory Endurance)

Aerobic exercise training, or cardiorespiratory endurance training, is augmentation of the energy utilization of the muscle by means of an exercise program.[2,11,12] The improvement of the muscle's ability to use energy is a direct result of increased levels of oxidative enzymes in the muscles, increased mitochondrial density and size, and an increased muscle fiber capillary supply.

- Training is dependent on exercise of sufficient frequency, intensity, and time.
- Training produces cardiovascular and/or muscular adaptation and is reflected in an individual's endurance.
- Training for a particular sport or event is dependent on the *specificity principle*[11,12]—that is, the individual improves in the exercise task used for training and may not improve in other tasks. For example, swimming may enhance one's performance in swimming events but may not improve one's performance in treadmill running.

Adaptation

The cardiovascular system and the muscles used *adapt* to the training stimulus over time.[11,12] Significant changes can be measured in as little as 10 to 12 weeks.

Adaptation results in increased efficiency of the cardiovascular system and the active muscles. Adaptation represents a variety of neurological, physical, and biochemical changes in the cardiovascular and muscular systems. Performance improves in that the same amount of work can be performed after training but at a lower physiological cost.

Adaptation is dependent on the ability of the organism to change and the training stimulus threshold (the stimulus that elicits a training response). The person with a low level of fitness has more potential to improve than the one who has a high level of fitness.

Training stimulus thresholds are variable. The higher the initial level of fitness, the greater the intensity of exercise needed to elicit a significant change.

Myocardial Oxygen Consumption

Myocardial oxygen consumption is a measure of the oxygen consumed by the myocardial muscle.[2,4,11,12] The need or demand for oxygen is determined by the heart rate (HR), systemic blood pressure, myocardial contractility, and afterload. Afterload is determined by the left ventricular wall tension and central aortic pressure. It is the ventricular force required to open the aortic valve at the beginning of systole. Left ventricular wall tension is primarily determined by ventricular size and wall thickness.

The ability to supply the myocardium with oxygen is dependent on the arterial oxygen content (blood substrate), hemoglobin oxygen dissociation, and coronary blood flow, which is determined by aortic diastolic pressure, duration of diastole, coronary artery resistance, and collateral circulation. In a healthy individual, a balance between myocardial oxygen supply and demand is maintained during maximum exercise. When the demand for oxygen is greater than the supply, myocardial ischemia results.

Because the myocardial muscle extracts 70% to 80% of the oxygen from the blood during rest, its main source of supply during exercise is through an increase in coronary blood flow. The clinical relevance is described in Box 7.1.

Deconditioning

Deconditioning occurs with prolonged bed rest, and its effects are frequently seen in the patient who has had an extended, acute illness or long-term chronic condition. Decreases in $VO_{2\ max}$, cardiac output (stroke volume), and muscular strength occur rapidly. These effects are also seen, although possibly to a lesser degree, in the individual who has spent a period of time on bed rest without any accompanying disease process and in the individual who is sedentary because of lifestyle and increasing age. Deconditioning effects associated with bed rest are summarized in Box 7.2.

FOCUS ON EVIDENCE

In a meta-analysis by Biswas et al,[5] increased time spent in sedentary activities, particularly sitting during the activities, was associated with an increased risk of all-cause mortality including cardiovascular disease incidence and mortality, cancer incidence and mortality, and type II diabetes incidence. When addressing the combined effect of sedentary time and physical activity with the noted risks, those with high levels of physical activity had a 30% lower risk of all-cause mortality.

Davis et al[7] assessed the amount of time spent in sedentary activities, the frequency of breaks in sedentary time, and the level of physical activity in 217 older adults (age ≥ 70 years) with lower extremity function. Less time spent in sedentary activities and more frequent breaks during sedentary time was associated with higher lower extremity function scores as measured by the Short Physical Performance Battery. An increase of 0.58 points in lower extremity function was reported with each additional break in sedentary time per hour.

BOX 7.1 Clinical Relevance—Exertional Angina

Persons who have coronary occlusion may not present with any type of chest pain/symptoms (angina) until they need to exert themselves. This is because when the body works harder the heart rate increases, diastolic filling time decreases, and increased coronary blood flow is sacrificed by the reduced time for filling the coronary arteries. Without an adequate blood supply, the underlying cardiac tissue no longer receives the oxygen needed for metabolic activity, resulting in anginal pain/symptoms.

BOX 7.2 Deconditioning Effects Associated With Bed Rest[8,10]

↓ Muscle mass
↓ Strength
↓ Cardiovascular function
↓ Total blood volume
↓ Plasma volume
↓ Heart volume
↓ Orthostatic tolerance
↓ Exercise tolerance
↓ Bone mineral density

Energy Systems, Energy Expenditure, and Efficiency

Energy Systems

Energy systems are metabolic systems involving a series of biochemical reactions resulting in the formation of adenosine triphosphate (ATP), carbon dioxide, and water.[11,12] The cell uses the energy produced from the conversion of ATP to adenosine diphosphate (ADP) and phosphate (P) to perform metabolic activities. Muscle cells use this energy for actin-myosin cross-bridge formation when contracting. There are three major energy systems. The intensity and duration of activity determine when and to what extent each metabolic system contributes.

Phosphagen, or ATP-PC, System

The adenosine triphosphate–phosphocreatine (ATP-PC) system has the following characteristics:

- PC and ATP are stored in the muscle cell.
- PC is the chemical fuel source.
- No oxygen is required (anaerobic).
- When muscle is rested, the supply of ATP-PC is replenished.
- The maximum capacity of the system is small (0.7 mol ATP).
- The maximum power of the system is great (3.7 mol ATP/min).
- The system provides energy for short, quick bursts of activity.
- It is the major source of energy during the first 30 seconds of intense exercise.

Anaerobic Glycolytic System

The anaerobic glycolytic system has the following characteristics:

- Glycogen (glucose) is the fuel source (glycolysis).
- No oxygen is required (anaerobic).
- ATP is resynthesized in the muscle cell.
- Lactic acid is produced (by-product of anaerobic glycolysis).
- The maximum capacity of the system is intermediate (1.2 mol ATP).

- The maximum power of the system is intermediate (1.6 mol ATP/min).
- The systems provide energy for activity of moderate intensity and short duration.
- It is the major source of energy from the 30th to 90th second of exercise.

Aerobic System

The aerobic system has the following characteristics:

- Glycogen, fats, and proteins are fuel sources and are utilized relative to their availability and the intensity of the exercise.
- Oxygen is required (aerobic).
- ATP is resynthesized in the mitochondria of the muscle cell. The ability to metabolize oxygen and other substrates is related to the number and concentration of the mitochondria and cells.
- The maximum capacity of the system is great (90.0 mol ATP).
- The maximum power of the system is small (1.0 mol ATP/min).
- The system predominates over the other energy systems after the second minute of exercise.

Recruitment of Motor Units

Recruitment of motor units is dependent on the rate of work. Fibers are recruited selectively during exercise.[11,12]

- *Slow-twitch fibers (type I)* are characterized by a slow contractile response, are rich in myoglobin and mitochondria, have a high oxidative capacity and a low anaerobic capacity, and are recruited for activities demanding endurance. These fibers are supplied by small neurons with a low threshold of activation and are used preferentially in low-intensity exercise.
- *Fast-twitch fibers (type IIB)* are characterized by a fast contractile response, have a low myoglobin content and few mitochondria, have a high glycolytic capacity, and are recruited for activities requiring power.
- *Fast-twitch fibers (type IIA)* have characteristics of both type I and type IIB fibers and are recruited for both anaerobic and aerobic activities.

Functional Implications

- *Bursts of intense activity* lasting only seconds develop muscle strength and stronger tendons and ligaments. ATP is supplied by the phosphagen system.
- *Intense activity* lasting 1 to 2 minutes repeated after 4 minutes of rest or mild exercise enhances anaerobic power. ATP is supplied by the phosphagen and anaerobic glycolytic system.
- Activity with *large muscles*, which is less than maximum intensity for 3 to 5 minutes repeated after rest or mild exercise of similar duration, may develop aerobic power and endurance capabilities. ATP is supplied by the phosphagen, anaerobic glycolytic, and aerobic systems.
- Activity of *submaximum intensity* lasting 20 to 30 minutes or more taxes a high percentage of the aerobic system and develops endurance.

Energy Expenditure

Energy is expended by individuals engaging in physical activity and is often expressed in kilocalories. Activities can be categorized as light, moderate, or heavy by determining the energy cost. The energy cost of any activity is affected by mechanical efficiency and body mass. Factors that affect both walking and running are terrain, stride length, and air resistance.[11,12]

Quantification of Energy Expenditure

Energy expended is computed from the amount of oxygen consumed. Units used to quantify energy expenditure are METs and kilocalories.

- A *MET* is defined as the oxygen consumed (milliliters) per kilogram of body weight per minute (mL/kg). It is equal to approximately 3.5 mL/kg per minute.[2,11,12]
- A *kilocalorie* is a measure expressing the energy value of food. It is the amount of heat necessary to raise 1 kilogram (kg) of water 1°C. A kilocalorie (kcal) can be expressed in oxygen equivalents. Five kilocalories equal approximately 1 liter of oxygen consumed (5 kcal = 1 liter O_2).[2,11,12]
- To convert METs to kcal per minute, use the following formula: [(METs x 3.5 mL/kg per minute x body weight in kg) ÷ 1000)] × 5.[2]

Classification of Activities

Activities are classified as light, moderate, or vigorous according to the energy expended or the oxygen consumed while accomplishing them.[2]

- *Light activity* is 2.0 to 2.9 METs or 3.5 to 10.15 mL/kg per minute.
- *Moderate activity* is 3.0 to 5.9 METs or 10.5 to 10.65 mL/kg per minute.
- *Vigorous activity* is 6 to 8.8 METs or 21 to 30.8 mL/kg per minute.

The energy expenditure necessary for most industrial jobs requires more than three times the energy expenditure at rest. Energy expenditure of certain physical activities can vary, depending on factors such as skill, pace, and fitness level (Box 7.3).

BOX 7.3 Energy Expenditure of Daily Tasks

MET	Type of Physical Activity
1.0–2.9	Sitting, standing, self-care, making the bed, food shopping, walking less than 2.5 mph
3.0–5.9	Walking downstairs, walking 2.5 mph to less than 3.5 mph, mowing the lawn (walking) with a power mower, playing golf
6.0–8.8	Walking faster than 3.5 mph, swimming laps (moderate effort), jogging, running at 5.0 mph, shoveling snow

Efficiency

Efficiency is usually expressed as a percentage:[11,12]

Percent efficiency = useful work output/ energy expended or work input × 100

Work output equals force times distance (W = F × D). It can be expressed in power units or work per unit of time (P = w/t). On a treadmill, work equals the weight of the subject times the vertical distance the subject is raised walking up the incline of the treadmill. On a bicycle ergometer, work equals the distance (which is the circumference of the flywheel times the number of revolutions) times the bicycle resistance.

Work input equals energy expenditure and is expressed as the net oxygen consumption per unit of time. With aerobic exercise, the resting volume of oxygen used per unit of time (VO_2 value) is subtracted from the oxygen consumed during 1 minute of the steady-state period.

- Steady state is reached within 3 to 4 minutes after exercise has started if the load or resistance is kept constant.
- In the steady-state period, VO_2 remains at a constant (steady) value.

Total net oxygen cost is multiplied by the total time in minutes the exercise is performed. The higher the net oxygen cost, the lower the efficiency in performing the activity. Efficiency of large muscle activities is usually 20% to 25%.

Physiological Response to Aerobic Exercise

The rapid increase in energy requirements during exercise requires equally rapid circulatory adjustments to meet the increased need for oxygen and nutrients to remove the end-products of metabolism, such as carbon dioxide, water, and lactic acid, and to dissipate excess heat. The shift in body metabolism occurs through a coordinated activity of all the systems of the body: neuromuscular, respiratory, cardiovascular, metabolic, and hormonal (Box 7.4). Oxygen transport and its utilization by the mitochondria of the contracting muscle are dependent on adequate blood flow in conjunction with cellular respiration.[11,12]

BOX 7.4 Factors Affecting the Response to Acute Exercise

Ambient temperature, humidity, and altitude can affect the physiological responses to acute exercise. Diurnal fluctuations as well as changes associated with a female subject's menstrual cycle can affect these responses as well. Therefore, researchers control these factors as much as possible when evaluating the response to exercise.

Cardiovascular Response to Exercise

Exercise Pressor Response

Stimulation of small myelinated and unmyelinated fibers in skeletal muscle involves a sympathetic nervous system (SNS) response. The central pathways are not known.[2,4,11,12]

- The SNS response includes generalized peripheral vasoconstriction in nonexercising muscles and increased myocardial contractility, an increased HR, and an increased systolic blood pressure. This results in a marked increase and redistribution of the cardiac output.
- The degree of the response equals the muscle mass involved and the intensity of the exercise.

Cardiac Effects

- The frequency of sinoatrial node depolarization increases, as does the HR.
- There is a decrease in vagal stimuli as well as an increase in SNS stimulation.
- There is an increase in the force development of the cardiac myofibers. A direct inotropic response of the SNS increases myocardial contractility.

Peripheral Effects

Net reduction in total peripheral resistance. Generalized vasoconstriction occurs that allows blood to be shunted from the nonworking muscles, kidneys, liver, spleen, and splanchnic area to the working muscles. A locally mediated reduction in resistance in the working muscle arterial vascular bed, independent of the autonomic nervous system, is produced by metabolites such as Mg^{2+}, Ca^{2+}, ADP, and PCO_2. The veins of the working and nonworking muscles remain constricted.

Increased cardiac output. The cardiac output increases because of the increase in myocardial contractility, with a resultant increase in stroke volume, HR, blood flow through the working muscle, and an increase in the constriction of the capacitance vessels on the venous side of the circulation in both the working and nonworking muscles, raising the peripheral venous pressure.

Increase in systolic blood pressure. The increase in systolic blood pressure is the result of the augmented cardiac output.

Respiratory Response to Exercise

- Respiratory changes occur rapidly, even before the initiation of exercise.[11,12] Gas exchange (O_2, CO_2) increases across the alveolar-capillary membrane by the first or second breath. Increased muscle metabolism during exercise results in more O_2 extracted from arterial blood, resulting in an increase in venous P_{CO_2} and H^+, an increase in body temperature, increased epinephrine, and increased stimulation of receptors of the joints and muscles. Any of these factors alone or in combination may stimulate the respiratory system. Baroreceptor reflexes, protective reflexes, pain, emotion, and voluntary control of respiration may also contribute to the increase in respiration.

- Minute ventilation increases as respiratory frequency and tidal volume increase.
- Alveolar ventilation, occurring with the diffusion of gases across the capillary-alveolar membrane, increases 10- to 20-fold during heavy exercise to supply the additional oxygen needed and excrete the excess CO_2 produced.

Responses Providing Additional Oxygen to Muscle

Increased Blood Flow

The increased blood flow to the working muscle previously discussed provides additional oxygen.

Increased Oxygen Extraction

There is also extraction of more oxygen from each liter of blood. There are several changes that allow for this.

- A decrease of the local tissue PO_2 occurs because of the use of more oxygen by the working muscle. As the partial pressure of oxygen decreases, the unloading of oxygen from hemoglobin is facilitated.
- The production of more CO_2 causes the tissue to become acidotic (the hydrogen ion concentration increases) and the temperature of the tissue to increase. Both situations increase the amount of oxygen released from hemoglobin at any given partial pressure.
- The increase of red blood cell 2,3-diphosphoglycerate (DPG) produced by glycolysis during exercise also contributes to the enhanced release of oxygen.

Oxygen Consumption

Factors determining how much of the oxygen is consumed are:

- Vascularity of the muscles.
- Fiber distribution.
- Number of mitochondria.
- Oxidative mitochondrial enzymes present in the fibers. The oxidative capacity of the muscle is reflected in the arteriovenous oxygen difference (a-vO_2 difference), which is the difference between the oxygen content of arterial and venous blood.

Testing as a Basis for Exercise Programs

Testing for physical fitness of healthy individuals should be distinct from graded exercise testing of convalescing patients, individuals with symptoms of coronary heart disease, or individuals who are 35 years or older but asymptomatic.[2-4] Regardless of the type of testing, the level of performance is based on the submaximum oxygen uptake, the $VO_{2\,max}$, or the symptom-limited oxygen uptake. The capacity of the individual to transport and utilize oxygen is reflected in the oxygen uptake. Readers are referred to publications by the ACSM[2-4] for additional information.

Fitness Testing of Healthy Subjects

Field tests for determining cardiovascular fitness include the time to run 1.5 miles or the distance run in 12 minutes. These measures correlate well with $VO_{2\,max}$, but their use is limited to young persons or middle-aged individuals who have been carefully screened and have been jogging or running for some time.[2,4] Other field tests include the 1-mile walk test, 6-minute walk test, and step tests. These tests are more suitable for individuals who are not as physically active.

Multistage testing can provide a direct measurement of $VO_{2\,max}$ by analyzing samples of expired air.[2,4] Testing is usually completed in four to six treadmill stages, which progressively increase in speed and or grade. Each stage is 3 to 6 minutes long. Electrocardiographic (ECG) monitoring is performed during the testing. Maximum oxygen uptake can be determined when the oxygen utilization plateaus despite an increase in workload.

Stress Testing for Convalescing Individuals and Individuals at Risk

Individuals undergoing stress testing should have a physical examination; be monitored by the ECG; and be closely observed at rest, during exercise, and during recovery (Fig. 7.1).

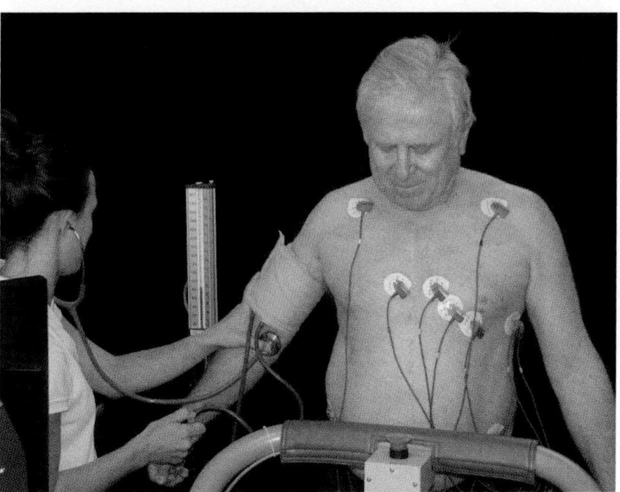

FIGURE 7.1 Treadmill stress test with electrocardiogram monitoring. *(From Porcari, J, Bryant, C, and Comana, F: Exercise Physiology. Philadelphia: F.A. Davis, 2015, p. 762, with permission.)*

Principles of Stress Testing

The principles of stress testing include:[2,4]

- Changing the workload by increasing the speed and/or grade of the treadmill or the resistance on the bicycle ergometer
- An initial workload that is low in terms of the individual's anticipated aerobic threshold

- Maintaining each workload for 1 minute or longer
- Terminating the test at the onset of symptoms or a definable abnormality of the ECG
- When available, measuring the individual's $VO_{2\ max}$

Purpose of Stress Testing

In addition to serving as a basis for determining exercise levels or the exercise prescription, the stress test:

- Helps establish a diagnosis of overt or latent heart disease.
- Evaluates cardiovascular functional capacity as a means of clearing individuals for strenuous work or exercise programs.
- Determines the physical work capacity in kilogram-meters per minute (kg-m/min) or the functional capacity in METs.
- Evaluates responses to exercise training and/or preventive programs.
- Assists in the selection and evaluation of appropriate modes of treatment for heart disease.
- Increases individual motivation for entering and adhering to exercise programs.
- Is used clinically to evaluate patients with chest sensations or a history of chest pain to establish the probability that such patients have coronary disease. It can also evaluate the functional capacity of patients with chronic disease.

Preparation for Stress Testing

All individuals who are taking a stress test should:

- Have had a physical examination
- Be monitored by ECG and closely observed at rest, during exercise, and during recovery
- Sign a consent form

PRECAUTIONS: Precautions to be taken are summarized in Box 7.5. They are applicable for both stress testing and the exercise program.[2,4]

Termination of Stress Testing

Endpoints requiring termination of the test period are[2]:

- Onset and/or progressive angina
- A significant drop (≥10 mm Hg) in systolic pressure in response to an increasing workload
- Lightheadedness, confusion, pallor, cyanosis, nausea, peripheral circulatory insufficiency, shortness of breath, wheezing, or leg cramps
- Excessive rise in blood pressure
- No increase in HR with an increase in exercise intensity
- Onset or change in heart rhythm
- Subject wishes to stop
- Observed or reported symptoms of severe fatigue

Multistage Testing

Each of the four to six stages lasts approximately 1 to 6 minutes. Differences in protocols involve the number of stages, magnitude of the exercise (intensity), equipment used (bicycle, treadmill), duration of stages, endpoints, position of body, muscle groups exercised, and types of effort.[2,4]

BOX 7.5 Precautions for Stress Testing and Exercise Program

Cardiopulmonary changes occur with stress testing and exercises. Monitor and recognize the following:

- Heart rate increases with exercise approximately 8–12 beats per minute per MET of physical activity. Monitor for abnormal increases in heart rate.
- Blood pressure increases with exercise approximately 8 to 12 millimeters (mm) of mercury (Hg) per MET of physical activity.
  - Systolic pressure should not exceed 250 mm Hg.
  - Diastolic pressure should not exceed 115 mm Hg.
- Rate and depth of respiration increase with exercise.
  - Respiration should not be labored.
  - The individual should have no perception of shortness of breath.
- The increase in blood flow while exercising, which regulates core temperature and meets the demands of the working muscles, results in changes in the skin of the cheeks, nose, and earlobes. They become pink, moist, and warm to the touch.

Protocols have been developed for multistage testing. The most popular treadmill protocol is the Bruce protocol. Treadmill speed and grade are changed every 3 minutes. Speed increases from 1.7 mph up to 5 mph, and the initial grade of 10% increases up to 18% during the five stages. A sample result of a stress test and referral for cardiac rehabilitation is available on the FA Davis website associated with this text.

Determinants of an Exercise Program

Just as testing for fitness should be distinct from stress testing for patients or individuals at high risk, training programs for healthy individuals are distinct from the exercise prescription for individuals with cardiopulmonary disease.

Effective endurance training for any population must produce a conditioning or cardiovascular response. Elicitation of the cardiovascular response is dependent on several critical elements of exercise. A recommendation by ACSM[2] and others[9,11,12] is to use the FITT-VP method: *F*requency, *I*ntensity, *T*ime (duration), and *T*ype of exercise, plus *V*olume (amount) and *P*rogression.

Frequency

While there is no clear-cut information provided on the most effective frequency of exercise for adaptation to occur, optimal frequency of training is generally three to four times a week. Frequency varies, dependent on the health and age of the individual, and may be a less important factor than intensity or duration in exercise training. If training is at a low intensity, greater frequency may be beneficial. A frequency of two times a week does not generally evoke cardiovascular changes, although older individuals and convalescing patients may benefit from a program of that frequency.

Intensity

Determination of the appropriate intensity of exercise to use is based on the overload principle and the specificity principle and is the most important component for successful changes to aerobic fitness.[2,4,11,12]

Overload Principle

Overload is stress on an organism that is greater than that regularly encountered during everyday life. To improve cardiovascular and muscular endurance, an overload must be applied to these systems. The exercise load (overload) must be above the training stimulus threshold (the stimulus that elicits a training or conditioning response) for adaptation to occur.

Once adaptation to a given load has taken place, the training intensity (exercise load) must be increased for the individual to achieve further improvement. Training stimulus thresholds are variable, depending on the individual's level of health, level of activity, age, and gender. The higher the initial level of fitness, the greater the intensity of exercise needed to elicit a change.

A conditioning response occurs generally at 60% to 90% maximum heart rate (HR_{max}; 50% to 85% $VO_{2\ max}$) depending on the individual and the initial level of fitness.

- Seventy percent HR_{max} is a minimal-level stimulus for eliciting a conditioning response in healthy young individuals.
- Sedentary or "deconditioned" individuals respond to a low exercise intensity, 40% to 50% of $VO_{2\ max}$.
- The exercise does not have to be exhaustive to achieve a training response.
- Determining the *HR_{max}* and the *exercise HR* for training programs provides the basis for the initial intensity of the exercise (Box 7.6).
- When the individual is young and healthy, the *HR_{max}* can be determined directly from a maximum performance multistage test; extrapolated from the HR achieved on a predetermined submaximum test; or, less accurately, calculated as 220 minus age.
- The *exercise HR* is determined in one of two ways: (1) as a percentage of the HR_{max} (the percentage used is dependent on the level of fitness of the individual) or (2) using the HR reserve (HRR; Karvonen's formula). Karvonen's formula is based on the HRR, which is the difference between the resting HR (HR_{rest}) and the HR_{max}. The exercise HR is determined as a percentage (usually 60% to 70%) of the HRR plus the HR_{rest} (see Box 7.6).
- When using Karvonen's formula, the exercise HR is higher than when using the HR_{max} alone.

BOX 7.6 Methods to Determine Maximum Heart Rate and Exercise Heart Rate

Determine Maximum Heart Rate (HR)
- From multistage test (for young and healthy)
- HR achieved in predetermined submaximum test
- 220 minus age (less accurate)

Determine Exercise HR
- Percentage of maximum HR (dependent on level of fitness)
- Karvonen's formula (HRR)

Exercise HR = HR_{rest}+ 60%–70% (HR_{max} - HR_{rest})

Individuals at Risk

HR_{max} and exercise HR used for the exercise prescription for individuals at risk for coronary artery disease, individuals with coronary artery disease or other chronic disease, and individuals who are elderly are ideally identified based on their performance on the stress test. The HR_{max} cannot be determined in the same manner as for the young and healthy.

- Assuming that an individual has an average HR_{max}, using the formula 220 minus age produces substantial errors in prescribing the exercise intensity for these individuals.
- HR_{max}, which may be symptom limited, is considered maximum. At no time should the exercise HR exceed the symptom-limited HR achieved on the exercise test.
- Individuals with cardiopulmonary disease may start exercise programs, depending on their diagnosis, as low as 40% to 60% of their HR_{max}.

Variables

Exercising at a high-intensity for a shorter period of time appears to elicit a greater improvement in $VO_{2\ max}$ than exercising at a moderate intensity for a longer period of time. However, as exercise approaches the maximum limit, there is an increase in the relative risk of cardiovascular complications and the risk of musculoskeletal injury.

- The higher the intensity and the longer the exercise intervals, the faster the training effect.
- $VO_{2\ max}$ is the best measure of exercise intensity. Aerobic capacity and HR are linearly related; therefore, the HR_{max} is a function of intensity.

Specificity Principle

The specificity principle as related to the specificity of training refers to adaptations in metabolic and physiological systems depending on the demand imposed. There is no overlap when training for strength-power activities and training for endurance activities. Workload and work-rest periods are selected so training results in:

- Muscle strength without a significant increase in total oxygen consumption.
- Aerobic or endurance training without training the anaerobic systems.

- Anaerobic training without training the aerobic systems.
- Aerobic training specific to the type of activity. When training for swimming events, the individual may not demonstrate an improvement in $VO_{2\,max}$ when running.

Time (Duration)

The optimal duration of exercise for cardiovascular conditioning is dependent on the total work performed, exercise intensity and frequency, and fitness level. Generally speaking, the greater the intensity of the exercise, the shorter the duration needed for adaptation, and the lower the intensity of exercise, the longer the duration needed.

A 20- to 30-minute session is generally optimal at 70% HR_{max}. When the intensity is below the HR threshold, a 45-minute continuous exercise period may provide the appropriate overload. With high-intensity exercise, 10- to 15-minute exercise periods are adequate; three 5-minute daily periods are effective in some deconditioned patients.

Type (Mode)

Many types of activity provide the stimulus for improving cardiorespiratory fitness. The important factor is that the exercise involves *large muscle groups* that are activated in a *rhythmic, aerobic* nature. However, the magnitude of the changes may be determined by the mode used.

For specific aerobic activities, such as cycling and running, the overload must use the muscles required by the activity and stress the cardiorespiratory system (specificity principle). If endurance of the upper extremities is needed to perform activities on the job, the upper extremity muscles must be targeted in the exercise program. The muscles trained develop a greater oxidative capacity with an increase in blood flow to the area. The increase in blood flow is due to increased microcirculation and more effective distribution of the cardiac output.

Training benefits are optimized when programs are planned to meet the individual needs and capacities of the participants. The skill of the individual, variations among individuals in competitiveness and aggressiveness, and variation in environmental conditions must be considered.

Volume

The volume or quantity of exercise completed weekly is the product of frequency, intensity, and time. Examples include MET-minute per week and kcal per week. The recommended volume of moderate intensity exercise needed for reaching health and fitness goals and to decrease the risk of cardiovascular disease for adults is ≥ 500 to 1,000 MET-min per week (approximately 1,000 kcal per week).[2,9]

Progression

How to progress the aerobic exercise prescription is dependent on an individual's overall health at the start of the program and what their fitness and health goals are. Generally, the time should be increased first, and then the frequency, with the intensity increased last.

Reversibility Principle

The beneficial effects of exercise training are transient and reversible.

- Detraining occurs rapidly when a person stops exercising. After only 2 weeks of detraining, significant reductions in work capacity can be measured, and improvements can be lost within several months. A similar phenomenon occurs with individuals who are confined to bed with illness or disability: the individual becomes severely deconditioned, with loss of the ability to carry out normal daily activities as a result of inactivity.
- The frequency or duration of physical activity required to maintain a certain level of aerobic fitness is less than that required to improve it.

CLINICAL TIP

The ACSM,[2,9] the American Heart Association, and the CDC and Surgeon General[6] have specified the amount of aerobic physical activity for children, adults, and older adults. The following are the general recommendations:

- ***Children age 6 to 17:*** 60 minutes of moderate to vigorous aerobic physical activity per day.
- ***Adults age 18 to 65:*** 30 minutes of moderate intensity activity (3–5.9 MET level) 5 days/week or 20 minutes of vigorous intensity activity (≥6 METs) 3 days/week, or a combination of moderate and vigorous intensity. The 30-minute total of moderate intensity can be accumulated in small bouts of continuous activity of at least 10 minutes. A volume of 500 to 1,000 MET-minutes per week or 1,000 kcal per week.
- ***Older adults age 65 or older (or adults 50 to 65 with chronic health conditions):*** 30 minutes of moderate intensity activity 5 days/week or 20 minutes of vigorous intensity activity 3 days/week, or a combination of moderate and vigorous intensity. The 30-minute total of moderate intensity can be accumulated in small bouts of continuous activity of at least 10 minutes. A volume of 500 to 1,000 MET-minutes per week or 1,000 kcal per week.

The adult criteria are based on MET level. The older adult criteria for moderate or vigorous intensity are based on a 10- point scale, where 0 is sitting and 10 is working as hard as you can. Moderate intensity activity would be a 5 to 6 and vigorous activity would be 7 to 8.

NOTE: Doing more than the minimum described above for adults and older adults is recommended for achieving additional health benefits.

Exercise Program

A carefully planned exercise program can result in higher levels of fitness for the healthy individual, slow the decrease in functional capacity of the elderly, and recondition those who have been ill or have chronic disease. There are three components of the exercise program: (1) a warm-up period; (2) the aerobic exercise period; and (3) a cool-down period. General guidelines for an aerobic training are summarized in Box 7.7.

Warm-Up Period

Physiologically, a time lag exists between the onset of activity and the bodily adjustments needed to meet the physical requirements of the body. The purpose of the warm-up period is to enhance the numerous adjustments that must take place before physical activity.

BOX 7.7 General Guidelines for an Aerobic Training Program

- Establish the target heart rate and maximum heart rate.
- Warm-up gradually for 5 to 10 minutes. Include stretching and repetitive motions at slow speeds, gradually increasing the effort.
- Increase the pace of the activity so the target heart rate can be maintained for 20 to 30 minutes. Examples include fast walking, running, bicycling, swimming, cross-country skiing, and aerobic dancing.
- Cool-down for 5 to 10 minutes with slow, total body repetitive motions and stretching activities.
- The aerobic activity should be undertaken three to five times per week.
- To avoid injuries from stress, use appropriate equipment, such as correct footwear, for proper biomechanical support. Avoid running, jogging, or aerobic dancing on hard surfaces such as asphalt and concrete.
- To avoid overuse syndromes in structures of the musculoskeletal system, proper warm-up and stretching of muscles to be used should be performed. Progression of activities should be within the tolerance of the individual. Overuse commonly occurs when there is an increase in time or effort without adequate rest (recovery) time between sessions. Increase the repetitions or the time by no more than 10% per week. If pain begins while exercising or lasts longer than 2 hours after exercising, heed the warning and reduce the stress.
- Individualize the program of exercise. All people are not at the same fitness level and therefore cannot perform the same exercises. Any one exercise has the potential to be detrimental if attempted by someone not able to execute it properly. During recovery following an injury or surgery, choose an exercise that does not stress the vulnerable tissue. Begin at a safe level for the individual and progress as the individual meets the desired goals.

Physiological Responses

During this period there is:

- An increase in muscle temperature. The higher temperature increases the efficiency of muscular contraction by reducing muscle viscosity and increasing the rate of nerve conduction.
- An increased need for oxygen to meet the energy demands for the muscle. Extraction from hemoglobin is greater at higher muscle temperatures, facilitating the oxidative processes at work.
- Dilatation of the previously constricted capillaries with increases in the circulation, augmenting oxygen delivery to the active muscles and minimizing the oxygen deficit and the formation of lactic acid.
- Adaptation in sensitivity of the neural respiratory center to various exercise stimulants.
- An increase in venous return. This occurs as blood flow is shifted centrally from the periphery.

Purposes

In addition to the physiological responses, the warm-up also prevents or decreases the susceptibility of the musculoskeletal system to injury and the occurrence of ischemic ECG changes and arrhythmias.

Guidelines

The warm-up should be gradual and sufficient to increase muscle and core temperature without causing fatigue or reducing energy stores. Characteristics of the period include:

- A 10-minute period of total body movement exercises, such as calisthenics and walking slowly
- Attaining a HR that is within 20 beats/min of the target HR

Aerobic Exercise Period

The aerobic exercise period is the training part of the exercise program. Attention to the determinants of frequency, intensity, time, and type of the program, as previously discussed, has an impact on the effectiveness of the program. The main consideration when choosing a specific method of training is that the intensity be great enough to stimulate an increase in stroke volume and cardiac output and to enhance local circulation and aerobic metabolism in the appropriate muscle groups. The exercise period must be within the person's tolerance, above the threshold level for adaptation to occur, and below the level of exercise that evokes clinical symptoms.

In aerobic exercise, submaximal, rhythmic, repetitive, dynamic exercise of large muscle groups is emphasized.

There are four methods of training that challenge the aerobic system: continuous, interval (work relief), circuit, and circuit interval.

Continuous Training

- A submaximum energy requirement, sustained throughout the training period, is imposed.

- Once the steady state is achieved, the muscle obtains energy by means of aerobic metabolism. Stress is placed primarily on the slow-twitch fibers.
- The activity can be prolonged for 20 to 60 minutes without exhausting the oxygen transport system.
- The work rate is increased progressively as training improvements are achieved. Overload can be accomplished by increasing the exercise duration.

Interval Training

With this type of training, the work or exercise is followed by a properly prescribed relief or rest interval. Interval training is perceived to be less demanding than continuous training.

- The relief interval is either a rest relief (passive recovery) or a work relief (active recovery), and its duration ranges from a few seconds to several minutes. Work recovery involves continuing the exercise but at a reduced level from the work period. During the relief period, a portion of the muscular stores of ATP and the oxygen associated with myoglobin that were depleted during the work period are replenished by the aerobic system; an increase in $VO_{2\,max}$ occurs.
- The longer the work interval, the more the aerobic system is stressed. With a short work interval, the duration of the rest interval is critical if the aerobic system is to be stressed (a work/recovery ratio of one to one to one to five is appropriate). A rest interval equal to one and a half times the work interval allows the succeeding exercise interval to begin before recovery is complete and stresses the aerobic system. With a longer work interval, the duration of the rest is not as important.
- A significant amount of high-intensity work can be achieved with interval or intermittent work if there is appropriate spacing of the work-relief intervals. The total amount of work that can be completed with intermittent work is greater than the amount of work that can be completed with continuous training.

Circuit Training

Circuit training employs a series of exercise activities. At the end of the last activity, the individual starts from the beginning and again moves through the series. The series of activities is repeated several times.

- Several exercise modes can be used involving large and small muscle groups and a mix of static or dynamic effort.
- Use of circuit training can improve strength and endurance by stressing both the aerobic and anaerobic systems.

Circuit-Interval Training

- Combining circuit and interval training is effective because of the interaction of aerobic and anaerobic production of ATP.
- In addition to the aerobic and anaerobic systems being stressed by the various activities, with the relief interval, there is a delay in the need for glycolysis and the production of lactic acid prior to the availability of oxygen supplying the ATP.

Cool-Down Period

The cool-down period is similar to the warm-up period in that it should last 5 to 10 minutes and consist of total-body movements and static stretching.

The purpose of the cool-down period is to:

- Prevent pooling of the blood in the extremities by continuing to use the muscles to maintain venous return
- Prevent fainting by increasing the return of blood to the heart and brain as cardiac output and venous return decreases
- Enhance the recovery period with the oxidation of metabolic waste and replacement of the energy store
- Prevent myocardial ischemia, arrhythmias, or other cardiovascular complications

Physiological Changes That Occur With Training

Changes in the cardiovascular and respiratory systems as well as changes in muscle metabolism occur following endurance training. These changes are reflected both at rest and with exercise. It is important to note that all of the following training effects cannot result from one training program.

Cardiovascular Changes

Changes at Rest

- *A reduction in the resting pulse rate* occurs in some individuals because of a decrease in sympathetic drive, with decreasing levels of norepinephrine and epinephrine; a decrease in atrial rate secondary to biochemical changes in the muscles and levels of acetylcholine, norepinephrine, and epinephrine in the atria; and an apparent increase in parasympathetic (vagal) tone secondary to decreased sympathetic tone.
- *A decrease in blood pressure* occurs in some individuals with a decrease in peripheral vascular resistance. The largest decrease is in systolic blood pressure and is most apparent in hypertensive individuals.
- *An increase in blood volume and hemoglobin* may occur. This facilitates the oxygen delivery capacity of the system.

Changes During Exercise

- A reduction in the pulse rate occurs in some individuals because of the mechanisms listed earlier in this section.
- *Increased stroke volume* may occur because of an increase in myocardial contractility and an increase in ventricular volume.
- *Increased cardiac output* may occur as a result of the increased stroke volume that occurs with maximum exercise but not with submaximum exercise. The magnitude of the change is directly related to the increase in stroke volume and the magnitude of the reduced HR.
- *Increased extraction of oxygen by the working muscle* occurs in some individuals because of enzymatic and biochemical changes in the muscle, as well as increased $VO_{2\,max}$. Greater

$VO_{2\,max}$ results in a greater work capacity. The increased cardiac output increases the delivery of oxygen to the working muscles. The increased ability of the muscle to extract oxygen from the blood increases the utilization of the available oxygen.
- *Decreased blood flow per kilogram of the working muscle* may occur even though increasing amounts of blood are shunted to the exercising muscle. The increase in extraction of oxygen from the blood compensates for this change.
- *Decreased myocardial oxygen consumption (pulse rate times systolic blood pressure) for any given intensity of exercise* may occur as a result of a decreased pulse rate with or without a modest decrease in blood pressure. The product can be decreased significantly in the healthy subject without any loss of efficiency at a specific workload.

Respiratory Changes

Changes at Rest

- *Larger lung volumes* develop because of improved pulmonary function, with no change in tidal volume.
- *Larger diffusion capacities* develop because of larger lung volumes and greater alveolar-capillary surface area.

Changes During Exercise

- Larger diffusion capacities occur for the same reasons as those listed previously; the maximum capacity of ventilation is unchanged.
- A smaller amount of air is ventilated at the same oxygen consumption rate; maximum diffusion capacity is unchanged.
- The maximal minute ventilation is increased.
- Ventilatory efficiency is increased.

Metabolic Changes

Changes at Rest

- Muscle hypertrophy and increased capillary density occurs.
- The number and size of mitochondria are increased, increasing the capacity to generate ATP aerobically.
- The muscle myoglobin concentration increases, increasing the rate of oxygen transport and possibly the rate of oxygen diffusion to the mitochondria.

Changes During Exercise

- A decreased rate of depletion of muscle glycogen at submaximum work levels may occur. Another term for this phenomenon is glycogen sparing. It is due to an increased capacity to mobilize and oxidize fat and increased fat-mobilizing and fat-metabolizing enzymes.
- Lower blood lactate levels at submaximal work may occur. The mechanism for this is unclear; it does not appear to be related to decreased hypoxia of the muscles.
- Less reliance on PC and ATP in skeletal muscle and an increased capability to oxidize carbohydrate may result because of an increased oxidative potential of the mitochondria and an increased glycogen storage in the muscle.

NOTE: Ill health may influence metabolic adaptations to exercise.

Other System Changes

Changes in other systems that occur with training include:

- Decrease in body fat
- Decrease in blood cholesterol and triglyceride levels
- Increased heat acclimatization
- Increase in the breaking strength of bones and ligaments and the tensile strength of tendons

Application of Principles of an Aerobic Training Program for the Patient With Coronary Disease

Employing the principles of aerobic training, in addition to secondary prevention and risk factor modification, is a dominant part of cardiac rehabilitation for individuals following a coronary event such as myocardial infarction (MI), revascularization, valve replacement, coronary artery bypass surgery, heart transplant, or heart failure.[8,10]

Inpatient Cardiac Rehabilitation[1]

The inpatient phase of the program occurs in the hospital following stabilization of the patient's cardiovascular status, such as MI, valve replacement, or coronary bypass surgery, and generally lasts 3 to 5 days.

Purpose

The purpose of the early portion of cardiac rehabilitation is to:

- Initiate risk factor education and address future modification of certain behaviors, such as eating habits and smoking.
- Initiate self-care activities and progress from sitting to standing to minimize deconditioning (1 to 3 days post event).
- Provide an orthostatic challenge to the cardiovascular system (3 to 5 days post event). This is usually accomplished by supervised ambulation. Ambulation is usually monitored electrocardiographically, as well as manually monitoring the HR, ventilation rate, and blood pressure. The intensity level of activity starts at 1 to 2 MET and is progressed to 3 to 4 MET by discharge if tolerated.
- Prepare patients and family for continued rehabilitation and for life at home after a cardiac event.

Outpatient Cardiac Rehabilitation: Early Exercise Program

The early outpatient exercise program is initiated within 1 to 3 weeks of discharge from the hospital and lasts up to 36 sessions. Participants are monitored via telemetry to determine

HR and rhythm responses; blood pressure is recorded at rest and during exercise, and ventilation responses are noted A description of a cardiac rehabilitation referral is available on the FA Davis website associated with this text.

Purpose

The purpose of the program is to:

- Increase the person's exercise capacity in a safe, progressive manner so adaptive cardiovascular and muscular changes occur. The early part of the program might be considered by some as "low-level" exercise training.
- Enhance cardiac functions and reduce the cardiac cost of work. This may help eliminate or delay symptoms such as angina and ST-segment changes in the patient with coronary heart disease.
- Produce favorable metabolic changes.
- Determine the effect of medications on increasing levels of activity.
- Relieve anxiety and depression.
- Progress the patient to an independent exercise program.

Guidelines[2]

Frequency. Participants often attend sessions offered three times per week.

Intensity. Multiple methods may be used to determine the intensity of the aerobic activity. The training intensity may be prescribed using the exercise capacity of HRR and may range from 40% to 80%. Another method is using the Rate of Perceived Exertion scale and should be between 11 and 16 on the 6-20 scale (see Box 25.4 in Chapter 25). The starting intensity is dictated by the severity of the diagnosis in concert with the individual's age and prior fitness level. The intensity is progressed as the individual responds to the training program.

Time. The duration of the exercise session may be limited to 10 to 15 minutes at the start, progressing to 20 to 60 minutes as the patient's status improves. Each session usually includes 5 to 10-minute warm-up and cool-down periods.

Type. The mode of exercise is usually continuous, using large muscle groups, such as stationary bike, rower, stepper, elliptical, or treadmill walking.

Volume. As noted previously the volume of exercise is the product of frequency, intensity, and time.

Progression. The progression of aerobic training is dependent on the patients' response to the activities and their goals for treatment.

Maintenance Program[1]

The outpatient phase of cardiac rehabilitation includes a supervised exercise conditioning program, which is often continued in a hospital or community setting. HR and rhythm are no longer monitored via telemetry. Participants are reminded to monitor their own pulse rate, and a supervisory person is available to monitor blood pressure.

Purpose

The purpose of the program is to continue to improve or maintain fitness levels achieved during early outpatient cardiac rehabilitation and to continue secondary prevention activities to assist with behavior change and risk factor modification.

CLINICAL TIP[1]

The number of visits completed in early outpatient cardiac rehabilitation and whether a patient is monitored with ECG (and for how long) depends on the risk for participating in aerobic training. Low-risk patients participate in 6 to 18 sessions which start with continuous ECG monitoring and then decrease its use within 6 to 12 visits. Moderate-risk patients participate in 12 to 24 sessions which start with continuous ECG monitoring decreasing to intermittent or no monitoring within 12 to 18 sessions if appropriate based on ECG results during exercise. High-risk patients participate in 28 to 36 sessions and start with continuous ECG monitoring and decreasing to intermittent if appropriate.

Special Considerations

There are special considerations related to types of exercise and patient needs that must be recognized when developing conditioning programs for patients with coronary disease. Arm exercises elicit different responses than leg exercises.

- Mechanical efficiency based on the ratio between output of external work and caloric expenditure is lower than with leg exercises.
- Oxygen uptake at a given external workload is significantly higher for arm exercises than for leg exercises.
- Myocardial efficiency is lower with leg exercises than with arm exercises.
- Myocardial oxygen consumption (HR × systolic blood pressure) is higher with arm exercises than with leg exercises.

PRECAUTION: Patients with coronary disease complete 35% less work with arm exercises than with leg exercises before symptoms occur.

Adaptive Changes

Adaptive changes following training of individuals with cardiac disease include:

- Increased myocardial aerobic work capacity.
- Increased maximum aerobic or functional capacity by predominantly widening the a-vO_2 difference.

- Increased stroke volume following high-intensity training 6 to 12 months into the training program.
- Decreased myocardial demand for oxygen.
- Increased myocardial supply by the decreased HR and prolongation of diastole.
- Increased tolerance to a given physical workload before angina occurs.
- Significantly lower HR at each submaximum workload and, therefore, a greater HRR. When muscles are used that are not directly involved in the activity, the reduction in HR is not as great.
- Improved psychological orientation and, over time, an impact on depression scores, scores for hysteria, hypochondriasis, and psychoasthenia on the Minnesota Multiphasic Personality Inventory.

Applications of Aerobic Training for the Deconditioned Individual and the Patient With Chronic Illness

Deconditioned individuals, including those with chronic illness and the elderly, may have major limitations in pulmonary and cardiovascular reserves that severely curtail their daily activities.

Deconditioning

Implications of the changes due to deconditioning brought on by inactivity resulting from any illness or chronic disease are important to remember.[8,10,11]

- There is decreased work capacity, which is a result of decreased maximum oxygen uptake and decreased ability to use oxygen and perform work. There is also decreased cardiac output, which is the major limiting factor.
- There is decreased circulating blood volume that can be as much as 700 to 800 mL. For some individuals, this results in tachycardia along with orthostatic hypotension, dizziness, and episodes of syncope when initially attempting to stand.
- There is a decrease in plasma and red blood cells, which increases the likelihood of life-threatening embothrombolic episodes and prolongation of the convalescent period.
- There is a decrease in lean body mass, which results in decreased muscle size and decreased muscle strength and ability to perform activities requiring large muscle groups. For example, the individual may have difficulty walking with crutches or climbing stairs.
- There is increased excretion of urinary calcium, which results from a decrease in the weight-bearing stimulus critical in maintaining bone integrity, in bone loss or osteoporosis, and in an increased likelihood of fractures upon falling because of osteoporosis.

Reversal of Deconditioning

Through an exercise program, the negative cardiovascular, neuromuscular, and metabolic functions can be reversed. This results in:

- A decrease in the HR_{rest}, the HR with any given exercise load, and urinary excretion of calcium
- An increase in stroke volume at rest, stroke volume with exercise, cardiac output with exercise, total heart volume, lung volume (ventilatory volume), vital capacity, maximum oxygen uptake, circulating blood volume, plasma volume and red blood cells, and lean body mass
- A reversal of the negative nitrogen and protein balance
- An increase in levels of mitochondrial enzymes and energy stores
- Less use of the anaerobic systems during activity

Adaptations for Those With Activity Limitations and Participation Restrictions

Individuals who have participation or activity restrictions should not be excluded from a training program that can increase their fitness level. This includes individuals in wheelchairs or persons who have problems ambulating, such as those with paraplegia, hemiplegia, or amputation, and those with an orthopedic problem, such as arthrodesis.

- Adaptations must be made when testing the physically disabled using a wheelchair treadmill or, more frequently, using the upper extremity ergometer.
- Exercise protocols may emphasize upper extremities and manipulation of the wheelchair.
- It is important to remember that energy expenditure is increased when the gait is altered, and wheelchair use is less efficient than walking without impairment.

Impairments, Goals, and Plan of Care

The goals of an aerobic exercise program are dependent on the initial level of fitness of the individual and on his or her specific clinical needs. The general goals are to decrease the deconditioning effects of disease and chronic illness and to improve the individual's cardiovascular and muscular fitness.

Common Impairments

- Increased susceptibility to thromboembolic episodes, pneumonia, atelectasis, and the likelihood of fractures
- Tachycardia, dizziness, and orthostatic hypotension when moving from sitting to standing

- A decrease in general muscle strength, with difficulty and shortness of breath in climbing stairs
- A decrease in work capacity that limits distances walked and activities tolerated
- Increased HR and blood pressure responses (rate-pressure product) to various activities
- A decrease in the maximum rate-pressure product tolerated with angina or other ischemic symptoms appearing at low levels of exercise

Goals

- Prevent thromboembolic episodes, pneumonia, atelectasis, and fractures
- Decrease the magnitude of the orthostatic hypotensive response
- Improve ability to climb stairs safely and without shortness of breath
- Develop tolerance for walking longer measured distances and completing activities without fatigue or symptoms
- Decrease HR and blood pressure (rate-pressure product) at a given level of activity
- Increase the maximum rate-pressure product tolerated without ischemic symptoms

Outcomes

- Improved pulmonary, cardiovascular, and metabolic response to various levels of exercise
- Improved ability to complete selected activities with appropriate HR and blood responses to exercise

Guidelines

Guidelines for establishing a safe program of intervention for the deconditioned individual and the convalescent patient with chronic illness are summarized in Boxes 7.8 and 7.9.

BOX 7.8 Guidelines for Initiating an Aerobic Exercise Program for the Deconditioned Individual and the Patient With Chronic Illness

- Determine the exercise heart rate response that can be safely reached using the Karvonen formula as a guide, accounting for medical conditions, medications, and the individual's perceived exertion.
- Initiate a program of activities for the patient that does not elicit a cardiovascular response over the exercise heart rate (e.g., walking, repetitive activities, easy calisthenics).
- Provide patients with clearly written instructions about any activity they perform on their own.
- Initiate an educational program that provides the patient with information about effort symptoms and exercise precautions, monitoring the heart rate, and making modifications when indicated.

BOX 7.9 Guidelines for Progression of an Aerobic Training Program

- Determine the maximum heart rate or symptom-limited heart rate by multistage testing with ECG monitoring.
- Decide on the threshold stimulus (percentage of maximum or symptom-limited heart rate) that elicits a conditioning response for the individual tested and that can be used as the exercise heart rate.
- Determine the frequency, intensity, and time of exercise that results in attaining the exercise heart rate and a training response.
- Determine the type of exercise to be used based on the individual's physical capabilities and interest.
- Initiate an exercise program with the patient and provide clearly written instructions regarding the details of the program.
- Discuss how to progress the activity: increase time first, then increase frequency, and then increase the intensity.
- Educate the patient about:
  - Effort symptoms and the need to cease or modify exercise when these symptoms appear and to communicate with the physical therapist and/or physician about these problems.
  - Monitoring heart rate at rest as well as during and following exercise.
  - The importance of exercising within the guidelines provided by the physical therapist.
  - The importance of consistent long-term follow-up with the exercise program so it can be progressed within safe limits.
  - The importance of modifying risk factors related to cardiac problems.

Age Differences

Differences in endurance and physical work capacity among children, young adults, and middle-aged or elderly individuals are evident. Some comparisons are made between maximum oxygen uptake and the factors influencing it and among blood pressure, respiratory rate, vital capacity, and maximum voluntary ventilation in the different age categories. It is important when developing aerobic conditioning programs that these age-related differences are taken into consideration.

Children

Between the ages of 5 and 15, there is a three-fold increase in body weight, lung volume, heart volume, and maximum oxygen uptake.

Heart rate. HR_{rest} is on the average above 125 (126 in girls and 135 in boys) at infancy. HR_{rest} drops to adult levels at puberty. HR_{max} is age related (220 minus age).

Stroke volume. Stroke volume is closely related to size. Children 5 to 16 years of age have a stroke volume of 30 to 40 mL.

Cardiac output. Cardiac output is related to size. Cardiac output increases with increasing stroke volume. The increase in cardiac output for a given increase in oxygen consumption is a constant throughout life: it is the same in the child as in the adult.

Arteriovenous oxygen difference. Children tolerate a larger arteriovenous oxygen difference (a-VO_2) than adults. The larger a-VO_2 difference makes up for the smaller stroke volume.

Maximum oxygen uptake. The VO_{2max} increases with age up to 20 years (expressed as liters per minute). Before puberty, girls and boys show no significant difference in maximum aerobic capacity. Cardiac output in children is the same as in the adult for any given oxygen consumption. Endurance times increase with age until 17 to 18 years.

Blood pressure. Systolic blood pressure increases from 40 mm Hg at birth to 80 mm Hg at age 1 month to 100 mm Hg several years before puberty. Adult levels are observed at puberty. Diastolic blood pressure increases from 55 to 70 mm Hg from 4 to 14 years of age, with little change during adolescence.

Respiration. Respiratory rate decreases from 30 breaths per minute at infancy to 16 breaths per minute at 17 to 18 years of age. Vital capacity and maximum voluntary ventilation are correlated with height, although the greater increase in boys than girls at puberty may be due to an increase in lung tissue.

Muscle mass and strength. Muscle mass increases through adolescence, primarily owing to muscle fiber hypertrophy and the development of sarcomeres. Sarcomeres are added at the musculotendinous junction to compensate for the required increase in length. Girls develop peak muscle mass between 16 and 20 years, whereas boys develop peak muscle mass between 18 and 25 years. Strength gains are associated with increased muscle mass in conjunction with neural maturation.

Anaerobic ability. Children generally demonstrate a limited anaerobic capacity. They produce less lactic acid which may be due to a limited glycolytic capacity.

Young Adults

There are more data on the physiological parameters of fitness for the young and middle-aged adult than for children or the elderly.

Heart rate. HR_{rest} reaches 60 to 65 beats per minute at 17 to 18 years of age (75 beats per minute in a sitting, sedentary young man). HR_{max} is age related (190 beats per minute in the same sedentary young man).

Stroke volume. The adult values for stroke volume are 60 to 80 mL (75 mL in a sitting, sedentary young man). With maximum exercise, stroke volume is 100 mL in that same sedentary young man.

Cardiac output for the sedentary young man at rest. Cardiac output at rest is 75 beats per minute × 75 mL, or 5.6 liters per minute. With maximum exercise, cardiac output is 190 beats per minute × 100 mL, or 19 liters per minute.

Arteriovenous oxygen difference. Approximately 25% to 30% of the oxygen is extracted from blood as it runs through the muscles or other tissues at rest. In a normal, sedentary young man, it increases three-fold (5.2 to 15.8 mL/dL blood) with exercise.

Maximum oxygen uptake. The difference in $VO_{2\ max}$ between males and females is greatest in the adult. Differences in $VO_{2\ max}$ between the sexes is minimal when $VO_{2\ max}$ is expressed relative to lean body weight. In the sedentary young man, maximum oxygen uptake equals 3,000 mL/min (oxygen uptake at rest equals 300 mL/min).

Blood pressure. Systolic blood pressure is 120 mm Hg (average). At peak effort during exercise, values may range from as low as 190 mm Hg to as high as 240 mm Hg. Diastolic blood pressure is 80 mm Hg (average). Diastolic pressure does not change markedly with exercise.

Respiration. Respiratory rate is 12 to 15 breaths per minute. Vital capacity is 4,800 mL in a man 20 to 30 years of age. Maximum voluntary ventilation varies considerably from laboratory to laboratory and is dependent on age and the surface area of the body.

Muscle mass and strength. Muscle mass increases with training as a result of hypertrophy. This hypertrophy can be the result of an increased number of myofibrils or increased actin and myosin, sarcoplasm, and/or connective tissue. As the nervous system matures, increased recruitment of motor units or decreased autogenic inhibition by Golgi tendon organs appears also to dictate strength gains.

Anaerobic ability. Anaerobic training increases the activity of several controlling enzymes in the glycolytic pathway and enhances stored quantities of ATP and PC. Anaerobic training increases the muscle's ability to buffer the hydrogen ions released when lactic acid is produced. Increased buffering allows the muscle to work anaerobically for longer periods of time.

Older Adults

(See Chapter 24 for additional information on exercise in the older adult population.)

Heart rate. HR_{rest} is not influenced by age. HR_{max} is age related and decreases with age (in very general terms, 220 minus age). The average HR_{max} for men 20 to 29 years of age is 190 beats/min. For men 60 to 69 years of age, it is 164 beats/min. The amount that the HR increases in response to static and maximum dynamic exercise (hand grip) decreases in the elderly.

Stroke volume. Stroke volume decreases in the aged and results in decreased cardiac output.

Cardiac output. Cardiac output decreases with age as the result of a decrease in stroke volume and other age-related health changes which affect preload and afterload.

Arteriovenous difference. Arteriovenous oxygen difference decreases as a result of decreased lean body mass and low oxygen-carrying capacity.

Maximum oxygen uptake. According to cardiorespiratory fitness classification, if men 60 to 69 years of age of average fitness level are compared with men 20 to 29 years of age of the same fitness level, the maximum oxygen uptake for the older man is lower (20 to 29 years is 31 to 37 mL/kg per minute; 60 to 69 years is 18 to 23 mL/kg per minute). Aerobic capacity decreases about 10% per decade when evaluating sedentary men. $VO_{2\ max}$ decreases on an average from 47.7 mL/kg per minute at age 25 years to 25.5 mL/kg per minute at age 75 years. This decrease is not directly the result of age; athletes who continue exercising have significantly less decrease in $VO_{2\ max}$ when evaluated over a 10-year period.

Blood pressure. Blood pressure increases because of increased peripheral vascular resistance (average systolic blood pressure of the aged is 150 mm Hg; average diastolic blood pressure is 90 mm Hg).

Respiration. Respiratory rate increases with age. Vital capacity decreases with age. There is a 25% decrease in the vital capacity of the 50- to 60-year-old man compared with the 20- to 30-year-old man with the same surface area. Maximum voluntary ventilation decreases with age.

Muscle mass and strength. Generally, the strength decline with age is associated with a decrease in muscle mass and physical activity. The decrease in muscle mass is primarily due to a decrease in protein synthesis, in concert with a decline in the number of fast-twitch muscle fibers. Aging may also affect strength by slowing the nervous system's response time. This may alter the ability to recruit motor units effectively. Continued training as one ages appears to reduce the effects of aging on the muscular system.

Independent Learning Activities

Critical Thinking and Discussion

1. The clinic in which you work has developed an outpatient program to help overweight young adults lose weight and improve their cardiorespiratory fitness. Your first client is a 13-year-old male who is 5 feet, 3 inches tall and weighs 250 pounds.
   - Describe several methods of assessing this individual's current aerobic fitness level.
   - Outline an aerobic training program using the FITT-VP model. Be specific as to the type of aerobic exercise this client will do.
   - What precautions will you take working with this client?
2. You are an invited speaker at a senior citizen center for a lunchtime discussion of lifetime fitness and establishing an appropriate exercise program for individuals in this age category.
   - Discuss the definition of physical activity, fitness, and endurance.
   - Discuss the benefits of aerobic training and the effect of training on HR, blood pressure, stroke volume, and cardiac output.
   - Discuss the deleterious effects of sitting too much and what an older adult could do to decrease these effects.
   - Describe the necessary precautions when dealing with the older population (both the older athlete and the untrained individual).
3. Explain the concepts of energy expenditure, oxygen consumption, and efficiency with regard to ambulating with an assistive device in the following weight bearing scenarios: nonweight bearing, partial weight bearing, and weight bearing as tolerated. Consider the use of a walker and crutches. How would energy expenditure change ambulating upstairs with crutches?
4. Design an exercise program for the local firefighters. Utilize the concepts of the aerobic energy systems, anaerobic energy system, and strength training. What type of training activities would you prescribe keeping in mind the specificity principle?
5. You have been invited to speak to a group of parents about the importance of aerobic exercise for children. Explain the basic physiological differences between children and adults at rest with regard to HR, respiratory rate, and metabolism and their response to exercise.

REFERENCES

1. American Association of Cardiovascular and Pulmonary Rehabilitation: *Guidelines for Cardiac Rehabilitation and Secondary Prevention Programs,* ed. 5. Champaign: Human Kinetics, 2013.
2. American College of Sports Medicine: *ASCM's Guidelines for Exercise Testing and Prescription,* ed. 9. Philadelphia: Lippincott Williams, & Wilkins, 2014.
3. American College of Sports Medicine: *Exercise Management for Persons With Chronic Diseases and Disabilities,* ed. 3. Champaign, IL: Human Kinetics, 2009.
4. American College of Sports Medicine: *Resource Manual for Guidelines for Exercise Testing and Prescription,* ed. 7. Philadelphia: Lippincott Williams & Wilkins, 2013.
5. Biswas A, et al: Sedentary time and its association with risk for disease incidence, mortality, and hospitalization in adults: a systematic review and meta-analysis. *Ann Intern Med* 162:123–132, 2015.
6. Centers for Disease Control and Prevention: Physical activity for everyone. Available at http://www.cdc.gov/physicalactivity/everyone/guidelines/index.html. Accessed June 7, 2015.
7. Davis, M, Fox, K, Stathi, A, Trayers, T, Thompson, J, and Cooper, A: Objectively measured sedentary time and its association with physical function in older adults. *J Aging Phys Act* 22:474–481, 2014.
8. Frownfelter, D, and Dean, E: *Cardiovascular and Pulmonary Physical Therapy—Evidence and Practice,* ed. 5. St. Louis: Elsevier, 2012.
9. Garber, CE et al: American College of Sports Medicine Position Stand. The quantity and quality of exercise for developing and maintaining cardiorespiratory, musculoskeletal, and neuromuscular fitness in apparently healthy adults: guidance for prescribing exercise. *Med Sci Sports Exerc* 43:1334–1359, 2011.
10. Hillegass, S: *Essentials of Cardiopulmonary Physical Therapy,* ed. 3. St. Louis: Elsevier, 2011.
11. McArdle, WD, Katch, FI, and Katch, VL: *Essentials of Exercise Physiology,* ed. 4. Philadelphia: Lippincott Williams & Wilkins, 2011.
12. McArdle, WD, Katch, FI, and Katch, VL: *Exercise Physiology: Energy, Nutrition, and Human Performance,* ed. 8. Philadelphia: Lippincott Williams & Wilkins, 2015.

CHAPTER

8

Exercise for Impaired Balance

ANNE D. KLOOS, PT, PHD, NCS ▪ DEBORAH L. GIVENS, PT, PHD, DPT

Loss of balance and falling are problems that affect individuals with a wide range of diagnoses. Physical therapists commonly evaluate balance and use balance training/exercises as either primary or secondary interventions for patients undergoing many types of rehabilitation programs. The purpose of this chapter is to present an overview of key background terms and concepts related to balance, how balance control is normally achieved in humans for a variety of conditions, possible causes of balance impairments, and evidence-based assessments and interventions for enhancing all aspects of an individual's balance control.

Background and Concepts

Balance: Key Terms and Definitions

Balance, or *postural stability*, is a generic term used to describe the dynamic process by which the body's position is maintained in equilibrium. Equilibrium means that the body is either at rest (static equilibrium) or in steady-state motion (dynamic equilibrium). Balance is greatest when the body's center of mass (COM) or center of gravity (COG) is maintained over its base of support (BOS).

Center of mass. The COM is a point that corresponds to the center of the total body mass and is the point at which the body is in perfect equilibrium. It is determined by finding the weighted average of the COM of each body segment.[15]

Center of gravity. The COG refers to the vertical projection of the COM to the ground. In the anatomical position, the COG of most adult humans is located slightly anterior to the second sacral vertebra,[15] or approximately 55% of a person's height.[63]

Momentum. Momentum is the product of mass times velocity. Linear momentum relates to the velocity of the body along a straight path, for example, in the sagittal or transverse planes. Angular momentum relates to the rotational velocity of the body.

Base of support. The BOS is defined as the perimeter of the contact area between the body and its support surface; foot placement alters the BOS and changes a person's postural stability.[118] A wide stance, such as is seen with many elderly individuals, increases stability, whereas a narrow BOS, such as tandem stance or walking, reduces it. As long as a person maintains the COG within the limits of the BOS, referred to as the *limits of stability*, he or she does not fall.

Limits of stability. "Limits of stability" refers to the sway boundaries in which an individual can maintain equilibrium without changing his or her BOS (Fig. 8.1).[118] These boundaries are constantly changing depending on the task, the individual's biomechanics, and aspects of the environment.[159] For example, the limits of stability for a person during quiet stance is the area encompassed by the outer edges of the feet in contact with the ground. Any deviations in the body's COM position relative to this boundary are corrected intermittently, producing a random

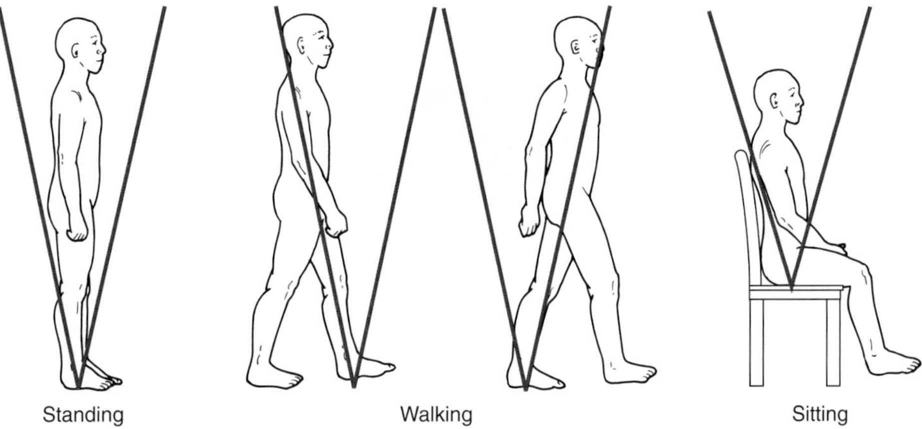

FIGURE 8.1 Boundaries of the limits of stability while standing, walking, and sitting.

swaying motion. For normal adults, the anteroposterior sway limit is approximately 12° from the most posterior to most anterior position.[121] Lateral stability varies with foot spacing and height; adults standing with 4 inches between the feet can sway approximately 16° from side to side.[120] However, a person sitting without trunk support has much greater limits of stability than when standing because the height of the COM above the BOS is less and the BOS is much larger (i.e., perimeter of the buttocks in contact with a surface).

Ground reaction force and center of pressure. In accordance with Newton's law of reaction, the contact between our bodies and the ground due to gravity (action forces) is always accompanied by a reaction from it, the so-called ground reaction force.

The *center of pressure* (COP) is the location of the vertical projection of the ground reaction force.[181] It is equal and opposite to the weighted average of all the downward forces acting on the area in contact with the ground. If one foot is on the ground, the net COP lies within that foot. When both feet are on the ground, the net COP lies somewhere between the two feet, depending on how much weight is taken by each foot. When both feet are in contact, the COP under each foot can be measured separately. To maintain stability, a person produces muscular forces to continually control the position of the COG, which in turn changes the location of the COP. Thus, the COP is a reflection of the body's neuromuscular responses to imbalances of the COG.[182] A force plate is traditionally used to measure ground reaction forces (in Newton's [N]) and COP movements (in meters [m]).

Balance Control

Balance is a complex motor control task involving the detection and integration of sensory information to assess the position and motion of the body in space and the execution of appropriate musculoskeletal responses to control body position within the context of the environment and task. Thus, balance control requires the interaction of the nervous and musculoskeletal systems and contextual effects (Fig. 8.2).

- The *nervous system* provides the (1) sensory processing for perception of body orientation in space provided mainly by the visual, vestibular, and somatosensory systems; (2) sensorimotor integration essential for linking sensation to motor responses and for adaptive and anticipatory (i.e., centrally programmed postural adjustments that precede voluntary movements) aspects of postural control; and (3) motor strategies for planning, programming, and executing balance responses.[67]
- *Musculoskeletal contributions* include postural alignment, musculoskeletal flexibility such as joint range of motion (ROM), joint integrity, muscle performance (i.e., muscle strength, power, and endurance), and sensation (touch, pressure, vibration, proprioception, and kinesthesia).
- *Contextual effects* that interact with the two systems are the environment, whether it is closed (predictable with no distractions) or open (unpredictable and with distractions); the support surface (i.e., firm versus slippery, stable versus unstable, and type of shoes); the amount of lighting; effects of gravity and inertial forces on the body; and task characteristics (i.e., well learned versus new, predictable versus unpredictable, and single versus multiple tasks).

Even if all elements of the neurological and musculoskeletal systems are operating effectively, a person may fall if contextual effects force the balance control demands to be so high that the person's internal mechanisms are overwhelmed.

Sensory Systems and Balance Control

Perception of one's body position and movement in space require a combination of information from peripheral receptors in multiple sensory systems, including the visual, somatosensory (proprioceptive, joint, and cutaneous receptors), and vestibular systems.

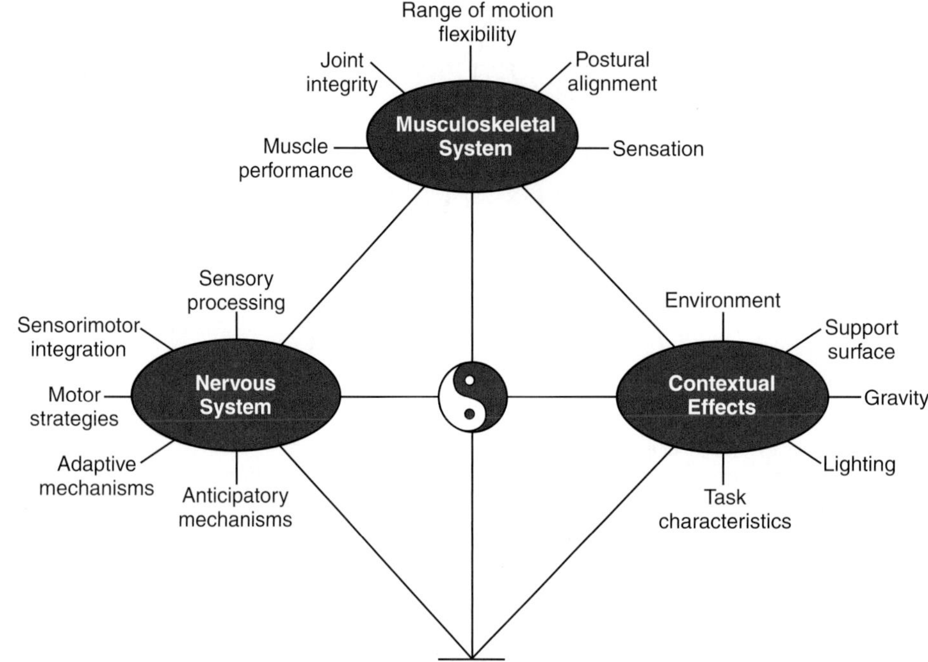

FIGURE 8.2 Interactions of the musculoskeletal and nervous systems and contextual effects for balance control.

Visual System

The visual system provides information regarding (1) the position of the head relative to the environment, (2) the orientation of the head to maintain level gaze, and (3) the direction and speed of head movements because as a person's head moves, surrounding objects move in the opposite direction. Visual stimuli can be used to improve a person's stability when proprioceptive or vestibular inputs are unreliable by fixating the gaze on an object. Conversely, visual inputs sometimes provide inaccurate information for balance control, such as when a person is stationary and a large object, such as a nearby bus, starts moving, causing the person to have an illusion of movement.

Somatosensory System

The somatosensory system provides information about the position and motion of the body and body parts relative to each other and the support surface. Muscle proprioceptors, including muscle spindles and Golgi tendon organs (sensitive to muscle length and tension), joint receptors (sensitive to joint position, movement, and stress), and skin mechanoreceptors (sensitive to vibration, light touch, deep pressure, and skin stretch), are the dominant sensory inputs for maintaining balance when the support surface is firm, flat, and fixed. However, when standing on a surface that is moving (e.g., on a boat) or on a surface that is not horizontal (e.g., on a ramp), inputs about body position with respect to the surface are not appropriate for maintaining balance; therefore, a person must rely on other sensory inputs for stability in these conditions.[159]

Information from joint receptors does not contribute greatly to conscious joint position sense. It has been demonstrated that local anesthetization of joint tissues and total joint replacement does not impair joint position awareness.[56,57] Muscle spindle receptors appear to be mostly responsible for providing joint position sense, whereas the primary role of joint receptors is to assist the gamma motor system in regulating muscle tone and stiffness to provide anticipatory postural adjustments and to counteract unexpected postural disturbances.[131]

Vestibular System

The vestibular system provides information about the position and movement of the head with respect to gravity and inertial forces. Receptors in the semicircular canals (SCCs) detect angular acceleration of the head, whereas the receptors in the otoliths (utricle and saccule) detect linear acceleration and head position with respect to gravity. The SCCs are particularly sensitive to fast head movements, such as those made during walking or during episodes of imbalance (slips, trips, and stumbles), whereas the otoliths respond to slow head movements, such as during postural sway.[66,159]

By itself, the vestibular system can give no information about the position of the body. For example, it cannot distinguish a simple head nod (head movement on a stable trunk) from a forward bend (head movement in conjunction with a moving trunk).[66] Consequently, additional information, particularly from mechanoreceptors in the neck, must be provided for the central nervous system (CNS) to have a true picture of the orientation of the head relative to the body.[131]

The vestibular system uses motor pathways originating from the vestibular nuclei for postural control and coordination of eye and head movements. The vestibulospinal reflex brings about postural changes to compensate for tilts and movements of the body through vestibulospinal tract projections to antigravity muscles at all levels of the spinal cord. The vestibulo-ocular reflex stabilizes vision during head and body movements through projections from the vestibular nuclei to the nuclei that innervate extraocular muscles.

Sensory Organization for Balance Control

Vestibular, visual, and somatosensory inputs are normally combined seamlessly to produce our sense of orientation and movement.[131] Incoming sensory information is integrated and processed in the cerebellum, basal ganglia, and supplementary motor area.[180] Somatosensory information has the fastest processing time for rapid responses, followed by visual and vestibular inputs.[180] When sensory inputs from one system are inaccurate owing to environmental conditions or injuries that decrease the information-processing rate, the CNS must suppress the inaccurate input and select and combine the appropriate sensory inputs from the other two systems. This adaptive process is called *sensory organization*. Most individuals can compensate well if one of the three systems is impaired; therefore, this concept is the basis for many treatment programs.

Types of Balance Control

Functional tasks require different types of balance control, including (1) static balance control to maintain a stable antigravity position while at rest, such as when standing and sitting; (2) dynamic balance control to stabilize the body when the support surface is moving or when the body is moving on a stable surface, such as sit-to-stand transfers or walking; and (3) automatic postural reactions to maintain balance in response to unexpected external perturbations, such as standing on a bus that suddenly accelerates forward.

- *Feedforward (open loop motor control)* is utilized for movements that occur too fast to rely on sensory feedback (e.g., reactive responses) or for anticipatory aspects of postural control.
- *Anticipatory control* involves activation of postural muscles in advance of performing skilled movements, such as activation of posterior leg and back extensor muscles prior to a person pulling on a handle when standing[32] or planning how to navigate to avoid obstacles in the environment.
- *Closed loop control* is utilized for precision movements that require sensory feedback (e.g., maintaining balance while sitting on a ball or standing on a balance beam).

Motor Strategies for Balance Control

To maintain balance, the body must continually adjust its position in space to keep the COM of an individual over the BOS or to bring the COM back to that position after a perturbation. Horak and Nashner[68] described three primary movement strategies used by healthy adults to recover balance in response to sudden perturbations of the supporting surface (i.e., brief anterior or posterior platform displacements) called ankle, hip, and stepping strategies (Fig. 8.3). Factors that determine which strategy most effectively addresses a balance disturbance are identified in Box 8.1. Results of research examining the patterns of muscle activity underlying these movement strategies suggest that preprogrammed muscle synergies comprise the fundamental movement unit used to

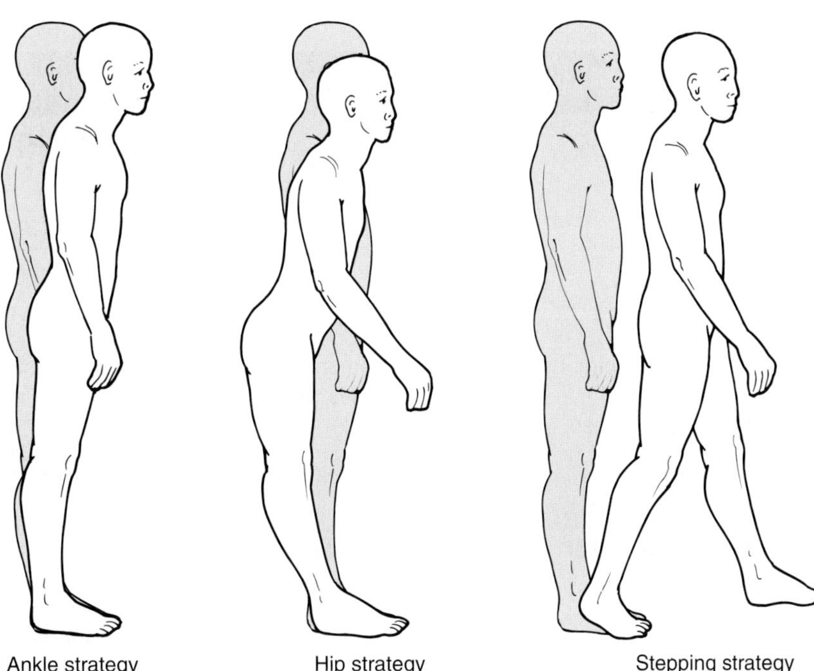

FIGURE 8.3 Ankle, hip, and stepping strategies used by adults to control body sway.

BOX 8.1 Factors Influencing Selection of Balance Strategies

- Speed and intensity of the displacing forces
- Characteristics of the support surface
- Magnitude of the displacement of the center of mass
- Subject's awareness of the disturbance
- Subject's posture at the time of perturbation
- Subject's prior experiences

restore balance.[68,122,123] A *synergy* is a functional coupling of groups of muscles, so they must act together as a unit; this organization greatly simplifies the control demands of the CNS.

The CNS uses three movement systems to regain balance after the body is perturbed: reflex, automatic, and voluntary systems. Table 8.1 summarizes the key characteristics of reflexes, automatic postural responses, and voluntary movements.[120]

- "*Stretch*" *reflexes* mediated by the spinal cord comprise the first response to external perturbations. They have the shortest latencies (<70 ms), are independent of task demands, and produce stereotyped muscle contractions in response to sensory inputs.
- *Voluntary responses* have the longest latencies (>150 ms), are dependent on task parameters, and produce highly variable motor outputs (e.g., reach for a nearby stable support surface or walk away from a destabilizing condition).
- *Automatic postural reactions* have intermediate latencies (80 to 120 ms) and are the first responses that effectively prevent falls. They produce quick, relatively invariant movements among individuals (similar to reflexes), but they require coordination of responses among body regions and are modifiable depending on the demands of the task (similar to voluntary responses).

The reflex, automatic, and voluntary movement systems interact to ensure that the response matches the postural challenge.

Ankle Strategy (Anteroposterior Plane)

In quiet stance and during small perturbations (i.e., slow-speed perturbations usually occurring on a large, firm surface), movements at the ankle act to restore a person's COM to a stable position. For small external perturbations that cause loss of balance in a forward direction (i.e., platform displacements in a backward direction), muscle activation usually proceeds in a distal to proximal sequence: gastrocnemius activity beginning about 90 to 100 ms after perturbation onset, followed by the hamstrings 20 to 30 ms later, and finally paraspinal muscle activation.[119,120] In response to backward instability, muscle activity begins in the anterior tibialis, followed by the quadriceps and abdominal muscles.

Weight-Shift Strategy (Lateral Plane)

The movement strategy utilized to control mediolateral perturbations involves shifting the body weight laterally from one leg to the other. The hips are the key control points of the weight-shift strategy. They move the COM in a lateral plane primarily through activation of hip abductor and adductor muscles, with some contribution from ankle invertors and evertors.[120]

TABLE 8.1 Characteristics of the Three Movement Systems for Balance Control Following Perturbations

Characteristic	Reflex	Automatic	Voluntary
Mediating pathway	Spinal cord	Brain stem/subcortical	Cortical
Mode of activation	External stimulus	External stimulus	External stimulus or self-stimulus
Comparative latency of response	Fastest	Intermediate	Slowest
Response	Localized to point of stimulus and highly stereotyped	Coordinated among leg and trunk muscles; stereotypical but adaptable	Coordinated and highly variable
Role in balance	Muscle force regulation	Resist disturbances	Generate purposeful movements
Factors modifying the response	Musculoskeletal or neurological abnormalities	Musculoskeletal or neurological abnormalities; configuration of support; prior experience	Musculoskeletal or neurological abnormalities; conscious effort; prior experience; task complexity

Adapted from Nashner, LM: Sensory, neuromuscular, and biomechanical contributions to human balance. In Duncan, PW (ed): *Balance Proceedings of the APTA Forum.* Alexandria, VA: American Physical Therapy Association, 1990: 5-12.[120]

Suspension Strategy

The suspension strategy is observed during balance tasks when a person quickly lowers his or her body COM by flexing the knees, causing associated flexion of the ankles and hips.[118] The suspension strategy can be combined with the ankle or the weight-shift strategy to enhance the effectiveness of a balance movement.[118]

Hip Strategy

For rapid and/or large external perturbations or for movements executed with the COG near the limits of stability, a hip strategy is employed.[118] The hip strategy uses rapid hip flexion or extension to move the COM within the BOS.[181] As the trunk rotates rapidly in one direction, horizontal (shear) forces are generated against the support surface in the opposite direction, moving the COM in the opposite direction as the trunk.[118] The muscle activity associated with the hip strategy has been studied by having a person stand crosswise on a narrow balance beam while the support surface suddenly moves backward (i.e., person sways forward) or forward (i.e., person sways backward).[68] In response to a forward body sway, muscles are typically activated in a proximal to distal sequence: Abdominals beginning about 90 to 100 ms after perturbation onset followed by activation of the quadriceps. Backward body sway results in activation first of the paraspinals followed by the hamstrings. A person cannot use the hip strategy to restore balance while walking on slippery surfaces because the large horizontal forces generated cause the feet to slip.

Stepping Strategy

If a large force displaces the COM beyond the limits of stability, a forward or backward step is used to enlarge the BOS and regain balance control. The uncoordinated step that follows a stumble on uneven ground is an example of a stepping strategy.

Combined Strategies

Research has shown that movement response patterns to postural perturbations are more complex and variable than originally described by Nashner.[87] Most healthy individuals use combinations of strategies to maintain balance depending on the control demands. Balance control requirements vary depending on the task and the environment. For example, standing on a bus that is moving has higher control demands than standing on a fixed surface. Therefore, it is important during treatment of balance disorders to vary the task and environment so the person develops movement strategies for different situations.

Balance Control Under Varying Conditions

Balance During Stance

In quiet stance, the body sways like an inverted pendulum about the ankle joint.[181] The balance goal is to keep the body's COM safely within the BOS. To accomplish this goal, an ankle strategy is utilized in which ankle muscles (i.e., ankle plantarflexors/dorsiflexors, invertors/evertors) are automatically and selectively activated to counteract body sway in different directions. Other muscles that are tonically active during quiet stance to maintain an erect posture are the gluteus medius and tensor fasciae latae, the iliopsoas to prevent hyperextension of the hip, and the thoracic paraspinals (with some intermittent abdominal activation).[7] Body alignment contributes to stability in quiet stance. Standing with the body in optimal body alignment allows the body to maintain balance with the least amount of muscle energy expenditure.[159]

Balance With Perturbed Standing

Perturbations to balance in standing can be either internal (i.e., voluntary movement of the body) or external (i.e., forces applied to the body). Both types of perturbations involve activation of muscle synergies, but the response timing is proactive (i.e., anticipatory) for internally generated perturbations and reactive for externally generated perturbations.[181]

Moving platform experiments have provided much information about the motor strategies (i.e., ankle, hip, and stepping strategies) and associated muscle activation patterns that result when a person is standing on a surface that unexpectedly translates or tilts.[88,117-119] With repetition of a platform perturbation, learning adaptation occurs that is characterized by a significant reduction in the reactive response.[106,117] For example, Nashner[117] found that upward rotation of a platform initially elicited reflex contractions of the gastrocnemius muscles of subjects, giving them the false impression that their bodies were falling forward; with repeated tilts, the gastrocnemius response diminished, and by the fourth repetition, it was completely absent. Thus, prior experience and feedforward anticipatory control have an important influence on balance responses.

Balance During Whole-Body Lifting

One of the most common ways that balance is challenged during everyday life is when lifting boxes or other large objects that are resting on the floor or at a level that is low relative to the person's COM (Fig. 8.4). Loss of balance during lifting may result in a fall, slip, or back injury.[4,141,155]

COM shift. During lifting, the movement of the body toward the load disturbs the position of the COM. When a load is lifted in front of the body, the COM is shifted forward during flexion of the trunk and legs, which is an internal disturbance to balance. The COM is further displaced forward when the load is added to the hands, creating an external disturbance to balance. In this case, anticipatory postural adjustments are needed to match whole-body backward momentum (horizontal linear and angular) to the displacement of the body and magnitude of the expected load.[31,61,62] The CNS estimates the amount of momentum necessary for lifting the load based on previous experience

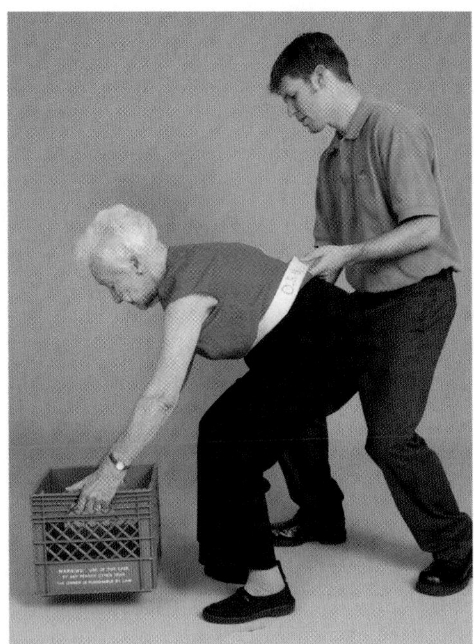

FIGURE 8.4 Balance during forward lifting with knees flexed.

with the load or other objects of similar physical properties (e.g., size, weight, and density).[62] The generation of backward horizontal linear momentum serves to keep the COM of the body within the base of support. The generation of angular momentum is essential for movement of the person with the load toward the upright posture.

Anticipated weight and momentum. The amount of whole-body momentum and the lifting force generated are scaled to the anticipated weight of the load.[62] When a heavy load is expected, sufficient levels of backward horizontal and angular momentum are needed to counteract the additional load, which tends to pull and rotate the body COM forward. Subtle differences in lifting posture, which reflect the underlying differences in momentum, occur when subjects lift a light load versus a heavy load (Fig. 8.5). Subjects tend to flex their hips and knees more and shift their weight back when lifting a heavy load (dark circles) than when lifting a light load (light circles).

Loss of balance. Loss of balance during lifting can occur when subjects overestimate or underestimate the weight of the load.[61] When the load weight is overestimated, too much momentum is generated and the body tends to topple backward. Most subjects compensate for this loss of balance by taking a step backward. When the load weight is underestimated, too little momentum is generated and the body tends to topple forward, resulting in the load quickly coming back to the ground.

Lifting style. The lifting style does appear to affect the challenges to balance. Keeping the knees more extended during lifting (Fig. 8.6) reduces the risk of balance loss, especially when the quadriceps are weak. Research comparing lifting styles has found that loss of balance was more common when subjects used a style of lifting in which the knees were more flexed compared to when the knees were straighter.[27,30,61,167]

Lifting instructions. Clinicians frequently instruct patients to use the leg lifting style, with the knees bent and the trunk erect, when lifting loads (Fig. 8.7).[112,162] This recommendation is based on the assumption that leg lifting imposes lower compression loads on the spine than other styles of lifting, such as the stoop lift, with the knees straight and the trunk flexed.[95] This assumption is likely true when the

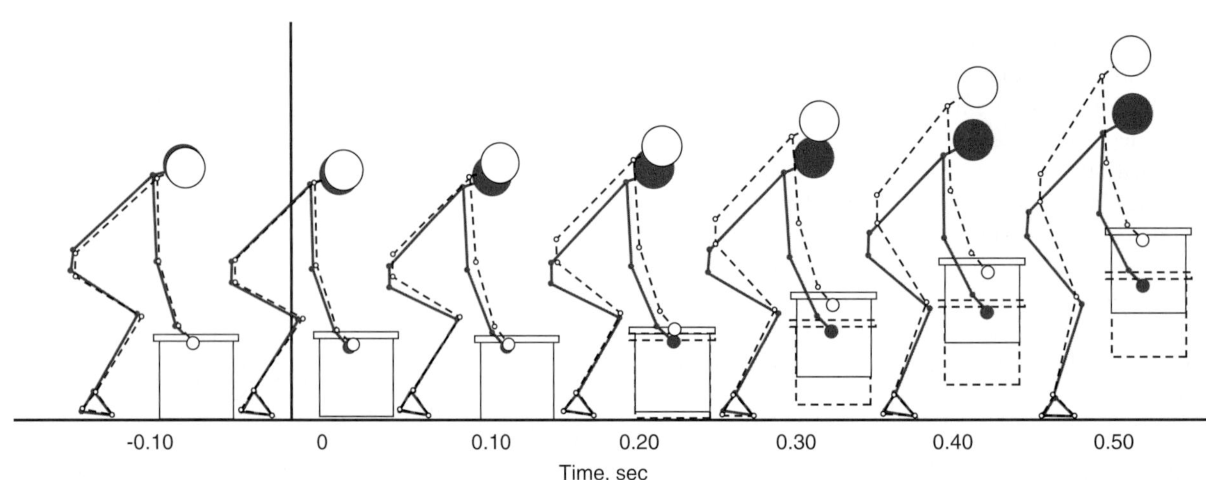

FIGURE 8.5 Postural adjustments for lifting a heavy versus a light load. When subjects approach a load (indicated by the vertical bar at time 0), early in the lift subtle differences in the anticipatory postural adjustments are evident. When a heavy load is expected (dark circles) there is greater flexion of the trunk, hips, and knees compared to when a light load is expected (light circles). *(Adapted from Heiss, DG, Shields, RK, and Yack, HJ: Anticipatory control of vertical lifting force and momentum during the squat lift with expected and unexpected loads.* J Orthop Sports Phys Ther *31(12):708–723; discussion 724–709, 2001.*[61]*)*

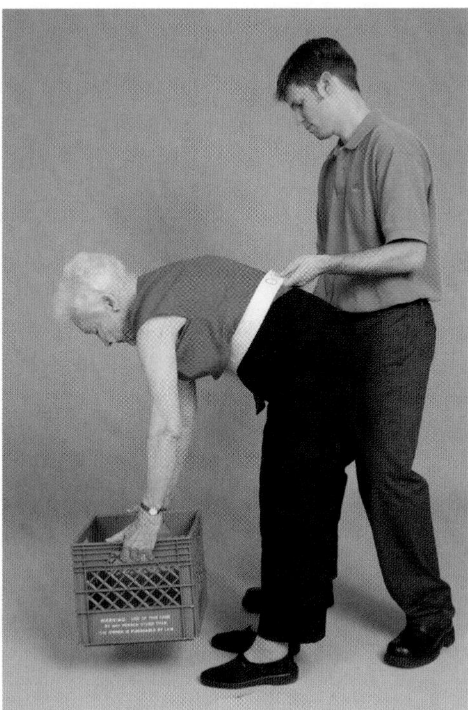

FIGURE 8.6 Balance during forward lifting with knees extended.

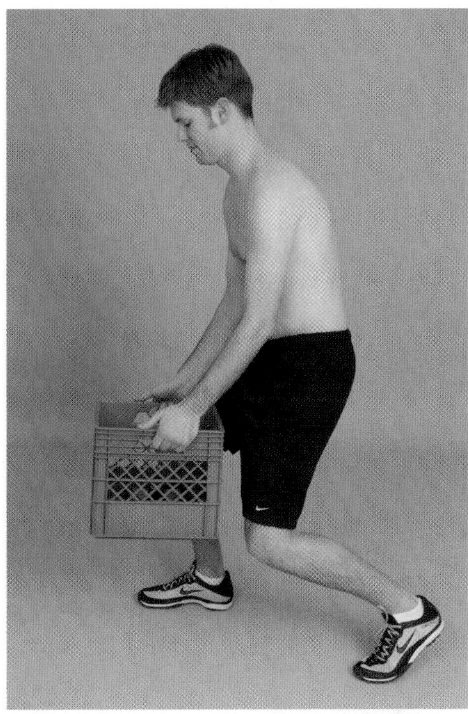

FIGURE 8.8 Straddle lift with trunk erect and object placed between the feet.

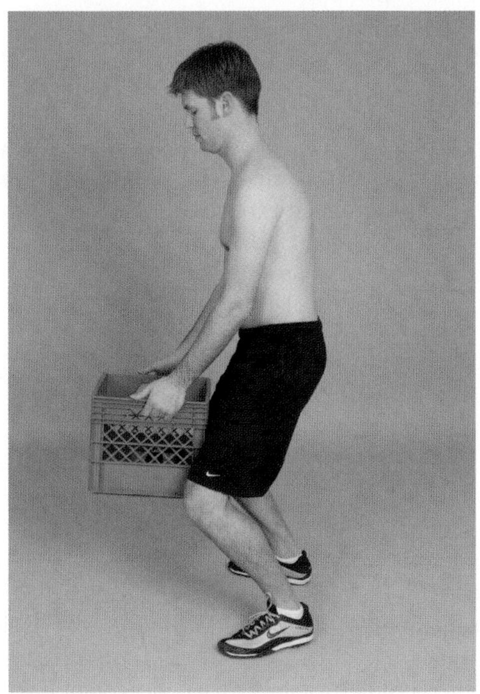

FIGURE 8.7 Squat lift with trunk erect and object placed between the feet.

load to be lifted can be placed between the feet (Figs. 8.7 and 8.8). However, van Dieen and colleagues[171] found little evidence in the biomechanical literature to support that leg lifting generally results in lower loads on the spine than back lifting. Recent research, using sophisticated biomechanical models, indicates that leg lifting results in higher compression forces on the spine compared to back lifting when the load is not positioned between the legs.[23,36,89,139] Although researchers have consistently found that bending moments and fascial strain are substantially greater with the back lift compared to the squat lift,[36,37] the magnitude of the bending moments on the spine appear to be well below the threshold for injury.[2,36,172]

Based on the current literature, it appears that if the objective of training for lifting is to reduce the load on the lumbar spine, other factors that have a more substantial effect on reducing the load on the lumbar spine should be emphasized over the selection of a lifting style, especially when placing the load between the legs is not feasible.

CLINICAL TIP

Important factors for safe lifting include maintaining a neutral spine, slowing the lifting speed, optimizing the horizontal and vertical position of the load, avoiding asymmetrical lifts (because of the increased lateral and twisting moments on the spine) (Fig. 8.9), and reducing the load weight.[172]

If maintaining balance is a concern—especially in the elderly—lifting styles in which the knees are more extended, such as with the semi-squat and stoop lift, are probably safer. In younger individuals with strong quadriceps, the straddle lift with one leg in front of the other to widen the base of support would reduce the risk of balance loss.

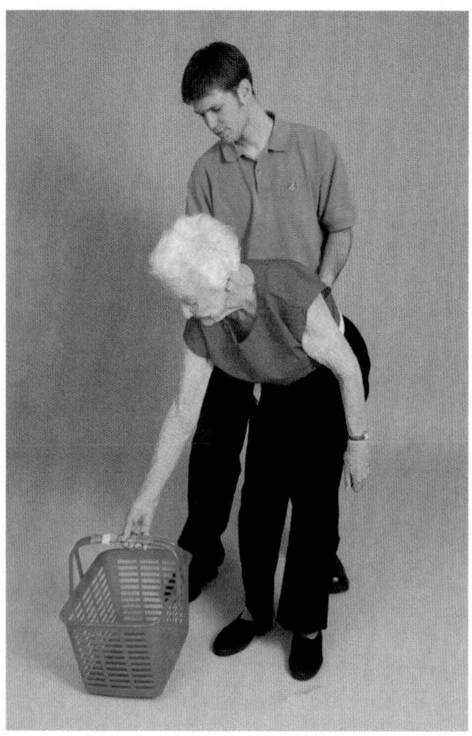

FIGURE 8.9 Side lift with the right trunk in lateral flexion and rotation results in high loads on the lumbar spine and should be avoided.

Balance in Unperturbed Human Gait

During walking, the COM is always outside the BOS except during the short double support period.[181] Therefore, the balance goal is to move the body outside the BOS by letting the body fall forward and yet prevent a fall. To accomplish this goal, a person must be able to maintain balance and posture of the upper body (i.e., head, arms, and trunk) and vertical alignment of the body against gravity. Trunk and hip muscles (flexors/extensors in the sagittal plane; abductors/adductors in the frontal plane) keep the upper body balanced, and extensor muscles of the lower extremities prevent vertical collapse.[181,182] The ankle muscles control anterior/posterior or medial/lateral acceleration of the body's COG but are not able to prevent falls.[181] Fine motor control of the foot during the swing phase involving anticipatory activation of the ankle dorsiflexors ensures minimum toe clearance (0.55 cm) to prevent trips.[135]

Impaired Balance

Impaired balance can be caused by injury or disease to any structures involved in the three stages of information processing—sensory input, sensorimotor integration, and motor output generation.

Sensory Input Impairments

Proprioceptive deficits have been implicated as contributing to balance impairments following lower extremity and trunk injuries or pathologies. Decreased joint position sense has been reported in individuals with recurrent ankle sprains,[14,46,49,54] knee ligamentous injuries,[6,134,148] degenerative joint disease,[6] and low back pain (LBP).[17,51,94] These same conditions have been associated with increased postural sway compared to that of controls.[3,33,46,49,94,113,129,178] It is unclear whether decreased joint position sense is due to changes in joint receptors or in muscle receptors.

Somatosensory, visual, or vestibular deficits may impair balance and mobility.

- Reduced somatosensation in the lower extremities caused by peripheral polyneuropathies in the aged and in individuals with diabetes is associated with balance deficits[143,144,160,169] and an increased risk for falls.[76,144] These individuals tend to rely more heavily on a hip strategy to maintain balance than do those without somatosensory deficits.[69]
- Visual loss or specific deficits in acuity, contrast sensitivity, peripheral field vision, and depth perception caused by disease, trauma, or aging can impair balance and lead to falls.[25,80]
- Individuals with damage to the vestibular system due to viral infections, traumatic brain injury (TBI), or aging may experience vertigo (a feeling of spinning) and postural instability. Black and colleagues[12] found that patients with severe bilateral loss of vestibular function are unable to use hip strategies even when standing crosswise on a narrow beam, although ankle strategies are unaffected.

Sensorimotor Integration Impairments

Damage to the basal ganglia, cerebellum, or supplementary motor area impairs processing of incoming sensory information, resulting in difficulty adapting sensory information in response to environmental changes and in disruption of anticipatory and reactive postural adjustments.[70,120,159] When stance is perturbed by platform translations, patients with Parkinson's disease tend to have a smaller than normal amplitude of movement due to co-activation of muscles on both sides of the body, whereas patients with cerebellar lesions typically demonstrate larger response amplitudes.[159]

Sensory organization problems that manifest as overreliance on one particular sense for balance control or a more generalized inability to select an appropriate sense for balance control when one or more senses give inaccurate information have been demonstrated in patients with a wide variety of neurological conditions.[159] Individuals who rely heavily on visual inputs (visually dependent) or somatosensory inputs (surface dependent) become unstable or fall under conditions in which the preferred sense is either absent or inaccurate, whereas those with generalized adaptation problems are unstable in any condition in which a sensory input is not accurate.

Biomechanical and Motor Output Impairments

Deficits in the motor components of balance control can be caused by musculoskeletal (i.e., poor posture, joint ROM limitations, and decreased muscle performance) and/or neuromuscular system (i.e., impaired motor coordination, and pain) impairments. Postural malalignment, such as the typical thoracic kyphosis of the elderly, that shifts the COM away from the center of the BOS increases a person's chance of exceeding his or her limits of stability.[120] Because each segment within the legs exerts forces on its adjunct segments, impaired ROM or muscle strength at one joint can alter posture and balance movements throughout the entire limb. For example, restriction of ankle motion by contractures or wearing ankle-foot orthoses and/or ankle dorsiflexor weakness eliminates the use of an ankle strategy, resulting in increased use of hip and trunk muscles for balance control.[19,150]

In individuals with neurological conditions (e.g., stroke, TBI, and Parkinson's disease), failure to generate adequate muscle forces due to abnormal tone or impaired coordination of motor strategies may limit the person's ability to recruit muscles required for balance.[159]

Pain can alter movements; reduce a person's normal stability limits; and, if persistent, produce secondary strength and mobility impairments.

Deficits With Aging

Falls are common and are a major cause of morbidity, mortality, reduced functioning, and premature nursing home admissions in persons over age 65.[25,38,126,147,149] The most common risk factors associated with falls in the elderly are listed in Box 8.2. Most falls by the elderly are likely due to complex interactions between multiple risk factors. Clinicians are encouraged to follow published guidelines for the prevention of falls by older persons when prescribing fall prevention interventions.[1]

Declines in all sensory systems (somatosensory, vision, and vestibular) and all three stages of information processing (i.e., sensory processing, sensorimotor integration, and motor output) are found with aging.[96,159] In comparison to young adults, older adults have more difficulty maintaining balance when sensory inputs from more than one system are greatly reduced, particularly when they must rely solely on vestibular inputs for balance control.[144,184] Studies of response patterns to platform perturbations in older adults have demonstrated the following motor strategy changes compared to those of young adults.

- Slower-onset latencies[161,184]
- More frequent use of a hip strategy for balance control[71]
- Limitations in the ability to maintain balance when challenged with perturbations of increasing magnitude and velocity[97]

Impaired anticipatory postural adjustments prior to making voluntary movements have been demonstrated in older individuals and may explain the high incidence of falls during activities such as walking, lifting, and carrying objects.[45,79] Valid and reliable outcome measures for assessing fall risk in the elderly are listed in Table 8.2. The BESTest, mini-BESTest, and Brief-BESTest are emerging fall risk assessments that have primarily been studied in the Parkinson's disease population.[40]

BOX 8.2 Most Common Risk Factors for Falls Among the Elderly

- Muscle weakness
- History of falls
- Gait deficit
- Balance deficit
- Use of assistive device
- Visual deficit
- Arthritis
- Impaired activities of daily living
- Depression
- Cognitive impairment
- Age >80 years

(From American Geriatrics Society British Geriatrics Society, American Academy of Orthopaedic Surgeons Panel on Fall Prevention: Guidelines for the prevention of falls in older persons. *J Am Geriatr Soc* 49:664–672, 2001.[1])

CLINICAL TIP

Divided attention as when a person is doing two tasks simultaneously (i.e., walking while doing a secondary cognitive or motor task) can lead to postural instability and falls, particularly in the elderly.[142,158] Modified versions of the Timed Up-and-Go Test[138] with secondary cognitive and motor tasks can be used by clinicians to assess the influence of divided attention on balance control.[104,156] If deficits are found, patients should be allowed to practice walking while doing a secondary task and progress to doing multiple tasks according to their improvements in performance.

Elderly individuals who have experienced one or more falls may develop fear of falling, which leads to a loss of confidence in a person's ability to perform routine tasks, restricted activity, social isolation, functional decline, depression, and decreased quality of life.[25,91] The fear of falling arises more often from a person's fear of institutionalization than a fear of injury.[75] Individuals with fear of falling demonstrate perceived stability limits that are reduced from their actual stability limits and gait changes, including decreased stride length, reduced speed, increased stride width, and increased double-support time.[24,105] It is important that clinicians screen patients for fear of falling with instruments, such as the Activities-Specific Balance Confidence (ABC) Scale[140] or the Fall Efficacy Scale,[166] so evidence-based interventions that reduce fear of falling and promote physical, social, and functional activity are implemented.[16,164,175]

Deficits From Medications

There is an increased risk of falling among older individuals who take four or more medications and among those taking certain medications (i.e., hypnotics, sedatives, tricyclic

TABLE 8.2 Outcome Measures for Fall Risk Assessment

Outcome Measure	Perfect Score	Cut-off Score (Sensitivity, Specificity)*
Berg Balance Test	56	<46 (25%, 87% for predicting any fall and 42%, 87% for multiple falls)[115]
Tinetti Performance-Oriented Mobility Assessment	28 (Balance subscale 16, Gait subscale 12)	<20 for elderly (64%/66%)**[42] and individuals with Parkinson's disease (76%, 66%)[86]
Timed Up-and-Go Test	N/A (timed test)	>13.5 seconds (87%, 87%)[156]
Four-Square Step Test	N/A (timed test)	>15 seconds (89%, 85%)[35]
Dynamic Gait Index	24	<20 (67%, 86%)[185]
Functional Gait Assessment	30	<23 (100%, 72%)[185]
Five-Times-Sit-to-Stand Test	N/A (timed test)	>15 seconds (55%, 65%)[18]
ABC Scale	100%	<67% (84%, 88%)[92]

*Sensitivity and specificity values are given for community-dwelling elderly.
**Sensitivity and specificity values are for elderly in long-term self-care and nursing care facilities.

antidepressants, tranquilizers, and antihypertensive drugs) due to dizziness or other side effects.[1,25] Individuals who have fallen should have their medications reviewed and altered or stopped as appropriate to prevent future falls.

Management of Impaired Balance

Examination and Evaluation of Impaired Balance

The key elements of a comprehensive evaluation of individuals with balance problems include the following:

- A thorough history of falls (whether onset of falls is sudden versus gradual; the frequency and direction of falls; the environmental conditions, activities, and presence of dizziness, vertigo, or lightheadedness at time of the fall; current and past medications; and presence of fear of falling)
- Assessments to identify sensory input (proprioceptive, visual, and vestibular), sensory processing (sensorimotor integration, anticipatory and reactive balance control), and biomechanical and motor (postural alignment, muscle strength and endurance, joint ROM and flexibility, motor coordination, and pain) impairments contributing to balance deficits
- Tests and observations to determine the impact of balance control system deficits on functional performance
- Environmental assessments to determine fall risk hazards in a person's home.[25]

Commonly used tests and measures for each of the three categories of balance assessment are presented in Table 8.3. Clinicians should carefully select a variety of tests and measures that assess all of the various types of balance control.

Static Balance Tests

Static balance can be assessed by observing the patient's ability to maintain different postures.

- The Romberg Test[127] tests the patient's ability to stand with the feet parallel and together with the eyes open and then closed for 30 seconds.
- The sharpened Romberg, also known as the tandem Romberg,[127] requires the patient to stand with the feet in a heel-to-toe position with arms folded across the chest and eyes closed for 1 minute. The Romberg and sharpened Romberg tests are screening tools that help the therapist to decide if more specific testing is needed to determine the cause of imbalance or to establish a person's balance status.
- The Single-Leg Balance Stance Test[173] (SLB) asks the patient to stand on one leg without shoes with arms crossed or hands on hips without letting the legs touch each other. Three 30-second trials are performed for each leg, and a best or a mean time of the three trials is recorded. The SLB is reliable and has been found to predict injurious falls in community-dwelling elderly[173] and ankle sprains in athletes.[168]
- The Stork Stand Test[84] is performed by having the patient stand on both feet with hands on the hips, then lift one leg and place the toes of that foot against the knee of the other leg. On command from the tester, the patient then raises the heel to stand on the toes and tries to balance for as long as possible without letting either the heel touch the ground or the other foot move away from the knee. Normal adults should be able to balance for 20 to 30 seconds on each leg.

Dynamic Balance Tests

Dynamic balance control can be assessed by observations of how well the patient is able to stand or sit on unstable surfaces (e.g., foam or Swiss ball); transition from one position to another (e.g., supine-to-sit or sit-to-stand transfers); and

TABLE 8.3 Balance Assessments and Interventions

Category of Balance Assessment	Clinical Tests/Measures*	Interventions if Deficits Present
Static	Observations of patient maintaining different postures; Romberg Test[127]; sharpened (tandem) Romberg[127]; Single-Leg Stance Test[173]; Stork Stand Test[84]	Vary postures Vary support surface Incorporate external loads
Dynamic	Observations of patient standing or sitting on unstable surface or performing postural transitions and functional activities; Five-times-sit-to-stand test (5 × STS)[34]	Moving support surfaces Move head, trunk, arms, legs Transitional and locomotor activities
Anticipatory (feedforward)	Observations of patient catching ball, opening doors, lifting objects of different weights; Functional Reach Test[39]; Multidirectional Reach Test[128]; Star Excursion Balance Test[132]; Y-Balance Test[152]	Reaching Catching Kicking Lifting Obstacle course
Reactive (feedback)	Observation of patient's responses to pushes (small or large, slow or rapid, anticipated and unanticipated); Pull Test[116]; Push and Release Test (PRT)[81]; Postural Stress Test[183]	Standing sway Ankle strategy Hip strategy Stepping strategy Perturbations
Sensory organization	Clinical Test of Sensory Integration on Balance Test (CTSIB)[157] or modified CTSIB, Balance Error Scoring System (BESS)[58]	Reduce visual inputs Reduce somatosensory cues
Balance during functional activities	Berg Balance Scale (BBS)[11]; Timed Up and Go Test (TUG)[138]; Tinetti Performance-Oriented Mobility Assessment (POMA)[165]; Balance Evaluation Systems Test (BESTest) or mini-BESTest[72]; Four Square Step Test (4SST)[35]; Dynamic Gait Index (DGI)[159]; Functional Gait Assessment (FGA)[186]; Community Balance and Mobility Scale[73]; High Level Mobility Assessment (HiMat)[179]; Dizziness Handicap Inventory (DHI)[82]	Functional activities Dual or multitask activities (e.g., walking with secondary cognitive or motor task)
Safety during gait, locomotion, or balance	Observations; home assessments; Falls Efficacy Scale[166]; Activities-Specific Balance Confidence (ABC) Scale [140]	Balance within stability limits, environmental modifications, assistive devices, external support

*Tests are listed in relative order of least to most difficult to perform.

perform activities such as walking, jumping, hopping, and skipping.

- The Five-times-sit-to-stand test (5 × STS) can be used to evaluate balance control when moving between sitting and standing.[34] The person is seated in a chair with the arms across the chest and then stands up and sits back down as quickly as possible five times consecutively while being timed. A score of >15 seconds on the 5 × STS was found to predict recurrent falls (sensitivity 55%, specificity 65%) in 2,735 community-dwelling elderly individuals.[18]

Anticipatory Postural Control Tests

Anticipatory postural control is evaluated by having the patient perform voluntary movements that require the development of a postural set to counteract a predicted postural disturbance. The patient's ability to catch balls, open doors, lift objects of different weights, and reach without losing balance is indicative of adequate anticipatory control.

- The Functional Reach Test[39] and the Multi-Directional Reach Test[128] require the patient to reach in different directions as far as possible without changing the BOS. Normative data are available, and the tests are reliable and valid.[128]
- The Star Excursion Balance Test (SEBT) is a test of lower extremity reach that challenges an individual's limits of stability.[132] The patient is instructed to reach as far as possible with one leg in each of eight prescribed directions while maintaining balance on the contralateral leg. The test is reliable[64,90] and has validity to detect dynamic balance deficits in individuals with chronic ankle instability, anterior cruciate ligament deficiency, or patellofemoral pain syndrome; to predict risk of lower extremity injury in high school athletes; and to show improvement in performance

after balance training in patients with chronic ankle instability and healthy adults .[8,55,137] A more time-efficient test based on research suggesting redundancy in the eight directions of the SEBT is the Y-Balance Test (YBT).[152] The patient reaches with one leg in only three directions (anterior, posteromedial, and posterolateral). The YBT has been found to be reliable and valid and is predictive of lower extremity injury in athletes.[93,136,137,152]

Reactive Postural Control Tests

Automatic postural responses or reactive control can be assessed by the patient's response to external perturbations.

- Pushes (small or large, slow or rapid, and anticipated and unanticipated) applied in different directions to the sternum, posterior trunk, or pelvis are used widely, but they are not quantifiable or reliable. The clinician subjectively rates the responses as normal, good, fair, poor, or unable.
- The Pull Test,[116] Push and Release Test,[81] and Postural Stress Test[183] are more objective and reliable measures of reactive postural control.

Sensory Organization Tests

The Clinical Test of Sensory Integration on Balance Test (CTSIB), also called the "Foam and Dome" Test,[157] measures the patient's ability to balance under six different sensory conditions:

1. Standing on a firm surface with the eyes open (visual, somatosensory, and vestibular information accurate)
2. Standing on a firm surface with the eyes closed (somatosensory and vestibular information accurate)
3. Standing on a firm surface wearing a dome made from a modified Japanese lantern (somatosensory and vestibular information accurate, visual information inaccurate)
4. Standing on a foam cushion with the eyes open (visual and vestibular information accurate, somatosensory inaccurate)
5. Standing on foam with the eyes closed (vestibular information accurate, somatosensory information inaccurate)
6. Standing on foam wearing the dome (vestibular information accurate, somatosensory and visual information inaccurate).

The patient stands with feet parallel and arms at sides or hands on hips. A minimum of three 30-second trials of each condition are performed.

- Individuals who rely heavily on visual inputs for balance (i.e., visual dependent) will become unstable or fall in conditions 2, 3, 5, and 6.
- Those who rely heavily on somatosensory inputs (i.e., surface dependent) will show deficits with conditions 4, 5, and 6.
- Individuals with generalized adaptation problems will be unstable in conditions 3, 4, 5, and 6.
- Individuals with vestibular loss will be very unstable in conditions 5 and 6.

NOTE: Because no difference was found in scores between conditions 2 and 3 and conditions 5 and 6,[29] the dome portions have been removed from the CTSIB. The modified version consists of the four conditions of eyes open and closed while standing on the floor and then on a piece of foam. A computerized version of the CTSIB using a moveable force plate and visual surround is called the Sensory Organization Test.[120]

The Balance Error Scoring System (BESS) is a clinical test of postural stability that requires an individual to assume three different stance positions (double leg, single leg, and tandem) while standing on a firm surface and then standing on a piece of foam with eyes closed for a total of six 20-second trials.[58] The tester observes for six types of errors in performance such as opening the eyes, steps, stumbles, or falls. Performance is scored by adding one error point for each error committed. The BESS has moderate to good interrater reliability and is useful for identifying balance deficits in individuals with concussion, functional ankle instability, external ankle bracing, fatigue, and older age.[9,58]

Functional Tests

Functional tests are used to determine activity limitations and participation restrictions and to identify tasks that a patient needs to practice. Four mobility scales (i.e., Tinetti Performance-Oriented Mobility Assessment [POMA],[165] Timed Up and Go Test [TUG],[138] Berg Balance Scale, and Four Square Step Test [4SST[35]]) and two gait scales (i.e., Dynamic Gait Index[159] and Functional Gait Assessment[186]) can be easily used to assess balance performance during functional activities. Most of these tests were designed to assess fall risk in the elderly, with the exception of the Functional Gait Assessment, which was developed specifically for use with patients with vestibular disorders. The most comprehensive clinical balance tool currently available is the Balance Evaluation Systems Test (BESTest), a 36-item test consisting of balance tasks borrowed from several balance measures that assesses 6 systems underlying balance control (i.e., biomechanical constraints, stability limits/verticality, anticipatory postural adjustments, postural responses, sensory orientation, and stability in gait).[72] The BESTest was shortened to 14 items (mini-BESTest) and then to 6 items (brief-BESTest) to increase its use in the clinical setting.[44,133] The Community Balance and Mobility Scale[73] and the High Level Mobility Assessment Tool[179] can be used to evaluate balance and mobility in people who are ambulatory and functioning at a high level, yet have some balance deficits. The 25-item Dizziness Handicap Scale is a questionnaire that can evaluate the self-perceived impact of dizziness and unsteadiness on functional activities in people with vestibular disorders.[82]

Balance Training

There are many factors to consider when developing an intervention program for balance impairments. Most balance intervention programs require a multisystem approach. For example, an individual who has experienced prolonged bed rest or inactivity following an illness may require a program that includes stretching the lower extremities and trunk to improve postural alignment and mobility; strengthening exercises to improve motor performance; and dynamic, functional balance activities to improve the ability to perform daily activities safely.

The focus of attention is important when improving balance performance through training. An *external focus of attention* means that the performer is attending to the external environment when practicing balance control.[26,188] For example, if balancing on a tilt board, the instruction would be to keep the board horizontal; or, if holding a bar in an outstretched hand, the instruction would be to keep the bar horizontal.[10,26] An external focus of attention is more effective for motor learning than instruction or feedback that promotes an *internal focus of attention,* which directs the learner to focus on body movements or positions—for example, keeping the feet horizontal on a tilt board or keeping the trunk posture straight. It is suggested that an external focus of attention facilitates the use of unconscious, fast, and reflexive control processes (e.g., automaticity) and speeds up the learning process.[26,187,189]

The following elaborates on the interventions suggested previously (see Table 8.3), which are based on identified deficits in static, dynamic, anticipatory, and reactive control, as well as problems involving sensory organization, function, and safety. For specific procedures to address musculoskeletal problems such as strength, joint mobility, flexibility, or posture, refer to the chapters of this textbook addressing these interventions or to chapters focused on specific regions of the body.

Because balance training often involves activities that challenge the patient's limits of stability, it is important that the therapist takes steps to ensure the patient's safety. Box 8.3 lists safety measures that should be considered and utilized to prevent falls and injuries during therapy.

BOX 8.3 Safety During Balance Training

1. Use a gait belt any time the patient practices exercises or activities that challenge or destabilize balance.
2. Stand slightly behind and to the side of the patient with one arm holding or near the gait belt and the other arm on or near the top of the shoulder (on the trunk, not the arm).
3. Perform exercises near a railing or in parallel bars to allow patient to grab when necessary.
4. Do not perform exercises near sharp edges of equipment or objects.
5. Have one person in front and one behind when working with patients at high risk of falling or during activities that pose a high risk of injury.
6. Check equipment to ensure that it is operating correctly.
7. Guard patient when getting on and off equipment (such as treadmills and stationary bikes).
8. Ensure that the floor is clean and free of debris.

CLINICAL TIP

Cognitive deficits can considerably impact the success of balance training programs. If deficits are moderate to severe and a person is unable to follow directions, then performance of specific balance exercises may be unsafe and have limited success. In these cases, repetitive practice of common functional activities is advised.

Static Balance Control

Activities to promote static balance control include having the patient maintain sitting, half-kneeling, tall kneeling, and standing postures on a firm surface.

- To promote an *external focus of attention,* have the patient hold a bar in the outstretched hand and instruct him/her to maintain the bar in a horizontal position.
- More challenging activities include practice in the tandem and single-leg stance (Fig. 8.10), lunge, and squat positions.
- Progress these activities by working on soft surfaces (e.g., foam, sand, and grass), narrowing the base of support, moving the arms, or closing the eyes.
- Provide resistance via handheld weights or elastic resistance (Figs. 8.11 and 8.12).
- Add a secondary task (i.e., catching a ball or mental calculations) to further increase the level of difficulty (Fig. 8.13).

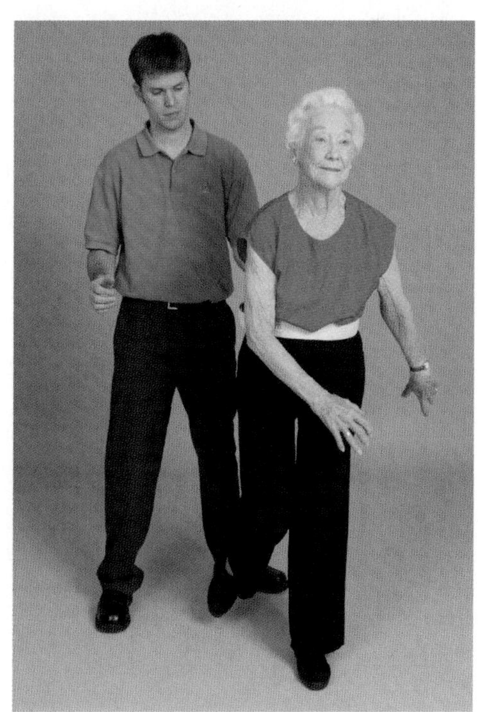

FIGURE 8.10 Balance during single leg stance.

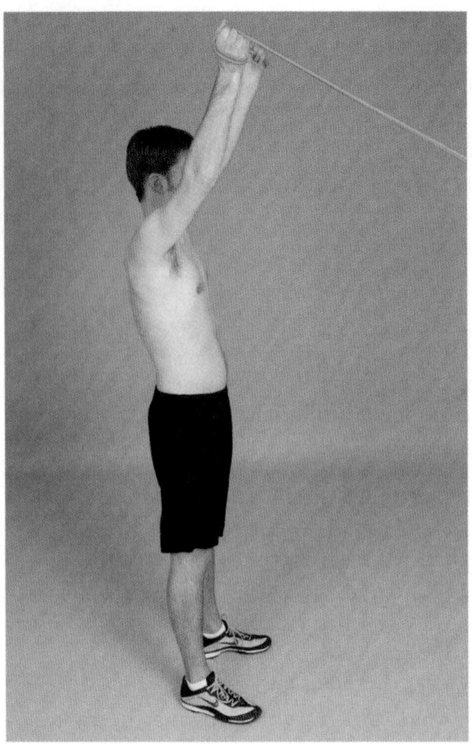

FIGURE 8.11 Balance while standing with resistance provided to the arms via elastic resistance.

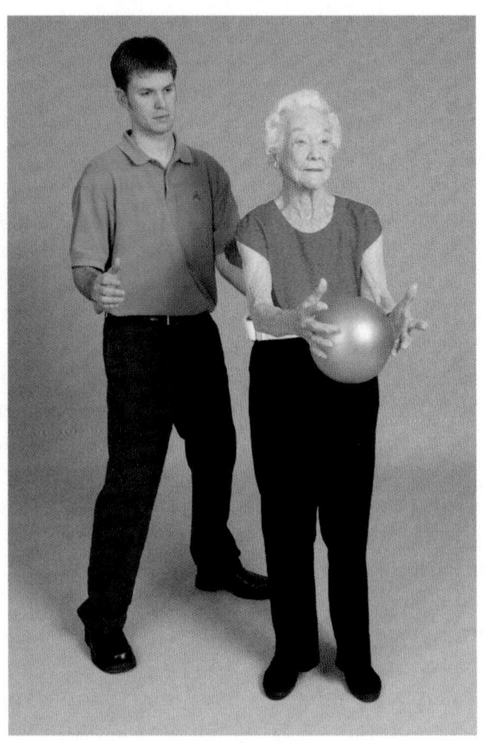

FIGURE 8.13 Balance while standing and catching a ball.

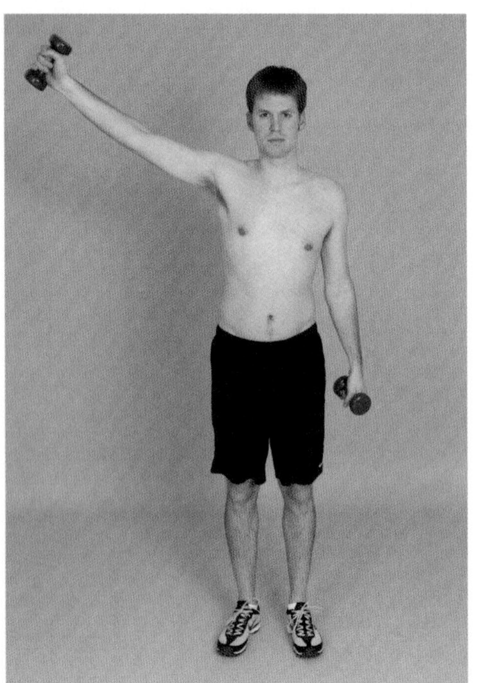

FIGURE 8.12 Balance while standing with arm abducting and holding a weight.

Dynamic Balance Control

To promote dynamic balance control, interventions may involve the following:

- Have the patient practice balance control while on moving surfaces, such as sitting on a therapeutic ball, standing on wobble boards (Fig. 8.14), or bouncing on a mini-trampoline. To promote an external focus, instruct the patient to focus on keeping the ball from rolling or the wobble board level.
- Progress the activities by superimposing movements such as shifting the body weight, rotating the trunk, and moving the head or arms (Fig. 8.15).
- Vary the position of the arms from out to the side to above the head (Fig. 8.16).
- Practice stepping exercises starting with small steps and then mini-lunges to full lunges. For external focus, imagine you have a plank against your back and push as hard as you can on the floor underneath the stance leg.
- Progress the exercise program to include hopping, skipping, rope jumping, and hopping down from a small stool while maintaining balance.
- Have the patient perform arm and leg exercises while standing with normal stance, tandem stance, and single-leg stance (Fig. 8.17).

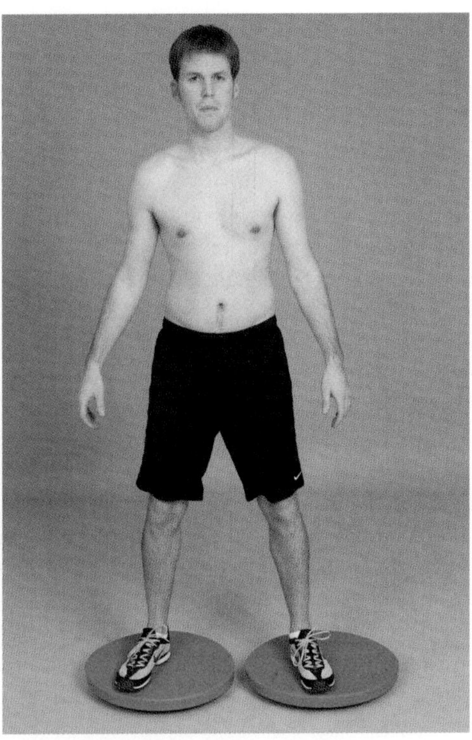

FIGURE 8.14 Balance while standing on wobble boards.

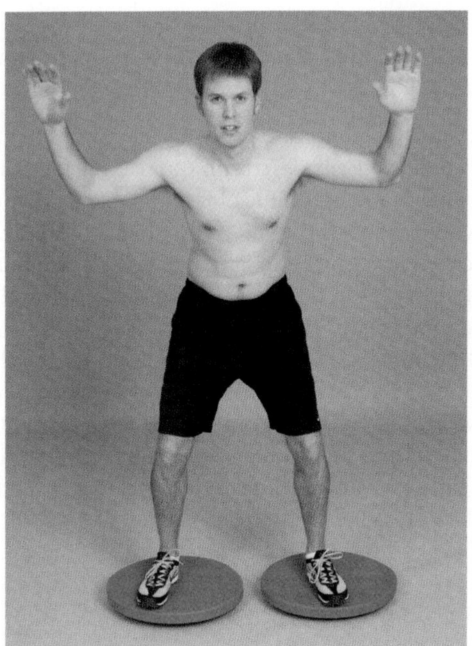

FIGURE 8.16 Balance while standing on wobble boards with arms above the head.

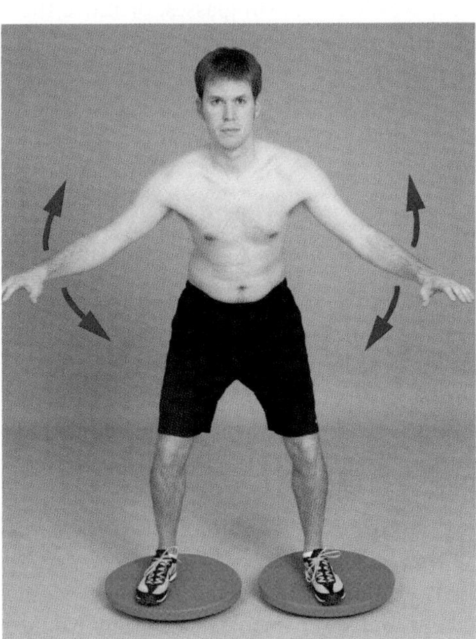

FIGURE 8.15 Balance while standing on wobble boards with arm movements.

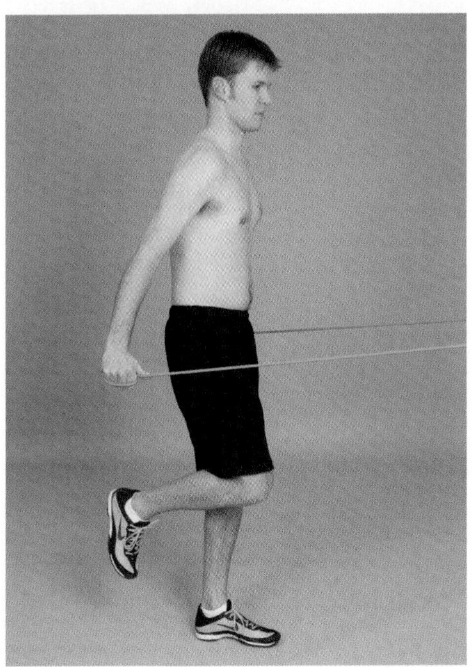

FIGURE 8.17 One-legged stance with resisted shoulder extension using elastic resistance.

Anticipatory Balance Control

Practice anticipatory balance control by performing the following:

- Reach in all directions to touch or grasp objects, catching a ball, or kicking a ball. To promote external focus, instruct the patient to focus on the object. For example, touch the object lightly, catch the ball softly, or kick the ball far.
- Use different postures for variation (e.g., sitting, standing, and kneeling) and throwing or rolling the ball at different speeds and heights (Fig. 8.18).
- Use functional tasks that involve multiple parts of the body to increase the challenge to anticipatory postural control by having the patient lift objects of varying weight in different postures at varying speeds, open and close doors with different handles and heaviness, or maneuver through an obstacle course.

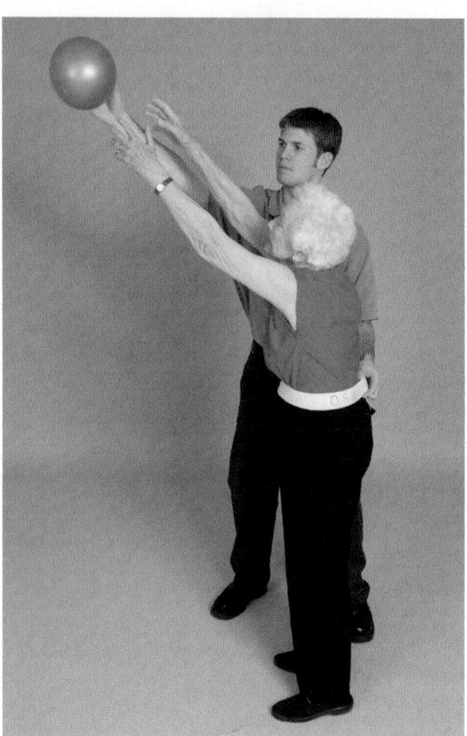

FIGURE 8.18 Balance when standing while reaching and catching the ball overhead.

Reactive Balance Control

Train reactive balance control by using the following activities:

- Have the patient work to gradually increase the amount of sway in different directions while standing on a firm, stable surface. Have the patient concentrate on how much force the feet are pushing on the floor to promote an external focus of attention.
- To emphasize training of the *ankle strategy*, have the patient practice while standing on one leg with the trunk erect.
- To emphasize training of the *hip strategy*, have the patient walk on balance beams or lines drawn on the floor; perform tandem stance and single-leg stance with trunk bending; or stand on a mini-trampoline, rocker balance, or sliding board.
- To emphasize the *stepping strategy*, have the patient practice stepping up onto a stool or stepping with legs crossed in front or behind other leg (e.g., weaving or braiding).
- To increase the challenge during these activities, add anticipated and unanticipated external forces. For example, have the patient lift boxes that are identical in appearance but of different weights; throw and catch balls of different weights and sizes; or while on a treadmill, suddenly stop/start the belt or increase/decrease the speed.

Sensory Organization

Many of the activities previously described can be utilized while varying the reliance on specific sensory systems.

- To reduce or destabilize the *visual inputs*, have the patient close the eyes, wear prism glasses, or move the eyes and head together during the balance activity.
- To decrease reliance on *somatosensory cues*, patients can narrow the BOS, stand on foam, or stand on an incline board.

Balance During Functional Activities

Focus on activities similar to the functional limitations identified in the evaluation. For example:

- If reaching is limited, have the patient work on activities, such as reaching for a glass in a cupboard, reaching behind (as putting arm in a sleeve), or catching a ball off center. To promote an external focus, instruct the patient to focus on the object (e.g., keep the water in the glass level or catch the ball softly).
- Perform two or more tasks simultaneously to increase the level of task complexity.
- Practice recreational activities the patient enjoys, such as golf, to increase motivation while challenging balance control (Fig. 8.19).

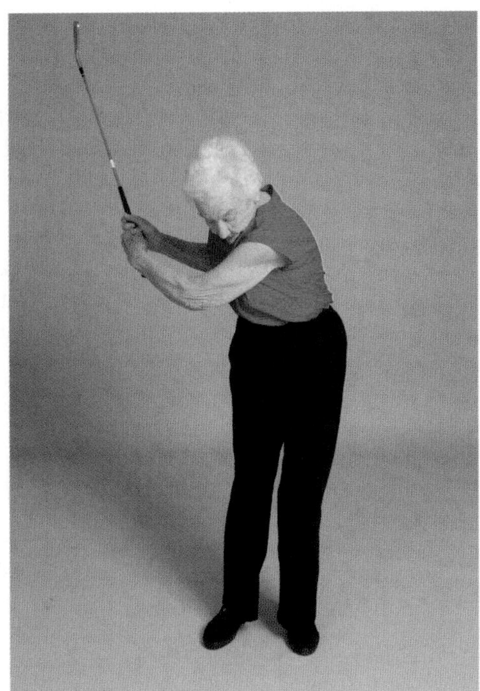

FIGURE 8.19 Functional balance during a golf swing.

Safety During Gait, Locomotion, or Balance

To emphasize safety, have the patient practice postural sway activities within the person's actual stability limits and progress dynamic activities with emphasis on promoting function and an external focus of attention. If balance deficits cannot be changed, environmental modifications, assistive devices, and increased family or external support may be required to ensure safety.

CLINICAL TIP

Assistive devices, such as rollator walkers, are often appropriately prescribed as a compensatory measure for people with a variety of balance impairments. However, clinicians should be aware that assistive devices that are incorrectly fitted or used by a patient can precipitate falls. Therefore, clinicians must properly adjust and provide instruction on proper use of assistive devices to prevent unnecessary falls.

Health and Environmental Factors

In addition to exercise and balance training activities, clinicians should address several other factors affecting balance to reduce the risk of falls.[102]

Low Vision

To address low vision issues, encourage regular eye examinations with adjustments to lens prescriptions and cataract surgery, if necessary. Wearing a hat and sunglasses in bright sunlight, taking extra precautions when it is dark, and making sure lights are on when walking about the house at night are other recommendations. Advise patients to avoid using bifocal glasses when walking, because single lens glasses are safest for improving depth perception and contrast sensitivity, especially on stairs.[101]

Sensory Loss

For individuals with sensory loss in the legs, caution them to take extra care when walking on soft carpet or uneven ground and use a cane or other device if necessary. Recommend that they wear firm rubber shoes with low heels. Regular medical examinations should be encouraged to ensure that a patient's blood glucose levels and other factors (i.e., cholesterol, lipids) are under control to minimize damage to sensory nerves from diseases such as diabetes and peripheral vascular disease. Advise patients to seek medical attention if they experience any symptoms of dizziness.

Medications

Patients should be educated about the influence of certain medications, such as sedatives and antidepressants, on their risk of falling. For example, if such medications are used at night as a sleep aid, an individual should take extra precautions when getting up to use the bathroom.

Evidence-Based Balance Exercise Programs for Fall Prevention in the Elderly

With at least one-third of people aged 65 years or more falling at least once each year, physical therapists can play a major role in the prevention of falls. Mounting evidence from randomized clinical trials indicates that therapeutic exercise is an effective tool in the prevention of falls, especially if it is incorporated with a comprehensive strategy targeting health, environmental, and behavioral risk factors that contribute to falls.[52,111] The selection of exercises and activities for balance training should be based on two major factors: the person's fall risk and the setting in which the training will take place. Economic and transportation factors also play a role in these decisions. Since people can fall while participating in balance training and exercise programs, it is critical that adequate protections are in place to prevent falls. Based on these issues, the following guidelines are proposed.

- Elderly individuals who have no history of falls and do not have scores that are within the "at risk" category on standardized balance tests should participate in an individual or community-based group exercise program incorporating muscle strengthening, balance, and coordination exercises.
- Individuals who are at risk of falls, based on standardized balance tests, but have not developed a history of falls should participate in individual or group exercise programs in which there are well-trained leaders and support staff who appropriately supervise and guard the person during the activities that challenge balance.

- People who are at risk of falls and have a history of falls require an individually tailored, supervised, exercise program by a physical therapist or physical therapist assistant and, if appropriate, a caregiver who is trained to supervise and guard the person during the home exercise activities. This program may take place in a clinic- or home-based setting.

CLINICAL TIP

According to current best evidence, an exercise program to reduce risk of falls should include at least 2 hours per week devoted to exercises and activities to improve balance.[154]

Exercise programs that incorporate multiple types of exercise, such as balance training, strength/resistance training, and constant repetitive movements through all 3 planes (e.g., tai chi or square stepping), are effective for reducing both rate of falls and risk of falling.[53]

Although walking has many health benefits, the time devoted to a walking exercise program should be *in addition* to time spent in balance training and not a substitute for it.

Home Exercise Program for Reducing Risk of Falls for People at High Risk

The home setting may be the best option for an exercise-based falls prevention program for some people who are at high risk of falls. Reasons why the home may be the best location for such programs include (1) the person functions most often in this environment, and therefore the training takes place in the location where falls are most likely to occur, and (2) the person may participate more fully to his or her physical capacity without the stress and fatigue that may be associated with transportation issues.

Otago Home Exercise Program

The Otago Exercise Program[20,48,145] is a cost-effective home program supervised by a physical therapist that reduces falls in frail older adults. This program consists of a series of 17 strength and balance exercises that are individually tailored and performed at least three times per week. The 30-minute exercise program is complemented with a walking plan with the goal of walking 30 minutes at least twice per week. The program is designed to be performed for 1 year under the supervision of physical therapists or health professionals trained by the physical therapist.[48] The first 2 months of the Otago program is the Physical Therapy Management Phase during which the physical therapist conducts the initial evaluation, instructs the patient in the exercises, and progresses the exercise and walking program.[22] The Self-Management Phase follows in which the patient carries out the program with assistance of a caregiver, if necessary. Follow-up visits by the physical therapist are scheduled at 6, 9, and 12 months. Physical therapists can obtain online training and free resources for implementing the Otago Exercise Program through the Carolina Geriatric Education Center at the University of North Carolina at Chapel Hill.[22]

- The patient receives a manual with illustrations and instructions on each exercise. Videos are also available online.
- Ankle weights are used to provide resistance during the leg strengthening exercises that target the muscles that extend and abduct the hip and flex and extend the knee.[48]
  - The amount of resistance should be based on the amount of weight that the person can lift for 8 to 10 repetitions of the exercise before fatiguing. Most people start with 1- or 2-kg (2.2- or 4.4-lb) cuff weights.
  - The goal is for the person to be able to do 2 sets of 10 repetitions before the amount of weight is increased.
  - The ankle dorsiflexor and plantarflexor muscles are strengthened using body weight as the resistance (Fig. 8.20 and Fig. 8.21).
  - Box 8.4 provides a list of the strengthening exercises in the Otago program.
- The balance training component of the Otago Exercise Program is also tailored to the individual and emphasizes dynamic exercises that are closely related to functional activities (Fig 8.22).[48] Depending on the ability of the individual, the balance exercises may be performed by holding on to a large, stable piece of furniture or a kitchen counter and progressed by performing the exercises without support (Fig 8.23). Balance training exercises are listed in Box 8.4.
- A walking program is part of the Otago Exercise Program.[48] People are told to walk for at least 30 minutes per day at their usual pace. The walking plan may be accomplished by taking walks of smaller intervals (e.g., 10 minutes) throughout the day.

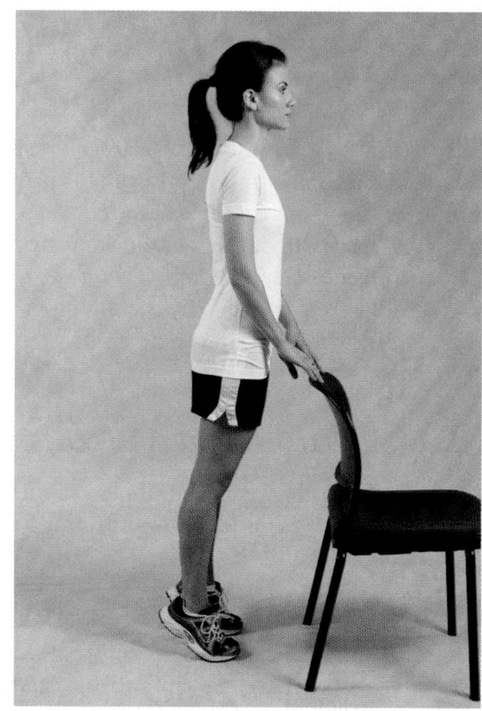

FIGURE 8.20 Rising up on toes to strengthen plantarflexors.

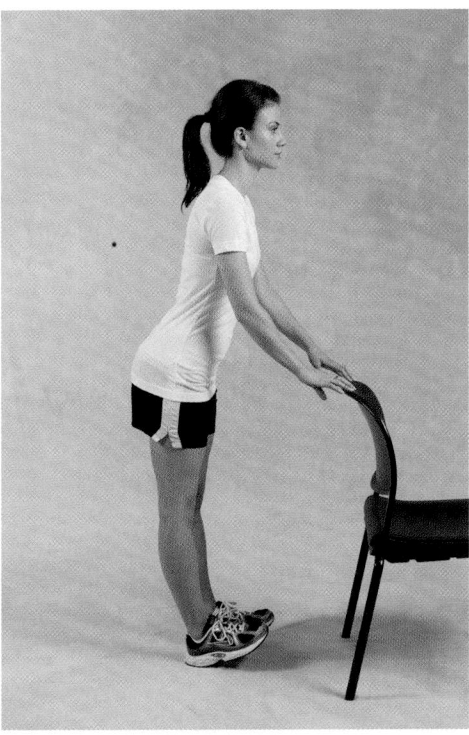

FIGURE 8.21 Rocking back onto the heels while raising the toes to strengthen dorsiflexors.

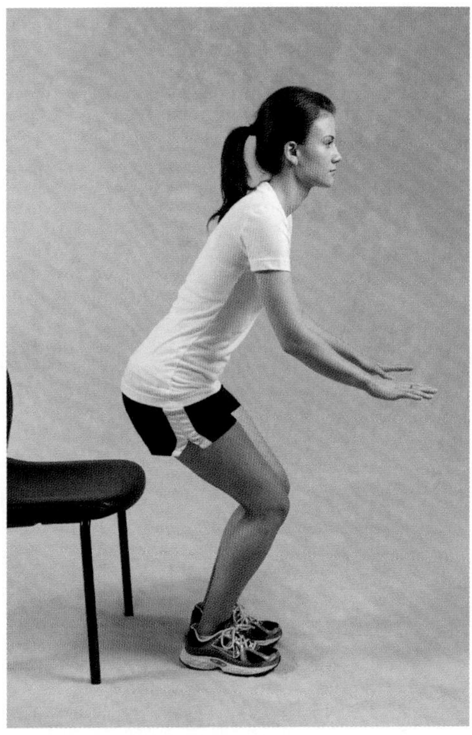

FIGURE 8.22 Practicing the sit-to-stand transfer is an important functional activity to strengthen the legs and improve dynamic balance.

BOX 8.4 The Otago Home Exercise Program[22,48]

Warm Up Exercises

Perform five repetitions of each of the following flexibility exercises:

- Stand up tall and look ahead. Turn head slowly to the right and then to the left as far as possible.
- Stand up tall and look straight ahead. Place one hand on the chin. Guide the head straight back (tuck chin).
- Stand up tall with feet shoulder width apart. Place the hands on the small of the lower back. Gently arch the back (extension).
- Stand up tall and place the hands on the hips. Do not move the hips. Turn as far as possible to the right, comfortably. Turn as far as possible to the left, comfortably.
- Either sit or stand. Point the foot up and then point the foot down.

Lower Extremity Strengthening*

Balance Training**

With the person sitting in a straight-back chair with the back well supported:

- Add appropriate ankle cuff weight. Have the patient perform unilateral knee extension. Repeat for the opposite leg.

With the person standing up tall and facing a table with both hands on the table:

- Add appropriate ankle cuff weight and have patient perform unilateral knee flexion. Repeat for the opposite leg.
- Adjust cuff weight if necessary and have patient perform unilateral hip abduction. Repeat for the opposite leg.
- Calf raises—raise up on toes to strengthen ankle plantarflexors.
- Toe raises - rock back on heels for ankle dorsiflexors.
- Knee bends—10 repetitions, 3 times.
- Backwards walking—10 steps, 5 times.
- Walking and turning around—Make a figure "8" 2 times.
- Sideways walking—10 steps, 5 times.
- Heel toe standing—10 seconds with each foot.
- Heel toe walking—10 steps, 5 times.
- One leg stand – hold up to 30 seconds, repeat for the opposite leg.
- Heel walking—10 steps, 5 times.
- Toe walking—10 steps, 5 times.
- Heel toe walking backwards—10 steps, 5 times.
- Sit to stand—with two hands, with one hand, or with no support based on ability. Repeat 5 or 10 times.
- Stair walking—using handrail, go up and down 12 steps.

*Each exercise is to be done slowly (e.g., 2–3 seconds to lift the weight and 4–6 seconds to lower the weight) and through the full functional range of motion. The goal is to perform each exercise for 2 sets of 10 repetitions. To advance the calf raises and toe raises, have the patient try the exercise without having the hands on the table.

**The easiest level for the balance exercises is to use two hands for support. Progression to harder levels (to one hand support and no hands for support) depends on the ability to complete the targeted number of repetitions or amount of time using smooth, controlled movements. To progress to exercises without holding onto support, the instructor must be confident that the person can safely recover balance using lower-body strategies such as stepping. The number of repetitions listed represents the most advanced level.

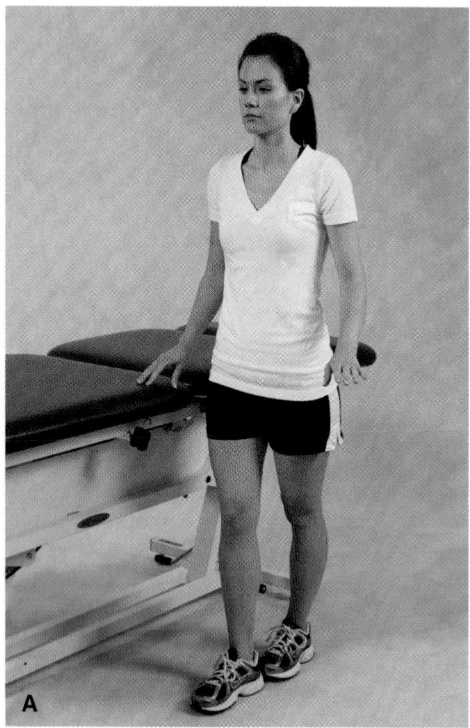

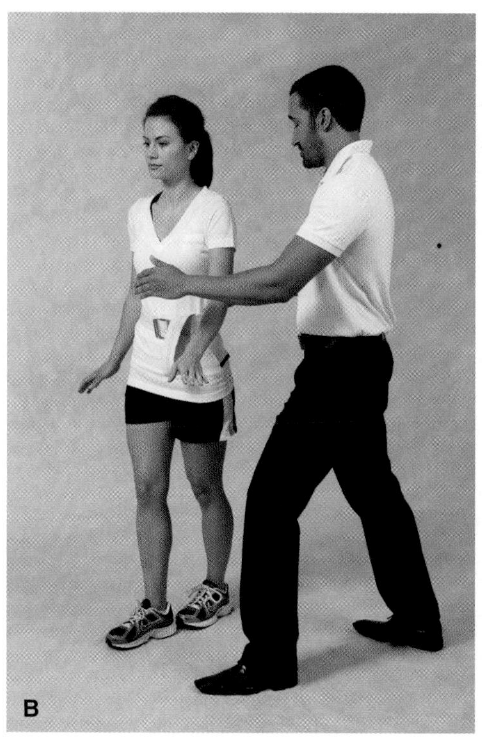

FIGURE 8.23 Tandem walking **(A)** performed with light touch on a firm surface for support and **(B)** performed without external support. Note that the therapist closely guards the patient for safety.

Supervised Group Program Incorporating Strengthening, Walking, and Functional Activities

Multimodal exercise programs incorporating muscle strengthening, gait, balance, coordination, and functional exercises have beneficial effects on balance, at least in the short term.[74] The more effective programs for improving balance are carried out three times per week for at least three months and include dynamic exercises in standing.[74]

FOCUS ON EVIDENCE

One example of a supervised group program comes from a study by Means and colleagues[111] that investigated the effects of a program designed to improve balance in community-residing elders with or without a history of falls. The program incorporated activities such as stretching, strengthening, coordination exercises, body mechanics, balance training, survival training maneuvers, and walking for endurance. The participants attended 90-minute exercise sessions three times per week in groups of six to eight. The exercises were performed under the direction of a physical therapist. Initially, participants were encouraged to exercise at a "fairly light" level (equal to 11 on the 6- to 20-point Borg perceived exertion scale[13]). After the first week, participants were encouraged to exercise at a level of intensity that was "somewhat hard" (equal to 13 on the Borg scale). The participants who attended this 6-week comprehensive exercise program showed a reduction in the time to complete an obstacle course (e.g., walking, climbing stairs, opening doors, getting up from a chair, and stepping over objects) and in the number of fall and fall-related injuries for up to 6 months after participation.

Box 8.5 provides general guidelines for exercise repetitions, duration of endurance walking, and progression of a supervised group program.[111]

Multisystem Group Exercise Program Incorporating a Circuit of Activities to Address Balance Impairments and Function

Nitz and Choy[130] investigated the efficacy of a balance training program that integrated individual and group exercises targeting strength, coordination, sensory systems (vision, perception, vestibular), cognition, reaction time, and static and dynamic stability. Community-residing elderly individuals with a recent history of falls were randomly assigned to two groups. One group participated in the balance training program that addressed multisystem activities. The control group participated in a more traditional group exercise program. Participants in both groups received an educational booklet on how to prevent falls in the home and attended a 1-hour exercise session once a week for 10 weeks. The exercises were led by a physical therapist assisted by one or two students when small group activities (six participants per group) were performed.

After the intervention, both groups reported a reduction in the number of falls. The reduction in falls was greater in

BOX 8.5 Balance Exercise Program Incorporating Strengthening, Walking, and Functional Activities

Week 1

Flexibility exercises (5 repetitions, 15-second hold)
Hamstring stretch
Gluteus maximus and hip flexor stretch
Gastrocnemius and soleus stretch
Paraspinal stretch
Strengthening exercises (baseline determination of preferred elastic-band strengths for lower limb exercises—1 repetition maximum)
Lower limb muscles (elastic band: 1 set of 8–10 repetitions for each leg)
Quadriceps (sitting and straight leg raises)
Hamstrings
Gluteus maximus
Gluteus medius
Upper limb muscles (5–10 repetitions)
Push-ups
Abdominal muscles (5 repetitions)
Curl-ups with arms behind head

Instruction in body mechanics for:

Standing
Sitting
Lying
Lifting
Reaching
Carrying
Arising from floor
Ascending/descending stairs
Baseline walking evaluation (determine maximum comfortable distance)

Week 2

Flexibility exercises (as above)
Strengthening exercises: lower limb muscles (elastic band: 1 set of 10 repetitions, each leg), upper limb muscles (10 repetitions), abdominal muscles (5–10 repetitions)
Postural exercises (10 repetitions, 10-second hold)
Head and neck
Trunk

Coordination exercises

Reciprocal leg movements (10 repetitions, eyes closed)
Bridging (10 repetitions)
Sitting/standing (5 repetitions)
Braiding exercises (2 repetitions)
Reciprocal ankle motion (10 repetitions)
Rung ladder: forward stepping (2 repetitions)

"Survival" maneuvers

Floor recovery exercises—"how to get up if you should fall"
Ascending and descending stairs safely (individual practice)
Endurance walking (begin at 75%–100% of baseline minutes walked; increase at comfortable pace)

Week 3

Flexibility exercises (5 repetitions, 20-second hold)
Strengthening exercises: lower limb (2 sets of 10 repetitions), upper limb (push-ups, 10–15 repetitions), abdominals (curl-ups, 10–15 repetitions)
Postural exercises (15 repetitions, 10-second hold)
Coordination exercises (repetitions increased)
Survival maneuvers: practice (floor recovery/stairs)
Endurance walking (0–6 minutes, comfortable pace)

Week 4

Flexibility exercises (5 repetitions, 25-second hold)
Strengthening exercises: lower limb (2–3 sets of 10 repetitions), upper limb (push-ups, 15 repetitions), abdominals (curl-ups, 15 repetitions)
Postural exercises (20 repetitions, 10-second hold)
Coordination exercises (repetitions increased)
Reciprocal legs (eyes closed)
Braiding (no holding, eyes open)
Rung ladder (forward, side, and backward stepping)
Survival maneuvers: practice (floor recovery/stairs)
Endurance walking (3–8 minutes, comfortable pace)

Week 5

Flexibility exercises (5 repetitions, 30-second hold)
Strengthening exercises: lower limb (3 sets of 10 repetitions), upper limb (push-ups, 15–20 repetitions), abdominals (curl-ups, 15–20 repetitions)
Postural exercises (25 repetitions, 10-second hold)
Coordination exercises: as above with increased repetitions, plus:
Braiding (no holding, eyes closed)
Reciprocal ankle dorsi/plantar flexion (25 repetitions)
Survival maneuvers: practice (floor recovery/stairs)
Endurance walking (6–10 minutes, comfortable pace)

Week 6

Flexibility exercises (5 repetitions, 30-second hold)
Strengthening exercises: lower limb (3 sets of 10 repetitions), upper limb (push-ups, 20 repetitions), abdominals (curl-ups, 15–20 repetitions)
Postural exercises (25 repetitions, 10-second hold)
Coordination exercises (as above with increased repetitions)
Endurance walking (8–12 minutes, comfortable pace)
Survival maneuvers: practice (floor recovery/stairs)

the group that performed the circuit training program; they also showed greater improvements in functional tests of the ability to perform activities of daily living. Although the circuit training program devised by Nitz and Choy[130] clearly incorporates many important activities to address multiple systems affecting balance, the results should be interpreted with caution because there was a small sample size and a high proportion of dropouts throughout the study.

Table 8.4 provides the details of the balance exercise program, consisting of circuit training and group activities, from the Nitz and Choy study.[130]

TABLE 8.4 Circuit Training Program to Address Balance Impairments and Function[130]

Activity	Responses Targeted	Progression of Activity
Sit-to-stand-to-sit	Lower limb strength Functional ability Multiple tasks	Lower the height of the chair Add/remove upper limb assistance Hold an item in the hands, balance a cup with/without water on a saucer/tray Add a cognitive task to the manual task
Stepping in all directions (forward, side, back)	Choice step reaction time Lower limb strength and coordination	Increase speed of step Perform stepping on a soft surface Close eyes
Reaching to limits of stability	Challenging limits of stability Vestibular stimulation and integration Upper and lower limb strengthening	Stick objects on a wall in the front by reaching to limits in all directions up and down while keeping feet in one position Lunge forward to pick up objects that are shifted to a high shelf to the side and behind; progress by reaching further and increasing the weight and size of objects
Step up and down	Lower limb strengthening and endurance Step reaction time	Step up forward, backward, and sideways over blocks of various heights; increase height, repetitions, and speed of stepping
Ankle, hip, and upper limb balance strategy practice	Lower limb strengthening Balance strategy training	Stand in front of a wall with toe touching a line 0.5 meter from the wall. Lean back toward the wall, keeping balance and dorsiflexing the feet and using arm movement to balance while lowering toward the wall
Sideways reach task	Mediolateral muscle strengthening in lower limbs Vestibular stimulation and integration Challenging limits of stability Multiple tasks and confounded proprioceptive input	Stand between a high and a low table positioned on either side; pick up objects from one table and transfer to other table Move the tables farther apart and increase the weight and size of the objects to increase the challenge Perform task while standing on an exercise mat on the floor
Ball games	Multiple tasks Hand-eye coordination Vestibular stimulation Ballistic upper and lower limb activity	Use inflated beach balls and progress to smaller or harder balls or two or three balls at once Add a cognitive task such as naming an animal that starts with a G, while throwing and catching or kicking the ball
Card treasure hunt/sort into suits	Coping strategies with visual conflict Vestibular stimulation and challenge of limits of stability	Prior to the session, hide playing cards in the room such that to collect the cards the participants have to bend and look under furniture, reach up high, or detect the card from a visually confounding background. Red and black teams are possible, and the team with the most cards returned to a collecting point inside 5 minutes is the winner Add the cognitive challenge of finding/sorting cards into order according to suit

Tai Chi for Balance Training

Tai chi has become a popular form of exercise for balance training. Tai chi is a traditional Chinese exercise program consisting of a sequence of whole-body movements that are performed in a slow, relaxed manner with an emphasis on awareness of posture alignment and synchronized breathing. The four styles of tai chi are Yang, Sun, Chen, and Wu, and they differ in terms of principles, forms, and function. Yang style tai chi is the most popular and widely practiced style today and consists of 24 forms (postures and movements).[103] Tai chi programs for the elderly may adopt a short form of tai chi with only 6 to 12 forms.[103] During tai chi training, participants learn to control the displacement of the body COM while standing and increase their lower extremity strength and flexibility during the regimens of physical movement.[28]

Some of the characteristics of tai chi exercise and the therapeutic rationale for why tai chi may affect posture and balance include the following:[176]

- The slow, continuous, even rhythm of the movements facilitates sensorimotor integration and awareness of the external environment (see Fig. 8.2).
- The emphasis on maintaining a vertical posture enhances postural alignment and perception of orientation.
- The continuous weight shifting from one leg to the other facilitates anticipatory balance control, motor coordination, and lower extremity strength.
- Finally, the large dynamic, flowing, and circular movements of the extremities promote joint ROM and flexibility (Fig 8.24). These characteristics should be considered when recommending tai chi classes to patients to ensure that instructors are following these principles and that the patients are appropriate for these activities.

FOCUS ON EVIDENCE

The effectiveness of tai chi training depends on the duration of the program, which may range from 4 weeks to 1 year, and the targeted populations. Studies have shown that tai chi improves standing balance control through performing head, trunk, and arm movements simultaneously with weight shifting.[5,77] Elderly individuals who participated in a tai chi group program had significant reductions in reported fear of falling compared to those who did not exercise, perhaps because the training leads to an increased self-awareness of balance.[5,151,191]

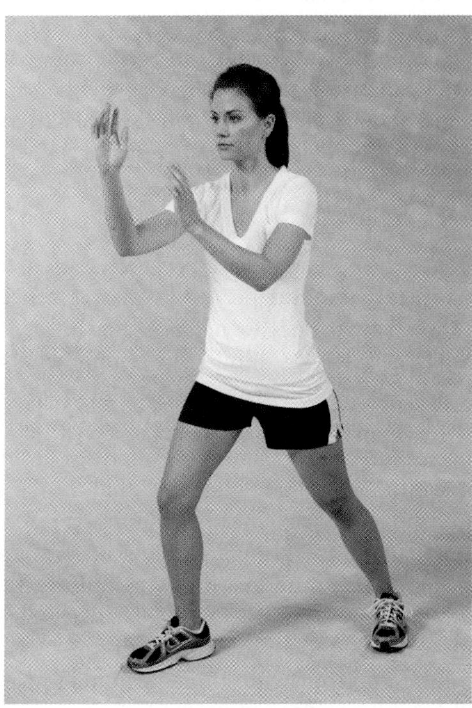

FIGURE 8.24 In this tai chi form, the participant shifts the bodyweight toward one leg while moving the arms.

However, tai chi training has shown less robust improvements in dynamic balance during functions such as gait and turning.[5,77,98,151] This may explain why there is conflicting evidence as to whether tai chi reduces falls or the risk of falls among people over the age of 50.[59,98,103] For this reason, Tai Chi should be considered as only one part of a comprehensive fall prevention program rather than being advocated as the sole exercise intervention.

Evidence-Based Balance Exercise Programs for Specific Musculoskeletal Conditions

Evidence is growing that specific balance exercise programs can effectively prevent and/or treat balance control deficits associated with lower extremity and trunk injuries and pathologies.

Ankle Sprains

Therapeutic activities such as single-leg balance training on unstable surfaces are recommended in the postacute phase of rehabilitation for ankle sprains for their potential to improve static and dynamic balance control.[107] Because of the interdependency between the segments of the lower extremity and trunk, especially during sports activities where energy is transferred from the legs through the trunk to the arms, or vice versa, it is also important to consider the regions above the ankle when designing a program for rehabilitation of ankle sprains.[83,125] Therefore, training for balance control should incorporate activities that require recruitment and coordination of the hip and trunk musculature. The BESS test, SEBT, or the YBT have been used to document deficits in balance control and improvements in performance with ankle injuries.[107]

Systematic reviews have concluded that balance training programs can improve static and dynamic balance and reduce the risk of ankle sprains in individuals with a history of ankle sprains.[65,78,109,177] Successful programs utilized wobble or unstable balance platforms, single-leg stance progressions, and resisted kicks of the uninvolved leg against an elastic band or tubing.[41,60,108,114,146,174] Programs typically were conducted for at least three times per week throughout a competitive season for prevention or two to three times per week for approximately 6 to 8 weeks post injury. Refer to Chapter 22 for additional information on rehabilitation following ankle sprain.

FOCUS ON EVIDENCE

A balance program developed by McGuine and Keene[108] reduced the risk of ankle sprains by 38% in male (n = 112) and female (n = 261) high school soccer and basketball players, especially in those with a history of ankle sprains. Participants performed the single-leg stance (Fig. 8.25), progressing from standing on the floor to standing on a wobble board with and

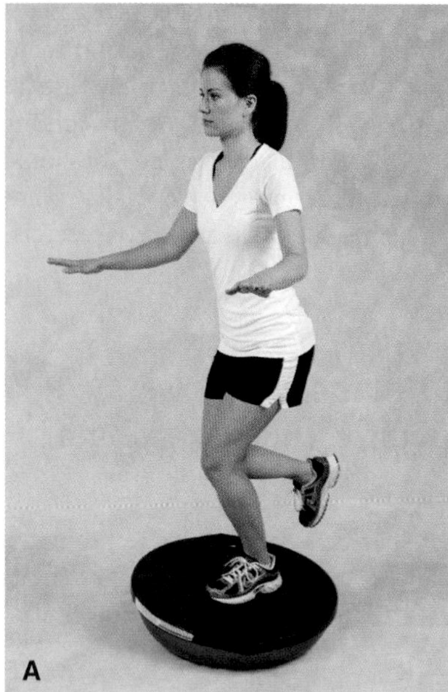

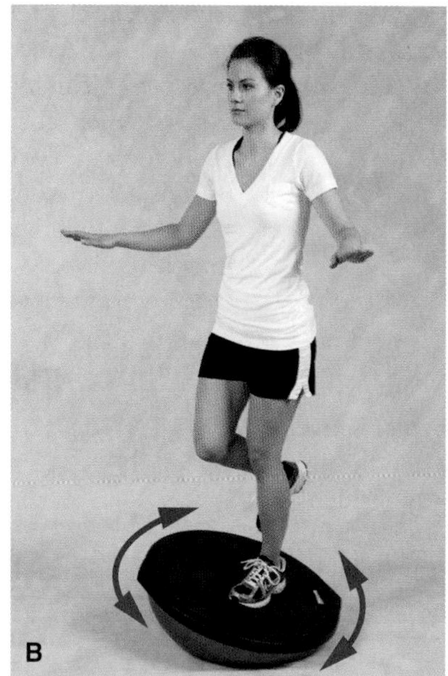

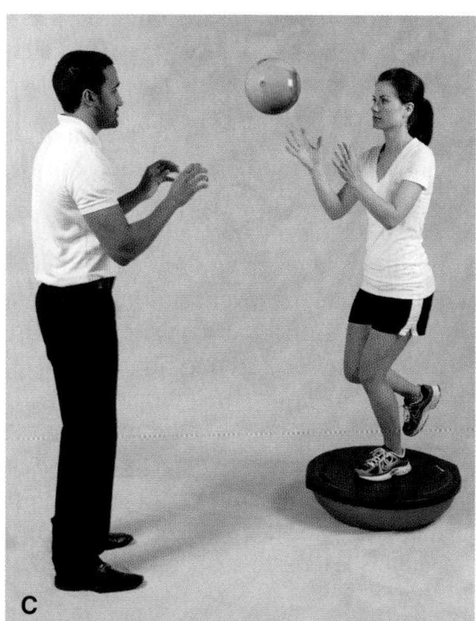

FIGURE 8.25 Balance program for reducing the incidence of ankle sprains in athletes using a wobble board: **(A)** single-leg squat (knee bent 30° to 45°), **(B)** single-leg stance while rotating the board, and **(C)** single-leg stance while performing functional activities (i.e., catching a ball).

without eyes open. They performed the balance activities 5 days a week for the first 5 weeks and then 3 days a week for the rest of the season. Each exercise was performed for a duration of 30 seconds per leg, and legs were alternated during a rest period of 30 seconds between repetitions.

Anterior Cruciate Ligament Injuries

Proprioceptive and balance training programs either alone or in combination with neuromuscular training that includes lower extremity plyometrics (as described in Chapter 23), trunk stabilization and strengthening (refer to Chapter 16), and sport-specific functional training (refer to Chapters 21 and 23) have been shown to reduce the incidence of anterior cruciate ligament (ACL) injuries by about 50% in adolescents and adults.[47,163] These proprioceptive and balance training programs frequently consisted of double and single leg balance exercises progressing from firm to unstable surfaces, such as ankle disks, tilt boards, or foam, with variations such as squatting or catching a ball.[21,43,50,110] Balance exercises usually were done 10 to 15 minutes daily during preseason training and 3 times a week during the season for prevention. Neuromuscular training sessions longer than 20 minutes appear to be more effective than shorter sessions for reducing ACL injuries in female athletes.[163]

Benjaminse and colleagues[10] have recently proposed novel techniques to enhance balance training for ACL injury prevention. These techniques build on the concept that motor learning is enhanced when instructional strategies incorporate an external focus of attention, especially for complex motor skills required for sports. One easy technique to implement in the clinical setting is the use of dyad training, where athletes practice in pairs, observing and providing feedback of each other's performance. For example, one athlete performs an exercise such as the single leg hop in forward-backward and side-to-side directions and ends by landing on two feet. The second athlete observes the performance, provides feedback after one set of hops, and then performs the exercise while the first athlete plays the role of observer and coach.[10] Alternating back and forth between the role of performer and observer, promoting dialog between learners, seems to encourage more cognitive effort and processing, which may explain why studies have shown enhanced retention and transfer of the motor skill when dyad training is employed compared to other forms of individual or group practice.[153,190]

Low Back Pain

Individuals with LBP show altered postural responses in laboratory studies that induce perturbations to balance.[85,99] In response to disturbances to balance, the most common compensatory strategy exhibited by people with chronic LBP is to co-contract the trunk muscles in order to stiffen the spine.[124,170] Deficits in postural control may be detected by balance testing such as the SEBT described in this chapter.[132] Since the trunk makes up about half of the mass of the body, from a biomechanical standpoint, it is reasonable to propose that balance training should be incorporated into a comprehensive, multimodal intervention for LBP as described in Chapters 15 and 16. Evidence to date suggests that interventions designed to improve neuromuscular control of the trunk in persons with LBP contribute to patient reports of reduced pain and improved function; however, demonstrated improvements in balance or postural reactions remain elusive.[99,100,124]

Independent Learning Activities

Critical Thinking and Discussion

1. A person is experiencing falls when rising from a chair. Using biomechanical principles of balance, what adjustments can the person immediately make to increase his or her stability and prevent falls?
2. Differentiate and describe several balance movements that rely primarily on feedforward or open-loop motor control versus those that utilize closed-loop control.
3. Review the ankle, hip, and stepping strategies and discuss how the strategies are elicited and what key muscles are activated to control balance.
4. Think about the times you have fallen in the past. What activity were you doing at the time that you fell? What musculoskeletal, neurological, and/or contextual factors contributed to the fall occurrence? What were the consequences of the fall? What differences would you expect between your falls and those experienced by an elderly person?
5. Differentiate and discuss treatment activities that you would use to train static, dynamic, anticipatory, reactive, and sensory organization aspects of balance control. Provide examples of how you would progress each of the activities.
6. For an elderly person with a history of falls, what aspects of the home environment might need to be modified to maximize the individual's safety and independence?
7. Differentiate between internal versus external focus of attention. Provide examples of verbal cues that you would use to promote external focus of attention for training static, dynamic, anticipatory, and reactive balance control.
8. The success of balance training programs depends on the compliance by the patient. What strategies would you use to increase the likelihood that a person would adhere to a home exercise program and ensure that his or her treatment outcomes are attained? Refer to Chapter 1 for discussion on teaching strategies for effective exercise.

Laboratory Practice

1. With a partner, mount a yardstick on the wall at the person's shoulder height. Measure the maximum amount of anterior and posterior sway by recording the maximum shoulder displacement during a 30-second period of quiet stance in each of the following conditions.
   - Standing on a firm surface with feet together, arms on hips, and eyes open
   - Standing on a firm surface with feet together, arms on hips, and eyes closed
   - Standing on a soft foam surface with feet together, arms on hips, and eyes open
   - Standing on a soft foam surface with feet together, arms on hips, and eyes closed

   For each of the conditions, what sensory inputs are available to the person for maintaining balance? How does the amount of sway vary with each condition and why?

2. With a partner, observe body movement during the following activities.
   - Standing with feet shoulder width apart, perform self-initiated forward and backward body sways progressing from small to large amplitudes.
   - Standing with feet apart, have your partner place his or her hand on your sternum and nudge you backward gently and then again with a larger force.
   - Standing with the feet placed heel to toe, have your partner gently nudge you backward.
   - Put on ankle-foot orthoses or ski boots that restrict ankle movements and have your partner gently nudge you backward.

   Which movement strategy is elicited with each activity and why?

3. Practice performing treatment activities that you would use to train static, dynamic, anticipatory, reactive, and sensory organization aspects of balance control as described in Table 8.2. Progress each of the activities to maximally challenge your balance. Practice performing treatment activities that promote external focus of attention during static, dynamic, anticipatory, and reactive balance.

Case Studies

1. A 20-year-old male soccer player sustained a right midtibial fracture in a motor vehicle accident and was required to wear a long-leg rigid cast for 6 weeks. You are seeing the patient 1 week after cast removal for physical therapy. He would like to return to playing soccer but is currently unable to maintain balance on his right leg to kick a soccer ball. What underlying impairments might be causing this individual's balance problems, and how would you design an exercise program that would allow him to reach his goals? How could you incorporate external focus of attention into his training program?
2. A 75-year-old woman fell in her bathtub and sustained a right pelvic fracture, requiring bed rest for 2 weeks. You are seeing the patient in her home following her hospital discharge. She has generalized weakness, deconditioning, is unsteady on her feet, and is fearful of falling. Currently, she is using a walker for ambulation. Prior to her fall, she was completely independent in all activities of daily living and enjoyed going on walks in her neighborhood in the evenings. Design a progressive balance program for this woman to restore her to her prior level of functioning.
3. A 70-year-old retiree has had bilateral knee replacement surgeries. He would like to resume his favorite hobby of

boating but lacks confidence in his ability to balance under dynamic conditions. Design an exercise and balance training program that will help him return to his recreational pursuits. What suggestions do you have to increase his safety when boating? What if his hobby was golfing instead of boating? Compare and contrast the activities and exercises you would prescribe for these two different issues. How can you incorporate external focus of attention to help him improve his golf swing?

4. A 56-year-old obese woman with diabetes is being treated for low back pain. She reports unsteadiness when walking, particularly in darkened environments. She has difficulty maintaining her balance during conditions 2, 3, 5, and 6 of the CTSIB test. What factors could be contributing to her unsteadiness? Design an exercise program that addresses her balance impairments.
5. An active, vibrant 70-year-old female seeks your advice on how to best maintain her health and fitness. What are the major components of a comprehensive exercise program for her? Give examples of exercises she should include.

REFERENCES

1. American Geriatrics Society British Geriatrics Society, American Academy of Orthopaedic Surgeons Panel on Fall Prevention: Guidelines for the prevention of falls in older persons. *J Am Geriatr Soc* 49:664–672, 2001.
2. Adams, MA, and Hutton, WC: Has the lumbar spine a margin of safety in forward bending? *Clin Biomech (Bristol, Avon)* 1(1):3–6, 1986.
3. Alexander, KM, and LaPier, TL: Differences in static balance and weight distribution between normal subjects and subjects with chronic unilateral low back pain. *J Orthop Sports Phys Ther* 28(6):378–383, 1998.
4. Andersson, GB: Epidemiologic aspects on low-back pain in industry. *Spine* 6(1):53–60, 1981.
5. Au-Yeung, SS, Hui-Chan, CW, and Tang, JC: Short-form tai chi improves standing balance of people with chronic stroke. *Neurorehabil Neural Repair* 23(5):515–522, 2009.
6. Barrack, RL, Skinner, HB, and Buckley, SL: Proprioception in the anterior cruciate deficient knee. *Am J Sports Med* 17(1):1–6, 1989.
7. Basmajian, JV, and DeLuca, CJ: *Muscles Alive: Their Functions Revealed by Electromyography*, ed. 5. Baltimore: Williams & Wilkins, 1985.
8. Basnett, CR, et al: Ankle dorsiflexion range of motion influences dynamic balance in individuals with chronic ankle instability. *Int J Sports Phys Ther* 8(2):121–128, 2013.
9. Bell, DR, Guskiewicz, KM, Clark, MA, and Padua, DA: Systematic review of the balance error scoring system. *Sports Health* 3(3):287–295, 2011.
10. Benjaminse, A, et al: Optimization of the anterior cruciate ligament injury prevention paradigm: novel feedback techniques to enhance motor learning and reduce injury risk. *J Orthop Sports Phys Ther* 45(3): 170–182, 2015.
11. Berg, KO, Wood-Dauphinee, SL, Williams, JI, and Maki, B: Measuring balance in the elderly: validation of an instrument. *Can J Public Health* 83 Suppl 2:S7–11, 1992.
12. Black, FO, Shupert, CL, Horak, FB, and Nashner, LM: Abnormal postural control associated with peripheral vestibular disorders. *Prog Brain Res* 76: 263–275, 1988.
13. Borg, G: Perceived exertion as an indicator of somatic stress. *Scand J Rehabil Med* 2(2):92–98, 1970.
14. Boyle, J, and Negus, V: Joint position sense in the recurrently sprained ankle. *Aust J Physiother* 44(3):159–163, 1998.
15. Braune, W, and Fischer, O: *On the Center of Gravity of the Human Body*. Berlin: Springer-Verlag, 1984.
16. Brouwer, BJ, Walker, C, Rydahl, SJ, and Culham, EG: Reducing fear of falling in seniors through education and activity programs: a randomized trial. *J Am Geriatr Soc* 51(6):829–834, 2003.
17. Brumagne, S, Cordo, P, Lysens, R, Verschueren, S, and Swinnen, S: The role of paraspinal muscle spindles in lumbosacral position sense in individuals with and without low back pain. *Spine* 25(8):989–994, 2000.
18. Buatois, S, et al: Five times sit to stand test is a predictor of recurrent falls in healthy community-living subjects aged 65 and older. *J Am Geriatr Soc* 56(8):1575–1577, 2008.
19. Burtner, PA, Woollacott, MH, and Qualls, C: Stance balance control with orthoses in a group of children with spastic cerebral palsy. *Dev Med Child Neurol* 41(11):748–757, 1999.
20. Campbell, AJ, et al: Randomised controlled trial of a general practice programme of home based exercise to prevent falls in elderly women. *BMJ* 315(7115):1065–1069, 1997.
21. Caraffa, A, Cerull,i G, Projetti, M, Aisa, G, and Rizzo, A: Prevention of anterior cruciate ligament injuries in soccer. A prospective controlled study of proprioceptive training. *Knee Surg Sports Traumatol Arthrosc* 4(1):19–21, 1996.
22. Centers for Disease Control and Prevention: *Tools to Implement the Otago Exercise Program: A Program to Reduce Falls*, ed. 1. Available at http://www.med.unc.edu/aging/cgec/exercise-program/tools-for-practice/ImplementationGuideforPT.pdf. Accessed July 23, 2015.
23. Chaffin, DB, and Page, GB: Postural effects on biomechanical and psychophysical weight-lifting limits. *Ergonomics* 37(4):663–676, 1994.
24. Chamberlin, ME, Fulwider, BD, Sanders, SL, and Medeiros, JM: Does fear of falling influence spatial and temporal gait parameters in elderly persons beyond changes associated with normal aging? *J Gerontol A Biol Sci Med Sci* 60(9):1163–1167, 2005.
25. Chandler, JM, and Duncan, PW: Balance and falls in the elderly: issues in evaluation and treatment. In Guccione, AA (ed): *Geriatric Physical Therapy*. St, Louis: Mosby, Inc, 1993, pp 237–251.
26. Chiviacowsky, S, Wulf, G, and Wally, R: An external focus of attention enhances balance learning in older adults. *Gait Post* 32(4):572–575, 2010.
27. Chow, DH, Cheng, IY, Holmes, AD, and Evans, JH: Postural perturbation and muscular response following sudden release during symmetric squat and stoop lifting. *Ergonomics* 48(6):591–607, 2005.
28. Christou, EA, Yang, Y, and Rosengren, KS: Taiji training improves knee extensor strength and force control in older adults. *J Gerontol A Biol Sci Med Sci* 58(8):763–766, 2003.
29. Cohen, H, Blatchly, CA, and Gombash, LL: A study of the clinical test of sensory interaction and balance. *Phys Ther* 73(6):346–351; discussion 351–344, 1993.
30. Commissaris, DA, and Toussaint, HM: Load knowledge affects low-back loading and control of balance in lifting tasks. *Ergonomics* 40(5): 559–575, 1997.
31. Commissaris, DA, Toussaint, HM, and Hirschfeld, H: Anticipatory postural adjustments in a bimanual, whole-body lifting task seem not only aimed at minimising anterior—posterior centre of mass displacements. *Gait Post* 14(1):44–55, 2001.
32. Cordo, PJ, and Nashner, LM: Properties of postural adjustments associated with rapid arm movements. *J Neurophysiol* 47(2):287–302, 1982.
33. Cornwall, MW, and Murrell, P: Postural sway following inversion sprain of the ankle. *J Am Podiatr Med Assoc* 81(5):243–247, 1991.
34. Csuka, M, and McCarty, DJ: Simple method for measurement of lower extremity muscle strength. *Am J Med* 78(1):77–81, 1985.
35. Dite, W, and Temple, VA: A clinical test of stepping and change of direction to identify multiple falling older adults. *Arch Phys Med Rehabil* 83(11):1566–1571, 2002.

36. Dolan, P, Earley, M, and Adams, MA: Bending and compressive stresses acting on the lumbar spine during lifting activities. *J Biomech* 27(10): 1237–1248, 1994.
37. Dolan, P, Mannion, AF, and Adams, MA: Passive tissues help the back muscles to generate extensor moments during lifting. *J Biomech* 27(8): 1077–1085, 1994.
38. Donald, IP, and Bulpitt, CJ: The prognosis of falls in elderly people living at home. *Age Ageing* 28(2):121–125, 1999.
39. Duncan, PW, Weiner, DK, Chandler, J, and Studenski, S: Functional reach: a new clinical measure of balance. *J Gerontol* 45(6):M192–197, 1990.
40. Duncan, RP, et al: Comparative utility of the BESTest, mini-BESTest, and brief-BESTest for predicting falls in individuals with Parkinson disease: a cohort study. *Phys Ther* 93(4):542–550, 2013.
41. Emery, CA, Rose, MS, McAllister, JR, and Meeuwisse, WH: A prevention strategy to reduce the incidence of injury in high school basketball: a cluster randomized controlled trial. *Clin J Sport Med* 17(1):17–24, 2007.
42. Faber, MJ, Bosscher, RJ, and van Wieringen, PC: Clinimetric properties of the performance-oriented mobility assessment. *Phys Ther* 86(7): 944–954, 2006.
43. Filipa, A, et al: Neuromuscular training improves performance on the star excursion balance test in young female athletes. *J Orthop Sports Phys Ther* 40(9):551–558, 2010.
44. Franchignoni, F, Horak, F, Godi, M, Nardone, A, and Giordano, A: Using psychometric techniques to improve the Balance Evaluation Systems Test: the mini-BESTest. *J Rehabil Med* 42(4):323–331, 2010.
45. Frank, JS, Patla, AE, and Brown, JE: Characteristics of postural control accompanying voluntary arm movement in the elderly. *Soci Neurosci Abstr* 13:335, 1987.
46. Freeman, MA, Dean, MR, and Hanham, IW: The etiology and prevention of functional instability of the foot. *J Bone Joint Surg Br* 47(4):678–685, 1965.
47. Gagnier, JJ, Morgenstern, H, and Chess, L: Interventions designed to prevent anterior cruciate ligament injuries in adolescents and adults: a systematic review and meta-analysis. *Am J Sports Med* 41(8):1952–1962, 2013.
48. Gardner, MM, Buchner, DM, Robertson, MC, and Campbell, AJ: Practical implementation of an exercise-based falls prevention programme. *Age Ageing* 30(1):77–83, 2001.
49. Garn, SN, and Newton, RA: Kinesthetic awareness in subjects with multiple ankle sprains. *Phys Ther* 68(11):1667–1671, 1988.
50. Gilchrist, J, et al: A randomized controlled trial to prevent noncontact anterior cruciate ligament injury in female collegiate soccer players. *Am J Sports Med* 36(8):1476–1483, 2008.
51. Gill, KP, and Callaghan, MJ: The measurement of lumbar proprioception in individuals with and without low back pain. *Spine* 23(3):371–377, 1998.
52. Gillespie, LD, et al: Interventions for preventing falls in elderly people. *Cochrane Database Syst Rev* (4):CD000340, 2003.
53. Gillespie, LD, et al: Interventions for preventing falls in older people living in the community. *Cochrane Database Syst Rev* 9:CD007146, 2012.
54. Glencross, D, and Thornton, E: Position sense following joint injury. *J Sports Med Phys Fitness* 21(1):23–27, 1981.
55. Gribble, PA, Hertel, J, and Plisky P: Using the Star Excursion Balance Test to assess dynamic postural-control deficits and outcomes in lower extremity injury: a literature and systematic review. *J Athl Train* 47(3):339–357, 2012.
56. Grigg, P: Articular neurophysiology. In Zachazewski, JE, and Quillen, WS (eds): *Athletic Injury Rehabilitation*. Philadelphia: WB Saunders, 1996: 152-169.
57. Grigg, P, Finerman, GA, and Riley, LH: Joint-position sense after total hip replacement. *J Bone Joint Surg Am* 55(5):1016–1025, 1973.
58. Guskiewicz, KM: Postural stability assessment following concussion: one piece of the puzzle. *Clin J Sport Med* 11(3):182–189, 2001.
59. Hackney, ME, and Wolf, SL: Impact of tai chi Chu'an practice on balance and mobility in older adults: an integrative review of 20 years of research. *J Geriatr Phys Ther* 37(3):127–135, 2014.
60. Han, K, Ricard, MD, and Fellingham, GW: Effects of a 4-week exercise program on balance using elastic tubing as a perturbation force for individuals with a history of ankle sprains. *J Orthop Sports Phys Ther* 39(4): 246–255, 2009.
61. Heiss, DG, Shields, RK, and Yack, HJ: Anticipatory control of vertical lifting force and momentum during the squat lift with expected and unexpected loads. *J Orthop Sports Phys Ther* 31(12):708–723; discussion 724–709, 2001.
62. Heiss, DG, Shields, RK, and Yack, HJ: Balance loss when lifting a heavier-than-expected load: effects of lifting technique. *Arch Phys Med Rehabil* 83(1):48–59, 2002.
63. Hellebrandt, FA, Tepper, RH, and Braun, GL: Location of the cardinal anatomical orientation planes passing through the center of weight in young adult women. *Am J Physiol* 121:465–470, 1938.
64. Hertel, J, Miller, SJ, and Denegar, CR: Intratester and intertester reliability during the Star Excursion Balance Tests. *J Sport Rehabil* 9:104–116, 2000.
65. Holmes, A, and Delahunt, E: Treatment of common deficits associated with chronic ankle instability. *Sports Med* 39(3):207–224, 2009.
66. Horak, F, and Shupert, C: The role of the vestibular system in postural control. In Herdman, S (ed): *Vestibular Rehabilitation*. New York: F.A. Davis, 1994.
67. Horak, FB: Postural orientation and equilibrium: what do we need to know about neural control of balance to prevent falls? *Age Ageing* 35 Suppl 2:ii7–ii11, 2006.
68. Horak, FB, and Nashner, LM: Central programming of postural movements: adaptation to altered support-surface configurations. *J Neurophysiol* 55(6):1369–1381, 1986.
69. Horak, FB, Nashner, LM, and Diener, HC: Postural strategies associated with somatosensory and vestibular loss. *Exp Brain Res* 82(1):167–177, 1990.
70. Horak, FB, Nutt, JG, and Nashner, LM: Postural inflexibility in parkinsonian subjects. *J Neurol Sci* 111(1):46–58, 1992.
71. Horak, FB, Shupert, CL, and Mirka, A: Components of postural dyscontrol in the elderly: a review. *Neurobiol Aging* 10(6):727–738, 1989.
72. Horak, FB, Wrisley, DM, and Frank J: The Balance Evaluation Systems Test (BESTest) to differentiate balance deficits. *Phys Ther* 89(5):484–498, 2009.
73. Howe, JA, Inness, EL, Venturini, A, Williams, JI, and Verrier, MC: The Community Balance and Mobility Scale—a balance measure for individuals with traumatic brain injury. *Clin Rehabil* 20(10):885–895, 2006.
74. Howe, TE, Rochester, L, Neil, F, Skelton, DA, and Ballinger, C: Exercise for improving balance in older people. *Cochrane Database Syst Rev* 11: CD004963, 2011.
75. Howland, J, et al: Fear of falling among the community-dwelling elderly. *J Aging Health* 5(2):229–243, 1993.
76. Huang, HC, Gau, ML, Lin, WC, and George, K: Assessing risk of falling in older adults. *Public Health Nurs* 20(5):399–411, 2003.
77. Huang, Y, and Lui, X: Improvement for balance control ability and flexibility in the elderly Tai Chi Chuan (TCC) practitioners: a systematic review and meta-analysis. *Arch Gernotol Geriatr* 60:233–238, 2015.
78. Hubscher, M, et al: Neuromuscular training for sports injury prevention: a systematic review. *Med Sci Sports Exerc* 42(3):413–421, 2010.
79. Inglin, B, and Woollacott, M: Age-related changes in anticipatory postural adjustments associated with arm movements. *J Gerontol* 43(4): M105–113, 1988.
80. Jack, CI, Smith, T, Neoh, C, Lye, M, and McGalliard, JN: Prevalence of low vision in elderly patients admitted to an acute geriatric unit in Liverpool: elderly people who fall are more likely to have low vision. *Gerontology* 41(5):280–285, 1995.
81. Jacobs, JV, Horak, FB, Van Tran, K, and Nutt, JG: An alternative clinical postural stability test for patients with Parkinson's disease. *J Neurol* 253(11):1404–1413, 2006.
82. Jacobson, GP, and Newman, CW: The development of the Dizziness Handicap Inventory. *Arch Otolaryngol Head Neck Surg* 116(4):424–427, 1990.
83. Jamison, ST, et al: Randomized controlled trial of the effects of a trunk stabilization program on trunk control and knee loading. *Med Sci Sports Exerc* 44(10):1924–1934, 2012.

84. Johnson, BL, and Nelso, JK: *Practical Measurements for Evaluation in Physical Education*, ed. 4. Minneapolis, MN: Burgess, 1979.
85. Jones, SL, Hitt, JR, DeSarno, MJ, and Henry, SM: Individuals with nonspecific low back pain in an active episode demonstrate temporally altered torque responses and direction-specific enhanced muscle activity following unexpected balance perturbations. *Exp Brain Res* 221(4): 413–426, 2012.
86. Kegelmeyer, DA, Kloos, AD, Thomas, KM, and Kostyk, SK: Reliability and validity of the Tinetti Mobility Test for individuals with Parkinson disease. *Phys Ther* 87(10):1369–1378, 2007.
87. Keshner, EA: Reflex, voluntary, and mechanical process in postural stabilization. In Duncan, PW (ed): *Balance Proceedings of the APTA Forum*. Alexandria, VA: American Physical Therapy Association, 1990.
88. Keshner, EA, Woollacott, MH, and Debu, B: Neck, trunk and limb muscle responses during postural perturbations in humans. *Exp Brain Res* 71(3):455–466, 1988.
89. Kingma, I, Bosch, T, Bruins, L, and van Dieen, JH: Foot positioning instruction, initial vertical load position and lifting technique: effects on low back loading. *Ergonomics* 47(13):1365–1385, 2004.
90. Kinzey, SJ, and Armstrong, CW: The reliability of the star-excursion test in assessing dynamic balance. *J Orthop Sports Phys Ther* 27(5):356–360, 1998.
91. Lachman, ME, et al: Fear of falling and activity restriction: the survey of activities and fear of falling in the elderly (SAFE). *J Gerontol B Psychol Sci Soc Sci* 53(1):P43–50, 1998.
92. Lajoie, Y, and Gallagher, SP: Predicting falls within the elderly community: comparison of postural sway, reaction time, the Berg balance scale and the Activities-specific Balance Confidence (ABC) scale for comparing fallers and non-fallers. *Arch Gerontol Geriatr* 38(1):11–26, 2004.
93. Lehr, ME, et al: Field-expedient screening and injury risk algorithm categories as predictors of noncontact lower extremity injury. *Scand J Med Sci Sports* 23(4):e225–232, 2013.
94. Leinonen, V, Kankaanpaa, M, Luukkonen, M, et al: Lumbar paraspinal muscle function, perception of lumbar position, and postural control in disc herniation-related back pain. *Spine* 28(8):842–848, 2003.
95. Leskinen, TP, Stalhammar, HR, Kuorinka, IA, and Troup JD: A dynamic analysis of spinal compression with different lifting techniques. *Ergonomics* 26(6):595–604, 1983.
96. Light, KE: Information processing for motor performance in aging adults. *Phys Ther* 70(12):820–826, 1990.
97. Lin, SI, Woollacott, MH, and Jensen, JL: Postural response in older adults with different levels of functional balance capacity. *Aging Clin Exp Res* 16(5):369–374, 2004.
98. Logghe, IH, Verhagen, AP, Rademaker, AC, et al: The effects of tai chi on fall prevention, fear of falling and balance in older people: a meta-analysis. *Prev Med* 51(3–4):222–227, 2010.
99. Lomond, KV, Henry, SM, Hitt, JR, DeSarno, MJ, and Bunn JY: Altered postural responses persist following physical therapy of general versus specific trunk exercises in people with low back pain. *Man Ther* 19(5):425–432, 2014.
100. Lomond, KV, et al: Effects of low back pain stabilization or movement system impairment treatments on voluntary postural adjustments: a randomized controlled trial. *Spine J* 15(4):596–606, 2015.
101. Lord, SR, Dayhew, J, and Howland A: Multifocal glasses impair edge-contrast sensitivity and depth perception and increase the risk of falls in older people. *J Am Geriatr Soc* 50(11):1760–1766, 2002.
102. Lord, SR, et al: The effect of an individualized fall prevention program on fall risk and falls in older people: a randomized, controlled trial. *J Am Geriatr Soc* 53(8):1296–1304, 2005.
103. Low, S, Ang, LW, Goh, KS, and Chew, SK: A systematic review of the effectiveness of tai chi on fall reduction among the elderly. *Arch Gerontol Geriatr* 48(3):325–331, 2009.
104. Lundin-Olsson, L, Nyberg, L, and Gustafson Y: Attention, frailty, and falls: the effect of a manual task on basic mobility. *J Am Geriatr Soc* 46(6): 758–761, 1998.
105. Maki, BE: Gait changes in older adults: predictors of falls or indicators of fear. *J Am Geriatr Soc* 45(3):313–320, 1997.
106. Maki, BE, Whitelaw RS: Influence of expectation and arousal on center-of-pressure responses to transient postural perturbations. *J Vestib Res* 3(1):25–39, 1993.
107. Martin, RL, Davenport, TE, Paulseth, S, Wukich, DK, and Godges, JJ, Orthopaedic Section American Physical Therapy A: ankle stability and movement coordination impairments: ankle ligament sprains. *J Orthop Sports Phys Ther* 43(9):A1–40, 2013.
108. McGuine, TA, and Keene, JS: The effect of a balance training program on the risk of ankle sprains in high school athletes. *Am J Sports Med* 34(7):1103–1111, 2006.
109. McKeon, PO, and Hertel, J: Systematic review of postural control and lateral ankle instability, part I: can deficits be detected with instrumented testing. *J Athl Train* 43(3):293–304, 2008.
110. McLeod, TC, Armstrong, T, Miller, M, and Sauers JL: Balance improvements in female high school basketball players after a 6-week neuromuscular-training program. *J Sport Rehabil* 18(4):465–481, 2009.
111. Means, KM, Rodell, DE, and O'Sullivan, PS: Balance, mobility, and falls among community-dwelling elderly persons: effects of a rehabilitation exercise program. *Am J Phys Med Rehabil* 84(4):238–250, 2005.
112. Miller, RL: When you lift, bend your knees. *Occup Health Saf* 45(3): 46–47, 1976.
113. Mizuta H, et al: A stabilometric technique for evaluation of functional instability in the anterior cruciate ligament deficient knee. *Clin J Sport Med* 2:235–239, 1992.
114. Mohammadi, F: Comparison of 3 preventive methods to reduce the recurrence of ankle inversion sprains in male soccer players. *Am J Sports Med* 35(6):922–926, 2007.
115. Muir, SW, Berg, K, Chesworth, B, and Speechley, M: Use of the Berg Balance Scale for predicting multiple falls in community-dwelling elderly people: a prospective study. *Phys Ther* 88(4):449–459, 2008.
116. Munhoz, RP, et al: Evaluation of the pull test technique in assessing postural instability in Parkinson's disease. *Neurology* 62(1):125–127, 2004.
117. Nashner, LM: Adaptations of human movement to altered environments. *Trends in Neurosci* 5:358–361, 1982.
118. Nashner, LM: The anatomic basis of balance in orthopaedics. In Wallman, HW (ed): *Orthopedic Physical Therapy Clinics of North America*. Philadelphia: W.B. Saunders, 2002.
119. Nashner, LM: Fixed patterns of rapid postural responses among leg muscles during stance. *Exp Brain Res* 30(1):13–24, 1977.
120. Nashner, LM: Sensory, neuromuscular, and biomechanical contributions to human balance. In Duncan, PW (ed): *Balance Proceedings of the APTA Forum*. Alexandria, VA: American Physical Therapy Association, 1990.
121. Nashner, LM, Shupert, CL, Horak, FB, and Black, FO: Organization of posture controls: an analysis of sensory and mechanical constraints. *Prog Brain Res* 80:411–418; discussion 395–417, 1989.
122. Nashner, LM, Woollacott, M, and Tuma, G: Organization of rapid responses to postural and locomotor-like perturbations of standing man. *Exp Brain Res* 36(3):463–476, 1979.
123. Nashner, LM, and Woollacott, MH: The organization of rapid postural adjustments of standing humans: an experimental-conceptual model. In Talbott, RE, and Humphrey, DR (eds): *Posture and Movement*. New York: Raven, 1979.
124. Navalgund, A, Buford, JA, Briggs, MS, and Givens, DL: Trunk muscle reflex amplitudes increased in patients with subacute, recurrent LBP treated with a 10-week stabilization exercise program. *Motor Control* 17(1):1–17, 2013.
125. Neptune, RR, Wright, IC, and van den Bogert, AJ: Muscle coordination and function during cutting movements. *Med Sci Sports Exerc* 31(2): 294–302, 1999.
126. Nevitt, MC: Falls in the elderly: risk factors and prevention. In Masdeu, JC, Sudarsky, L, and Wolfson, L (eds): *Gait Disorders of Aging: Falls and Therapeutic Strategies*. Philadelphia: Lippincott-Raven, 1997, pp 13–36.
127. Newton, RA: Review of tests of standing balance abilities. *Brain Inj* 3:335–343, 1989.
128. Newton, RA: Validity of the multi-directional reach test: a practical measure for limits of stability in older adults. *J Gerontol A Biol Sci Med Sci* 56(4):M248–252, 2001.

129. Nies, N, and Sinnott, PL: Variations in balance and body sway in middle-aged adults. Subjects with healthy backs compared with subjects with low-back dysfunction. *Spine (Phila Pa 1976)* 16(3):325–330, 1991.
130. Nitz, JC, and Choy, NL: The efficacy of a specific balance-strategy training programme for preventing falls among older people: a pilot randomised controlled trial. *Age Ageing* 33(1):52–58, 2004.
131. Nolte, J: *The Human Brain: An Introduction to Its Functional Anatomy*, ed. 5. St. Louis: Moby, Inc., 2002.
132. Olmsted, LC, Carcia, CR, Hertel, J, and Shultz SJ: Efficacy of the Star Excursion Balance Tests in detecting reach deficits in subjects with chronic ankle instability. *J Athl Train* 37(4):501–506, 2002.
133. Padgett, PK, Jacobs, JV, and Kasser, SL: Is the BESTest at its best? A suggested brief version based on interrater reliability, validity, internal consistency, and theoretical construct. *Phys Ther* 92(9):1197–1207, 2012.
134. Pap, G, Machner, A, Nebelung, W, and Awiszus, F: Detailed analysis of proprioception in normal and ACL-deficient knees. *J Bone Joint Surg Br* 81(5):764–768, 1999.
135. Patla, AE, et al: Identification of age-related changes in the balance-control system. In Duncan, PW (ed): *Balance Proceedings of the APTA Forum.* Alexandria, VA: American Physical Therapy Association, 1990.
136. Plisky, PJ, et al: The reliability of an instrumented device for measuring components of the star excursion balance test. *N Am J Sports Phys Ther* 4(2):92–99, 2009.
137. Plisky, PJ, Rauh, MJ, Kaminski, TW, and Underwood, FB: Star Excursion Balance Test as a predictor of lower extremity injury in high school basketball players. *J Orthop Sports Phys Ther* 36(12):911–919, 2006.
138. Podsiadlo, D, and Richardson, S: The timed "Up & Go": a test of basic functional mobility for frail elderly persons. *J Am Geriatr Soc* 39(2): 142–148, 1991.
139. Potvin, JR, McGill, SM, and Norman, RW: Trunk muscle and lumbar ligament contributions to dynamic lifts with varying degrees of trunk flexion. *Spine* 16(9):1099–1107, 1991.
140. Powell, LE, and Myers, AM: The Activities-specific Balance Confidence (ABC) Scale. *J Gerontol A Biol Sci Med Sci* 50A(1):M28–34, 1995.
141. Puniello, MS, McGibbon, CA, and Krebs, DE: Lifting characteristics of functionally limited elders. *J Rehabil Res Dev* 37(3):341–352, 2000.
142. Rankin, JK, Woollacott, MH, Shumway-Cook, A, and Brown, LA: Cognitive influence on postural stability: a neuromuscular analysis in young and older adults. *J Gerontol A Biol Sci Med Sci* 55(3):M112–119, 2000.
143. Resnick, HE, et al: Independent effects of peripheral nerve dysfunction on lower-extremity physical function in old age: the Women's Health and Aging Study. *Diabetes Care* 23(11):1642–1647, 2000.
144. Richardson, JK: Factors associated with falls in older patients with diffuse polyneuropathy. *J Am Geriatr Soc* 50(11):1767–1773, 2002.
145. Robertson, MC, Campbell, AJ, Gardner, MM, and Devlin, N: Preventing injuries in older people by preventing falls: a meta-analysis of individual-level data. *J Am Geriatr Soc* 50(5):905–911, 2002.
146. Ross, SE, and Guskiewicz, KM: Effect of coordination training with and without stochastic resonance stimulation on dynamic postural stability of subjects with functional ankle instability and subjects with stable ankles. *Clin J Sport Med* 16(4):323–328, 2006.
147. Rubenstein, LZ, Josephson, KR, and Robbins, AS: Falls in the nursing home. *Ann Intern Med* 121(6):442–451, 1994.
148. Safran, MR, et al: Proprioception in the posterior cruciate ligament deficient knee. *Knee Surg Sports Traumatol Arthrosc* 7(5):310–317, 1999.
149. Sattin, RW: Falls among older persons: a public health perspective. *Annu Rev Public Health* 13:489–508, 1992.
150. Schenkman, ML: Interrelationship of neurological and mechanical factors in balance control. In Duncan PW (ed.): *Balance Proceedings of the APTA Forum.* Alexandria, VA: American Physical Therapy Association, 1990.
151. Schleicher, MM, Wedam, L, and Wu, G: Review of tai chi as an effective exercise on falls prevention in elderly. *Res Sports Med* 20(1):37–58, 2012.
152. Shaffer, SW, et al: Y-balance test: a reliability study involving multiple raters. *Mil Med* 178(11):1264–1270, 2013.
153. Shea, CH, Wulf, G, and Whitacre, C: Enhancing training efficiency and effectiveness through the use of dyad training. *J Mot Behav* 31(2): 119–125, 1999.
154. Sherrington, C, and Tiedemann, A: Physiotherapy in the prevention of falls in older people. *J Physiother* 61(2):54–60, 2015.
155. Shu, Y, Southard, S, Shin, G, and Mirka, GA: The effect of a repetitive, fatiguing lifting task on horizontal ground reaction forces. *J Appl Biomech* 21(3):260–270, 2005.
156. Shumway-Cook, A, Brauer, S, and Woollacott, M: Predicting the probability for falls in community-dwelling older adults using the Timed Up & Go Test. *Phys Ther* 80(9):896–903, 2000.
157. Shumway-Cook, A, and Horak, FB: Assessing the influence of sensory interaction of balance. Suggestion from the field. *Phys Ther* 66(10): 1548–1550, 1986.
158. Shumway-Cook, A, and Woollacott, M: Attentional demands and postural control: the effect of sensory context. *J Gerontol A Biol Sci Med Sci* 55(1):M10–16, 2000.
159. Shumway-Cook, A, and Woollacott, MH: *Motor Control: Theory and Practical Applications*, ed. 2. Philadelphia: Lippincott, Williams & Wilkins, 2001.
160. Simoneau, GG, Ulbrecht, JS, Derr, JA, Becker, MB, and Cavanagh, PR: Postural instability in patients with diabetic sensory neuropathy. *Diabetes Care* 17(12):1411–1421, 1994.
161. Studenski, S, Duncan, PW, and Chandler, J: Postural responses and effector factors in persons with unexplained falls: results and methodologic issues. *J Am Geriatr Soc* 39(3):229–234, 1991.
162. Sturdevant, R: Prescription for workplace safety: bend and lift correctly to avoid back injuries! *J Tenn Med Assoc* 86(10):457, 1993.
163. Sugimoto, D, Myer, GD, Foss, KD, and Hewett, TE: Dosage effects of neuromuscular training intervention to reduce anterior cruciate ligament injuries in female athletes: meta- and sub-group analyses. *Sports Med* 44(4):551–562, 2014.
164. Taggart, HM: Effects of tai chi exercise on balance, functional mobility, and fear of falling among older women. *Appl Nurs Res* 15(4):235–242, 2002.
165. Tinetti, ME: Performance-oriented assessment of mobility problems in elderly patients. *J Am Geriatr Soc* 34(2):119–126, 1986.
166. Tinetti, ME, Richman, D, and Powell, L: Falls efficacy as a measure of fear of falling. *J Gerontol* 45(6):P239–243, 1990.
167. Toussaint, HM, Commissaris, DA, and Beek, PJ: Anticipatory postural adjustments in the back and leg lift. *Med Sci Sports Exerc* 29(9): 1216–1224, 1997.
168. Trojian, TH, and McKeag, DB: Single leg balance test to identify risk of ankle sprains. *Br J Sports Med* 40(7):610–613; discussion 613, 2006.
169. Uccioli, L, et al: Body sway in diabetic neuropathy. *Diabetes Care* 18(3):339–344, 1995.
170. van Dieen, JH, Cholewicki, J, and Radebold, A: Trunk muscle recruitment patterns in patients with low back pain enhance the stability of the lumbar spine. *Spine (Phila Pa 1976)* 28(8):834–841, 2003.
171. van Dieen, JH, Hoozemans, MJ, and Toussaint, HM: Stoop or squat: a review of biomechanical studies on lifting technique. *Clin Biomech (Bristol, Avon)* 14(10):685–696, 1999.
172. van Dieen, JH, and Visser, B: Estimating net lumbar sagittal plane moments from EMG data. The validity of calibration procedures. *J Electromyogr Kinesiol* 9(5):309–315, 1999.
173. Vellas, BJ, Wayne, SJ, Romero, L, Baumgartner, RN, Rubenstein, LZ, and Garry, PJ: One-leg balance is an important predictor of injurious falls in older persons. *J Am Geriatr Soc* 45(6):735–738, 1997.
174. Verhagen, E, et al: The effect of a proprioceptive balance board training program for the prevention of ankle sprains: a prospective controlled trial. *Am J Sports Med* 32(6):1385–1393, 2004.
175. Walker, JE, and Howland, J: Falls and fear of falling among elderly persons living in the community: occupational therapy interventions. *Am J Occup Ther* 45(2):119–122, 1991.
176. Wayne, PM, et al: Can tai chi improve vestibulopathic postural control? *Arch Phys Med Rehabil* 85(1):142–152, 2004.
177. Webster, KA, and Gribble, PA: Functional rehabilitation interventions for chronic ankle instability: a systematic review. *J Sport Rehabil* 19(1):98–114, 2010.

178. Wegener, L, Kisner, C, and Nichols, D: Static and dynamic balance responses in persons with bilateral knee osteoarthritis. *J Orthop Sports Phys Ther* 25(1):13–18, 1997.
179. Williams, GP, Greenwood, KM, Robertson, VJ, Goldie, PA, and Morris, ME: High-Level Mobility Assessment Tool (HiMAT): interrater reliability, retest reliability, and internal consistency. *Phys Ther* 86(3): 395–400, 2006.
180. Winstein, CJ, and Mitz, AR: The motor system. II Higher centers. In Cohen, H (ed): *Neuroscience for Rehabilitation*. Philadelphia: JB Lippincott, 1993.
181. Winter, DA: *A.B.C. (Anatomy, Biomechanics, and Control) of Balance During Standing and Walking*. Waterloo, Ontario: Waterloo Biomechanics, 1995.
182. Winter, DA, Patla, AE, Frank, JS, and Walt, SE: Biomechanical walking pattern changes in the fit and healthy elderly. *Phys Ther* 70(6):340–347, 1990.
183. Wolfson, LI, Whipple, R, Amerman, P, and Kleinberg, A: Stressing the postural response. A quantitative method for testing balance. *J Am Geriatr Soc* 34(12):845–850, 1986.
184. Woollacott, MH, Shumway-Cook, A, and Nashner, LM: Aging and posture control: changes in sensory organization and muscular coordination. *Int J Aging Hum Dev* 23(2):97–114, 1986.
185. Wrisley, DM, and Kumar, NA: Functional gait assessment: concurrent, discriminative, and predictive validity in community-dwelling older adults. *Phys Ther* 90(5):761–773, 2010.
186. Wrisley, DM, Marchetti, GF, Kuharsky, DK, and Whitney, SL: Reliability, internal consistency, and validity of data obtained with the functional gait assessment. *Phys Ther* 84(10):906–918, 2004.
187. Wulf, G: *Attention and motor skill learning*. Champaign, IL: Human Kinetics, 2007.
188. Wulf, G, Hoss, M, and Prinz, W: Instructions for motor learning: differential effects of internal versus external focus of attention. *J Mot Behav* 30(2):169–179, 1998.
189. Wulf, G, McNevin, N, and Shea, CH: The automaticity of complex motor skill learning as a function of attentional focus. *Q J Exp Psychol A* 54(4):1143–1154, 2001.
190. Wulf, G, Shea, C, and Lewthwaite, R: Motor skill learning and performance: a review of influential factors. *Med Educ* 44(1):75–84, 2010.
191. Zijlstra, GA, et al: Interventions to reduce fear of falling in community-living older people: a systematic review. *J Am Geriatr Soc* 55(4): 603–615, 2007.

CHAPTER 9

Aquatic Exercise

ELAINE L. BUKOWSKI, PT, DPT, MS, (D)ABDA EMERITUS

Aquatic therapy, the use of water for rehabilitation purposes, traces its origin back several centuries. The use of water for restorative purposes has grown in popularity and has gained increased use in facilitating therapeutic exercise. The unique properties of the aquatic environment provide clinicians with treatment options that may otherwise be difficult or impossible to implement on land. Using buoyant devices and varied depths of immersion, the practitioner has flexibility in positioning the patient (supine, seated, kneeling, prone, side-lying, or vertically) with any desired amount of weight bearing. Aquatic exercise has been successfully used for a wide variety of rehabilitation populations including pediatric,[8,30,39,49,55,73,78,84] orthopedic,[*] neurological,[41,54,56,61,63] and cardiopulmonary patients.[23,48,77]

Background and Principles for Aquatic Exercise

Definition of Aquatic Exercise

Aquatic exercise refers to the use of water (in multidepth immersion pools or tanks) that facilitates the application of established therapeutic interventions, including stretching, strengthening, joint mobilization, balance and gait training, and endurance training.

[*] 1,4,9,11,12,13,14,19,21,27,31,41,50,68,80

Goals and Indications for Aquatic Exercise

The specific purpose of aquatic exercise is to facilitate functional recovery by providing an environment that augments a patient's and/or practitioner's ability to perform various therapeutic interventions. Aquatic exercise can be used to achieve the following specific goals:

- Facilitate range of motion (ROM) exercise[33,82]
- Initiate resistance training[25,50,66,76,81]
- Facilitate weight-bearing activities[4]
- Enhance delivery of manual techniques[5,69]
- Provide three-dimensional access to the patient[16,69]
- Facilitate cardiovascular exercise[17,58,59,72]
- Initiate functional activity replication[53,57,76,82]
- Minimize risk of injury or re-injury during rehabilitation[29,82]
- Enhance patient relaxation[33,46]

Although research studies support these goals for aquatic exercise, Hall and associates[41] cited the need for more research with robust designs that address temperature, depth of immersion, and care settings.

Precautions and Contraindications to Aquatic Exercise

Most patients easily tolerate aquatic exercise. However, the practitioner must consider several physiological and psychological aspects of immersion that affect selection of an aquatic environment.

Precautions

Fear of Water

Fear of water can limit the effectiveness of any immersed activity. Fearful patients often experience increased symptoms during and after immersion because of muscle guarding, stress response, and improper form with exercise. Often patients require an orientation period designed to provide instruction regarding the effects of immersion on balance, control of the immersed body, and proper use of flotation devices.[57]

Neurological Disorders

Ataxic patients may experience increased difficulty controlling purposeful movements. Patients with heat-intolerant multiple sclerosis may fatigue with immersion in temperatures greater than 33°C.[12,59,61] Patients with controlled epilepsy require close monitoring during immersed treatment and must be compliant with medication prior to treatment.[16,47]

Respiratory Disorders

Water immersion may adversely affect the breathing of the patient with a respiratory disorder. Lung expansion tends to be inhibited due to hydrostatic pressure against the chest wall. Additionally, increased circulation in the chest cavity may further inhibit lung expansion due to increased circulation to the center of the body. Maximal oxygen uptake is lower during most forms of water exercise than during land exercise.[12,16]

FOCUS ON EVIDENCE

Although the above precautions have been cited, Kurabayashi and associates[48] compared nose and mouth immersion to non-immersion. Participants spent 30 minutes a day for 5 days a week for 2 months in the pool with water temperature set at 38°C. There was a significant difference in the immersion group with increased %FVC ($p = 0.058$), increased $FEV_{1.0\%}$ ($p = 0.018$), increased peak flow ($p = 0.039$), and increased P_{ao2} ($p = 0.010$). Based on their findings, they recommended the use of subtotal immersion to improve respiratory function for individuals with chronic pulmonary emphysema. Pechter and colleagues[59] compared 30 minutes of water-based aerobics to land-based aerobics done twice weekly for 12 weeks. The water-based group demonstrated increases in peak VO_2, peak O_2 pulse, peak ventilation, and peak load, as well as decreases in serum creatinine, glomerular filtration rate, cystatin-c in serum, protein/creatinine ratio, systolic and diastolic blood pressure, total serum cholesterol, and serum triglycerides. They recommended the use of low-intensity aquatic exercise to improve cardiorespiratory and renal function in individuals with chronic renal failure.

Cardiac Dysfunction

Patients with angina, abnormal blood pressure, heart disease, or compromised pump mechanisms also require close monitoring.[20,23,77,79] Cider and colleagues[24] demonstrated significant increases in work rate, VO_{2peak} and walking capacity, and muscle function in patients with congestive heart failure and type 2 diabetes mellitus. Teffaha and colleagues[74] demonstrated similar results of increased VO_{2peak} in patients with chronic heart failure or coronary artery disease with normal left ventricular function.

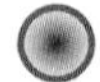

FOCUS ON EVIDENCE

Meyer and Leblanc[55] provided an algorithm for clinical decision-making when prescribing aquatic therapy for patients with left ventricular dysfunction and/or stable congestive heart failure. In their review of the literature, they suggested the following for rehabilitation and secondary prevention: (1) Temporary abnormal hemodynamic responses may be elicited by immersion to the neck; (2) water therapy is absolutely contradindicated in patients with decompensated congestive heart failure; (3) feeling good in water does not equate with left ventricular tolerance of increased volume loading caused by immersion; (4) if patients with previous severe myocardial infarctions and/or congestive heart failure can sleep supine, they may be able to tolerate bathing in a half-sitting position provided immersion does not exceed the xiphoid process; and (5) patients with Q-wave myocardial infarctions older than 6 weeks may exercise in a pool for orthopedic reasons provided they do so in an upright position and immersion does not exceed the xiphoid process.

Small, Open Wounds and Lines

Small, open wounds and tracheotomies may be covered by waterproof dressings. Patients with intravenous lines, Hickman lines, and other open lines require proper clamping and fixation.[16] Precautions should also be exercised with patients having G-tubes and suprapubic appliances. Observation for adverse reactions to aquatic therapy is essential.[18]

Contraindications

Contraindications to aquatic therapy include any situation creating the potential for adverse effects to either the patient or the water environment.[10] Such factors include:

- Incipient cardiac failure and unstable angina
- Respiratory dysfunction, vital capacity of less than 1 liter
- Severe peripheral vascular disease
- Danger of bleeding or hemorrhage
- Severe kidney disease (patients are unable to adjust to fluid loss during immersion)
- Open wounds without occlusive dressings, colostomy, and skin infections, such as tinea pedis and ringworm
- Uncontrolled bowel or bladder (bowel accidents require pool evacuation, chemical treatment, and possibly drainage)
- Menstruation without internal protection
- Water and airborne infections or diseases (examples include influenza, gastrointestinal infections, typhoid, cholera, and poliomyelitis)
- Uncontrolled seizures during the last year (they create a safety issue for both clinician and patient if immediate removal from the pool is necessary)[18]

Properties of Water

The unique properties of water and immersion have profound physiological implications in the delivery of therapeutic exercise. To utilize aquatics efficiently, practitioners must have a basic understanding of the clinical significance of the static and dynamic properties of water as they affect human immersion and exercise.

Physical Properties of Water

The properties provided by buoyancy, hydrostatic pressure, viscosity, and surface tension have a direct effect on the body in the aquatic environment.[12,35,40]

Buoyancy (Fig. 9.1)

Definition. Buoyancy is the upward force that works opposite to gravity.

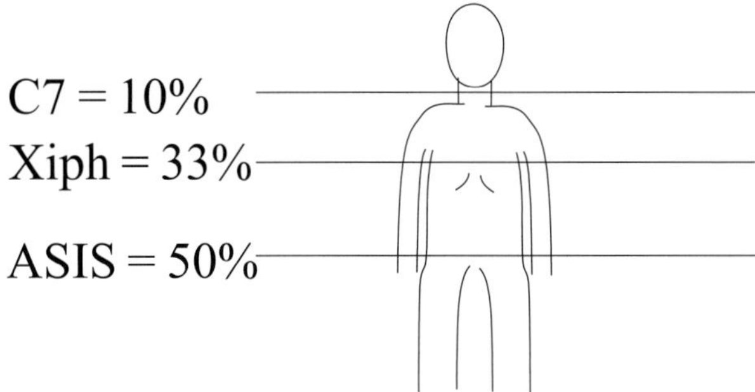

FIGURE 9.1 Percentage of weight bearing at various immersion depths.

Properties. Archimedes' principle states that an immersed body experiences upward thrust equal to the volume of liquid displaced.[40]

Clinical significance. The effects of buoyancy include the following:

- Buoyancy provides the patient with relative weightlessness and joint unloading by reducing the force of gravity on the body. In turn, this allows the patient to perform active motion with increased ease.
- Buoyancy provides resistance to movement when an extremity is moved against the force of buoyancy. This technique can be used to strengthen muscles.
- The amount of air in the lungs will affect buoyancy of the body. Buoyancy will be increased with fully inflated lungs and decreased with deflated lungs.
- Body composition will also affect buoyancy. Obese patients will have increased buoyancy due to fat tissue having a lower specific gravity. Patients with increased bone density will have less buoyancy than those with decreased bone density.
- Buoyancy allows the practitioner three-dimensional access to the patient.

CLINICAL TIP

Rotator cuff pathology. A patient recovering from rotator cuff repair can use the buoyancy force to increase range of motion in shoulder abduction and/or flexion while performing the motion in neck-deep water.[14] When performing shoulder extension from a 90° flexed position, the force of buoyancy becomes a resistance as the patient pulls the arm downward through the water.

Hydrostatic Pressure

Definition. Hydrostatic pressure is the pressure exerted by the water on immersed objects.

Properties. Pascal's law states that the pressure exerted by fluid on an immersed object is equal on all surfaces of the object. As the density of water and depth of immersion increase, so does hydrostatic pressure.

Clinical significance. The effects of hydrostatic pressure include the following:

- Increased pressure reduces or limits effusion, assists venous return, induces bradycardia, and centralizes peripheral blood flow.
- The proportionality of depth and pressure allows patients to perform exercise more easily when closer to the surface.

CLINICAL TIP

Regulation of performance. Barbosa and colleagues[6] compared the physiological adaptations of aquatic exercise with different levels of immersion to land exercise. Participants performed the same exercise on land, immersed to the hip, and immersed to the breast for 6 minutes. Physiological responses were higher when exercising immersed to the hip than when immersed to the breast and when exercising on land than immersed to either depth. The clinician should consider a progression from immersion to breast, to immersion to hip, to exercises on land in order to increase the physiological demands on the patient.

Viscosity

Definition. Viscosity is friction occurring between molecules of liquid resulting in resistance to flow.

Properties. Resistance from viscosity is proportional to the velocity of movement through liquid.

Clinical significance. Water's viscosity creates resistance with all active movements.

- Increasing the velocity of movement increases the resistance.
- Increasing the surface area moving through water increases resistance.

CLINICAL TIP

Lymphedema. Jamison[44,45] cited the effectiveness of hydrostatic pressure and viscosity for increasing lymph flow and reducing edema in patients with lymphedema. However, caution is needed as the dependent position of the extremity may cancel this effect. Recommended aquatic activities include Watsu® (a form of water Zen Shiatsu incorporating stretches that release blockages and produce relaxation), Jahara, Ai Chi (a form of water tai chi), water aerobics, the Halliwick Method® (a technique that increases balance, strength, coordination, and flexibility), and aquatic proprioceptive neuromuscular facilitation. The reader is referred to the following list of references for further information on these interventions:

- Watsu®: Dull, H: *WATSU® Freeing the Body in Water,* ed. 4. Victoria, BC: Trafford Publishing, 2008.
- Jahara: *Jahara Journal* 10th Anniversary Edition, 2007–2008. Available at http://www.jahara.com Accessed March 9, 2015.
- Ai Chi: Sova, R: *Ai Chi—Balance, Harmony and Healing.* Port Washington, WI: DSL, Ltd., 1999.
- Water aerobics: Sova, R: *Essential Principles of Aquatic Therapy and Rehabilitation.* Port Washington, WI: DSL, Ltd., 2003.
- Halliwick Method: Duffield, MH, Skinner, AT, and Thompson, AM: *Duffield's Exercise in Water.* Philadelphia: W.B. Saunders, 1983.
- Aquatic PNF: Jamison, L, and Ogden, D: *Aquatic Therapy Using PNF Patterns.* Tuscon, AZ: Therapy Skills Builders, 1994.

Surface Tension

Definition. The surface of a fluid acts as a membrane under tension. Surface tension is measured as force per unit length.

Properties. The attraction of surface molecules is parallel to the surface. The resistive force of surface tension changes proportionally to the size of the object moving through the fluid surface.

Clinical significance. The effect of surface tension includes the following:

- An extremity that moves through the surface performs more work than if kept under water.
- Using equipment at the surface of the water increases the resistance.

Hydromechanics

Definition. Hydromechanics comprise the physical properties and characteristics of fluid in motion.[40]

Components of flow motion. Three factors affect flow; they are laminar flow, turbulent flow, and drag.

- *Laminar flow.* Movement in which all molecules move parallel to each other, typically slow movement.
- *Turbulent flow.* Movement in which molecules do not move parallel to each other, typically faster movements.
- *Drag.* The cumulative effects of turbulence and fluid viscosity acting on an object in motion.

Clinical significance of drag. As the speed of movement through water increases, resistance to motion increases.[7]

- Moving water past the patient requires the patient to work harder to maintain his or her position in pool.
- Application of equipment (glove/paddle/boot) increases drag and resistance as the patient moves the extremity through water.[62]

CLINICAL TIP

Increasing resistance to motion. If the goal is to increase muscular force production during the early part of knee extension, the clinician should consider the use of a hydro-boot or similar device to increase the drag force on the leg/foot. Barbosa and associates[5] measured hydrodynamic drag in barefoot and hydro-boot conditions to determine the coefficients of drag on a human leg/foot model during simulated knee extension-flexion exercise. The influence of water resistance created higher drag force when using the hydro-boot during the early part of extension.

Thermodynamics

Water temperature has an effect on the body and therefore on performance in an aquatic environment.[16]

Specific Heat

Definition. Specific heat is the amount of heat (calories) required to raise the temperature of 1 gram of substance by 1°C.[40]

Properties. The rate of temperature change is dependent on the mass and the specific heat of the object.

Clinical significance. Water retains heat 1,000 times more than air. Differences in temperature between an immersed object and water equilibrate with minimal change in the temperature of the water.

Temperature Transfer

- Water conducts temperature 25 times faster than air.
- Heat transfer increases with velocity. A patient moving through the water loses body temperature faster than an immersed patient at rest.

Center of Buoyancy (Fig. 9.2)

Center of buoyancy, rather than center of gravity, affects the body in an aquatic environment.[33,39,40]

Definition. The center of buoyancy is the reference point of an immersed object on which buoyant (vertical) forces of fluid predictably act.

Properties. Vertical forces that do not intersect the center of buoyancy create rotational motion.

Clinical significance. In the vertical position, the human center is located at the sternum.

- In the vertical position, posteriorly placed buoyancy devices cause the patient to lean forward; anterior buoyancy causes the patient to lean back.
- During unilateral manual resistance exercises, the patient revolves around the practitioner in a circular motion.
- A patient with a unilateral lower extremity amputation leans toward the residual limb side when in a vertical position.
- Patients bearing weight on the floor of the pool (i.e., sitting, kneeling, or standing) experience aspects of both the center of buoyancy and center of gravity.

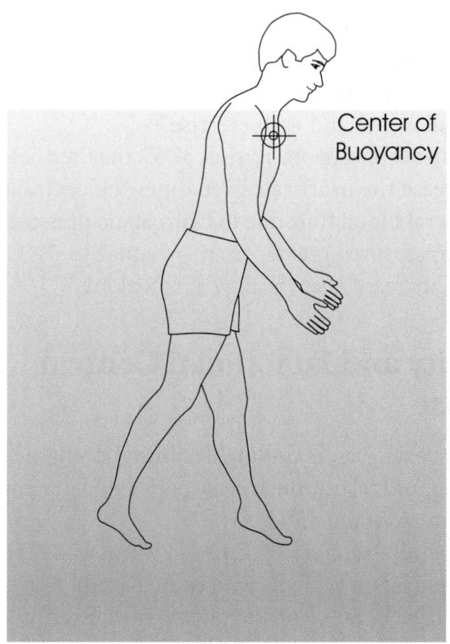

FIGURE 9.2 Center of buoyancy.

Aquatic Temperature and Therapeutic Exercise

A patient's impairments and the intervention goals determine the water temperature selection. In general, utilize cooler temperatures for higher intensity exercise and utilize warmer temperatures for mobility and flexibility exercise and for muscle relaxation.[12,16,18] The ambient air temperature should be 3°C higher than the water temperature for patient comfort. Incorrect water or ambient air temperature selection may adversely affect a patient's ability to tolerate or maintain immersed exercise.

Temperature Regulation

- Temperature regulation during immersed exercise differs from that during land exercise because of alterations in temperature conduction and the body's ability to dissipate heat.[2,12,16,18] With immersion there is less skin exposed to air, resulting in less opportunity to dissipate heat through normal sweating mechanisms.
- Water conducts temperature 25 times faster than air[12]—more if the patient is moving through the water and molecules are forced past the patient.
- Patients perceive small changes in water temperature more profoundly than small changes in air temperature.
- Over time, water temperature may penetrate to deeper tissues. Internal temperature changes are known to be inversely proportional to subcutaneous fat thickness.[12]
- Patients are unable to maintain adequate core warmth during immersed exercise at temperatures less than 25°C.[12,26]

- Conversely, exercise at temperatures greater than 37°C may be harmful if prolonged or maintained at high intensities. Hot water immersion may increase the cardiovascular demands at rest and with exercise.[67]
- In waist-deep water exercise at 37°C, the thermal stimulus to increase the heart rate overcomes the centralization of peripheral blood flow due to hydrostatic pressure.
- At temperatures greater than or equal to 37°C, cardiac output increases significantly at rest alone.[18]

Mobility and Functional Control Exercise

- Aquatic exercises, including flexibility, strengthening, gait training, and relaxation, may be performed in temperatures between 26°C and 35°C.[2,12,16,18]
- Therapeutic exercise performed in warm water (33°C) may be beneficial for patients with acute painful musculoskeletal injuries because of the effects of relaxation, elevated pain threshold, and decreased muscle spasm.[2,12,16,18]

Aerobic Conditioning

Cardiovascular training and aerobic exercise should be performed in water temperatures between 26°C and 28°C. This range maximizes exercise efficiency, increases stroke volume, and does not elevate the heart rate to the extent that warmer water does.[2,12,16,71]

- Intense aerobic training performed above 80% of a patient's maximum heart rate should take place in temperatures between 22°C and 26°C to minimize the risk of heat illness.[2,16,22,71]

CLINICAL TIP

There are several considerations for immersion times and pool temperatures.[12,15,16,65,79]

Because of the increased demands placed on the patient's temperature regulating systems when exercising in a pool the following are recommended:

- Generally, use a maximum immersion time of 20 minutes for patients with noncompromised cardiopulmonary systems. Begin with 10-minute sessions and increase the time as tolerated.
- Always monitor vital signs to ensure patient safety.
- Generally, water temperatures between 36°C and 37°C are considered high and temperatures between 26°C and 35°C are considered low. In addition to the following guidelines, the patient's fatigue factor needs to be considered.
- Higher temperatures are recommended for patients with rheumatoid arthritis except in the acute stage.
- Lower temperatures are recommended for patients with spasticity or for those whose immersion time lasts 20 to 45 minutes.
- For general flexibility, strengthening, gait training and relaxation, the range may be between 26°C and 35°C.[2,12,16,18]
- Cardiovascular training and aerobic exercise should be performed in water temperatures between 26°C and 28°C.

Pools for Aquatic Exercise

Pools used for aquatic therapy vary in shape and size. The rooms in which pools are housed need to be adequately ventilated to avoid the accumulation of condensation on walls, windows, and floors. A dressing room should be provided for changing clothes and showering.

Traditional Therapeutic Pools (Fig. 9.3)

Traditional therapeutic pools measure at least 100 feet in length and 25 feet in width. Depth usually begins at 3 to 4 feet with a sloping bottom, progressing to 9 or 10 feet.

- This larger type pool may be used for groups of patients and the therapists conducting the session while in the pool.
- Entrance to larger therapeutic pools includes ramps, stairs, ladders, or mechanical overhead lifts.
- These pools have built-in chlorination and filtration systems.

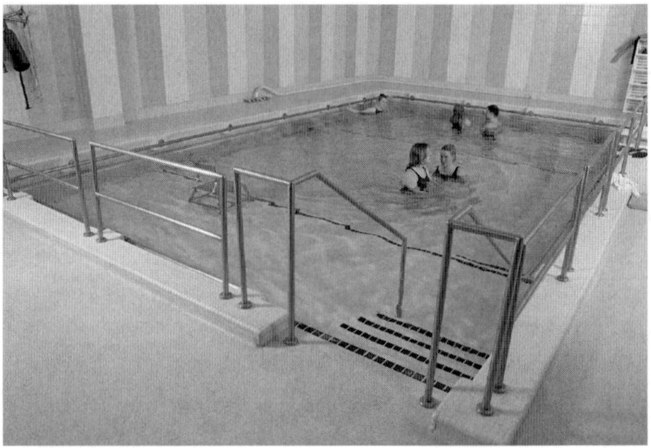

FIGURE 9.3 Traditional therapeutic pool. *(Courtesy of F.A. Davis Co., Philadelphia, PA.)*

Individual Patient Pools (Fig. 9.4)

Pools designed for individual patient use are usually smaller, self-contained units.

- These self-contained pools are entered via a door or one to two steps on the side of the unit.
- The therapist provides instructions or cueing from outside the unit.

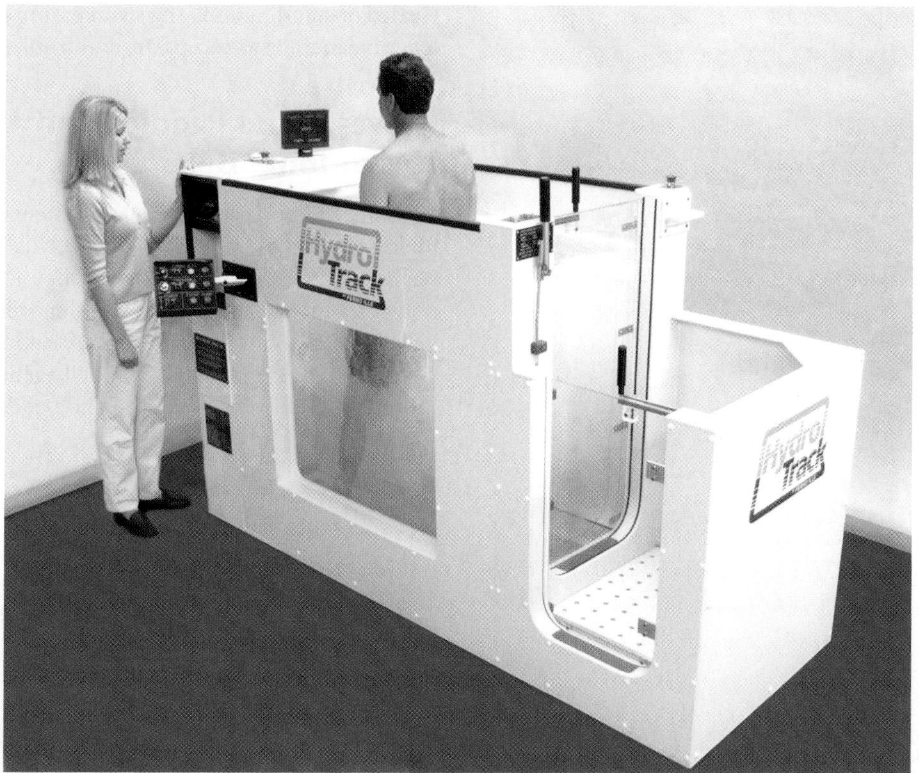

FIGURE 9.4 Hydro Track©, self-contained underwater treadmill system. *(Courtesy of Ferno-Washington, Inc., Wilmington, OH.)*

- In addition to built-in filtration systems, these units may include treadmills, adjustable currents, and varying water depths.

Special Equipment for Aquatic Exercise

A large variety of equipment exists for use with aquatic exercise. Aquatic equipment is used to provide buoyant support to the body or an extremity, challenge or assist balance, and generate resistance to movement. Resistive paddles, floats, paddle boards, and weighted stools and chairs are just a few of the many types of available equipment. By adding or removing equipment, the practitioner can progress exercise intensity. Type of equipment used is determined by the current functional level of the patient and the specific goals for the therapy session.

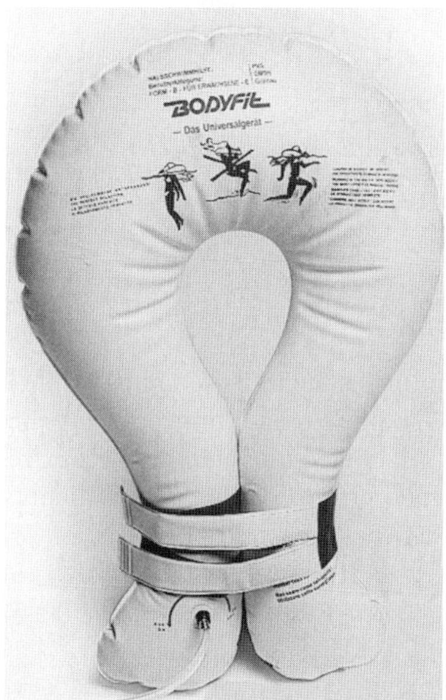

FIGURE 9.5 Cervical collar. *(Courtesy of Rothhammer International, Inc., San Luis Obispo, CA.)*

Collars, Rings, Belts, and Vests

Equipment designed to assist with patient positioning by providing buoyancy assistance can be applied to the neck, extremities, or trunk. Inflatable cervical collars are used for the supine patient to support the neck and maintain the head out of the water (Fig. 9.5). Flotation rings come in various sizes and are used to support the extremities in any immersed position (Fig. 9.6). Often the rings are used at the wrists and ankles during manual techniques to assist with patient positioning and relaxation. Several types of belts exist that may be used to assist with buoyancy of an extremity or the entire body (Fig. 9.7). Belts and vests are used to position patients supine, prone, or vertically for shallow and deep water activities.

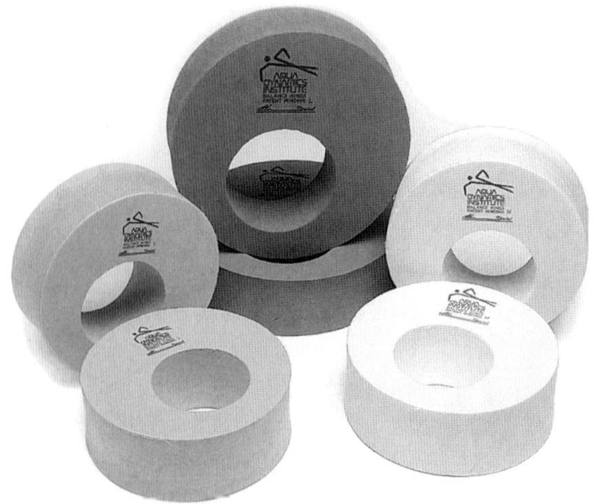

FIGURE 9.6 Flotation rings. *(Courtesy of Rothhammer International, Inc., San Luis Obispo, CA.)*

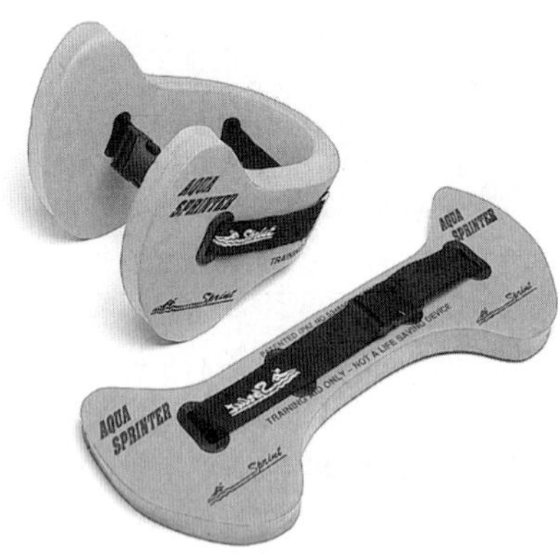

FIGURE 9.7 Buoyancy belts. *(Courtesy of Rothhammer International, Inc., San Luis Obispo, CA.)*

Swim Bars

Buoyant dumbbells (swim bars) are available in short and long lengths. They are useful for supporting the upper body or trunk in upright positions and the lower extremities in the supine or prone positions (Fig. 9.8). Patients can balance (seated or standing) on long swim bars in deep water to challenge balance, proprioception, and trunk strength.

Gloves, Hand Paddles, and Hydro-tone® Bells

Resistance to upper extremity movements is achieved by applying webbed gloves or progressively larger paddles to the hands (Fig. 9.9). These devices are not buoyant and therefore only resist motion in the direction of movement. Hydro-tone® bells are large, slotted plastic devices that increase drag during upper extremity motions. The bells generate substantially more resistance than gloves or hand paddles.

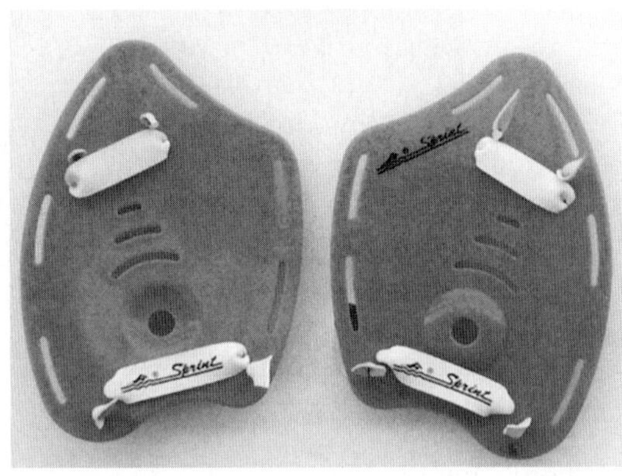

FIGURE 9.9 Hand paddles. *(Courtesy of Rothhammer International, Inc., San Luis Obispo, CA.)*

Fins and Hydro-tone® Boots

The application of fins or boots to the feet during lower extremity motions generates resistance by increasing the surface area moving through the water. Fins are especially useful for challenging hip, knee, and ankle strength. Hydro-tone® boots are most effective during deep water walking and running (Fig. 9.10).

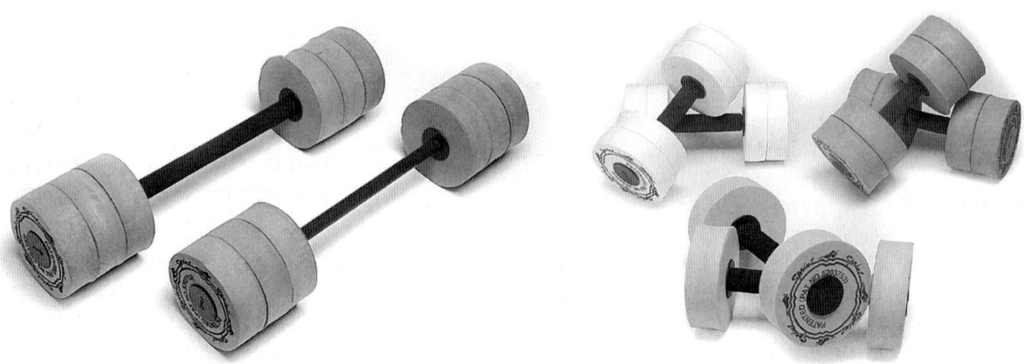

FIGURE 9.8 Swim bars. *(Courtesy of Rothhammer International, Inc., San Luis Obispo, CA.)*

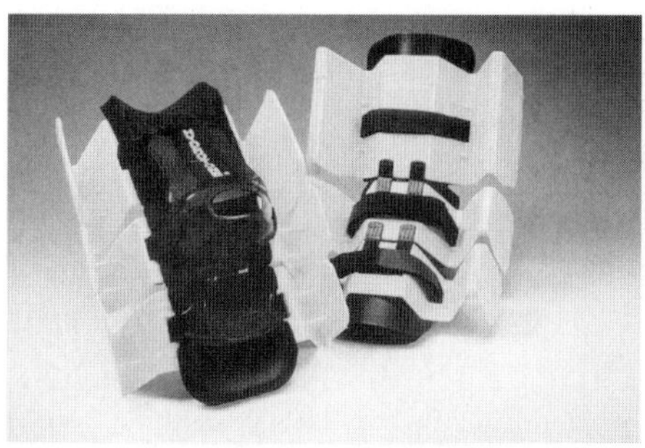

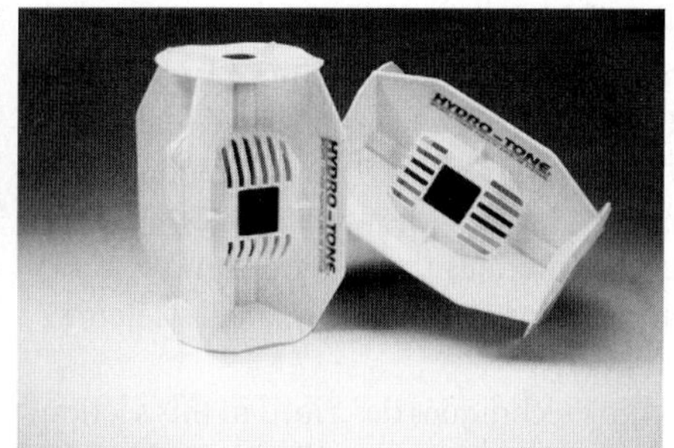

FIGURE 9.10 Hydro-tone® boots and bells. *(Courtesy of Rothhammer International, Inc., San Luis Obispo, CA.)*

Kickboards

The shapes and styles of kickboards (Fig. 9.11) vary extensively among manufacturers. Nevertheless, kickboards remain a versatile and effective aquatic tool for augmenting any exercise program. Kickboards may be used to provide buoyancy in the prone or supine positions; to create resistance to walking patterns in shallow water when held vertically; or to challenge seated, kneeling, or standing balance in the deep water.

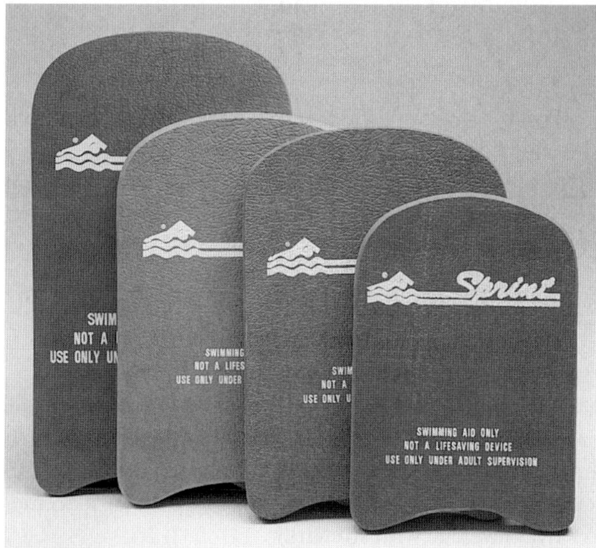

FIGURE 9.11 Kickboards. *(Courtesy of Rothhammer International, Inc., San Luis Obispo, CA.)*

Pool Care and Safety

Therapeutic pools require regular care and cleaning to avoid *Pseudomonas aeruginosa* (an infection causing folliculitis).[33,42,43,51] Frequent use increases the total organic carbon as well as ammonia and organic nitrogen found in the pool.

- Cleaning should occur at least twice weekly, and chlorine and pH level tests should be done twice daily.
- All walking surfaces near and around the pool should be slip-resistant and free of barriers. Water splashes should be dried immediately to prevent slips and falls.
- Safety rules and regulations are a must, as are emergency procedures, and should be posted and observed by all involved in therapeutic pool use.[83]
- Life preservers should be readily available, and at least one staff member who is CPR certified should be present at all times.

CLINICAL TIP

Prior to the first therapeutic session, the treatment schedule, procedures to be used, and proper pool attire should be discussed with the patient. This is a good time to review their previous pool experiences and their expectations for the sessions, any bowel or bladder problems, use of any assistive or adaptive equipment, and medications.

Exercise Interventions Using an Aquatic Environment

Stretching Exercises

Patients may tolerate immersed stretching exercises better than land stretching because of the effects of relaxation, soft tissue warming, and ease of positioning.[1,21,33,82] However, buoyancy creates an inherently less stable environment than the land. Therefore, careful consideration is warranted when recommending aquatic stretching.

Manual Stretching Techniques

Manual stretching is typically performed with the patient supine in waist depth water with buoyancy devices at the neck, waist, and feet. Alternatively, the patient may be seated on steps. The buoyancy-supported supine position improves (versus land techniques) both access to the patient and control by the practitioner, as well as the position of the patient.

However, turbulence from wave activity can adversely affect both the patient's and the practitioner's ability to perform manual stretching. Difficulties may be experienced maintaining and perceiving the subtleties of end-range stretching and scapular stabilization in the supine buoyancy supported position. Anecdotal evidence indicates that careful consideration of all factors is warranted prior to initiating manual stretching in an aquatic environment.[5,69]

The manual stretching techniques described in this section are considered passive techniques but may be adapted to utilize muscle inhibition techniques. The principles of stretching are the same as those discussed in Chapter 4.

The following terms are used to describe the stretching techniques:

- *Practitioner position.* Describes the orientation of the practitioner to the patient.
- *Patient position.* Includes buoyancy-assisted (BA) seated or upright positioning and buoyancy-supported (BS) supine positioning.
- *Hand placement.* The fixed hand, which stabilizes the patient, is typically the same (ipsilateral) hand as the patient's affected extremity, and it is positioned proximally on the affected extremity. The movement hand, which guides the patient's extremity through the desired motion and applies the stretch force, is typically the opposite (contralateral) hand as the patient's affected extremity and is positioned distally.
- *Direction of movement.* Describes the motion of the movement hand.

Spine Stretching Techniques

Cervical Spine: Flexion

Practitioner Position
Stand at the patient's head facing caudally.

Patient Position
BS supine without cervical collar.

Hand Placement
Cup the patient's head with your hands, the forearms supinated and thumbs placed laterally. Alternatively, place your hands in a pronated position with the thumbs at the occiput. This results in a more neutral wrist position at end-range stretch.

Direction of Movement
As you flex the cervical spine, the patient has a tendency to drift away from you if care is not taken to perform the motion slowly.

Cervical Spine: Lateral Flexion (Fig. 9.12)

Practitioner Position
Stand at the side facing the patient.

Patient Position
BS supine without a cervical collar.

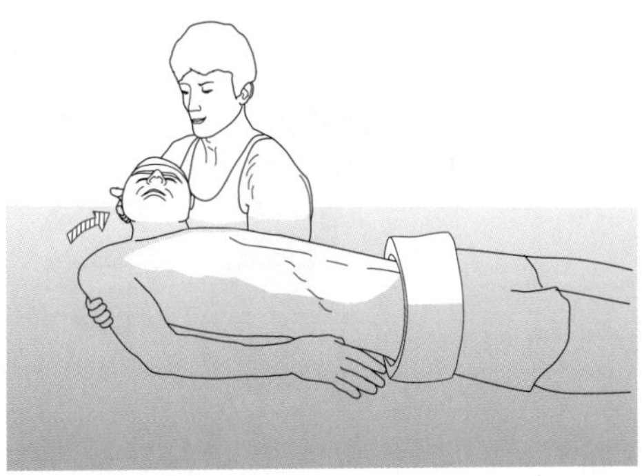

FIGURE 9.12 Hand placement and stabilization for stretching to increase cervical lateral flexion.

Hand Placement
Reach the fixed hand dorsally under the patient and grasp the contralateral arm; support the head with the movement hand.

Direction of Movement
Move the patient into lateral flexion and apply stretch force at desired intensity. This position prevents patient drift as the fixed hand stabilizes the patient against the practitioner.

Thoracic and Lumbar Spine: Lateral Flexion/Side Bending (Fig. 9.13)

Practitioner Position
Stand on the side opposite that to be stretched, facing cephalad with ipsilateral hips in contact (e.g., if stretching the left side of the trunk, the therapist's right hip is against patient's right hip).

Patient Position
BS supine, if tolerated. The patient's stretch side arm is abducted to end-range to facilitate stretch.

Hand Placement
Grasp the patient's abducted arm with the fixed hand; alternately, grasp at the deltoid if patient's arm is not abducted. The movement hand is at the lateral aspect of the lower extremity of the side to be stretched (more distal placement improves leverage with stretch).

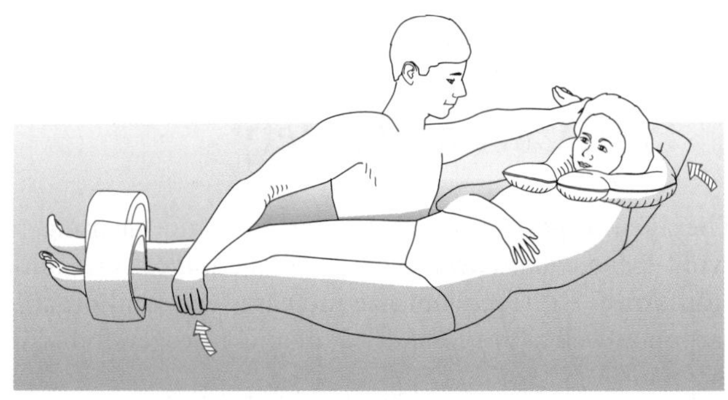

FIGURE 9.13 Hand placement and stabilization for stretching to increase lateral trunk flexion.

Direction of Movement

With the patient stabilized by your hip, pull the patient into lateral flexion. This technique allows variability in positioning and hand placement to isolate distinct segments of the spine.

Shoulder Stretching Techniques

Shoulder Flexion (Fig. 9.14)

Practitioner Position

Stand on the side to be stretched facing cephalad.

Patient Position

BS supine with the affected shoulder positioned in slight abduction.

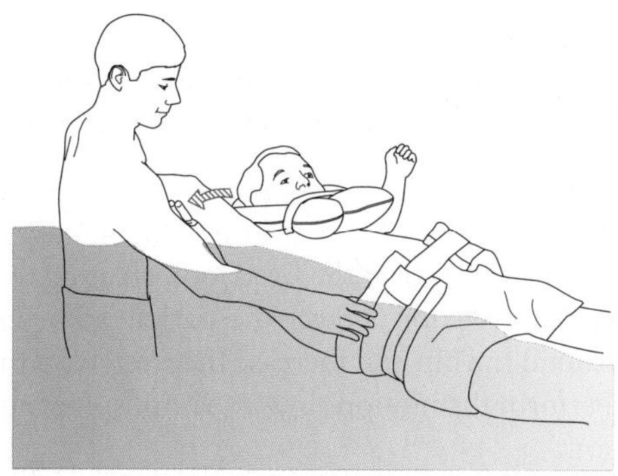

FIGURE 9.14 Hand placement and stabilization for stretching to increase shoulder flexion.

Hand Placement

Grasp the buoyancy belt with the fixed hand; the movement hand is at the elbow of the affected extremity.

Direction of Movement

After positioning the arm in the desired degree of abduction, direct the arm into flexion and apply the stretch force with the movement hand.

Shoulder Abduction

Practitioner Position

Stand on the affected side facing cephalad with your hip in contact with the patient's hip.

Patient Position

BS supine.

Hand Placement

Stabilize the scapula with the fixed hand; the movement hand grasps medially on the affected elbow joint.

Direction of Movement

Guide the arm into abduction and apply the stretch force. The hip contact provides additional stabilization as the stretch force is applied.

Shoulder External Rotation

Practitioner Position

Stand lateral to the affected extremity facing cephalad.

Patient Position

BS supine; position arm in desired degree of abduction with elbow flexed to 90°.

Hand Placement

Grasp the medial side of the patient's elbow with the palmar aspect of the fixed hand while fingers hold laterally; grasp the midforearm with the movement hand.

Direction of Movement

Movement hand guides forearm dorsally to externally rotate the shoulder and apply stretch force.

Shoulder Internal Rotation

Practitioner Position

Stand lateral to the patient's affected extremity facing caudally.

Patient Position

BS supine; position arm in desired degree of abduction with elbow flexed to 90°.

Hand Placement

Stabilize the scapula with the dorsal aspect of the fixed hand entering from the axilla; the movement hand is at the distal forearm.

Direction of Movement

Direct the forearm palmarward and apply the stretch force. Use care to observe the glenohumeral joint to avoid a forward thrust and substitution.

Hip Stretching Techniques

Hip Extension

Practitioner Position

Kneel on one knee at the patient's affected side.

Patient Position

BS supine with the hip extended and the knee slightly flexed.

Hand Placement

Stabilize the patient's affected extremity by hooking the top of the foot with your ipsilateral thigh. Grasp the buoyancy belt with the movement hand and guide the motion with the fixed hand on the knee.

Direction of Movement

Direct the patient caudally with the movement hand. To increase the stretch on the rectus femoris, lower the patient's knee in the water. Motion is performed slowly to limit spinal and pelvic substitution.

Hip External Rotation

Practitioner Position

Face the lateral aspect of the patient's thigh with your ipsilateral arm under the patient's flexed knee.

Patient Position
BS supine; hip flexed 70° and knee flexed 90°.

Hand Placement
Grasp the buoyancy belt with the contralateral (fixed) hand while the ipsilateral (movement) hand grasps the thigh.

Direction of Movement
Externally rotate hip with the movement hand as the patient's body lags through water to create stretch force.

Hip Internal Rotation

Practitioner Position
Face the lateral aspect of the involved thigh with the ipsilateral arm under the flexed knee.

Patient Position
BS supine, hip flexed 70° and knee flexed 90°.

Hand Placement
Stabilize the buoyancy belt with the contralateral (fixed) hand while grasping the thigh with the ipsilateral (movement) hand.

Direction of Movement
Internally rotate the hip as the patient's body lags through water to create the stretch force.

Knee Stretching Techniques

Knee Extension With Patient on Steps

Practitioner Position
Half-kneel lateral to the affected knee with the ankle of the affected extremity resting on your thigh.

Patient Position
Semi-reclined on pool steps.

Hand Placement
Place one hand just proximal and one just distal to the knee joint.

Direction of Movement
Extend the patient's knee.

Knee Flexion With Patient on Steps

Practitioner Position
Half-kneel lateral to the affected knee.

Patient Position
Semi-reclined on pool steps.

Hand Placement
Grasp the distal tibia with the ipsilateral hand; the contralateral hand stabilizes the lateral aspect of affected knee.

Direction of Movement
The stretch force into flexion.

Knee Flexion With Patient Supine (Fig. 9.15)

Practitioner Position
Half-kneel lateral to the affected knee with the dorsal aspect of the patient's foot hooked under the ipsilateral thigh.

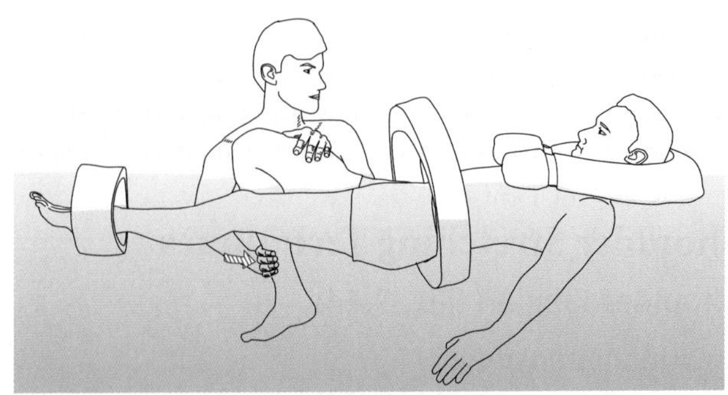

FIGURE 9.15 Hand placement and stabilization for stretching to increase knee flexion.

Patient Position
BS supine, affected knee flexed.

Hand Placement
Place the ipsilateral (fixed) hand on distal tibia and the contralateral (movement) hand on buoyancy belt to pull the body over the fixed foot.

Direction of Movement
Pull the patient's body over the fixed foot, creating the stretch to increase knee flexion. Lower the patient's knee into the water to extend the hip and increase the stretch on the rectus femoris. Perform the motion slowly to limit spinal and pelvic substitution.

Hamstrings Stretch

Practitioner Position
Face the patient and rest the patient's affected extremity on your ipsilateral shoulder.

Patient Position
BS supine, knee extended.

Hand Placement
Place both hands at distal thigh.

Direction of Movement
Start in the squatting position and gradually stand to flex the hip and apply the stretch force. Maintain knee extension by pulling the patient closer and increasing the stretch.

Self-Stretching With Aquatic Equipment

Often the intervention plan is to instruct the patient to perform independent stretching.[12,16,71,75] Self-stretching can be performed in either waist-deep or deep water. The patient frequently utilizes the edge of the pool for stabilization in both waist-deep and deep water.

Applying buoyancy devices may assist with stretching and increase the intensity of the aquatic stretch.[82] However, buoyancy devices are not required to achieve BA stretching—that is, as buoyancy acts on any submersed extremity, correct patient positioning adequately produces a gentle stretch. The following guidelines describe the use of equipment for mechanical stretching; the descriptions apply similarly for use without buoyancy equipment. Providing verbal cueing and visual demonstration for patient positioning and form aids in achieving the desired stretching effects.

Positioning for self-stretching of every body part is not described in this section. Typically, positioning for immersed self-stretches reflects traditional land positioning.

The following terms are used to describe the self-stretching techniques:

- *Patient position.* Includes BA (seated/upright), BS (supine), or vertical.
- *Buoyancy-assisted.* Using the natural buoyancy of water to "float" the extremity toward the surface.
- *Equipment-assisted.* Includes use of buoyancy devices attached or held distally on an extremity.

The following are some examples of self-stretching.

Shoulder Flexion and Abduction

Patient Position

Upright, neck level immersion.

Equipment

Small or large buoyant dumbbell or wrist strap.

Direction of Movement

Grasping the buoyant device with the affected extremity allows the extremity to float to the surface as the buoyancy device provides a gentle stretch.

Hip Flexion (Fig. 9.16)

Patient Position

Upright, immersed to waist, or seated at edge of pool/on steps with hips immersed.

Equipment

Small buoyant dumbbell or ankle strap. For hip flexion with knee flexion, place strap/dumbbell proximal to the knee. For hip flexion with knee extension (to stretch the hamstrings), place strap/dumbbell at the ankle.

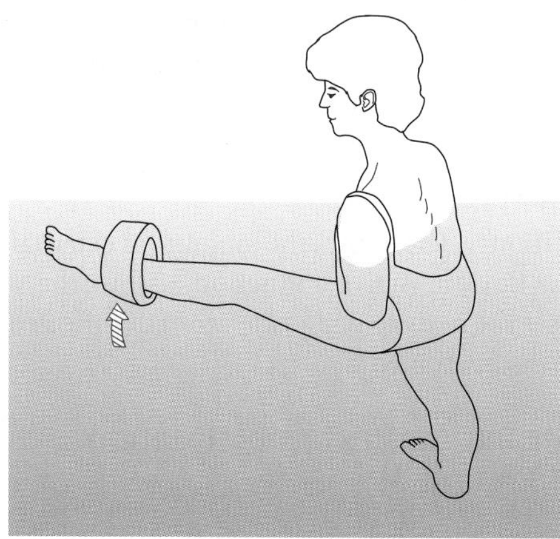

FIGURE 9.16 Self-stretching technique to increase hip flexion (stretch the hamstrings) using aquatic equipment.

Direction of Movement

Allow buoyancy device to float hip into flexion, applying stretch to hip extensors or hamstrings.

Knee Extension

Patient Position

Seated on steps/edge of pool with knee in a position of comfort.

Equipment

Small dumbbell or ankle strap.

Direction of Movement

Allow buoyancy device to extend knee toward the surface applying stretch to increase knee extension.

Knee Flexion

Patient Position

Stand immersed to waist with hip and knee in neutral position; increasing the amount of hip extension increases the stretch on the two joint knee extensors.

Equipment

Small dumbbell or ankle strap.

Direction of Movement

Allow buoyancy device to flex the knee toward the surface, applying stretch to knee extensors.

Strengthening Exercises

By reducing joint compression, providing three-dimensional resistance, and dampening perceived pain, immersed strengthening exercises may be safely initiated earlier in the rehabilitation program than traditional land strengthening exercises.[76,82] Both manual and mechanical immersed strengthening exercises typically are done in waist-deep water. However, some mechanical strengthening exercises may also be performed in deep water. Frequently, immersion alters the mechanics of active motion. For example, the vertical forces of buoyancy support the immersed upper extremity and alter the muscular demands on the shoulder girdle.[82] Furthermore, studies have demonstrated that lower extremity demand is inversely related to the level of immersion during closed-chain strengthening.[6,7]

Manual Resistance Exercises

Application of aquatic manual resistance exercises for the extremities typically occurs in a concentric, closed-chain fashion.[5,69] Manual aquatic resistance exercises are designed to fixate the distal segment of the extremity as the patient contracts the designated muscle group(s). The practitioner's hands provide primary fixation and guidance during contraction. As the patient contracts his or her muscles, the body moves over or away from the fixed distal segment (generally over the fixed segment for the lower extremity and away from the fixed segment for the upper extremity). The patient's movement through the viscous water generates resistance, and the patient's body produces the drag forces. Verbal cueing by the practitioner is essential to direct the patient when to contract and when to relax, thereby synchronizing practitioner and patient.

Stabilization of the distal extremity segment is essential for maintaining proper form and isolating desired muscles. However, appropriate stabilization is not possible in the BS supine position for eccentric exercises or rhythmic stabilization of the extremities. The patient's body will have a tendency to tip and rotate in the water. In addition, the practitioner will have difficulty generating adequate resistance force, and the patient's body will move easily across the surface of the water with minimal drag producing inadequate counterforce to the practitioner's resistance. When supine, some motions, including horizontal shoulder adduction and abduction, should be avoided because of the difficulty the patient may have isolating proper muscle groups. Nevertheless, for many motions, the aquatic environment allows closed-chain resistive training through virtually limitless planes of motion.

The following terms refer to manual resistance exercise in water.

- *Practitioner position.* Describes the orientation of the practitioner to the patient.
- *Patient position.* BS in the supine position.
- *Hand placement.* The guide hand is generally the ipsilateral hand as the patient's affected extremity and typically is positioned more proximally. It directs the patient's body as muscles contract to move the body through the water. The resistance hand is generally the contralateral hand and typically is placed at the distal end of the contracting segment. More distal placement increases overall resistance.
- *Direction of movement.* Describes the motion of the patient.

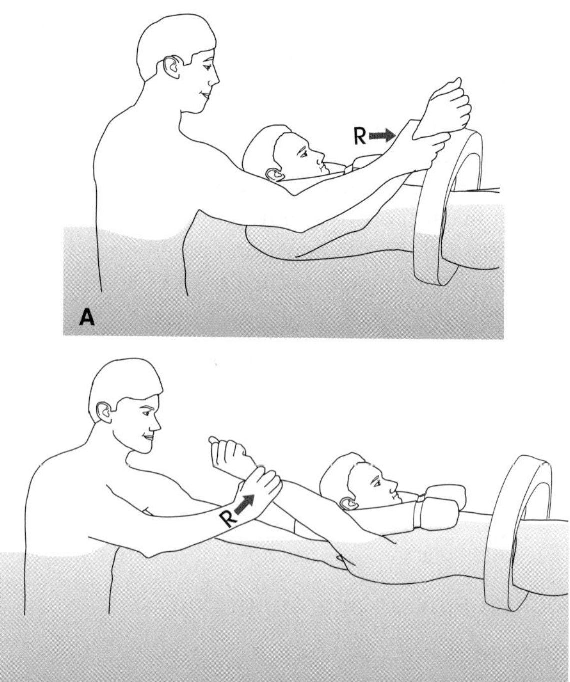

FIGURE 9.17 Manual resistance exercise for strengthening shoulder flexion; **(A)** start position and **(B)** end position.

Upper Extremity Manual Resistance Techniques

Shoulder Flexion/Extension (Fig. 9.17 A and B)

Practitioner Position

Face caudal, lateral to the patient's affected shoulder.

Patient Position

BS supine; affected extremity flexed to 30°.

Hand Placement

Place the palmar aspect of the guide hand at the patient's acromioclavicular joint. The resistance hand grasps the distal forearm. An alternative placement for the resistance hand may be the distal humerus; this placement alters muscle recruitment.

Direction of Movement

Active shoulder flexion against the resistance hand causes the body to move away from the practitioner. Active shoulder extension from a flexed position causes the body to glide toward the practitioner.

NOTE: The patient must be able to actively flex through 120° for proper resistance to be provided.

Shoulder Abduction

Practitioner Position

Face medially, lateral to the patient's affected extremity.

Patient Position

BS supine; affected extremity in neutral.

Hand Placement

Place the palmar aspect of guide hand at the proximal humerus as the thumb wraps anteriorly and the fingers wrap posteriorly. Place the resistance hand at the lateral aspect of distal humerus.

Direction of Movement

The practitioner determines the amount of external rotation and elbow flexion. Active abduction against the resistance hand causes the body to glide away from the affected extremity and the practitioner.

Shoulder Internal/External Rotation (Fig. 9.18 A and B)

Practitioner Position

Face medially on the lateral side of the patient's affected extremity.

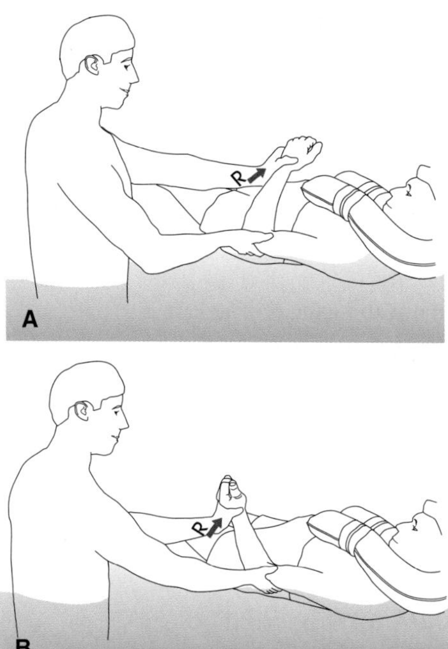

FIGURE 9.18 Manual resistance exercise for strengthening shoulder external rotation; **(A)** start position and **(B)** end position.

Patient Position

BS supine; affected extremity's elbow flexed to 90° with the shoulder in the desired amount of abduction and initial rotation.

Hand Placement

Place the palmar aspect of the guide hand at the lateral aspect of the elbow. The resistance hand grasps the palmar aspect of the distal forearm. An alternative method requires the practitioner to "switch" hands. The practitioner's ipsilateral hand becomes the guide hand and grasps the buoyancy belt laterally. The practitioner's contralateral hand becomes the resistance hand. This approach allows improved stabilization; however, the practitioner loses contact with the patient's elbow and must cue the patient to maintain the desired degree of shoulder abduction during the exercise.

Direction of Movement

Active internal rotation by the patient against the resistance hand causes the body to glide toward the affected extremity; active external rotation causes the body to glide away from the affected extremity.

Unilateral Diagonal Pattern: D_1Flexion/ Extension of the Upper Extremity

Practitioner Position

Stand lateral to the patient's unaffected extremity and face medially and caudally.

Patient Position

BS supine; affected extremity internally rotated and pronated with slight forward flexion.

Hand Placement

Secure the medial and lateral epicondyles of the distal humerus with the guide hand. Place the resistance hand on the dorsal surface of the distal forearm.

Direction of Movement

Prior to contraction, cue the patient to execute the specific joint motions expected in the diagonal patterns. Active contraction through the D_1flexion pattern causes the body to glide away from the practitioner. At the end position of D_1, secure the medial and lateral epicondyles of the distal humerus with the guide hand. The resistance hand will be on the palmar aspect of the distal forearm. From the flexed position, the practitioner cues the patient to contract through the D_1extension pattern.

Unilateral Diagonal Pattern: D_2Flexion/ Extension of the Upper Extremity (Fig. 9.19 A and B)

Practitioner Position

Stand lateral to the patient's affected shoulder; face medially and caudally.

Patient Position

BS supine; affected extremity adducted and internally rotated.

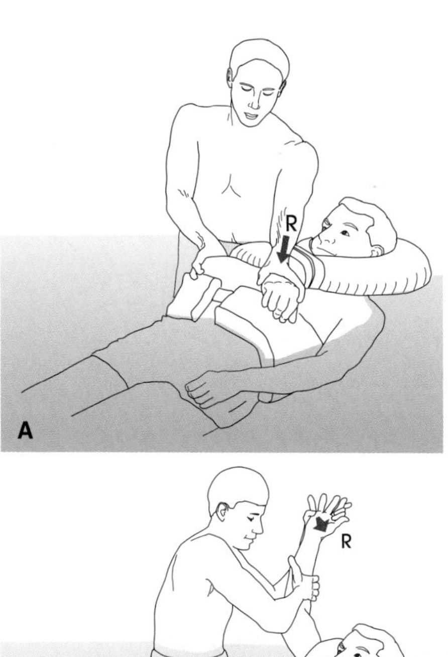

FIGURE 9.19 Manual resistance exercise for upper extremity unilateral diagonal D_2flexion pattern; **(A)** start position and **(B)** end position.

Hand Placement
Secure the medial and lateral epicondyles of the distal humerus with the guide hand. Wrap the palmar aspect of the resistance hand on the dorsal wrist medial to the palmar surface.

Direction of Movement
Active movement through the D_2flexion pattern causes the body to glide away from the practitioner. From the fully flexed position, cue the patient to then move into the D_2extension pattern. This causes the body to glide toward the practitioner.

Bilateral Diagonal Pattern: D_2Flexion/Extension of the Upper Extremities (Fig. 9.20 A and B)

Practitioner Position
Stand cephalad to patient, facing caudally.

Patient Position
BS supine; upper extremities adducted and internally rotated.

Hand Placement
Use both hands to provide resistance. Grasp the dorsal aspect of each of the patient's wrists, wrapping medially to the palmar surface.

Direction of Motion
Active contraction through the D_2flexion pattern causes the body to glide away from the practitioner. From the fully flexed position, cue the patient to contract through D_2extension, causing the patient to move toward the practitioner.

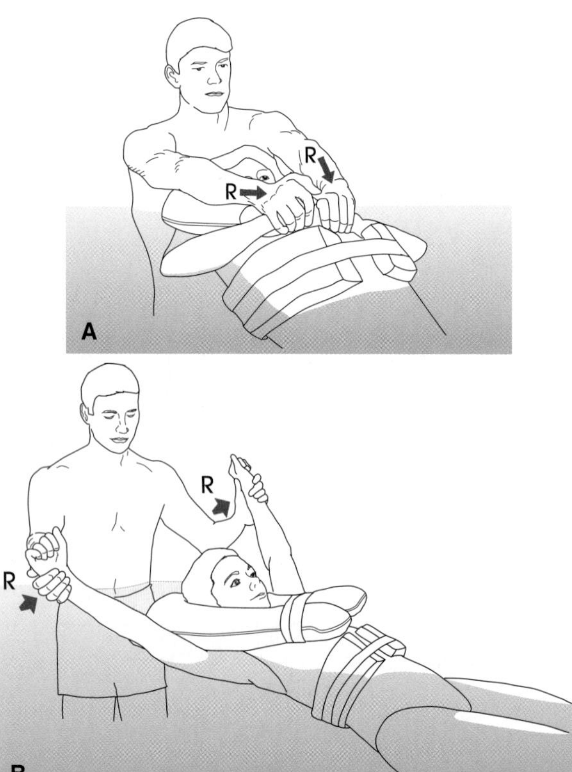

FIGURE 9.20 Manual resistance exercise for upper extremity bilateral diagonal D_2 pattern; **(A)** start position and **(B)** end position.

Lower Extremity Manual Resistance Techniques

Hip Adduction

Practitioner Position
Stand lateral to the patient's affected extremity and face medially.

Patient Position
BS supine; hip abducted.

Hand Placement
Place the guide hand on the buoyancy belt and the resistance hand on the patient's medial thigh.

Direction of Movement
Active contraction of the hip adductors causes the affected leg to adduct as the contralateral leg and body glides toward the affected leg and the practitioner.

Hip Abduction (Fig. 9.21)

Practitioner Position
Stand lateral to patient's affected extremity, facing medially.

Patient Position
BS supine; hip adducted.

Hand Placement
Place the guide hand on the buoyancy belt or lateral thigh and the thumb and base of the resistance hand on the patient's lateral leg.

Direction of Movement
Active contraction of the hip abductors causes the affected leg to abduct as the contralateral leg and body glide away from the affected leg and the practitioner.

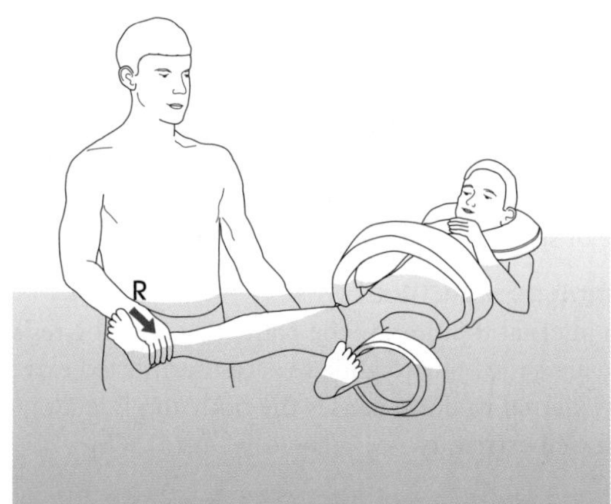

FIGURE 9.21 Manual resistance exercise for strengthening hip abduction with resistance applied to lateral aspect of the leg.

Hip Flexion With Knee Flexion (Fig. 9.22)

Practitioner Position
Stand at the side of the patient's affected extremity, facing cephalad.

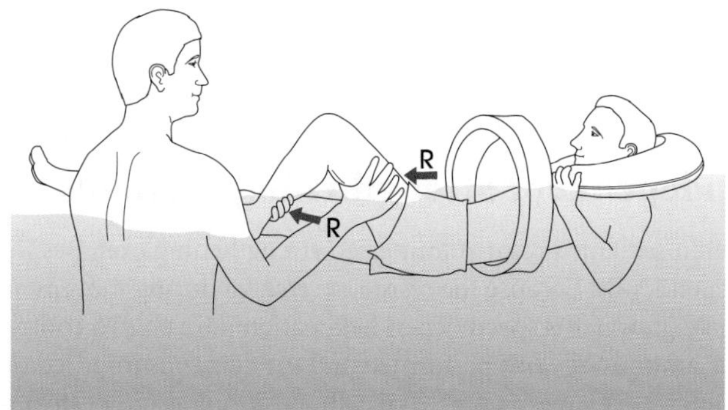

FIGURE 9.22 Manual resistance exercise for strengthening hip and knee flexion.

Patient Position

BS supine.

Hand Placement

Place the guide hand on the buoyancy belt or lateral hip. The resistance hand grasps proximal to the distal tibiofibular joint.

Direction of Movement

Active contraction of the hip and knee flexors causes the patient's body to glide toward the practitioner and fixed distal extremity.

Hip Internal/External Rotation

Practitioner Position

Stand lateral to the patient's affected extremity, facing medially.

Patient Position

BS supine; hip in neutral at 0° extension with knee flexed to 90°.

Hand Placement

Contact the distal thigh medially with the guide hand for resisted internal rotation and laterally for resisted external rotation. Place the resistance hand at the distal leg.

Direction of Movement

Active contraction of hip rotators (alternating between internal and external rotation) causes the patient's body to glide away from the distal fixed segment.

PRECAUTION: Avoid this exercise for patients with possible medial or lateral knee joint instability.

Knee Extension

Practitioner Position

Stand at the patient's feet, facing cephalad.

Patient Position

BS supine.

Hand Placement

Place the guide hand at the patient's lateral thigh and the resistance hand on the dorsal aspect of the distal tibiofibular joint.

Direction of Movement

Active contraction of the quadriceps against the practitioner's resistance hand directs the body away from the practitioner as the knee extends.

Ankle Motions

Practitioner Position

Stand lateral to the affected leg, facing caudally.

Patient Position

BS supine.

Hand Placement

The hand placement creates a short lever arm at the patient's ankle. As the patient moves through the resisted ankle motions, the patient's entire body moves through the water, producing a significant amount of drag and demand on the ankle complex.

PRECAUTION: For patients with ligamentous laxity and unstable ankles or compromised ankle musculature, the practitioner should cue the patient to avoid maximum effort during contraction to avoid potential injury.

Ankle Dorsiflexion and Plantarflexion

Hand Placement

Place the guide hand on the lateral aspect of the leg and the resistance hand over the dorsal aspect of the foot to resist dorsiflexion and on the plantar aspect to resist plantarflexion.

Direction of Movement

The body moves toward the practitioner during dorsiflexion and away from the practitioner during plantarflexion.

Ankle Inversion and Eversion

Hand Placement

Place the guide hand on the lateral aspect of the lower leg during inversion and on the medial aspect of tibia during eversion. To resist inversion, grasp the dorsal medial aspect of the foot and to resist eversion grasp the lateral foot.

Direction of Movement

During inversion, the body glides toward the practitioner, and during eversion, the body glides away from the practitioner.

Dynamic Trunk Stabilization

By applying concepts utilized for spinal stabilization exercises on land (see Chapters 15 and 16), the practitioner can challenge the dynamic control and strength of the trunk muscles in the aquatic environment. The BS supine position creates a unique perceptual environment for the patient.

Dynamic Trunk Stabilization: Frontal Plane (Fig. 9.23)

Practitioner Position

Hold the patient at the shoulders or feet.

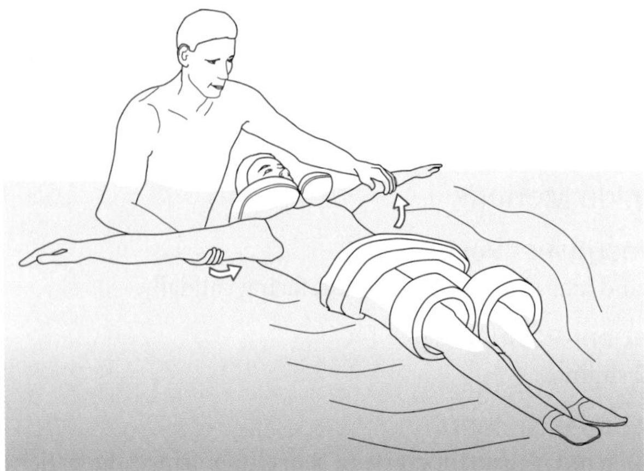

FIGURE 9.23 Isometric trunk stabilization exercise using side-to-side motions of the trunk.

Patient Position

Typically, the patient is placed in a supine position with buoyancy devices at the neck, waist, and legs.

Execution

Have the patient identify his or her neutral spine position, perform a "drawing-in maneuver" (see Chapter 16), and maintain the spinal position (isometric abdominal contraction). Move the patient from side to side through the water; monitor and cue the patient to avoid lateral trunk flexion, an indication that the patient is no longer stabilizing the spine.

Intensity

Moving the patient through the water faster increases drag and exercise intensity. Holding the patient more distally increases exercise intensity.

Dynamic Trunk Stabilization: Multidirectional

Practitioner Position

Stand at the shoulders or feet of the patient and grasp the patient's extremity to provide fixation as the patient contracts.

Patient Position

Typically, the patient is placed in a supine position with buoyancy devices at the neck, waist, and legs.

Execution

Instruct the patient to assume a neutral spine, perform the drawing-in maneuver, and "hold" the spine stable. Instruct the patient to perform either unilateral or bilateral resisted extremity patterns while maintaining a neutral spine and abdominal control. Monitor and cue the patient to avoid motion at the trunk, an indication that the patient is no longer stabilizing with the deep abdominal and global muscles. Upper extremity motions include shoulder flexion, abduction, and diagonal patterns. Lower extremity motions include hip and knee flexion and hip abduction and adduction.

Intensity

Unilateral patterns are more demanding than bilateral patterns. Increasing speed or duration increases exercise intensity.

Independent Strengthening Exercises

Often patients perform immersed strengthening exercises independently. Because the resistance created during movement through water is speed dependent, patients are able to control the amount of work performed and the demands imposed on contractile elements.[2,16,38] Typically, positioning and performance of equipment-assisted strengthening activities in water reflect that of traditional land exercise. However, the aquatic environment allows patients to assume many positions (supine, prone, side-lying, seated, and vertical). Attention to specific patient positioning allows the practitioner to utilize the buoyant properties of water and/or the buoyant and resistive properties of equipment that can either assist or resist patient movement.[2,14,16,62] Before initiating immersed strengthening activities, patients should be oriented to the effects of speed and surface area on resistance. Specific exercises for mechanical strengthening of every body part are not described. Only selected exercises are discussed and illustrated to reinforce major concepts and principles of application.

The following terms are used for equipment-assisted exercise.

- Buoyancy-assisted: Vertical movement directed parallel to vertical forces of buoyancy that assist motion (patient may use buoyant equipment to assist with motion).
- Buoyancy-supported: Horizontal movement with vertical forces of buoyancy eliminating or minimizing the need to support an extremity against gravity (patient may use buoyant equipment to assist with motion).
- Buoyancy-resisted: Movement directed against or perpendicular to vertical forces of buoyancy, creating drag (performed without equipment).
- Buoyancy-superresisted: Use of equipment generates resistance by increasing the total surface area moving through water by creating greater drag. Increasing the speed of motion through water generates further drag.

Extremity Strengthening Exercises (Fig. 9.24 A, B, C, D, and E)

The most common aquatic upper and lower extremity strengthening exercises are outlined in Table 9.1.[2,16] Typically, patients are positioned standing immersed to shoulder level for upper extremity strengthening and to midtrunk level for lower extremity strengthening. However, many exercises may be performed with the patient positioned vertically in deep water. The prone or supine position is useful when practitioners wish to progress patients or when patients require position-specific or sports-specific strengthening. Some exercises, most notably bilateral lower extremity diagonals, require the patient to be positioned supine, prone, or vertical in deep water.

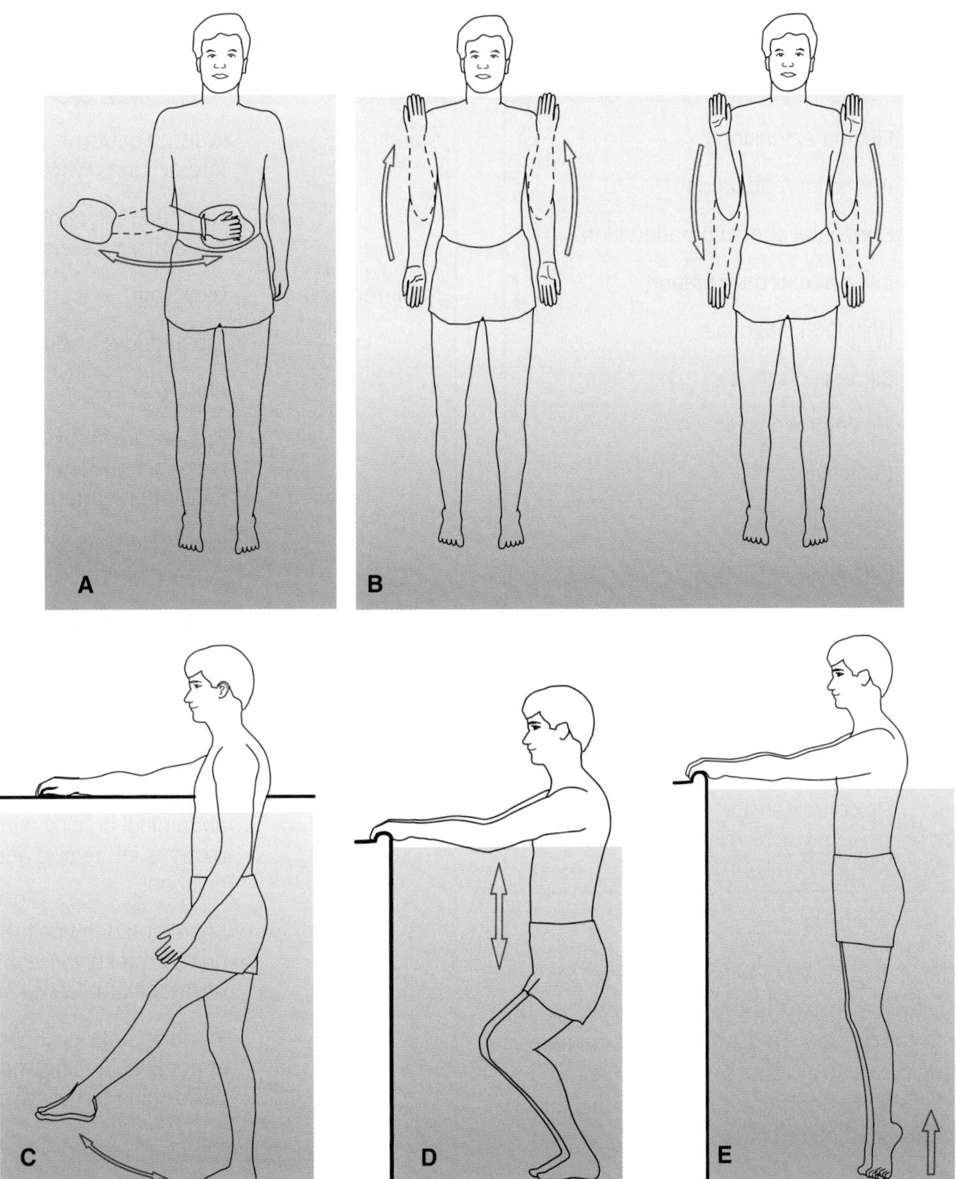

FIGURE 9.24 Mechanical resistance for strengthening **(A)** shoulder internal and external rotation, **(B)** elbow flexion and extension, **(C)** hip flexion and extension, **(D)** functional squatting, and **(E)** ankle plantarflexion.

Lumbar Spine Strengthening

Spinal stabilization may be performed in shallow, mid-depth, or deep water levels. Typically, patients are instructed to maintain a neutral spine with the drawing-in maneuver (see Chapter 16) while performing functional activities or moving the extremities. The patient's ability to stabilize the spine can be challenged by increasing the duration of the activity, the speed or surface area moving through water, and by the addition of buoyant devices in the deep water. The exercises are summarized in Table 9.2.

Trunk-Strengthening Exercises: Standing

- Have the patient hold a kickboard vertically in the water to increase resistance while walking in various patterns.
- Have the patient use unilateral or bilateral stance while performing upper extremity motions. The buoyant and turbulent forces of the water require co-contraction of the trunk muscles to stabilize the immersed body. Use equipment (Hydro-tone® bells, paddles, and resistive tubing) to increase resistance and the need for co-contraction of the trunk muscles.

Trunk-Strengthening Exercises: Semi-Reclined

Patients may use noodles, dumbbells, or kickboards for support. The practitioner can further challenge the patient by having him or her hold buoyant equipment, such as paddles, and then stabilize the trunk against the movement. A variety of lower extremity movements are suggested in Table 9.2.

TABLE 9.1 Summary of Motions Used for Upper and Lower Strengthening Exercises

Shoulder	Flexion/extension
	Abduction/adduction
	Horizontal abduction/adduction
	Internal/external rotation
	Unilateral diagonals
	Bilateral diagonals
Elbow	Flexion/extension
	Diagonals
	Push/pull
Hip	Flexion/extension
	Abduction/adduction
	Internal/external rotation
	Unilateral diagonals
	Bilateral diagonals
Knee	Flexion/extension
	Diagonals

Trunk-Strengthening Exercises: Supine

Various swimming kicks are used in the supine position. Instruct the patient to concentrate on the drawing-in maneuver and on maintaining the neutral spine position while moving the legs. Bridging while maintaining a neutral spine can be done with a long dumbbell placed at the knees.

Trunk-Strengthening Exercises: Prone

In the prone position, various swimming kicks, such as the flutter kick, are used while the patient performs the drawing-in maneuver and maintains a neutral spine.

Trunk-Strengthening Exercises in Deep Water

Stabilization exercises performed in deep water with the patient positioned vertically typically require the patient to brace with the abdominal muscles.[68,80] Emphasize identifying the neutral spine, activating the drawing-in maneuver, and holding the spine in the stable position while performing the various activities. Utilize any combination of unilateral or bilateral upper and/or lower extremity motions to further challenge the stabilization effort. Add equipment devices to the hands or legs for additional resistance and increased challenge when the patient can maintain good stabilization control. Variations include:

- Altering trunk positions such as the pike position or the iron-cross position.

TABLE 9.2 Summary of Lumbar Spine-Strengthening Exercises

Standing	Walking patterns: forward, backward, lateral, lunge walk, high stepping
	Unilateral/bilateral stance with upper extremity motions
Semi-reclined	Bicycling
	Hip abduction/adduction
	Flutter kick
	Bilateral lower extremity proprioceptive neuromuscular facilitation patterns
	Unilateral/bilateral hip and knee flexion/extension
Supine	Bridging with long dumbbell placed at knees
	Swimming kicks
Prone	Swimming kicks
Deep water	Vertical stabilization exercises; abdominal bracing with arm and leg motions in the pike and iron-cross positions
	Seated on dumbbell; abdominal bracing and balance while performing unilateral or bilateral arm motions
	Standing on a kickboard or dumbbell; abdominal bracing and balance while performing bicycling motions and/or arm motions

- Sitting on a dumbbell and bicycling forward or backward or moving the upper extremities through any combination of motions.
- Standing on a kickboard or dumbbell and moving the upper extremities through various combinations of motions, first without and then with equipment. Such standing activities typically induce obligatory abdominal bracing and challenges to balance.

Aerobic Conditioning

Aquatic exercise that emphasizes aerobic/cardiovascular conditioning can be an integral component of many rehabilitation programs.[58,81] Aerobic/cardiovascular exercise typically takes place with the patient suspended vertically in deep water pools without the feet touching the pool bottom. Alternative activities that may be performed in midlevel water, 4 to 6 feet in depth, include jogging, swimming strokes, immersed cycling, and immersed treadmill. Understanding the various treatment options, physiological responses, monitoring methods, proper form, and equipment selection allows the clinician to use this form of exercise effectively and safely in a rehabilitation program.

Treatment Interventions

Deep-water walking/running (Fig. 9.25). Deep water walking and running are the most common vertical deep-water cardiovascular endurance exercises. Alternatives include cross-country motions and high-knee marching. Deep-water cardiovascular training, which may be used as a precursor to midwater or land-based cardiovascular training, eliminates the effects of impact on the lower extremities and spine.

The patient can be tethered to the edge of the pool to perform deep-water running in those pools with limited space. Some small tanks provide resistance jets for the patient to move against.

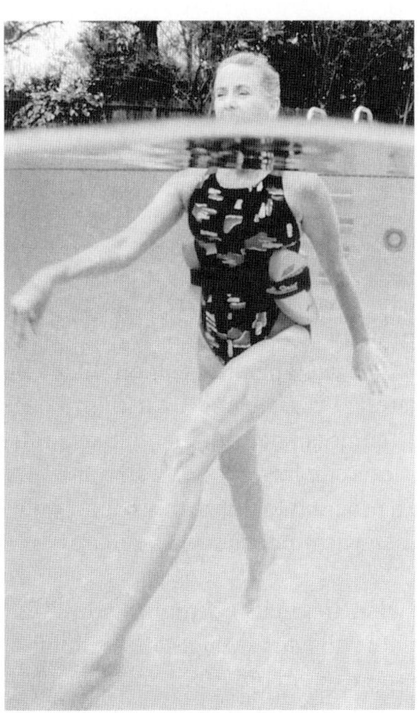

FIGURE 9.25 Deep-water walking/jogging. *(Courtesy of Rothhammer International, Inc., San Luis Obispo, CA.)*

Mid-water jogging/running (immersed treadmill running). Midwater aerobic exercise, which may be used as a precursor to land training, lessens the effects of impact on the spine and lower extremities. As a patient's tolerance to impact improves, midwater jogging may be performed in progressively shallower depths to provide increased weight bearing and functional replication. In pools with limited space, tethering with resistive tubing can provide resistance.

Immersed equipment. Immersed equipment includes an immersed cycle, treadmill, or upper body ergometer.

Swimming strokes. For patients able to tolerate the positions necessary to perform various swim strokes (neck and shoulder ROM and prone, supine, or side-lying positions), swimming can be an excellent tool to train and improve cardiovascular fitness. Swimming may elicit significantly higher elevations of heart rate, blood pressure, and VO_{2max} than other aquatic activities. Swimming contributes the added benefit of hip and trunk strengthening for some patients with spinal conditions.

PRECAUTION: Recommending swimming for poorly skilled swimmers with cardiac compromise may adversely challenge the patient's cardiovascular system.

Physiological Response to Deep-Water Walking/Running

Various physiological responses to deep-water walking and running have been reported.[3,17,28,36,37,64]

Cardiovascular response. Patients without cardiovascular compromise may experience dampened elevation of heart rate, ventilation, and VO_{2max} compared to similar land-based exercise. During low-intensity exercise, cardiac patients may experience lower cardiovascular stresses.[55] As exercise intensity increases, cardiovascular stresses approach those of related exercise on land.[6,77]

Training effect. Patients experience carryover gains in VO_{2max} from aquatic to land conditions.[43] Additionally, aquatic cardiovascular training maintains leg strength and maximum oxygen consumption in healthy runners.[36,37,47]

Proper Form for Deep-Water Running

Instruction for beginners. Proper instruction is important to ensure correct form because many beginners experience a significant learning curve.[12] Once immersed, the patient should maintain a neutral cervical spine and slightly forward flexed trunk with the arms at the sides. During running the hips should alternately flex to approximately 80° with the knee extended and then extend to neutral as the knee flexes.

Accommodating specific patient populations. For patients with positional pain associated with spinal conditions, a posterior buoyancy belt helps maintain a slightly forward flexed position, and a flotation vest helps maintain more erect posture and a relatively extended spine. Patients with unilateral lower extremity amputations may have difficulty maintaining a vertical position. Placing the buoyancy belt laterally (on the contralateral side of the amputation) allows the patient to remain vertical more easily.

Exercise Monitoring

Monitoring intensity of exercise. Monitor the rate of perceived exertion and heart rate.

- *Rate of perceived exertion.* Because skill may affect technique, subjective numerical scales depicting perceived effort may inadequately identify the level of intensity for novice deep-water runners. However, at both submaximal and maximal levels of exertion, subjective numerical rating of effort appears to correlate adequately with the heart rate during immersed exercise.[36]
- *Heart rate.* Because of the physiological changes that occur with neck level immersion, various adjustments have been suggested in the literature to lower the immersed maximum heart rate during near-maximum cardiovascular exercise.[3,17,64] The suggested decreases range from 7 to 20 beats per minute.[3,17,64] The immersed heart rate can be reliably monitored manually or with water-resistant electronic monitoring devices.

Monitoring beginners. Care should be taken to monitor regularly the cardiovascular response of novice deep-water runners or patients with known cardiac, pulmonary, or peripheral vascular disease.[55] Novice deep-water runners may experience higher levels of perceived exertion and VO_{2max} than they would during similar land exercise.[28]

Equipment Selection

Deep water equipment. Selection of buoyancy devices should reflect the desired patient posture, comfort, and projected intensity level. The most common buoyant device for deep-water running is the flotation belt positioned posteriorly (see Fig. 9.7). Patients presenting with injuries or sensitivity of the trunk may require an alternative buoyant device, such as vests, flotation dumbbells, or noodles. Providing the patient with smaller buoyant equipment (i.e., smaller belts, fewer noodles) requires the patient to work harder to maintain adequate buoyancy, thereby increasing the intensity of the activity. Fins and specially designed boots can be applied to the legs and feet to add resistance. Also, bells or buoyant dumbbells can be held in the hands to increase resistance (see Fig. 9.10).

Midwater equipment. Specially designed socks can help eliminate the potential problem of skin breakdown on the feet during impact activities, such as running. Patients can run against a forced current or tethered with elastic tubing for resistance. Using noodles around the waist or running while holding a kickboard increases the amount of drag and resistance against which the patient must move.

Independent Learning Activities

Case Studies

Postoperative Arthroscopic Knee Meniscectomy

Mike is a 54-year-old man who tore his right medial meniscus playing basketball. He is 2 weeks status postarthroscopic débridement of the torn piece of cartilage. Mike has returned to his desk job as a computer programmer but has a strong desire to return to his active workout schedule and weekend sports leagues. The surgeon has told Mike that he has no limitations except pain.

Past Medical History: Mike is healthy with no prior medical problems. He has never had an injury that made him miss more than a few days of sports participation.

Functional Status: Mike is ambulating without assistive devices, but he limps slightly because of a stiff knee. He is able to go up and down stairs but only one step at a time and has to lead with his left leg.

Musculoskeletal Status: Mike has only minimal swelling of the right knee. He rates his pain as a 1 out of 10 at rest and a 3 out of 10 with activity. His active knee ROM is 5° to 100°. He has normal ROM in the remaining joints of the right leg. Mike is able to perform a straight leg raise and has good quadriceps contraction. Manual muscle testing reveals 4/5 quadriceps strength and 4/5 hamstring and gastrocsoleus strength. He has good patellofemoral joint mobility.

Physician Referral: The prescription Mike's physician gave him states, "Evaluate and treat right knee, S/P arthroscopic meniscal débridement; may utilize land and aquatic exercise for ROM and strength."

- Formalize a program to utilize the shallow water (4-ft depth) to start Mike with independent exercises for strength and flexibility.
- Describe what manual techniques you might be able to perform with Mike for strength or flexibility.
- As Mike progresses to full ROM and near-normal strength, how could you use aquatics to replicate the demands of basketball?
- What can Mike do in the pool to maintain his cardiovascular fitness while his knee heals?

Calf Tear

Cecily is a 30-year-old weather anchor who happens to be an elite marathon runner. Four days ago, she was running up a hill and felt a "pulling" in her left calf just distal to the knee. She decided to run in a 10K race the next day but had to quit after about 5K because of a sharp pain in her calf. The doctor has told her to use crutches and remain 25% weight bearing for the next 3 days. After that she can gradually begin to increase the weight she puts through the leg over the next week. The doctor has told Cecily that she should be full weight bearing in 1 week and able to run in 3 weeks. Cecily is anxious to return to her intensive training schedule.

Past Medical History: Cecily is healthy with no prior medical problems. She has worn orthotic inserts in her shoes for "flat feet" for as long as she can remember. She says she has pulled her left calf several times during a running career that goes back to high school.

Functional Status: Cecily enters the facility ambulating with crutches. She is putting about 25% of her weight through her left foot. She is able to perform stairs without difficulty using the crutches and/or a railing.

Musculoskeletal Status: Cecily has a visible bruise at the medial head of the left gastrocnemius muscle belly. She is very tender to palpation there and has some swelling. She rates her pain at rest as 1 on a 10-point scale and her pain with activity as 2. Her ankle ROM is normal for all motions actively and passively with the exception of dorsiflexion. She dorsiflexes actively 5° and passively 8°. You grade her ankle strength as 5/5 except for plantarflexion, which you grade as a 4/5; this may be limited due to pain. You also notice that her left hip flexors, quadriceps, and hamstrings are all tight.

Physician Referral: The prescription that Cecily's doctor gives her states, "Aquatic therapy; evaluate and treat for left calf strain: gait training, ROM, strength. Progress to land as tolerated."

- Write up a program to address Cecily's dysfunctions and impairments utilizing the aquatic environment.
- At what depth of midwater does Cecily need to be to gait train in the water and still maintain 25% weight bearing?
- Write up a program for the deep water to help Cecily maintain her high level of cardiovascular fitness.
- What equipment might be useful to assist her with independent stretching in the deep water and for cardiovascular training in the deep water?

Chronic Low Back Pain

Develop an aquatic program for a patient who has chronic low back pain and needs a comprehensive flexibility and strengthening program for the legs and trunk. The patient has only one visit approved by the insurance company. However, the patient has a pool in his or her back yard that gradually goes from 3 feet to 7 feet in depth. The 7-foot deep area is only 10 feet long and 5 feet wide. The patient has no other medical problems that would limit his or her performance of the aquatic program.

REFERENCES

1. Al-Qubaeissy, KY, et al: The effectiveness of hydrotherapy in the management of RA: a systematic review. *Musculoskelet Care* 11:3–18, 2013.
2. Adams, HP, Norton, CO, and Tilden HM: *Aquatic Exercise Toolbox*, updated ed. Champaign, IL: Human Kinetics, 2006.
3. Assis, MR, et al: A randomized controlled trial of deep water running: clinical effectiveness of aquatic exercise to treat fibromyalgia. *Arthritis Rheum* 55(1):57–65, 2006.
4. Ay, A, and Yurtkuran, M: Influence of aquatic and weight-bearing exercises on quantitative ultrasound variable in postmenopausal women. *Am J Phys Med Rehab* 84(1):52–61, 2005.
5. Babb, R, and Simelson-Warr, A: Manual techniques of the lower extremities in aquatic physical therapy. *J Aquatic Phys Ther* 4(2):7–15, 1996.
6. Barbosa, TM, Garrido, MF, and Bragada, J: Physiological adaptations to head-out aquatic exercises with different levels of body immersion. *J Strength Cond Res* 21(4):1255–1259, 2007.
7. Barbosa, TM, et al: Effects of musical cadence in the acute physiologic adaptations to head-out aquatic exercises. *J Strength Cond Res* 24(1): 244–250, 2010.
8. Barczyk, K, et al: The influence of corrective exercises in a water environment on the shape of the anteroposterior curves of the spine and on the functional status of the locomotor system in children with lo scoliosis. *Orto Trauma Rehab* 11(3):209–211, 2009.
9. Bartels, EM, et al: Aquatic exercise for the treatment of knee and hip osteoarthritis. *Cochrane Database Syst Rev*, 2009.
10. Batavia, M: *Contraindications in Physical Rehabilitation: Doing No Harm.* St. Louis: Saunders Elsevier, 3:1–51, 2016.
11. Beana-Beato, PA, et al: Effects of different frequencies (203 days/week) of aquatic therapy program in adults with chronic low back pain. A non-randomized comparison trial. *Pain Med* 13:145–158, 2013.
12. Becker, BE: Aquatic therapy: scientific foundations and clinical rehabilitation applications. *Phys Med Rehab* 1(9):859–872, 2009.
13. Biscarini, A, and Cerulli, G: Modeling of the knee joint load in rehabilitative knee extension exercises under water. *J Biomech* 40(2):345–355, 2007.
14. Brady, B, et al: The addition of aquatic therapy to rehabilitation following surgical rotator cuff repair: a feasibility study. *Physiother Res Int* 13(3):153–161, 2008.
15. Broach, E, and Dattilo, J: The effect of aquatic therapy on strength of adults with multiple sclerosis. *Ther Recreation* 37:224–239, 2003.
16. Brody, LT, and Geigle, PR: *Aquatic Exercise for Rehabilitation and Training.* Champaign, IL: Human Kinetics, 2009.
17. Broman, G, et al: High intensity deep water training can improve aerobic power in elderly women. *Eur J Appl Physiol* 98(2):117–123, 2006.
18. Bukowski, EL, and Nolan, TP: Hydrotherapy: the use of water as a therapeutic agent. In Michlovitz, S, and Nolan, TP (eds): *Modalities for Therapeutic Intervention,* ed. 5. Philadelphia: F.A. Davis, 2011, pp 109–134.
19. Camilotti, BM, et al: Stature recovery after sitting on land and in water. *Manual Ther* 14(6):685–689, 2009.
20. Caminiti, G, et al: Hydrotherapy added to endurance training versus endurance training alone in elderly patients with chronic heart failure: a randomized pilot study. *Int J Cardiol* 148:199–203, 2011.
21. Cardoso, JR, et al: Aquatic therapy exercise for treating rheumatoid arthritis. *Cochrane Database Syst Rev*, 2009.
22. Choukroun, ML, and Varene, P: Adjustments in oxygen transport during head-out immersion in water at different temperatures. *J Appl Physiol* 68:1475–1480, 1990.
23. Cider, A, et al: Hydrotherapy—A new approach to improve function in older patients with chronic heart failure. *Eur J Heart Hail* 5:527–535, 2003.
24. Cider, A, et al: Aquatic exercise is effective in improving exercise performance in patients with heart failure and type 2 diabetes mellitus. *Evidence-Based Complementary and Alternative Medicine,* 2012.
25. Colado, JC, et al: Effects of a short-term aquatic resistance program on strength and body composition in fit young men. *J Strength Cond Res* 23:549–559, 2009.
26. Datta, A, and Tipton, M: Respiratory responses to cold water immersion: neural pathways, interactions, and clinical consequences awake and asleep. *J Appl Physiol* 100(6):2057–2064, 2006.

27. Delgado-Fernandez, M: Aquatic therapy improves pain, disability, quality of life, body composition and fitness in sedentary adults with chronic low back pain. *Clin Rehab* 28(4):350–360, 2014.
28. DeMaere, JM, and Ruby, BC: Effects of deep water and treadmill running on oxygen uptake and energy expenditure in seasonally trained cross country runners. *J Sports Med Phys Fitness* 37(3):175–181, 1997.
29. Devereux, K, Robertson, D, and Briffa, NK: Effects of a water-based program on women 65 years and over: a randomised controlled trial. *Aust J Physiother* 51:102–108, 2005.
30. Dumas, H, and Francesconi, S: Aquatic therapy in pediatrics: annotated bibliography. *Phys Occup Ther Pediatr* 20(4):63–78, 2001.
31. Eversden, L, et al: A pragmatic randomized controlled trial of hydrotherapy and land exercises on overall well being and quality of life in rheumatoid arthritis. *BMC Musculoskelet Disord* 8:23, 2007.
32. Fallon, RJ: *Pseudomonas aeruginosa* and whirlpool baths. *Lancet* 346(8978): 841, 1995.
33. Fappiano, M, and Gangaway, JMK: Aquatic physical therapy improves joint mobility, strength, and edema in lower extremity orthopedic injuries. *J Aquatic Phys Ther* 16(1):10–15, 2008.
34. Fatoye, FA, Goodwin, PC, and Yohannes, AM: The effectiveness of hydrotherapy in the management of RA: a systematic review. *Musculoskelet Care* 11:3–18, 2013.
35. Fischer-Cripps, AC: *The Physics Companion.* Philadelphia: Institute of Physics Publishing, 2003.
36. Frangolias, DD, and Rhodes, EC: Metabolic responses and mechanics during water immersion running and exercise. *Sports Med* 22(1):38–53, 1996.
37. Frangolias, DD, et al: Metabolic responses to prolonged work during treadmill and water immersion running. *J Sci Med Sports* 3(4):47–92, 2000.
38. Frey Law, LA, and Smidt, GL: Underwater forces produced by the Hydro-Tone® bell. *JOSPT* 23(4):267–271, 1996.
39. Getz, M, Jutzler, Y, and Vermeer, A: Effects of aquatic interventions in children with neuromotor impairments: a systematic review of the literature. *Clinic Rehab* 20:927–936, 2006.
40. Giancoli, DC: *Physics: Principles With Applications*, ed. 7. Upper Saddle River, NJ: Prentice Hall, 2014.
41. Hall, J, et al: Does aquatic exercise relieve pain in adults with neurologic or musculoskeletal disease? A systematic review and meta-analysis of randomized controlled trials. *Arch Phys Med Rehabil* 89:873–883, 2008.
42. Hollyoak, VA, and Freeman, R: *Pseudomonas aeruginosa* and whirlpool baths. *Lancet* 346:644–645, 1995.
43. Hollyoak, VA, Boyd, P, and Freeman, R: Whirlpool baths in nursing homes: use, maintenance, and contamination with *Pseudomonas aeruginosa. Commun Dis Rep CDR Rev* 5:R102–R104, 1995.
44. Jamison, LJ: Aquatic therapy for the patient with lymphedema. *J Aquatic Phys Ther* 13(1):9–12, 2005.
45. Jamison, LJ: The therapeutic value of aquatic therapy in treating lymphedema. Comprehensive decongestive physiotherapy. *Rehab Manage Interdiscipl J Rehab* 13(6):29–31, 2000.
46. Jentoft, ES, Kvalik, AG, and Mendshoel, AM: Effects of pool-based and land-based aerobic exercise on women with fibromyalgia/chronic widespread muscle pain. *Arthritis Rheum* 45:42–47, 2001.
47. Kaneda, K, et al: Lower extremity muscle activity during different types and speeds of underwater movement. *J Physiol Anthropol* 26(2):197–200, 2007.
48. Kurabayashi, H, et al: Breathing out into water during subtotal immersion: a therapy for chronic pulmonary emphysema. *Am J Phys Med Rehabil* 79:150–153, 2000.
49. Lai, C, et al: Pediatric aquatic therapy on motor function and enjoyment in children diagnosed with cerebral palsy of various motor severities. *J Child Neurol* pii:088307381453549, 2014. [Epub ahead of print].
50. Lima, T, et al: The effectiveness of aquatic physical therapy in the treatment of fibromyalgia: a systematic review with meta-analysis. *Clin Rehab* 27(10):892–908, 2013.
51. Lutz, JK, and Jiyoung, L: Prevalence and antimicrobial-resistance of pseudomonas aeruginosa in swimming pools and hot tubs. *Int J Environ Res Public Health* 8:554–564, 2011.
52. Mannerkorpi, K, et al: Pool exercise combined with an education program for patients with fibromyalgia syndrome. A prospective randomized study. *J Rheumatol* 27:2473–2481, 2000.
53. McManus, BM, and Kotelchuck, M: The effect of aquatic therapy on functional mobility of infants and toddlers in early intervention. *Pediatr Phys Ther* 19(4):275–282, 2007.
54. Mehrholz, J, Kugler, J, and Pohl, M: Water-based exercises for improving activities of daily living after stroke. *Cochrane Database of System Rev,* 1, 2011.
55. Meyer, K, and Leblanc, MC: Aquatic therapies for patients with compromised left ventricular function and heart failure. *Clin Invest Med* 31: E90–E97, 2008.
56. Noh, DK, et al: The effect of aquatic therapy on postural balance and muscle strength in stroke survivors: a randomized controlled pilot trial. *Clin Rehabil* 22:966–976, 2008.
57. O'Neill, DF: Return to function through aquatic therapy. *Athletic Ther Today* 5:14–16, 2000.
58. Pariser, G, Madras, D, and Weiss, E: Outcomes of an aquatic exercise program including aerobic capacity, lactate threshold, and fatigue in two individuals with multiple sclerosis. *J Neurol Phys Ther* 30:82–90, 2006.
59. Pechter, U, et al: Beneficial effects of water-based exercise in patients with chronic kidney failure. *Int J Rehabil Res* 26(2):153–156, 2003.
60. Peterson, C: Exercise in 94 degrees F water for a patient with multiple sclerosis. *Phys Ther* 81:1049–1058, 2001.
61. Plecash, AR, and Leavitt, BR: Aquatherapy for neurodegenerative disorders. *J Huntington's Dis* 3:5–11, 2014.
62. Poyhonen, T, et al: Determination of hydrodynamic drag forces and drag coefficients on human leg/foot model during knee exercise. *Clin Biomech* 15(4):256–260, 2000.
63. Poyhonen, T, et al: Neuromuscular function during therapeutic exercise under water and on dry land. *Arch Phys Med Rehabil* 82:1446–1452, 2001.
64. Reilly, T, Dowzer, CN, and Cable, NT: The physiology of deep-water running. *J Sports Sci* 21(12):959–972, 2003.
65. Resnick, B: Encouraging exercise in older adults with congestive heart failure. *Geriat Nurs* 25:204–211, 2004.
66. Robinson, LE, et al: The effects of land vs. aquatic plyometrics on power, torque, velocity, and muscle soreness in women. *J Strength Cond Res* 18(1):84–91, 2004.
67. Sagawa, S, et al: Water temperature and intensity of exercise in maintenance of thermal equilibrium. *J Appl Physiol* 65(6):2413–2419, 1988.
68. Saggini, R, et al: Efficacy of two microgravitational protocols to treat chronic low back pain associated with discal lesions: a randomized controlled trial. *Eura Medicophys* 40:311–316, 2004.
69. Schrepfer, R, and Babb, R: Manual techniques of the shoulder in aquatic physical therapy. *J Aquatic Phys Ther* 6(1):11–15, 1998.
70. Silva, LE, et al: Hydrotherapy versus conventional land-based exercise for the management of patients with osteoarthritis of the knee: a randomized clinical trial. *Phys Ther* 88:12–21, 2008.
71. Sova, R: *Essential Principles of Aquatic Therapy and Rehabilitation.* Port Washington, WI: DSL, 2003.
72. Takeshima, N, et al: Water-based exercise improved health-related aspects of fitness in older women. *Med Sci Sports Exerc* 34:544–551, 2002.
73. Takken, T, et al: Aquatic fitness for children with juvenile idiopathic arthritis. *Rheumatology* (Oxford) 42:1408–1414, 2003.
74. Teffaha, D, et al: Relevance of water gymnastics in rehabilitation programs in patients with chronic heart failure or coronary artery disease with normal left ventricular function. *J Cardiac Fail* 17:676–683, 2011.
75. Vargas, LG: *Aquatic Therapy: Interventions and Applications.* Enumclaw, WA: Idyll Arbor, 2004.
76. Villalta, EM, and Peiris, CI: Early aquatic physical therapy improves function and does not increase risk of wound-related adverse events for adults after orthopedic surgery: a systematic review and meta-analysis. *Arch Phys Med Rehabil* 94:138–148, 2013.
77. Volaklis, KA, Spassis, AT, and Tokmakidis, SP: Land versus water exercise in patients with coronary artery disease: effects on body composition, blood lipids, and physical fitness. *Am Heart J* 154:E1–E6, 2007.

78. Vonder Hulls, DS, Walker, LK, and Powell, JM: Clinicians' perceptions of the benefits of aquatic therapy for young children with autism: a preliminary study. *Phys Occup Ther in Pediatr* 26(1–2):13–22, 2006.
79. Wadell, K, et al: Muscle performance in patients with chronic obstructive pulmonary disease—effects of a physical training programme. *Adv Physiother* 7:51–59, 2005.
80. Waller, B, Lambeck, J, and Daly, D: Therapeutic aquatic exercise in the treatment of low back pain: a systematic review. *Clin Rehabil* 23:3–14, 2009.
81. Wang, TJ, et al: Effects of aquatic exercise on flexibility, strength, and aerobic fitness in adults with osteoarthritis of the hip or knee. *J Adv Nurs* 57: 141–152, 2007.
82. Watts, KE, and Gangaway, JMK: Evidence-based treatment of aquatic physical therapy in the rehabilitation of upper-extremity orthopedic injuries. *J Aquatic Phys Ther* 15(1):19–26, 2007.
83. Wykle, MO: Safety first. *Rehab Manage* 16(6):24–27, 50, 2003.
84. Yilmaz, I, et al: Effects of swimming training on physical fitness and water orientation in autism. *Pediatr Int* 46:624–626, 2004.

CHAPTER

10

Soft Tissue Injury, Repair, and Management

CAROLYN KISNER, PT, MS

The effective use of therapeutic exercise in the management of musculoskeletal disorders depends on sound clinical reasoning based on the best evidence available that supports the selection of the treatment interventions. Examination of the involved region is an important prerequisite to identify the impairments that are limiting or may be preventing full participation in desired activities. It is also important during the examination process to determine whether the tissues involved are in the acute, subacute, or chronic stage of recovery so that the type and intensity of exercises do not interfere with recovery but can most effectively facilitate healing for maximum return of functioning and prevention of further problems. This chapter and subsequent chapters in this book have been written with the assumption that the reader has a foundation of knowledge and skills in examination, evaluation, and program planning for orthopedically related problems in order to make effective choices of exercises that will meet the goals.

Utilizing the principles presented in this chapter, the reader should be able to design therapeutic exercise programs and choose techniques for intervention that are at an appropriate intensity for the stage of healing of connective tissue disorders. Specific joint, soft tissue, bony, and nerve lesions, as well as common surgical interventions, are presented in the remaining chapters.

Soft Tissue Lesions

Examples of Soft Tissue Lesions: Musculoskeletal Disorders

- Strain: Overstretching, overexertion, or overuse of soft tissue: tends to be less severe than a sprain, occurs from slight trauma or unaccustomed repeated trauma of a minor degree.[4] This term is frequently used to refer specifically to some degree of disruption of the musculotendinous unit.[13]
- Sprain: Severe stress, stretch, or tear of soft tissues, such as joint capsule, ligament, tendon, or muscle. This term is frequently used to refer specifically to injury of a ligament and is graded as a first (mild), second (moderate), or third (severe) degree sprain.[13]
- Dislocation: Displacement of a part, usually the bony partners in a joint, resulting in loss of the anatomical relationship and leading to soft tissue damage, inflammation, pain, and muscle spasm.
- Subluxation: An incomplete or partial dislocation of the bony partners in a joint that often involves secondary trauma to surrounding soft tissue.
- Muscle/tendon rupture or tear: If a rupture or tear is partial, pain is experienced in the region of the breach when the muscle is stretched or when it contracts against resistance.

If a rupture or tear is complete, the muscle does not pull against the injury, so stretching or contraction of the muscle does not cause pain.[6]

- Tendinopathy/tendinous lesions: *Tendinopathy* is the general term that refers to tendon injury affected by mechanical loading.[23,26] *Tenosynovitis* is inflammation of the synovial membrane covering a tendon. *Tendinitis* is inflammation of a tendon; there may be resulting scarring or calcium deposits. *Tenovaginitis* is inflammation with thickening of a tendon sheath. *Tendinosis* is degeneration of the tendon due to repetitive microtrauma.
- Synovitis: Inflammation of a synovial membrane; an excess of normal synovial fluid in a joint or tendon sheath caused by trauma or disease.
- Hemarthrosis: Bleeding into a joint, usually due to severe trauma.
- Ganglion: Ballooning of the wall of a joint capsule or tendon sheath. Ganglia may arise after trauma, and they sometimes occur with rheumatoid arthritis.
- Bursitis: Inflammation of a bursa.
- Contusion: Bruising from a direct blow, resulting in capillary rupture, bleeding, edema, and an inflammatory response.
- Overuse syndromes, cumulative trauma disorders, and repetitive strain injury: Repeated, submaximal overload and/or frictional wear to a muscle or tendon resulting in inflammation and pain.

Clinical Conditions Resulting From Trauma or Pathology

In many conditions involving soft tissue, the primary pathology is difficult to define or the tissue has healed with limitations, resulting in secondary loss of function. The following are examples of clinical manifestations resulting from a variety of causes, including those listed under the previous section.

- Dysfunction: Loss of normal function of a tissue or region. The dysfunction may be caused by adaptive shortening of the soft tissues, adhesions, muscle weakness, or any condition resulting in loss of normal mobility.
- Joint dysfunction: Mechanical loss of normal joint play in synovial joints; commonly causes loss of function and pain. Precipitating factors may be trauma, immobilization, disuse, aging, or a pathological condition such as rheumatoid arthritis.
- Contracture: Adaptive shortening of skin, fascia, muscle, or a joint capsule that prevents normal mobility or flexibility of that structure.
- Adhesion: Abnormal adherence of collagen fibers to surrounding structures during immobilization, after trauma, or as a complication of surgery, which restricts normal elasticity and gliding of the structures involved.
- Reflex muscle guarding: Prolonged contraction of a muscle in response to a painful stimulus. The primary pain-causing lesion may be in nearby or underlying tissue, or it may be a referred pain source. When not referred, the contracting muscle functionally splints the injured tissue against movement. Guarding ceases when the painful stimulus is relieved.
- Intrinsic muscle spasm: Prolonged contraction of a muscle in response to the local circulatory and metabolic changes that occur when a muscle is in a continued state of contraction. Pain is a result of the altered circulatory and metabolic environment, so the muscle contraction becomes self-perpetuating regardless of whether the primary lesion that caused the initial guarding is still irritable (Fig. 10.1). Spasm may also be a response of muscle to viral infection, cold, prolonged periods of immobilization, emotional tension, or direct trauma to muscle.

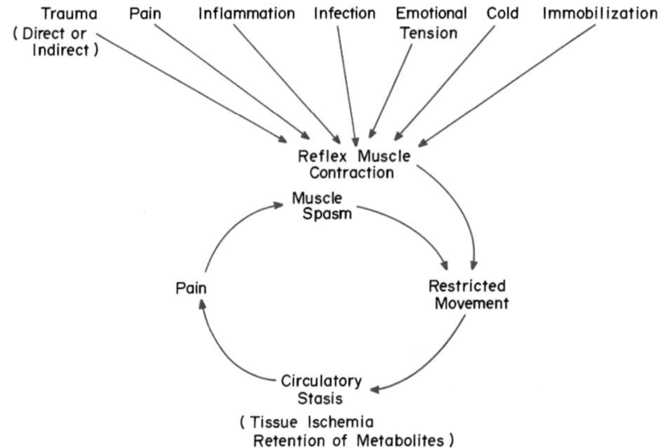

FIGURE 10.1 Self-perpetuating cycle of muscle spasm.

- Muscle weakness: A decrease in the strength of muscle contraction. Muscle weakness may be the result of a systemic, chemical, or local lesion of a nerve of the central or peripheral nervous system or the myoneural junction. It may also be the result of a direct insult to the muscle or simply due to inactivity.
- Myofascial compartment syndromes: Increased interstitial pressure in a closed, nonexpanding, myofascial compartment that compromises the function of the blood vessels, muscles, and nerves. It results in ischemia and irreversible muscle loss if there is no intervention.[11] Causes include, but are not limited to, fractures, repetitive trauma, crush injuries, skeletal traction, and restrictive clothing, wraps, or casts.

Severity of Tissue Injury

- *Grade 1 (first degree).* Mild pain at the time of injury or within the first 24 hours. Mild swelling, local tenderness, and pain occur when the tissue is stressed.[13,14]
- *Grade 2 (second degree).* Moderate pain that requires stopping the activity. Stress and palpation of the tissue greatly increase the pain. When the injury is to ligaments, some of the fibers are torn, resulting in some increased joint mobility.[13,14]
- *Grade 3 (third degree).* Near-complete or complete tear or avulsion of the tissue (tendon or ligament) with severe

pain. Stress to the torn tissue is usually painless; palpation may reveal the defect. A torn ligament results in instability of the joint.[13,14]

Irritability of Tissue: Stages of Inflammation and Repair

After any insult to connective tissue, whether it is from mechanical injury (including surgery) or chemical irritant, the vascular and cellular response is similar (Table 10.1).[16] Tissue irritability, or sensitivity, is the result of these responses and is typically divided into three overlapping stages of inflammation, repair, and maturation/remodeling.[16,27,29] The following table summarizes the clinical signs and symptoms.

Acute Stage (Reaction and Inflammation)

During the acute stage, the signs of inflammation develop; they are swelling, redness, heat, pain at rest, and loss of function.[16] When testing the range of motion (ROM), movement is painful and the patient usually guards against the motion before completion of the range is possible (Fig. 10.2 A). The pain and impaired movement are from the altered chemical state that irritates the nerve endings, increased tissue tension due to edema or joint effusion, and muscle guarding, which is the body's way of immobilizing a painful area. This stage usually lasts 4 to 6 days unless the insult is perpetuated.

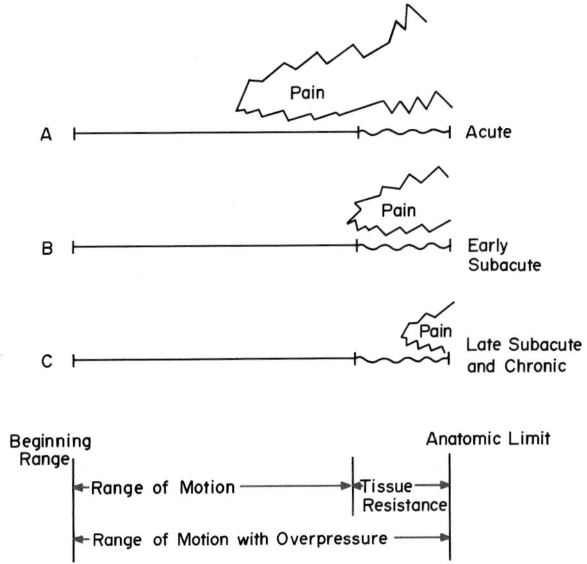

FIGURE 10.2 Pain experienced with ROM when involved tissue is in the **(A)** acute stage, **(B)** early subacute stage, and **(C)** late subacute or chronic stage.

TABLE 10.1 Stages of Tissue Healing: Characteristics, Clinical Signs, and Interventions

Acute Stage: Inflammation	Subacute Stage: Proliferation, Repair, and Healing	Chronic Stage: Maturation and Remodeling
Tissue responses and characteristics		
Vascular changes Exudation of cells and chemicals Clot formation Phagocytosis, neutralization of irritants Early fibroblastic activity	Removal of noxious stimuli Growth of capillary beds into area Collagen formation Granulation tissue Very fragile, easily injured tissue	Maturation of connective tissue Contracture of scar tissue Remodeling of scar Collagen aligns to stress
Clinical signs		
Inflammation Pain before tissue resistance	Decreasing inflammation Pain synchronous with tissue resistance	Absence of inflammation Pain after tissue resistance
Physical therapy goals and interventions for phases of rehabilitation		
Phase I Maximum Protection	***Phase II*** Moderate Protection/ Controlled-Motion	***Phase III*** Minimum to No Protection/ Return to Function
Control effects of inflammation: selective rest, ice, compression, elevation *Prevent deleterious effects of rest:* nondestructive movement: passive ROM, massage, and muscle setting with caution	*Develop mobile scar:* selective stretching, mobilization/manipulation of restrictions *Promote healing:* nondestructive active, resistive, open- and closed-chain stabilization, muscular endurance, and cardiopulmonary endurance exercises, carefully progressed in intensity and range	*Increase tensile quality of scar:* progressive strengthening and endurance exercises *Develop functional independence:* functional exercises and specificity drills

Subacute Stage (Proliferation, Repair, and Healing)

During the subacute stage, the signs of inflammation progressively decrease and eventually are absent. When testing ROM, the patient may experience pain synchronous with encountering tissue resistance at the end of the available ROM (Fig. 10.2 B). Pain occurs only when the newly developing tissue is stressed beyond its tolerance or when tight tissue is stressed. Muscles may test weak, and function is limited as a result of the weakened tissue. This stage usually lasts 10 to 17 days (14 to 21 days after the onset of injury) but may last up to 6 weeks in some tissues with limited circulation, such as tendons.[8,27,29]

Chronic Stage (Maturation and Remodeling)

There are no signs of inflammation during the chronic stage. There may be contractures or adhesions that limit range, and there may be muscle weakness limiting normal function. During this stage, connective tissue continues to strengthen and remodel in response to the stresses applied to it.[7,23,27,29] A stretch pain may be felt when testing tight structures at the end of their available range (Fig. 10.2C). Function may be limited by muscle weakness, poor endurance, or poor neuromuscular control. This stage may last 6 months to 1 year depending on the tissue involved and amount of tissue damage.

Chronic Inflammation

A state of prolonged inflammation may occur if injured tissue is continually stressed beyond its ability to repair. There are symptoms of increased pain, swelling, and muscle guarding that last more than several hours after activity. There are also increased feelings of stiffness after rest, loss of ROM 24 hours after activity, and progressively greater stiffness of the tissue as long as the irritation persists.

Chronic Pain Syndrome

Chronic pain syndrome is a state that persists longer than 6 months. It includes pain that cannot be linked to a source of irritation or inflammation resulting in activity limitations and participation restrictions that affect many parameters of function.

Management During the Acute Stage

Tissue Response: Inflammation

The inflammatory stage involves cellular, vascular, and chemical responses in the tissue. During the first 48 hours after insult to soft tissue, vascular changes predominate. Exudation of cells and solutes from the blood vessels takes place, and clot formation occurs. During this period, neutralization of the chemical irritants or noxious stimuli, phagocytosis (cleaning up of dead tissue), early fibroblastic activity, and formation of new capillary beds begin. These physiological processes serve as a protective mechanism as well as a stimulus for subsequent healing and repair.[16] Usually this stage lasts 4 to 6 days unless the insult is perpetuated.

Management Guidelines: Maximum Protection (Phase I)

The therapist's role during the protection phase of intervention is to control the effects of the inflammation, facilitate wound healing, and maintain normal functioning in unaffected tissues and body regions. The information provided here is summarized in Box 10.1.

Patient Education

Inform the patient about the expected duration of symptoms (4 to 6 days), what he or she can do during this stage, any precautions or contraindications, and what to expect when the symptoms lessen. Patients need reassurance that the acute symptoms are usually short-lived, and they need to learn what is safe to do during this stage of healing.

Protection of the Injured Tissue

To minimize musculoskeletal pain and promote healing, protection of the part affected by the inflammatory process is necessary during the first 24 to 48 hours. This is usually provided by rest (orthosis, tape, cast), cold (ice), compression, and elevation. Depending on the type and severity of the injury, manual methods of pain and edema control, such as massage and gentle (grade I) joint oscillations, may be beneficial. If a lower extremity is involved, protection with assistive devices for partial or nonweight-bearing ambulation may be required.

Prevention of Adverse Effects of Immobility

Complete or continuous immobilization should be avoided whenever possible as it can lead to adherence of the developing fibrils to surrounding tissue, weakening of connective tissue, and changes in articular cartilage.[6,24,25]

A *long-term goal of treatment* is the formation of a strong, mobile scar at the site of the lesion, so there is complete and painless restoration of activities. Initially, the network of fibril formation is random. It acquires an organized arrangement depending on the mechanical forces acting on the tissue.[15] To influence the development of an organized scar, begin treatment during the acute stage, when tolerated, with carefully controlled *passive movements.*

Tissue-specific movement. Tissue-specific movements should be directed to the structure involved to prevent abnormal adherence of the developing fibrils to surrounding tissue and thus avoid future disruption of the scar. Tissue-specific techniques are described below.

Intensity of movement. The intensity (dosage) of movement should be gentle enough so the fibrils are not detached from the site of healing. Too much movement too soon is painful

BOX 10.1 MANAGEMENT GUIDELINES—
Acute Stage/Maximum Protection

Impairments of Body Structure and Function:

- Inflammation, pain, edema, muscle spasm
- Impaired movement
- Joint effusion (if the joint is injured or if there is arthritis)
- Restricted use of associated areas

Plan of Care	Intervention (up to 1 week postinjury)
1. Educate the patient.	1. Inform patient of anticipated recovery time and how to protect the part while maintaining appropriate functional activities.
2. Control pain, edema, and spasm.	2. Cold, compression, elevation, and massage (48 hours). Immobilize the part (rest, orthosis, tape, cast). Avoid positions of stress to the part. Gentle (grade I or II) joint oscillations with joint in pain-free position.
3. Maintain soft tissue and joint integrity and mobility.	3. Appropriate dosage of passive movements within limit of pain, specific to structure involved. Appropriate dosage of intermittent muscle setting or electrical stimulation.
4. Reduce joint swelling if symptoms are present.	4. May require medical intervention if swelling is rapid (blood). Provide protection (orthosis, cast).
5. Maintain integrity and function of associated areas.	5. Active-assistive, free, resistive, and/or modified aerobic exercises, depending on proximity to associated areas and effect on the primary lesion. Adaptive or assistive devices as needed to protect the part during functional activities.

PRECAUTIONS: The proper dosage of rest and movement must be used during the inflammatory stage. Signs of too much movement are increased pain or increased inflammation.

CONTRAINDICATIONS: Stretching and resistance exercises should not be performed at the site of the inflamed or swollen tissue.

and reinjures the tissue. The dosage of passive movement depends on the severity of the lesion. Some patients tolerate no movement during the first 24 to 48 hours; others tolerate only a few degrees of gentle passive movement. Continuous passive movement (see Chapter 3) has been useful immediately after various types of surgery to joints—intra-articular, metaphyseal, and diaphyseal fractures; surgical release of extra-articular contractures and adhesions; and other select conditions.[24,25] Any movement tolerated at this stage is beneficial, but it must *not* increase the inflammation or pain. Active movement is usually *contraindicated* at the site of an active pathological process unless it is a chronic disease, such as rheumatoid arthritis.

General movement. Active movement is appropriate in neighboring regions to maintain integrity in uninjured tissue and to aid in circulation and lymphatic flow.

PRECAUTION: If movement increases pain or inflammation, it is either of too great a dosage or it should not be done. Extreme care must be used with movement at this stage.

Specific Interventions and Dosages

Passive ROM (PROM). PROM within the limit of pain is valuable for maintaining mobility in joints, ligaments, tendons, and muscles, as well as improving fluid dynamics and maintaining nutrition in the joints.[24,25] Initially, the range is probably very small.[31] Stretching at this stage is contraindicated. Any motion gained from the PROM techniques is because of decreased pain, swelling, and muscle guarding.

Low-dosage joint mobilization/manipulation techniques. Grade I or II distraction and glide techniques have the benefit of improving fluid dynamics in the joint to maintain cartilage health. These techniques may also reflexively inhibit or gate the perception of pain. Low-dosage joint mobilizations are beneficial with joint pathologies and any other connective tissue injury that affects joint motion during the acute stage.

Muscle setting. Gentle isometric muscle contractions performed intermittently and at a very low intensity so as not to cause pain or joint compression have several purposes. The pumping action of the contracting muscle assists the circulation and, therefore, fluid dynamics. If there is muscle damage or injury, the setting techniques are done with the muscle in the shortened position to help maintain mobility of the actin-myosin filaments without stressing the breached tissue. If there is joint injury, the position during the setting techniques is dictated by pain; usually the resting position for the joint is most comfortable. If tolerated, the intermittent setting techniques are performed in several positions.

Massage. Massage serves the purpose of moving fluid, and if it is applied cautiously and gently to injured tissue, it may assist in preventing adhesions. Tendinous lesions are treated with a gentle dosage applied transverse to the fibers to smooth roughened surfaces or to maintain mobility of the tendon in its sheath. When applied, the tendon is kept taut. When treating muscle lesions, the muscle is usually kept in its shortened position so as not to separate the healing breach.[6] Massage to manage the effects of edema is discussed in Chapter 26.

Interventions for Associated Areas

During the protection phase, maintain as normal a physiological state as possible in related areas of the body. Include techniques to maintain or improve the following areas.

Range of motion. These techniques may be done actively or passively, depending on the proximity to and the effect on the injured tissue.

Resistance exercise. Resistance exercises may be applied at an appropriate dosage to muscles not directly related to the injured tissue to prepare the patient for use of assistive devices, such as crutches or a walker, and to improve ability to perform needed activities.

Functional activities. Supportive or adaptive devices may be necessary depending on area of injury and expected activities.

CLINICAL TIP

It is important to prevent vascular stasis, which may occur due to swelling and immobility. Circulation is helped by encouraging activities within safe parameters and by using supportive elastic wraps, elevating the part, and using appropriate massage and muscle-setting techniques. In the lower extremities, active ankle and toe ROM should be performed if possible.

Management During the Subacute Stage

Tissue Response: Proliferation, Repair, and Healing

During the second to fourth days after tissue injury, the inflammation begins to decrease, the clot starts resolving, and repair of the injured site begins. This usually lasts an additional 10 to 17 days (14 to 21 days after the onset of injury) but may last up to 6 weeks.

The synthesis and deposition of collagen characterize this stage. Noxious stimuli are removed, and capillary beds begin to grow into the area. Fibroblastic activity, collagen formation, and granulation tissue development increase. Fibroblasts are present in tremendous numbers by the fourth day after injury and continue in large number until about day 21.[28] The fibroblasts produce new collagen, and this immature collagen replaces the exudate that originally formed the clot. In addition, myofibroblastic activity begins about day 5, causing scar shrinkage (contraction).[28,29] Depending on the size of injury, wound closure usually takes 5 to 8 days in muscle and skin and 3 to 6 weeks in tendons and ligaments.[8,29]

During this stage of healing, the immature connective tissue that is produced is thin and unorganized. It is extremely fragile and easily injured if overstressed, yet proper growth and alignment can be stimulated by appropriate tensile loading in the line of normal stresses for that tissue. At the same time, adherence to surrounding tissues can be minimized.[5]

Management Guidelines: Moderate Protection/Controlled Motion (Phase II)

The therapist's role during this stage of healing is critical. The patient feels much better because the pain is no longer constant, and active movement can begin. It is easy to begin too much movement too soon or, conversely, to be tempted to approach intervention cautiously and not progress rapidly enough. Understanding the healing process and tissue response to stresses underlies the critical decisions that are made throughout this phase of intervention. The key is to initiate and progress *nondestructive* exercises and activities, that is to perform exercises and activities that are within the tolerance of the healing tissues, which can then heal without re-injury or inflammation.[7] The information that follows is summarized in Box 10.2.

Patient Education

Inform the patient about what to expect at this stage, the time frame for healing, and what signs and symptoms indicate that he or she is pushing beyond tissue tolerance.

- Encourage the patient to return to normal activities that do not exacerbate symptoms, but caution against participating in recreational, sports, or work-related activities at this time that would be detrimental to the healing process.

BOX 10.2 MANAGEMENT GUIDELINES—
Subacute Stage/Controlled Motion

Impairments of Body Structure and Function:

- Pain when end of available ROM is reached
- Edema (decreasing but may still be present)
- Joint effusion (decreasing but may still be present if joints are involved)
- Soft tissue, muscle, and/or joint contractures (developing in immobilized region)
- Muscle weakness from reduced usage or pain
- Restricted ADLs and IADLs related to involved tissues

Plan of Care	Intervention (up to 3 weeks postinjury)
1. Educate the patient.	1. Inform patient of anticipated healing time and importance of following guidelines. Teach home exercises and encourage functional activities consistent with plan; monitor and modify as patient progresses.
2. Promote healing of injured tissues.	2. Monitor response of tissue to exercise progression; decrease intensity if pain or inflammation increases. Protect healing tissue with assistive devices, orthoses, tape, or wrap; progressively increase amount of time the joint is free to move each day and decrease use of assistive device as strength in supporting muscles increases.
3. Restore soft tissue, muscle, and/or joint mobility.	3. Progress from passive to active-assistive to active ROM within limits of pain. Gradually increase mobility of scar, specific to structure involved. Progressively increase mobility of related structures if limiting ROM; use techniques specific to tight structure.
4. Develop neuromuscular control, muscle endurance, and strength in involved and related muscles.	4. Initially, progress multiple-angle isometric exercises within patient's tolerance; begin cautiously with mild resistance. Initiate AROM, protected weight bearing, and stabilization exercises. As ROM, joint play, and healing improve, progress isotonic exercises with increased repetitions. Emphasize control of exercise pattern and proper mechanics. Progress resistance later in this stage.
5. Maintain integrity and function of associated areas.	5. Apply progressive strengthening and stabilizing exercises, monitoring effect on the primary lesion. Resume low-intensity activities involving the healing tissue that do not exacerbate the symptoms.

PRECAUTIONS: The signs of inflammation or joint swelling normally decrease early in this stage. Some discomfort will occur as the activity level is progressed, but it should not last longer than a couple of hours. Signs of too much motion or activity are resting pain, fatigue, increased weakness, and spasm lasting beyond 24 hours.

- Teach the patient a home exercise program and help him or her adapt work and recreational activities that are consistent with intervention strategies so the patient becomes an active participant in the recovery process.

Management of Pain and Inflammation

Pain and inflammation decrease as healing progresses.

- Criteria for initiating active exercises and stretching during the early subacute stage include decreased swelling, pain that is no longer constant, and pain that is not exacerbated by motion in the available range.
- As new exercises are introduced or as the intensity of exercises is progressed, monitor the patient's response. Exercises progressed too vigorously or activities begun too early can be injurious to the fragile, newly developing tissue and may delay recovery, cause pain, and perpetuate the inflammatory response.[7,27] If symptoms increase, modify the intensity of exercises.

Initiation of Active Exercises

Because of the restricted use of the injured region, there is muscle weakness even in the absence of muscle pathology.

The subacute stage of healing is a transition period during which active exercises within the pain-free range of the injured tissue can begin and be progressed to muscular endurance and strengthening exercises with care, keeping within the tolerance of the healing tissues (nondestructive motion). If activity is kept within a safe intensity and frequency, symptoms of pain and swelling progressively decrease each day. Patient response is the best guide to how quickly or vigorously to progress. Clinically, if signs of inflammation increase or the ROM progressively decreases, the intensity of the exercise and activity must decrease, because chronic inflammation has developed and a retracting scar will become more limiting.[2,3,17] Signs of excessive stress with exercise or activities are highlighted in Box 10.3.

Multiple-angle, submaximal isometric exercises. Submaximal isometric exercises are used during the early subacute stage to initiate control and strengthening of the muscles in the involved region in a nonstressful manner. They may also help the patient become aware of using the correct muscles. The intensity and angles for resistance are determined by the absence of pain.

- To initiate isometric exercise in an injured, healing muscle, place it in the shortened or relaxed position so the new scar is not pulled from the breached site.[5,27]
- To initiate isometric exercises when there is joint pathology, the resting position for the joint may be the most comfortable position. The intensity of contraction should be kept below the perception of pain.

Active ROM (AROM) exercises. AROM activities in pain-free ranges are used to develop control of the motion.

- Initially, use isolated, single plane motions. Emphasize control of the motion using light-resistive, concentric exercises of involved muscle and muscles needed for proper joint mechanics.
- Use combined motions or diagonal patterns to facilitate contraction of the desired muscles, but do not use patterns of motion that are dominated by stronger muscles with the weaker muscles not effectively participating at this early stage. Do not stress beyond the ability of the involved or weakened muscles to participate in the motion.

Muscular endurance exercises. Exercises for muscle endurance are emphasized during the subacute phase because slow-twitch muscle fibers are the first to atrophy when there is joint swelling, trauma, or immobilization.

- Initially, use only active ROM, with emphasis on control. Later during the healing phase, low-intensity, high-repetition exercise with light resistance is used rather than high-intensity resistance.
- Be certain that the patient is using correct movement patterns without substitution and is informed of the importance of stopping the exercise or activity when the involved muscle fatigues or involved tissue develops symptoms. For example, if the patient is doing shoulder flexion or abduction activities, substitution with scapular elevation should be avoided, or if the patient is doing leg-lift exercises, proper stabilization of the pelvis and the spine is important to ensure safety and correct motor learning.

Protected weight-bearing exercises. Partial weight bearing within the tolerance of the healing tissues may be used early to load the region in a controlled manner and stimulate stabilizing co-contractions in the muscles.

- Provide reinforcement to help develop awareness of appropriate muscle contractions and to help develop control while the patient shifts his or her weight in a side-to-side or anterior-to-posterior motion. As tolerated by the patient, progress by increasing the amplitude of movement or by decreasing the amount of support or protection.
- Add resistance to progress strength in the weight-bearing and stabilizing muscles.

PRECAUTION: Eccentric and heavy-resistance exercises, including progressive resistance exercise may cause added trauma to muscle and are not used in the early subacute stage after muscle injury when the weak tensile quality of the healing tissue could be jeopardized.[18] For nonmuscular injuries, eccentric exercises may not reinjure the part, but the resistance should be limited to a low intensity at this stage to avoid delayed-onset muscle soreness. (This is in contrast to using eccentric exercises to facilitate and strengthen weak muscles when there has been no injury to take advantage of greater tension development with less energy in eccentric contractions, which is described in Chapter 6.)

BOX 10.3 Signs of Excessive Stress With Exercise or Activities

- Exercise or activity soreness that does not decrease after 4 hours and is not resolved after 24 hours
- Exercise or activity pain that comes on earlier or is increased over the previous session
- Progressively increased feelings of stiffness and decreased ROM over several exercise sessions
- Swelling, redness, and warmth in the healing tissue
- Progressive weakness over several exercise sessions
- Decreased functional usage of the involved part

Exercise progressions may cause some temporary soreness that can last 4 hours, but if the above signs and symptoms occur, the activity, exercise, or stretching maneuvers are too stressful and should be modified or reduced in intensity.

Initiation and Progression of Stretching

Restricted motion during the acute stage and adherence of the developing scar usually cause decreased flexibility in the healing tissue and related structures in the region. To increase mobility and stimulate proper alignment of the developing scar, initiate stretching techniques that are specific to the tissues involved. More than one technique may have to be used to regain the ROM.

Warm the tissues. Use modalities or active ROM to increase the tissue temperature and relax the muscles for ease in stretching.

Muscle relaxation techniques. Muscles that are not relaxed interfere with joint mobilization and passive stretching of inert tissue. If necessary, utilize hold-relax techniques first to be able to take the tissues to the end of their available range.

Joint mobilization/manipulation. If there is decreased joint play restricting range, it is important to begin stretching with specific joint techniques. Use grade III sustained or grade III and IV oscillation techniques to restore some of the joint slide prior to physiological stretching so as to minimize excessive compression of vulnerable cartilage. Joint distraction and gliding techniques are applied to stretch restricting capsular tissue. (See Chapter 5 for the principles and techniques of joint mobilization.)

Stretching techniques. Passive stretching techniques, self-stretching, and prolonged mechanical stretching are used to increase the extensibility of inert connective tissue, which permeates every structure in the body. These techniques are interspersed with neuromuscular inhibition techniques to relax and elongate the muscles crossing the joints. (See Chapter 4 for the principles and techniques of stretching.)

Massage. Various types of massage can be used for their soft tissue mobilizing effects. For example, cross-fiber friction massage is used to mobilize ligaments and incision sites so they move freely across the joint. Cross-fiber massage is also used at the site of muscle scar tissue or tendon adhesions to gain mobility of the scar tissue. The intensity and duration of the technique is progressively increased as the tissue responds.

Use of the new range. The patient must use the new range to maintain any extensibility gained with the stretching maneuvers and to develop control of the new range. Teach home exercises that include light resistance using the agonist in the new range as well as self-stretching techniques. Also encourage the patient to incorporate the new range into his or her daily activities.

Correction of Contributing Factors

Continue to maintain or develop as normal a physiological and functional state as possible in related areas of the body. Address any postural or biomechanical impairments in stability, connective tissue and muscle flexibility, or strength that may have precipitated the problem or that may prevent full recovery. Resume low-intensity activities as the patient tolerates without exacerbating symptoms. Continue to reassess the patient's progress and understanding of the controlled activities.

Management During the Chronic Stage

Tissue Response: Maturation and Remodeling

Scar retraction from activity of the myofibroblasts is usually complete day 21 and the scar stops increasing in size, so from day 21 to day 60, there is a predominance of fibroblasts that are easily remodeled.[27] The process of maturation begins during the late subacute stage and continues for several months. The maturation and remodeling of the scar tissue occur as collagen fibers become thicker and reorient in response to stresses placed on the connective tissue. Remodeling time is influenced by factors that affect the density and activity level of the fibroblasts, including the amount of time immobilized, stress placed on the tissue, location of the lesion, and vascular supply.

Maturation of Tissue

The primary differences in the state of the healing tissue between the late subacute and chronic stages are the improvement in quality (orientation and tensile strength) of the collagen and the reduction of the wound size during the chronic stages. The quantity of collagen stabilizes, and there is a balance between synthesis and degradation. Depending on the size of the structure or degree of injury or pathology, healing with progressively increasing tensile quality in the injured tissue may continue for 12 to 18 months.[8,19,28]

Remodeling of Tissue

Because of the way immature collagen molecules are held together (hydrogen bonding) and adhere to surrounding tissue, they can be easily remodeled with gentle and persistent treatment. This is possible for up to 10 weeks. If not properly stressed, the fibers adhere to surrounding tissue and form a restricting scar. As the structure of collagen changes to covalent bonding and thickens, it becomes stronger and resistant to remodeling. At 14 weeks, the scar tissue is unresponsive to remodeling. Consequently, an old scar has a poor response to stretch.[5] Treatment under these conditions requires either adaptive lengthening in the tissue surrounding the scar or surgical release.

Management Guidelines: Minimum to No Protection/Return to Function (Phase III)

The therapist's role during this phase is to design a progression of exercises that safely stresses the maturing connective tissue in terms of both flexibility and strength so the patient can return to his or her regular activities and participate in life situations including work, community mobility, and recreation/sports. Individuals returning to high-intensity work and sport activities require more intense exercises to prepare the tissues to withstand the stresses and train the neuromuscular system to respond to the demands of the activity (this may be referred to as Phase IV).

Because remodeling of the maturing collagen occurs in response to the stresses placed on it, it is important to use controlled forces that replicate normal stresses on the tissue.[7,15,23] Maximum strength of the collagen develops in the direction of the imposed forces. Pain that the patient now experiences arises only when stress is placed on restrictive contractures or adhesions or when there is soreness due to increased stress of resistive exercise. To avoid chronic or recurring pain, the contractures must be stretched or the adhesions broken up and mobilized. Excessive or abnormal stress leads to re-injury and chronic inflammation, which can be detrimental to the return of function. The information that follows is summarized in Box 10.4.

BOX 10.4 MANAGEMENT GUIDELINES—
Chronic Stage/Return to Function

Impairments of Body Structure and Function:

Soft tissue and/or joint contractures and adhesions that limit normal ROM or joint play

Decreased muscle performance—weakness, poor endurance, poor neuromuscular control

Decreased usage of the involved part

Inability to participate normally in an expected activity

Plan of Care	Interventions (>3 weeks postinjury)
1. Educate the patient.	1. Instruct patient in safe progressions of exercises and stretching. Monitor understanding and compliance. Teach ways to avoid reinjuring the part. Teach safe body mechanics. Provide ergonomic counseling.
2. Increase soft tissue, muscle, and/or joint mobility.	2. Stretching techniques specific to tight tissue: ▪ Joint and selected ligaments (joint mobilization/manipulation) ▪ Ligaments, tendons, and soft tissue adhesions (cross-fiber massage) ▪ Muscles (neuromuscular inhibition, passive stretch, massage, and flexibility exercises)
3. Improve neuromuscular *control,* strength, and muscle endurance.	3. Progress exercises: ▪ Submaximal to maximal resistance ▪ Specificity of exercise using resisted concentric and eccentric, weight bearing and nonweight bearing ▪ Single plane to multiplanar motions ▪ Simple to complex motions, emphasizing movements that simulate functional activities ▪ Controlled proximal stability, superimpose distal motion ▪ Safe biomechanics ▪ Low repetitions to high repetitions at slow speeds; progress complexity and time; progress speed and time.
4. Improve cardiopulmonary endurance.	4. Progress aerobic exercises using safe activities.
5. Progress activities and participation in life situations.	5. Continue using supportive and/or assistive devices until the ROM is functional with joint play and strength in supporting muscles is adequate. Progress functional training with simulated activities from protected and controlled to unprotected and variable. Continue progressive strengthening exercises and advanced training activities until the muscles are strong enough and able to respond to the required demands.

PRECAUTIONS: There should be no signs of inflammation. Some discomfort will occur as the activity level is progressed, but it should not last longer than a couple of hours. Signs that activities are progressing too quickly or with too great a dosage are joint swelling, pain that lasts longer than 4 hours or that requires medication for relief, a decrease in strength, or fatiguing more easily.

Patient Education

Unless there is restrictive scar tissue requiring manual techniques for intervention, the patient becomes more responsible for carrying out the exercises in the plan of treatment.

- Instruct the patient in biomechanically safe progressions of resistance and self-stretching and how to self-monitor for detrimental effects and signs of excessive stress (see Box 10.3).
- Establish guidelines for what must be attained to return safely to recreational, sport, or work-related activities.
- Re-examine and evaluate the patient's progress and modify the exercises as progress is noted or if problems develop.
- Recommend modifications in daily living, work, or sport activities if they are contributing to the patient's impairments and preventing return to desired activities.

Considerations for Progression of Exercises

Free joint play within a useful (or functional) ROM is necessary to avoid joint trauma. If joint play is restricted, joint-mobilization/manipulation techniques should be used. These stretching techniques can be vigorous so long as no signs of increased irritation result.

Adequate muscle support is necessary to protect the joint. If there is weakness, faulty neuromuscular patterns may develop as activities are attempted. Poor support or faulty patterns of movement may result in microtrauma. The criterion for strength should be a muscle test grade of 4 on a 5-point scale in lower extremity musculature before discontinuing use of supportive or assistive devices for ambulation.

- To increase strength when there is a loss of joint play, use multiple-angle isometric exercises in the available range.
- Once joint play within the available ROM is restored, use resistive dynamic exercises within the available range. This does not imply that normal ROM needs to be present before initiating dynamic exercises but that joint play within the available range should be present. (See Chapter 5 for information on joint play.)
- In summary, joint dynamics and muscle strength and flexibility should be balanced as the injured part is progressed to functional exercises.

Progression of Stretching

Stretching of any restricting contractures or adhesions should be specific to the tissue involved using manual techniques, such as joint mobilization/manipulation, myofascial massage, proprioceptive neuromuscular facilitation stretching, and passive stretching in addition to instruction in self-stretching. (See Chapters 4 and 5 and the self-stretching exercises described in Chapters 16 to 22.) At this stage, progress the intensity and duration of the stretching maneuvers so long as no signs of increased irritation persist beyond 24 hours.

Progression of Exercises for Muscle Performance: Developing Neuromuscular Control, Strength, and Endurance

As the patient's tissues heal, not only does treatment progress to stimulate proper maturation and remodeling in the healing tissue, but emphasis is also placed on controlled progressive exercises designed to prepare the patient to meet the outcome goals.

- If the patient is not using some of the muscles because of inhibition, weakness, or dominance of substitute patterns, isolate the desired muscle action or use unidirectional motions to develop awareness of muscle activity and control of the movement.
- Progress exercises from isolated, unidirectional, simple movements to complex patterns and multidirectional movements requiring coordination with all muscles functioning for the desired activity.[30]
- Progress strengthening exercises to simulate specific demands including both weight-bearing and nonweight-bearing (closed- and open-chain) and both eccentric and concentric contractions.[22]
- Progress trunk stabilization, postural control, and balance exercises and combine with extremity motions for effective total body movement patterns.[30]
- Teach safe body mechanics and have the patient practice activities that replicate his or her work environment.
- Often overlooked but of importance in preventing injury associated with fatigue is developing muscular endurance in the prime mover muscles and stabilizing muscles as well as cardiopulmonary endurance.

Return to High-Demand Activities

Patients who must return to activities with greater than normal demand, such as is required in sports participation and heavy work settings, are progressed further to more intense exercises including plyometrics, agility training, and skill development.

- Develop exercise drills that simulate the work[12] or sport[2,30] activities using a controlled environment with specific, progressive resistance and plyometric drills.
- As the patient demonstrates capabilities, increase the repetitions and speed of the movement.
- Progress by changing the environment and introducing surprise and uncontrolled events into the activity.[1,30]

The importance of proper education to teach a safe progression of exercises and how to avoid damaging stresses cannot be overemphasized. To return to the activity that caused the injury prior to regaining functional pain-free motion, strength, endurance, and skill to match the demands of the task would probably result in recurring injury and pain.

Cumulative Trauma: Chronic Recurring Pain

Tissue Response: Chronic Inflammation

When connective tissue is injured, it goes through a healing process of repair, which was described in the preceding sections. However, in connective tissue that is repetitively stressed beyond the ability to repair itself, the inflammatory process is perpetuated. Proliferation of fibroblasts with increased collagen production and degradation of mature collagen leads to a predominance of new, immature collagen. This has an overall weakening effect on the tissue. In addition, myofibroblastic activity continues, which may lead to progressive limitation of motion.[27]

Causes of Chronic Inflammation

Prolonged or recurring pain and resulting limitations in activity and function occur as a result of stress being imposed on tissues that are unable to respond to the repetitive or excessive nature of the stress.

Overuse, cumulative trauma, repetitive strain. These are terms descriptive of the repetitive nature of the precipitating event.[9] Repetitive microtrauma or repeated strain overload over time results in structural weakening, or fatigue breakdown, of connective tissue, with collagen fiber cross-link breakdown and inflammation. Initially, the inflammatory response from the microtrauma is subthreshold but eventually builds to the point of perceived pain and resulting dysfunction.

Repetitive microtrauma to tendons may lead to tendon degeneration.[29] It has been reported that inflammation occurs in the early stages of tendinopathy, but when tendons become degenerative, inflammation largely disappears, leading some to state that this is not an inflammatory condition.[23,27,29] Histological findings in tendinopathy have shown a poor healing response with collagen degeneration, fiber thinning and disorientation, hypercellularity, and scattered vascular ingrowth.[26,27] The underlying abnormalities resulting in a weakened tendon are not quickly resolved resulting in loss of function.[26]

Trauma. Trauma that is followed by superimposed repetitive trauma results in a condition that never completely heals. This may be the result of too early return to high-demand functional activities before the original injury has properly healed. The continued re-injury leads to the symptoms of chronic inflammation and dysfunction.

Reinjury of an "old scar." Scar tissue is not as compliant as surrounding, undamaged tissue. If the scar adheres to the surrounding tissues or is not properly aligned to the stresses imposed on the tissue, there is an alteration in the force transmission and energy absorption. This region becomes more susceptible to injury with stresses that normal, healthy tissue could sustain.

Contractures or poor mobility. Faulty postural habits or prolonged immobility may lead to connective tissue contractures that become stressed with repeated or vigorous activity.

Contributing Factors

By the nature of the condition, there is usually some factor that perpetuates the problem. Not only should the tissue at fault and its stage of pathology be identified, but the *mechanical cause* of the repetitive trauma needs to be defined. Evaluate for faulty mechanics or faulty habits that may be sustaining the irritation. Possibilities include:

- *Imbalance between the length and strength of the muscles* around the joint, leading to faulty mechanics of joint motion or abnormal forces through the muscles
- *Rapid or excessive repeated eccentric demand* placed on muscles not prepared to withstand the load, leading to tissue failure, particularly in the musculotendinous region[18]
- *Muscle weakness* or an inability to respond to excessive strength demands that results in muscle fatigue with decreased contractility and shock-absorbing capabilities and increased stress to supporting tissues[18]
- *Bone malalignment or weak structural support* that causes faulty joint mechanics of force transmission through the joints (poor joint stability as in a flat foot)[20]
- *Change in the usual intensity or demands* of an activity such as an increase or change in an exercise or a training routine or change in job demands[18]
- *Returning to an activity too soon after an injury* when the muscle-tendon unit is weakened and not ready for the stress of the activity[7,10]
- *Sustained awkward postures or motions*, placing parts of the body at a mechanical disadvantage, leading to postural fatigue or injury
- *Environmental factors* such as a work station not ergonomically designed for the individual, excessive cold, continued vibration, or inappropriate weight-bearing surface (for standing, walking, or running), which may contribute to any of the previous factors
- *Age-related factors* such that a person attempts activities that could be done when younger but his or her tissues are no longer in condition to withstand the sustained stress[21]
- *Training errors*, such as using improper methods, intensity, amount, or equipment, or the condition of the participant, which lead to abnormal stresses.[20]
- *A combination of several contributing factors* are frequently seen that cause the symptoms

Management Guidelines: Chronic Inflammation

When the patient has symptoms and signs of chronic inflammation, it is imperative that treatment begins by controlling the inflammation—in other words, treat it as an acute condition. Once the inflammation is under control, treatment progresses to dealing with the impairments and functional limitations. Management guidelines are summarized in Box 10.5.

Chronic Inflammation: Acute Stage

When the inflammatory response is perpetuated because of continued tissue irritation, the inflammation must be controlled to avoid the negative effects of continued tissue breakdown and excessive scar formation.

- In addition to the use of modalities and resting the part, it is imperative to identify and then modify the mechanism

BOX 10.5 MANAGEMENT GUIDELINES—
Chronic Inflammation/Cumulative Trauma Syndromes

Impairments of Body Structure and Function:

Pain in the involved tissue of varying degrees:

- Only after doing repetitive activities
- When doing repetitive activities as well as after
- When attempting to do activities; completion of activity is prevented
- Continued and unremitting

Soft tissue, muscle, and/or joint contractures or adhesions that limit normal ROM or joint play

Connective tissue weakness in painful region

Muscle weakness and poor muscular endurance in postural or stabilizing muscles as well as primary muscle at fault

Imbalance in length and strength between antagonistic muscles; biomechanical dysfunction

Faulty position or movement pattern perpetuating the impairment

Decreased use of the region for activities and participation in desired life situation

Plan of Care	Interventions During Chronic Inflammation
1. Educate the patient.	1. Counsel as to cause of chronic irritation and need to avoid stressing the part while inflamed. Adapt the environment to decrease tissue stress. Implement a home exercise program to reinforce therapeutic interventions.
2. Promote healing; decrease pain and inflammation.	2. Cold, compression, massage Rest to the part (stop mechanical stress, orthosis, tape, cast)
3. Maintain integrity and mobility of involved tissue.	3. Nonstressful passive movement, massage, and muscle setting within limits of pain
4. Develop support in related regions	4. Posture training Stabilization exercises

Plan of Care	Interventions—Controlled Motion and Return to Function Phases
1. Educate the patient.	1. Ergonomic counseling in ways to prevent recurrence Home instruction in safe progression of stretching and strengthening exercises. Instruction on signs of too much stress (see Box 10.3)
2. Develop strong, mobile scar.	2. Friction massage Soft tissue mobilization
3. Develop a balance in length and strength of the muscles.	3. Correct cause of faulty muscle and joint mechanics with appropriately graded stretching and strengthening exercises.
4. Progress functional independence.	4. Train muscles to function according to demand; provide alternatives or support if they cannot. Train coordination and timing. Develop endurance.
5. Analyze job/activity.	5. Adapt home, work, and sport environment/tools.

PRECAUTION: If there is progressive loss of ROM as the result of stretching, do not continue to stretch. Reevaluate the condition and determine if there is still a chronic inflammation with contracting scar or if there is protective muscle guarding. Emphasize stabilizing the part and training in safe adaptive patterns of motion.

of chronic irritation with appropriate biomechanical counseling. This requires cooperation from the patient. Describe to the patient how the tissue reacts and breaks down under continued inflammation and explain the strategy of intervention.

CLINICAL TIP

Use of illustrations to help the patient understand the mechanism of tissue breakdown with cumulative trauma syndromes—such as what happens when a person repeatedly hits a thumbnail with a hammer or repeatedly irritates or scrapes a skin area before it heals—helps the patient visualize the repeated trauma occurring in the musculoskeletal problem and understand the need to quit "hitting or irritating the sore."

- Initially, allow only nonstressful activities.
- Initiate exercises at safe, nonstressful intensities in the involved tissues, as with any acute lesion, and at appropriate corrective intensities in related regions without stressing the involved tissues.

Subacute and Chronic Stages of Healing Following Chronic Inflammation

Once the constant pain from the chronic inflammation has decreased, progress the patient through an exercise program with controlled stresses until the connective tissue in the involved region has developed the ability to withstand the stresses imposed by the functional activities.

- Locally, if there is a chronic, contracted scar that limits range or continually becomes irritated with microruptures, mobilize the scar in the tissue using friction massage, soft tissue manipulation, or stretching techniques. If inflammation results from the stretching maneuvers, treat it as an acute injury. Because chronic inflammation can lead to proliferation of scar tissue and contraction of the scar, progressive loss of range is a warning sign that the intensity of stretching is too vigorous.
- Muscle guarding could be a sign that the body is attempting to protect the part from excessive motion. In this case, the emphasis is on developing stabilization of the part and training in safe adaptive patterns of motion.
- Identify the cause of the faulty muscle and joint mechanics. Strengthening and stabilization exercises, in conjunction with working or recreational adaptations, are necessary to minimize the irritating patterns of motion.
- Because chronic irritation problems frequently result from an inability to sustain repetitive activities, muscle endurance is an appropriate component of the muscle re-education program. Consider endurance in the postural stabilizers as well as in the prime movers of the desired functional activity.
- As when treating patients in the chronic stage of healing, progress exercises to develop functional independence. The exercises become specific to the demand and include timing, coordination, and skill.
- Work-conditioning and work-hardening programs may be used to prepare the person for return to work; training in sports-specific exercises is important for returning an individual to sports.

NOTE: Specific overuse syndromes are covered in detail in the respective chapters associated with the involved region.

Independent Learning Activities

Critical Thinking and Discussion

1. Your patient has experienced an injury to a muscle. Describe the symptoms that he or she will experience during each stage of inflammation and repair and describe the principles of the exercise intervention that should be used during each stage. Once you have identified the principles, choose a commonly injured muscle, such as the hamstrings, and describe the symptoms, test results, goals, treatment plan, and actual interventions that you would use for each stage of intervention.
2. Repeat Activity 1, except use a ligamentous injury, such as strain of the humeroulnar ligament or anterior talofibular ligament.
3. Describe the mechanism of injury for common overuse syndromes, such as lateral epicondylitis or shin splints, and explain the differences between such an injury and an acute traumatic injury.

REFERENCES

1. Arnheim, DD, and Prentice, WE: *Principles of Athletic Training,* ed. 3. Boston: McGraw-Hill, 1997.
2. Bandy, WD: Functional rehabilitation of the athlete. *Orthop Phys Ther Clin North Am* 1:269–281, 1992.
3. Barrick, EF: Orthopedic trauma. In Kauffman, TL (ed): *Geriatric Rehabilitation Manual.* New York: Churchill Livingstone, 1999.
4. Cailliet, R: *Soft Tissue Pain and Disability,* ed. 3. Philadelphia: F.A. Davis, 1996.
5. Cummings, GS, and Tillman, LJ: Remodeling of dense connective tissue in normal adult tissues. In Currier, DP, and Nelson, RM (eds): *Dynamics of Human Biologic Tissues.* Philadelphia: F.A. Davis, 1992, p 45.
6. Cyriax, J: *Textbook of Orthopaedic Medicine, Vol 1. Diagnosis of Soft Tissue Lesions,* ed. 8. London: Bailliere & Tindall, 1982.
7. Davenport, TE, et al: The EdUReP model for nonsurgical management of tendinopathy. *Phys Ther* 85(10):1093–1103, 2005.
8. Enwemeka, CS: Connective tissue plasticity: ultrastructural, biomechanical, and morphometric effects of physical factors on intact and regenerating tendons. *J Orthop Sports Phys Ther* 14(5):198–212, 1991.
9. Guidotti, TL: Occupational repetitive strain injury. *Am Fam Physician* 45:585–592, 1992.
10. Hawley, DJ: Health status assessment. In Wegener, ST (ed): *Clinical Care in the Rheumatic Diseases.* Atlanta: American College of Rheumatology, 1996.
11. Helgeson, K: Soft-tissue, joint, and bone disorders. In Goodman, CC, and Fuller, KS (eds): *Pathology: Implications for the Physical Therapist,* ed. 4, St. Louis, Elsevier/Saunders, 2015, p. 1285.
12. Isernhagen, SJ: Exercise technologies for work rehabilitation programs. *Orthop Phys Ther Clin North Am* 1:361–374, 1992.
13. Keene, J, and Malone, TR: Ligament and muscle-tendon unit injuries. In Malone, TR, McPoil, TG, and Nitz, AJ (eds): *Orthopaedic and Sports Physical Therapy,* ed. 3. St. Louis: CV Mosby, 1997, p 135.
14. Kellet, J: Acute soft tissue injuries: a review of the literature. *Med Sci Sports Exerc* 18:489–500, 1986.
15. Khan, JM, and Scott, A: Mechanotherapy: how physical therapists' prescription of exercise promotes tissue repair. *Br J Sports Med* 43:247–252, 2009.
16. Lazaro, RT and Bkurke-Doe, A: Injury, inflammation, healing, and repair. In Goodman, CC, and Fuller, KS (eds): *Pathology: Implications for the Physical Therapist,* ed. 4, St. Louis, Elsevier/Saunders. 2015, p 216.
17. McGinty, JB (ed): *Operative Arthroscopy.* Philadelphia: Lippincott-Raven, 1996.
18. Noonan, TJ, and Garrett, WE: Injuries at the myotendinous junction. *Clin Sports Med* 11:783–806, 1992.
19. Noyes, FR, et al: Advances in understanding of knee ligament injury, repair, and rehabilitation. *Med Sci Sports Exerc* 16:427–443, 1984.
20. Pease, BJ: Biomechanical assessment of the lower extremity. *J Orthop Phys Ther Clin North* Am 3:291–325, 1994.
21. Puffer, JC, and Zachazewski, JE: Management of overuse injuries. *Am Fam Physician* 38:225–232, 1988.
22. Rabin, A: Evidence in practice: is there evidence to support the use of eccentric strengthening exercises to decrease pain and increase function in patients with patellar tendinopathy? *Phys Ther* 86(3):450–456, 2006.
23. Riley, G: Tendinopathy—from basic science to treatment. *Nat Clin Pract Rheumatol* 4(2):82–89, 2008.
24. Salter, RB: *Continuous Passive Motion, A Biological Concept.* Baltimore: Williams & Wilkins, 1993.
25. Salter, RB: *Textbook of Disorders and Injuries of the Musculoskeletal System,* ed. 3. Baltimore: Williams & Wilkins, 1999.
26. Scott, A, Backman, L, and Speed, C: Tendinopathy: update on pathophysiology. *J Orthop Sports Phys Ther* 45(11):833–841, 2015.
27. Sharma, P, and Maffulli, N: Biology of tendon injury: healing, modeling, and remodeling. *J Musculoskelet Neuronal Interact* 6(2):181–190, 2006.
28. Tillman, LJ, and Cummings, GS: Biologic mechanisms of connective tissue mutability. In Currier, DP, and Nelson, RM (eds): *Dynamics of Human Biologic Tissues.* Philadelphia: FA Davis, 1992, p 1.
29. Wang, J: Mechanobiology of tendon. *J Biomech* 39(9):1563–1582, 2006.
30. Wilk, KE, and Arrigo, C: An integrated approach to upper extremity exercises. *J Orthop Phys Ther Clin North Am* 1:337–360, 1992.
31. Wynn Parry, CB, and Stanley, JK: Synovectomy of the hand. *Br J Rheumatol* 32:1089–1095, 1993.

CHAPTER 11

Joint, Connective Tissue, and Bone Disorders and Their Management

CAROLYN KISNER, PT, MS ■ JACOB N. THORP, PT, DHS, OCS, MTC ■ KAREN HOLTGREFE, PT, DHS, OCS

General guidelines and principles for developing exercise interventions for patients with soft tissue lesions were presented in the previous chapter. The purpose of this chapter is to present principles of management of selected pathologies that affect joints, connective tissue, and bone. Characteristics of arthritis, fibromyalgia, myofascial pain syndrome, osteoporosis, and fractures are described in conjunction with the effects of therapeutic exercise on impairments associated with these pathological conditions.

Arthritis: Arthrosis

Arthritis is inflammation of a joint. There are many types of arthritis, both inflammatory and noninflammatory, that affect joints and other connective tissues in the body. The most common types treated by therapists are rheumatoid arthritis and osteoarthritis. *Arthrosis* is limitation of a joint without inflammation. Unless the cause of the joint problems is known, such as recent trauma or immobility, medical intervention is necessary to diagnose and medically manage the pathology. Traumatic arthritis may require aspiration if there is bloody effusion.

The therapist examines, integrates, and evaluates the presenting information and then develops a plan of care by selecting interventions to safely meet the goals. Knowledge of the underlying pathology is important in order to understand the prognosis and safely manage the patient's impairments, activity limitations, and participation restrictions.[61,75]

Clinical Signs and Symptoms

Signs and symptoms common to all types of arthritic conditions generally include the following.

Impaired Mobility

The patient usually presents with signs typical of joint involvement that include a characteristic pattern of limitation (called a capsular pattern), usually a firm end-feel (unless acute—then the end-feel may be guarded), decreased and possibly painful joint play, and joint swelling (effusion).[79] Additional signs and symptoms may be present depending on the specific disease process. Table 11.1 summarizes the characteristic signs and symptoms of osteoarthritis and rheumatoid arthritis.

Arthrosis may be present if the individual is recovering from a fracture or other problem requiring immobilization. There is limited joint play along with other connective tissue and muscular contractures limiting range of motion (ROM).

Impaired Muscle Performance

Weakness from disuse or reflex inhibition of stabilizing muscles occurs when there is joint swelling or pain. Muscle weakness or inhibition leads to imbalances in strength and flexibility and poor support for the involved joints. Asymmetry in muscle pull may be a deforming force to the joints, and poor muscle support allows the joint to be more susceptible to trauma; conversely, good muscle support helps protect an arthritic joint.

TABLE 11.1 Comparison of Osteoarthritis and Rheumatoid Arthritis[6,23,68,140]

Characteristics	Osteoarthritis	Rheumatoid Arthritis
Age of onset	Usually after age of 40	Usually begins between age 15 and 50
Progression	Usually develops slowly over many years in response to mechanical stress	May develop suddenly, within weeks or months
Manifestations	Cartilage degradation, altered joint architecture, osteophyte formation	Inflammatory synovitis and irreversible structural damage to cartilage and bone
Joint involvement	Affects a few joints (usually asymmetrical); typically: —DIP, PIP, 1st CMC of hands —Cervical and lumbar spine —Hips, knees, 1st MTP of feet	Usually affects many joints, usually bilateral; typically: —MCP and PIP of hands, wrists, elbows, shoulders —Cervical spine —MTP, talonavicular and ankle
Joint signs and symptoms	Morning stiffness (usually < 30 min), increased joint pain with weight-bearing and strenuous activity; crepitus and loss of ROM	Redness, warmth, swelling, and prolonged morning stiffness; increased joint pain with activity
Systemic signs and symptoms	None	General feeling of sickness and fatigue, weight loss, and fever; may develop rheumatoid nodules; may have ocular, respiratory, hematological, and cardiac symptoms

Impaired Balance

Patients may develop balance deficits because of altered or decreased sensory input from joint mechanoreceptors and muscle spindle. This is particularly a problem with weight-bearing joints.[99,155]

Activity Limitations and Participation Restrictions

The ability to carry out home, community, work-related, or social activities may be minimally to significantly restricted. Adaptive and assistive devices may be used by the patient to improve function or help prevent possible deforming forces. A variety of classification systems and functional instruments have been developed for use in clinical studies as well as routine practice to measure patient function and outcomes in response to interventions.[65]

Rheumatoid Arthritis

Rheumatoid arthritis (RA) is an autoimmune, chronic, inflammatory, systemic disease primarily of unknown etiology affecting the synovial lining of joints as well as other connective tissue. It is characterized by a fluctuating course, with periods of active disease and remission. The onset and progression vary from mild joint symptoms with aching and stiffness to abrupt swelling, stiffness, and progressive deformity.[4,6,87,97,124] The revised criteria for classification of RA are summarized in Box 11.1. This classification criteria was

BOX 11.1 Criteria for Diagnosis of Rheumatoid Arthritis[2]

1. Confirmed presence of synovitis in at least one joint, absence of an alternative diagnosis
2. Achievement of a total score ≥ 6 out of 10 from the following 4 domains:
   A. Number and site of involved joints.
      - 1 large joint = 0
      - 2–10 large joints = 2
      - 1–3 small joints = 2
      - 4–10 small joints = 3
      - >10 joints (at least 1 small) = 5
   B. Serology (at least 1 test result required)
      - Negative RF and negative ACPA = 0
      - Low-positive RF or low-positive ACPA = 2
      - High-positive RF or high-positive ACPA = 3
   C. Acute-phase reactants (at least 1 test is needed)
      - Normal CRP and normal ESR = 0
      - Abnormal CRP and abnormal ESR = 1
   D. Duration of Symptoms
      - < 6 weeks = 0
      - ≥ 6 weeks = 1

RF = rheumatoid factor; ACPA = anti-citrullinated protein; CRP = C-reactive protein; ESR = erythrocyte sedimentation rate.

developed in order to focus on identification of the disease at earlier stages rather than features present in late stages of the disease.[2]

Characteristics of RA

- This disease is characterized by symmetric, erosive synovitis[4] with periods of exacerbation (flare) and remission.[6,87,97] Joints are characteristically involved with early inflammatory changes in the synovial membrane, peripheral portions of the articular cartilage, and subchondral marrow spaces. In response, granulation tissue (pannus) forms, covers, and erodes the articular cartilage, bone, and ligaments in the joint capsule. Adhesions may form, restricting joint mobility. With progression of the disease, cancellous bone becomes exposed. Fibrosis, ossific ankylosis, or subluxation may eventually cause deformity and disability (Figs. 11.1, 11.2, and 11.3).[6,124]

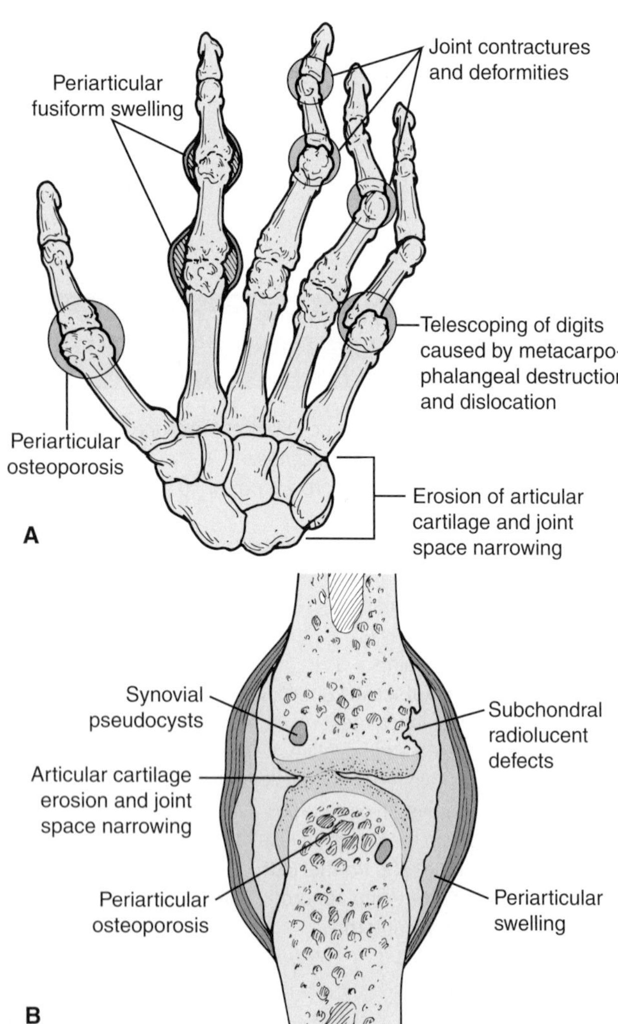

FIGURE 11.1 (A) Radiographic hallmarks and typical joint deformities with rheumatoid arthritis in small joints of the wrist and hand. **(B)** Radiographic hallmarks of rheumatoid arthritis in large joints.

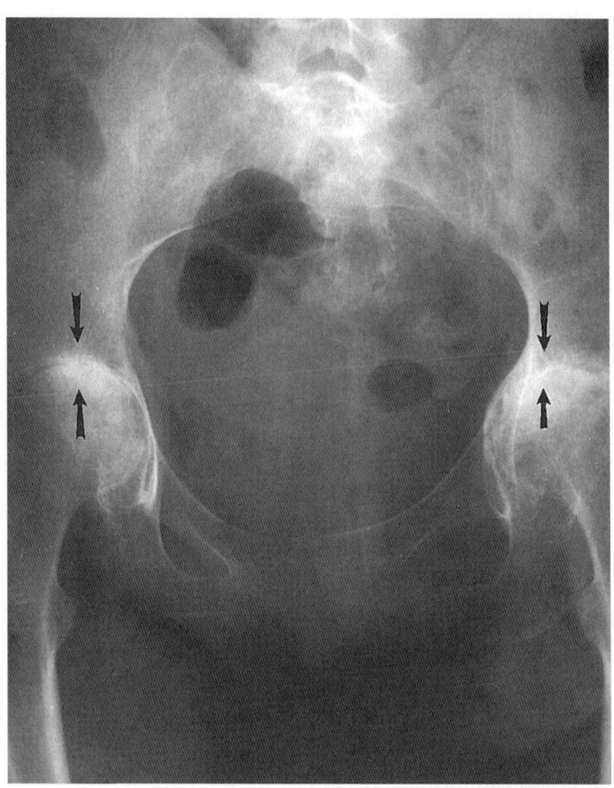

FIGURE 11.2 Advanced rheumatoid arthritis of the hip joints. Note that the destruction caused by rheumatoid arthritis involves the entire joint space and the bone on both sides of the joint. This causes concentric joint space narrowing. The arrows point to small areas of sclerosis on the weight-bearing superior joint surfaces. Although not a primary characteristic of RA, sclerotic repair (primary in degenerative joint disease) can occur over the years in between episodes of RA exacerbations. *(From McKinnis, LN:* Fundamentals of Musculoskeletal Imaging, *ed. 4. Philadelphia: F.A. Davis, 2014, p 53, with permission.)*

- Inflammatory changes also occur in tendon sheaths (tenosynovitis); if subjected to recurring friction, the tendons may fray or rupture.
- Extra-articular pathological changes sometimes occur; they include rheumatoid nodules, atrophy and fibrosis of muscles with associated muscular weakness, fatigue, and mild cardiac changes.
- Progressive deterioration and decline in the functional level of the individual attributed to the muscular changes and progressive muscle weakness is often seen,[35] leading to major economic loss and significant impact on families.[4]
- The degree of involvement varies. Some individuals experience mild symptoms that require minor lifestyle changes and mild anti-inflammatory medications. Others experience significant pathological changes in the joints that require major adaptations in lifestyle. Loss of joint function is irreversible, and often surgery is needed to decrease pain and improve function. Early recognition is essential during the initial stages, with referral to a rheumatologist for diagnosis and

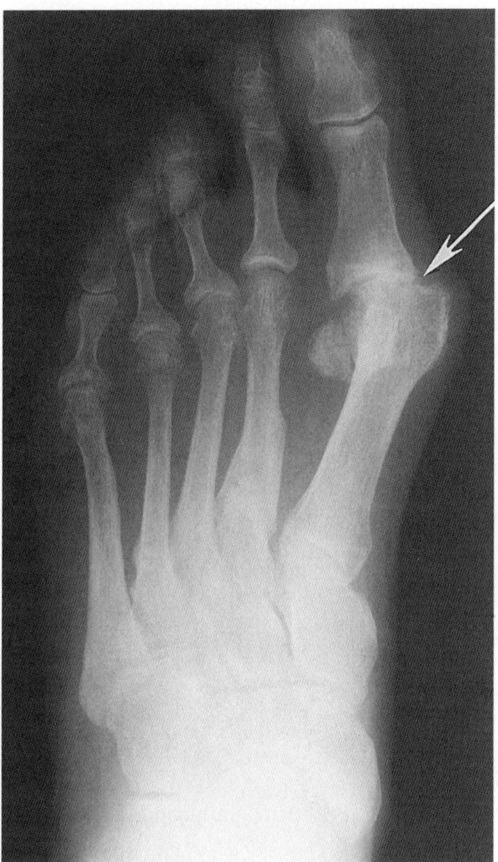

FIGURE 11.3 Rheumatoid arthritis of the foot. First metatarsophalangeal joint shows severe *erosion* of the joint surface with *subluxation* of the metatarsal (arrow). *(From McKinnis, LN:* Fundamentals of Musculoskeletal Imaging, *ed. 4. Philadelphia: F.A. Davis, 2014, p 57, with permission.)*

medical management to control the inflammation and minimize joint damage.[23]

Signs and Symptoms: Periods of Active Disease

- With synovial inflammation, there is effusion and swelling of the joints, which cause aching and limited motion. Joint stiffness is prominent in the morning. Usually there is pain on motion, and a slight increase in skin temperature can be detected over the joints. Pain and stiffness worsen after strenuous activity.
- Onset is usually in the smaller joints of the hands and feet, most commonly in the proximal interphalangeal joints. Usually symptoms are bilateral.
- With progression, the joints become deformed and may ankylose or subluxate.
- Pain is often felt in adjoining muscles, and eventually muscle atrophy and weakness occur. Asymmetry in muscle strength and alterations in the line of pull of muscles and tendons add to the deforming forces.
- The person often experiences nonspecific symptoms such as low-grade fever, loss of appetite and weight, malaise, and fatigue.

Principles of Management: Active Inflammatory Period of RA

Management guidelines are summarized in Box 11.2.

- *Patient education.* Because periods of active disease may last several months to more than a year, begin education in the overall treatment plan, safe activity, and joint protection (Box 11.3) as soon as possible.[100] It is imperative to involve the patient in the management, so he or she learns how to conserve energy and avoid potential deforming stresses during activities and when exercising.
- *Joint protection and energy conservation.* It is important that the patient learns to respect fatigue and, when tired, rests to minimize undue stress to all the body systems. Because inflamed joints are easily damaged and rest is encouraged to protect the joints, teach the patient how to rest the joints in nondeforming positions and to intersperse rest with ROM.
- *Joint mobility.* Use gentle grade I and II distraction and oscillation techniques to inhibit pain and minimize fluid stasis. Stretching techniques are not performed when joints are swollen.
- *Exercise.* The type and intensity of exercise vary depending on the symptoms. Encourage the patient to do active exercises through as much ROM as possible (not stretching). If active exercises are not tolerated owing to pain and swelling, passive ROM is used. Once symptoms of pain and signs of swelling are controlled with medication, progress exercises as if subacute.

CLINICAL TIP

Therapeutic exercises cannot positively alter the pathological process of RA, but if administered carefully, they can help prevent, retard, or correct the mechanical limitations and deforming forces that occur and, therefore, help maintain function.

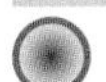

FOCUS ON EVIDENCE

The ***Clinical Practice Guidelines (CPGs) for Therapeutic Exercise in the Management of Rheumatoid Arthritis in Adults*** recommend therapeutic exercise based on the strength of evidence from comparative controlled trials.[18]

- *Functional training.* Modify any activities of daily living (ADL) needed in order to protect the joints. If necessary, use orthoses and assistive devices to provide protection.

PRECAUTIONS: Secondary effects of steroidal medications may include osteoporosis and ligamentous laxity, so use exercises that do not cause excessive stress to bones or joints.

CONTRAINDICATIONS: Do not perform stretching techniques across swollen joints. When there is effusion, limited motion is the result of excessive fluid in the joint space. Forcing motion on the distended capsule overstretches it, leading to

BOX 11.2 MANAGEMENT GUIDELINES—
Rheumatoid Arthritis/Active Disease Period

Impairments, Activity Limitations, and Participation Restrictions:

Tenderness and warmth over the involved joints with joint swelling
Muscle guarding and pain on motion
Joint stiffness and limited motion
Muscle weakness and atrophy
Potential deformity and ankylosis from the degenerative process and asymmetric muscle pull
Fatigue, malaise, and sleep disorders
Restricted ADLs and IADLs

Plan of Care	Interventions
1. Educate the patient.	1. Inform the patient on importance of rest, joint protection, energy conservation, and performance of ROM. Teach home exercise program and activity modifications that conserve energy and minimize stress to vulnerable joints.
2. Relieve pain and muscle guarding and promote relaxation.	2. Modalities Gentle massage Immobilize in orthoses Relaxation techniques Medications as prescribed by physician
3. Minimize joint stiffness and maintain available motion.	3. Passive or active-assistive ROM within limits of pain; gradual progression as tolerated. Gentle joint techniques using grade I or II oscillations.
4. Minimize muscle atrophy.	4. Gentle isometrics in pain-free positions, progression to ROM when tolerated.
5. Prevent deformity and protect the joint structures.	5. Use of supportive and assistive equipment for all pathologically active joints. Good bed positioning while resting. Avoidance of activities that stress the joints.

PRECAUTIONS: Respect fatigue and increased pain; do not overstress osteoporotic bone or lax ligaments.

CONTRAINDICATIONS: Do not stretch swollen joints or apply heavy resistance exercise that cause joint stress or place deforming forces on the joint.

subsequent hypermobility (or subluxation) when the swelling abates. It may also increase the irritability of the joint and prolong the joint reaction.

Principles of Management: Subacute and Chronic Stages of RA

As the intensity of pain, joint swelling, morning stiffness, and systemic effects diminish, the disease is considered subacute. Often medications can decrease the acute symptoms, so the patient can function as if in the subacute stage. The chronic stage occurs between exacerbations. This may be very short in duration, or it may last many years.

- *Treatment approach.* The treatment approach is the same as with any subacute and chronic musculoskeletal disorder, except appropriate precautions must be taken because the pathological changes from the disease process make the tissues more susceptible to damage.
- *Joint protection and activity modification.* Continue to emphasize the importance of protecting the joints by adapting the environment, and by modifying activity, using orthoses, and assistive devices.
- *Flexibility and strength.* To improve function, exercises should be aimed at improving flexibility, muscle strength, and muscle endurance within the tolerance of the joints.[35]
- *Cardiopulmonary endurance.* Nonimpact or low-impact conditioning exercises—such as aquatic exercise, cycling, aerobic dancing, and walking/running—performed within the tolerance of the individual improve aerobic capacity and physical activity and decrease depression and anxiety.[10,105,132,159] Group activities, such as water aerobics, also provide social support in conjunction with the activity. One randomized review suggested that aerobic training also has a positive impact on the cardiovascular status of patients with RA.[104]

BOX 11.3 Principles of Joint Protection and Energy Conservation[88,123]

- Monitor activities and stop when discomfort or fatigue begins to develop.
- Use frequent but short episodes of exercise (three to five sessions per day) rather than one long session.
- Alternate activities to avoid fatigue.
- Decrease level of activities or omit provoking activities if joint pain develops and persists for more than 1 hour after activity.
- Maintain a functional level of joint ROM and muscular strength and endurance.
- Balance work and rest to avoid muscular and total body fatigue.
- Increase rest during flares of the disease.
- Avoid deforming positions.
- Avoid prolonged static positioning; change positions during the day every 20 to 30 minutes.
- Use stronger and larger muscles and joints during activities whenever possible.
- Use appropriate adaptive equipment.

PRECAUTIONS: The joint capsule, ligaments, and tendons may be structurally weakened by the rheumatic process (also as a result of using steroids), so the dosage of stretching and joint mobilization techniques used to counter any contractures or adhesions must be carefully graded.

CONTRAINDICATIONS: Vigorous stretching or high-velocity thrust manipulative techniques.

FOCUS ON EVIDENCE

Several systematic reviews looking at best evidence for the use of therapeutic exercise in the treatment of RA have been published.[18,34,38,104] Although there are few randomized well-controlled studies looking at the outcome of exercise, studies of various strength do support that therapeutic exercise, including functional strengthening and aerobic exercise, is beneficial for patients with RA, demonstrating relief of pain, improved muscle strength, and functional status. In one of the reviews,[38] investigators found that moderate- or high-intensity exercise in patients with RA had a minimal effect on disease activity and radiological evidence of damage in the hands and feet, and that there is insufficient radiological evidence to determine the effect in large joints. The reviewers also reported that long-term moderate- or high-intensity exercises (individualized to protect radiologically damaged joints) improve aerobic capacity, muscle strength, functional ability, and psychological well-being in patients with RA.[38] A more recent systematic review of randomized research studies on the effect of aerobic exercise in adults with RA found that aerobic exercise improved the quality of life, decreased pain, increased function, and did not exacerbate the disability or radiologic indicators.[136]

Osteoarthritis: Degenerative Joint Disease

Osteoarthritis (OA) is a chronic degenerative disorder primarily affecting the articular cartilage of synovial joints, with eventual bony remodeling and overgrowth at the margins of the joints (spurs and lipping) (Fig. 11.4). There is also progression of synovial and capsular thickening and joint effusion. The impairments from OA lead to activity limitations and participations restrictions in a substantial number of people with a significant social and financial impact as a result of surgical and medical interventions.[19]

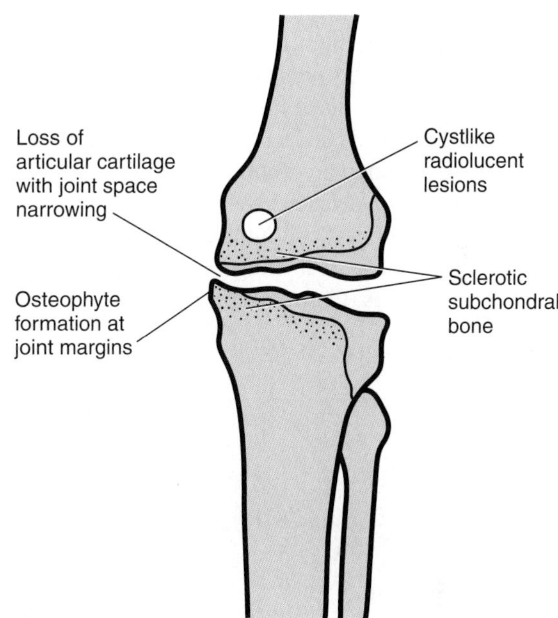

FIGURE 11.4 Radiographic hallmarks of osteoarthritis. *(From McKinnis, LN:* Fundamentals of Musculoskeletal Imaging, *ed. 4. Philadelphia: F.A. Davis, 2014, p 60, with permission.)*

Although the etiology of OA is not known, mechanical injury to the joint due to a major stress or repeated minor stresses and poor movement of synovial fluid when the joint is immobilized are possible causes. Rapid destruction of articular cartilage occurs with immobilization because the cartilage is not being bathed by moving synovial fluid and is thus deprived of its nutritional supply.[66,87]

OA is also genetically related, especially in the hands and hips and, to some degree, in the knees.[42] Other risk factors that show a direct relationship to OA are obesity, weakness of the quadriceps muscles, joint impact, sports with repetitive impact and twisting (e.g., soccer, baseball pitching, and football), and occupational activities such as jobs that require kneeling and squatting with heavy lifting.[42]

The perception of pain in OA is complex in that it is influenced not only by local factors, but also activation of central pain-producing pathways and psychological fear avoidance behaviors in some individuals.[84,146]

Characteristics of OA

- With degeneration, there may be capsular laxity as a result of bone remodeling and capsule distention, leading to hypermobility or instability in some ranges of joint motion. With pain and decreased willingness to move, contractures eventually develop in portions of the capsule and overlying muscle, so as the disease progresses, motion becomes more limited.[42,68]
- The cartilage splits and thins out, losing its ability to withstand stress. As a result, crepitation or loose bodies may occur in the joint. Eventually, subchondral bone becomes exposed. There is increased density of the bone along the joint line, with cystic bone loss and osteoporosis in the adjacent metaphysis. During the early stages, the joint is usually asymptomatic because the cartilage is avascular and aneural, but pain becomes constant in later stages.
- Affected joints may become enlarged. Heberden's nodes (enlargement of the distal interphalangeal joints of the fingers) and Bouchard's nodes (enlargement of the proximal interphalangeal joints) are common.
- Most commonly involved are weight-bearing joints (hips and knees), the cervical and lumbar spine, and the distal interphalangeal joints of the fingers and carpometacarpal joints of the thumbs (Figs. 11.5 and 11.6).

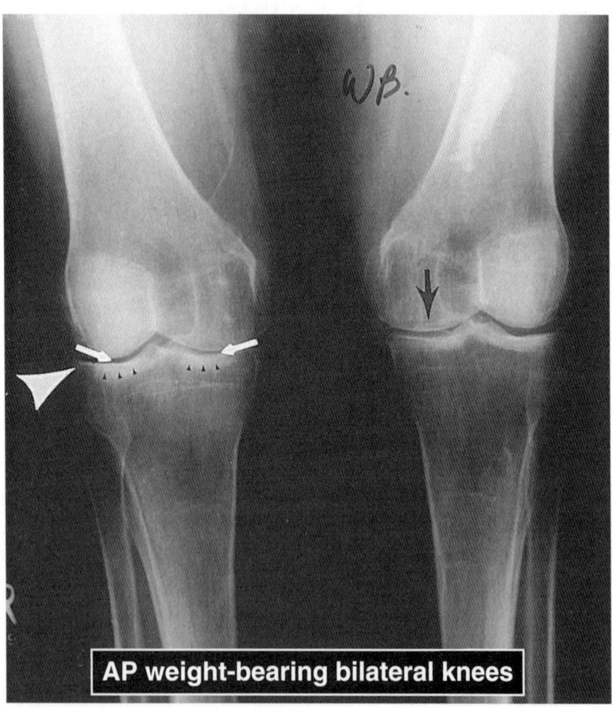

FIGURE 11.5 Osteoarthritis of the knees in a 66-year-old woman. This film was made with the patient weight-bearing. At the patient's right knee, osteoarthritis is evidenced by narrowed joint space (white arrows), osteophyte formation at the joint margins (large white arrowhead), and sclerotic subchondral bone (small black arrowheads) of both the medial and lateral tibial plateaus. At the patient's left knee, it is interesting to note that in the area of minimal weight-bearing stress, the subchondral bone has lost density, and rarefaction is present on the medial aspect of the joint. *(From McKinnis, LN:* Fundamentals of Musculoskeletal Imaging, *ed. 4. Philadelphia: F.A. Davis, 2014, p 60, with permission.)*

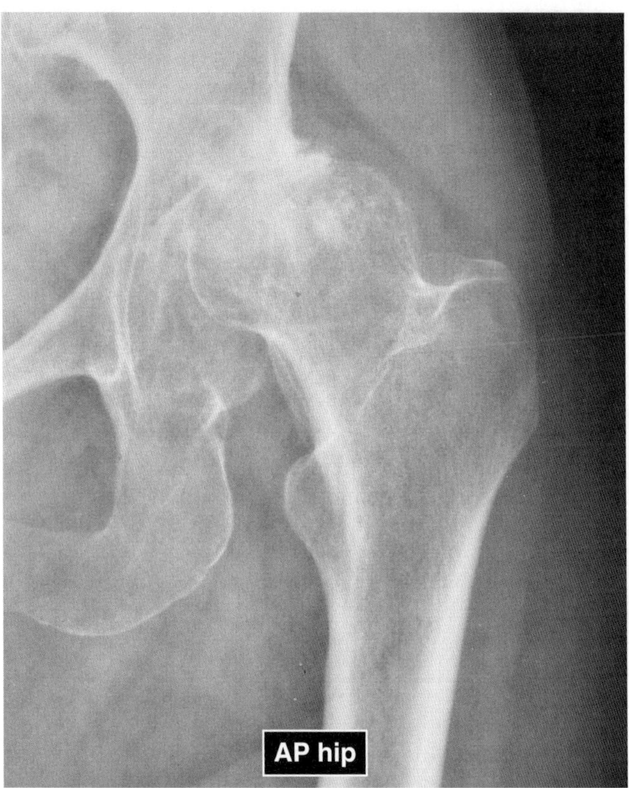

FIGURE 11.6 Severe osteoarthritis of the hip with pseudocysts. The radiolucent cyst-like areas (*ovals*) are caused by intrusion of synovial fluid into areas of subchondral bone that have become weakened by microfractures. *(From McKinnis, LN:* Fundamentals of Musculoskeletal Imaging, *ed. 4. Philadelphia: F.A. Davis, 2014, p 61, with permission.)*

Principles of Management: OA

Pain, joint stiffness, decreased muscle performance, and decreased aerobic capacity affect the quality of life and increase the risk for disability for the individual with OA.[43] Therapeutic exercise and manual therapy interventions are important in the comprehensive management of OA.[116] Management guidelines are summarized in Box 11.4.

- *Patient instruction.* Education includes teaching the patient about the disease of OA, how to protect the joints while remaining active, and how to manage the symptoms. Instruct the patient in a home program of safe exercises to improve muscle performance, ROM, and endurance.
- *Pain management—early stages.* Pain and feelings of "stiffness" are common complaints during the early stages. Pain usually occurs because of excessive activity and stress on the involved joint and is relieved with rest. Brief periods of stiffness occur in the morning or after periods of inactivity. This is due to gelling of the involved joints after periods of inactivity.[3] Movement relieves the stasis and feelings of stiffness. Help the patient find a balance between activity and rest and correct biomechanical stresses in order to prevent, retard, or correct the mechanical limitations.
- *Pain management—late stages.* During the late stages of the disease, pain is often present at rest. The pain may be from

BOX 11.4 MANAGEMENT GUIDELINES—
Osteoarthritis

Impairments, Activity Limitations, and Participation Restrictions:

Pain with mechanical stress or excessive activity
Pain at rest in the advanced stages
Stiffness after inactivity
Limitation of motion
Muscle weakness
Decreased proprioception and balance
Functional limitations in ADLs and IADLs

Plan of Care	Intervention
1. Educate the patient.	1. Teach about deforming forces and prevention. Teach home exercise program to reinforce interventions and minimize symptoms.
2. Decrease effects of stiffness.	2. Active ROM Joint-play mobilization techniques
3. Decrease pain from mechanical stress and prevent deforming forces.	3. Orthoses and/or assistive equipment to minimize stress or to correct faulty biomechanics, strengthen supporting muscles. Alternate activity with periods of rest.
4. Increase ROM.	4. Stretch muscle, joint, or soft tissue restrictions with specific techniques.
5. Improve neuromuscular control, strength, and muscle endurance.	5. Low-intensity resistance exercises and muscle repetitions.
6. Improve balance.	6. Balance training activities.
7. Improve physical conditioning.	7. Nonimpact or low-impact aerobic exercise.

PRECAUTIONS: When strengthening supporting muscles, increased pain in the joint during or following resistive exercises probably means that too great a weight is being used or stress is being placed at an inappropriate part of the ROM. Analyze the joint mechanics and at what point during the range the greatest compressive forces are occurring. Maximum resistance exercise should not be performed through that ROM.

involvement of subchondral bone, synovium, and the joint capsule with local inflammatory and molecular stimuli or from psychological or neurophysiological influences.[84,146] In the spine, if bony growth encroaches on the nerve root, there may be radicular pain (see Chapter 15). Emphasize activity modification and use of assistive devices and/or orthoses to minimize joint stress. Pain that cannot be managed with activity modification (as described in the following bullet) and analgesics is usually an indication for surgical intervention.

- *Assistive and supportive devices and activity.* With progression of the disease, the bony remodeling, swelling, and contractures alter the transmission of forces through the joint, which further perpetuates the deforming forces and creates joint deformity. Functional activities become more difficult. Adaptive or assistive devices, such as a raised toilet seat, cane, or walker, may be needed to decrease painful stresses and maintain function. Shock-absorbing footwear may decrease the stresses in OA of the knees.[42] Aquatic therapy and group-based exercise in water decreases pain and improves physical function in patients with lower extremity OA.[36,154]
- *Resistance exercise.* Progressive weakening in the muscle occurs either from inactivity or from inhibition of the neuronal pools. Weak muscles may add to the joint dysfunction.[3] Strong muscles protect the joint. Use resistance exercises, within the tolerance of the joint, as part of the patient's exercise program. Avoid deforming forces and heavy weights that the patient cannot control or that cause joint pain. Adaptations include the use of multiple-angle isometrics in pain-free positions, applying resistance only through arcs of motion that are not painful, and use of a pool to decrease weight-bearing stresses and improve functional performance.[52]
- *Stretching and joint mobilization.* Use stretching and joint mobilization techniques to increase mobility. Teach the patient self-stretching/flexibility exercises and the importance of movement through the full available ROM to counteract the developing restrictions.

FOCUS ON EVIDENCE

In a single-blind, randomized clinical trial of 109 patients with OA of the hip, specific manipulations and mobilizations of the hip joint were reported to have a greater success rate than active exercise for improving muscle function and joint motion. Outcomes measured were perceived improvement after treatment (81% vs. 50%), pain, stiffness, hip function, and ROM.[69]

- *Balance activities.* Joint position sense may be impaired.[155] (See Chapter 8 for principles and description of balance exercises.) Nontraditional forms of exercise, such as tai chi, have been found to be effective for improving balance in patients with OA.[147]
- *Aerobic conditioning.* Instruct the patient in exercises designed to improve cardiopulmonary function.[17] It is also proposed that aerobic exercise be used to improve pain and treat underlying depression and anxiety that may be comorbidities in OA.[120,146] The choice of exercise should have low impact on the joints, such as walking, biking, or swimming. Avoid activities that cause repetitive intensive loading of the joints, such as jogging and jumping.

FOCUS ON EVIDENCE

The ***CPGs for Therapeutic Exercises and Manual Therapy in the Management of Osteoarthritis***, which is based on a systematic review of randomized controlled and observational studies, highlight the importance of therapeutic exercise and physical activity to increase strength, manage pain, and improve aerobic capacity and functional status in patients with OA.[19]

The ***CPGs for the Management of Osteoarthritis in Adults Who Are Obese or Overweight*** identified that diet programs combined with physical activity (both aquatic and land-based exercises that include endurance, strength, ROM, and aerobic training) are more beneficial showing improved clinical outcomes of pain relief, improved strength, functional status, and quality than physical activity alone or diet alone and therefore recommends that physical therapists work with an interdisciplinary team that includes dietitians when treating this population.[20]

Two systematic reviews of studies designed to examine evidence of the effects of exercise in the management of hip and knee OA describe support for aerobic exercise and strengthening exercises to reduce pain and disability.[127,128] The consensus of expert opinion cited by Roddy[123] is that there are few contraindications and that exercise is relatively safe in patients with OA but that exercise should be individualized and patient-centered with consideration for age, comorbidity, and general mobility.

A systematic review of 15 randomized controlled trials that looked at therapies to improve balance and reduce falls in older individuals with OA of the knee concluded that strength training, tai chi, and aerobic exercises improved balance and reduced the risk of falls in this population and that balance outcomes were not significantly improved with water-based exercises.[99]

In another study that followed 285 patients with knee OA for 3 years, investigators found that factors that protected the individuals from poor functional outcomes included strength and activity level, as well as factors such as mental health, self-efficacy, and social support.[138]

Fibromyalgia and Myofascial Pain Syndrome

Fibromyalgia (FM) and myofascial pain syndrome (MPS) are chronic pain syndromes that are often confused and interchanged. Each has a distinct proposed etiology. Individuals with FM process nociceptive signals differently from individuals without FM,[131,148] and individuals with MPS have localized changes in the muscle.[45,56,57,137,141,148] Although there are some similarities, the differences are significant and determine the method of treatment. They are summarized in Table 11.2.

Fibromyalgia

FM, as defined by the American College of Rheumatology in 1990,[158] is a chronic condition characterized by widespread pain that affects multiple body regions (right or left side, upper or lower half of the person) plus the axial skeleton and that has lasted for more than 3 months. Additional symptoms include 11 of 18 tender points at specific sites throughout the body (Fig. 11.7), nonrestorative sleep, and morning stiffness. A final common problem is fatigue with subsequent diminished exercise tolerance.

TABLE 11.2 Similarities and Differences Between Fibromyalgia and Myofascial Pain Syndrome

Similarities	
Pain in muscles Decreased ROM Postural stresses	
Differences	
Fibromyalgia	**Myofascial Pain Syndrome**
Tender points at specific cites	Trigger points in muscle
No referred patterns of pain	Referred patterns of pain
No tight band of muscle	Tight band of muscle
Fatigue and waking unrefreshed	No related fatigue complaints

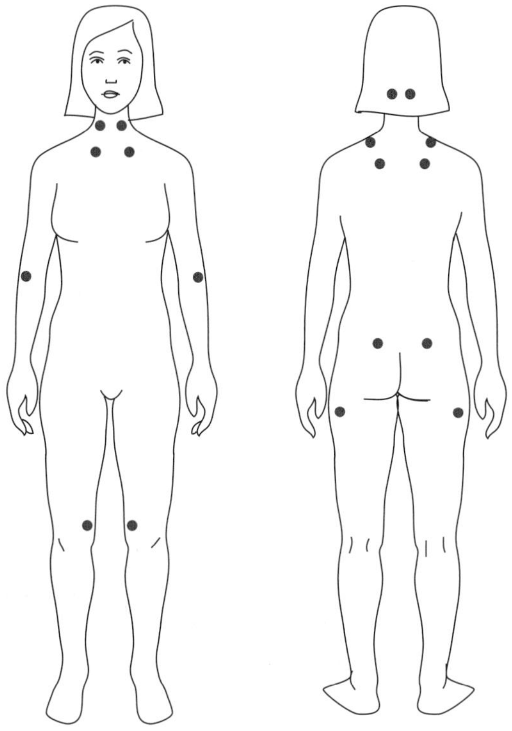

FIGURE 11.7 Fibromyalgia tender points.

FOCUS ON EVIDENCE

In 2010, Wolfe and associates[157] developed preliminary diagnostic criteria to complement the ACR-specific criteria, including the measurement of symptom severity. The authors recommend the following: widespread pain index (WPI) ≥ 7 _and_ symptom severity (SS) scale ≥ 5, *OR* WPI 3 to 6 _and_ SS ≥ 9. These criteria correctly classified 88.1% of individuals with FM determined from the ACR classification without tender point palpation. The SS scale includes items such as somatic symptoms, not feeling refreshed after sleeping, fatigue, and cognition.

Prevalence of FM

It is estimated that 2% of the population—nearly 5 million adults 18 years old or older—have FM, with women affected far more than men (3.4% to 0.5%). In addition, the prevalence increases with age, with 7.4% of women ages 70 to 79 affected.[86] While women have also been shown to have greater pain intensity, men report a longer duration of symptoms of FM.[30]

Characteristics of FM

The characteristics of FM include the following:[148]

- The first symptoms of FM can occur at any age but usually appear during early to middle adulthood.
- For many of those diagnosed, the symptoms develop after physical trauma such as a motor vehicle accident or a viral infection.
- Although the symptoms vary from individual to individual, there are several hallmark complaints. Pain is usually described as muscular in origin and is predominantly reported in the scapula, head, neck, chest, and low back.
- Another common report is a significant fluctuation in symptoms. Some days an individual may be pain free, whereas other days the pain is markedly increased. Most individuals report that when they are in a cycle in which the symptoms are diminished, they try to do as much as possible. This is usually followed by several days of worsening symptoms and an inability to carry out their normal daily activities. This is often the response to exercise.
- Individuals with FM have a higher incidence of tendonitis, headaches, irritable bowel, temporal mandibular joint dysfunction, restless leg syndrome, mitral valve prolapse, anxiety, depression, and memory problems.

Factors Contributing to a Flare

Although FM is a noninflammatory, nondegenerative, nonprogressive disorder, several factors may affect the severity of symptoms. These factors include environmental stresses, physical stresses, and emotional stresses. FM is not caused by these various stresses, but it is aggravated by them.

- Environmental stresses include weather changes, especially significant changes in barometric pressure, cold, dampness, fog, and rain.
- Physical stresses include repetitive activities, such as typing, playing piano, vacuuming; prolonged periods of sitting and/or standing; and working rotating shifts.
- Emotional stresses are any normal life stresses.

Principles of Management: FM

Individuals with FM typically have lower tolerance for activities and exercise. People often report "good" and "bad" days in which they have more or less energy, respectively. Learning to pace activities throughout the day so as to not push too hard or too little is an important component of the intervention plan.

CLINICAL TIP

The Fibromyalgia Impact Questionnaire (FIQ), originally developed in 1991,[24] includes 10 items that assess the patient's overall function status. A higher score is correlated with lower function. It has been used in many studies to report progress[90, 96,152] and predict successful outcomes.[121,152] The FIQ has been modified in 1997, 2002, and 2009 and has been shown to be valid and reliable. The minimal clinically important difference has been estimated to be 14%.

- *Exercise.* Research supports the use of exercise, particularly aerobic exercise, to reduce the most common symptoms associated with FM.[21,22,25,26,41,95]

FOCUS ON EVIDENCE

The ***CPGs for Aerobic Fitness Exercises in the Management of Fibromyalgia: Part 1***[21] and the ***CPGs for Strengthening Exercises in the Management of Fibromyalgia: Part 2***[22] show emerging evidence that aerobic fitness and strengthening exercises are beneficial in the overall management of FM for pain relief, muscle strength, quality of life, self-efficacy, and decreased depression and that progressive strengthening programs do not cause an exacerbation of exercise-induced FM symptoms. The guidelines also recommend individualized programs with multiple treatment regimens be used due to the variability in FM symptoms.[22]

An updated evidence report from the Cochrane Collaborative[27] summarized the findings of five randomized trials related to FM and exercise. The reviewers concluded that while moderate-intensity and moderate- to high-intensity resistance training can improve function, pain, strength, and tenderness in people with FM, an 8-week aerobic program has even better outcomes. Furthermore, the authors reported that a 12-week low-intensity exercise program was superior to flexibility training for improving pain and function.

While these findings are supported elsewhere in the literature,[28] some evidence suggests aerobic activity is sufficient.[62,76,78] In a randomized controlled trial, 199 participants with FM tracked their daily steps. It was determined that people averaging at least 5,000 steps each day had better functional outcomes after 12 weeks as compared with those individuals with less than 5,000 steps a day.[78] Still other research promotes a combination of strength and flexibility training for improved functional outcomes and decreased pain.[55,58,71,82,134,135]

- *Additional interventions*[64]
  - Prescription medication
  - Over-the-counter medication
  - Instruction in pacing activities, in an attempt to avoid fluctuations in symptoms
  - Cognitive behavior therapy
  - Avoidance of stress factors
  - Decreasing alcohol and caffeine consumption
  - Diet modification
  - Manual therapy[29,160]

CLINICAL TIP

When beginning any type of exercise with individuals with FM, it is best to begin at lower levels than recommended by the American College of Sports Medicine[5] for aerobic and strengthening and to slowly increase the activity. If the exercise leads to an increase in FM symptoms, reduce the intensity, while encouraging continued participation in the exercise.[21,22,25,70]

Myofascial Pain Syndrome

Myofascial pain syndrome (MPS) is defined as a chronic, regional pain syndrome.[56,141] The hallmark classification of MPS comprises the myofascial trigger points (MTrPs) in a muscle that have a specific referred pattern of pain (Fig. 11.8), along with sensory, motor, and autonomic symptoms.[40,45,56,142,143]

The *trigger point* is defined as a hyperirritable area in a tight band of muscle.[45,48,49,56,74] The pain from these points is described as dull, aching, and deep.

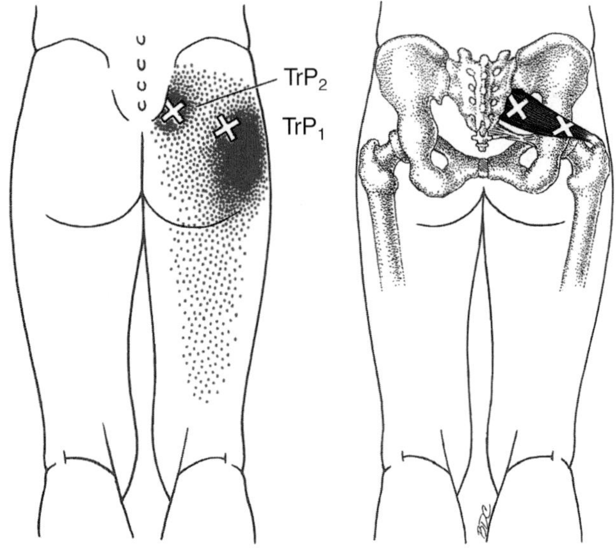

FIGURE 11.8 Composite pattern of pain (dark red) referred from trigger points (TrPs) (Xs) in the right piriformis muscle (medium red). The lateral X (TrP$_1$) indicates the most common TrP location. The red stippling locates the spillover part of the pattern that may be felt as less intense pain than that of the essential pattern (solid red). The spillover pain may be absent. *(From Travell, JG, Simmons, DG:* Myofascial Pain and Dysfunction: The Trigger Point Manual: The Lower Extremities, Vol 2. *Baltimore: Williams & Wilkins, 1992, p 188, with permission.)*

Possible Causes of Trigger Points

Although the etiology of trigger points is not completely understood, some potential causes are:[56,141-143]

- Chronic overload of the muscle that occurs with repetitive activities or that maintain the muscle in a shortened position.
- Acute overload of muscle, such as slipping and catching oneself, picking up an object that has an unexpected weight, or following trauma such as in a motor vehicle accident.
- Poorly conditioned muscles compared to muscles that are exercised on a regular basis.

- Postural stresses such as sitting for prolonged periods of time, especially if the workstation is not ergonomically correct, and leg length differences.
- Poor body mechanics with lifting and other activities.

FOCUS ON EVIDENCE

Recently researchers have looked at the contribution of MTrPs as a contributing factor in chronic headaches,[133] tension type headaches,[46,47] mechanical neck pain,[31,44,122,161] and shoulder disorders.[31,67,92,133] Additionally, Iglesias-Gonzalez and associates[74] compared active and latent trigger points (LTrPs) in participants with non-specific low back pain. The authors reported direct correlation with increased number of trigger points and high pain intensity ($p < 0.001$) and worse quality of sleep ($p = 0.03$).

Lucas and associates[91] investigated the muscle activation pattern (MAP) of scapular muscles during arm elevation in pain-free individuals without trigger points and pain-free individuals with LTrPs. The LTrP group had a significant difference in MAP ($p < 0.05$). These individuals were then treated with either a placebo or active intervention to deactivate the trigger point, and the MAP was reassessed. There was a significant difference ($p < 0.05$) in MAP after deactivation of the LTrPs.

Principles of Management: Myofascial Pain Syndrome

Pain from trigger points is described as dull, aching, and deep. Additional impairments from the trigger points include decreased ROM when the muscle is being stretched, decreased strength in the muscle, and increased pain with muscle stretching. The trigger points may be active (producing a classic pain pattern) or latent (asymptomatic unless palpated).

Treatment consists of three main components:[1,16,45,80,94,141-143,150]

- *Correct chronic overload.* Correct contributing factors that cause chronic overload of the muscle, such as faulty posture, repetitive activity, or poor lifting techniques. The correction is often done with education including stressing the importance of taking intermittent mini-breaks. If indicated, an ergonomic assessment of the work environment is performed.
- *Eliminate the trigger point.* Several techniques are used to eliminate trigger points
  - Contract-relax-passive stretch done repeatedly until the muscle lengthens
  - Contract-relax-active stretch also done in repetition
  - Trigger point release
  - Spray and stretch
  - Modalities
  - Dry needling or injection
- *Strengthen muscle.* Exercise prescription, using a muscle endurance protocol, is typically indicated for core and scapular stabilizing muscle groups to improve overall muscle performance.

FOCUS ON EVIDENCE

Dry needling (DN) has been shown to be a low-risk intervention that can decrease pain severity and pain pressure threshold as well as improve functional outcomes in people with MTrPs.[16,83,125,149,161] In a recent randomized controlled trial, Ziaeifar and associates found that DN significantly decreased pain intensity when compared with trigger point compression technique of the upper trapezius.[161] Additionally, a meta-analysis showed both an immediate and 4 week follow-up improvement in pain in the cervicothoracic region when using DN as the intervention.[83]

CLINICAL TIP

If the cause of the trigger point in myofascial pain syndrome is a chronic overload of the muscle, eliminate the contributing factor prior to addressing the trigger point. Initiate muscle strengthening when ROM is restored and the trigger point has been addressed.

Osteoporosis

Osteoporosis is a disease of bone that leads to decreased mineral content and weakening of the bone. This weakening may lead to fractures, especially of the spine, hip, and wrist. Approximately 10 million Americans have osteoporosis, 80% of them women, and an additional 34 million individuals are at increased risk due to decreased bone mass.[109] The diagnosis of osteoporosis is determined by the T-score of a bone mineral density (BMD) scan. The T-score is the number of standard deviations above or below a reference value (young, healthy Caucasian women). The World Health Organization has established the following criteria:[110,151]

- Normal: –1.0 or higher
- Osteopenia: –1.0 to –2.4
- Osteoporosis: –2.5 or less

A decrease of 1 standard deviation represents a 10% to 12% loss of BMD.

Risk Factors

Primary osteoporosis. Risk factors for developing primary osteoporosis include being postmenopausal, Caucasian or Asian descent, family history, low body weight, little or no physical activity, diet low in calcium and vitamin D, and smoking.[51,59,111] Additional risk factors include prolonged bed rest and advanced age. (Refer to Chapter 24 for additional information on osteoporosis in the older population.)

Secondary osteoporosis. Secondary osteoporosis develops owing to other medical conditions (i.e., gastrointestinal diseases, hyperthyroidism, chronic renal failure, and excessive alcohol consumption) and the use of certain medications such as glucocorticoids.[51,112,151] Regardless of etiology, osteoporosis is detected radiographically by cortical thinning, osteopenia (increased bone radiolucency), trabecular changes, and fractures (Figs. 11.9 and 11.10).[102]

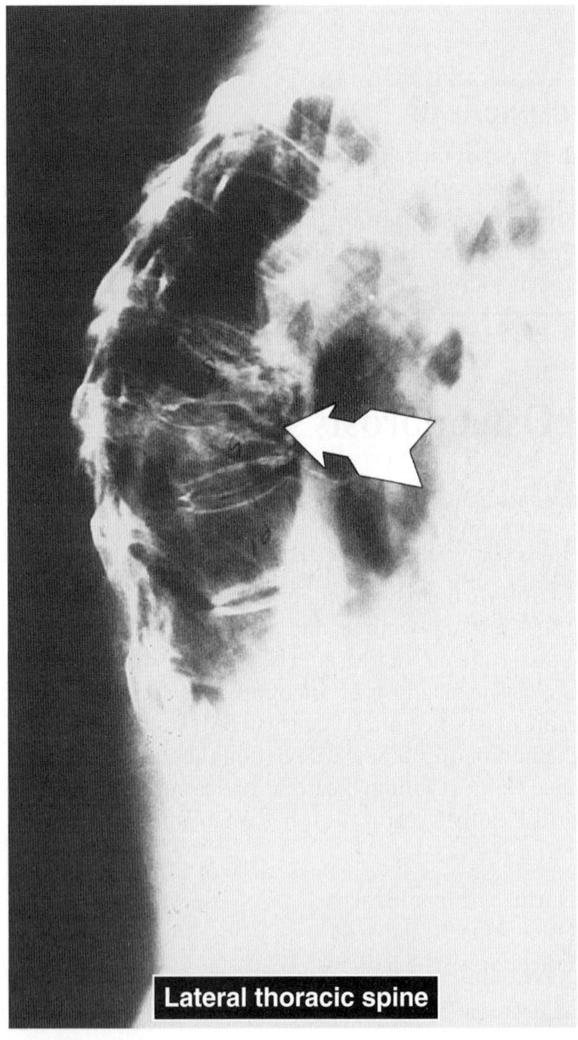

FIGURE 11.9 Osteoporosis of the spine with multiple compression fractures. The arrow points to the T8-T9 disc space, which is deformed by the collapse of these two vertebrae from multiple compression fractures. This 94-year-old woman has severe kyphosis of the thoracic spine (also known as a gibbous deformity) accentuated by vertebral collapse at multiple levels. The whitish area of the lower half of this lateral radiograph is the combined radiodensities of the pelvis and the abdominal organs. *(From McKinnis, LN:* Fundamentals of Musculoskeletal Imaging, *ed. 4. Philadelphia: F.A. Davis, 2014, p 63, with permission.)*

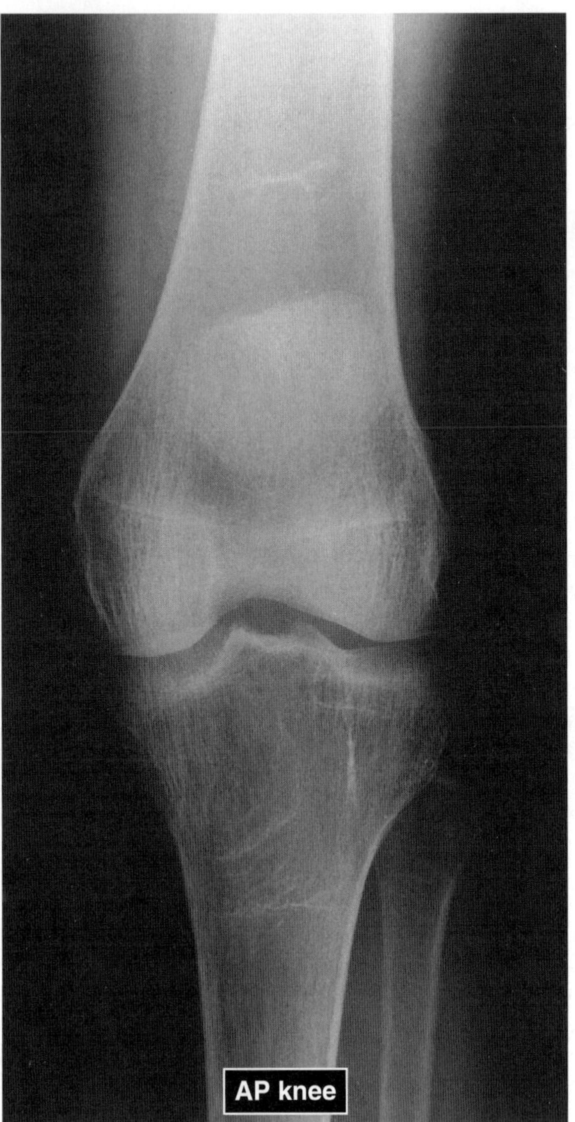

FIGURE 11.10 Osteoporosis is evident in this knee by the accentuation of the remaining trabeculae. The trabeculae have diminished in number and thickness, and the remaining vertically oriented trabeculae stand out as thin, delicate line images. *(From McKinnis, LN:* Fundamentals of Musculoskeletal Imaging, *ed. 4. Philadelphia: F.A. Davis, 2014, p 63, with permission.)*

Prevention of Osteoporosis

The National Osteoporosis Foundation (NOF) recommends four ways to prevent osteoporosis.[113]

- Eating foods that are good for bone health, such as fruits and vegetables
- Maintaining a balanced diet that is rich in calcium and vitamin D
- Performing regular weight-bearing exercise
- Following a healthy lifestyle with moderate alcohol consumption (limit 2-3 drinks per day) and no smoking

Bone is living tissue that is continually replacing itself in response to the daily demands placed on it. Normally, this continual replacement keeps our bone at its optimum strength.

Cells in bone called osteoclasts resorb bone, especially if calcium is needed for particular body functions and not enough is obtained in the diet. Another type of cell, the osteoblast, builds bone. This cycle is usually kept in balance with bone resorption equaling bone replacement until the third decade of life. At this point, peak bone mass should be reached. With increasing age, there is a shift to greater resorption. For women, resorption is accelerated during menopause owing to the decrease in estrogen.[114,116,117,151] Both exercise and pharmacological therapy have been shown to be effective in the prevention of decreased bone mass density.[54,72,89] Bleicher et al[11] tracked the bone density of 1,100 men, aged 70 to 97 years, for 2 years. They concluded that walking, improved balance, and the use of beta blockers were found to retard the bone absorption process.

Physical Activity

Physical activity has been shown to have a positive effect on bone remodeling. In children and adolescents, this activity may increase the peak bone mass. In adults, it has been shown to maintain or increase bone density; in the elderly, it has been shown to reduce the effects of age-related or disuse-related bone loss.[51,115] Maintenance of, or an increase in, bone density is important for preventing fractures associated with osteoporosis. Weak bones due to osteoporosis have been attributed to causing more than 1.5 million fractures per year at a cost of $19 billion dollars. Many of these individuals never return to their previous functional level.[151]

Effects of Exercise

Muscle contraction (e.g., strengthening exercises and resistance training) and mechanical loading (weight bearing) deform bone. This deformation stimulates osteoblastic activity and improves BMD.[144]

 **FOCUS ON EVIDENCE**

Martyn-St James and Carroll[98] completed a meta-analysis of prescribed walking programs on BMD at the hip and spine in postmenopausal women. Results reported no increase in BMD at the spine, but a significant increase at the femoral neck.

Huntoon, Schmidt, and Sinaki[73] completed a retrospective analysis of medical records comparing the refracture rate following vertebral compression fractures in patients instructed in a back extension program following percutaneous vertebroplasty to those who did not perform the exercises. The nonexercise group refractured within an average of 4.5 months, whereas the exercise group average time to refracture was 20.4 months.

An evidence report from the Cochrane Collaborative[14] summarized the findings of 18 randomized trials related to exercise and osteoporosis in women. The reviewers concluded that exercise, particularly fast walking, was effective on the BMD of the spine and hip. Resistance and weight-bearing exercises were also beneficial on the BMD of the spine.

In a meta-analysis, it was concluded that lower extremity exercises decreased bone loss in postmenopausal women. Those participants that exercised for either longer duration (12 months) or early postmenopause showed the most significant changes.[126]

Recommendations for Exercise

The NOF recommends weight-bearing exercise in the prevention of osteoporosis but does not specify what type of exercise or how often it should be done. Based on current research, the following recommendations are made.*

- Weight-bearing exercise, such as walking, jogging, climbing stairs, and jumping
- Nonweight-bearing exercise, such as with a bicycle ergometer
- Resistance (strength) training of 8 to 10 exercises that target major muscle groups

Mode: Aerobic

Frequency. Five or more days per week.

Intensity. Thirty minutes of moderate intensity (fast walking) or 20 minutes of vigorous intensity (running). Doing three short bouts per day of 10 minutes of activity is acceptable.

Mode: Resistance

Frequency. Two to three days per week with a day of rest in between each bout of exercise.

Intensity. Eight to 12 repetitions that lead to muscle fatigue.

 **FOCUS ON EVIDENCE**

Weighted vests or backpacks have been shown to improve bone mass density.[129,156] The increased weight has been shown to alter the spinal muscle imbalance and focus more weight bearing to the osseous structures of the spine.[156] If there is a history of vertebral fracture, recommendations are that up to 1 kg can be carried on the back or up to 2 kg on the front.[156] A study by Roghani et al[125] followed three groups of women for 6 weeks that exercised 3 times per week. The groups included a control population and two exercise groups; one with and one without a weighted vest (4%-8% of body weight). It was reported that while both exercise groups had increased bone synthesis and decreased bone resorption, the weighted exercise group also demonstrated improved balance.(See Fig 24.10A & B for pictures of a weighted vest.)

Precautions and Contraindications

- Because osteoporosis changes the shape of the vertebral bodies (they become more wedge shaped), leading to kyphosis, flexion activities and exercise, such as supine curl-ups and sit-ups, as well as the use of sitting abdominal machines, should be avoided. Stress into spinal flexion increases the risk of a vertebral compression fracture.

---

*8,9,12,13,14,14,32,33,50,51,53,60,63,73,77,81,85,98,103,107,108,115,118, 119,130,139,145,151

- Avoid combining flexion and rotation of the trunk to reduce stress on the vertebrae and the intervertebral discs.
- When performing resistance exercise, it is important to increase the intensity progressively but within the structural capacity of the bone.

NOTE: Refer to Chapter 6 for a discussion of pathological fractures and precautions that should be taken during resistance exercise, identified in Box 6.14.

CLINICAL TIP

Utilizing a multimodal program of weight-bearing exercise, balance activities, and strengthening may help reduce the risk of falls and subsequent hip fractures in individuals with osteoporosis.[39,106,141] Walking has good cardiopulmonary benefits, but an exercise program that involves only walking does not appear to have a significant effect on increasing bone density in people that have been diagnosed with osteoporosis.[93,157]

Fractures and Posttraumatic Immobilization

A fracture is a structural break in the continuity of a bone, an epiphyseal plate, or a cartilaginous joint surface.[132] When there is a fracture, some degree of injury also occurs to the soft tissues surrounding the bone. Depending on the site of the fracture, the related soft tissue injury could be serious if a major artery or peripheral nerve is also involved. If the fracture is more central, the brain, spinal cord, or viscera could be involved. Causes and types of fractures are summarized in Table 11.3 and are illustrated in Figures 11.11, 11.12, and 11.13.

TABLE 11.3 Causes and Types of Fractures[132]

Force	Effect on Bone	Type of Fracture
Bending (angulatory)	Long bone bends causing failure on convex side of bend	Transverse or oblique fracture; Greenstick fracture in children
Twisting (torsional)	Spiral tension failure in long bone	Spiral fracture
Straight pulling (traction)	Tension failure from pull of ligament or muscle	Avulsion fracture
Crushing (compression)	Usually in cancellous bone	Compression fracture; Torus (buckle) fracture in children
Repetitive microtrauma	Small crack in bone unaccustomed to the repetitive/rhythmic stress	Fatigue fracture or stress fracture
Normal force on abnormal bone	Such as with osteoporosis, bony tumor, or other diseased bone	Pathological fracture

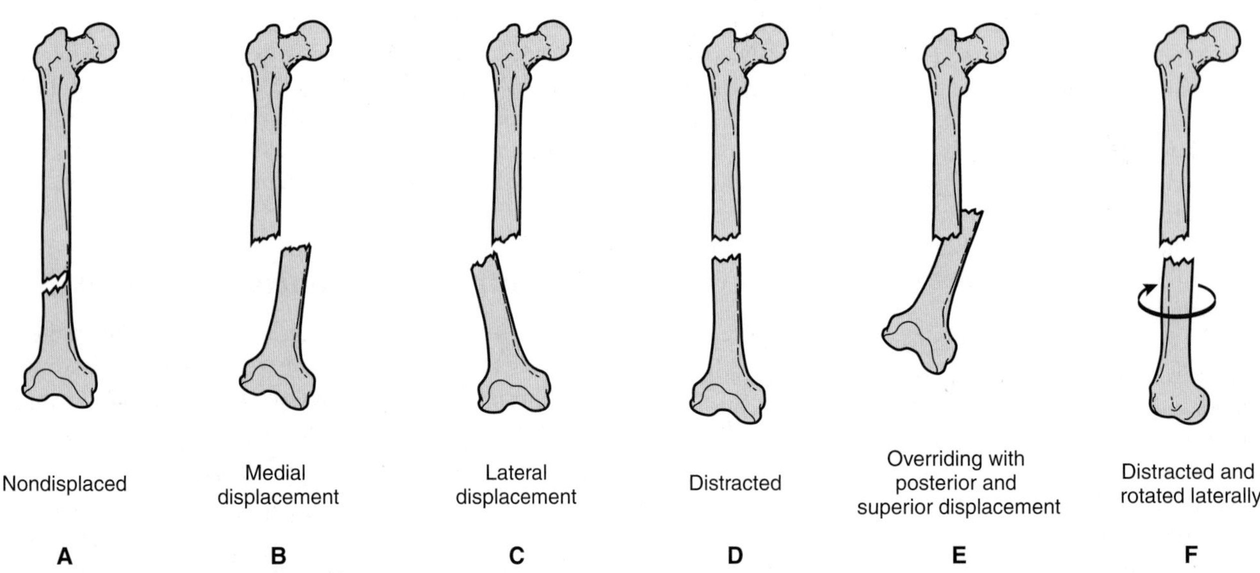

FIGURE 11.11 (A–F) The *position* of fracture fragments may be described by how the *distal* fragment displaces in relationship to the *proximal* fragment. *(From McKinnis, LN:* Fundamentals of Musculoskeletal Imaging, *ed. 4. Philadelphia: F.A. Davis, 2014, p 82, with permission.)*

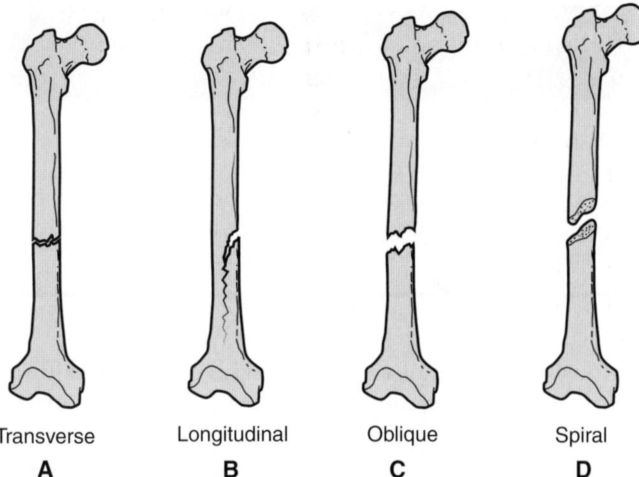

FIGURE 11.12 (A–D) Directions of fracture lines are described in reference to the longitudinal axis of the bone. *(From McKinnis, LN:* Fundamentals of Musculoskeletal Imaging, *ed. 4. Philadelphia: F.A. Davis, 2014, p 83, with permission.)*

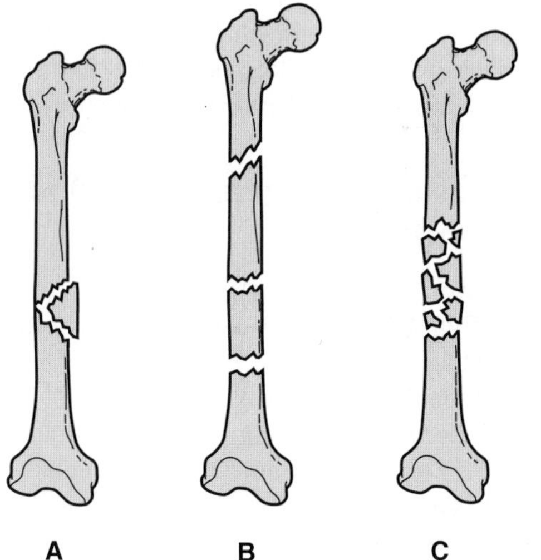

FIGURE 11.13 *Comminuted* fractures are fractures with more than two fragments. Some frequently occurring comminuted fracture patterns are **(A)** the wedge-shaped or butterfly pattern and **(B)** a two- or three-segmented level fracture. **(C)** Other fractures with multiple fragments, be it several or several hundred, are still described as comminuted. *(From McKinnis, LN:* Fundamentals of Musculoskeletal Imaging, *ed. 4. Philadelphia: F.A. Davis, 2014, p 83, with permission.)*

A fracture is identified by:[132]

- *Site:* diaphyseal, metaphyseal, epiphyseal, intra-articular
- *Extent:* complete, incomplete
- *Configuration:* transverse, oblique or spiral, comminuted (two or more fragments)
- *Relationship of the fragments:* undisplaced, displaced
- *Relationship to the environment:* closed (skin intact), open (fracture or object penetrated the skin)
- *Complications:* local or systemic; related to the injury or to the treatment

The diagnosis, reduction, alignment, and immobilization for healing of a fracture are medical procedures and are not discussed in this text. There are times, though, when the therapist provides the initial screening following a traumatic event or examines a patient following repetitive microtrauma; moreover, a patient may sustain an injury while at a therapy session. Hence, the therapist must be aware of symptoms and signs of a potential fracture. If a fracture is suspected, refer the patient for radiographic examination, medical diagnosis, and management. Box 11.5 summarizes the typical symptoms and signs of a possible fracture.

Risk Factors

Risk factors for fracture include:[66]

- Sudden impact (e.g., trauma, accidents, abuse, or assault)
- Osteoporosis (women more than men)
- History of falls (especially with increased age, low body mass index, and low levels of physical activity)
- Repetitive stress (repeated microtrauma)
- Pathology (abnormal fragile bone from neoplastic, poor health, or disease conditions)

(See Chapter 24 for additional information on risk factors in the older population.)

Bone Healing Following a Fracture

Fracture healing has (1) an *inflammatory phase* in which there is hematoma formation and cellular proliferation, (2) *a reparative phase* in which there is callous formation uniting the breach and ossification, and (3) a *remodeling phase* in which there is consolidation and remodeling of the bone.[87]

Cortical Bone Healing

Inflammatory Phase

When the dense cortical bone of the shaft of a long bone is fractured, the tiny blood vessels are torn at the site, resulting in internal bleeding followed by normal clotting. The amount of bleeding depends on the degree of fracture displacement and amount of soft tissue injury in the region.

BOX 11.5 Symptoms and Signs of a Possible Fracture

The following should alert the therapist to a possible fracture.

- History of a fall, direct blow, twisting injury, or accident
- Localized pain aggravated by movement and on weight bearing
- Muscle guarding with passive movement
- Decreased functional use of the part
- Swelling, deformity, or abnormal movement (may or may not be obvious)
- Sharp, localized tenderness at the site

Reparative Phase

The early stages of healing take place in the hematoma. Osteogenic cells proliferate from the periosteum and endosteum to form a thick callus, which envelopes the fracture site. At this stage, the callus does not contain bone and is therefore radiolucent.

As the callus starts to mature, the osteogenic cells differentiate into osteoblasts and chondroblasts. Initially, the chondroblasts form cartilage near the fracture site, and the osteoblasts form primary woven bone.

Remodeling Phase

- *Stage of clinical union.* When the fracture site is firm enough that it no longer moves, it is clinically united. This occurs when the temporary callus consisting of the primary woven bone and cartilage surrounds the fracture site. The callus gradually hardens as the cartilage ossifies (endochondral ossification). On radiographic examination, the fracture line is still apparent, but there is evidence of bone in the callus. Usually at this stage, immobilization is no longer required. Movement of the related joints is allowed with the caution of avoiding deforming forces at the site of the healing fracture. When assessing the site, no movement of the fracture site or pain should be felt by the patient or therapist.
- *Stage of radiological union.* The bone is considered radiographically healed, or consolidated, when the temporary callus has been replaced by mature lamellar bone. The callus is resorbed, and the bone returns to normal.

Rigid Internal Fixation

Sometimes it is necessary to surgically apply an internal fixation device, such as a rod or a plate with screws, to protect a healing bone. This allows the bone to be kept stable as it heals, but disuse osteoporosis of the bone under the device occurs because normal stresses are transmitted through the device and bypass the bone. Usually the fixation device is removed once the fracture is united in order to reverse the osteoporosis. Following removal of the rod or plate, the bone must be protected from excessive stress for several months until the osteoporosis is reversed.

Healing Time

Healing time varies with age of the patient, the location and type of fracture, whether it was displaced, whether surgical repair was needed, amount of soft tissue injury, and the blood supply to the fragments. Healing is assessed by the physician using radiological and clinical examinations. The prognosis for healing is influenced by many factors including health of the individual, age, and use of tobacco. Generally, children heal within 4 to 6 weeks, adolescents within 6 to 8 weeks, and adults within 10 to 18 weeks.[66] Several types of abnormal healing may occur. These are summarized in Box 11.6.

BOX 11.6 Types of Abnormal Healing of Fractures[66]

Malunion: The fracture heals in an unsatisfactory position resulting in a bony deformity.
Delayed union: The fracture takes longer than normal to heal.
Nonunion: The fracture fails to unite with a bony union. There may be a *fibrous union* or a *pseudarthrosis*.

Cancellous Bone Healing

When the sponge-like lattice of the trabeculae of cancellous bone fractures (in the metaphysis of long bones and bodies of short bones and flat bones), healing occurs primarily through formation of an internal callus (endosteal callus). There is a rich blood supply and a large area of bony contact, so union is more rapid than in dense cortical bone.

Cancellous bone is more susceptible to compression forces, resulting in crush or compression fractures. If the surfaces of the fracture are pulled apart, which may occur during reduction of the fracture, healing is delayed.

Epiphyseal Plate Healing

If a fracture involves the epiphyseal plate, there may be growth disturbances and bony deformity as the skeleton continues to mature. The prognosis for growth disturbances depends on the type of injury, age of the child, blood supply to the epiphysis, method of reduction, and whether it is a closed or open injury.

Principles of Management: Period of Immobilization

Local Tissue Response

With immobilization, there is connective tissue weakening, articular cartilage degeneration, muscle atrophy, and contracture development as well as sluggish circulation.[37,66,101] In addition, there is soft tissue injury with bleeding and scar formation.[132] Because immobilization is necessary for bone healing, the soft tissue scar cannot become organized along lines of stress as it develops (described in Chapter 10). Early, nondestructive motion within the tolerance of the fracture site is ideal but usually not feasible unless there is some type of internal fixation to stabilize the fracture site. It is important to keep structures in the related area in a state as near normal as possible by using appropriate exercises without jeopardizing alignment of the fracture site while it is healing. The therapist must be alert to complications that can occur following a fracture (summarized in Box 11.7).

Immobilization in Bed

If bed rest or immobilization in bed is required, as with skeletal traction, secondary physiological changes occur systematically throughout the body. General exercises for the uninvolved portions of the body are initiated to minimize these problems.

Functional Adaptations

If there is a lower extremity fracture, alternative modes of ambulation, such as the use of crutches or a walker, are taught to the patient who is allowed out of bed. The choice of device

BOX 11.7 Complications of Fractures[66]

- *Swelling* that is contained within a compartment (fascial compartment or tight cast) leading to nerve and circulatory compromise.
- *Fat embolism* (may occur with fracture in bones with the most marrow, such as long bones and the pelvis) that migrates to the lungs and blocks pulmonary vessels. This is potentially life-threatening.
- *Skin ulceration, nerve injury, or vascular compromise*
- *Problems with fixation devices* such as displacement of screws and breakage of wires
- *Infection* that occurs locally or systemically
- *Refracture*
- *Delayed union or malunion*

and gait pattern depends on the fracture site, the type of immobilization, and the functional capabilities of the patient. The patient's physician should be consulted to determine the amount of weight bearing allowed. Management guidelines are summarized in Box 11.8.

Postimmobilization

Impairments

- Decreased ROM, joint play, and muscle flexibility.
- Muscle atrophy with weakness and poor muscle endurance.
- Initially, the patient experiences pain as movement begins, but it should progressively decrease as joint movement, muscle strength, and ROM improve.
- If there was soft tissue damage at the time of the fracture, an inelastic scar restricts tissue mobility in the region of the scar.

Management: Postimmobilization

Management guidelines are summarized in Box 11.9.

Consultation with the referring physician is necessary to determine if there is clinical or radiological healing. Until the fracture site is radiologically healed, care should be used any time stress is placed across the fracture site, such as when applying resistance or a stretch force or during weight-bearing activities. Once radiologically healed, the bone has normal structural integrity and can withstand normal stress.

The patient is examined to identify impairments and determine the current functional status, activity level, and desired outcome. ROM, joint mobility, and muscle performance, as well as any other impairments, are measured and documented. Usually all of the joint and periarticular tissues are affected in the region that was immobilized.

Typical interventions include:

- ***Joint mobilization.*** Joint mobilization techniques are effective for regaining lost joint play without traumatizing the articular cartilage or stressing the fracture site.[79] Intervention begins with grade I and II techniques and progresses to more aggressive grades as joint reaction becomes predictable and progresses in intensity as joint reaction becomes predictable.

BOX 11.8 MANAGEMENT GUIDELINES—
Postfracture/Period of Immobilization

Impairments, Activity Limitations, and Participation Restrictions:

Initially, inflammation and swelling

Progressive muscle atrophy, contracture formation, cartilage degeneration, and decreased circulation in the immobilized area

Potential overall body weakening/complications if confined to bed (deep vein thrombosis, pulmonary embolism, pneumonia)

Limited activity and restricted participation in ADLs, IADLs, and work imposed by the fracture site and method of immobilization used

Plan of Care	Intervention
1. Educate the patient.	1. Teach functional adaptations. Teach safe ambulation, bed mobility.
2. Decrease effects of inflammation during acute period.	2. Ice, elevation
3. Decrease effects of immobilization.	3. Intermittent muscle setting. Active ROM to joints above and below immobilized region.
4. If patient is confined to bed, maintain ROM and strength in major muscle groups.	4. ROM activities to all areas not immobilized Resistive exercises to major muscle groups not immobilized, especially in preparation for future ambulation

BOX 11.9 MANAGEMENT GUIDELINES—Postfracture/Postimmobilization

Impairments:

- Pain with movement, which progressively decreases
- Decreased ROM
- Decreased joint play
- Scar tissue adhesions
- Decreased strength and endurance

Plan of Care	Interventions
1. Educate the patient.	1. Inform patient of limitations until fracture site is radiologically healed. Teach home exercises that reinforce interventions.
2. Provide protection until radiologically healed.	2. Use partial weight bearing in lower extremity and nonstressful activities in the upper extremity.
3. Initiate active exercises.	3. Active ROM, gentle multi-angle isometrics
4. Increase joint and soft tissue mobility.	4. Initiate joint play stretching techniques (using grades III and IV) with the force applied proximal to the healing fracture site. For muscle stretching, apply the force proximal to the healing fracture site until radiologically healed.
5. Increase strength and muscle endurance.	5. As the ROM increases and the bone heals, initiate resistive and repetitive exercises.
6. Improve cardiorespiratory fitness.	6. Initiate safe aerobic exercises that do not stress the fracture site until it is healed.

PRECAUTIONS: No stretch or resistive forces distal to the fracture site until the bone is radiologically healed. No excessive joint compression or shear for several weeks after the period of immobilization. Use protected weight bearing until the site is radiologically healed.

- ***PNF Stretching.*** Hold-relax and agonist-contraction techniques are used during the postimmobilization period because the intensity can be controlled by the patient. It is important to monitor the intensity of contraction and to not apply the resistive or stretch force beyond the fracture site until there is radiological healing of the bone in order to avoid a bending force across the fracture site. Once the bone is radiologically healed, the stretch force can be applied beyond the fracture site.
- ***Functional activities.*** The patient can resume normal activities with caution. During the early postimmobilization period, it is important to not traumatize the weakened muscle, cartilage, bone, and connective tissue. Partial weight bearing must be continued for several weeks after a lower extremity fracture until the fracture site is completely healed and able to tolerate full weight bearing.
- ***Muscle performance: Strengthening and muscle endurance.*** For 2 to 3 weeks following immobilization, because neither the bone nor cartilage can tolerate excessive compressive or bending forces, exercises are initiated with light isometrics. As joint play and ROM improve, progression is made to light resistance through the available range. The resistive force should be applied proximal to the fracture site until the bone is radiologically healed. Once healed, PRE and other more intense dynamic exercises can be initiated.
- ***Scar tissue mobilization.*** If there is restricting scar tissue, manual techniques to mobilize the scar are used. The choice of technique depends on the tissue involved.

Independent Learning Activities

Critical Thinking and Discussion

1. Your patient sustained a traumatic knee joint injury in an automobile accident. There is joint effusion, limited ROM, and decreased joint play 2 days after the accident. X-rays have cleared the area of any fractures. The patient guards against motion as you approach the end of the available range. Identify the principles of treatment, the goals, and plan of care for this patient. Describe and practice specific therapeutic techniques that you would use for intervention and describe how you would progress the techniques through the stages of healing.
2. Develop a program of interventions for a patient with OA in the knees who has pain when ascending and descending steps and has difficulty standing up from a chair. What examination procedures do you want to do? What functional tests do you want to document? How would the program differ for an individual with symptoms of RA during a period of active disease (the acute phase)? During a period of remission (the chronic phase)?
3. Describe your plan of care and list specific interventions for a 55-year-old woman who is postmenopausal and has early signs of osteoporosis. What patient instructions would be important to include?
4. An individual sustained a fracture 6 weeks ago, and the limb was just removed from the cast. How does treatment differ from that of other traumatic conditions 6 weeks post injury? Describe what precautions you will follow and why they are important.
5. Your patient was involved in a motor vehicle accident 6 months ago. You saw her 3 months ago, but now she has returned with a diagnosis of FM. Her physician recommends exercise. Describe your treatment program, taking into consideration the characteristics of FM and the benefits and problems of exercise in this population.
6. Your new patient is a secretary who presents with upper back and neck pain. She describes a gradual onset. She reports sitting at a computer for 6 to 8 hours each day and having to take phone calls on a regular basis as well. You examine the patient and find several active MTrPs. Describe your course of treatment for this patient. How will you address the effect her work has on her problem?

REFERENCES

1. Aguila, FJ, et al: Immediate effect of ultrasound and ischemic compression techniques for the treatment of trapezius latent myofascial trigger points in healthy subjects: a randomized controlled study. *J Manipulative Physiol Ther* 32:515–520, 2009.
2. Aletaha, D, et al: 2010 Rheumatoid arthritis classification criteria: an American College of Rheumatology/European League Against Rheumatism collaborative initiative. *Ann Rheum Dis* 69:1580–1588, 2010.
3. American College of Rheumatology Subcommittee on Osteoarthritis Guidelines: Recommendations for the medical management of osteoarthritis of the hip and knee: 2000 update. *Arthritis Rheum* 43(9): 1905–1915, 2000.
4. American College of Rheumatology Subcommittee on Rheumatoid Arthritis Guidelines: 2002 Update. *Arthritis Rheum* 46(2):328–346, 2002.
5. American College of Sports Medicine: *American College of Sports Medicine's Guidelines for Exercise Testing and Prescription,* ed. 8. Philadelphia: Lippincott Williams & Wilkins, 2010.
6. Anderson, RJ: Rheumatoid arthritis: clinical and laboratory features. In Klippel, JH (ed): *Primer on the Rheumatic Diseases,* ed. 12. Atlanta: Arthritis Foundation, 2001, p 218.
7. Bennett, RM, et al: The revised Fibromyalgia Impact Questionnaire (FIQR): validation and psychometric properties. *Arthritis Res Ther* 11(5):R120, 2009.
8. Bergland, A, Thorsen, H, and Kåresen, R: Effect of exercise on mobility, balance, and health-related quality of life in osteoporotic women with a history of vertebral fracture: a randomized, controlled trial. *Osteoporos Int* 22(6):1863–1871, 2011.
9. Bergstrom, I, et al: Physical training preserves bone mineral density in postmenopausal women with forearm fractures and low bone mineral density. *Osteoporos Int* 19:177–183, 2008.
10. Bilberg, A, Ahlmen, M, and Mannerkorpi, K: Moderately intensive exercise in a temperate pool for patients with rheumatoid arthritis: a randomized controlled study. *Rheumatology* (Oxford) 44(4):502–508, 2005.
11. Bleicher, K, et al: Predictors of the rate of BMD loss in older men: findings from the CHAMP study. *Osteoporos Int* 24(7):1951–1963, 2013.
12. Bocalini, DS, et al: Strength training preserves the bone mineral density of postmenopausal women without hormone replacement therapy. *J Aging Health* 21:519–527, 2009.
13. Bolam, KA, van Uffelen, JG, and Taaffe, DR: The effect of physical exercise on bone density in middle-aged and older men: a systematic review. *Osteoporos Int* 24(11):2749–2762, 2013.
14. Bonaiuti, D, et al: Exercise for preventing and treating osteoporosis in postmenopausal women. *Cochrane Database Syst Rev* 2002(3):CD000333.
15. Borg, G, Hassmen, P, and Lagerstrom, M: Perceived exertion related to heart rate and blood lactate during arm and leg exercise. *Eur J Appl Physiol* 65:679–685, 1987.
16. Borg-Stein, J and Iaccarino, MA: Myofascial pain syndrome treatments. *Phys Med Rehabil Clin N Am* 23:357–375, 2014.
17. Brosseau, L, et al: Intensity of exercise for the treatment of osteoarthritis. *Cochrane Database Syst Rev* 2003(2):CD004259.
18. Brosseau, L, et al: Ottawa panel evidence-based clinical practice guidelines for therapeutic exercise in the management of rheumatoid arthritis in adults. *Phys Ther* 84(10):934–972, 2004.
19. Brosseau, L, et al: Ottawa panel evidence-based clinical practice guidelines for therapeutic exercises and manual therapy in the management of osteoarthritis. *Phys Ther* 85(9):907–971, 2005.
20. Brosseau, L, et al: Ottawa panel evidence-based clinical practice guidelines for the management of osteoarthritis in adults who are obese or overweigh. *Phys Ther* 91(6):843–861, 2011.
21. Brosseau, L, et al: Ottawa panel evidence-based clinical practice guidelines for aerobic fitness exercises in the management of fibromyalgia: part 1. *Phys Ther* 88:857–871, 2008.
22. Brosseau, L, et al: Ottawa panel evidence-based clinical practice guidelines for strengthening exercises in the management of fibromyalgia: part 2. *Phys Ther* 88:873–886, 2008.
23. Bruce, ML, and Peck, B: New rheumatoid arthritis treatments. *Holistic Nurs Pract* 19(5):197–204, 2005.

24. Burckhardt, CS, Clark, SR, and Bennett, RM: The Fibromyalgia Impact Questionnaire: development and validation. *J Rheumatol* 18:728–733, 1991.
25. Busch, A, et al: Exercise for treating fibromyalgia syndrome. *Cochrane Database Syst Rev* 2007(4):CD003786.
26. Busch, A, et al: Exercise for fibromyalgia: a systematic review. *J Rheumatol,* 35:1130–1144, 2008.
27. Busch, AJ, et al: Resistance exercise training for fibromyalgia. *Cochrane Database Syst Rev* 2013 (20):CD010884.
28. Carbonell-Baeza, A, et al: Does a 3-month multidisciplinary intervention improve pain, body composition and physical fitness in women with fibromyalgia? *Br J Sports Med*45(15):1189–1195, 2011.
29. Castro-Sánchez, AM, et al: Short-term effects of a manual therapy protocol on pain, physical function, quality of sleep, depressive symptoms, and pressure sensitivity in women and men with fibromyalgia syndrome: a randomized controlled trial. *Clin J Pain* 30(6):589–597, 2014.
30. Castro-Sánchez, AM, et al: Gender differences in pain severity, disability, depression, and widespread pressure pain sensitivity in patients with fibromyalgia syndrome without comorbid conditions. *Pain Med* 13(12): 1639–1647, 2012.
31. Catarero-Villanueva, I, et al: Effectiveness of water physical therapy on pain, pressure pain sensitivity, and myofascial trigger points in breast cancer survivors: a randomized, controlled clinical trial. *Pain Med* 13(11): 1509–1519, 2012.
32. Centers for Disease Control and Prevention: Physical activity for everyone. Available at http://www.cdc.gov/physicalactivity/everyone/guidelines/index.html. Accessed June 3, 2015.
33. Chodzko-Zajko, W, Proctor, D, and Singh, M: American College of Sports Medicine position stand on exercise and physical activity for older adults. *Med Sci Sports Exerc* 41:1510–1530, 2009.
34. Christie, A, et al: Effectiveness of nonpharmacological and nonsurgical interventions for patients with rheumatoid arthritis: an overview of systematic reviews. *Phys Ther* 87(12):1697–1715, 2007.
35. Clark, SR, Burckhardt, CS, and Bennett, RM: The use of exercise to treat rheumatic disease. In Goldberg, L, and Elliot, DL (eds): *Exercise for Prevention and Treatment of Illness.* Philadelphia: F.A. Davis, 1994, p 83.
36. Cochrane, T, Davey, RC, and Matthes Edwards, SM: Randomised controlled trial of the cost-effectiveness of water-based therapy for lower limb osteoarthritis. *Health Technol Assess* 9(31):1–114, 2005.
37. Cummings, GS, and Tillman, LJ: Remodeling of dense connective tissue in normal adult tissues. In Currier, DP, and Nelson, RM (eds): *Dynamics of Human Biologic Tissues.* Philadelphia: F.A. Davis, 1992, p 45.
38. De Jong, Z, and Vlieland, TP: Safety of exercise in patients with rheumatoid arthritis. *Curr Opin Rheumatol* 17(2):177–182, 2005.
39. de Kam, D, Smulders, E, and Weerdesteyn, V: Exercise interventions to reduce fall-related fractures and their risk factors in individuals with low bone density: a systematic review of randomized controlled trials. *Osteoporos Int* 20:2111–2125, 2009.
40. Dommerholt, J, Bron, C, and Franssen, J: Myofascial trigger points: an evidence-informed review. *J Manual Manip Ther* 14:203–221, 2006.
41. Evcik, D, et al: Effectiveness of aquatic therapy in treatment of fibromyalgia syndrome: a randomized controlled open study. *Rheumatol Int* 28: 885–890, 2008.
42. Felson, DT, et al: Osteoarthritis: new insights. Part 1: the disease and its risk factors. *Ann Intern Med* 133(8):635–646, 2000.
43. Felson, DT, et al: Osteoarthritis: new insights. Part 2: treatment approaches. *Ann Intern Med* 133(9):726–737, 2000.
44. Fernandes-de-las-Penas, C, Alonso-Blanco, C, and Miangolarra, JC: Myofascial trigger points in subjects presenting with mechanical neck pain: a blinded, controlled study. *Manual Ther* 12:29–33, 2007.
45. Ferández-de-Las-Peñas, C, and Dommerholt, J: Myofascial trigger points: peripheral or central phenomenon? *Curr Rheumatol Rep* 16(1):1–6, 2014.
46. Fernandes-de-las-Penas, C, Cuadrado, M, and Pareja, J: Myofascial trigger points, neck mobility, and forward head posture in episodic tension-type headache. *Headache* 47:662–672, 2007.
47. Fernandes-de-las-Penas, C, et al: Myofascial trigger points and sensitization: an updated pain model for tension-type headache. *Cephalagia* 27:383–393, 2007.
48. Fernández-de-Las-Peñas, C, et al: Referred pain from myofascial trigger points in head, neck, shoulder, and arm muscles reproduces symptoms in blue-collar (manual) and white-collar (office) workers. *Clin J Pain* 28(6):511–518, 2012.
49. Fernández-Pérez, AM, et al: Muscle trigger points, pressure pain threshold, and cervical range of motion in patients with high level of disability related to acute whiplash injury. *J Orthop Sports Phys Ther* 42(7): 634–641, 2012.
50. Fiatorone, M, et al: Exercise training and nutritional supplementation for physical frailty in very elderly people. *N Engl J Med* 30(25):1769–1775, 1994.
51. Fletcher, JA: Canadian Academy of Sport and Exercise Medicine position statement: osteoporosis and exercise. *Clin J Sport Med* 23(6):504, 2013.
52. Foley, A, et al: Does hydrotherapy improve strength and physical function in patients with osteoarthritis—a randomized controlled trial comparing a gym based and a hydrotherapy based strengthening programme. *Ann Rheum Dis* 62(12):1162–1167, 2003.
53. Frontera, W, et al: Strength conditioning in older men: skeletal muscle hypertrophy and improved function. *J Appl Physiol* 64(3):1038–1044, 1988.
54. Gammage, KL, and Klentrou, P: Predicting osteoporosis prevention behaviors: health beliefs and knowledge. *Am J Health Behav* 35(3):371–383, 2011.
55. Gavi, MB, et al: Strengthening exercises improve symptoms and quality of life but do not change autonomic modulation in fibromyalgia: a randomized clinical trial. *PLoS One* Mar 20:9(3):e90767, 2014.
56. Gerwin, RD: Diagnosis of myofascial pain. *Phys Med Rehabil Clin N Am* 25:341–355, 2014.
57. Gerwin, R: The taut band and other mysteries of the trigger point: an examination of the mechanisms relevant to the development and maintenance of the trigger point. *J Musculoskel Pain* 16:115–121, 2008.
58. Giannotti, E, et al: Medium-/long-term effects of a specific exercise protocol combined with patient education on spine mobility, chronic fatigue, pain, aerobic fitness and level of disability in fibromyalgia. *Biomed Res Int* Epub Jan 29, 2014.
59. Gouveia, ER, et al: Functional fitness and bone mineral density in the elderly. *Arch Osteoporos* 7(1-2):75–85, 2012.
60. Guadalupe-Grau, A, et al: Exercise and bone mass in adults. *Sports Med* 39:439–468, 2009.
61. *Guide to Physical Therapist Practice 3.0.* Alexandria, VA: American Physical Therapy Association; 2014. Available at http://guidetoptpractice.apta.org/. Accessed May 6, 2015.
62. Harden, RN, et al: Home-based aerobic conditioning for management of symptoms of fibromyalgia: a pilot study. *Pain Med* 13(6):835–842, 2012.
63. Haskell, W, et al: Physical activity and public health: updated recommendations for adults from the American College of Sports Medicine and the American Heart Association. *Circulation* 116:1081–1093, 2007.
64. Hawkins, RA: Fibromyalgia: a clinical update. *J Am Osteopath Assoc* 113(9):680–689, 2013.
65. Hawley, DJ: Health status assessment. In Wegener, ST (ed): *Clinical Care in the Rheumatic Diseases.* Atlanta: American College of Rheumatology, 1996.
66. Helgeson, K: Soft-tissue, joint, and bone disorders. In Goodman, CC, and Fuller, KS (eds): *Pathology, Implications for the Physical Therapist,* ed. 4. St. Louis: Elsevier/Saunders, 2015, p 1285.
67. Hidalgo-Losano, A, et al: Muscle trigger points and pressure hyperalgesia in the shoulder muscles in patients with unilateral shoulder impingement: a blinded, controlled study. *Exp Brain Res* 202:915–925, 2010.
68. Hockberg, MC: Osteoarthritis: clinical features and treatment. In Klippel, JH (ed): *Primer on the Rheumatic Diseases,* ed. 11. Atlanta: Arthritis Foundation, 1997, p 218.
69. Hoeksma, HL, et al: Comparison of manual therapy and exercise therapy in osteoarthritis of the hip: a randomized clinical trial. *Arthritis Rheum* 51(5):722–729, 2004.
70. Holtgrefe, K, McCloy, C, and Rome, L: Changes associated with a quota-based approach on a walking program for individuals with fibromyalgia. *JOSPT* 37:717–724, 2007.

71. Hooten, WM, et al: Effects of strength vs aerobic exercise on pain severity in adults with fibromyalgia: a randomized equivalence trial. *Pain* Apr;153(4):915-023, 2012.
72. Hower, TE, et al: Exercise for preventing and treating osteoporosis in postmenopausal women. *Cochrane Database Syst Rev* 2011(7): CD000333.
73. Huntoon, E, Schmidt, C, and Sinaki, M: Significantly fewer refractures after vertebroplasty in patients who engage in back-extensor-strengthening exercises. *Mayo Clin Proc* 83:54–57, 2008.
74. Iglesias-González, JJ, et al: Myofascial trigger points, pain, disability, and sleep quality in patients with chronic nonspecific low back pain. *Pain Med* 14(12):1964–1970, 2013.
75. Iversen, MD: Physical therapy for older adults with arthritis: what is recommended? *Int J Clin Rheumatol* 5(1):37–51, 2010.
76. Jones, KD: Nordic walking in fibromyalgia: a means of promoting fitness that is easy for busy clinicians to recommend. *Arthritis Res Ther* Feb 16;13(1):103, 2011.
77. Kaelin, ME, et al: Cardiopulmonary responses, muscle soreness, and injury during the one repetition maximum assessment in pulmonary rehabilitation patients. *J Cardiopulm Rehabil* 19(6):366–372, 1999.
78. Kaleth, AS, Slaven, JE, and Ang, DC: Does increasing steps per day predict improvement in physical function and pain interference in adults with fibromyalgia? *Arthritis Care Res* 66(12):1887–1894, 2014.
79. Kaltenborn, FM, et al: *Manual Mobilization of the Joints: Joint Examination and Basic Treatment, Vol I. The Extremities,* ed. 8. Oslo, Norway: Norli, 2014.
80. Kannan, P: Management of myofascial pain of upper trapezius: a three group comparison study. *Glob J Health Sci* 4(5):46–52, 2012.
81. Karlsson, M, Nordqvist, A, and Karlsson, C: Sustainability of exercise induced increase in bone density and skeletal structure. *Food Nutr Res* 2008:52. DOI: 10.3402/fnr.v52i0.1872.
82. Kayo, AH, et al: Effectiveness of physical activity in reducing pain in patients with fibromyalgia: a blinded randomized clinical trial. *Rheumatol Int* Aug;32(8):2285–2292, 2012.
83. Kietrys, DM, et al: Effectiveness of dry needling for upper quarter myofascial pain: a systemic review and meta-analysis. *J Orthop Sports Phys Ther* 43(9):620–634, 2013.
84. Kittelson, AJ, et al: Future directions in painful knee osteoarthritis: harnessing complexity in a heterogeneous population. *Phys Ther* 94(3): 422–432, 2014.
85. Kukuljan, S, et al. Effects of a multi-component exercise program and calcium-vitamin-D_3-fortified milk on bone mineral density in older men: a randomized controlled trial. *Osteoporos Int* 20:1241–1251, 2009.
86. Lawrence, RC, et al: Estimates of the prevalence of arthritis and other rheumatic conditions in the United States: Part II. *Arthritis Rheum* 58: 26–35, 2008.
87. Lazaro, RT, and Burke-Doe, A: Injury, inflammation, healing, and repair. In Goodman, CC, and Fuller, KS (eds): *Pathology, Implications for the Physical Therapist,* ed. 4. St. Louis: Elsevier/Saunders, 2015, p 216.
88. Leonard, JB: Joint protection for inflammatory disorders. In Lichtman, DM, and Alexander, AH (eds): *The Wrist and Its Disorders,* ed. 2. Philadelphia: WB Saunders, 1997, p 1377.
89. Levine, JP: Identification, diagnosis, and prevention of osteoporosis. *Am J Manag Care* 17 Suppl 6:S170–S176, 2011.
90. Lima, TD, et al: The effectiveness of aquatic physical therapy in the treatment of fibromyalgia: a systematic review with meta-analysis. *Clin Rehabil* 27(10):892–908, 2013.
91. Lucas, K, Polus, B, and Rich, P: Latent myofascial trigger points: their effects on muscle activation and movement efficiency. *J Body Movt Ther* 8:160–166, 2004.
92. Lucas, K, Rich, P, and Polus, B: How common are latent myofascial trigger points in the scapular positioning muscles? *J Musculoskel Pain* 16:279–286, 2008.
93. Ma, D, Wu, L, and He, Z: Effects of walking on the preservation of bone mineral density in perimenopausal and postmenopausal women: a systematic review and meta-analysis. *Menopause* 20(11):1216–1226, 2013.
94. Majlesi, J, and Unalan, H: High power pain threshold ultrasound technique in the treatment of active myofascial trigger points: a randomized, double blind, case-control study. *Arch Phys Med Rehabil* 85: 833–836, 2004.
95. Mannerkorpi, K, et al: Pool exercise for patients with fibromyalgia or chronic widespread pain: a randomized controlled trial and subgroup analyses. *J Rehabil Med* 41:751–760, 2009.
96. Marcus, DA, et al: Including a range of outcome targets offers a broader view of fibromyalgia treatment outcome: results from a retrospective review of multidisciplinary treatment. *Musculoskel Care* 12(2):74–81, 2014.
97. Margolis, S, and Flynn, JA: *Arthritis: The Johns Hopkins White Papers.* Baltimore: The Johns Hopkins Medical Institutions, 2000.
98. Martyn-St James, M, and Carroll, S: Meta-analysis of walking for preservation of bone mineral density of postmenopausal women. *Bone* 43:521–531, 2008.
99. Mat, S, et al: Physical therapies for improving balance and reducing fall risk in osteoarthritis of the knee: a systematic review. *Age Ageing* 44(1):16–24, 2015.
100. Matteson, EL: Rheumatoid arthritis: treatment. In Klippel, JH (ed): *Primer on the Rheumatic Diseases,* ed. 12. Atlanta: Arthritis Foundation, 2001, p 225.
101. McDonough, A: Effect of immobilization and exercise on articular cartilage: a review of literature. *J Orthop Sports Phys Ther* 3(1):2–5, 1981.
102. McKinnis, LN: *Fundamentals of Musculoskeletal Imaging,* ed. 4. Philadelphia: F.A. Davis, 2014.
103. McNamara, AJ, Pavol, MJ, and Gunter, KB: Meeting physical activity guidelines through community-based group exercise: "better bones and balance." *J Aging Phys Act* 21(2):155–166, 2013.
104. Metsios, GS, et al: Rheumatoid arthritis, cardiovascular disease, and physical exercise: a systematic review. *Rheumatology* 47(3):239–248, 2007.
105. Minor, MA, et al: Efficacy of physical conditioning exercise in patients with rheumatoid arthritis and osteoarthritis. *Arthritis Rheum* 32(11):1396–1405, 1989.
106. Moayyeri, A: The association between physical activity and osteoporosis fractures: a review of the evidence and implications for future research. *Ann Epidemiol* 18:827–835, 2008.
107. Mosti, MP, et al: Maximal strength training in postmenopausal women with osteoporosis or osteopenia. *J Strength Cond Res* 27(10):2879–2886, 2013.
108. Morganti, C, et al: Strength improvements with 1 yr of progressive resistance training in older women. *Med Sci Sports Exerc* 27(6):906–912, 1995.
109. National Osteoporosis Foundation. Available at http://nof.org/articles/235. Accessed June 3, 2015.
110. National Osteoporosis Foundation. Available at http://nof.org/articles/8. Accessed June 3, 2015.
111. National Osteoporosis Foundation. Available at http://nof.org/articles/2. Accessed June 3, 2015,
112. National Osteoporosis Foundation. Available at http://nof.org/articles/6. Accessed June 3, 2015,
113. National Osteoporosis Foundation. Available at http://nof.org/learn/prevention. Accessed June 3, 2015,
114. National Osteoporosis Foundation. Available at http://nof.org/learn/bonebasics. Accessed June 3, 2015,
115. National Osteoporosis Foundation. Available at http://nof.org/exercise. Accessed June 3, 2015.
116. Nedergaard, A, Henriksen, K, Karsdal, MA, and Christian, C: Musculoskeletal ageing and primary prevention. *Best Pract Clin Obstet Gynaecol* Oct;27(5):673–688, 2013.
117. Nelson, M, and Wernick, S: *Strong Women, Strong Bones, Updated.* New York: Berkley Publishing Group, 2006.
118. Nelson, M, et al: Physical activity and public health in older adults: recommendation from the American College of Sports Medicine and the American Heart Association. *Circulation* 116:1094–1105, 2007.
119. Nelson, M, et al: Physical activity and public health in older adults: recommendation from the American College of Sports Medicine and the American Heart Association. *Med Sci Sports Exerc* 39:1435–1445, 2007.

120. NICE: Osteoarthritis: care and management. Available at http://www.nice.org.uk/guidance/cg177/chapter/1-recommendations, 2011. Accessed May, 9, 2015.
121. Oh, TH, et al: Predictors of clinical outcome in fibromyalgia treatment program: single center experience. *PM R* Apr;4(4):257–263, 2012.
122. Olveira-Campelo, N, de Melo, CA, Alburquerue-Sendin, F, and Machado, JP: Short- and medium-term effects of manual therapy on cervical active range of motion and pressure pain sensitivity in latent myofascial pain of the upper trapezius muscle: a randomized controlled trial. *J Manipulative Physiol Ther* 36(5):300–309, 2013.
123. Phillips, CA: Therapist's management of patients with RA. In Lichtman, DM, and Alexander, AH (eds): *The Wrist and Its Disorders*, ed. 2. Philadelphia: WB Saunders, 1997, p 1345.
124. Pincus, T: Rheumatoid arthritis. In Wegener, ST (ed): *Clinical Care in the Rheumatic Diseases.* Atlanta: American College of Rheumatology, 1996, p 147.
125. Rayegani, SM, Bayat, M, Bahrami, MH, Raeissadat SA, and Kargozar, E: Comparison of dry needling and physiotherapy in treatment of myofascial pain syndrome. *Clin Rheumatol* 34:859–864, 2014.
126. Polidoulis, I, Beyene, J, and Cheung, AM: The effect of exercise on pQCT parameters of bone structure and strength in postmenopausal women—a systematic review and meta-analysis of randomized controlled trials. *Osteoporos Int* 23(1):39–51, 2012.
127. Roddy, E, et al: Evidence-based recommendations for the role of exercise in the management of osteoarthritis of the hip or knee—the MOVE consensus. *Rheumatology* 44(1):67–73, 2005.
128. Roddy, E, Zhang, W, and Doherty, M: Aerobic walking or strengthening exercise for osteoarthritis of the knee? A systematic review. *Ann Rheum Dis* 64(4):544–548, 2005.
129. Roghani, T, et al: Effects of short-term aerobic exercise with and without external loading on bone metabolism and balance in postmenopausal women with osteoporosis. *Rheumatol Int* 33(2):291–298, 2013.
130. Rotstein, A, Harush, M, and Vaisman, N: The effect of a water exercise program on bone density of postmenopausal women. *J Sports Med Phys Fitness* 48:352–359, 2008.
131. Russel, IJ: Fibromyalgia syndrome. In Mense, S, and Simons, D (eds): *Muscle Pain, Understanding its Nature, Diagnosis, and Treatment.* Philadelphia: Lippincott Williams & Wilkins, 2001, pp 289–337.
132. Salter, RB: *Textbook of Disorders and Injuries of the Musculoskeletal System*, ed. 3. Baltimore: Williams & Wilkins, 1999.
133. Sanita, P, and de Alencar, F: Myofascial pain syndrome as a contributing factor in patients with chronic headaches. *J Musculoskel Pain* 17:15–25, 2009.
134. Sañudo, B, et al: Effects of exercise training and detraining in patients with fibromyalgia syndrome: a 3-yr longitudinal study. *Am J Phys Med Rehabil* 91(7):561–569, 2012.
135. Sañudo, B, et al: Effects of a prolonged exercise program on key health outcomes in women with fibromyalgia: a randomized controlled trial. *J Rehabil Med* 43(6):521–526, 2011.
136. Scarvell, J, and Elkins, M: Aerobic exercise is beneficial for people with rheumatoid arthritis. *Br J Sports Med* 45(12): 1008–1009, 2011.
137. Shah, J, and Gilliams, E: Uncovering the biochemical milieu of myofascial trigger points using in vivo microdialysis: an application of muscle pain concepts to myofascial pain syndrome. *J Bodywork Movt Ther* 12:371–384, 2008.
138. Sharma, L, et al: Physical functioning over three years in knee osteoarthritis: role of psychosocial, local mechanical, and neuromuscular factors. *Arthritis Rheum* 48(12):3359–3370, 2003.
139. Shaw, C, McCully, K, and Posner, J: Injuries during the one repetition maximum assessment in the elderly. *J Cardiopulm Rehabil* 15(4): 283–287, 1995.
140. Simon, LS: Arthritis: new agents herald more effective symptom management. *Geriatrics* 54(6):37–42, 1999.
141. Simons, D: Myofascial pain caused by trigger points. In Mense, S, and Simons, D (eds): *Muscle Pain, Understanding its Nature, Diagnosis, and Treatment.* Philadelphia: Lippincott Williams & Wilkins, 2001, pp 205–288.
142. Simons, D, Travell, J, and Simons, L: *Myofascial Pain and Dysfunction: The Trigger Point Manual, Vol 1*, ed. 2. Baltimore: Williams & Wilkins, 1999.
143. Simons, D: Review of enigmatic MTrPs as a common cause of enigmatic musculoskeletal pain and dysfunction. *J Electromyogr Kinesiol* 14: 95–107, 2004.
144. Sinaki, M: Effect of physical activity on bone mass. *Curr Opin Rheumatol* 8:376–383, 1996.
145. Sinaki, M: Exercise for patients with osteoporosis: management of vertebral compression fractures and trunk strengthening for fall prevention. *PM R* 4(11):882–888, 2012.
146. Sofaat, N, Ejindu, V, and Kiely, P: What makes osteoarthritis painful? The evidence for local and central processing. *Rheumatology* 50(12):22157–2165, 2011.
147. Song, R, et al: Effect of tai chi exercise on pain, balance, muscle strength, and perceived difficulties in physical functioning in older women with osteoarthritis: a randomized clinical trial. *J Rheumatol* 30(9):2039–2044, 2003.
148. Starlanyl, D, and Copeland, M: *Fibromyalgia and Chronic Myofascial Pain*, ed. 2. Oakland: New Harbinger Publications, 2001.
149. Tekin, L, et al: The effect of dry needling in the treatment of myofascial pain syndrome: a randomized double-blinded placebo-controlled trial. *Clin Rheumatol* 32(3):309–319, 2013.
150. Tough, E, White, A, and Cummings, TM: Acupuncture and dry needling in the management of myofascial trigger point pain: a systematic review and meta-analysis of randomized controlled trials. *Eur J Pain* 13:3–10, 2009.
151. United States Department of Health and Human Services: Bone health and osteoporosis: a report by the Surgeon General (2004). Available at http://www.surgeongeneral.gov/library/bonehealth/content.html. Accessed March 20, 2015.
152. Van Abbema, R, Van Wilgen, CP, Van Der Schans, CP, and Van Ittersum, MW: Patients with more severe symptoms benefit the most from an intensive multimodal programme in patients with fibromyalgia. *Disabil Rehabil* 33(9):7430750, 2011.
153. Waddington, G, Dickson, T, Trathen, S, and Adams, R: Walking for fitness: is it enough to maintain both heart and bone health? *Aust J Prim Health* 17(1):86–88, 2011.
154. Waller, B, et al: Effect of therapeutic aquatic exercise on symptoms and function associated with lower limb osteoarthritis: systematic review with meta-analysis. *Phys Ther* 94(10):1383–1395, 2014.
155. Wegener, L, Kisner, C, and Nichols, D: Static and dynamic balance responses in persons with bilateral knee osteoarthritis. *J Orthop Sports Phys Ther* 25:13–18, 1997.
156. Wendlova, J: The importance of carrying a backpack in the rehabilitation of osteoporotic patients (biomechanical analysis). *Bratisl Lek Listy* 112(1):41–43, 2011.
157. Wolfe, F, Clauw, D, and Fitzcharles, M: The American College of Rheumatology preliminary diagnostic criteria for fibromyalgia and measurement of symptom severity. *Arthritis Care Res* 62:600–610, 2010.
158. Wolfe, F, Smythe, HA, and Yunus, MB: The American College of Rheumatology 1990 criteria for the classification of fibromyalgia: report of the Multicenter Criteria Committee. *Arthritis Rheum* 33:160–172, 1990.
159. Ytterberg, SR, Mahowald, ML, and Krug, HE: Exercise for arthritis. *Baillieres Clin Rheumatol* 8(1):161–189, 1994.
160. Yuan, SL, Berssaneti, AA, and Marques, AP. Effects of shiatsu in the management of fibromyalgia symptoms: a controlled pilot study. *J Manipulative Physiol Ther* Sept;26(7):426–443, 2013.
161. Ziaeifar, M, Arab, AM, Karimi, N, and Nourbakhsh, MR: The effect of dry needling in patients with a myofascial trigger point in the upper trapezius muscle. *J Bodyw Mov Ther* 18(2):298–305, 2014.

CHAPTER

12

Surgical Interventions and Postoperative Management

LYNN COLBY, PT, MS ■ JOHN BORSTAD, PT, PHD

Many injuries, diseases, and disorders of the musculoskeletal system can be associated with levels of impairment so significant that surgical intervention is required. These impairments can affect all musculoskeletal tissues—muscles, tendons, ligaments, cartilage, fascia, joint capsules, or bones—of the upper or lower extremities or spine. Ideally, surgery is preceded by a comprehensive examination and evaluation of the patient's impairments and functional status, coupled with preoperative patient education. Following surgery, a planned course of postoperative rehabilitation is usually warranted.

This chapter provides an overview of the indications for surgical intervention for musculoskeletal pathology, describes considerations for preoperative management, notes factors that influence the outcomes of surgery, provides general rehabilitation guidelines following surgery, and identifies potential complications that may interfere with the achievement of optimal functional outcomes. The chapter concludes with an overview of several orthopedic surgical procedures that may be undertaken for the management of musculoskeletal conditions

Descriptions of selected surgical procedures for common injuries or disorders of each region of the extremities are provided in Chapters 17 through 22. In these chapters, guidelines and progressions for postoperative management of specific surgeries are presented that are based on the principles of tissue healing and exercise prescription addressed in Chapter 10, rather than adherence to specific protocols. These principles can be applied by the therapist when designing exercise interventions for patients undergoing current surgical procedures and can also be applied as a foundation for future rehabilitation strategies as surgical interventions change and evolve.

Indications for Surgical Intervention

Many acute, recurring, and chronic musculoskeletal conditions are managed successfully with conservative measures, such as rest, protection with splinting or use of assistive devices, medication, therapeutic exercise, manual therapy, functional training, and the use of physical agents or electrotherapy. However, surgical intervention is the best treatment option when a conservative program has not been successful in adequately modifying impairments or restoring function, or if the severity of a patient's condition is beyond the level that is appropriate for conservative management. Indications for a variety of musculoskeletal surgeries are identified in Box 12.1.[11,13,16,62]

Guidelines for Preoperative and Postoperative Management

Although surgical intervention can correct or reduce the adverse conditions and impairments associated with musculoskeletal pathology, a carefully planned and progressed

BOX 12.1 Indications for Surgery for Musculoskeletal Disorders of the Extremities and Spine

- Incapacitating pain at rest or with functional activities
- Marked limitation of active or passive motion
- Gross instability of a joint or bony segments
- Joint deformity or abnormal joint alignment
- Significant structural degeneration
- Chronic joint swelling
- Failed conservative (nonsurgical) or prior surgical management
- Significant loss of function leading to disability as the result of any of the preceding factors

rehabilitation program is essential for the patient to achieve optimal functional outcomes after surgery. Ideally, rehabilitation begins with patient education and "prehabilitation" exercises or functional skill development before surgery and continues with direct intervention from a therapist and long-term self-management by the patient after surgery.

Considerations for Preoperative Management

Direct communication with the patient prior to pre-planned, elective surgery is advisable, preferably on a one-to-one basis between therapist and patient, but a group setting can also be used. In the current health-care environment, authorization for reimbursable preoperative consultations with individual patients is often difficult. However, preoperative contact with a group of patients scheduled for similar surgeries may be possible. The benefits of preoperative communication and instruction with a patient include the ability to assess their preoperative functional status, to discuss their goals and expectations following surgery, to establish rapport, and to educate the patient regarding postoperative rehabilitation.

There are several elements of preoperative management, including a comprehensive examination and evaluation of a patient's preoperative status, patient education, an opportunity for the patient to ask questions about the procedure, instruction regarding postoperative care, and providing a preoperative exercise program if appropriate.

Preoperative Examination and Evaluation

When a preoperative visit is approved for an individual patient, the therapist can perform a comprehensive examination to determine the patient's impairments and functional status prior to surgery.[61,74] The therapist can evaluate the findings of the examination to identify the patient's needs and goals, document the pre-surgical level of function, and generate a prognosis regarding the expected functional outcomes following surgery.

Examination of specific factors is particularly important for developing realistic goals and estimating functionally relevant outcomes of surgery and postoperative rehabilitation.[74] These factors are also emphasized in the postoperative examination and in subsequent evaluations during rehabilitation.

- *Pain.* Quantitatively measure the patient's level of pain with a visual analog scale or a scale that identifies the degree of pain with specific functional activities.
- *Range of motion and joint integrity.* Measure both active and passive range of motion (ROM) of the involved joint or extremity and compare it to the ROM of the uninvolved areas. Evaluate the quality of active joint motion. Assess joint stability using passive accessory mobility testing and special tests specific to passive restraints.
- *Skin integrity.* Note the presence of scars from previous injuries or surgeries, particularly those that are adherent and restrict mobility of skin or underlying connective tissue and joints.
- *Muscle performance.* Evaluate muscle strength of the affected areas, recognizing that pain adversely affects strength. Assess the functional strength of unaffected body segments in anticipation of postoperative needs such as ambulation with assistive devices, transfers, and activities of daily living (ADLs).
- *Posture.* Identify the patient's preferred positions for comfort and any postural abnormalities that may affect ROM and function.
- *Gait analysis.* Analyze the gait characteristics, type of supportive or protective devices currently used, and degree of weight bearing tolerated during ambulation.
- *Functional status.* Identify the patient's preoperative functional activity limitations and functional abilities and his or her perception of disability associated with participation restrictions using a quantitative, self-report measurement tool. A valid and reliable outcome measure should be used if available and specific to the body region.

Preoperative Patient Education: Methods and Rationale

Patient education can begin preoperatively during an individual instruction session with a patient or in a group setting with patients planning to undergo similar surgeries. Some large, acute-care facilities have education programs for patients scheduled for joint replacement surgery that use group instruction by team members from several disciplines, including nursing, physical therapy, and occupational therapy.[28,46,52] The group programs may also include a tour of the operating and recovery rooms. Programs such as these may help a patient understand what to expect the day of surgery and during the early postoperative phase, possibly alleviating some of a patient's anxiety about the surgery and hospital experience.

Preoperative instruction gives a patient an opportunity to learn about factors associated with surgery such as wound care, special precautions that must be followed after surgery, and the use of assistive or supportive equipment such as crutches, an immobilizer, or a sling.[61,74] Of equal importance, the patient can learn and practice early postoperative exercises without being hampered by postoperative pain or the side effects of pain medication, such as disorientation and drowsiness.[61,74] If surgery is scheduled as an outpatient procedure, preoperative instruction teaches the patient skills needed to be safe at home and the postoperative exercises they can perform at home before formal rehabilitation with the therapist begins.

Components of Preoperative Patient Education

- *Overview of the plan of care.* Explain the overall plan of care the patient can expect during the postoperative period.
- *Postoperative precautions.* Advise the patient of any precautions or contraindications to positioning, movement, or weight bearing that must be followed postoperatively.
- *Bed mobility and transfers.* Teach the patient how to move in bed or perform wheelchair transfers safely, incorporating the necessary postoperative precautions.
- *Initial postoperative exercises.* Teach the patient any exercises that will be started during the very early postoperative period. These exercises often include:
  - *Deep-breathing and coughing exercises.* Explain the rationale for periodically performing deep-breathing exercises throughout the day.
  - *Active ankle exercises (pumping exercises).* Teach the patient how to reduce postoperative venous stasis and decrease the risk of deep vein thrombosis (DVT).
  - *Gentle muscle-setting exercises of immobilized joints.*
- *Gait training.* Teach the patient to use supportive devices that may be needed for protected weight bearing during ambulation after surgery, such as crutches or a walker.
- *Wound care.* Explain or reinforce postoperative care of the incision for optimal wound healing.
- *Pain management.* Educate on the correct use of cryotherapy for postoperative pain management.

FOCUS ON EVIDENCE

Although preoperative education is considered a valuable component of the preparation and recovery from surgery, evidence supporting its effectiveness is limited. McDonald et al reviewed 18 randomized or quasi-randomized trials evaluating the effectiveness of preoperative patient education prior to hip or knee arthroplasty and found no added benefit with respect to reducing anxiety, or for improved surgical outcomes like pain, function, or number of adverse events.[58]

An Extended Preoperative Exercise Program

The rationale for implementing an exercise program prior to a planned surgical procedure is to limit further progression of impairments, such as long-standing strength and ROM deficits, that have developed as the result of the musculoskeletal condition requiring surgery, to improve the likelihood that learning will carry over and exercises will be performed correctly following surgery, and to increase the likelihood of achieving optimal postoperative functional outcomes.[47,75]

A preoperative exercise program may be particularly beneficial if a prolonged period of immobilization or reduced weight bearing is necessary after surgery.

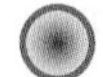

FOCUS ON EVIDENCE

Studies evaluating the effectiveness of an exercise program initiated prior to a planned orthopedic surgical procedure have reported mixed results. Kean and colleagues[47] studied the functional impact of a strengthening program initiated prior to high tibial osteotomy in a relatively young, active group of patients with medial compartment osteoarthritis. Fourteen individuals (13 men and 1 woman, mean age 48 years) participated in a supervised isokinetic resistance training program for the quadriceps and hamstrings muscle groups 3 times a week for 12 weeks prior to surgery, leading to significant gains in strength. They also participated in postoperative rehabilitation. The functional status of the experimental group was compared with a matched control group of patients who also had undergone high tibial osteotomy and postoperative rehabilitation, but no preoperative resistance training. At 6 months postsurgery, the preoperative resistance training group scored significantly better than the control group on ADL and recreational/sports participation subscales of a quantitative measurement tool assessing function in individuals with knee arthritis.

In contrast, Rooks and associates[75] found that despite a 20% increase in lower extremity strength as the result of a preoperative exercise program in a group of patients scheduled to undergo total hip or knee arthroplasty, there were no significant improvements in postoperative functioning compared with that of a control group. Key differences in these studies were the type of preoperative resistance training programs, the mean ages of the participants, and degree of joint arthritis.

A recent systematic review of seventeen studies that provided prehabilitation prior to surgery demonstrated no benefit to patients over usual care at any time point following surgery. Prehabilitation programs consisted of aerobic exercises, strength training, and/or functional task training, and main outcome measures included quality of life, pain, hospital readmission, and nursing home placement. The majority of studies (13) included patients planning hip or knee arthroplasty. The lone positive finding was that a dose of over 500 hours of prehabilitation minimized the need for postoperative rehabilitation.[15]

Considerations for Postoperative Management

A well-planned rehabilitation program, composed of a carefully progressed sequence of therapeutic exercise, functional training, and ongoing patient education, is fundamental to the patient's postoperative care. Appropriate rehabilitative management must consider many factors, all of which will affect the components, the progression, and the outcomes of a patient's postoperative program. These factors are noted in Box 12.2. Ultimately, the success of the surgical procedure is closely linked with the effectiveness of the postsurgical rehabilitation.

To design a safe, effective, efficient rehabilitation program for a patient, the therapist must understand the indications and rationale for a particular surgical procedure; become familiar with the procedure itself; be aware of special precautions related to the surgery; and communicate effectively with the patient, surgeon, and other members of the rehabilitation team.[31]

Postoperative Examination and Evaluation

Every postoperative rehabilitation program must be based on initial and ongoing examinations of the individual patient. In addition to the components of a preoperative examination noted previously in this section, an assessment of integumentary integrity is important after surgery. The incision should be inspected before and after each exercise session to identify any evidence of wound infection or delayed healing. Inspection of the surgical site includes the items noted in Box 12.3.

Phases of Postoperative Rehabilitation

Postoperative rehabilitation is most often divided into phases, with each phase containing goals and suggested interventions. Phases can be distinguished in several ways: by the transitional sequences of tissue healing (acute/inflammatory, subacute/proliferative, chronic/remodeling), by the permitted level activity (initial, intermediate, advanced), by the degree of protection of healing tissues (maximum, moderate, minimum protection), or simply by sequential numbering (e.g., I, II, III).

As with non-operative management of musculoskeletal pathology, the phase descriptions all reflect to some extent the stages of healing of involved soft tissue and bone. In addition, phases of postoperative rehabilitation must account for particular elements of the surgical procedure, such as the type of surgical approach or tissue fixation.

In general, the goals and interventions across the phases of postoperative rehabilitation are established to safely progress the patient toward functional recovery. Early after surgery, the emphasis of management focuses on minimizing pain, preventing postoperative complications, and resuming a safe level of functional mobility while protecting the surgical site. Later, as tissues heal and the patient recovers from surgery, interventions are directed toward restoring or improving range of motion (ROM), strength, neuromuscular control, stability, balance, and muscular and cardiopulmonary endurance, as well as the patient's ability to perform all necessary and desired functional activities.

Phases of postoperative rehabilitation do not take into account the individual qualities, needs, and abilities of each patient, nor do they consider how a modification to the normal surgical procedure may impact care. Therefore, the phases are intended as general guidelines for management rather than prescriptive programs. To develop an individualized rehabilitation program for the patient, the suggested guidelines for each phase should be modified based on the results of ongoing postoperative examination of the patient.

Recognizing the differences among various surgical procedures and the fact that each patient's recovery after surgery is unique, guidelines for postoperative rehabilitation in this section are divided into three broad, overlapping phases based on the degree of protection of operated structures. The characteristics of these three phases are as follows.

- ***Maximum protection phase.*** This is the initial postoperative period when protection of operated tissues is paramount in the presence of tissue inflammation and pain. After some surgeries, immobilization of the operated area is necessary during this phase. After other surgeries, it is advisable to

BOX 12.2 Factors That Influence the Components, Progression, and Outcomes of a Postoperative Rehabilitation Program

- Extent of tissue pathology or damage
  - Size or severity of the lesion
- Type and unique characteristics of the surgical procedure
- Patient-related factors
  - Age, extent of preoperative impairments, and functional limitations
  - Health history, particularly use of medications and diabetes
  - Lifestyle history, including use of tobacco
  - Needs, goals, expectations, and social support
  - Level of motivation and ability to adhere to an exercise program
- Stage of healing of involved tissues
- Characteristics of types of tissues involved
  - Response to immobilization and remobilization
- Integrity of structures adjacent to involved tissues
- Philosophy of the surgeon

BOX 12.3 Inspection of the Surgical Incision

- Check for signs of redness or tissue necrosis along the incision(s) and around sutures.
- Palpate along the incision and note signs of tenderness and edema.
- Palpate to determine evidence of increased heat.
- Check for signs of drainage; note color and amount of drainage on the dressing.
- Note the integrity of an incision across a joint *during and after* exercise.
- As the incision heals, check the mobility of the scar.

place low-level stresses on operated tissues soon after surgery, making early passive or assisted ROM within a protected range or within a patient's tolerance permissible. In both situations, muscle-setting exercises to prevent muscle disuse atrophy also are indicated. The time frame for maximum protection ranges from a few days to 6 weeks depending on the type of surgery and the tissues involved.

- ***Moderate protection phase.*** This is the intermediate phase of rehabilitation when inflammation has subsided, pain and tenderness are minimal, and tissues are able to withstand gradually increasing levels of stress. Criteria for progression to this phase often include the absence of pain at rest and the availability of at least limited pain-free movement of the operated extremity. There is an emphasis on restoring ROM and normal arthrokinematics while tissues continue to heal and remodel, improving neuromuscular control and stability, and gradually increasing strength during this phase. Depending on the healing characteristics of the operated tissues, this phase typically begins around 4 to 6 weeks postoperatively and continues for an additional 4 to 6 weeks.
- ***Minimum protection/return to function phase.*** During this advanced phase, little to no protection of operated tissues is required. To progress to this phase, full (or almost full) pain-free active ROM should be available and the joint capsule (if involved) should be clinically stable. Strength requirements to begin this phase vary widely depending on the procedure. Rehabilitation focuses on restoring functional strength and gradually progressing the patient's functional activities. This phase begins anywhere from 6 to 12 weeks postoperatively and may continue until 6 months postoperatively or beyond.

Box 12.4 summarizes general management guidelines for postoperative rehabilitation, including the common structural and functional impairments that must be addressed and a plan of care with suggested goals and interventions for each phase of rehabilitation. Postsurgical guidelines for specific surgeries at each region are provided in Chapter 15 and Chapters 17 through 22.

Time-Based and Criterion-Based Progression

Time frames for each phase of rehabilitation can vary dramatically depending on the procedure. For example, immediately after an arthroscopic meniscectomy, the maximum protection phase during which movement of the operated

BOX 12.4 MANAGEMENT GUIDELINES—
Postoperative Rehabilitation

Structural and Functional Impairments:

Postoperative pain because of disruption of soft tissue
Postoperative swelling
Potential circulatory and pulmonary complications
Joint stiffness or limitation of motion because of injury to soft tissue and necessary postoperative immobilization
Muscle disuse atrophy because of immobilization
Loss of strength for functional activities
Limitation of weight bearing
Potential loss of strength and mobility of non-operated joints

Maximum Protection Phase

Plan of Care	Interventions
1. Educate the patient in preparation for self-management.	1. Instruction in safe positioning and limb movements and special postoperative precautions or contraindications.
2. Decrease postoperative pain, muscle guarding, or spasm.	2. Relaxation exercises. Use of modalities such as transcutaneous electrical nerve stimulation (TENS), cold, or heat. Continuous passive motion (CPM) during the early postoperative period.
3. Prevent wound infection.	3. Instruction or review of proper wound care (cleaning and dressing the incision).
4. Minimize postoperative swelling.	4. Elevation of the operated extremity. Active muscle pumping exercises at the distal joints. Use of compression garment. Gentle distal-to-proximal massage.

Continued

BOX 12.4 MANAGEMENT GUIDELINES—
Postoperative Rehabilitation—cont'd

Plan of Care	Interventions
5. Prevent circulatory and pulmonary complications, such as deep vein thrombosis, pulmonary embolus, or pneumonia.	5. Active exercises to distal musculature. Deep-breathing and coughing exercises.
6. Prevent unnecessary, residual joint stiffness or soft tissue contractures.	6. CPM or passive or active-assistive ROM initiated in the immediate postoperative period.
7. Minimize muscle atrophy across immobilized joints.	7. Muscle-setting exercises.
8. Maintain motion and strength in areas above and below the operative site.	8. Active and resistive ROM exercises to nonoperated areas.
9. Maintain functional mobility while protecting the operative site.	9. Adaptive equipment and assistive devices.

Moderate Protection/Controlled Motion Phase

Plan of Care	Interventions
1. Educate the patient.	1. Teach the patient to monitor the effects of the exercise program and make adjustments if swelling or pain increases.
2. Gradually restore soft tissue and joint mobility.	2. Active-assistive or active ROM within limits of pain. Joint mobilization procedures.
3. Establish a mobile scar.	3. Gentle massage across and around the maturing scar.
4. Strengthen involved muscles and improve joint stability.	4. Multiple-against increasing resistance. Alternating isometrics and rhythmic stabilization procedures. Dynamic exercise against light resistance in open- and closed-chain positions. Light functional activities with operated limb.

Minimum Protection/Return to Function Phase

Plan of Care	Interventions
1. Continue patient education.	1. Emphasize gradual but progressive incorporation of improved muscle performance, mobility, and balance into functional activities.
2. Prevent re-injury or postoperative complications.	2. Reinforce self-monitoring and review the signs and symptoms of excessive use; identify unsafe activities.
3. Restore full joint and soft tissue mobility, if possible.	3. Joint stretching (mobilization) and self-stretching techniques.
4. Maximize muscle performance, dynamic stability, and neuromuscular control.	4. Progressive strengthening exercises using higher loads and speeds and combined movement patterns. Integrate movements and positions into exercises that simulate functional activities.

BOX 12.4 MANAGEMENT GUIDELINES—
Postoperative Rehabilitation—cont'd

Plan of Care	Interventions
5. Restore balance and coordinated movement.	5. Progressive balance and coordination training.
6. Acquire or relearn specific motor skills.	6. Apply principles of motor learning (appropriate practice and feedback during task-specific training).

PRECAUTIONS: In addition to the precautions already addressed that relate to the stages of tissue repair and healing, there are several additional precautions that are of particular importance to the postoperative patient.

- Avoid positions, movements, or weight bearing that could compromise the integrity of the surgical repair.
- Keep the wound clean to avoid postoperative infection. Monitor for wound drainage and signs of systemic or local infection, such as elevated temperature.
- Avoid vigorous/high-intensity stretching or resistance exercises with soft tissues, such as muscles, tendons, or joint capsules that have been repaired or reattached for at least 6 weeks to ensure adequate healing and stability.
- Modify level and selection of physical activities, if necessary, to prevent premature wear and tear of repaired or reconstructed soft tissues and joints.

joint is limited to passive or assisted motion within a protected range may extend for only 1 day postoperatively. However, after a complex tendon repair in the hand, maximum protection may be required for several weeks.

Although published descriptions of postoperative rehabilitation typically include estimated time frames for each phase of a program, these time periods must be considered general guidelines. Determining the patient's readiness to advance from one phase of postoperative rehabilitation to the next should not be based solely on time but also on the patient's attainment of predetermined criteria, such as the absence of pain or restoration of a particular amount of ROM or level of strength. However, at this time most published guidelines and protocols are time based and provide little or no information for making criterion-based decisions.

Putting Postoperative Rehabilitation Into Perspective

Postoperative rehabilitation after an orthopedic surgical procedure is often a lengthy process. Given the limited number of justifiable therapy sessions available for postoperative management, it is highly unlikely for a therapist to have direct, ongoing contact with a patient through all phases of a rehabilitation program. Consequently, the key to successful postoperative outcomes is effective, long-term patient self-management. This approach includes therapist-directed, early postoperative patient education, followed by a home program of selected interventions—in particular, a progression of exercises that have been carefully taught and are periodically monitored and modified by the therapist during each phase of rehabilitation.[38]

Potential Postoperative Complications and Risk Reduction

There are a number of serious complications that a patient may encounter after surgery, any one of which can adversely affect the outcomes of surgery and postoperative rehabilitation. Complications can manifest early (within 6 months after surgery) and/or late, and some aspects of preoperative patient education and postoperative interventions are included to reduce the risk of developing complications. Potential complications are described here and noted in Box 12.5.[3,13,45,79]

Pulmonary Complications

The risk of pneumonia or atelectasis (collapse of the lung caused by bronchial obstruction) is highest during the early postoperative period. General anesthesia and use of pain medication increase the risk of these complications, as does extended confinement to bed. Deep breathing exercises initiated on the day of surgery and early standing and ambulation following surgery may reduce this risk.

DVT and Pulmonary Embolism

Although there is an increased risk of development of a DVT and a subsequent pulmonary embolism in all patients who have undergone surgery, this risk is particularly increased after total joint replacement surgery of the hip or knee.[21,89] A therapist must be familiar with signs and symptoms and risk factors for these complications, as well as interventions for prevention or management. The next section of this chapter contains more detailed information about DVT and pulmonary embolism.

BOX 12.5 Potential Postoperative Complications

- Pulmonary dysfunction, including pneumonia or atelectasis
- Local or systemic infection
- Deep vein thrombosis or pulmonary embolism
- Delayed wound healing
- Muscle function deficits secondary to tourniquet compression and resulting ischemia or nerve compression
- Failure, loosening, or displacement of internal fixation devices
- Delayed union of bone after fracture, osteotomy, or joint fusion
- Rupture of incompletely healed soft tissue after repair or reconstruction
- Subluxation or dislocation of joint surfaces or implants
- Nerve entrapment from scar tissue formation resulting in pain or sensory changes
- Adhesions and scarring leading to contractures of soft tissues and joint hypomobility
- Loosening of joint implants secondary to periprosthetic osteolysis or infection

Joint Subluxation or Dislocation

If a joint capsule has been incised during surgery, as is the case for total joint replacement or an open labrum repair, there is an increased risk of postoperative joint dislocation. This risk can be reduced through patient education and exercise instruction. For example, a preoperative or postoperative program typically includes teaching a patient proper use of a removable immobilization device, such as a splint or sling, and the joint positions to avoid during exercises and ADL so that the incision site is protected from increased loading.

Restricted Motion From Adhesions and Scar Tissue Formation

Postoperative contractures can develop as incised or repaired tissues progress through the healing process. Movement of the operated area as early as possible after surgery with ROM exercises or continuous passive motion (CPM) within a safe range is directed at maintaining the extensibility of soft tissues and preventing contractures.

Failure, Displacement, or Loosening of Internal Fixation Device

Excessive or premature weight bearing prior to bony healing after open reduction and internal fixation of a fracture can cause loss of bone-to-bone apposition of the fracture site. Heavy lifting or strong muscle recruitment after a soft tissue repair in the upper extremity can cause rupture of sutured, but incompletely healed, tissues. Proper use of supportive devices, such as crutches or a walker, to control weight bearing during ambulation and appropriate progression of exercises and functional activities can reduce the risk of these postoperative complications.

Deep Vein Thrombosis and Pulmonary Embolism: A Closer Look

A thrombosis is a bolus of coagulated blood in the circulatory system. Lower extremity venous thrombosis can occur in the superficial or deep vein systems (Fig. 12.1).[35] A thrombus in one of the superficial veins in the calf usually is small and resolves without serious consequences.[73] In contrast, thrombus formation in a deep vein in the calf, thigh, or pelvic region, known as DVT, tends to be larger and can cause serious complications. When a clot breaks away from the wall of a vein and travels proximally, it is called an *embolus*. When an embolus affects pulmonary circulation, it is called a *pulmonary embolism*, which is a potentially life-threatening disorder.[35,73]

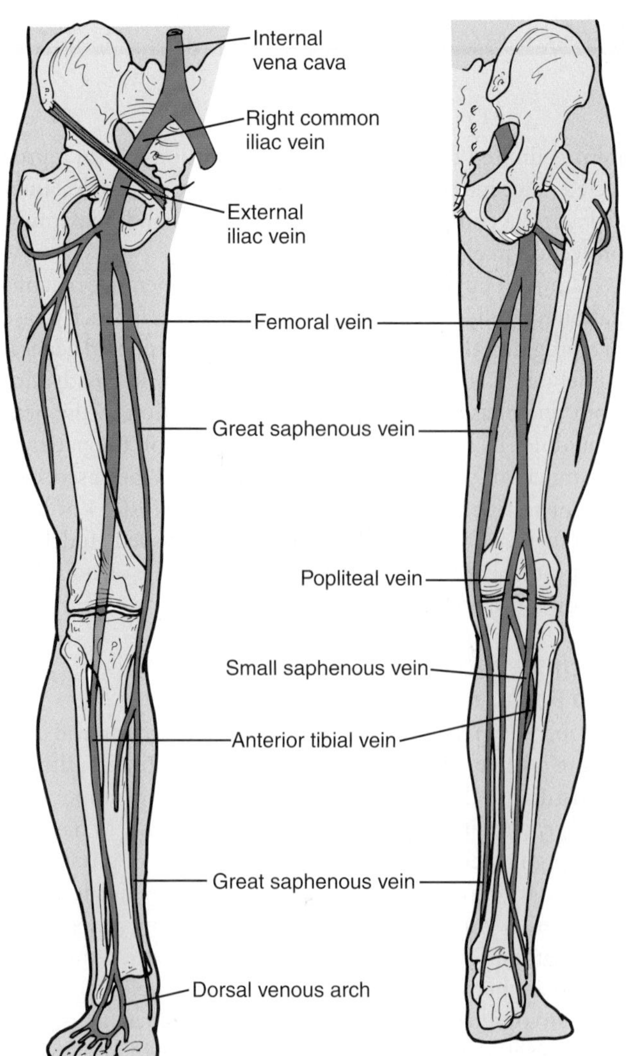

FIGURE 12.1 Veins of the lower extremity.

Risk Factors for DVT

A lower extremity DVT is a common complication after musculoskeletal injury or surgery, prolonged limb immobilization, or bed rest and is attributed to venous stasis, injury to and inflammation of the walls of a vein, or a hypercoagulable state of the blood.[39,87] Risk factors for DVT are listed in Box 12.6.[32,35,39,73]

DVT: Signs and Symptoms

During the early stages of a DVT, only 25% to 50% of cases can be recognized by clinical manifestations, such as dull aching or severe pain, swelling, or changes in skin temperature and color, specifically heat and redness.[2,35,39,73]

The Wells Criteria[88] provide the clinician with a tool to establish the likelihood of a lower extremity DVT when the condition is suspected. The criteria include both patient history and physical signs, and the presence of two or more clinical features indicate that a DVT is likely, while fewer than two suggests a DVT is unlikely.[88] Box 12.7 lists the Wells criteria. When a DVT is likely based on the clinical features present, medical testing should be initiated to confirm or rule out the condition. Only diagnostic imaging, such as ultrasonography, venous duplex screening, or venography, can confirm a DVT.[2,87]

BOX 12.7 Wells Criteria for Likelihood of Deep Vein Thrombosis[88] (A score of 2 or more points indicates a DVT is likely)

Clinical Feature	Points
Active cancer (treatment ongoing, within 6 months, or palliative care)	1
Paralysis, paresis, or recent plaster immobilization of the lower extremities	1
Recently bedridden for 3 days or longer, or major surgery requiring general or regional anesthesia within 12 weeks	1
Localized tenderness along the distribution of the deep venous system	1
Entire leg swollen	1
Calf swelling at least 3 cm larger than asymptomatic side	1
Pitting edema confined to symptomatic leg	1
Collateral superficial veins	1
Previously documented DVT	1
Alternative diagnosis at least as likely as DVT	-2

Pulmonary Embolism: Signs and Symptoms

As described previously, pulmonary embolism is a possible consequence of DVT. Risk factors for pulmonary embolism are similar to those already identified for DVT (see Box 12.6).

The signs and symptoms of pulmonary embolism vary considerably depending on the size of the embolus, the extent of lung involvement, and the presence of coexisting cardiopulmonary conditions.[93] The hallmark signs and symptoms are a sudden onset of shortness of breath (dyspnea), rapid and shallow breathing (tachypnea), and chest pain located at the lateral aspect of the chest that intensifies with deep breathing and coughing. Other signs and symptoms include swelling in the lower extremities, anxiety, fever, excessive sweating (diaphoresis), a cough, and blood in the sputum (hemoptysis).[93]

If a patient presents with signs or symptoms of possible pulmonary embolism, immediate medical referral is warranted for a definitive diagnosis and management.

BOX 12.6 Risk Factors for Deep Vein Thrombosis and Thrombophlebitis

- Postoperative or postfracture immobilization
- Prolonged bed rest
- Sedentary lifestyle or extended episode of sitting
- Prolonged standing (>6 hours)
- Trauma to venous vessels
- Limb paralysis
- Active malignancy (within past 6 months)
- History of deep vein thrombosis or pulmonary embolism
- Advanced age
- Obesity
- Congestive heart failure
- Use of oral contraceptives
- Pregnancy

Reducing the Risk of DVT

Every effort should be made to reduce the risk of a DVT and subsequent thrombophlebitis in patients who have undergone a surgical procedure, particularly a lower extremity procedure. The following medical/pharmacological and exercise-related interventions are implemented for risk reduction.[21,43,87,89]

- Prophylactic use of anticoagulant therapy (high molecular weight heparin) for the high-risk patient because of a lower extremity surgery or extended bed rest
- Elevating the legs when lying supine or when sitting
- No prolonged periods of sitting, especially for the patient with a long-leg cast
- Initiating ambulation as soon as possible after surgery, preferably no more than a day or two postoperatively
- Active "pumping" exercises (active dorsiflexion, plantarflexion, and circumduction of the ankle) regularly throughout the day when lying supine
- Use of compression stockings to support the walls of the veins and minimize venous pooling
- Use of a sequential pneumatic compression unit for patients on bed rest

CLINICAL TIP

In addition to medical/pharmacological management with administration of early postoperative, anticoagulant drugs,[21,89] 1 minute of active ankle pumping exercises performed at regular intervals during the day has been shown to increase venous blood flow (for up to 30 minutes after exercise) and decrease venous stasis in the calf after total hip replacement surgery.[60] Therefore, ankle pumping exercises are thought to decrease the risk of developing a DVT. Early ambulation (before day 2) after surgery also promotes circulation and reduces the risk of a DVT.[89]

Management of DVT

Acute care management. If the presence of DVT and resulting thrombophlebitis is confirmed, immediate medical intervention is essential to reduce the risk of pulmonary embolism. Initial management includes administering anticoagulant medication, placing the patient on bed rest, elevating the involved extremity, and using graduated compression stockings. The reported time frame for bed rest varies from 2 days to more than a week.[1] Box 12.8 summarizes the guidelines for management of acute DVT and thrombophlebitis.[1,54]

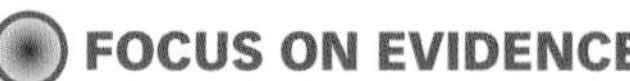

FOCUS ON EVIDENCE

A ***clinical practice guideline*** (CPG) for management of individuals at risk for or diagnosed with venous thromboembolism, developed by the APTA, provides 14 key action statements for therapists to consider in making decisions regarding care of patients with this condition.[42] The overall main points are that physical therapists:

- Are an integral part of the health care team in identifying those at risk for venous thromboembolism and lower extremity DVT;
- Should advocate for preventive measures in those determined to be at risk; should use the Wells criteria for assessing the degree of DVT risk;
- Should mobilize patients with a confirmed lower extremity DVT once therapeutic levels of anticoagulation medication are reached; and
- Can minimize future complications for patients after DVT through education, mechanical compression, and exercise.[42]

During the period of bed rest, exercises usually are contraindicated because movement of the involved extremity may cause pain and is thought to increase congestion in the venous channels when tissues are inflamed. It is currently suggested that ambulation can begin after anticoagulant therapy reaches

BOX 12.8 MANAGEMENT GUIDELINES—Deep Vein Thrombosis and Thrombophlebitis

Structural and Functional Impairments

Dull ache or pain usually in the calf

Tenderness, warmth, and swelling with palpation

Plan of Care	Interventions
1. Relieve pain during the acute inflammatory period.	1. Bed rest, pharmacological management (systemic anticoagulant therapy); elevation of the affected lower extremity, maintaining slight knee flexion.
2. Begin mobility when therapeutic levels of anticoagulant medication have been administered.	2. Progressively increasing ambulation and functional activity training while graded compression stockings are worn by patient.
3. As acute symptoms subside, regain functional mobility.	3. Continue graded ambulation with legs in pressure-gradient support stockings.
4. Prevent recurrence of the acute disorder.	4. Continuation of appropriate medical and pharmacological management. Use of strategies to prevent DVTs.

CONTRAINDICATIONS: Passive or active motion or application of moist heat; use of a sequential pneumatic compression pump.

PRECAUTIONS: Following discharge but while continuing anticoagulant medication, avoid contact sports and high fall risk physical activities.

therapeutic levels, and the therapist should consult the medical team regarding the timing of initiating this intervention.[42]

 **FOCUS ON EVIDENCE**

Aldrich and colleagues[1] conducted a systematic review of the literature to determine when a patient with DVT should be allowed to begin walking. The review revealed a limited number of studies (a total of five, three of which were randomized, controlled trials) that addressed this issue. Results of these studies suggest that early ambulation, begun within the first 24 hours after initiating anticoagulant therapy, does not increase the incidence of pulmonary embolism in patients without an existing pulmonary embolism and who have adequate cardiopulmonary reserve. However, if a patient has a known pulmonary embolism, an ambulation program must be initiated more cautiously. It is important to note that in the studies reviewed all patients who participated in an early ambulation program wore compression garments.

The results also revealed that early ambulation is associated with more rapid resolution of pain and swelling. The authors of the review were unable to identify studies that investigated the initiation and progression of other forms of exercise for patients with DVT.

Posthospitalization precautions. Following discharge, a patient typically continues on an anticoagulant medication for about 6 months. During that time period, the patient must avoid contact sports, running, and skiing; however, treadmill walking or jogging and use of an elliptical trainer is permitted. Mandatory helmet use also is advisable during participation in high "fall risk" activities.[32]

Overview of Common Orthopedic Surgeries and Postoperative Management

Surgical management of musculoskeletal conditions encompasses a wide variety of procedures. Orthopedic surgery procedures can be divided into several broad categories, including repair, reattachment, reconstruction, stabilization, replacement, realignment, transfer, release, resection (excision), fixation, and fusion.[17,37,77] Examples of specific procedures in these categories are identified in Table 12.1.

The purpose of this final chapter section is to provide brief descriptions of some surgical procedures in these categories and a broad overview of the place of therapeutic exercise in postoperative rehabilitation. Factors such as duration of immobilization following surgery and the timing, intensity and progression of exercise will vary based on the surgical techniques used, the surgeon's philosophy, and patient's response to surgery and postoperative therapy. Chapters 17 through 22 contain more extensive descriptions of selected surgical procedures and progressions of postoperative management for each region of the upper and lower extremities. For more detailed descriptions of specific surgeries and operative techniques for musculoskeletal conditions from the orthopedic surgeon's perspective, many textbooks and journals are available for reference.[17,33,37,59,66,80,90] The specific aspects of an individual patient's surgical procedure should be known prior to designing and implementing a safe and effective postoperative exercise program and this information is available in the operative report in the patient's medical record and through communication with the surgeon.

Surgical Approaches

Open Procedures

An open surgical procedure involves an incision of adequate length and depth through the necessary superficial and deep layers of skin, fascia, muscles, and joint capsule that allows the operative field to be fully visualized by the surgeon during the procedure.[57,77] The term *arthrotomy* is used to describe an open procedure in which the joint capsule is incised to expose joint structures. Open approaches are necessary for surgeries such as joint replacement, arthrodesis, or internal fixation of fractures and for some soft tissue repairs and reconstruction such as tendon or ligament tears. Open procedures result in extensive disturbance of soft tissues and require a lengthy period of rehabilitation to allow soft tissue healing.

Arthroscopic Procedures

Arthroscopy is used as a diagnostic tool and as a means of treating a variety of intra-articular disorders.[29,59,72,82] Arthroscopic procedures are typically performed on an outpatient basis and often under local anesthesia.

Arthroscopy involves several very small incisions (portals) in the skin, muscle, and joint capsule for insertion of an endoscope to visualize the interior of the joint by means of a camera, and of miniature, motorized surgical tools used for the procedures. Arthroscopic techniques are most often used for surgical procedures at the shoulder and knee[57,59,72,82] but are being used increasingly more frequently for hip joint disorders.[20,29]

Arthroscopic procedures include ligament, tendon, and capsule repairs or reconstruction, joint débridement, meniscectomy, articular cartilage repair, and synovectomy. Because the incisions for the portals are so small, there is minimal disturbance of soft tissues during arthroscopic procedures. Therefore, rehabilitation usually—but not always—can proceed more quickly than after an open procedure.

Arthroscopically Assisted Procedures

An arthroscopically assisted procedure uses arthroscopy for a portion of the procedure but also requires an open surgical field for selected aspects of the operative procedure.[57,59] This approach is sometimes referred to as a "mini-open" procedure.[31]

TABLE 12.1 General Methods and Examples of Musculoskeletal Surgeries

Surgical Methods	Examples of Procedures
Repair	Tenorrhaphy, tendon repair; meniscus or ligament repair; articular cartilage repair
Release or decompression	Myotomy, tenotomy, fasciotomy; capsulotomy; tenolysis; muscle-tendon lengthening; retinacular release; arthroscopic subacromial decompression
Resection or removal	Synovectomy, meniscectomy, capsulectomy; débridement and lavage; laminectomy; excision of soft tissue or boney neoplasms
Realignment or stabilization	Tendon transfer, tenodesis; extensor mechanism realignment; capsulorrhaphy, capsular shift; osteotomy
Reconstruction or replacement	Tenoplasty; capsulolabral reconstruction; ligamentous reconstruction; chondroplasty; arthroplasty
Fusion or fixation for bony union	Arthrodesis; open reduction with internal fixation

Tissue Grafts

In a number of orthopedic procedures to repair damaged structures, tissue grafts are implanted during the repair process. For example, soft tissue grafts are routinely used to reconstruct ligaments of the knee or ankle. Grafts are also used in articular cartilage repair procedures and many bony procedures.

Types of Grafts

Tissue grafts can be placed into several categories: autografts, allografts, and synthetic grafts.[51]

Autograft. An autograft, also referred to as an autogenous or autologous graft, uses a patient's own tissue harvested from a donor site in the body. Patellar tendon grafts, for example, have been used for more than 4 decades for intra-articular anterior or posterior cruciate ligament reconstruction.[69] More recently, autografts have been used for osteochondral implantation for repair of small, localized femoral condyle articular defects.[19] Risks associated with autografts include the need for two surgical procedures and the potential for negative consequences at the donor site.

Allograft. An allograft uses fresh or cryopreserved tissue that comes from a source other than the patient, typically from a cadaveric donor. This type of graft is used when an autograft in a previous surgery has failed or when an appropriate autograft is not available. Allografts are associated with several risks, such as disease transmission from the donor, compromised graft strength resulting from sterilization, and failure secondary to immunological rejection. Allograft is not an option for articular cartilage implantation because cryopreservation destroys articular chondrocytes.

Synthetic grafts. Materials such as Gore-Tex® and Dacron offer an alternative to human tissue and have been used on a limited basis for ligament reconstruction in the knee. However, synthetic ligaments, to date, have had a high rate of failure and have not maintained their integrity over time.[19] Implantation of synthetic ligaments has also been associated with chronic synovitis of the knee.

Repair, Reattachment, Reconstruction, Stabilization, or Transfer of Soft Tissues

Surgical repair, reattachment, or reconstruction of soft tissues may be necessary after severe injury of a muscle, tendon, or ligament.[37,48,55,62] Surgical reconstruction and stabilization of a joint capsule may be indicated to reduce excessive capsular laxity contributing to instability of the joint.[56,91] Transfer of a muscle-tendon unit may be required to improve stability of an unstable joint or to enhance neuromuscular control and function.

Although there are numerous surgeries that fall into this category, a therapist must always consider the effects of immobilization and remobilization and the healing characteristics of the soft tissues involved when designing a postoperative exercise program.

Muscle Repair

A complete tear or rupture of a muscle is unusual but may occur if a muscle that is in a state of contraction takes a direct blow or is forcibly stretched.[17]

Procedure

Immediate surgical repair of a severe tear or even complete rupture of a muscle is uncommon because inflammation affects the texture of muscle tissue, making it difficult to hold sutures in place. A patient can achieve a more satisfactory outcome with a late repair (approximately 48 to 72 hours after injury) after acute symptoms have decreased. For repair, the muscle is re-opposed, sutured, and immobilized in a shortened position as healing begins.[62,77]

Postoperative Management

- Gradual muscle-setting exercise of the sutured muscle may be initiated immediately after surgery.
- When the immobilization is removed, active ROM, emphasizing controlled motion within a protected range, may begin to restore joint mobility and prevent contractures.
- Weight bearing is partially restricted until the patient achieves a functional level of strength and flexibility in the repaired muscle.
- Low-load, high-repetition resistance exercises should not elicit pain and be progressed very gradually to protect the healing muscle.
- Vigorous stretching or the return to full activity level are contraindicated until soft tissue healing is complete—as long as 6 to 8 weeks postoperatively.

Tendon Repair

When a tendon tears or ruptures in a young person, it is usually the result of severe trauma.[68] In an elderly person, tears are usually the result of progressive deterioration of a tendon coupled with a sudden and unusual or forceful motion.[6] Tendons usually rupture at musculotendinous or tendo-osseous junctions.[68] Common sites of acute tear or rupture are the bicipital tendon at the shoulder and the Achilles tendon.[49]

In patients with chronic tenosynovitis of the hand and wrist, the extensor tendons can erode over time and may eventually rupture along the dorsum of the hand.[7,13] The superficial tendons of the hand and foot also are vulnerable to lacerations that may require surgical repair. The flexor tendons of the fingers, for example, are commonly severed as the result of a deep laceration to the palm of the hand.

Aside from the acute pain that occurs at the time of injury, a complete tendon tear, rupture, or laceration causes an inability to generate tension in the muscle-tendon unit and results in weakness but little pain. With a partial tear, there is significant pain during an active muscle contraction or stretch of the muscle-tendon unit.

Procedure

A complete tear or laceration of a tendon should be repaired immediately or within a few days after injury. If not repaired within this time the tendon begins to retract, making reattachment difficult. After the tendon is sutured, the repaired muscle-tendon unit is maintained in a shortened position, as with a complete tear of a muscle. A longer immobilization period may be required for a repaired tendon than for a repaired muscle because the vascular supply to tendons is poor.[26,24] However, remobilization involving a limited degree of tensile forces on the repaired tendon is initiated as early as possible to prevent or minimize adhesions that can hinder tendon gliding.

Postoperative Management

- Muscle setting is begun immediately after surgery to prevent adhesions of the tendon to the sheath or surrounding tissues and to promote alignment of healing tissue. If it is possible to remove the immobilization for brief periods of exercise, passive motion or active contraction of a muscle group that is an antagonist of the repaired muscle tendon within a protected range also may be permissible within a few days after surgery.[7,14]
- Controlled antigravity motions are initiated after the repaired tendon has had several weeks to heal.
- Weight bearing may be restricted after an upper or lower extremity tendon repair, and heavy lifting activities are often contraindicated for as long as 6 to 8 weeks after an upper extremity repair.
- Because the muscle-tendon unit must be held in a shortened position for several weeks, regaining full range may be difficult. However, vigorous stretching and high-intensity resistance exercise should not be initiated for at least 8 weeks after repair, when healing of the tendon has occurred.[14]

NOTE: For detailed information on postoperative rehabilitation after repair of tendons in the shoulder, fingers, or ankle, refer to Chapters 17, 19, and 22, respectively.

Ligament Repair or Reconstruction

After a large or complete ligament tear or when a ligament cannot be approximated for healing through closed reduction, surgical intervention through repair or reconstruction is warranted. Repair involves approximating and suturing the torn ligament, whereas reconstruction is accomplished with a tissue graft taken from a donor site. The knee, ankle, and elbow joints are the more common sites of ligament injury and surgical intervention.[33,48,50,90]

Procedure

There are many surgical procedures that involve ligamentous repair or reconstruction. What is common to these surgeries is that, postoperatively, the joint is held in a position that places a safe level of tension on the sutured or reconstructed ligament during the healing process.[50,55] The duration of immobilization varies with the site and severity of injury and the type of repair or reconstruction that was done.[11,16,77,90]

Postoperative Management

Rehabilitation after ligament surgery emphasizes early but protected motion and progressive strengthening and weight-bearing activities to load the healing tissues consistently but safely.[50,69,90] The rate of progression depends on many factors, such as the type of repair or reconstruction that was done. For example, rehabilitation after anterior cruciate ligament reconstruction utilizing a patellar tendon graft and bone-to-bone fixation can be progressed more rapidly than after a soft tissue stabilization procedure involving a hamstring graft.[16,27,55] The rate of advancement also depends on the site of the repair or reconstruction. For example, if the repair is at a potentially unstable joint, external support such as a brace should be worn and weight bearing restricted until muscular control can adequately protect the joint.

Generally, postoperative rehabilitation after ligamentous surgery is a lengthy process. For patients wishing to return to high-demand work or sports activities, it may take at least 6 months or as long as a year of rehabilitation until they are ready.[27,55]

NOTE: Rehabilitation after reconstruction of ligaments of the knee and ankle is addressed in Chapters 21 and 22.

Capsule Stabilization and Reconstruction

A joint capsule with excessive laxity loses the capacity to provide passive stability to the joint. Hypermobility of the capsule can therefore be an underlying cause of symptomatic joint instability ranging from subluxation to gross instability and recurrent dislocation. Joints particularly vulnerable to instability are those with minimal inherent stability, most notably the glenohumeral joint.

In some instances, an individual is predisposed to instability at many joints because capsular laxity and joint hypermobility are congenital.[76] More often, joint instability results from an acute capsular injury suffered during a traumatic dislocation or from repetitive stresses applied to the capsule with the joint in extreme positions.[56] The latter is seen most often in athletes participating in sports such as baseball and tennis that involve repetitive, end-range shoulder motions.[84]

Surgical stabilization or reconstruction of a joint capsule is indicated for a patient with traumatic dislocation with associated capsular or labral avulsion or fracture, recurrent dislocation or symptomatic subluxation despite a course of nonoperative treatment, or an irreducible (fixed) dislocation.[56,72,84,94]

Procedure

Surgical procedures designed to reduce capsular laxity and joint volume and restore or improve joint stability fall into several categories and are performed using open or arthroscopic approaches. An open procedure with arthrotomy is used if an open reduction of the joint is required or if there is extensive damage to the labrum, avulsion of the capsule, or a fracture. An arthroscopic approach is most often used to reduce capsular laxity and for some reconstructive procedures.[56,94]

Examples of stabilization and reconstruction procedures at the glenohumeral joint used for anterior, posterior, inferior, or multidirectional instabilities are described here.

Capsulorrhaphy (capsular shift). For capsulorrhaphy using an arthroscopic or open approach, a specific portion of the capsule is incised and tightened by imbrication/plication (overlapping and then suturing) of the redundant tissue.

Capsulolabral reconstruction. Capsulolabral reconstruction involves arthroscopic or open repair of a capsular lesion and labral tear by reattaching the labrum to the rim of the glenoid in combination with capsule stabilization.

Electrothermally assisted capsulorrhaphy. For electrothermally assisted capsulorrhaphy using an arthroscopic approach, thermal energy (laser or radiofrequency) is delivered to the capsule to shrink identified regions of laxity.[91]

Postoperative Management

After any joint stabilization or reconstruction procedure, the emphasis of postoperative management is to restore the balance among joint stability and functional motion while protecting the joint capsule and other repaired tissues during healing. The duration of the immobilization period and the selection and progression of postoperative exercises and functional activities depend on factors such as the preoperative direction of the instability, the surgical approach, the type of stabilization or reconstruction procedure and tissue fixation used, and the quality of the patient's tissue.

Postoperative exercises focus on the following:

- Restoring ROM, emphasizing active motions within a protected range during early rehabilitation. Movements that place stress on the portion of the capsule that was tightened or repaired are progressed cautiously.
- Strengthening exercises, when permissible, emphasizing the function of the dynamic joint stabilizers.

NOTE: Detailed progressions of postoperative exercises after surgical stabilization of the shoulder are presented in Chapter 17.

Tendon Transfer or Realignment

The transfer or realignment of a muscle-tendon unit alters the line of pull, potential force generation, and excursion of the muscle.[71] Transfers may be indicated, for example, to improve the stability of an unstable shoulder joint or to stabilize a chronically dislocating patella. Although a realignment procedure alters the line of pull, it does not change the action of the muscle-tendon unit. For instance, after realignment of the extensor mechanism for recurrent patellar dislocation, the quadriceps muscle remains a knee extensor.

A tendon transfer from one bony surface to another is sometimes indicated for the patient with a significant neurological deficit to prevent deformity and improve functional control.[71] With this type of procedure, not only is the line of pull of the muscle-tendon unit altered, but the action of the muscle is also changed. For example, transfer of the distal attachment of the flexor carpi ulnaris to the dorsal surface of the wrist changes the action of the muscle-tendon unit from a wrist flexor to a wrist extensor. This procedure may be indicated for a child with cerebral palsy to prevent wrist flexion contracture and improve active wrist extension for functional grasp.[71]

Procedure

During a typical tendon transfer or realignment procedure, the distal attachment of the muscle-tendon unit is removed from its bony insertion and reattached to a different bone, to a different location on the same bone, or to adjacent soft tissues.[62,71,77] The realigned muscle-tendon unit is then immobilized in a shortened position for a period of time.

Postoperative Management

- As with a tendon repair, early muscle setting and protected motion are important to maintain tendon gliding. Resisted movements are progressed cautiously and gradually to protect the reattached tendon.
- If the purpose of the transfer was to change the function of the muscle, biofeedback and electrical muscle stimulation are often used to help a patient learn to control the new actions of the transferred muscle-tendon unit.[77]

NOTE: Rehabilitation after tendon transfer for rheumatoid arthritis of the hand and wrist is described in Chapter 19. Chapter 21 contains information on rehabilitation after realignment of the patellar tendon for chronic patellofemoral dysfunction.

Release, Lengthening, or Decompression of Soft Tissues

Soft tissues may be incised or sectioned to improve ROM, prevent or minimize progressive deformity, or relieve pain. Procedures include myotomy, tenotomy, or fasciotomy.[11,62,77]

Surgical release of soft tissues may be indicated for a young patient with severe arthritis and resulting contractures in whom joint replacement is not advisable or as a preliminary procedure in adults prior to joint replacement.[13] Releases are also performed in patients with myopathic and neuropathic diseases, such as muscular dystrophy and cerebral palsy, to improve functional mobility.[77] Release of soft tissues to achieve decompression of tissues and relieve pain may be indicated for a patient with an impingement or compartmental syndrome, such as shoulder impingement or carpal tunnel syndrome.[11,62]

Procedure

During release or lengthening of a shortened muscle group, a portion of the muscle-tendon unit is surgically sectioned and fibrotic tissues are incised. A tendon also can be partially incised, as in a Z-lengthening to allow greater extensibility. The incised structures are then immobilized in a lengthened position except during exercise.[62,77] Some form of splinting or bracing in the corrected position in conjunction with exercise is always used postoperatively to maintain the ROM gained by the procedure.

During decompression procedures, fasciae that are compressing muscles, tendons, or nerves may be released or removed. Some decompression procedures also involve removal of osteophytes or alteration of bony structures that are contributing to the excessive pressure on soft tissues.

Postoperative Management

- CPM and/or active-assistive ROM is typically initiated within a day or two after surgery. As soft tissue healing progresses, this is followed by active ROM through the gained ranges.[11,77]
- Strengthening of the antagonists of the lengthened muscle and functional use within the available ROM are also started early to maintain active control of movement within the newly gained range.

Joint Procedures

Orthopedic surgery involving the joints of the upper and lower extremities is most frequently used for pain management and for dysfunction associated with arthritis or acute injury. Surgical interventions for arthritis range from arthroscopic joint débridement and lavage or repair of a small chondral lesion to total joint replacement arthroplasty or joint fusion. An overview of these procedures follows.

Arthroscopic Débridement and Lavage

Joint débridement and lavage involves arthroscopic removal of fibrillated cartilage, unstable chondral flaps, and fragments of cartilage or bone from a joint.[13] Osteophytes also may be excised. This procedure is most often indicated to relieve joint pain and "clicking," "ratcheting," or "catching" during joint movement.

Synovectomy

Synovectomy involves removal of the synovial lining of the joint in the presence of chronic joint inflammation. Typically, it is performed in patients who have rheumatoid arthritis with chronic proliferative synovitis but minimal articular changes.[13,41,61,92] It is indicated when medical management has failed to alleviate joint inflammation for 4 to 6 months.

Procedure

Synovectomy is usually performed using an arthroscopic approach and is most commonly performed on the knee, elbow, wrist, and metacarpophalangeal (MCP) joints.[7,13,41,61,92] When synovium proliferates in the synovial sheaths of tendons, it is referred to as tenosynovitis. Removal of excessive synovium from tendon sheaths is known as a tenosynovectomy. This procedure is most often done for chronic synovitis of the wrist to clear synovium from the extensor tendons of the hand and is also called a dorsal clearance procedure.[13,61,92]

Although synovium tends to regenerate, resection of the inflamed synovium temporarily relieves pain and swelling and is thought to protect articular cartilage or tendons from enzymatic damage secondary to the tenosynovitis.[13,41]

Postoperative Management

- If an arthroscopic approach is used, passive or assisted ROM exercises (or CPM) and muscle-setting exercises are begun immediately or within 24 hours after surgery. Exercises quickly progress to active ROM. After synovectomy of the knee, for example, partial weight bearing as tolerated during ambulation progresses to full weight bearing by 10 to 14 days. After wrist or elbow synovectomy, lifting heavy objects is restricted for several weeks.
- After open synovectomy, progression of exercises and ADLs proceeds more slowly than after arthroscopic synovectomy.
- Progression of the rehabilitation program is based on the patient's response to exercise combined with their response to medication for the primary inflammatory disease. Every effort should be made to avoid excessive exercise or activity that could increase joint pain or swelling.[7,61,92]

Articular Cartilage Procedures

Surgical intervention for repair of articular cartilage defects, or osteochondral lesions, has proven to be particularly challenging because of the limited capacity of this type of connective tissue to heal.[19,64] However, several procedures for a symptomatic extremity joint have been developed. Selection criteria for one procedure over another are based on the size of the chondral lesion and patient-related factors, such as age and the ability to participate in the rehabilitation process.

Procedure

Abrasion arthroplasty, subchondral drilling, and microfracture. Several arthroscopic procedures are used to promote healing of small chondral defects in symptomatic joints. These procedures stimulate a bone marrow-based response that leads to local ingrowth of fibrocartilage.[19,64,82] Lesions of the medial femoral condyle and the posterior aspect of the patella are most often treated with these procedures.

Abrasion arthroplasty, also known as abrasion chondroplasty, and subchondral drilling involve mechanical disruption of the articular surface down to the superficial layer of subchondral bone using a motorized, arthroscopic burr or drill. The positive effects of these procedures have been questionable, at best, and possibly no more effective for symptom relief than arthroscopic débridement alone.[19]

FOCUS ON EVIDENCE

A long-term assessment of abrasion arthroplasty for full-thickness medial femoral condyle cartilage lesions noted that at 20 years' post procedure, 68% of the patients reported Knee Society Scores ≥ 70 or no secondary operation on their knee. All patients had CPM until hospital discharge, 6 to 8 hours of CPM per day following discharge, and protected weight bearing for a minimum of 6 weeks.[78] Outcomes at a mean of 38.1 months for subchondral drilling of the talus demonstrated improvements in pain and two separate standardized outcome measures. Weight bearing in a walking boot was limited to tolerance for 2 weeks, followed by full weight-bearing and active exercises.[18]

NOTE: Despite evidence supporting long-term functional outcomes after abrasion arthroplasty or subchondral drilling,[18,78] the local, tissue-specific benefits may be short-lived. Because the fibrocartilage replacement tissue lacks the qualities of the original hyaline cartilage, the new tissue tends to deteriorate readily after ingrowth.[11,19]

A newer technique, microfracture of articular cartilage, is designed to repair osteochondral defects smaller than 1.5 cm^2. This procedure involves the use of a nonmotorized arthroscopic awl to systematically penetrate the subchondral bone and expose the bone marrow. Initial studies of this procedure suggested that microfracture relieved symptoms more effectively than abrasion arthroplasty or subchondral drilling, possibly because using the nonmotorized instrument reduces the potential for tissue damage due to thermal necrosis.[19,64] However, a recent comparison of microfracture and subchondral drilling for talus osteochondral defects did not find long-term differences in outcomes between the two procedures.[18] A recent systematic review of level I and II studies of microfracture suggests that this procedure provides good short-term benefit for younger patients and those with small defects but that osteoarthritis and failures requiring additional surgical procedures were frequently reported at long-term follow-up.[36]

Chondrocyte transplantation. Chondrocyte transplantation, also known as autologous chondrocyte implantation (ACI),[34,64] is designed to stimulate growth of hyaline cartilage for repair of articular cartilage focal defects and to prevent progressive deterioration of joint cartilage leading to osteoarthritis.[12,19,34,63,64] It was introduced during the mid-1990s as an alternative to abrasion arthroplasty for full-thickness, symptomatic focal chondral and osteochondral defects (2.5 to 4.0 cm^2) of the knee, specifically lesions of the femoral condyles or patella.[12]

Chondrocyte transplantation occurs in two stages. First, healthy articular cartilage is harvested arthroscopically from the patient. Chondrocytes are extracted from this articular cartilage, cultured for several weeks, and processed in a laboratory to increase the volume of healthy tissue. The second stage, currently an open procedure, involves debridement of the defect sites, covering the site with a periosteal patch, and injecting millions of autologous chondrocytes into the covered defect.[19] Long-term success for function and patient satisfaction have been reported in up to 82% of patients following ACI.[70]

Osteochondral autografts and allografts. Unlike transplantation of chondrocytes, osteochondral grafts involve transplantation of intact articular cartilage along with some underlying bone, resulting in a bone-to-bone graft.[64] An autogenous osteochondral graft procedure harvests a patient's own articular cartilage and bone from a donor site.[19] As noted previously (see Box 12.10), a drawback to this type of articular graft is damage to the donor site, specifically the creation of an osteochondral defect. To minimize damage to the patient's donor site, osteochondral mosaicplasty was developed where small-diameter osteochondral plugs are retrieved from a donor site and press-fit into the chondral defect.[9]

In contrast, an osteochondral allograft procedure transplants intact articular cartilage and bone from a cadaveric donor. However, only fresh, intact grafts, which are in limited supply and can be stored for only a few days, can be used. This is because freezing the graft material prior to storage for later use destroys the articular chondrocytes and results in graft failure.

Postoperative Management

Rehabilitation after all of the articular cartilage procedures described in this section, with the exception of arthroscopic débridement, is a slow and arduous process.[12,19,34,44,63,64] Exercise is an important aspect of postoperative management at each stage of rehabilitation. Early passive motion, sometimes with CPM, and protected weight bearing are essential to promote the maturation and maintain the health of implanted chondrocytes or an osteochondral graft. Full weight bearing is allowable by 8 to 9 weeks. A well-controlled program of progressive exercises continues for 6 months to a year to achieve optimal functional outcomes.[334,44]

NOTE: More detailed information on rehabilitation after procedures to repair articular cartilage and osteochondral lesions is presented in Chapter 21.

Arthroplasty

Any reconstructive joint procedure designed to relieve pain and improve function is referred to broadly as arthroplasty. This definition encompasses excision, interposition, and replacement arthroplasty, procedures that may or may not include a joint implant.

Procedure

Excision arthroplasty. Excision arthroplasty, also known as resection arthroplasty, involves removing periarticular bone from one or both articular surfaces. A space is maintained between the new surfaces that is filled with fibrotic scar tissue during the healing process.[13,61] Excision arthroplasty is performed to relieve pain in many joints, including the hip, elbow, wrist, and foot. Although an older and less frequently used procedure, this type of arthroplasty is still considered appropriate in select cases. Resection of the head of the radius for late-stage arthritis of the humeroradial joint[22] or a severe comminuted fracture of the radial head[65] and resection of the distal ulna (Darrach procedure) for late-stage arthritis of the distal radioulnar joint[24] are still used as primary excision procedures to reduce pain. However, excision arthroplasty of the hip (Girdlestone procedure) is only used now as a salvage procedure after a failed total hip replacement when revision arthroplasty is not feasible.[13]

Despite the usefulness of excision arthroplasty, there are also a number of disadvantages:

- Possible joint instability
- In the hip, significant leg length discrepancy and poor cosmetic result because of shortening of the operated extremity
- Persistent muscular imbalance and weakness

NOTE: Rehabilitation after excision arthroplasty of the radial head is discussed in Chapter 18.

Excision arthroplasty with implant. For excision arthroplasty with implant, an artificial implant is inserted to help in the remodeling of a new joint. This is sometimes called implant resection arthroplasty.[22,61] The implant usually is made of a flexible silicone material that becomes encapsulated by fibrous tissue as the joint reforms.

Interposition arthroplasty. Interposition arthroplasty is biological resurfacing of a joint to provide a new articulating surface. After the involved joint surfaces are débrided, a foreign material is placed, or interposed, between the two joint surfaces.[5,61] A variety of materials including fascia tendon, silicone material, or metal may be inserted between the joint surfaces.

This type of arthroplasty is used most often in young patients with incapacitating pain and loss of function from severe articular surface deterioration who are not appropriate for replacement arthroplasty. Some examples of interpositional arthroplasty are resurfacing of the glenoid fossa with fascia[5] and tendon interposition arthroplasty of the carpometacarpal (CMC) joint of the thumb.[23]

Joint replacement arthroplasty. Joint replacement arthroplasty includes total joint replacement arthroplasty and hemireplacement arthroplasty. Total joint replacement is a common reconstructive procedure to relieve pain and improve function in patients with severe joint degeneration associated with late-stage arthritis (Fig. 12.2).[13,57,61,66]

Total joint replacement arthroplasty involves resecting both articular surfaces and replacing them with artificial components. Hemireplacement arthroplasty involves resection and replacement of only one of the articular surfaces.[13,61,66] Hemireplacement is used when only one articulating surface of a joint has deteriorated and is also an option after femoral neck and proximal humeral fractures.[13]

- ***Materials, designs, and methods of fixation.*** Prosthetic components have been developed and refined for almost every extremity joint but are used more frequently and successfully at the hip and knee than at the smaller joints of the foot and hand.[13,61,66] The materials, designs, and fixation methods used for replacement arthroplasty are summarized in Box 12.9. Prosthetic implants are made of inert materials, specifically metal alloys, high-density polyethylenes (plastics), and sometimes ceramics. Component designs range from unconstrained (resurfacing) with no inherent stability to semiconstrained and fully constrained (articulated) designs that provide stability to the joint. In almost all designs, one articular surface is metal and the other is plastic. The choice of fixation is based in part on the anticipated loading that will be normally placed on the components over time. Cemented fixation, using an acrylic-based

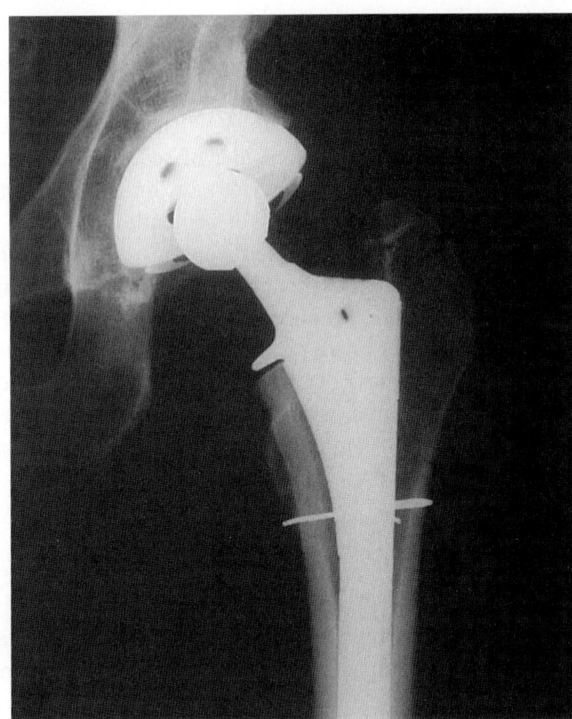

FIGURE 12.2 Total hip replacement arthroplasty. Both the acetabular and femoral portions of the joint have been replaced with prosthetic components. *(From McKinnis, LN:* Fundamentals of Musculoskeletal Imaging, *ed. 4. Philadelphia: F.A. Davis, 2014, p 387, with permission.)*

BOX 12.9 Materials, Designs, and Methods of Fixation for Joint Replacement Arthroplasty

Implant Materials
- Rigid: inert metal (cobalt-chrome alloy, titanium alloy, or ceramic)
- Semirigid: plastic (high-density polymers such as polyethylene)

Implant Designs
- Unconstrained (resurfacing): no inherent stability
- Semiconstrained
- Fully constrained (articulated): inherent stability

Methods of Fixation
- Cemented
  - Acrylic cement (polymethylmethacrylate)
- Noncemented
  - Biological fixation (microscopic ingrowth of bone into a porous-coated prosthetic surface)
  - Macrointerlock between a nonporous component and bone with a bioactive compound applied to the component to improve osseous integration
  - Press fit (tight fit between bone and implant)
  - Screws, bolts, or nails
- Hybrid
  - Noncemented component for one joint surface and cemented component for opposing joint surface

cement (polymethylmethacrylate), tends to eventually break down at the bone-cement interface, resulting in mechanical loosening of the implant and pain.[13,66,79] Therefore, cemented fixation is used primarily for older or sedentary patients who are unlikely to place high stresses on the implants. Bio-ingrowth fixation, a form of cementless fixation, is achieved by growth of bone into the porous-coated exterior surface of an implant. It is thought that this form of fixation, which is advocated for younger, more active patients, is less likely to loosen over time.[13,66,79] Most recently, a nonporous, cementless prosthetic implant has been developed that is used with a bioactive compound that stimulates bone growth. Fixation is achieved by a macrointerlock between the implant and adjacent bone.[66]

NOTE: Descriptions of implants are reviewed, joint by joint, in Chapters 17 through 22.

- ***Minimally invasive versus traditional arthroplasty.*** A recent advance in joint replacement arthroplasty that may have a significant impact on postoperative rehabilitation and outcomes is the development of minimally invasive surgical techniques with less soft tissue disruption than traditional arthroplasty. Currently, minimally invasive procedures are being used for total hip and total knee replacement.[4,10,85] Although traditional hip and knee replacement procedures have provided excellent results for several decades,[13,67,79] they impose substantial trauma to skin, muscles, and joint capsule, leading to significant postoperative pain and prolonged postoperative recovery. Compared to surgical techniques for traditional hip and knee replacement, minimally invasive procedures use smaller skin incisions, less muscle splitting to expose the joint, and less capsule disruption in preparation for insertion of prosthetic implants. For example, a minimally invasive hip replacement surgery uses one or two small incisions (<10 cm in length) rather than a single longer incision (15 to 30 cm long involving extensive muscle splitting).[10] A 2-year follow-up study indicates that patients who underwent minimally invasive total knee replacement had less pain, better early motion, and a shorter hospital stay than patients who had standard knee replacement surgery.[85] These early patient benefits of minimally invasive surgery for knee arthroplasty have not translated to improved functional performance, pain, ROM, or surgical outcomes at either 8 or 12 weeks when compared to those having a conventional open technique.[81,86]
- ***Contraindications to joint replacement arthroplasty.*** Despite the positive functional outcomes after joint replacement arthroplasty, not every patient with advanced joint disease is a candidate for these procedures. Contraindications are noted in Box 12.10.[13,61,66] Although opinions vary as to which of these contraindications are absolute versus relative, there is general agreement that infection is of the utmost concern.

Postoperative Management

Postoperative management, including therapeutic exercise interventions, after selected types of joint replacement arthroplasty of major joints of the extremities is described in detail in Chapters 17 through 22.

Arthrodesis

Arthrodesis is surgical fusion of the joint surfaces. It is indicated as a primary surgical intervention in cases of severe joint pain associated with late-stage arthritis and joint instability in which mobility of the joint is a lesser concern.[8,83] Arthrodesis of the extremity joints is also reserved for patients with significant weakness of muscles surrounding a joint as the result of neurological abnormalities, such as a peripheral neuropathy of the ankle or a severe brachial plexus injury.[62,77] In addition,

BOX 12.10 Contraindications to Total Joint Arthroplasty

- Active infection in the joint
- Chronic osteomyelitis
- Systemic infection
- Substantial loss of bone or malignant tumors that prohibit adequate implant fixation
- Significant paralysis of muscles surrounding the joint
- Neuropathic joint
- Inadequate patient motivation

it may be the only salvage procedure available for a patient with a failed total joint arthroplasty when revision arthroplasty is not an option.[53]

Arthrodesis is used most frequently in the cervical or lumbar spine, wrist, thumb, and ankle but also has been used in the shoulder and hip joints. For example, arthrodesis of one or more joints of the ankle and foot (Fig. 12.3) is the procedure most often used to relieve pain associated with severe arthritis.[83]

The optimal joint position for arthrodesis is somewhat dependent on the functional needs or goals of each patient and may vary slightly in some joints, such as the elbow and ankle. For example, the optimal position for elbow fusion in the dominant upper extremity usually is between 70° and 90°. However, in the nondominant limb, the elbow must be in more extension for assistive activities.[8] For a woman, the optimal position for arthrodesis of the ankle might be in slightly greater plantarflexion than for a man to allow a woman to wear shoes with a slightly higher heel height.[77] Optimal positions for arthrodesis are listed in Table 12.2.

Although arthrodesis eliminates pain and creates stability in the involved joint, it is not without disadvantages. Because loads and motions needed for functional activities are transferred to joints above and below the fused joint, there is the potential that excessive stresses may lead to pain and hypermobility at these joints over time.

TABLE 12.2 Optimal Positions for Arthrodesis

Joint	Position
Shoulder	At 15°–30° of abduction and flexion and 45° of internal rotation: a position so the hand can reach the mouth
Elbow	Dominant upper extremity: 70°–90° of flexion and midposition of forearm pronation/supination; Nondominant limb: greater elbow extension than the dominant extremity
Wrist	Slight extension
MCP of the thumb	At 20° of flexion
Hip	At 10°–15° of flexion to allow ambulation and comfortable sitting
Ankle	
Tibiotalar joint	Neutral (90°) or slight equinus for women who wear low heels
Subtalar joint	Neutral to valgus
Spine	Neutral so normal lordosis or kyphosis is maintained

Procedure

Fusion of joint surfaces in the position of maximum function is achieved with internal fixation (i.e., pins, nails, screws, plates, and bone grafts). Initially, the joint is immobilized in a cast above and below the site of arthrodesis for 6 to 12 weeks postoperatively. Later, an orthotic device is used until complete bony healing and joint ankylosis has occurred.[8]

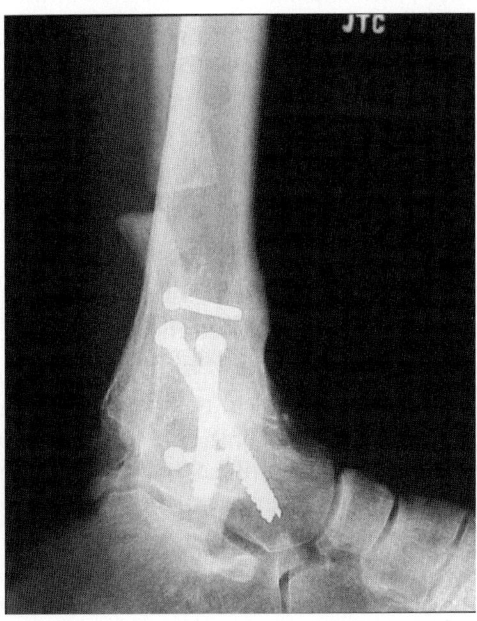

FIGURE 12.3 Arthrodesis (surgical fusion with internal fixation of the ankle). *(From Logerstedt, DS, Smith, HL:* Postoperative Management of the Foot and Ankle. Independent Study Course 15.2. Postoperative Management of Orthopedic Surgeries. Orthopedic Section. *La Crosse, WI: APTA, Inc., 2005, with permission.)*

Postoperative Management

- Because no movement is possible in the fused joint, ROM and strength must be maintained above and below the operated joint.
- Weight bearing is restricted until there is evidence of bony healing.

Extra-articular Bony Procedures

Two of the more common reasons for surgical intervention involving bony structures outside a joint are fractures that require open reduction combined with internal fixation and deformity or malalignment of bone, sometimes associated with arthritis.

Open Reduction and Internal Fixation of Fractures

Fractures are managed with either closed or open reduction. The process of bone healing and fracture management, addressed in Chapter 11, applies regardless of the method of reduction. In most instances in which open reduction is required, some type of internal fixation device is used to stabilize and maintain the alignment of the fracture site as it heals.

Procedure

After exposing the fracture site during surgery, any number of internal fixation devices such as pins, nails, screws, plates, or rods, may be used to align and stabilize the bone fragments.[17,77] Intertrochanteric fracture of the femur, for example, is commonly stabilized with a compression plate and screws, as shown in Figure 12.4. After the fracture has healed, a second surgery may be necessary to remove some or all of the internal fixation devices because they tend to migrate over time.

Postoperative Management

Maintaining stability of the fracture site so bony healing can occur and getting the patient up and out of bed as early as possible are the main postoperative priorities. The progression of rehabilitation after surgical stabilization of a fracture is dependent not only on factors such as the type and severity of fracture and the patient's age and health status but also on the method(s) of internal fixation used.

Some fixation methods eliminate the need for additional external stabilization of the fracture site thereby enabling the patient to begin assisted or active movement of the involved limb and protected weight bearing shortly after surgery. With other fractures, however, external stabilization and restricted weight bearing are necessary even with the use of internal fixation.[17,77]

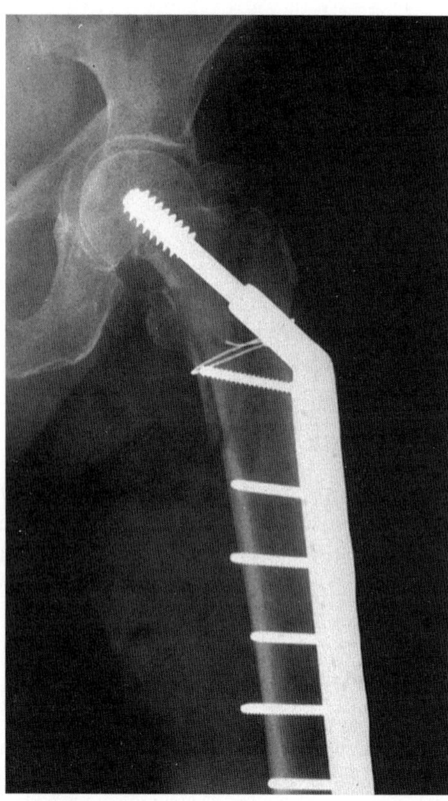

FIGURE 12.4 Intertrochanteric fracture of the left femur, fixed with compression plate and screws. *(From McKinnis, LN:* Fundamentals of Musculoskeletal Imaging, *ed. 4. Philadelphia, FA Davis, 2014, p 64, with permission.)*

During postoperative management, not only must the fracture site be protected as it heals, soft tissues injuries associated with the fracture or the surgery must also be managed appropriately as they heal.

NOTE: Surgical interventions and postoperative management after hip fracture are discussed in Chapter 20.

Osteotomy

Osteotomy—the surgical cutting and realignment of bone—is an extra-articular procedure indicated for the management of impairments associated with a number of musculoskeletal disorders. It is most often performed at the knee or hip.[13] For example, osteotomy is used to reduce pain and correct deformity in a young adult with moderate, focal articular degeneration in the medial compartment and a varus deformity of the knee as the result of osteoarthritis[40,61] or in a child with severe hip joint deterioration and pain secondary to congenital dysplasia or Legg-Calvé-Perthes disease (avascular necrosis of the head of the femur).[62]

Cutting and realigning bone near the involved joint shifts weight-bearing loads to intact joint surfaces, reducing joint pain and preventing further deterioration of the involved articular cartilage.[13,77] It is also thought that redistributing loads on joint surfaces may stimulate the growth of fibrocartilage in the unloaded compartment of the joint.[25] A successful osteotomy delays the need for total joint replacement in patients who will most likely require revision arthroplasty sooner than the average patient with degenerative arthritis.

Osteotomy is also used to correct angular or rotational deformities of bone occurring in congenital or developmental disorders, such as congenital dislocation of the hip, acquired hip dislocation in cerebral palsy, or congenital foot deformities.[77] Osteotomy is also used when surgically shortening or lengthening a bone to correct a severe leg length discrepancy.[17,77]

Procedure

Numerous procedures are classified as osteotomies. Several examples are:

- High tibial, medial or lateral opening, wedge osteotomy with screw-plate fixation, which is a procedure to correct varus or valgus deformities, change the mechanical axis of the knee, and shift the load on joint surfaces in a patient with unicompartmental degenerative arthritis of the knee.[40,47]
- Medial wedge osteotomy of the distal femur to correct a valgus deformity of the knee and shift weight-bearing loads away from the deteriorated cartilage in the lateral compartment of the knee.[61]
- Intertrochanteric osteotomy of the proximal femur, which repositions the femoral head to change the area in which weight bearing occurs for a patient with arthritis or avascular necrosis of the hip.[61]
- Periacetabular osteotomy, which repositions the acetabulum, to improve coverage of the head of the femur for a patient with congenital dysplasia of the hip and recurrent

dislocation that could not be managed effectively by nonoperative methods, such as splinting.[77]

During an osteotomy, muscles and other soft tissues may have to be reflected to expose the operative field and then reattached or repositioned. As with any type of soft tissue repair, muscle-tendon units disturbed during surgery must be protected from excessive stress postoperatively.

Postoperative Management

The primary concern of postoperative management is maintaining bone-to-bone apposition for healing of the osteotomy site. Some procedures allow early joint motion and protected weight bearing because internal fixation maintains apposition of the osteotomy fragments. Others require additional external (cast) stabilization of the joints above and below the osteotomy site until bony union occurs, which may take as long as 8 to 12 weeks.[25,61] Full functional recovery after osteotomy may take as long as 6 months.

Postoperative exercises, when permissible, include the following:

- If cast stabilization is necessary, the patient can begin active ROM of the joints above and below the site of the osteotomy to prevent joint stiffness and muscle weakness.
- When motion and weight bearing are allowed, either immediately after surgery or when the cast is removed, active-assistive and active exercise progressing to light resistive exercise is performed to restore joint ROM and strength. (See the discussion of management of fractures after immobilization in Chapter 11.)
- Weight bearing is typically protected for 4 to 6 weeks or more.

Independent Learning Activities

Critical Thinking and Discussion

1. You have been asked to develop two preoperative patient education programs for groups of individuals scheduled for surgery—a total hip arthroplasty group and a total knee arthroplasty group. What topics should be covered in your presentations? Why are these topics important for prospective patients to understand? How will the two programs be similar? How will the programs differ?
2. You are treating an elderly patient for the first time who underwent an open reduction with internal fixation of a proximal femur fracture 24 hours ago. What are the priorities of your initial examination of this patient? What is the general emphasis of postoperative management, including goals and interventions, during the maximum, moderate, and minimum protection phases of recovery?
3. What is the role of the physical therapist in the overall prevention or management of a lower extremity DVT? What are the signs and symptoms of DVT that a patient at risk for this problem must learn to recognize? If you suspect that a patient you are treating has developed a DVT following lower extremity orthopedic surgery, what questions should you ask the patient? What should you do before contacting the patient's physician?
4. Briefly describe the various surgical interventions for repair of articular cartilage. Describe the pros and cons of each intervention and the long-term results.
5. Differentiate among the following types of soft tissue or bony surgeries primarily used in the management of arthritis: arthrodesis, arthroplasty, articular cartilage repair, débridement, and osteotomy. Briefly describe each surgery and compare and contrast the postoperative management with respect to the use of therapeutic exercise.
6. Discuss the similarities and differences of postoperative management for the following soft tissue surgeries: muscle repair, tendon repair, tendon transfer, ligament reconstruction, repair of a joint capsule, tenotomy or myotomy, and decompression.

REFERENCES

1. Aldrich, D, and Hunt, DP: When can the patient with deep vein thrombosis begin to ambulate? *Phys Ther* 84(3):268–273, 2004.
2. Anand, SS, et al: Does this patient have a deep vein thrombosis? *JAMA* 279:1094–1099, 1998.
3. Armstrong, AD, and Galatz, LM: Complications of total elbow arthroplasty. In Williams, GR, et al (eds): *Shoulder and Elbow Arthroplasty.* Philadelphia: Lippincott Williams & Wilkins, 2005, pp 459–473.
4. Baerga-Varela, L, and Malanga, GA: Rehabilitation and minimally invasive surgery. In Hozack, M, et al (eds): *Minimally Invasive Total Joint Arthroplasty.* Heidelberg: Springer Verlag, 2004, pp 2–5.
5. Ball, CM, and Yamaguchi, K: Interpositional arthroplasty. In Williams, GR, et al (eds): *Shoulder and Elbow Arthroplasty.* Philadelphia: Lippincott Williams & Wilkins, 2005, pp 49–56.
6. Metzger, PC, Lombardi, M, and Barrick, EF: Orthopedic trauma. In Kauffman, TL (ed): *Geriatric Rehabilitation Manual,* ed. 2. New York: Churchill Livingstone, 2007, pp 167–171.
7. Batts Shanku, CD: Rheumatoid arthritis. In Hansen, RA, and Atchison, B (eds): *Conditions in Occupational Therapy,* ed. 2. Philadelphia: Lippincott Williams & Wilkins, 2000.
8. Beckenbaugh, RD: Arthrodesis. In Morrey, BF, and Sanchez-Sotelo, J (eds): *The Elbow and Its Disorders,* ed. 4. Philadelphia: WB Saunders, 2009, pp 949–955.
9. Berlet, GC, Mascia, A, and Miniaci, A: Treatment of unstable osteochondritis dessicans lesions of the knee using autogenous osteochondral grafts (mosaicplasty). *Arthroscopy* 15:312–316, 1999.
10. Berry, DJ, et al: Minimally invasive total hip arthroplasty: Development, early results, and critical analysis. *J Bone Joint Surg Am* 85:2235–2246, 2003.

11. Brinker, M, and Miller, M: *Fundamentals of Orthopedics.* Philadelphia: WB Saunders, 1999.
12. Brittberg, M, et al: Treatment of deep cartilage defects in the knee with autologous chondrocyte transplantation. *N Engl J Med* 331:889–895, 1994.
13. Buckwalter, JA, and Ballard, WT: Operative treatment of arthritis. In Klippel, JH, et al (eds): *Primer on the Rheumatic Diseases,* ed. 13. Atlanta: Arthritis Foundation, 2008, pp 613–623.
14. Burks, R, Burke, W, and Stevanovic, M: Rehabilitation following repair of a torn latissimus dorsi tendon. *Phys Ther* 86(3):411–423, 2006.
15. Cabilan, CJ, Hines, S, and Munday, J: The effectiveness of prehabilitation or preoperative exercise for surgical patients: a systematic review. *JBI Database System Rev Implement Rep* 13(1):146–187, 2015.
16. Canavan, PK: *Rehabilitation in Sports Medicine: A Comprehensive Guide.* Stamford, CT: Appleton & Lange, Stamford, 1998.
17. Chapman, M: *Chapman's Orthopaedic Surgery, Vols 1–4,* ed. 3. Philadelphia: Lippincott Williams & Wilkins, 2004.
18. Choi, J-I, and Lee, K-B: Comparison of clinical outcomes between arthroscopic subchondral drilling and microfracture for osteochondral lesions of the talus. *Knee Surg Sports Traumatol Arthrosc* DOI 10.1007/s00167-015-3511-1, 2015.
19. Chu, CR: Cartilage therapies: Chondrocyte transplantation, osteochondral allografts, and autografts. In Pedowitz, RA, O'Connor, JJ, and Akeson, WH (eds): *Daniel's Knee Injuries: Ligament and Cartilage Structure, Function, Injury, and Repair,* ed. 2. Philadelphia: Lippincott Williams & Wilkins, 2003, pp 227–237.
20. Colvin, AC, Harrast, J, and Harner, C: Trends in hip arthroplasty. *J Bone Joint Surg* 94(4):e23, 2012.
21. Comp, PC, et al: Prolonged enoxaparin therapy to prevent venous thromboembolism after primary hip or knee replacement. *J Bone Joint Surg Am* 83:336–343, 2001.
22. Cooney, WP: Elbow arthroplasty: historical perspective and current concepts. In Morrey, BF (ed): *The Elbow and Its Disorders,* ed. 3. Philadelphia: WB Saunders, 2000, p 581.
23. Cooney III, WP: Arthroplasty of the thumb axis. In Morrey, BF (ed): *Reconstructive surgery of the joints,* ed. 2. New York: Churchill Livingstone, 1996, pp 313–339.
24. Cooney III, WP, and Berger, RA: The distal radioulnar joint. In Morrey, BF (ed): *Joint Replacement Arthroplasty,* ed. 3. Philadelphia: Churchill Livingstone, 2003, pp 226–243.
25. Coventry, MB, Ilstrup, DM, and Wallrichs, SL: Proximal tibial osteotomy: a critical long-term study of eighty-seven cases. *J Bone Joint Surg Am* 75:196–201, 1993.
26. Cummings, GS, and Tillman, LJ: Remodeling of dense connective tissue in normal adult tissues. In Currier, DP, and Nelson, RM (eds): *Dynamics of Human Biologic Tissues.* Philadelphia: F.A. Davis, 1992, p 45.
27. D'Amato, M, and Bach, BR: Knee injuries. In Brotzman, SB, and Manske, RC (eds): *Clinical Orthopedic Rehabilitation,* ed. 3. Philadelphia: Mosby, 2011, pp 211–314.
28. D'Lima, DD, et al: The effect of preoperative exercise on total knee replacement outcomes. *Clin Orthop* 326:174–182, 1996.
29. Enseki, JR, et al: The hip joint: arthroscopic procedures and postoperative rehabilitation. *J Ortho Sports Phys Ther* 36(7):516–525, 2006.
30. Enwemeka, CS: Connective tissue plasticity: ultrastructural, biomechanical, and morphometric effects of physical factors on intact and regenerating tendons. *J Orthop Sports Phys Ther* 14(5):198–212, 1991.
31. Fealey, S, Kingham, TP, and Altchek, DW: Mini-open rotator cuff repair using a two-row fixation technique: outcomes analysis in patients with small, moderate, and large rotator cuff tears. *Arthroscopy* 18(6):665–670, 2002.
32. Fink, NL, and Stoneman, PD: Deep vein thrombosis in an active military cadet. *J Orthop Sports Phys Ther* 36(9):686–697, 2006.
33. Galatz, LM (ed): *Orthopedic Knowledge Update: Shoulder and Elbow,* ed. 3. Rosemont, IL: American Academy of Orthopedic Surgeons, 2008.
34. Gillogly, SD, Voight, M, and Blackburn, T: Treatment of articular cartilage defects of the knee with autologous chondrocyte implantation. *J Orthop Sports Phys Ther* 28(4):241–251, 1998.
35. Smirnova, IV: The cardiovascular system. In Goodman, CC, and Fuller, KS (eds): *Pathology: Implications for the Physical Therapist,* ed. 4. Philadelphia: Elsevier, 2015, pp 538–665.
36. Goyal, D, et al: Evidence-based status of microfracture technique: A systematic review of level I and II studies. *Arthroscopy* 29(9):1579–1588, 2013.
37. Green, DP, et al (eds): *Green's Operative Hand Surgery,* ed. 6. Philadelphia: Churchill Livingstone, 2011.
38. Grotle, M, et al: What's in team rehabilitation care after arthroplasty for osteoarthritis? Results of a multicenter, longitudinal study assessing structure, process, and outcome. *Phys Ther* 40(1):121–131, 2010.
39. Hansen, M: *Pathophysiology: Foundations of Disease and Clinical Intervention.* Philadelphia: WB Saunders, 1998.
40. Hart, JA, and Sekel, R: Osteotomy of the knee: is there a seat at the table? *J Arthoplasty* 4(Suppl 1):45–49, 2002.
41. Hatrup, SJ: Synovectomy. In Morrey, BF (ed): *Reconstructive Surgery of the Joints,* ed. 2. New York: Churchill Livingstone, 1996, p 1599.
42. Hillegass, E, et al: Role of physical therapists in the management of individuals at risk for or diagnosed with venous thromboembolism: Evidence-based clinical practice guideline. *Phys Ther* 96(2): 143–166, 2016.
43. Hull, RD, et al: Extended out-of-hospital low-molecular-weight heparin prophylaxis against deep venous thrombosis in patients after elective hip arthroplasty. *Ann Intern Med* 1355:858–869, 2001.
44. Irrgang, JJ, and Pezzullo, D: Rehabilitation following surgical procedures to address articular cartilage lesions in the knee. *J Orthop Sports Phys Ther* 28(4):232–240, 1998.
45. Jacobson, MD, et al: Muscle function deficits after tourniquet ischemia. *Am J Sports Med* 22(3):372–377, 1994.
46. Jones, RE, and Blackburn, WD: Joint replacement surgery preoperative management. *Bull Rheum Dis* 47(4):5–8, 1998.
47. Kean, CO, et al: Preoperative strength training for patients undergoing high tibial osteotomy: a prospective cohort study with historical controls. *J Orthop Sports Phys Ther* 41(2):52–59, 2011.
48. Keene, J, and Malone, TR: Ligament and muscle-tendon unit injuries. In Malone, TR, McPoil T, and Nitz, AJ (eds): *Orthopaedic and Sports Physical Therapy,* ed. 3. St. Louis: Mosby, 1997, p 135.
49. Khan, RJK, et al: Treatment of acute Achilles tendon rupture: a meta-analysis of randomized controlled trials. *J Bone Joint Surg AM* 87(10): 2202–2210, 2005.
50. Khatod, M, and Akerson, WH: Ligament injury and repair. In Pedowitz, RA, O'Connor, JJ, and Akeson, WH (eds): *Daniel's Knee Injuries: Ligament and Cartilage Structure, Function, Injury, and Repair,* ed. 2. Philadelphia: Lippincott Williams & Wilkins, 2003, pp 185–201.
51. Kim, CW, and Pedowitz, RA: Principles of surgery. Part A. Graft choice and the biology of graft healing. In Pedowitz, RA, O'Connor, JJ, and Akeson, WH (eds): *Daniel's Knee Injuries: Ligament and Cartilage Structure, Function, Injury, and Repair,* ed. 2. Philadelphia: Lippincott Williams & Wilkins, 2003, pp 435–455.
52. King, L: Case study: physical therapy management of hip osteoarthritis prior to total hip arthroplasty. *J Orthop Sports Phys Ther* 26(1):35–38, 1997.
53. Kitaoka, HB: Complications of replacement arthroplasty of the ankle. In Morrey, BF (ed): *Joint Replacement Arthroplasty,* ed. 3. Philadelphia: Churchill Livingstone, 2003, pp 1151–1171.
54. Knight, CA: Peripheral vascular disease and wound care. In O'Sullivan, SB, and Schmitz, TJ (eds): *Physical Rehabilitation: Assessment and Treatment,* ed. 4. Philadelphia: FA Davis, 2001, p 583.
55. Laimins, PD, and Powell, SE: Principles of surgery. Part C. Anterior cruciate ligament reconstruction: Techniques past and present. In Pedowitz, RA, O'Connor, JJ, and Akeson, WH (eds): *Daniel's Knee Injuries: Ligament and Cartilage Structure, Function, Injury, and Repair,* ed. 2. Philadelphia: Lippincott Williams & Wilkins, 2003, pp 227–223.
56. Matsen, FA, et al: Glenohumeral instability. In Rockwood, Jr, et al (eds): *The Shoulder, Vol 2,* ed. 3. Philadelphia: Saunders, 2004, p 655.
57. Matsen, FA, et al: Glenohumeral arthritis and its management. In Rockwood, Jr, CA, et al (eds): *The Shoulder, Vol 2,* ed. 3. Philadelphia: Saunders, 2004, p 879.

58. McDonald, S, et al: Preoperative education for hip or knee replacement. *Cochrane Database Syst Rev* 13, 2014.
59. McGinty, JB (ed): *Operative Arthroscopy,* ed. 3. Philadelphia: Lippincott Williams & Wilkins, 2003.
60. McNally, MA, and Mollan, RAB: The effect of active movement of the foot on venous blood flow after total hip replacement. *J Bone Joint Surg Am* 79:1198–1201, 1997.
61. Melvin, JL, and Gall, V (eds): *Rheumatologic Rehabilitation Series, Vol 5: Surgical Rehabilitation.* Bethesda, MD: American Occupational Therapy Association, 1999.
62. Mercier, LR: *Practical Orthopedics,* ed. 6. St. Louis: Mosby, 2008
63. Minas, T, and Nehrer, S: Current concepts in the treatment of articular cartilage defects. *Orthopedics* 20:525–538, 1997.
64. Mirzayan, R: *Cartilage Injury in the Athlete.* New York: Thieme, 2006.
65. Morrey, BF: Radial head fracture. In Morrey, BF, and Sanchez-Sotelo, J (eds): *The Elbow and Its Disorders,* ed. 4. Philadelphia: WB Saunders, 2009, pp 381–388.
66. Morrey, BF (ed): *Joint Replacement Arthroplasty,* ed. 4. Philadelphia: Wolthers Kluwer Health/Lippincott Williams & Wilkins, 2010.
67. NIH Consensus Development Panel on Total Hip Replacement. *JAMA* 273:1950–1956, 1995.
68. Noonan, TJ, and Garrett, WE: Injuries at the myotendinous junction. *Clin Sports Med* 11:783–806, 1992.
69. Noyes, FR, et al: Biomechanical analysis of human ligament grafts used in knee ligament repairs and reconstructions. *J Bone Joint Surg Am* 66:334–352, 1984.
70. Pareek, A, et al: Long-term outcomes after autologous chondrocyte implantation: a systematic review at mean follow-up of 11.4 years. *Cartilage* doi:10.1177/1947603516630786, 2016.
71. Peljovich, A, Ratner, JA, and Marino, J: Update of the physiology and biomechanics of tendon transfer surgery. *J Hand Surg* 35A:1365–1369, 2010.
72. Peterson, CA, Alteck, DW, and Warren, RE: Shoulder arthroscopy. In Rockwood, CA, and Matsen, FA (eds): *The Shoulder, Vol 2,* ed. 2. Philadelphia: WB Saunders, 1998, p 290.
73. Riddle, DL, et al: Diagnosis of lower extremity deep vein thrombosis in outpatients with musculoskeletal disorders: a national survey study of physical therapists. *Phys Ther* 84(8):717–728, 2004.
74. Roach, JA, Tremblay, LM, and Bowers, DL: A preoperative assessment and education program: implementation and outcomes. *Patient Educ Couns* 25:83–88, 1995.
75. Rooks, DS, et al: Effect of preoperative exercise on measures of functional status in men and women undergoing total hip and knee arthroplasty. *Arthritis Rheum* 55:700–708, 2006.
76. Saccomanno, MR, et al: Generalized joint laxity and multidirectional instability of the shoulder. *Joints* 1(4):171–179, 2013.
77. Salter, RB: *Textbook of Disorders and Injuries of the Musculoskeletal System,* ed. 3. Baltimore: Williams & Wilkins, 1999.
78. Sansone, V, et al: Long-term results of abrasion arthroplasty for full-thickness cartilage lesions of the medial femoral condyle. *Arthroscopy* 31(3):396–403, 2015.
79. Scott, RD: *Total Knee Arthroplasty,* ed. 2. Philadelphia: Saunders, 2015.
80. Scott, WN (ed): *Insall & Scott Surgery of the Knee,* ed. 5. Philadelphia: Churchill Livingstone, 2012.
81. Stevens-Lapsley, JE, et al: Minimally invasive total knee arthroplasty: surgical implication for recovery. *J Knee Surg* 26(3):195–201, 2013.
82. Tasto, JP, et al: Surgical decisions and treatment alternatives—meniscal tears, malalignment, chondral injury and chronic arthrosis. In Pedowitz, RA, O'Connor, JJ, and Akeson, WH (eds): *Daniel's Knee Injuries: Ligament and Cartilage Structure, Function, Injury, and Repair,* ed. 2. Philadelphia: Lippincott Williams & Wilkins, 2003, pp 567–586.
83. Thomas, RH, and Daniels, TR: Ankle arthritis. *J Bone Joint Surg Am* 85:923–936, 2003.
84. McMahon, PJ, Lee, TQ, and Tibone, JE: Biomechanics and pathologic lesions in the overhead athlete. In Iannotti, JP, and Williams, GR (eds): *Disorders of the Shoulder: Diagnosis and Management,* ed. 2. Philadelphia: Lippincott Williams & Wilkins, 2007.
85. Tria, Jr, AJ: Advances in minimally invasive total knee arthroplasty. *Orthopedics* 26(8 Suppl):859–863, 2003.
86. Wegrzyn, J, et al: No benefit of minimally invasive TKA on gait and strength outcomes. A randomized controlled trial. *Clin Orthop Relat Res* 471:46–55, 2013.
87. Weinmann, EE, and Salzman, EW: Deep vein thrombosis. *N Engl J Med* 331:1630–1641, 1994.
88. Wells, PS, et al: Evaluation of D-dimer in the diagnosis of suspected deep-vein thrombosis. *N Eng J Med* 349:1227–1235, 2003.
89. White, RH, et al: Predictors of rehospitalization for symptomatic venous thromboembolism after total hip arthroplasty. *N Engl J Med* 343: 1758–1764, 2000.
90. Wiesel, BB, et al: *Orthopedic Surgery: Principles of Diagnosis and Treatment.* Philadelphia: Wolthers Kluwer Health/Lippincott Williams & Wilkins, 2011.
91. Wilk, KE, and Andrews, JR: Rehabilitation following thermal assisted capsular shrinkage of the glenohumeral joint: current concepts. *J Orthop Sports Phys Ther* 32(6):268–287, 2002.
92. Wynn Parry, CB, and Stanley, JK: Synovectomy of the hand. *Br J Rheumatol* 32:1089–1095, 1993.
93. Young, BA, and Flynn, TW: Pulmonary embolism: the differential diagnosis dilemma. *J Orthop Phys Ther* 35(10):637–642, 2005.
94. Zazzali, MS, and Vad, VB: Shoulder instability. In Donatelli, RA (ed): *Physical Therapy of the Shoulder,* ed. 4. St. Louis: Churchill Livingstone, 2004, pp 483–505.

CHAPTER

13

Peripheral Nerve Disorders and Management

CAROLYN KISNER, PT, MS
CINDY JOHNSON ARMSTRONG PT, DPT, CHT

Therapeutic exercise and related manual therapy techniques would not be possible without the nervous system and all its components activating, controlling, and modifying motor responses as well as receiving and interpreting feedback from the variety of sensory receptors throughout the body. Because of their intimate proximity to all the structures in the trunk and extremities, nerves may become stressed or injured with various musculoskeletal conditions, postures, and repetitive microtraumas, resulting in neurological symptoms, structural and functional impairments, activity limitations, and participation restrictions. Highlights of the anatomy and results of injury to the peripheral nervous system are reviewed in the first section of this chapter for the purpose of laying the foundation for management guidelines, including therapeutic exercise and manual therapy interventions, that are described in the remainder of the chapter. In the treatment of patients with musculoskeletal impairments, often the therapist does not think of the components of the central nervous system. Even though this chapter primarily deals with the peripheral nervous system, acknowledgment that the central nervous system plays a key role in the initiation and control of movement is a must. The reader is referred to Chapter 8 for consideration of motor control in the total rehabilitation of the individual with musculoskeletal involvement.

The development of a plan of care and intervention techniques differs for patients with impairments due to nerve involvement. Nerve injuries may result in significant activity limitations and participation restrictions due to paralysis and resulting deformity. Utilizing the principles presented in this chapter, along with the knowledge and skills of examination and evaluation of the neural, muscular, and skeletal systems, the reader should be able to design therapeutic exercise programs for patients with limitations due to injury or mobility restrictions of the peripheral nervous system. Several peripheral nerve entrapment conditions are described in order to illustrate therapeutic interventions, including thoracic outlet syndrome and carpal tunnel syndrome. Also included in this chapter is a section on complex regional pain syndrome (CRPS).

Review of the Peripheral Nervous System

Nerve Structure

Peripheral components of the neuromuscular system include the alpha and gamma motor neurons, their axons, and the skeletal muscles they innervate; the sensory neurons and their receptors located in the connective tissues, joints, and blood vessels; and the neurons of the autonomic nervous system. Connective tissue surrounds each axon (endoneurium) as well as fascicles (perineurium) and entire nerve fibers (epineurium).[3,78] The axolemma is the surface membrane of an axon. Schwann cells lie between the axolemma and endoneurium; they form myelin, which functions to insulate the axon as well as speed the conduction of action potentials along the nerve fiber. The exceptions are very small fibers that are unmyelinated. A peripheral nerve may consist of a single fascicle or consist of several fascicles. The structure of a peripheral nerve with its connective tissue and vascular layers is illustrated in Figure 13.1, and the location of their cell bodies and structures innervated are summarized in Box 13.1.

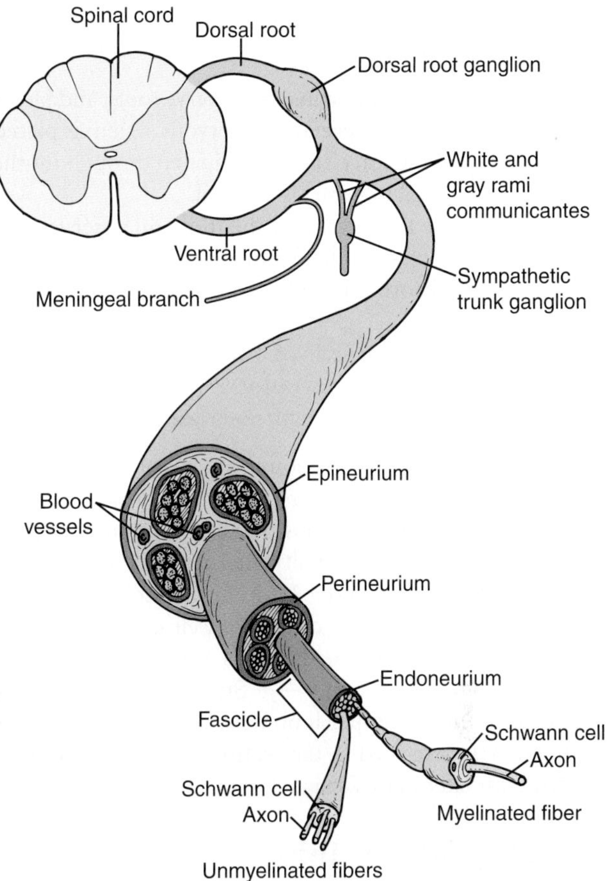

FIGURE 13.1 Peripheral nerve and its connective tissue coverings.

BOX 13.1 Content of Peripheral Nerves and Location of Their Cell Bodies

Peripheral nerves contain a mix of motor, sensory, and sympathetic neurons.

- *Alpha motor neurons (somatic efferent fibers)*: cell bodies located in anterior column of spinal cord; innervate skeletal muscles
- *Gamma motor neurons (efferent fibers)*: cell bodies located in lateral columns of spinal cord; innervate intrafusal muscle fibers of the muscle spindle
- *Sensory neurons (somatic afferent fibers)*: cell bodies located in the dorsal root ganglia; innervate sensory receptors
- *Sympathetic neurons (visceral afferent fibers)*: cell bodies located in sympathetic ganglia; innervate sweat glands, blood vessels, viscera, and glands

Mobility Characteristics of the Nervous System

In 1991, David Butler,[15] one of the original therapists to study neurodynamics, described the peripheral and central nervous systems as a continuous tissue tract; simply stated, the tract is like an H on its side. Structurally and functionally, there is continuity of the connective tissues, the impulse transmission between the neurons, and the chemical flow of neurotransmitters. The nervous system is designed to move as well as withstand mechanical forces, while at the same time conduct impulses.

Nerves slide and glide relative to the adjacent tissue, both longitudinally and transversely. Excursion of the nerve is critical to neural function because it serves to dissipate tension within the neural system. Initially, excursion occurs adjacent to the moving joint, but excursion of the nerve progresses more distally from the moving joint as limb movement continues.[61,71,79]

Substantial mobility in the nervous system is needed for an individual to move during functional activities. With movement of an extremity, before there is increased tension in the nerve itself, the whole peripheral nerve moves, and there is movement between connective tissues and neural tissues. This mobility is allowed without undue stress on the nerve tissue because:

- The arrangement of the spinal cord, nerve roots, and plexes allows mobility. If any part of the nervous system is placed under tension, the force can be dissipated throughout the system and neural ischemia is avoided.
- The connective tissue around the individual nerves and bundles of nerves (epineurium, perineurium, and endoneurium) absorb tensile forces before the nerve itself stretches.
- The perineurium specifically, the primary guard against excessive tension, allows for 18% to 22% strain before failure due to its longitudinal strength and elasticity.

Cadaveric and in vivo ultrasound studies of median nerve mobility and strain have shown nerve movement of 0.1 and 12.5 mm depending on the position and motion of each of the joints in the upper extremity and neck, 0.1 and 4.0 mm for the ulnar nerve, 0.7 and 5.2 mm for the tibial nerve, and 0.1 and 3.5 mm for the sciatic nerve, as well as a wavy appearance when on a slack (unloaded) and a straightening of the nerve when under tension.[19,25,72] Strain calculated in the stretch position (see upper limb neurodynamic test for the median nerve described in the section on peripheral nerve impairments later in this chapter) was 2.5% to 3.0%.[25,72]

Common Sites of Injury to Peripheral Nerves

Compression and/or injury to the nerves of the peripheral nervous system can occur anywhere along the pathway from the nerve roots to their termination in the tissues of the trunk and extremities. As each nerve courses from the intervertebral foramina to its peripheral destination, there are sites that increase its susceptibility to either tension or compression. Symptoms and signs of nerve impairments are sensory changes or loss and motor weakness in the distribution of the involved nerve fibers. Because nerves are composed of innervated connective tissue and because blood vessels surround the axons, ischemic pain or tension pain may occur when these tissues are stressed. Also, because peripheral nerves include sympathetic fibers, autonomic responses might occur. Whenever neurological symptoms and signs are present, the entire nerve should be tested for mobility and signs of compression at key points along its pathway.

In this section, primary sites of compression, stress, or injury are identified for the peripheral nerves in the upper and lower quarter regions including their origins at the nerve roots and pathways through each of the plexuses.

Nerve Roots

Nerve roots emerge from the spinal canal and traverse the foramina of the spine, where they can become impinged as a result of various pathologies of the spine that reduce the space in the foramina, such as degenerative disc disease, degenerative joint disease, disc lesions, and spondylolisthesis. With reduced spinal canal or foraminal space (stenosis), extension, side bending, or rotation of the vertebra to the side of the stenosis further decreases the space where the nerve root courses and may cause or perpetuate symptoms. If adhesions place compression or stress on a nerve root, nerve mobility tests (described later in this chapter) can reproduce symptoms when the spine is side-bent (laterally flexed) away from the side causing the symptoms. When involved, symptoms and signs include sensory changes and/or loss of motor function in the respective dermatome and myotome patterns (Fig. 13.2 and Box 13.2). Nerve roots of the upper quarter include C5 through T1 and those of the lower quarter L1 through S3. Management guidelines for individuals with nerve root symptoms are described in Chapter 15.

Brachial Plexus

After emerging from the foramina, the nerve fibers divide into anterior and posterior primary rami. Vasomotor fibers from the sympathetic trunk join the anterior primary rami to course within the brachial plexus and peripheral nerves to the extremities. The brachial plexus is formed by the anterior primary divisions of the C5–T1 nerve roots (Fig. 13.3). The plexus functions as the distribution center for organizing the contents of each peripheral nerve. In addition, Butler[16] suggested that the weave pattern in the brachial plexus contributes to the mobility of the nerves such that when tension is placed on any one peripheral nerve, the tension is transmitted to several cervical nerve roots rather than just one nerve root.

The brachial plexus courses through the region known as the thoracic outlet. There are three primary sites for compression or entrapment of the neurovascular structures in this region (see Fig. 13.19 later in this chapter).

- *Interscalene triangle*: bordered by the anterior and middle scalene muscles and first rib. It contains the subclavian artery and the upper, middle, and lower trunks of the brachial plexus.
- *Costoclavicular space*: between the clavicle, the subclavius muscle, and the costocoracoid ligament anteriorly and the first rib and the anterior and middle scalene muscles posteriorly. This space contains the subclavian vessels and the divisions of the brachial plexus.
- *Retropectoralis minor space*: inferior to the coracoid process, anterior to the second through fourth ribs, and posterior to the pectoralis minor. This space contains the cords of the brachial plexus and the axillary artery and vein.
- Structural anomalies, such as a cervical rib, an elongated C7 transverse process, or malunion of a clavicular fracture, may compress or entrap a portion of the plexus as well.

When vascular and/or neurological symptoms are caused by compression in the thoracic outlet, it is commonly referred to as thoracic outlet syndrome. Characteristics of this syndrome and management guidelines are described later in the chapter.

Other injuries to the brachial plexus include:

- **Upper plexus injuries (C5, 6):** The most common injury to the plexus involves compression or tearing of the upper trunk. The mechanism involves shoulder depression and lateral flexion of the neck to the opposite side. There is loss

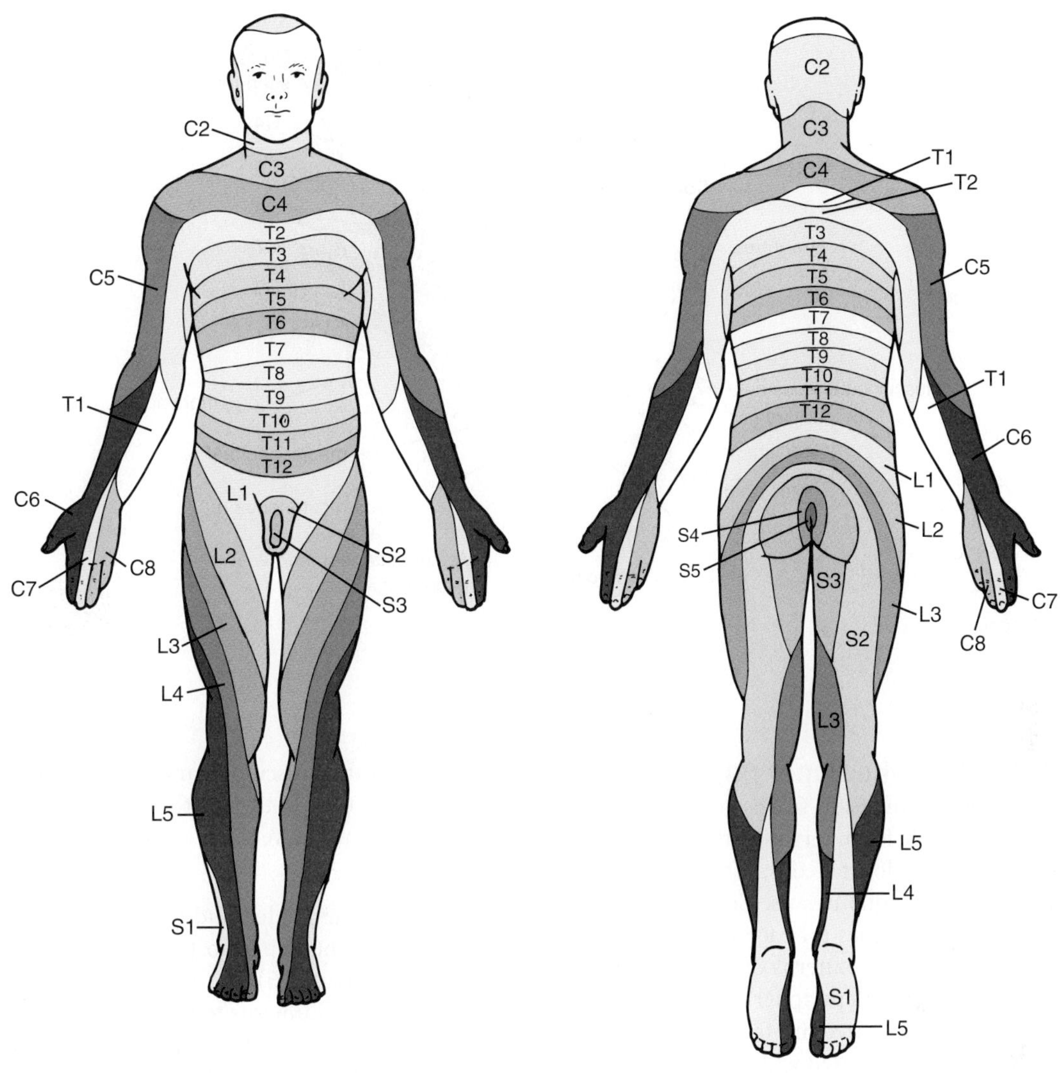

FIGURE 13.2 Dermatomes—anterior and posterior views.

BOX 13.2 Key Muscles for Testing Upper and Lower Quarter Myotomes[52]

Upper Quarter

C1–2	Cervical flexion
C3	Cervical side flexion
C4	Scapular elevation
C5	Shoulder abduction
C6	Elbow flexion and wrist extension
C7	Elbow extension and wrist flexion
C8	Thumb extension
T1	Finger abduction

Lower Quarter

L1–2	Hip flexion
L3	Knee extension
L4	Ankle dorsiflexion
L5	Big toe extension
S1	Ankle eversion and plantar flexion, hip extension
S2	Knee flexion
S3	No specific test action; intrinsic foot muscles (except abductor hallucis)

of abduction and lateral rotation of the shoulder and weakness in elbow flexion and forearm supination (waiter's tip position). Erb's palsy occurs with birth injuries when the shoulder is stretched downward, although Benjamin[5] cautioned that there are maternal and infant factors that could contribute to this injury in addition to the forces applied during delivery. A "stinger" occurs with injuries that might be sustained when a football player lands on the upper torso and shoulder with the head/neck laterally flexed in the opposite direction.

- **Middle plexus injuries (C7):** Rarely seen alone.
- **Lower plexus injuries (C8, T1):** Usually due to compression by a cervical rib or stretching the arm overhead. Klumpke's paralysis (paralysis of the intrinsics of the hand) occurs in birth injuries when the baby presents with its arm overhead.[5]
- **Complete or total injury of the plexus:** Complete paralysis from a total brachial plexus injury may occur as a complication of birth; it is known as Erb-Klumpke's paralysis and is associated with Horner's syndrome in one-third of those severely affected.[5]

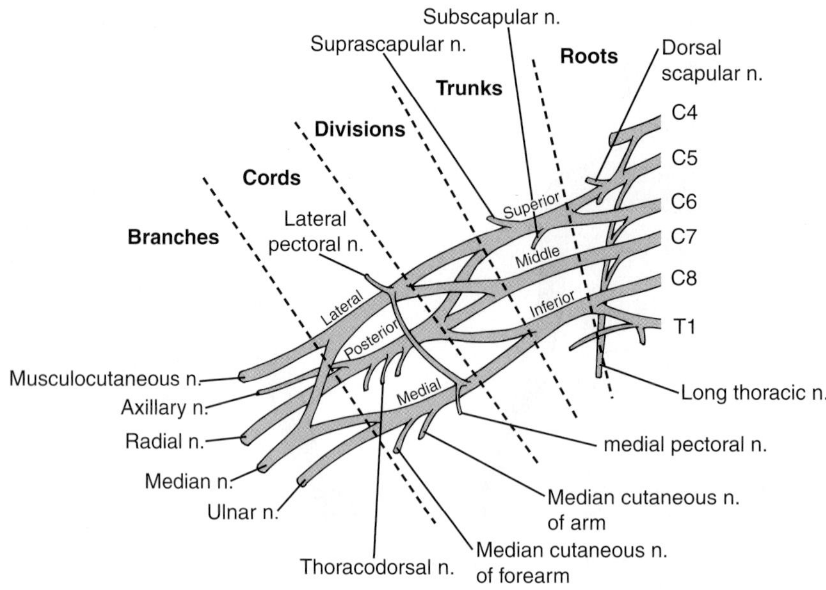

FIGURE 13.3 Brachial plexus.

Peripheral Nerves in the Upper Quarter

The brachial plexus terminates in five primary peripheral nerves that are responsible for innervating the tissues of the upper extremity: (1) musculocutaneous, (2) axillary, (3) median, (4) ulnar, and (5) radial nerves. Common sites for compression or tension injuries for each of the nerves are described in this section. The patterns of muscle weakness and primary impairments with peripheral nerve injuries in the upper quarter are summarized in a table that is available on the FA Davis web site associated with this text (see ONL Table 13.1)

Axillary Nerve: C5, 6

The axillary nerve (Fig. 13.4) emerges from the posterior cord of the brachial plexus; it passes laterally through the axilla, sends a branch to the teres minor muscle, courses behind the surgical neck of the humerus, and innervates the deltoid muscle and overlying skin. The axillary nerve is vulnerable to injury with dislocation of the shoulder and fractures of the surgical neck of the humerus. If the upper trunk of the brachial plexus is stretched or injured, it affects the function of the axillary nerve. Shoulder abduction and lateral rotation are impaired when this nerve is affected.

Musculocutaneous Nerve: C5, 6

The musculocutaneous nerve (Fig. 13.4) emerges from the lateral cord of the brachial plexus and crosses the axilla with the median nerve; it pierces and innervates the coracobrachialis and then travels distally to innervate the biceps and brachialis muscles. It continues between these muscles to the flexor surface of the elbow; after emerging from the deep fascia at the elbow, it becomes the lateral cutaneous nerve of the forearm. Isolated impingement of this nerve is not common; injury to the lateral cord or the upper trunk of the brachial plexus affects the musculocutaneous nerve. When affected, the patient is unable to flex the elbow with the forearm supinated and may have some instability in the shoulder.

Median Nerve: C6–8

Bundles from the medial and lateral cords of the brachial plexus unite in the uppermost part of the arm to form the median nerve (Fig. 13.5). The median nerve courses the medial aspect of the humerus to the elbow, where it is deep in the cubital fossa under the bicipital aponeurosis, medial to the tendon of the biceps and brachial artery; it then moves into the forearm between the two heads of the pronator teres muscle. Hypertrophy of this muscle can compress the median nerve, producing symptoms that mimic carpal tunnel syndrome except that the forearm muscles (pronator teres, wrist flexors, extrinsic finger flexors) are involved in addition to the intrinsic muscles.

To enter the hand, the median nerve passes through the carpal tunnel at the wrist with the flexor tendons. The carpal tunnel is covered by the thick, relatively inelastic transverse carpal ligament. Entrapment of the median nerve in the tunnel, called carpal tunnel syndrome, causes sensory changes and progressive weakness in the muscles innervated by the median nerve distal to the wrist. Characteristics of this syndrome and management guidelines are described later in the chapter.

Ulnar Nerve: C8, T1

The ulnar nerve (Fig. 13.6) emerges from the medial cord of the brachial plexus at the lower border of the pectoralis minor and descends the arm along the medial side of the humerus. It passes posterior to the elbow joint in the groove between the medial epicondyle of the humerus and the olecranon of the ulna. The groove is covered by a fibrous sheath that forms

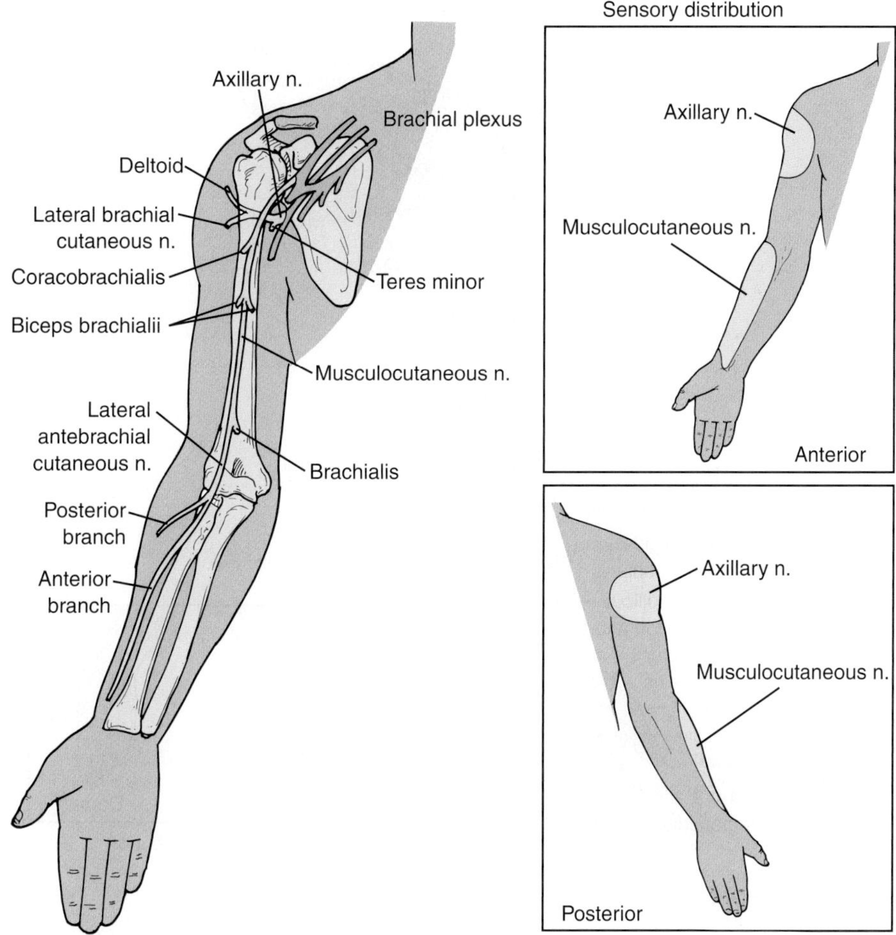

FIGURE 13.4 Sensory and motor innervations of the axillary (C5, 6) and musculocutaneous (C5, 6) nerves.

the cubital tunnel. The nerve possesses considerable mobility to stretch around the elbow as it flexes, although the nerve can be easily irritated or entrapped at the elbow owing to its superficial location and anatomic arrangement.[28] It then passes between the humeral and ulnar heads of the flexor carpi ulnaris muscle, another site where impingement could occur.[28] The extrinsic muscles innervated by the ulnar nerve are the flexor carpi ulnaris and ulnar half of the flexor digitorum profundus.

The ulnar nerve enters the hand through a trough formed by the pisiform bone and hook of the hamate bone and is covered by the volar carpal ligament and palmaris brevis muscle, forming the tunnel of Guyon. Trauma or entrapment in this region causes sensory changes and progressive weakness of muscles innervated distal to the site, resulting in a partial claw-hand deformity. Injury to the nerve after it bifurcates leads to partial involvement, depending on the site of injury.[27,28] Characteristics of ulnar nerve impingement in the tunnel and management guidelines are described later in the chapter.

Radial Nerve: C6–8, T1

The radial nerve (Fig. 13.7) emerges directly from the posterior cord of the brachial plexus at the lower border of the pectoralis minor. As it descends the arm, it winds around the posterior aspect of the humerus in the spiral groove between the lateral and medial heads of the triceps muscle and continues to the radial aspect of the elbow. In the arm it innervates the triceps, anconeus, and upper portion of the extensor and supinator group of the forearm. Injury to this nerve may occur with shoulder dislocations and midshaft humeral fractures. Also known to all therapists is "crutch palsy," a condition of nerve compression caused by leaning on axillary crutches. "Saturday night palsy" occurs when sleeping with the person's head on the arm that is slung over the back of a chair or open car window. The triceps is involved only if the compression or injury to the nerve occurs close to the axilla. At the elbow, the radial nerve pierces the lateral muscular septum anterior to the lateral epicondyle and passes under the origin of the extensor carpi radialis brevis; it then divides into a superficial and a deep branch. The deep branch may become entrapped as it passes under the edge of the extensor carpi radialis brevis and the fibrous slit in the supinator, causing progressive weakness in the wrist and finger extensor and supinator muscles (except the extensor carpi radialis longus, which is innervated proximal to the bifurcation). Impingement may occur here and may be erroneously called tennis elbow (lateral epicondylosis—see

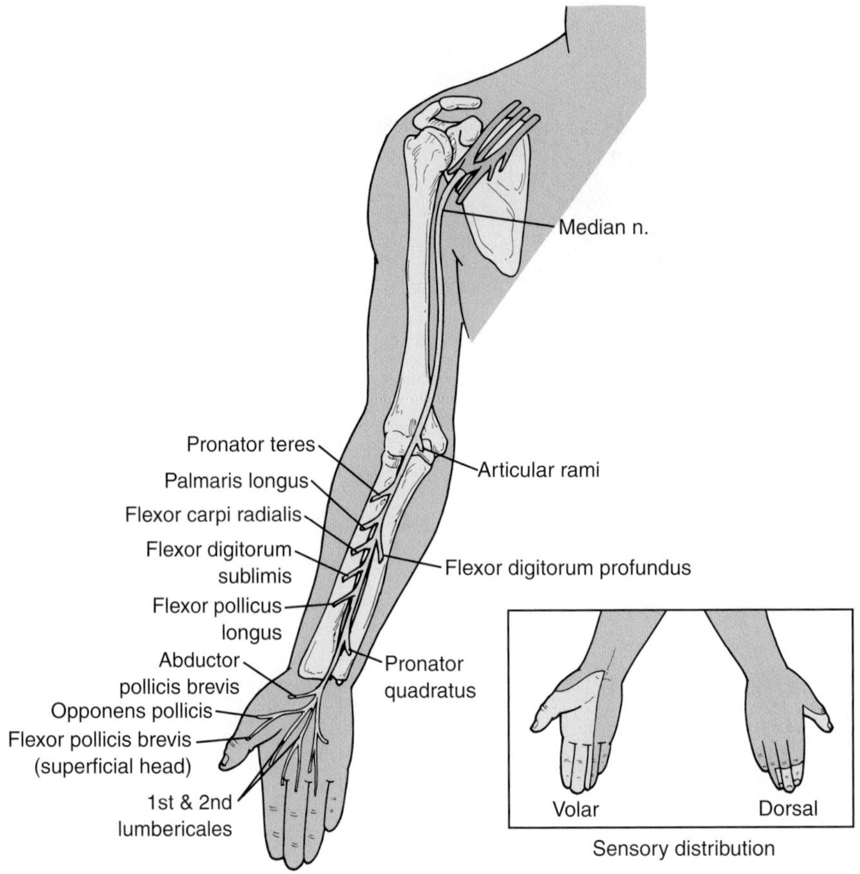

FIGURE 13.5 Sensory and motor innervations of the median nerve (C6–8, T1).

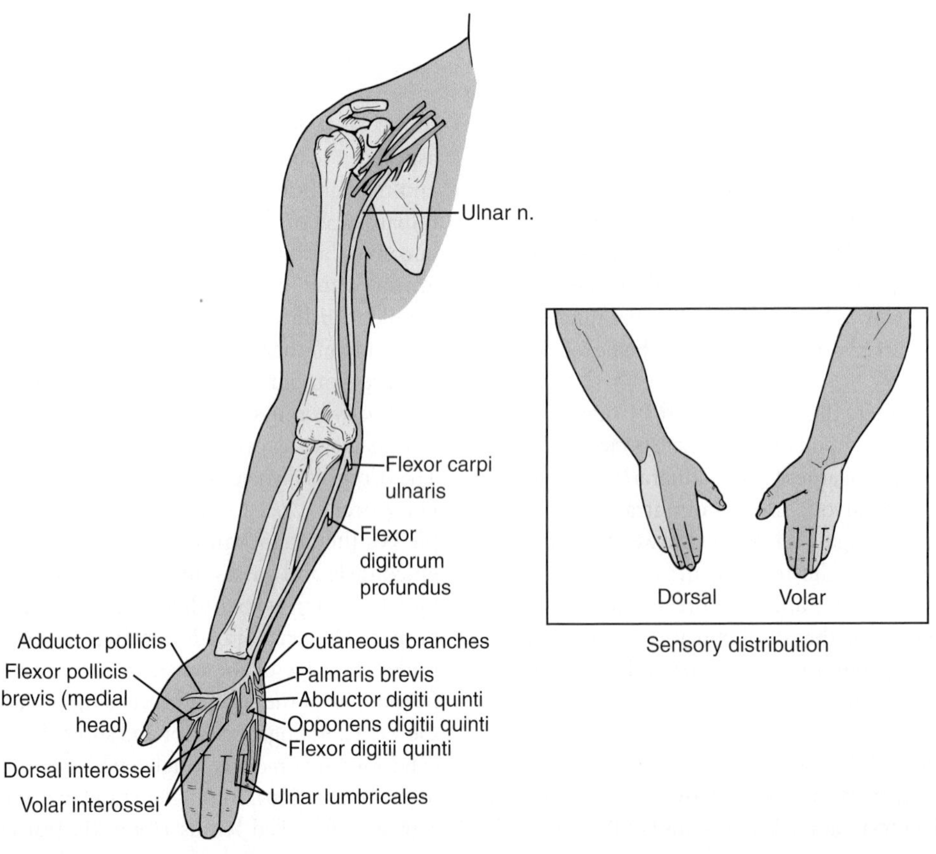

FIGURE 13.6 Sensory and motor innervations of the ulnar nerve (C8, T1).

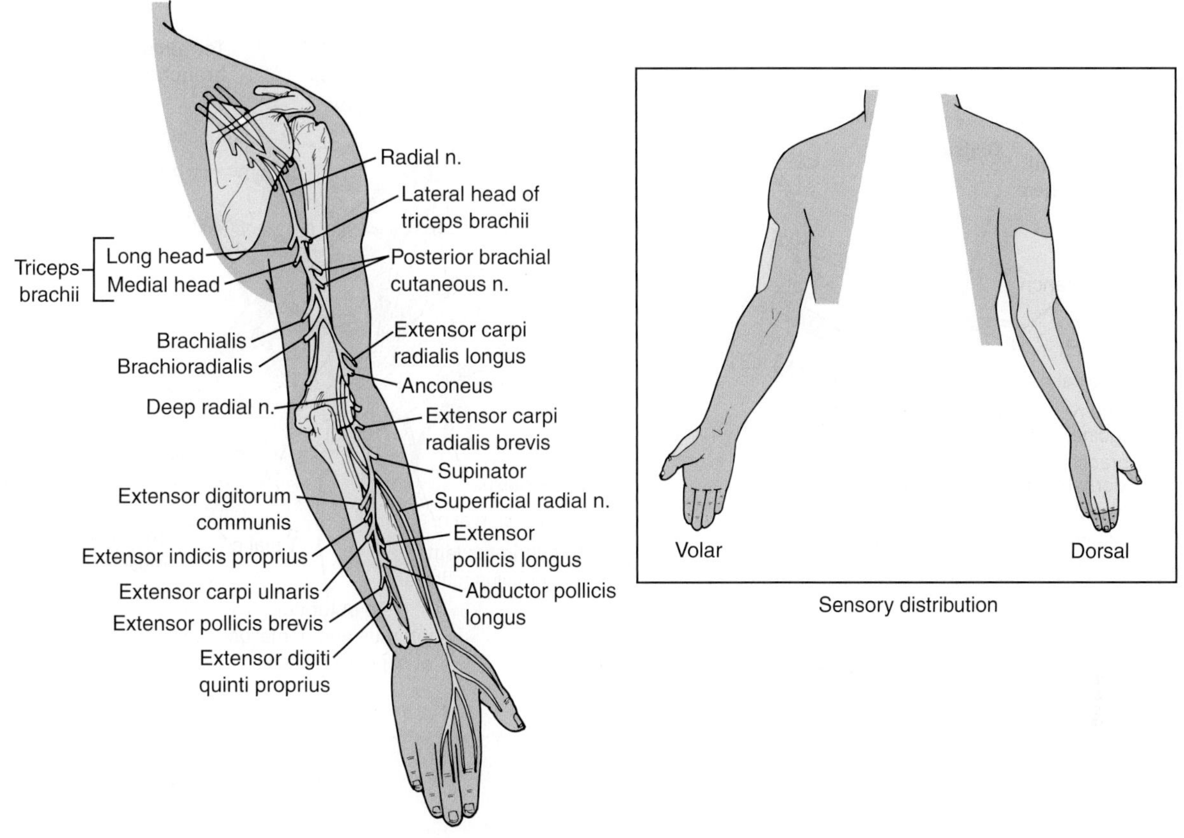

FIGURE 13.7 Sensory and motor innervations of the radial nerve (C6–8, T1).

Chapter 18). The deep branch passes around the neck of the radius and may be injured with a radial head fracture. The superficial radial nerve may undergo direct trauma that causes sensory changes in the distribution of the nerve.

The radial nerve enters the hand on the dorsal surface as the superficial radial nerve, which is sensory only; therefore, injury to it in the wrist or hand does not cause any motor weakness. The influence of the radial nerve on hand musculature is entirely proximal to the wrist. Injury proximal to the elbow results in wrist drop and inability to actively extend the wrist and fingers. This affects the length-tension relationship of the extrinsic finger flexors, resulting in an ineffective grip unless the wrist is splinted in partial extension. Injury to the radial nerve in the proximal forearm affects only the supinator muscle and extrinsic abductor and extensor pollicis longus muscles.[47]

Lumbosacral Plexus

The lumbar plexus is formed by the anterior primary divisions of the nerve roots L1, L2, L3, and part of L4 (Fig. 13.8 A); the sacral plexus is formed from L4, L5, S1, and parts of S2 and S3 (Fig. 13.8 B). As with the brachial plexus, the branches and divisions of the lumbosacral plexus organize the content of each of the peripheral nerves coursing into the lower extremity. In addition, the anterior primary rami of the plexus receive postganglionic sympathetic fibers from the sympathetic chain that innervate blood vessels, sweat glands, and piloerector muscles in the lower extremity. Isolated injuries to the lumbar plexus or sacral plexus are not common; symptoms more commonly arise from disc lesions or spondylitic deformities that affect one or more nerve roots or from tension or compression of specific peripheral nerves.

Peripheral Nerves in the Lower Quarter

The lumbosacral plexus terminates in three primary peripheral nerves, which are responsible for innervating the tissues of the lower extremity. They are the femoral and obturator nerves from the lumbar plexus and the sciatic nerve from the sacral plexus. Common sites for compression or tension injuries are described in this section. The patterns of muscle weakness with peripheral nerve injuries in the lower quarter and primary impairments are summarized in a table that is available on the FA Davis website associated with this text (see ONLINE Table 13.2).

Femoral Nerve: L2–4

The femoral nerve (Fig. 13.9) arises from the three posterior divisions of the lumbar plexus. It emerges from the lateral border of the psoas muscle superior to the inguinal ligament and descends underneath the ligament to the

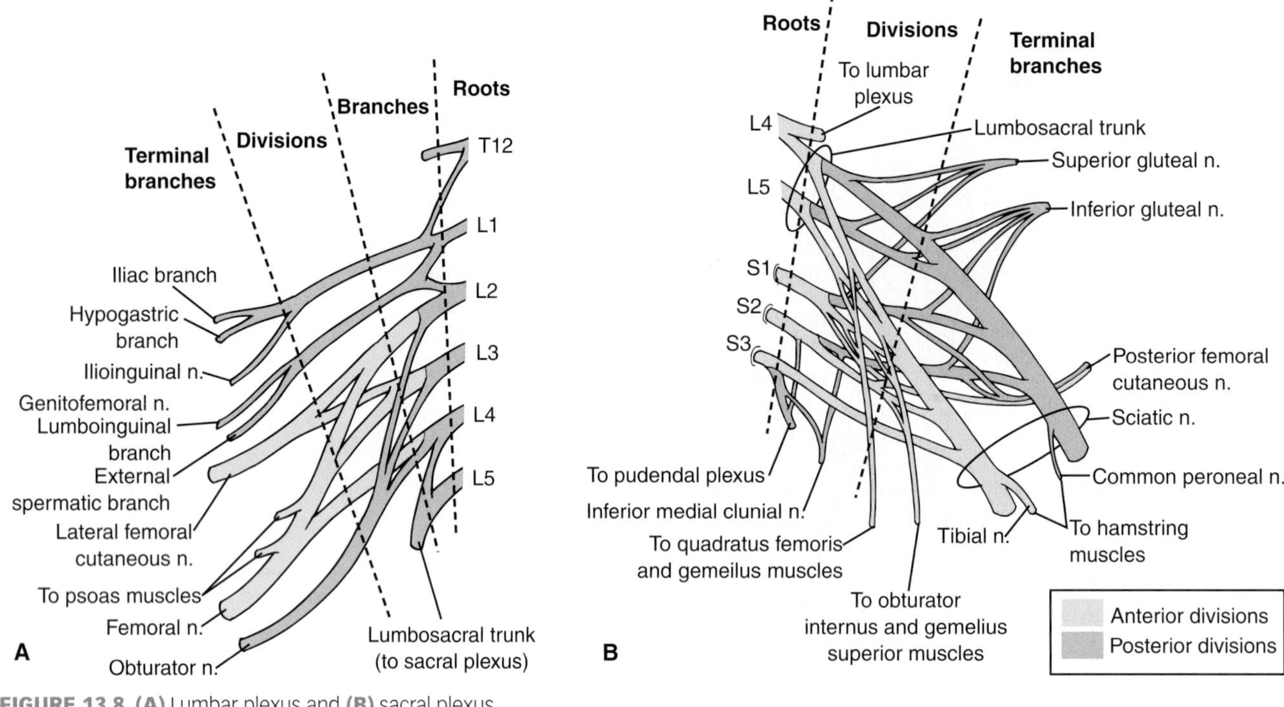

FIGURE 13.8 **(A)** Lumbar plexus and **(B)** sacral plexus.

femoral triangle, lateral to the femoral artery, to innervate the sartorius and quadriceps muscle group. The iliopsoas is supplied superior to the ligament. Injuries to the nerve may occur with trauma, such as fractures of the upper femur or pelvis, during reduction of congenital dislocation of the hip, or from pressure during a forceps labor and delivery—resulting in weakness of hip flexion and loss of knee extension. Symptoms may occur from neuritis in diabetes mellitus.

Obturator Nerve: l2–4

The obturator nerve (Fig. 13.9) arises from the three anterior divisions of the lumbar plexus. It descends through the obturator canal in the medial obturator foramen to the medial side of the thigh to innervate the adductor muscle group and obturator externus. Isolated injury to this nerve is rare, although uterine pressure and damage during labor may cause the injury. If damaged, adduction and external rotation of the thigh are impaired, with the individual having difficulty crossing his or her legs.

Sciatic Nerve: l4, 5; S1–3

The sciatic nerve (Fig. 13.10) emerges from the sacral plexus as the largest nerve in the body; its component parts—the tibial and common peroneal nerves—can be differentiated in the common sheath. Muscles in the buttock region (external rotators and gluteal muscles) are innervated by small nerves from the sacral plexus, which emerge proximal to formation of the sciatic nerve. The sciatic nerve exits the pelvis through the greater sciatic foramen and typically courses below, although sometimes through, the piriformis muscle. Piriformis syndrome may occur from a shortened muscle, causing compression and irritation of the nerve at this site. The nerve is protected under the gluteus maximus as it courses between the ischial tuberosity and greater trochanter, although injury may occur in this region with hip dislocation or reduction. The tibial portion of the sciatic nerve innervates the biarticular hamstring muscles and a portion of the adductor magnus; the common peroneal portion innervates the short head of the biceps femoris. Proximal to the popliteal fossa, the sciatic nerve terminates when the tibial and common peroneal nerves emerge as separate structures.

Tibial/Posterior Tibial Nerve: L4, 5; S1–3

The tibial nerve (Fig. 13.10) forms from the anterior primary rami of the sacral plexus, courses with the common peroneal nerve as the sciatic nerve, and then emerges as a separate nerve proximal to the popliteal fossa. After coursing through the popliteal fossa, it sends a branch that joins a branch from the common peroneal nerve to form the sural nerve and continues on as the posterior tibial nerve. In the leg, it innervates the muscles of the posterior compartment, including the plantar flexors, popliteus, tibialis posterior, and extrinsic toe flexors.

In its approach to the foot, the nerve occupies a groove behind the medial malleolus along with the tendons of the tibialis posterior, flexor hallucis longus, and flexor digitorum longus; the groove is covered by a ligament, forming a tunnel. Entrapment, usually from a space-occupying lesion, is known as *tarsal tunnel syndrome*. The nerve then divides into the medial and lateral plantar and calcaneal nerves.

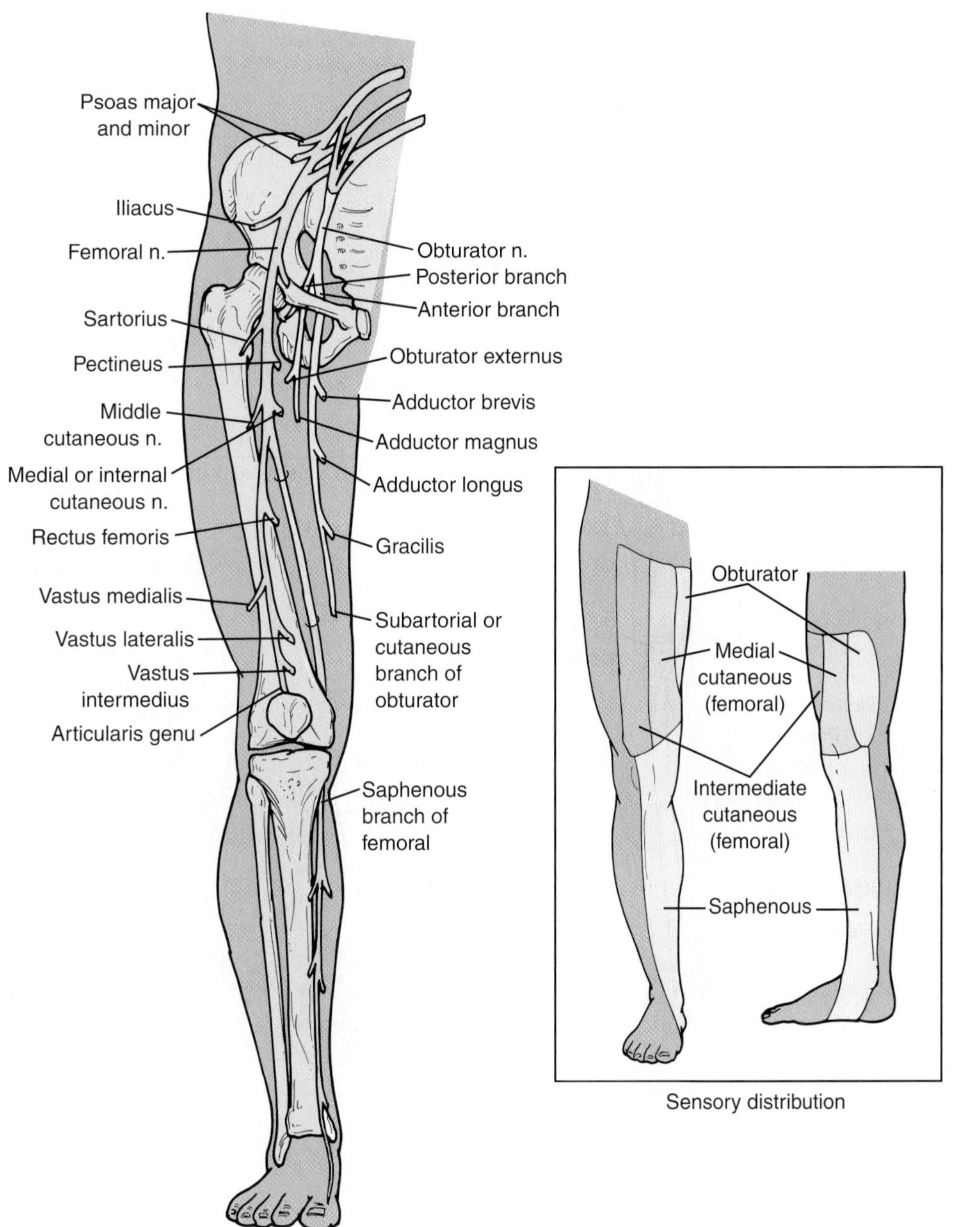

FIGURE 13.9 Sensory and motor innervations of the femoral (L2–4) and obturator (L2–4) nerves.

Plantar and calcaneal nerves. The plantar and calcaneal nerves may become entrapped as they turn under the medial aspect of the foot and pass through openings in the abductor hallucis muscle, especially with overpronation of the foot, which stresses the nerves against the fibrous-edged openings in the muscle. Symptoms elicited are similar to acute foot strain (tenderness at the posteromedial plantar aspect of the foot), painful heel (inflamed calcaneal nerve), and pain in a pes cavus foot. The medial and lateral plantar nerves innervate all the intrinsic muscles of the foot except the extensor digitorum brevis. The innervation pattern of the lateral plantar nerve in the foot corresponds to the ulnar nerve in the hand, and the medial plantar nerve corresponds to the median nerve. Weakness and postural changes in the foot, such as pes cavus and clawing of the toes, may occur with nerve compression or injury.

Common Peroneal Nerve: L4, 5; S1, 2

After it bifurcates from the sciatic nerve in the knee region, the common peroneal nerve (Fig. 13.11) passes between the biceps femoris tendon and lateral head of the gastrocnemius muscle, sends a branch to join the tibial nerve and form the sural nerve, and then comes laterally around the fibular neck and passes through an opening in the peroneus longus muscle. Pressure or force against the nerve in this region can cause neuropathy, including sensory changes and weakness in the

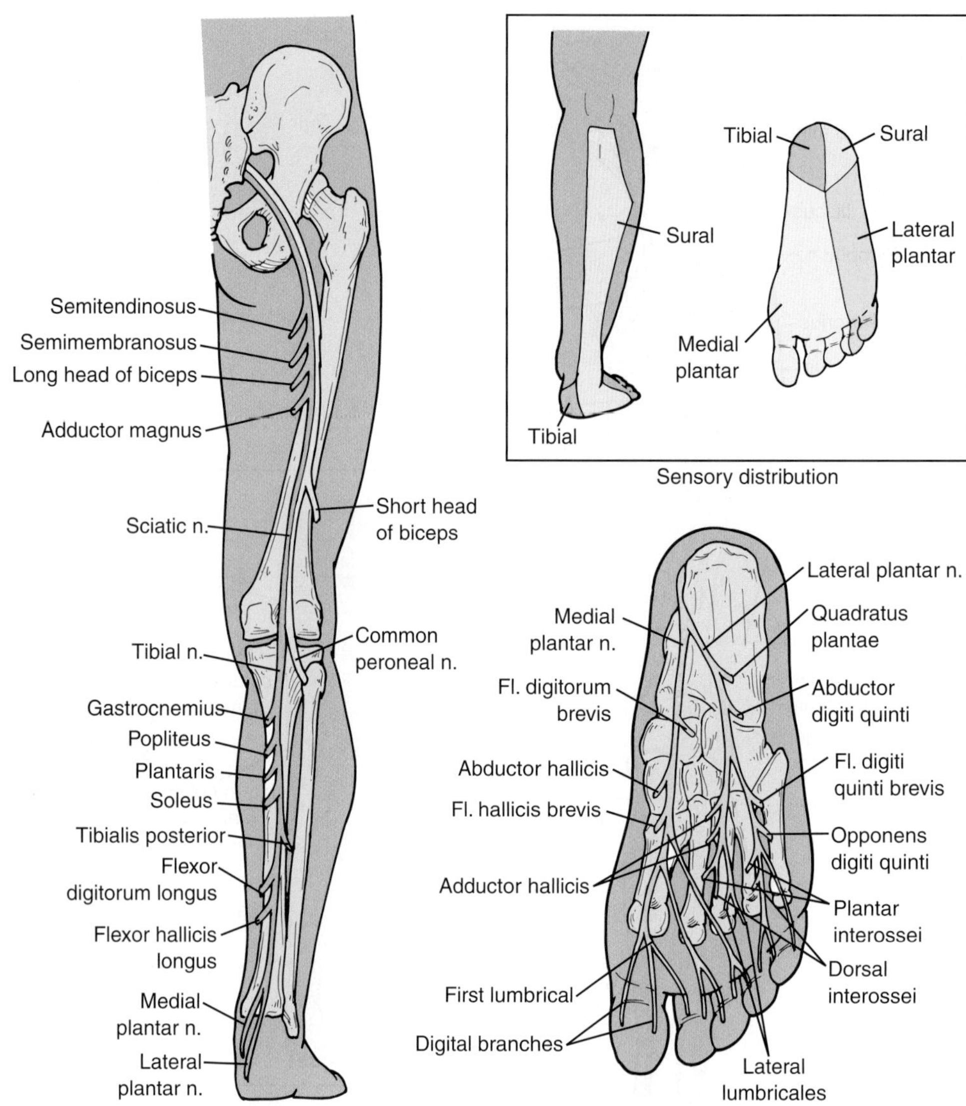

FIGURE 13.10 Sensory and motor innervations of the sciatic nerve (L4, 5, S1–3) and tibial nerve (L4, 5, S1–3).

muscles of the anterior and lateral compartments of the leg. Injury also occurs subsequent to fracture of the head of the fibula, from rupture of the lateral collateral ligament of the knee, or from a tightly applied cast. Also, most people have experienced their foot "falling asleep" from sustained pressure when crossing their legs. The common peroneal nerve bifurcates just below the neck of the fibula into the superficial and deep peroneal nerves.

Superficial peroneal nerve. The superficial peroneal nerve descends along the anterior part of the fibula, innervating the peroneus longus and brevis muscles, and continues on with cutaneous innervations. Injury to just this nerve primarily affects eversion. Over time, equinovarus may develop from unopposed inversion.

Deep peroneal nerve. The deep peroneal nerve descends the leg along the interosseous membrane and distal tibia, innervating the ankle dorsiflexors, toe extensors, and peroneus tertius. In the foot, it innervates the extensor digitorum brevis. Injury to the deep peroneal nerve results in foot drop and unopposed eversion during gait. Over time, pes valgus may develop.

Impaired Nerve Function

Nerve Injury and Recovery

Peripheral nerve injury may result in motor, sensory, and/or sympathetic impairments. In addition, pain may be a symptom of nerve tension or compression because the connective tissue and vascular structures surrounding and in the peripheral nerves are innervated and the peripheral nerve function is sensitive to hypoxic states. Knowing the mechanism of injury and the clinical signs and symptoms helps the clinician

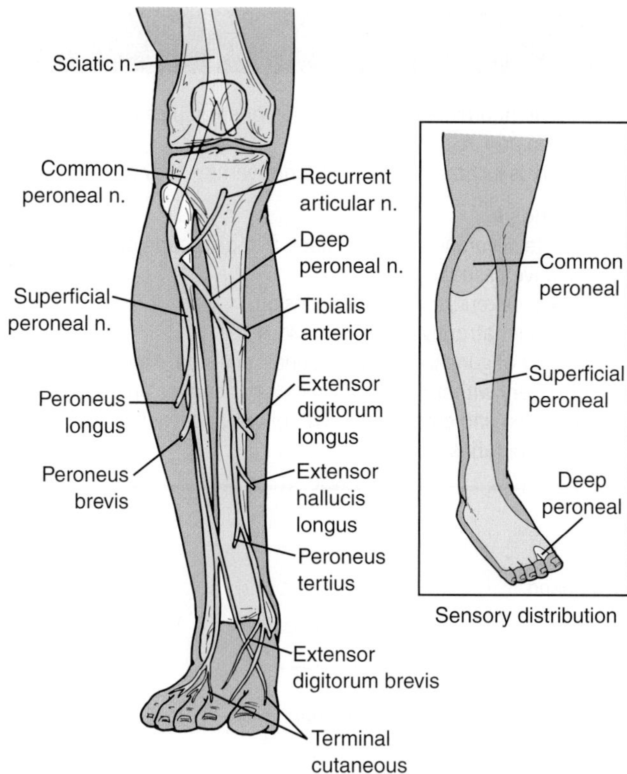

FIGURE 13.11 Sensory and motor innervations of the peroneal nerve (L4, 5, S1, 2).

determine the potential outcome for the patient and develop a plan of care.[38,71,74]

Mechanisms of Nerve Injury

Nerves are mobile and capable of withstanding considerable torsion and lengthening owing to their arrangement. Yet, they are susceptible to various types of injury and malfunction including:[13,71,74]

- Compression (sustained pressure applied externally, such as tourniquet, or internally, such as from bone, tumor, edema, or soft tissue impingement resulting in mechanical or ischemic injury).
- Laceration (knife, gunshot, surgical complication, or injection injury).
- Stretch (excessive tension or tearing from traction forces).
- Radiation.
- Electricity (lightning strike or electrical malfunction).
- Injection (local anesthesia, steroids, or antibiotics).

Injury may be complete or partial and produces symptoms based on the location of the insult.

Biomechanical injuries to the peripheral nervous system are most commonly the result of friction, compression, and stretch.[13,16,71] Secondary injury can be from blood or edema. Compressive forces can affect the microcirculation of the nerve, causing venous congestion and reduction of axoplasmic transport,[53,71] thus blocking nerve impulses; if sustained, the compression can cause nerve damage. The endoneurium helps maintain fluid pressure and may provide cushioning for nerves, especially when the nerves are close to the surface and subject to greater pressure.

The insult can be acute from trauma or chronic from repetitive trauma or entrapment. Sites where a peripheral nerve is more vulnerable to compression, friction, or tension include tunnels (soft tissue, bony, fibro-osseus), branches of the nervous system (especially if the nerve has an abrupt angle), points at which a nerve is relatively fixed when passing close to rigid structures (across a bony prominence), and at specific tension points.

Response to injury can be pathophysiological or pathomechanical, leading to symptoms derived from adverse tension on the nervous system. Results may be intraneural and/or extraneural.[16]

- ***Intraneural.*** Pathology that affects the conducting tissues (e.g., hypoxia or demyelination) or connective tissues of the nerve (e.g., scarring of epineurium or irritation of dura mater) may restrict the elasticity of the nervous system itself.
- ***Extraneural.*** Pathology that affects the nerve bed (e.g., blood), adhesions of epineurium to another tissue (e.g., a ligament), and swelling of tissue adjacent to a nerve (e.g., foraminal stenosis) may restrict the gross movement of the nervous system in relation to surrounding tissues.

Classification of Nerve Injuries

Nerve injuries are classified using either the Seddon or Sunderland classification systems; both are based on structural and functional changes that occur in the nerve with various degrees of damage.[3,33,38,62,75,78] These systems describe the degree of injury to nerve substructures and the effect on prognosis. Seddon's system describes three levels of pathology: neuropraxia, axonotmesis, and neurotmesis. Sunderland's classification details five levels of injury and potential for recovery. The characteristics of Seddon's classification of nerve injuries are summarized in Box 13.3 and are compared with Sunderland's classification in Figure 13.12.

Recovery From Nerve Injuries

Nerve tissue that has become irritated from tension, compression, or hypoxia may not have permanent damage and shows signs of recovery when the irritating factors are eliminated.[16] When the nerve has been injured, recovery is dependent on several factors, including the extent of injury to the axon and its surrounding connective tissue sheath, the nature and level of the injury, the timing and technique of the repair (if necessary), and the age and motivation of the person.[13,74]

- ***Nature and level of injury.*** The more damage to the nerve and tissues, the more tissue reaction and scarring occur. Also, the proximal aspect of a nerve has greater combinations of motor, sensory, and sympathetic fibers, so disruption there

BOX 13.3 Seddon's Classification and Characteristics of Nerve Injury[3,33,38,61,75,78]

Neuropraxia
- Segmental demyelination
- Action potential slowed or blocked at point of demyelination; normal above and below point of compression
- Muscle does not atrophy; temporary sensory symptoms
- The result of mild ischemia from nerve compression or traction
- Recovery is usually complete

Axonotmesis
- Loss of axonal continuity but connective tissue coverings remain intact
- Wallerian degeneration distal to lesion
- Muscle fiber atrophy and sensory loss
- The result of prolonged compression or stretch causing infarction and necrosis
- Recovery is incomplete—surgical intervention may be required

Neurotmesis
- Complete severance of nerve fiber with disruption of connective tissue coverings
- Wallerian degeneration distal to lesion
- Muscle fiber atrophy and sensory loss
- The result of gunshot or stab wounds, avulsion, rupture
- No recovery without surgery—recovery depends on surgical intervention and correct regrowth of individual nerve fibers in endoneural tubes

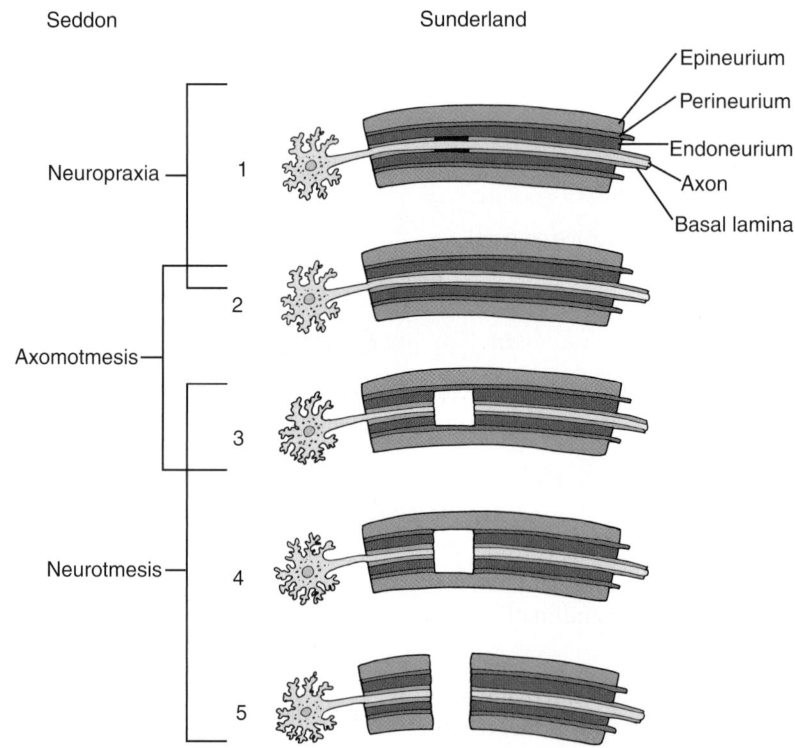

FIGURE 13.12 Comparison of Sunderland's and Seddon's classifications of nerve injuries. **(1)** First degree injury (neuropraxia): minimal structural disruption—complete recovery; **(2)** second degree (axonotmesis): complete axonal disruption with wallerian degeneration—usually complete recovery; **(3)** third degree (may be either axonotmesis or neurotmesis): disruption of axon and endoneurium—poor prognosis without surgery; **(4)** fourth degree (neurotmesis): disruption of axon, endoneurium, and perineurium—poor prognosis without surgery; **(5)** fifth degree (neurotmesis): complete structural disruption—poor prognosis without microsurgery.[74]

results in a greater chance of mismatching the fibers, thus affecting regeneration. Regeneration is often said to occur at a rate of 1 mm per day, but rates from 0.5 to 9.0 mm per day have been reported based on the nature and severity of the injury, duration of denervation, condition of the tissues, and whether surgery is required.[3,13,62]

- ***Timing and technique of repair.*** Laceration or crush injuries that disrupt the integrity of the entire nerve require surgical repair. For optimal nerve regeneration, timing of the repair is critical, as are the skill of the surgeon and the technique used to align the segments accurately and avoid tension at the suture line. Different regenerative potential outcomes following nerve repair have also been reported based on groupings of specific nerves.[3,38,74]
  - Excellent regenerative potential: radial, musculocutaneous, and femoral nerves

- Moderate regenerative potential: median, ulnar, and tibial nerves
- Poor regenerative potential: peroneal nerve

- ***Age and motivation of the patient.*** The nervous system must adapt and relearn use of the pathways once regeneration occurs. Motivation and age play a role in this, especially in the very young and the elderly.[74]

Outcomes of Nerve Regeneration

Smith[74] described five possible outcomes of nerve regeneration.

1. Exact reinnervation of its native target organ with return of function
2. Exact reinnervation of its native target organ but no return of function due to degeneration of the end organ
3. Wrong receptor reinnervated in the proper territory; therefore, improper input
4. Receptor reinnervation in wrong territory causing false localization of input
5. No connection with an end organ

Management Guidelines: Recovery from Nerve Injury

In general, recovery from nerve injury can be viewed as occurring in three phases.

- ***Acute phase.*** This is early after injury or surgery when the emphasis is on healing and prevention of complications.
- ***Recovery phase.*** This is when reinnervation occurs. Emphasis is on retraining and re-education.
- ***Chronic phase.*** This occurs when the potential for reinnervation has peaked, and there are significant residual deficits. The emphasis is training compensatory function.

Effective management must consider not only nerve healing, but also connective tissue healing in general (see Chapter 10). Management guidelines for the three phases of recovery from peripheral nerve injury are summarized in Box 13.4.

Acute Phase

Following injury or immediately after surgery (e.g., following decompression and release or following repair of a lacerated nerve), there may be a period of immobilization for a minimum of 3 weeks to protect the nerve, minimize inflammation, and minimize compression or traction at the injured/repaired site. The specific orthosis or position of the orthosis will depend on the nerve injured or repaired. Encourage active movement of uninvolved joints immediately. As soon as allowed, begin:

- ***Pain and edema management.*** Elevation, compression, and use of modalities (transcutaneous electrical nerve stimulation [TENS], high voltage galvanic stimulation [HVGS]) to wean off medications.
- ***Movement.*** Begin range of motion (ROM) of uninvolved joints to minimize joint and connective tissue contractures.
- ***Orthosis management.*** Use of an orthosis may be necessary to prevent deformities due to strength imbalances (e.g., use of a radial nerve orthosis to prevent wrist drop; a median nerve orthosis to position the thumb in opposition; a plantarflexion orthosis to prevent foot drop), to prevent undue stress on the healing nerve tissue, and to facilitate new movement as reinnervation occurs.
- ***Patient education.*** Teach the patient safe movements and ways to protect the injured nerve and to avoid injury due to loss of sensation.

Recovery Phase

The recovery phase begins with signs of reinnervation (volitional muscle contraction and hypersensitivity). With nerve regeneration and recovery, begin:[26]

- ***Motor retraining.*** When signs of volitional muscle contraction occur, begin place and hold exercises by positioning the

BOX 13.4 MANAGEMENT GUIDELINES—
Recovery from Peripheral Nerve Injury

***Acute phase*: immediately after injury or surgery**
- *Immobilization*: time dictated by surgeon
- *Movement*: amount and intensity dictated by type of injury and surgical repair
- *Orthosis*: may be necessary to prevent deformities
- *Patient education*: protection of the part (see Box 13.5)

***Recovery phase*: signs of reinnervation (muscle contraction, increased sensitivity)**
- *Motor retraining*: muscle "hold" in the shortened position
- *Desensitization*: multiple textures for sensory stimulation; vibration
- *Discriminative sensory reeducation*: identification of objects with, then without, visual cues

***Chronic phase*: reinnervation potential peaked with minimal or no signs of neurological recovery**
- *Compensatory function*: compensatory function is minimized during the recovery phase but is emphasized when full neurological recovery does not occur
- *Preventive care*: emphasis on lifelong care to involved region (see Box 13.5)

muscle in its shortened position; then ask the patient to hold. Provide assistance as needed to prevent the part from "falling" out of the shortened position.

- Use neuromuscular electrical stimulation to reinforce this active effort.
- When the muscles demonstrate control of some range, begin gravity-eliminated, active-assistive ROM. Continue to protect the weak muscles with an orthosis as needed.

- ***Desensitization.*** As nerves regenerate, the person experiences increased sensitivity (hypersensitivity) in the area that had previously been without sensation. Use a graded series of multisensory procedures to decrease the irritability, increase cortical representation, and increase reintegration of sensory input.[26] Suggestions are described in Box 13.5.
- ***Discriminative sensory re-education.*** This is the process of retraining the brain to recognize a stimulus once the hypersensitivity diminishes. Techniques are summarized in Box 13.5.
- ***Patient education.*** Instruct the patient to resume use of the extremity gradually while monitoring pain, swelling, or any discoloration; if necessary, modify or temporarily avoid any aggravating activities. While the nerve is recovering or if nerve recovery is incomplete, teach the patient preventive care to avoid injury (Box 13.6).

Chronic Phase

When the potential for reinnervation has peaked and there are minimal or no signs of reinnervation, emphasize training for compensatory function. The person will probably have to continue to wear the supportive orthosis and preventive care must continue indefinitely.

BOX 13.5 Desensitization and Sensory Re-education Techniques

Suggestions for graded modalities and procedures for desensitizing:

- Use multiple types of textures or contact for sensory stimulation, such as cotton, rough material, sandpaper of various grades, and Velcro. The textures can be wrapped around dowel rods for finger manipulation or to stroke along the skin for 1-3 minutes.
- Place contact particles, such as cotton balls, beans, macaroni, sand, or other material, with various degrees of roughness in tubs or cans, so the patient can run the involved hand or foot through the material. Have the patient begin by manipulating or placing the extremity in the least irritating texture for 1-3 minutes. As tolerance improves, progress to the next texture of slightly more irritating but tolerable stimulus. Maximum progress occurs when the most irritating texture is tolerated.
- Use vibration. Pattern of recovery after nerve injury is pain (hypersensitivity), perception of slow vibration (30 cps), moving touch, constant touch, rapid vibration (256 cps), and awareness from proximal to distal.[74]

Suggestions for retraining the brain to recognize a stimulus:

- Begin by using a moving touch stimulus, such as the eraser end of a pencil, and stroke over the area. The patient first watches, then closes his or her eyes, and tries to identify *where* touch occurred.
- Progress from stroking to using constant touch.
- When the patient is able to localize constant touch, progress to identification of familiar objects of various sizes, shapes, and textures.
- For the hand, use familiar household and personal care objects, such as keys, coins, eating utensils, blocks, toothbrush, and safety pins.
- For the feet, have the patient walk on various surfaces, such as grass, sand, wood, pebbles, and uneven surfaces.

BOX 13.6 Patient Instructions for Preventive Care After Nerve Injury

While the nerve is regenerating, or if nerve recovery is incomplete:

- Inspect skin regularly; provide prompt treatment of wounds or blisters.
- Compensate for dryness with massage creams or oils.

In the upper extremity:

- Avoid handling hot, cold, sharp, or abrasive objects.
- Avoid sustained grasps; change use of tools frequently.
- Redistribute hand pressure by building up the size of the handles.
- Wear protective gloves.

In the lower extremity:

- Wear protective shoes that fit properly.
- Inspect feet regularly for pressure points (reddened area) and modify shoes or provide protection if they occur.
- Do not walk barefoot, especially in the dark or on rough surfaces.
- Shift weight frequently when standing for long periods.

Neural Tension Disorders

Normally, the nervous system has considerable mobility to adapt to the wide range of movements imposed on it by daily activities. Still, there are sites where nerves are vulnerable to increased pressure or tension, especially when excessive or repetitive stresses or strains are imposed on the tissues surrounding the nerves or on the nerves themselves. If a nerve is compressed as it passes near a bony structure or through a confined space, undue deformation may occur as movement occurs proximal or distal to that site. This may be magnified if there is adhesive scar tissue or swelling that restricts elongation and mobility. When examining a patient, the therapist needs to be alert to symptoms described by the patient and able to understand and interpret positive signs detected with testing maneuvers.

This section summarizes the tests of provocation and describes the techniques that have been reported to mobilize components of the nervous system in order to improve the patient's outcome.[16,62,71]

Symptoms and Signs of Impaired Nerve Mobility

History

Vascular and mechanical factors can lead to nerve pathology. Pain is the most common symptom. Sensory responses, reported as stretch pain or paresthesia, occur when tissues are in the neural stretch position.[21] Clinical reasoning is used to understand the possible mechanism of injury, such as pathological insult to the nervous tissue or surrounding tissues or symptoms from movement patterns that place compression or tension on the neural tissues and reproduce symptoms.[71]

Tests of Provocation

Neurodynamic test maneuvers are performed to detect tension or compression in the neural tissue. The upper limb neurodynamic test (ULNT), straight leg raise (SLR), and slump test are familiar terms that describe various tests and procedures that will be described later in this chapter.[16,71] Points regarding the tests:

- Because the test positions elongate the nerves across multiple joints, every joint in the chain must be examined separately for limitations in ROM, mobility, and symptom provocation prior to neurodynamic testing so that any restriction that occurs during the test is not the result of joint or periarticular tissue limitations.[16,71] Coppieters and associates[21] demonstrated that the stretch position altered the available ROM and sensory responses in 35 normal male subjects during neurodynamic testing and reiterated the importance of looking at other influences prior to neurodynamic testing.
- Additional tests for nerve function include nerve palpation, sensation testing, reflex testing, dexterity testing, and muscle testing.[16,26,71]
- The test positions and maneuvers used to detect nerve mobility are the same as the treatment positions and maneuvers.
- Test the uninvolved or least symptomatic side first. If testing of the uninvolved side produces symptoms, sensitivity of the nerve roots or central sensitization should be considered.[16]
- Perform the tests actively before passively to decrease the patient's anxiety about performing the maneuver. If the active test is found to be sensitive, determine whether a passive test is also needed. A positive active test will also inform the therapist that neurodynamic glides would be an appropriate adjunct to the plan of care.
- For a test to be considered positive it must (1) reproduce the patient's symptoms (pain or paresthesias) within the nerve distribution being tested, plus (2) demonstrate differences from side to side and to known normal responses, plus (3) support findings from the full examination including symptom pattern and location, physical findings (i.e., strength, ROM, joint mobility), plus (4) the sensitizing maneuvers alter the patient's symptoms.[11,71] Sensitizing maneuvers produce either pain or paresthesias when the neurological system is elongated across multiple joints or is relieved when one of the joints (usually the most proximal or distal) is moved out of the elongated position.

General testing procedure: Slowly and carefully elongate the nerve across each joint in succession until there is symptom provocation or tissue restriction is felt (described in detail in the techniques section). When symptoms occur, note the final position. Once symptoms are provoked or limitation in motion occurs, sensitize the maneuver by moving one of the joints out of the elongated position or moving one of the joints proximal or distal into a more elongated position to see if the symptoms are relieved or provoked respectively.

Causes of Symptoms

Butler[15] originally proposed that symptoms are the result of tension being placed on some component of the nervous system, thus referring to these set of tests as "neural tension tests." He thought that if compression is preventing normal mobility, tension signs occur when the nerve is stressed either proximal or distal to the site of compression. Restriction of movement could be from inflammation and scarring between the nerve and the tissue through which it runs or from actual changes in the nerve itself. More recently, Butler has embraced the concept of "neurodynamics" introduced by Shacklock in 1995. The thought is that "dynamics" is more encompassing, moving away from strictly mechanical causes to include physiological issues as well as changes in plasticity in the nervous system.[16,71]

FOCUS ON EVIDENCE

Cadavaric and in vivo ultrasound imaging studies have demonstrated that ROM of the moving joint, distance from the moving joint to the site of the lesion, position of adjacent joints, number of moving joints, and whether joint movement elongates or shortens the nerve bed all have an impact on nerve excursion[18-20,25,39,72] and that elongation or shortening of the sciatic, tibial, and plantar nerves occur to various degrees with hip, knee, ankle, and toe movements.[1,11,18,20] In addition, Coppieters[18] demonstrated greater sciatic nerve excursion occurs with simultaneous hip/knee movement than with any of the tensioning techniques.

As with many manual testing techniques, the sensitivity and validity of the tests have yet to be determined. Although the volume of evidence continues to be limited, more recent studies demonstrate the reliability and validity of ULNT to be promising.[60,68,81] In addition, there is emerging evidence that ULNT testing may not only be for brachial plexus and peripheral nerve testing and treatment, but that it may also be effective for pathology in the cervical region including cervical radiculopathy, entrapment neuropathies, and thoracic outlet syndrome.[48]

The efficacy of interventions based on the neurodynamic maneuvers has been presented in the literature.[17,29,42] A systematic review of research on therapeutic efficacy of neural mobilization evaluated 10 randomized controlled studies.[29] Even though the majority of the studies described positive benefits, the review questioned the quality of the studies and expressed the need for more homogeneity and control in future studies in order to provide evidence for the use of neural mobilization as a therapeutic intervention.

Principles of Management

The principles of neural mobilization are based on the anatomic and biomechanical properties of peripheral nerves and their response to stress and strain. The goal of neural mobilization is to maximize the excursion of the nerve while minimizing the strain. Strain is defined as the change in nerve length induced by a longitudinal tensile stress.[67] For the nervous system to move normally, it must withstand tensile stress, slide in its container, and be compressible.[71]

The principles of treatment are similar to those of any mobilization technique; however, the greatest error clinicians make with these techniques is being too aggressive and doing too much, too fast.[16,61,71]

- The intensity of the maneuver should be related to irritability of the tissue, patient response, and change in symptoms. The greater the irritability, the gentler the technique.
- The technique, when applied properly, should be symptom free, slow, and rhythmic, utilizing an oscillatory motion.
- ***Neural sliding, flossing technique.*** Position the patient at the point of tissue resistance or onset of symptoms, then move two joints in the chain simultaneously so that the neural tissue glides proximally or distally. For example, to glide the median nerve proximally once at the position of tissue resistance or onset of symptoms, perform elbow flexion simultaneously with cervical contralateral flexion or wrist flexion simultaneously with elbow flexion.
- ***Neural glide technique:*** Position the patient at the same point as in the sliding technique. Offload the nerve by placing the neural tissue on slack either by laterally flexing the proximal segment toward the involved side or by releasing the position of the distal segment. Then slowly and in an oscillatory fashion using large movements, gently move one segment in and out of the point of tissue resistance.
- After performing several treatments and determining the tissue response, teach the patient self-mobilization techniques.

Precautions and Contraindications to Neurodynamic Testing and Treatment

There is incomplete scientific understanding of the pathology and mechanisms that occur when mobilizing the nervous system. The clinician should always perform a thorough subjective and physical examination which includes a systems review and screening for "red flag" conditions prior to neurodynamic testing and treatment. Caution should be used when loading the neurological system during performance of these techniques. Neurological symptoms of tingling or increased numbness should not last when the position is released.[16,67,71]

PRECAUTIONS:

- Know what other tissues are affected by the positions and maneuvers.
- Recognize the irritability of the tissues involved and do not aggravate the symptoms with excessive stress or repeated movements.
- Identify whether the condition is worsening and the rate of worsening. A rapidly worsening condition requires greater care than a slowly progressing condition.
- Use care if there is an active disease or other pathology affecting the nervous system.
- Watch for signs of vascular compromise. The vascular system is in close proximity to the nervous system and at no time should show signs of compromise when mobilizing the nervous system.

CONTRAINDICATIONS:

- Acute or unstable neurological signs
- Cauda equina symptoms related to the spine including changes in bowel or bladder control and perineal sensation
- Spinal cord injury or symptoms
- Neoplasm and infection

Neural Testing and Mobilization Techniques for the Upper Quadrant

Median Nerve—ULNT 1 (Passive) (Fig. 13.13)

This maneuver is used when examining and treating symptoms related to median nerve distribution, including carpal tunnel syndrome.[16]

Patient position and procedure: Begin with the patient in supine position close to your side (no pillows at the head or knees) with the patient's upper arm on your thigh. Place your hand closest to the patient in a fist and position it at the superior aspect of the patient's shoulder, pushing it into the table to control elevation of the shoulder during abduction of the arm (maintaining equal shoulder positions). Abduct the arm to approximately 110° keeping the elbow at 90° flexion. Maintain the shoulder and elbow position, extend the wrist and fingers including the thumb (using your thumb and index finger). Supinate the forearm followed by lateral rotation of the shoulder. Slowly extend the elbow, keeping the wrist and shoulder position constant. Stop the elbow extension when either the patient reports symptoms or you feel tension in the tissue.

To sensitize the maneuver: Ask the patient to laterally flex their cervical spine away from the test side and inquire if this movement increases their symptoms. Then ask the patient to laterally flex their cervical spine toward the test side and inquire

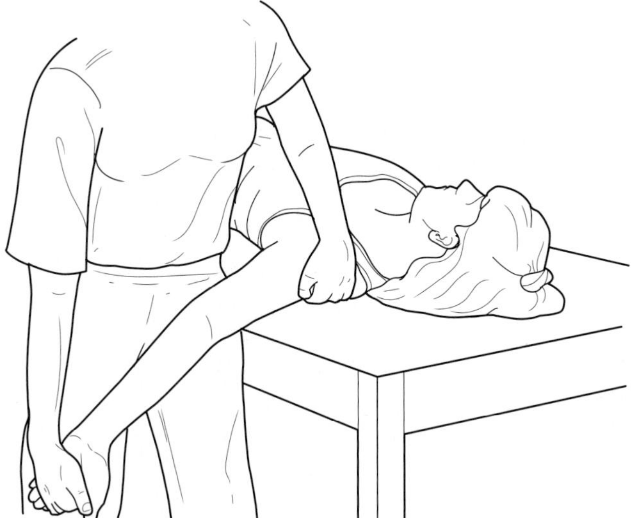

FIGURE 13.13 Position of maximum elongation of the median nerve includes shoulder abduction to 110°; elbow extension; shoulder external rotation and supination of the forearm; wrist, finger, and thumb extension; and finally contralateral cervical side flexion.

if this movement alleviates or lessens their symptoms (if there is concern about "leading" the patient to a particular answer, the clinician can inquire if the movement increases, decreases, or if the symptoms remain unchanged) during the particular sensitizing movement.[16]

FOCUS ON EVIDENCE

Using ultrasound imaging, Coppieters and associates[20] examined the longitudinal excursion of the median nerve, using several variations of cervical and elbow movements that caused either sliding or tensioning of the median nerve. For the sliding technique, elbow flexion and cervical side flexion were performed simultaneously in the same direction; for one tensioning technique, elbow extension and cervical side flexion were performed simultaneously in opposite directions; and for four techniques, only one joint (elbow or neck) was moved after prepositioning the other joint.

Results showed significant differences in the amount of nerve movement with the various techniques ($P < .0001$). Greatest excursion occurred with the sliding technique when the two joints were moved in the same direction (10.2 +/ -2.8 mm); the smallest excursion occurred with the tensioning technique when the two joints were moved in opposite directions (1.8 +/ -4.0 mm). Techniques in which only one joint moved demonstrated larger excursions when the elbow moved (5.6 and 5.5 mm) than when the neck moved (3.3 and 3.4 mm). These tests were performed on healthy volunteers and therefore cannot be generalized to therapeutic effects for patients with different pathologies affecting the median nerve.

Radial Nerve—ULNT 2 (Fig. 13.14)

This maneuver is important when examining and treating symptoms that are related to shoulder girdle depression, radial nerve distribution, and differentiating between tennis elbow and radial tunnel syndrome, as well as de Quervain's syndrome and superficial sensory radial nerve involvement.[16]

Patient position and procedure: Begin with the patient supine; sequentially apply gentle shoulder girdle depression, then slightly abduct the shoulder to about 10°, extend the elbow, and then medially rotate the whole arm (including forearm pronation). Keep the elbow in extension and add wrist, finger, and thumb flexion and finally ulnar deviation of the wrist. Maintaining this position, slowly abduct the shoulder until reproduction of symptoms or tension is felt in the tissue. The full elongated position includes lateral flexion of the cervical spine away from the test side. Have the patient then laterally flex the cervical spine toward the test side, noting increase or decrease of symptoms.

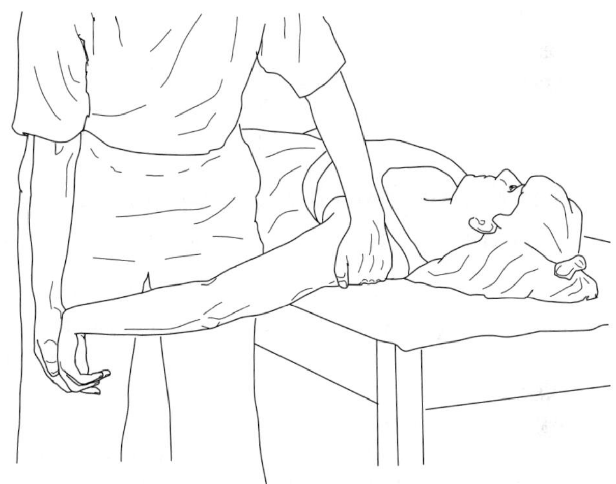

FIGURE 13.14 Position of maximum elongation of the radial nerve includes shoulder girdle depression; shoulder abduction; elbow extension; shoulder medial rotation and forearm pronation; wrist, finger, and thumb flexion; wrist ulnar deviation; and finally contralateral cervical side flexion.

Ulnar Nerve—ULNT 3 (Fig. 13.15)

This maneuver is used when symptoms are related to the lower brachial plexus or ulnar nerve and differentiating between medial epicondylosis and pronator syndrome.[16]

Patient position and procedure: Begin with the patient supine. Extend the wrist and fingers, pronate the forearm and flex the elbow. While maintaining this position laterally rotate the shoulder and depress the shoulder girdle. Finally abduct the shoulder to about 110° or until symptoms are felt. The full elongated position includes lateral flexion of the cervical spine away from the test side. Have the patient then laterally flex the cervical spine toward the test side noting increase or decrease of symptoms.

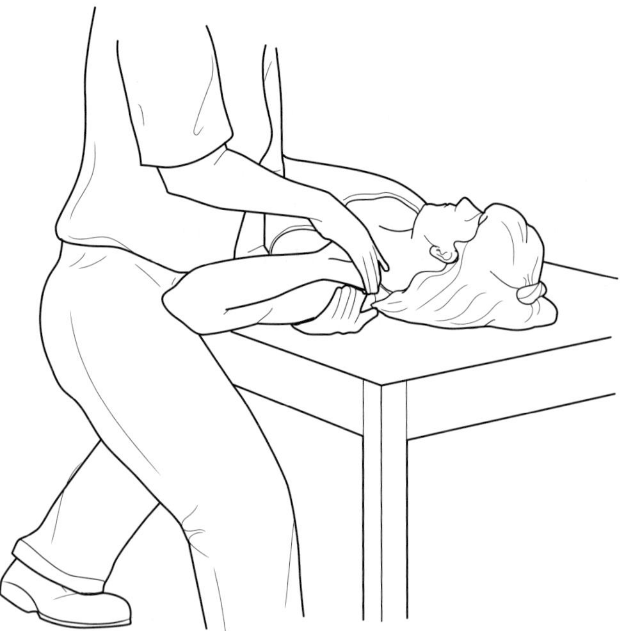

FIGURE 13.15 Position of maximum elongation on the ulnar nerve includes shoulder girdle depression; shoulder external rotation and abduction; elbow flexion; forearm pronation and wrist extension; and finally contralateral cervical side flexion.

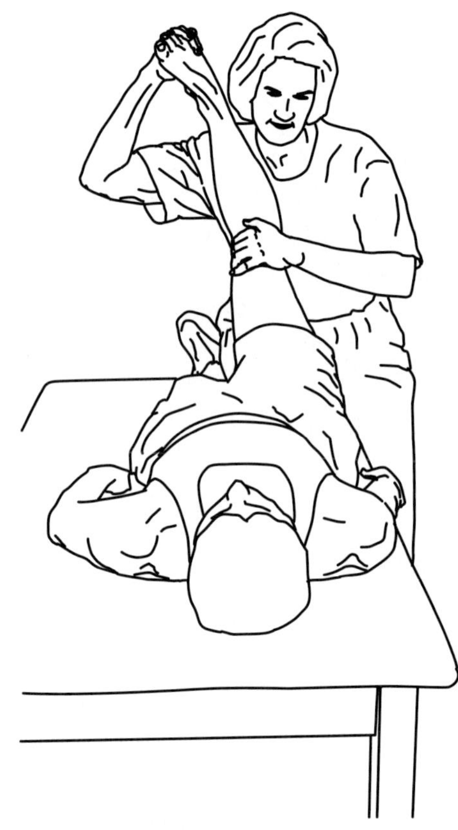

FIGURE 13.16 Position of stretch on the sciatic nerve includes straight-leg raising with adduction and internal rotation of the hip and dorsiflexion of the ankle.

Neural Testing and Mobilization Techniques for the Lower Quadrant

Sciatic Nerve: Straight Leg Raising (Fig. 13.16)

Patient position and procedure: The patient is supine. Lift the lower extremity in the straight leg raise (SLR) position and add ankle dorsiflexion. Several variations may be done to assist with differentiating the neural load; ankle dorsiflexion, dorsiflexion with eversion, ankle plantar flexion with inversion, hip adduction, hip medial rotation, and passive neck flexion.[16] The maneuver may also be performed long-sitting (slump-sitting position—see below) and side-lying. These various positions of the lower extremity and neck are used to differentiate tight or strained hamstrings from possible sites of restriction or nerve mobility in the lumbosacral plexus and sciatic nerve.[11,34,73] Changing positions of the ankle in conjunction with variations in the hip and knee positions are used to differentiate foot impairments, such as plantar fasciitis and tarsal tunnel syndrome.[1]

Once the position that places tension on the involved neurological tissue is found, maintain the stretch position and then move one of the joints a few degrees in and out of the stretch position, such as ankle plantarflexion and dorsiflexion or knee flexion and extension.

- Ankle dorsiflexion with eversion places more tension on the tibial tract.
- Ankle dorsiflexion with inversion places tension on the sural nerve.
- Ankle plantarflexion with inversion places tension on the common peroneal tract.
- Adduction of the hip while doing SLR places further tension on the nervous system, because the sciatic nerve is lateral to the ischial tuberosity; medial rotation of the hip while doing SLR also increases tension on the sciatic nerve (see Fig. 13.16).
- Passive neck flexion while doing SLR pulls the spinal cord cranially and places the entire nervous system on a stretch.[16]
- Strain on the medial and lateral plantar nerves increases with toe extension and is larger with ankle dorsiflexion than plantarflexion.[1]

Neural slide (flossing) technique: Beginning with the hip and knee in flexion, simultaneously extend the hip and knee to obtain maximum sliding of the sciatic nerve (knee extension loads the tibial and sciatic nerve; hip extension unloads the sciatic nerve).[18]

FOCUS ON EVIDENCE

A study using ultrasound imaging of the sciatic nerve under different hip and knee movements demonstrated the following biomechanics on the nerve: greatest sliding occurred with simultaneous hip/knee extension (approximately five times larger than with the tensioning techniques of hip flexion with knee extension and two times larger than during isolated hip and knee movements).[18]

Slump-Sitting Maneuver (Fig. 13.17)

NOTE: The slump test is simply the SLR performed in sitting with the addition of spinal flexion for greater overall neural tension.

Patient position and procedure: Begin with the patient sitting upright. Have the patient slump by flexing the spine and neck. Apply gentle overpressure guidance to cervical spine flexion. As a sensitizing maneuver, dorsiflex the ankle and then extend the knee as much as possible to the point of tissue resistance and symptom reproduction. Release the overpressure on the spine and have the patient actively extend the neck to see if symptoms decrease. Increase and release the stretch force by moving one joint in the chain a few degrees, such as knee flexion and extension or ankle dorsiflexion and plantarflexion and note response.

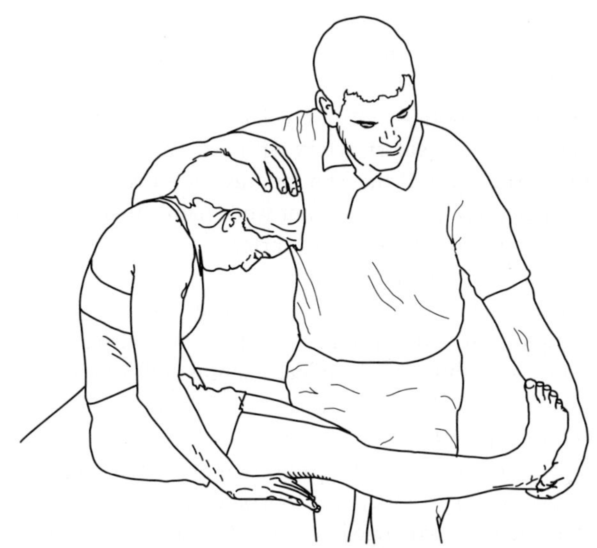

FIGURE 13.17 Slump-sitting with neck, thorax, and low back flexed, knee extended, and ankle dorsiflexed just to the point of tissue resistance and symptom reproduction.

FOCUS ON EVIDENCE

A study evaluating the accuracy of the slump test in patients with low back pain found the test was highly sensitive in identifying those with neuropathic pain and that adding the criterion of pain distal to the knee during the maneuver improved specificity.[80]

Femoral Nerve: Prone Knee Bend (PKB) (Fig. 13.18)

Patient position and procedure: Prone with the spine neutral (not extended) and the hips extended to 0°. Flex the knee

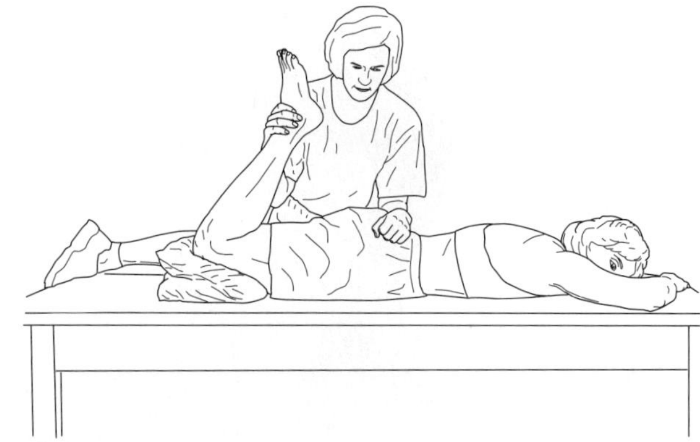

FIGURE 13.18 Position of stretch on the femoral nerve; prone lying with the spine neutral, hip extended to zero degrees, and knee flexed. It is important to maintain the spine in neutral and not allow it to extend.

to the point of resistance and symptom reproduction. Pain in the low back or neurological signs (change in sensation in the anterior thigh) are considered positive for upper lumbar nerve roots and femoral nerve tension. Thigh pain could be rectus femoris tightness. It is important not to hyperextend the spine to avoid confusion with nerve root pressure from decreased foraminal space or facet pain from spinal movement. Flex and extend the knee a few degrees to apply and release tension.

Alternate position and procedure: Side-lying with the involved leg uppermost. Stabilize the pelvis and extend the hip with the knee flexed until symptoms are reproduced. Maintain knee flexion, release, and apply tension across the hip by moving it a few degrees at a time.

Musculoskeletal Diagnoses Involving Impaired Nerve Function

Thoracic Outlet Syndrome

The thoracic outlet is the region along the pathway of the brachial plexus from just distal to the nerve roots where they exit the intervertebral foramen to the lower border of the axilla (Fig. 13.19). The outlet is bordered medially by the anterior and middle scalene muscles and the first rib; posteriorly by the upper trapezius and scapula; anteriorly by the clavicle, coracoid, pectoralis minor, and deltopectoral fascia; and laterally by the axilla. The plexus enters the outlet between the anterior and middle scalene muscles; the subclavian artery runs posterior to the anterior scalene; and the subclavian vein runs anterior to the anteriorscalene muscle. The blood vessels join the brachial plexus and course together under the clavicle, over the first rib, and under the coracoid process posterior

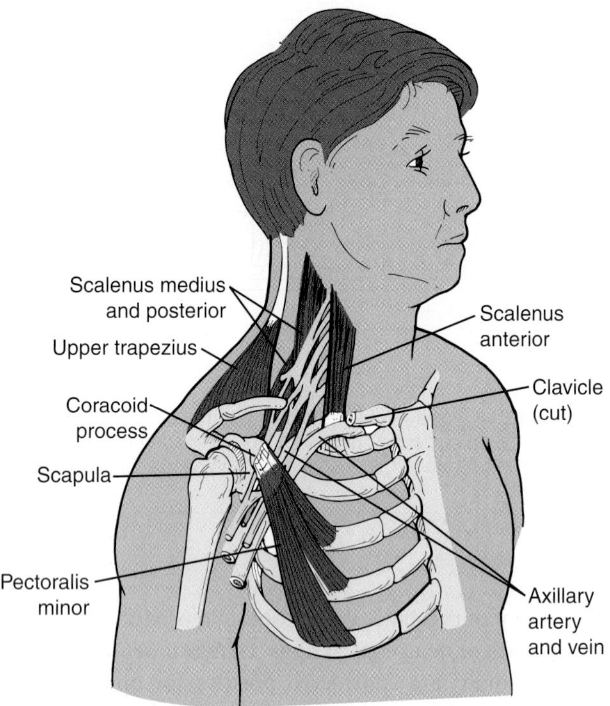

FIGURE 13.19 Region of the thoracic outlet bordered medially by the scalene muscle and first rib; posteriorly by the upper trapezius and scapula; anteriorly by the clavicle, coracoid, pectoralis minor, and deltopectoral fascia; and laterally by the axilla.

to the pectoralis minor muscle. Vascular and/or upper extremity neurological symptoms that are not consistent with nerve root or peripheral nerve dermatome and myotome patterns should lead the therapist to suspect thoracic outlet problems.[45]

NOTE: Sites of impingement of the brachial plexus and vascular structures within the thoracic outlet are described later in this section.

Related Diagnoses

Thoracic outlet syndrome (TOS) encompasses a variety of clinical problems in the shoulder girdle region. The diagnosis itself is controversial because of the clinical complexity and variability in presentation that involves upper extremity neurological and vascular symptoms, including pain, paresthesia, numbness, weakness, discoloration, swelling, and loss of pulse. Patients may also complain of headaches, which may be related to posture, tension, or vascular compromise. Diagnoses that have been used to describe TOS include cervical rib, scalenus anticus syndrome, costoclavicular syndrome, subcoracoid-pectoralis minor syndrome, droopy shoulder syndrome, and hyperabduction syndrome.[37,43,45,76,83] TOS is categorized into two specific clinical entities: vascular TOS and neurological or neurogenic TOS. Vascular TOS is further subcategorized into arterial and venous, while neurogenic TOS is further subdivided into "true" neurogenic or disputed TOS. It is estimated that over 90% of cases are neurogenic in origin, whereas 1% are arterial and approximately 3% to 5% are venous.[37,43,76,83,84]

- ***True Neurogenic TOS.*** This condition is rare. The patient presents with an anatomical abnormality, such as cervical rib or elongated C7 transverse process. The patient describes paresthesias and pain along the medial border of the arm and experiences muscle weakness; there is atrophy in the intrinsic muscles of the hand. There are also positive electromyographic (EMG) findings.[76]
- ***Disputed, symptomatic or nonspecific neurogenic TOS.*** This is the most common form of TOS. Symptoms are similar to true neurogenic TOS, however there is no definitive radiologic evidence of bony anomaly. There is no evidence of muscle atrophy, and EMG testing is negative. Disputed TOS involves intermittent compression of the neurovascular bundle due to poor posture (especially in those with large amounts of breast tissue), occupation, or sporting incidents. Symptoms are aggravated by repetitive, suspensory, or sustained overhead activity, forward or elevation of the shoulder and/or activities that depress the shoulder girdle. Symptoms are present at rest and at night.[76,83,84]
- ***Vascular TOS—arterial.*** This condition is rare and is usually the result of structural abnormalities such as cervical rib or other bony abnormality. There is compression of the subclavian or axillary artery with arm motion, especially overhead usage. If the arm fatigues with overhead usage, the person may have to adapt work habits that avoid risk from repetitive trauma to the artery.
- ***Vascular syndromes—venous.*** Compression of the subclavian or axillary vein does not typically occur in TOS; venous symptoms would be from some other cause, such as thrombosis. Acute thrombosis (sudden, painful swelling with bluish discoloration of the arm) is usually dealt with medically, but the therapist should always be suspicious of unexplained swelling of the arm. Effort thrombosis could occur from sudden maximal arm use, or there could be insidious onset of swelling with prolonged use. If these occur, an immediate referral to an appropriate physician is warranted.

Etiology of Symptoms

Three causative factors for TOS have been identified that could be interrelated or exist separately: compressive neuropathy, faulty posture, and entrapment.

- ***Compressive neuropathy.*** Compression of the neurovascular structures can occur if there is a decrease in the size of the area through which the brachial plexus and subclavian vessels pass. Compression can result from muscle hypertrophy in the scalenes or pectoralis minor muscles, anatomical anomalies such as cervical rib or fractured clavicle, adaptive shortening of fascia, or a space-occupying lesion.
- ***Faulty posture.*** Changes in posture, particularly a forward head with increased thoracic kyphosis, protracted scapulae, and forward shoulders, narrow the spaces through which the neurovascular structures pass. Specifically, adaptive

shortening of the scalene and pectoralis minor muscles can potentially compress the neurovascular tissues or can cause repetitive trauma and adhesions with overuse.[61] If the angle of the clavicle falls below the level of the sternoclavicular joint, the shoulder girdle causes traction on the plexus. In addition, the clavicle can compress the neurovascular structures against the first rib. Hypertrophy of breast tissue may cause postural fatigue or pressure from undergarment support straps, Carrying a heavy briefcase, suitcase, backpack, or shoulder purse may cause pressure across the shoulder girdle, fatigue in the scapular stabilizers, or traction across the shoulder girdle tissues and brachial plexus.

FOCUS ON EVIDENCE

A study reported by Pascarelli and Hsu[65] of 485 patients with work-related upper quarter pain and symptoms indicated that 70% of patients displayed posture-related neurogenic TOS as a key factor in a series of cascading events, including 78% with protracted shoulders, 71% with forward head posture, 50% with hyperlaxity of fingers and elbows, 20% with sympathetic dysfunction, 64% with cubital tunnel, 60% with medial epicondylitis, 70% with peripheral muscle weakness, and other miscellaneous conditions such as carpal tunnel syndrome. Wood and Biondi[86] pointed out that, among 165 patients with TOS, 44% also had compression of a nerve distally, most commonly in the carpal tunnel (41 cases).

A surgical study reported findings that pathological adhesions of the brachial plexus to the scalene muscles led to nerve fiber distraction as the mechanism behind the symptoms and suggested that the restrictive adhesions were directly related to long-standing postural deviations and myofascial pain syndrome.[22]

- ***Entrapment of neural tissue from scar tissue or pressure.*** Entrapment affects the ability of nerve tissue of the brachial plexus to tolerate tension as it courses through the various tissues in the thoracic outlet. A possible explanation was offered in a review article by Crotti[23] wherein the pain-immobility-fibrosis loop that occurs after trauma (e.g., following an acceleration-extension motor vehicle injury) leads to the development of adhesions, which cause or perpetuate TOS symptoms. The Halstead test[52] and the upper limb neurodynamic test for the median nerve[16] (see Fig. 13.14) place the brachial plexus and median nerve on stretch and symptoms may indicate restricted nerve gliding. The Halstead test also may obliterate the radial pulse indicating vascular entrapment. Lohman and associates[48] performed a cadaver study that demonstrated strain placed on cervical nerve roots during upper limb neurodynamic testing. They suggested that this could be used in the clinical evaluation of cervical pathology including thoracic outlet syndrome.

Contributing factors in the development of TOS are summarized in Box 13.7.

BOX 13.7 Summary of Contributing Factors to Thoracic Outlet Syndrome

There is wide latitude of motion in the various joints of the shoulder complex that may result in compression or impingement of the nerves or vessels in TOS.

- *Postural variations*, such as a forward head or round shoulders, lead to associated muscle shortening in the scalene, levator, subscapularis, and pectoralis minor muscles and a depressed clavicle.
- *Postural stress*, such as narrow bra straps, carrying a heavy suitcase, backpack, briefcase, or purse, can place stress across the shoulder girdle, creating pressure in the thoracic outlet or traction on the brachial plexus.
- *Respiratory patterns* that continually use the action of the scalene muscles to elevate the upper ribs lead to hypertrophy of these muscles. Also, the elevated upper ribs decrease the space under the clavicle.
- *Congenital factors*, such as an accessory rib, a long transverse process of the C-7 vertebra, or other anomalies in the region, can reduce the space for the vessels. A traumatic or arteriosclerotic insult can also lead to TOS symptoms.
- *Traumatic injuries*, such as clavicular fracture or subacromial dislocations of the humeral head, can injure the plexus and vessels, leading to TOS symptoms.
- *Hypertrophy or scarring* in the pectoralis minor muscles can lead to TOS symptoms.
- *Injuries* that result in inflammation, scar tissue formation, and adhesions can restrict nerve tissue mobility when the nerve is elongated. This may occur anywhere from the intervertebral foramina at the spine to the distal-most portion of the peripheral nerve.

Sites of Compression or Entrapment

There are three primary sites for compression or entrapment of the neurovascular structures.[43,45]

- **Interscalene triangle:** *bordered by the anterior and middle scalene muscles and the first rib.* If these muscles are hypertrophied, tight, or have anatomical variations, or if the first rib is elevated, they may compress the subclavian artery or the upper, middle or lower trunks of the brachial plexus and impair normal mobility of the neural tissues with head and arm movements.

Symptoms from dysfunction in this area are reproduced with the Adson maneuver, which decreases the space for the neurovascular bundle. If the artery is compressed, there is also a decreased pulse.[45,52] Palpation of the scalene muscles may also provoke symptoms.

- **Costoclavicular space:** *between the clavicle, the subclavius muscle, and the costocoracoid ligament anteriorly and the first rib posteriorly.* Compression of the neurovascular bundle can occur between the clavicle and first rib, especially if the clavicle is depressed for periods of time, as occurs when carrying a heavy suitcase, a backpack or shoulder bag, or with a slouched posture. A fractured clavicle or anomalies in the region can also lead to symptoms. An elevated first rib, which can occur with first rib subluxation or upper thoracic breathing (as with asthma or chronic emphysema), also narrows the costoclavicular space.

Symptoms caused by a depressed clavicle are reproduced when the shoulders are retracted and depressed as with the Military Brace Test.[52] If a patient is asked to take in a breath while in this posture and symptoms are reproduced, the rib elevation is causing the symptoms. The mobility of the clavicle and first rib should also be examined.

- **Rectropectoralis minor space:** *between the second through fourth ribs anteriorly, posterior to the pectoralis minor muscle, and inferior to the coracoid process.* Compression or restricted movement of the neurovascular structures may occur in this region if the pectoralis minor muscle is tight owing to faulty posture with the scapula tipped forward or from repetitive overuse.

Holding the arms in an elevated position compresses the cords of the brachial plexus and axillary artery and vein. Compression of the neurovascular bundle in this space may be tested utilizing Roos test.[52] Palpation pressure against the pectoralis minor may also reproduce the neurological symptoms if the muscle is tight.

Common Impairments of Structure and Function in TOS

- Intermittent brachial plexus and vascular symptoms of pain, paresthesia, numbness, weakness, discoloration, and swelling
- Muscle length–strength imbalance in the shoulder girdle with tightness in anterior and medial structures and weakness in posterior and lateral structures
- Faulty postural awareness in the upper quarter
- Poor endurance in the postural muscles
- Poor scapular control
- Shallow respiratory pattern characterized by upper thoracic breathing
- Poor clavicular and first rib mobility
- Neurological symptoms when the brachial plexus is placed on stretch

Common Activity Limitations and Participation Restrictions

- Sleep disturbances that could be from excessive pillow thickness or arm position
- Inability to carry briefcase, backpack, suitcase, purse with shoulder strap, or other weighted objects on the involved side
- Inability to maintain prolonged overhead reaching position
- Inability to do sustained computer or desk work, cradle a telephone receiver between head and involved shoulder, or drive a car for prolonged periods
- Inability to do sustained overhead work such as electrical work or painting a ceiling

Nonoperative Management of TOS

Conservative management is often recommended for all types of TOS in the absence of any acute or progressive neurological or vascular lesion. The primary emphasis of management may involve medication, injection therapy, rest, and activity modification in addition to physical therapy. Physical therapy management often involves postural education, strengthening and endurance exercises, scapular stabilization, and manual therapy.[81,84]

A program is developed utilizing interventions that specifically address the presenting impairments, activity limitations, and participation restrictions (Box 13.8). Also, secondary or associated complaints, such as myofascial trigger points, glenohumeral joint pathology, cervical pathology, or distal peripheral neuropathies, should be identified, and appropriate interventions incorporated into the program.[45,84] Consider the following precautions and interventions.

PRECAUTIONS: Shoulder girdle exercises may cause worsening of symptoms in some patients with venous or arterial TOS, or they may be progressing favorably and then symptoms worsen. Worsening of neurological or vascular symptoms may indicate axonal disruption or vascular compromise. Refer the patient to his or her physician; surgical decompression may be indicated.

BOX 13.8 Summary of Guidelines for Management of Thoracic Outlet Syndrome

Educate the patient.
- Teach posture correction.
- Teach how to modify provoking stresses.
- Teach safe exercises for home exercise program.

Correct impaired posture.
- See Chapter 14

Mobilize restricted neurological tissue.
- Nerve mobilization techniques if testing is positive for restricted mobility

Mobilize restricted joints, connective tissue, and muscle.
- Tissue-specific manual techniques to restricted structures if testing is positive for restricted mobility
- Self-stretching exercises for restricted muscle flexibility

Improve muscle performance.
- Develop control and endurance in postural muscles.
- Progress strengthening exercises.

Correct faulty breathing patterns.
- Relax upper thorax.
- Teach abdominal diaphragmatic or bi-basilar breathing patterns.

Progress functional independence.
- Involve patient in all aspects of program.

- ***Patient education.*** Teach the patient how to modify or eliminate provoking postures and activities and provide a home exercise program that includes flexibility, muscle performance, and postural exercises (see Chapter 14). Emphasize the importance of compliance to reduce the stresses on the nerve and vascular structures.
- ***Nerve tissue mobility.*** Use nerve mobilization maneuvers if neurodynamic tests are positive.[16,71,85] These are described earlier in this chapter.
- ***Joint, muscle, and connective tissue mobility.*** Use manual and self-stretching techniques to address any mobility impairments. Restricted joint mobility might be present in the upper thoracic, scapulothoracic, glenohumeral, sternoclavicular, or first costotransverse articulations. Common muscle restrictions with an impaired postural component include but are not limited to the scalene, levator scapulae, pectoralis minor, pectoralis major, anterior portion of the intercostals, and suboccipital muscles. Stretching exercises to increase mobility in these muscles are described in Chapter 14 (section on posture exercises) and Chapter 17.
- ***Muscle performance.*** Develop a program to improve control and endurance in the postural muscles. Common weaknesses include but are not limited to scapular adductors and upward rotators, shoulder lateral rotators, deep cervical flexor muscles, and thoracic extensors. Identification of postural exercises to improve muscle performance are listed in Chapter 14 (section on posture exercises).
- ***Respiratory patterns and elevated upper ribs.*** If the patient tends to use apical breathing patterns and has increased tension in the scalene muscles, teach abdominodiaphragmatic or bi-basilar breathing patterns and relaxation of the upper thorax.
- ***Functional independence.*** Increase patient awareness and ability to manage symptoms through education. Have patients actively involved in all aspects of their program and interventions.

Carpal Tunnel Syndrome

The carpal tunnel is a confined space between the carpal bones dorsally and the transverse carpal ligament (flexor retinaculum) volarly (Fig. 13.20). In this region, the median nerve is susceptible to pressure as it courses through the tunnel along with the extrinsic finger flexor tendons on their way into the hand. Carpal tunnel syndrome (CTS) is characterized by the sensory loss and motor weakness that occur when the median nerve is compromised in the carpal tunnel. Anything that decreases the space in the carpal tunnel or causes the contents of the tunnel to enlarge could compress or restrict the mobility of the median nerve, causing a compression or traction injury, ischemia, and neurological symptoms distal to the wrist.[2,7,53,54]

Etiology of Symptoms

Etiology is multifactorial, including both local and systematic factors.[54] Local factors include synovial thickness and scarring in the tendon sheaths (tendinosis) or irritation, inflammation,

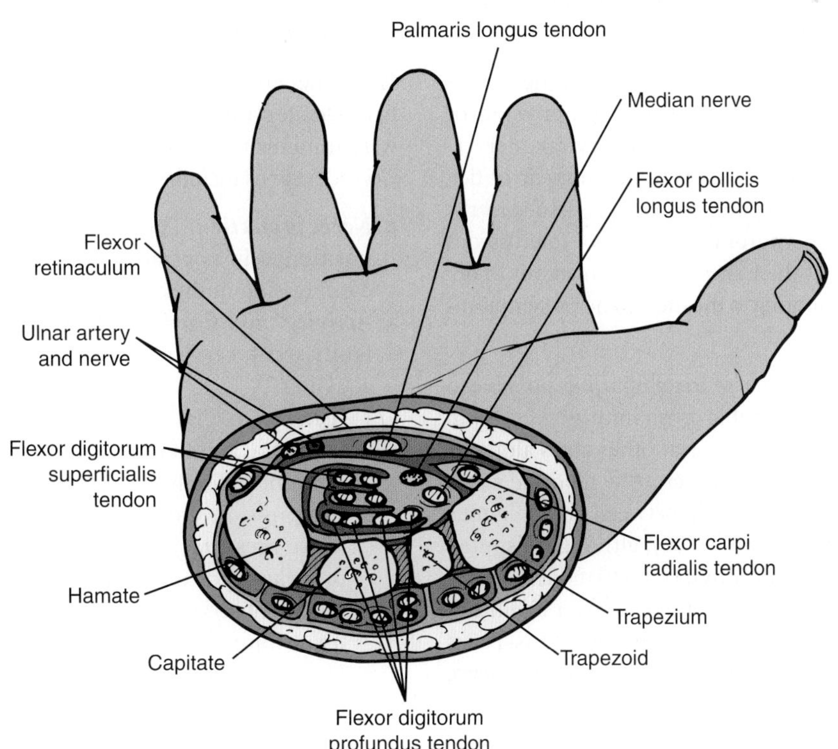

FIGURE 13.20 Boundaries of the carpal tunnel.

and swelling of the tendons (tendinitis) as a result of repetitive or sustained wrist flexion, extension, or gripping activities. Because of this, CTS is frequently classified as a cumulative trauma or overuse syndrome. Swelling in the wrist area due to local trauma (e.g., a fall or blow to the wrist, with or without a carpal or distal radius fracture), carpal dislocation, or osteoarthritis or systematic factors, such as pregnancy (hormonal changes and water retention), rheumatoid arthritis, or diabetes, could decrease the carpal tunnel space. Awkward wrist postures (flexion or extension), compressive forces from sustained equipment usage, and vibration against the carpal tunnel could also lead to median nerve compression and trauma.[2,7,54]

Examination

In a review on the sensitivity and specificity of the various tests used when screening for CTS, MacDermid and Doherty[50] summarized the key signs and symptoms that increase the probability of diagnosing CTS.

History. The patient describes sensory changes in the median nerve distribution of the hand (excluding the palm, which is innervated by the palmar cutaneous branch of the median nerve arising proximal to the carpal tunnel) and nocturnal numbness and pain that is relieved by flicking the wrists.

Positive clinical findings. Depending on severity, there may be atrophy of the thenar eminence. Results of tests include thenar muscle weakness, positive Phalen's test (sustained wrist flexion), loss of two-point discrimination, positive carpal compression test, and positive Tinel's sign (tapping the median nerve).[7,54] Electrophysiological studies (nerve conduction and electromyography) are used to assist with a differential diagnosis.[2,7,54]

Associated areas to clear. Because there can be other causes of median nerve symptoms, such as tension, compression, or restricted mobility of the nerve roots in the cervical intervertebral foramen, of the brachial plexus in the thoracic outlet, or of the median nerve as it courses through tissues in the forearm region (pronator syndrome and anterior interosseous nerve syndrome); each of these sites must be ruled out to determine if they are contributing to the median nerve symptoms (see Fig. 13.5).[39,46,54]

Double crush injury. With nerve irritability, it is possible to develop what is known as a double crush injury[16,40,51,55,61] in which the nerve develops symptoms at other areas along its course as well as at the primary site. Seror[69,70] reported a lack of evidence supporting a relationship between unambiguous CTS in true neurogenic TOS (< 1/100), although disputed neurogenic TOS was frequently found (mild to moderate clinical symptoms and signs) even when there were no significant findings on electrodiagnostic tests. Fernández-de-Las-Peñas and colleagues[31] demonstrated increased mechanical nerve pain sensitivity of the entire median nerve in subjects with CTS, as measured by pressure pain thresholds. They suggested that there is both central and peripheral sensitization of the entire nerve trunk in this condition.

Common Impairments of Structure in CTS

- Increasing pain and paresthesias in the hand with repetitive use
- Progressive weakness or atrophy in the thenar muscles and first two lumbricals
- Irritability or sensory loss in the median nerve distribution (see Fig. 13.5)
- Possible decreased joint mobility in the wrist and metacarpophalangeal joints of the thumb and digits 2 and 3
- Sympathetic nervous system changes may develop
- Faulty forward head posture and decreased cervical ROM[24]

Common Impairments of Function, Activity Limitations, and Participation Restrictions

- Decreased prehension in tip-to-tip, tip-to-pad, and pad-to-pad activities requiring fine neuromuscular control of thumb opposition, such as buttoning clothes and manipulating small objects
- Avoidance of using the area of the hand where there is decreased sensation
- Inability to perform provoking sustained or repetitive wrist or finger motion, such as cashier checkout scanning, assembly line work, fine tool manipulation, cutting/styling hair, or typing
- Sleep disturbances

Nonoperative Management of CTS

Guidelines are summarized in Box 13.9. In patients with mild to moderate symptoms, conservative intervention is directed toward minimizing or eliminating the causative factor.[4,7,50,53,54 64] Considerations include:

- ***Nerve protection.*** The use of a static wrist orthosis at night positioned in neutral is highly recommended to reduce compression in the carpel tunnel.[4,7,50,53,54,64]
- ***Activity modification and patient education.*** Identify faulty wrist, cervical, and upper extremity postures and activities.
  - *Activity modification.* Modify activities to keep the wrist in neutral and to reduce forceful prehension.
  - *Education.* Teach the patient about the mechanisms of compression and their effect on the circulation and nerve pressure, as well as how to modify or eliminate provoking postures and activities. Also, instruct the patient to observe areas with decreased sensitivity to avoid tissue injury (see Box 13.6).
  - *Home exercise program.* Teach the patient safe exercises for a home exercise program. Emphasize the importance of compliance to reduce stresses on the nerve and tendinous structures. Incorporate postural exercises for the spinal and shoulder girdle regions.

BOX 13.9 Summary of Guidelines for Nonoperative Management of Carpal Tunnel Syndrome

Protect the nerve
- Place in static wrist orthosis, in neutral position at night
- Protect areas that have decreased sensitivity

Modify activity and educate the patient
- Teach patient about provoking activities and how to modify them
- Teach safe exercises for home exercise program
- Teach patient how to protect areas of decreased sensitivity in the hand (see Box 13.5)

Mobilize restricted joints, connective tissue, and muscle/tendon
- Mobilize carpals if restricted
- Tendon gliding exercises
- Median nerve mobilization exercises

Improve muscle performance
- Gentle multi-angle muscle setting
- Progress to resistance and endurance
- Fine-finger dexterity

Progress functional independence
- Involve patient in all aspects of program
- Self-monitoring of symptoms

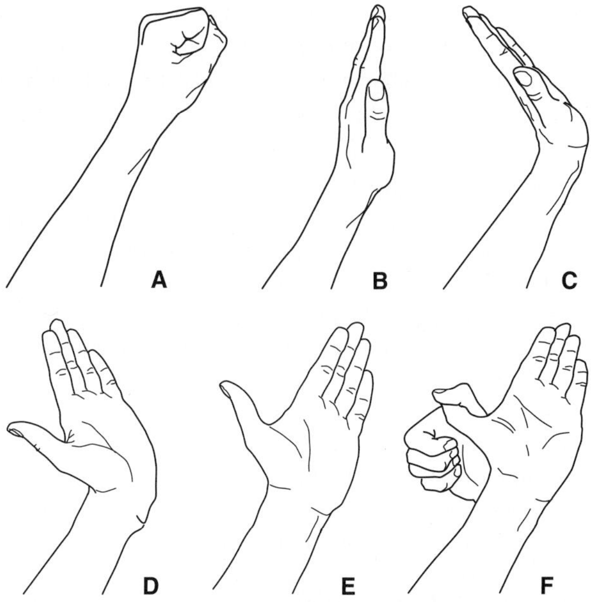

- ***Mobility techniques***
  - *Joint mobilization.* If there is restricted joint mobility, mobilize the carpals for increased carpal tunnel space (see Fig. 5.39 and its description in Chapter 5).
  - *Tendon-gliding exercises.* Teach the patient tendon-gliding exercises for mobility in the extrinsic tendons; they should be performed gently to prevent increased swelling (see Figure 19.17 and the description in the exercise section of Chapter 19[4]).
  - *Median nerve mobilization.*[4,16,30,54,64] The six positions for median nerve mobilization in the wrist and hand are illustrated in Figure 13.21. Begin with position A and slowly progress to each succeeding position until the median nerve symptoms just begin to be provoked (tingling). That is the maximum position to use. Alternate between that position and the preceding position. When the patient can be moved into that position without symptoms, progress to the next position and repeat the mobilizing routine. The mobilization exercise should be done three or four times per day unless symptoms are exacerbated then the intensity and frequency should be reduced but not eliminated.

Additional median nerve mobilization techniques, including the entire upper extremity and neck, is recommended and if symptoms warrant (see Fig. 13.14 and the description of principles earlier in this chapter under upper limb neurodynamics).

A B C D E F

FIGURE 13.21 Positions for median nerve glides and mobilization in the hand: **(A)** wrist neutral with fingers and thumb flexed; **(B)** wrist neutral with fingers and thumb extended; **(C)** wrist and fingers extended, thumb neutral; **(D)** wrist, fingers, and thumb extended; **(E)** wrist, fingers, and thumb extended and forearm supinated; **(F)** wrist, fingers, and thumb extended, forearm supinated, and thumb stretched into extension.

FOCUS ON EVIDENCE

Bialosky and associates[6] compared a group treated with median nerve mobilization techniques and a group with a sham technique that did not place the entire median nerve on a stretch; wrist and finger flexion/extension was consistent in both groups. A series of tests was conducted at the beginning and after 3 weeks of treatment (two times per week for up to six treatments); both groups received orthoses to wear at night. There was no control group. The only significant difference between groups was a reduction of temporal summation of symptoms in the group receiving the mobilization to the median nerve. The authors speculated that improved outcomes in most of the measures seen in both groups were related to receiving manual therapy and were independent of the specific mechanical force on the median nerve. Oskouei and associates[64] compared two groups of patients with CTS. Twenty patients and a total of 32 hands were assigned to either routine physical therapy (control group) or routine physical therapy plus neuromobilization (treatment group). Symptom severity scale, VAS, functional status scale, Phalen's test, median nerve neurodynamic test, and EMG (distal sensory and motor latency) were assessed. Routine physical therapy included the use of an orthosis positioned in neutral, TENs, and ultrasound. Improvements in both groups were noted with the symptom severity scale, VAS, median nervy neurodynamic test, and Phalen's test; however, the functional status scale and EMG studies were significantly improved in only the treatment group. The authors concluded that the combination of routine physical therapy and neuromobilization is an effective noninvasive treatment for patients with CTS.

- ***Muscle performance***
  - *Gentle multiple-angle muscle-setting exercises.* Initially, gentle muscle-setting exercises are the only resistance exercises done. It is important that they do not provoke symptoms.
  - *Strengthening and endurance exercises.* Add proximal stabilization, postural strengthening, and endurance exercises.[53] Utilize exercises that prepare the patient for a return to functional activities.
  - *Speed, coordination, endurance, and fine finger dexterity.* Emphasize these activities when the symptoms are no longer provoked. Utilize activities that develop tip-to-tip and tip-to-pad prehension in order to improve use of the thenar muscles.
- ***Functional independence.*** Teach the patient how to monitor his or her hand for recurrence of symptoms and the provoking factors and how to modify activities to decrease nerve injury. Usually, sustained wrist flexion, ulnar deviation, and repetitive wrist flexion and extension combined with gripping and pinching are the most aggravating motions.

FOCUS ON EVIDENCE

In a Cochrane review of 21 trials involving 884 people, a hand brace significantly alleviated symptoms of CTS after 4 weeks; in one trial involving 21 people, symptoms were significantly diminished after 3 weeks with carpal bone mobilization (compared to no intervention). Other evidence supported the use of oral steroids, ultrasound, and yoga.[63]

Surgical and Postoperative Management for CTS

If conservative measures do not relieve the nerve symptoms or the neurological symptoms are severe (persistent numbness, weakness, pain, and decreased functional use of the hand),[2,7,50,54] surgical decompression involving transection of the transverse carpal ligament and excision of scar tissue is performed to increase the volume of the carpal tunnel and relieve the compressive forces on the median nerve. Surgery may be an open carpal tunnel release or endoscopically assisted carpal tunnel release.[2,7,54] Postoperative therapy is open to debate, especially following an uncomplicated carpal tunnel release; however, it may be initiated after surgery if there are postoperative complications. The most important contribution following surgery is wound management and patient education regarding proper exercises, activity restrictions, and return to activity.[30]

Pillar pain is a relatively uncommon complication of unknown etiology following carpal tunnel surgery. The pain is localized in the thenar and hypothenar eminences and should be distinguished from incisional pain or scar tenderness. Usually the pain decreases over time and may be treated with neuromodulation using a local anesthetic.[30,56]

Maximum Protection Phase

Usually a bulky dressing or orthosis is used following surgery. The protective orthosis is removed during therapy.

PRECAUTION: Avoid active wrist flexion and extension for the first 2 weeks after surgery.

- ***Patient education.*** Educate the patient on expectations for recovery. Initial decreases in grip and pinch strength should gradually resolve with normal use of the hand.[53] Neurological symptoms should resolve with time, with light touch returning first.
- ***Wound management, control of edema and pain.***
- ***Active tendon-gliding.*** Tendon-gliding (see Fig. 19.17 in Chapter 19) exercises are important to prevent adhesion formation from restricting motion in the carpal tunnel.[4]
- ***Exercises for related areas.*** Active forearm, elbow, and shoulder exercises are important to initiate in the initial phase following surgery.

Moderate and Minimum Protection Phases

Sutures are removed between the 10th to 12th postoperative day, and more active treatment is allowed.[30] The patient should be able to return to full activity by 6 to 12 weeks. Residual impairments may include weakness, and sensory deficits, persistent edema, limited motion, hypersensitivity, and pain.

Suggested interventions include:

- ***Scar tissue mobilization.*** Use soft tissue mobilization techniques to the palmar fascia and scar.
- ***Progressive neuromobilization.*** Begin gentle neuromobilization techniques for the median nerve once symptoms have resolved and the scar is completely healed. (2-3 weeks post operatively)
- ***Muscle performance.*** Begin isometric strengthening exercises approximately 4 weeks after surgery. Progress to grip and pinch exercises by 6 weeks. Emphasize strength, coordination, and endurance toward functional goals. Wrist and hand exercises are described and illustrated in detail in Chapter 19.
- ***Dexterity exercises.*** Begin as soon as signs of motor recovery occur. Suggestions include picking up small objects using pad-to-pad, tip-to-tip, and tip-to pad prehension patterns; turning over cards; stacking checkers; writing; and holding the perimeter of a jar lid and having the thumb move around the edge in a circumduction motion.
- ***Desensitization and discriminative sensory reeducation.*** Desensitization of hypersensitive scar tissue and skin is a priority. As the nerve recovers, help desensitize and reprogram awareness.[30] These techniques were described earlier in this chapter. Educate the patient about the progression of nerve recovery such that an area that had absence of

sensation may have increased sensitivity and pain as it recovers. Symptoms typically subside within 1 to 6 months.

Ulnar Nerve Compression in the Tunnel of Guyon

Entrapment of the ulnar nerve in the Tunnel of Guyon, also referred to as Guyon's canal or ulnar tunnel, is second only to entrapment at the elbow. There are three sites (zones) where entrapment can occur.[27,28]

- Zone 1 is proximal to the bifurcation of the nerve; compression causes combined motor and sensory loss.
- Zone 2 is just distal to the bifurcation of the nerve; compression causes loss of motor function in ulnar-innervated muscles in the hand.
- Zone 3 encompasses the sensory branch; compression causes sensory loss to the hypothenar eminence, small finger, and part of the ring finger.

Etiology of Symptoms

Injury or irritation of the ulnar nerve in the tunnel between the hook of the hamate and pisiform is the result of sustained pressure, such as prolonged handwriting or leaning forward onto extended wrists while biking; from repetitive gripping with the fourth and fifth fingers, as with knitting, tying knots, or using pliers and staplers; from trauma, such as falling on the ulnar border of the wrist (with or without a fracture to the hook of the hamate); or from a space-occupying lesion, such as a ganglion or aneurysm of the ulnar artery.[27]

Examination

History. The patient describes sensory symptoms in the little finger and ulnar side of the ring finger and may complain of fatigue or weakness in the hand with repetitive motions and difficulty with activities, such as opening jars or turning doorknobs.

Positive clinical findings. Depending on severity, there may be atrophy of the hypothenar eminence and intrinsic muscles and a partial claw hand posture. Results of tests include intrinsic muscle weakness and positive Tinel's sign over the tunnel of Guyon (tapping the ulnar nerve).[27,28]

Associated areas to clear. There can be other causes of ulnar nerve symptoms, such as tension, compression, or restricted mobility of the nerve roots in the cervical intervertebral foramen, the brachial plexus in the thoracic outlet, or the ulnar nerve as it courses through the bicipital groove, or there could be impingement between the heads of the flexor carpi ulnaris muscle. Each of these sites must be examined and ruled out as the cause of the symptoms[28,61] (see Fig. 13.6). In addition, with nerve irritability it is possible to develop what is known as a double crush injury,[40] where the nerve develops symptoms at other areas along its course as well as at the primary site.

Common Impairments of Structure

- Pain and paresthesia along the ulnar side of the palm and in the 4th and 5th digits in the distribution of the ulnar nerve (see Fig. 13.6)
- Progressive weakness or atrophy in the intrinsic muscles innervated by the ulnar nerve
- Restricted mobility in the flexor carpi ulnaris and extensor carpi ulnaris
- Possible adhesions and restricted mobility of the pisiform

Common Impairments of Function, Activity Limitations, and Participation Restrictions

- Decreased grip strength
- Fatigue in the hand with repetitive or sustained activities
- Inability to use fourth and fifth digits for spherical or cylindrical power grips
- Decreased ability to perform provoking activity

Nonoperative Management

- Follow the same guidelines as for CTS. Modify the provoking activity, avoid pressure to the base of the palm of the hand, and provide rest with a hand-based ulnar gutter orthosis.
- Ulnar nerve mobilization: Move the wrist into extension and radial deviation, then apply overpressure stretch into extension against the ring and little finger. Include forearm pronation and elbow flexion to move the nerve in a proximal direction. To test and mobilize the entire ulnar nerve, see Figure 13.15.

Surgical Release and Postoperative Management

If the patient's symptoms do not improve with 6 to 12 weeks of conservative treatment, or if there is progressive paralysis, long-standing muscle wasting, and clawing of the digits, surgical release of the ulnar tunnel is performed.[27] After release, the wrist is immobilized 3 to 5 days; then treatment begins with gentle ROM. Follow the same guidelines as with carpal tunnel surgery but with ulnar nerve mobilization techniques.

Complex Regional Pain Syndrome

Complex regional pain syndrome (CRPS) is a painful, disabling, and often chronic condition with a prevalence of an estimated 50,000 new cases diagnosed in the United States every year.[77] The most frequent causes of CRPS involve surgery and trauma, and it occurs acutely in about 7% of patients who have limb fractures, limb surgery, or other injuries, with hand surgery being a particularly relevant factor.[12,77] CRPS is diagnosed purely on the basis of clinical signs and symptoms. There are two key elements in the diagnosis of CRPS, the first being that there is continuing pain disproportionate to the inciting event and the second being that there is no other diagnosis that explains the signs and symptoms.[8] It is widely accepted that there are three forms of CRPS as summarized in Box 13.10. CRPS Type I is caused by an initiating noxious event, such as a crush or soft tissue injury, immobilization, a tight cast or surgery, and involves the absence of an identified nerve lesion. CRPS Type II involves the presence of an identifiable nerve lesion, and CRPS-NOS (not otherwise specified) is where symptoms are consistent with CRPS but a specific injury or lesion has not been determined as the cause. Regardless, multidisciplinary clinical care, which centers on a functionally based approach, is recommended.[9,12,14,32,36,44,59]

Signs and Symptoms of CRPS

CRPS is distinguished from other chronic pain conditions by the presence of signs indicating prominent autonomic and inflammatory changes in the region of pain. Pain is a key feature; however, other signs and symptoms may include sensory abnormalities (burning pain and allodynia), trophic changes, impairment of motor function, and emotional/psychological responses[12,36,49,77] (see Box 13.10).

BOX 13.10 Classification and Clinical Features of Complex Regional Pain Syndromes

CRPS type I
- Develops after an initiating noxious event
- Spontaneous pain or allodynia/hyperalgesia
- Edema, vascular abnormalities
- Abnormal sudomotor activity
- Non-nerve origin

CRPS type II
- Develops after nerve injury
- Not limited to territory of injured nerve
- Edema; skin blood flow abnormality
- Abnormal sudomotor activity

CRPS-NOS (not otherwise specified)
- Specific injury or lesion has not been determined as the cause of symptoms

Clinical features of CRPS (in addition to the differences listed above)
- Symptoms more marked distally in an extremity
- Symptoms progress in intensity and spread proximally
- Symptoms vary with time
- Disproportion of symptoms in relation to the causing event
- A specific diagnosis, such as diabetes or fibromyalgia, has been excluded

Etiology of Symptoms

The underlying mechanism that stimulates the onset of these syndromes is unclear; however, there has been significant progress over the past few years in understanding the various pathophysiological aspects of CRPS.[8] After trauma or surgery, the presence of inflammation is physiological; however, in CRPS the inflammation lasts indefinitely. There is an abundance of inflammatory mediators with a lack of anti-inflammatory mediators. This proinflammatory response sensitizes the peripheral and spinal nociceptive systems facilitating the release of neuropeptides inducing the signs of inflammation and stimulates bone cell and fibroblast proliferation and endothelial dysfunction leading to vascular changes. During this inflammatory stage, sensory-motor integration becomes disturbed, leading to loss of motor function and distortion of body representation, leading to autonomic disturbances.[8,77]

Clinical Course

Clinical signs and symptoms seem to be dynamic in nature, where the impacted limb evolves from an acute warm phase (limb is sensitive, swollen, and displays an elevated temperature) to a chronic cold phase (resolution of inflammatory appearance, decreased temperature, pain and disability persist). In general, the evolution of CRPS is characterized by the transition from an acute state with prominent peripheral characteristics (Fig. 13.22) to a chronic state characterized by central changes (such as central sensitization), including persistent pain along with significant cognitive and mood alterations.[12,49,77]

CLINICAL TIP

It is important to recognize the early symptoms of CRPS when the limb is in the acute warm stage because early intervention may prevent progression to the cold chronic stage.[12]

Common Impairments of Structure in CRPS

- Pain or hyperesthesia in the extremity disproportionate to any inciting event
- Limitation of motion and/or motor dysfunction (weakness tremor, dystonia)
- Sudomotor/edema: Edema and/or sweating changes and/or sweating asymmetry (hyper or hypohydrosis)
- Vasomotor instability: temperature asymmetry and/or skin color changes and/or asymmetry
- Trophic changes: increased or decreased hair and nail growth and/or skin changes (thin or shiny)

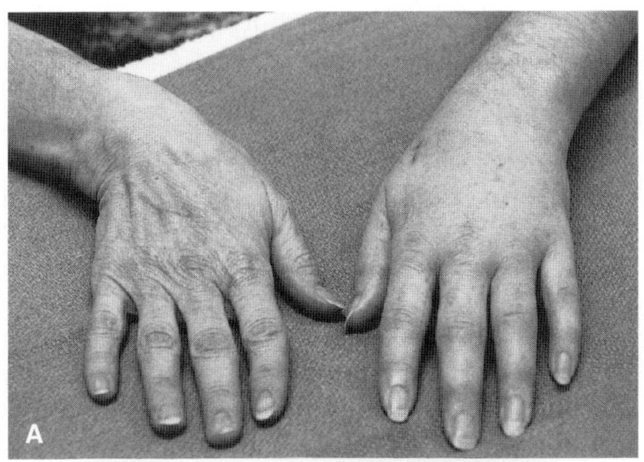

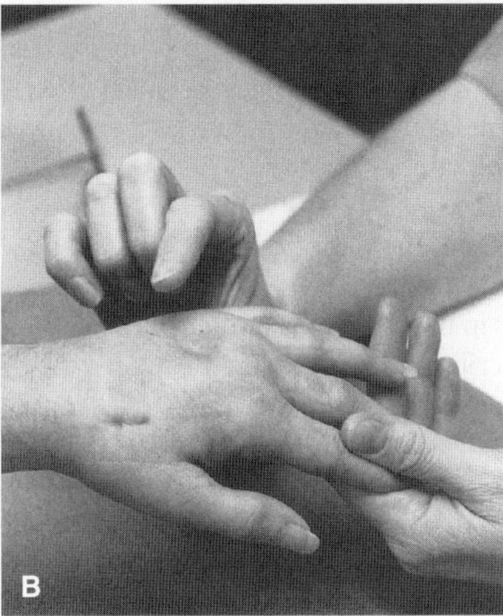

FIGURE 13.22 (A) In the early stages of complex regional pain syndrome, generalized edema is present. This edema is often localized over the dorsum of the hand in the metacarpal and proximal interphalangeal joint areas. **(B)** The edema is usually of a pitting nature, as indicated by the indentation that remains once the pressure is removed.

Common Impairments of Function, Activity Limitations, and Participation Restrictions

- Pain avoidance behaviors, resulting in decreased use of the involved limb in ADLs, which may cause muscle atrophy or osteoporosis/ osteopenia in chronic stages
- Slower at initiating movement and/or slower and more inaccurate in executing targeted movement with the involved limb
- Gait abnormalities (when the lower extremity is involved)
- Limitations in ability to participate in gainful employment and/or housework
- Limitations in ability to participate in leisure activities

Management

Effective treatment for CRPS requires recognition and prompt intervention. Of patients with CRPS treated within the first year of injury, 80% will show significant improvement and only 50% of those treated after 1 year will show signs of improvement.[44] It requires that the therapist is aware of pain responses that exceed the normally expected reaction following seemingly minor injuries as well as to be in tune with common diagnoses that have a higher incidence for the development of CRPS. It also requires the therapist to be alert to the development of adverse symptomatology, which can be addressed early despite the possibility of an incorrect or incomplete diagnosis.[44,82]

There is no gold standard for the treatment of CRPS, although there is significant evidence to support the integration of physical therapy focusing on functional restoration in combination with pharmacotherapy and psychotherapy.[10,32,36,59] Functional restoration is based on a gradual and steady progression from activation of presensorimotor cortices (motor imagery) to very gentle active movements such as progressing from active ROM to weight-bearing activities as described below.[36] The emphasis is on early diagnosis, early treatment, and avoidance of implementing drug therapy independently in order to prevent disuse of the affected limb and the psychological consequences of living in pain.[59]

Medical management. Medical management and pharmacology are most effective in combination with functional restoration. If a patient is unable to participate in therapy due to pain or other associated symptoms, medication can help facilitate their progress. In the acute inflammatory phase, oral corticosteroids are often beneficial. To address mild to moderate pain a simple analgesic or opioids may be used to provide relief while interventional blocks may be necessary to manage excruciating or intractable pain. For neuropathic pain, anticonvulsants or tricyclic antidepressants may be prescribed. Because there is often an emotional or psychological component, medical intervention may include medications to manage this area (sedatives, antidepressants, antianxiety) in addition to psychotherapy.[12,32,59] As with all medical interventions, but especially with CRPS, it is critical for the physical therapist to have a thorough understanding of medication in order anticipate their impact on their patient's plan of care.

Physical therapy management. The goals for treating patients with CRPS include minimizing edema, desensitizing the painful limb, normalizing sensation, promoting normal positioning, decreasing muscle guarding, and increasing functional use of the extremity.[33,66] There is very little evidence to support the effectiveness of physical therapy despite the fact that most literature on CRPS cites the use and critical importance for therapy intervention.[9,12,66,73,82] Therefore, a practical, common sense approach can be taken based on the patient's presenting signs and symptoms including tissue irritability, vasomotor status, and identified impairments. The guidelines for management of CPRS are summarized in Box 13.11.

- ***Pain and edema control.*** Use modalities such as HVGS, TENS, or heat or ice (depending on vasomotor status). Fluidotherapy is particularly beneficial (despite the lack of

BOX 13.11 Summary of Guidelines for Management of Complex Regional Pain Syndrome Type I

Early intervention

Relieve pain and control edema
- Modalities
- Retrograde massage
- Elevate, compression sleeve or glove

Correct sensorimotor incongruence
- Mirror therapy
- Graded motor imagery

Increase mobility (specific to involved tissues)
- Gentle active motion specific to involved extremity

Improve muscle performance
- Active loading (closed chain activities)
- Distraction

Improve total body circulation
- Low impact aerobic exercise
- Aquatic exercise

Desensitize the area
- Desensitization techniques for brief periods 5×/day

Educate the patient
- Teach interventions that deal with variable vasomotor responses; when to use heat, cold, gentle exercises

Chronic stage

Manage pain
- Modalities prior to or in conjunction with exercise as needed
- Desensitize the area
- Progress desensitization techniques to increase tolerance of various textures
- Progress mirror therapy

Increase mobility (specific to involved tissues)
- Joint mobilization/ manipulation of the upper thoracic or lumbar spine (location of sympathetic ganglia) and soft tissue mobilization/ manipulation as indicated
- Neuromobilization
- Passive and self-stretching techniques

Improve functional performance
- Carefully monitor and progress strength, endurance, and functional exercises

empirical evidence) as active exercise may be combined with this modality and has been shown to decrease pain.[82] Utilize retrograde massage (as tolerated), elevation, compression sleeves or gloves, and pneumatic compression treatment for edema management.[82]

- ***Mobility.*** In the early stages, use gentle, active exercises to manage stiffness.[82] It is important to avoid increasing painful reactions that would decrease mobility. Have the patient actively move each joint for a short period of time. They should follow this program of brief motion frequently throughout the day.
  - In the hand, include tendon glide exercises (see Chapter 19, Fig. 19.17)
  - In the feet, include towel curls, sitting balance board progressing to gradual weight bearing, weight shifting, and balancing on the involved limb during gait training.[32,36]
  - Aquatic therapy has also been shown to facilitate early weight bearing.[32]
- ***Muscle performance.*** Facilitate active muscle contractions. Include joints proximal to the symptoms (shoulder/hip); they often develop restrictions due to pain or lack of use. Use active load bearing, utilizing closed chain techniques for the upper and lower extremity. Distraction activities such as carrying a light bag for the upper extremity should be included for neuromuscular control as well as afferent fiber stimulation. The objective is to provide tissue stress with minimal joint motion.
- ***Mirror therapy.*** Patients with CRPS have an altered body perception of their affected limb. They are slower to "connect" with their affected limb before movement, and disruptions in their motor planning and processing have been well described in the literature. Patient's with CRPS often closely guard their affected limb and disengage from normal activities due to pain. The purpose of mirror therapy is to correct the sensorimotor incongruence by visualizing the unaffected limb in the felt position of the affected limb. Mirror therapy is an inexpensive and easily accessible tool that brings significant pain relief to some patient's with CRPS, especially in the early stages.[57,58]
  - Position the involved limb inside the box with the uninvolved limb parallel to mirror. Be sure and remove all jewelry, watches, or other objects that might confuse the brain.
  - Have the patient look into the mirror to see the reflection of the limb, which will give the illusion that they are looking at the limb that is hidden.
  - Begin by keeping both limbs still, progress to moving the limb outside the box while keeping the hidden one still. To progress further, move the hidden limb within its limit while taking the uninvolved limb through large movements. The final progression would be to move the limbs equally.
- ***Graded motor imagery.*** This approach targets the activation of different brain regions in a graded manner. Treatment consists of three components that include left/right discrimination of the affected area, motor imagery rehearsal, and mirror therapy. (Refer to the work by Moseley for detailed instruction.[57,58])
  - Left/right discrimination links the unconscious brain representation of a person's body part and/or movement of it. It is to be done as quickly as possible in order to access deep movement planning areas in the brain.
  - Explicit motor imagery is an imagined movement. Start by having the patient imagine a movement away from the affected area so that they can experience the task and

obtain feedback on how it should feel. Progress by working toward the affected area.
- Mirror therapy is as described on page 412.

- ***Total body circulation and cardiac output.*** Initiate a program of low-impact aerobic exercises. Consider aquatic exercises to facilitate activity while minimizing the load in early stages.
- ***Desensitization.*** Utilize desensitization techniques (as described earlier in this chapter) for brief periods five times per day, such as having the patient work with various textures, percussion, pressure, and vibration. The therapist should initiate desensitization techniques outside of the area of hypersensitivity gradually narrowing the area toward the area of greatest sensitivity.[36,82]
- ***Patient education.*** Emphasize the importance of using the affected limb in daily activity, even if it involves mild increases in pain or associated symptoms. Care must be taken, and working within the patient's tolerance is essential so as not to reinforce anxiety and passive coping, which can lead to further functional impairment.[9]
  - Teach the patient interventions that deal with the variable vasomotor responses with the use of gentle heat, gentle exercises for short periods throughout the day, and use of associated parts of the extremity.
  - Patient education involves explaining fear avoidance using the patient's individual symptoms, beliefs, and behaviors. Patients are taught to view their various autonomic and vasomotor disturbances as a condition that can be self-managed, rather than a disease where the affected limb needs to be protected. During therapy, the patient identifies painful or threatening situations and the therapist gradually increases their exposure to these activities until anxiety levels have decreased.[32]

CLINICAL TIP

Pain continues to be a variable throughout a patient's recovery, and therefore the initiation of any therapeutic exercise or manual therapy technique should be carefully monitored and adapted to the patient at each visit to minimize exacerbation of symptoms.[82]

FOCUS ON EVIDENCE

Evidence supports effective use of physical therapy for CRPS with early intervention (acute stage), but there is contradictory evidence for its effectiveness during the later stages.[35,41] In one study, the primary predictors for success and satisfaction with patients during the chronic phase after 6 months of therapy (evaluated at 12 months) was with the patient group that began therapy at a higher baseline of function, higher baseline ROM and strength, and less baseline pain.[41]

Independent Learning Activities

Critical Thinking and Discussion

1. Your patient describes intermittent sensory changes in the index and middle finger. What are the possible causes? What tests would you use to examine this patient? What results would lead you to determine nerve mobility restrictions?
2. You have a new client who describes intermittent tingling and sensations of heaviness in his hands whenever working with his hands in an overhead position. He is an auto mechanic and frequently has to work this way. Identify possible causes of these symptoms. What is usually the source of "tingling" sensations? What may be the source of the "heaviness" feelings? Why would the overhead position cause both vascular and neurological symptoms? Identify possible sites that could cause these symptoms. What tests would you use to confirm or rule out your hypotheses?
3. A 19-year-old patient presents with the medical diagnosis of complex regional pain syndrome type I and the following history.
   - Three-month history of midfoot pain that increases with standing more than 5 minutes or running. Symptoms have increased over the past 3 weeks.
   - Stress fracture to the navicular was detected on radiography, so patient was placed in a BK nonweight-bearing cast.
   - Foot discomfort increased and became more diffuse, radiating into the lateral forefoot and digits even after pain medications were prescribed.
   - Symptoms increased with burning or stinging pain, edema, and discoloration of the digits.
   - Examination 3 weeks after cast applied: digits cool, edematous, hyperesthetic, and hyperhidrotic. Passive and active motions of ankle and toes were moderately painful. Radiographs showed diffuse osteoporosis.

   What would be your goals for this patient? Develop a program of interventions.
4. Identify and describe everyday activities and/or positions that mimic the neurodynamic test positions. These activities/positions may be patient complaints that indicate further neurodynamic testing. For example, getting into a car by straightening the leg and ducking the head mimics the "slump" position.

Laboratory Practice

1. With your laboratory partner, practice each of the neurodynamic positions. Demonstrate how you would mobilize restrictions for each of the nerves.
2. Practice each of the thoracic outlet tests and describe the mechanics of each test. Identify and practice techniques you could use to increase mobility or reduce compression on the brachial plexus at each of the sites where compression or tension might occur. Design an exercise program and progression for managing impairments that could cause TOS symptoms.
3. Practice desensitization and sensory reeducation techniques by doing each of the following.
   - Gather 10 pieces of material of various textures. Place them in order of least irritating to most irritating. Practice sensory stimulation techniques by gently rubbing each material across your fingers.
   - Use five plastic tubs or buckets. Place each of the following in a container: dry peas or beans, spiral macaroni, sand, fine gravel, and seeds. Practice sensory stimulation by moving your hand (or foot) through each of the textures.
   - Have your laboratory partner place several familiar household items in a bag (e.g., key, dime, penny, can opener). Without looking, attempt to identify each one.

REFERENCES

1. Alshami, AM, et al: Strain in the tibial and plantar nerves with foot and ankle movements and the influence of adjacent joint positions. *J Applied Biomech* 24:368–376, 2008.
2. Amadio, PC: Carpal tunnel syndrome: surgeon's management. In Skirven, TM, Osterman, AL, Fedorczyk, JM, and Amadio, PC (eds): *Rehabilitation of the Hand and Upper Extremity, Vol I,* ed. 6. Philadelphia, PA: Elsevier Mosby, 2011, pp 657–665.
3. Bathen, M, and Gupta, R: Basic science of peripheral nerve injury and repair. In Skirven, TM, Osterman, AL, Fedorczyk, JM, and Amadio, PC (eds): *Rehabilitation of the Hand and Upper Extremity, Vol I,* ed. 6. Philadelphia, PA: Elsevier Mosby, 2011, pp 591–600.
4. Baysal, O, et al: Comparison of three conservative treatment protocols in carpal tunnel syndrome. *J Clin Pract* 60:820–828, 2006.
5. Benjamin, K: Injuries to the brachial plexus: mechanisms of injury and identification of risk factors. *Adv Neonatal Care* 5(4):181–189, 2005.
6. Bialosky, JE, et al: A randomized sham-controlled trial of a neurodynamic technique in the treatment of carpal tunnel syndrome. *J Orthop Sports Phys Ther* 39(10):709–723, 2009.
7. Bickel, KD: Carpal tunnel syndrome. *J Hand Surg* 35A:147–152, 2010.
8. Birklein, F, and Schlereth, T: Complex regional pain syndrome—significant progress in understanding. *Pain* 156:S94–S103, 2015.
9. Birklein, F, O'Neill D, and Schlereth, T: Complex regional pain syndrome: An optimistic perspective. *Neurology* 84:89–96, 2015.
10. Borchers, AT, and Gershwin, ME: Complex regional pain syndrome: A comprehensive and critical review. *Autoimmun Rev* 13:241–265, 2014.
11. Boyd, BS, et al: Mechanosensitivity of the lower extremity nervous system during straight-leg raise neurodynamic testing in healthy individuals. *J Orthop Sports Phys Ther* 39(11):780–790, 2009.
12. Bruehl, S: Complex regional pain syndrome. *BMJ* 350:1–13, 2015.
13. Burnett, MG, and Zager, EL: Pathophysiology of peripheral nerve injury: a brief review. *Neurosurg Focus* 16(5):1–7, 2004.
14. Bussa, M, et al: Complex regional pain syndrome type I: a comprehensive review. *Acta Anaesthesiologica Scandinavica* 59:685–697, 2015.
15. Butler, DS: *Mobilization of the Nervous System.* New York: Churchill Livingstone, 1991.
16. Butler, DS: *The Sensitive Nervous System.* Adelaide, Australia: Noigroup Publications, 2000.
17. Coppieters, MW, Alshami, AM, and Babri, AS: Strain and excursion of the sciatic, tibial, and plantar nerves during a modified straight leg raising test. *J Orthop Res* 24:1883–1889, 2006.
18. Coppieters, MW, et al: Excursion of the sciatic nerve during nerve mobilization exercises: an in vivo cross-sectional study using dynamic ultrasound imaging. *J Orthop Sports Phys Ther* 45(10):731–737, 2015.
19. Coppieters, MW, and Butler, DS: Do "sliders" slide and "tensioners" tension? An analysis of neurodynamic techniques and considerations regarding their application. *Man Ther* 13:213–221, 2008.
20. Coppieters, MW, Hough, AD, and Dilley, A: Different nerve-gliding exercises induce different magnitudes of median nerve longitudinal excursion: an in vivo study using dynamic ultrasound imaging. *J Orthop Sports Phys Ther* 39(3):164–171, 2009.
21. Coppieters, MW, et al: Addition of test components during neurodynamic testing: effect on range of motion and sensory responses. *J Orthop Sports Phys Ther* 31(5):226–237, 2001.
22. Crotti, FM, et al: TOS pathophysiology and clinical features. *Acta Neurochir Suppl* 92:7–12, 2005.
23. Crotti, FM, et al: Post-traumatic thoracic outlet syndrome (TOS). *Acta Neurochir Suppl* 92:13–15, 2005.
24. De-La-Llave-Rincán, A, et al: Increased forward head posture and restricted cervical range of motion in patients with carpal tunnel syndrome. *J Orthop Sports Phys Ther* 39(9):658–664, 2009.
25. Dilley, A, et al: Quantitative in vivo studies of median nerve sliding in response to wrist, elbow, shoulder, and neck movements. *Clin Biomech* 18:899–907, 2003.
26. Duff, SV, and Estilow, T: Therapist's management of peripheral nerve injury. In Skirven, TM, Osterman, AL, Fedorczyk, JM, and Amadio, PC (eds): *Rehabilitation of the Hand and Upper Extremity, Vol I,* ed. 6. Philadelphia, PA: Elsevier Mosby, 2011, pp 619–633.
27. Earp, BE, Floyd, WE, Louie, D, Koris, M, and Protomastro, P: Ulnar nerve entrapment at the wrist. *J Am Acad Orthop Surg* 22:699–706, 2014.
28. Elhassan, B, and Steinmann, SP: Entrapment Neuropathy of the Ulnar Nerve. *J Am Acad Orthop Surg* 15:672–681, 2007.
29. Ellis, RF, and Hing, WA: Neural mobilization: a systematic review of randomized controlled trials with an analysis of therapeutic efficacy. *J Man Manip Ther* 16(1):8–22, 2008.
30. Evans, RB: Therapist's management of carpal tunnel syndrome: a practical approach. In Skirven, TM, Osterman, AL, Fedorczyk, JM, and Amadio, PC (eds): *Rehabilitation of the Hand and Upper Extremity, Vol I,* ed. 6. Philadelphia, PA: Elsevier Mosby, 2011, pp 666–677.
31. Fernández-de-Las-Peñas, C, et al: Specific mechanical pain hypersensitivity over peripheral nerve trunks in women with either unilateral epicondylalgia or carpal tunnel syndrome. *J Orthop Sports Phys Ther* 40(11):751–760, 2010.

32. Freedman, M, Greis, AC, Marino, L, Sinha, AN, and Henstenburg, J: Complex regional pain syndrome: diagnosis and treatment. *Phys Med Rehabil Clin N Am* 25:291–303, 2014.
33. Freedman, M, et al: Electrodiagnostic evaluation of compressive nerve injuries of the upper extremities. *Orthop Clin N Am* 43:409–416, 2012.
34. George, SZ: Differential diagnosis and treatment for a patient with lower extremity symptoms. *J Orthop Sports Phys Ther* 30(8):468–472, 2000.
35. Guisel, A, Gill, JM, and Witherell, P: Complex regional pain syndrome: which treatments show promise? *J Fam Pract* 54(7):599–603, 2005.
36. Harden, RN, et al: Complex regional pain syndrome: practical diagnostic and treatment guidelines, ed. 4. *Pain Med* 14:180–229, 2013.
37. Hooper, TL, Denton, J, McGalliard, MK, Brismee, JM, and Sizer, PS: Thoracic outlet syndrome: a controversial clinical condition. Part 1: anatomy, and clinical examination/ diagnosis. *J Man Manip Ther* 18: 74–83, 2010.
38. Jacoby, SM, Eichenbaum, MD, and Osterman, AL: Basic science of nerve compressions. In Skirven, TM, Osterman, AL, Fedorczyk, JM, Amadio, PC (eds): *Rehabilitation of the Hand and Upper Extremity, Vol I*, ed. 6. Philadelphia, PA: Elsevier Mosby, 2011, pp 649–656.
39. Julius, A, et al: Shoulder posture and median nerve sliding. *BMC Musculoskel Disord* 5:23, 2004.
40. Kane, PM, Daniels, AH, and Akelman, E: Double crush syndrome. *J Am Acad Orthop Surg* 23:558–562, 2015.
41. Kemler, MA, Rijks, CP, and de Vet, HC: Which patients with chronic reflex sympathetic dystrophy are most likely to benefit from physical therapy? *J Manipulatiave Phys Ther* 24(4):272–278, 2001.
42. Kietrys, DM: Neural mobilization: an appraisal of the evidence regarding validity and efficacy. *Orthop Pract* 15(4):18–20, 2003.
43. Klaassen, Z, et al: Thoracic outlet syndrome: a neurological and vascular disorder. *Clin Anat* 27:724–732, 2014.
44. Koman, LA, Li, Z, Smith BP, and Smith, TL: Complex regional pain syndrome: types I and II. In Skirven, TM, Osterman, AL, Fedorczyk, JM, and Amadio, PC (eds): *Rehabilitation of the Hand and Upper Extremity, Vol I*, ed. 6. Philadelphia, PA: Elsevier Mosby, 2011, pp 1470–1478.
45. Kuhn, JE, Lebus, GF, and Bible, JE: Thoracic outlet syndrome. *J Am Acad Orthop Surg* 23:222–232, 2015.
46. Lee, MJ, and LaStayo, PC: Pronator syndrome and other nerve compressions that mimic carpal tunnel syndrome. *J Orthop Sprots Phys Ther* 34(10):601–609, 2004.
47. Ljungquist, KL, Martineau, P, and Allan, C: Radial nerve injuries. *J Hand Surg Am* 40:166–172, 2015.
48. Lohman, CM, et al: 2015 Young Investigator Award winner: cervical nerve root displacement and strain during upper limb neural tension testing. *Spine* 40(11):793–800, 2015.
49. Lohnberg, JA, and Altmaier, EM: A review of psychosocial factors in complex regional pain syndrome. *J Clin Psychol Med Settings* 20: 247–254, 2013.
50. MacDermid, JC, and Doherty, T: Clinical and electrodiagnostic testing of carpal tunnel syndrome: a narrative review. *J Orthop Sports Phys Ther* 34(10):565–588, 2004.
51. Mackinnon, SE: Pathophysiology of nerve compression. *Hand Clin* 18:231–241, 2002.
52. Magee, DJ: *Orthopedic Physical Assessment*, ed. 5. Missouri: Saunders Elsevier, 2008.
53. Michlovitz, SL: Conservative interventions for carpal tunnel syndrome. *J Orthop Sports Phys Ther* 34(10):589–600, 2004.
54. Middleton, SD, and Anakwe, RE: Carpal tunnel syndrome. *BMJ* 349: 1–7, 2014.
55. Molinari, WJ, and Elfar, JC: The double crush syndrome. *J Hand Surg* 38A(4):799–801, 2013.
56. Monacelli, G, et al: The pillar pain in the carpal tunnel's surgery. Neurogenic inflammation? A new therapeutic approach with local anaesthetic. *J Neurosurg Sci* 52(1):11–15, 2008.
57. Moseley, GL: Graded motor imagery is effective for long-standing complex regional pain syndrome: a randomised controlled trial. *Pain* 108: 192–198, 2004.
58. Moseley, GL, Butler, DS, Beames, TB, and Giles, TJ: *The Graded Motor Imagery Handbook*. Adelaide, Australia: Noigroup Publications, 2012.
59. Murakami, M, Kosharskyy, B, Gritsenko, K, and Shaparin, N: Complex regional pain syndrome: update and review of management. *Topics in Pain Management* 30(7):1–10, 2015.
60. Nee, RJ, Jull, GA, Vincenzino, B, and Coppieters, MW: The validity of upper-limb neurodynamic tests for detecting peripheral neuropathic pain. *J Orthop Sports Phys Ther* 42(5):413–424, 2012.
61. Novak, CB: Upper extremity work-related musculoskeletal disorders: a treatment perspective. *J Orthop Sports Phys Ther* 34(10):628–637, 2004.
62. Novak, CB, and Mackinnon, SE: Evaluation of nerve injury and nerve compression in the upper quadrant. *J Hand Ther* 18:230–240, 2005.
63. O'Connor, D, Marshall, S, and Massy-Westropp, N: Non-surgical treatment (other than steroid injection) for carpal tunnel syndrome. *Cochrane Database Syst Rev* 1:CD003219, 2003.
64. Oskouei, AE, Talebi, GA, Shakouri, SK, and Ghabili, K: Effects of neuromobilization maneuver on clinical and electrophysiological measures of patients with carpal tunnel syndrome. *J Phys Ther Sci* 26:1017–1022, 2014.
65. Pascarelli, EF, and Hsu, YP: Understanding work-related upper extremity disorders: clinical findings in 485 computer users, musicians, and others. *J Occup Rehabil* 11(1):1–21, 2001.
66. Pollard, C: Physiotherapy management of complex regional pain syndrome. *NZJ Physiother* 41(2):65–72, 2013.
67. Porretto-Loehrke, A, and Soika, E: Therapist's management of other nerve compressions about the elbow and wrist. In Skirven, TM, Osterman, AL, Fedorczyk, JM, and Amadio, PC (eds): *Rehabilitation of the Hand and Upper Extremity, Vol I*, ed. 6. Philadelphia, PA: Elsevier Mosby, 2011, pp 695–709.
68. Schmid, AB, et al: Reliability of clinical tests to evaluate nerve function and mechanosensitivity of the upper limb peripheral nervous system. *BMC Musculoskelet Disord* 10:1–9, 2009.
69. Seror, P: Frequency of neurogenic thoracic outlet syndrome in patients with definite carpal tunnel syndrome: an electrophysiological evaluation in 100 women. *Clin Neurophysiol* 116(2):259–263, 2005.
70. Seror, P: Symptoms of thoracic outlet syndrome in women with carpal tunnel syndrome. *Clin Neurophysiol* 116(10):2324–2329, 2005.
71. Shacklock, M: *Clinical Neurodynamics: A New System of Musculoskeletal Treatment.* Philadelphia: Elsevier, 2005.
72. Silva, A, et al: Quantitative in vivo longitudinal nerve excursion and strain in response to joint movement: A systematic literature review. *Clin Biomech* 29:839–847, 2014.
73. Smart, KM, Wand, BM, and O'Connell, NE: Physiotherapy for pain and disability in adults with complex regional pain syndrome (CRPS) types I and II (review). *Cochrane Database Syst Rev* 2:1–101, 2016.
74. Smith, KL: Nerve response to injury and repair. In Skirven, TM, Osterman, AL, Fedorczyk, JM, and Amadio, PC (eds): *Rehabilitation of the Hand and Upper Extremity, Vol I*, ed. 6. Philadelphia, PA: Elsevier Mosby, 2011, pp 601–610.
75. Smith, MB: The peripheral nervous system. In Goodman, CC, Fuller, KS, and Boissonnault, WG: *Pathology: Implications for the Physical Therapist.* Philadelphia: Saunders, 2003, pp 1140–1173.
76. Stewman, C, Vitanzo, PC, and Harwood, MI: Neurologic thoracic outlet syndrome: summarizing a complex history and evolution. *Curr Sports Med Rep: ACSM* 13(2):100–106, 2014.
77. Tajerian, M, and Clark, JD: New concepts in complex regional pain syndrome. *Hand Clinics* 32:41–49, 2016.
78. Topp, KS, and Boyd, BS: Structure and biomechanics of peripheral nerves: nerve responses to physical stresses and implications for physical therapist practice. *Phys Ther* 86(1):92–109, 2006.

79. Turl, SE, and George, KP: Adverse neural tension: a factor in repetitive hamstring strain. *J Orthop Sports Phys Ther* 27:16–21, 1998.
80. Urban, LM, and Macneil, BJ: Diagnostic accuracy of the slump test for identifying neuropathic pain in the lower limb. *J Orthop Sports Phys Ther* 45(8):596–603, 2015.
81. Vanti, C, et al: The upper limb neurodynamic test I: intra- and intertester reliability and the effect of several repetitions on pain and resistance. *J Manip Physiol Ther* 33:292–299, 2010.
82. Walsh, MT: Therapist's management of complex regional pain syndrome. In Skirven, TM, Osterman, AL, Fedorczyk, JM, and Amadio, PC (eds): *Rehabilitation of the Hand and Upper Extremity, Vol I*, ed. 6. Philadelphia, PA: Elsevier Mosby, 2011, pp 1479–1492.
83. Watson, LA, Pizzari, T, and Balster, S: Thoracic outlet syndrome part 1: clinical manifestations, differentiation and treatment pathways. *Man Ther* 14:586–595, 2009.
84. Watson, LA, Tizzari, T, and Balster, S: Thoracic outlet syndrome part 2: conservative management of thoracic outlet. *Man Ther* 15:305–314, 2010.
85. Wehbe, MA, and Schlegel, JM: Nerve gliding exercises for thoracic outlet syndrome. *Hand Clin* 20(1):51–55, 2004.
86. Wood, VE, and Biondi, J: Double-crush nerve compression in thoracic-outlet syndrome. *J Bone Joint Surg Am* 72(1):85–87, 1990.

CHAPTER 14

The Spine: Structure, Function, and Posture

CAROLYN KISNER, PT, MS ■ JACOB N. THORP, PT, DHS, OCS, MTC

Posture is alignment of the body parts whether upright, sitting, or recumbent. It is described by the positions of the joints and body segments and also in terms of the balance between the muscles crossing the joints.[46] Impairments in the joints, muscles, or connective tissues may lead to faulty postures, or, conversely, faulty postures may lead to impairments in the joints, muscles, and connective tissues as well as symptoms of discomfort and pain. Many musculoskeletal complaints can be attributed to stresses that occur from repetitive or sustained activities when in a habitually faulty postural alignment. This chapter reviews the structural relationships of the spine and extremities to normal and abnormal posture and describes the mechanisms that control posture. Common postural impairments and general guidelines for their management are described. Specific exercises for the various body regions are highlighted in this chapter and are described in detail in the succeeding chapters in Part IV of the text. Chapter 15 describes the common pathologies associated with the spine and details management guidelines, and Chapter 16 describes spinal exercises and manual interventions in detail.

Structure and Function of the Spine

Structure

The structure of the spinal column consists of 33 vertebrae (7 cervical, 12 thoracic, 5 lumbar, 5 fused sacral, and 3 or 4 coccygeal) and their respective intervertebral discs. Articulating with the spine are the 12 pair of ribs in the thoracic region, the cranium at the top of the spine at the occipital-atlas joint, and the pelvis at sacroiliac joints (Fig. 14.1).

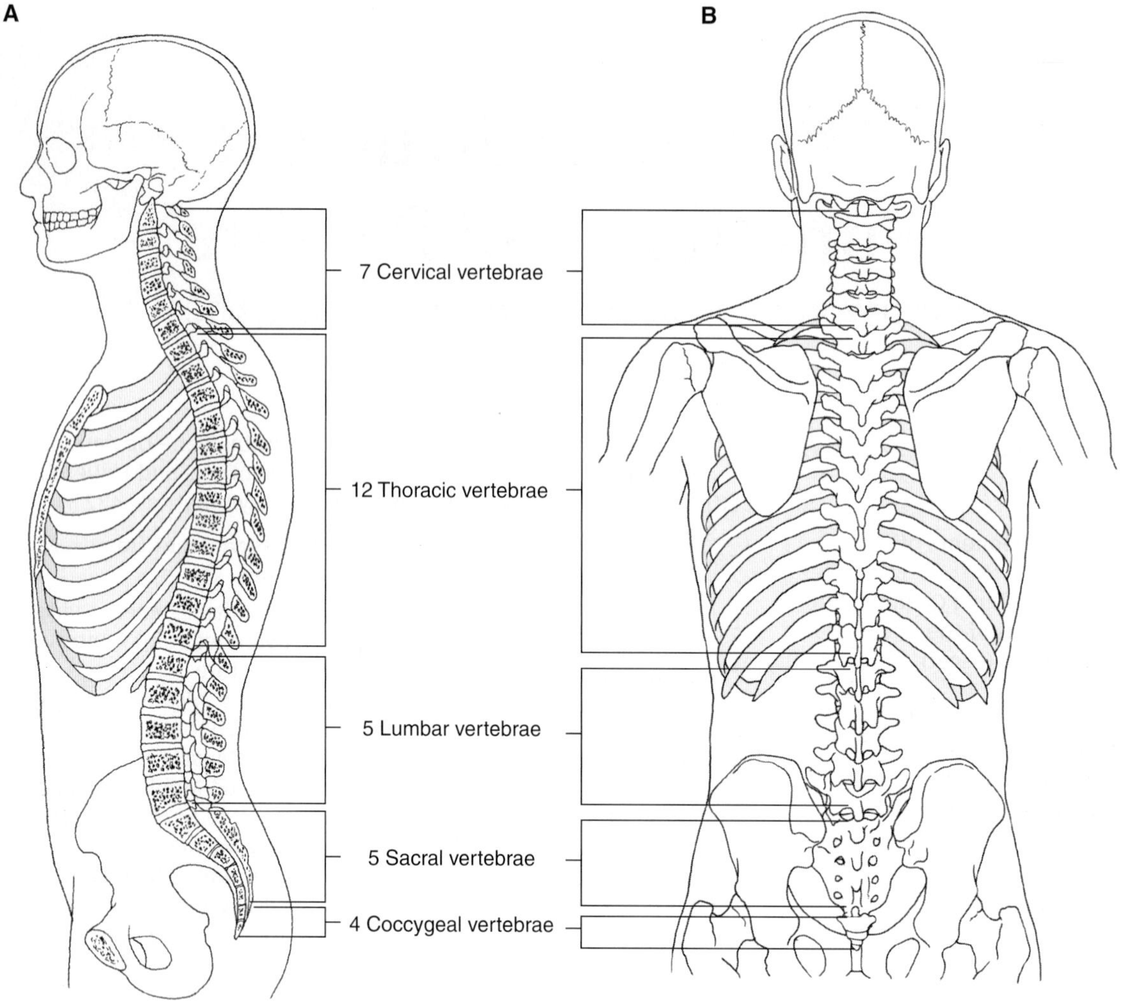

A

B

7 Cervical vertebrae

12 Thoracic vertebrae

5 Lumbar vertebrae

5 Sacral vertebrae

4 Coccygeal vertebrae

FIGURE 14.1 **(A)** Lateral and **(B)** posterior views showing the five regions of the spinal column. *(From Levangie, P, and Norkin, C [eds]:* Joint Structure and Function: A Comprehensive Analysis, *ed. 5. Philadelphia: F.A. Davis, 2011, p 141 with permission.)*

Functional Components of the Spine

Functionally, the spinal column is divided into anterior and posterior pillars (Fig. 14.2).[16]

- The *anterior pillar* is made up of the vertebral bodies and intervertebral discs and is the hydraulic, weight-bearing, shock-absorbing portion of the spinal column. The size of the disc influences the amount of motion available between two vertebrae.
- The *posterior pillar*, or vertebral arch, is made up of the articular processes and facet joints, which provide the gliding mechanism for movement. The orientation of the facets influences the direction of motion. Also part of the posterior unit are the boney levers, the two transverse processes, and the spinous process to which the muscles attach and function to cause and control motions and provide spinal stability.

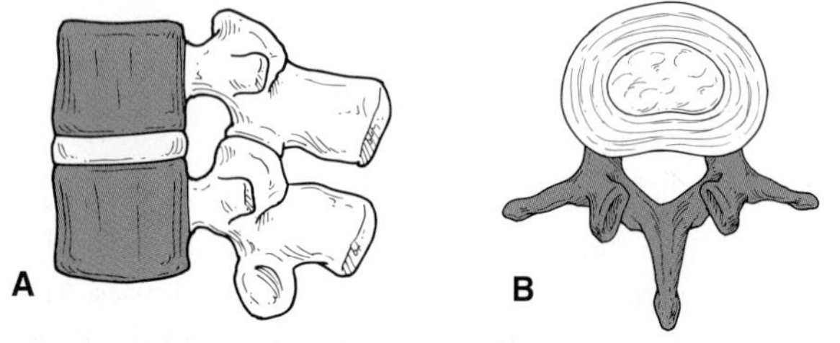

FIGURE 14.2 Spinal segment showing **(A)** the anterior weight-bearing, shock-absorbing portion and **(B)** the posterior gliding mechanism and lever system for muscle attachments.

Motions of the Spinal Column

Motion of the spinal column is described both globally and at the functional unit or motion segment. The functional unit is comprised of two vertebrae and the joints in between (typically, two zygapophyseal facet joints and one intervertebral disc). Generally, the axis of motion for each unit is in the nucleus pulposus of the intervertebral disc. Because the spine can move from top down or bottom up, motion at a functional unit is defined by what is occurring with the anterior portion of the body of the superior vertebra (Fig. 14.3).

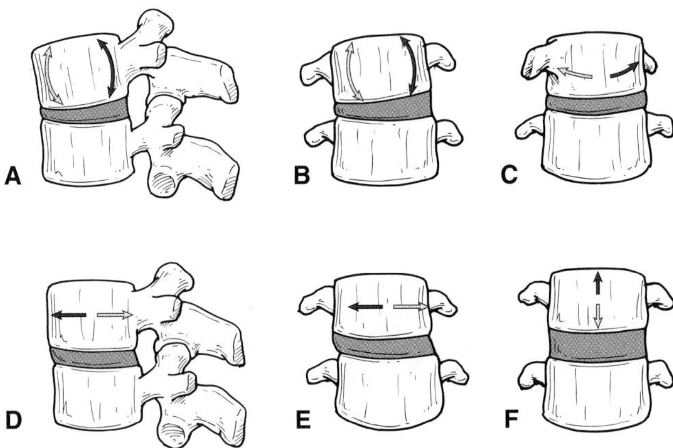

FIGURE 14.3 Motions of the spinal column. **(A)** Flexion/extension (forward/backward bending). **(B)** Lateral flexion (side bending). **(C)** Rotation. **(D)** Anterior/posterior shear. **(E)** Lateral shear. **(F)** Distraction/compression.

The Six Degrees of Motion

Flexion/extension. Motion in the sagittal plane results in flexion (forward bending) or extension (backward bending). With flexion, the anterior portion of the bodies approximate and the spinous processes separate; with extension, the anterior portion of the bodies separate and the spinous processes approximate.

Side bending. Motion in the frontal plane results in side bending (lateral flexion) to the left or right. With side bending, the lateral edges of the vertebral bodies approximate on the side toward which the spine is bending and separate the opposite side.

Rotation. Motion in the transverse plane results in rotation. Rotation to the right results in relative movement of the body of the superior vertebrae to the right and its spinous process to the left; the opposite occurs with rotation to the left. If movement occurs from the pelvis upward, the motion is still defined by the relative motion of the top vertebra.

Anterior/posterior shear. Forward or backward shear (translation) occurs when the body of the superior vertebra translates forward or backward on the vertebra below.

Lateral shear. Lateral shear (translation) occurs when the body of the superior vertebra translates sideways on the vertebra below.

Compression/distraction. Separation or approximation occurs with a longitudinal force, either away from or toward the vertebral bodies.

Arthrokinematics of the Zygapophyseal (Facet) Joints

Each region of the spine has its own special considerations as pertains to arthrokinematic movement and function. The arthrokinematics of the craniovertebral (suboccipital) area are described below. The remainder of the cervical spine and all the thoracic facets have relatively flat articular surfaces and glide on the adjacent facet joint.[16] The superior facets of the lumbar spine are concave and articulate with the adjacent inferior convex facets.[65] The arthrokinematics that are described in this section are summarized in ONLINE Table 14.1 available on the FA Davis website associated with this text.

Coupled motions typically occur at a segmental level when a person side bends or rotates their spine. *Coupled motion* is defined as "consistent association of one motion about an axis with another motion around a different axis"[16] and varies depending on the region, the spinal posture, the orientation of the facets, and factors such as extensibility of the soft tissues. When motions of side bending and rotation are coupled, foraminal opening is dictated by the side bending component.

Cervical spine. The cervical spine can be divided into the craniovertebral region and the "typical" cervical region.

- The *craniovertebral region* is composed of the occiput, atlas, and superior facets of the axis.
- The occipito-atlanto (OA) joint is considered a ball and socket joint; the convex facets of the occiput articulate with the concave facets of the atlas. Its primary motions are forward and backward nodding (flexion and extension) (Fig. 14.4). There is a small amount of side bending available at the OA joint; rotation and side bending are coupled in opposite directions in this region.
- The atlanto-axial (AA) joint consists of convex articulating surfaces of the atlas articulating on the convex articulating surfaces of the axis; its primary motion is rotation as the atlas pivots around the dens of the axis. It is important to note that, during rotation, one side of the AA joint complex is behaving as though it is flexing (moving forward) and the other side as though it is extending (moving backward) (Fig. 14.5).
- The *typical cervical* region includes the inferior facets of the axis and rest of the cervical spine; it features facet joints that are angled at 45° from the horizontal plane. Side bending and rotation typically couple toward the same side.
- Another unique characteristic of the cervical spine is the *joints of Luschka*. These bony projections provide lateral stability to the spine and reinforce the vertebral disc posterolaterally.

Thoracic spine. The thoracic facets begin in a frontal plane orientation and transition to a sagittal plane orientation as they near the lumbar spine. The ribs articulate with the thoracic spine at the transverse processes as well as the vertebral bodies and IV discs. In the upright posture, side bending and rotation typically couple in the same direction in the upper thoracic spine and in the opposite directions in the lower thoracic region,[16] although variability has been described.[78]

Lumbar spine. As the lumbar facets transition from a sagittal plane to a frontal plane orientation, some of the facets have a biplanar orientation.[16] Coupling varies in that with lateral flexion, rotation occurs to the same side, but with rotation,

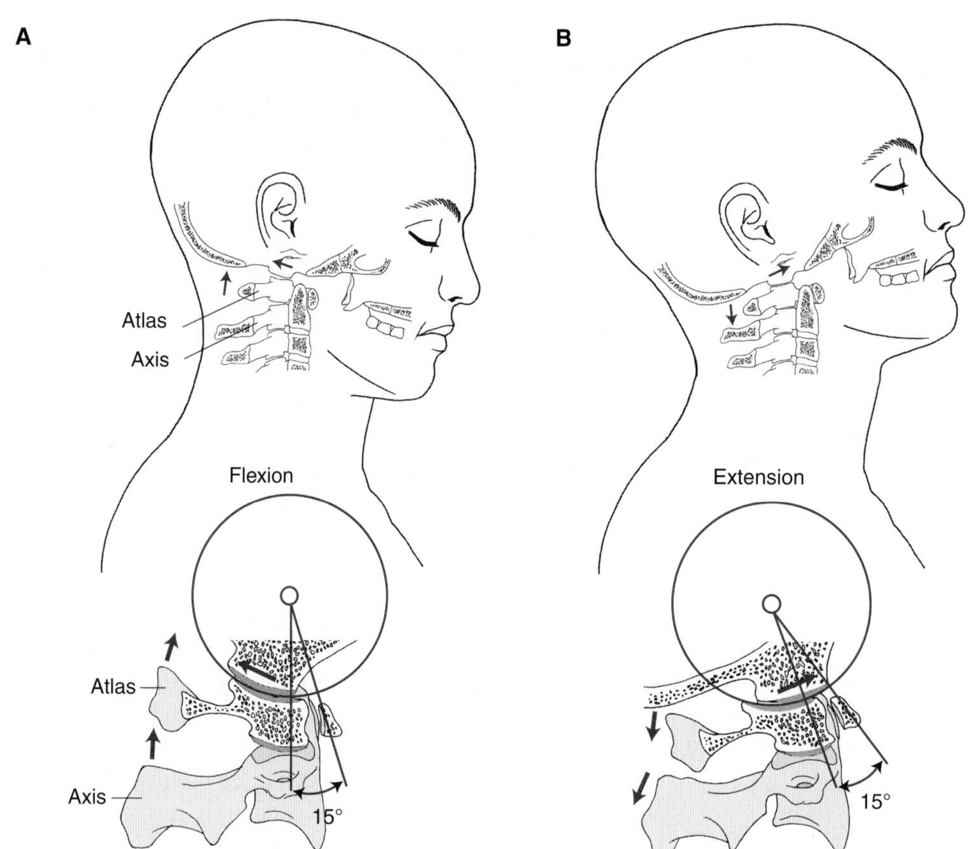

FIGURE 14.4 Nodding motions of the atlanto-occipital joints. (A) Flexion. (B) Extension. *(From Levangie, P, and Norkin, C [eds]:* Joint Structure and Function: A Comprehensive Analysis, *ed. 5. Philadelphia: F.A. Davis, 2011, p 141 with permission.)*

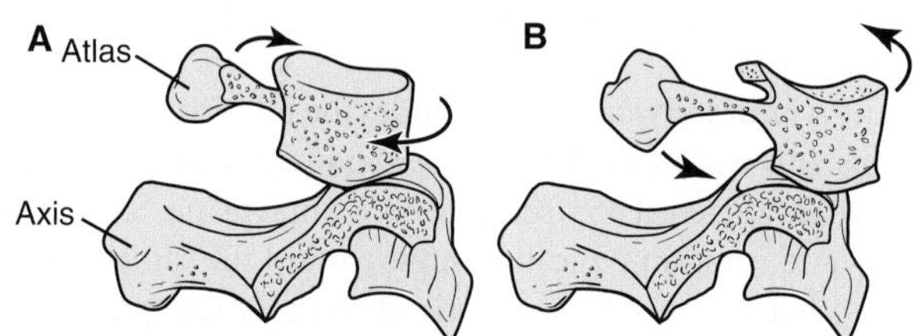

FIGURE 14.5 Rotation of the atlas-axis joints (view from the side). (A) Right rotation showing backward movement of the right articulating surface of C1 on C2. (B) Left rotation showing forward movement of the right articulating surface of C1 on C2.

lateral flexion occurs opposite[16]; there is variability with flexion and extension.

Structure and Function of Intervertebral Discs and Cartilaginous End-Plates

The intervertebral disc, consisting of the annulus fibrosus and nucleus pulposus, is one component of a three-joint complex between two adjacent vertebrae and cartilaginous end-plates of the vertebral bodies. The structure of the disc dictates its function (Fig. 14.6).[16,50]

Annulus fibrosus. The outer portion of the disc is made up of dense layers of type I collagen fibers. The collagen fibers in any one layer are parallel and angled around 60° to 65° to the axis of the spine, with the tilt alternating in successive layers.[31,47] Because of the orientation of the fibers, tensile strength is provided to the disc by the annulus when the spine is distracted, rotated, or bent. This structure helps restrain the various spinal motions as a complex ligament. The annulus is firmly attached to adjacent vertebrae, and the layers are firmly bound to one another. Fibers of the innermost layers blend with the matrix of the nucleus pulposus. The annulus fibrosus is supported by the anterior and posterior longitudinal ligaments.

Nucleus pulposus. The central portion of the disc is a gelatinous mass that normally is contained within, but whose loosely aligned type II collagen fibers merge with the inner layer of the annulus fibrosus. It is located centrally in the disc except in the lumbar spine, where it is situated closer to the posterior border than the anterior border of the annulus. Aggregating proteoglycans, normally in high concentration

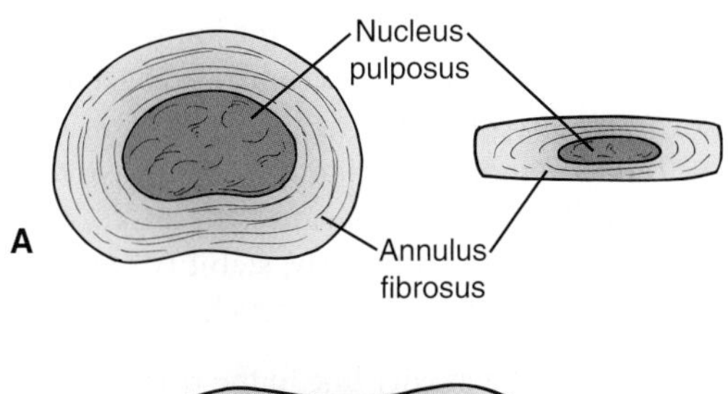

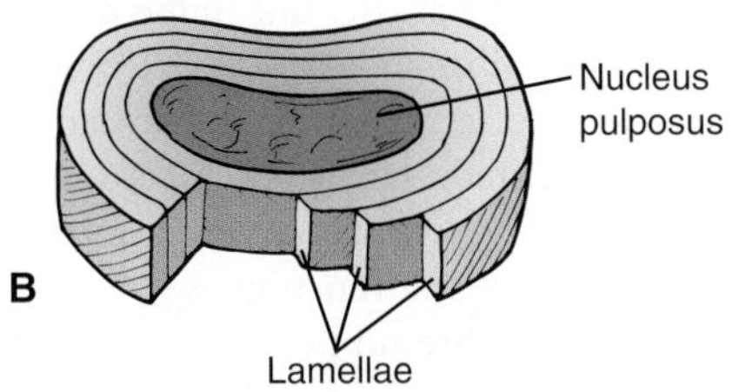

FIGURE 14.6 Intervertebral disc. **(A)** The annular rings enclose the nucleus pulposus, providing a mechanism for dissipating compressive forces. **(B)** Orientation of the layers of the annulus provides tensile strength to the disc with motions in various directions.

in a healthy nucleus, have great affinity for water. The resulting fluid mechanics of the confined nucleus functions to distribute pressure evenly throughout the disc and from one vertebral body to the next under loaded conditions. Because of the affinity for water, the nucleus imbibes water when pressure is reduced on the disc and squeezes water out under compressive loads. These fluid dynamics provide transport for nutrients and help maintain tissue health in the disc.

With flexion (forward bending) of a vertebral segment, the anterior portion of the disc is compressed, and the posterior is distracted. The nucleus pulposus generally does not move in a healthy disc but may have slight distortion with flexion, potentially to redistribute the load through the disc.[48] Asymmetrical loading in flexion results in distortions of the nucleus toward the contralateral posterolateral corner, where the fibers of the annulus are more stretched.

Cartilaginous end-plates. End-plates cover the nucleus pulposus superiorly and inferiorly and lie between the nucleus and vertebral bodies. Each is encircled by the apophyseal ring of the respective vertebral body.[16] The collagen fibers of the inner annulus fibrosus insert into the end-plate and angle centrally, thus encapsulating the nucleus pulposus. Nutrition diffuses from the marrow of the vertebral bodies to the disc via the end-plates.[16] The end-plates are also responsible for containing the nucleus from migrating superior/inferior.

Intervertebral Foramina

The intervertebral foramina are between each vertebral segment in the posterior pillar. Their anterior boundary is the intervertebral disc, the posterior boundary is the facet joint, and the superior and inferior boundaries are the pedicles of the superior and inferior vertebrae of the spinal segment. The mixed spinal nerve exits the spinal canal via the foramen along with blood vessels and recurrent meningeal or sinuvertebral nerves. The size of the intervertebral foramina is affected by spinal motion, being larger with forward bending and contralateral side bending and smaller with extension and ipsilateral side bending.

Biomechanical Influences on Postural Alignment

Curves of the Spine

The adult spine is divided into four curves: two *primary*, or posterior, curves, so named because they are present in the infant and the convexity is posterior, and two *compensatory*, or anterior, curves, so named because they develop as the infant learns to lift the head and eventually stand, and the convexity is anterior.

- Posterior curves are in the thoracic and sacral regions. *Kyphosis* is a term used to denote a posterior curve. Kyphotic posture refers to an excessive posterior curvature of the thoracic spine.[46]
- Anterior curves are in the cervical and lumbar regions. *Lordosis* is a term also used to denote an anterior curve, although some sources reserve the term lordosis to denote abnormal conditions such as those that occur with a sway back.[46]
- The curves and flexibility in the spinal column are important for withstanding the effects of gravity and other external forces.[16,56]
- The structure of the bones, joints, muscles, and inert tissues of the lower extremities are designed for weight bearing; they support and balance the trunk in the upright posture. Lower extremity alignment and function are described in greater detail in each of the extremity chapters (see Chapters 20 to 22).

Gravity

When looking at posture and function, it is critical to understand the influence of gravity on the structures of the trunk and lower extremities. Gravity places stress on the structures responsible for maintaining the body upright and therefore provides a continual challenge to stability and efficient movement. For a weight-bearing joint to be stable, or in equilibrium, the gravity line of the mass must fall exactly through the axis of rotation, or there must be a force to counteract the moment caused by gravity.[49] In the body, the counterforce is provided by either muscle or inert structures. In addition, the standing posture usually involves a slight anterior/posterior swaying of the body of about 4 cm, so muscles are necessary to control the sway and maintain equilibrium.

In the upright posture, the line of gravity transects the spinal curves, which are balanced anteriorly and posteriorly, and it is close to the axis of rotation in the lower extremity joints. The following describes the standard of a balanced upright posture (Fig. 14.7).

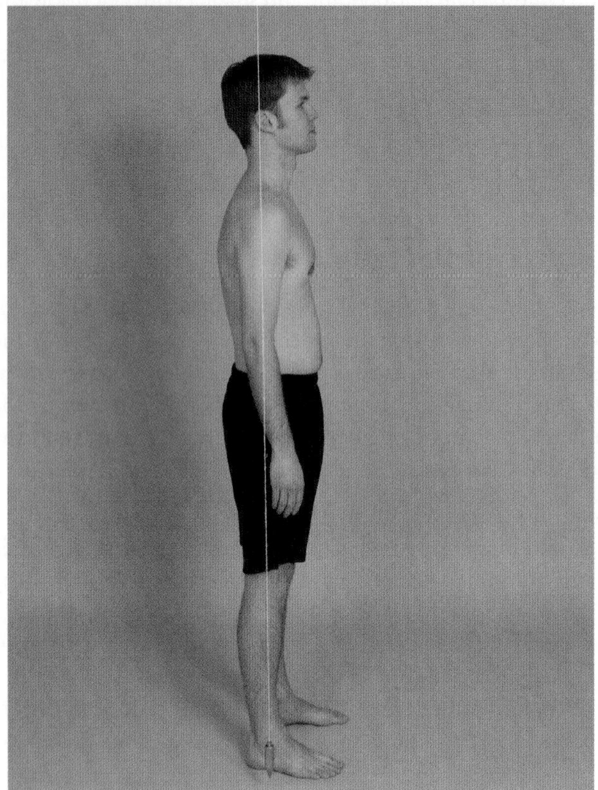

FIGURE 14.7 Lateral view of standard postural alignment. A plumb line is typically used for reference and represents the relationship of the body parts with the line of gravity. Surface landmarks are slightly anterior to the lateral malleolus, slightly anterior to the axis of the knee joint, through the greater trochanter (slightly posterior to the axis of the hip joint), through the bodies of the lumbar and cervical vertebrae, through the shoulder joint, and through the lobe of the ear.

Ankle. For the ankle, the gravity line is anterior to the joint, so it tends to rotate the tibia forward about the ankle. Stability is provided by the plantarflexor muscles, primarily the soleus muscle.

Knee. The normal gravity line is anterior to the knee joint, which tends to keep the knee in extension. Stability is provided by the anterior cruciate ligament, posterior capsule (locking mechanism of the knee), and tension in the muscles posterior to the knee (the gastrocnemius and hamstring muscles). The soleus provides active stability by pulling posteriorly on the tibia. With the knees fully extended, no muscle support is required at that joint to maintain an upright posture; however, if the knees flex slightly, the gravity line shifts posterior to the joint, and the quadriceps femoris muscle must contract to prevent the knee from buckling.

Hip. The gravity line at the hip varies with the swaying of the body. When the line passes through the hip joint, there is equilibrium, and no external support is necessary. When the gravitational line shifts posterior to the joint, some posterior rotation of the pelvis occurs but is controlled by tension in the hip flexor muscles (primarily the iliopsoas). During relaxed standing, the iliofemoral ligament provides passive stability to the joint, and no muscle tension is necessary. When the gravitational line shifts anteriorly, stability is provided by active support of the hip extensor muscles.

Trunk. Normally, the gravity line in the trunk goes through the bodies of the lumbar and cervical vertebrae, and the curves are balanced. Some activity in the muscles of the trunk and pelvis helps maintain the balance. (This is described in greater detail in the following sections.) As the trunk shifts, contralateral muscles contract and function as guy wires. Extreme or sustained deviations are supported by inert structures.

Head. The center of gravity of the head falls anterior to the atlanto-occipital joints. The posterior cervical muscles contract to keep the head balanced.

Stability

When standing, the center of gravity typically falls slightly anterior to S2 in the pelvis. So long as the line of gravity from the center of mass falls within the base of support, a structure is stable. Stability is improved by lowering the center of gravity or increasing the base of support. In the upright position, the body is relatively unstable because it is a tall structure with a small base of support. When the center of gravity falls outside the base of support, either the structure falls or some force must act to keep the structure upright. Both inert and dynamic structures support the body against gravitational and other external forces. The inert osseous and ligamentous structures provide passive tension when a joint reaches the end of its range of motion (ROM). Muscles act as dynamic guy wires, responding to perturbations by providing counterforces to the torque of gravity as well as stability within the ROM so stresses are not placed on the inert tissues.

Postural Stability in the Spine

Spinal stability is described in terms of three subsystems: passive (inert structures/bones and ligaments), active (muscles), and neural control.[24,64] The three subsystems are interrelated and can be thought of as a three-legged stool; if any one of the legs is not providing support, it affects the stability of the whole structure.[64] Instability of a spinal segment is often a combination of inert tissue damage, insufficient muscular strength or endurance, and poor neuromuscular control.[3,24]

Inert Structures: Influence on Stability

Penjabi[63,64] described the ROM of any one segment as being divided into an elastic zone and a neutral zone. When spinal segments are in the neutral zone (midrange/neutral range), the inert joint capsules and ligaments provide minimal passive resistance to motion and therefore minimal stability. As a segment moves into the elastic zone, the inert structures provide restraint as passive resistance to the motion occurs. When a structure limits movement in a specific direction, it provides stability in that direction. In addition to the inert tissues providing passive stability when limiting motion, the sensory receptors in the joint capsules and ligaments sense position and changes in position. Stimulation of these receptors provides feedback to the central nervous system, thus influencing the neural control system.[64,66] The stabilizing features of the inert tissues in the spine are summarized in ONLINE Table 14.2 available on the FA Davis website associated with this text.

Muscles: Influence on Stability

The muscles of the trunk not only act as prime movers or as antagonists to movement caused by gravity during dynamic activity; they are important stabilizers of the spine.[3,9,11,27,39,54,66] Without the dynamic stabilizing activity from the trunk muscles, the spine would collapse in the upright position.[14]

Role of Global and Segmental Muscle Activity

Both superficial (global) and deep (segmental) muscles play critical roles in providing stability and maintaining the upright posture. Table 14,1 summarizes the stabilizing characteristics of these two muscle groups.

Global muscle function. In the lumbar spine, the global muscles, being the more superficial of the two groups, are the large guy wires that respond to external loads imposed on the trunk that shift the center of mass (Fig. 14.8 A). Their reaction is direction specific to control spinal orientation.[3,39] The global muscles are unable to stabilize individual spinal segments except through compressive loading because they have little or no direct attachment to the vertebrae. If an individual segment is unstable, compressive loading from the global guy wires may lead to or perpetuate a painful situation as stress is placed on the inert tissues at the end of the range of that segment (Fig. 14.8 B).

Deep/segmental muscle function. The deeper, segmental muscles, which have direct attachments across the vertebral segments, provide dynamic support to individual segments in the spine and help maintain each segment in a stable position, so the inert tissues are not stressed at the limits of motion (Fig. 14.9).[39,43,44,55]

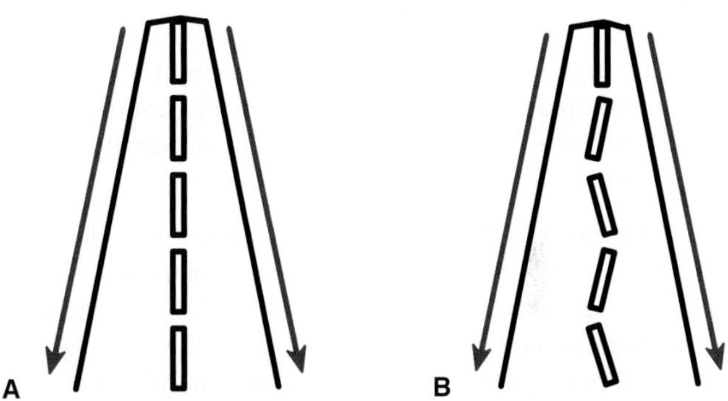

FIGURE 14.8 (A) Guy wire function of global trunk muscles provides overall stability against perturbations. **(B)** Instability in the multisegmental spine cannot be controlled by the global trunk muscle guy wires. Compressive loading from the long guy wires leads to stress on the inert tissues at the end-ranges of the unstable segment.

TABLE 14.1 Stabilizing Features of Muscles Controlling the Spine

Global Muscles	Deep Segmental Muscles
Characteristics	
▪ Superficial: farther from axis of motion ▪ Cross multiple vertebral segments ▪ Produce motion and provide large guy wire function ▪ Compressive loading with strong contractions	▪ Deep: closer to axis of motion ▪ Attach to each vertebral segment ▪ Control segmental motion; segmental guy wire function ▪ Greater percentage of type I muscle fibers for muscular endurance
Lumbar region	
▪ Rectus abdominis ▪ External and internal obliques ▪ Quadratus lumborum (lateral portion) ▪ Erector spinae ▪ Iliopsoas	▪ Transversus abdominis ▪ Multifidus ▪ Quadratus lumborum (deep portion) ▪ Deep rotators
Cervical region	
▪ Sternocleidomastoid ▪ Scalene ▪ Levator scapulae ▪ Upper trapezius ▪ Erector spinae	▪ Rectus capitis anterior and lateralis ▪ Longus colli

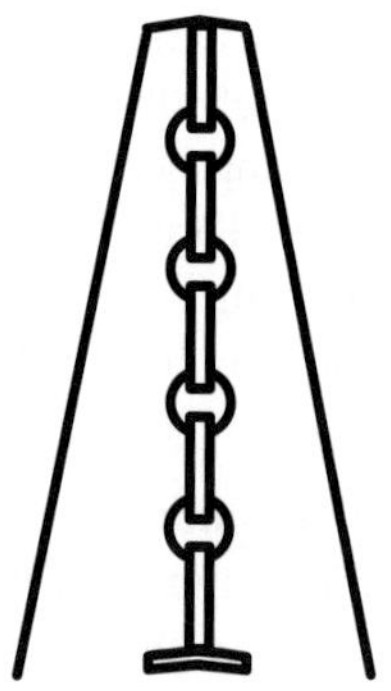

FIGURE 14.9 Deep muscles attached to each spinal segment provide segmental stability.

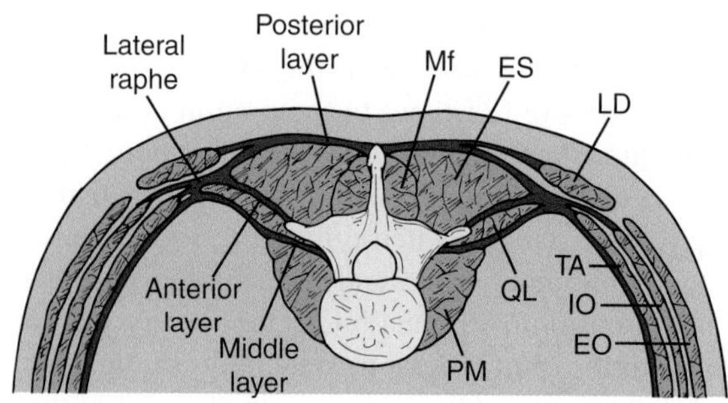

FIGURE 14.11 Transverse section in the lumbar region shows the relationships of the three layers of the thoracolumbar fascia to the muscles in the region and their attachments to the spine. (ES, erector spinae; MF, multifidus; TA, transversus abdominis; IO, internal obliques; EO, external obliques; LD, latissimus dorsi; PM, psoas major; QL, quadratus lumborum muscles)

Muscle Control in the Lumbar Spine

General muscle function and stabilizing actions of the muscles of the spine described in this section are summarized in ONLINE Table 14.3 available on the FA Davis website associated with this text.

Abdominal muscles (Fig. 14.10). The rectus abdominis (RA), external oblique (EO), and internal oblique (IO) muscles are large, multisegmental global trunk flexor muscles and are important guy wires for stabilizing the spine against postural perturbations. The transversus abdominis (TrA) is the deepest of the abdominal muscles and responds uniquely to postural perturbations. It attaches posteriorly to the lumbar vertebrae via the posterior and middle layers of the thoracolumbar fascia (Figs. 14.11 and 14.12) and through its action develops tension that acts like a girdle of support around the abdomen and lumbar vertebrae. Only the TrA is active with both isometric trunk flexion and extension, whereas the other abdominal muscles have decreased activity with resisted extension. This is attributed to the stabilization function of the TrA.[13,41]

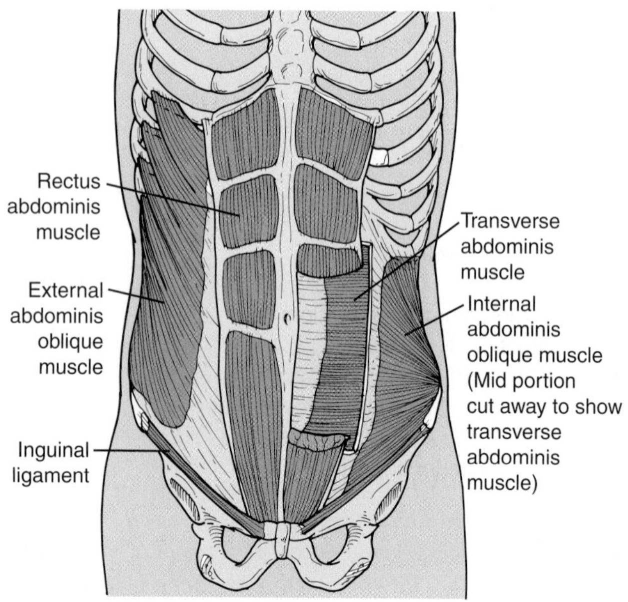

FIGURE 14.10 Abdominal muscles.

Transversus abdominis stabilization activity. Early electromyographic research studies of the activity of the deeper abdominal muscles in their stabilization function were done with surface electrodes and did not discriminate activity between the TrA and IO. By using ultrasound imaging techniques, insertion of fine-needle electrodes into the various muscles has produced evidence of differing functions between these two muscles with perturbations to balance in healthy individuals as well as those who have low back pathology.[37]

The TrA responds with anticipatory activity and with rapid arm and leg movements (before the other abdominals) and coordinates with respiration during these activities.[39,43,44] The TrA also has a coordinated link with the perineum and pelvic floor muscle function (see Chapter 25),[7,15,57,69,70] as well as with the deep fibers of the multifidi.[39,42-44,55] The "drawing-in" maneuver is used to activate the TrA voluntarily and, with training, produces the most independent activity of this muscle.[67,76] Training the TrA for postural control and stability has been shown to improve the long-term outcome in patients experiencing their first episode of low back pain.[32] (See Chapter 16 for a description of this maneuver.)

FOCUS ON EVIDENCE

In a study involving 42 healthy controls and 56 people with back pain, the thickness of the TrA and LM muscle groups measured with ultrasound imaging was calculated at rest and then during a stabilizing contraction with no resistance. The results were expressed as a percentage of change in thickness during these times of measurement. It was found that the healthy group average increase was 60% for the TrA and 30% for the LM. This was compared with 40% and 20%, respectively, for the group with LBP.[19] However, a systematic review reported conflicting evidence for a relationship in percentage of change in LM thickness and functional outcomes following various conservative interventions.[80]

Erector spinae muscles (Fig. 14.13). The erector spinae muscles are the long, multisegmental extensors that begin as a large musculotendinous mass over the sacral and lower

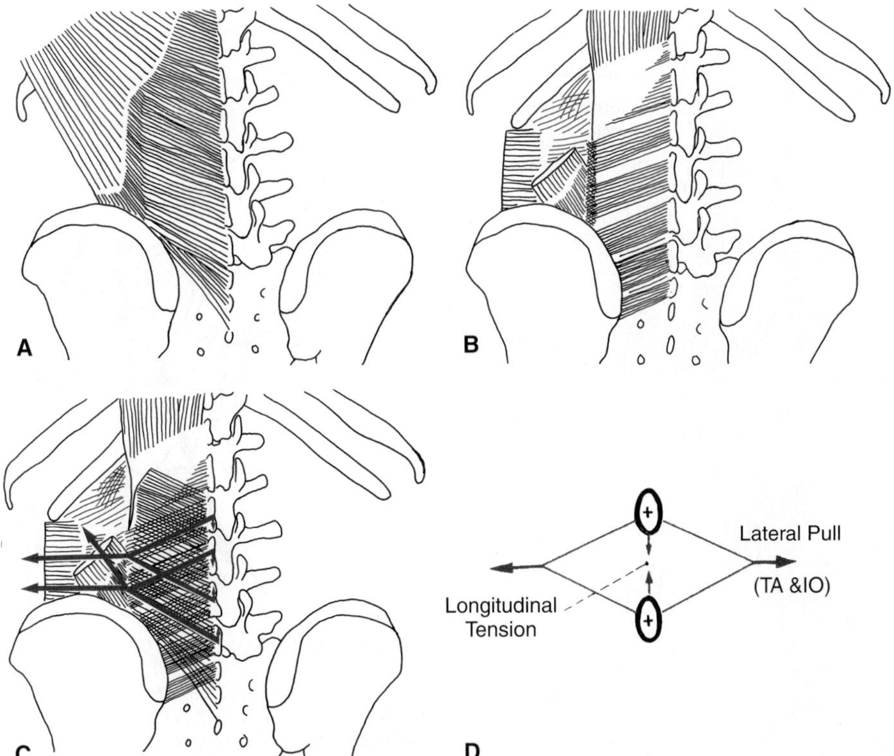

FIGURE 14.12 Orientation and attachments of the posterior layer of the thoracolumbar fascia. From the lateral raphe, **(A)** the fibers of the superficial lamina are angled inferiorly and medially and **(B)** the fibers of the deep lamina are angled superiorly and medially. **(C)** Tension in the angled fibers of the posterior layer of the fascia is transmitted to the spinous processes in opposing directions, resisting separation of the spinous processes. **(D)** Diagrammatic representation of a lateral pull at the lateral raphe, resulting in tension between the lumbar spinous processes that oppose separation, thus providing stability to the spine. *(A–C: adapted from Bogduk, N, and MacIntosh, JE: The applied anatomy of the thoracolumbar fascia.* Spine *9:164–170, 1984, pp 166–167, 169, with permission; D: adapted from Gracovetsky, S, Farfan, H, and Helleur, C: The abdominal mechanism.* Spine *10:317–324, 1985, p 319, with permission.)*

lumbar vertebrae. They are important global guy wires for controlling the trunk against postural perturbations.

Multifidus stabilization activity. The multifasciculed multifidi muscle group has a high distribution of type I fibers and large capillary network, emphasizing its role as a tonic stabilizer. Its segmental attachments are able to control movement of the spinal segments as well as increase spinal stiffness. The multifidus, along with the erector spinae, are encased by the posterior and middle layers of the lumbodorsal fascia (see Fig. 14.11), so bulk and muscle contraction increase tension on the fascia, adding to the stabilizing function of the fascia (see below for a description of this mechanism).

In patients with low back impairment, the fibers of the multifidi quickly atrophy at the spinal segment,[6,33] and a moth-eaten appearance has been reported in patients undergoing surgery for lumbar disc disease.[66] Additionally, it has been reported that individuals with LBP have been shown to have significantly more fatty infiltration in the LM when compared with healthy controls.[10,18] This reflects that muscle quality might be a precursor in reoccurring LBP. Evidence supports the idea that training with specific exercises increases the function of the multifidi as well as the erector spinae in general.[17,32,34] Other deep muscles that theoretically play a role in segmental stability but to this point in time have been difficult to assess because of their depth include the intersegmental muscles (rotators and intertransversarii muscles) and deep fibers of the quadratus lumborum.

FOCUS ON EVIDENCE

Inactivity has been shown to increase the risk of high fat content in the multifidus as well as higher pain intensity and disability.[73] Additionally, it has been reported in a systematic review that the paraspinal muscles are significantly smaller in patients with chronic LBP.[22] However, no significant correlation has been associated with decreased physical activity and a decreased cross-sectional area of the multifidi or erector spinae.[73] Conversely, in another systematic review, strong evidence was identified that changes in TrA thickness during contraction were unrelated to low back pain intensity and changes in the multifidi muscles and clinical outcomes were uncertain.[79]

Thoracolumbar (lumbodorsal) fascia. The thoracolumbar fascia is an extensive fascial system in the back that consists of several layers.[8,9,27-29] It surrounds the erector spinae, multifidi, and quadratus lumborum, thus providing support to these muscles when they contract[28] (see Fig. 14.11). Increased bulk in these muscles increases tension in the fascia, perhaps contributing the stabilizing function of these muscles.

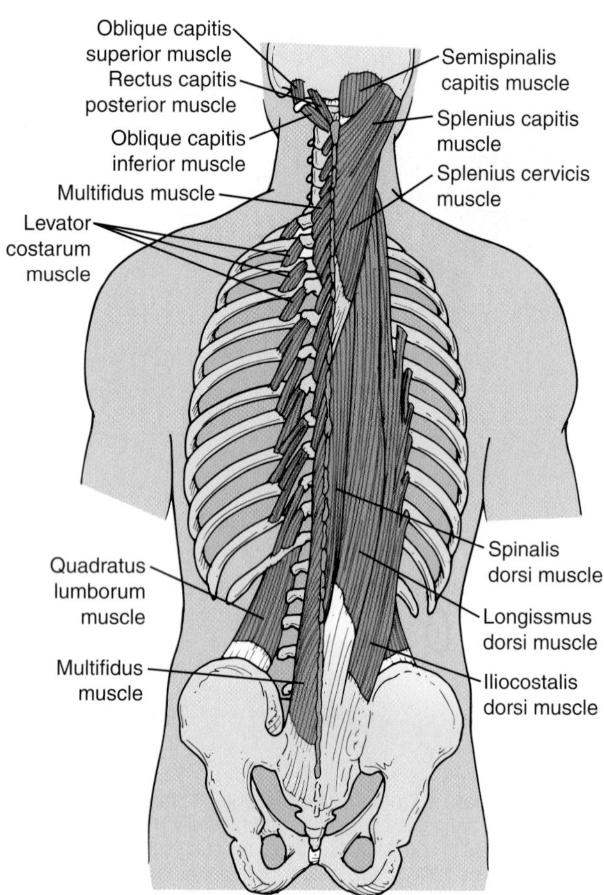

FIGURE 14.13 Muscles of the back.

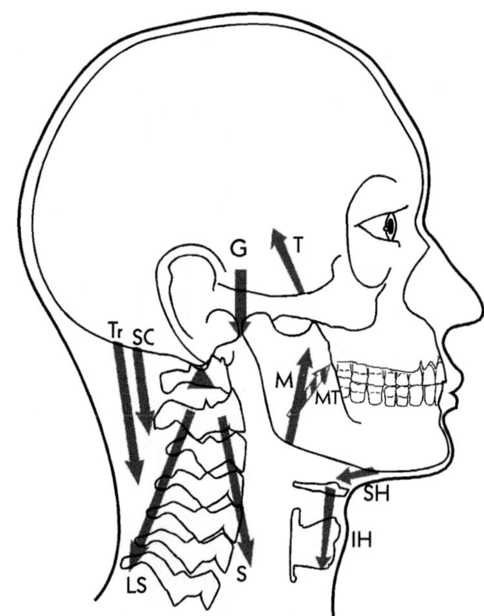

FIGURE 14.14 Head balance on the cervical spine. The posterior cervical muscles (trapezius and semispinalis capitis) counter the weight of the head. The mandibular elevating muscles (masseter, temporalis, medial pterygoid) maintain jaw elevation opposing the mandibular depression force of gravity and tension in the anterior throat muscles (suprahyoid and infrahyoid groups). The scalene and levator muscles stabilize against the posterior and anterior translatory forces on the cervical vertebrae. (TR, trapezius; SC, semispinalis capitis; M, masseter; T, temporalis; MT, medial pterygoid; SH, suprahyoid; IH, infrahyoid; S, scalene; LS, levator scapulae; G, center of gravity; ▲, axis of motion.)

The aponeurosis of the latissimus dorsi and fibers from the serratus posterior inferior, internal oblique, and transverse abdominis muscles blend together at the lateral raphe of the thoracolumbar fascia, so contraction in these muscles increases tension through the angled fascia, providing stabilizing forces for the lumbar spine[28] (see Fig. 14.12). In addition, the "X" design of the latissimus dorsi and contralateral gluteus maximus has the potential to provide stability to the lumbosacral junction.

Muscle Control in the Cervical Spine

The fulcrum of the head on the spine is through the occipital/atlas joints. The center of gravity of the head is anterior to the joint axis and therefore has a flexion moment. The weight of the head is counterbalanced by the cervical extensor muscles (upper trapezius and cervical erector spinae). Tension and fatigue in these muscles, as well as in the levator scapulae (which supports the posture of the scapulae), is experienced by most people who experience postural stress to the head and neck (Fig. 14.14). The position of the mandible and the tension in the muscles of mastication are influenced by the postural relationship between the cervical spine and head.

Mandibular elevator group. The mandible is a movable structure that is maintained in its resting position with the jaw partially closed through action of the mandibular elevators (masseter, temporalis, and medial pterygoid muscles).

Suprahyoid and infrahyoid group. The anterior throat muscles assist with swallowing and balancing the jaw against the muscles of mastication. These muscles also function to flex the neck when rising from the supine position. With a forward head posture, they, along with the longus colli, tend to be stretched and weak so the person lifts the head with the sternocleidomastoid (SCM) muscles. In addition, with a forward head posture, the suprahyoid muscles have a tendency to pull the mandible into depression due to their orientation and attachments at the hyoid and mandible. This is counteracted by the mandibular elevator muscle group, which creates a sustained contraction in order to keep the mouth closed.

Rectus capitis anterior and lateralis, longus colli, and longus capitis (Fig. 14.15). The deep craniocervical flexor muscles have segmental attachments and provide dynamic support to the cervical spine and head.[30] The longus colli is important in the action of axial extension (retraction) and works with the SCM for cervical flexion. Without the segmental influence of the longus colli, the SCM would cause increased cervical lordosis when attempting flexion.[5]

Multifidus. With its segmental attachments, the multifidus is thought to have a local stabilizing function in the cervical spine similar to its function in the lumbar region (see Fig. 14.13).[30]

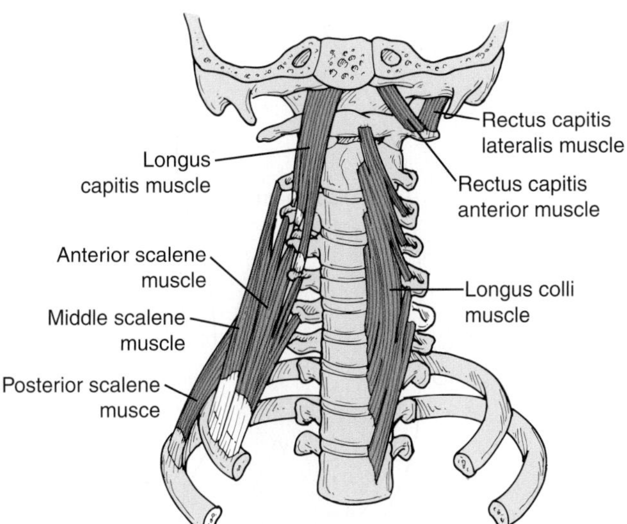

FIGURE 14.15 Deep segmental musculature in the cervical spine: rectus capitis anterior and lateralis, longus colli, longus capitis, and scalene muscles.

Role of Muscle Endurance

Strength is critical for controlling large loads or responding to large and unpredictable loads (such as during laborious activities, sports, or falls), but only about 10% of maximum contraction is needed to provide stability in usual situations.[3] Slightly more might be needed in a segment damaged by disc disease or ligamentous laxity when muscles are called on to compensate for the deficit in the passive support.[3] In a study that looked at 17 mechanical factors and the occurrence of low back pain in 600 subjects (ages 20 through 65), poor muscular endurance in the back extensors muscles had the greatest association with low back pain.[59]

Greater percentages of type I fibers than type II fibers are found in all back muscles, which is reflective of their postural and stabilization functions.[58]

Neurological Control: Influence on Stability

The muscles of the neck and trunk are activated and controlled by the nervous system, which is influenced by peripheral and central mechanisms in response to fluctuating forces and activities. Basically, the nervous system coordinates the response of muscles to expected and unexpected forces at the right time and by the right amount by modulating stiffness and movement to match the various imposed forces.[3,20,39]

Feedforward control and spinal stability. The central nervous system activates the trunk muscles in anticipation of the load imposed by limb movement to maintain stability in the spine.[44] Research has demonstrated that there are feedforward mechanisms that activate postural responses of all trunk muscles preceding activity in muscles that move the extremities[39,42,44] and that anticipatory activation of the transversus abdominis and deep fibers of the multifidus is independent of the direction or speed of the postural disturbance.[37,38,43,55] The more superficial trunk muscles vary in response depending on the direction of arm and leg movement, reflective of their postural guy wire function, which controls displacement of the center of mass when the body changes configuration.[39,44] There are reported differences in patterns of muscle recruitment in patients with low back pain with delayed recruitment of the transversus abdominis in all movement directions and delayed recruitment of the rectus abdominis, erector spinae, and oblique abdominal muscles specific to the direction of movement compared to healthy subjects.[40]

FOCUS ON EVIDENCE

A study by Allison and associates[1] collected data from muscle activity of the TrA, internal obliques, erector spinae, and multifidus muscle groups bilaterally in seven subjects and provided evidence that challenges the concept of bilateral feed forward symmetry in the activation of the TrA and that also contradicts previously published studies that contraction of the TrA is independent of the direction of arm movement causing trunk perturbations. The data support the motor control strategy of feed-forward activity but challenge the influence of support to the spine through symmetrical force generation due to the asymmetry in activation patterns dependent on side and direction of arm movement and thus direction of trunk perturbations. The authors acknowledge the value of TrA training but suggest further research is needed to provide explanation for the mechanism of its stabilizing action.

Effects of Limb Function on Spinal Stability

Without adequate stabilization of the spine, contraction of the limb-girdle musculature transmits forces proximally and causes motions of the spine that place excessive stresses on spinal structures and the supporting soft tissue.

CLINICAL TIP

- Stabilization of the pelvis and lumbar spine by the abdominal muscles against the pull of the iliopsoas muscle is necessary during active hip flexion to avoid increased lumbar lordosis and anterior shearing of the vertebrae.
- Stabilization of the ribs by the intercostal and abdominal muscles is necessary for an effective pushing force from the pectoralis major and serratus anterior muscles.
- Stabilization of the cervical spine by the longus colli muscle is necessary to prevent excessive lordosis from contraction of the upper trapezius as it functions with the shoulder girdle muscles in lifting and pulling activities.

Localized muscle fatigue. Localized fatigue in the stabilizing spinal musculature may occur with repetitive activity or heavy exertion or when the musculature is not utilized effectively due to faulty postures. There is a greater chance of injury in the supporting structures of the spine when the stabilizing muscles fatigue. Marras and Granata[52] reported significant changes in motion patterns between the spine and lower extremity joints as well as significant changes in muscle recruitment patterns with repetitive lifting during an extended period of time, resulting in increased anterior/posterior shear in the lumbar spine.

Muscle imbalances. Imbalances in the flexibility and strength of the hip, shoulder, and neck musculature cause asymmetrical forces on the spine and affect posture. Common problems are described in the section later in this chapter on "Common Faulty Postures."

Effects of Breathing on Posture and Stability

Inspiration and thoracic spine extension elevate the rib cage and assist with posture. The intercostal muscles function as postural muscles to stabilize and move the ribs. They act as a dynamic membrane between the ribs to prevent sucking in and blowing out of the soft tissue with the pressure changes during respiration.[4] The stabilizing function of the TrA also works in conjunction with the diaphragm in a feed-forward response to rapid arm motions. Contraction of the diaphragm and increased intra-abdominal pressure (IAP) occur prior to rapid arm movement, irrespective of the phase of respiration or the direction of the arm motion.[39,41] The tonic activities of the TrA and diaphragm are modulated to meet respiratory demands during both inspiration and expiration and provide stability to the spine when there are repetitive limb movements.[35,36]

Effects of Intra-abdominal Pressure and the Valsalva Maneuver on Stability

During the Valsalva maneuver, contraction of the TrA, IO, and EO muscles increase IAP.[13] Contraction of the TrA alone pushes the abdominal contents up against the diaphragm; therefore, to complete the enclosed chamber, the diaphragm and pelvic floor muscles contract in synchrony with the TrA.[57] There are several ideas that explain how IAP improves spinal stability. The increased pressure in the enclosed chamber may act to unload the compressive forces on the spine as well as increase the stabilizing effect by pushing out against the abdominal muscles, increasing their length-tension relationship and tension on the thoracolumbar fascia (Figs. 14.16 and 14.17).[69] It is also suggested that the IAP may act to prevent buckling of the spine and thus prevent tissue strain or failure.[12]

The Valsalva maneuver is a technique frequently used by individuals lifting heavy loads and potentially has cardiovascular risks (see Chapter 6), so it is recommended that individuals be taught to exhale while maintaining the abdominal contractions to decrease the risks. In addition, Hodges and associates[41] found that if a static expulsive effort is maintained

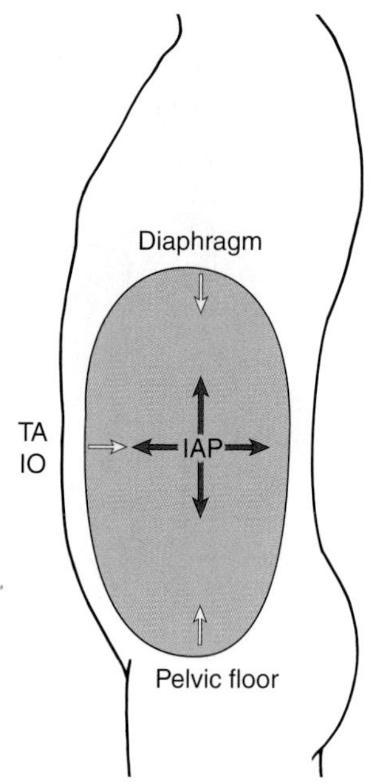

FIGURE 14.16 Coordinated contraction of the transversus abdominis, diaphragm, and pelvic floor musculature increases intra-abdominal pressure, which unloads the spine and provides stability.

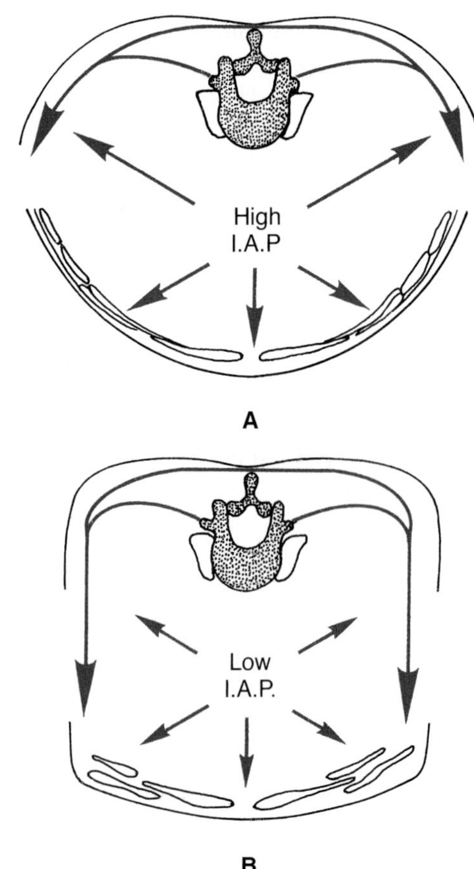

FIGURE 14.17 (A) Increased intra-abdominal pressure (IAP) pushes outward against the transversus abdominis and internal obliques, creating increased tension on the thoracolumbar fascia, resulting in improved spinal stability. **(B)** Reduced pressure decreases the stabilizing effect. *(Adapted from Gracovetsky, S:* The Spinal Engine. *New York: Springer-Verlag Wein, 1988, p 114, with permission.)*

(holding the breath while contracting the abdominal muscles), activation of the transverse abdominis is delayed. Because activation of the transversus abdominis is necessary for segmental spinal stability, expiration during exertion reinforces this stabilizing function.

Impaired Posture

In order to make sound clinical decisions when managing patients with activity or participation restrictions due to spinal impairments, it is necessary to understand the underlying effects of faulty posture on flexibility, strength, and the pain experienced by the individual. Impaired posture may be the underlying cause of the patient's pain or may be the result of some traumatic or pathological event. In this section, the etiology of pain and common faulty postures are described in detail followed by guidelines for developing therapeutic exercise interventions.

Etiology of Pain

The ligaments, facet capsules, periosteum of the vertebrae, muscles, anterior dura mater, dural sleeves, epidural areolar adipose tissue, and walls of blood vessels are innervated and responsive to nociceptive stimuli.[16]

Effect of Mechanical Stress

Mechanical stress to pain-sensitive structures, such as sustained stretch to ligaments or joint capsules or compression of blood vessels, causes distention or compression of the nerve endings, which leads to the experience of pain. This type of stimulus occurs in the absence of an inflammatory reaction. It is not a pathological problem but a mechanical one because signs of acute inflammation with constant pain are not present.

Relieving the stress to the pain-sensitive structure relieves the pain stimulus, and the person no longer experiences pain. If the mechanical stresses exceed the supporting capabilities of the tissues, breakdown ensues. If it occurs without adequate healing, musculoskeletal disorders or overuse syndromes with inflammation and pain affect function without an apparent injury (see Chapter 10). Relieving the mechanical stress (i.e., correcting the posture) along with decreasing the inflammation is important.

CLINICAL TIP

To illustrate the mechanical effects of prolonged stress on tissues, have your patient/client take one of their fingers to the end of the range in extension and hold the position with their other hand. After a brief period of time when they begin to feel some discomfort, have them move out of the end range position and note relief. Point out that this is what is happening to their joints and ligaments when they are in a sustained faulty posture.

Effect of Impaired Postural Support From Trunk Muscles

Little muscle activity is required to maintain upright posture, but with total relaxation of muscles, the spinal curves become exaggerated and passive structural support is called on to maintain the posture. When there is continued end-range loading, strain occurs with creep and fluid redistribution in the supporting tissues, making them vulnerable to injury.[74]

Continual exaggeration of the curves leads to postural impairment and muscle strength and flexibility imbalances as well as other soft tissue restrictions or hypermobility. Muscles that are habitually kept in a stretched position tend to test weaker because of a shift in the length-tension curve; this is known as *stretch weakness*.[46] Muscles kept in a habitually shortened position tend to lose their elasticity. These muscles test strong only in the shortened position but become weak as they are lengthened. This condition is known as *tight weakness*.[26]

Effect of Impaired Muscle Endurance

Endurance in muscles is necessary to maintain postural control. Sustained postures require continual, small adaptations in the stabilizing muscles to support the trunk against fluctuating forces. Large, repetitive motions also require muscles to respond so as to control the activity. In either case, as the muscles fatigue, the mechanics of performance change and the load is shifted to the inert tissues supporting the spine at the end-ranges.[71] With poor muscular support and a sustained load on the inert supporting tissues, creep and distention occur, causing mechanical stress. In addition, injuries occur more frequently after a lot of repetitive activity or long periods of work and play when there is muscle fatigue.

Pain Syndromes Related to Impaired Posture

Postural fault. A postural fault is a posture that deviates from normal alignment but has no structural impairments.

Postural pain syndrome. Postural pain syndrome refers to the pain that results from mechanical stress when a person maintains a faulty posture for a prolonged period; the pain is usually relieved with activity. There are no impairments in functional strength or flexibility, but if the faulty posture continues, strength and flexibility imbalances eventually develop.

Postural dysfunction. Postural dysfunction differs from postural pain syndrome in that adaptive shortening of soft tissues and muscle weakness are involved. The cause may be prolonged poor postural habits, or the dysfunction may be a result of contractures and adhesions formed during the healing of tissues after trauma or surgery. Stress to the shortened structures causes pain. In addition, strength and flexibility imbalances may predispose the area to injury or overuse syndromes that a normal musculoskeletal system could sustain.

Postural habits. Good postural habits in the adult are necessary to avoid postural pain syndromes and postural dysfunction. Also, careful follow-up in terms of flexibility and posture training exercises is important after trauma or surgery to prevent impairments from contractures and adhesions. In the child, good postural habits are important to avoid abnormal stresses on growing bones and adaptive changes in muscle and soft tissue.

Common Faulty Postures: Characteristics and Impairments

The head, neck, thorax, lumbar spine, and pelvis are all interrelated, and deviations in one region affect the other areas. For clarity of presentation, the lumbopelvic (or lower quarter) and cervicothoracic (or upper quarter) regions and typical muscle length-strength impairments for each region are described separately in this section and illustrated in Figure 14.18.

Pelvic and Lumbar Region

Lordotic Posture

Lordotic posture (see Fig. 14.18 A) is characterized by an increase in the lumbosacral angle (the angle that the superior border of the first sacral vertebral body makes with the horizontal, which optimally is 30°), an increase in lumbar lordosis, and an increase in the anterior pelvic tilt and hip flexion. It is often seen with increased thoracic kyphosis and forward head and is called kypholordotic posture.[46]

Potential Muscle Impairments

- Mobility impairment in the hip flexor muscles (iliopsoas, tensor fasciae latae, rectus femoris) and lumbar extensor muscles (erector spinae)
- Impaired muscle performance due to stretched and weak abdominal muscles (rectus abdominis, internal and external obliques, and transversus abdominis) and hip extensors (gluteus maximus and hamstrings)

Potential Sources of Symptoms

- Stress to the anterior longitudinal ligament.
- Narrowing of the posterior disc space and narrowing of the intervertebral foramen. This may compress the dura and blood vessels of the related nerve root or the nerve root itself, especially if there are degenerative changes in the vertebra or intervertebral disc.
- Approximation of the articular facets. Weight bearing through the facets may increase, which may cause synovial irritation and joint inflammation and may eventually accelerate degenerative changes if not corrected.

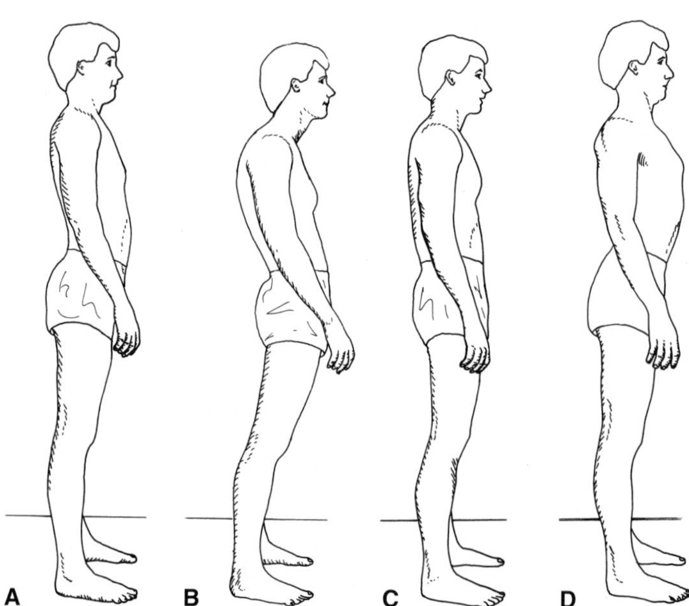

FIGURE 14.18 (A) Lordotic posture characterized by an increase in the lumbosacral angle, increased lumbar lordosis, increased anterior tilting of the pelvis, and hip flexion. **(B)** Relaxed or slouched posture characterized by excessive shifting of the pelvic segment anteriorly, resulting in hip extension, and shifting of the thoracic segment posteriorly, resulting in flexion of the thorax on the upper lumbar spine. A compensatory increased thoracic kyphosis and forward head placement are also seen. **(C)** Flat low-back posture characterized by a decreased lumbosacral angle, decreased lumbar lordosis, and posterior tilting of the pelvis. **(D)** Flat upper back and cervical spine characterized by a decrease in the thoracic curve, depressed scapulae, depressed clavicle, and an exaggeration of axial extension (flexion of the occiput on the atlas and flattening of the cervical lordosis).

Common Causes

Sustained faulty posture, pregnancy, obesity, and weak abdominal muscles are common causes.

Relaxed or Slouched Posture

The relaxed or slouched posture (see Fig. 14.18 B) is also called swayback.[46] The amount of pelvic tilting is variable, but usually there is a shifting of the entire pelvic segment anteriorly, resulting in hip extension, and shifting of the thoracic segment posteriorly, resulting in flexion of the thorax on the upper lumbar spine. This results in increased lordosis in the lower lumbar region, increased kyphosis in the thoracic region, and usually a forward head. The position of the mid and upper lumbar spine depends on the amount of displacement of the thorax. When standing for prolonged periods, the person usually assumes an asymmetrical stance in which most of the weight is borne on one lower extremity with pelvic drop (lateral tilt) and hip abduction on the unweighted side. This affects frontal plane symmetry.

A sitting slouched posture occurs when there is an overall kyphotic curve throughout the entire thoracic and lumbar spine.

Potential Muscle Impairments

- Mobility impairment in the upper abdominal muscles (upper segments of the rectus abdominis and obliques), internal intercostal, hip extensor, and lower lumbar extensor muscles and related fascia
- Impaired muscle performance due to stretched and weak lower abdominal muscles (lower segments of the rectus abdominis and obliques), extensor muscles of the lower thoracic region, and hip flexor muscles

Potential Sources of Symptoms

- Stress to the iliofemoral ligaments, the anterior longitudinal ligament of the lower lumbar spine, and the posterior longitudinal ligament of the upper lumbar and thoracic spine. With asymmetrical postures, there is also stress to the iliotibial band on the side of the elevated hip. Other frontal plane asymmetries may also be present and are described in the following section.
- Narrowing of the intervertebral foramen in the lower lumbar spine that may compress the blood vessels, dura, and nerve roots, especially with arthritic conditions.
- Approximation of articular facets in the lower lumbar spine.

Common Causes

As the name implies, this is a relaxed posture in which the muscles are not used to provide support. The person yields fully to the effects of gravity, and only the passive structures at the end of each joint range (e.g., ligaments, joint capsules, bony approximation) provide stability. Causes may be attitudinal (the person feels comfortable when slouching), fatigue (seen when required to stand for extended periods), or muscle weakness (the weakness may be the cause or the effect of the posture). A poorly designed exercise program—one that emphasizes thoracic flexion without balancing strength with other appropriate exercises and postural training—may perpetuate these impairments.

Flat Low-Back Posture

Flat low-back posture (see Fig. 14.18 C) is characterized by a decreased lumbosacral angle, decreased lumbar lordosis, hip extension, and posterior tilting of the pelvis.

Potential Muscle Impairments

- Mobility impairment in the trunk flexor (rectus abdominis, intercostals) and hip extensor muscles
- Impaired muscle performance due to stretched and weak lumbar extensor and possibly hip flexor muscles

Potential Sources of Symptoms

- Lack of the normal physiological lumbar curve, which reduces the shock-absorbing effect of the lumbar region and predisposes the person to injury
- Stress to the posterior longitudinal ligament
- Increase of the posterior disc space, which allows the nucleus pulposus to imbibe extra fluid and, under certain circumstances, may protrude posteriorly when the person attempts extension. This increased weight bearing on the disc may lead to degenerative changes.

Common Causes

Common causes include habitual slouching in flexion when sitting or standing and overemphasis on flexion exercises in general exercise programs.

Cervical and Thoracic Region

Round Back (Increased Kyphosis) With Forward Head

The round back with forward head posture (see Fig. 14.18 B) is characterized by an increased thoracic curve, protracted scapulae (round shoulders), and forward (protracted) head. A forward head involves increased flexion of the lower cervical and the upper thoracic regions, increased extension of the upper cervical vertebra, and extension of the occiput on C1. There also may be temporomandibular joint dysfunction with protrusion and depression of the mandible.

Potential Muscle Impairments

- Mobility impairment in the muscles of the anterior thorax (intercostal muscles), muscles of the upper extremity originating on the thorax (pectoralis major and minor, latissimus dorsi, serratus anterior), muscles of the cervical spine and head that attached to the scapula and upper thorax (levator scapulae, sternocleidomastoid, scalene, upper trapezius), and muscles of the suboccipital region (rectus capitis posterior major and minor, obliquus capitis inferior and superior)
- Impaired muscle performance due to stretched and weak lower cervical and upper thoracic erector spinae and scapular retractor muscles (rhomboids, middle and lower trapezius), anterior throat muscles (suprahyoid and infrahyoid muscles), and capital flexors (rectus capitis anterior and lateralis, superior oblique longus colli, longus capitis)
- With temporomandibular joint symptoms, the muscles of mastication (pterygoid, masseter, temporalis muscles) may experience increased tension

Potential Sources of Symptoms

- Stress to the anterior longitudinal ligament in the upper cervical spine and to the posterior longitudinal ligament and ligamentum flavum in the lower cervical and thoracic spine
- Fatigue of the thoracic erector spinae and scapular retractor muscles
- Irritation of facet joints in the upper cervical spine
- Narrowing of the intervertebral foramina in the upper cervical region, which may impinge on the blood vessels and nerve roots, especially if there are degenerative changes
- Impingement on the neurovascular bundle from anterior scalene or pectoralis minor muscle tightness (see "Thoracic Outlet Syndrome" in Chapter 13)
- Strain on the neurovascular structures of the thoracic outlet from scapular protraction[45]
- Impingement of the cervical plexus from levator scapulae muscle tightness
- Impingement on the greater occipital nerves from a tight or tense upper trapezius muscle, leading to tension headaches
- Temporomandibular joint pain from joint compression due to mandibular malalignment and tension headaches resulting from associated muscle tension in the mandibular elevator muscle group (see section on "Temporomandibular Joint Dysfunction" in Chapter 15).
- Lower cervical disc lesions from the faulty flexed posture

Common Causes

- The effects of gravity, slouching, and poor ergonomic alignment in the work or home environment. Occupational or functional postures requiring leaning forward or tipping the head backward for extended periods; faulty sitting postures, such as working at an improperly placed computer keyboard or screen, relaxed postures, or the end result of a faulty pelvic and lumbar spine posture are common causes of forward head posture. Causes are similar to the relaxed lumbar posture or the flat low-back posture in which there is continued slouching and overemphasis on flexion exercises in general exercise programs.

Flat Upper Back and Neck Posture

The flat upper back and neck posture (see Fig. 14.18 D) is characterized by a decrease in the thoracic curve, depressed scapulae, depressed clavicles, and decreased cervical lordosis with increased flexion of the occiput on atlas. It is associated with an exaggerated military posture but is not a common postural deviation. There may be temporomandibular joint dysfunction with protraction of the mandible.

Potential Muscle Impairments

- Mobility impairment in the anterior neck muscles, thoracic erector spinae, and scapular retractors, and potentially restricted scapular movement, which decreases the freedom of shoulder elevation
- Impaired muscle performance in the scapular protractor and intercostal muscles of the anterior thorax

Potential Sources of Symptoms

- Fatigue of muscles required to maintain the posture
- Compression of the neurovascular bundle in the thoracic outlet between the clavicle and ribs
- Temporomandibular joint pain and occlusive changes
- Decrease in the shock-absorbing function of the kypholordotic curvature, which may predispose the neck to injury

Common Causes

As noted, this is not a common postural deviation and occurs primarily with exaggeration of the military posture.

Frontal Plane Deviations: Scoliosis and Lower Extremity Asymmetries

Scoliosis

Scoliosis is defined as a lateral curvature in the spine. It usually involves the thoracic and lumbar regions. Typically, in right-handed individuals, there is a mild right thoracic, left lumbar S-curve, or a mild left thoracolumbar C-curve. There may be asymmetry in the hips, pelvis, and lower extremities.

Structural scoliosis. *Structural scoliosis* involves an irreversible lateral curvature with fixed rotation of the vertebrae (Fig. 14.19 A). Rotation of the vertebral bodies is toward the convexity of the curve. In the thoracic spine, the ribs rotate with the vertebrae, so there is prominence of the ribs posteriorly on the side of the spinal convexity and prominence anteriorly on the side of the concavity. A posterior rib hump is detected on forward bending in structural scoliosis (Fig. 14.19 B).[49]

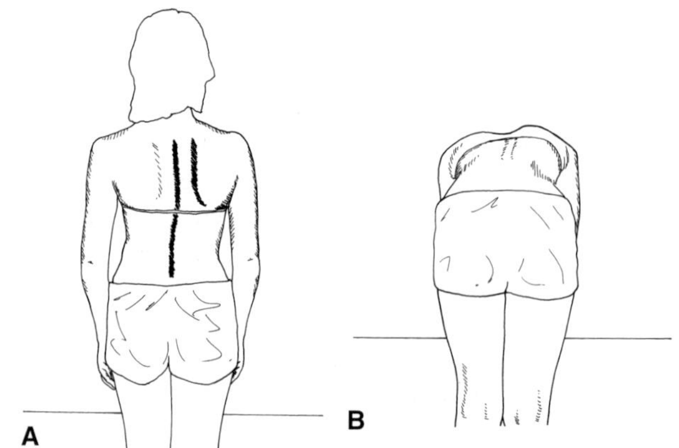

FIGURE 14.19 (A) Mild right thoracic left lumbar structural scoliosis with prominence of the right scapula. **(B)** Forward bending produces a slight posterior rib hump, indicating fixed rotation of the vertebrae and rib cage.

Nonstructural scoliosis. *Nonstructural scoliosis* is reversible and can be changed with forward or side bending and with positional changes, such as lying supine, realignment of the pelvis by correction of a leg-length discrepancy, or with muscle contractions. It is also called *functional* or *postural scoliosis.*

Potential Impairments

- Mobility impairment in joints, muscles, and fascia on the concave side of the curves.
- Impaired muscle performance due to stretch and weakness in the musculature on the convex side of the curves.
- If one hip is adducted, the adductor muscles on that side have decreased flexibility, and the abductor muscles are stretched and weak. The opposite occurs on the contralateral extremity.[46]
- With advanced structural scoliosis, there is decreased rib expansion; cardiopulmonary impairments may result in difficulty breathing.

Potential Sources of Symptoms

- Muscle fatigue and ligamentous strain on the side of the convexity
- Nerve root irritation on the side on the concavity
- Joint irritation from approximation of the facets on the side of the concavity

Common Causes: Structural Scoliosis

Neuromuscular diseases or disorders (e.g., cerebral palsy, spinal cord injury, progressive neurological or muscular diseases), osteopathic disorders (e.g., hemivertebra, osteomalacia, rickets, fracture), and idiopathic disorders in which the cause is unknown are common causes of structural scoliosis.

Common Causes: Nonstructural Scoliosis

Leg-length discrepancy (structural or functional), muscle guarding or spasm from a painful stimuli in the back or neck, and habitual or asymmetrical postures are common causes of nonstructural scoliosis.

Frontal Plane Deviations From Lower Extremity Asymmetries

Any lower extremity inequality has an effect on the pelvis that, in turn, affects the spinal column and structures supporting it.[23] When dealing with spinal posture, it is imperative to assess lower extremity alignment, symmetry, foot posture, ROM, muscle flexibility, and strength. (See Chapters 20 through 22 for principles, procedures, and techniques for treating the hip, knee, ankle, and foot.) Frontal plane deviations may also be seen with faulty postural habits such as perpetually standing with a pelvic drop on one side as frequently seen with relaxed postures. This may result in muscle imbalances in the hip and spine and an apparent leg-length discrepancy.

Characteristic Deviations

When standing with weight equally distributed to both lower extremities, an elevated ilium on the long leg (LL) side and lowered on the short leg (SL) side typically results in the following deviations (Fig. 14.20).

- The LL side is in hip adduction with greater shear stress, and the SL side is in hip abduction with greater compression stress.
- The sacroiliac (SI) joint on the LL side is more vertical with greater shear stress; on the SL side, it is more horizontal with greater compression stress.

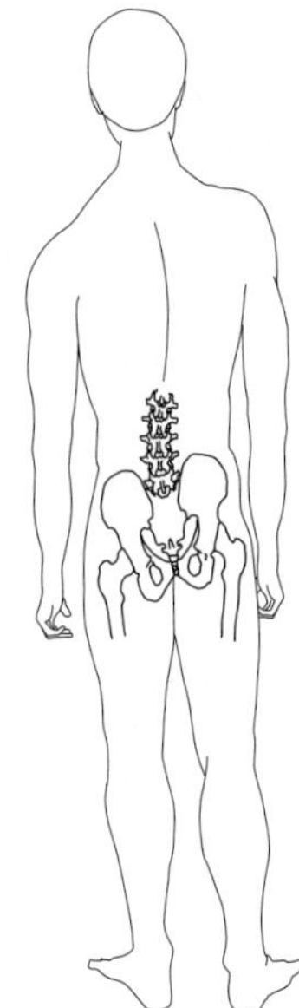

FIGURE 14.20 Frontal plane asymmetries. Pictured is an individual with a long leg and elevated ilium on the right side. Typically, hip adduction, vertical sacroiliac (SI) joint, side bending toward and rotation opposite that of the lumbar spine, and compensations in thoracic and cervical spine are seen on the long-leg side.

- There is side bending of the lumbar spine toward the LL side coupled with rotation in the opposite direction.
- The vertebral side bending and rotation compresses the intervertebral disc on the LL side and distracts the disc on the SL side; it also causes torsional stress.
- There is extension and compression of the lumbar facets on the LL side (concave portion of the curve) and flexion and distraction of the lumbar facets on the SL side (convex portion of the curve).
- There is narrowing of the intervertebral foramina on the LL side.
- The thoracic and cervical spine has compensatory scoliosis in the opposite direction.

Potential Muscle Impairments

- Mobility impairment from decreased flexibility in the hip adductors on the LL side and abductors on the SL side. There may also be asymmetrical differences in the iliopsoas, quadratus lumborum, piriformis, erector spinae, and multifidus muscles, with those on the concave side of the curve or the LL side having decreased flexibility.
- Impaired muscle performance from stretched and weakened muscles that typically includes hip adductors on the SL side, abductors on the LL side, and in general muscles on the convex side of the curve.

Potential Sources of Symptoms

- Greater shear forces occur in the hip and SI joints on the LL side, which increases stress in the supporting ligaments and decreases the load-bearing surface in the joint. Degenerative changes occur more frequently in hips on the LL side.[21]

- Stenosis in the lumbar intervertebral foramina on the LL side may cause vascular congestion or nerve root irritation.
- Lumbar facet compression and irritation on the LL side leading to early degenerative changes.
- Intervertebral disc breakdown from torsional and asymmetrical forces.
- Muscle tension, fatigue, or spasm in response to asymmetrical loading and response.
- Lower extremity overuse syndromes.

Common Causes

Asymmetry in the lower extremities may result from structural or functional deviations at the hip, knee, ankle, or foot. Common functional problems include unilateral flat foot and imbalances in the flexibility of muscles. The resulting asymmetrical ground reaction forces transmitted to the pelvis and back may lead to tissue breakdown and overuse, particularly as a person ages, becomes overweight, or is generally deconditioned from inactivity.

Management of Impaired Posture

Faulty posture underlies many spinal and extremity disorders and functional restrictions. Often by simply correcting the underlying postural stresses, the primary symptoms can be minimized or even alleviated. Because of this the following guidelines may become part of most rehabilitation programs. Exercises for use with postural impairments are identified in this section and are described in detail in the respective chapters that follow.

General Management Guidelines

Before developing a plan of care and selecting interventions for management, evaluate the findings from the examination of the patient, including the history, review of systems, and specific tests and measures, and document the findings.

- Postural alignment (sitting and standing), balance, and gait
- ROM, joint mobility, and flexibility
- Muscular strength and endurance for repetitions and holding
- Ergonomic assessment, if indicated
- Body mechanics
- Cardiopulmonary endurance/aerobic capacity, breathing pattern

Common impairments and a summary of the information that follows on management of patients with impaired posture are summarized in Box 14.1.

BOX 14.1 MANAGEMENT GUIDELINES—Impaired Posture

Structural and Functional Impairments

- Pain from mechanical stress to sensitive structures and from muscle tension
- Impaired mobility from muscle, joint, or fascial restrictions
- Impaired muscle performance associated with an imbalance in muscle length and strength between antagonistic muscle groups
- Impaired muscle performance associated with poor muscular endurance
- Insufficient postural control of scapular and trunk stabilizing muscles
- Decreased cardiopulmonary endurance
- Altered kinesthetic sense of posture associated with poor neuromuscular control and prolonged faulty postural habits
- Lack of knowledge of healthy spinal control and mechanics

Plan of Care	Intervention
1. Develop awareness and control of spinal posture	1. Kinesthetic training; cervical and scapular motions, pelvic tilts, control of neutral spine. Utilize procedures to develop and reinforce control of posture when sitting, standing, walking, and performing targeted functional activities
2. Educate the patient about the relationship between faulty posture and symptoms	2. Practice positions and movements to experience control of symptoms with various postures
3. Increase mobility in restricting muscles, joints, fascia	3. Manual stretching and joint mobilization/manipulation; teach self-stretching

BOX 14.1 MANAGEMENT GUIDELINES—Impaired Posture—cont'd

Plan of Care	Intervention
4. Develop neuromuscular control, strength, and endurance in postural and extremity muscles	4. Stabilization exercises; progress repetitions and challenge with extremity motions; progress to dynamic trunk strengthening exercises
5. Teach safe body mechanics	5. Functional exercises to prepare for safe mechanics (squatting, lunges, reaching, pushing/pulling, lifting and turning loads with stable spine)
6. Ergonomic assessment of home, work, recreational environments	6. Adapt work, home, recreational environment
7. Stress management/relaxation	7. Relaxation exercises and postural stress relief
8. Identify safe aerobic activities	8. Implement and progress an aerobic exercise program
9. Promote healthy exercise habits for self-maintenance	9. Integration of a fitness program, regular exercise, and safe body mechanics into daily life

Awareness and Control of Spinal Posture

Initially, good spinal posture may be prevented because of restricted mobility of muscle, connective tissue, or vertebral segment, but developing patient awareness of balanced posture and its effects should begin as soon as possible in the treatment program in conjunction with stretching and muscle-training maneuvers.

Posture Training Techniques

Isolate each body segment and train the patient to properly move that segment. If one region is out of alignment, it is likely that there are compensatory deviations in the alignment throughout the spine. Therefore, total posture correction, including upper and lower extremity alignment, should be emphasized. Direct the patient's attention to the feel of proper movement and muscle contraction and relaxation. Another technique is to have the patient assume an extreme corrected posture, then ease away from the extreme toward mid-position, and finally hold the corrected posture. Use verbal, tactile, and visual reinforcement cues such as:

- ***Verbal reinforcement.*** As you interact with the patient, frequently interpret the sensations of muscle contraction and spinal positions that he or she should be feeling.
- ***Tactile reinforcement.*** Help the patient position the head and trunk in correct alignment and touch the muscles that need to contract to move and hold the parts in place.
- ***Visual reinforcement.*** Use mirrors so the patient can see how he or she looks, what it takes to assume correct alignment, and then how it feels when properly aligned.

Axial Extension (Cervical Retraction) to Decrease a Forward Head Posture

Patient position and procedure: Sitting or standing, with arms relaxed at the side. Lightly touch above the lip under the nose and ask the patient to lift the head up and away as if a string was pulling their head upward (Fig. 14.21 A). Verbally reinforce the correct posture and draw attention to the way it feels. Have the patient move to the extreme of the correct posture and then return to midline.

Scapular Retraction

Patient position and procedure: Sitting or standing. For tactile and proprioceptive cues, gently resist movement of the inferior angle of the scapulae and ask the patient to pinch them together (retraction). Suggest that the patient imagine "holding a quarter between the shoulder blades" or imagine

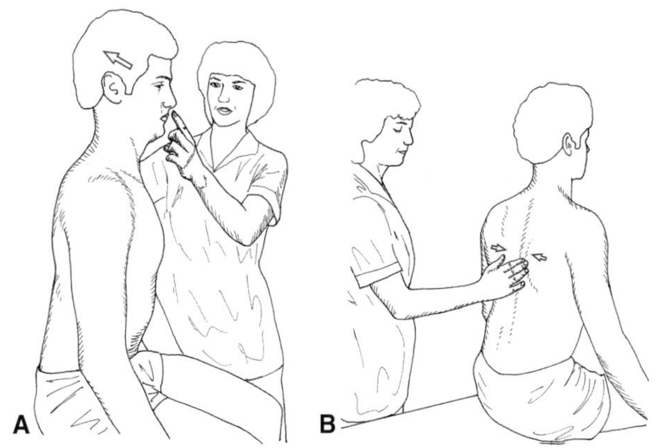

FIGURE 14.21 Training the patient to correct **(A)** forward-head posture and **(B)** protracted scapulae.

"putting their elbows in their back pockets" The patient should not extend the shoulders or elevate the scapulae (Fig. 14.21 B).

Pelvic Tilt and Neutral Spine

Patient position and procedure: Sitting, then standing with the back against a wall. Teach the patient to roll the pelvis forward and backward to isolate an anterior and posterior pelvic tilt. After the patient has learned to isolate the movement, instruct him or her to practice control of the pelvis and lumbar spine by moving from extreme lordosis to extreme flat back and then assume mild lordosis. Identify the midposition as the "neutral spine" so the patient becomes familiar with the term. Show that the hand should be able to easily slip between the back and the wall and that he or she can then feel the back with one side of the hand and the wall with the other side. If the patient has difficulty tilting the pelvis, suggest that he or she imagine that the pelvis is a bushel basket with a rounded bottom and the waist is the rim of the basket. Have the patient then imagine and practice tipping the "basket" forward and backward and then finding the neutral spine position.

Thoracic Spine

Patient position and procedure: Standing. The position of the thorax affects the posture of the lumbar spine and pelvis; consequently, the feel of thoracic movement is incorporated in posture training for the lumbar spine. As the patient assumes a mildly lordotic posture, have him or her breathe in and lift the rib cage (extension). Guide him or her to a balanced posture, not an extremely extended posture. Standing with the back against a wall (as in the pelvic tilt training above) encourages thoracic extension.

Total Spinal Movement and Control

Patient position and procedure: Sitting or standing. Instruct the patient to curl the entire spine by first flexing the neck, then the thorax, and then the lumbar spine. Give cues for unrolling by first touching the lumbar spine as the patient extends it, then the thoracic spine as he or she extends it and takes in a breath to elevate the rib cage. Then direct attention to adducting the scapulae while you gently resist the motion and then lifting the head in axial extension while you give slight pressure against the upper lip (see Fig. 14.21). If the patient overcorrects his or her posture, have them relax slightly to a neutral spinal position. Verbally and visually reinforce the correct posture when it is obtained.

Reinforcement techniques. It is not possible for a person always to maintain good posture. Therefore, to reinforce proper performance, teach the patient to use cues throughout the day to check posture. For example, instruct the patient to check the posture every time he or she walks past a mirror, waits at a red traffic light while driving a car, sits down for a meal, enters a room, or begins talking with someone. Find out what daily routines the patient has that could be used for reinforcement or reminders; instruct the patient to practice and report the results. Provide positive feedback as the patient becomes actively involved in the relearning process.

Postural support. If necessary, provide external support with a postural splint or tape to prevent the extreme posture of round shoulders and protracted scapulae. These supports help train correct muscle functioning by acting as a reminder for the patient to assume correct posture when he or she slouches. Also, by preventing the position of stretch from occurring, stretch weakness can be corrected. These devices should be used only on a temporary basis for training so the patient does not become dependent on them.

Posture, Movement, and Functional Relationships

Once the patient has learned how to assume correct postures, it is important to have him or her experience the effect sustained or repetitive faulty postures have on pain and function, followed by their ability to alter these affects by correcting their posture.

Relationship of impaired posture and pain. Have the patient assume the faulty posture and wait. When he or she begins to feel discomfort, point out the posture and then instruct how to correct it and notice the feeling of relief. Many patients do not accept such a simple relationship between stress and pain, so draw their attention to noticing what posture they are in (including when at work, home, driving/riding in a car, or in bed), when their symptoms develop, and how they can control the discomfort with the following techniques.

Relationship of impaired posture and extremity function. Have the patient assume their faulty posture and attempt a functional activity such as reaching upward with their upper extremity, moving their lower extremity, or opening and closing their jaw. They then assume a corrected posture, repeat the same activity, and note the difference. Once the improved range and quality of movement are experienced, reinforce them so the patient can understand the value of developing and maintaining good alignment when performing functional activities.

Joint, Muscle, and Connective Tissue Mobility Impairments

Common muscle imbalances in length and strength were described in the previous section on impaired postures. It is critical that specific mobility restrictions are identified so that stretching techniques can be selective. For example, the transition areas between the cervicothoracic, thoracolumbar, and lumbosacral regions typically have greater mobility. When faulty postural habits dominate, the segmental mobility in these areas tends to become exaggerated in the direction of the faulty posture. Stretching should proceed cautiously so as not to accentuate the problem while attempting to correct the tissues with decreased mobility. Stretching techniques for the cervical, thoracic, and lumbar regions are described in Chapter 16. Specific spinal mobilization/manipulation techniques directed at specific hypomobile segments are described in Chapters 15 and 16. Although any structure could be involved, particularly following an injury or pathological condition, the muscle flexibility impairments most typically seen are identified in Box 14.2. Included are references for self-stretching/flexibility exercises for each muscle group. Specific instructions and precautions are described in the text accompanying the pictures in the respective chapters.

Impaired Muscle Performance

Typically impaired postural muscles that support the body in sustained postures succumb to the effects of gravity, become less active,[61] and develop stretch weakness.[46] Strengthening alone does not correct this problem, so any exercises must be done in conjunction with posture training for control, as described earlier in this section. In addition, exercises for muscular endurance are necessary to prepare the muscles to function over an extended period of time. Finally, environmental adaptations must be made to minimize the stresses of sustained and repetitive postures. Muscles that typically demonstrate stretch weakness or poor postural endurance are identified in Box 14.3. In-depth descriptions of the exercises are in the chapters identified.

BOX 14.2 Self-Stretching Techniques for Common Mobility Impairments

- *Suboccipital region*: self-stretch with capital nodding; apply a gentle self-stretch against the occiput with the lateral border of the hand
- *Levator scapulae*: self-stretch with scapular depression and cervical flexion and rotation to the opposite side (see Fig. 17.35 in Chapter 17)
- *Scalenes*: self-stretch with axial extension, side bend neck opposite and then rotate neck toward side of restriction (see position Fig. 16.3 in Chapter 16)
- *Pectoralis major and anterior thorax*: self-stretch with corner stretches (see Fig. 17.31 in Chapter 17) or while lying supine on a foam roll placed longitudinally under the spine (see Fig. 16.1 B in Chapter 16)
- *Latissimus dorsi*: self-stretch lying supine on a foam roll, reach arms overhead (see Fig. 16.1 A in Chapter 16)
- *Lumbar and hip extensors*: self-stretch lying supine, bring knees to chest; or quadruped position, move buttocks back over the feet (see Figs. 16.13 and 16.14 in Chapter 16)
- *Lumbar flexors*: self-stretch with prone press-ups or standing back bends (see Fig. 16.15 in Chapter 16)
- *Hip flexors*: self-stretch lying supine in Thomas position or standing in modified fencer's squat (see Figs. 20.10 and 20.11 in Chapter 20)
- *Tensor fascia lata*: self-stretch either supine, side-lying, or standing; extend, laterally rotate, then adduct the hip (see Figs. 20.19, 20.20, and 20.21 in Chapter 20)
- *Iliotibial band foam roll stretch*: side-lie on a foam roll placed perpendicular to the thigh, gently roll the thigh back and forth with body weight applying the stretch force (see Fig. 21.22 in Chapter 21)
- *Pyriformis:* self-stretch lying supine or sitting and bringing the flexed knee toward the opposite shoulder. Flex, adduct, and internally rotate the hip (see Fig. 20.15 in Chapter 20)
- *Hamstrings*: self-stretch with a straight-leg maneuver either lying supine or long-sitting (see Figs. 20.17 and 20.18 in Chapter 20)
- *Gastrocsoleus (heel cords)*: self-stretch in a forward stride position with the heel of the back leg maintained on the floor, or stand on an incline board or edge of a step (see Fig. 22.9 in Chapter 22)

Body Mechanics

Muscle strengthening for safe body mechanics includes not only strengthening specific muscles, but also functional activities that prepare the body for specific stresses that it is required to do for a particular function, as identified in Box 14.4. Instruction in body mechanics is described in detail in Chapter 16 in the section "Functional Training."

Ergonomics: Relief and Prevention

It is critical to help the patient adapt postures and activities that are performed on a sustained or repetitive basis at work, at home, recreationally, or socially if they are contributing to

BOX 14.3 Training and Strengthening Techniques for Common Muscle Impairments

- Activate and learn control of the longus colli and deep capital flexors (see Figs. 16.39 B and 16.59 in Chapter 16)
- Lower cervical extension (see Fig. 16.40 in Chapter 16)
- Scapular retraction and shoulder lateral rotation (see Fig. 16.45 in Chapter 16 and Figs. 17.46 and 17.47 in Chapter 17)
- Lumbar spinal stabilization (see Figs. 16.47 through 16.56 plus accompanying text in Chapter 16)
- Hip abduction; posterior gluteus medius; begin side-lying, progress to standing. Place emphasis on maintaining the hip in extension with slight lateral rotation while abducting (see Fig. 20.26 B in Chapter 20)

BOX 14.4 Functional Exercises in Preparation for Safe Body Mechanics

- Upper extremity pulling and pushing (see Fig. 17.58 in Chapter 17)
- Wall slides—progress to squatting and squatting with lifting (see Fig. 20.29 in Chapter 20)
- Lunges—progress to lunges with lifting and with pushing and pulling (see Fig. 20.32 in Chapter 20 and Figs. 23.31 and Fig. 23.36 in Chapter 23)

the postural stresses and musculoskeletal disorders.[60] It may be necessary to use a lumbar pillow for support or to modify the work environment (workstation) to relieve sustained stressful postures. There are many resources, such as the Occupational Safety and Health Administration website (http://www.osha.gov/SLTC/ergonomics/) and others (http://ergo.human.cornell.edu/) that provide information on ergonomic assessment and adaptation to work environments to relieve postural stress and musculoskeletal disorders. Principles of ergonomic interventions are listed in Box 14.5.

FOCUS ON EVIDENCE

There is strong evidence, documented in a 3-year prospective study of 632 newly hired computer users, that a computer workstation may be the source of symptoms if the chair, desk, keyboard, mouse, and monitor are improperly positioned for the individual.[25,51] There is also mixed evidence, summarized in a systematic study of the literature on the relationship of posture and repetitive stresses in the work environment, regarding the development of low back pain.[77] In a 3-year follow-up study that involved 12,550 workers, it was determined that prolonged standing, awkward lifting, and squatting/kneeling were the top mechanical factors related to job related low back pain.[72]

Stress Management/Relaxation

A component of the educational process is to teach the individual how to relax tense muscles and relieve postural stress. Muscle relaxation techniques can be incorporated throughout the day to relieve postural stress, and conscious relaxation training increases patient awareness and control over tension in the muscles.

PRECAUTION: These techniques are not appropriate for managing acute pain due to inflammation, joint swelling, or disc derangements. If the patient is recovering from a pathologic condition in the spine, caution him or her that these techniques should not increase symptoms (other than a stretching sensation in chronic conditions), especially radicular symptoms. Caution should also be used with flexion in patients with a medical diagnosis of herniated disc so that symptoms should not peripheralize.

BOX 14.5 Basic Principles of Ergonomic Interventions

- Set up work station to keep everything within easy reach and at the proper height so that joints function in neutral positions and neutral postures can be maintained
- Minimize excessive repetitive motions
- Reduce excessive forces
- Minimize need to maintain a static hold on objects or maintain a static posture leading to fatigue
- Minimize pressure points
- Maintain adequate clearance around work station for safe movement
- Move head, spine, and extremities through their ROM frequently
- Use adequate lighting

Muscle Relaxation Techniques

Whenever discomfort develops from maintaining a constant posture or from sustaining muscle contractions for a period of time, active ROM in the opposite direction aids in taking stress off supporting structures, promoting circulation, and maintaining flexibility. All motions are performed slowly, through the full range, with the patient paying particular attention to the feel of the muscles. Repeat each motion several times. Suggest to the patient that these are mini rest breaks or micro breaks to be done at work, home, or whenever tension, stress, or postural pain is experienced.

Cervical and Upper Thoracic Region

Patient position and procedure: Sitting with the arms resting comfortably on the lap, or standing. Instruct the patient to:

- Bend the neck forward and backward. (Backward bending is contraindicated with symptoms of nerve root compression—if numbness or pain radiates down the arm, examine to identify cause; see Chapter 15 for interventions to treat nerve root compression.)
- Side bend the head in each direction; then rotate the head in each direction.
- Roll the shoulders; protract, elevate, retract, and then relax the scapulae (in a position of good posture).
- Circle the arms (shoulder circumduction). This is accomplished with the elbows flexed or extended, using either small or large circular motions with the arms pointing either forward or out to the side. Both clockwise and counterclockwise motions should be performed, but conclude the circumduction by going forward, up, around, and then back so the scapulae end up in a retracted position. This has the benefit of helping retrain proper posture.

Lower Thoracic and Lumbar Region

Patient position and procedure: Sitting or standing. If standing, the feet should be shoulder-width apart with the knees slightly bent. Have the patient place the hands at the waist with the fingers pointing backward. Instruct the patient to:

- Extend the lumbar spine by leaning the trunk backward (see Fig. 16.15 B). This is particularly beneficial when the person must sit or stand in a forward-bent position for prolonged periods.
- Flex the lumbar spine by contracting the abdominal muscles, causing a posterior pelvic tilt; or bend the trunk forward while sitting, dangling the arms toward the floor. This motion is beneficial when the person stands in a lordotic or swayback posture for prolonged periods.
- Side bend in each direction.

- Rotate the trunk by turning in each direction while keeping the pelvis facing forward.
- Stand up and walk around at frequent intervals when sitting for extended periods.

Conscious Relaxation Training for the Cervical Region

Specific techniques in guided imagery for the cervical region develop the patient's kinesthetic awareness of a tensed or relaxed muscle and how consciously to reduce tension in the muscle. In addition, if done with posture training techniques in mind, as described earlier in the chapter, the patient can be helped to recognize decreased muscular tension when the head is properly balanced and the cervical spine is aligned in midposition.

Patient position and procedure: Sitting comfortably with arms relaxed, such as resting on a pillow placed on the lap; the eyes are closed. Position yourself next to the patient to use tactile cues on the muscles and help position the head as necessary. Have the patient perform the following activities in sequence.

- Use diaphragmatic breathing and breathe in slowly and deeply through the nose, allowing the abdomen to relax and expand; then relax and allow the air to be expired through the relaxed open mouth. This breathing is reinforced after each of the following activities.
- Next, relax the jaw. The tongue rests gently on the hard palate behind the front teeth with the jaw slightly open. If the patient has trouble relaxing the jaw, have him or her click the tongue and allow the jaw to drop. Practice until the patient feels the jaw relax and the tongue rests behind the front teeth. Follow with relaxed breathing.
- Slowly flex the neck. As the patient does so, direct the attention to the posterior cervical muscles and the sensation of how the muscles feel. Use verbal cues such as, "Notice the feeling of increased tension in your muscles as your head drops forward."
- Then slowly raise the head to neutral, inhale slowly, and relax. Help the patient position the head properly and suggest that he or she note how the muscles contract to lift the head, and then relax once the head is balanced.
- Repeat the motion; again, direct the patient's attention to the feeling of contraction and relaxation in the muscles as he or she moves. Imagery can be used with the breathing such as "fill your head with air and feel it lift off your shoulders as you breathe in and relax."
- Then go through only part of the range, noting how the muscles feel.
- Next, just think of letting the head drop forward and then tightening the muscles (setting); then think of bringing the head back and relaxing. Reinforce to the patient the ability to influence the feeling of contraction and relaxation in the muscles.
- Finally, just think of tensing the muscles and relaxing, letting the tension go out of the muscles even more. Point out that he or she feels even greater relaxation. Once the patient learns to perceive tension in muscles, he or she can then consciously think of relaxing the muscles. Emphasize the fact that the position of the head also influences muscle tension. Have the patient assume various head postures and then correct them until the feeling is reinforced.

Modalities and Massage

Once acute symptoms are under control, the use of modalities and massage are minimized or decreased so the patient learns self-management through exercises, relaxation, and posture retraining and does not become dependent on external applications of interventions for comfort.

Healthy Exercise Habits

It is important to integrate a progression of postural control into all exercises, aerobic conditioning, and functional activities (see Chapter 16). The patient is carefully observed as greater challenges to activities are performed, and, if necessary, reminders are provided to find the neutral spinal position and to initiate contraction of the stabilizing muscles prior to the activity. For example, when reaching overhead, the patient learns to contract the abdominal muscles to maintain a neutral spine position and not allow the spine to extend into a painful or unstable range. This is incorporated into body mechanics, such as when going from picking up and lifting to placing an object on a high shelf, or into sport activities when reaching up to block or throw a ball. Once developed under your guidance, encourage the patient to continue with a healthy lifestyle, fitness level, and body mechanics.

Independent Learning Activities

Critical Thinking and Discussion

1. What are the functional differences between the way the cervical spine and lumbar spine are used in daily activities?
2. Explain how faulty posture can cause painful symptoms.
3. Explain why a "one-size-fits-all" exercise program for posture correction cannot benefit everyone, or how it may be detrimental to some individuals. Discuss this in relation to each of the faulty postures described in this chapter.

Laboratory Practice

1. Practice identifying the effects various postures have on the various regions of the spine—that is, what happens to the cervical and lumbar spine when in supine, prone, side-lying, sitting, and standing postures; does the spine tend to move into flexion or extension? Determine what is needed to change the position; that is, if flexion is emphasized in a particular posture, what is needed to move the spine into a more neutral (midrange) position?
2. Identify and feel what happens to the various portions of the spine when moving from one position to another (i.e., rolling supine to prone and return, moving from supine to sit, sit to stand and reverse). What happens to the lumbar spine and pelvis when walking; how is this affected if the person has a hip-flexion contracture or a contracture in the external rotators of the hip?
3. Examine the standing posture of a classmate; then examine the joint ROM, muscle flexibility, and muscle strength. Identify any muscle imbalances in length and strength; then design an intervention program to influence change in the impairments. Use the guidelines presented in this chapter and summarized in Box 14.1 as well as Chapters 16 through 22 for suggested exercises and their safe application.
4. Identify and compare the similarities and differences in flexibility and muscle weakness between a person with excessive lumbar lordosis and an anterior pelvic tilt and a person with a slouched posture who stands with the pelvis shifted forward and the thorax flexed. What effect does each pelvic posture have on the hip position, and what muscles would develop restricted mobility? Usually in the slouched posture the thorax and upper lumbar spine are flexed; would the curl-up exercise be beneficial, or would it contribute to this problem? Develop an exercise program that addresses the common flexibility and strength impairments without reinforcing the faulty posture.

Case Studies

Case 1

Your patient is a 35-year-old computer programmer who is referred to you because of pain symptoms in the right cervical, posterior shoulder, and arm regions. The symptoms get progressively worse when at work; usually the pain begins within 1 hour, and it is 6/10 by lunchtime. The same cycle occurs in the afternoon. There is occasional "tingling" in the thumb and index finger. The symptoms have progressively worsened over the last 3 months, ever since being placed in a priority job. Recreational activities include tennis and reading; the tennis does not cause symptoms, but reading makes the neck pain worse.

Examination reveals forward head and round shoulder posture. Capital flexion 50% range, cervical rotation and side bending are each 80% range, shoulder external rotation is 75°. There is restricted flexibility in the pectoralis major, pectoralis minor, levator scapulae, and scalene muscles. Cervical quadrant test reproduces the tingling in the right hand; all other neurological tests are negative. Strength of the suprahyoid and infrahyoid muscles, scapular retractors, and shoulder lateral rotators is 4/5.

- What is provoking the patient's symptoms and signs? What are the functional limitations? What is the prognosis?
- Identify impairment and functional outcome goals.
- Establish a program of intervention. How can you progress this person to functional independence?

Case 2

A 51-year-old auto mechanic is referred to physical therapy because of pain symptoms in the left buttock and posterior thigh. The symptoms are worse when standing and reaching overhead for more than 15 minutes, which is what he does when working on a car that is up on the racks. Carrying heavy objects (> 50 lb), standing, and walking for more than a half-hour increase the symptoms. There is no precipitating incident, but the symptoms have been recurrent over the past year. Symptoms also increase with the recreational activity of backpacking. Symptoms ease when in the rocker recliner, lying on a couch with knees bent, or when hugging knees to chest.

Examination reveals swayback posture when standing; decreased flexibility in the low back, gluteus maximus, hamstrings (straight leg raising to 60°), and upper abdominals; and increased pain with backward bending. Strength of the lower abdominals is 3/5. He is able to do repetitive lunges and partial squats for a maximum of 20 seconds.

- What is provoking the patient's symptoms and signs? What are the functional limitations? What is the prognosis?
- Identify impairment and functional outcome goals.
- Establish a program of intervention. Use the taxonomy of motor tasks discussed in Chapter 1 (see Figs. 1.6 and 1.7 and accompanying text) to develop a progression of exercises and tasks to progress this person to functional independence.

REFERENCES

1. Allison, GT, Morris, SL, and Lay, B: Feedforward responses of transversus abdominis are directionally specific and act asymmetrically: implications for core stability theories. *J Orthop Sports Phys Ther* 38(5):228–237, 2008.
2. Andersson E, et al: The role of the psoas and iliacus muscles for stability and movement of the lumbar spine, pelvis, and hip. *Scand J Med Sci Sports* 5:10–16, 1995.
3. Barr, KP, Griggs, M, and Cadby, T: Lumbar stabilization: core concepts and current literature. Part 1. *Am J Phys Med Rehabil* 84:473–480, 2005.
4. Basmajian, JV: *Muscles Alive,* ed. 4. Baltimore: Williams & Wilkins, 1979.
5. Beazell, JR: Dysfunction of the longus colli and its relationship to cervical pain and dysfunction: a clinical case presentation. *J Manual Manipulative Ther* 6(1):12–16, 1998.
6. Beneck, GJ, and Kulig K. Multifidus atrophy is localized and bilateral in active persons with chronic unilateral low back pain. *Arch Phys Med Rehabil* 93(2):300–306, 2012.
7. Bo, K, Sherburn, M, and Allen, T: Transabdominal ultrasound measurement of pelvic floor muscle activity when activated directly or via a transverse abdominis muscle contraction. *Neurourol Urodyn* 22:582–588, 2003.

8. Bogduk, N, and MacIntosh, JE: The applied anatomy of the thoracolumbar fascia. *Spine* 9:164–170, 1984.
9. Bogduk, N, and Twomey, LT: *Clinical Anatomy of the Lumbar Spine and Sacrum,* ed. 4. New York: Elsevier Churchill-Livingston, 2005.
10. Chen, YY, Pao, JL, Liam, CK, Hsu, WL, and Yang, RS. Image changes of paraspinal muscles and clinical correlations in patients with unilateral lumbar spinal stenosis. *Eur Spine J* 23(5):999–1006; 2014.
11. Cholewicki, J, Panjabi, MM, and Khachatryan, A: Stabilizing function of trunk flexor-extensor muscle around a neutral spine posture. *Spine* 22(19):2207–2212, 1997.
12. Cholewicki, J, et al: Intra-abdominal pressure mechanism for stabilizing the lumbar spine. *J Biomech* 32:13–17, 1999.
13. Cresswell, AG, Grundstrom, H, and Thorstensson, A: Observations on intra-abdominal pressure and patterns of abdominal intra-muscular activity in man. *Acta Physiol Scand* 144:409–418, 1992.
14. Crisco, J: Stability of the human ligamentous lumbar spine. *Clin Biomech* 7:19–32, 1992.
15. Critchley, D: Instructing pelvic floor contraction facilitates transversus abdominis thickness increase during low-abdominal hollowing. *Physiother Res Int* 7(2):65–75, 2002.
16. Dalton, D: The vertebral column. In Levangie, P, and Norkin, C (eds): *Joint Structure and Function: A Comprehensive Analysis,* ed. 5. Philadelphia: F.A. Davis, 138–187, 2011.
17. Danneels, L, et al: The effects of three different training modalities on the cross-sectional area of the paravertebral muscles. *Scand J Med Sci Sports* 11:335–341, 2001.
18. D'hooge, R, et al: Increased intramuscular fatty infiltration without differences in lumbar muscle cross-sectional area during remission of recurrent low back pain. *Man Ther* 19(6):584–588, 2012.
19. Djordjevic, O, Djordjevic, A, and Konstantinovic, L. Interrater and intrarater reliability of transverse abdominal and lumbar multifidus muscle thickness in subjects with and without low back pain. *J Orthop Sports Phys Ther* 44(12):979–988, 2014.
20. Ebenbichler, GR, et al: Sensory-motor control of the lower back: implications for rehabilitation. *Med Sci Sports Exerc* 33(11):1889–1898, 2001.
21. Farfan, HF, et al: The effects of torsion on the lumbar intervertebral joints: the role of torsion in the production of disc degeneration. *J Bone Joint Surg Am* 52(3):468–497, 1970.
22. Fortin, M, and Macedo, LG. Multifidus and paraspinal muscle group cross-sectional areas of patients with low back pain and control patients: a systematic review with a focus on blinding. *Phys Ther* 93(7):873–888, 2013.
23. Friber, O: Clinical symptoms and biomechanics of lumbar spine and hip joint in leg length inequality. *Spine* 8:643–651, 1983.
24. Fritz, JM, Erhard, RD, and Hagen, BF: Segmental instability of the lumbar spine. *Phys Ther* 78(8):889–896, 1998.
25. Gerr, F, et al: A prospective study of computer users. I. Study design and incidence of musculoskeletal symptoms and disorders. *Am J Ind Med* 41:221–235, 2002.
26. Gossman, M, Sahrmann, S, and Rose, S: Review of length-associated changes in muscle. *Phys Ther* 62:1799–1808, 1982.
27. Gracovetsky, S, Farfan, H, and Helleur, C: The abdominal mechanism. *Spine* 10:317–324, 1985.
28. Gracovetsky, S, and Farfan, H: The optimum spine. *Spine* 11:543–573, 1986.
29. Gracovetsky, S: *The Spinal Engine.* New York: Springer-Verlag Wein, 1988.
30. Grant, R, Jull, G, and Spencer, T: Active stabilization training for screen-based keyboard operators—a single case study. *Aust Physiother* 43(4): 235–232, 1997.
31. Hickey, DS, and Hukins, DW: Aging changes in the macromolecular organization of the intervertebral disc: an x-ray diffraction and electron microscopic study. *Spine* 7(3):234–242, 1982.
32. Hides, JA, Jull, GA, and Richardson, CA: Long-term effects of specific stabilizing exercises for first-episode low back pain. *Spine* 26:E243–E248, 2001.
33. Hides, JA, et al: Evidence of lumbar multifidus muscle wasting ipsilateral to symptoms in patients with acute/subacute low back pain. *Spine* 19(2):165–172, 1994.
34. Hides, JA, Richardson, CA, and Jull, GA: Multifidus muscle recovery is not automatic after resolution of acute, first-episode low back pain. *Spine* 21:2763–2769, 1996.
35. Hodges, P, and Gandevia, SC: Changes in intra-abdominal pressure during postural and respiratory activation of the human diaphragm. *J Appl Physiol* 89:967–976, 2000.
36. Hodges, P, and Gandevia, SC: Activation of the human diaphragm during a repetitive postural task. *J Physiol* 522:165–175, 2000.
37. Hodges, PW, and Richardson, CA: Altered trunk muscle recruitment in people with low back pain with upper limb movement at different speeds. *Arch Phys Med Rehabil* 80(9):1005–1012, 1999.
38. Hodges, PW, and Richardson, CA: Transversus abdominis and the superficial abdominal muscles are controlled independently in a postural task. *Neurosci Lett* 265(2):91–94, 1999.
39. Hodges, P, Cresswell, A, and Thorstensson, A: Preparatory trunk motion accompanies rapid upper limb movement. *Exp Brain Res* 134: 69–79, 1999.
40. Hodges, PW, and Richardson, CA: Delayed postural contraction of transversus abdominis in low back pain associated with movement of the lower limb. *J Spinal Disord* 11(1):46–56, 1998.
41. Hodges, PW, Gandevia, SC, and Richardson, CA: Contractions of specific abdominal muscles in postural tasks are affected by respiratory maneuvers. *J Appl Physiol* 83(3):753–760, 1997.
42. Hodges, PW, and Richardson, CA: Relationship between limb movement speed and associated contraction of the trunk muscles. *Ergonomics* 40(11):1220–1230, 1997.
43. Hodges, PW, and Richardson, CA: Feedforward contraction of transversus abdominis is not influenced by direction of arm movement. *Exp Brain Res* 114(2):362–370, 1997.
44. Hodges, PW, and Richardson, CA: Contraction of the abdominal muscles associated with movement of the lower limb. *Phys Ther* 77(2): 132–142, 1997.
45. Julius, A, et al: Shoulder posture and median nerve sliding. *BMC Musculoskel Disord* 5:23, 2004.
46. Kendall, FP, et al: *Muscles: Testing and Function, with Posture and Pain,* ed. 5. Baltimore: Lippincott Williams & Wilkins, 2005.
47. Klein, JA, and Hukins, DW: Collagen fiber orientation in the annulus fibrosus of intervertebral disc during bending and torsion measured by x-ray defraction. *Biochim Biophys Acta* 719:98–101, 1982.
48. Krag, MH, et al: Internal displacement distribution from in vitro loading of human thoracic and lumbar spinal motion segments: experimental results and theoretical predictions. *Spine* 12:1001–1007, 1987.
49. Levangie, P, and Norkin, C: *Joint Structure and Function: A Comprehensive Analysis,* ed. 5. Philadelphia: F.A. Davis, 2011.
50. Lundon, K, and Bolton, K: Structure and function of the lumbar intervertebral disc in the health, aging, and pathologic conditions. *J Orthop Sports Phys Ther* 31(6):291–306, 2001.
51. Marcus, M, et al: A prospective study of computer users. II. Postural risk factors for musculoskeletal symptoms and disorders. *Am J Ind Med* 41:236–249, 2002.
52. Marras, WS, and Granata, KP: Changes in trunk dynamics and spine loading during repeated trunk exertions. *Spine* 22(21):2564–2570, 1997.
53. McGill, SM: Low back exercises: evidence for improving exercise regimens. *Phys Ther* 78(7):754–765, 1998.
54. McGill, SM, and Norman, RW: Low back biomechanics in industry: the prevention of injury through safer lifting. In Grabiner, M (ed): *Current Issues in Biomechanics.* Champaign, IL: Human Kinetics, 1993.
55. Moseley, GL, Hodges, PW, and Gandevia, SC: Deep and superficial fibers of the lumbar multifidus muscle are differently active during voluntary arm movements. *Spine* 27:E29–36, 2002.
56. Neumann, DA: *Kinesiology of the Musculoskeletal System: Foundations for Physical Rehabilitation.* St. Louis: Mosby, 2002.
57. Neumann, P, and Gill, V: Pelvic floor and abdominal muscle interaction: EMG activity and intra-abdominal pressure. *Int Urogynecol J* 13:125–132, 2002.
58. Ng, JK-F, et al: Relationship between muscle fiber composition and functional capacity of back muscles in healthy subjects and patients with back pain. *J Orthop Sports Phys Ther* 27(6):389–402, 1998.
59. Nourbakhsh, MR, and Arab, AM: Relationship between mechanical factors and incidence of low back pain. *J Orthop Sports Phys Ther* 32(9): 447–460, 2002.

60. Novak, CB: Upper extremity work-related musculoskeletal disorders: a treatment perspective. *J Orthop Sprots Phys Ther* 34(10):628–637, 2004.
61. O'Sullivan, PB, et al: The effect of different standing and sitting postures on trunk muscle activity in a pain-free population. *Spine* 27(11): 1238–1244, 2002.
62. Park, RJ, et al: Changes in regional activity of the psoas major and quadratus lumborum with voluntary trunk and hip tasks and different spinal curvatures in sitting. *J Orthop Sports Phys Ther* 43(2): 74–83, 2013.
63. Penjabi, MM: The stabilizing system of the spine. Part I. Function, dysfunction, adaptation, and enhancement. *J Spinal Disord* 5:383–389, 1992.
64. Penjabi, MM: The stabilizing system of the spine. Part II. Neutral zone and instability hypothesis. *J Spinal Disord* 5:390–397, 1992.
65. Porterfield, JA, and DeRosa, C: *Mechanical Low Back Pain: Perspectives in Functional Anatomy,* ed. 2. Philadelphia: WB Saunders, 1998.
66. Richardson, C, Hodges, P, and Hides, J: *Therapeutic Exercise for Lumbopelvic Stabilization: A Motor Control Approach for the Treatment and Prevention of Low Back Pain,* ed. 2. Edinburgh: Churchill Livingstone, 2004.
67. Richardson, CA, et al: Techniques for active lumbar stabilisation for spinal protection: a pilot study. *Aust J Physiother* 38:105–111, 1992.
68. Richardson, CA, Toppenberg, R, and Jull, G: An initial evaluation of eight abdominal exercises for their ability to provide stabilisation for the lumbar spine. *Aust J Physiother* 36:6–11, 1990.
69. Sapsford, RR, et al: Co-activation of the abdominal and pelvic floor muscles during voluntary exercises. *Neurol Urodynam* 20:31–42, 2001.
70. Sapsford, RR, and Hodges, PW: Contraction of the pelvic floor muscles during abdominal maneuvers. *Arch Phys Med Rehabil* 82:1081–1088, 2001.
71. Sparto, PJ, et al: The effect of fatigue on multijoint kinematics, coordination, and postural stability during a repetitive lifting test. *J Orthop Sports Phys Ther* 25(1):3–11, 1997.
72. Sterud, T, and Tynes, T. Work-related psychosocial and mechanical risk factors for low back pain: a 3-year follow-up study of the general working population in Norway. *Occup Environ Med* 70(5):296–302, 2013.
73. Teichtahl, AL, et al: Physical inactivity is associated with narrower lumbar intervertebral discs, high fat content of paraspinal muscles and low back pain and disability. *Arthritis Res Ther*. May 17(1):114, 2015.
74. Twomey, LT: A rationale for the treatment of back pain and joint pain by manual therapy. *Phys Ther* 72:885–892, 1992.
75. Twomey, T, and Taylor, JR: Sagittal movements of the human lumbar vertebral column: a quantitative study of the role of the posterior vertebral elements. *Arch Phys Med Rehabil* 64:322–325, 1983.
76. Urquhart, DM, et al: Abdominal muscle recruitment during a range of voluntary exercises. *Manual Ther* 10(2):144–153, 2005.
77. Waddell, G, and Burton, AK: Occupational health guidelines for the management of low back pain at work: evidence review. *Occup Med* 51(2):124–135, 2001.
78. White, AA, and Panjabi, MM: *Clinical Biomechanics of the Spine,* ed. 2. Philadelphia: JB Lippincott, 1990.
79. Wong, AY, Parent, EC, Funabashi, M, and Kawchuk, GN. Do changes in transversus abdominis and lumbar multifidus during conservative treatment explain changes in clinical outcomes related to nonspecific low back pain? A systematic review. *J Pain* 15(4):377.e1–35, 2014.
80. Wong, AY, Parent, EC, Funabashi, M, Stanton, TR, and Kawchik, GN. Do various baseline characteristics of transversus abdominis and lumbar multifidus predict clinical outcomes in nonspecific low back pain? A systematic review. *Pain* 154(12):2589–2602, 2013.

CHAPTER 15

The Spine: Management Guidelines

CAROLYN KISNER, PT, MS ■ JACOB N. THORP, PT, DHS, OCS, MTC

In theory, treating impairments and activity limitations related to the tissues of the spinal column and trunk is the same as treating tissue injuries of the extremities. The major complicating factor in the spine is the close proximity of key structures to the spinal cord and nerve roots. The challenge for the therapist is to recognize the complex functional relationships of the facet joints, the intervertebral joints, the muscles, the fascia, and the nervous system and know how to examine and evaluate the individual who presents with pain and activity limitations. Activity, rather than prolonged bed rest, has long been accepted as important in the management of patients with spinal and postural pain[2,242] but defining what are beneficial and safe activities during the process of healing and rehabilitation is the task of the therapist.

The medical model of diagnosis does not lend itself to direct therapeutic exercise intervention strategies, particularly because patients' complaints of back or neck pain often do not relate to specific pathologies. Efforts are being made to determine the most effective way to categorize patients with symptoms affecting spine and trunk function in order to be more accurate with outcome research.[37,49,73,158,159,204,214] In addition, results from research studies have provided some criteria for predicting outcomes in subgroups of patients with back and neck pain so therapists can better identify the interventions that are more likely to result in positive outcomes.[9,14,38,42,103,145,198,200,233,249] The approach described in this text supports the importance of treatment based on the presenting structural and functional impairments that result in activity limitations while respecting the pathomechanics, pathophysiology, and precautions of specific medical diagnoses.

The content of this chapter has three major emphases. The first section reviews the pathology and pathomechanics of spinal structures. The focus of the second section is on principles and guidelines for managing patients with impaired function in the spine. This section includes principles of interventions for the broad categories of acute, subacute, and chronic spinal conditions and also expands on specific interventions for impairment-based diagnostic categories and their relationship to the Clinical Practice Guidelines.[37,48] Techniques geared toward treating specific impairments are described in these sections.

The third major section contains medical diagnoses unique to the thoraco-lumbopelvic and upper thoraco-craniocervical regions. Because the function of the temporomandibular joint (TMJ) is closely related to the cervical spine, physical therapy management guidelines for impairments related to the TMJ conclude the chapter.

General therapeutic exercise techniques of intervention for all spinal and postural impairments are described in Chapter 16. Chapters 14, 15, and 16 are written with the assumption that the reader has completed or is concurrently taking a course in examination and evaluation of the spine and posture.

Spinal Pathologies and Impaired Spinal Function

Pathology of the Intervertebral Disc

Normal structure and function of the intervertebral (IV) disc are described in Chapter 14. Trauma, as well as normal aging, can lead to degeneration of the disc and affect the mechanics of the entire spine.[91,195]

Injury and Degeneration of the Disc

Various authors have defined the terms herniation, protrusion, and extrusion differently.[23,65,148,158,213] The following definitions are used in this text (Fig. 15.1):

- *Herniation*: displacement of disc material beyond the normal limits of the IV disc space. It may include the nucleus pulposus, cartilage, fragmented apophyseal bone, or annulus fibrosus. Herniated discs are further described as *protrusions* or *extrusions*, based on the shape of material outside the disc space.[88]
- *Protrusion*: the displaced disc material is continuous with the material within the disc. This is also described as the nuclear material being contained by the outer layers of the annulus and supporting ligamentous structures.
- *Extrusion*: extension of nuclear material beyond the confines of the posterior longitudinal ligament or above and below the disc space, as detected on magnetic resonance imaging (MRI),[213] but may still be in contact with the disc,[158] or may be completely sequestrated.[65]
- *Sequestration*: the extruded disc material is no longer contained by the outer annulus and has separated and moved away from the IV disc.[65,158]

Fatigue Breakdown and Traumatic Rupture

A decrease in the continuity and integrity of structure of the annulus fibrosus may be a consequence of the normal aging process resulting in annular fissures or may be caused by fatigue breakdown or traumatic rupture

Fatigue breakdown. Over time, the annulus breaks down as a result of repeated overloading of the spine in flexion with asymmetrical forward bending and torsional stresses.[3,4,66]

- With torsional stresses, the annulus becomes distorted, most obviously at the posterolateral corner opposite the direction of rotation. The layers of the outer annulus fibrosus lose their cohesion and begin to separate from each other. Each layer then acts as a separate barrier to the nuclear material. Eventually, radial tears occur, and there is communication of the nuclear material between the layers.[66]
- With repeated forward bending and lifting or prolonged postural stresses, the layers of the annulus are strained.

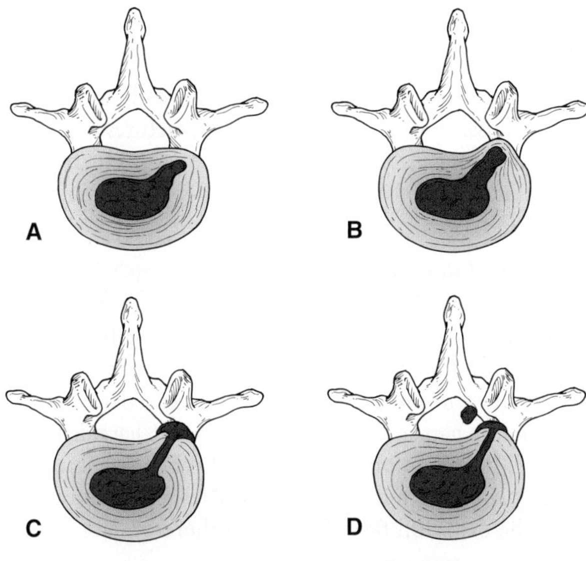

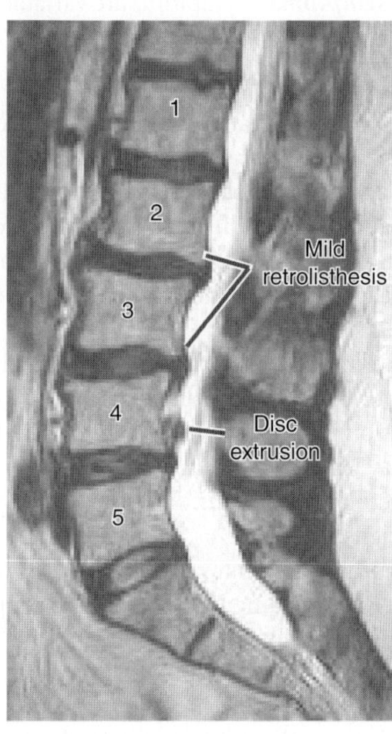

FIGURE 15.1 Disc breakdown, showing **(A)** breakdown and compression of fibrous layers of the annulus and displacement of disc material; **(B)** radial fissures with nuclear material bulging against the outer annulus; **(C)** extrusion of nuclear material through the outer annulus but still in contact with the disc; **(D)** sequestration of nuclear material beyond the annulus; and **(E)** MRI scan of a 61-year-old patient with low back pain and symptoms radiating into the leg. The scan demonstrates moderate multilevel degenerative disc disease of T12–L1 through L4–5 with mild retrolisthesis of L2 on L3 and L3 on L4. At the L4–5 level, note a small diffuse disc herniation with large paracentral disc extrusion dissecting cranially.

They become tightly packed together in the posterolateral corners, radial fissures develop, and the nuclear material migrates down the fissures.[3,4] Outer layers of annular fibers can contain the nuclear material so long as they remain a continuous layer.[3] After injury, there is a tendency for the nucleus to swell and distort the annulus. Distortion is more severe in the region in which the annular fibers are stretched.[4] If the outer layers rupture, nuclear material may herniate through the fissures.

- Healing is attempted, but there is poor circulation in the disc.[17] There may be self-sealing of a defect with nuclear gel or proliferation of cells of the annulus. Any fibrous repair is weaker than normal and takes a long time because of the relative avascular status of the disc.

Traumatic rupture. Rupture of the annulus can occur as a one-time event, or it can be superimposed on a disc where there has been gradual breakdown of the annular rings. This is seen most commonly in traumatic hyperflexion injuries.[4]

Axial Overload

Axial overload (compression) of the spine usually results in end-plate damage or vertebral body fracture before there is any damage to the annulus fibrosus.[25] Scheuermann's disease occurs when the nucleus migrates either superior or inferior through a cracked end-plate. When there is a compression fracture, flexion and axial loading usually causes increased pain. Pain may occur without nerve root involvement, although there may be referred pain in the extremities. Scheuermann's disease and compression fracture are discussed in the third section of this chapter.

Age

Individuals are most susceptible to symptomatic disc injuries between the ages of 30 and 45 years. During this time the nucleus is still capable of imbibing water, but the annulus weakens owing to fatigue loading over time and therefore is less able to withstand increased pressures when there are disproportionately high or repetitive stresses. The nuclear material may protrude into the tears of fissures, which most commonly are posterolateral and, with increased pressures, may bulge against the outer annular fibers, causing annular distortion. The nuclear material may also extrude from the disc through complete fissures in the annulus.[3,17,66,148]

Degenerative Changes

Any loss of integrity of the disc from infection, disease, herniation, or an end-plate defect becomes a stimulus for degenerative changes in the disc.[17] A strong genetic component has been linked to disc degeneration, whereas smoking and a history of heavy lifting appear to have little effect on this disease process.[16] Battie[16] identified people who were diagnosed with a disc injury prior to turning age 21 and found they were four to five times more likely to have a significant family history of IV disc pathologies.

- Degeneration is characterized by progressive fibrous changes in the nucleus, loss of the organization of the rings of the annulus fibrosus, and loss of cartilaginous end-plates.[14]
- As the nucleus becomes more fibrotic, it loses its capacity to imbibe fluid. Water content decreases, and there is an

associated decrease in the size of the nucleus. Acute disc protrusions caused by a bulging nucleus pulposus against the annulus or extrusions of the nucleus through a torn annulus are rare in older people.

- It is possible to have protrusions of the annulus fibrosus without bulging from nuclear pressure. Myxomatous degeneration with annular protrusion has been demonstrated in disc lesions in older people.[248]

Effect on Spinal Mechanics

Injury or degeneration of the disc affects spinal mechanics in general.[187] During the early stages, there is increased mobility of the segment with greater than normal flexion/extension and forward and backward translation of the vertebral body, leading to segmental instability. Force distribution through the entire segment is altered, causing abnormal forces in the facets and supporting structures.[31,66]

Disc Pathologies and Related Conditions

Disc herniation, tissue fluid stasis, discogenic pain, and swelling from inflammation are conditions that may result from prolonged flexion postures, repetitive flexion microtrauma, or traumatic flexion injuries. Initially, symptoms may be exacerbated when attempting extension but then may be decreased when using carefully controlled extension motions. Several studies have documented that patients with a herniated nucleus pulposus (HNP) who have symptom reduction with an extension approach to treatment respond favorably to conservative nonsurgical treatment.[9,26,48,133,201,220]

Tissue Fluid Stasis

During sustained end-range flexed postures in the spine, the discs, facet joints, and ligaments are placed under sustained loading.[23] The intradiscal pressure increases, and there is compression loading on the cartilage of the facets and a distractive tension on the posterior longitudinal ligament and posterior fibers of the annulus fibrosus. Ligamentous creep and fluid transfer occur. Sudden movement into extension does not allow for redistribution of the fluids and so increases the vulnerability of the distended tissue to injury and inflammation.[234] Symptoms may be similar to those described for disc lesions because they lessen with repeated extension motions and respond to treatment described in the management section (under Extension Bias) later in the chapter.

Signs and Symptoms of Disc Lesions and Fluid Stasis

Etiology of Symptoms

The disc is innervated by the mixed spinal nerve and the gray ramus communicans. Since only the outer one-third of the annulus has nerve innervation,[189] not all disc protrusions are symptomatic.

Pain. Symptoms of pain arise from pressure of a swollen disc or swollen tissues against pain-sensitive structures (ligaments, dura mater, blood vessels around nerve roots) or from the chemical irritants of inflammation if there is herniated disc material.[17,197]

Neurological signs and symptoms. Neurological signs arise from pressure against the spinal cord or nerve roots. The only true neurological signs and symptoms are specific myotome weaknesses and specific dermatome sensory changes. Radiating pain in a dermatomal pattern, increased myoelectric activity in the hamstrings, decreased straight-leg raising, and depressed deep tendon reflexes can also be associated with referred pain stimuli from spinal muscles, interspinous ligaments, the disc, and facet joints and therefore are not true signs of nerve root pressure.[126,164]

Variability of symptoms. Symptoms are variable depending on the degree and direction of the protrusion as well as the spinal level of the lesion.

- Posterior or posterolateral protrusions are most common. With a small posterior or posterolateral lesion, there may be pressure against the posterior longitudinal ligament or against the dura mater or its extensions around the nerve roots. The patient may describe a severe midline backache or pain spreading across the back into the buttock and thigh.
- A large posterior protrusion may cause spinal cord signs such as loss of bladder control and saddle anesthesia. If a large protrusion is untreated or undiagnosed in the cervical region, it may lead to cervical myelopathy.
- A large posterolateral protrusion may cause partial cord or nerve root signs.
- An anterior protrusion may cause pressure against the anterior longitudinal ligament, resulting in back pain. There are no neurological signs.
- The most common levels of protrusion are the segments between the fourth and fifth lumbar vertebrae and between the fifth lumbar vertebra and sacrum,[149,190,191,217] although a protrusion may occur at any level, including the cervical spine. Disc herniations in the thoracic spine are extremely rare (only 1 in 1,000[190,191]) due in part to the small disc to vertebrae ratio and the stable osseous anatomy of the thoracic region. They are most common at T11 and T12 because of the increased mobility in this area. A herniation in the thoracic region is much more severe than a herniation in the lumbar spine because if the disc herniates directly posterior, this will place the person at risk for spinal cord compression.

Shifting symptoms. Symptoms from a disc lesion may shift if there is integrity of the annular wall because the hydrostatic mechanism is still intact.[158,159]

Inflammation. Contents of the nucleus pulposus in the neural canal may cause an inflammatory reaction and irritate the dural sac, its nerve root sleeves, or the nerve roots. The symptoms may persist for extended periods and are not responsive to purely mechanical changes. The back pain may be worse than leg pain on the straight-leg raising test. Poor resolution of this inflammatory stimulus may lead to fibrotic reactions, nerve mobility impairments, and chronic pain.[155,209,212] Early medical intervention with anti-inflammatory agents is usually necessary.[209] However, patients with large sequestration fragments have better success with surgery.[127,226]

Onset and Behavior of Symptoms From Disc Lesions

Onset. Onset is usually between 20 and 55 years of age but most frequently from the mid-30s to 40s. Except in cases of trauma, symptomatic onset in the lumbar spine is usually associated simply with bending, bending and lifting, or attempting to stand up after having been in a prolonged recumbent, sitting, or forward-bent posture. The person may or may not have the sensation of something tearing.[159] Although cervical disc lesions are not as prevalent, a prolonged flexed spinal position as in a forward head posture may lead to or exacerbate symptoms from a protrusion. Many patients have a predisposing history of a faulty flexion posture.

Pain behavior. Pain may increase gradually when the person is inactive, such as when sitting or after a night's rest. The patient often describes increased pain when attempting to get out of bed in the morning or when first standing up. Symptoms are usually aggravated with activities that increase the intradiscal pressure, such as sitting, forward bending, coughing, straining, or when attempting to stand after being in a flexed position. Usually, symptoms are lessened when walking except when the bulge is large or the nuclear material has prolapsed and moved beyond the confines of the annulus.[159]

Acute pain. When there is inflammation during the acute phase, pain is almost always present but varies in intensity, depending on the person's position or activity.

When there is a lumbar disc lesion, initially discomfort is noticed in the lumbosacral or buttock region. Some patients experience aching that extends into the thigh or leg. In the cervical spine, initially pain is noticed in the midscapular and shoulder area. Numbness or muscle weakness (neurological signs) is not noted unless the protrusion has progressed to a degree to which there is nerve root, spinal cord, or cauda equina compression.

Objective Clinical Findings in the Lumbar Spine

NOTE: The following information relates to a contained posterior or posterolateral nuclear protrusion in the lumbar spine.[159] The impairments are summarized in Box 15.1.

- The patient usually prefers standing and walking to sitting.

BOX 15.1 Summary of Common Impairments Related to Disc Protrusions in the Lumbar Spine

- Pain, muscle-guarding
- Flexed posture and deviation away from (usually) the symptomatic side
- Neurological symptoms in dermatome and possibly myotome of affected nerve roots
- Increased symptoms (peripheralization) with sitting, prolonged flexed postures, transition from sit to stand, coughing, straining
- Limited nerve mobility, such as straight-leg raising (usually between 30° and 60°)
- Peripheralization of symptoms with repeated forward-bending (spinal flexion) tests

- The patient may have a decrease in or loss of lumbar lordosis and may have some lateral shifting of the spinal column.
- Forward bending is limited. When repeating the forward-bending test, the symptoms increase or peripheralize. *Peripheralization* means the symptoms are experienced farther down the leg (Fig. 15.2).
- Backward bending is limited; when repeating the backward-bending test, the pain lessens or centralizes.[140,146,250] *Centralization* means that the symptoms recede up the leg or become localized to the back. If the protrusion cannot be mechanically reduced, backward bending peripheralizes or increases the symptoms.
- If there is a *lateral shift* of the spinal column, backward bending increases the pain. If the lateral shift is first corrected, repeated backward bending lessens or centralizes the pain (see Figs. 15.6 and 15.7 in the management section of this chapter).
- Testing passive lumbar flexion in the supine position (double knees-to-chest) and passive extension in the prone position (press-ups) usually produces signs similar to those of the standing tests, but results may not be as dramatic because gravity is eliminated.
- Pain between 30° and 60° of straight-leg raising is considered positive for interference of dural mobility but not pathognomonic for a disc protrusion.[235]
- Contained nuclear protrusion can be influenced by movement because the hydrostatic mechanism is still intact. A complete tear of the outer layers of the annulus disrupts the hydrostatic mechanism, so the herniated or prolapsed nuclear material cannot be influenced by movement.[158] Anti-inflammatory intervention by a physician is important during the acute phase. Patients with disc extrusions may respond to conservative measures owing to resolution of the inflammation and resorption of the disc material.[213]

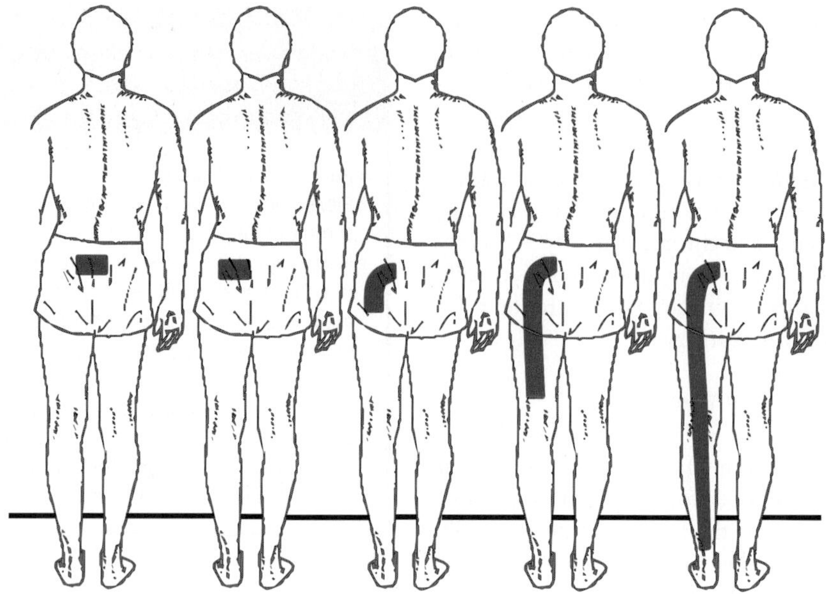

FIGURE 15.2 Examples of peripheralization and centralization of lower-quarter symptoms. Viewing the images left to right illustrates peripheralization of symptoms; from right to left illustrates centralization.

Objective Clinical Findings in the Cervical Spine

- Findings are similar to those in the lumbar spine except they are displayed in the respective dermatomes and myotomes of the cervical nerve roots.
- Initially, the patient may present with a faulty forward head posture and may hold the head in a guarded side-bent or rotated position away from the symptomatic side.
- Cervical flexion peripheralizes the symptoms; neck retractions (axial extension) followed by extension may centralize the symptoms of a contained nuclear bulge.
- There may be nerve mobility impairments in the upper extremity.
- Manual distraction may relieve or centralize the symptoms.
- In severe cases, the patient may present with bilateral symptoms or cervical myelopathy characterized by gait abnormalities, upper motor neuron lesions, and/or leg weakness and paresthesia due to pressure on or irritation of the spinal cord.

Pathomechanical Relationships of the Intervertebral Disc and Facet Joints

The disc and facets make up a three-joint complex between two adjoining vertebrae and are biomechanically interrelated. An asymmetrical disc injury affects the kinematics of the entire unit plus the joints above and below, resulting in asymmetrical movements of the facets, abnormal stresses, and eventually cartilage degeneration.[188]

Disc Degeneration

As the disc degenerates, there is a decrease in both water content and disc height. The vertebral bodies approximate, and the IV foramina and spinal canal narrow.[31] This is called degenerative disc disease.

Initial Changes

Initially, there is increased slack with increased mobility and translation in the spinal segment. Opposition of the facet surfaces changes and the capsules are strained, resulting in irritation, swelling, and muscle spasm.

Altered Muscle Control

Altered joint receptor function negatively affects muscle recruitment in swollen joints.[212] Pain has also been cited as a factor for altered and diminished recruitment patterns in the stabilizing muscles of the spine.[108,109,112] Increasing shear forces from poor midrange stabilization places increased stresses on the osteoligamentous support structures, which is thought to contribute to segmental hypermobility or instability.[72]

Progressive Bony Changes

Eventually, with the repeated irritation due to the faulty mechanics, there are progressive bony changes in the facet and vertebral body margins. This is known as spondylosis, osteoarthritis (OA), or degenerative joint disease (DJD). Osteophyte formation along the facets and spondylitic lipping and spurring along the vertebral bodies occur, and hypomobility develops.[165] These changes lead to additional narrowing of the associated foramina and spinal canal. In the cervical spine, the uncovertebral joints thicken, roughen, and distort.[207]

Related Pathologies

Segmental (Clinical) Instability

Segmental instability has been described as poor control in the neutral zones within the physiological range of spinal movement because of a decrease in the capacity of the neuromuscular stabilizing system to control the movement.[72,188] Clinically, patients demonstrate difficulty moving in the midranges of spinal motion and may demonstrate shifting or fluctuation in movement (see the section on pathomechanics of spinal instability in this chapter).

Stenosis

Stenosis is narrowing of a passage or opening. In the spine, stenosis is any compromise of the space in the spinal canal (central stenosis), nerve root canal, or foramen (lateral stenosis); it can be congenital or acquired and can occur at any age. The narrowing may be caused by soft tissue structures, such as a disc protrusion, fibrotic scars, or joint swelling; by bony narrowing as with spondylitic osteophyte formation or spondylolisthesis; or by faulty posture. With progression, neurological symptoms develop. Extension exacerbates the symptoms.[175]

 **FOCUS ON EVIDENCE**

The report of a study in which patients with four or more of the following variables identified a specificity of 0.98 for central stenosis: bilateral LE symptoms, leg pain that is worse than back pain, pain during walking and/or standing, pain relief with sitting, and more than 48 years old.[44]

Neurological Symptoms: Radiculopathy

Spinal nerve root or spinal cord symptoms may occur:

- When protrusion of the disc compresses against the cord or nerve roots.
- When there is decreased disc height due to degenerative changes[196] or excessive translation of the vertebra from shear forces resulting in decreased foraminal space. The nerve root becomes impinged between the tip of the superior articulating facet and the pedicle.
- When there is an inflammatory response due to trauma, degeneration, or disease with accompanying edema and stenosis.
- When spondylosis results in osteophytic growth on the articular facets or along the disc borders of the vertebral bodies that decreases spinal canal or IV foraminal size.
- When there is spondylolisthesis or when there is scarring or adhesion formation after injury or spinal surgery.

Dysfunction

The cycle of dysfunction caused by injury, pain, and muscle splinting leads to further restriction of movement, pain, and muscle splinting unless appropriate therapy is introduced. There are additional descriptions of facet joint pathologies in the following section.

Pathology of the Zygapophyseal (Facet) Joints

Facet joints are synovial articulations that are enclosed in a capsule and supported by ligaments; they respond to trauma and arthritic changes similar to any peripheral joint.

Various types of meniscoid-like structures or invaginations of the facet capsules are present in the zygapophyseal joints of the spine. They are synovial reflections containing fat and blood vessels. In some cases, dense fibrous tissue develops as a result of mechanical stresses.[23] Some people describe entrapment of these structures between the articulating surfaces with sudden or unusual movement as a source of pain and limited motion via tension on the well-innervated capsule.[23,228] Bogduk[23] describes the *locked-back mechanism* as being "extrapment" of the meniscoids in the supracapsular or infracapsular folds, which then blocks the return to extension from the flexed position. It is called an "extrapment" because the meniscoid fails to re-enter the joint cavity; consequently, it becomes a space-occupying lesion in the capsular folds, causing pain as it impacts against and stretches the capsules.

Common Diagnoses and Impairments From Facet Joint Pathologies

The etiology of facet joint pathologies may be a result of trauma, degeneration, or a systemic disease. Box 15.2 summarizes the impairments and functional limitations.

Facet Sprain/Joint Capsule Injury

There is usually a history of trauma, such as falling or a motor vehicle accident. The joints react with effusion (swelling), limited range of motion (ROM), and accompanying muscle guarding. The swelling may cause foraminal stenosis and neurological signs.

Spondylosis, Osteoarthritis, and Degenerative Joint Disease

Spondylosis and OA are synonymous terms. This pathology may also be referred to as DJD. Osteoarthritis involves degeneration of the IV disc as well as the facet joints. Usually, there is a history of faulty posture, prolonged immobilization after injury, or severe or repetitive trauma.

- During the early stages of degenerative changes, there is greater play, or hypermobility/instability, in the three-joint

BOX 15.2 Summary of Common Impairments and Activity Limitations Related to Facet Joint Pathology

- *Pain*: When acute, there is pain and muscle guarding with all motions; pain when subacute and chronic is related to periods of immobility or excessive activity.
- *Impaired mobility*. Usually hypomobility and decreased joint play in affected joints; there may be hypermobility or instability during early stages.
- *Impaired posture.*
- *Impaired spinal extension:* Extension may cause or increase neurological symptoms due to foraminal stenosis; therefore, may be unable to sustain or perform repetitive extension activities without exacerbating symptoms.
- *Any activity that requires flexibility or prolonged repetition of trunk motions*, such as repetitive lifting and carrying of heavy objects, may exacerbate symptoms in the arthritic spine.

complex. Over time, stress from the altered mechanics leads to osteophyte formation with spurring and lipping along the joint margins and vertebral bodies. Progressive hypomobility with bony stenosis results. The encroachment of osteophytes on the spinal canal and IV foramina may cause neurological signs, especially with spinal extension and side bending.

- Usually, when there is hypomobility, compensatory hypermobility occurs in neighboring spinal segments.
- Pain with movement and/or joint stiffness following periods of rest are the primary reasons people seek physical therapy.
- Pain may result from the stresses of excessive mobility or from stretch to hypomobile structures. Pain may also be a result of the encroachment of developing osteophytes against pain-sensitive tissue or of swelling and irritation because of excessive or abnormal mobility of the segments.
- The degenerating joint is vulnerable to facet impingement, sprains, and inflammation, as is any arthritic joint.
- In some patients, movement relieves the symptoms; in others, movement irritates the joints, and painful symptoms increase.

Rheumatoid Arthritis

Symptoms of rheumatoid arthritis (RA) can affect any of the synovial joints of the spine and ribs. There is pain and swelling.

- RA in the cervical spine presents special problems. There are neurological symptoms wherever degenerative change or swelling impinges against neurological tissue. There is increased fragility of tissues affected by RA, such as osteoporosis with cyst formation, erosion of bone, and instabilities from ligamentous necrosis. Most common of the serious lesions are atlantoaxial subluxation and C4–5 and C5–6 vertebral dislocations.[163]
- Pain or neurological signs originating in the spine may or may not be related to subluxation. Therefore, these signs should be used as a precaution whenever dealing with this disease because of the potential damage to the spinal cord.[163]
- Radiograph or CT scan examinations are important in ruling out instabilities; signs and symptoms alone are not conclusive.

PRECAUTION: Inappropriate movements of the spine in patients with RA, such as performing cervical manipulation, could be life-threatening or extremely debilitating because of the potential to cause damage to the cervical cord or vertebral artery.[163]

Ankylosing Spondylitis

Ankylosing spondylitis (AS) is a rheumatic disease characterized by chronic inflammation of the ligaments in the lumbar and spinal areas.[80] The inflamed cartilage/bony junction will fuse in approximately 20% of the population.[241]

- The prevalence of this pathology is approximately 1 to 3 per 1,000 people, and the diagnosis peaks in the mid-20s.[59]
- This pathology appears to begin in the lumbar spine and progress cephalad. The sacroiliac (SI) joints are affected nearly 100% of the time, followed by the neck (75%), lumbosacral area (50%), and hips and heels (30%).[80,141]
- There is a gradual loss of motion and the person will complain of general stiffness. The patient may initially complain of bilateral pain in his or her SI joints, thoracic spine, or shoulders. The person will wake up early with pain and stiffness and have difficulty standing up straight.
- In advanced cases, radiographs will reveal a "bamboo" spine. This imaging identifies where the anterior longitudinal ligament has fused to the vertebral bodies. Decreased joint spaces may also be identified on the film.[80,141]

FOCUS ON EVIDENCE

Rudwaleit and associates[206] identified four variables that were often seen in people with ankylosing spondylitis. The variables were stiffness greater than 30 minutes in duration, back pain that improved with exercise but not rest, back pain that wakes a person up in the second half of the night, and alternating buttock pain. If three or more of these parameters were met, this yielded a positive likelihood ratio of 12.4 and specificity and sensitivity of .97 and .34, respectively.

PRECAUTION: Atlanto-axial subluxation is the hallmark of cervical spine involvement. Extreme caution should be used when assessing and manipulating the cervical spine region to avoid causing serious or fatal injury.[80,141,239]

Facet Joint Impingement (Blocking, Fixation, Extrapment)

With a sudden or unusual movement, the meniscoid of a facet capsule may be extrapped, impinged (entrapped), or stressed, which causes pain and muscle guarding. The onset is sudden and usually involves forward bending and rotation.[23,234]

- There is loss of specific motions and attempted movement induces pain. At rest, the individual has no pain.
- There are no true neurological signs, but there may be referred pain in the related dermatome.
- Over time, stress is placed on the contralateral joint and on the disc, leading to problems in these structures.

Pathology of the Vertebrae

Axial overload (compression) of the spine may cause end-plate damage or vertebral body fracture. Compression fracture is a complication of osteoporosis.

Compression Fracture Secondary to Osteoporosis

The prevalence, risk factors, prevention, recommendations for general exercise, and exercise precautions for osteoporosis are described in detail in Chapter 11, with information related to the older population in Chapter 24. Vertebral compression fractures most often occur in the thoracolumbar region as the result of a fall or trauma or from performing basic activities of daily living (ADLs) that require forward bending of the trunk.

- Fractures usually occur during the sixth or seventh decade of life in the anterior vertebral body.
- Pain may be referred to the low back or abdominal region with or without lower extremity radiculopathy.
- Patients present with increased thoracic kyphosis (sometimes called dowager's hump) and lumbar lordosis secondary to instability, bony changes (wedging), and muscle weakness.
- Exercise prescription is based on the person's pain tolerance.
- Surgical interventions, such as vertebroplasty, may be indicated in severe cases or to prevent progression.
- The risk of low back pain (LBP) caused by a serious pathology, in the absence of trauma is less than 1% in the general population.[99] The physical therapist is encouraged to be concerned when multiple red flags are present versus a single outlying sign or symptom.

FOCUS ON EVIDENCE

Henske et al[98] identified five major factors that may incriminate a spinal fracture. These variables include >50 years old, female gender, history of major trauma, pain and tenderness, and/or co-occurring distraction/painful injury. Additionally, this same study reported that a person with ≥3 of the following variables had a posttest probability of 52% for a vertebral compression fracture. The variables were: >70 years old, female gender, significant trauma, and prolonged use of corticosteroids.

Scheuermann's Disease

Scheuermann's disease is a rare congenital and/or degenerative weakening of the vertebral endplates, typically seen at T10–L2.[149] The nucleus pulposus can protrude vertically into the vertebral end-plate, which can lead to a bony necrosis or Schmorl's nodes. Scheuermann's disease may also be caused by insufficient blood supply to the growing bone. This pathology is usually seen in the second decade of life and may be diagnosed as "growing pains." Intervention should be related to presenting signs with the caution to minimize compressive forces on the vertebrae.

Pathology of Muscle and Soft Tissue Injuries: Strains, Tears, and Contusions

Common impairments and functional limitations are summarized in Box 15.3.

General Symptoms From Trauma

Often more than one tissue is injured as a result of trauma. The extent of the tissue involvement may not be detectable during the acute phase.

- There is pain, localized swelling, tenderness on palpation, and protective muscle guarding regardless of whether the injured tissue is inert or contractile. Muscle guarding serves the immediate purpose of immobilizing the region. If the muscle contraction is prolonged, it results in the buildup of metabolic waste products and sluggish circulation. This altered local environment results in irritation of the free nerve endings, so the muscle continues to contract and becomes the source of additional pain (see Fig. 10.1).
- Ligamentous strains cause pain when the ligament is stressed. If torn, there is hypermobility of the segment.
- As healing of the involved structures occurs, there may be adaptive shortening or scar tissue adhering to surrounding tissue and restricting tissue mobility and postural alignment.

Common Sites of Lumbar Strain

A common site for injury in the lumbar region is along the iliac crest. This is where many forces converge around the attachment of the lateral raphe of the lumbodorsal fascia, quadratus lumborum, erector spinae, and iliolumbar ligament (see Fig. 14.12). Injury to this region frequently occurs with falls and with repeated loading of the region during lifting or twisting motions.

BOX 15.3 Summary of Common Impairments and Activity Limitations Associated With Muscle and Soft Tissue Injuries

Acute Stage

- Pain and muscle guarding
- Pain with contraction of the muscle or stretch on the muscle
- Interference with ADLs (rolling over, turning, sitting, sit to stand, standing, walking)

Subacute and Chronic Stages

- Impaired muscle performance
- Impaired mobility—may have contractures in muscle and related connective tissue or may have adhesions at site of tissue injury
- Impaired spinal control and stabilization during functional activities
- Impaired postural awareness
- Limited IADLs, work, and recreational activities (difficulty with repetitive or sustained postures, lifting, pushing, pulling, reaching, and holding loads)

Common Sites of Cervical Strain

Common injuries in the neck and upper thoracic region occur with flexion/extension trauma. Serious cervical trauma may result in vertebral fractures and spinal cord injury. Discussion of vertebral fractures and spinal cord injury is beyond the scope of this text.

Extension injuries. When the head rapidly accelerates into extension, if nothing stops it (such as a headrest in a car), the occiput is stopped by the thorax. The posterior structures, especially the joints, are compressed. The anterior structures (longus colli, suprahyoid, and infrahyoid muscles) are stretched. The mandible is pulled open; the condylar head of the TMJ translates forward, stressing the joint structures, and the muscles (masseter, temporalis, medial pterygoids) controlling jaw elevation are stretched.

Flexion injuries. When the head rapidly accelerates into flexion and nothing stops it (such as the steering wheel or air bag in a car), the chin is stopped by the sternum. The mandible is forced posteriorly so the condylar head is forced into the retrodiscal pad in the joint. The posterior cervical muscles, ligaments, fasciae, and joint capsules are stretched.

Postural Strain

Strain to the posterior cervical, scapular, and upper thoracic muscles and fasciae is common with postural stresses such as prolonged sitting at a computer terminal, a desk, or focused on a tablet or other electronic device. Structures in the low back region are strained with faulty standing and sitting postures. Postural stresses are described in detail in Chapter 14.

Emotional Stress

Emotional stress is often expressed as increased tension in the posterior cervical or lumbar region.

Activity Limitations and Participation Restrictions

Impaired muscle function underlies most spinal problems that demonstrate pain or poor spinal control and stabilization during functional activities.

Acute. During the acute phase, muscle guarding interferes with basic activities, such as bed mobility, sitting, standing, and walking, as well as ability to participate in family, work, and recreational demands.

Subacute and chronic. With the subacute and chronic conditions, muscle impairments result in poor stabilization and spinal control in prolonged upright postures and activities. Stability of the spine is imperative for most activities and needs to be addressed to minimize restrictions and improve function.

Pathomechanics of Spinal Instability

Spinal stability was defined and described in Chapter 14. The mechanical model of stability in which stability is maintained over the base of support by the guy wire function of the global and segmental musculature was reviewed, as was the functional model proposed by Panjabi and colleagues[185-187] in which stability is visualized as a three-legged stool that requires not only the active muscle function, but also the passive osteoligamentous structures and neural control from the central nervous system to program muscle response for spinal stability. All three legs of the stool are necessary for stability; instability results when one (or more) of the legs does not function properly.

There are various grades of instability. Patients who have severe symptoms and radiographic evidence of excessive motion and who do not respond to conservative treatment become candidates for spinal fusion.[72] Surgical fusion of the cervical and lumbar regions are discussed later in this chapter. Clinical instability that can be managed by therapeutic exercise interventions is defined by an increase in the neutral zone.

Neutral Zone

The *neutral zone*[185,186] is the area that is midrange in the ROM of a spinal segment in which no stress is placed on the passive osteoligamentous structures. In the spine, the neutral zone is relatively small (usually only several degrees of range is possible between any two vertebrae before the elastic zone of the inert tissues is reached) and is controlled by dynamic tension in the deep segmental musculature that attaches to each of the spinal segments.

The neutral zone can be visualized as a ball lying on the bottom of a bowl. The sides of the bowl represent the osteoligamentous structures that provide passive support of the spinal segment. When the ball is disturbed, it rolls back and forth and up against the sides of the bowl and eventually settles back in the middle. A deep bowl has a smaller region in which the ball can roll back and forth and therefore, less motion or more stability; a shallow bowl has a larger region in which the ball can roll, so there is greater displacement or more mobility (less stability) (Fig. 15.3 A and B). Muscles added to this visualization are depicted as bungee cords that are attached to the ball and go outward to the edges of the bowl; they help center the ball in the middle of the bowl when perturbations occur (Fig. 15.3 C). In a structure in which there is less stability (more segmental movement), the muscles have greater responsibility to maintain the neutral zone (ball in the middle of the bowl).

Neutral spine. The term neutral spine is used clinically to define the midrange of motion.

Instability

If there is an increase in the neutral zone, the segment may show signs of instability.[72,185-187] More segmental movement may occur owing to disc degeneration, spondylolysis, spondylolisthesis, or ligamentous laxity; or it may be due to poor neuromuscular control of the deep segmental stabilizing muscles

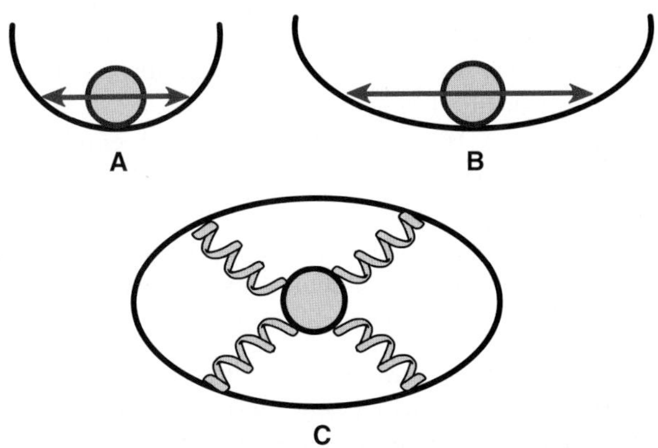

FIGURE 15.3 Neutral zone of a spinal segment depicted as a bowl, with the sides of the bowl representing the osteoligamentous tissues and the moving ball representing the segmental mobility. **(A)** In a deep bowl, when perturbations disturb the ball, there is little motion as the ball rolls back and forth and settles in the center of the bowl—representing stability. **(B)** In a shallow bowl, there is greater motion—representing greater segmental mobility or instability. **(C)** Viewing the bowl from above, bungee cords attached to the ball and the sides of the bowl represent the dynamic function of segmental muscles. Appropriately graded tension in the bungee cords stabilizes the ball when perturbations disturb the unit.

in maintaining the neutral zone because of fatigue, altered recruitment pattern, reflex inhibition from pain, or some pathology.[72,186,187,236] The individual may experience neck or back pain when aberrant movement occurs at the segment or stresses are imposed at the end of the range (relaxed postures for a period of time or sudden stress that the muscles cannot control).

FOCUS ON EVIDENCE

It has been shown that activation and function in the transversus abdominis (TrA) changes (delayed and more phasic) in patients with LBP;[110,111] there may be atrophy, structural change, and altered electromyographic activity in the multifidus at the painful spinal level as well, [46,105,203] possibly indicating less effective stabilizing action from these muscles. Studies have also documented that training the deep segmental muscles for postural control and stability improves the long-term outcome in patient populations with acute[104] and chronic[183] LBP as well as pelvic girdle pain following pregnancy.[223] In the cervical region, studies have documented that training the stabilizing function of the deep cervical musculature for postural control decreases the frequency and intensity of symptoms of cervical headaches.[121]

Management Guidelines Based on Stages of Recovery and Diagnostic Categories

Principles of Management for the Spine

At the time of a spinal injury, impairments, activity limitations, and participation restrictions are not known. Up to 60% of acute back injuries resolve within 1 week and up to 90% resolve within 6 weeks[129] with a recurrence rate of less than 25%.[22,222,243] Participation restrictions are dependent on the extent of the injury. If it involves the spinal cord, levels of complete paralysis may occur requiring rehabilitative interventions to develop adaptations for participation in daily activities. If it involves the nerve roots (also the cauda equina), varying degrees of sensory loss in specific dermatomes and muscle weakness in specific myotomes may occur, which may or may not interfere with the individual's daily personal and work-related activities. Upper-quarter nerve roots affect function of the arms and hands; lower-quarter nerve roots affect function of the lower extremities, especially during weight-bearing activities. Studies on chronic pain syndromes as a result of spinal injuries seem to conclude that the degree of participation restrictions is related to psychological, economic, and sociological factors and prior incidence of injury more than the actual tissues involved.[135] Nerve root involvement and pain provocation with active movements in several directions are more common in patients who develop chronic pain. Discussion of treatment for spinal cord injuries and chronic pain syndromes is beyond the scope of this book.

Examination and Evaluation

History, systems review, and testing. A history and systems review of the patient is conducted to rule out any serious conditions, determine if the patient should be referred to another practitioner, or determine if the patient's condition is appropriate for physical therapy intervention. Then, if it is safe, tests and measures are conducted to determine if the source of symptoms can be influenced by mechanical changes in position or movement and to establish a baseline from which changes can be documented. Examination techniques and procedures are beyond the scope of this text, but a brief summary of concerns in the spinal area is listed to help focus on critical decisions prior to establishing an intervention strategy.

- *Serious "red flag" conditions related to orthopedic conditions* that should be referred to a physician for management include spinal cord symptoms and signs (upper motor neuron lesions), recent trauma in which spinal fracture or instabilities have not been ruled out, and serious pain (especially pain that awakens the individual) that cannot be explained mechanically.
- *Psychological distress* may interfere with a patient's recovery; therefore, referral to an appropriate professional may be indicated for a multidisciplinary approach in the patient's care. Several psychosocial questionnaires, including the Patient Health Questionnaire for Depression and Anxiety (PHQ-4)[138] and the Graded Chronic Pain Scale,[178,237] can be used to determine if referral is indicated.
- *Neurological symptoms* should be explored in an attempt to relate them to spinal cord, nerve root, spinal nerve, plexus, or peripheral nerve patterns. Causes of nerve root signs frequently seen by physical therapists include IV disc protrusions; bony, soft tissue, or vascular stenosis in the spinal canal or IV foramina; facet joint swelling; and nerve root tension from restricted mobility or inflammation.
- *Pain patterns* should be explored to determine if they relate to a known musculoskeletal pattern or signal a medical condition. It should be recognized that pain is interpreted in many ways and has various meanings for different people; therefore, the information is interpreted as only one factor when determining cause of the symptoms.

FOCUS ON EVIDENCE

Based on strong evidence, the ***Clinical Practice Guidelines (CPGs) for Low Back Pain***[48] and for ***Neck Pain***[37] support utilizing self-report questionnaires (such as the Oswestry Disability Index or Roland-Morris Disability Questionnaire for the low back and the Neck Disability Index or Patient-Specific Functional Scale for neck pain) for identifying the baseline status of pain, function, and disability to monitor change. Based on expert opinion, the ***CPGs for Low Back*** and ***Neck Pain*** recommend monitoring activity limitations and participation restrictions by using reproducible and validated measures.[37,48]

Stage of recovery. Time frames for each recovery stage vary depending on the reference used. In general, the acute stage usually lasts less than 4 weeks, the subacute stage is 4 to 12 weeks, and the chronic stage is greater than 12 weeks.[2] Chronic pain syndromes generally are conditions that extend beyond 6 months.

- ***Acute inflammatory stage.*** The patient experiences constant pain, and there are signs of inflammation. No position or movement completely relieves the symptoms. Medical intervention with anti-inflammatory medications is usually warranted.
- ***Acute stage without signs of inflammation.*** Symptoms are intermittent and related to mechanical deformation. There may be signs of nerve irritability when the nerve root or spinal nerve is compressed or placed under tension. The patient may be categorized into an extension bias, a flexion bias, or a nonweight-bearing bias based on the presenting posture, movement impairments, or positions of symptom relief. These categories are described in greater detail in the next section. Delitto and associates[49] classified patients as being at this stage if they cannot stand longer than 15 minutes, sit longer than 30 minutes, or walk more than one-quarter of a mile without their status worsening.
- ***Subacute stage.*** Usually at this stage, certain movements and postures with some instrumental ADLs (IADLs) still provoke symptoms, such as lifting, vacuuming, gardening, and other activities requiring repetitive movement of loads, so a basic lifestyle cannot fully be resumed. A more thorough examination is conducted to identify specific impairments, activity limitations, and participation restrictions that could be interfering with recovery.
- ***Chronic stage.*** When this stage is reached, emphasis is placed on returning the patient to high-level demand activities that require handling repetitive loads on a sustained basis over a prolonged period of time (from heavy material handling, to repetitive household activities that include lifting small children, to strenuous athletic activities).

Diagnosis, prognosis, and plan of care. As mentioned in the introduction to this chapter, specific pathologies and medical diagnoses often do not guide the therapist when choosing appropriate treatment interventions, and various systems of patient classification for treating musculoskeletal impairments and functional limitations are present in the literature.[2,49,50,73,158,204,214] Several validation studies supporting clinical prediction rules are available to assist the therapist in making decisions when developing and modifying interventions.[14,38,41,42,75,103,145,200,233] In addition, the ***CPGs for Neck Pain***[37] and for ***Low Back Pain***[48] have organized recommendations in relation to the International Classification of

Functioning, Disability, and Health (ICF) categories. These classifications are available in ONLINE Box 15.1 on the FA Davis website associated with this text,

The material in the remainder of this section is organized to integrate impairment-based diagnostic categories with the medical model of spinal pathologies in order to help the therapist choose an intervention strategy that best enhances the patient's recovery. Specific medical diagnoses with unique regional features and interventions are described in the last section of this chapter. A table that summarizes the interventions for the spinal and related pathologies described in this chapter is available on the FA Davis website associated with this text (ONLINE Table 15.1)

The decisions concerning the approach to treatment are determined by the patient's responses to the examination maneuvers and the maneuvers that provide the greatest relief of symptoms. Adjustments in the intervention occur as the patient progresses through the healing process. The categories described in this and the following sections are summarized in Box 15.4.

 **FOCUS ON EVIDENCE**

In two separate, but similar systematic reviews, using directional preference for treatment (the direction of movement that decreased symptoms at the initial evaluation) was shown to be an effective approach when centralization occurred[154] or when compared with other treatment options.[224] This approach was further substantiated in a study by Donelson et al[55] that included 71 patients with acute to chronic LBP with and without leg radicular pain. Each person was treated for 2 weeks according to their directional preference. At the follow-up, 91% to 100% of participants reported significant improvement or complete resolve in their pain location, pain duration, or neurological status.

Based on strong evidence for patients with acute LBP and related lower extremity pain, the ***CPGs for Low Back Pain*** recommend utilizing repeated movements, exercises, or procedures that promote centralization of symptoms.[48]

General Guidelines for Managing Acute Spinal Impairments: Maximum Protection Phase

Use of modalities, myofascial release, and massage to decrease pain and swelling from acute symptoms is appropriate during this stage. It is also important that the patient becomes an active participant in his or her program. Kinesthetic training of neutral or functional spinal posture, nondestructive movements in the pain-free range, awareness and activation of deep segmental musculature, and basic functional training maneuvers are taught if they do not exacerbate the symptoms. Specific interventions for various impairments, specific biases, or syndromes and common pathologies in the spinal region are described in the remaining sections of this chapter. Specific techniques for kinesthetic training, deep segmental muscle

BOX 15.4 Impairment-Based Diagnostic Categories That Direct Intervention[49,73,158,204]

General: Stage of Recovery
- Acute with inflammation (0–4 weeks).
- Acute without inflammation (0–4 weeks): intermittent symptoms with acute nerve root symptoms.
- Subacute (4–12 weeks).
- Chronic (>12 weeks).
- Chronic pain syndrome (>6 months).

Nonweight-Bearing Bias: Traction Approach
- Patient does not tolerate being upright for basic ADLs and IADLs.
- Movement testing makes symptoms worse.
- Traction (or other nonweight-bearing procedures) relieves symptoms.

Extension Bias: Extension Approach
- Patient usually presents with flexed posture—a *lateral shift* may also be present.
- Extension tests decrease or centralize symptoms.
- Diagnosis may include intervertebral disc lesions, impaired flexed posture, fluid stasis.

Flexion Bias: Flexion Approach
- Patient usually presents with flexed posture and is more comfortable when flexed.
- Extension tests exacerbate or peripheralize symptoms.
- Diagnoses may include spondylosis, stenosis, extension load injuries, swollen facet joints.

Hypermobility/Functional Instability: Stabilization/ Immobilization Approach
- Patients present with hypermobile spinal segment(s); poor spinal stability (segmental or global).
- Diagnoses may include trauma, ligamentous laxity, spondylolysis, or spondylolisthesis.

Hypomobility: Mobilization/Manipulation Approach
- Restricted mobility in one or more spinal segments.

Muscle and Soft Tissue Lesions: Exercise Approach
- Patient usually presents with guarded posture or increased muscle tension.
- Diagnoses may include strains, tears, contusions, or overuse.

Postural Pain Syndrome: Exercise and Conditioning Approach
- Patient presents with faulty posture; symptoms increase with sustained position.
- Diagnoses may include postural strain, cervico-genic headache, thoracic outlet syndrome, poor physical condition
- Movement, posture correction, and exercise decrease symptoms

activation, stabilization training, joint manipulation, and functional training activities for the acute stage in the cervical and lumbar spinal regions are described in Chapter 16. Management guidelines for treating the patient with acute symptoms are summarized in Box 15.5. The following points are fundamental to all interventions.

Patient Education

It is important to engage patients in all aspects of intervention, including information about anticipated progress and outcome, the healing time of inflamed tissues or reduction of symptoms due to nerve root pressure (if indicated), and precautions and contraindications.

FOCUS ON EVIDENCE

Based on moderate evidence, the ***CPGs for Low Back Pain*** recommend providing education and counselling that includes promoting the importance of remaining active (including resumption of normal and vocational activities), self-care options, and avoiding bed rest during the acute phase, as well as an explanation of the natural history of back pain, the inherent strength of the spine, and use of pain coping strategies.[48]

Symptom Relief or Comfort

If a patient is experiencing acute inflammation from a traumatic injury, there is constant pain; yet, often an optimal position of comfort or symptom reduction can be determined in which there is the least amount of stress on the inflamed, irritated, or swollen region. The terms *functional position* or *functional range* are used to describe this position.[167] (Neutral position is midrange.) The functional range may change for the individual as the tissues heal and the person gains mobility and strength in the region. Some pathological conditions typically tend to cause symptoms in one portion of the range and are relieved in another range.[167] The following terms, describing subcategories of diagnoses or syndromes, have been popularized based on the work of Morgan,[167] Saal and associates,[209,211] Delitto and colleagues,[49] and Fritz and George.[73]

CLINICAL TIP

For patients with acute or chronic LBP with or without leg radicular pain, utilizing exercises that emphasize directional preference (flexion, extension, or side glide rotation) results in greater improvement in outcome than using nondirectional or general exercises.[14,55,224]

BOX 15.5 MANAGEMENT GUIDELINES— Acute Spinal Impairments/Protection Phase

Impairments, Activity Limitations, and Participation Restrictions

Pain and/or neurological symptoms
Inflammation
Guarded posture (prefers flexion, extension, or nonweight bearing)
Limited ability to perform ADLs and IADLs

Plan of Care	Intervention
1. Educate the patient.	1. Engage patient in all activities to learn self-management. Inform patient of anticipated progress and precautions.
2. Decrease acute symptoms.	2. Modalities, massage, traction, or mobilization/manipulation as needed. Rest only for first couple days if needed.
3. Teach awareness of neck and pelvic position and movement.	3. Kinesthetic training: cervical and scapular motions, pelvic tilts, neutral spine.
4. Demonstrate safe postures.	4. Practice positions and movement and experience effect on spine. Help patient find the functional spinal position of comfort in supine, sitting, standing.
5. Initiate neuromuscular activation and control of stabilizing muscles.	5. Deep segmental muscle activation techniques: ▪ Lumbar spine: drawing-in maneuver, multifidus contraction. ▪ Cervical spine: gentle head nods Basic stabilization: with arm and leg motions (passive support if needed, progress to active control).
6. Teach safe performance of basic ADLs; progress to IADLs.	6. Roll, sit, stand, and walk with safe postures. Progress tolerance to sitting longer than 30 minutes, standing longer than 15 minutes, and walking > 1 mile.

Extension bias-extension syndrome. The patient's symptoms are lessened in positions of extension (lordosis). Sustained flexed postures or repetitive flexion motions load the anterior disc region, causing fluid redistribution from the compressed areas and swelling and creep in the distended areas. This is frequently the mechanism of symptom production with posterior or posterolateral IV disc lesions or injury to the posterior longitudinal ligament. Whether the pathology is an injured disc or stressed and swollen tissues, repeated extension motions and positions relieve the symptoms by moving the fluid to reverse the stasis (these techniques are described in the Extension Bias section of this chapter). Some patients present with a lateral shift, which usually requires correction before extension relieves the symptoms.[158-160]

Flexion bias-flexion syndrome. The patient's symptoms are lessened in positions of spinal flexion and provoked in extension. This is often the case when there is compromise of the facets, IV foramen, or spinal canal, as in bony spinal stenosis, spondylosis, and spondylolisthesis (these techniques are described in the Flexion Bias section of this chapter).

Nonweight-bearing bias-traction syndrome. The patient's symptoms are lessened when in nonweight-bearing positions, such as when lying down or in traction. Symptoms also lessen when spinal pressure is reduced by leaning on the upper extremities (using arm rests to unweight the trunk), by leaning the trunk against a support, or when in a pool. The condition is considered *gravity sensitive* because the symptoms worsen during standing, walking, running, coughing, or similar activities that increase spinal pressure. Often, traction and aquatic therapy are the only interventions that minimize symptoms during the acute phase.

Kinesthetic Awareness of Safe Postures and Effects of Movement

The patient is taught how to identify and assume the spinal position that is most comfortable and reduces the symptoms, using pelvic tilts for lumbar positioning and head nods and chin tucks for cervical spine positioning, and is taught how to use passive positioning to help maintain the functional position during the acute state (Box 15.6). If necessary (usually only in severe cases for a limited time or following surgery), a corset or cervical collar may be used to provide support.

Muscle Performance: Deep Segmental Muscle Activation and Basic Stabilization

Whether the patient has a cervical or lumbar problem, as soon as tolerated, the patient is taught how to activate the deep segmental muscles.

Lumbar Region: Deep Segmental Muscle Activation

For the lumbar region, the "*drawing-in*" maneuver is used to activate the TrA and a gentle bulging contraction of the multifidus muscle. Facilitation techniques, which are described in detail in the Segmental Activation section of Chapter 16, may be necessary.

Cervical Region: Deep Segmental Muscle Activation

For the patient with cervical pain, gentle head nods and slight flattening of the cervical lordosis in the supine position are used for activation of the longus colli and multifidus.

Basic Stabilization

Once the patient learns to activate the segmental muscles, simple upper and lower extremity motions with the spine stabilized are added to the intervention to initiate training of the global stabilizers. *Passive prepositioning* is used if the patient is unable actively to maintain his or her functional position, as described in Box 15.6. For both cervical and lumbar problems, the patient is instructed first to do the drawing-in maneuver followed by gentle arm motions within a range that does not exacerbate symptoms. Leg motions require greater lumbopelvic control and are introduced if the patient is able to demonstrate pelvic control and the symptoms are not exacerbated with the movements. Suggestions for determining the exercise progressions are detailed in the Stabilization section of Chapter 16.

Basic Functional Movements

The patient is taught to perform simple movements for ADLs while protecting the spine in the functional position. These movements include rolling from prone to supine and reverse, lying to sitting and reverse, sitting to standing and reverse, and walking. Descriptions of these maneuvers are in the Functional Activities section of Chapter 16.

PRECAUTIONS: Review any special precautions for the condition with the patient. Condition-specific precautions are described in the remaining sections of this chapter.

BOX 15.6 Examples of Passive Positioning of the Spine

- *Supine:* Hook-lying flexes the lumbar spine; extended legs extends the lumbar spine. A pillow under the head flexes the neck; a small roll under the neck stabilizes a mild lordosis with the head neutral.
- *Prone:* Use of a pillow under the abdomen flexes the lumbar spine; no pillow extends the spine. To maintain the cervical spine in neutral alignment without rotation, a split table or a small towel roll placed under the forehead provides space for the nose, so the patient does not turn the head.
- *Sitting:* Usually causes spinal flexion, especially if the hips and knees are flexed. To emphasize flexion, the feet are propped up on a small footstool; to emphasize extension, a lumbar pillow or towel roll is placed in the low-back region. To unweight the spine, the arms are placed on an armrest, or a reclining chair is used.
- *Standing:* Usually causes spinal extension; to emphasize flexion, one foot is placed on a small stool.

General Guidelines for Managing Subacute Spinal Impairments: Controlled Motion Phase

When the signs and symptoms of the inflammatory process are under control and pain is no longer constant, the patient is progressed through a program of safe muscle endurance and strengthening exercises to prepare the tissue for functional activities and rehabilitation training. Functional activities that can be performed safely are resumed. Pain may still interfere with some daily activities, but it should no longer be constant. Poor neuromuscular control and stabilization, poor postural awareness and body mechanics, decreased flexibility and strength, and generalized deconditioning may be the underlying impairments at this stage. Intervention during this stage is critical, because either the patient feels good and tends to overdo activities and reinjures the tissues or the patient is fearful and does not adequately resume safe movements, leading to further participations restrictions. Either extreme may slow down the recovery process.

Management guidelines for cervical and lumbar problems that require controlled motion interventions are summarized in Box 15.7. The specific techniques and progressions of intervention outlined here are described in detail in Chapter 16.

Pain Modulation

At this stage, use of modalities to modulate pain is not recommended. Emphasis is placed on increasing patient awareness of posture, strength, mobility, and spinal control and their relationship to modulating pain.

BOX 15.7 MANAGEMENT GUIDELINES—
Subacute Spinal Problems/Controlled Motion Phase

Impairments, Activity Limitations, and Participation Restrictions

Pain: only when excessive stress is placed on vulnerable tissues
Impaired posture/postural awareness
Impaired mobility
Impaired muscle performance: poor neuromuscular control of stabilizing muscles; decreased muscle endurance and strength
General deconditioning
Limited ability to perform IADLs for extended periods of time
Poor body mechanics

Plan of Care	Intervention
1. Educate the patient in self-management and how to decrease episodes of pain.	1. Engage patient in all activities emphasizing safe movement and postures. Home exercise program. Ergonomic adaptation of work or home environment.
2. Progress awareness and control of spinal alignment.	2. Practice active spinal control in pain-free positions and with all exercises and activities. Practice posture correction.
3. Increase mobility in restricted muscles/joint/fascia/nerve.	3. Joint mobilization/manipulation, neuromobilization, muscle inhibition, self-stretching.
4. Teach techniques to develop neuromuscular control, strength, and endurance.	4. Progress stabilization exercises; increase repetitions (emphasize muscle endurance). Initiate extremity-strengthening exercises in conjunction with spinal stabilization.
5. Develop cardiopulmonary endurance.	5. Low to moderate intensity aerobic exercises; emphasize spinal bias.
6. Teach techniques of stress relief/relaxation.	6. Relaxation exercises and postural stress relief.
7. Teach safe body mechanics and functional adaptations.	7. Practice stable spine lifting, pushing/pulling, and reaching practice activities specific to desired outcome emphasizing spinal control, endurance, and timing.

Kinesthetic Training

Kinesthetic training is progressed by using reinforcement techniques. Feed-forward control of the deep segmental musculature, active control of the spinal position, and correct posture are reinforced in a variety of ways until activation and control become habitual. Kinesthetic training overlaps the stabilization exercises.

Stretching/Manipulation

Decreased flexibility in joints, muscles, and fascia may restrict the patient's ability to assume normal spinal alignment. Manual techniques and safe self-stretching techniques are used to increase muscle, joint, and connective tissue mobility.

Muscle Performance

Exercises are progressed with increased challenges for control, muscular endurance, and strength in the spinal stabilizing muscles; these exercises include activities that increase control and strength in the extremity musculature in conjunction with spinal stabilization.

CLINICAL TIP

If a patient continues to display a flexion or extension bias, adapt exercises to emphasize that particular bias and prevent stresses in the symptom-producing direction.

- Stabilization exercises are used to emphasize movement and resistance to the extremities while maintaining control of the spinal position. Increasing the time and number of repetitions builds muscle endurance at each level of performance.
- Wall slides, partial squats, partial lunges, pushing, and pulling against resistance are used to strengthen the extremities to prepare for lifting, reaching, pushing, and pulling activities.
- When the patient learns effective spinal control with the stabilizing muscles in a variety of stabilization exercise routines, dynamic trunk and neck strengthening exercises, such as curl-ups, back extension, and cervical motions, are introduced. Care is taken to monitor symptoms and modify any activities that exacerbate the problem.

Cardiopulmonary Conditioning

Aerobic capacity is usually compromised after injury. It is important to guide the patient in the initiation of or safe return to an aerobic conditioning program. Help the patient identify activities that do not exacerbate spinal symptoms and set goals and progressions to achieve desired outcome.

Postural Stress Management and Relaxation Exercises

It is common that a patient's symptoms are exacerbated with sustained postural stresses such as sitting at a computer, talking on the phone (head tilted), utilizing a digital mobile device, or repetitive forward bending (shoe salesman); therefore, analysis of work, home, or recreational postures and activities is a necessary component of the patient's program. The patient is then advised about methods to correct the sustained or repetitive postural stresses. In addition, frequent changes of position and movement through the pain-free ROMs should be encouraged. It may be necessary to teach the patient how to consciously relax tension in muscles to relieve stress. Relaxation exercises are described in Chapter 14.

Functional Activities

Once the patient has learned spinal control and stabilization and has developed adequate flexibility and strength for specific tasks, components of the task are incorporated into the exercise program and then into the patient's daily lifestyle. Safe body mechanics are included in all aspects of care.

General Guidelines for Managing Chronic Spinal Impairments: Return to Function Phase

Patients who have been treated through the acute and subacute phases of healing with appropriately graded exercises should have minimal structural or functional impairments that prevent or restrict daily activities. Individuals who must do heavy material handling (e.g., a manual laborer, firefighter, or caregiver of patients or of small children) or who participate in high-demand sports activities may require additional rehabilitative training to return safely to these high-demand activities and to avoid further injury. Impairments in strength, endurance, neuromuscular control, and skill are related to the functional goals of the individual. At this stage, conditioning and spinal control during high-intensity and repetitive activities are emphasized. Any underlying impairments that interfere with the desired outcomes must be remediated. Management guidelines for return to function are summarized in Box 15.8. Suggestions for progressing exercise intervention techniques from the subacute through chronic stages are described in Chapter 16.

Management Guidelines: Nonweight-Bearing Bias

During examination, some patients do not respond to extension, flexion, or even midrange spinal positions or motions due to the acuity of or mechanical stimuli from their condition. The person is often more comfortable lying down and may have partial or full relief with a traction test maneuver to the painful region of the spine.

For these patients, use of traction procedures or unweighting the body in a pool may be the interventions of choice until the symptoms stabilize.

BOX 15.8 MANAGEMENT GUIDELINES—
Chronic Spinal Problems/Return to Function Phase

Impairments, Activity Limitations, and Participation Restrictions

Pain: only when excessive stress is placed on vulnerable tissues in repetitive or sustained nature for prolonged periods
Poor neuromuscular control and endurance in high-intensity or destabilized situations
Flexibility and strength imbalances
Generalized deconditioning
Limited ability to perform high-intensity physical demands for extended periods of time

Plan of Care	Intervention
1. Emphasize spinal control in high-intensity and repetitive activities.	1. Practice active spinal control in various transitional activities that challenge balance.
2. Increase mobility in restricted muscles/joints/fascia/nerve.	2. Joint mobilization/manipulation, neuromobilization, muscle inhibition, self-stretching.
3. Improve muscle performance; dynamic trunk and extremity strength, coordination, and endurance.	3. Progress dynamic trunk and extremity resistance exercises emphasizing functional goals.
4. Increase cardiopulmonary endurance.	4. Progress intensity of aerobic exercises.
5. Emphasize habitual use of techniques of stress relief/relaxation and posture correction.	5. Motions and postures to relieve stress.
6. Teach safe progression to high-level/high-intensity activities.	6. Apply any ergonomic changes to work/home environment.
7. Teach healthy exercise habits for self-maintenance.	7. Progressive practice using activity-specific training consistent with desired functional outcome, emphasizing spinal control, endurance, balance, agility, timing, and speed.

Management of Acute Symptoms

Traction

- Various references have reported the benefits of traction in patients meeting this criteria.[27,40,74,193,217] Traction has the mechanical benefit of temporarily separating the vertebrae, causing mechanical sliding of the facet joints in the spine, and increasing the size of the IV foramina. If done intermittently, this motion may help reduce circulatory congestion and relieve pressure on the dura, blood vessels, and nerve roots in the IV foramina. Improving circulation also may help decrease the concentration of noxious chemical irritants due to swelling and inflammation.
- There may be a neurophysiological response via stimulation of the mechanoreceptors that may modulate the transmission of nociceptive stimuli at the spinal cord or brain stem level.

Pool

If a person is not fearful of being in a pool, supporting the individual with a buoyant life belt in deep water reduces the effects of gravity on the lumbar spine. If symptoms are reduced, it may be possible to begin and progress gentle stabilization exercises in this buoyant environment to meet some of the goals during the acute and subacute phases. Exercises can also be progressed by using the properties of water for resistance and stretching (see description of aquatic exercises in Chapter 9).

Progression

As healing occurs, the patient should begin to tolerate weight bearing. After re-examination and assessment, identify the impairments and activity and participation restrictions. If a bias toward flexion or extension is determined, or if there are areas of hypermobility or hypomobility, plan the interventions accordingly.

Management Guidelines: Extension Bias

Patients with an extension bias often assume a flexed posture or a flexed posture with lateral deviation of the trunk or neck, but during the examination, sustained or repetitive extension maneuvers reduce or relieve their symptoms. These patients would benefit from early interventions that emphasize extension of the involved segments. The impairments may be due to a contained IV disc lesion, fluid stasis, a flexion injury, or muscle imbalances from a faulty flexed posture. McKenzie[158-160] developed a method of categorizing these patients based on the extent of their pain and/or neurological symptoms. He also described the phenomena of peripheralization and centralization that accompany an expanding and receding lesion, frequently attributed to IV disc lesions (see Fig. 15.2).

Many of the techniques that were originally described by McKenzie[158-160] to manage a patient with an acute disc lesion have been found to be beneficial in the management of patients who have a cluster of signs and symptoms that categorize them into the extension bias (extension syndrome) category.[71,73,145,211]

Principles of Management

Because patients with signs and symptoms of a bulging IV disc often fit into the "extension bias" category, a brief discussion of the response of the IV disc is presented here.

Effects of Postural Changes on IV Disc Pressure

Relative changes in posture and activities affect intradiscal pressure. When compared to the level of pressure when standing, intradiscal pressure is least when lying supine, increases by almost 50% while sitting with hips and knees flexed, and almost doubles if leaning forward while sitting.[217] Sitting with a back rest inclination of 120° and lumbar support 5 cm in depth provides the lowest load to the disc while sitting.[11] Therefore, sitting with the hips and knees flexed or leaning forward should be avoided when there is an acute disc lesion. If sitting is necessary, there should be support for the lumbar spine by reclining the trunk 120°.

Effects of Bed Rest on the IV Disc

When a person is lying down, compression forces to the disc are reduced, and with time, the nucleus potentially can absorb more water to equalize pressures (imbibition). When lying down with the spine in flexion, the imbibed fluid accumulates posteriorly in the disc where there is greater space. Then, upon rising, body weight compresses the disc with the increased fluid, and intradiscal pressure greatly increases. The pain or symptoms from a disc protrusion are accentuated. To avoid exacerbating symptoms, absolute bed rest during the acute phase should be avoided.[48] Bed rest during the first 2 days (when symptoms are highly irritable) may be needed to promote early healing, but it should be interspersed with short intervals of standing, walking, and appropriately controlled movement.[242]

Effects of Traction on the IV Disc

Traction may relieve symptoms from a disc protrusion, although there is conflicting evidence as to whether traction in general is beneficial.[40,48] It is proposed that separating the vertebral bodies may have the effect of placing tension on the annular fibers and posterior longitudinal ligament, thus having a flattening effect on the bulge; or it may decrease the intradiscal pressure.[217] If traction relieves symptoms, the time of application must be short because with the reduced pressure fluid imbibition may occur to equalize the pressure. Then, when the traction is released, the pressure increases and symptoms are exacerbated.

Effects of Flexion and Extension on the IV Disc and Fluid Stasis

Rest in a slightly forward-bent position often lessens pain because of the space potential for the nucleus pulposus of the IV disc. The patient may also deviate laterally to minimize pressure against a nerve root. Movement into extension initially causes increased symptoms. With acute disc lesions in which there is protective lateral shifting and lumbar flexion, techniques that cause lateral shifting of the spine opposite to the deviation followed by passive spinal extension (sustained or repetitive) to compress the protrusion mechanically have been found to relieve the clinical signs and symptoms in many patients.[133,159]

Patients experiencing pain due to fluid stasis after being in a sustained flexed posture also experience relief with movement into extension.

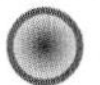

FOCUS ON EVIDENCE

In a study of 20 subjects with LBP who were candidates for extension-based treatment, those who experienced an immediate decrease in pain intensity (N = 10) of at least 2/10 after treatment (posterior to anterior mobilization followed by prone press-ups) demonstrated a mean increase in diffusion coefficient of 4.2% of the nuclear region of the L5-S1 IV disc measured by MRI. Those who did not experience pain reduction (N = 10) did not have a change in diffusion (mean decrease of 1.6%; $P < .005$).[18]

Effects of Isometric and Dynamic Exercise

Isometric activities (resisted pelvic tilt exercises, straining, Valsalva maneuver) and active back flexion or extension exercises increase intradiscal pressures above normal. They therefore must be avoided during the acute stage of a disc lesion. Strong muscle contractions also exacerbate symptoms if a muscle has been injured. Therefore, active and resistive extension exercises are avoided during the acute stage.

Effects of Muscle Guarding

Reflex muscle guarding or splinting often accompanies an acute disc lesion and adds to the compressive forces on the disc. Modalities and gentle oscillatory traction to the spine may help decrease the splinting.

Indications, Precautions, and Contraindications for Interventions: Extension Approach

Indications. Extension is used if pain and/or neurological symptoms centralize (decrease or move more proximally) during repeated extension testing maneuvers and peripheralize (worsen) during flexion.[158] Extension is also indicated for flexed postural dysfunctions with limited range into extension. If no test movements decrease the symptoms, this mechanical approach to treatment should not be used. This was illustrated in a randomized control trial by Hosseinifar et al,[114] where patients with nonspecific LBP were placed into either a McKenzie (extension) or stabilization exercise group. After 18 visits, the stabilization group reported a significant decrease in their pain and functional outcomes compared with the McKenzie group.

PRECAUTION: A patient with acute pain in the spinal region that is not influenced by changing the patient's position or by movement must be screened by a physician for signs of serious pathology.

CONTRAINDICATIONS: When there is an acute disc lesion, any form of exercise or activity that increases intradiscal pressure, such as the Valsalva maneuver, active trunk flexion, or trunk rotation, is contraindicated during the protection phase of treatment. Any movement that peripheralizes the symptoms signals a movement that is contraindicated during the acute and early subacute period of treatment. Peripheralization with extension motions may indicate stenosis, a large lateral disc protrusion, or pathology in a posterior element.[210] Contraindications to specific movements are summarized in Box 15.9.

BOX 15.9 Contraindications to Specific Spinal Movements

Extension of the spine is contraindicated:[100]

- When no position or movement decreases or centralizes the described pain
- When saddle anesthesia and/or bladder weakness is present (could indicate spinal cord or cauda equina lesion)
- When a patient is in such extreme pain that he or she rigidly holds the body immobile with any attempted correction

Flexion of the spine should be avoided:

- When extension relieves the symptoms
- When flexion movements increase the pain or peripheralize the symptoms

Interventions Using an Extension Approach in the Lumbar Spine

Management of Acute Symptoms

If symptoms are severe, bed rest is indicated with short periods of walking at regular intervals. Walking usually promotes lumbar extension and stimulates fluid mechanics to help reduce swelling in the disc or connective tissues. If the patient cannot stand upright, he or she should use crutches or a walker to help relieve the increased pressure of the forward-bent posture.

If repeated flexion test movements increase the symptoms and if repeated extension test movements decrease or centralize the symptoms, all flexion activities should be avoided during the early phases of intervention. Treatment begins with the following maneuvers.

Extension

Patient position and procedure: Prone. If the flexion posture is severe, place pillows under the abdomen for support. Gradually increase the amount of extension by removing the pillows, and then progress by having the patient prop himself or herself up on the elbows, allowing the pelvis to sag (Fig. 15.4 A). When propping, pillows placed under the thorax help take strain off the shoulders. Wait 5 to 10 minutes between each increment of extension to allow reduction of the water content and the size of the bulge. There should be an accompanying centralization of or decrease in symptoms. Progress to having the patient prop himself or herself up on the hands, allowing the pelvis to sag (Fig. 15.4 B).

If the sustained position of prone propping is not well tolerated, have the patient perform passive lumbar extension intermittently by repeating the *prone press-ups,* at least 10 times, attempting to go into greater extension with each repetition. If possible, have the patient maintain the end position (as in Fig. 15.4 B) after the 10th repetition as long as tolerated.

PRECAUTION: Carefully monitor the patient's symptoms. They should lessen peripherally (i.e., decreased foot and leg symptoms or decreased thigh and buttock symptoms) but may increase (centralize) in the low back. If the symptoms progress down the lower extremity (peripheralize), immediately stop the exercises and reassess.[159]

Alternate positions and procedure: if the patient does not tolerate the prone position, alternate positions may be effective:

- Sitting with a lumbar roll (or towel roll) placed behind the low back. Include repetitive extension motions while sitting, either with pelvic rocking or by extending the thorax over the stable pelvis.
- Standing and performing repetitive back extensions (Fig. 15.5).
- Standing with hands placed on a counter or table and then sagging the pelvis forward to create lumbar extension. This can be a sustained posture or performed repetitively

Lateral Shift Correction

If the patient has lateral shifting of the spine (Fig. 15.6), extension alone cannot reduce a nuclear protrusion of the disc

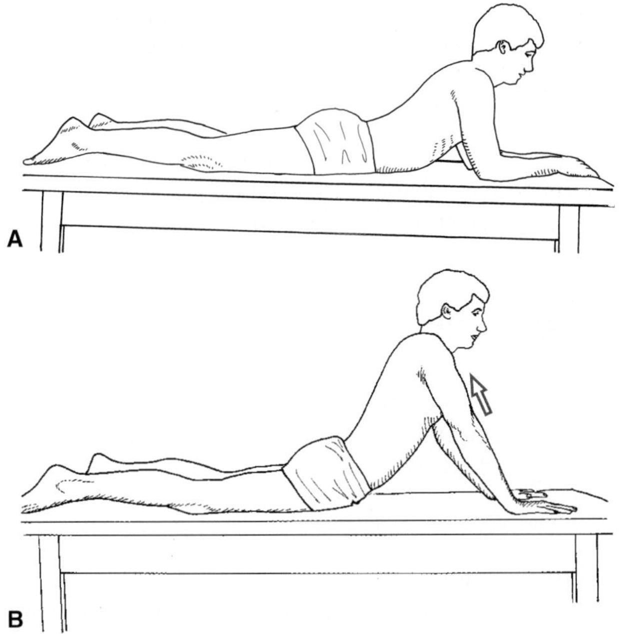

FIGURE 15.4 Lumbar extension is accomplished **(A)** by having the patient prop up on the elbows and **(B)** by propping on hands and allowing the pelvis to sag.

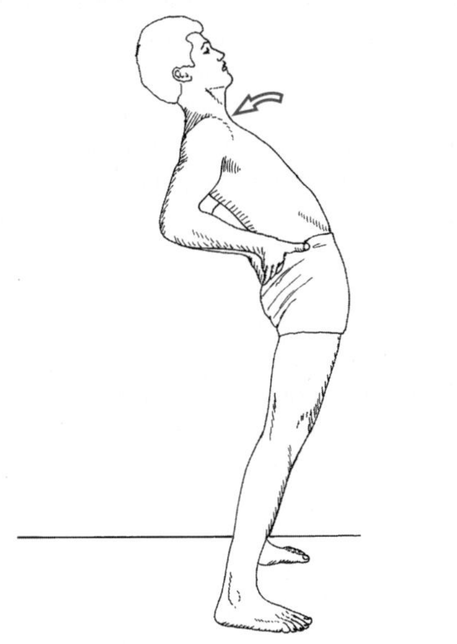

FIGURE 15.5 Standing back extension.

until the shift is corrected. Once the shift is corrected, the patient must extend (as described above) to maintain the correction.

Patient position and procedure: Standing with flexed elbow against the side of the deviated rib cage. Stand on the side to which the thorax is shifted and place your shoulder against the patient's elbow. Then wrap your arms around the patient's pelvis on the opposite side and simultaneously pull the pelvis toward you while pushing the patient's thorax away (Fig. 15.7).

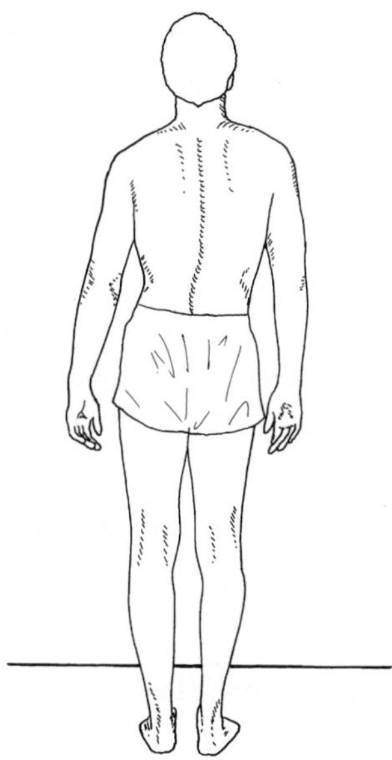

FIGURE 15.6 Patient with lateral shift of the thoracic cage toward the right. The pelvis is shifted toward the left.

This is a gradual maneuver. Continue with the lateral shifting if centralization of the symptoms occurs. If there is overcorrection, the pain and lateral shift may move to the contralateral side, which is corrected by shifting the thorax back. The purpose is to centralize the pain and correct the lateral shift. Once the shift is corrected, *immediately* have the patient backward-bend (see Fig. 15. 5). Again, allow time. Progress to passive extension with prone propping and prone press-ups as previously described.

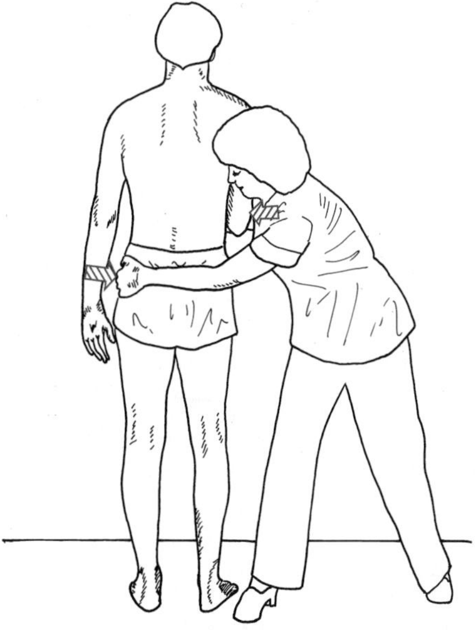

FIGURE 15.7 A lateral gliding technique used to correct a lateral shift of the thorax is applied against the patient's elbow and thoracic cage as the pelvis is pulled in the opposite direction.

Alternate patient positions and procedures:

- Side-lying on the side to which the thorax is shifted. Place a small pillow or towel roll under the thorax. The patient remains in this position until the pain centralizes; he or she then rolls prone and begins passive extension with prone propping and prone press-ups.
- Prone-lying. Attempt to side-glide the thorax and pelvis toward the midline with manual pressure. The forces are in equal and opposite directions. Once the symptoms centralize, instruct the patient to begin passive extension with prone propping and prone press-ups.

Teach self-correction of the lateral shift. The patient places the hand on the side of the shifted rib cage on the lateral aspect of the rib cage and places the other hand over the crest of the opposite ilium and then gradually pushes these regions toward the midline and holds (Fig. 15.8).

Patient Education

- Help the patient recognize what positions and motions increase or decrease the pain or other symptoms by performing them under supervision. Teach safe movement patterns to protect the back as described in the guidelines for treating acute spinal problems (see Box 15.5).
- Instruct the patient to repeat the extension activities frequently, such as 10 times every hour with lateral shift correction if necessary, during the first couple of days. The more severe the symptoms, the more frequently the extension exercises should be completed. In addition, they should be performed immediately upon waking up and after periods of prolonged sitting and/or bending.
- Caution the patient to stop the activity immediately if the pain worsens or peripheralizes during exercises.
- Instruct the patient to maintain an extended posture with passive support while the lesion is healing. For example, have the patient use a towel roll or lumbar pillow while sitting. This is especially important when riding in a car or sitting in a soft chair. When going to bed, have the patient pin a towel, folded lengthwise four times, around the waist.

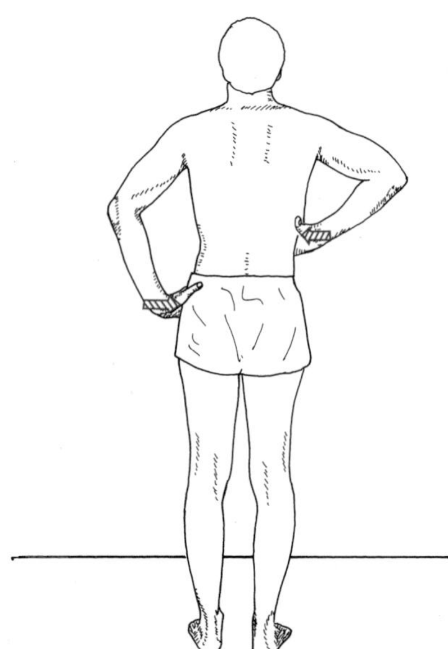

FIGURE 15.8 Self-correction of a lateral shift.

Instruct the patient to use extreme caution if needing to perform flexion activities, such as lifting, or during any other functions that increase intradiscal pressure such as straining.

CLINICAL TIP

If your patient must do an activity that requires flexion or straining, instruct them to first preset the spine in extension by extending the spine, and then after completing the activity to do repeated extensions.

Lumbar Traction

Traction may be tolerated by the patient during the acute stage and has the benefit of widening the disc space and possibly reducing the nuclear protrusion by decreasing the pressure on the disc or by placing tension on the posterior longitudinal ligament.[217]

- Time of the traction should be short; osmotic forces soon equalize. However, upon release of the traction force, there could be an increase in disc pressure, leading to increased pain. Use less than 15 minutes of intermittent traction or less than 10 minutes of sustained traction.
- High poundage; more than half the patient's body weight is necessary for separating the lumbar vertebrae.
- If there is complete relief initially, often there is an exacerbation of symptoms later.
- If the symptoms are relieved with mechanical traction, instruct a family member or caregiver in the application of a unilateral leg pull of the involved extremity for home treatment. This manual traction technique is applied intermittently for 10 to 15 seconds with enough force to decrease symptoms and may be performed throughout the day.

Joint Manipulation

Grades I through IV joint mobilization/manipulation may be utilized preceding the prone press ups, but high-velocity thrust (HVT) should not be performed as this may promote inflammation at the segment. HVTs also require a rotation component, and this may place further stress on the disc.

Kinesthetic Training, Stabilization, and Basic Functional Activities

Once the patient learns to control the symptoms, the following should be emphasized.

- Teach simple spinal movements in pain-free ranges using gentle pelvic tilts. The patient is taught to be aware of how far forward and backward he or she can rock the pelvis and move the spine without increasing the symptoms. The pelvic rocking is done in supine, sitting, hand-knee all-fours (quadruped), prone-lying, side-lying, and standing positions. It is important to stay within the patient's ability to control the symptoms.

- Instruct the patient to finish all exercise routines with the pelvis tilted anteriorly and the spine in extension.
- Teach the patient basic stabilization techniques utilizing the deep trunk muscles while maintaining control of the extended spinal position and performing simple extremity motions. It is important to caution against holding the breath and causing the Valsalva maneuver, which would excessively increase the intradiscal pressure.
- Encourage activities, such as walking or swimming, within the tolerance of the individual.
- Initiate passive, straight-leg raising with intermittent dorsiflexion and plantarflexion to maintain mobility in the nerve roots of the lumbar spine.

Management When Acute Symptoms Have Stabilized

Signs of Improvement

Improvement is noted with loss of spinal deformity, increased motion in the back, and negative dural mobility signs. Loss of back pain with an increase in true neurological signs is an indication of worsening. The patient is tested to determine that the symptoms have stabilized; this is accomplished by performing repeated flexion and extension tests with the patient standing and then lying supine and prone as done initially. The tests may be positive for structural impairments (restricted motion, weakness, and tension), but should not cause peripheralization of the symptoms, as when the condition was acute.[159]

Intervention

The emphases during this stage are *recovery of function, development of a healthy back care plan,* and *teaching the patient how to prevent recurrences.* The pain from adaptive shortening decreases as normal flexibility, neural mobility, strength, and endurance are restored.

In addition to general exercise instruction, teach the patient these principles:

- Following any flexion exercises, perform extension exercises, such as prone press-ups or standing back extension (see Figs. 15.4 and 15.5).
- If being in a prolonged flexed posture is necessary, interrupt the flexion with backward bending at least once every hour. Also, perform intermittent pelvic tilts every hour throughout the day.
- If symptoms of a protrusion develop and are felt, immediately perform press-ups in the prone position, anterior pelvic tilts in the quadruped position, or backward bending while standing to prevent progression of the symptoms.

CLINICAL TIP

It is important that the patient understands they should continue with their daily activities and that symptoms can often be managed with lumbar extension postures and pelvic tilt motion. Instruct them to perform repeated lumbar extension in sitting, standing, or prone position every hour that they are awake, in addition to lumbar ROM via pelvic tilting.

Interventions to Manage a Disc Lesion in the Cervical Spine

Disc lesions in the cervical spine are less common than in the lumbar spine. Herniated discs are most common between the C6 and C7 vertebrae; this is likely due to the increased mobility at this transitional section between the cervical lordosis to the thoracic kyphosis. It may also be the result of degeneration, osteophytes, or poor posture. Patients may present with peripheral neuropathy and forward-head posture without a diagnosis of disc pathology. Symptoms increase with activities and postures that increase flexion in the lower cervical and upper thoracic spine and decrease with extension in that region (axial extension or neck retraction).[1]

Conservative management is similar to that in the lumbar spine and follows the same principles described in the previous section. Medical management includes pharmacological pain and inflammation control measures. Often disc extrusions are an indication for surgery because of potential compromise of the spinal canal and pressure on the spinal cord.[213] These procedures are described in the next section.

Acute Phase

Passive Axial Extension (Cervical Retraction)

Patient position and procedure: Begin with the patient supine, with no pillow under the head or neck. Gently nod the patient's head and allow the neck to flatten against the treatment table. If the neck is deviated or rotated to one side, moving the head and neck back toward the midline must be done first. This may require gentle, progressive positioning and may take 10 to 20 minutes to accomplish.

Progression: Progress the retraction to hyperextension of the cervical spine and then progress to rotation. Use caution and carefully monitor the signs and symptoms; do not progress if symptoms peripheralize down the arm.

Patient Education

Teach the patient to retract his or her head and neck in the sitting position. The patient may gently push against the chin (caution not to push so hard as to cause joint compression of the TMJ) to direct the motion. This technique has been shown to improve the H-reflex amplitude and may be useful for improving mobility and decreasing symptoms of radiculopathy by decompressing nerve roots in the lower cervical spine.[1]

Traction

Cervical traction may relieve the patient's symptoms. As described for lumbar traction, during the acute phase, sustained traction should be no longer than 10 minutes and intermittent traction no longer than 15 minutes in duration. The dosage is at an intensity that causes vertebral separation (at least 15 lb).

CLINICAL TIP

A family member or caregiver may be instructed in performing home traction. The provider gently cradles the patient's head and applies enough distraction force to decrease the symptoms. This can be done in increments of 10 to 30 seconds and can be performed throughout the day.

Kinesthetic Training for Posture Correction

Instruct the patient in safe mechanics for maintaining the head position. It is important to help the patient identify the posture that centralizes the symptoms and to adjust the collar to maintain that position.

Progression as Symptoms Stabilize

Follow the guidelines described in Box 15.7. Faulty cervical, thoracic, and scapular posture may be present. Emphasize kinesthetic training for postural awareness, stabilization exercises for postural control with emphasis on the scapular and shoulder muscles, environmental adaptations to reduce postural stresses, and functional activities with safe spinal mechanics.[89,139]

FOCUS ON EVIDENCE

Kjellman and Oberg[130] randomly placed 77 people with neck pain into one of the following three groups: general exercise, McKenzie extension exercise, and a control group (ultrasound and education). Outcome measures were pain intensity and the Neck Disability Index. After 12 months, all groups showed significant improvement with no significant difference between the three groups, with nearly 70% of patients reporting they were better or completely restored. The authors did note, though, that in the short term (during the first 3 weeks of treatment), those in the extension exercise group had more favorable response to treatment than the general exercise group or the control group, and there was a tendency that those in the extension exercise group used the health-care system less frequently during the 6- to 12-month period. Analysis showed significant improvement between the extension exercise group and control group at 3 weeks and at 6 months ($P < 0.05$).

Disc Lesions: Surgery and Postoperative Management

Indications for Surgery

Patients with upper or lower extremity radiculopathy caused by nerve root irritation and who have failed conservative measures, including physical therapy, medications, and steroid injections, may be appropriate surgical candidates.[33,34,36,78,131,151,184,194,240]

Common Surgeries

The two most common surgical procedures in the spine are laminectomy and fusion of one of more vertebrae.[152]

Laminectomy. A laminectomy is the removal of the lamina. A partial or hemi-laminectomy is a removal of only part of the lamina; a complete laminectomy is the excision of the entire lamina, the spinous process, and the ligamentum flavum that attached to the lamina. The primary disadvantage to a complete laminectomy is that the surgical segment loses its anatomical stabilization.[34,36,100] A laminectomy is typically indicated over a fusion in patients with a small unilateral disc protrusion. The benefits of a laminectomy are that the patients retain segmental mobility while experiencing symptom relief.

Fusions. Fusions are indicated when the patient presents with axial pain combined with instability, severe arthritic degenerative changes, or peripheral pain that is not controlled.[33,36,78,94,131,151,184,194,240] The advantages of a spinal fusion are that it reduces or eliminates segmental motion, reduces mechanical stress at the degenerated disc area, and reduces the incidence of additional herniations at the affected disc site.[240] However, effects of a fusion may expedite the degenerative processes, create a hypermobility at adjacent spinal segments, and alter overall spinal mechanics.[19,62,100,106]

Procedures

Anterior cervical disc fusion. Anterior cervical disc fusion (ACDF) involves a horizontal incision at the level(s) of the cervical vertebrae that are to be fused. Both the platysma and longus coli muscles are interrupted during this procedure. Once the disc is excised, the adjacent vertebrae are then internally fixated with a single unilateral plate and screws attaching directly to the vertebral bodies. Although complications are rare, they can include sore throat, hoarseness, and difficulty swallowing.[81] Medical complications involving the heart, lungs, and other organs affect approximately 5% of surgical patients following ACDF.[152] Neurological or more serious complications, including myelopathy, radiculomyelopathy, and recurrent laryngeal nerve palsy, have been reported as ranging from 1% to 4% of the postsurgical population.[20,33,69] Complications are more likely in elderly patients (≥ 65 years old).[30]

Outcomes

Pain has been reported to significantly decrease following ACDF.[78,107,131,144,168,184,247] Good to excellent outcomes have been reported as high as 92%.[100]

Transforaminal lumbar interbody fusion. Transforaminal lumbar interbody fusion (TLIF) involves a vertical incision centrally along the posterior spine.[94] The paraspinals muscles, including the multifidi, are refracted prior to the removal of the lamina, spinous process, and ligamentum flavum. The vertebrae are fused together using bone from the facetetomy and autologous bone from the iliac crest.[94] Complications, occurring in 2% to 5% of patients, include infection, epidural bleeding, neural injury, postsurgical instability, epidural fibrosis, and arachnoiditis.[19,76,86,194,246] Surgical site infection and wound complications have been cited as the most common complications after surgery.[6] Hayashi et al[96] reported adjacent segment degeneration in 40% of people at 121 month follow-up. Re-operation rates range from 8% to 14%.[96,216] The fusion rate has been reported to range from 70% to 96%.[76,143,170]

Outcomes

Significant improvement in VAS, Oswestry Disability scores, and other functional outcomes have been reported.[12,76,86,90,102,216] Berg and associates[19] identified that 84% of people reported improvement and/or complete resolution of pain at 1 year postoperative and 86% at 2 years. The authors also reported that 71% of people returned to work after 1 year. In a similar study, Fujimori and colleagues[76] reported a 3.4 point decrease in pain on the visual analogue scale and a 14 point improvement in the Oswestry Disability Index at 1.3 years postoperative.

Laminectomy. Laminectomies can be performed in either the lumbar or cervical spine regions. Both involve a posterior approach and are performed similarly to a posterior fusion with the exception that the vertebrae are not internally fixated to each other. The recovery time and return to work time are usually much quicker as compared with a fusion. However, similar rehabilitation guidelines are followed as described in the next section. The need for re-operation following a laminectomy has been reported to range between 14% and 33.8%,[32,216] and lifetime risk of fusion after laminectomy is 8%.[32]

Postoperative Management

Postoperative management is similar for all of these surgical procedures.

Maximum Protection Phase

- ***Patient education.*** Educate the patient on the expectations of the surgeon, the surgical procedure, and the rehabilitation involved in the process. Also, instruct the patient on any restrictions as detailed by the surgeon. These restrictions typically include no heavy lifting (>10 lb) for up to 3 months. Limitations in active motions may also be imposed depending on the surgeon's preference and type of procedure.
- ***Wound management and pain control.*** Teach the patient to look for signs of inflammation such as redness, swelling, or nonclosure of the wound.
- ***Bed mobility.*** The patient must relearn how to perform bed mobility as they may be wearing a spinal orthosis that prevents normal movement.
- ***Bracing.*** To promote healing, patients who have undergone either an ACDF or TLIF are typically placed in a Philadelphia collar and then a soft collar or a chairback brace, respectively, for up to 3 months. The patient may be allowed to remove the brace to shower but must immediately don the orthosis upon getting dressed.
- ***Exercises.*** Encourage walking and gentle ROM exercises (assisted if necessary) that can be completed in the supine position. Include heel slides, short-arc quads, quad and gluteal isometrics, and ankle pumps. Patients who have undergone a laminectomy are instructed to avoid excessive spinal extension due to the weakened bony neural arch.

CONTRAINDICATIONS: Patients are to avoid a shower or getting the incision wet until it is completely closed. This is usually 1 to 2 weeks following surgery. As described above, the patient is instructed to follow the surgeon's guidelines regarding limitations with movement and lifting.

Moderate and Minimum Protection Phases

- ***Scar tissue mobilization.*** After the incision site is healed, initiate scar mobilization to improve connective tissue mobility and decrease pain at the surgical site.
- ***Progressive stretching and joint mobilization/manipulation of restricted tissue.*** Gentle (grade I to II) joint techniques at adjacent segments are indicated for pain modulation and improved ROM.
- ***Muscle performance***
  - Initiate segmental and progress to global stabilization exercises to patient tolerance.[97]
  - Address patient goals directed at minimizing specific activity restrictions and impairments.
  - Begin with single plane exercises and progress complexity as patient tolerates.
- ***Gait training.*** Once the patient is allowed to ambulate, an assistive device is usually indicated to facilitate an erect posture and unload some of the stress to the surgical area.

CONTRAINDICATIONS:
- The patient must continue to follow the surgeon's contraindications to promote optimal healing.
- Joint manipulations at the level(s) of the fusion are contraindicated.
- Extension exercises, including prone press-up, are contraindicated in patients who have undergone a laminectomy.

FOCUS ON EVIDENCE

Multiple research studies report improved functional status in patients who begin rehabilitation at 12 weeks following lumbar spine surgery (with or without fusion).[157,176,177,208] Several authors report that beginning rehabilitation at 6 weeks has inferior outcomes compared to waiting until 12 weeks.[176,177,208]

Management Guidelines: Flexion Bias

Patients may present with a flexed posture and be unable to extend because of increased neurological symptoms and decreased mobility; these patients would benefit from early interventions that emphasize flexion of the involved segments to relieve symptoms. The patients may have a medical diagnosis of spondylosis or spinal stenosis (central or lateral), an extension load injury, or capsular impingement or swollen facet joints, so symptoms increase with extension. The flexed position reduces or relieves the symptoms.

NOTE: Cervical radiculopathy is discussed in the section on Management of Regional Diagnoses later in this chapter.

Principles of Management

Physical therapy interventions focus on increasing the diameter of the foramen and minimizing nerve root irritation.

Effect of position. Flexion widens the IV foramina, whereas extension decreases the size of the foramina. Any compromise of the foraminal opening, such as encroachment from bony spurs or lipping or swollen tissue, reduces the space. The patient may describe intermittent nerve root symptoms (intermittent numbness or tingling) whenever the involved segment extends, indicating mechanical compression. Constant nerve root symptoms could be caused by inflammation and swollen tissue.

Effect of traction. Traction has been demonstrated to widen the IV foramina. Positioning the spine in flexion prior to the application of traction provides the greatest increased space.[145,193] Positional traction, in which the patient is placed in side bending away from the side of pain and rotation toward the pain, may also be beneficial to increase the diameter of the lateral foramen.

Effect of trauma and repetitive irritation. Swelling in the facet joints from macrotrauma or microtrauma leads to a compromised foraminal space. With degeneration and increased mobility in a spinal segment, instability could be the cause of repetitive microtrauma, leading to swelling and pain.

Effect of meniscoid tissue. The meniscoid tissue of the joint capsule may become impinged with sudden movements. This blocks specific movements, such as extension and side bending to the involved side. Manipulation and traction usually relieve the symptoms.

Indications and Contraindications for Intervention: Flexion Approach

Indications. Flexion is used if neurological and/or pain symptoms are eased with flexion and worsened with extension positions or motions.

CONTRAINDICATIONS: Extension and extension with rotation positions, motions, and exercises are contraindicated if neurological symptoms or pain worsen with these motions. Flexion exercises are contraindicated if neurological or pain symptoms peripheralize with flexion or repeated flexion maneuvers (see Box 15.9).

Techniques Utilizing a Flexion Approach

In general, spinal flexion postures and exercises are taught following the guidelines described in Boxes 15.5, 15.7, and 15.8. The following suggestions should also be considered for special conditions.

Management of Acute Symptoms

Patient Education

- As described in the general acute section earlier in this chapter, once the functional position for comfort is identified, encourage the patient to move within pain-free ranges and maintain daily activities that do not exacerbate the symptoms.
- Passive support, such as use of a cervical collar or lumbar corset, is typically not utilized or discussed with the patient except when managing patients with RA or other disorders associated with hypermobility or instability.

Functional Position for Comfort

- For flexion bias in the lumbar spine, the position is usually with the hips and knees flexed so the lumbar spine flexes.
- In the cervical spine, the position is toward axial extension (upper cervical flexion) with some flexion also in the lower cervical region.
- If there are neurological signs, the position provides maximal opening of the IV foramina to minimize impingement of the nerve root.

Traction

- Gentle intermittent joint distraction and gliding techniques may inhibit painful muscle responses and provide synovial fluid movement in the joint for healing.
- Dosages must be very gentle grade I or II to avoid stretching the capsules and are best applied with manual techniques during the acute stage.
- With spondylosis or stenosis, if a patient does not have signs of acute joint inflammation but does have signs of nerve root irritation, stronger traction forces may be beneficial to cause opening of the IV foramina, which helps relieve the pressure.

CONTRAINDICATION: If a patient has RA, traction and joint mobilizations/manipulations in the spine are potentially dangerous because of ligamentous necrosis and vertebral instability; therefore, they should not be performed.[163]

Correction of Lateral Shift

If the patient has a lateral shift of the thoracic region along with symptom relief when in flexion, he or she may be taught self-correction.

Patient position and procedure: Standing with the leg opposite the shift on a chair so the hip is in about 90° of flexion. The leg on the side of the lateral shift is kept extended. Have the patient then flex the trunk onto the raised thigh and apply pressure by pulling on the ankle (Fig. 15.9).

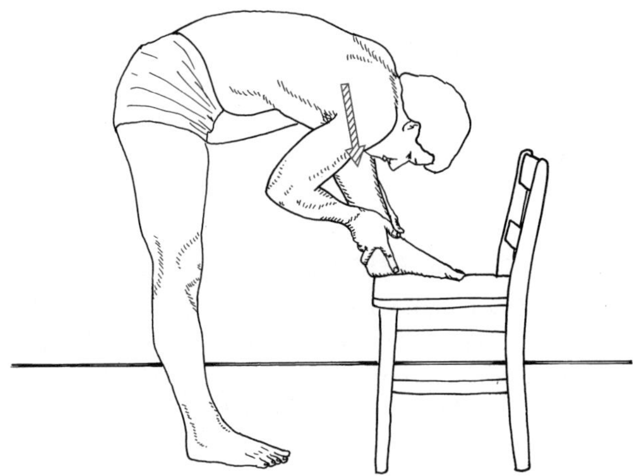

FIGURE 15.9 Self-correction of a lateral shift when there is deviation of the trunk as it flexes.

Correction of Meniscoid Impingements

If there is entrapped synovial or meniscoid tissue in a facet joint that blocks motion into extension, release of the trapped meniscoid relieves the pain and the accompanying muscle guarding. The joint surfaces need to be separated and the joint capsules made taut.[23] General techniques include traction and manipulation.

- Traction to the spine may be applied manually or mechanically. The patient also can be taught self-traction and positional traction techniques. Traction applied longitudinally along the axis of the spine has the effect of sliding the facets' joint surfaces and thus placing tension on the facet capsules. Traction with contralateral side bending and rotation of the spine has the effect of distracting the facet joint surfaces as well as placing tension on the capsules.
- Techniques of manual traction, self-traction, and positional traction with rotation and manipulations are described in the stretching section of Chapter 16.

Management When Acute Symptoms Have Stabilized

General guidelines for subacute and chronic spinal problems are summarized in Boxes 15.7 and 15.8. Specific emphasis when treating patients with mobility impairments due to hypomobile or hypermobile facet joints should include the following:

- Hypomobile joints require stretching but not if the techniques stress a hypermobile region. Traction techniques may be effective if the hypermobile region is stabilized during stretching. For those trained in joint mobilization/manipulation techniques, these techniques are effective for selective facet joint stretching and have been found to be an effective part of a total treatment approach when there is instability in specific areas and restricted mobility in neighboring facet joints.[182] Emphasis is on developing dynamic stability through muscle control in the hypermobile regions while gaining mobility in the restricted regions.
- Strength and flexibility of the trunk, hip, and shoulder girdle musculature require selective stretching and strengthening.
- If there are bony changes and osteophytic spurs, the patient should avoid postures and activities of hyperextension, such as reaching or looking overhead for prolonged periods of time. Adaptations in the environment might include using a stepstool so reaching is at shoulder level. Postures and motions emphasizing flexion of the spine that increase the size of the IV foramina are usually preferred.
- For patients with RA, emphasis is on stabilization and control. Because of the potential instabilities from necrotic tissue and bone erosion, subluxations and dislocations may cause damage to the spinal cord or vascular supply and can be extremely debilitating or life-threatening.

Management Guidelines: Stabilization

Patients with segmental instability—including hypermobility; ligamentous laxity; and diagnoses such as spondylolysis, spondylolisthesis, or poor neuromuscular control of the deep segmental and global stabilizing musculature—require interventions that improve stability. Some of the patients may have a history of trauma, repeated manipulations, or early signs of spondylosis. Mobility testing of the spinal segments reveals increased mobility at one or more segments. There may be decreased activity in the stabilizing musculature, particularly in response to postural perturbations, and there may be faulty respiratory patterns. (Additional information on spondylolisthesis is in the final section of this chapter.)

Identification of Clinical Instability

Stress radiographs are typically used by the medical profession to identify instability. Those with more than 4 mm of translation or 10° of rotation are considered candidates for surgery.[72] Radiographs can identify problems only in the passive structures. To identify impairments in the musculature and the ability to control movement, techniques have been developed that specifically address deep segmental muscle activation and endurance and global muscle stabilization. The following may be used:

- *Quality of movement.* Observe spinal ROM (standing) and note if there is a catch or aberrant movement. Patients may demonstrate difficulty moving smoothly in the midranges as well as a shifting or fluctuation in movement.[75]
- *Control of deep segmental musculature.* In the lumbar region, palpate the TrA and multifidus muscles while the patient attempts to contract them. Devices to measure activation, such as using a biopressure feedback unit or ultrasound imaging, have been developed for both research and clinical usage[113] (see the next section titled Principles of Management as well as Chapter 16).

- *Control of the global musculature.* Several protocols have been developed to test the stabilizing function of the global musculature.[79,92,203] They primarily challenge the isometric holding capability of the anterior, posterior, and lateral trunk musculature under various loads. The passive lumbar extension test, the lumbar extension load test, and the active straight leg raise test have all been shown to be good predictors of patients that may need lumbar stabilization exercises.[199]

Principles of Management

Passive Support

Although not usually recommended, braces or corsets may be necessary for support to provide stability and reduce pain when instability is significant.[72] If needed, these devices should be used in conjunction with training the deep segmental musculature for dynamic control.

Deep Segmental Muscle Activation

Activation of segmental musculature may not be automatic in patients with pain or instability. In addition to verbal and tactile cues, techniques used to instruct patients include use of a biofeedback pressure cuff (Chattanooga®) and ultrasound imaging. Ultrasound imaging is primarily used in research settings because of the cost of the units. The pressure cuff has been shown to have clinical relevance in providing immediate feedback to patients.[113] Use of the cuff for testing and instruction in deep segmental muscle activation of the cervical and lumbar regions is described in detail in the Muscle Performance section of Chapter 16.

Once the patient learns to activate the segmental muscles, emphasis is placed on sustaining the contraction over a period of time and on increasing the repetitions of the static hold to reinforce the postural function. These contractions are of low-intensity to minimize the compressive activity of the global muscles.[83]

CLINICAL TIP

"Strengthening the core" has become a popular phrase in general exercise programs, with its meaning being applied to any exercise that focuses attention on the trunk musculature (usually the abdominals). For *therapeutic purposes* when managing patients with segmental instability, the emphasis is initially directed toward training activation of the deep segmental muscles, followed by the global trunk muscles, and helping the patient become aware of the difference in the actions and functions of these muscles. These techniques are described in detail in Chapter 16.

Lumbar Region

Initially, the patient is taught to find and maintain a neutral spinal position using pelvic tilts (midrange). The patient is then instructed in the "drawing-in maneuver" to activate the TrA, and he or she learns to contract the multifidus by bulging out the muscle. Gentle co-activation of the muscles of the perineum facilitates contraction of these segmental muscles.[173]

FOCUS ON EVIDENCE

A review of systematic reviews from 2000 to 2011 on core stabilization exercises for chronic LBP summarized that stabilization exercise programs benefit people with nonspecific LBP.[93] Additionally, it is reported that core stabilization is more effective in reducing LBP and improving functional outcomes when compared with conventional exercises.[29,119]

Cervical Region

The patient is taught to activate the segmental musculature with gentle capital nodding and slight flattening of the cervical lordosis.[83]

Progression of Stabilization Exercises

- Progress from segmental muscle activation to general stabilization exercises using the global musculature to emphasize cervical and pelvic control while superimposing extremity motions. Include weight-bearing activities, such as wall slides, partial lunges, and partial squats, with emphasis on the "drawing-in" maneuver and spinal control in the neutral spinal position while doing the activities.
- Incorporate functional activities into the stabilization exercise routines. Encourage the patient to activate the segmental musculature consciously and maintain a neutral spinal position until it becomes habitual.

Management Guidelines: Mobilization/Manipulation

NOTE: The terms *manipulation* and *mobilization* are currently being used interchangeably, with a trend toward using the term *manipulation* (see Chapter 5). The authors of this chapter are using *manipulation* to mean graded oscillation techniques and *HVT* to mean high-velocity, small-amplitude motion performed at the end of the pathological limit of the joint. When describing or documenting manipulation techniques used, the clinician is reminded to define the intensity (grade I–IV or HVT) as well as spinal level (target), direction of force application, and patient position.

Some patients benefit from spinal manipulation during the early stages of intervention.[39,43,161] Hypomobile spinal segments may add to stress of hypermobile segments and require a combined approach of manipulation as well as stabilization exercises.[116,182] Manipulation techniques for the cervical, thoracic, and lumbar spines are described in Chapter 16.

Management: Lumbar Spine

Following determination of a hypomobile segment in the lumbar spine, perform the general manipulation (using the lumbar roll technique) up to two times followed by instruction in ROM exercises. This is repeated for two sessions, after which the patient is instructed in stabilization exercises and progressed through treatment as summarized in Boxes 15.7 and 15.8.

The lumbopelvic technique used in validation studies[38,39] as well as an alternate technique[43] are described in Chapter 16. The traction procedures described in the nonweight-bearing section earlier in this chapter may also be beneficial.

 **FOCUS ON EVIDENCE**

In a randomized controlled trial of 71 subjects with LBP, Flynn and associates[68] determined that patients most likely to benefit from spinal manipulation prior to stabilization exercises were those who met four of five of the following criteria: symptom duration less than 16 days; no symptoms distal to the knee; score less than 19 on a fear-avoidance measure; at least one hypomobile lumbar segment; and at least one hip with more than 35° internal rotation. This was validated by Childs and colleagues[38] in a multicenter randomized, controlled trial of 131 consecutive patients.

Fritz and associates[75] reported that those who had positive tests for spinal hypomobility had more successful outcomes if manipulation was included in the interventions and those with hypermobility were more successful if stabilization was included.

The *CPGs for Low Back Pain*[48] cite strong evidence for use of manipulation procedures when treating patients with mobility deficits and acute, subacute, and chronic LBP and back-related buttock or thigh pain in order to reduce pain and improve mobility.

Management: Cervical Spine

Cervical manipulation, in combination with exercise, has been shown to significantly decrease neck pain[7,63,64,87] as well as increase ROM, upper extremity and neck strength, and endurance.[27] Gross and associates[87] completed a Cochrane review and identified strong evidence in favor of manipulation combined with exercise to decrease pain when compared with a control group.

NOTE: The risk of serious or life-threatening injuries has been reported from 1 in 20,000 to 5 in 10 million.[88] In spite of the potential risks,[53,118] many authors have reported there is no risk to damage of the vertebra-basilar artery as a result of cervical thrust joint manipulation.[15,35,101,227] Additionally, cervical thrust joint manipulation has been shown to decrease pain when compared with traction,[251] to decrease pain and disability, and to improve patient outcomes when compared with nonthrust manipulations.[58,225]

It is important that the thoracic spine is assessed in patients with cervical impairments.[120,132] Not only does the thoracic spine move during cervical motion, but it is prone to mobility impairments. In addition, there are common muscle attachments in both regions. Performing joint manipulation and HVT of the thoracic spine often improves outcomes in patients with cervical complaints.[41,42,120,132,153]

 **FOCUS ON EVIDENCE**

Cleland and Childs[41] performed thoracic manipulation, exercise, and patient education on 78 patients with neck pain. An 86% success rate was found for patients with three or more of the following criteria: symptoms <30 days; no symptoms distal to the shoulder, cervical extension did not aggravate the symptoms; Fear-Avoidance Belief Questionnaire-Physical Activity Score of <12; diminished upper thoracic kyphosis (T3–5); and cervical extension <30°.

Puentedura and associates[198] identified four clinical variables that predicted success following cervical thrust joint manipulation. The variables were symptom duration less than 38 days, patient expectation that thrust manipulation would be effective, rotation left and right had a difference of greater than or equal to 10°, and pain with posterior to anterior midcervical mobility testing. If three or more variables were identified, there was a 90% chance of short-term success. Additionally, Bishop and associates[21] found that patients who believed manipulation would be successful had better outcomes.

Management Guidelines: Soft Tissue Injuries

As previously described, symptoms in soft tissues, including muscles, can occur as a result of direct trauma (tears/contusions), strain from sustained or repetitive activities, or as a protective mechanism (guarding/spasm) from injury to joints or other tissues. General guidelines for management are summarized in Boxes 15.5, 15.7, and 15.8. In addition, specific considerations when treating muscle injury are described in this section.

Management During the Acute Stage: Protection Phase

Pain and Inflammation Control

Use appropriate modalities and myofascial release techniques to control pain and inflammation.

Cervical Region

For serious injuries, cervical collars provide passive support to relieve the muscles from the job of supporting or controlling the injured part. Cervical collars are usually reserved for severe and acute whiplash injuries or postoperative intervention per the physician's recommendations. The length of time a collar is worn during the day relates to the severity of the condition and the amount of protection required. Wean the patient from this form of passive support as soon as possible to minimize dependency on its use.

Lumbar Region

Corsets provide passive support of the lumbar region and may be used following serious injury or postsurgically. As with the cervical region, the length of time that a corset is worn should be related to the amount of protection required. Some patients tend to become dependent on the corset and continue to wear it even after healing when it no longer serves its intended purpose. During healing, it is better to strengthen the body's natural corset (deep abdominal muscles) and develop effective spinal mechanics (see Chapter 16) than to have the patient rely on passive support.

Muscle Function

When evaluating muscle function, identify the functional position in which the patient has a decrease in the intensity of symptoms. With a muscle injury, this is often with the muscle in its shortened position. In this position, begin gentle muscle-setting techniques. Dosage is critical; resistance is minimal. Use only enough to generate a setting contraction.

Cervical Region

Patient position and procedure: Supine. Stand at the head of the treatment table, supporting the patient's head with your hands. Start with the guarding muscle in its shortened position. Ask the patient to hold as you apply gentle resistance (light enough to barely move a feather). Both the contraction and the relaxation should be gradual. There should be no neck movement or jerky resistance.

- If there has been muscle injury, the technique is repeated with the muscle kept in the shortened range for several days before beginning to lengthen it.
- As the muscle heals or if there is no muscle injury, progress the treatment by gradually lengthening the guarding muscle after each contraction and relaxation. Movement is performed only within the patient's pain-free range; no stretching is performed when there is muscle guarding.

Alternate procedure: Reverse muscle action. These exercises are valuable for gentle muscle performance activity when neck motions cause pain and muscle guarding. The neck is not moved, but the muscles are called on to contract and relax. The motions include active scapular elevation, depression, adduction, and rotation. If symptoms are not exacerbated, active shoulder flexion, extension, abduction, adduction, and rotation are used to stimulate the stabilizing function of the cervical musculature.

Lumbar Region

Patient position and procedure: Prone, with arms resting at the side. Have the patient lift the head. This initiates a setting (stabilizing) contraction of the lumbar erector spinae muscles. A stronger contraction of the lumbar extensor muscles occurs if the head and thorax are extended. Alternate hip extension also causes a setting contraction of the lumbar extensor muscles.

- When there is muscle injury, the muscle is kept in this shortened range for several days.
- For progression as the muscle heals or if there is no muscle injury, gradually allow the muscle to elongate after each contraction by putting a pillow under the abdomen and having the patient extend the thorax on the lumbar spine through a greater range. Elongation is performed only within tolerance during the early healing phase. There should be no increase in symptoms.

Alternate position and procedure: Supine. Have the patient gently press the head and neck into the bed, causing a setting contraction of the spinal extensors.

Traction

Gentle oscillating traction may reflexively inhibit the pain and help maintain synovial fluid and joint-play motion during the acute stage when the muscles do not allow full ROM. Gentle techniques are most effectively applied using manual traction. Position the part with the injured tissue in a shortened position and use a dosage less than that which causes vertebral separation.

PRECAUTION: Traction techniques may aggravate a muscle or soft tissue injury if the tissue is placed in a lengthened position during the setup or with a high dosage of pull during treatment.[169]

Environmental Adaptation

If there are activities or postures that caused the trauma or are continuing to provoke symptoms, identify the mechanism and modify the activity or environment to eliminate the potential of recurrence of the problem.

Management in the Subacute and Chronic Stages of Healing: Controlled Motion and Return to Function Phases

Once acute symptoms are under control, re-examine the patient and determine the impairments and activity limitations. Refer to the general guidelines for management as presented in Boxes 15.7 and 15.8.

Management of Regional Diagnoses

Most spinal pathologies may affect any region in the spine and tend to cluster in the diagnostic categories that are described in the previous section. There are several pathologies unique to the thoracic and lumbopelvic region and several unique to the craniocervical and upper thoracic region; the interventions for these pathologies are described in this section.

Lower Thoracic and Lumbopelvic Region

Compression Fracture Secondary to Osteoporosis

As described earlier in this chapter, compression fractures of the vertebral bodies, secondary to osteoporosis, commonly occur in the thoracolumbar region as a result of axial loading or trunk flexion. Symptoms are provoked with flexion activities.

Interventions

- Teach stabilization exercises to promote a neutral thoracolumbar junction and develop spinal stability.
- Teach scapular stabilization exercises to assist with correct posture and decrease the progression of a thoracic kyphosis, commonly seen in people with osteoporosis.
- Stretch the antagonist muscles. These muscles include the shoulder horizontal adductors, internal rotators, hip flexors, and internal rotators.
- Instruct in correct lifting techniques and advise to avoid extreme and prolonged trunk flexion when possible.
- Whenever possible, instruct patients who have osteoporosis in preventative measures and safe exercises as described in the osteoporosis section of Chapter 11.

CONTRAINDICATIONS: Avoid trunk flexion activities and exercises, such as bending forward to lift heavy objects and performing toe touch and sit up (crunch) exercises.

Spondylolisthesis

Spondylolisthesis is defined as an anterior slippage of one vertebra on the one directly below it. It is graded according to the amount the superior vertebra moves in relation to the one directly below it as identified on a radiograph. Grade I includes all films that demonstrate up to a 25% slippage, grade II is reserved for patients who have a slippage from 26% to 50%, grade III indicates a 51% to 75% slip, and grade IV is more than 75% slippage.[85,245] This pathology can occur at any age and is associated with instability at the involved segment. Spondylolisthesis can be the result of either a congenital malformation in the pars interarticularis, a traumatic fracture of the vertebral arch, or degenerative changes associated with age or obesity.

Physical Therapy Interventions

- Use the flexion approach described in the previous section.
- Stabilization exercises: include both segmental and global stabilization.
- Stretch the hip flexors.
- Gentle manipulations (grades I and II) for pain modulation. Avoid HVT techniques, as they may further exacerbate the symptoms or instability.

Ankylosing Spondylitis

This is a rheumatic disorder that results in the eventual ossification of both the anterior and posterior longitudinal spinal ligaments and the facet joints. Ankylosing spondylitis first appears in adolescence and "peaks" in the mid-20s.[80,120,239,241] People with this pathology complain of pain at the bilateral SI joints, thoracic or lumbar spine, shoulder, or foot regions.

Rudwaleit and associates[206] identified the following characteristics in people with ankylosing spondylitis: stiffness >30 minutes of duration, back pain that improves with exercise but not rest, back pain that wakes a person up only during the second half of the night, and alternating buttock pain. It was determined, that if at least three of four of these were present, the positive likelihood ratio was 12:4.

Interventions

The primary physical therapy intervention for this pathology is patient education. Patients must have a good understanding of the disease progress (may require a referral to a rheumatologist).

- Educate the patient about the proper, or "functional," posture before the spine becomes ankylosed. An exaggerated lumbar lordosis is required to facilitate a functional thoracic kyphosis and prevent the person from fusing in a posture in which the entire spine is in a kyphotic posture. This can be accomplished by instructing patients to sleep in a prone position and to use a pillow or towel roll behind their lumbar spine during all sitting activities.
- Gentle manipulations (grades I and II) for pain modulation at the non-ankylosed segments
- Segmental and global trunk stabilization and scapular stabilization exercises are mandatory to strengthen the muscles surrounding the spine.
- Stretch to maintain hip extension and shoulder flexion, as lumbar and thoracic extension may eventually be lost.

Scheuermann's Disease

This pathology is similar to HNP except the nucleus pulposus migrates either superior or inferior versus posterior or posterolateral. Scheuermann's disease is the result of a weakened vertebral end-plate. This weakness causes a crack and a breakdown in the weight-bearing ability of the vertebra. The nucleus pulposus then travels to the path of least resistance. Typically, patients with Scheuermann's disease do not have any radicular symptoms as the nerve roots are not involved.

Interventions

- Segmental and global stabilization exercises
- Stretching of tight muscles
- Posture education
- Joint manipulation may be used either for pain modulation or to improve ROM.[125] However, use caution with high-velocity techniques.

Rib Subluxation

The ribs articulate with the thoracic spine and move with all arm and thoracic activities. The place/location where the rib articulates with the thoracic spine is called a costovertebral joint. These joints can become sprained, or displaced, during twisting activities (unloading the trunk of a car or swinging a golf club), trauma (motor vehicle collision or fall), or following a period of prolonged sickness in which repetitive or aggressive coughing was involved. Radicular pain (intercostal nerve) may or may not be involved depending on the mechanism and severity of the injury. Muscle energy (ME) techniques may be used to correct either a posterior or anterior rib hypomobility.

Interventions VIDEO 15.1

ME technique to correct a rib that has been forced and stuck in a posterior position.

- *Patient position:* sitting.
- *Technique:* Stand on the involved side. Place one hand lateral to the rib angle while resisting horizontal adduction (isometrically) with the other hand (Fig 15.10). During the isometric contraction, elicit an anteromedial force at the rib, attempting to improve movement. Hold the contraction and force for 3 to 5 seconds and repeat three to five times.

ME to correct a rib that has been forced and stuck in an anterior position.

- *Patient position:* sitting.
- *Technique:* Stand on the uninvolved side. Place hand medial to the rib angle while resisting horizontal abduction with the other hand (Fig. 15.11). During the isometric contraction, elicit a posterolateral force at the rib attempting to improve movement. The contraction and force are held for 3 to 5 seconds and repeated three to five times. A thorough assessment of the thoracic facet and IV facet joints is also indicated.

CLINICAL TIP

In addition to ME techniques to correct rib dysfunctions, examine thoracic IV mobility and scapular muscular strength since the function of these areas may also be affected with impairments of the costovertebral joints. Thoracic IV manipulations are described in Chapter 16; scapular stabilization exercises are presented in Chapter 17.

Sacroiliac Joint Dysfunction

SI joint sprain has been shown to occur in 10% to 33% of the patient population.[8,23,56,57,150,219] Impairments can be either traumatic or insidious onset. Patients will frequently complain of pain localized to the SI joint region with or without radiculopathy depending on the involvement of the sciatic nerve. Pain is usually relieved with rest and/or by unweighting the joint. Unresolved inflammation or a traumatic etiology may yield a hypomobile SI joint. It is beyond the scope of this textbook to discuss all the hypomobility impairments as they pertain to the sacrum and innominate. Four common impairments include pubic symphysis hypomobility, an anterior rotated innominate, a posterior rotated innominate, and an upslipped innominate (Fig. 15.12). The first three can be corrected with ME techniques, while the fourth may require a HVT.

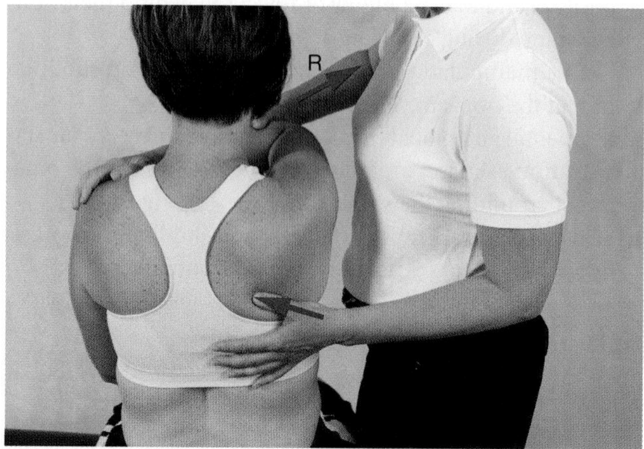

FIGURE 15.10 ME technique to correct a posterior rib.

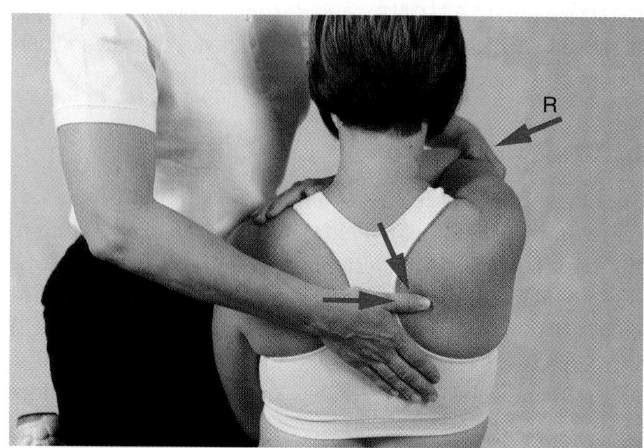

FIGURE 15.11 ME technique to correct an anterior rib.

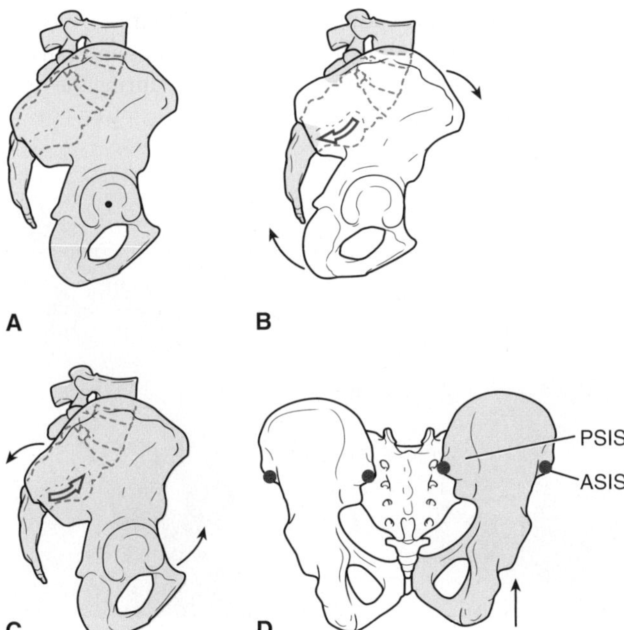

FIGURE 15.12 (A) Normal relationship of the sacrum and innominate, (B) anterior rotated innominate showing the ASIS inferior and PSIS superior, (C) posterior rotated innominate showing the ASIS superior and PSIS inferior, (D) upslipped innominate showing ASIS and PSIS superior on the right compared to contralateral side.

Identification of SI Joint Impairments

- *Observation and findings.* With the patient standing, view from the posterior aspect. Look for symmetry in the heights of the iliac crests, posterior superior iliac spines, and anterior superior iliac spines. With your hands on these bony landmarks, have the patient march in place (March Test) and observe movement of the innominate. If there are positive signs, conduct additional tests, supine and prone lying, to verify SI joint involvement.[56,149,197]
- *General SI joint hypomobility.* The pelvis will "rise up" on the restricted side during the March Test.
- *Anterior rotated innominate.* The posterior superior iliac spine (PSIS) with be higher and the anterior superior iliac spine (ASIS) will be lower on the involved side.
- *Posterior rotated innominate.* The PSIS will be lower and the ASIS will be higher on the involved side.
- *Upslipped innominate.* All bony landmarks of the pelvis will be higher on the side of the upslip.

Interventions VIDEO 15.2

"Shot-gun" technique. The "shot-gun" technique is used to treat both pubic symphysis and general SI joint hypomobility. The idea used to describe the mechanics of this technique is that it creates a gapping followed by a compression of the pubic symphysis joint to improve mobility, although no known studies have confirmed this concept.

- *Patient position:* Supine in a hook-lying position.
- *Technique:* Instruct the patient to contract against your resistance to submaximal contractions, alternating between hip abduction and adduction for a series of three to five repetitions holding each contraction for 3 to 5 seconds (Fig. 15.13).

ME techniques to correct an anterior rotated innominate. ME techniques to correct an anterior rotated pelvis use the force generated by the contracting gluteus maximus to rotate the innominate posteriorly.

- *Patient position:* Supine.
- *Technique:* Flex the involved hip to the point of pain and/or restriction, then resists a series of submaximal isometric hip extension contractions (Fig. 15.14).

ME technique to correct a posterior rotated innominate. A patient that has a posterior rotated innominate can be treated with ME techniques using the rectus femoris muscle.

- *Patient position:* Prone.
- *Technique:* Passively extend the involved extremity to the restriction or point of pain, then resists a series of submaximal isometric hip flexion contractions (Fig. 15.15). With one hand on the pelvis, assist gliding the pelvis anteriorly by pushing on the posterior superior iliac spine when the other hand lifts the femur.

HVT to treat an upslipped innominate. An upslip is usually the result of trauma (such as a fall) or scoliosis. Treatment utilizes a HVT rather than an ME technique. VIDEO 15.3

- *Patient position:* Supine.
- *Technique:* Hold the ankle on the side of the involved pelvis. Place the extremity in slight hip extension, abduction, and internal rotation. This will place the SI joint in a loose pack

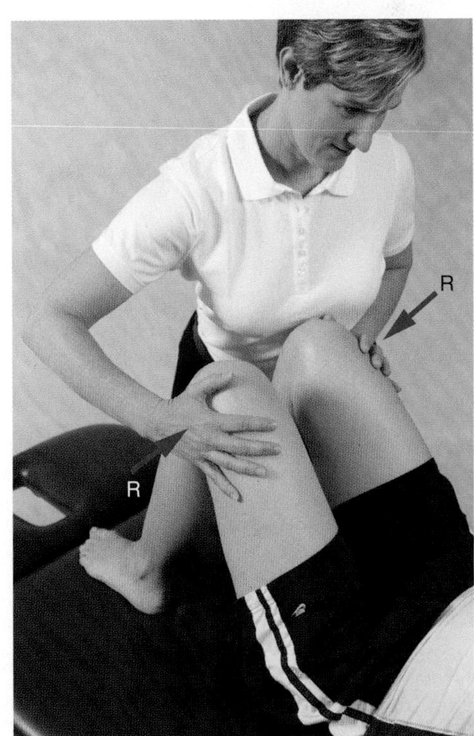

FIGURE 15.13 "Shot-gun" ME technique.

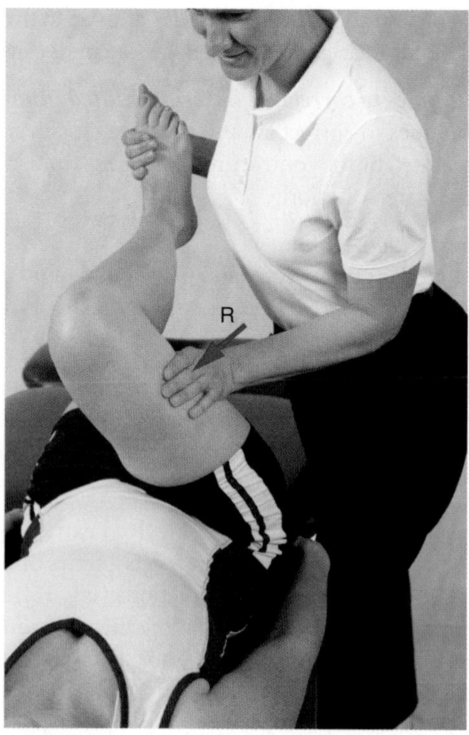

FIGURE 15.14 ME technique of the gluteus maximus to correct an anteriorly rotated innominate bone.

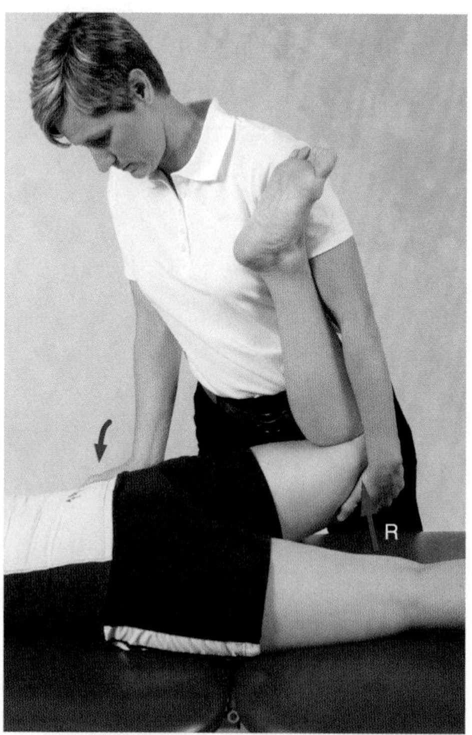

FIGURE 15.15 ME technique of the rectus femoris to correct a posteriorly rotated innominate bone.

position while providing maximum stability to the hip joint. After a series of two to three inhalations and exhalations by the patient, provide a quick "tug" during the final exhalation (Fig. 15.16).

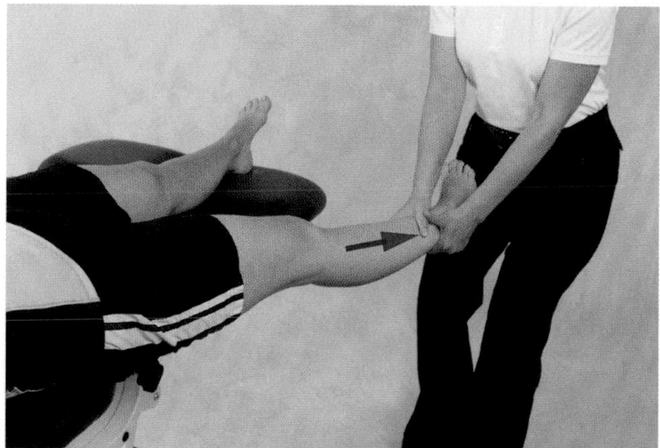

FIGURE 15.16 HVT to correct an upslip of the innominate bone.

Cervical and Upper Thoracic Region

The anatomy and arthrokinematics of the craniocervical region are described in Chapter 14, and physical therapy interventions are discussed in Chapter 16. It is, however, necessary to discuss the significance of this region as both a transitional area from the neck to the head and the precautions needed with respect to the vertebral artery as it courses through this region.

This region is important because the *greater occipital nerve* (sensory branch of C2) pierces the semispinalis capitis muscle prior to providing innervation to the posterior scalp. Irritation of this nerve can be a major cause of headaches.

This craniovertebral area is also important, as it pertains to the vulnerability of the *vertebral artery*. The two vertebral arteries arise from the subclavian arteries prior to entering the transverse foramen of C6, bilaterally, and traveling up through C1. These arteries are responsible for providing 20% of the blood to the brain. After they pass through C1, the arteries travel along the superior surface of the atlas before entering the brain through the foramen magnum.

PRECAUTIONS AND CONTRAINDICATIONS: Extreme caution should be used during grade IV manipulations, HVT, ME techniques, and manual traction so as not to occlude these arteries. Only 45° of rotation is enough to "kink" the artery, and the lumen can narrow up to 90% of its original size with contralateral side bending.[85,192] This can be exaggerated when coupled with backward bending. If the patient has a history of instability, such as RA or long-term steroid use, or complains of dizziness or balance impairments, manipulative movements of the cranio-vertebral region should not be done.

Additional risk factors include cervical trauma in the past month, recent infection, hypertension, migraine headaches without aura, low cholesterol, and low body mass index.[47] Cervical arterial dissection, which is a tear or hematoma in the wall of the vertebral or internal carotid artery, has been reported as a potential complication in a very small population of individuals. Early warning signs of dissection were summarized in a prospective case control study; they include transient ischemic neurological features, blurred vision, and imbalance, as well as dizziness, dysphasia, and paresthesia and weakness in the arm.[230]

CLINICAL TIP

If a patient reports dizziness that is associated with movement, be cautious with examination and intervention techniques that use rotation or extension of the upper cervical spine.

Specific treatment of headaches and selected cervical impairments are discussed in the following sections.

Tension Headache/Cervical Headache

According to the International Headache Society, the three categories of headaches are primary (migraine, cluster, or tension), secondary (headaches caused by another disorder), and cranial neuralgias.[229] Secondary headaches include those that result from cervical spine impairments (musculoskeletal) or temporomandibular dysfunction (TMD). Musculoskeletal headaches are a common complaint with impaired posture. About 15% to 20% of chronic and recurrent headaches are diagnosed as cervical headaches and are related to musculoskeletal impairments.[122] Often, there is associated tension in the posterior cervical muscles and pain at the attachment of the cervical extensors, at the cervicothoracic junction, and/or radiating across the top, side, or back of the scalp.

Etiology

There are many factors that may cause a cervical headache.[156] Headaches may follow soft tissue injury or may be caused by faulty or sustained postures, greater occipital nerve irritation or impingement, or sustained muscle contraction (from faulty posture or emotional tension) leading to ischemia. Cervical muscle trigger points can all contribute to pain in the craniofacial region.[10,123,142,232,244] With cervical headaches, the joints, ligaments, and neuronal structures of the upper cervical spine are often inflamed or in dysfunction.[13,61,77,181] This includes inflammation of cranial nerves V, VII, IX, X, and XI as they descend into the grey matter of C1–3 and provide sensation to the face, forehead, orbit, sinuses, and TMJ region.[192]

Headaches may be related to TMJ dysfunction[147,180] or other conditions, including cardiovascular,[70,136] systemic inflammation,[24,137,205] allergies, or sinusitis.[5] Cervical impairments, which may lead to headaches, can also arise from faulty thoracic joint mobility.[120,132] Whatever the cause, there usually is a cycle of pain, muscle contraction, decreased circulation, and more pain, which leads to decreased function and potential soft tissue and joint impairments.

Presenting Signs and Symptoms

Therapists can effectively treat headaches if they were caused by trauma or stress or if function triggers the onset and/or pain begins in the neck and becomes a headache.[218] Differentiating cervical headaches and related impairments in the musculoskeletal system from other kinds of headaches, such as cluster or migraine headaches, is important for developing a plan of care that effectively manages the headaches. Box 15.10 identifies common history and symptoms associated with cervical headaches as well as red flags that require referral to a physician.[122]

BOX 15.10 History and Symptoms of Cervical Headaches

- Unilateral headaches or bilateral headaches with one side predominant
- Pain in the neck or suboccipital region that spreads into the head
- Intensity can fluctuate between mild, moderate, or severe
- Precipitated by sustained neck postures or movements
- May be precipitated by stress (also common with other types of headache)
- May be related to trauma, DJD, or a sedentary lifestyle and postural stresses
- More prevalent in females but no familial tendency
- Pain or altered sensation in the face or TMJ region

Red Flags and Precautions

A referral to a physician is indicated if the patient complains of any of the following, as the headache is probably not of musculoskeletal origin.

- States this is either the first or worst headache they have ever experienced
- Reports sharp pain or spikes in intensity
- Reports headaches come in bunches; i.e., throughout the day or over several hours, the headaches come and go
- A change in personality or behavior is reported

Refer to a specialist with the following reported history and headache[88]

- Positive cardiac history or signs, send to a cardiologist
- Bilateral pain or in multiple joints, send to a rheumatologist
- Sinusitis, facial pain, nasal congestion or pressure, send to ENT
- Vision loss/disturbances or pain with eye movement, send to ophthalmologist
- TMD symptoms, send to pain center or dentist

Musculoskeletal Impairments

Musculoskeletal impairments include:

- Joint impairments in the upper cervical spine and craniovertebral region (pain and motion restrictions).
- Impaired muscle performance (impaired tonic postural control and endurance in upper and deep cervical flexors and possibly multifidus and small posterior suboccipital muscles).[122]
- Impaired shoulder girdle/scapular posture with related muscle imbalances.
- Impaired lumbar posture with related muscle imbalances.[156]
- Impaired neural tissue from pressure or inflammation in the upper cervical/craniovertebral region.
- Impaired neuromotor control.
- Impaired upper thoracic mobility.

General Management Guidelines

Management is directed toward reversing physical impairments, including posture correction, stress management, and prevention of future episodes.[122]

Pain Management

Modalities, massage, and muscle-setting exercises are used to break into the cycle of pain and muscle tension.

Soft tissue techniques and myofascial release. Various forms of soft tissue mobilization, myofascial release, and trigger point release have been reported to decrease pain intensity and improve cervical ROM.[67,115,117,166]

Dry needling. This manual therapy intervention has been reported to decrease pain both immediately and for a 4-week follow-up.[124,128]

NOTE: The inclusion of soft tissue, myofascial release, and dry needling techniques are beyond the scope of this textbook.

Mobility and Muscle Performance

Examine the flexibility and strength of the muscles in the cervical, upper thoracic, shoulder girdle, and lumbar spine and design an exercise program to regain a balance in flexibility and neuromuscular control in conjunction with posture correction and training as described in Chapter 14 (see Boxes 14.2 and 14.3). Interventions that have been reported to decrease the intensity and incidence of cervical headaches include the following.[28,67,115,117,122,124,128,156,166]

Mobility and flexibility. Increase joint mobility in the cervical spine and flexibility in the suboccipital muscles to relieve tension in that region as well as to activate and train the deep cervical flexors for control of capital flexion and cervical retraction (described in Chapter 16). Control and support from the deep segmental muscles are the foundation of management.

Cervical stabilization. Utilize cervical stabilization exercises as described in detail in Chapter 16, emphasizing tonic holding of the deep segmental muscles in isolation from the global muscles.[122]

Scapular stabilization and posture. Train the lower trapezius, rhomboids, and serratus anterior muscles in tonic holding postures to improve control of scapulothoracic posture (described in Chapter 17). Exercise prescription should focus on the endurance aspects of these muscles.[28]

Stress Management

If the person is in tension-producing situations, relaxation techniques, ROM and muscle-setting techniques, and proper spinal mechanics are taught.

FOCUS ON EVIDENCE

Jull and associates[121] conducted a multicenter, randomized, controlled study of 200 individuals with cervicogenic headache. They looked at the effectiveness of manipulative therapy and a low-load exercise program alone and in combination compared to a control group and found that both interventions reduced headache frequency and intensity and reduced neck pain compared to that in the control group and that the effects were maintained at the 12-month follow-up. The exercise intervention primarily consisted of training postural control of the longus colli and other deep neck flexors as well as the serratus anterior and lower trapezius muscles and increasing muscular endurance. (See Chapter 16 for a description of the cervical stabilization exercises and Chapter 17 for a description of the scapular stabilizing exercises.) Postural correction exercises were also performed throughout the day and progressed to isometric resistance and flexibility exercises.

Prevention. Underlying the prevention of future episodes of cervical headaches is the education of the patient to correct postural stresses; maintain a healthy balance in the length and strength of the postural muscles; and adapt the home, work, or recreational environment to minimize sustained or repetitive faulty postural alignment.

Neck Pain

It is estimated that 22% to 70% of the American population will have neck pain in their life. Prevalence increases with age, and nearly 37% of people have neck pain that lasts longer than 12 months. Almost 25% of all patients seen in outpatient physical therapy clinics have this complaint.[37]

Therapy interventions for cervical pain follow the same guidelines described earlier (see Management Guidelines in Boxes 15.5, 15.7, and 15.8). As identified in the Hypomobility: Manipulation section, it is important to assess and treat the thoracic spine in people with cervical impairments[132] because not only does the thoracic spine move during cervical motions, influence cervical posture, and have common muscle attachments, but also because the thoracic spine is prone to hypomobility impairments. Performing joint manipulation and HVT to the thoracic spine will often improve outcomes in people with cervical symptoms.[41,120,132] Patients with neck pain also report more symptoms of TMJ dysfunction than healthy controls (see management guidelines for TMJ Dysfunction later in this chapter).[52]

FOCUS ON EVIDENCE

The summary recommendations for interventions in the treatment of neck pain published in the ***CPGs for Neck Pain***[37] include:

- cervical mobilization/manipulation based on strong evidence;
- thoracic mobilization/manipulation based on weak evidence;
- targeted stretching exercises based on weak evidence;
- coordination, strengthening, and endurance exercises based on strong evidence;
- upper quarter and nerve mobilization based on moderate evidence;
- traction based on moderate evidence; and
- patient education and counselling based on strong evidence.

Raney and colleagues[200] applied mechanical traction to 68 patients with neck pain for 15 minutes each session. Mechanical traction was found to be 90% successful in 90% of the patients if they met four of the five following criteria: (1) patient reported peripheralization with C4–7 mobility testing; (2) patient had a positive abduction sign; (3) patient was age 55 years or older; (4) patient returned a positive median nerve tension test; and (5) patient experienced relief of symptoms with manual distraction.

Tseng[233] followed 100 patients with neck pain and identified six variables for patient success with manipulation. The authors concluded that if the patients met four of the following criteria their chance for success using cervical manipulation was 89%. The variables were (1) initial Neck Disability index <11.5, (2) bilateral involvement pattern, (3) not performing sedentary work >5 hours each day, (4) feeling better while moving neck, (5) did not feel worse with neck extension, and (6) diagnosis of spondylosis without radiculopathy.

Cervical Radiculopathy

Neck pain with pain and/or neurologic symptoms extending into the arm can be the result of several pathologic conditions, including narrowing of the IV foramen from inflammation and/or degenerative changes in the facets or the IV discs. Thus, foraminal stenosis with accompanying neurologic signs require careful examination as to what positions, motions, and activities lead to symptom production as well as symptom relief. Interventions are then directed toward relieving the symptoms. Interventions typically include:

- Cervical traction
- Cervical stabilization exercises that emphasize training, strengthening, and developing endurance in the deep cervical flexors, axial extension/cervical retraction, and scapular posture (these are described in detail in Chapter 16)
- Posture training with emphasis on postures that relieve symptoms (Chapter 14)

FOCUS ON EVIDENCE

Fritz and associates[74] randomized 86 people with cervical radiculopathy into three different intervention groups for 4 weeks of treatment and followed them for 12 months after the conclusion of therapy. All patients were told to remain active and perform exercises every day. The groups were: exercise alone, exercise with intermittent mechanical traction (performed supine, and exercise with over the door traction (for home use). The mechanical traction group had significantly improved Neck Disability Index scores at both 6 and 12 months with respect to the other groups. The exercises used in the study included scapular strengthening and cervical stabilization exercises to the deep cervical flexors.

A systematic review[231] summarized that patients with cervical radiculopathy have a favorable natural course of recovery. The review identified that use of a collar was no more effective than physical therapy or traction. It was also reported that traction was no more effective than placebo traction.

Cleland and associates[42] identified 96 consecutive patients with cervical radiculopathy. Patients had a 90% success rate using an intervention manual therapy, traction, and deep neck flexor strengthening exercises if they met the following criteria: <54 years old; dominant hand not affected; looking down did not worsen the symptoms; and ME and/or thrust, traction, and deep neck flexor muscle strengthening used ≥50% of the time during PT sessions.

Cervical Myelopathy

Cervical myelopathy is a disease of the spinal cord.[192] It results from degeneration or stenosis of the central spinal canal. The prevalence of this disease is unknown. A person with cervical myelopathy may experience neurological symptoms in both his hands and feet. In addition to an uncoordinated gait, people who have cervical myelopathy may experience a variety of upper motor neuron lesions, including bowel and bladder impairments. Myelomalacia, seen on a MRI film, is the gold standard for the accurate diagnosis of this pathology.[45] There are no neurologic tests or signs that offer both a high sensitivity and specificity.[45]

Therapy interventions are based on the associated impairments and identifying the cause. As this pathology is caused by degeneration, stenosis, or spondylosis, the intervention sequence for cervical myelopathy will follow the same guidelines as described under those pathologies. This includes scapular stabilization, posture education, and cervical and thoracic joint manipulations.

 **FOCUS ON EVIDENCE**

Rhee and associates[202] conducted a systematic review of the literature from January 1956 through November 2012 that compared conservative treatment with surgery for outcomes of patients with myelopathy. Only 1 randomized control trial was identified that favored conservative care over surgery in patients with mild myelopathy. Since cervical myelopathy is typically a progressive disorder, the overall recommendation is that patients need to be monitored for neurological deterioration. Additionally, patients with moderate to severe symptoms need to be counselled that even a minor traumatic event could significantly worsen their neurologic status.

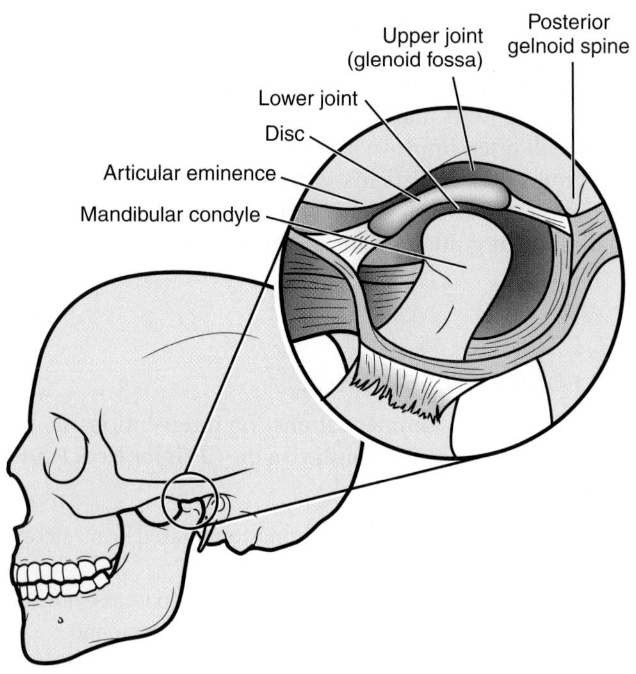

FIGURE 15.17 Structure of the TMJ.

Temporomandibular Joint Dysfunction

The function of the TMJ is closely related to the function of the upper cervical spine and posture. In 44% of patient cases, neck pain is associated with TMD.[238] Because of this close relationship and co-occurrence of neck pain and jaw dysfunction, a brief description of the structure, function, impairments, and interventions related to the TMJ are included.

Structure and Function

Each TMJ is described as a ginglymoarthrodial joint (combination of a hinge and plane joint), consisting of the mandibular condyle articulating with the TM disc and glenoid fossa of the temporal bone (Fig. 15.17). Together, these joints perform tasks such as chewing, talking, and yawning.

Motions of the TMJs. The motions available at the TMJs include mandibular depression (mouth opening), lateral deviation, and protrusion.

- During mandibular depression, the condyle both rolls and slides anterior on the TM disc while the disc also slides anterior to maintain a congruent surface with the fossa (Fig. 15.18). Mouth opening is primarily facilitated by gravity with minimal assistance from the anterior digastric and the lateral pterygoid muscles.
- Protrusion occurs when both TMJs slide anteriorly.
- Lateral excursion involves the ipsilateral TMJ spinning in place with the contralateral TMJ sliding anterior. Both protrusion and lateral excursion are needed when grinding small foods, like lettuce.

Signs and Symptoms

The three cardinal (main) signs of TMJ impairments are:[51,60,82,162,171,172,179]

- Pain in the TMJ region that is affected by movement.
- Joint noise during movement.
- Restrictions or limitations with jaw movement.

Pain from a variety of sources is often cited as part of the TM joint syndrome.[174]

- Pain may occur locally in the TMJ, in the richly vascularized and highly innervated retrodiscal pad located in the posterior region of the joint or in the ear.
- Pain from muscle spasm or myofascial pain in the masseter, temporalis, or the medial or lateral pterygoid muscles may be described as a headache or facial pain.
- Tension in the muscles of the cervical spine may itself be painful or cause referenced pain from irritation of the greater occipital nerve that may be described as a tension headache.

Etiology of Symptoms

TM joint impairments and pain are usually the result of trauma, poor posture, or faulty movement patterns. Additionally, symptoms can result from:

- Poor oral hygiene
- Gum chewing
- Heavy kissing
- Bruxism (grinding the teeth)
- Smoking

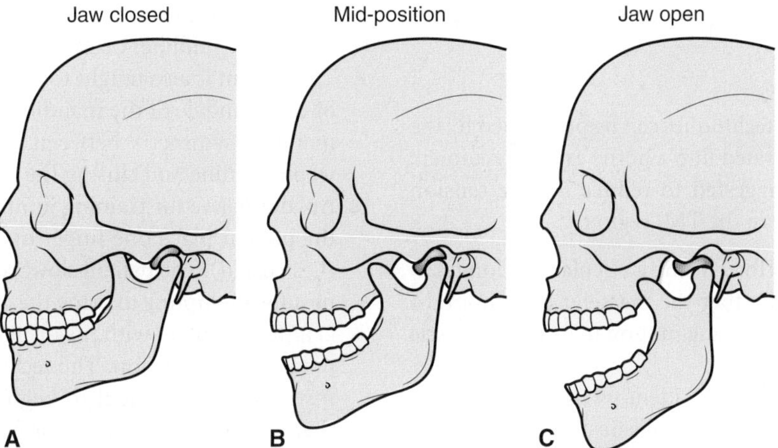

FIGURE 15.18 Mandibular depression: **(A)** relationship of the condyle, TM disc and glenoid fossa with jaw closed; **(B)** as the jaw opens the condyle rolls on the TM disc, then **(C)** the disc and condyle slid anterior on the articular eminence.

- Inflammatory conditions such as RA
- Open mouth breathing

Relationship to Neck Pain

Two theories have been proposed as to why neck pain may cause TMJ discomfort.[215] Causes may be:

- A result of the neurophysiological influences from pain in masticatory muscles via the tonic neck reflex and/or the agonist/antagonist relationship of the anterior and posterior cervical muscles.
- Patients with neck pain respond by bruxing (grinding the teeth), which may lead to muscle or TMJ pain.

Mechanical Imbalances

Imbalance that occurs between the head, jaw, neck, and shoulder girdle may also precipitate TMD signs and symptoms. Causes may be:

- Malocclusion, decreased vertical dimension of the bite, or other dental problems.[134]
- Faulty joint mechanics from inflammation, subluxation of the meniscus (disc), dislocation of the condylar head, joint contractures, or asymmetrical forces from jaw and bite imbalances. Restricted motion results from periods of immobilization after reconstructive surgery or fracture of the jaw.
- Muscle spasm in the muscles of mastication, causing abnormal or asymmetrical joint forces. Muscle spasm can be the result of emotional tension, faulty joint mechanics, direct or indirect injury, or a postural dysfunction.
- Sinus problems, resulting in mouth breathing, which indirectly affects posture and jaw position.
- Forward-head posture resulting in retraction of the mandible, which places the anterior throat muscles in a lengthened position. Consequently, there is increased activity in the muscles that close the jaw to counter the mandibular depression force caused by the digastric muscles. Extension of the head on the upper cervical spine places the muscles and soft tissue in the suboccipital region in a shortened position, so they lose flexibility. Also, the nerves and joints in the upper cervical region become compressed or irritated.
- Sudden trauma, such as a flexion/extension accident in which the jaw forcefully opens when the head whips back into hyperextension; a direct blow from an auto accident, boxing, a fall, or similar trauma.
- Sustained trauma associated with prolonged dental surgery in which the mouth is held open for a lengthy period of time may initiate symptoms in the TMJ or supporting tissue. Excessive stresses, such as biting or chewing on large pieces of hard food, may also traumatize the joints.

Principles of Management and Interventions

The approach to management depends on the cause of symptoms and/or functional limitations. It is important to remember that "aggressive and irreversible treatments" should be avoided if possible.[84] In simple cases in which posture, joint dysfunction, or muscle imbalances are the source of the problem, intervention with therapeutic exercise can directly address the impairments. In most cases, a dental referral, otolaryngology referral, or psychological support may be necessary to deal with related pathology.[95] A complete evaluation is necessary prior to initiation of any treatment. Successful management of TMJ impairments is directly related to the accuracy of diagnosing the underlying pathology.[54]

Reduction of Pain and Muscle Guarding

Use of modalities for pain modulation and relaxation are often indicated during acute and painful episodes. Extra- and intra-oral myofascial techniques are indicated to improve joint and muscle mobility and decrease pain. In addition, the person should eat soft foods and avoid items requiring excessive jaw opening (i.e., apple, corn on the cob, large sandwich) or firm biting (i.e., carrots) and repetitive chewing motions (i.e., gum).

Soft Tissue Techniques

The following soft tissue techniques can be performed by the therapist and/or incorporated into a home exercise regimen. These techniques are suggested to reduce muscle tension and/or improve mobility in the TMJ region:

- *Extra-oral massage.* Perform using a circular motion technique in the region of either the masseter or temporalis muscle. Use a gentle massaging motion to facilitate muscle relaxation.
- *Intra-oral trigger point release.* Identify a point of muscle tension within either the temporalis or masseter tendons. Maintain gentle finger point pressure until the muscle is felt to relax. Repeat at multiple areas of the muscle where muscle tension is identified.
- *A petrous sinus release.* This technique is indicated in patients with TMJ pain and limitations due to muscle guarding and/or sinus involvement. Place one finger on the buccal side of the maxillary teeth and move posterior and cephalad. Once resistance is met, then maintain pressure until a "release" or softening of the muscle occurs. It is judicious to advise the patient that this technique may be a little uncomfortable.

Fascial Muscle Relaxation and Tongue Proprioception and Control

The following are suggested techniques:

- Place the tip of the tongue on the hard palate behind the front teeth and draw little circles or letters on the palate. For additional stimulus, place a Lifesaver® between the tongue and palate; then follow the circular edge with the tip of the tongue.
- Place the tip of the tongue on the hard palate and blow air out to vibrate the tongue, making an "r r r r" sound.
- Fill the cheeks with air (mouth closed); then let the air out in a puff.
- Make a "clicking" sound with the tongue on the roof of the mouth. When doing so, the jaw drops open quickly and returns with the teeth slightly apart, and the tongue usually rests on the hard palate behind the front teeth. This is the resting position of the jaw and is also the first step in teaching relaxation exercises. (Relaxation exercises are described in Chapter 14.)

Control of Jaw Muscles and Joint Proprioception

First, teach recognition of the resting position of the jaw. The lips are closed, teeth slightly apart, and tongue resting lightly on the hard palate behind the front teeth. The patient should breathe in and out slowly through the nose, using diaphragmatic breathing. Resting position of the jaw should be maintained throughout the day.

- Teach control while opening and closing the jaw through the first half of the ROM. With the tongue on the roof of the mouth, the patient opens the mouth, trying to keep the chin in the midline. Use a mirror for visual reinforcement. The patient is also taught to lightly palpate the lateral pole of each condyle of the mandible bilaterally and attempt to maintain symmetry between movement of the two sides when opening and closing the mouth.
- An alternative for training joint proprioception is to have the patient place one finger on a maxillary canine tooth (i.e., cuspid). The patient slowly opens and closes his or her mouth, attempting to bring the corresponding mandibular canine in contact with his or her finger during end-range mandibular elevation. The technique can be advanced by instructing the patient to begin in lateral excursion and then attempt to return his or her mandible to the correct position.
- If the jaw deviates while opening or closing, have the patient practice lateral deviation to the opposite side. The lateral motion should not be excessive or cause pain.
- Progress to applying gentle resistance with the thumb against the chin. Do not overpower the muscles.

Stretching Techniques

If there is restricted jaw opening, determine if it is from hypomobile tissues or a dislocated meniscus. Passive stretching and joint mobilization/manipulation are used to stretch tight tissues. Joint distraction can be used to reposition a meniscus that is blocking opening.

Passive Stretching

Stretch to increase jaw opening if indicated. Begin by placing layered tongue depressors between the central incisors. The patient can gradually work to increase the amount of tongue depressors used until he or she can open approximately far enough to insert the knuckles of the index and middle fingers.

- Self-stretching is carried out by placing each thumb under the upper teeth and the index or middle fingers over the lower teeth and pushing the teeth open.

Joint Manipulation Techniques **VIDEO 15.4**

Patient position and procedures: Supine or sitting, with the head supported and stabilized. Perform joint techniques with a gloved hand or hands. Determination of dosages and precautions for administration of manipulative techniques are described in Chapter 5.

- *Unilateral distraction* (Fig. 15.19 A). Use the hand opposite the side on which you are working. Place your thumb in the patient's mouth on the back molars; the fingers are outside and wrapped around the jaw. The force is in a downward (caudal) direction.
- *Unilateral distraction with glide* (Fig. 15.19 B). After distracting the jaw as described above, pull it in a forward (anterior) direction with a tipping motion. The other hand can be placed over the TMJ to palpate the amount of movement.
- *Bilateral distraction* (Fig. 15.20). If the patient is supine, stand at the head of the treatment table. If the patient is

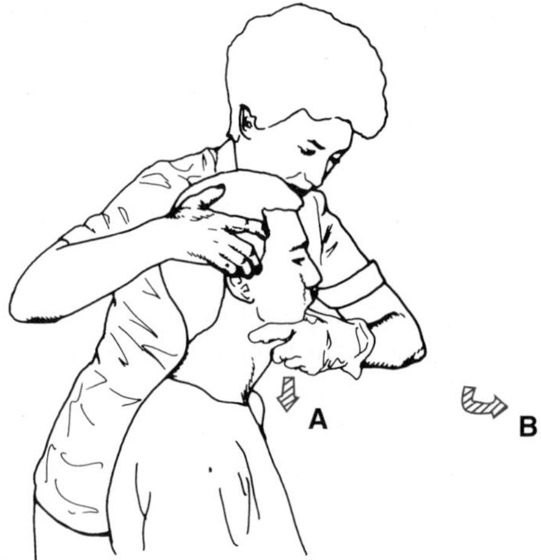

FIGURE 15.19 Unilateral mobilization of the temporomandibular joint. **(A)** Distraction is in a caudal direction. **(B)** Arrow indicates distraction with glide in a caudal, then anterior direction.

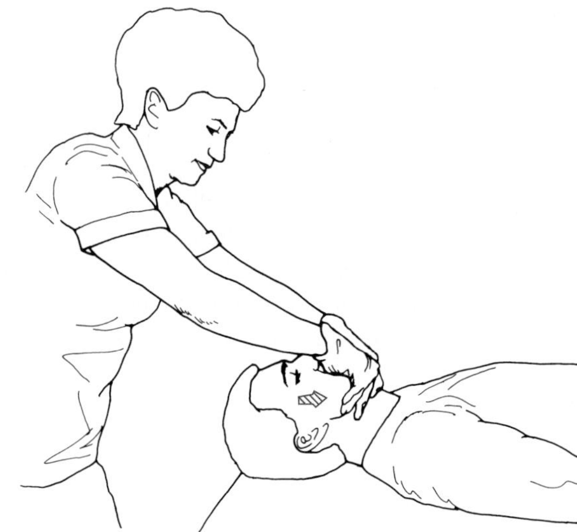

FIGURE 15.20 Bilateral distraction of the temporomandibular joint with the patient supine.

sitting, stand in front of the patient. Use both thumbs, placing them on the molars on each side of the mandible. The fingers are wrapped around the jaw. The force from the thumbs is equal in a caudal direction.

- *Self-manipulation.* Place cotton dental rolls between the back teeth and have the patient bite down. This distracts the condyles from the fossae in the joints.

Reduction of Upper Quarter Muscle Imbalances

Identify flexibility and strength imbalances in the upper quarter. Stretch restricting postural muscles, teach relaxation, and then retrain for proper muscle control. Cervical and shoulder postural stretching and retraining exercises are described in Chapters 16 and 17, respectively.

Independent Learning Activities

Critical Thinking and Discussion

1. What are the functional differences between the way the cervical spine and lumbar spine are used in daily activities?
2. Explain how different individuals who sustain back injuries can experience different symptoms of radiating pain down the leg, numbness and tingling into the foot, deep aching down the leg, or no leg symptoms at all. What does each of these symptoms mean?
3. Explain why some people experience diminished symptoms and improved function if the emphasis of intervention is spinal extension, whereas others improve if the emphasis of intervention is spinal flexion.
4. Identify three common causes of musculoskeletal headaches. What are the indications of headaches that could be identified that would warrant a referral to a medical physician?

Laboratory Practice

1. Practice identifying cervical and lumbar spine positions when in the supine, prone, side-lying, sitting, and standing positions. Determine what is needed to change the position. For instance, if flexion is emphasized, what is needed to cause extension?
2. Identify and feel what happens to the various portions of the spine when moving from one position to another, such as rolling supine to prone and return, moving from supine to sit, moving from sit to stand, and reverse.
3. Practice methods for developing gentle isometric muscle contractions that could be used during the acute phase of treatment for both the cervical and lumbar spines.
4. Practice the various proprioceptive exercises and manipulation techniques for the TMJ region.
5. Create a list of pros/cons comparing and contrasting cervical mobilizations with high velocity thrust techniques. What are the safety precautions associated with these techniques? Perform the vertebral artery test on a lab partner. Given a low sensitivity, how does this affect your interpretation of the test results?

Case Studies

Case 1

A 45-year-old man sustained injuries in a rear-end collision 4 days ago (a car hit him going approximately 45 mph while he was stopped at a stop light). He was in an older car without an air bag or properly positioned headrest, although he was wearing a seatbelt. Initially, he hit the headrest at the mid-cervical spine as his neck extended, and then his head flexed forward but did not hit anything. He has been cleared of cervical fractures or instability. Medical history is unremarkable; he is a social drinker and gave up smoking 5 years ago. He is an accountant and usually works long hours at a computer but has been unable to work since the accident. He presents wearing a cervical collar and has a facial expression of distress. He states he has had difficulty sleeping because the pain wakes him whenever he moves.

Pain: constant posterior cervical pain, headaches, and pain radiating into the shoulder region bilaterally; intermittent tingling in the right thumb, index, and middle finger. Pain rated at 8/10 when at rest, 10/10 when attempting to move.

Positive findings: guarded forward-head posture. He is unwilling to move more than 10° into flexion or extension, 25° into side bending bilaterally; minimal rotation. Gentle traction to the head relieves the neurological symptoms. Palpation tenderness in upper trapezius and posterior cervical and anterior throat muscles bilaterally. Increased tenderness along facet margins of C4–5, 5–6 and 6–7, right > left.

- Based on the above impairments and functional limitations, identify goals and interventions for this patient. Describe the techniques you would use and practice them on a lab partner.
- How long do you anticipate the patient will have these symptoms? At what point will you change your goals?

Case 2

Assume you did not see the patient described in Case Study 1 until 4 weeks after the accident. He no longer has constant pain and has returned to work. His complaints are an inability to sit at the computer for more than 30 minutes before his hand starts to tingle. Numbness occurs after 1 hour of work. Headaches begin within 2 hours of work. Neck and shoulder pain is 6/10 by midday at which time he takes NSAIDs so he can continue working. Positive tests include forward-head posture with forward shoulders; decreased flexibility in the suboccipital muscles, anterior thorax, and internal rotators of the shoulder. Cervical flexion is 75%, extension 50%, and side bending and rotation 75% bilaterally. Sustained extension of the cervical spine causes tingling in the thumb, index, and middle finger of the right hand. Strength of scapular adductors and lateral rotators of the shoulder is 4/5; myotome testing is normal bilaterally.

- What are your goals and interventions for this patient at this stage?
- After studying the techniques described in Chapter 16, describe the techniques you would use with this patient and practice them on a laboratory partner.
- For each therapeutic exercise technique, practice progressions and determine how you would progress this patient so he could work without exacerbation of symptoms.

Case 3

A 55-year-old woman presents with early signs of degenerative joint disease of the lumbar spine. She has been an active runner since college. Occasionally, she has participated in aerobic dance classes. Her history is unremarkable. She has three grown children and had no complaints of back pain related to the pregnancies.

Current symptoms: intermittent periods of pain extending from the mid-lumbar spine, through the right buttock and posterior thigh. The pain begins 15 minutes into her running and progresses to an 8/10 by 25 to 30 minutes. She also complains of increased stiffness after sitting > 1 hour, standing > 15 minutes, as well as when waking in the morning and getting out of bed. She is a middle-school teacher and track coach for a girls' high school team.

Key findings: lordotic posture, with tight low back, hip flexors, and tensor fasciae latae. Strength of lower abdominals is 4/5. Forward bending of the spine increases tension in low back, repeated backward bending and prone press-ups increase buttock pain. Side bending is decreased 25%, with some discomfort with overpressure into right side bending.

- Based on these impairments and limitations, identify the irritability of the condition and determine goals and intervention.
- What are the most important factors to emphasize with this individual to help her manage her symptoms?
- After studying the exercises in Chapter 16, practice the techniques you would have this patient do. Also, practice how you would progress the techniques and what criteria you would use for progressions.

Case 4

A 42-year-old man presents with a medical diagnosis of HNP at the L5–S1 area. Present symptoms began 4 days ago when rising out of bed. He is a sedentary person who plays social golf on the weekends (rides in a cart) and is 50 lb overweight. He has had occasional episodes of LBP over the past 15 years, but "nothing like this."

Medical history: smokes one pack of cigarettes per day and is on blood pressure medication. He describes the symptoms as a sharp pain beginning in the left buttock region and radiating down the back of the thigh; there is intermittent paresthesia along the lateral border of his foot, which is noticeable when sitting. He describes a considerable increase in symptoms when attempting to rise from bed or from a chair or when straining. He has been unable to walk because he cannot stand upright. On observation, you note that the patient is standing with a posterior pelvic tilt and forward-bend of the trunk and the thorax is deviated to the right.

Examination maneuvers: all spinal flexion motions increase symptoms; side gliding of the thorax to the left followed by lumbar extension centralizes the symptoms primarily to buttock and LBP.

- Based on this information, identify the impairments and functional limitations. What type of intervention should be used?
- Develop a sequence of treatment techniques that you would use during the first visit. Include instructions and precautions. Practice the techniques.

Case 5

A 61-year-old male underwent a transforminal lumbar interbody fusion at the levels of L4–S1 approximately 8 weeks ago. He is a retired high school teacher and would like to return to working in his yard and playing golf. He states his pain is localized to his low back region with a 3/10 with activity. His current complaints include difficulty standing from low surfaces, such as the commode and the couch. He also feels he has decreased endurance, as he is unable to walk his dog more than 10 minutes in the morning. He would like to be able to walk for up to 1 hour.

Medical history: patient reports he drinks one glass of wine with dinner and does not smoke. He has a positive history for hypertension. All other medical history is unremarkable.

Examination: patient has full trunk ROM with pain reported at end-range in all directions. Patient has bilateral 4/5 knee extension and 3+/5 hip flexion strength. Abdominals are 3/5. Sensation is intact to light touch bilaterally throughout his lower extremities. Patient ambulates without an assistive device but is still wearing a removable lumbar orthotic (chair-back brace) for the next 4 weeks. The physician has told the patient not to lift anything heavier than 20 pounds.

- What are your goals and interventions for this patient at this stage?
- After studying the techniques described in Chapter 16, describe what you would use with this patient at his current level of function and practice the regimen on a lab partner. What criteria would you use to progress his exercises? How would you incorporate functional progressions in his exercise routines?
- How would you discuss with your patient the resumption of his activities of yard work and golf? What modifications/precautions should he make?

Case 6

A 22-year-old female presents with left side TMJ pain with an onset of approximately 6 months ago. She is a graduate student (law school) and reports she has been extremely busy in school. She also reports she is planning her wedding, which will occur in 3 months. She cannot recall any previous trauma. She has been to the dentist, and he cleared her from any dental pathologies (abscess, fracture, etc.). The current complaint is pain with chewing and limited opening, especially with yawning. Her past medical history is unremarkable.

Examination: she has forward head posture with increased cervical lordosis and no deviation in the frontal plane. Bilateral upper extremity strength and sensation are normal and symmetrical. Cervical range of motion is approximately 25% limited with flexion and bilateral rotation. Patient demonstrates TMJ opening 50% of normal and lateral excursion 75% of normal. There is pain with palpation at the muscle bellies of the masseter and temporalis.

- Based on this information, identify the impairments and functional limitations. What type of intervention should be used?
- Develop a sequence of treatment techniques that you would use during the first visit. Include instructions and precautions. Practice the techniques.
- Identify methods the patient can use to manage and/or decrease her stress.

REFERENCES

1. Abdulwahab, SS, and Sabbahi, M: Neck retractions, cervical root decompression, and radicular pain. *J Orthop Sports Phys Ther* 30(1):4–9, 2000.
2. Abenhaim, L, et al: The role of activity in the therapeutic management of back pain: report of the international Paris task force on back pain. *Spine* 25(4Suppl):S1–S33, 2000.
3. Adams, MA, and Hutton, WC: Gradual disc prolapse. *Spine* 10(6): 524–531, 1985.
4. Adams, MA, and Hutton, WC: The effect of fatigue on the lumbar intervertebral disc. *J Bone Joint Surg Br* 65(2):199–203, 1983.
5. Ah-See KW, and Evans AS: Sinusitis and its management. *Br Med J* 334 (7589):358, 2007.
6. Akamnonu, C, et al: Unplanned hospital readmission after surgical treatment of common lumbar pathologies: rates and causes. *Spine* 15:40(6): 423–428, 2015.
7. Akhter, S, et al: Role of manual therapy with exercise regime versus exercise regime alone in the management of non-specific chronic neck pain. *Pak J Pharm Sci* 27(6 Suppl):2125–2128, 2014.
8. Albert, H, Godskesen, M, and Westergaard, JG: Incidence of four syndromes of pregnancy-related pelvic joint pain. *Spine* 27(24):2831–2834, 2002.
9. Alexander, AH, Jones, AM, and Rosenbaum, DH: Nonoperative management of herniated nucleus pulposus: patient selection by the extension sign. *Orthop Rev* 21:181–188, 1992.
10. Amiri M, et al: Cervical musculoskeletal impairment in frequent intermittent headache. Part 2: subjects with concurrent headache types. *Cephalalgia* 27(8):891–898, 2007.
11. Anderson, B, et al: The influence of backrest inclination and lumbar support on lumbar lordosis. *Spine* 4:52–58, 1979.
12. Anderson, T, et al: The effect of electrical stimulation on lumbar spinal fusion in older patients: a randomized, controlled, multi-center trial. *Spine* 34(21):2241–2247, 2009.

13. Aprill C, Dwyer A, and Bogduk N: Cervical zygapophyseal joint pain patterns II. *Spine* 15(6):458–461, 1990.
14. Audrey, L, Donelson, R, and Fung, T: Does it matter which exercise? A randomized control trial of exercise for low back pain. *Spine* 29(23): 2593–2602, 2004.
15. Austin N, DiFrancesco LM, and Herzog W: Microstructural damage in arterial tissue exposed to repeated tensile strains. *J Manipulative Physiol Ther* 33(1):14–19, 2010.
16. Battie, MC, and Videman, T: Lumbar disc degeneration: epidemiology and genetic influences. *Spine* 29:2679–2690, 2004.
17. Beattie, PF: Current understanding of lumbar intervertebral disc degeneration: a review with emphasis upon etiology, pathophysiology, and lumbar magnetic resonance imaging findings. *J Orthop Sports Phys Ther* 38(6):329–340, 2008.
18. Beattie, PF, et al: The immediate reduction in low back pain intensity following lumbar joint mobilization and prone press-ups is associated with increased diffusion of water in the L5–S1 intervertebral disc. *J Orthop Sports Phys Ther* 40(5):256–264, 2010.
19. Berg, S, et al: Total disc replacement compared to lumbar fusion: a randomized controlled trial with 2-year follow-up. *Eur Spine J* 18:1512–1519, 2009.
20. Beutler, WJ, Sweeney, CA, and Connolly, PJ: Recurrent laryngeal nerve injury with anterior cervical spine surgery. *Spine* 26(12):1337–1342, 2001.
21. Bishop, MD, et al: Patient expectations of benefit from interventions for neck pain and resulting influence on outcomes. *J Orthop Sports Phys Ther* 43(7):457–465, 2013.
22. Bogduk, N: Management of chronic low back pain. *Med J Aust* 180(2): 79–83, 2004.
23. Bogduk, N, and Twomey, LT: *Clinical Anatomy of the Lumbar Spine and Sacrum,* ed. 4. New York: Elsevier Churchill-Livingston, 2005.
24. Boissonnault, WG: *Primary Care for the Physical Therapist-E-book: Examination and Triage.* St. Louis: Saunders, 2010.
25. Brinckmann, P: Injury of the annulus fibrosus and disc protrusions. *Spine* 11(2):149–153, 1986.
26. Broetz, D, Burkard, S, and Weller, M: A prospective study on mechanical physiotherapy for lumbar disk prolapse: five year follow-up and final report. *Neurorehabilitation* 26:155–158, 2010.
27. Bronfort, G, et al: A randomized clinical trial of exercise and spinal manipulation for patients with chronic neck pain. *Spine* 26(7):788–799, 2001.
28. Bronfort G, et al: Non-invasive physical treatments for chronic/recurrent headache. *Cochrane Database Syst Rev* (8), 2004. Art. No: CD001878, DOI: 10.1002/14651858.CD001878.pub3.
29. Brumitt, J, Matheson, JW, and Meira, EP: Core stabilization exercise prescription, part 2: a systematic review of motor control and general (global) exercise rehabilitation approaches for patients with low back pain. *Sports Health* 5(6):510–513, 2013.
30. Buerba, R, et al: Increased risk of complications after anterior cervical discectomy and fusion in the elderly: analysis of 6253 patients in the American College of Surgeons National Surgical Quality Improvement Program database. *Spine* 39(25):2062–2069, 2014.
31. Butler, D, et al: Discs degenerate before facets. *Spine* 15:111–113, 1990.
32. Bydon, M, et al: Clinical and surgical outcomes after lumbar laminectomy: an analysis of 500 patients. *Surg Neurol Int* 6(4):S190–193, 2015.
33. Carragee, EJ, et al: Injections and surgical interventions: results of the bone and joint decade 2000–2010 task force on neck pain and its associated disorders. *Spine* 33(45):S153–S169, 2008.
34. Carragee, EJ: The increasing morbidity of elective spinal stenosis surgery. *J Am Med Assn* 303(13):1309–1310, 2010.
35. Cassidy JD, et al: Risk of vertebrobasilar stroke and chiropractic care: results of a population-based case-control and case-crossover study. *Spine* 33(4):S176–183, 2008.
36. Chen, WJ, et al: Surgical treatment of adjacent instability after lumbar spine fusion. *Spine* 26(22):E519–E524, 2001.
37. Childs, JD, et al: Neck pain: clinical practice guidelines linked to the International Classification of Functioning, Disability, and Health from the orthopedic section of the American Physical Therapy Association. *J Orthop Sports Phys Ther* 38(9):A1–A34, 2008. DOI:10.2519/jospt.2008.0303.
38. Childs, JD, et al: A clinical prediction rule to identify patients with low back pain most likely to benefit from spinal manipulation: a validation study. *Ann Intern Med* 141(12):920–928, 2004.
39. Childs, JD, et al: Clinical decision making in the identification of patients likely to benefit from spinal manipulation: a traditional versus an evidence-based approach. *J Orthop Sports Phys Ther* 33(5):259–275, 2003.
40. Clarke, JA, et al: Traction for low back pain with or without sciatica. *Cochrane Database Syst Rev* (2), 2007. Art.No:CD003010. DOI: 10.1002/14561858.CD003010. pub4.
41. Cleland, JA, et al: Development of clinical prediction rule for guiding treatment of a subgroup of patients with neck pain: use of thoracic spine manipulation, exercise, and patient education. *Phys Ther* 87(1):9–23, 2007.
42. Cleland, JA, et al: Predictors of short-term outcome in people with a clinical diagnosis of cervical radiculopathy. *Phys Ther* 87(12):1619–1632, 2007.
43. Cleland, JA, et al: The use of a lumbar spine manipulation technique by physical therapists in patients who satisfy a clinical prediction rule: a case series. *J Orthop Sports Phys Ther* 36(4):209–214, 2006.
44. Cook, C, et al: The clinical value of a cluster of patient history and observational findings as a diagnostic support tool for lumbar spine stenosis. *Physiother Res Int* 16(3):170–178, 2011.
45. Cook, C, et al: Reliability and diagnostic accuracy of clinical special tests for myelopathy in patients seen for cervical dysfunction. *J Orthop Sports Phys Ther* 39(3):172–178, 2009.
46. Danneels, LA, et al: Differences in electromyographic activity in the multifidus muscle and the iliocostalis lumborum between healthy subjects and patients with sub-acute and chronic low back pain. *Eur Spine J* 11: 13–19, 2002.
47. Debette, S: Pathophysiology and risk factors of cervical artery dissection: what have we learnt from large hospital-based cohorts? *Curr Opin Neurol* 27(1):20–28, 2014.
48. Delitto, A, et al: Low Back Pain: Clinical practice guidelines linked to the International Classification of Functioning, Disability, and Health from the orthopaedic section of the American Physical Therapy Association. *J Orthop Sports Phys Ther* 42(4):A1–A57, 2012. DOI:10.2519/jospt.2012.0301.
49. Delitto, A, Erhard, RE, and Bowling, RW: A treatment-based classification approach to low back syndrome: identifying and staging patients for conservative treatment. *Phys Ther* 75(6):470–485, 1995
50. DeRosa, CP, and Porterfield, JA: A physical therapy model for the treatment of low back pain. *Phys Ther* 72:261–269, 1992.
51. De Wijer, A, et al: Reliability of clinical findings in temporomandibular disorders. *J Orofac Pain* 9(2):181–191, 1995.
52. De Wijer, A: Temporomandibular and cervical spine disorders. Thesis. Utrecht University. Utrecht, The Netherlands: Elinkwijk BV, 1995, as cited in De Wijer, A, et al: Reliability of clinical findings in temporomandibular disorders. *J Orofac Pain* 9(2):181–191, 1995.
53. DiFabio, RP: Manipulation of the cervical spine; risks and benefits. *Phys Ther* 79:50–65, 1999.
54. Dimitroulis, G, Dolwick, M, and Gremillion, H: Temporomandibular disorders. 1. Clinical evaluation. *Aust Dent J* 40(5):301–305, 1995.
55. Donelson, R, Long, A, Spratt, K, and Fung, T: Influence of directional preference on two clinical dichotomies: acute versus chronic pain and axial low back pain versus sciatica. *PM R* 4(9):667–681, 2012.
56. Dreyfuss, P, et al: Positive sacroiliac screening tests in asymptomatic adults. *Spine* 19(10):1138–1143, 1994.
57. Dreyfuss, P, et al: The value of medical history and physical examination in diagnosing sacroiliac joint pain. *Spine* 21(22):2594–2602, 1996.
58. Dunning JR, et al: Upper cervical and upper thoracic thrust manipulation versus non-thrust mobilization in patients with mechanical neck pain: multicenter randomized clinical trial. *J Ortho Sports Phys Ther* 42(1):5–21, 2012.
59. Dutton, M: *Orthopedic Examination, Evaluation, and Intervention,* ed. 2, New York: McGraw Hill Co, 2008.

60. Dworkin, SF, et al: A randomized clinical trial using research diagnostic criteria for temporomandibular disorders-Axis II to target clinic cases for tailored self-care TMD treatment programs. *J Orofac Pain* 16(1): 48–63, 2002.
61. Dwyer, A, Aprill, C, and Bogduk, N: Cervical zygapophyseal joint pain patterns I: A study in normal volunteers. *Spine* 15(6):453–457, 1990.
62. Ekman, P, et al: A prospective randomised study on the long-term effect of lumbar fusion on adjacent disc degeneration. *Eur Spine J* 18: 1175–1186, 2009.
63. Evans, R, et al: Supervised exercise with and without spinal manipulation performs similarly and better than home exercise for chronic neck pain: a randomized controlled trial. *Spine* 37(11):903–914, 2012.
64. Evans, R, et al: Two-year follow-up of a randomized clinical trial of spinal manipulation and two types of exercise for patients with chronic neck pain. *Spine* 27(21):2383–2389, 2002.
65. Fardon, DF, et al: Lumbar disc nomenclature: version 2.0. Recommendations of the combined task forces of the North American Spine Society, the American Society of Spine Radiology, and the American Society of Neuroradiology. *Spine* 39(24):E1448–E1465, 2014.
66. Farfan, HF, et al: The effects of torsion on the lumbar intervertebral joints: the role of torsion in the production of disc degeneration. *J Bone Joint Surg Am* 52(3):468–497, 1970.
67. Fernández de las Peñas C, et al: Predictor variables for identifying patients with chronic tension-type headache who are likely to achieve short-term success with muscle trigger point therapy. *Cephalagia* 28: 264–275, 2008.
68. Flynn, T, et al: A clinical prediction rule for classifying patients with low back pain who demonstrate short-term improvement with spinal manipulation. *Spine* 27(24):2835–2843, 2002.
69. Flynn, TB: Neurologic complications of anterior cervical interbody fusion. *Spine* 7(6):536–539, 1982.
70. Franco, AC, Siqueira, JT, and Mansur, AJ: Facial pain of cardiac origin: A case report. *Sao Paulo Med J* 124(3):163–164, 2006.
71. Fritz, JM: Use of a classification approach to the treatment of 3 patients with low back syndrome. *Phys Ther* 78(7):766–777, 1998.
72. Fritz, JM, Erhard, RE, and Hagen, BF: Segmental instability of the lumbar spine. *Phys Ther* 78(8):889–896, 1998.
73. Fritz, JM, and George, S: The use of a classification approach to identify subgroups of patients with acute low back pain. Interrater reliability and short-term outcomes. *Spine* 25(1):106–114, 2000.
74. Fritz, JM, Thackeray, A, Brennan, GP, and Childs, JD: Exercise only, exercise with mechanical traction, or exercise with over-door traction for patients with cervical radiculopathy, with or without consideration of status on a previously described subgrouping rule: a randomized clinical trial. *J Orthop Sports Phys Ther* 44(2):45–57, 2014.
75. Fritz, JM, Whitman, JM, and Childs, JD: Lumbar spine segmental mobility assessment: an examination of validity for determining intervention strategies in patients with low back pain. *Arch Phys Med Rehabil* 86: 1745–1752, 2005.
76. Fujimori, T, et al: Does transforaminal lumbar interbody fusion have advantages over posterolateral lumbar fusion for degenerative spondylolisthesis? *Global Spine J* 5(2):102–109, 2015.
77. Fukui, S, Ohseto, K, Shiotani, M, et al: Referred pain distribution of the cervical zygapophyseal joints and cervical dorsal rami. *Pain* 68(1):79–83, 1996.
78. Garvey, TA, et al: Outcome of anterior cervical discectomy and fusion as perceived by patients treated for dominant axial-mechanical cervical spine pain. *Spine* 27(17):1887–1895, 2002.
79. Gilleard, WL, and Brown, MM: A electromyographic validation of an abdominal muscle test. *Arch Phys Med Rehabil* 75:1002–1007, 1994.
80. Goodman, C, Boissonnault, W, and Fuller, K: *Pathology: Implications for the Physical Therapist,* ed. 2. Philadelphia: Elsevier Science, 2003.
81. Gore, DR, and Sepic, SB: Anterior cervical fusion for degenerated or protruded discs. A review of one hundred forty-six patients. *Spine* 9: 667–671, 1984.
82. Goulet, JP, and Clark, GT: Clinical TMJ examination methods. *J Calif Dental Assoc* 18(3):25–33, 1990.
83. Grant, R, Jull, G, and Spencer, T: Active stabilization training for screen based keyboard operators—a single case study. *Aust Physiother* 43(4): 235–242, 1997.
84. Greene, CS: The etiology of temporomandibular disorders: implications for treatment. *J Orofac Pain* 15(2):93–105, 2001.
85. Greenspan, A: *Orthopedic Imaging: A Practical Approach,* ed. 4. Philadelphia: Lippincott Williams and Wilkins, 2004.
86. Grob, D, et al: A prospective, cohort study comparing translaminar screw fixation with transforminal lumbar interbody fusion and pedicle screw fixation for fusion of the degenerative lumbar spine. *J Bone J Surg Br* 91(10):1347–1353, 2009.
87. Gross, AR, et al: A Cochrane review of manipulation and mobilization for mechanic neck disorders. *Spine* 29(14):1541–1548, 2004.
88. Gross, AR, et al: Clinical practice guidelines on the use of manipulation or mobilization in the treatment of adults with mechanical neck disorders. *Man Ther* 7:193–205, 2002.
89. Gross, A, et al: Exercises for mechanical neck disorders. *Cochrane Database Syst Rev* 28;1, 2015. CD:004250. DOI:10/1002/14561858.
90. Gu, G, et al: Clinical and radiological outcomes of unilateral versus bilateral instrumentation in two-level degenerative lumbar disease. *Eur Spine J*. May 23, 2015.
91. Hadjipavlou, AG, et al: The pathophysiology of disc degeneration: a critical review. *J Bone Joint Surg Br* 90(10):1261–1270, 2008.
92. Hagins, M, et al: Effects of practice on the ability to perform lumbar stabilization exercises. *J Orthop Sports Phys Ther* 29(9):546–555, 1999.
93. Haladay, DE, et al: Quality of systematic reviews on specific spinal stabilization exercise for chronic low back pain. *J Orthop Sports Phys Ther* 43(4):242–250, 2013.
94. Harms, JG, and Jeszenszky, D: The unilateral transforaminal approach for posterior lumbar Interbody fusion. *Orthop Traumatol* 6:88–99, 1998. In Schizas, D, et al: Minimally invasive versus open transforaminal lumbar interbody fusion: evaluation initial experience. *Int Orthop* 33: 1683–1688, 2009.
95. Harrison, AL, Thorp, JN, and Ritzline, PD. A proposed diagnostic classification of patients with temporomandibular disorders: implications for physical therapists. *J Orthop Sports Phys Ther* 44(3):182–197, 2014
96. Hayashi, H, et al: Outcome of posterior lumbar interbody fusion for L4-L5 degenerative spondylolisthesis. *Indian J Orthop* May-Jun;49(3): 284–288, 2015.
97. Hebert, JJ, et al: Postoperative rehabilitation following lumbar discectomy with quantification of trunk muscle morphology and function: a case report and review of the literature. *J Orthop Sports Phys Ther* 40(7):402–412, 2010.
98. Henschke N, Maher CG, and Refshauge KM: A systematic review identifies five "red flags" to screen for vertebral fracture in patients with low back pain. *J Clin Epidemiol.* 61:110–118, 2008.
99. Henschke N, et al: Prevalence of and screening for serious spinal pathology in patients presenting to primary care settings with acute low back pain. *Arthritis Rheum* 60:3072– 3080, 2009.
100. Herkowitz, HN: A comparison of anterior cervical fusion, cervical laminectomy, and cervical laminoplasty for the surgical management of multiple level spondylitic radiculopathy. *Spine* 13(7):774–780, 1988.
101. Herzog W, Leonard TR, Symons B, Tang C, and Wuest S. Vertebral artery strains during high-speed, low amplitude cervical spinal manipulation. *J Electromyogr Kinesiol* Oct 22(5):740–746, 2012.
102. Hey, HQ and Hee, HT: Open and minimally invasive transforaminal lumbar interbody fusion: comparison of intermediate results and complications. *Asian Spine J* Apr;9(2):185–193, 2015.
103. Hicks, GE, et al: Preliminary development of a clinical prediction rule for determining which patients with low back pain will respond to a stabilization exercise program. *Arch Phys Med Rehabil* 86:1753–1762, 2005.
104. Hides, JA, Jull, GA, and Richardson, CA: Long-term effects of specific stabilizing exercises for first-episode low back pain. *Spine* 26: E243–E248, 2001.
105. Hides, JA, et al: Evidence of lumbar multifidus muscle wasting ipsilateral to symptoms in patients with acute/subacute low back pain. *Spine* 19(2):165–172, 1994.

106. Hisey, MS, et al: Prospective, randomized comparison of cervical total disk displacement versus anterior cervical fusion: results at 48 months follow-up. *J Spinal Disorder Tech* 28(4):E237–243, 2015.
107. Hisey, MS, et al: Multi-center, prospective, randomized, controlled investigational device exemption clinical trial comparing Mobi-C cervical artificial disc to anterior discectomy and fusion in the treatment of symptomatic degenerative disc disease in the cervical spine. *Int J Spine Sur* 1(8), eCollection, 2014.
108. Hodges, PW, and Moseley, GL: Pain and motor control of the lumbopelvic region: effect and possible mechanisms. *J Electromyogr Kinesth* 13:361–370, 2003.
109. Hodges, PW, et al: Experimental muscle pain changes feedforward postural responses of the trunk muscles. *Exp Brain Res* 151:262–271, 2003.
110. Hodges, PW, and Richardson, CA: Altered trunk muscle recruitment in people with low back pain with upper limb movement at different speeds. *Arch Phys Med Rehabil* 80(9):1005–1012, 1999.
111. Hodges, PW, and Richardson, CA: Delayed postural contraction of transversus abdominis in low back pain associated with movement of the lower limb. *J Spinal Disord* 11(1):46–56, 1998.
112. Hodges, PW, and Richardson, CA: Contraction of the abdominal muscles associated with movement of the lower limb. *Phys Ther* 77(2): 132–142, 1997.
113. Hodges, P, Richardson, C, and Jull, G: Evaluation of the relationship between laboratory and clinical tests of transversus abdominis function. *Physiother Res Int* 1(1):30–40, 1996.
114. Hosseinifar, M, et al: The effects of stabilization and McKenzie exercises on transverse abdominis and multifidus muscle thickness, pain, and disability: A randomized controlled trial in non specific chronic low back pain. *J Phys Ther Sci.* 25(12):1541–1545, 2013.
115. Hou, CR, Tsai, LC, Cheng, KF, Chung, KC, and Hong, CZ: Immediate effects of various physical therapeutic modalities on cervical myofascial pain and trigger-point sensitivity. *Arch Phys Med Rehabil* Oct;83(10): 1406–14, 2002.
116. Hoving, JL, et al: Manual therapy, physical therapy, or continued care by a general practitioner for patients with neck pain. *Ann Intern Med* 136:713–722, 2002.
117. Hsueh, TC, et al: The immediate effectiveness of electrical nerve stimulation and electrical muscle stimulation on myofascial trigger points. *Am J Phys Med Rehabil* 76(6):471–476, 1997.
118. Hurwitz, EL, et al: Frequency and clinical predictors of adverse reactions to chiropractic care in the UCLA neck pain study. *Spine* 30:1477–1484, 2005.
119. Inani, SB, and Selkar, SP: Effect of core stabilization exercises versus conventional exercises on pain and functional status in patients nonspecific low back pain: a randomized clinical trial. *J Back Musculoskeletal Rehabil* 26(1):37–43, 2013.
120. Johansson, H, and Sojka, P: Pathophysiological mechanisms involved in genesis and spread of muscular tension in occupation muscle pain and in chronic musculoskeletal pain syndromes: a hypothesis. *Med Hypotheses* 35:196–203, 1991.
121. Jull, G, et al: A randomized controlled trial of exercise and manipulative therapy for cervicogenic headache. *Spine* 27(17):1835–1834, 2002.
122. Jull, G: Management of cervical headache. *Manual Ther* 2(4):182–190, 1997.
123. Jull, G, et al: Cervical musculoskeletal impairment in frequent intermittent headache. Part 1: subjects with single headaches. *Cephalalgia* 27(7):793–802, 2007.
124. Kalichman, L, and Vulfsons, S: Dry needling in the management of musculoskeletal pain. *J Am Board Fam Med.* Sep-Oct;23(5):640–646, 2010.
125. Kaltenborn, FM: *The Spine: Basic Evaluation and Mobilization Techniques.* Oslo: Olaf Norlis Bokhandel, 1993.
126. Kellegren, J: Observations on referred pain arising from muscle. *Clin Sci* 3:175–190, 1983.
127. Kerr, D, Zhao, W, and Lurie, JD: What are long-term predictors of outcomes for lumbar disc herniation? A randomized and observational study. *Clin Orthop Relat Res* 473(6):1920–1030, 2015.
128. Kietrys, DM, et al: Effectiveness of dry needling for upper-quarter myofascial pain: a systematic review and meta-analysis. *J Orthop Sports Phys Ther* 43(9):620–634, 2013.
129. Kinkade, S: Evaluation and treatment of acute low back pain. *Am Fam Physician* 75:1181–1188, 2007.
130. Kjellman, G, and Oberg, B: A randomized clinical control trial comparing general exercise, McKenzie treatment, and a control group in patients with neck pain. *J Rehab Med* 34:183–190, 2002.
131. Klein, GR, Vaccaro, AR, and Albert, TJ: Health outcome assessment before and after anterior cervical discectomy and fusion for radiculopathy: a prospective analysis. *Spine* 25(7):801–803, 2000.
132. Knutson, GA: Significant changes in systolic blood pressure post vectored upper cervical adjustment vs resting control groups: a possible effect of the cervicosympathetic and/or pressor reflex. *J Man Phy Ther* 24:101–109, 2001.
133. Kopp, JR, et al: The use of lumbar extension in the evaluation and treatment of patients with acute herniated nucleus pulposus. *Clin Orthop* 202:211–218, 1986.
134. Kraus, SL: *TMJ Craniomandibular Cervical Complex: Physical Therapy and Dental Management.* Atlanta: Clinical Education Associates, 1986.
135. Krause, N, and Ragland, DR: Occupational disability due to low back pain: a new interdisciplinary classification based on a phase model of disability. *Spine* 19:1011–1120, 1994.
136. Kreiner, M, et al: A quality difference in craniofacial pain of cardiac vs. dental origin. *J Dent Res* 89(9):965–9, 2010.
137. Kretapirom, K, et al: MRI characteristics of rheumatoid arthritis in the temporomandicular joint. *Dentomaxillofac Radiol* 42:3, 2013. Available at http://www.birpublications.org/doi/full/10.1259/dmfr/31627230. Accessed October 8, 2015.
138. Kroenke, K, et al: An ultra-brief screening scale for anxiety and depression: The PHQ–4. *Psychosomatics* 50(6):613–621, 2009.
139. Langevin, P, et al: Comparison of 2 manual therapy and exercise protocols for cervical radiculopathy: a randomized clinical trial evaluating short-term effects. *J Orthop Sports Phys Ther* 45(1):4–17, 2015.
140. Laslett, M, et al: Diagnosing painful sacroiliac joints: a validity study of a McKenzie evaluation and sacroiliac provocation tests. *Aust J Physiotherapy* 49:89–97, 2003.
141. Lee, HS, et al: Radiologic changes of cervical spine in ankylosing spondylitis. *Clin Rheum* 20:262–266, 2001.
142. Leeuw, R, and Klasser, G: *Orofacial Pain: Guidelines for Assessment, Diagnosis, and Management,* ed. 5. Chicago: American Academy of Orofacial Pain, Quintessence Pub Co, 2013.
143. Liang, Y, et al: Clinical outcomes and sagittal alignment of single-level unilateral instrumented transforaminal lumbar interbody fusion with a 4 to 5-year follow-up. *Eur Spine* Apr 14, 2015.
144. Liu, J, et al: Anterior cervical discectomy and fusion versus corpectomy and fusion in treating two-level adjacent cervical spondylotic myelopathy: a minimum 5-year follow-up study. *Arch Orthop Trauma Surg* 135(2):149–153, 2015.
145. Long, AL: The centralization phenomenon: its usefulness as a predictor of outcome in conservative treatment of chronic low back pain (a pilot study). *Spine* 20(23):2513–2521, 1995.
146. Long, A, Donelson, R, and Fung, T. Does it matter which exercise? A randomized control trial of exercise for low back pain. *Spine* 29(23): 2593–2602, 2004.
147. Louw, A, et al: The effect of neuroscience education on pain, disability, anxiety, and stress in chronic musculoskeletal pain. *YAPMR Arch Phys Med Rehab* 92(12):2041–56, 2011.
148. Lundon, K, and Bolton, K: Structure and function of the lumbar intervertebral disc in the health, aging, and pathologic conditions. *J Orthop Sports Phys Ther* 31(6):291–306, 2001.
149. Magee, DJ: *Orthopedic Physical Assessment,* ed. 5. St. Louis: Saunders Elsevier, 2008.
150. Maigne, JY, Aivaliklis, A, and Pfefer, F: Results of sacroiliac joint double block and value of sacroiliac pain provocation tests in 54 patients with low back pain. *Spine* 21(16):1889–1892, 1996.

151. Malter, AD, et al. Five-year reoperation rates after different types of lumbar spine surgery. *Spine* 23:814–820, 1998.
152. Marawar, S, et al: National trends in anterior cervical disc fusion procedures. *Spine* 35(15):1454–1459, 2010.
153. Masaracchio, M, et al: Short-term combined effects of thoracic spine thrust manipulation and cervical spine nonthrust manipulation in individuals with mechanical neck pain: a randomized clinical trial. *J Orthop Sports Phys Ther*. 43(3):118–127, 2013.
154. May, S, and Aina, A: Centralization and directional preference: a systematic review. *Man Ther* 17(6):497–506, 2012.
155. McCarron, RF, et al: The inflammatory effect of nucleus pulposus: a possible element in the pathogenesis of low-back pain. *Spine* 12: 760–764, 1987.
156. McDonnell, MK, Sahrmann, SA, and Van Dillen, L: A specific exercise program and modification of postural alignment for treatment of cervicogenic headache: a case report. *J Orthop Sports Phys Ther* 35(1): 3–15, 2005.
157. McGregor, AH, et al: Rehabilitation following surgery for lumbar spinal stenosis. *Cochrane Database Syst Rev*. Dec 9;12:CD009644, 2013. DOI: 10.1002/145651858.
158. McKenzie, R, and May, S: *The Lumbar Spine: Mechanical Diagnosis and Therapy, Vol 1,* ed. 2. Waikanae, NZ: Spinal Publications, 2003.
159. McKenzie, R, and May, S: *The Lumbar Spine: Mechanical Diagnosis and Therapy, Vol 2,* ed. 2. Waikanae, NZ: Spinal Publications, 2003.
160. McKenzie, R: Manual correction of sciatic scoliosis. *N Z Med J* 89:22, 1979.
161. Mintken, PE, et al: Some factors predict successful short-term outcomes in individuals with shoulder pain receiving cervicothoracic manipulation: a single-arm trial. *Phys Ther* 90(1):26–42, 2010.
162. Mohl, ND: The anecdotal tradition and the need for evidence-based care for temporomandibular disorders. *J Orofac Pain* 13(4):227–231, 1999.
163. Moneur, C, and Williams, HJ: Cervical spine management in patients with rheumatoid arthritis. *Phys Ther* 68:509–515, 1988.
164. Mooney, V, and Robertson, J: The facet syndrome. *Clin Orthop* 115: 149–156, 1976.
165. Mooney, V: The syndromes of low back disease. *Orthop Clin North Am* 14(3):505–515, 1983.
166. Moraska, A, and Chandler, C: Changes in clinical parameters in patients with tension-type headache following massage therapy: a pilot study. *J Man Manip Ther* 16(2):106–112, 2008.
167. Morgan, D: Concepts in functional training and postural stabilization for the low-back injured. *Top Acute Care Trauma Rehabil* 2:8–17, 1988.
168. Muheremu, A, et al: Comparison of the sort- and long-term treatment effect of cervical disk replacement and anterior cervical disk fusion: a meta-analysis. *Eur J Orthop Surg Traumatol* May 5, Epub, 2014.
169. Murphy, MJ: Effects of cervical traction on muscle activity. *J Orthop Sports Phys Ther* 13:220–225, 1991.
170. Nam, WD, and Cho, JH: The importance of proximal fusion level selection for outcomes of multi-level lumbar posterolateral fusion. *Clin Orthop Surg* May;7(1):77–84, 2015.
171. Nassif, NJ, and Talic, YF: Classic symptoms in temporomandibular disorder patients: a comparative study. *J Craniomandibular Pract* 19(1): 33–41, 2001.
172. National Institutes of Health Technology Assessment Conference on Management of Temporomandibular Disorders, pp 15–120. Bethesda, MD. April 29–May 1, 1996.
173. Neuman, P, and Gill, V: Pelvic floor and abdominal muscle interaction: EMG activity and intra-abdominal pressure. *Int Urogynecol J* 13:125–132, 2002.
174. Nicholson, GG, and Gaston, J: Cervical headache. *J Orthop Sports Phys Ther* 31(4):184–193. 2001.
175. Nowakowski, P, Delitto, A, and Erhard, RE: Lumbar spinal stenosis. *Phys Ther* 76:187, 1996.
176. Oestergaard, LG, et al: Early versus late initiation of rehabilitation after lumbar spinal fusion: economic evaluation alongside a randomized controlled trial. *Spine* 38(23):1979–1985, 2013.
177. Oestergaard, LG, et al: The effect of early initiation of rehabilitation after lumbar spinal fusion: a randomized clinical study. *Spine* 37(21): 1803–1809, 2012.
178. Ohrbach, R, et al: The research diagnostic criteria for temporomandibular disorders. IV: evaluation of psychometric properties of the axis II measures. *Orofac Pain* 24(1):48–62, 2010.
179. Okeson, JP (ed): *Orofacial Pain: Guidelines for Assessment, Diagnosis, and Management.* Chicago: Quintessence Publishing Co, 1996.
180. Okeson, JP: *Management of Temporomandibular Disorders and Occlusion.* St. Louis: Elsevier/Mosby, 2013.
181. Oliveira-Campelo, NM, et al: The immediate effects of atlanto-occipital joint manipulation and suboccipital muscle inhibition technique on active mouth opening and pressure pain sensitivity over latent myofascial trigger points in the masticatory muscles. *J Orthop Sports Phys Ther* 40(5):310–307, 2010.
182. Olson, KA, and Dustin, J: Diagnosis and treatment of cervical spine clinical instability. *J Orthop Sports Phys Ther* 31(4):194–206, 2001.
183. O'Sullivan, PB, Twomey, LT, and Allison, GT: Altered abdominal muscle recruitment in patients with chronic low back pain following a specific exercise intervention. *J Orthop Sports Phys Ther* 27(2):114–124, 1998.
184. Palit, M, et al: Anterior discectomy and fusion for the management of neck pain. *Spine* 24(21):2224–2228, 1999.
185. Panjabi, MM: The stabilizing system of the spine. Part I. Function, dysfunction, adaption, and enhancement. *J Spinal Disord* 5:383–389, 1992.
186. Panjabi, MM: The stabilizing system of the spine. Part II. Neutral zone and instability hypothesis. *J Spinal Disord* 5:390–396, 1992.
187. Panjabi, MM, et al: On the understanding of clinical instability. *Spine* 19:2642–2650, 1994.
188. Panjabi, MM, Krag, MH, and Chung, TQ: Effects of disc injury on mechanical behavior of the human spine. *Spine* 9:707–713, 1984.
189. Paris, SV: Anatomy as related to function and pain. *Ortho Clin North Am* 14:475–489, 1983.
190. Paris, SV: *S1-Introduction to Spinal Evaluation and Manipulation (Course Manual).* St. Augustine, FL: University of St. Augustine, 2002.
191. Paris, SV, Irwin, ML, and Yack, L: *S2-Advanced Evaluation and Manipulation of Pelvis, Lumbar, and Thoracic Spine (Course Manual).* St. Augustine, FL: University of St. Augustine, 2004.
192. Paris, SV: *S3-Advanced Evaluation & Manipulation of CranioFacial, Cervical & Upper Thoracic Spine (Course Manual).* St. Augustine, FL: University of St. Augustine, 2000.
193. Pellechia, GL: Lumbar traction: a review of the literature. *J Orthop Sports Phys Ther* 20:262–267, 1994.
194. Phillips, FM, and Cunningham, B: Intertransverse lumbar interbody fusion. *Spine* 27:E37–E41, 2002.
195. Podichetty, VK: The aging spine: the role of inflammatory mediators in intervertebral disc degeneration. *Cell Mol Biol* 53(5):4–18, 2007.
196. Porter, RW, Hibbert, C, and Evans, C: The natural history of root entrapment syndrome. *Spine* 9:418–421, 1984.
197. Porterfield, JA, and DeRosa, C: *Mechanical Low Back Pain: Perspectives in Functional Anatomy,* ed. 2. Philadelphia: Saunders Company, 1998.
198. Puentedura, EJ, et al: Development of a clinical prediction rule to identify patients with neck pain likely to benefit from thrust joint manipulation to the cervical spine. *J Orthop Sports Phys Ther* 42(7):577–592, 2012.
199. Rabin, A, et al: The interrater reliability of physical examination tests that may predict the outcome or suggest the need for lumbar stabilization exercises. *J Orthop Sports Phys Ther* 43(2):83–90, 2013.
200. Raney, NH, et al: Development of a clinical prediction rule to identify patients with neck pain likely to benefit from cervical traction and exercise. *Eur Spine J* 18(3):382–391, 2009.
201. Rhee, JM, Schaufele, M, and Abdu, WA: Radiculopathy and the herniated lumbar disc. *J Bone Joint Surg* 88(9):2077–2080, 2006.
202. Rhee, JM, et al: Nonoperative management of cervical myelopathy: a systematic review. *Spine* 38(22):S55–67, 2013.
203. Richardson, C, Hodges, PW, and Hides, J: *Therapeutic Exercise for Lumbopelvic Stabilization,* ed. 2. Edinburgh: Churchill Livingstone, 2004.

204. Riddle, DL: Classification and low back pain: a review of the literature and critical analysis of selected systems. *PHYS Ther* 78(7):708–737, 1998.
205. Ringold, S, Tzaribachev, N, and Cron, RQ: Management of temporomandibular joint arthritis in adult rheumatology practices: a survey of adult rheumatologists. *Pediatr Rheumatol Online J* 10:(1):26, 2012.
206. Rudwaleit, M, et al: Inflammatory back pain in ankylosing spondylitis: a reassessment of the clinical history for application as classification and diagnostic criteria. *Arthritis Rheum* 54(2):569–578, 2006.
207. Russell, EJ: Cervical disc disease. *Radiology* 177(2):313–325, 1990.
208. Ruston, A, et al: Physiotherapy rehabilitation following lumbar spinal fusion: a systematic review and meta-analysis of randomized controlled trials. *Brit Med J Open* 2(4), 2012.
209. Saal, JA, Saal, JS, and Herzog, RJ: The natural history of lumbar intervertebral disc extrusions treated nonoperatively. *Spine* 15:683–686, 1990.
210. Saal, JA, and Saal, JS: Nonoperative treatment of herniated lumbar intervertebral disc with radiculopathy. An outcome study. *Spine* 14: 431–437, 1989.
211. Saal, JA: Dynamic muscular stabilization in the nonoperative treatment of lumbar pain syndromes. *Orthop Rev* 19:691–700, 1990.
212. Saal, JS, et al: High levels of inflammatory phospholipase A2 activity in lumbar disc herniations. *Spine* 15:674–678, 1990.
213. Saal, JS, Saal, JA, and Yurth, EF: Nonoperative management of herniated cervical intervertebral disc with radiculopathy. *Spine* 21(16):1877–1883, 1996.
214. Sahrmann, SA: *Diagnosis and Treatment of Movement Impairment Syndromes.* St. Louis: Mosby, 2002.
215. Santander, H, et al: Effects of head and neck inclination on bilateral sternocleidomastoid EMG activity in health subjects in patients with myogenic cranio-cervical-mandibular dysfunction. *J Craniomandular Pract* 18(3):181–191, 2000.
216. Sato, S, et al: Reoperation rate and risk factors of elective spinal surgery of degenerative spondylolisthesis: minimum 5-year follow-up. *Spine J.* Feb 11, 2015.
217. Saunders, HD, and Ryan, RS. *Evaluation, Treatment, and Prevention of Musculoskeletal Disorders. Vol 1,* ed. 4. Chaska, MN: The Saunders Group, 2004.
218. Schoensee, SK, et al: The effect of mobilization on cervical headaches. *J Orthop Sports Phys Ther* 21(4):184–196, 1995.
219. Schwarzer, A, Aprill, CN, and Bogduk, N. The sacroiliac joint in chronic low back pain. *Spine* 20:31–37, 1995.
220. Skytte, L, May, S, and Petersen, P: Centralization: its prognostic value in patients with referred symptoms and sciatica. *Spine* 30(11): 293–299, 2005.
221. Spencer, JD, Hayes, KC, and Alexander, IJ: Knee joint effusion and quadriceps reflex inhibition in man. *Arch Phys Med Rehabil* 65:171–177, 1984.
222. Stanton, TR, et al: After an episode of acute low back pain, recurrence is unpredictable and not as common as previously thought. *Spine* 33: 2923–2928, 2008.
223. Stuge, B, et al: The efficacy of a treatment program focusing on specific stabilizing exercises for pelvic girdle pain after pregnancy. *Spine* 29(4): 351–359, 2004.
224. Surkitt, LD, et al: Efficacy of directional preference management for low back pain: a systematic review. *Phys Ther* 92(5):652–665, 2012.
225. Survarnnato, T, et al: The effects of thoracic manipulation versus mobilization for chronic neck pain: a randomized controlled trial pilot study. *J Phys Ther Sci* 25:865–871, 2013
226. Sutheerayongprasert, C, et al: Factors predicting failure of conservative treatment in lumbar-disc herniation. *J Med Assoc Thai* 95(5):674–680, 2012.
227. Symons BP, Leonard T, and Herzog W: Internal forces sustained by the vertebral artery during spinal manipulative therapy. *J Manipulative Physiol Ther* 8:504–510, 2002.
228. Taylor, JR, and Twomey, LT: Age changes in lumbar zygapophyseal joints. *Spine* 11(7):739–745, 1986.
229. The International Headache Society: H.C.S. The international classification of headache disorders. *Cephalagia* 24:1–160, 2004.
230. Thomas, LC, et al: Risk factors and clinical presentation of cervical arterial dissection: preliminary results of a prospective case-control study. *J Orthop Sports Phys Ther* 45(7):503511, 2015.
231. Thoomes, EJ, et al: The effectiveness of conservative treatment for patients with cervical radiculopathy: a systematic review. *Clin J Pain* 29(12): 1073–1086, 2013.
232. Travell, JG, Simons, DG, and Simons, LS: *Myofascial Pain and Dysfunction: The Trigger Point Manual.* Baltimore: Lippincott Williams & Wilkins, 1998.
233. Tseng, YL, Wang, WT, and Chen, WY: Predictors for the immediate responders to cervical manipulation in patients with neck pain. *Man Ther* 11:306–315, 2006.
234. Twomey, LT: A rationale for the treatment of back pain and joint pain by manual therapy. *Phys Ther* 72:885–892, 1992.
235. Urban, L: The straight-leg-raising test: a review. *J Orthop Sports Phys Ther* 2:117–133, 1981.
236. Van Dieen, JH, Cholewicki, J, and Radeboid, A: Trunk muscle recruitment patterns in patients with low back pain enhance the stability of the lumbar spine. *Spine* 28(8):834–841, 2003.
237. Von Korff M, et al: Grading the severity of chronic pain. *Pain* 50(2): 133–149, 1992.
238. von Piekartz, H, and Ludtke, K: Effect of treatment of temporomandibular disorders (TMD) in patients with cervicogenic headache: a single-blind, randomized controlled study. *Cranio* 29(1):43–56, 2011.
239. Vinje, O, Dale, K, and Moller, P: Radiographic evaluation of patients with Bechterew's syndrome (ankylosing spondylitis) and their first-degree relatives. *Scand J Rheumatology* 14:119–132, 1985.
240. Vishteh, AG, and Dickman, CA: Anterior lumbar microdiscectomy and interbody fusion for the treatment of recurrent disc herniation. *Neurosurgery* 48:334–337, 2001.
241. Vlam, K, Mielants, H, and Veys, E: Involvement of the zygapophyseal joint in ankylosing spondylitis: relation to the bridging syndesmophyte. *J Rheumotolgy* 26:1738–1745, 1999.
242. Waddell, G: A new clinical model for the treatment of low back pain. *Spine* 12:632–644, 1987.
243. Wasiak R, et al: Recurrence of low back pain: definition-sensitivity analysis using administrative data. *Spine* 28:2283–2291, 2003.
244. Watson, DH, and Drummond, PD: Head pain referral during examination of the neck in migraine and tension-type headache. *Headache: J Head Face Pain* 52(8):1226–35, 2012.
245. Wiltse, LL, Newman, PH, and MacNab, I: Classification of spondylolisthesis and spondylolysis. *Clin Orthop* 117:23–29, 1976.
246. Wong, AP, et al: Intraoperative and perioperative complications in minimally invasive transforaminal lumbar interbody fusion: a review of 513 patients. *J Neurosurg Spine* 22(5):487–495, 2015.
247. Xiao, SW, et al: Anterior cervical discectomy versus corpectomy for multilevel cervical spondylotic myelopathy: a meta-analysis. *Eur Spine J* 2491:31–30, 2015.
248. Yasuma, T, et al: Histological development of intervertebral disc herniation. *J Bone Joint Surg Am* 68(7):1066–1072, 1986.
249. Young, IA, et al: Manual therapy, exercise, and traction for patients with cervical radiculopathy: a randomized clinical trial. *J Orthop Sports Phys Ther* 89(7):632–642, 2009.
250. Young, S, Aprill, C, and Laslett, M: Correlation of clinical examination characteristics with three sources of chronic low back pain. *Spine J* 3(6): 460–465, 2003.
251. Zhu, L, Wei, X, and Wang, S: Does cervical spine manipulation reduce pain in people with degenerative cervical radiculopathy? A systematic review of the evidence, and a meta-analysis. *Clin Rehabil* Feb 12, 2013.

CHAPTER 16

The Spine: Exercise and Manipulation Interventions

CAROLYN KISNER, PT, MS ■ JACOB N. THORP, PT, DHS, OCS, MTC

Continued

Basic spinal anatomy, mechanics, and posture are presented in Chapter 14. In Chapter 15, the pathomechanics, common pathologies, and management guidelines related to the spine are presented. The management guidelines are outlined based on stages of healing as well as subgroupings based on diagnostic categories that reflect impairments and movement disorders. Chapter 16 is a continuation of this material in which the techniques of intervention using therapeutic exercise and mobilization/manipulation for management of neck and trunk impairments are described.

This chapter is divided into six main sections. The first section describes the underlying concepts and approaches to exercise interventions for spinal impairments. Each of the remaining five sections describes components of exercise interventions for the neck and trunk. The topics covered include exercises for kinesthetic awareness, mobility/flexibility (including manipulation), muscle performance (including stability, muscle endurance, and strength), cardiopulmonary endurance, and functional activities. Stress relief and relaxation principles and techniques, important components of total rehabilitation, are covered in detail in Chapter 14.

Basic Concepts of Spinal Management With Exercise

It is important to recognize that even though the material in this chapter is presented in separate sections, there is an overlap in the use of the techniques described in each section, and there are fundamental interventions basic to all exercise programs.

Fundamental Interventions

When patients seek treatment from a physical therapist, they come with different diagnoses, impairments, and activity limitations and are at different stages of tissue healing. Yet the treatment plan for each patient must begin with fundamental interventions in order to lay the foundation on which to build an effective therapeutic exercise program. *Fundamental interventions* are defined as exercises or skills that all patients with spinal impairments should learn regardless of their functional level at the time of examination and initial treatment. The interventions include basic kinesthetic training, basic spinal stabilization training, and functional training of basic body mechanics. These interventions are summarized in Box 16.1.

BOX 16.1 Fundamental Exercise Interventions for Spinal Rehabilitation

These fundamental interventions are adapted or modified based on patient abilities and responses.

Kinesthetic Training
- Awareness and control of safe spinal motion: head nodding and pelvic tilts
- Awareness of neutral spinal position (if needed begin in the patient's spinal bias) while supine, prone, sitting, and standing
- Awareness of effects of activities of daily living and extremity motion on the spine (see Functional Training)

Stabilization Training
- *Deep segmental muscle* activation and sustained contraction
  - Cervical region: controlled axial extension (cervical retraction) with craniocervical flexion and lower cervical/upper thoracic extension
  - Lumbar region: drawing-in maneuver and multifidus muscle activation techniques
- *Superficial multi-segmental (global) muscle* control of spinal posture with extremity loading
- Passive support of spinal posture only if needed; progress to active control
- Coordinate segmental muscle activation with maintenance of a stable spine in neutral spinal position (or position of bias) with all arm and leg motions

Functional Training (Basic Body Mechanics With Stable Spine)
- Log roll supine to prone, prone to supine
- Transition from supine to side-lying to sitting and return
- Transition from sit to stand and return
- Walking

Once the fundamental skills are learned, exercise interventions then progress on a continuum at the level of the patient's abilities and willingness to learn. For example, a patient beginning treatment with chronic symptoms several months after the onset of symptoms must first become aware of positions or activities that increase the symptoms and then learn how to move the spine safely as well as learn what effects the various postures and movements have on symptoms (*fundamental* kinesthetic awareness). The patient must learn how to activate the deep segmental stabilizing musculature and then how to use the deep stabilizers with the global musculature to stabilize the spine against various extremity loading exercises (*fundamental* muscle performance). Finally, the patient must learn basic body mechanics (*fundamental* functional activities) in order to minimize stresses to the spine during daily activities before progressing to exercises that can be tolerated at the chronic stage of healing and returning to desired functional activities.

The fundamental exercises are described in detail preceding the exercise progressions in each of the respective sections of this chapter. The principles of management are similar for the cervical and lumbar spinal regions, and many of the same techniques may be used or modified for both regions.

Patient Education

Patient education is the key component of every goal and intervention. It encompasses several ideas. First, the patient is an active participant in identifying the desired goals; education as to potential outcomes is part of this process. Second, the patient may need to be informed about limitations at each stage of healing, so he or she will not become concerned that the acute symptoms will be forever disabling, but also will not "overdo" exercises and activities during the early subacute phase that cause exacerbation of symptoms. The patient may then need to be challenged to progress beyond perceived limitations during the later stages of recovery.

To ensure that each individual develops control over and learns to manage the symptoms and any impairments, it is important that the patient is engaged in all activities at each stage of recovery and is not just a passive recipient of "treatment." Instruct the patient on how to safely progress self-management beyond the time spent under professional supervision so he or she can reach the maximum level of functional return with minimal activity or participation restrictions.

Finally, the patient needs instruction in prevention. This includes safe ways to exercise, safe body mechanics for return to high-intensity activities, modification of the work and home environment, and activities to minimize stresses.

FOCUS ON EVIDENCE

The ***Clinical Practice Guidelines (CPGs) for Low Back Pain,*** based on moderate evidence, recommend patient education and counselling to include promoting the inherent anatomical/structural strength of the spine, the explanation of pain, the favorable prognosis of low back pain (LBP), use of pain coping strategies, early resumption of normal activities, and improvement of activity levels.[17]

General Exercise Guidelines

Therapeutic exercise is an important intervention in the management of impairments in the spinal region. Although this text does not deal with specific examination techniques, it is critical to emphasize the importance of identifying each patient's structural and functional impairments, their activity and participation restrictions, and the stage of tissue healing or stage of rehabilitation in order to establish a baseline for the initiation of intervention techniques and to measure progress toward the outcome goals.

In general, the following components of physical function are used in all intervention programs for spinal problems. These five areas are listed in Table 16.1 with interventions outlined for each phase of rehabilitation. The interventions are described in detail in the remaining sections of this chapter. Prior to developing an exercise program, it is important that the reader has knowledge of various spinal pathologies and the special precautions and contraindications (see Chapter 15), so each patient can safely achieve his or her maximum potential.

Kinesthetic Awareness

One of the fundamental interventions for spinal rehabilitation is for the patient to develop awareness of safe spinal positions and spinal movement as well as what effect the supine, prone, side-lying, sitting, and standing positions have on the spine. Awareness of what postures make the symptoms better or worse and identifying the neutral spinal position or position of bias are important in helping patients manage their symptoms. Awareness and control of spinal posture and movement are progressed and incorporated into all the exercises described in the remaining sections of this chapter and underlie exercises for the extremities as well.

Mobility/Flexibility

Stretching and flexibility exercises as well as mobilization/manipulation techniques are used to increase mobility of restricting tissues so the patient can assume an effective position of the spine when exercising to improve muscle performance and functional outcomes. For patients who fit the Mobilization/Manipulation diagnostic category (described in Chapter 15), spinal manipulation techniques or specific high-velocity thrust (HVT) techniques may be indicated during the early intervention period and then followed with stretching exercises. Nerve mobilization may be indicated in either the cervical/upper

TABLE 16.1 Intervention for Each Phase of Rehabilitation

Phases of Rehabilitation Intervention	Phase I: Early Training Maximum to moderate protection of injured area, pathologically involved tissues, or painful region	Phase II: Basic Training: Controlled motion with moderate to minimum protection	Phase III: Intermediate to Advanced Training Return to function with minimum to no protection
Five components of exercise intervention			
Kinesthetic awareness ■ Proprioception training of safe movement and postures	■ Pelvic tilt /cervical retraction: passive —> active assist —> active in comfortable positions* ■ Awareness of what makes symptoms better vs. worse* ■ Learn neutral spine (or bias)*	■ Active spinal control in supine, prone, quadruped, sitting, standing ■ Dynamic maintenance of pain-free position with activities	■ Habitual use of neutral spine in all functional activities
Mobility/flexibility ■ Move, stretch, manipulate restricting tissues	■ Movement to relieve fluid stasis ■ Trunk stretching: only in pain-relieving positions ■ Extremity stretching: stretch U/LE if no stress to the spine ■ Manipulation: grades I and II ■ High-velocity thrust if indicated	■ Gentle spinal movement into painful range ■ Stretch U/LE muscles; stabilize spine in position of bias ■ Manipulation: progress to grade III	■ Move into painful ranges to stretch and manipulate as indicated
Muscle performance ■ Stabilization training (deep muscles for segmental stability, global muscles for general stability) ■ Muscle endurance ■ Strength and power	■ Activation of deep musculature* ■ Stabilization exercises with extremity loading (use of passive positioning of spine with pillows, splints, corsets if necessary)*	■ Stabilization exercises with extremity loading (active control of spine position) ■ Emphasize muscle endurance ■ Perturbation training ■ Low-intensity dynamic spinal exercises	■ Stabilization with transitional motions and functional activities; emphasize strength ■ Progression to dynamic trunk strengthening ■ Progress trunk and extremity strengthening exercises in patterns that reinforce activity goals
Cardiopulmonary Endurance ■ Aerobic training	■ Only if tolerated with maximum protection in position of comfort	■ Low to moderate intensity with moderate to minimal protection. ■ Use activities that emphasize spinal bias	■ High-intensity (target heart rate), multiple times per week
Functional Activities ■ Body mechanics ■ Skill in home, community, work, recreation, sport activities	■ Safe postures for recumbent, sitting, and standing* ■ Stable-spine techniques while rolling over, moving supine to sit, sit to stand*	■ Strengthen U/LE while stabilizing spine ■ Stable spine body mechanics ■ Environmental and ergonomic adaptations	■ High-intensity functional activities ■ Endurance and strengthening activities that replicate return to desired activities ■ Practice prevention

*Fundamental interventions for all patients.

extremity or lumbar/lower extremity regions. Indications and techniques are described in Chapter 13.

NOTE: The terms *mobilization* and *manipulation* are used interchangeably (see Chapter 5). The authors of this chapter are using *manipulation* to refer to graded oscillation techniques and HVT to refer to high-velocity, small-amplitude techniques performed at the end of the pathological limit of the joint.

Muscle Performance

In the spine, muscle performance involves not only strength, power, and endurance, but also stability. Activation of the deep segmental muscles as well as the superficial/global multisegmental muscles of the neck and trunk are fundamental techniques for developing spinal stability. Initially, emphasis is placed on awareness of muscle contraction and control of spinal position while moving the extremities and performing basic functional activities. Exercises are then progressed to challenge the holding capacity of the stabilizing muscles, emphasizing muscle endurance, balance, and strength. Once the individual learns effective stabilization and management of symptoms, dynamic neck and trunk strengthening exercises are initiated to emphasize strength in the full range of motion (ROM). Most people are familiar with trunk curls, "crunches," and back lifts. The emphasis of therapeutic exercise is safe execution of the exercises combined with respect of the biomechanics of the spine. Exercises should be chosen with the functional outcome goals in mind and integrated with the principles discussed in the Functional Activities section of this chapter.

Cardiopulmonary Endurance

Aerobic conditioning exercises are initiated as soon as the patient tolerates repetitive activity without exacerbating symptoms. Emphasis is placed on using safe spinal postures while exercising. Aerobic activity increases the patient's feeling of well-being and improves cardiovascular and pulmonary fitness. Principles of aerobic conditioning are detailed in Chapter 7 and summarized in this chapter, along with suggestions for safe application of aerobic exercises when there are spinal impairments.

Functional Activities

Fundamental functional activities include training the basic body mechanics of rolling, supine to sit, sit to stand (and reverse), and walking. These activities are coordinated with kinesthetic training and segmental muscle activation and stabilization exercises. When the patient is able, stabilization exercises, muscle endurance, and strengthening exercises are integrated with skills for body mechanics (lifting, pushing, pulling, carrying), safe work habits (ergonomic adaptations), and effective recreational or sport activities to meet the goals of the individual.

FOCUS ON EVIDENCE

The ***CPGs for Neck Pain***[12] and for ***Low Back Pain***[17] identify strong evidence for manipulation and thrust techniques to reduce pain and disability with mobility impairments; strong evidence for trunk coordination, strengthening, and endurance exercise; and strong evidence for progressive endurance and fitness activities when treating patients with back and neck pain. There is also strong evidence supporting interventions for subgroups that respond with centralization and directional preference exercises.

Kinesthetic Awareness

Goal. To develop proprioception of spinal positioning, safe movement, and postural control.

Elements of Functional Training: Fundamental Techniques

Position of Symptom Relief

It is important that the patient learn how to move the spine and find the range or position in which symptoms are minimized. The position of symptom relief is called the *position of bias* or *the resting position*. The *neutral* spine position is midrange; the patient may or may not feel most comfortable in that position initially. See Chapter 15 for a discussion on spinal bias as it relates to relief of symptoms and common pathologies.

Cervical Spine

Patient position and procedure: Begin supine; progress to sitting and other functional postures as tolerated.

- If the patient is experiencing a lot of pain and is not able to, or not wanting to, move their head, begin with passive movements. Passively move the head and neck with gentle nodding motions of the head into flexion and extension, side bending, and/or rotation to find the most comfortable position for the patient. If necessary, prop the head and neck with pillows.
- Describe the mechanics of what you are doing to the patient.
- Have the patient identify the change in symptoms as movement occurs in and out of the position of bias.
- Have the patient practice moving into and out of that position to develop control.
- If the patient cannot maintain this position while sitting and standing, wearing a cervical collar may be appropriate during the acute stage following an injury or postsurgically, but it is important to use judiciously, so the patient does not become dependent on it.

Lumbar Spine

Patient position and procedure: Begin supine or hook-lying, then sitting, standing, and quadruped.

- Teach the patient to move his or her pelvis into an anterior and posterior pelvic tilt through the range that is comfortable.
- Once the patient has moved the pelvis and spine through a safe range of motion (ROM), instruct him or her to find the position of greatest symptom relief.
- If active movement and control are not possible, teach *passive positioning* (see Chapter 15, Box 15.6). Have the patient assume each of the following positions, and draw the association between the spinal position and what is felt. While supine, passively position the pelvis in posterior tilt and lumbar spine in flexion by placing the lower extremities in the hook-lying position or anterior tilt and lumbar spine extension by placing a small pillow or folded towel under the lumbar spine. If prone lying is tolerated, position the lumbar spine in extension when lying flat or in flexion by placing one or two pillows under the abdomen. Sitting encourages spinal flexion; if extension is more comfortable, instruct the person to use a lumbar pillow for support. Standing usually causes spinal extension; if flexion is desired, instruct the person to place one foot up on a stool while standing.

Effects of Movement on the Spine

Once the functional spinal position is determined, it is important for the patient to feel and learn what motions make the symptoms better or worse. In general, movement of the extremities away from the trunk (shoulder flexion and abduction, hip extension and abduction) causes spinal extension; movement of the extremities toward the trunk (shoulder extension and adduction, hip flexion and adduction) causes spinal flexion.

- Have the patient find the neutral or functional spine position (bias); then move the arms and then the legs to feel the effect on the spine. Control of the spinal position is emphasized; have the patient practice the arm and leg motions and attempt to maintain control of the spinal position. These motions are the same as the basic stabilization exercises and are described in detail in the muscle performance section.
- If the patient cannot maintain control or the symptoms are made worse, he or she requires passive support or passive positioning when initiating the stabilization exercises.

Blending of Kinesthetic Training, Stabilization Exercises, and Fundamental Body Mechanics

Once awareness of safe positions and movement is learned, teach the patient the fundamental stabilization techniques for developing neuromuscular control of the position (see the Muscle Performance section of this chapter) and teach the fundamental body mechanics of rolling, moving supine to sit, sit to stand, and ambulation (see the Functional Activities section of this chapter).

Progression to Active and Habitual Control of Posture

Awareness and control of posture is described in detail in Chapter 14 (see General Management Guidelines for Impaired Posture and Box 14.1). The use of reinforcement techniques (verbal, visual, tactile) is described, as are activities to train cervical, scapular, thoracic, and lumbopelvic alignment and control. It is important to reinforce the relationship between faulty posture and the development of painful symptoms and to identify a need for postural support (temporary or long term).

Integrate the awareness of posture and control of the spinal segments into all stabilization exercises, aerobic conditioning, and functional training activities. Observe the patient as greater challenges to activities are performed and, if necessary, provide reminders to find the neutral spinal position and to initiate contraction of the stabilizing muscles prior to the activity. For example, when reaching overhead, help the patient become aware of the need to contract the abdominal muscles to maintain a neutral spine position and not allow the spine to extend into a painful or unstable range; this is practiced until the stabilization becomes habitual. This principle is also incorporated into body mechanics, such as when going from picking up and lifting to placing an object on a high shelf, or into sport activities when reaching up to block or throw a ball.

Mobility/Flexibility

Goal. To increase ROM of specific structures that affect alignment and mobility in the neck and trunk.

In general, stretching is contraindicated in the region of inflamed tissue. However, if there are postures that relieve symptoms but are difficult to assume because of tissue restriction or fluid stasis, stretching or repetitive movement into the restricted range may be appropriate. For example, repetitive lumbar extension has been shown to relieve symptoms of fluid stasis or a disc lesion, yet a patient may not be able to get into an extended posture because of flexed postural dysfunction or swollen tissue. Prone propping and press-ups may stretch the tight tissue or may compress and massage swollen disc material or fluid stasis to reduce symptoms (see Fig. 15.4 and the section on Management Guidelines: Extension Bias in Chapter 15.)

Acute nerve root irritation from bony spurs or lipping in an arthritic spine is another situation in which acute symptoms may be relieved with stretching. Reducing pressure on the nerve roots with a stretch traction force, which widens the intervertebral foramina, or with procedures that help position the spine in its optimal spinal position may relieve the symptoms.[1]

Decreased mobility in structures in the upper and lower extremities that restrict normal postural alignment may be stretched or mobilized if the techniques do not stress the area of inflammation.

Stretching is done on a continuum. Critical judgment is used to determine the intensity and duration of stretch based on proximity to the healing tissue and the integrity and tolerance of the tissue. Principles of stretching for impaired mobility are described in Chapter 4.

Joint manipulation techniques and specific HVT techniques may be used to stretch a hypomobile facet joint capsule. Principles of joint manipulation are described in Chapter 5; indications for their use in the spine are identified in Chapter 15 in the Management Guidelines: Mobilization/Manipulation section.

If indicated, the patient is also taught general stress-relieving movements to reduce fluid stasis after being in prolonged postures. These movements are described in Chapter 14 in the Management of Impaired Posture section.

CLINICAL TIP

In general, stretching is contraindicated in the region of inflamed tissues.

Exceptions:

- Fluid stasis that restricts movement may respond to repetitive motion or sustained positioning into restricted range.
- Acute nerve root impingement may be relieved with traction or flexion to widen the intervertebral foramina.

Use clinical judgment to determine intensity and duration of stretch based on proximity to healing tissue, integrity, and tolerance of the tissue.

Cervical and Upper Thoracic Region: Stretching Techniques

Techniques to Increase Thoracic Extension

Self-Stretching

- *Patient position and procedure:* Hook-lying, with the hands behind the head and the elbows resting on the mat. Progress with both arms elevated overhead while maintaining back flat on the mat. To increase the stretch, place a pad or rolled towel lengthwise under the thoracic spine between the scapulae. Incorporate breathing exercises to increase mobility of the rib cage and assist with thoracic extension. Have the patient start with the elbows together in front of the face and then inhale as the elbows are brought down to the mat; hold the stretch position; then exhale as the elbows are brought together again.
- *Patient position and procedure:* Supine, with a foam roll placed longitudinally down the length of the spine. If the patient cannot balance on the roll or experiences tenderness along the spinous processes from pressure, tape two foam rolls together. The patient elevates both arms overhead in a "touchdown" position and allows gravity to apply the stretch force (Fig. 16.1 A). The patient then abducts and laterally rotates both shoulders (90/90 position) so the hands are facing the ceiling (Fig. 16.1 B). This position also stretches the pectoralis major and subscapularis muscles. Breathing exercises can be added to mobilize the ribs.

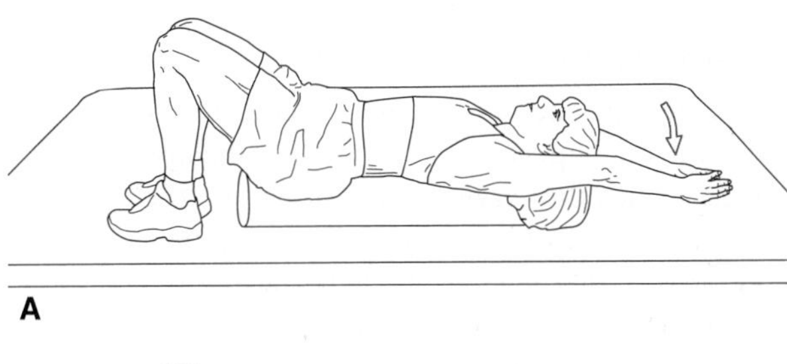

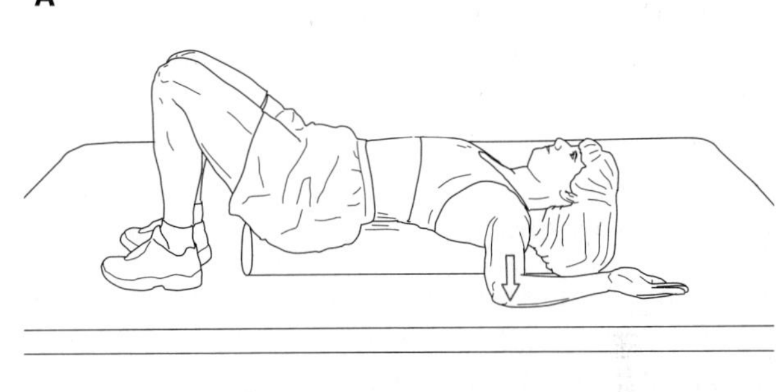

FIGURE 16.1 Foam roll stretch to increase flexibility of anterior thorax. **(A)** In the "touchdown" position, the shoulder extensors are also stretched. **(B)** With the shoulders abducted and laterally rotated, the pectoralis major and other internal rotators are also stretched. For a less intensive stretch, use a rolled towel placed longitudinally under the spine.

- *Patient position and procedure:* Sitting on a firm, straight-backed chair with the hands behind the head or held abducted and externally rotated 90°. The patient then brings the elbows out to the side as the scapulae are adducted and the thoracic spine is extended (head held neutral, not flexed). To combine with breathing, have the patient inhale as he or she takes the elbows out to the side and exhale as the elbows are brought in front of the face (Fig. 16.2).

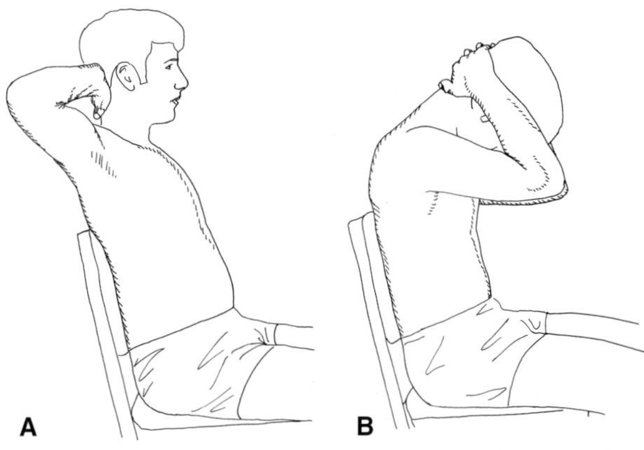

FIGURE 16.2 **(A)** Increase flexibility of anterior thorax and pectoralis muscles by adducting the scapula and extending the thoracic spine against the back of the chair. Inspiration increases the stretch; **(B)** facilitate expiration by bringing the elbows together and flexing the spine.

Techniques to Increase Cervical Retraction (Axial Extension): Scalene Muscle Stretch

CLINICAL TIP

Because the scalene muscles are attached to the transverse processes of the upper cervical spine and the upper two ribs, they either flex the cervical spine or elevate the upper ribs when they contract bilaterally. Unilaterally, the scalenes side bend the cervical spine to the same side and rotate it to the opposite side. To effectively stretch this muscle, stabilize the head and apply the stretch force against the upper portion of the rib cage.

Manual Stretching

Patient position and procedure: Sitting. The patient first performs axial extension (tucks the chin and straightens the neck) and then side bends the neck opposite and rotates it toward the tight muscles. Stand behind the patient and stabilize the head with the one hand around the side of the patient's head and face, holding the head against your trunk or shoulder. Place the other hand across the top of the rib cage on the side of tightness (Fig. 16.3). Instruct the patient to inhale and exhale; apply a downward pressure (resisting elevation of the rib cage) as the patient inhales again. As the patient relaxes (exhales), take up the slack. Repeat. This is a gentle, hold-relax stretching maneuver. This technique can also be done in supine.

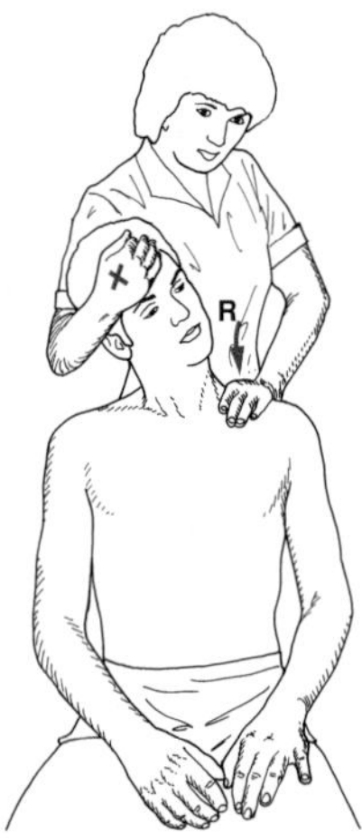

FIGURE 16.3 Unilateral active stretching of the scalenus muscles (manual stretch). The patient first performs axial extension, then side-bends the neck opposite and rotates it toward the tight muscles. The therapist stabilizes the head and upper thorax as the patient breathes in, contracting the muscle against the therapist's resistance. As the patient relaxes, the rib cage lowers and stretches the muscle.

Self-Stretching

Patient position and procedure: Standing next to a table and holding onto its underside. The patient positions the head in axial extension, side bends opposite, and rotates toward the same side as the muscle being stretched. To stretch, he or she leans away from the table, inhales, exhales, and holds the stretch position.

Techniques to Increase Upper Cervical Flexion: Suboccipital Muscle Stretch

Manual Stretching

Patient position and procedure: Sitting. Identify the spinous process of the second cervical vertebra and stabilize it with your thumb or with the second metacarpophalangeal joint (and the thumb and index finger around the transverse processes). Have the patient slowly nod, doing just a tipping motion of the head on the upper spine (Fig. 16.4). Guide the movement by placing the other hand across the patient's forehead.

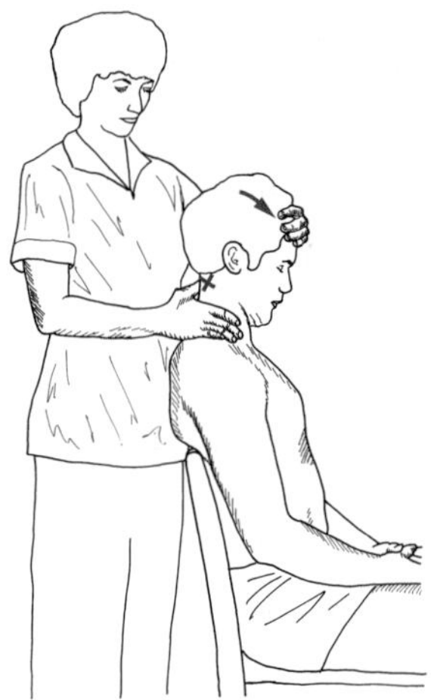

FIGURE 16.4 Stretching the short suboccipital muscles. The therapist stabilizes the second cervical vertebra as the patient slowly nods the head.

Self-Stretching

Patient position and procedure: Supine or sitting. Instruct the patient to first perform a chin tuck (axial extension), then nod the head, bringing the chin toward the larynx until a stretch is felt in the suboccipital area.

- Have the patient put a light pressure under the occipital region with the palm of his or her hand while tipping the head forward to reinforce the motion.
- For a *unilateral stretch*, instruct the patient to first perform a chin tuck, rotate slightly (up to 45°) to the left or right, and then nod.

NOTE: The weight of the head is enough stretch force in these exercises; the patient should not pull on the head when there is cervical pathology.

CLINICAL TIP

Shoulder girdle posture is directly related to cervical and thoracic posture. Techniques to increase flexibility in the shoulder girdle muscles are described in Chapter 17. Of primary importance:

- Pectoralis major (see Figs. 17.30 to 17.32)
- Pectoralis minor (see Fig. 17.33)
- Levator scapulae (see Figs. 17.34 and 17.35)
- Shoulder internal rotator muscles (see Fig. 17.26)

Traction as a Stretching Technique

Manual Traction: Cervical Spine

Traction techniques can be used for the purposes of stretching the muscles and the facet joint capsules and widening the intervertebral foramina.[72] The value of manual traction is that the angle of pull, head position, and placement of the force (via specific hand placements) can be controlled by the therapist; thus, the force can be specifically applied with minimum stress to regions that should not be stretched.

Patient position: Supine on a treatment table. The patient should be as relaxed as possible.

Therapist position and hand placement: Standing at the head of the treatment table, supporting the weight of the patient's head in the hands. Hand placement depends on comfort, the size of the patient's head and the therapist's hands. Suggestions include:

- Place the fingers of both hands under the occiput (Fig. 16.5 A), or with the hands on the sides of the face (not covering the ears).
- Place one hand over the forehead and the other hand under the occiput (Fig. 16.5 B).
- Place the index fingers around the spinous process above the vertebral level to be moved. This hand placement provides a specific traction only to the vertebral segments below the level at which the fingers are placed. A belt around the therapist's hips can be used to reinforce the fingers and increase the ease of applying the traction force (Fig. 16.5 C).

Procedure: Vary the patient's head position in flexion, extension, side bending, and side bending with rotation until the tissue to be stretched is taut; then apply a traction force by assuming a stable stance and leaning backward in a controlled manner. If a belt is used, the force is transmitted through the belt. The force is usually applied intermittently with smooth and gradual building and releasing of the force. The intensity and duration are usually limited by the therapist's strength and endurance.

CLINICAL TIP

When applying cervical traction, the more a person's head is flexed, the lower in the cervical spine the traction force is directed. When side bending, caution should be used because the position may cause facet and foramen approximation on the side of the concavity, which, in turn, may cause radicular or facet joint symptoms on that side.

Self-Traction: Cervical Spine

Patient position and procedure: Sitting or lying down. Have the patient place his or her hands behind the neck with the fingers interlocking; the ulnar border of the fingers and hands are under the occiput and mastoid processes. The patient then gives a lifting motion to the head. The head and spine may be placed in flexion, extension, side bending, or rotation for more isolated effects. He or she may apply the traction intermittently or in a sustained manner throughout the day.

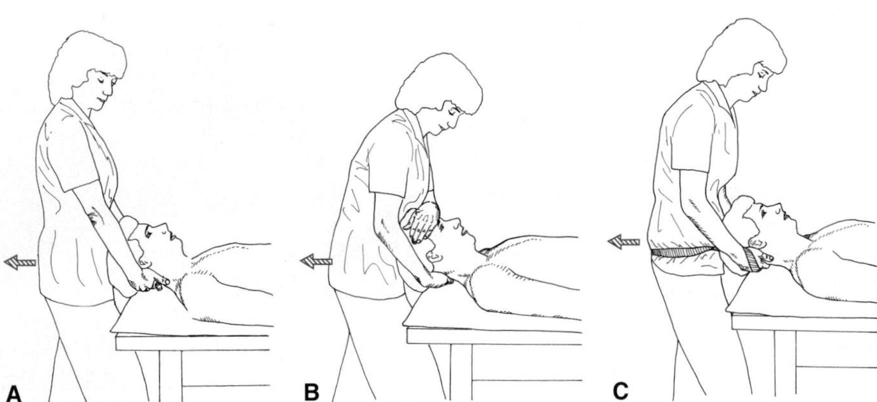

FIGURE 16.5 Manual cervical traction: **(A)** with the fingers of both hands under the occiput; **(B)** with one hand over the frontal region and the other hand under the occiput; and **(C)** using a belt to reinforce the hands for the traction force.

NOTE: Various forms of mechanical traction can be used in the clinical setting and at home. The position, dosage, and duration of traction are determined by the therapist. Instruction for use of the equipment is not described in this text.

Cervical Joint Manipulation Techniques

As previously noted, the principles of joint mobilization/manipulation are discussed in detail in Chapter 5 and their indications for use with specific impairments are identified in Chapter 15. Spinal manipulative techniques are indicated for pain modulation and to improve joint motion.

CLINICAL TIP

Spinal manipulations are graded I–V. All spinal and rib manipulations, with the exception of HVT techniques, are performed for 1 to 2 minutes and then reassessed for increased motion or decreased pain. Intervention is terminated once the desired result is achieved or to patient tolerance.

- Grade I—small-amplitude oscillations are used for pain modulation, typically during the acute stage following injury.
- Grade II—large-amplitude oscillations are also used for pain modulation. Dosage and indications are similar to grade I manipulations.
- Grade III—large-amplitude oscillations that go up to the restrictive joint barrier are designed to improve joint ROM and can be used during the subacute or chronic stages of healing.
- Grade IV—small-amplitude oscillations that go through the restrictive joint barrier. These manipulations are designed to improve joint ROM and should be used only during the chronic stages of healing.
- Grade V (HVT)—high-velocity and low-amplitude thrust applied at the physiologic limit of joint motion. These manipulations are performed only one time and designed solely to improve ROM.

PRECAUTIONS:
- If a manipulation procedure causes a change in sensation or an increased pain to radiate down an extremity, or if a patient reports a feeling of dizziness or light-headedness, do not perform additional manipulations.
- Use extreme caution if the patient reports either a current history of corticosteroid use or excessive pain.

CONTRAINDICATIONS:
- Unhealed fracture
- History of joint or ligamentous laxity caused by trauma or systemic diseases, such as rheumatoid arthritis
- Vertebral artery disease or occlusion
- Acute joint inflammation/irritation
- Cauda equina symptoms

Manipulation to Increase Cervical Flexion (Fig. 16.6)

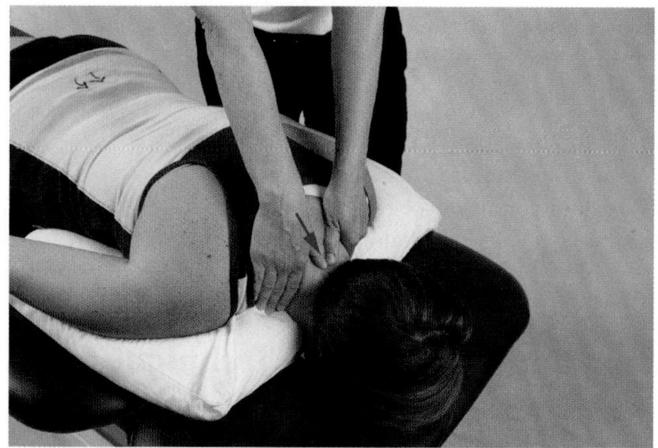

FIGURE 16.6 Cervical Flexion Manipulation—prone

Patient position: Prone with arms resting comfortably at patient's side. Place a pillow under the clavicular region for patient comfort and to promote a neutral cervical-thoracic curve.

Therapist position and hand placement: Stand on one side of the patient with your body facing toward his or her head. Use a two-thumb contact on the spinous process of the superior restricted segment of the three-joint complex.

Manipulation force: Using force through the thumbs, slide the superior vertebra in a cephalad-anterior direction.

Manipulation to Increase Cervical Extension (Fig. 16.7)

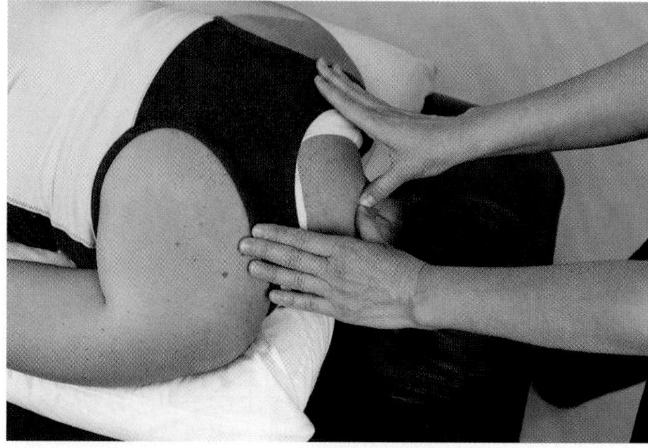

FIGURE 16.7 Cervical Extension Manipulation—prone

Patient position: Prone with arms resting comfortably at patient's side, use a pillow for patient comfort and to promote a neutral cervical-thoracic curve.

Therapist position and hand placement: Stand at the head of the patient with your body facing toward his or her feet. Use a two-thumb contact on the spinous process of the superior restricted segment of the restricted three-joint complex.

Manipulation force: Using force through the thumbs, slide the superior vertebra in a caudal-posterior direction.

Manipulation to Increase Cervical Rotation (Fig. 16.8)

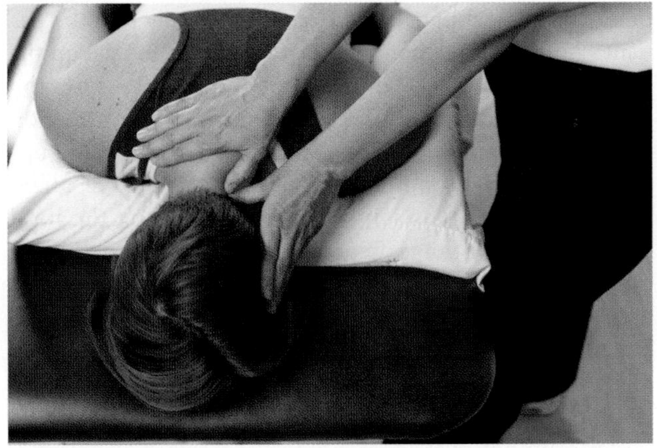

FIGURE 16.8 Cervical Rotation Manipulation—prone

Patient position: Prone with arms resting comfortably at patient's side, use a pillow for patient comfort and to promote a neutral cervical-thoracic curve.

Therapist position and hand placement: Stand on one side of the patient with your body facing toward their head. Use a two-thumb contact on the transverse process on the superior restricted vertebrae of the three-joint complex to cause rotation toward the direction of restriction.

Manipulation force: Using force through the thumbs, slide the superior vertebra in a cephalad-anteromedial direction.

Manipulation to Increase Cervical Rotation and Side Bending (Fig. 16.9)

VIDEO 16.1

This technique increases the diameter of the ipsilateral foramen, as seen with contralateral rotation and side bending.

Patient position: Supine.

Therapist position and hand placement: Stand at the head of the patient with one hand (the hand opposite the side of restriction) supporting the head and the other hand in contact with the lateral aspect of the verterbra to be manipulated.

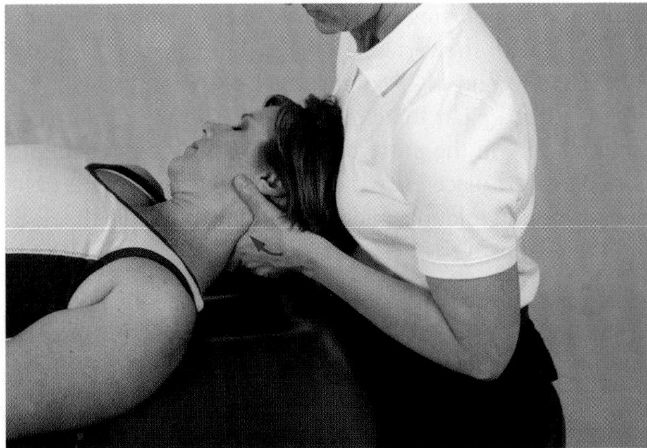

FIGURE 16.9 Cervical Rotation and Side-Bending Upglide Manipulation—supine

The medial side of the second MCP joint should be in contact with the edge of the facet and pillar to be manipulated and the rest of your hand relaxed on the postero-lateral portion of the patient's neck. Passively place the patient's head and neck into flexion, contralateral rotation, and side bending to take up the slack until the segment to be treated is identified.

Manipulation force: Using force through the metacarpal joint of the second digit, slide (or upglide) the cervical facet in an anterior-superior-medial direction at a 45° angle.

Manipulation to Increase Cervical Rotation and Side Bending: Alternate Technique (Fig. 16.10) VIDEO 16.1

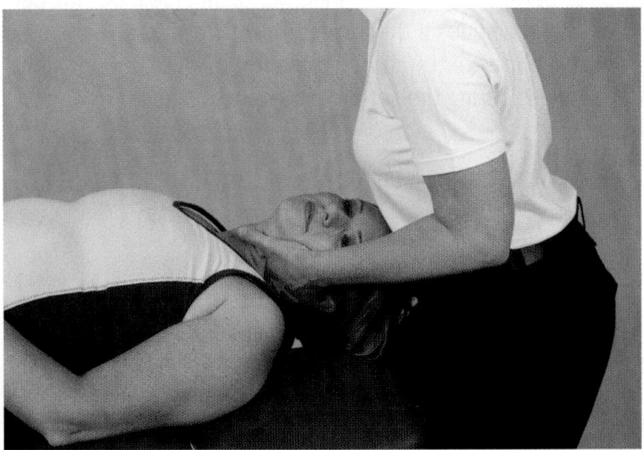

FIGURE 16.10 Cervical Rotation and Side-Bending Downglide Manipulation—supine

This technique decreases the diameter of the ipsilateral foramen, as seen with ipsilateral rotation and side bending.

Patient position: Supine.

Therapist position and hand placement: Stand at the head of the patient with one hand (the hand opposite the side of restriction) supporting the patient's head and the other hand in contact with the vertebra to be manipulated. The medial side of the second MCP joint should be in contact with the edge facet and pillar to be manipulated and the rest of your hand relaxed on the postero-lateral portion of the patient's neck. Passively place the patient's head and neck into extension, ipsilateral rotation, and side bending to take up the slack until the segment to be treated is identified.

Manipulation force: Using force through the MCP joint of the second digit, slide (or downglide) the cervical facet in an inferior-medial direction at a 45° angle.

Muscle Energy Techniques to Increase Craniocervical Mobility

Muscle energy (ME) uses the application of submaximum, isometric contractions of muscles whose line of pull can cause the desired accessory motion of a joint; ME techniques are designed to improve joint mobility (see Chapter 5). The patient holds the gentle muscle contraction against the therapist's graded resistance for 3 to 5 seconds and then relaxes. This process is repeated for three to five repetitions. When performed correctly, ME techniques are extremely safe and are indicated for most joint restrictions resulting from musculoskeletal disorders at any stage of healing.

PRECAUTION: Great care should be used when applying the following techniques so as not to occlude the vertebral artery. The therapist should test the integrity of the vertebral artery prior to performing the following ME techniques. Do not perform ME techniques if the patient reports an altered sensation in either upper extremity or a feeling of dizziness or lightheadedness during the set-up of these techniques.

Techniques to Increase Craniocervical Flexion (Fig. 16.11) VIDEO 16.2

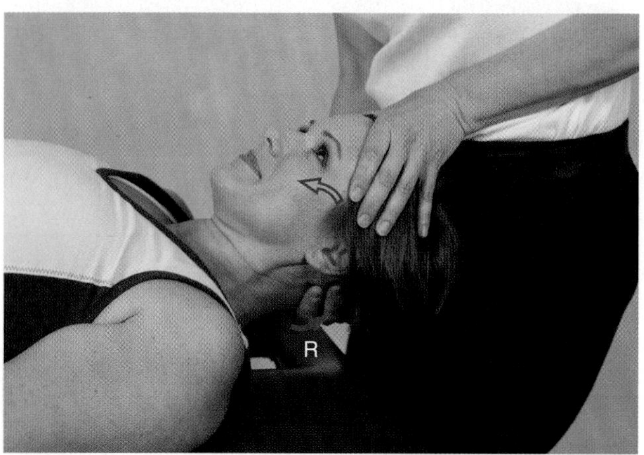

FIGURE 16.11 Muscle Energy: Craniocervical Flexion

Patient position: Supine, with hands placed comfortably at the side.

Therapist position, hand placement, and patient effort: Stand at the head of the treatment table. Support the occiput with one hand and place the other hand across the forehead. Ask the patient to look upward gently as if nodding the head backwards and apply resistance against the patient's occiput, creating a gentle isometric contraction in the suboccipital muscles. When the patient relaxes, take up the slack by passively nodding the head through any new range.

Alternate technique: Sit on a stool at the head of patient with your forearms resting on the treatment table. One hand stabilizes the C2 vertebra by grasping the transverse processes between the proximal portions of the thumb and index finger; the other hand supports the occiput. Passively nod the patient's head with the hand under the occiput to take up the slack of the suboccipital muscles; then ask the patient to roll the eyes upward. This causes a gentle isometric contraction of the suboccipital muscles. The patient keeps looking upward for 3 to 5 seconds and then relaxes. After the patient relaxes, take up the slack by passively nodding the head through any new range. Repeat this procedure three to five times or until the desired outcome is achieved. Only motion between the occiput and C2 should occur. The contraction is gentle in order not to cause overflow into the multisegmental erector spinae and upper trapezius muscles. This technique uses a gentle hold-relax, of the rectus capitis posterior minor muscle.

Techniques to Increase Craniocervical Rotation (Fig. 16.12) VIDEO 16.2

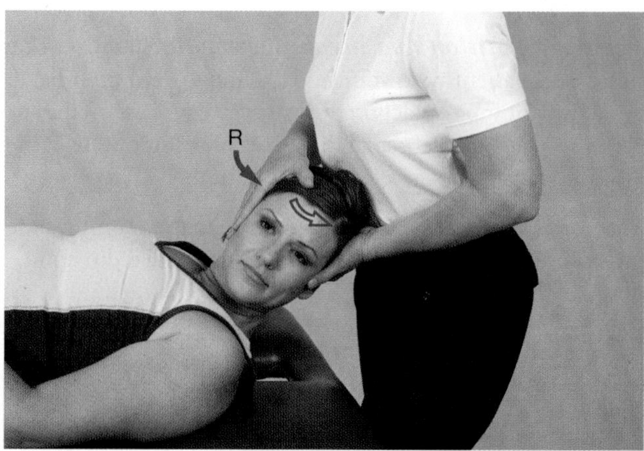

FIGURE 16.12 Muscle Energy: Craniocervical Rotation

Patient position: Supine, with hands placed comfortably at the side.

Therapist position, hand placement, and patient effort: Stand at the head of the patient. Wrap hands around the side of the patient's head with fingers under the occiput. Place the patient's head in end-range cervical flexion. Next, rotate his or her head in the direction of the restriction (for example, with restricted rotation to the left, place head in end-range left rotation). Once the patient is at end-range, instruct the patient to look in the opposite direction (example, toward the right) while you resist this movement with gentle pressure against the side of the head. After a 3- to 5-second hold, have the patient relax and move the head into greater rotation. Repeat as needed.

Mid and Lower Thoracic and Lumbar Regions: Stretching Techniques

Techniques to Increase Lumbar Flexion

PRECAUTION: Do not perform if flexion causes a change in sensation or causes pain to radiate down the lower extremity.

Self-Stretching

- *Patient position and procedure:* Hook-lying. Have the patient first bring one knee and then the other toward the chest, clasp the hands around the thighs and pull them to the chest, elevating the sacrum off the mat (Fig. 16.13). The patient should not grasp around the tibia; it places stress on the knee joints as the stretch force is applied.

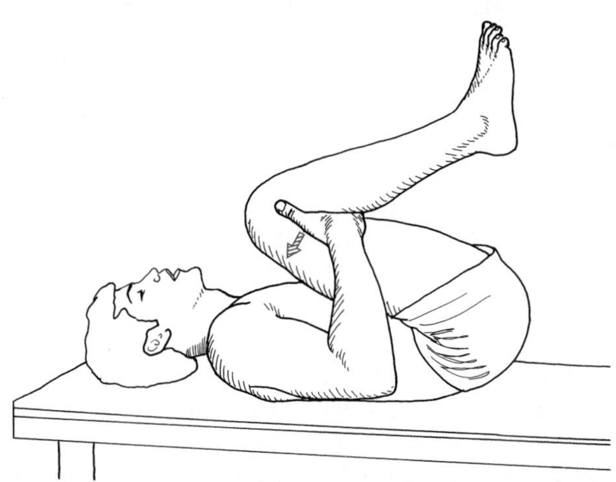

FIGURE 16.13 Self-stretching the lumbar erector spinae muscles and tissues posterior to the spine. The patient grasps around the thighs to avoid compression of the knee joints.

- *Patient position and procedure:* Quadruped (on hands and knees). Have the patient perform a posterior pelvic tilt without rounding the thorax (concentrate on flexing the lumbar spine, not the thoracic spine), hold the position, then relax (Fig. 16.14 A). Repeat; this time bring the hips back to the feet, hold, and then return to the hands and knees position (Fig. 16.14 B). This also stretches the gluteus maximus, quadriceps femoris, and shoulder extensor muscles.

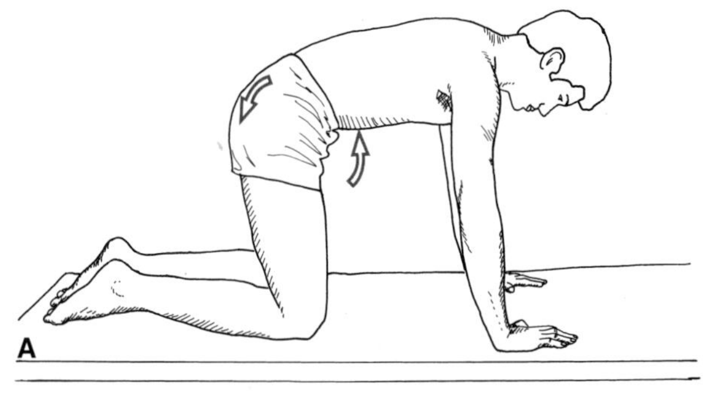

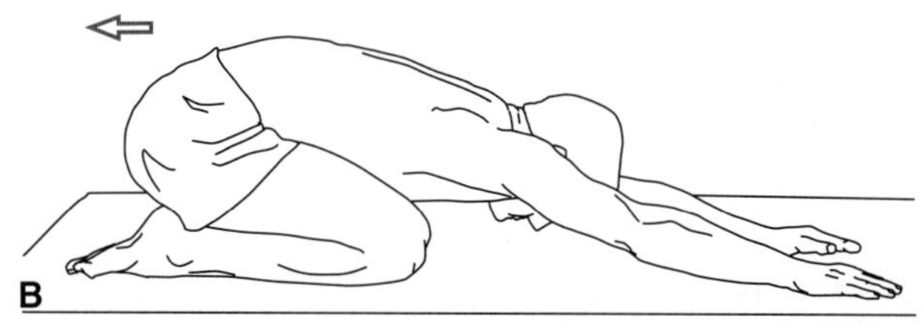

FIGURE 16.14 Stretching of the lumbar spine. **(A)** The patient performs a posterior pelvic tilt without rounding the thorax. **(B)** The patient moves the buttocks back over the feet for a greater stretch.

Techniques to Increase Lumbar Extension

PRECAUTION: Do not perform if extension causes a change in sensation or causes pain to radiate down the lower extremity.

Self-Stretching

- *Patient position and procedure:* Prone, with hands placed under the shoulders. Have the patient extend the elbows and push the thorax up off the mat but keep the pelvis down on the mat. This is a prone press-up (Fig. 16.15 A). To increase the stretch force, the pelvis can be strapped to the treatment table. This exercise also places the hip flexor muscles and soft tissue anterior to the hips in an elongated position, although it does not selectively stretch these tissues.
- *Patient position and procedure:* Standing, with the hands placed in the low back area. Instruct the patient to lean backward (Fig. 16.15 B).
- *Patient position and procedure:* Quadruped (hands and knees). Instruct the patient to allow the spine to sag, creating lumbar extension. Alternating between this motion and a posterior pelvic tilt (as in Fig. 16.14) can be used to teach the patient how to control pelvic motion.

Techniques to Increase Lateral Flexibility of the Spine

Stretching techniques to increase lateral flexibility are used for intervention when there is asymmetrical flexibility in side bending as well as in the management of scoliosis. It is important to note that stretching has not been shown to correct or halt progression of structural scoliosis, although they may be beneficial in gaining some flexibility prior to surgical fusion of

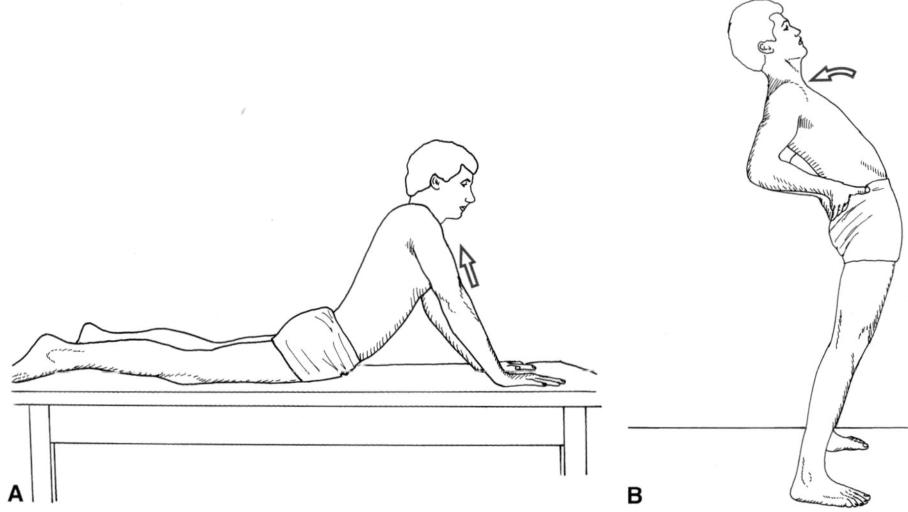

FIGURE 16.15 Self-stretching of the soft tissues anterior to the lumbar spine and hip joints with the patient **(A)** prone (using a press-up) and **(B)** standing.

the spine for correcting a scoliotic deformity. They may also be used to regain flexibility in the frontal plane when muscle or fascial tightness is present with postural dysfunction. All of the following exercises are designed to stretch hypomobile structures on the concave side of the lateral curvature.

When stretching the trunk, it is necessary to stabilize the spine either above or below the curve. If the patient has a double curve, one curve must be stabilized while the other is stretched.

- *Patient position and procedure:* Prone. Stabilize the patient (manually or with a belt) at the iliac crest on the side of the concavity. Have the patient reach toward the knee with the arm on the convex side of the curve while stretching the opposite arm up and overhead (Fig. 16.16). Instruct the patient to breathe in and expand the rib cage on the side being stretched.
- *Patient position and procedure:* Prone. Have the patient stabilize the upper trunk (thoracic curve) by holding onto the edge of the mat table with the arms. Lift the hips and legs and laterally bend the trunk away from the concavity (Fig. 16.17).

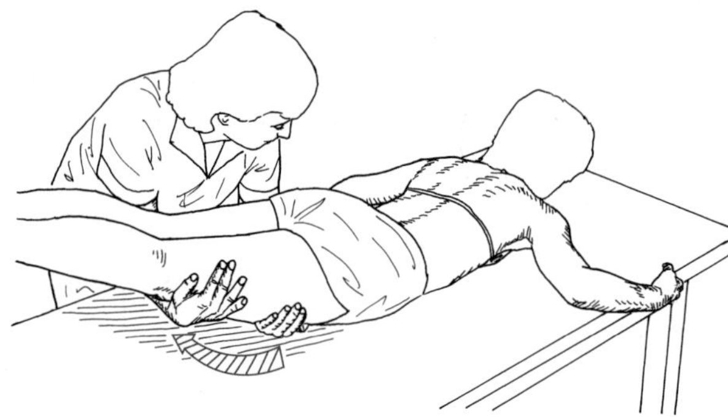

FIGURE 16.17 Stretching hypomobile structures on the concave side of a left lumbar curve. The patient stabilizes the upper trunk and thoracic curve as the therapist passively stretches the lumbar curve.

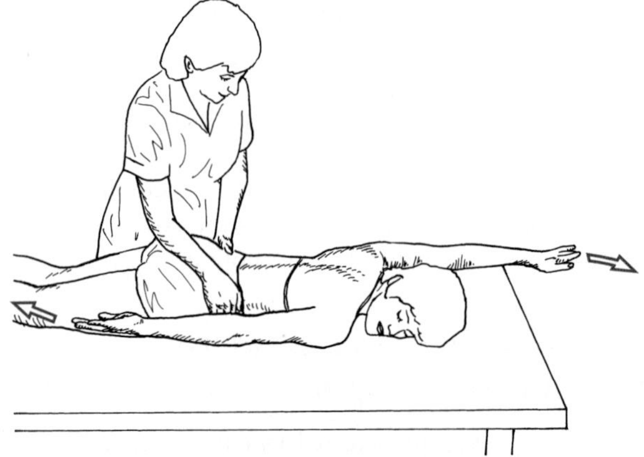

FIGURE 16.16 Stretching hypomobile structures on the concave side of the thoracic curve. Illustrated is a patient with a right thoracic left lumbar curve. The therapist stabilizes the pelvis and lumbar spine while the patient actively stretches the thoracic curve by reaching upward on side of concavity and downward on side of convexity.

- *Patient position and procedure:* Heel-sitting. Have the patient lean forward so the abdomen rests on the anterior thighs (Fig. 16.18 A); the arms are stretched overhead bilaterally; and the hands are flat on the floor. Then have the patient laterally bend the trunk away from the concavity by walking the hands to the convex side of the curve. Hold the position for a sustained stretch (Fig. 16.18 B).
- *Patient position and procedure:* Side-lying on the convex side of the curve. Place a rolled towel at the apex of the curve, and have the patient reach overhead with the top arm. Stabilize the patient at the iliac crest. Do not allow the patient to roll forward or backward during the stretch. Hold this position for a sustained period of time (Fig. 16.19).
- *Patient position and procedure:* Side-lying over the edge of a mat table with a rolled towel at the apex of the curve and the top arm stretched overhead. Stabilize the iliac crest. Hold this head-down position as long as possible (Fig. 16.20).

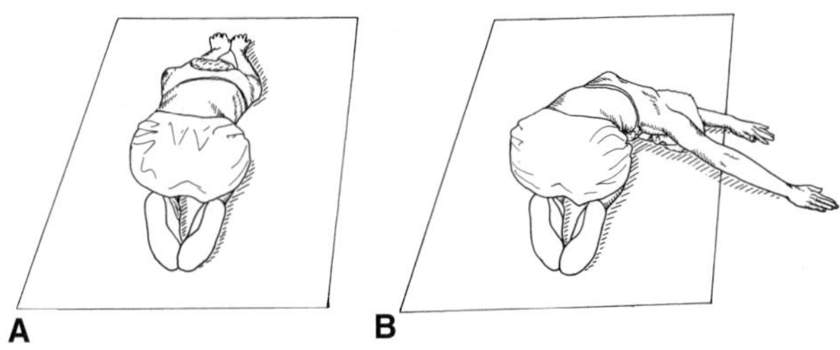

FIGURE 16.18 (A) Heel-sitting to stabilize the lumbar spine. (B) Hypomobile structures on the concave side of a right thoracic curve are stretched by having the patient reach the arms overhead and then walk the hands toward the convex side.

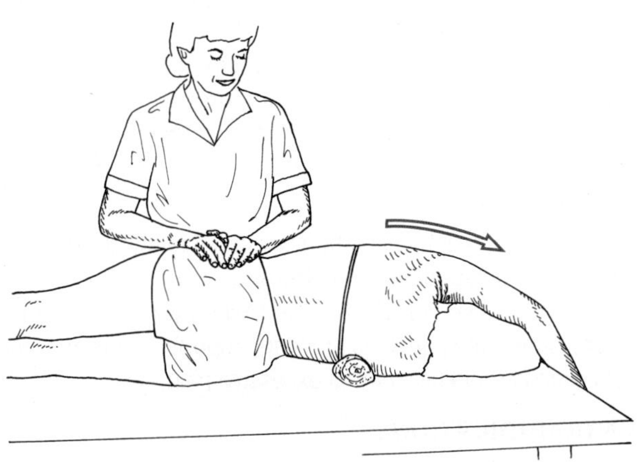

FIGURE 16.19 Stretching tight structures on the concave side of a right thoracic curve. The patient is positioned side-lying with a rolled towel at the apex of the convexity. The lumbar spine is stabilized by the therapist.

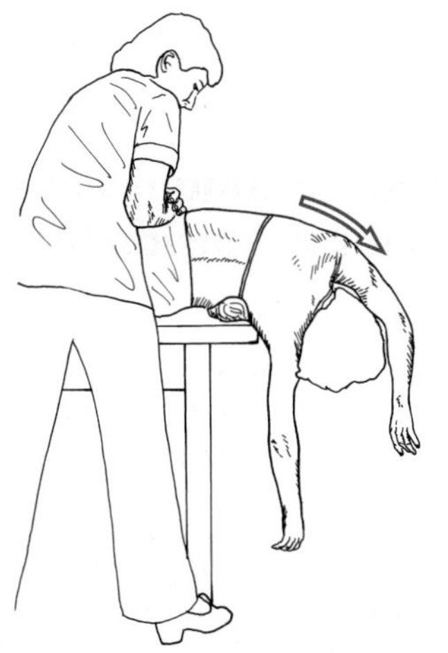

FIGURE 16.20 Side-lying over the edge of a mat table to stretch hypomobile structures of a right thoracic scoliosis. The therapist stabilizes the pelvis.

CLINICAL TIP

Hip muscles have a direct effect on spinal posture and function because of their attachment on the pelvis. It is important that they have adequate flexibility for proper pelvic and spinal alignment. In addition to manual stretching techniques described in Chapter 4 (see Figs. 4.25 to 4.30), see Chapter 20 for specific self-stretching techniques in the hip. Of primary importance:

- Hip extension (see Figs. 20.10 and 20.11)
- Hip flexion (see Fig. 20.12, also knee to chest as in Fig. 20.10)
- Hip rotation (see Figs. 20.14 and 20.15)
- Hamstrings (See Figs. 20.17 and 20.18)
- Tensor fascia lata (See Figs. 20.19 to 20.21)

Traction as a Stretching Technique

Manual Traction: Lumbar Spine

Manual traction is not as easily applied in the lumbar region as in the cervical region. At least one-half of the patient's body weight must be moved, and the coefficient of friction of the part to be moved also must be overcome to cause vertebral distraction and stretching. It is helpful to place the patient on a split-traction table for ease in moving and stretching the spine.

Patient position: Supine or prone. Stabilize the thorax with a harness secured to the head end of the table or have an assistant stabilize the patient by standing at the head of the table and holding the patient's arms. Position the patient so there is maximal stretch on the hypomobile tissue.

- To stretch into extension, extend the hips.
- To stretch into flexion, flex the hips.
- To stretch into side bending, move the lower extremities to one side.

Therapist position and procedures: Position yourself so effective body mechanics and body weight can be used.

- If the lower extremities are extended to emphasize spinal extension, exert the pull at the ankles.
- If the lower extremities are flexed to emphasize spinal flexion, drape both of the legs over your shoulder that is closest to the mid-line of the table and exert the stretch force with your arms wrapped across the patient's thighs. As an alternative, place a pelvic belt with straps around the patient and manually pull on the straps.
- For unilateral impairments, pull on one extremity.

Positional Traction: Lumbar Spine

The value of positional traction is that the primary traction force can be directed to the side on which symptoms occur, or it can be isolated to a specific facet, making it beneficial for selective stretching.

Patient position: Side-lying, with the side to be stretched uppermost. A rolled blanket or thick towel is placed under the spine at the level where the traction force is desired; this causes side bending away from the side to be treated and, therefore, an upward gliding of the facets (Fig. 16.21 A).

Therapist position: Standing, at the side of the treatment table facing the patient. Determine the segment that is to receive most of the traction force and palpate the spinous processes at that level and the level above.

Procedure: The patient relaxes in the side-bent position. Rotation is added to isolate a distraction force to the desired level. Rotate the upper trunk by gently pulling on the arm on which the patient is lying while simultaneously palpating the spinous processes with your other hand to determine when rotation has arrived at the level just above the joint to be distracted. Then flex the patient's uppermost thigh, again palpating the spinous processes until flexion of the lower portion of the spine occurs at the desired level. The segment at which these two opposing forces meet now has maximum positional distraction force (Fig. 16.21 B).

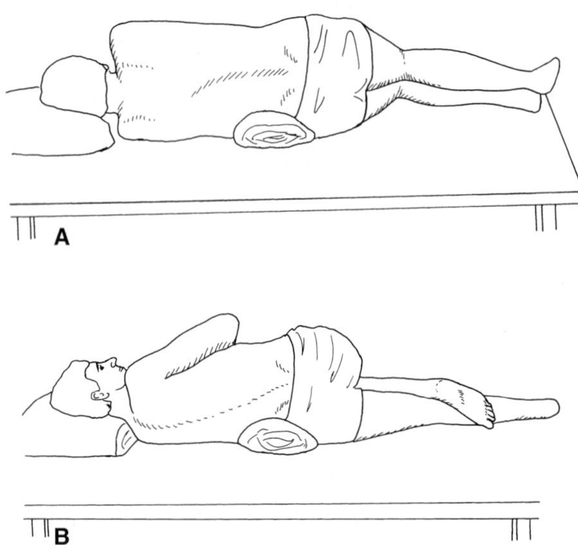

FIGURE 16.21 Positional traction for the lumbar spine. **(A)** Side bending over a 6- to 8-inch roll causes longitudinal traction to the segments on the upward side. **(B)** Side-bending with rotation adds a distraction force to the facets on the upward side.

CLINICAL TIP

Mechanical traction units can provide considerable stretch force to the tissues of the thoracic and lumbar spine. Positioning considerations are as described for manual traction. Instructions for use of the equipment are not part of this text.

Thoracic and Lumbar Joint Manipulation and HVT Techniques

Joint manipulation and HVT techniques have been shown to have minimal risk to patients[8,21] and also to be an effective intervention for spinal pain.[8,11,14,17,21] Although HVT has been practiced in physical therapy since the 1920s,[62] these techniques should not be performed by physical therapist assistants or physical therapy aides.[4,62] The indications for joint manipulation and HVT are discussed in Chapter 5.

HVT techniques may be easier to perform if the application of the force is coordinated with the patient's breathing. Instruct the patient to breathe deeply several times, and on the final exhalation, a high-velocity, low-amplitude force is delivered. Use caution that the patient does not hyperventilate during these procedures.

CLINICAL TIP

When applying spinal manipulation techniques:

- Modify the application force for pain modulation.
- Coordinate stretch manipulation and HVT techniques with patient breathing.
- HVT is a low-amplitude, high-velocity technique.
- HVT is applied with one repetition only.

PRECAUTIONS:

- Do not perform if manipulation causes a change in sensation or pain to radiate down an extremity.
- Extreme caution should be used when performing these techniques if the patient is pregnant, reports a current history of corticosteroid use, or has excessive pain.

CONTRAINDICATIONS:

- Unhealed fracture
- History of joint or ligamentous laxity caused by trauma or systemic diseases
- Spondylolisthesis
- Acute joint inflammation/irritation
- Cauda equine symptoms
- HVT is contraindicated in persons with a history of osteoporosis or osteopenia.

Manipulation Technique to Increase Thoracic Spine Extension (Fig. 16. 22)

VIDEO 16.3

Patient position: Prone with arms resting comfortably at patient's side. Place a pillow under the thoracic region for increased patient comfort and to promote a neutral cervical-thoracic curve.

Therapist position and hand placement: Stand on one side of the patient with your body facing toward the head of the patient. Place the distal phalanx of your second and third fingers on the transverse processes of the superior vertebral segment to be manipulated (Fig. 16.22 A). This is also referred to as the "V-spread technique." Place the hypothenar eminence of your other hand on top of the two-finger contact (Fig. 16.22 B).

Manipulation force: Apply an anterior glide. The contact points on the transverse processes serve as a point of reference. Your other hand exerts a force through the hypothenar eminence in an anterior direction.

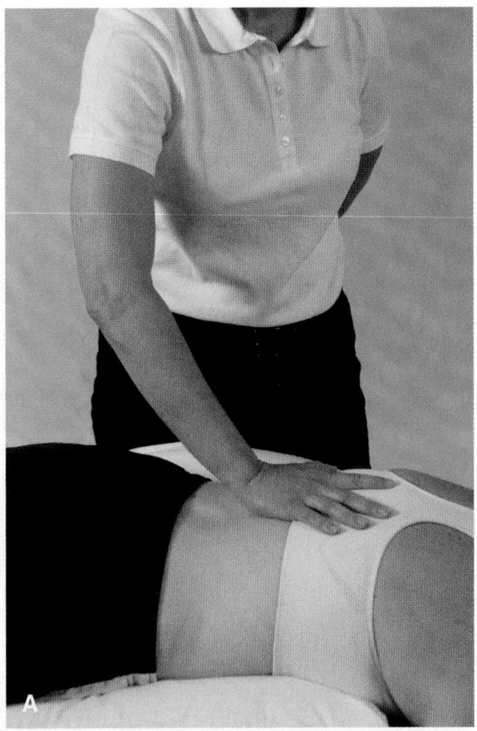

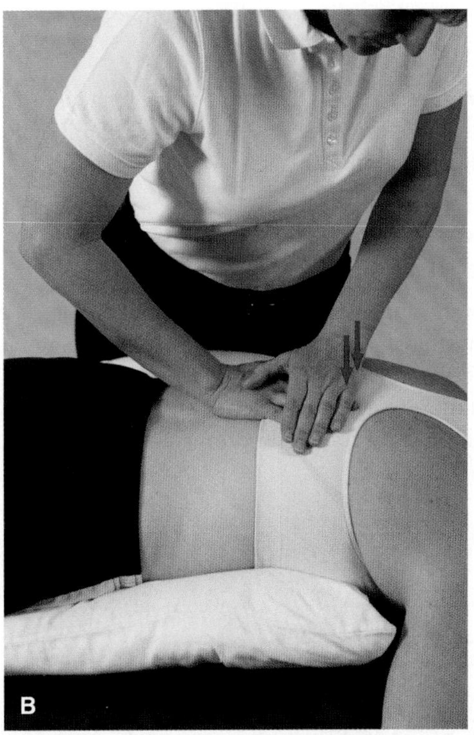

FIGURE 16.22 Thoracic Spine Extension Manipulation or HVT—prone: **(A)** "V-spread" finger placement on transverse processes and **(B)** force application with hypothenar eminence.

Manipulation Technique to Increase Thoracic Spine Flexion

Patient position: Prone with arms resting comfortably at patient's side. Place a pillow under the thoracic region for increased patient comfort and to promote a neutral cervical-thoracic curve.

Therapist position and hand placement: Same as for thoracic extension except the V-spread contact is on the transverse processes of the inferior vertebral segment to be mobilized.

Manipulation force: Apply an anterior glide. The contact points on the transverse processes serve as a point of reference. The other hand exerts a force through the hypothenar eminence in an anterior direction. Modify your forces for pain modulation or to improve motion.

Manipulation to Increase Thoracic Spine Rotation (Fig. 16.23)

VIDEO 16.3

Patient position: Prone with arms resting comfortably at patient's side. Place a pillow under the thoracic region for increased patient comfort and to promote a neutral cervical-thoracic curve.

Therapist position and hand placement: Using the V-spread contact, place one finger on the superior transverse process and the second finger on the contralateral inferior transverse process

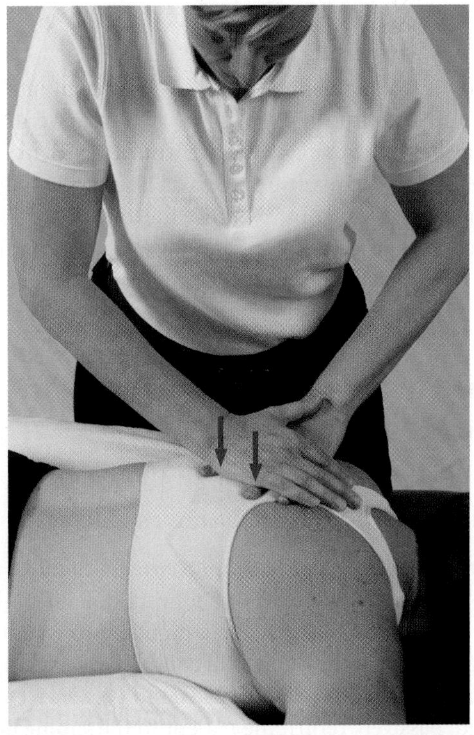

FIGURE 16.23 Thoracic Spine Left Rotation Manipulation or HVT—prone.

to be mobilized. The finger placement follows the "Rule of the Lower Finger" (see Clinical Tip).

Manipulation force: Apply an anteriorly directed force against the transverse processes with the contralateral hand pressing through the contact fingers.

CLINICAL TIP

Rule of the Lower Finger

When applying the V-spread contact on the contralateral transverse processes for thoracic rotation assessment or manipulation, rotation of a segment occurs in the direction of the finger on the inferior transverse process.

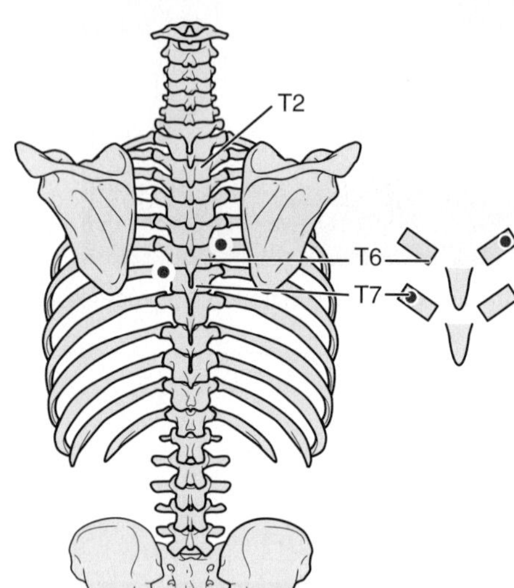

Example: Manipulation of the T6–7 segment into left rotation. The superior finger is on the right transverse process of T6, facilitating rotation to the left. Concurrently, the inferior finger on the left transverse process of T7 is facilitating a right rotation force (see Fig. 16.23). Since the lower finger is on the left transverse process, the "rule of the lower finger" makes it easy to remember this is a left rotation manipulation.

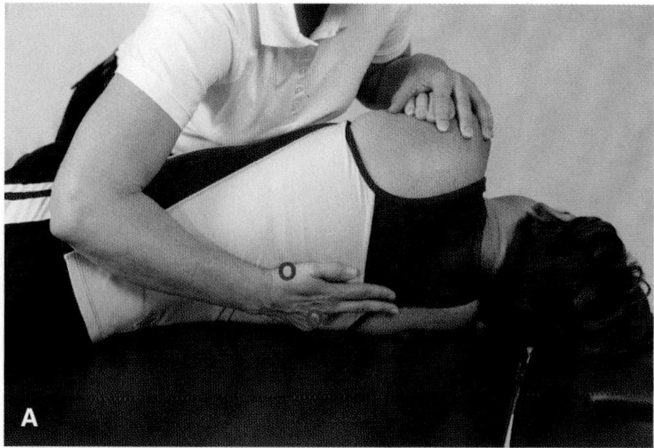

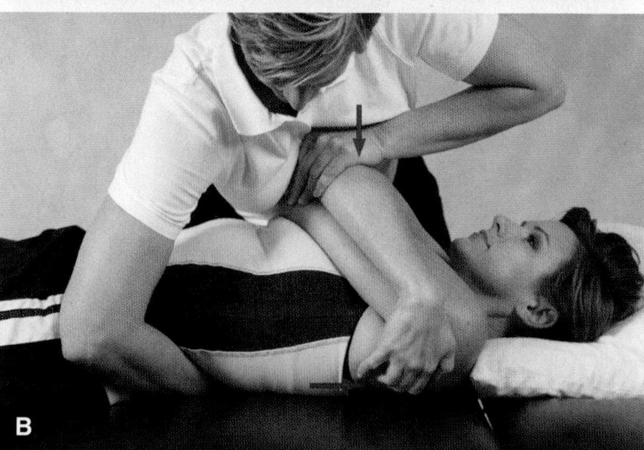

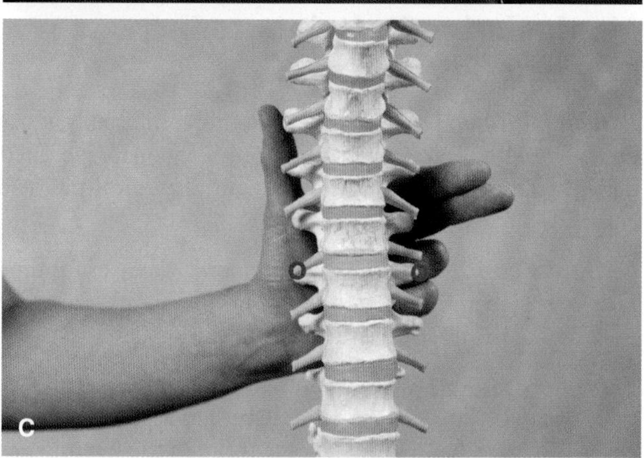

FIGURE 16.24 Thoracic spine manipulation: **(A)** hand placement on thoracic spine using a "pistol grip" and **(B)** manipulation force against patient's crossed arms. **(C)** Pistol grip on a spinal model, showing carpometacarpal joint of thumb on one transverse process and flexed middle phalanx on opposite transverse process.

Pistol Thrust to Increase Thoracic Spine Mobility (Fig. 16.24)

VIDEO 16.4

Patient position: Supine with arms crossed.

Therapist position and hand placement: Stand at the patient's side facing toward his or her head. Roll the patient toward you and reach across the patient's body; contact the inferior vertebra of the three-joint complex to be manipulated using the "pistol grip" (Fig. 16.24 A and C). Once contact is achieved, passively return the patient to the supine position. To improve rotation, use the rule of the lower finger as described in the clinical tip above.

Manipulation force: Place your trunk directly over the segment to be manipulated. A cephalad distraction force is initiated with the patient's body weight at the segment to be manipulated; this is followed by a high-velocity, posterior force against the patient's crossed arms toward the table (Fig. 16.24 B).

Cross-Arm Thrust to Increase Thoracic Spine Mobility (Fig. 16.25)

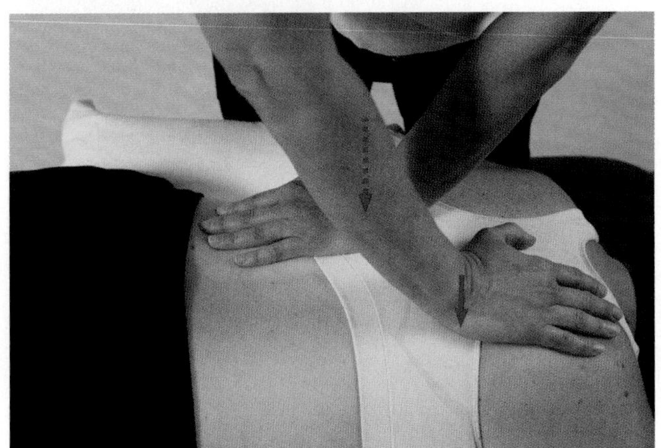

FIGURE 16.25 Thoracic spine manipulation using cross-arm thrust

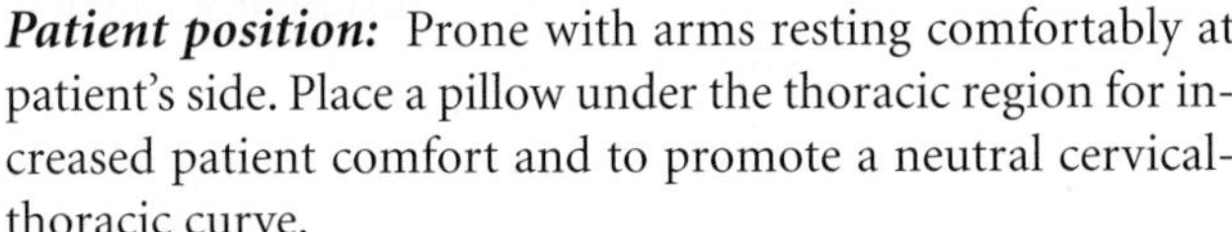

Patient position: Prone with arms resting comfortably at patient's side. Place a pillow under the thoracic region for increased patient comfort and to promote a neutral cervical-thoracic curve.

Therapist position and hand placement: Stand beside the patient. Cross your arms and place the pisiform (hypothenar eminence) of one hand on a left and one on a right transverse process of the segment to be manipulated. Modify transverse process contact to promote flexion, extension, or rotation by placing the pisiform on the superior, inferior, or "rule of the lower finger" transverse processes as described in the preceding sections.

Manipulation force: An anterior force is applied simultaneously by the hypothenar eminences. This may be used as either a manipulation or HVT intervention.

Fall Thrust to Increase Thoracic Spine Mobility (Fig. 16.26) VIDEO 16.5

Patient position: Standing with arms crossed.

Therapist position and hand placement: Stand behind the patient and wrap your arms around the patient. Place a mobilization wedge or folded towel at the desired spinal level to direct the force to a specific thoracic segment. Grasp patient's elbows (left hand grasps patient's right elbow and right hand grasps left elbow). If unable to grasp the elbows, interlock your fingers in front of the patient.

Manipulation force: Lean backwards on your heels while applying an extension force on the patient's spine, then quickly drop down so your feet are flat on the floor.

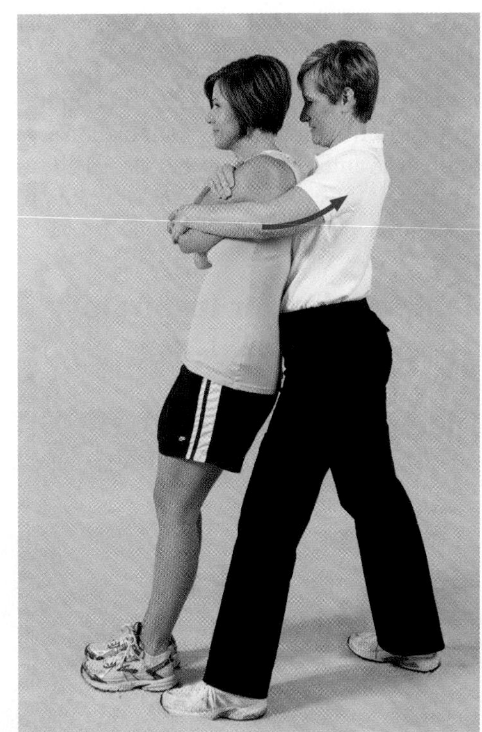

FIGURE 16.26 Thoracic spine manipulation using a fall thrust

Rib Manipulation for Expiratory Restriction (Fig. 16.27) VIDEO 16.6

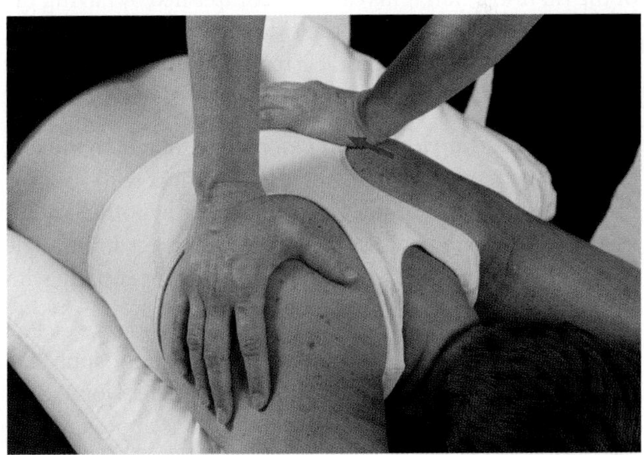

FIGURE 16.27 Expiratory restriction rib manipulation

Patient position: Prone with arms resting comfortably at the patient's side or overhead. Place a pillow under the thoracic region for increased patient comfort and to promote a neutral cervical-thoracic curve.

Therapist position and hand placement: Stand beside the patient. The hypothenar eminence of your caudal facing hand is placed on the rib angle at the level of the hypomobility, and the rest of the hand relaxes on the patient's back. The other hand is placed on the opposite rib to stabilize the rib cage.

Manipulation force: During active patient expiration, exert a series of four to five progressive manipulations against the restricted rib in an anterior, caudal, and medial direction during the last half of the expiratory phase. Use caution that the patient does not hyperventilate.

Rib Manipulation for Inspiratory Restriction (Fig. 16.28)

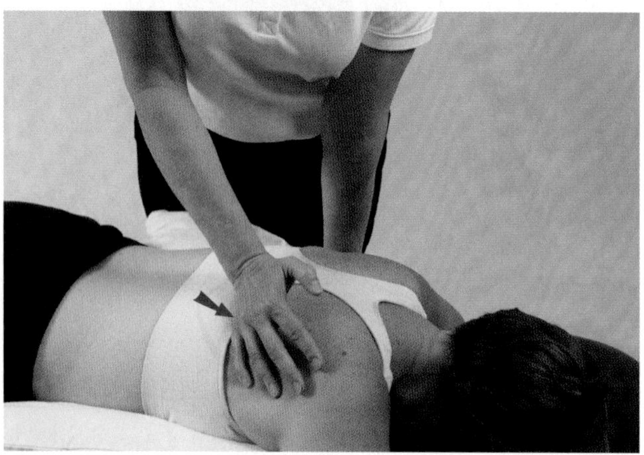

FIGURE 16.28 Inspiratory restriction rib manipulation

Patient position: Prone with scapula protracted on the side of the rib restriction. This can be accomplished by having the patient dangle the arm off the side of the treatment table. Place a pillow under the thoracic region for increased patient comfort and to promote a neutral cervical-thoracic curve.

Therapist position and hand placement: Stand on the side opposite the restriction; reach across the thorax with your inferior extremity and contact the pisiform or hypothenar eminence of your hand on the inferio-medial aspect at the angle of the rib to be manipulated. Stabilize your upper body with the contralateral hand leaning on the table.

Manipulation force: During patient exhalation, apply the force to remove all the slack from the costovertebral joint; continue with four to five progressive oscillations approximately half-way through the inspiratory phase. Apply the force perpendicular to the rib angle (in an anterior, caudal, and medial direction). Use caution that the patient does not hyperventilate.

Elevated First Rib Manipulation (Fig. 16.29) VIDEO 16.7

Patient position: Sitting in a firm chair with his or her back supported. The head and neck are laterally flexed towards and rotated away from the side of restriction to stabilize the facets in the closed-pack position and relax the scalene muscle.

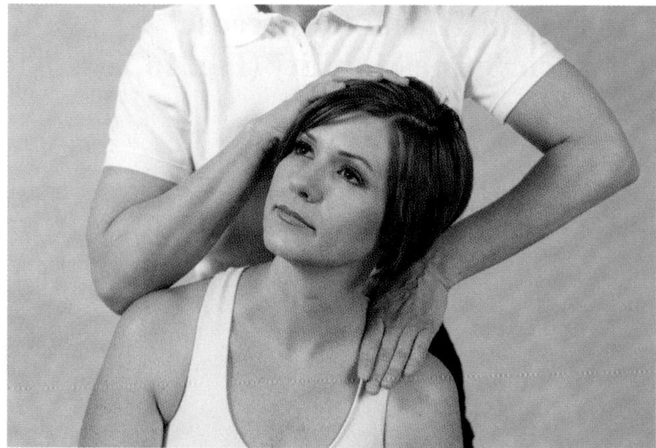

FIGURE 16.29 Elevated first rib manipulation

Alternate head/neck position: The head and cervical spine are rotated toward the side of restriction to bring the transverse process posterior and place the first costotransverse articulation at end-range stretched position.

Therapist position and hand placement: Stand behind the patient and stabilize the head against your thorax. Place the second MCP of your other hand on the first rib just lateral to the costotransverse joint.

Manipulation force: Exert the manipulation force or HVT through the rib in a caudal and medial direction during patient exhalation.

Manipulation Techniques to Increase Lumbar Spine Extension (Fig. 16.30)

VIDEO 16.8

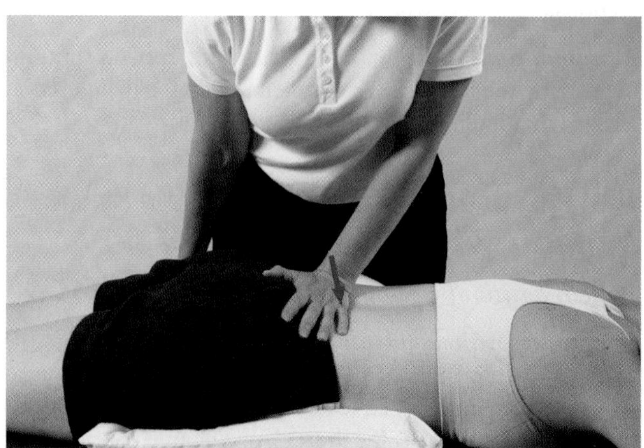

FIGURE 16.30 Lumbar spine extension manipulation/HVT—prone

Patient position: Prone. Place a pillow under the abdominal region for patient comfort and to provide a neutral lumbosacral curve.

Therapist position and hand placement: Place your pisiform (hypothenar eminence) over the spinous process. Relax the rest of your hand on the patient's back.

Anterior glide manipulation force: Push with your hypothenar eminence in an anterior direction. Align your trunk directly over the segment, so the force is directed downward and not at an angle.

Manipulation to Increase Lumbar Spine Rotation (Fig. 16.31)

VIDEO 16.8

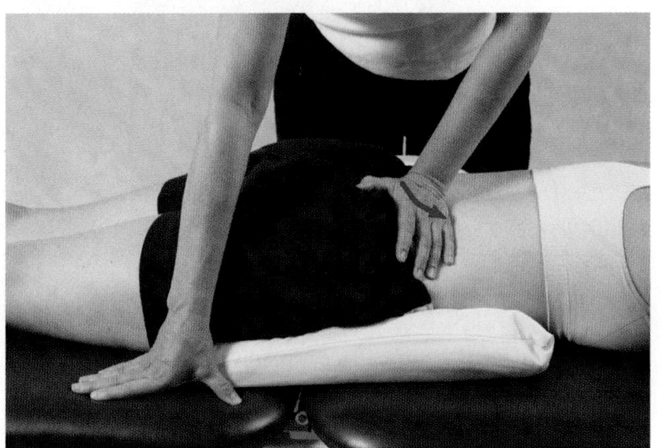

FIGURE 16.31 Lumbar spine left rotation manipulation/HVT—prone

Patient position: Prone. Place a pillow under the abdominal region for patient comfort and to provide a neutral lumbosacral curve.

Therapist position and hand placement: Place your pisiform (hypothenar eminence) over one transverse process on the side opposite of the direction of the motion you wish to facilitate (i.e., if wanting to promote left rotation, place your hypothenar eminence on the right transverse process). Relax the rest of your hand on the patient's back.

Anterior glide manipulation force: Push with your hypothenar eminence in an anterior and medial direction.

Manipulation to Increase Lumbar Intervertebral Side Bending (Fig. 16.32) VIDEO 16.9

Patient position: Side-lying with the restricted side down. Position the patient as close to the edge of the bed as possible and flex the hips and knees to 90°.

Therapist position and hand placement: Stand facing the patient. Place the finger tip from your caudal hand on the superior spinous process to monitor motion. Passively rotate the patient's trunk backward to "take up the slack" until just

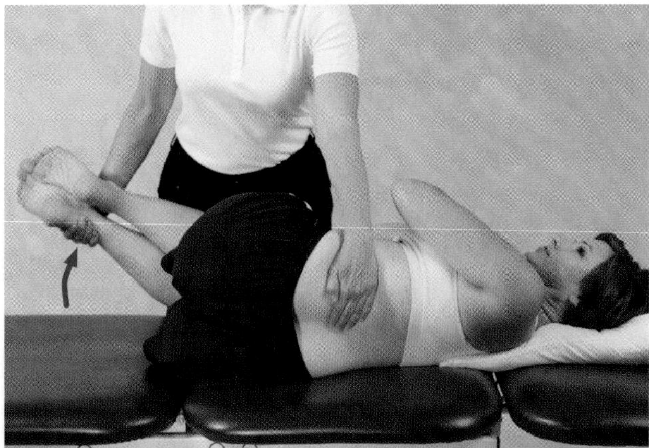

FIGURE 16.32 Lumbar spine side-bending manipulation—side-lying

before you feel the vertebral segment move. Now, place the finger tip of your cephlad hand on the superior spinous process to monitor motion. Flex both of the patient's legs (hips) until just before you feel the vertebral segment move. The patient's legs can then be supported either on the plinth or your thigh.

Manipulation force: Lift the patient's legs into hip rotation, causing the lumbar spine to side bend in the same direction as the lifted legs.

HVT Lumbar Roll to Increase Lumbar Rotation (Fig. 16.33)

VIDEO 16.10

Patient position: Side-lying with the restricted side up. Position the patient as close to the edge of the bed as possible and flex the hips and knees to 90°. Provide a pillow for the patient to hold that can act as a physical barrier.

Therapist position and hand placement: Stand facing the patient. Place the fingertips of your cephalad hand on the inferior spinous process to monitor motion. Move the patient's top leg into hip flexion until just before you feel the inferior vertebral segment move. Maintain the patient's hip flexion by stabilizing the leg between the therapist's body and the treatment table, and move your cephalad hand to the superior spinous process to monitor motion (Fig. 16.33 A).

Passively rotate the patient's trunk backward to "take up the slack" until just before you feel the superior vertebral segment move, and rest the forearm on the patient's torso. The therapist's torso should be directly over the segment to be manipulated (Fig. 16.33 B).

Manipulation force:

- Therapist exerts a downward rotational thrust toward the table with the cephalad forearm and hand while exerting a rotational force through the caudal forearm by pulling

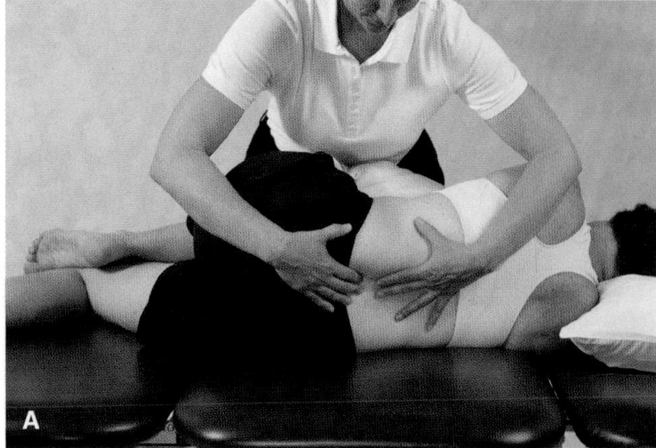

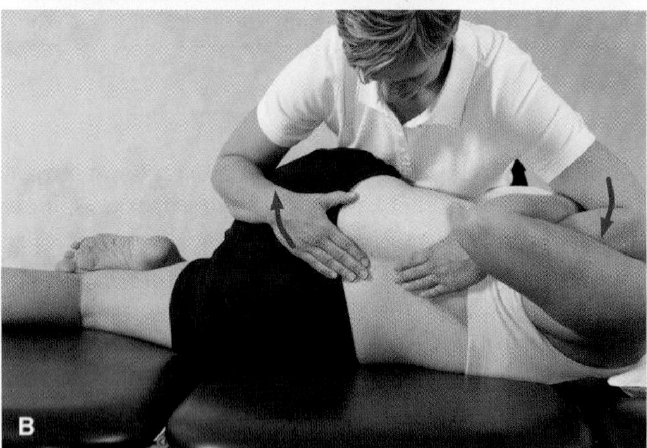

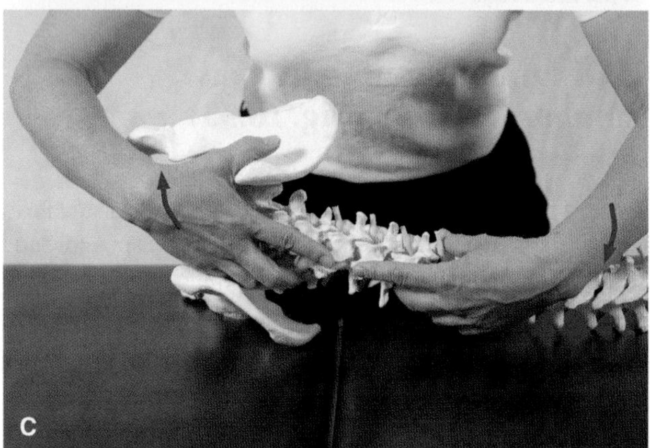

FIGURE 16.33 Lumbar roll HVT: **(A)** monitor motion at the spine as the hip is flexed then stabilized by the therapist's trunk; **(B)** rotate the patient's trunk backward to take up the slack, and apply a rotational force through the lower spine by moving the innominate forward; **(C)** rotational forces applied to the segment above and below, including the innominate, demonstrated on a spine model.

the patient's lower trunk toward your body (Fig. 16.33 B and C).

- Alternative method is to use the caudal forearm and apply a rotational force through the patient's innominate. This technique (patient contact) is particularly useful if attempting to increase rotation at L5–S1.

SI Joint Manipulation Technique to Increase Sacral Nutation (Flexion) (Fig. 16.34) VIDEO 16.11

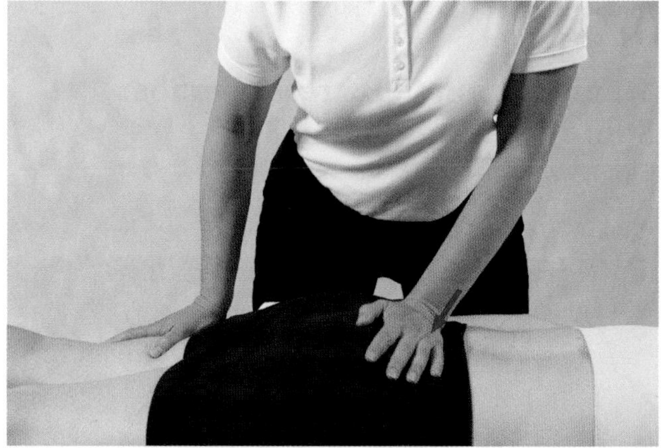

FIGURE 16.34 SI Nutation (Flexion) Manipulation.

Patient position: Prone. Place a pillow under the abdominal region for patient comfort and to provide a neutral lumbosacral curve.

Therapist position and hand placement: Place your pisiform (hypothenar eminence) over the sacral base (S1) region. Relax the rest of your hand on the patient's back.

Anterior glide manipulation force: Push with your hypothenar eminence in an anterior-inferior direction.

SI Joint Manipulation Technique to Increase Sacral Counternutation (Extension) (Fig. 16.35) VIDEO 16.11

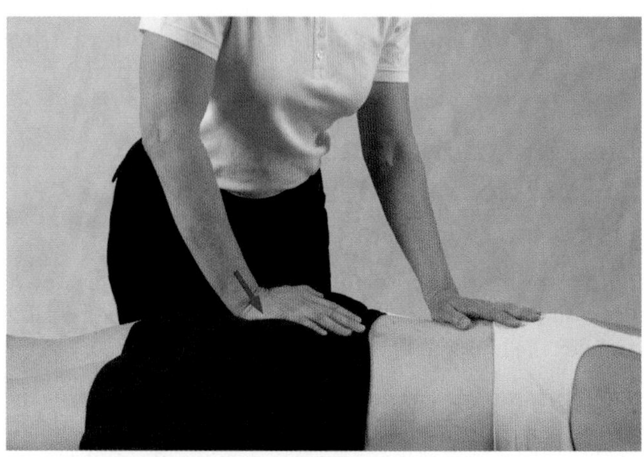

FIGURE 16.35 SI Counternutation (Extension) Manipulation

Patient position: Prone. Place a pillow under the abdominal region for patient comfort and to provide a neutral lumbosacral curve.

Therapist position and hand placement: Place your pisiform (hypothenar eminence) over the apex of the sacrum (S5) region. Relax the rest of your hand on the patient's sacrum.

Anterior glide manipulation force: Push with your hypothenar eminence in an anterior-inferior direction.

Posterior Rotation Manipulation to Innominate (Fig. 16.36)

VIDEO 16.11

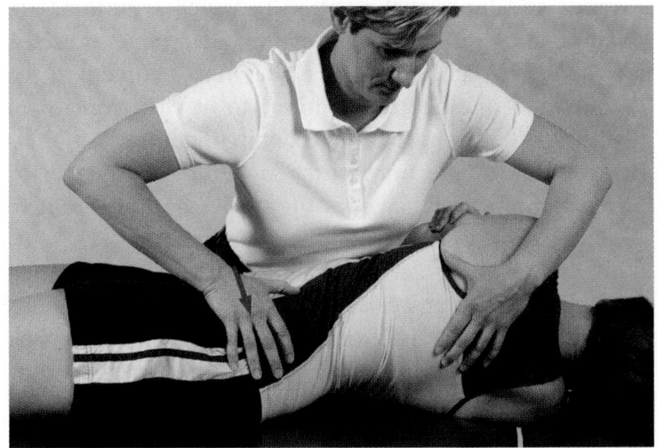

FIGURE 16.36 Posterior Rotation Innominate Manipulation

Patient position: Supine with arms crossed over chest. Move the patient's trunk and legs toward the side of the restriction to create side-bending in the lumbar spine.

Therapist position and hand placement: Stand on the side opposite the restriction. Contact the patient's opposite anterior superior iliac spine (ASIS) with your caudal hand. With the cephalad, roll the patient's trunk toward you.

Manipulation force: Exert a progressive oscillation or HVT force posterior through the hand contact at the innominate.

Muscle Performance: Stabilization, Muscle Endurance, and Strength Training

Goals. To (1) activate and develop neuromuscular control of deep segmental and global spinal stabilizing muscles to support the spine against external loading; (2) develop endurance and strength in the muscles of the axial skeleton for functional activities; and (3) develop control of balance in stable and unstable situations.

This section is divided into two main sections. The first section presents principles and techniques of stabilization exercises for the cervical and lumbar spinal regions with a subsection on motor control exercises for segmental muscle activation and a subsection on global muscle stabilization. The second section presents principles and techniques of general isometric, dynamic, and functional exercises for the neck and trunk.

Stabilization Training: Fundamental Techniques and Progressions

"Proximal stability for distal mobility," a well-known phrase, is an underlying principle of intervention with therapeutic exercise. "Strengthening the core" has become a popular phrase in general exercise programs and classes, supporting the importance of focusing exercises on the trunk musculature to support the spine, even if not differentiating the specific functions of the various muscle groups. The primary functions of the muscles of the trunk are to provide stability so upright posture can be maintained against a variety of forces that disturb balance, to provide a stable base so the muscles of the extremities can execute their function efficiently and without undue stress to the spinal structures, and to move and control trunk motions during functional activities.

In Chapter 14, the two muscle systems that provide spinal stability and control are identified and described in detail: the deep segmental and superficial global (multi-segmental) musculature (see Figs. 14.10 to 14.15). Several studies have demonstrated altered or delayed neuromuscular recruitment patterns in the deep stabilizing muscles of the lumbar spine during active movement in individuals with LBP.[31,34,35,55,61] Results of other studies have shown improved ability to recruit these muscles with specific training[9,60] and improved outcomes compared with individuals not receiving the training.[30,60,61] Studies have also demonstrated improved outcomes in patients with cervical pain and cervicogenic headaches with recruitment of the deep stabilizing musculature in the cervical spine in conjunction with total trunk stabilization.[40,46,50,53]

Therefore, one of the primary areas of emphasis for rehabilitation of individuals with spinal problems is teaching them how to recruit the segmental muscles and then how to use them to respond along with the global musculature to various forces and demands imposed on the spine to improve coordination of their overall function. Activation of the stabilizing musculature is then reinforced when progressing to muscular endurance and strengthening exercises, when performing aerobic exercises, and when practicing functional activities throughout the rehabilitative process with the anticipation that muscle activation for stabilization will become automatic during all daily activities and functional challenges (Fig. 16.37).

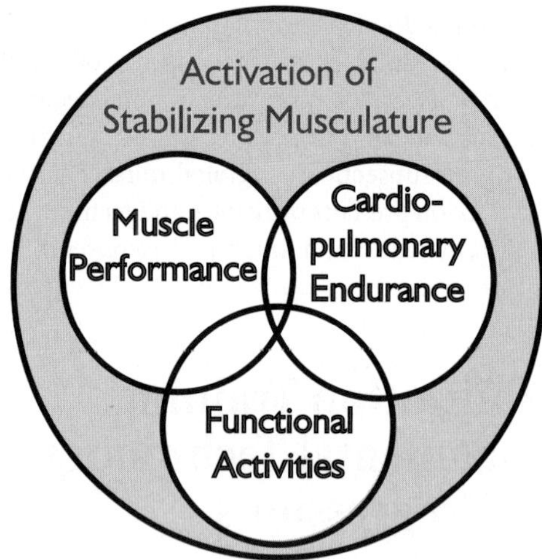

FIGURE 16.37 Exercises to improve muscle performance, cardiopulmonary endurance, and functional activities are integrated over a background of activating the deep segmental and global multi-segmental spinal stabilizing musculature.

Stabilization training follows the basic principles of learning motor control first by developing awareness of muscle contractions and spinal position, then by developing control in simple patterns and exercises, then progressing to complex exercises, and finally by demonstrating automatic maintenance of spinal stability and control in a progression of simple functional activities to complex and unplanned situations.[75] Many of the exercises can be used to accomplish more than one purpose; there is definite overlap with kinesthetic training, muscle performance, and functional training. The choice and progression of exercises described in each of the sections rely on clinical judgment of the patient's response and attainment of goals, not on a strict, time-based protocol or number of days from injury. The ability of the patient to control the spine in a neutral or non-stressful position is paramount for all the exercises.

CLINICAL TIP

Stabilization training follows basic principles of learning motor control.

1. Patient develops awareness of muscle contractions and spinal positions.
2. Patient develops control of spine when performing simple extremity patterns and exercises.
3. Patient demonstrates control of spine when progressing to complex exercises.
4. Patient demonstrates automatic maintenance of spinal stability and control in a progression of simple functional activities to complex and unplanned situations.

There is considerably more research on muscle function and its stabilization action in the lumbar spine than the cervical spine. The cervical spine requires more mobility to position the head, yet relies on the thoracic and lumbar spinal regions to provide a base for stability and postural control. Even though there are unique anatomical considerations in the cervical spine, there is overlap between stabilization training for cervical and lumbar problems.

Guidelines for Stabilization Training

It is important to understand and use the principles and progression of stabilization training for effective instruction.[7,56,69-71] The following guidelines are summarized in Box 16.2.

1. *Kinesthetic training* for awareness of safe motion and positions must precede stabilization training. The functional range and functional position in which symptoms are minimal or absent are used for stabilization exercises.[56] When the condition is not acute, most people find the midrange (the neutral position) to be their functional position. It is important to recognize that this position or range is not static, nor is it the same for every person. In addition, it may change as the tissues heal, nociceptive stimuli decrease, and flexibility improves.[56]
2. *Activation* of the deep segmental muscles of the trunk, specifically the transversus abdominis (TrA) and multifidus (Mf), is often delayed or absent in patients with back pain.[31,35,61] In addition, ultrasound and MR imaging studies on individuals with unilateral LBP have shown decreased activation and atrophy of these deep muscles on the side of symptoms compared to the uninvolved side when performing voluntary contractions.[22,79]

BOX 16.2 Guidelines for Stabilization Training: Principles and Progression

1. Begin training with awareness of safe spinal motions and the neutral spine position or bias.
2. Have patient learn to activate the deep stabilizing musculature while in the neutral position.
3. Add extremity motions to load the superficial global musculature while maintaining a stable neutral spine position (*dynamic stabilization*).
4. Increase repetitions to improve holding capacity (endurance) in the stabilizing musculature; increase load (change lever arm or add resistance) to improve strength while maintaining a stable neutral spine position.
5. Use alternating isometric contractions and rhythmic stabilization techniques to enhance stabilization and balance with fluctuating loads.
6. Progress to movement from one position to another in conjunction with extremity motions while maintaining a stable neutral spine (*transitional stabilization*).
7. Use unstable surfaces to improve the stabilizing response and improve balance.

Learning conscious activation of the deep segmental muscles without contracting the global trunk musculature is the first step in developing habitual activation for spinal stability in patients with pain related to poor spinal control and segmental instability. Once the individual learns correct activation of the segmental stabilizers using the "drawing-in" maneuver, this maneuver is used prior to all exercises and activities to develop the activation and stabilizing function and eventually automatic feedforward stabilization from the muscles.[36] A study involving 42 subjects demonstrated that it is possible to alter abdominal muscle activation consciously and automatically with specific exercises.[60]

In the cervical region, the deep cervical flexors, the longus colli and longus capitis, and the deep cervical and upper thoracic extensors are activated to stabilize the cervical spine in a neutral spinal position (axial extension with mild lordosis).

3. *Extremity motions* are added to the stabilization program to coordinate segmental muscle activity with the global stabilizing musculature. Loading via the extremities increases the stabilizing challenge to the musculature. The patient positions the spine in the neutral position (using pelvic tilt motions in the lumbar region and gentle head nodding in the cervical region), performs the drawing-in maneuver, and then begins moving one or several extremities while maintaining the neutral position. Extremity motions are performed within the tolerance of the trunk or neck muscles to control the neutral or functional position. This is called *dynamic stabilization*, because the stabilizing muscles in the spinal area must respond to the changing forces coming from the dynamic movement of the extremities. Exercises that require stabilization against transverse plane rotational forces on the pelvis more consistently activate the oblique abdominal and deep spinal stabilizers than sagittal plane resistive forces.[68]
4. *Increase muscular endurance and strength* once control of the spinal position is established and the patient can activate the stabilizing muscles. Repetitions of extremity motions are increased, and resistance is applied to the extremities. The intent is to challenge the trunk muscles to stabilize against these increased forces yet stay within their tolerance and ability to control the spinal position. Repetitions also help develop *habit*; therefore, it is important to use careful instructions and provide feedback. Fatigue is determined by the inability of the trunk or neck muscles to stabilize the spine in its functional position or by increased pain. For example:
   - Begin at a resistance force that the patient can repeat for 30 to 60 seconds and maintain the neutral position of the spine; progress the repetitions to 3 minutes.
   - Progress by adding resistance to or increasing the lever arm of the extremities; initially, reduce the time and again progress to doing the new activity for 1 to 3 minutes.
   - Another way to develop endurance in the trunk muscles is to begin exercising at the most difficult level for that patient, then shift to simpler levels of resistance as fatigue begins in order to keep moving. It is important that the patient does not lose control of the functional position or experience increased symptoms.
5. *Alternating isometric contractions* between antagonists and *rhythmic stabilization* of the trunk muscles against manual resistance also enhance stabilizing contractions. When performed while sitting and standing, the alternating contractions and co-contractions also develop control of balance.
6. *Transitional stabilization* develops as the patient moves from one position to another in conjunction with extremity motions. This requires graded contractions and adjustments between the trunk flexors and extensors and requires greater awareness and concentration.[7,56] For example, any motion of the arms or legs away from the trunk tends to cause the spine to extend. The abdominals (trunk flexors) must contract to maintain control of the functional spinal position. This occurs, for example, when lifting a load from the floor to overhead. Then, as the arms or legs move anteriorly toward the center of gravity, the spine tends to flex, which requires the extensors to contract to maintain the functional position (as would occur when lowering a weight to the floor). Greater concentration on maintaining the functional spinal position is necessary when doing more advanced functional activities.
7. *Perturbation (balance) training*, exercising against destabilizing forces or on unstable surfaces, develops neuromuscular responses to improve balance.

Deep Segmental Muscle Activation and Training

The function of the deep musculature (TrA and Mf in the lumbar spine and longus colli and other deep musculature in the cervical spine) is described in Chapter 14, and the results of impaired function in these muscles are described in Chapter 15. Techniques for activation of the segmental musculature are described in this section.

FOCUS ON EVIDENCE

Methods for testing and training activation of the deep segmental musculature have been developed and used in both research and clinical settings.[48,65] Placement of fine-wire electrodes with ultrasound guidance has provided valuable information regarding the muscle function and recovery in research settings,[36,37,63] and ultrasound imaging has provided a valuable tool for biofeedback in training.[28,32,33,80] Use of ultrasound biofeedback imaging has been prohibitively expensive to use clinically for training activation of the deep musculature. As an alternative device, a pressure biofeedback unit (Stabilizer™; © 2006 Encore Medical, L.P.) was developed and has been shown to have clinical usage in training activation and control of the stabilizing musculature of the trunk and neck.[38,76]

Cervical Musculature

In the cervical region, the goal is to activate and control the muscles that control axial extension (cervical retraction). This requires capital flexion, slight flattening of the cervical lordosis, and flattening of the upper thoracic kyphosis (Fig. 16.38).

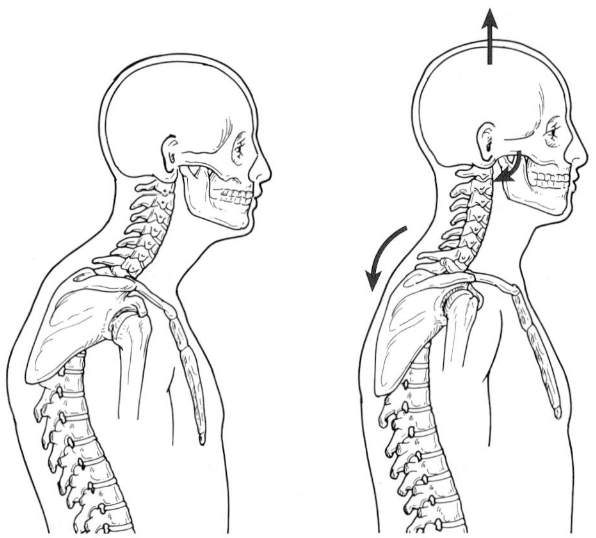

FIGURE 16.38 Axial extension (cervical retraction) involves the motion of capital flexion and movement of the lower cervical and upper thoracic spine toward extension, resulting in slight flattening of the cervical lordosis and "lifting" of the head.

Deep Neck Flexors: Activation and Training (Fig 16.39) VIDEO 16.12

Patient position and procedure: Supine. For craniocervical flexion and gentle axial extension, teach the patient to perform slow, controlled nodding motions of the head on the upper cervical spine ("yes" motion). If the patient has a significant forward head posture, place a folded towel under the occipital area so extension of the head on the neck does not occur. Facilitate the motion with manual cues to ensure the longus colli is contracting, or the sternocleidomastoid is at a relative state of rest. Once the patient is able to activate the motion, the Stabilizer™ (or blood pressure cuff) may be used to monitor the amount of cervical flattening and measure the muscular endurance for holding the contraction (Fig. 16.39).

The protocol for use of the Stabilizer™ is summarized in Box 16.3.

FOCUS ON EVIDENCE

Jull and associates[41] reported that the controlled performance of upper cervical flexion increases the pressure in the Stabilizer™ to 30 mm Hg and that the test-retest reliability of the craniocervical flexion test (conducted on 50 asymptomatic subjects 1 week between tests) was an ICC of 0.81 for the activation score and 0.93 for the performance index (see Box 16.3).

Lower Cervical and Upper Thoracic Extensor Activation and Training

Patient position and procedure: Prone with forehead on the treatment table and arms at the sides. Have the patient lift the forehead off the treatment table, keeping the chin tucked and eyes focused on the table to maintain the neutral spinal position (reinforces the craniocervical flexion motion learned in the supine position). Lifting the head is a small motion (Fig. 16.40).

Progression

Once the patient learns to activate the deep musculature and assume the neutral posture in the cervical spine, practice throughout the day is encouraged in order to develop good postural control. Stabilization training is initiated by

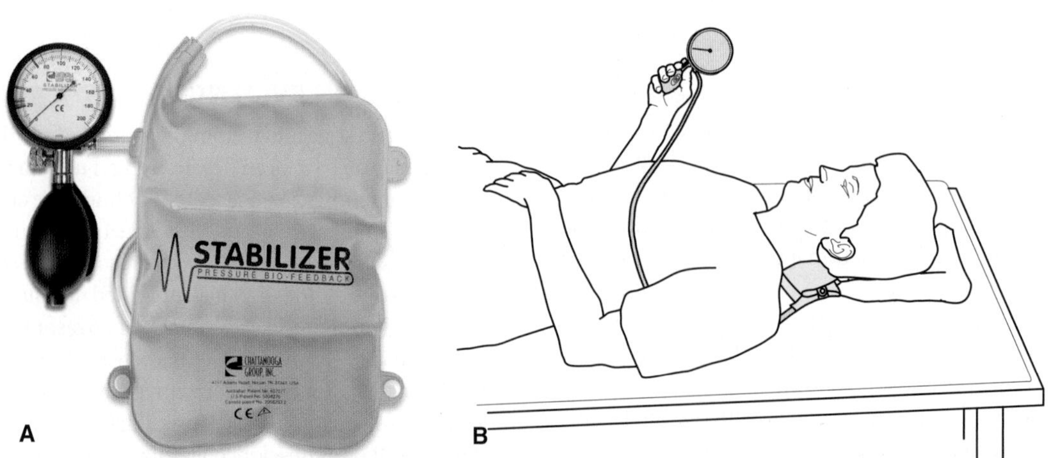

FIGURE 16.39 **(A)** The Stabilizer™ pressure biofeedback unit (© 2006 Encore Medical, L.P.) is used to provide visual feedback to the patient while training for spinal stabilization; **(B)** Stabilizer folded into thirds under the cervical spine to test and train capital flexion with neutral spine axial extension.

BOX 16.3 Testing and Training Deep Segmental Muscle Activation in the Cervical Spine

- Place blood pressure cuff or the folded Stabilizer™ pressure biofeedback unit (folded into thirds) under the upper cervical spine and inflate to 20 mm Hg.
- Instruct the patient to nod and increase pressure on the cuff to 22 mm Hg and hold the pressure steady for 10 seconds.
- If the patient is successful (i.e., can hold the position with minimal superficial muscle activity), have him or her relax and repeat the flexion, this time increasing pressure to 24 mm Hg. Repeat this incremental activation up to 30 mm Hg (total 10 mm Hg increase).
- The final pressure is the one at which the patient can hold steady for 10 seconds.
- Muscle endurance (holding or tonic capacity) of the deep neck flexors is measured by the number of 10-second holds (up to 10) at the final pressure.

A *performance index* can be used to document an objective measure. Multiply the pressure increase by the number of times the patient can repeat the 10-second holds—with 100 reflecting the holding of a 10 mm Hg increase for 10 repetitions.[41]

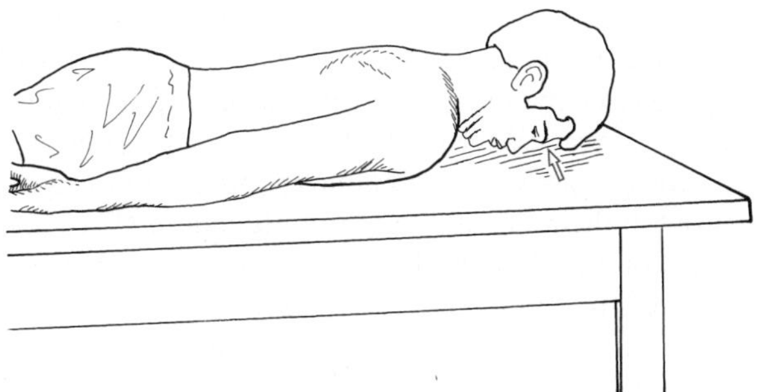

FIGURE 16.40 Prone lying axial extension (cervical retraction) exercises.

coordinating control of the neutral spinal position with upper extremity loading. The extremity motions are used to stimulate muscular endurance as well as strengthen the stabilizing musculature in the spine. These exercises are described in the next section (Global Muscle Stabilization Exercises).

Lumbar Musculature

Three techniques for abdominal muscle activation have been described and used in clinical practice: the drawing-in maneuver, abdominal bracing, and posterior pelvic tilt (Fig. 16.41). Each technique differs in the stabilization activity of the

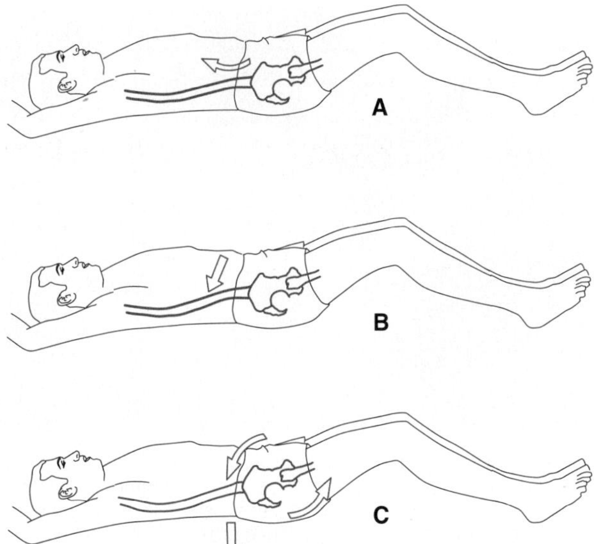

FIGURE 16.41 Three methods to activate the stabilizing musculature in the lumbar spine. **(A)** Drawing-in maneuver in which the patient hollows the abdominal region ("draws" the belly button toward the spine). **(B)** Abdominal bracing in which setting the abdominal muscles results in flaring laterally around the waist. **(C)** Posterior pelvic tilt in which the pelvis is actively tilted posteriorly and the lumbar spine flattens.

abdominal and Mf muscles.[67] Studies have demonstrated that the drawing-in maneuver is more selective in co-activating the TrA and Mf muscles than the abdominal bracing and posterior pelvic tilt techniques[38,67] and that the drawing-in maneuver leads to improvement in feedforward postural strategies.[82] The drawing-in maneuver also functions to increase intra-abdominal pressure by inwardly displacing the abdominal wall. Because of this, the drawing-in maneuver is recommended for stabilization training; the other two methods are also described, primarily so the reader can recognize the differences.

Drawing-In Maneuver (Abdominal Hollowing Exercise) for TrA Activation VIDEO 16.13

Patient positions: Training may be easiest in the quadruped position in order to use the effects of gravity on the abdominal wall. Hook-lying (with knees 70° to 90° and feet resting on an exercise mat), prone-lying, or semi-reclined positions may be used if more comfortable for the patient. It is important to progress training to sitting and standing as soon as possible.[51,54]

Procedure: Teach the patient using demonstration, verbal cues, and tactile facilitation. Explain that the muscle encircles the trunk, and when activated, the waistline draws inward.

- Palpate the TrA muscle just distal to the ASIS and lateral to the rectus abdominis (RA) (Fig. 16.42). When the internal oblique (IO) contracts, a bulge of the muscle is felt; when the TrA contracts, flat tension is felt. The goal is to activate the TrA with minimal or no contraction of the IO. This is a gentle contraction.
- Have the patient assume a neutral spinal position and attempt to maintain it while gently drawing in and hollowing

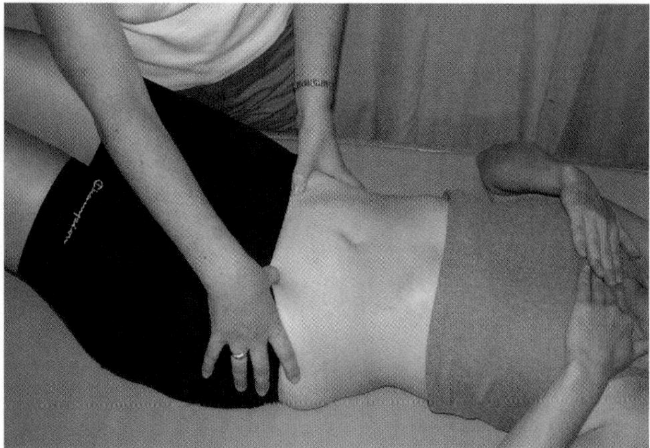

FIGURE 16.42 Palpation of the transversus abdominis (TrA) muscle just distal to the anterior superior iliac spine and lateral to the rectus abdominis muscle. The TrA feels like a tense sheet (a bulge is the internal oblique) when performing a gentle drawing-in maneuver.

the abdominal muscles.[65] Instruct the patient to breathe in, breath out, and then gently draw the belly button in toward the spine to hollow out the abdominal region. Once activated, have the patient maintain the contraction and resume breathing. When done properly, there are no substitute patterns; that is, there is minimal to no movement of the pelvis (posterior pelvic tilting), no flaring or depression of the lower ribs, no inspiration or lifting of the rib cage, no bulging out of the abdominal wall, and no increased pressure through the feet. Performing the drawing-in maneuver with the spine in a neutral position results in increased TrA response (measured as increased thickness in ultrasound imaging) compared to slouched sitting or slouched standing postures.[64]

If a patient has difficulty activating the TrA, the following two feedback techniques have been shown to assist with learning.[25,66,67]

- *Pressure biofeedback for clinical testing and visual feedback.* With the patient prone, the Stabilizer™ (or blood pressure cuff) is placed horizontally under the abdomen (centered under the navel). Inflate the Stabilizer™ to 70 mm Hg. Have the patient perform a drawing-in maneuver, as described above. A decrease of 6 to 10 mm Hg during the drawing-in maneuver (without substitutions) indicates proper activation of the deep abdominal muscles. The dial on the unit is large and easily read by the patient for immediate feedback.
- *Biofeedback with surface electrodes.* Surface electrodes placed over the RA and external obliques (EOs), near its attachment on the eighth rib, may be used in conjunction with the inflatable cuff. There should be minimal to no activation of these muscles if the drawing-in maneuver is done correctly.

As with the cervical spine, the Stabilizer™ can be used not only to train and reinforce activation of the TrA but also to measure control for a measured period of time as well as number of repetitions. The protocol is summarized in Box 16.4.

BOX 16.4 Testing and Training Deep Segmental Muscle Activation (Transversus Abdominis) in the Lumbar Spine

- Patient is prone lying.
- Place a blood pressure cuff or the Stabilizer™ pressure biofeedback unit horizontally under the abdomen with the lower edge just below the anterior superior iliac spine (navel at center of unit).
- Inflate to 70 mm Hg and instruct the patient to perform the drawing-in maneuver.
- If done properly, the pressure drops 6 to 10 mm Hg.
- Have the patient maintain the gentle contraction while resuming relaxed breathing.
- See if the patient can maintain the pressure drop for up to 10 seconds.
- Muscle endurance (holding or tonic capacity) of the transversus abdominis is measured by the number of 10-second holds (up to 10).

Adapted from the instruction manual that accompanies the Stabilizer™ © 2006 Encore Medical, L.P., with permission.

Abdominal Bracing

In contrast to the drawing-in maneuver, abdominal bracing occurs by setting the abdominals and actively flaring out laterally around the waist (see Fig. 16.41 B). There is no head or trunk flexion, no elevation of the lower ribs, no protrusion of the abdomen, and no pressure through the feet. The patient should be able to hold the braced position while breathing in a relaxed manner. This technique has been taught for a number of years as the method to stabilize the spine; it has been shown to activate the oblique abdominal muscles consistent with their global stabilization function.[48,67] In addition, abdominal bracing has been reported to activate a stronger contraction in the IOs than with sagittal plane exercises including various dynamic trunk flexion exercises.[48] Instructions to brace frequently during the day, whether combined with a strengthening or stretching exercise program, has been shown improved outcomes in managing LBP over a 10-year period.[2]

Posterior pelvic tilt

Posterior pelvic tilt exercises (see Fig. 16.41 C) principally activate the RA muscle, which is used primarily for dynamic trunk flexion activity. It is a superficial muscle that does not have segmental attachments; therefore, it is not emphasized in the training for stabilization.[67] Pelvic tilt exercises are used to teach awareness of the movement of the pelvis and lumbar spine as the patient explores his or her lumbar ROM to find the functional spinal range and the neutral position.

Mf Activation and Training VIDEO 16.14

Patient position and procedure: Prone or side-lying. Place your palpating digits (thumbs or index fingers) immediately lateral to the spinous processes of the lumbar spine (Fig. 16.43).

- Palpate each spinal level so comparisons in the activation of the Mf muscle can be made between each segment as well as from side-to-side.
- Instruct the patient to "swell the muscle" out against your digits. Palpate for consistency of muscle contraction at each level.
- Facilitation techniques include using the drawing in maneuver and gently contracting the pelvic floor muscles (as in Kegel exercises, described in Chapter 24).
- In the side-lying position, facilitate by gently applying manual resistance to the thorax or pelvis to activate the rotation function of the Mf.
- The patient may be taught to self-palpate a Mf contraction in the following manner. Sit and rock the pelvis to find the neutral position; with the fingers or thumbs placed along the lumbar spinous processes, lean forward a couple degrees. The Mf is thus activated. Differentiate a Mf contraction from tension in the aponeurosis of the global erector spinae.

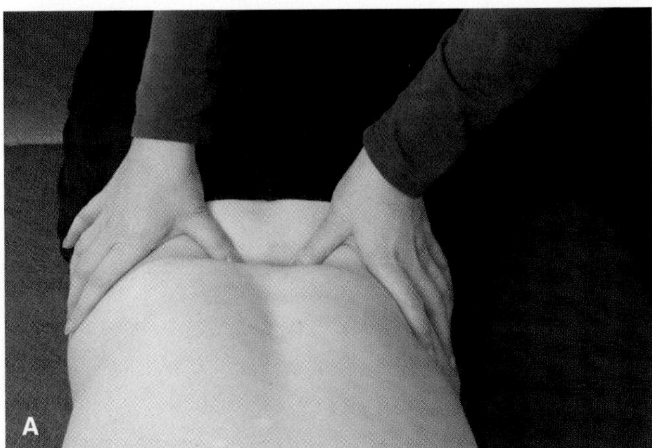

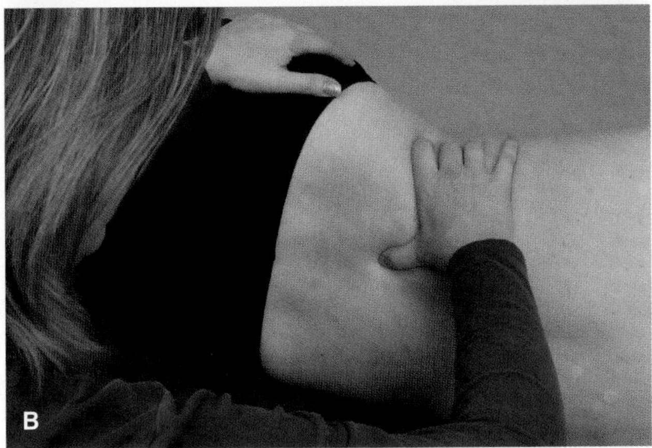

FIGURE 16.43 Palpation of the multifidus muscle lateral to the spinous processes in the lumbar spine, **(A)** bilaterally in the supine position and **(B)** unilaterally in the side-lying position.

Progression

Once the patient learns to activate the deep segmental musculature, practice throughout the day is encouraged. Segmental muscle activation is then coordinated with stabilization training, using the global musculature and extremity loading. Extremity motions are added and used to stimulate muscle endurance as well as strengthen the trunk muscles. Global stabilization exercises are described in the next section.

Global Muscle Stabilization Exercises

Even though this section is divided into cervical and lumbar regions, many of the same exercises may be used for impairments in either region because of the functional relationships of the entire axial skeleton.

Stabilization Exercises for the Cervical Region

Stabilization With Progressive Limb Loading

In general, stabilization exercises begin in the recumbent position and progress to quadruped with the trunk supported on a large gym ball, sitting, sitting on a large gym ball, standing with the back supported against a wall, and finally standing without support. For advanced training, exercises are progressed to standing on an unstable surface.

- Begin all exercises with gentle craniocervical nods and axial extension to the neutral spinal position to activate the deep segmental muscles as described in the previous section. During the early phases of training, if the patient has difficulty maintaining a neutral spinal position, a small towel roll may be placed under the neck for passive support.
- Initially, the only resistance load comes from simple upper extremity movements. When the patient can perform multiple repetitions of the upper extremity motions without losing control of the spinal position or causing an increase in symptoms, resistance is added with handheld weights or elastic resistance.
- The principles of muscle endurance and strengthening described in Chapter 6 are used to challenge the spinal stabilizing musculature.
- Table 16.2 summarizes limb-loading exercises that emphasize the flexor muscles, and Figure 16.44 illustrates the basic exercise progression in the supine position.
- Table 16.3 summarizes limb-loading exercises that emphasize the lower cervical/upper thoracic extensor muscles, and Figure 16.45 illustrates a basic exercise progression in the prone position. It is important to note that these exercises do not isolate the flexors or extensors, but the designation is primarily for emphasis due to the effects of gravity.

Variations and Progressions in the Stabilization Program

Remind the patient to find and maintain the neutral spinal position when doing these exercises.

TABLE 16.2 Cervical Stabilization With Progressive Limb Loading—Emphasis on Cervical Flexors VIDEO 16.15

Instructions: Determine amount of support needed and amount of protection. Begin each exercise with axial extension to the neutral spinal position and maintain it while exercising; increase extremity repetitions, then increase resistance before progressing to a new challenge.	**Maximum Support ←——→ Minimum Support**			
	Supine	Sitting (sitting on ball for less stability)	Standing with wall support	Standing with no support (standing on unstable surface for less stability)

Limb loading	Phase	Exercise
Deep Segmental Activation		Gentle craniocervical flexion/axial extension hold 10 seconds × 10 repetitions
Minimum limb loading ↕	***Maximum to moderate protection phase***	Shoulder flexion to 90°
		Shoulder abduction 90°
		Shoulder external rotation with arms at sides
	Moderate to minimum protection phase	Shoulder flexion to end of range
		Shoulder abduction combined with external rotation to end of range
		Diagonal patterns
Maximum limb loading	***Minimum to no protection phase***	Reaching forward, outward, upward in functional patterns
		Pushing/pulling and lifting activities

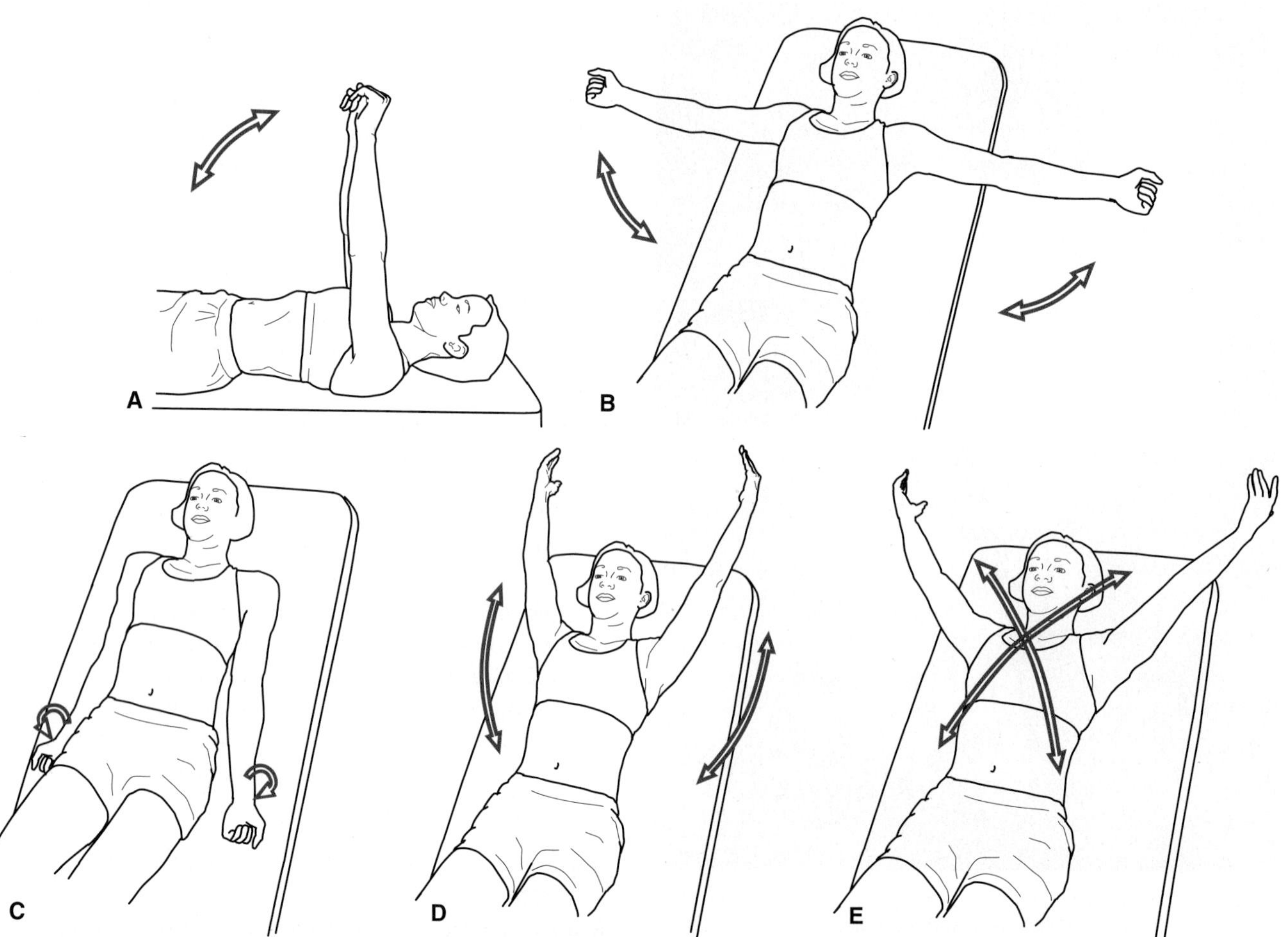

FIGURE 16.44 Limb loading for basic stabilization progression of cervical musculature in the supine position. Maximum protection phase: **(A)** shoulder flexion to 90°; **(B)** shoulder abduction to 90°; **(C)** shoulder external rotation arms at the side. Moderate protection phase: **(D)** shoulder flexion and abduction to end-range; **(E)** diagonal patterns.

TABLE 16.3 Cervical Stabilization With Progressive Limb Loading—Emphasis on Cervical and Thoracic Extensors VIDEO 16.16

<table>
<tr><td colspan="2" rowspan="2">Instructions: Determine amount of support needed and amount of protection. Begin each exercise with axial extension to the neutral spinal position and maintain it while exercising; increase extremity repetitions, then increase resistance before progressing to a new challenge.</td><td colspan="4">Maximum Support ⟷ Minimum Support</td></tr>
<tr><td>Prone forehead on treatment table—lift forehead off table (Fig. 16.40)</td><td>Quadruped over padded stool or gym ball—maintain eyes focused on floor</td><td>Standing back supported by wall (ball behind head for less stability)</td><td>Standing, no support, (standing on unstable surface for less stability)</td></tr>
<tr><td colspan="2">Deep segmental muscle activation—gentle craniocervical flexion/axial extension</td><td colspan="4">Lift forehead off exercise mat; hold 10 seconds × 10 repetitions</td></tr>
<tr><td rowspan="7">Minimum limb loading
↕
Maximum limb loading</td><td rowspan="2">Maximum to moderate protection phase</td><td colspan="4">Arms at side: laterally rotate shoulders and adduct scapulae</td></tr>
<tr><td colspan="4">Arms in 90/90 position (abducted and laterally rotated), horizontally abduct shoulders and adduct scapulae</td></tr>
<tr><td rowspan="3">Moderate to minimum protection phase</td><td colspan="4">Elevate shoulder in full flexion</td></tr>
<tr><td colspan="4">Arms abducted to 90° and laterally rotated, elbows extended: horizontally abduct shoulders and adduct scapulae</td></tr>
<tr><td colspan="4">Upper extremity diagonal patterns</td></tr>
<tr><td rowspan="2">Minimum to no protection phase</td><td colspan="4">Standing, no support → standing on unstable surface:
■ Reaching forward, outward, upward in functional patterns
■ Pushing/pulling and lifting activities</td></tr>
<tr><td colspan="4">Standing on unstable surface:
■ Reaching, pushing, pulling</td></tr>
</table>

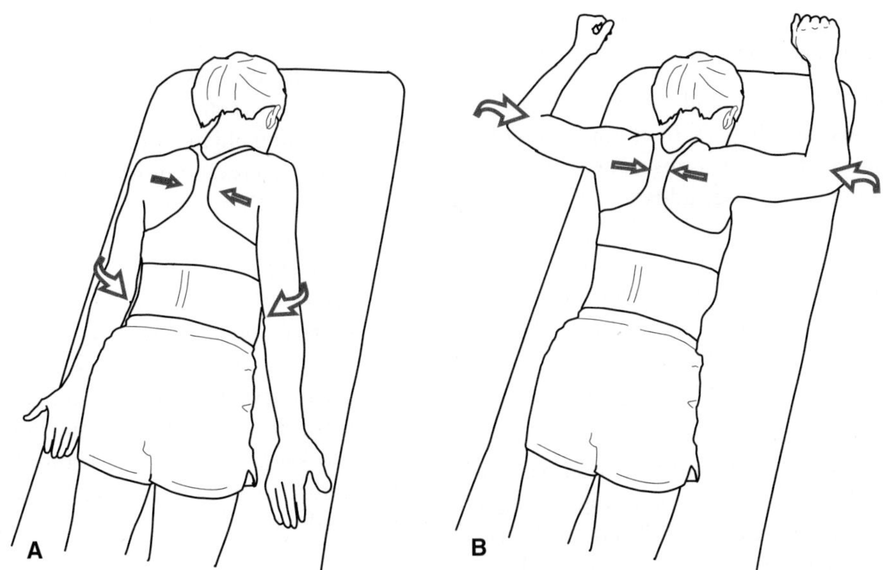

FIGURE 16.45 Limb loading for basic stabilization progression of cervical musculature in prone position. Maximum protection phase: **(A)** arms at side, shoulder lateral rotation, and scapular adduction; **(B)** arms at 90/90, horizontal abduction, and scapular adduction. Moderate protection phase:

Continued

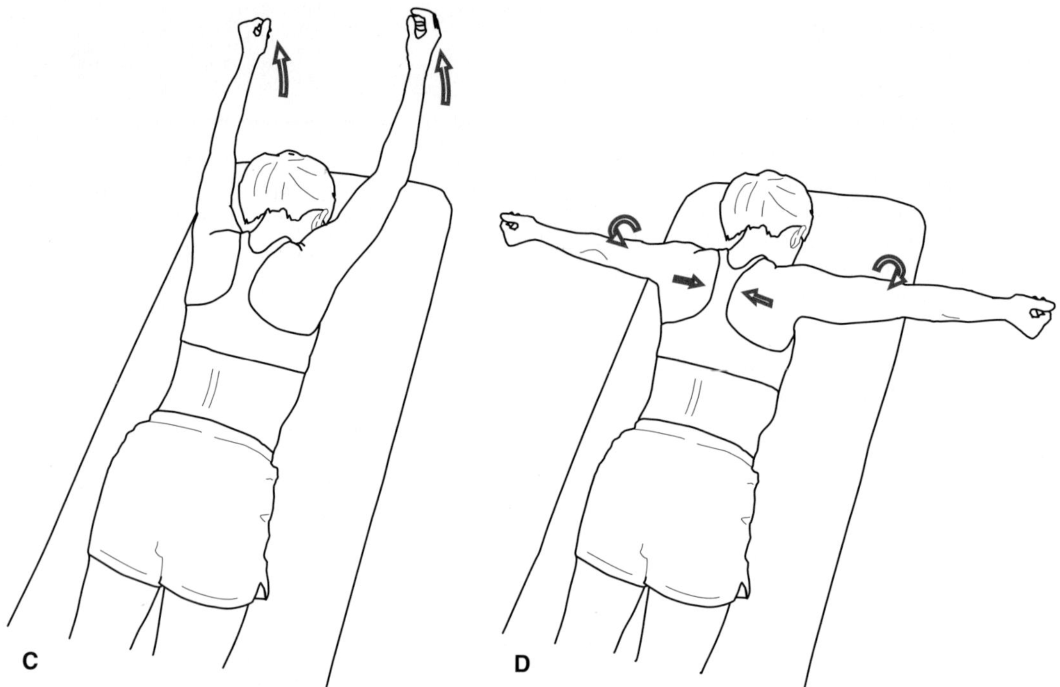

FIGURE 16.45—cont'd **(C)** shoulder elevation full range, **(D)** shoulders 90° with lateral rotation and elbow extended, horizontal abduction, and scapular adduction.

Extremity loading. During the early phases of training, limit shoulder flexion to 90° flexion and abduction. Once the patient can maintain stability and symptoms are not provoked, greater challenges occur with elevating the upper extremity full ROM. Unilateral and asymmetrical upper extremity motion require greater control than bilateral motion.

External resistance. Tables 16.2 and 16.3 summarize progressions based on position changes. In addition, use of resistance loads (free weights, elastic resistance, or manual resistance) to any of the exercises adds to the stabilizing challenge. Even though external resistance applied through the extremities has the benefit of increasing strength in the extremity musculature, the primary goal is to increase the stabilizing response of the cervical musculature. Therefore, any loss of the neutral spinal posture or increase in cervical symptoms signals the need to decrease the intensity of the resistance force.

Unstable surfaces. The application of external resistance while on an unstable surface, such as sitting on a large ball (Fig. 16.46 A), lying prone over a ball (Fig. 16.46 B), or standing supporting the ball between the head and the wall (Fig. 16.46 C), provides additional challenges to the muscles as they respond to perturbations. Many variations of these exercises can be used to challenge the stabilizing muscles so long as the patient is able to maintain control.

Muscular endurance and strength. Determine the maximum level of resistance tolerated by the cervical-stabilizing musculature that does not reproduce symptoms. Decrease the intensity and have the patient exercise with multiple repetitions at that level (20 to 30 repetitions or for 1 minute). Resistance can then be added for strengthening (decrease the number of repetitions) at that level before progressing to endurance training at the next level.

Integration of Stabilization Exercises and Posture Training

Good postural alignment of the neck begins with the pelvis and lumbar spine and moves up to the scapular and thoracic regions. The thorax must be lifted up from the pelvis and scapula retracted in a comfortable position for the cervical spine to assume an efficient position of axial extension (cervical retraction). Therefore, begin with lumbopelvic control if necessary and develop thoracic extension and scapular retraction. While the patient is performing the extremity motions to develop stability, reinforce good scapulohumeral alignment. It is important to remember that strengthening alone does not correct faulty posture and, therefore, to utilize the reinforcement techniques and environmental adaptations that are discussed in Chapter 14.

Progression of Isometric and Dynamic Strengthening in Conjunction With Functional Activities

When the patient demonstrates good cervical stabilization and response to various upper extremity resistance changes, isometric and dynamic exercises are integrated into the program. These are described in the Isometric and Dynamic Exercise section following this section.

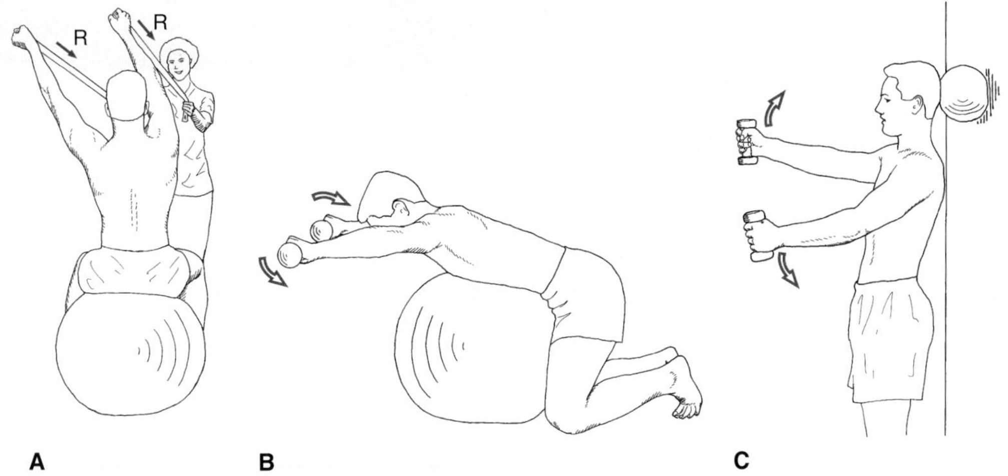

FIGURE 16.46 Unstable surfaces provide increased challenges to the cervical stabilizing musculature, requiring greater control. Examples include performing upper extremity motions, such as diagonal patterns **(A)** while sitting on a gym ball, **(B)** while quadruped over a gym ball, and **(C)** while pressing a ball against the wall. Use of external resistance is also illustrated.

Stabilization Exercises for the Lumbar Region

Once the patient learns to activate the deep segmental muscles in the lumbar region, explain that prior to each exercise the patient is to find the neutral spinal position, perform the drawing-in maneuver, and then maintain control while applying an exercise load with extremity motions. The drawing-in maneuver develops the pattern of setting the deep abdominal and Mf muscles in a feedforward pattern and then trains their holding capacity in coordination with the global muscles.[25]

Stabilization With Progressive Limb Loading

Begin with the patient supine for greatest support, adding quadruped exercises when able. If the patient cannot control the position, pre-position him or her using pillows or supports (see Box 15.6 in Chapter 15).

- To improve the holding capacity of the stabilizing muscles, increase the amount of time the patient does the exercises. It is important that no exercise is continued if the patient cannot maintain the stable position. If the deep abdominals cannot stabilize, substitute patterns in the superficial muscles that override the deep muscle activation.
- The Stabilizer™ Pressure Biofeedback unit (or blood pressure cuff) may be used for feedback during this early training (see Box 16.5 for guidelines).
- Table 16.4 summarizes basic limb-loading exercises in the supine position that emphasize the abdominal muscles, and Figures 16.47 and 16.48 illustrate the exercise progression.
- Table 16.5 summarizes limb-loading exercises in the quadruped and prone positions that emphasize the extensor muscles, and Figure 16.49 illustrates a basic exercise progression.

TABLE 16.4 Basic Lumbar Stabilization With Progressive Limb Loading—Emphasis on Abdominals

Instructions: Patient position hook lying (knees 90°). Place pressure cuff under lumbar spine and inflate to 40 mm Hg. Begin each exercise with drawing-in maneuver to activate deep segmental muscles. Determine level at which patient can maintain pressure constant (stable pelvis) while performing either A, B, or C limb load activity. For endurance, decrease load and perform repetitive motion for 1 minute or longer. For strength, progress load.		**Progressive Limb Loading →**		
		A. Lift bent leg to 90° hip flexion	B. Slide heel to extend knee	C. Lift straight leg to 45°
Lower intensity	*Level 1: deep segmental muscle activation*	Draw in and hold 10 seconds		
↓	*Level 2:*	Opposite LE on mat; bent leg fall out		
	Level 3: A, B, or C	Opposite LE is on table		
	Level 4: A, B, or C	Hold opposite LE @ 90° of hip flexion with UE		
	Level 5: A, B, or C	Hold opposite LE @ 90° of hip flexion (no UE assistance)		
Greater intensity	*Level 6: A, B, or C*	Bilateral LE movement		

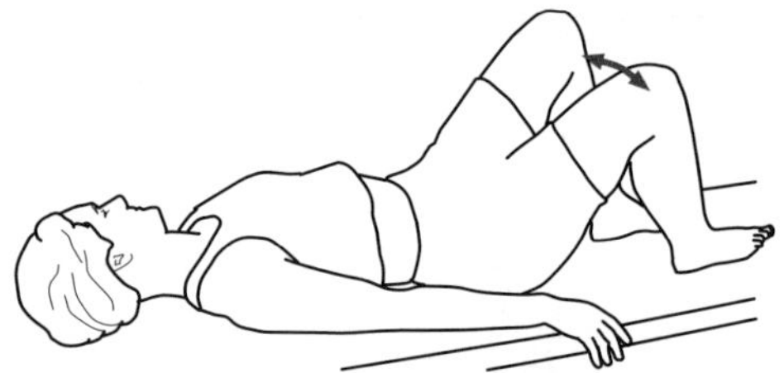

FIGURE 16.47 Bent-leg fall out. Level 2 limb loading for basic stabilization of the abdominal muscles in the supine position. This requires control to prevent pelvic rotation; stability is assisted by the opposite lower extremity while hook-lying. **VIDEO 16.17**

BOX 16.5 Instructions for Use of Stabilizer™ for Stabilization Training With Leg Loading

Patient position: Supine, hook lying.

- Place the three-chamber pressure cell under the lumbar spine horizontally across low back area.
- Position the spine in neutral.
- Inflate the pressure cell to a baseline of 40 mm Hg.
- Draw in the abdominal wall without moving the spine or pelvis.
- Pressure should remain at 40 mm Hg (±10 mm Hg) while performing the lower extremity loading exercises.

Adapted from the instruction manual that accompanies the Stabilizer™ © 2006 Encore Medical, L.P., with permission.

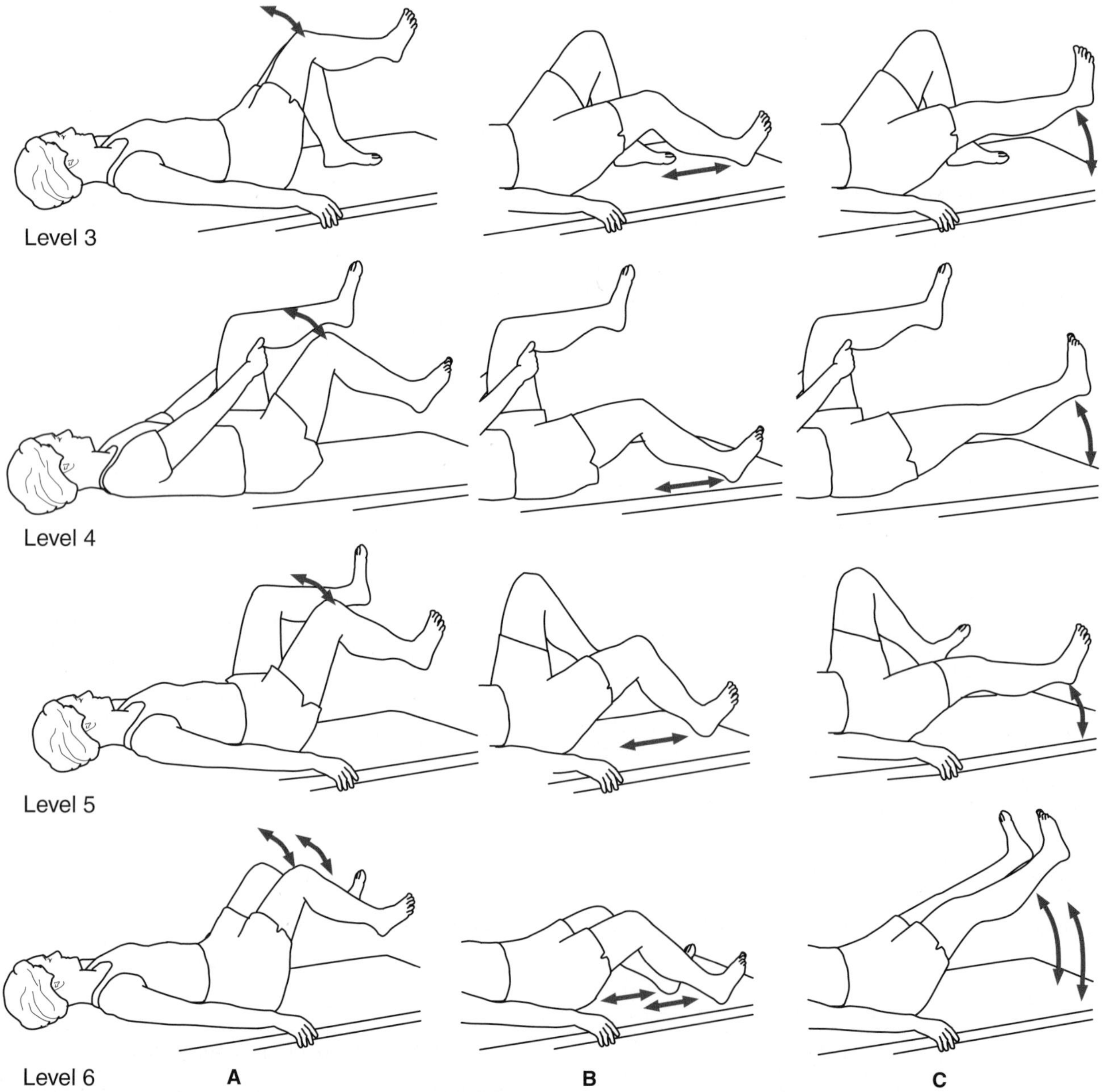

Level 3

Level 4

Level 5

Level 6

A B C

FIGURE 16.48 Limb loading for basic stabilization progression of the abdominal muscles in the supine position, levels 3 to 6: level 3, stability assisted by opposite extremity in hook-lying position; level 4, stability assisted by patient holding opposite leg at 90°; level 5, stability challenged by patient actively holding opposite leg at 90°; level 6, stability challenged with both lower extremities moving. **(A)** Bent leg lift to 90°. **(B)** Heel slide to extend knee. **(C)** Straight-leg lift to 45°. **VIDEO 16.18**

TABLE 16.5 Basic Lumbar Stabilization With Progressive Limb Loading: Emphasis on Trunk Extensors

		Position	Load
Instructions: Patient position quadruped or prone. Patient assumes neutral spine in lumbar and cervical regions (keeping eyes focused toward floor or exercise mat), performs drawing-in maneuver, and moves extremities. Motions are repeated or alternated from side to side.	Lower intensity	Quadruped position	Flex one UE
	↓		Extend one LE by sliding it along the exercise mat
	↓		Extend one LE and lift 6–8 inches off exercise mat
	↓		Flex one UE and extend contralateral LE
	Greater intensity and spinal compression	Prone lying position—near end of range of motion, requiring greater control of neutral spine	Extend one LE
			Extend both LE
			Lift head, arms, and LE

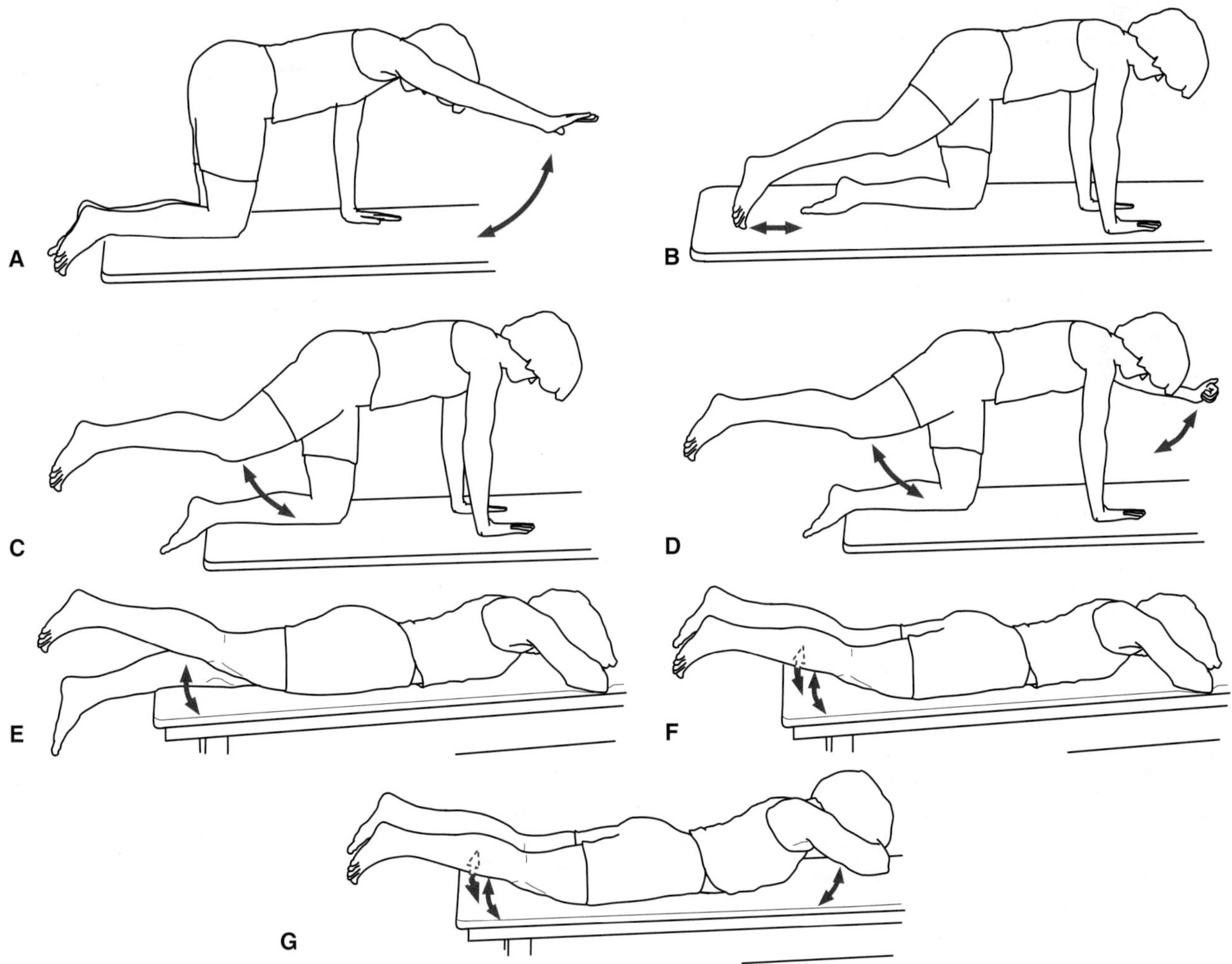

FIGURE 16.49 Limb loading for basic stabilization progression of the lumbar extensors. Begin in the quadruped position and progress the intensity by **(A)** flexing one UE; **(B)** extending one LE with a leg slide; **(C)** extending one LE by lifting it off the mat; **(D)** flexing one UE while extending contralateral LE and then alternate to opposite extremities. Progress to prone: **(E)** extending one LE; **(F)** extending both LE; and **(G)** lifting head, arms, and trunk. **VIDEO 16.19**

CLINICAL TIP

Performance of extremity loading in the prone position places a greater compressive load on the lumbar spine[5,52] and is not possible if there are hip flexion contractures; therefore, initiate extension exercises in the quadruped position so the lumbar spine can be positioned more easily in neutral and the patient can learn control.

If the patient cannot bear weight on the extremities or maintain balance in the quadruped position, use a padded stool or large gym ball for additional support.

It is important to maintain the cervical spine in its neutral position during quadruped exercises. The patient should be able to align the head and focus the eyes on the floor. As the exercises progress, there is a greater challenge on co-activation of all of the stabilizing musculature.

NOTE: The exercise progressions described in Table 16.4 are adapted from several research studies that investigated the reliability, validity, and sensitivity to change one exercise level with abdominal muscle stabilizing ability using lower-limb loading.[23,25,39] The exercise progressions described in Table 16.5 are adapted from electromyography (EMG) studies that documented extensor activity with limb loading in the quadruped and prone-lying positions.[6,52]

Variations and Progressions in the Stabilization Exercise Program

For all exercises, reinforce the importance of first finding the neutral spine (cervical and lumbar regions), performing the drawing-in maneuver, and then maintaining the neutral spine while superimposing any extremity motions. It is critical to instruct the patient to stop the exercises (or decrease the intensity) as soon as loss of control of the stable spinal position is sensed. In order to develop the desired muscle response it is important not to progress the patient beyond what he or she is able to control. The emphasis is first on improving the static holding capacity (endurance) of the trunk muscles followed by strengthening. Endurance training of the trunk extensor muscles is related to decreased pain and improving function during the early stages of recovery in patients with subacute LBP.[13]

Emphasis on muscle endurance. Determine a level of exercise that the patient can perform for several repetitions while maintaining a stable spine in the neutral position. Have the patient exercise at that level with the goal of increasing the number of repetitions or the time. Once the patient can perform repetitions for 1 minute, add weights, decrease the repetitions, and emphasize strength. Progress to the next level of difficulty for muscular endurance.

Use of external props. Use of the Stabilizer™ pressure biofeedback unit to help the patient learn control while doing the abdominal stabilization exercises was described earlier (see Box 16.5). For exercises in the quadruped position, if the patient has difficulty controlling the trunk rotation, use a prop, such as a dowel rod, placed along the spine. Have the patient attempt to keep it balanced while performing the arm and leg exercises (Fig. 16.50). It may be helpful to cue the patient not to shift his or her weight as the extremity is moved—this is difficult to do but is effective in bringing in the stabilizing trunk muscles.

Extremity loading. Boxes 16.5 and 16.6 identify a progression of exercises in supine and quadruped/prone positions with extremity loading. Initially, have the patient do the motions repetitively; then progress to alternating the extremities or moving all four extremities simultaneously (Fig. 16.51).

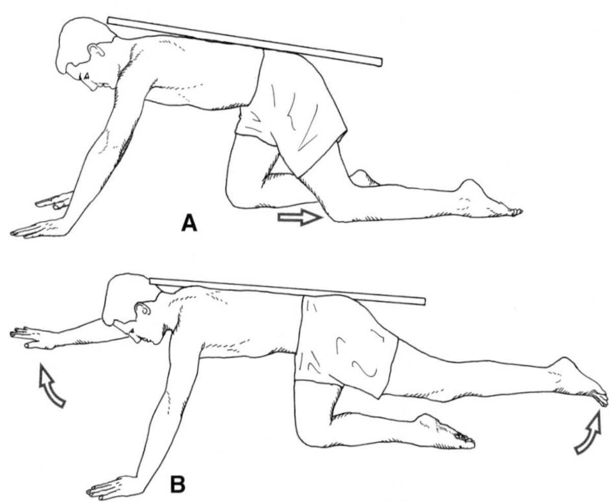

FIGURE 16.50 Balancing a rod on the back while doing quadruped exercises provides reinforcement that the trunk is not twisting. **(A)** Single leg slides. **(B)** Lifting the opposite arm and leg simultaneously, then alternating extremities.

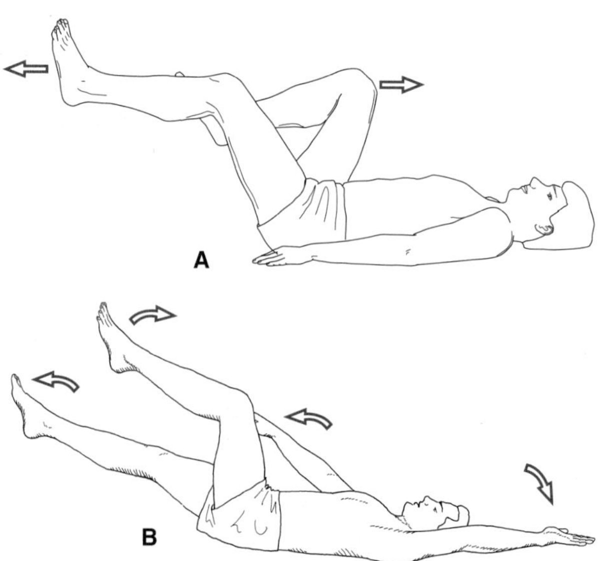

FIGURE 16.51 **(A)** Alternating LE motions with the "modified bicycle" or **(B)** reciprocal and alternating patterns using the UE and LE simultaneously require a strong controlling action in the abdominals.

This requires the stabilizing musculature to adjust to the shifting loads. Motions begin in the sagittal plane and then progress to the transverse plane and diagonal patterns (unilateral and bilateral), in which movement away from the midline adds a rotational component and increases the challenge to the stabilizing musculature.

External resistance. Use weights, elastic resistance, or pulleys for strengthening. Several suggestions are illustrated in Figures 16.52, 16.53, and 16.54. Even though the extremities benefit from the exercises, the primary purpose is to improve performance in the stabilizing muscles of the trunk; therefore, when signs of fatigue occur, such as poor control of spinal stability (seen as movement of the pelvis or lumbar spine), reduce the intensity or stop the exercise and allow recovery.

Position changes. Apply the extremity-loading exercises in the sitting (supported then unsupported), kneeling, and standing positions. Also, use modified bridging and plank exercises to challenge the stabilizing function of the trunk musculature.

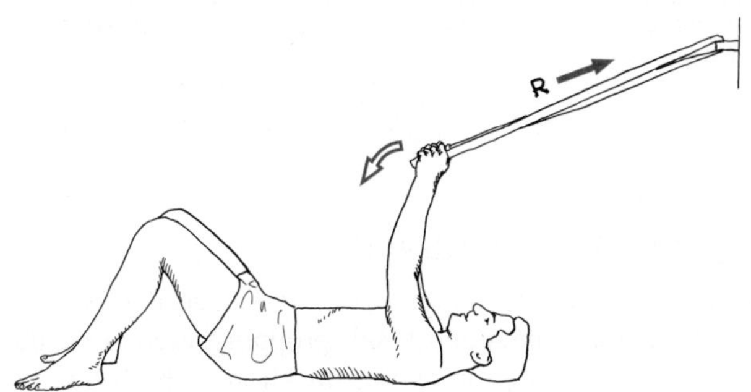

FIGURE 16.52 Developing the stabilizing action of the abdominal muscles by using pull-down activities against a resistive force from pulleys or elastic bands. This exercise can also be done sitting or standing to increase the challenge to the muscles in less stable positions.

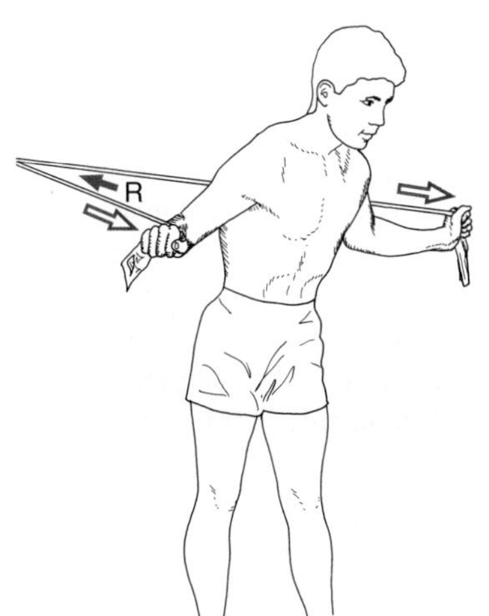

FIGURE 16.53 Using elastic resistance to train and strengthen the abdominal muscles in the upright position. The drawing-in maneuver to set the deep segmental stabilizing muscles precedes the movement of the arms forward against the resistance.

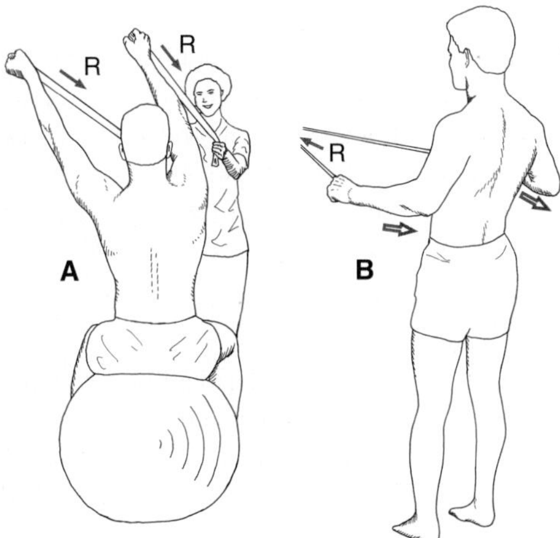

FIGURE 16.54 Using elastic resistance to train and strengthen the back extensor muscles to stabilize in the upright position **(A)** diagonal patterns while sitting on an unstable surface and **(B)** while standing.

These exercises are described in the following Isometric and Dynamic Exercises section.

Functional activities. Exercises, such as wall slides and partial lunges and bridging with extremity motions, use the extremities and trunk during weight bearing and prepare the muscles for functional activities. These exercises are described in the final section under Functional Activities but also serve the purpose of challenging the stabilizing muscles.

Unstable surfaces. Use a large gym ball, foam roller, or wobble board to challenge the patient's balance and develop the stabilizing musculature. Scott et al[73] documented increased cross sectional area of the Mf when sitting on a large gym ball when compared with sitting on a firm surface. With the ball, a variety of positions can be used, such as sitting upright on the ball with the feet on the floor (Fig. 16.55), lying supine with

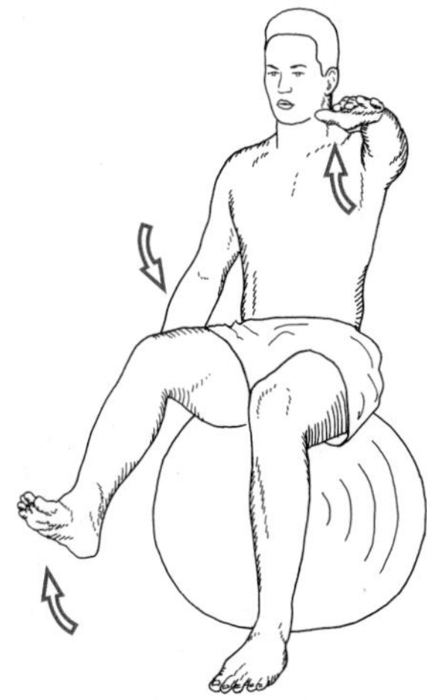

FIGURE 16.55 Strength, balance, and coordination are required to maintain spinal stabilization while sitting on a gym ball and moving the extremities. This activity is progressed by adding weights to the extremities.

the trunk on the ball and feet on the floor (see Fig. 16.60 B), or with the feet on a low mat or wobble board. The foam roller can be used with the patient supine (Fig. 16.56), kneeling, quadruped (with hands on one roller and knees on another), or standing. Use handheld weights or elastic or pulley resistance secured at various heights (see Fig. 16.54) to increase the challenge. **VIDEOS 16.20 AND 16.21**

Quadratus Lumborum: Stabilization Exercises

VIDEO 16.22

The quadratus lumborum has been identified as an important stabilizer of the spine in the frontal and transverse planes.[52,63] Strongest activation of this muscle occurs with the side propping (side plank) position. The EOs are also activated in this position.[48,52]

Patient position and procedure: Begin side-lying. Have the patient prop up on the elbow and then lift the pelvis off the mat, supporting the lower body with the lateral side of the knee on the downward side. The position can be maintained for an isometric hold or performed intermittently (Fig. 16.57 A). Progress by having the patient support the upper body with the hand (with the elbow extended) and lateral aspect of the foot on the downward side (Fig. 16.57 B). Arm and leg movements (without then with weights) are added to increase the challenge.

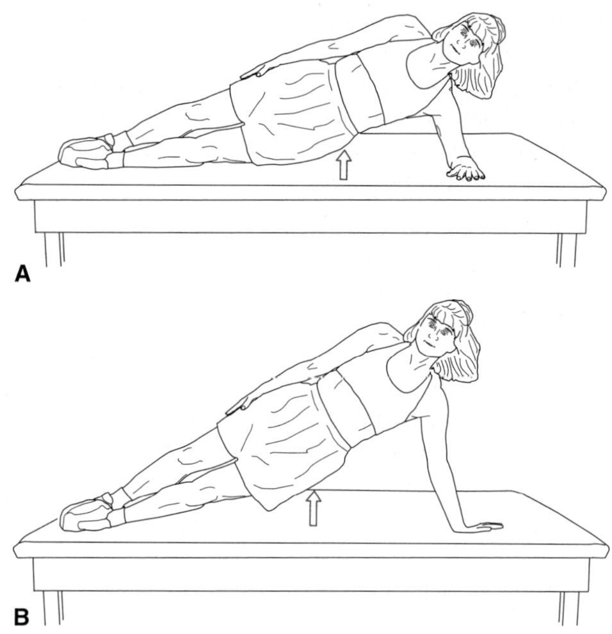

FIGURE 16.57 Quadratus lumborum stabilization training using side-propping (side plank) **(A)** on the elbow and knee and **(B)** on the hand and foot.

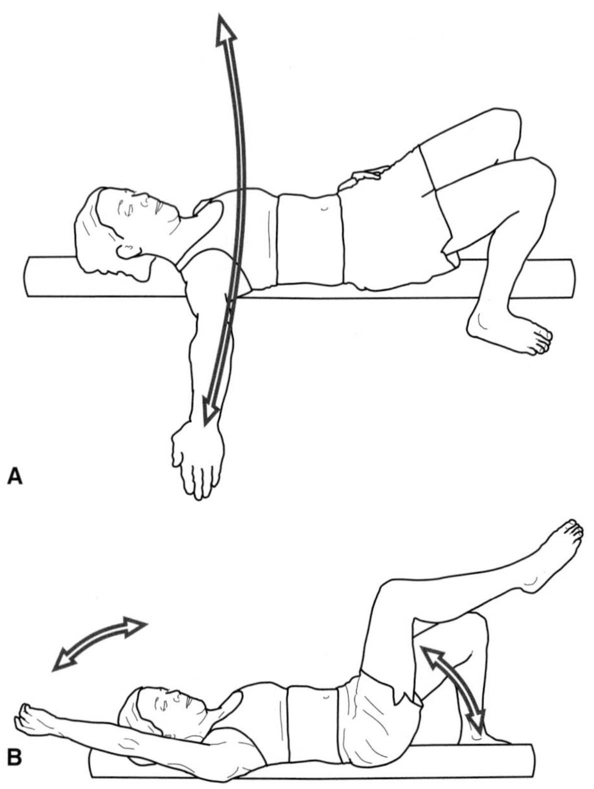

FIGURE 16.56 Activation of the stabilizing trunk muscles occurs to maintain balance on a foam roll while the extremities move in various planes: **(A)** shoulder horizontal abduction/adduction and **(B)** ipsilateral hip and shoulder flexion/extension are shown. Weights are added to increase the challenge.

FOCUS ON EVIDENCE

Using ultrasound imaging, Teyhen and associates[81] demonstrated that the side support (side propping) exercise resulted in the greatest change in muscle thickness of the TrA and IO muscles with the least amount of lumbar loading compared to five other trunk exercises (abdominal crunch, drawing-in maneuver, quadruped opposite upper extremity and lower extremity lift, supine lower extremity extender, and abdominal sit back).

Progression to Dynamic Exercises

When the patient has developed control, endurance, and strength in the stabilizing muscles in weight-bearing and nonweight-bearing positions, dynamic trunk strengthening exercises are initiated at a low intensity (see the following section). The emphasis is on control and safety.

As the patient returns to his or her instrumental activities of daily living (IADLs) and limited work activities, instruct him or her to incorporate the deep segmental activation and global stabilization techniques into the activities.

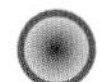

FOCUS ON EVIDENCE

In a 10-year follow up study of individuals with recurring LBP, half of whom were taught to incorporate abdominal bracing in daily activities in addition to either a strengthening or flexibility exercise program, it was reported that regardless of exercise intervention, those who regularly used abdominal bracing when doing functional activities had fewer recurrences of LBP, suggesting that abdominal bracing adds to the exercise effect and improves long-term prevention of recurrent LBP.[2]

Isometric and Dynamic Exercises

Isometric exercises may be considered stabilizing exercises, as there is little or no movement of the spinal segments. They are included in this section with dynamic exercises, however, because of the method of application of the resistive force; that is, the resistive force is applied directly to the axial skeleton rather than through limb loading, as described in the spinal stabilization section. The decision to use the isometric exercises described in this section must be based on the goals of intervention. The exercises may be combined with the stabilization exercises in a home exercise program.

Dynamic exercises with spinal movement are introduced into the patient's exercise program when the patient demonstrates effective segmental and global stabilization techniques and has developed endurance in the stabilizing musculature. Dynamic exercises should not be a substitute for stabilization exercises. Because of the load imposed on the spine, they may exacerbate the patient's symptoms if introduced prior to effective stabilization and control. They are important in the total rehabilitation of the individual with neck, thoracic, or LBP, as dynamic muscle endurance and strength is required for many daily activities as well as manual labor and athletic performance.

Exercises for the Cervical Region

PRECAUTION: Use of external weights via a cable or pulley system applied directly to the head are contraindicated for cervical strength training due to the compressive loading on the spine and the potential loss of control during the exercise.

Isometric Exercises: Self-Resistance

The intensity of the isometric exercises can range from low to high, depending on the patient's symptoms and tolerance.

Patient position and procedure: Sitting.

- *Flexion.* Have the patient place both hands on the forehead and press the forehead into the palms in a nodding fashion while not moving (Fig. 16.58 A).
- *Side bending.* Have the patient press one hand against the side of the head and attempt to side bend, as if trying to bring the ear toward the shoulder but not allowing motion.
- *Extension.* Have the patient press the back of the head into both hands, which are placed in the back, near the top of the head (Fig. 16.58B).

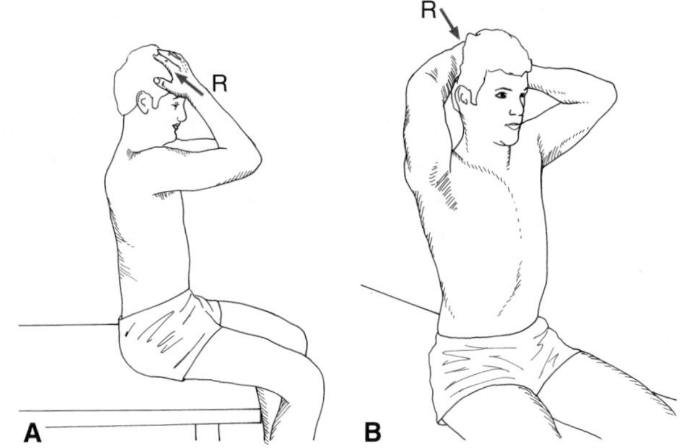

FIGURE 16.58 Self-resistance for isometric **(A)** cervical flexion and **(B)** axial extension.

- *Rotation.* Have the patient press one hand against the region just superior and lateral to the eye and attempt to turn the head to look over the shoulder without allowing motion.

Isometric Resistance Activities

Patient position and procedure: Standing with a basketball-sized inflatable ball between the forehead and a wall. Have the patient keep the chin tucked and not go into a forward-head posture. The patient maintains the functional position while superimposing arm motions. Progress by adding weights to the arm motions (see Fig. 16.46 C).

Dynamic Cervical Flexion

Patient position and procedure: Supine. If the patient cannot tuck the chin and curl the neck to lift the head off the mat, begin with the patient on a slant board or large wedge-shaped bolster under the thorax and head to reduce the effects of gravity (Fig. 16.59). Have the patient practice tucking the chin and curling the head up. Use assistance until the correct pattern is learned. Progress by decreasing the angle of the board or wedge and then adding manual resistance if the patient does not substitute with the sternocleidomastoid (SCM) muscles.

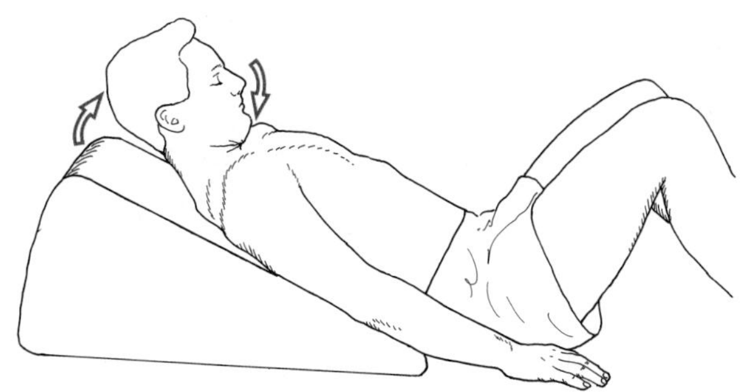

FIGURE 16.59 Training the short cervical flexors while de-emphasizing the sternocleidomastoid for cervical flexion to regain a balance in strength for anterior cervical stabilization.

> **CLINICAL TIP**
>
> Often with faulty forward-head postures, the patient substitutes using the SCM muscles to lift the head when getting up from the supine position rather than the overstretched, weak, deep cervical flexors. To correct this muscle imbalance, begin training capital flexion as described in the stabilization section (deep segmental muscle activation). For home exercise and when rising from a bed, emphasize "curling" the head and neck, not lifting the head up.

Manual Resistance: Cervical Muscles

Patient position and procedures: Supine. Stand at the head end of the treatment table, supporting the patient's head for each exercise.

- Place one hand on the patient's head to resist opposite the motion. Do not resist against the mandible lest force be transmitted to the temporomandibular joint. Resistance is given to isolated muscle actions or to general ROMs, whichever best gains muscle balance and function.
- Isometric resistance can be applied with the head in any desired position before applying resistance. Avoid jerking the neck when applying or releasing the resistance by gradually building up the intensity, telling the patient to match your resistance, holding, and then gradually releasing and asking the patient to relax.

Intermediate and Advanced Training

As the patient progresses in the rehabilitation program, greater challenges to the musculature to stabilize and control motion are emphasized, especially for those individuals returning to work, sports, or recreational activities that place greater demands on the cervical structures.

Transitional Stabilization for the Cervical and Upper Thoracic Regions

- *Patient position and procedure:* Standing with a basketball-sized inflatable ball between the head and the wall. Have the patient roll the ball along the wall, using the head. This requires the patient to turn the body as he or she walks along.
- *Patient position and procedure:* Sitting on a large gym ball. Have the patient walk the feet forward so the ball rolls up the back and the thorax is resting on the ball (Fig. 16.60 A and B). The head and neck are maintained in neutral position, and the cervical flexors are emphasized. Have the patient then walk the ball farther, so it is under the head. The extensors are now emphasized (Fig. 16.60 C). The patient walks the feet forward and backward, alternating stabilization between the flexors and extensors. Progress to advanced training by adding arm motions and then arm motions with weights in each of the positions.

NOTE: This activity requires considerable strength in the cervical extensors to support the body weight and should be performed only with advanced training with patients who have been properly progressed to tolerate the resistance.

Functional Exercises

Design exercises that simulate patient-specific functional activities. Identify what activities stress that individual's neck and have the patient practice modifications of those activities with the spine kept in neutral position. Include pushing, pulling, reaching, and lifting (see the Functional Training section later in this chapter). Challenge the patient with increased repetitions and weight and by using patterns that replicate functional demands.

Exercises for the Thoracic and Lumbar Regions

Alternating Isometric Contractions and Rhythmic Stabilization VIDEO 16.23

Patient positions and procedures: Begin with the patient supine in the most stable position (Fig. 16.61). Progress to sitting kneeling, and then standing. Sitting, brings in the hip muscles, kneeling adds the knee muscles, and standing requires stabilizing action in the hip, knee, and ankle musculature

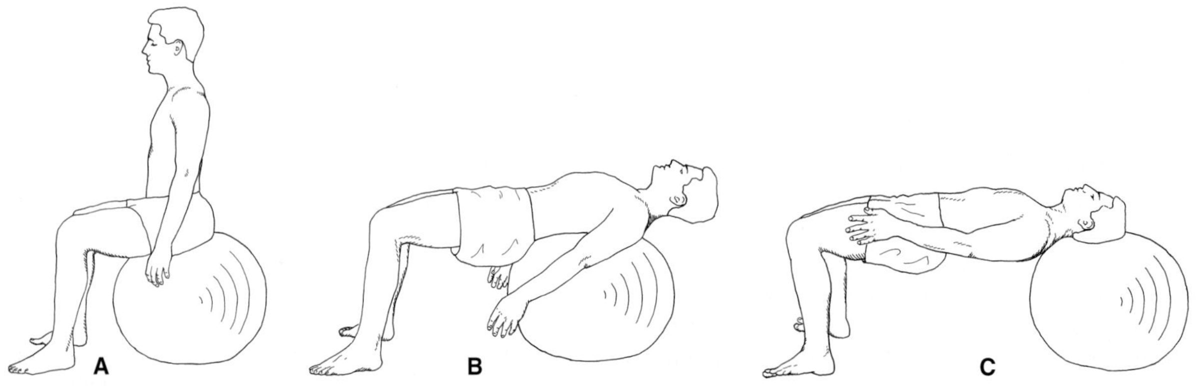

FIGURE 16.60 Advanced exercises for strengthening the cervical and upper thoracic flexors and extensors as stabilizers. Begin by **(A)** sitting on a large gym ball, then **(B)** walking forward while rolling the ball up the back. With the ball behind the midthoracic area, the cervical flexors must stabilize. Continue walking forward until the ball is **(C)** under the head; the cervical extensors now must stabilize. Walk back and forth between the two positions (B and C) to alternate control between the flexors and extensors. Progress by adding arm motions or arm motions with weights to increase resistance.

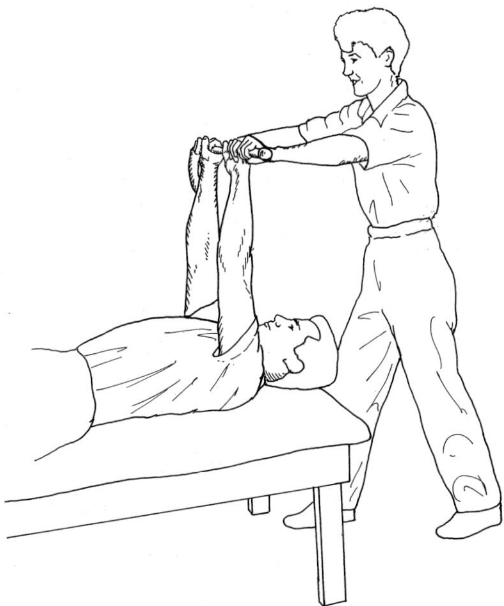

FIGURE 16.61 Alternating isometric resistance applied in the sagittal, frontal, and horizontal planes with the patient supine to stimulate the stabilizing function of the trunk musculature.

as well as the spinal muscles. Apply resistance directly against the patient's shoulders or pelvis, against a rod that is held by the patient (as in Fig. 16.61), or against the patient's outstretched arms.

- Have the patient find the neutral spine position and then activate the stabilizing muscles with the drawing-in maneuver prior to applying the resistive force. Then instruct the patient to "meet my resistance" while applying a force to stimulate isometric contractions. Apply the resistance in alternating directions at a controlled speed while the patient learns to maintain a steady position.
- Initially, provide verbal cues, such as "hold against my resistance, but do not overpower me. Feel your abdominal muscles contracting. Now, I'm pulling in the opposite direction. Match the resistance and feel your back muscles contracting."
- Progress by shifting the directions of resistance without the verbal cues and then by increasing the speed and force.
- Begin with alternating resistance in the sagittal plane; progress to side-to-side and then transverse plane resistance. Isometric resistance to trunk rotation (transverse plane resistance) has been shown to be the most effective in stimulating the oblique abdominals, TrA, and deep spinal extensor muscles.[68]
- Increase the challenge by having the patient sit on a large gym ball while stabilizing against the alternating resistance.
- Alternating resistance to pelvic rotation can also be done by having the patient assume a modified bridge position. Apply resistance directly to the pelvis to stimulate rotation while the patient isometrically holds the pelvis and spine in a stable position.

Isometric and Dynamic Strengthening: Abdominal Muscles

NOTE: Dynamic and high intensity isometric exercises of the trunk musculature are not initiated until late during the rehabilitation process and not until after the patient has learned to activate the drawing-in maneuver automatically for stabilization in all functional activities.

No one abdominal exercise equally challenges all of the abdominal muscles;[52] therefore, a variety of exercises should be included in the patient's exercise program to include the entire region.

FOCUS ON EVIDENCE

EMG studies have looked at abdominal muscle recruitment with various abdominal exercises.[5,20,45,48,52,83] Although there is some variation in outcomes, based on the study design and method of recording, in general the following can be summarized:

- Curl-ups (various types) recruit primarily the RA, with lower activity in the obliques, TrA, and psoas.
- Sit-ups (straight-leg and bent-knee) show high rectus and EO activity, high psoas activity, and high low back compression. Heel press sit-ups increase psoas activity.
- Hanging-leg raises show high EO and high spinal compression.
- Supine single-leg lifts show negligible global abdominal muscle activity (opposite lower extremity provides stability). Primarily, these exercises are used early in the stabilization exercise routines to train the deep stabilizing muscles under progressive extremity loading.
- Supine-bilateral leg lifts show increased activity in the RA, EO, and IO during the first part of the range of hip flexion and increased load on the spine.
- Curl-ups on a labile surface doubled the activity of the RA and increased the activity of the EOs four-fold compared with curl-ups on a stable surface.[83]
- V-sits show the greatest EMG muscle activity in the RA and EO.[48]
- Prone bridges (planks)[15,43] and pike with legs on a large gym ball show high activity in the RA, EO, and IO.[20,43]

Rectus abdominis. There is no clinically significant selective difference between the upper and lower RA function.[45] Both portions contract strongly in all trunk curl-type and leg lift exercises.[45,52] Strongest contraction occurs in V-sits, curl-ups, and sit-ups.[48]

External obliques. EOs contract strongest in sit-ups and diagonal sit-ups to the opposite side,[50] as well as v-sits.[48]

Internal obliques. IOs contract strongest in diagonal sit-ups to the same side and horizontal side propping (see Fig. 16.57),[52] as well as with abdominal bracing and hollowing.[48]

Transversus abdominis. Use of the drawing-in maneuver prior to the abdominal crunch, abdominal sit-back, and lateral side propping activates increased muscle thickness in the TrA (demonstrated with ultrasound imaging).[81]

Trunk Flexion (Abdominals): Supine

Patient position and procedures: Supine or hook-lying with the lumbar spine neutral. McGill[52] suggested supporting the low back with the hands to maintain slight lordosis. The spine should not be allowed to go into an increased lordosis during the exercise—this indicates weakness of the abdominals and consequently lifting of the trunk occurs from hip flexor action only.[42] When training the abdominals, curl-up exercises should be performed at a slow, controlled rate to activate the stabilizing function of the abdominals.[84]

PRECAUTIONS: If a patient experiences pain or increased radicular symptoms with trunk flexion, these exercises should not be done. Use the stabilization exercises, as described in the previous section, with the spine maintained in a neutral position (slight lordosis).

Curl-ups. First, instruct the patient to perform the drawing-in maneuver to cause a stabilizing contraction of the abdominal muscles.[81] Progress by lifting the shoulders until the scapulae and thorax clear the mat, keeping the arms horizontal (Fig. 16.62). A full sit-up is not necessary, because once the thorax clears the mat, the rest of the motion is performed by the hip flexor muscles.

- Further progress the difficulty of the curl-up by having the patient change the arm position from horizontal to folded across the chest and then to behind the head, and then by holding a weight or medicine ball.

Curl-downs. If the patient is unable to perform the curl-up, begin with curl-downs by having the patient start in the hook-sitting or long-sitting position and lower the trunk only to the point at which he or she can maintain a flat low back and then return to the sitting position.

- Once the patient can curl-down full range, reverse and perform a curl-up.

Diagonal curl-ups. Have the patient reach one hand toward the outside of the opposite knee while curling up, then alternate. Reverse the muscle action by bringing one knee up toward the opposite shoulder, then repeat with the other knee. Diagonal exercises emphasize the oblique muscles.

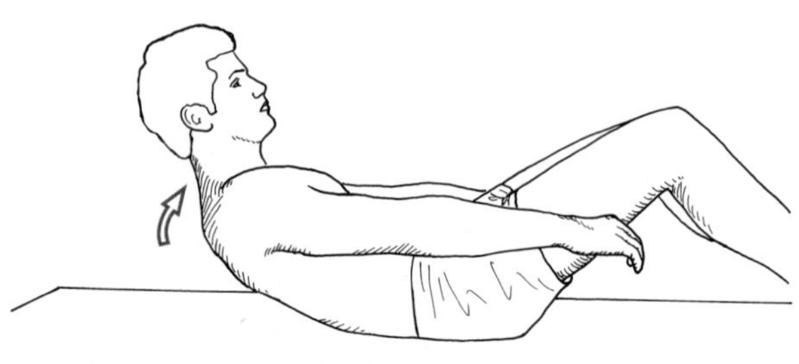

FIGURE 16.62 The curl-up exercise to strengthen the abdominal muscles. The thorax is flexed on the lumbar spine. The arms are shown in the position of least resistance. Progress by crossing the arms across the chest and then behind the head.

Curl-ups on an unstable surface. Progress the above curl-up exercises on an unstable surface, such as a large gym ball (Fig. 16.63), foam roller, or a biomechanical ankle platform system (BAPS) board.

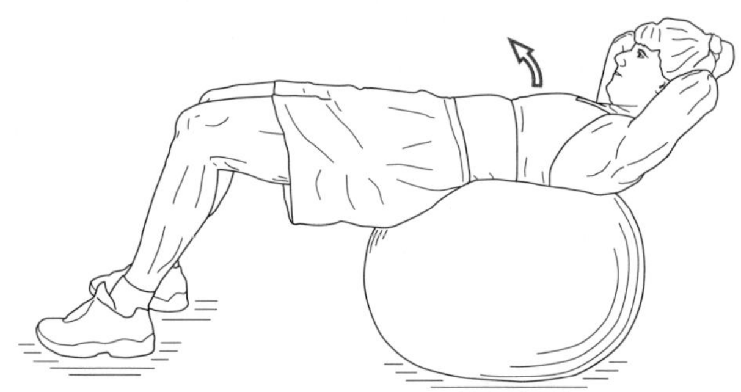

FIGURE 16.63 Curl-ups on an unstable surface. The unstable surface increases activity in the oblique and rectus abdominis muscles.

FOCUS ON EVIDENCE

Both healthy adults[24] and patients with chronic LBP[3,29] have been shown to have impaired balance. Using unstable surfaces, such as a gym ball or a balance board, while doing abdominal curl-up exercises has been shown to increase activity in the IOs and EOs and the RA.[83] The presumption is that these muscles generate increased activity to maintain balance on the unstable surfaces.

Double knee-to-chest. To emphasize the lower RA and oblique muscles, have the patient set a posterior pelvic tilt, bring both knees to the chest, and return. Progress the difficulty by decreasing the angle of hip and knee flexion (Fig. 16.64).

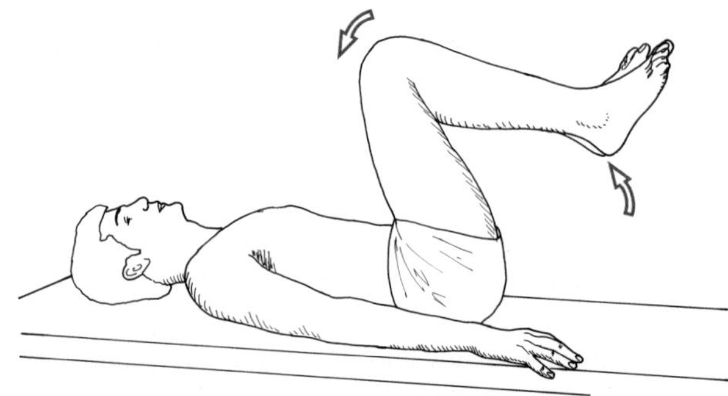

FIGURE 16.64 Strengthening the abdominal muscles by flexing the hip and pelvis on the lumbar spine. The legs are shown in the position for least resistance. Progress by decreasing the angle of hip flexion until the legs can be lifted with the knees extended, as in the pelvic lift.

Pelvic lifts. Have the patient begin with the hips at 90° and the knees extended; then lift the buttocks upward off the mat (small motion). The feet move upward toward the ceiling (Fig. 16.65). The patient should not push against the mat with the hands.

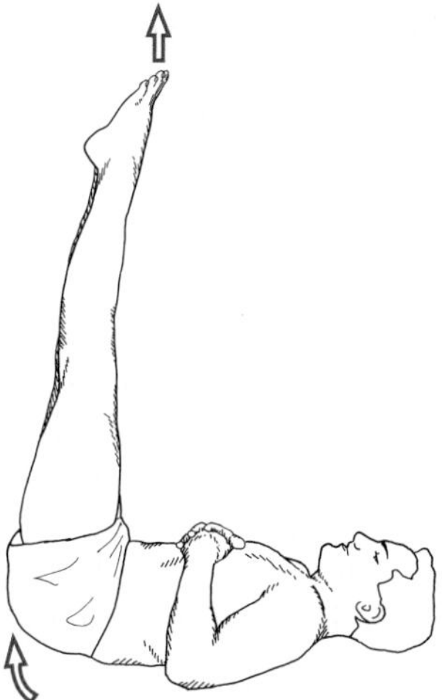

FIGURE 16.65 Pelvic lifts. Elevating the legs upward toward the ceiling by raising the buttocks off the floor emphasizes strengthening the lower abdominal muscles.

Bilateral straight-leg raising. Have the patient begin with legs extended; then perform a posterior pelvic tilt followed by flexing both hips, keeping the knees extended. If the pelvis and spine cannot be kept stable, the knees should be flexed to a degree that allows control. If the hips are abducted before initiating this exercise, greater challenge is placed on the oblique abdominal muscles.

Bilateral straight-leg lowering. Bilateral straight-leg lowering can be performed if the bilateral straight-leg raising is difficult. Have the patient begin with the hips at 90° and knees extended; then, lower the extremities as far as possible while maintaining stability in the lumbar spine (should not increase the lordosis), followed by raising the legs back to 90°. See the Precaution under the bilateral SLR exercise.

PRECAUTIONS:

- The strong pull of the psoas major causes shear forces on the lumbar vertebrae. Also, the bilateral straight-leg raising and lowering exercises cause increased spinal compression loads.
- If there is any LBP or discomfort, especially with spinal hypermobility or instability, the bilateral straight-leg raising and lowering exercises should not be performed even if the abdominals are strong enough to maintain a posterior pelvic tilt.
- Be sure the patients avoid holding their breath (Valsalva maneuver) as they may try to use their diaphragm to provide the stabilization.

Trunk Flexion (Abdominals): Sitting or Standing

Patient position and procedures: Sitting or standing. Pulleys or elastic material are secured at shoulder level behind the patient. Progress the resistance as the patient's abdominal strength increases.

- Have the patient hold the handles or ends of the elastic material with each hand and then flex the trunk, with emphasis on bringing the rib cage down toward the pubic bone and performing a posterior pelvic tilt (Fig. 16.66).
- Have the patient perform diagonal motions by bringing one arm down toward the opposite knee with emphasis on moving the rib cage down toward the opposite side of the pelvis. Repeat the diagonal motion in the opposite direction.

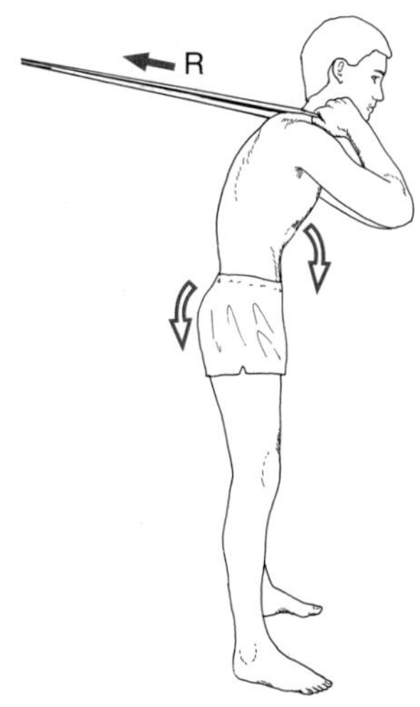

FIGURE 16.66 Standing trunk flexion against elastic material to strengthen the abdominal muscles. The patient performs a posterior pelvic tilt and then approximates the ribs toward the pubis.

Trunk Flexion (Abdominals): Prone

Patient position and procedures: Prone lying and with variations using a large gym ball.

Planks (prone bridging). Have the patient support self on elbows and knees and elevate the pelvis off the floor while maintaining a neutral spinal position (Fig. 16.67A). If tolerated, progress to supporting self on elbows and toes, hands and knees, or hands and toes. If able, have the patient alternately lift

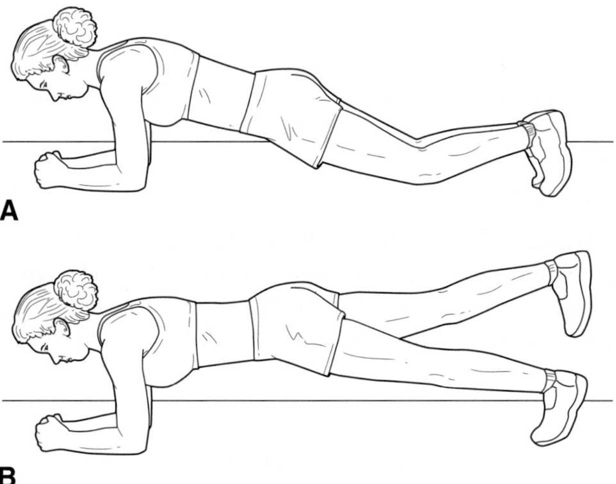

FIGURE 16.67 Plank position **(A)** on elbows and knees, and **(B)** on elbows and toes; shown is a progression with alternating lower extremity extension while in the elbow-toe position.

one leg then the other (Fig. 16.67B), and then one arm with opposite leg. Planks with either arms on a large gym ball, or legs on the ball require high stabilization activity in the abdominal muscles.[15,20]

Roll-out on gym ball. Have the patient begin with knees on the floor and hands on the ball, and then have the patient roll the ball outward away from the knees until the forearms are on the ball, and then return upright while maintaining a neutral spinal position (Fig. 16.68 A and B).

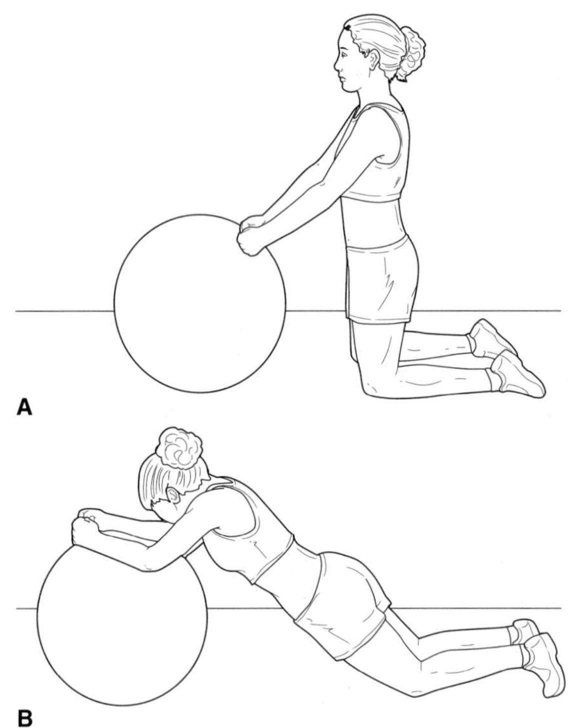

FIGURE 16.68 Beginning **(A)** and end positions **(B)** for roll-out on a large gym ball to strengthen the abdominal muscles.

Pike on a gym ball. Have the patient begin with legs supported on the gym ball and hands on the floor then roll the legs along the ball while elevating the pelvis upward in a pike position. This is a difficult exercise requiring high activity in the abdominal muscles.[20]

Advanced planks with push-ups. Advanced variations of prone exercises that challenge the abdominal muscles combined with upper extremity push-ups, are depicted in the Functional Activities section later in this chapter (see Fig. 16.74) and in Chapter 23 (see Figs. 23.23 and 23.24).

Isometric and Dynamic Strengthening: Erector Spinae and Multifidus Muscles

Strengthening the extensor muscles and an improved extensor/flexor ratio of the trunk muscles have been found to be important in decreasing symptoms in patients with chronic LBP.[78]

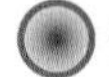 **FOCUS ON EVIDENCE**

Lee and associates[44] determined that the trunk extensor/flexor ratio is a sensitive parameter for predicting LBP. After following 67 asymptomatic individuals for 5 years, they found an increased incidence of LBP in those who had lower extensor strength than flexor muscle strength. Danneels and colleagues[16] demonstrated that intensive lumbar resistance training (isometric or dynamic) is necessary to develop paravertebral muscle strength and bulk. The following is a summary of specific exercise outcomes studies:

- Dynamic prone extension (prone arch), isometric trunk extension, and isometric leg extensions: result in high activity in both the Mf and erector spinae,[59] trunk extensor muscles activated at a higher level with trunk extension than with leg extension exercises,[18] and stronger contractions in the extensors when both lower extremities are stabilized during trunk extension.[19]
- Quadruped and prone upper and lower extremity lifts: stronger contractions than bridging (including bridging with feet on gymnastic ball or shoulders on gymnastic ball).[19]
- Isolated training of Mf: requires a low-intensity focus, as described in the Stabilization section.[65]

Extension Exercises in Prone or Quadruped Position

Resistance can be applied to any of the following recumbent exercises by having the patient hold weights in the hands or by strapping weights around the patient's legs.

PRECAUTIONS: Extension exercises in the prone position (prone arch) are performed at the end of the ROM in spinal extension and therefore may not be appropriate for individuals with symptoms from conditions, such as arthritis, spondylolisthesis, nerve root compression, or other flexion bias conditions, or patients who develop symptoms under loaded conditions (e.g., with disc lesions). Modify the positioning toward more neutral spinal positions by using the quadruped position and emphasize stabilization with isometric holds rather than moving into full extension (see Figs. 16.49 A through D, 16.50, and 16.54).

Thoracic elevation. Begin with the arms at the sides, progress to behind the head or reaching overhead as strength improves. Have the patient tuck in the chin and lift the head and thorax. The lower extremities must be stabilized (Fig. 16.69).

Leg lifts. Initially, have the patient lift only one leg, alternate with the other leg, and, finally, lift both legs and extend the spine (see Fig 16.49 E through G). Stabilize the thorax by having the patient hold onto the side of the treatment table.

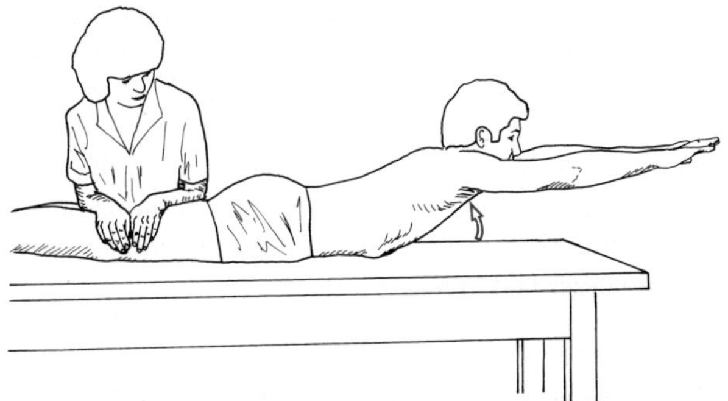

FIGURE 16.69 Strengthening the back extensors with the arms in position to provide maximal resistance. Additional resistance can be provided by holding weights in the hands.

Variations. Patient positioned prone on a large gym ball; combine spinal extension with upper extremity and/or lower extremity resistance, similar to exercises described in the stabilization exercise section (see Fig. 16.46 B).

Extension Exercises Sitting or Standing

Elastic resistance or weighted pulleys. Secure pulleys or elastic resistance in front of the patient at shoulder level. Have the patient hold onto the ends of the material or handles and extend the spine (Fig. 16.70).

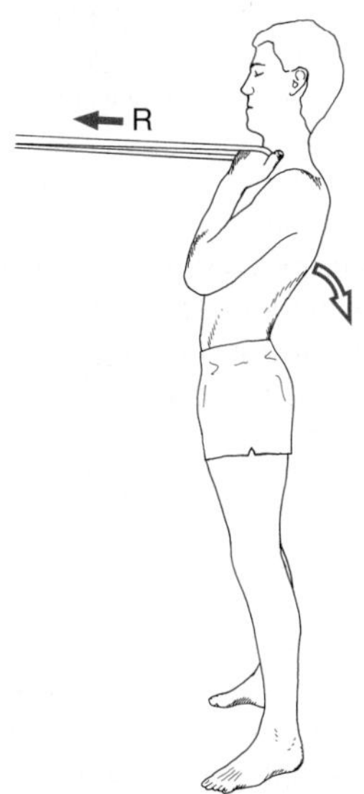

FIGURE 16.70 Using elastic resistance for concentric eccentric back extension.

For trunk rotation, use a pulley or elastic resistance secured under the foot or to a stable object opposite the side being exercised. Have the patient pull against the resistance, extending and rotating the back. Change the angle of pull of the resistance to recreate functional patterns specific to the patient's needs (Fig. 16.71).

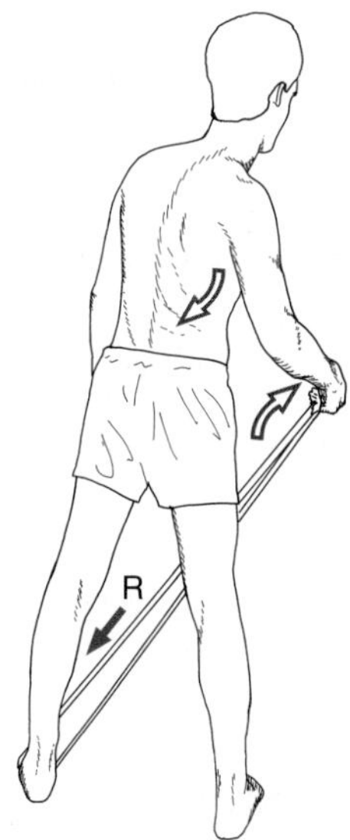

FIGURE 16.71 Rotation with extension strengthens the back extensors in functional patterns.

Trunk Side Bending (Lateral Abdominals, Erector Spinae, Quadratus Lumborum)

Trunk side-bending exercises are used for general strengthening of the muscles that side bend the trunk.

FOCUS ON EVIDENCE

McGill[52] identified the quadratus lumborum as one of the most important stabilizers of the spine and documented the isometric horizontal side support (side plank) as an effective exercise to strengthen this muscle (see discussion in the Stabilization section and Fig. 16.57).

Side-bending exercises are also used if there is scoliosis, although exercise alone has not been shown to halt or change the progression of a structural scoliosis curve. Exercise in conjunction with other methods of correction, such as bracing, is often employed.[10,57,58] When there is a lateral curve, the muscles on the convex side are usually stretched and weakened. The following exercises are described for use as strengthening exercises on the side of the convexity, although they may be used bilaterally for symmetrical strengthening. Stabilization exercises for spinal control, as previously described, may be beneficial for strengthening and conditioning when there is scoliosis.

- *Patient position and procedure:* Standing. Place elastic resistance under the foot or have the patient hold a weight in the hand on the side of the concavity; then have him or her side bend the trunk in the opposite direction.
- *Patient position and procedure:* Side-lying on the concave side of the curve with the apex at the edge of the table or

mat so the thorax is lowered. If you have access to a split table with one end that can be lowered, begin with the apex of the curve at the bend of the table. Have the patient place the lower arm folded across the chest and upper arm along the side of the body and side bend the trunk up against gravity. Progress by having the patient clasp both hands behind the head (Fig. 16.72). Stabilization of the pelvis and lower extremities must be provided.

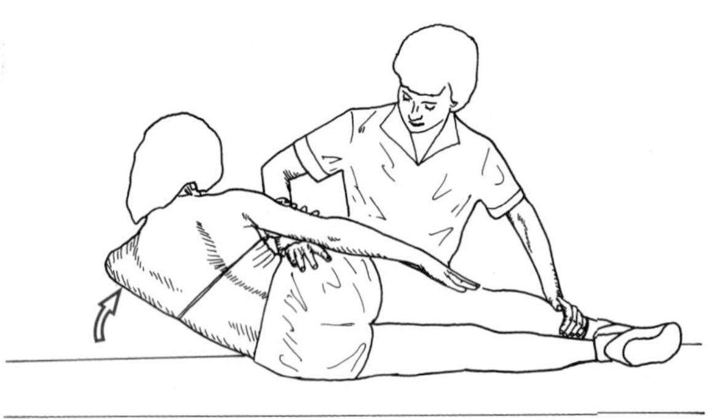

A

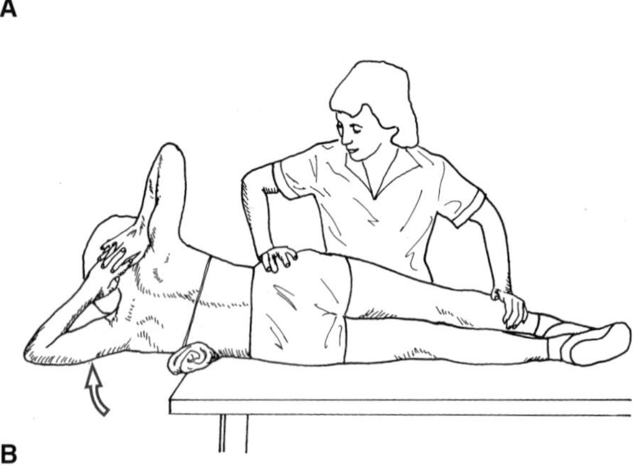

B

FIGURE 16.72 Antigravity strengthening of the lateral trunk musculature. **(A)** There is less resistance if the top arm is at the side and the bottom arm is folded across the chest. **(B)** Increase resistance by positioning the arms behind the head.

Cardiopulmonary Endurance

Goal. To develop cardiopulmonary fitness for overall endurance and well-being.

Aerobic conditioning exercises provide many benefits for the patient with spinal symptoms. The activity not only improves cardiopulmonary endurance, but also stimulates feelings of well-being and relief of symptoms. Chapter 7 describes cardiopulmonary conditioning principles and procedures. Specific precautions and suggestions for medical conditions are also explained. For patients recovering from spinal injuries, surgery, or postural dysfunction, aerobic exercises may be initiated once signs of inflammation no longer exist. Begin with low to moderate intensity and work with the patient to choose activities that do not place added stress on the recovering spinal structures. If a particular spinal bias has been identified (see Chapter 15), choose aerobic exercises that emphasize that spinal bias. A brief summary of the principles is reviewed in Box 16.6. Guidelines for safe application of common conditioning exercises when there are spinal impairments are described in this section.

Common Aerobic Exercises and Effects on the Spine

Some aerobic exercises place the spine in end-range positions. They are reviewed so the reader understands why some activities may be inappropriate for patients with specific conditions. If modifications are possible, they should be considered.

BOX 16.6 Summary of Aerobic Conditioning Principles

1. Establish the target heart rate and maximum heart rate.
   - The maximum heart rate is generally 220 minus the individual's age or may be the symptom-limiting heart rate (the rate at which cardiovascular symptoms appear).
   - Target heart rate is between 60% and 80% of the maximum heart rate.
2. Perform warm-up exercises for 10 to 15 minutes, including active movements of the neck and trunk.
3. Individualize the program of exercise.
   - Select activities that emphasize the patient's spinal bias if necessary (see information in the text).
   - Not all people are at the same fitness level and therefore cannot perform the same exercises. Any one exercise has the potential to be detrimental if attempted by someone not able to execute it properly.
   - To avoid overuse syndromes to structures of the musculoskeletal system, appropriate equipment, such as correct footwear, should be used for biomechanical support with weight-bearing exercises.
4. Increase the pace of the activity to reach the target heart rate and maintain it for 20 to 30 minutes.
5. Cool down for 5 to 10 minutes with slow, total body, repetitive motions and stretching activities.
6. Frequency of aerobic exercise should be three to five times per week.
7. Always stay within the tolerance of the individual. Overuse commonly occurs when there is an increase in time or effort without adequate rest (recovery) time between sessions. Increase repetitions or time by no more than 10% per week.[47] If pain begins while exercising, heed the warning and reduce the stress.

Cycling

Road bikes place the thoracolumbar spine in flexion and the upper cervical spine in hyperextension. Use this exercise for patients who have a flexion bias in the lumbar region so long as there are no upper cervical symptoms. Modifications include using a bike that positions the body in a more upright posture, such as a mountain bike or hybrid bike. Many stationary bikes also position the individual in upright postures and therefore are less likely to precipitate cervical problems.

Walking and Running

The upright posture emphasizes normal spinal curves, and lumbar extension is emphasized with walking and running (terminal stance). Emphasize the importance of identifying the neutral spine, activating the drawing-in maneuver, and stabilizing the spine while walking or running. Because conscious control is not possible during the entire exercise time, coach the patient to check his or her posture and muscle control frequently, such as each time he or she crosses an intersection or passes another individual or if symptoms develop in the spinal region. Walking or running with the cervical spine in retraction (axial extension) and the scapulae comfortably adducted, along with a rhythmic arm swing, reinforces cervical stabilization. Easy access to treadmills, tracks, or roads and trails makes these activities popular. Running is a high-impact activity and may not be tolerated by individuals with intervertebral disc lesions or degenerative joint conditions.

Stair Climbing

Commercial devices that replicate stepping with various grades of resistance are used for strengthening and aerobic conditioning. Regular steps can also be used for aerobic conditioning. This activity requires pelvic control of the reciprocating lower extremities, because lifting the leg on one side emphasizes spinal flexion while the contralateral lower extremity and spine are extending. Coach the patient to maintain the neutral spine with the stabilizing muscles against the rotational forces.

Cross-Country Skiing and Ski Machines

Cross-country skiing, whether out in the cold or on a commercial machine, is a high-intensity aerobic activity. The kicking motion that accompanies the backward motion of the leg emphasizes spinal extension. It is important to coach the patient to maintain the neutral spine and contract the stabilizing abdominal muscles.

Swimming

Breast stroke. The breaststroke emphasizes extension in the cervical and lumbar spinal regions when taking a breath. Coach the patient not to extend the neck full range but to keep it neutral and lift the head out of the water as a "solid" unit with the thorax just enough to clear the mouth for breath.

Freestyle. The freestyle stroke may exacerbate cervical problems because of the repetitive cervical rotation while taking a breath; this stroke also emphasizes lumbar extension with the flutter kick. Teach the patient to breathe using a "log-roll" technique in which the whole body rolls toward one side while breathing and then rolls back to the face-down position for the stroke. This requires good spinal stabilization.

Backstroke. The backstroke emphasizes spinal extension via kicking the lower extremities and the arm motions.

Butterfly stroke. The butterfly stroke moves the spine through a full ROM; emphasis is placed on controlling the range with the stabilizing muscles.

Upper Body Ergometers

Ergometry machines provide upper extremity resistance and can also be used for aerobic training. Forward motions emphasize spinal flexion and shoulder girdle protraction; backward motions emphasize spinal extension and shoulder girdle retraction. Coach the patient to assume the neutral spinal posture and use the stabilizing muscles prior to and during the use of the ergometer to enhance postural responses. If the machine can be used standing, progression to the standing position stimulates a total body response.

Step Aerobics and Aerobic Dancing

Stepping is similar to using stairs or a stair machine except for the jumping and bouncing that is usually added to the more advanced step aerobics programs.

Dancing moves take on many forms, and classes are taught that address various fitness levels and age groups. If possible, review safe movement patterns and help the patient recognize the safe limits of his or her spinal range and abilities.

Cross Fit

This high intensity and variable strength training program has become increasingly popular since the early part of the century. It yields the benefits of aerobic exercise combined with team building. Smith et al[74] followed 43 participants in a 10-week program. Pre and post VO_{2max} and body fat percentage both showed improvement. To determine if people are at increased risk for injury, Hak et al[26] distributed online questionnaires to international Cross Fit forums. One hundred thirty-two people responded, with 97 reporting an injury that was caused by training, 9 of which required surgery. This yielded an injury rate of 3.1 per 1,000 hours of Cross Fit training. This injury rate is similar to Olympic sports such as weight lifting and gymnastics. As with all exercise programs, it is important to provide proper instruction for safe use of equipment and application of each exercise related to specific abilities or limitations of each person.

"Latest Popular Craze"

People like variety and may be attracted to charismatic and energetic figures who demonstrate "new" workout techniques and routines or new exercise machines. Patients may ask for advice as to the value of the activities and techniques. Knowledge and skill in analyzing the biomechanics of the activity and the forces that are imposed through the spine should be used to provide advice about exercise safety. End-of-range postures and high-velocity stresses (such as vigorous kicking and ballistic motions) may be damaging to vulnerable tissues in the spine and should not be attempted by patients recovering from spinal problems.

Functional Activities

Goal. To progress to independence safely.

NOTE: Achieving the maximum level of independence underlies all the goals of therapeutic exercise. The patient develops segmental and global spinal stability; develops flexibility, muscle endurance, and strength; learns how exercise and posture correction relieve stress; and develops cardiopulmonary endurance—all to be able to function safely in daily activities, including work, recreation, and athletic pursuits.

Early Functional Training: Fundamental Techniques

Early functional training consists of teaching basic maneuvers needed for ADL, such as safely rolling over, moving from lying down to sitting (and reverse), and going from sitting to standing (and reverse). These techniques follow the early kinesthetic training instruction in which the patient learns to find his or her neutral spine and experiences the effect that simple arm and leg motions have on the spine, as well as early muscle performance training in which the patient learns how to activate the core musculature for segmental stabilization. If the examination reveals problems with basic ADL activities, the following are included in the early training program.

Rolling. Rolling with a neutral spine requires that the patient first find the neutral spine, perform the drawing-in maneuver, and then roll the trunk as a unit.

- It may be helpful to suggest that the patient "imagine a solid rod connecting the shoulders and pelvis so as not to twist" or suggest that he or she "roll like a log."
- Encourage the patient to use the arms and top leg to assist the roll.

Supine to sit/sit to lying down. Have the patient use the log roll maneuver (as described above) to roll from supine to side-lying while simultaneously flexing the hips and knees and pushing up with the arms.

- Help the patient focus on stabilizing the trunk with commands such as "push up your trunk as if it is a board; do not allow it to twist or bend."
- The reverse is practiced by coaching the patient to lower to the side-lying position as a unit first onto the elbow and then shoulder. Once down, the patient can roll to supine or prone-lying using the log-roll technique.

Sit to stand/stand to sit. The patient's level of function dictates how much assistance from the upper extremities is needed to accomplish "sit to stand" or "stand to sit." If the hip and knee extensors are not strong enough to elevate the body, the patient requires a chair with armrests, so there is some leverage for pushing up; alternatively, a firm seat or elevated seat may be necessary.

- To use the stable spine technique, instruct the patient to find the neutral spine by rolling the pelvis forward and backward, activate the drawing-in maneuver, and then bend forward at the hips while maintaining the neutral spine position.
- Help the patient focus on the hip motion while keeping the spine "solid like a board." The reverse is also practiced.

In and out of a car. Getting in and out of a car is often symptom-provoking for patients with low back or sacroiliac joint pain. Once sit to stand can be safely performed, have the patient practice the following:

- Approach the open car door and seat with the back toward the seat; stabilize the spine in its neutral position with the drawing-in maneuver; then bend at the hips and sit down.
- Once seated, flex both hips and knees and pivot the whole body around as a unit, maintaining a stable spine.
- When exiting a car, keep both knees together and pivot the legs and trunk outward as a unit. Once the feet are on the ground, bend at the hips and elevate the trunk as a unit.

Walking. For some patients, walking may provoke symptoms.

- Remind the patient to use the neutral spine and drawing-in maneuvers to stabilize the spine while walking.
- It is not possible to maintain conscious control for long, so remind the patient to check the spinal posture and reactivate the drawing-in maneuver whenever the symptoms recur.

Preparation for Functional Activities: Basic Exercise Techniques

Once the patient has learned to manage his or her symptoms and the symptoms of inflammation diminish, exercises are initiated that prepare the extremities and trunk for functional activities, such as safely lifting, carrying, pushing, pulling, and reaching in various directions. In the subacute or controlled motion phase of rehabilitation, emphasis is placed on strengthening the extremities in functional patterns while maintaining a stable spine. The patient should be able to perform IADLs and limited work activities at this stage. Evaluate the patient's performance and modify what he or she is doing to include safe spinal postures and correct stabilization. Use the activities in this section to prepare for or advance the patient's function.

Many of the strengthening exercises described in the extremity chapters are appropriate to use in preparation for functional training. With postural problems and recovery from back or neck injuries, it is critical to emphasize the neutral (functional) spinal posture before and during total body exercises. Many of the stabilization and movement patterns described earlier in this chapter can also be progressed in intensity, repetition, speed, and coordination to prepare for return to functional activities.

Weight-Bearing Exercises

Modified Bridging Exercises

Modified bridging exercises require stabilization with the trunk flexor and extensor muscles in conjunction with strengthening the gluteus maximus and quadriceps muscles in preparation for lifting activities. The abdominals function with the gluteus maximus to control the pelvic tilt, and the lumbar extensors stabilize the spine against the pull of the gluteus maximus.

Patient position and procedures: Begin with the patient hook-lying. Have the patient concentrate on maintaining the neutral spinal position while raising and lowering the pelvis (flexing and extending at the hips) (see Fig. 20.28). Hold the bridge for isometric control.

- Alternate arm motions; progress by adding weights to the hands.
- Alternate lifting one foot and then the other by marching in place (Fig. 16.73 A); progress by extending the knee as each leg is lifted. When the patient tolerates greater resistance, add ankle weights and coordinate with arm motions (Fig. 16.73 B).
- Abduct and adduct the thighs without letting the pelvis sag. Progress by placing the feet on a stool, chair, or large gym ball and repeating the bridging activities, or by placing the large gym ball under the shoulder/neck region with feet on the floor.

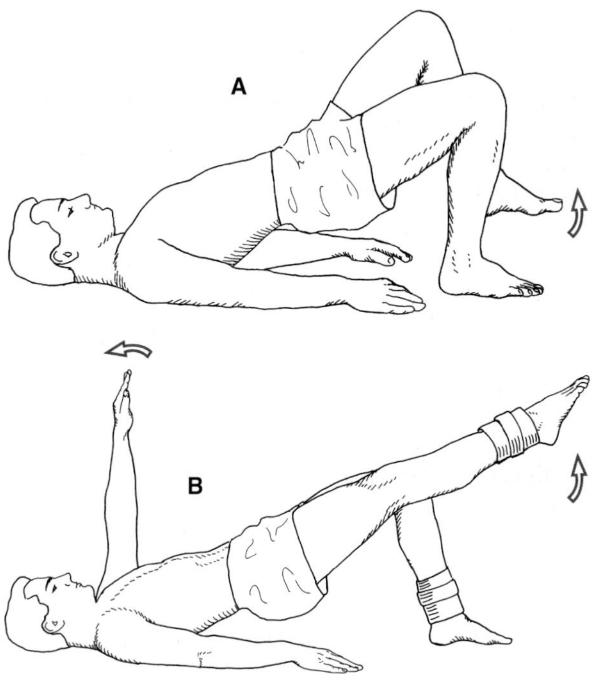

FIGURE 16.73 Holding a modified bridge to develop trunk control and gluteus maximus strength while superimposing extremity motions by **(A)** marching in place and **(B)** extending the extremities. Adding weights to the arms or legs requires greater strength and control.

Push-Ups With Trunk Stabilization

Push-ups use the body weight to strengthen the triceps and shoulder girdle musculature in preparation for pushing activities. The trunk musculature must stabilize against the pull of the shoulder girdle musculature as well as control the neutral spinal position as the body is raised and lowered.

Patient positions and procedures: Standing facing a wall or prone-lying with hands placed against the wall or floor in front of the shoulders. Remind the patient to find and maintain the neutral spinal position while performing the exercise.

- These exercises may begin as wall push-ups if the patient is not strong enough to push up from the floor.
- Prone-lying on the floor, the patient may push up with the pivot point being the knees or may perform full body push-ups with the pivot point being the feet.
- To challenge the patient on an unstable surface, he or she begins prone on a large gym ball. Have the patient walk forward with the hands on the floor until just the thighs are supported by the ball, maintain a stable spinal posture, and perform push-ups with the arms. To progress, walk out farther with the hands until just the legs are supported by the ball (Fig. 16.74). Additional advanced push up activities are described and illustrated in Chapter 23 (see Figs. 23.21 to 23.24).

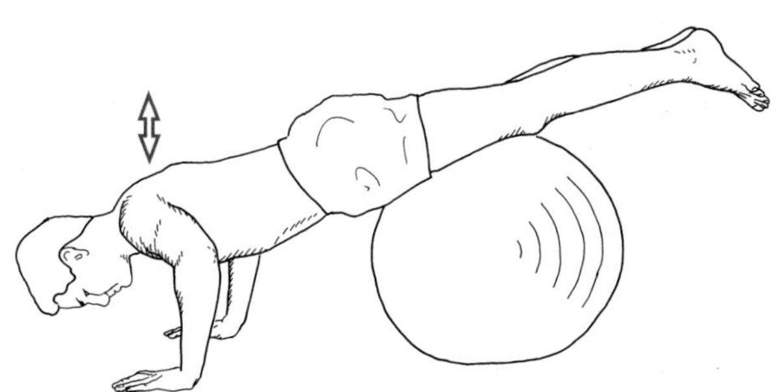

FIGURE 16.74 Push-up activities with the lower extremities balanced on a gym ball for strengthening the arms and developing trunk control.

Wall Slides

Wall slides develop strength in the hip and knee extensor muscles to prepare the lower extremities for squatting activities and training in safe body mechanics.

Patient position and procedure: Standing with the back to a wall and the spine held in its neutral position. Place a towel behind the back, so it slides easier along the wall. The exercise is more challenging if a large gym ball is placed between the back and the wall (Fig. 16.75). Have the patient slide his or

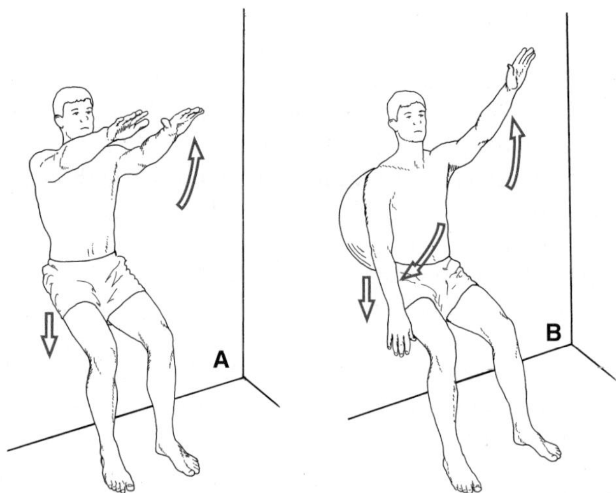

FIGURE 16.75 Wall slides/partial squats to develop LE strength and coordinate with trunk stability in preparation for training body mechanics. **(A)** The back sliding down a wall, with bilateral arm motion for added resistance. **(B)** Rolling a gym ball down the wall, with antagonistic arm motion to develop coordination.

her back down the wall into a partial squat and hold the position for isometric strengthening of the hip and knee extensors or move up and down for concentric/eccentric strengthening.

- Superimpose arm motions such as alternating or bilateral shoulder flexion/extension.
- Progress strengthening by incorporating single leg movements with marching steps or alternate knee extension.
- Use handheld weights to add resistance for upper and lower extremity strengthening.

Partial Lunges, Partial Squats, and Steps

Partial lunges and squats are described in Chapters 20 and 21. They are beneficial for strengthening total body movement in preparation for learning body mechanics. If necessary, begin by having the patient balance by holding onto the side of a treatment table or other stable object and then progress to balancing with a cane (see Fig. 20.32). Once able to perform multiple repetitions without holding on, add weights to the upper extremities for resistance.

- Add arm motions that are synchronized with the leg motions, such as reaching forward and downward to develop coordination and control.
- Progress to lunging onto an unstable surface and return upright.
- Add step-up/step-down activities, beginning with a low step and progressing the height.

Walking Against Resistance

Secure a weighted pulley or elastic resistance around the patient's pelvis with a belt, or the patient can hold the handles. Have the patient walk forward, backward, or diagonally against the resistive force. Emphasis is placed on spinal control (see Fig. 23.34).

Progress by having the patient push and pull weighted objects, such as a cart or a box on a table. Place emphasis on maintaining a stable spinal position while the extremities are loaded (see Figs. 17.58, 18.21 A, 23.18, and 23.36).

Transitional Stabilization Exercises

Exercises that cause movement into spinal flexion and then extension (and vice versa) challenge the patient to control the neutral spine position. The patient learns to stabilize the spine against alternating trunk and extremity motions.

Quadruped Forward/Backward Shifting

Patient position and procedure: Quadruped. Have the patient rock back to rest the buttocks on the heels; then shift the body forward onto the hands in the press-up position. The patient concentrates on controlling the pelvis in its neutral position rather than allowing full spinal flexion when shifting toward the heels or full spinal extension when shifting forward toward the press-up position.

Squatting and Reaching

Patient position and procedure: Begin standing. Have the patient reach downward while partially squatting. The tendency is for the spine to flex, so have the patient concentrate on maintaining a neutral spinal position with the spinal extensors. The patient then stands up and reaches overhead. This causes the spine to extend, so have the patient concentrate on using the trunk flexors to stabilize in the neutral position. Progress by lifting and reaching with weights while controlling the neutral posture of the spine.

Shifting Weight and Turning

Have the patient practice shifting weight forward/backward and side-to-side while maintaining the neutral spinal position and absorbing the forces with the hip and knee muscles. Practice turning using small steps and rotating at the hips rather than the back. Instruct the patient to imagine two rigid poles connecting each shoulder to each hip that do not allow the spine to twist. Even though some movement in the spine occurs, the activity helps the patient focus on a stable spine rather than rotating full range. Progress by using weights and having the patient lift, turn, and then place the weight at a new location.

Body Mechanics and Environmental Adaptations

Principles of Body Mechanics: Instruction and Training

When teaching safe body mechanics, it is advisable not to overwhelm the patient with too many instructions. Most people "know" they are to lift with their legs rather than their back, but they still have faulty techniques. Initiate training by suggesting that the patient find his or her neutral spine, perform the drawing-in maneuver, and then lift. Observe the technique they use and suggest modifications if needed. Squatting is often taught as the preferred method, yet not all patients are able to squat if they have impairments, such as knee pain or weakness. Under some circumstances, an individual may be more stable lifting with a lunge technique rather than the squat technique.

Lumbar Spine Position

The position of the lumbar spine, whether it is flexed, extended, or in midrange, raises several issues. Of the three postures, lifting with a neutral spinal posture provides greater stability of the spine[27] and uses both the ligamentous and muscular system for stabilization and control.[77] After a back injury, the preferred lifting posture may have to be adapted, depending on the type of injury and the response of the tissues when stressed.[77]

Spinal flexion. When lifting with a flexed lumbar spine (posterior pelvic tilt), support for the spine is primarily from inert structures (ligaments, lumbodorsal fasciae, posterior annulus fibrosus, and facets); there is little muscle activity.

- Flexion occurs when stooping to the floor. Some have suggested that it may also be the posture of choice for a patient who has injured the back muscles because the muscles are "quiet" when the spine is in flexion since the ligaments provide support.[77]
- Lifting with the lumbar spine in flexion may pose some problems. When lifting slowly with a flexed spine, the load is maintained on the ligaments, and creep of the inert tissues occurs; this increases the chance of injury if the tissue is already weakened. In addition, with the muscles lengthened and relaxed, they may be at an unfavorable length-tension relationship to respond quickly with appropriate force to resist a sudden change in load. There is greater chance of ligamentous strain when a person lifts with a flexed spine.[77]

Spinal extension. When lifting with an extended (lordotic) lumbar spine, the muscles supporting the spine are more active than when flexed, which increases the compressive forces on the disc. Also, the facets are approximated (close-pack position). This posture relieves stress on the ligaments, but for an individual whose back muscles are in poor condition and fatigue quickly, this posture may jeopardize the spine when repeated lifts are performed because the ligaments are not providing support.[77]

Load Position

Reinforce the concept of lifting and carrying objects as close to the center of gravity as possible.

- Have the patient practice carrying objects close to his or her center of gravity and draw attention to the feel of balance and control as well as less stress on the neck and back compared to the feel when carrying objects in more stressful positions. Point out that when lifting, the closer the object is held to the center of gravity, the less stress is placed on the supporting structures.
- Have the patient practice shifting the load from side-to-side and turning. Have the patient practice turning with hip rotation and minimal trunk rotation. The action should be directed by the legs while the spine is kept stable.
- Replicate the mechanics of the patient's job setting and practice safe mechanics.
- Teach the "golfer's lift" for picking up light objects, such as keys, pencils, and small toys. This is done by flexing the trunk forward over one hip while the other hip extends. It allows the patient to maintain a neutral spine and places the majority of the work on the lower extremities.

Environmental Adaptations

Ergonomic assessment and modification of the home and working environments are necessary to correct stresses as well as prevent future recurrence of symptoms.

Home, Work, and Driving Considerations

- Chairs and car seats should have lumbar support to maintain slight lordosis. Use a towel roll or lumbar pillow if necessary.
- Chair height should allow knees to flex to take tension off the hamstring muscles, support the thighs, and allow the feet to rest comfortably on the floor.
- Arm rests should be used if prolonged sitting is required in order to take the stress off shoulders and the cervical spine.
- Desk or table height should be adequate to keep the person from having to lean over the work.
- Work and driving habits should allow frequent changing of posture. If normally sedentary, the patient should get up and walk every hour.

Sleeping Environment

- The mattress needs to provide firm support to prevent any extreme stresses. If it is too soft, the patient sags and stresses ligaments; if it is too firm, some patients cannot relax.
- Pillows should be of a comfortable height and density to promote relaxation but should not place joints in an extreme position. Foam rubber pillows tend to cause increased tension in muscles because of the constant resistance they provide.
- Whether the person should sleep prone, side-lying, or supine is something that must be analyzed for each individual patient. Ideally, a comfortable posture is one that is in the midrange and that does not place stress on any supporting structure. Pain that is experienced when waking up in the morning is often related to sleeping posture; if this is the case, listen carefully to the patient's description of postures when sleeping and see if it relates to the pain. Then, attempt to modify the sleep position accordingly. Remind the patient that it takes several weeks to change habits.

Intermediate to Advanced Exercise Techniques for Functional Training

As the patient learns spinal control while doing the exercises, repetitions are increased to develop muscular endurance, and resistance is added to develop strength. If coordination, agility, and balance are required, they are emphasized. By this stage, it is recognized that the individual already knows the basic spinal stabilization techniques and is habitually assuming the neutral spinal position and activating the drawing-in maneuver. Reinforce the importance of this when doing the following exercises. It is also recognized that the patient should be able to control greater spinal ROM without experiencing symptoms. Adapt the exercises to replicate return to work or sport-related activities. Some examples include the following.

Repetitive Lifting

The ability to do repetitive lifting throughout the workday is necessary for many jobs and may result in symptom recurrence. To prepare for returning to work, progressively increase the repetitions of lifting activities the patient must do to improve muscle endurance. Marras and Granta[49] demonstrated that with repetitive lifting (over a 5-hour period) subjects had a significant change in their lifting pattern and in the muscle recruitment patterns, so there was a decrease in spine stabilization (decreased compression) and an increase in anterior/posterior shear in the lumbar spine. To reduce the risk of recurrence of low back disorders, a patient needs to learn to monitor these changes and be conscious of correcting faulty patterns. Help the patient modify and adapt the stable spine body mechanics that were initiated under basic techniques to replicate the type of lifting he or she will be doing at home or on the job. Include variations in the lifting tasks to prepare for unexpected situations.

Repetitive Reaching

Repetitive reaching requires that the patient learn to assume a comfortable stride and then practice shifting his or her weight forward and backward on the lower extremities rather than bending forward and backward with the spine. Preparatory exercises should include partial lunging forward, sideways, and backward. During practice, have the patient use a weight comparable to that in the real-life situation and go through the action on a repetitive basis, concentrating on spinal control and resting only when control is no longer possible.

Repetitive Pushing and Pulling

Repetitive pushing and pulling require strong upper extremities and a stable spine. Preparatory activities should include pushing and pulling against elastic resistance or pulley resistance set at heights that replicate the work environment. Progress to pushing and pulling a weighted cart or a weighted box across a table. Reinforce the importance of activating the spinal stabilizers.

Rotation or Turning

Turning with a load is a component of most work activity. A person may rotate the spine to reach around to place a load to the side or behind. Rotation may create an unstable situation or may be damaging to the spinal structures. Therefore, it is important to take the rotation out of turning. Have the patient practice a "stable spine turn," which requires motion and control in the hips or taking steps into the direction of the turn rather than twisting and rotating the back.

Transitional Movements

Most functional activities require transitional motions, such as reaching downward to pick up something (spinal flexion), then reaching overhead to place it on a high shelf (spinal extension). In sports activities, the activity may require moving quickly from a forward-bent position to an extended position with arms overhead (such as dribbling a basketball and then shooting). Set up drills that replicate the speed and movements of the desired outcome; have the patient practice moving through the patterns while attempting to maintain control of his or her functional spinal position and range.

Transfer of Training

Ideally, each patient is progressed through rehabilitation to the level of being able to transfer skills learned to closely related but new situations. Provide variable learning opportunities from simple to complex and then help the patient analyze successful adaptations to each new experience. (See Fig. 1.8 and accompanying text in Chapter 1 for examples of how to vary tasks from simple to complex.)

Patient Education for Prevention

Education occurs on a continual basis. Before discharge, review the following relationships of posture and pain with the patient.

- When experiencing pain or the recurrence of symptoms, check posture. Avoid any one posture for prolonged periods. Change positions before pain or discomfort is experienced.
- If sustained postures are necessary, take frequent breaks and perform appropriate ROM exercises at least every half hour. Finish all exercises by assuming a well-balanced posture.
- Avoid hyperextending the neck or being in a forward-head posture or forward-bent position for prolonged periods.

Find ways to modify a task so it can be accomplished at eye level or with proper lumbar support.

- If in a tension-producing situation, perform conscious relaxation exercises.
- Use common sense and follow good safety habits.
- Review the home exercise program and explain how to safely progress and vary the exercises to maintain interest.
  - Teach flexibility, muscle endurance, and strengthening exercises appropriate for the patient to maintain ROM, muscle endurance, and strength.
  - Address any misconceptions the patient may have about exercise and management of the spine.
  - Teach the patient to safely progress the aerobic exercise program. Reinforce the importance of maintaining cardiopulmonary endurance and its effect on managing symptoms.

Independent Learning Activities

Critical Thinking and Discussion

1. Observe a homemaker or worker doing an activity that requires pushing, pulling, reaching, lifting, or some other repetitive pattern. Analyze what component motions are part of the total pattern and decide if strength, range, endurance, balance, or coordination (or a combination) is necessary in the upper extremities, lower extremities, and trunk. Decide what is necessary to make the spine safe while doing this activity and design an exercise program that encompasses all the components.
2. Go to a health club or exercise class and observe how individuals are performing the exercises. Note the activities that cause stress to the spine or pelvis. How would you modify each exercise? Consider safe use of the equipment, safe biomechanics, and appropriate instruction for the audience. Can you tell the purpose of each exercise (strength, stretch, endurance, balance)? Are the directions appropriately given for the level of participants?
3. What is the law in your state as it pertains to physical therapists performing manipulation and HVT? What are some situations in which you would perform a manipulation rather than an HVT technique? What are some situations in which you would perform an HVT technique rather than a manipulation technique?

Laboratory Practice

1. With a laboratory partner practice the kinesthetic training techniques and deep segmental muscle activation techniques for the cervical spine and the lumbar spine until you become proficient at performing them and recognizing when they are done correctly. Then practice teaching them to a family member or friend and see how well they understand what they are to do.
2. Practice the progression of spinal stabilization exercises described in the muscle performance section. Start at the easiest level and progress the leg and arm movements until you feel you are at your maximum resistance for stabilization. After resting, time yourself for 1 minute, beginning at the most difficult level of movement. The idea is to keep the spine stable during the entire minute. If you begin to feel you are losing control, decrease the amount of extremity resistance (e.g., going from moving both lower extremities in a reciprocal pattern to moving just one extremity while the other is on the floor). This can also be done for 3 minutes. Were you able to meet the challenge yet keep the spine stable? Did you feel your stabilizing muscles "working"?
3. Practice doing wall slides, partial squats, and partial lunges with a stable spine. When you can do the squat comfortably with a stable spine, practice lifting a box from the floor to table height, then from the floor to shoulder height, then place it on a shelf at each height. Feel what is happening to your spine. Then repeat the maneuvers with a stable spine, and see if you can control the spinal position with the drawing-in maneuver. When you can do the lunge comfortably, practice lifting small objects from the floor with a lunging technique and stable spine. Finally, practice lifting objects from the floor and turning (using legs and hips to change direction, not spinal rotation) to place the objects on a table or shelf. Feel what is happening to the spine and repeat the activities with a stable spinal posture.
4. Review the indications and contraindications for spinal manipulation. Practice the cervical manipulations with your laboratory partner in both the supine and prone positions. In which position do you have better control (patient supine or prone)?
5. Several HVT techniques were discussed in this chapter. What are the contraindications for HVT in the spine? Practice three HVTs to improve thoracic flexion. How would you change the technique if your goal was to improve rotation to the left?

Case Studies

Review the cases described in Chapters 14 and 15 and modify your answers based on the information presented in this chapter.

REFERENCES

1. Abdulwahab, SS: Treatment based on H-reflexes testing improves disability status in patients with cervical radiculopathy. *Int J Rehabil Res* 22(3): 207–214, 1999.
2. Aleksiev, AR: Ten-year follow-up of strengthening versus flexibility exercises with or without abdominal bracing in recurrent low back pain. *Spine* 39(13), 997–1003, 2014.
3. Alexander, KM, and LaPier, TL: Differences in static balance and weight distribution between normal subjects and subjects with chronic unilateral low back pain. *J Orthop Sports Phys Ther* 28(6):378–383, 1998.
4. American Physical Therapy Association: Position on thrust joint manipulation provided by physical therapists: White paper-manipulation. Available at http://www.apta.org/uploadedFiles/APTAorg/Advocacy/State/Issues/Manipulation/WhitePaperManipulation.pdf#search=%22http%2f%2fwww.apta.org%2fAM%2fTemplate.cfm%3fSection%ef%80%bdHome%22. Accessed September 30, 2015.
5. Andersson, EA, et al: Abdominal and hip flexor muscle activation during various training exercises. *Eur J App Physiol* 75:115–123, 1997.
6. Arokoski, JP, et al: Back and abdominal muscle function during stabilization exercises. *Arch Phys Med Rehabil* 82(8):1089–1098, 2001.
7. Bondi, BA, and Drinkwater-Kolk, M: Functional stabilization training. Workshop notes, Northeast Seminars, October 1992.
8. Bronfort, G, et al: Efficacy of spinal manipulation and mobilization for low back pain and neck pain: a systemic review and best evidence synthesis. *Spine J* 4:335–356, 2004.
9. Byström, MG, Rasmussen-Barr, E, and Grooten, WJ: Motor control exercises reduces pain and disability in chronic and recurrent low back pain: a meta-analysis. *Spine* 38(6):E350–358, 2013.
10. Cassella, MC, and Hall, JE: Current treatment approaches in the nonoperative and operative management of adolescent idiopathic scoliosis. *Phys Ther* 71:897–909, 1991.
11. Childs, JD, et al: A clinical prediction rule to identify patients with low back pain most likely to benefit from spinal manipulation: a validation study. *Ann Intern Med* 141(12):920–928, 2004.
12. Childs, JD, et al: Neck pain: clinical practice guidelines linked to the international classification of functioning, disability, and health from the Orthopaedic Section of the American Physical Therapy Association. *J Orthop Sports Phys Ther* 38(9):A1–A34, 2008
13. Chok, B, et al: Endurance training of the trunk extensor muscles in people with subacute low back pain. *Phys Ther* 79(11):1032–1042, 1999.
14. Cleland, JA, et al: The use of lumbar spine manipulation technique by physical therapists in patients who satisfy a clinical prediction rule: a case series. *J Orthop Sports Phys Ther* 36:209–214, 2006.
15. Czaprowski, D, et al: Abdominal muscle EMG-activity during bridge exercises on stable and unstable surfaces. *Phys Ther Sport* 15(3):162–168, 2014.
16. Danneels, LA, et al: The effects of three different training modalities on the cross-sectional area of the paravertebral muscles. *Scand J Med Sci Sports* 11:335–341, 2001.
17. Delitto, A, et al: Low back pain: clinical practice guidelines linked to the International Classification of Functioning, Disability, and Health from the orthopaedic section of the American Physical Therapy Association. *J Orthop Sports Phys Ther* 42(4):A1–A52, 2012.
18. De Ridder, E, et al: Posterior muscle chain activity during various extension exercises: an observational study. *BMC Musculoskelet Disord* 14:204, 2013.
19. Ekstrom, RA, Osborn, RW, and Haver, PL: Surface electromyographic analysis of the low back muscles during rehabilitation exercises. *J Orthop Sports Phys Ther* 38(12)736–745, 2008.
20. Escamilla, RF, et al: Core muscle activation during Swiss ball and traditional abdominal exercises. *J Ortho Sports Phys Ther* 40(5), 265–276, 2010.
21. Flynn, TM, Fritz, JM, and Wainner, RS: Spinal manipulation in physical therapist professional degree education: a model for teaching and integration into clinical practice. *J Orthop Sports Phys Ther* 36(8):577–587, 2006.
22. Fortin, M, and Macedo, LG: Multifidus and paraspinal muscle group cross-sectional areas of patients with low back pain and control patients: a systematic review with a focus on blinding. *Phys Ther* 93(7):873–888, 2013.
23. Gilleard, WL, and Brown, JM: An electromyographic validation of an abdominal muscle test. *Arch Phys Med Rehabil* 75:1002–1007, 1994.
24. Granacher, U, et al: The importance of trunk muscle strength for balance, functional performance, and fall prevention in seniors: a systematic review. *Sports Med* 43:627–641, 2013.
25. Hagins, M, et al: Effects of practice on the ability to perform lumbar stabilization exercises. *J Orthop Sports Phys Ther* 29(9):546–555, 1999.
26. Hak, PT, Hodzovic, E, and Hickey, B: The nature and prevalence of injury during CrossFit training. *J Strength Cond Res* Nov 22, 2013.
27. Hart, DL, Stobbe, TJ, and Jaraiedi, M: Effect of lumbar posture on lifting. *Spine* 12(2):138–145, 1987.
28. Henry, SM, and Westervelt, KC: The use of real-time ultrasound feedback in teaching abdominal hollowing exercises to healthy subjects. *J Orthop Sports Phys Ther* 35(6):338–345, 2005.
29. Hicks, GE, et al: Trunk muscle composition as a predictor of reduced functional capacity in the health, aging and body composition: the moderating role of back pain. *J Gerontol* 60A(11):1420–1424, 2005.
30. Hides, JA, Jull, GA, and Richardson, CA: Long-term effects of specific stabilizing exercises for first-episode low back pain. *Spine* 26(11): E243–E248, 2001.
31. Hides, JA, Richardson, CA, and Gwendolen, AJ: Multifidus muscle recovery is not automatic after resolution of acute, first-episode low back pain. *Spine* 21(23):2763–2769, 1996.
32. Hides, JA, et al: Ultrasound imaging in rehabilitation. *Aust J Physiother* 41:187–193, 1995.
33. Hides, JA, Richardson, CA, and Jull, GA: Use of real-time ultrasound imaging for feedback in rehabilitation. *Manual Ther* 3:125–131, 1993.
34. Hodges, PW, and Richardson, CA: Transversus abdominis and the superficial abdominal muscles are controlled independently in a postural task. *Neurosci Lett* 265:91–94, 1999.
35. Hodges, PW, and Richardson, CA: Delayed postural contraction of transversus abdominis in low back pain associated with movement of the lower limb. *J Spinal Disord* 11(1):46–56, 1998.
36. Hodges, PW, and Richardson, CA: Contraction of the abdominal muscles associated with movement of the lower limb. *Phys Ther* 77(2):132–142, 1997.
37. Hodges, PW, and Richardson, CA: Feedforward contraction of transversus abdominis is not influenced by the direction of arm movement. *Exp Brain Res* 114:362–370, 1997.
38. Hodges, PW, Richardson, CA, and Jull, G: Evaluation of the relationship between laboratory and clinical tests of transversus abdominis function. *Physiother Res Int* 1(1):30–40, 1996.
39. Hubley-Kozey, CL, and Vezina, MJ: Muscle activation during exercises to improve trunk stability in men with low back pain. *Arch Phys Med Rehabil* 83:1100–1108, 2002.
40. Jull, G, et al: A randomized controlled trial of exercise and manipulative therapy for cervicogenic headache. *Spine* 27(17):1835–1843, 2002.
41. Jull, G, et al: Further clinical clarification of the muscle dysfunction in cervical headache. *Cephalalgia* 19:179–185, 1999.
42. Kendall, FP, et al: *Muscles: Testing and Function, With Posture and Pain*, ed. 5. Baltimore, MD: Lippincott Williams & Wilkins, 2005.
43. Kong, YS, Cho, YH, Park, and JW: Changes in the activities of the trunk muscles in different kinds of bridging exercises. *Phys Ther Sci* 25(12): 1609–1612, 2013.
44. Lee, FH, et al: Trunk muscle weakness as a risk factor for low back pain. *Spine* 24(1):54–57, 1999.
45. Lehman, GJ, and McGill, SM: Quantification of the differences in electromyographic activity magnitude between the upper and lower portions of the rectus abdominis muscle during selected trunk exercises. *Phys Ther* 81(5):1096–1101, 2001.
46. Lluch, E, et al: Effects of deep cervical flexor training on pressure pain thresholds over myofascial trigger points in patients with chronic neck pain. *J Manip Phys Ther* 36(9):604–611, 2013.

47. Lubell, A: Potentially dangerous exercises: are they harmful to all? *Phys Sports Med* 17:187–192, 1989.
48. Maeo, S, et al: Trunk muscle activities during abdominal bracing: comparison among muscles and exercises. *J Sports Sci Med* 12(3):467–474, 2013.
49. Marras, WS, and Granata, KP: Changes in trunk dynamics and spine loading during repeated trunk exertions. *Spine* 22(21):2564–2570, 1997.
50. McDonnell, KM, Sahrmann, SA, and Van Dillen, L: A specific exercise program and modification of postural alignment for treatment of cervicogenic headache: a case report. *J Orthop Sports Phys Ther* 35(1):3–15, 2005.
51. McGalliard, MK, et al: Changes in transversus abdominal thickness with use of the abdominal drawing in maneuver during a functional task. *Phys Med and Rehab* 2(3):187–194, 2010.
52. McGill, SM: Low back exercises: evidence for improving exercise regimens. *Phys Ther* 78(7):754–765, 1998.
53. McLean, SM, et al: A randomised controlled trial comparing graded exercise treatment and usual physiotherapy for patients with non-specific neck pain (the GET UP neck pain trial). *Man Ther* 18(3):199–205, 2013.
54. Mew, R: Comparison of changes in abdominal muscle thickness between standing and crook lying during active abdominal hollowing using ultrasound imaging. *Man Ther* 14(6):690–695, 2009.
55. Miura, T, et al: Individuals with chronic low back pain do not modulate the level of transversus abdominis muscle contraction across different postures. *Man Ther* 19(6):534–540, 2014.
56. Morgan, D: Concepts in functional training and postural stabilization for the low-back injured. *Top Acute Care Trauma Rehabil* 2:8–17, 1988.
57. Monticone, M, et al: Active self-correction and task-oriented exercises reduce spinal deformity and improve quality of life in subjects with adolescent idiopathic scoliosis. Results of a randomized controlled trial. *Eur Spin J* 23:1204–1214, 2014.
58. Negrini, S, et al: 2011 SOSORT Guidelines: orthopaedic and rehabilitation treatment of idiopathic scoliosis during growth. *Scoliosis* 7:3, 2102.
59. Ng, JK, and Richardson, CA: EMG study of erector spinae and multifidus in two isometric back extension exercises. *Aust J Physiother* 40:115–121, 1994.
60. O'Sullivan, PT, Twomey, L, and Allison, GT: Altered abdominal muscle recruitment in patients with chronic back pain following a specific exercise intervention. *J Orthop Sports Phys Ther* 27(2):114–124, 1998.
61. O'Sullivan, PT, et al: Altered patterns of abdominal muscle activation in patients with chronic low back pain. *Aust Physiother* 43(2):91–98, 1997.
62. Paris, SV: A history of manipulative therapy. *JMMT* 8(2):66–67, 2000.
63. Park, RJ, et al: Changes in regional activity of the psoas major and quadratus lumborum with voluntary trunk and hip tasks and different spinal curvatures in sitting. *J Ortho Sport Phys Ther* 43(2):74–82, 2013.
64. Reeve, A, and Dilley, A: Effects of posture on the thickness of transversus abdominis in pain-free subjects. *Man Ther* 14(6):679–684, 2009.
65. Richardson, C, Hodges, P, and Hides, J: *Therapeutic Exercise for Lumbopelvic Stabilization: A Motor Control Approach for the Treatment and Prevention of Low Back Pain,* ed. 2. Philadelphia: Churchill Livingstone, 2004.
66. Richardson, C, and Jull, G: A historical perspective on the development of clinical techniques to evaluate and treat the active stabilising system of the lumbar spine. *Aust J Physiother Monogr* 1:5–13, 1995.
67. Richardson, C, et al: Techniques for active lumbar stabilisation for spinal protection: a pilot study. *Aust J Physiother* 38:105, 1992.
68. Richardson, C, Toppenberg, R, and Jull, G: An initial evaluation of eight abdominal exercises for their ability to provide stabilisation for the lumbar spine. *Aust J Physiother* 36:6, 1990.
69. Robinson, R: The new back school prescription: stabilization training. Part I. *Occup Med* 7:17–31, 1992.
70. Saal, JA: The new back school prescription: stabilization training. Part II. *Occup Med* 7:33–42, 1992.
71. Saal, JA: Dynamic muscular stabilization in the nonoperative treatment of lumbar pain syndromes. *Orthop Rev* 19:691–700, 1990.
72. Saunders, HD, and Ryan, RS: Spinal traction. In Saunders, HD, and Ryan, RS (eds): *Evaluation, Treatment and Prevention of Musculoskeletal Disorders, Vol 1. Spine,* ed. 4. Chaska, MN: Saunders Group, 2004.
73. Scott, IR, Vaughan, ARS, and Hall, J: Swiss ball enhances lumbar multifidus activity in chronic low back pain. *Phys Ther in Sport* 16(1):40–44, 2015.
74. Smith, MM, et al: Crossfit-based high-intensity power training improves maximal aerobic fitness and body composition. *J Strength Cond Res* Nov;27(11):3159–3172, 2013.
75. Stevans, J, and Hall, KG: Motor skill acquisition strategies for rehabilitation of low back pain. *J Orthop Sports Phys Ther* 28(3):165–167, 1998.
76. Storheim, K, et al: Intra-tester reproducibility of pressure biofeedback in measurement of transversus abdominis function. *Physiother Res Int* 7(4): 239–249, 2002.
77. Sullivan, MS: Back support mechanisms during manual lifting. *Phys Ther* 69:38–45, 1989.
78. Takemasa, R, Yamamoto, H, and Tani, T: Trunk muscle strength in and effect of trunk muscle exercises for patients with chronic low back pain. *Spine* 20(23):2522–2530, 1995.
79. Teyhen, DS, et al: Changes in lateral abdominal muscle thickness during the abdominal drawing-in maneuver in those with lumbopelvic pain. *J Orthop Sports Phys Ther* 39(11):791–798, 2009.
80. Teyhen, DS, et al: The use of ultrasound imaging of the abdominal drawing-in maneuver in subjects with low back pain. *J Orthop Sports Phys Ther* 35(6):346–355, 2005.
81. Teyhen, DS, et al: Changes in deep abdominal muscle thickness during common trunk-strengthening exercises using ultrasound imaging. *J Ortho Sports Phys Ther* 38(10):596–605, 2008.
82. Tsao, H, and Hodges, PW: Immediate changes in feedforward postural adjustments following voluntary motor training. *Exp Brain Res* 181(4): 537–546, 2007.
83. Vera-Garcia, FJ, Grenier, SG, and McGill, SM: Abdominal muscle response during curl-ups on both stable and labile surfaces. *Phys Ther* 80(6): 564–569, 2000.
84. Wohlfahrt, D, Jull, G, and Richardson, C: The relationship between the dynamic and static function of abdominal muscles. *Aust J Physiother* 39:9–13, 1993.

CHAPTER 17

The Shoulder and Shoulder Girdle

CAROLYN KISNER, PT, MS ■ LYNN COLBY, PT, MS ■ JOHN D. BORSTAD, PT, PHD

The shoulder complex design enables great mobility of the upper extremity. As a result, the hand can be placed almost anywhere within a sphere of movement, its range limited primarily by the length of the arm and the space taken up by the body. The combined mechanics of the three synovial and two functional joints with the many muscles that comprise the shoulder complex interact to provide and control the mobility. When establishing a therapeutic exercise program for impaired function of the shoulder region, as with any other body region, the unique anatomical and kinesiological features must be considered along with the state of pathology and functional limitations imposed by the impairments.

This chapter is divided into three main sections. The first section reviews the structure and function of the shoulder complex. The second section describes common shoulder disorders and provides guidelines for conservative and postsurgical management. The last section describes exercise techniques commonly used to meet the goals of treatment during the stages of tissue healing and phases of rehabilitation.

Structure and Function of the Shoulder Girdle

The shoulder girdle has only one bony articulation with the axial skeleton (Fig. 17.1). The clavicle articulates with the sternum via the small sternoclavicular (SC) joint, and this reduced articular contact area is an important reason for the considerable mobility of the upper extremity. Stability, however, is hampered by this articular arrangement and relies on an intricate balance among the scapular and glenohumeral (GH) muscles and the soft tissue structures of the joints in the shoulder complex.

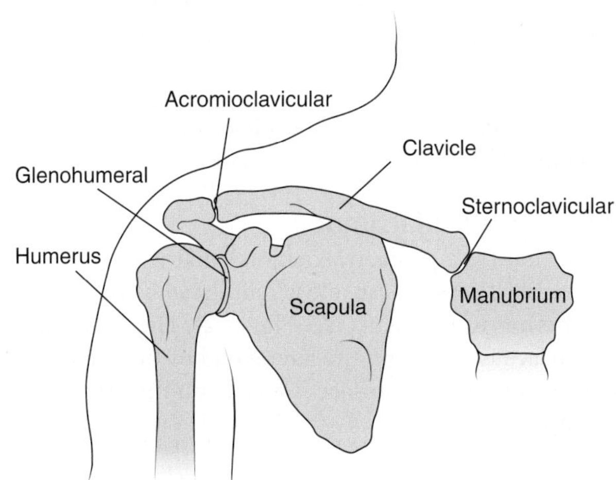

FIGURE 17.1 Bones and joints of the shoulder girdle complex.

Joints of the Shoulder Complex

Three synovial joints (GH, acromioclavicular [AC], and SC) and two functional articulations (scapulothoracic and suprahumeral) make up the shoulder complex.

Synovial Joints

Glenohumeral Joint

The GH joint is an incongruous, ball-and-socket (spheroidal) triaxial joint with a lax joint capsule. It is supported by the tendons of the rotator cuff and the GH (superior, middle, inferior) and coracohumeral ligaments (Fig. 17.2). The concave

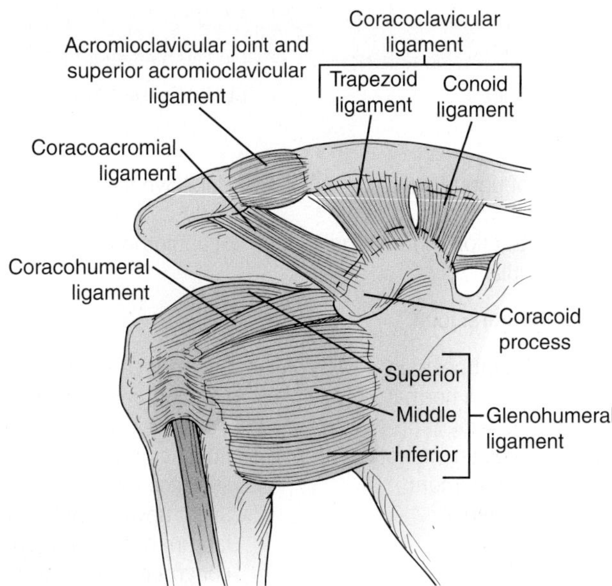

FIGURE 17.2 Ligaments of the glenohumeral (GH) and acromioclavicular (AC) joints.

joint surface, the glenoid fossa, is located on the superior-lateral margin of the scapula. It faces primarily laterally, somewhat anteriorly, and slightly upward, providing minimal stability to the joint. A fibrocartilagenous lip, the glenoid labrum, deepens the fossa to increase joint congruity and stability and serves as the attachment site for the capsule. The convex joint surface is the hemispheric head of the humerus. Only a small portion of the head contacts the fossa at any time, allowing for considerable joint movement but also the potential for instability.[155]

Arthrokinematics

According to the convex-concave theory of joint motion (see Chapter 5), with motions of the humerus (physiological motions), the convex head rolls in the same direction and slides in the opposite direction on the glenoid fossa. The arthrokinematics of the GH joint are summarized in ONLINE Box 19.1 on the FA Davis website that supports this textbook.

Stability

Both static and dynamic restraints provide GH joint stability (Table 17.1).[28,44,180,218,221] The structural relationships among the joint morphology, ligaments, and glenoid labrum, along with adhesive and cohesive forces in the joint, provide static stability. The tendons of the rotator cuff blend with the ligaments and glenoid labrum at their sites of attachment, so muscle contractions provide dynamic stability by tightening the static restraints (Fig. 17.3). The coordinated response of the muscles of the cuff and tension in the ligaments provide varying degrees of support depending on the position and motion of the humerus.[170,180,204] In addition, the long head of the biceps and the long head of the triceps brachii reinforce the capsule with their attachments and provide superior and inferior shoulder joint support, respectively, when functioning with

TABLE 17.1 Static and Dynamic Stabilizers of the Scapula and Glenohumeral Joint

Description	Static Stabilizers	Muscular Stabilizers
Scapula		
Weight of upper extremity creates downward rotation and protraction moment on the scapula	▪ Cohesive forces of subscapular bursa, SC, and AC joint ligaments ▪ Scapulothoracic fascia	Scapulothoracic musculature, especially upper, middle, and lower trapezius, serratus anterior, levator scapula, and rhomboids
Glenohumeral joint		
In dependent position: if scapula is in normal alignment, weight of arm creates an inferior translation moment on the humerus	▪ Superior capsule, superior GH ligament, and coracohumeral ligament are taut ▪ Adhesive and cohesive forces of synovial fluid and negative joint pressure hold surfaces together ▪ Slight upward inclination of glenoid and labrum deepens fossa and improves congruency; acts as inferior barrier	Rotator cuff, deltoid, long head of biceps brachii, pectoralis major, latissimus dorsi, and teres major
When the humerus is elevating and the scapula is rotating upward	▪ Tension placed on static restraints by the rotator cuff ▪ Glenohumeral ligaments limit excessive translations of humeral head	▪ Rotator cuff and deltoid; elbow action brings in two-joint muscle support ▪ Long head of biceps stabilizes against humeral elevation

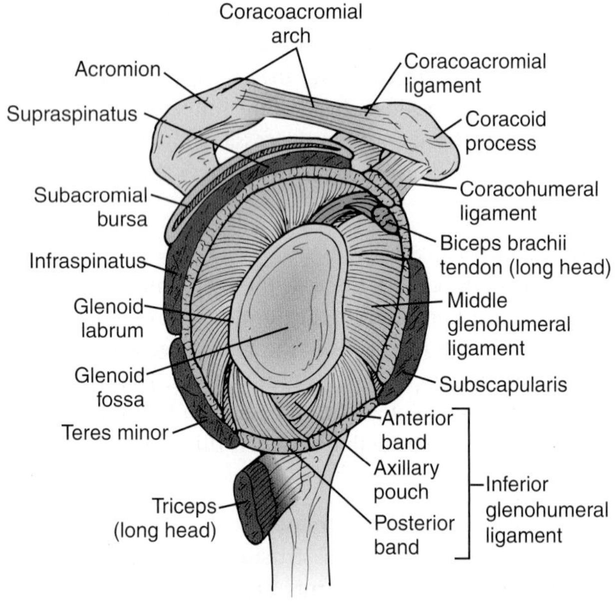

FIGURE 17.3 Lateral aspect of the glenoid fossa (interior view), showing attachments of the glenoid labrum, capsule, and ligaments as well as their relationship to the rotator cuff and long head of the biceps brachii musculature.

elbow motions.[105] The long head of the biceps, in particular, stabilizes against humeral elevation[105] and contributes to anterior stability of the GH joint by resisting torsional forces when the shoulder is abducted and externally rotated.[9,170] Neuromuscular control, including movement awareness and motor response, underlies coordination of the dynamic restraints.[218,221]

Acromioclavicular Joint

The AC joint is a plane, triaxial joint that may or may not have a disk. The weak capsule is reinforced by the superior and inferior AC ligaments (see Fig. 17.2). The convex articular surface is a facet on the lateral end of the clavicle and the concave articular surface is a facet on the acromion of the scapula.

Arthrokinematics

With motions of the scapula, the concave acromial surface slides in the same direction in which the scapula moves. Motions affecting this joint include upward rotation (the scapula turns so the glenoid fossa rotates upward), downward rotation, winging of the vertebral border (also called internal/external rotation), and tilting of the inferior angle.

Stability

The AC ligaments are supported by the strong coracoclavicular ligament. No muscles directly cross this joint for dynamic support.

Sternoclavicular Joint

The SC joint is an incongruent, triaxial, saddle-shaped joint with a disk. The joint is supported by the anterior and posterior SC ligaments and the interclavicular and costoclavicular ligaments (Fig. 17.4). The medial end of the clavicle is convex superior to inferior and concave anterior to posterior. The joint disk attaches superiorly. The superior-lateral portion of

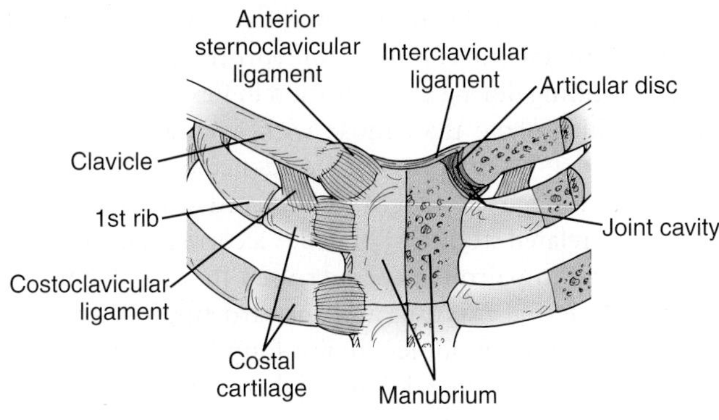

FIGURE 17.4 Ligaments of the sternoclavicular (SC) joint.

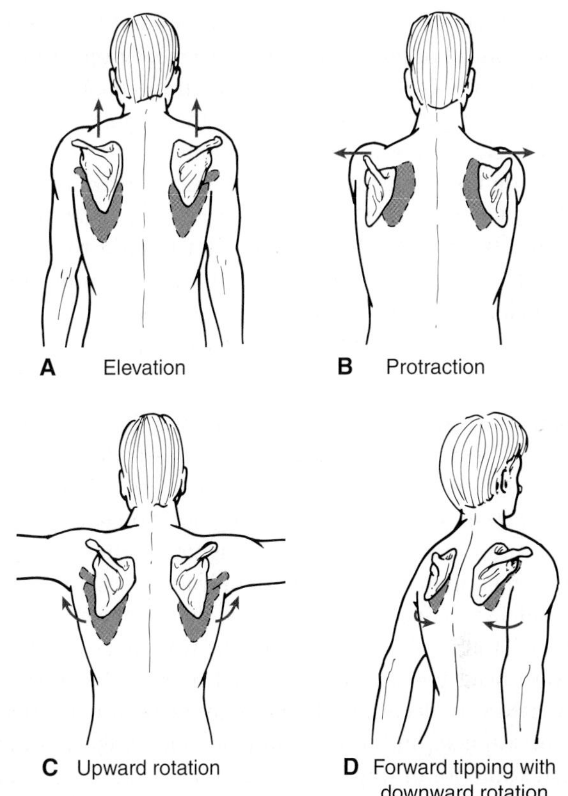

FIGURE 17.5 Scapular motions. **(A)** Elevation occurs with clavicular elevation at the SC joint when shrugging. **(B)** Protraction (abduction) occurs with clavicular abduction at the SC joint when reaching forward. **(C)** Upward rotation occurs with clavicular rotation at the SC and AC joints when flexing and abducting the shoulder. **(D)** Forward tilting (along with downward rotation) occurs at the AC joint when extending and internally rotating the shoulder.

the manubrium and first costal cartilage is concave superior to inferior and convex anterior to posterior.

Arthrokinematics

The motions of the clavicle occur as a result of the scapular motions of elevation, depression, protraction (abduction), and retraction (adduction). Rotation of the clavicle occurs as an accessory motion when the humerus is elevated above the horizontal position and the scapula upwardly rotates; it cannot occur as an isolated voluntary motion. The arthrokinematics of the SC joint are summarized in ONLINE Box 17.2 on the FA Davis website that supports this textbook.

Stability

The ligaments crossing the joint provide static stability. There are no muscles crossing the joint for dynamic stability.[40]

Functional Articulations

Scapulothoracic Articulation

Normally, there is considerable soft tissue flexibility, allowing the scapula to slide along the thorax and contribute to all upper extremity motions.

Motions of the Scapula

- *Elevation, depression, protraction, and retraction*: These motions are seen with clavicular motions at the SC joint (Fig. 17.5 A and B). Elevation and depression occur in the frontal plane as the scapula moves upward and downward, respectively; protraction/retraction occur in the transverse plane as the scapula moves away from or toward the spinal column. They are also component motions when the humerus moves.
- *Upward and downward rotation:* These motions are seen with clavicular motions at the SC joint and rotation at the AC joint and occur concurrently in various planes with motions of the humerus (Fig. 17.5 C). Upward rotation along with posterior tilting and external rotation of the scapula are component motions that occur with full shoulder range of motion (ROM) of elevation (flexion, scapular plane abduction, and frontal-plane abduction of the humerus).[60,131]
- *Internal and external rotation and tilting:* These motions are seen with motion at the AC joint concurrently with motions of the humerus (Fig. 17.5 D). Internal and external rotations are transverse plane motions in which the medial border lifts away from (wings) or approximates the rib cage, respectively. Anterior tilting of the scapula occurs in conjunction with internal rotation and extension of the humerus when reaching the hand behind the back, while posterior tilting occurs during humeral elevation.[64,133]

Scapular Stability

Postural relationship. In the dependent position, the scapula is stabilized primarily through a balance of forces. The weight of the arm creates a downward rotation, protraction, and forward tilting moment on the scapula. These moments are balanced by the support of the upper trapezius, serratus anterior, rhomboids, and middle trapezius[116,181] (see Table 17.1).

Active arm motions. With active arm motions, the muscles of the scapula function in synchrony to stabilize and control the position of the scapula, so the scapulohumeral muscles can maintain an effective length-tension relationship as they function to stabilize and move the humerus. Without the positional control of the scapula, the efficiency of the humeral muscles decreases. The upper and lower trapezius along with the serratus anterior upwardly rotate the scapula whenever the arm elevates, and the serratus anterior protracts the scapula on the thorax to align the scapula during flexion or pushing activities. During arm extension or during pulling activities, the rhomboids function to downwardly rotate and retract the scapula in synchrony with the latissimus dorsi, teres major, and rotator cuff muscles. These stabilizing muscles also eccentrically control acceleration of upward rotation and protraction of the scapula.[157]

Faulty posture. A slouched posture significantly alters scapular kinematics. Specifically, sitting or standing with increased thoracic kyphosis decreases posterior tilting and external rotation of the scapula during elevation of the arm.[60] Furthermore, with faulty scapular alignment, muscle length and strength imbalances occur not only in the scapular muscles, but also in the humeral muscles, altering the mechanics of the GH joint. A forward tilt of the scapula (seen with a forward head posture and increased thoracic kyphosis) is associated with decreased flexibility in the pectoralis minor, levator scapulae, and scalenus muscles and weakness in the serratus anterior or trapezius muscles. This scapular posture also changes the posture of the humerus in the glenoid, which assumes a relatively abducted and internally rotated position with respect to the scapula (Fig. 17.6). The GH internal rotators may become less flexible, and external rotators may weaken, affecting the mechanics of the joint.

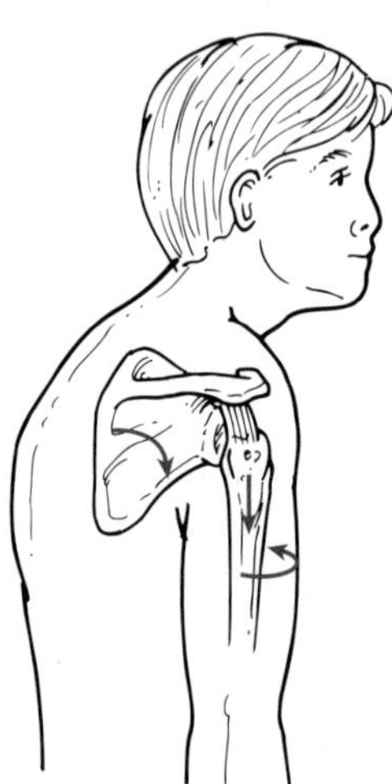

FIGURE 17.6 Faulty forward head, thoracic kyphosis, and shoulder girdle posture result in a forward tilt and downward rotation of the scapula with relative abduction and internal rotation of the humerus when the arm is in a dependent position.

FOCUS ON EVIDENCE

A study by Borstad and Ludewig,[15] which looked at the effect of pectoralis minor resting length on scapular kinematics in subjects without shoulder pain, documented that those individuals with a shorter pectoralis minor ($n = 25$) had greater scapular internal rotation (protraction) and less posterior tilting during arm elevation in flexion, abduction, and scapular plane than those with a longer pectoralis minor ($n = 25$), thus providing evidence for altered pectoralis minor muscle length and altered scapular movement. In a related study by Borstad,[16] a correlation between the postural impairments of increased thoracic kyphosis, scapular internal rotation and forward tipping, and decreased pectoralis minor length was found to be significant, further supporting the relationship between muscle length and posture.

Suprahumeral (Subacromial) Space

The coracoacromial arch, composed of the acromion and coracoacromial ligament, overlies the subacromial/subdeltoid bursa, the supraspinatus tendon, and a portion of the muscle (Fig. 17.7).[116] These structures allow for and participate in normal shoulder function. Compromise of this space from faulty muscle function, faulty postural relationships, faulty joint mechanics, injury to the soft tissue in this region, or structural anomalies of the acromion lead to impingement syndromes.[15,101,109,114,130,233] After a rotator cuff tear, the bursa may communicate with the GH joint cavity.[44]

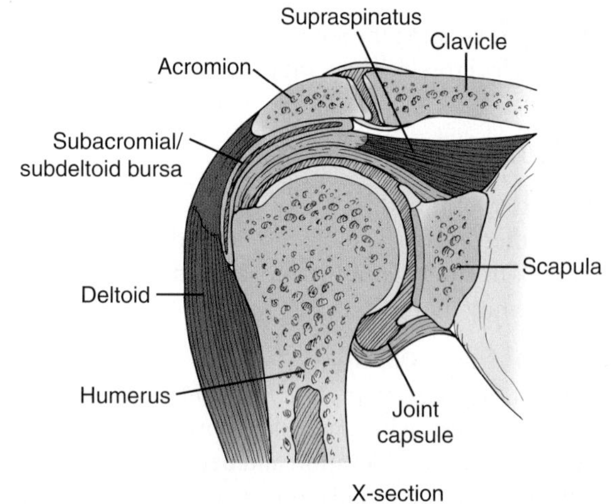

FIGURE 17.7 The supraspinatus and subacromial/subdeltoid bursa lie in the suprahumeral space.

Shoulder Girdle Function

Scapulohumeral Rhythm

Motion of the scapula, synchronous with motions of the humerus, allows for 150° to 180° of shoulder ROM into flexion or abduction with elevation. The ratio has considerable variation among individuals but is commonly accepted to average 2:1 (2° of GH motion to 1° of scapular rotation) at the end of full arm elevation. During the setting phase (0° to 30° abduction, 0° to 60° flexion), motion is primarily at the GH joint, whereas the scapula seeks a stable position. During the midrange of humeral motion, the scapula has greater motion, approaching a 1:1 ratio with the humerus; later in the range, the GH joint again dominates the motion.[38,116,187]

- Early studies analyzed only upward rotation of the scapula. More recent three-dimensional research demonstrated component scapular motions to be upward rotation, posterior tilting, and scapular external rotation with full shoulder elevation (flexion, scapular plane abduction, and frontal-plane abduction of the humerus).[101,131]
- During humeral elevation, the synchronous motion of the scapula allows the muscles moving the humerus to maintain an effective length-tension relationship throughout the activity and helps maintain congruency between the humeral head and fossa while decreasing shear forces.[38,116,187]
- The upper and lower trapezius and the serratus anterior muscles create upward rotation of the scapula. Weakness or complete paralysis of these muscles results in the scapula rotating downward by the contracting deltoid and supraspinatus as abduction or flexion is attempted. These two muscles then reach active insufficiency, and functional elevation of the arm cannot be reached, even though there may be normal passive ROM and normal strength in the shoulder abductor and flexor muscles.[187]
- During elevation of the humerus, the pectoralis minor is lengthened as the scapula upwardly rotates, retracts, and tips posteriorly. Restricted scapular movement during humeral elevation from a shortened pectoralis minor results in patterns similar to those seen in patients with impingement symptoms and could be a risk factor for development of the syndrome.[15]

Clavicular Elevation and Rotation With Humeral Motion

It is commonly accepted that the first 30° of upward rotation of the scapula occurs with elevation of the clavicle at the SC joint. Then, as the coracoclavicular ligament becomes taut, the clavicle rotates 38° to 55° about its longitudinal axis, which elevates its acromial end (because it is crank shaped). This motion allows the scapula to rotate an additional 30° at the AC joint.[116] Loss of any of these functional components decreases the amount of scapular rotation and thus the ROM of the upper extremity.

FOCUS ON EVIDENCE

A three-dimensional study[115] of clavicular motion during humeral flexion, scapular plane elevation of the arm, and abduction to 115° using surface electromagnetic sensors on 30 asymptomatic subjects and 9 individuals with shoulder pathology documented 11° to 15° of clavicular elevation, 15° to 29° of retraction, and 15° to 31° of posterior long axis rotation, showing similar patterns but different ranges from previously reported studies. Ranges of clavicular motion above 115° were not reliable, owing to movement of the clavicle under the skin.

External Rotation of the Humerus With Elevation

During elevation of the arm, the humerus externally rotates; this allows the greater tubercle of the humerus to clear the coracoacromial arch. Weak infraspinatus and teres minor muscles or inadequate external rotation may result in impingement of the soft tissues in the suprahumeral space, causing pain, inflammation, and eventually loss of function.

FOCUS ON EVIDENCE

An *in vivo* study of elevation in flexion, in the plane of the scapula, and in abduction demonstrated approximately 55° external rotation in all planes.[189] During abduction, external rotation occurred up to 125° followed by some internal rotation; during forward flexion, external rotation occurred until 50° and then plateaued. Lastly, external rotation occurred again from 110° to 160°. During elevation in the scapular plane, external rotation occurred throughout.

Deltoid–Short Rotator Cuff and Supraspinatus Mechanisms

Most of the force produced by the deltoid muscle causes upward translation of the humerus; if unopposed, it leads to impingement of the soft tissues in the suprahumeral space between the humeral head and the coracoacromial arch.

- The combined effect of the short rotator muscles (infraspinatus, teres minor, and subscapularis) produces stabilizing compression and downward translation of the humerus in the glenoid.
- The combined actions of the deltoid and short rotators result in a balance of forces that elevate the humerus and control the humeral head.
- The supraspinatus muscle has a significant stabilizing, compressive, and slight upward translation effect on the humerus during arm elevation. It functions with the deltoid in humeral elevation.
- Interruption of the coordinated function of these mechanisms may lead to tissue microtrauma and shoulder complex dysfunction.

Referred Pain and Nerve Injury

For a detailed description of referred pain patterns, peripheral nerve injuries in the shoulder, thoracic outlet syndrome (TOS), and complex regional pain syndromes and their management, see Chapter 13.

Common Sources of Referred Pain in the Shoulder Region

Cervical Spine

- Vertebral joints between C3 and C4 or between C4 and C5
- Nerve roots C4 or C5

Referred Pain From Related Tissues

- Dermatome C4 is over the trapezius to the tip of the shoulder.
- Dermatome C5 is over the deltoid region and lateral arm.
- Diaphragm: pain perceived in the upper trapezius region.
- Heart: pain perceived in the left axilla and pectoral region.
- Gallbladder: pain perceived at the tip of shoulder and scapular region.

Nerve Disorders in the Shoulder Girdle Region

Brachial plexus in the thoracic outlet. Common sites for compression are the scalene triangle and the costoclavicular space and under the coracoid process and pectoralis minor muscle.[104]

Suprascapular nerve in the suprascapular notch. This injury occurs from either direct compression or from nerve stretch, such as when carrying a heavy book bag over the shoulder.

Radial nerve in the axilla. Compression occurs from continual pressure, such as when leaning on axillary crutches.

Management of Shoulder Disorders and Surgeries

To make sound clinical decisions when managing patients with shoulder disorders, it is necessary to understand the various pathologies, surgical procedures, and associated precautions and to identify impairments, functional limitations, and possible disabilities. In this section, common pathologies and surgeries are presented, and the conservative and postoperative management of these conditions are described.

Joint Hypomobility: Nonoperative Management

Glenohumeral Joint

Restricted mobility of the GH joint may occur as a result of pathology, such as rheumatoid arthritis (RA) or osteoarthritis (OA); from prolonged immobilization; or from unknown causes (idiopathic frozen shoulder). Concurrent impairments in muscle performance and connective tissue mobility in the cervical and shoulder girdle region may also be present.

Related Pathologies and Etiology of Symptoms

RA and OA (degenerative arthritis). These disorders follow the clinical pictures described in Chapter 11.

Traumatic arthritis. This disorder occurs in response to a fall or high force blow to the shoulder.

Postimmobilization arthritis or stiff shoulder. This disorder occurs with lack of movement or as a secondary effect from conditions such as heart disease, stroke, or diabetes mellitus.

Idiopathic frozen shoulder. This disorder, which is also called *adhesive capsulitis* or *periarthritis,* is characterized by the development of dense adhesions, capsular thickening, and capsular restrictions, especially in the dependent folds of the capsule, rather than arthritic changes in the cartilage and bone, as seen with RA or OA. The onset is insidious and usually occurs between the ages of 40 and 65 years; there is no known cause (primary frozen shoulder), although problems already mentioned in which there is a period of pain and/or restricted motion, such as with RA, OA, trauma, or immobilization, may lead to a frozen shoulder (secondary frozen shoulder). With primary frozen shoulder, the pathogenesis may be a provoking chronic inflammation in musculotendinous or synovial tissue, such as the rotator cuff, biceps tendon, or joint capsule.[40,70,100,145,148] Patients with diabetes mellitus and thyroid disease are at increased risk for developing the disorder.[97]

Clinical Signs and Symptoms

GH joint arthritis. The following characteristics are typically associated with GH joint arthritis that leads to hypomobility.

- *Acute phase.* Pain and protective muscle guarding limit motion, usually external rotation and abduction. Pain frequently radiates distal to the elbow and may disturb sleep. Owing to the depth of the GH capsule, joint swelling is not detected, although tenderness can be elicited by palpating in the sulcus immediately below the edge of the acromion process between the attachments of the posterior and middle deltoid.
- *Subacute phase.* Capsular tightness, consistent with a capsular pattern (external rotation and abduction are most limited, and internal rotation and flexion are least limited), often begins to develop. The patient may feel pain as the

end of the limited range is reached. Passive accessory motion testing reveals limited joint play. If the patient can be treated as the acute condition begins to subside by gradually increasing shoulder motion and activity, the complication of joint and soft tissue contractures can usually be minimized.[139,145]

- *Chronic phase.* Progressive restriction of the GH joint capsule magnifies the signs of limited motion in a capsular pattern and decreased joint play. There is significant loss of function with an inability to reach overhead, outward, or behind the back. Pain is often localized to the deltoid region.

Idiopathic frozen shoulder. This clinical entity progresses through a series of four stages following a classic continuum.[40,70,100,144,145,148]

- **Stage 1.** Characterized by a gradual onset of pain that increases with movement and is present at night. Loss of external rotation motion with intact rotator cuff strength is common. The duration of this stage is usually less than 3 months.
- **Stage 2** (Often referred to as the *"Freezing" Stage).* Characterized by persistent and more intense pain even at rest. Motion is limited in all directions and cannot be fully restored with an intra-articular injection. This stage is typically between 3 and 9 months after onset.
- **Stage 3** (*"Frozen" Stage).* Characterized by pain only with movement, significant adhesions, and limited GH motions. Excessive scapulothoracic movement is a typical compensation. Atrophy of the deltoid, rotator cuff, biceps, and triceps brachii muscles may be noted. This stage occurs between 9 and 15 months after onset.
- **Stage 4** (*"Thawing" Stage).* Characterized by minimal pain and no synovitis but significant capsular restrictions from adhesions. Motion may gradually improve during this stage. This stage lasts from 15 to 24 months after onset, although some patients never regain normal ROM.

Some references indicate that spontaneous recovery occurs, on average, 2 years from onset,[70] although others report long-term limitations without spontaneous recovery.[173] Inappropriately aggressive therapy at the wrong time may prolong the symptoms.[13] Management guidelines are progressed based on the continuum of stages[100] and are the same as for acute (maximum protection during stages 1 and 2), subacute (controlled motion during stage 3), and chronic (return to function during stage 4) joint pathology described in this section.

Common Impairments of Structure and Function

- Night pain and disturbed sleep during acute flares
- Pain on motion and often at rest during acute flares
- Mobility: decreased joint play and ROM, usually limiting external rotation and abduction with some limitation of internal rotation and flexion
- Posture: possible faulty postural compensations with protracted and anteriorly tilted scapula, rounded shoulders, or guarding the painful shoulder in a position of scapula elevation and arm adduction
- Decreased arm swing during gait
- Muscle performance: general muscle weakness and poor endurance in the GH muscles with overuse of the scapular muscles leading to pain in the trapezius, levator scapulae, and posterior cervical muscles
- Increased scapulothoracic motion during arm movements to compensate for limited GH mobility

Common Activity Limitations and Participation Restrictions

- Inability to reach overhead, behind head, out to the side, and behind back leading to difficulty dressing (putting on a jacket or coat or in the case of women, fastening undergarments behind their back), reaching hand into back pocket of pants (to retrieve wallet), reaching out a car window (to use an ATM machine), self-grooming (combing hair, brushing teeth, washing face), and bringing eating utensils to the mouth
- Difficulty lifting heavy objects above shoulder level
- Limited ability to sustain repetitive activities

GH Joint Hypomobility: Management—Protection Phase

See General Guidelines for Management When Symptoms Are Acute in Chapter 10 and Box 10.1.

Educate the Patient

- Provide information about what to expect regarding the stages of healing.
- Instruct patient in safe motions and activity modifications that minimize joint stress.

Control Pain, Edema, and Muscle Guarding

- The joint may be immobilized in a sling to provide rest and minimize pain.
- Intermittent periods of passive or assisted motion within the pain free/protected ROM and gentle joint oscillation techniques to minimize further adhesions are initiated as soon as the patient tolerates movement.
- Gentle soft tissue mobilization of the cervical and periscapular muscles may improve patient comfort and minimize protective guarding, as may cervical ROM and/or cervical grade I or II passive intervertebral mobilizations.

Maintain Soft Tissue and Joint Integrity and Mobility

PRECAUTION: If there is increased pain or irritability in the joint after use of the following techniques, either the dosage was too strong or the techniques should be modified by decreasing the range of passive movement or delaying joint glides.

CONTRAINDICATION: If there are mechanical restrictions causing limited motion, appropriate tissue stretching should be initiated only *after* the inflammation subsides.

- *Passive ROM (PROM)* in all ranges of pain-free motion (see Chapter 3). As pain decreases, the patient is progressed to active ROM with or without assistance, using activities such as rolling a small ball or sliding a rag on a smooth table top. Planar, multiplanar and circular motions can be given to move the shoulder to the end range of its available motions. Be sure the patient is taught proper mechanics and to avoid faulty patterns, such as scapular elevation or a slumped posture.

- *Passive joint distraction and glides, grade I and II* with the joint placed in a pain-free position (see Chapter 5).
- *Pendulum (Codman's) exercises* are techniques that use the effects of gravity to distract the humerus from the glenoid fossa.[28,31] They help relieve pain through gentle traction and oscillating movements (grade II) and provide early motion of joint structures and synovial fluid. No weight is used during this phase of treatment (see Fig. 17.22).

CLINICAL TIP

Many patients perform pendulum exercises incorrectly by using the GH muscles to initiate shoulder motion and by performing large excursion of motion. The technique must be taught as small, gentle pendular motions initiated with body swaying while keeping the shoulder muscles relaxed.[113]

- *Gentle muscle setting* to all muscle groups of the shoulder and adjacent regions, including cervical and elbow muscles because of their close association with the shoulder complex. Instructions are given to the patient to gently contract a group of muscles while slight manual resistance is applied—just enough to stimulate a muscle contraction without provoking pain. The emphasis is on rhythmic contracting and relaxing of the muscles to stimulate blood flow and prevent circulatory stasis.

Maintain Integrity and Function of Associated Regions

- Complex regional pain syndrome type I is a potential complication after shoulder injury or immobility. Therefore, additional exercises, such as having the patient repetitively squeeze a ball or other soft object, may be given for the hand.
- The patient is educated on the importance of keeping the joints distal to the shoulder complex as active and mobile as possible. The patient or family member is taught to perform ROM exercises of the elbow, forearm, wrist, and fingers several times each day while the shoulder is immobilized. If tolerated, active or gentle resistive ROM is preferred to passive ROM for a greater effect on circulation and muscle integrity.
- If edema is noted in the hand, instruct the patient to elevate the hand above the level of the heart whenever possible.
- Cervical ROM (active and/or passive), intervertebral joint mobilizations, and soft tissue mobilization should also be considered.

CLINICAL TIP

For conditions in which there is potential for a prolonged acute/inflammatory stage, such as with RA and during stages I or II of idiopathic frozen shoulder, it is critical to teach the patient active-assistive exercises to maintain muscle and joint integrity and as much mobility as possible without exacerbating the symptoms.

GH Joint Hypomobility: Management—Controlled Motion Phase

When symptoms are subacute, follow the guidelines as described in Chapter 10, Box 10.2, emphasizing joint mobility, neuromuscular control, and instructions to the patient for self-care.

Control Pain, Edema, and Joint Effusion

- *Functional activities.* It is important to carefully monitor activities. If the joint is immobilized, the amount of time the shoulder is free to move each day is progressively increased.
- *ROM.* GH and scapula motions are progressed up to the point of pain. The patient is instructed in the use of self-assistive ROM techniques, such as wand exercises or hand slides on a table.

PRECAUTION: With increased pain or decreased motion after these techniques, the activity may be too intense or the patient may be using faulty mechanics. Reassess the technique and modify it by restricting the joint to a safer ROM, correcting faulty movements, or altering the intensity, frequency, and/or duration of the technique.

Progressively Increase Joint and Soft Tissue Mobility

- *Passive joint mobilization techniques.* Grade III sustained or grade III and IV oscillations that focus on the restricted capsular tissue at the end of the available ROM are used to increase joint capsule mobility[94,207] (see Figs. 5.15 to 5.20 in Chapter 5 and ONLINE Box 17.1). End-of-range techniques include rotating the humerus and then applying either a grade III distraction or a grade III glide to stretch the restrictive capsular tissue or adhesions (see Figs. 5.17, 5.21, and 17.20).
  - Use a grade I distraction with all gliding techniques. If the joint is irritable and gliding in the direction of restriction is not tolerated, glide in the opposite direction. As pain and irritability decrease, begin to glide in the direction of restriction.[94]

FOCUS ON EVIDENCE

Evidence supporting joint mobilization techniques is limited. A multiple-subject case study, using seven subjects with adhesive capsulitis of the GH joint (mean disease duration 8.4 months, range 3 to 12 months) treated with end-range mobilization techniques twice a week for 3 months, showed increased active and passive range and increased capacity of the joint capsule at the end of treatment and at the 9-month follow-up. No control groups were used; therefore, the natural course of the disease could not be excluded as the explanation for improvement.[207]

A follow-up study by the same author randomly assigned 100 subjects with stage II adhesive capsulitis to a group receiving high-grade mobilization techniques (end-range stretching using Maitland grade III or IV) or a group receiving low-grade mobilization techniques (Maitland grade I or II). After 3 months of treatment, both groups exhibited clinically significant improvement, with the group receiving the high-grade mobilization techniques showing greater improvement than the low-grade mobilization group. Because there was no control group, natural progression could not be ruled out.[208]

A study exploring the effect of the direction of joint mobilization demonstrated that a posterior glide was more effective than an anterior glide to increase GH external rotation ROM. Patients with stage II to IV primary adhesive capsulitis received distraction plus grade III sustained mobilizations, held for at least 1 minute, with treatment duration of 15 minutes, for six treatment sessions. Anterior mobilizations were progressed by placing the humerus at end-range abduction and external rotation, while posterior mobilizations were progressed by placing the humerus at end-range flexion and external rotation. At the end of the sixth visit, subjects in the anterior mobilization group (n = 10) increased external rotation ROM by 3.0°, while those in the posterior mobilization group (n = 8) increased by 31.3°, a difference that was statistically significant.[93]

PRECAUTION: Carefully monitor the joint reaction to the mobilization stretches; if irritability increases, grade III or IV techniques should not be undertaken until the chronic stage of healing.

- *Self-mobilization techniques.* The following self-mobilization techniques may be used for a home program.
  - CAUDAL GLIDE. *Patient position and procedure:* Sitting on a firm surface and grasping the fingers under the edge. The patient then leans the trunk away from the stabilized arm (Fig. 17.8).
  - ANTERIOR GLIDE. *Patient position and procedure:* Sitting with both arms behind the body or lying supine supported on a solid surface. The patient then leans the body weight between the arms (Fig. 17.9).
  - POSTERIOR GLIDE. *Patient position and procedure:* Prone, propped up on both elbows. The body weight shifts downward between the arms (Fig. 17.10).
- *Manual stretching.* Manual stretching techniques are used to increase mobility in shortened muscles and related connective tissue.
- *Self-stretching exercises.* As the joint reaction becomes predictable and the patient begins to tolerate stretching, self-stretching techniques are taught (see Figs. 17.24 through 17.29 in the Exercise section).

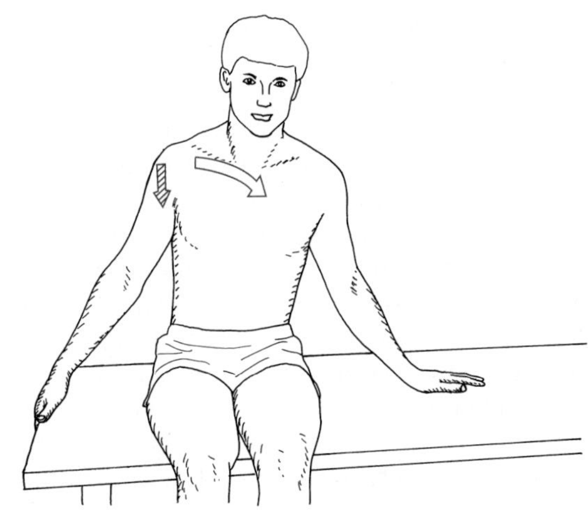

FIGURE 17.8 Self-mobilization. Caudal glide of the humerus occurs as the person leans away from the fixed arm.

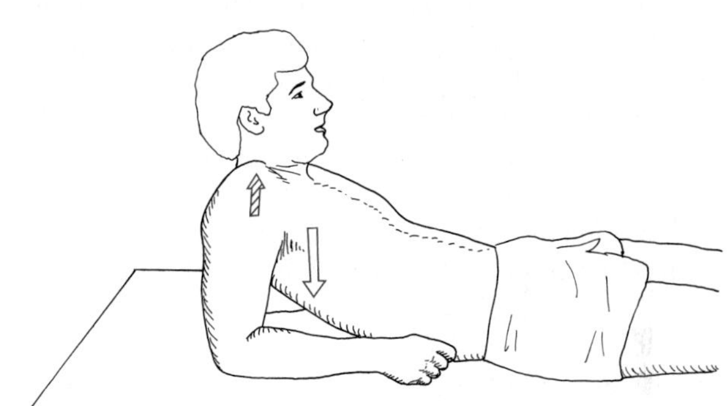

FIGURE 17.9 Self-mobilization. Anterior glide of the humerus occurs as the person leans between the fixed arms.

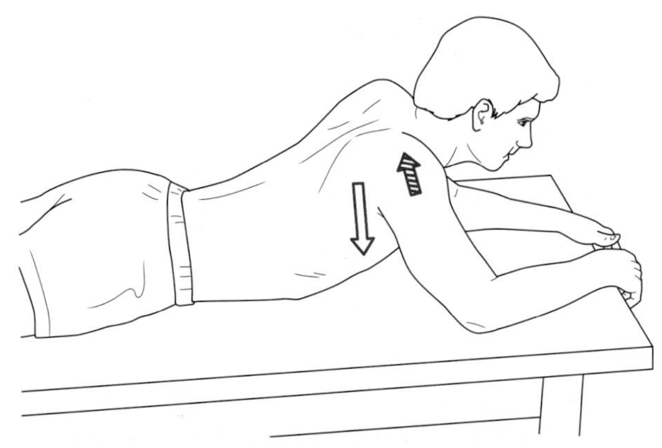

FIGURE 17.10 Self-mobilization. Posterior glide of the humerus occurs as the person shifts his weight downward between the fixed arms.

Inhibit Muscle Spasm and Correct Faulty Mechanics

Muscle spasm may lead to a faulty deltoid-rotator cuff mechanism and altered scapulohumeral rhythm when the patient attempts arm elevation (Fig. 17.11). Greater relative deltoid activation may result in superior humeral head translation and impingement of the greater tuberosity on the coracoacromial arch, making it difficult and/or painful to elevate the arm. In this case, repositioning the humeral head with a caudal glide is necessary before proceeding with any other form of shoulder exercise. The patient must also learn to recognize and avoid "hiking the shoulder" when at rest or when elevating the arm. The following techniques may address these problems. See also Mobilization with Movement Techniques in the next section.

- Gentle joint oscillation techniques (grade I or II) to help decrease the muscle spasm.
- Sustained caudal glide joint techniques to reposition the humeral head in the glenoid fossa.
- Protected weight bearing, such as leaning hands against a wall or on a table, to stimulate rotator cuff and scapula stabilizer co-contraction and improve synovial fluid movement through hyaline cartilage compression. Techniques are progressed by gentle rocking forward/backward and side to side, moving from bilateral to unilateral, increasing the angle of the joint, or adding perturbations.
- GH internal/external rotation strengthening to facilitate stabilization of the humeral head (see Fig. 17.52).
- Movement retraining to minimize the substitution pattern of scapular elevation can be initiated by providing the visual feedback of a mirror or the tactile feedback of the opposite hand placed on the ipsilateral upper trapezius.

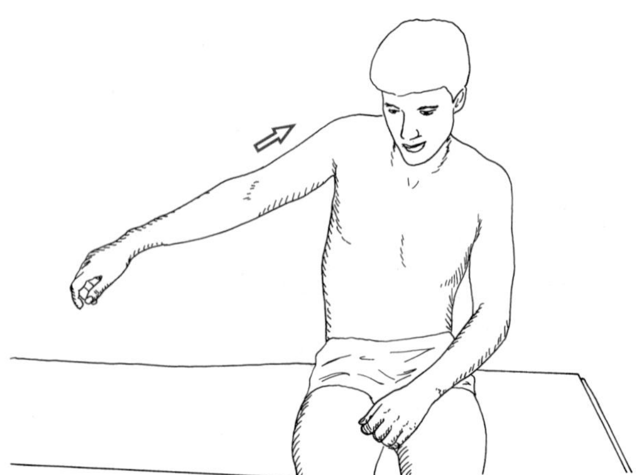

FIGURE 17.11 Poor mechanics with the patient hiking the shoulder while attempting to abduct the arm. This results in limited scapula upward rotation and increased superior humeral head translations.

Improve Joint Tracking

Mobilization with movement (MWM) techniques may assist with retraining muscle function for proper tracking of the humeral head.[136]

- *Shoulder MWM for painful restriction of shoulder external rotation* (Fig. 17.12).
  - *Patient position:* Supine lying with folded towel under the scapula; the elbow is near the side and flexed to 90°. A cane is held in both hands.

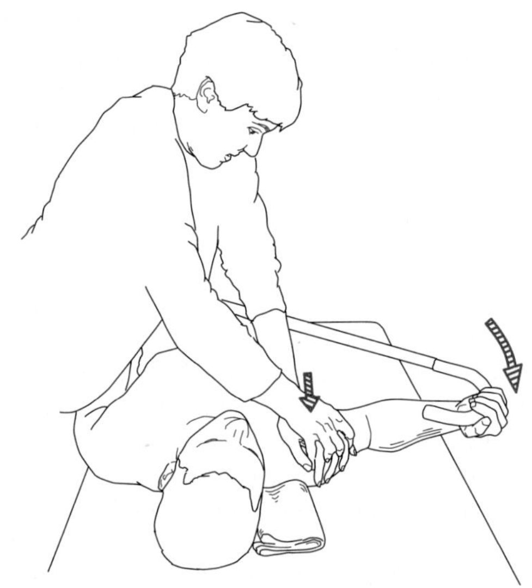

FIGURE 17.12 Mobilization with movement (MWM) to improve GH joint external rotation. A posterolateral glide is applied to the humeral head while the patient pushes the arm into the end-range of external rotation with a cane.

  - *Therapist position and procedure:* Stand on the opposite side of the bed facing the patient and reach across the patient's torso to cup the anteromedial aspect of the head of the humerus with reinforced hands. Apply a pain-free graded posterolateral glide of the humeral head on the glenoid. Instruct the patient to use the cane to push the affected arm into the previously restricted range of external rotation. Sustain the movement for 10 seconds and repeat in sets of 5 to 10. It is important to maintain the elbow near the side of the trunk and ensure that no pain is experienced during the procedure. Adjust the grade and direction of the glide as needed to achieve pain-free function.
- *Shoulder MWM for painful restriction of internal rotation* and inability to reach the hand behind the back (Fig. 17.13).
  - *Patient position:* Standing with a towel draped over the unaffected upper trapezius and affected hand at current range of maximum pain-free position behind back. The patient's hand on the affected side grasps the towel behind the back.

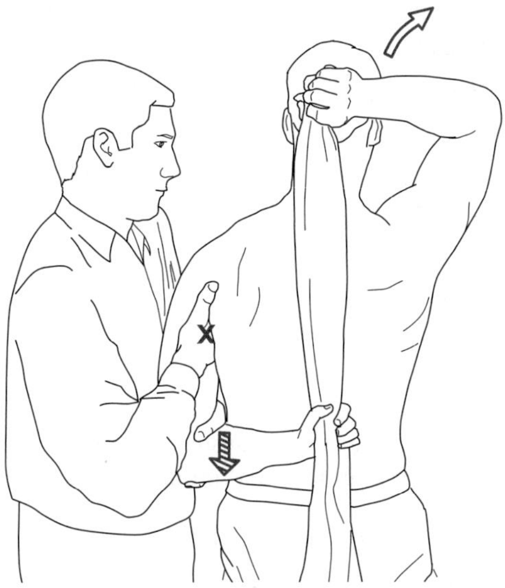

FIGURE 17.13 MWM to improve GH joint internal rotation. An inferior glide is applied to the humerus while the patient pulls the hand up the back with a towel.

- *Therapist position and procedure:* Stand facing the patient's affected side. Place the hand closest to the patient's back high up in the axilla with the palm facing outward to stabilize the scapula with an upward and inward pressure. With the hand closest to the patient's abdomen, hook the thumb in the cubital fossa and grasp the lower humerus to provide an inferior glide. Your abdomen is in contact with the patient's elbow to provide an adduction force to the arm. Have the patient pull on the towel with the unaffected hand to draw the affected hand up the back while the mobilization force is being applied in an inferior direction. Ensure that no pain is experienced during the procedure. Adjust the grade and direction of glide as needed to achieve pain-free function. Maximal glide should be applied to achieve end-range loading.

- *Shoulder MWM for painful arc or impingement signs.* If impingement signs are present in addition to the capsular restrictions, the MWM active elevation technique may be appropriate. (See Fig. 17.17 and description in the impingement section.)

Improve Muscle Performance

- Faulty postures or shoulder girdle mechanics when moving the upper extremity, such as scapula elevation or protraction or excessive trunk movement, should first be identified and corrected. Manual techniques, stretches, and strengthening exercises are initiated to correct muscle length or strength imbalances, followed by an emphasis on developing active control of weak musculature. As the patient learns to activate the weak muscles, progress to strengthening in functional patterns.
- Because faulty postures or shoulder girdle mechanics may be impacted by impaired trunk strength or control, an emphasis on trunk stability should also be considered. Exercises to manage faulty spinal posture are described in Chapter 16, with active cervical retraction and thoracic extension especially important for shoulder function.
- After proper mechanics are restored, the patient should perform active ROM of all shoulder motions daily and return to functional activities to the extent tolerated.

GH Joint Hypomobility: Management—Return to Function Phase

For joint impairments in the chronic stage, follow the guidelines described in Chapter 10, Box 10.4.

Progressively Increase Flexibility and Strength

- Stretching and strengthening exercises are progressed as the joint tissue tolerates. The patient should be actively involved in self-stretching and strengthening by this time, so emphasis during treatment is on maintaining correct mechanics, safe progressions, and exercise strategies for return to function. Progressions may include increasing resistance and repetitions, performing exercises through multiple planes, adding perturbations, and incorporating regional muscle groups (such as the trunk) into dynamic exercises.
- If capsular tissue is still restricting ROM, vigorous manual stretching and joint mobilization techniques are applied.

Prepare for Functional Demands

If the patient is involved in repetitive heavy lifting, pushing, pulling, carrying, or reaching, exercises are progressed to replicate these demands. See the last section of this chapter and Chapter 23 for suggestions.

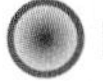

FOCUS ON EVIDENCE

The ***Clinical Practice Guidelines (CPGs) for Shoulder Pain and Mobility Deficits from Adhesive Capsulitis*** published by the Orthopaedic Section of the American Physical Therapy Association summarizes research and makes treatment recommendations supporting patient education (moderate evidence), GH joint mobilization (weak evidence), modalities (weak evidence), translational manipulation (weak evidence), and stretching exercises (moderate evidence) for treating this patient population.[97]

GH Joint Management: Postmanipulation Under Anesthesia

Occasionally, no progress is made and the physician chooses to perform manipulation under anesthesia. Following this procedure there is an inflammatory reaction and the joint is treated as an acute lesion. If possible, joint mobility and passive ROM techniques are initiated while the patient is still in the recovery room. Surgical intervention with incision of the dependent capsular fold may be used if the adhesions are not broken with the manipulation. Postoperative treatment is the same with the following considerations.[148]

- The arm is kept elevated overhead in abduction and external rotation during the inflammatory reaction stage; treatment principles progress as with any joint lesion.
- Therapeutic exercises are initiated the same day while the patient is still in the recovery room, with emphasis on internal and external rotation in the 90° (or higher) abducted position.
- Joint mobilization procedures are used, particularly a caudal glide, to prevent re-adherence of the inferior capsular fold.
- When sleeping, the patient may be required to position the arm in abduction for up to 3 weeks after manipulation.

Acromioclavicular and Sternoclavicular Joints

Related Pathologies and Etiology of Symptoms

Overuse syndromes. Overuse syndromes of the AC joint may result from repeated stressful joint movements with the arm at waist level, such as with grinding, packing assembly, and construction work,[71] or repeated diagonal extension, adduction, and internal rotation motions, as when spiking a volleyball or serving in tennis. The AC joint is susceptible to overuse syndromes in conjunction with arthritis or following a traumatic injury.

Subluxation or dislocation. Subluxation or dislocation of either the AC or SC joints is usually caused by falling on the shoulder or an outstretched arm. At the AC joint, the distal end of the clavicle often displaces posteriorly and superiorly on the acromion, and the ligaments supporting the AC joint may rupture.[147] After trauma and associated overstretching of the capsules and ligaments of either joint, hypermobility is usually permanent because there are almost no muscles that provide direct stability to these joints.

Hypomobility. Decreased clavicular mobility may occur with SC joint OA and may contribute to TOS by compromising the space available for the neuromuscular bundle as it courses between the clavicle and first rib (described in Chapter 13).

Common Impairments of Structure and Function

- Pain localized to the involved joint or ligament.
- Painful arc toward the end-range of shoulder elevation.
- Pain with shoulder horizontal adduction or abduction.
- Hypermobility if trauma or overuse is involved.
- Hypomobility if sustained posture, arthritis, or immobility is involved.

Common Activity Limitations and Participation Restrictions

- Limited ability to sustain repeated forceful movements of the arm, such as with grinding, packing, assembly, and construction work.[71]
- Inability to reach overhead or perform repetitive overhead activities without pain.

Nonoperative Management of AC or SC Joint Strain or Hypermobility

- Minimize joint loading by supporting the weight of the arm with a sling.
- Cross-fiber massage to the capsule or ligaments.
- Maintain ROM of the GH joint and scapulothoracic articulation.
- Instruction in self-application of cross-fiber massage if joint symptoms occur after excessive activity.
- Increase strength of shoulder complex, trunk, and legs.
- Gradually return to functional activities.

Nonoperative Management of AC or SC Joint Hypomobility

Joint mobilization techniques are used to increase joint mobility (see Figs. 5.22 through 5.24).

Glenohumeral Joint Surgery and Postoperative Management

Severe deterioration of one or both surfaces of the GH joint or an acute or nonunion fracture of the proximal humerus often must be managed with surgical intervention. Underlying pathologies that cause advanced joint destruction include late-stage OA, RA, traumatic arthritis, cuff tear arthropathy, and osteonecrosis (avascular necrosis) of the head of the humerus.

The most common surgical procedure used to treat advanced shoulder joint pathology is *GH arthroplasty,* often simply referred to as *shoulder arthroplasty.*[34] In rare situations, *arthrodesis* (surgical ankylosis) of the GH joint may be necessary as an alternative to arthroplasty or as a salvage procedure.[124]

The goals of these surgical procedures and the postoperative rehabilitation program are to (1) relieve pain, (2) improve shoulder mobility or stability, and (3) restore or improve strength and functional use of the upper extremity. The extent to which these goals are achieved is predicated on the patient's participation in postoperative rehabilitation, the distinguishing features and severity of the underlying pathology; the prosthetic design and surgical techniques; the integrity of the rotator cuff mechanism and other soft tissues; and the age, overall health, and anticipated activity level of the patient.[33,124,179,185]

Glenohumeral Arthroplasty

GH arthroplasty falls into several categories, the most common of which are *total shoulder arthroplasty (TSA)*,[124,141,179,185] in which both the glenoid and humeral surfaces are replaced (Fig. 17.14), and *hemireplacement arthroplasty (hemiarthroplasty)*, in which only the humeral head is replaced.[59,124,143,179,234] *Reverse total shoulder arthroplasty (rTSA)* is another type of arthroplasty, typically used when rotator cuff integrity is compromised.[37,127,211] Other categories of shoulder arthroplasty include interpositional and resurfacing arthroplasties, which involve less extensive removal of bone.[124,179,185,202]

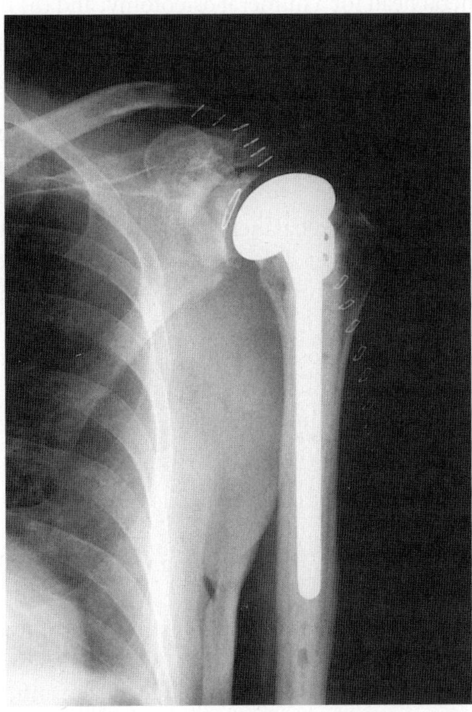

FIGURE 17.14 Postoperative anterior-posterior view of the shoulder showing a Neer II type of cemented humeral prosthesis and a nonmetal backed polyethylene glenoid. *(From Tovin, BJ, and Greenfield, BH:* Evaluation and Treatment of the Shoulder—An Integration of the Guide to Physical Therapist Practice. *Philadelphia: F.A. Davis, 2001, p 266, with permission.)*

Indications for Surgery

The following structural and functional impairments associated with these pathologies are widely accepted indications for GH arthroplasty.[33,49,123,124,141,143,179,185,194,215]

- Persistent and incapacitating pain (at rest or with activity) secondary to GH joint destruction is the primary indication for GH arthroplasty.
- Secondary indications include loss of shoulder mobility or stability and/or loss of upper extremity strength with an inability to perform functional tasks.

Procedures

Background

Implant design, materials, and fixation. Since the pioneering work of Neer during the 1960s and 1970s[141,143] prosthetic designs and surgical techniques for replacing the shoulder joint have continued to evolve. The designs of contemporary TSA hardware, composed of a high-density polyethylene glenoid component (usually all plastic) and a modular inert metal humeral component, closely approximate the biomechanical characteristics of the human shoulder.[227] The exception to this is the rTSA, the design of which reverses the native shoulder ball and socket relationship. Specifically, the glenoid fossa is replaced with a convex, "glenospherical" component attached to a glenoid base and the humeral head is replaced with a stemmed concave cup.[209] Fixation of the prosthetic components is achieved with cement, , bio-ingrowth, or a press fit. The type of fixation selected by the surgeon depends on the component, the underlying pathology, and the quality of the bone stock. Cement fixation is most often necessary in patients with osteoporosis.[33,123,124,227]

The designs of total shoulder replacements, ranging from *unconstrained* to *semiconstrained* to *constrained,* provide varying amounts of mobility and stability to the GH joint. Box 17.1 summarizes the characteristics of each of these designs.[33,123,124,176,179,185,202]

Selection of procedure. Controversy exists over the specific criteria for selection of TSA versus rTSA versus hemiarthroplasty, but in general it depends on the etiology and severity of joint deterioration and the condition of the periarticular soft tissues, particularly the rotator cuff mechanism.[124,186] Several examples that follow underscore the complexity of the clinical decision-making process involved in the choice of operative procedure and prosthetic design.

In patients with late-stage primary OA, the GH joint typically exhibits loss or thinning of the articular cartilage of the head of the humerus and the posterior portion of the glenoid fossa. The rotator cuff is intact in approximately 90% to 95% of these patients, making them good candidates for either TSA or hemiarthroplasty.[33,123,176,179,185] A recent meta-analysis found better functional outcomes in those receiving a TSA, but no differences in instability or revision rates between TSA and hemiarthroplasty.[48] Chronic synovitis associated with RA or other types of synovium-based arthritis tends to erode periarticular soft tissues in addition to joint articular surfaces. As a consequence, a full-thickness rotator cuff tendon tear (typically the supraspinatus) develops in 25% to 40% of these patients and a biceps tendon rupture in an even greater percentage.[59,176,185,202] If the soft tissues can be repaired and their functions improved, a semiconstrained TSA may be indicated. If an effective repair cannot be achieved, an rTSA is usually indicated. When there is insufficient bone stock for fixation of a glenoid implant, hemiarthroplasty is usually the procedure of choice.[59,124,176,179,186,202]

Hemiarthroplasty is often used when the articular surface and underlying bone of the humeral head have deteriorated,

BOX 17.1 Designs of Prosthetic Implants for Total Shoulder Arthroplasty

Unconstrained
- Anatomical design with a small, shallow glenoid component combined with a stemmed humeral component
- The most frequently used prosthetic design
- Provides the greatest freedom of shoulder motion but no inherent stability
- Indicated when the rotator cuff mechanism is intact or can be repaired to provide dynamic stability to the GH joint

Semiconstrained
- A larger glenoid component that is hooded or cup-shaped
- Some degree of joint stability inherent in the design
- Indicated when erosion of the glenoid fossa can be compensated for by reaming the fossa in conjunction with a functional rotator cuff; although deficient preoperatively, fossa can be improved by repair

Reversed Ball and Socket
- Small humeral socket that slides on a larger ball-shaped glenoid component
- Combines moderate stability with mobility for rotator cuff-deficient shoulders that cannot be repaired
- Provides an alternative to standard, semiconstrained total shoulder arthroplasty (TSA) and hemiarthroplasty

Constrained
- Fixed fulcrum, ball-in-socket designs with congruency of the glenoid and humeral components
- Greatest amount of inherent joint stability but less mobility than other designs
- Once thought to be an alternative to hemiarthroplasty for the selected patient with a deficient rotator cuff, cuff tear arthropathy, or chronic/recurrent GH joint dislocation after a previous TSR
- Rarely used today owing to high rate of loosening or failure of the components

but the glenoid fossa is reasonably intact, as seen with osteonecrosis.[33,124,185] For the patient with severe, chronic pain and loss of function as the result of a massive, irreparable cuff tear and subsequent *cuff tear arthropathy,* rTSA is usually indicated. (First used by Neer, the term "cuff tear arthropathy" refers to deterioration and eventual collapse of the head of the humerus, an infrequent but debilitating long-term result of a primary, massive, and irreparable tear of the rotator cuff.[124,176,215,234])

Chronic deficiency of the rotator cuff mechanism often leads to superior migration of the humeral head on the glenoid fossa. If a glenoid TSA component is inserted under these conditions, superior migration creates an incongruous articulation that can increase the risk of component loosening and premature wear of the glenoid implant.[32,79,176] The rTSA was developed to overcome this complication by minimizing translation between the glenosphere and humeral articular surfaces. Other features of the rTSA include reduced forces on the glenoid component, inherent stability owing to the congruency of the components, and increased deltoid moment arms. One limitation of the rTSA design is decreased GH ROM.[20,127,209]

Operative Procedures

TSA, rTSA, and hemiarthroplasty are open surgical procedures performed with the patient in a semi-reclining position. These operative procedures involve the following components:[33,59,124,179,185] (1) anterior approach using a deltopectoral incision that extends from the AC joint to the deltoid insertion for adequate surgical exposure; (2) release (tenotomy) of the subscapularis tendon from its proximal attachment on the lesser tuberosity; (3) anterior capsulotomy; (4) exposure of the humeral head for a humeral osteotomy; and (5) preparation of the humeral canal for insertion of the prosthetic implant. The glenoid fossa is either débrided or contoured to accept the implant for a TSA. After component placement, the subscapularis is then reattached and may be lengthened (medial advancement or Z-plasty) if external rotation ROM is limited.

Reconstruction and balancing of soft tissues is critical for optimal function after TSA, rTSA, and hemiarthroplasty. "Balancing" refers to the intraoperative lengthening or tightening of soft tissues to restore as near-normal resting tension in the tissues as possible, particularly in the rotator cuff, biceps, and deltoid muscle-tendon units.

Concurrent procedures that may be necessary during shoulder arthroplasty include:

- Repair of a deficient rotator cuff if the quality of the cuff tissue is sufficient.
- Capsular plication and tightening for chronic GH joint subluxation or dislocation.
- Anterior acromioplasty for a history of impingement syndrome.
- Bone graft of the glenoid if bone stock is insufficient for fixation of the glenoid implant.

After implantation of the prosthetic component(s) and repair of soft tissues but before closure of the skin incision, the shoulder is passively moved through all planes of motion to visually evaluate the stability of the prosthetic joint and the integrity of the repaired soft tissues. This determines the anatomical ROM possible after surgery and the aggressiveness of the postoperative program.[33,124]

Complications

Although the incidence of intraoperative and postoperative complications after current-day arthroplasty is low, even a single complication can adversely affect functional outcomes. The incidence of complications after TSA tends to be higher in patients with a deficient rotator cuff mechanism, osteoporosis, or a history of chronic GH joint instability.[78] Aside from medical complications such as infection or a deep vein thrombosis, complications specific to shoulder arthroplasty are noted in Box 17.2.[32,78]

BOX 17.2 Complications Specific to Glenohumeral Arthroplasty

Intraoperative Complications
- Insufficient lengthening of a tight subscapularis muscle-tendon unit
- Intraoperative damage to the axillary or suprascapular nerves, affecting the deltoid and supraspinatus/infraspinatus muscles, respectively
- Humerus fracture

Postoperative Complications Related to Soft Tissue
- Re-tearing a repaired rotator cuff mechanism
- Disruption or failure of the repaired subscapularis
- Chronic GH joint instability or dislocation
- Dislocation (higher after rTSA than TSA)
- Progressive erosion of the glenoid fossa articular surface (after hemiarthroplasty)

Postoperative Complications Related to the Implants
- After TSA mechanical (aseptic) loosening, premature wear, or fracture of the polyethylene glenoid implant
  - Most often seen in a rotator cuff-deficient shoulder
  - Due to excessive stresses at the bone–prosthesis interface
  - Low incidence with unconstrained designs but higher with early-generation constrained designs
- Loosening of the humeral prosthesis after hemiarthroplasy

Postoperative Management

NOTE: Effective patient education and close communication among the therapist, surgeon, and patient are the basis of an effective and safe rehabilitation program. Postoperative management is individualized to address the specific surgical procedures used and to meet the unique needs of each patient.

Special Considerations

Integrity of the rotator cuff. Regardless of the underlying cause of late-stage GH arthritis, the goals, components, and rate of progression of a rehabilitation program after TSA or hemiarthroplasty are influenced by the preoperative and postoperative integrity of the rotator cuff mechanism. The rehabilitation program for the patient with an intact rotator cuff prior to shoulder arthroplasty can be progressed more rapidly than the program for a patient with rotator cuff deficiency that requires repair at the time of shoulder arthroplasty.

When the rotator cuff is intact prior to surgery, the emphasis of postoperative rehabilitation is to restore shoulder mobility and functional use of the arm as soon as possible while protecting soft tissues as they heal. In contrast, with a tenuous repair or preoperative history of recurrent GH dislocation, rehabilitation will emphasize improving or maintaining joint stability rather than mobility.[42,49,54,99,124]

Intraoperative ROM. Goals for safe, stable postoperative ROM are based on intraoperative ROM measurements taken prior to closing the surgical incision. For a patient with an unconstrained TSA and sufficient postoperative shoulder stability, the goal at the conclusion of rehabilitation is to achieve active ROM equal to intraoperative ROM—ideally, 140° to 150° of shoulder elevation and 45° to 50° of external rotation.[42,124] For the patient with a more constrained TSA, a deficient rotator cuff mechanism, or GH laxity, intraoperative ROM is typically less, and postoperative goals focus more on dynamic stability and less on shoulder mobility. Following rTSA, ROM is limited to 0° to 20° external rotation and 90° to 120° elevation for 3 months.[20,127]

Posture. When increased thoracic kyphosis and scapular protraction are present,[103] it is important to emphasize an erect sitting or standing posture during elevation of the arm and to incorporate spinal extension and scapular retraction exercises into the postoperative program.

Immobilization and Postoperative Positioning

At the close of the surgical procedure, the operated arm is placed in some type of shoulder immobilizer, usually a sling or sometimes a splint, for comfort and to protect reattached and repaired soft tissues.[33,124,176,185,204] Early postoperative positioning that protects the operated shoulder is detailed in Box 17.3.

Initially, the immobilizer is removed only for exercise and bathing. A patient who did not require repair of the rotator cuff is weaned from the sling during the day as quickly as possible to prevent postoperative stiffness. However, a patient who has undergone a cuff repair or other soft tissue reconstruction may need to wear the sling while in crowded areas or during sleep for approximately 4 to 6 weeks to protect the repaired tissues until sufficient healing has occurred.[21,23,33,42,49,50,99,124,194]

BOX 17.3 Positioning After Shoulder Arthroplasty: Early Postoperative (Maximum Protection) Phase

Supine
- Arm immobilized in sling that is worn continuously
  - Elbow flexed to 90°
  - Forearm and hand resting on abdomen
- Arm supported at the elbow on a folded blanket or pillow slightly away from the side and anterior to the midline of the trunk
  - Forward flexion (10° to 20°), slight abduction, and internal rotation of the shoulder
  - Head of bed elevated about 30°

Sitting
- Arm supported in sling or resting on a pillow in the patient's lap or on the armrest of a chair

With Tenuous Rotator Cuff Repair
- In some cases, if a sling does not provide adequate protection of a repaired cuff, an abduction splint must be worn

A patient who has undergone an rTSA wears a shoulder immobilizer (sling and swathe) continuously for 3 to 4 weeks following surgery except for daily personal hygiene and periodic PROM during the day.[127]

Exercise Progression

The guidelines for progression of exercises during each phase of rehabilitation after TSA, rTSA, or hemiarthroplasty presented in this section are primarily drawn from the limited number of published protocols available, most of which are based on clinical experience rather than evidence from controlled studies and none of which has been shown to be more effective than another.[21,23,34,42,49,98,99,103,124,194,215] Although most of the protocols are time-based, a handful of more recent criteria-based protocols are now available.[20,34,49,209,215] It is important to note that these criteria and suggested timelines for progression of exercises and functional activities must be adapted to each patient based on periodic evaluations of the patient's status and ongoing communication between the therapist and the surgeon.

NOTE: The exercise guidelines in this section are for patients *without* preoperative rotator cuff deficiency and who *did not* undergo a cuff repair during TSA or hemiarthroplasty. For patients with a poor quality rotator cuff mechanism or who underwent rTSA, modifications in guidelines are noted. A comparison of postoperative exercise guidelines and precautions following TSA versus rTSA is summarized in Table 17.2.

TABLE 17.2 Comparison of Exercise Guidelines and Precautions Following Total Shoulder Arthroplasty and Reverse Total Shoulder Arthroplasty

	Total Shoulder Arthroplasty (Intact Rotator Cuff)	Reverse Total Shoulder Arthroplasty
Progression of rehab	Phase 1: postop weeks 0–4 Phase 2: postop weeks 4–12 Phase 3: postop weeks 12+	Phase 1: postop weeks 0–6 Phase 2: postop weeks 6–12 or 16 Phase 3: postop weeks 12+ or 16+
Immobilization	▪ No immobilizer unless rotator cuff repaired ▪ Sling worn for comfort when shoulder unsupported and when in crowded, public areas or during sleep for about 4 weeks ▪ Sling removed for exercise soon after surgery as directed by surgeon	▪ Abduction splint (shoulder in scapular plane) ▪ Worn 24 hours/day for first 3–4 or up to 6 weeks ▪ Removed for pendulum exercises 3–4 times/day and personal hygiene
ROM restrictions	*Limit from 0–4 weeks:* ▪ Elevation of the arm: up to 120° ▪ External rotation up to 30° (arm at side) *Limit for 4–6 weeks:* ▪ No GH extension past neutral *After 6–12 weeks:* ▪ Combined adduction, internal rotation, extension permitted	*Limit for 12 weeks or more:* ▪ No GH extension or internal rotation past neutral ▪ No combined GH extension, adduction, internal rotation ▪ 0°–20° external rotation and up to 90°–120° arm elevation in scapular plane
ROM exercises, stretching, and joint mobilization	*During Phase 1:* ▪ Grade I /II joint oscillations ▪ AROM: scapula and distal extremity joints only ▪ Pendulum exercises ▪ PROM→A-AROM GH joint —Perform in *supine* (0–3 weeks) —Progress to A-AROM in sitting and standing ▪ AROM of GH joint by 4–6 weeks ▪ No *active* internal rotation for at least 6 weeks (to protect subscapularis repair) *During Phase 2:* ▪ Continue AROM ▪ Gradually increase GH rotation ▪ Gentle stretching after 6–8 weeks, if needed	*During Phase 1* (when immobilizer can be removed): ▪ Grade I /II joint oscillations ▪ AROM: scapula and distal extremity joints only ▪ Pendulum exercises ▪ PROM only of GH joint ▪ Observe ROM restrictions *During Phase 2:* ▪ Increase PROM while observing motion restrictions ▪ A-AROM→AROM of GH joint —Begin in supine; progress to sitting, standing —Gradually increase internal rotation past neutral

TABLE 17.2 Comparison of Exercise Guidelines and Precautions Following Total Shoulder Arthroplasty and Reverse Total Shoulder Arthroplasty—cont'd

	Total Shoulder Arthroplasty (Intact Rotator Cuff)	Reverse Total Shoulder Arthroplasty
	During Phase 3: ▪ Progress end-range self-stretching	*During Phase 3:* ▪ Gentle stretching, if needed within motion restrictions
Resistance exercises	*During Phase 1:* ▪ Only light, NWB isometrics of ST and deltoid muscles with shoulder in scapular plane *During Phase 2:* ▪ Emphasis on improving function of rotator cuff and ST muscles ▪ Submaximal isometrics of GH muscles combined with light weight bearing (closed-chain) through UE ▪ Delay resisted rotation for several weeks (to protect repaired rotator cuff) ▪ Progress to low-resistance dynamic strengthening of elbow and wrist; ST and GH joints if mechanics during AROM allow *During Phase 3:* ▪ Progress PRE in functional patterns ▪ Progress closed-chain stabilization exercises	*During Phase 1:* ▪ Only light, NWB isometrics of ST and deltoid muscles with shoulder in scapular plane *During Phase 2:* ▪ Emphasis on improving function of deltoid and ST muscles ▪ Submaximal isometrics (NWB only) of GH and ST muscles ▪ Delay resisted rotation for several weeks (to protect repaired subscapularis and teres minor, if preserved) ▪ Progress to low-resistance, dynamic strengthening of elbow and wrist; ST and GH joints if mechanics during AROM allow —NWB positions only (through week 12) *During Phase 3:* ▪ Begin closed-chain stabilization exercises ▪ Progress UE PRE in functional patterns
ADL precautions	*For first 4 to 6 weeks:* ▪ Observe ROM restrictions: —Do not reach behind the back or into hip pocket —When supine, support arm on pillow to avoid GH extension past neutral —Light ADL permitted with *elbow at waist level* (writing, eating, washing face) ▪ Do not lean on involved arm (rising from or sitting down in chair) ▪ Lifting limit: 1 lb (cup of coffee or glass of water) *From 6–12 weeks:* ▪ Limit *unilateral* lifting to 3 lb *After 12 weeks:* ▪ Ultimate *bilateral* lifting limit: 10–15 lb ▪ Gradual return to light functional activities	*For first 12 weeks:* ▪ Observe ROM restrictions during functional activities —Do not reach behind the back or into hip pocket —When supine, support arm on pillow to avoid GH extension past neutral ▪ By 5–7 *weeks* light ADL permitted with elbow at waist level (writing, eating, washing face) ▪ Do not lean on involved arm (rising from or sitting down in chair ▪ Restrict lifting with operated arm for 12–16 weeks (no heavier than cup of coffee or glass of water) *After 12–16 weeks* ▪ Limit *unilateral* lifting to 6 lb ▪ Ultimate *bilateral* lifting limit: 10–15 lb ▪ Gradual return to light functional activities

A-AROM = active-assistive ROM; AROM = active ROM; ADL = activities of daily living; GH = glenohumeral; NWB = nonweight bearing; ST = scapulothoracic; UE = upper extremity

CLINICAL TIP

Remember, regardless of implant design, pain relief is the primary goal of shoulder arthroplasty, with improvement in functional mobility a secondary goal. Although improvements in surgical techniques and implant technology allow more accelerated progression of postoperative rehabilitation than was possible several decades ago, it is still important to proceed judiciously during each phase of rehabilitation to avoid damage to the healing soft tissues, implant loosening, or excessive muscle fatigue or irritation.

Exercise: Maximum Protection Phase

The maximum protection phase of rehabilitation following TSA begins on the first postoperative day and extends for 4 to 6 weeks. The emphasis of this phase is patient education, pain control, and initiation of ROM exercises to prevent tissue adhesions and restore shoulder mobility to the ranges achieved during surgery as early as possible. Early motion is permissible after uncemented and cemented fixation.

While the patient is hospitalized, patient education includes reviewing early postoperative precautions and teaching the initial exercises of the patient's home program. Precautions during the first 4 to 6 weeks after TSA, when protection of soft tissues is crucial, are summarized in Box 17.4. A patient's adherence to these precautions is critical during this phase of rehabilitation.

Goals and interventions. The maximum protection phase of rehabilitation includes the following:[21,23,34,42,49,50,98,99,124,194]

- ***Control pain and inflammation.***
  - Use a sling or splint for comfort.
  - Use prescribed analgesic and anti-inflammatory medication.
  - Use cryotherapy, especially after exercise.
- ***Maintain mobility of adjacent joints.***
  - Active movements of the spine and scapula (while wearing the shoulder sling and when it is removed for exercise) to maintain motion and minimize muscle guarding and spasm. Incorporate "shoulder rolls" by elevating, retracting, and then relaxing the scapulae to reinforce an erect posture of the trunk. Emphasize active scapular retraction and spinal extension.
  - Active ROM of the hand, wrist, and elbow when the arm is removed from the sling.
- ***Restore shoulder mobility.***
  - Passive or therapist-assisted shoulder motions *within the safe ROM limits determined during surgery.* With the patient lying supine and the arm slightly away from the side of the trunk on a folded towel and the elbow flexed, perform elevation of the arm in the plane of the scapula to tolerance, external rotation to no more than 30° to 45°, and internal rotation until the forearm rests on the chest.
  - Pendulum (Codman's) exercises. In addition, encourage the patient to periodically remove the sling and swing the arm gently during ambulation at home.
  - Later in this phase, progress to *supine self-assisted* shoulder ROM (elevation and rotation) by first assisting with the sound hand and later with a wand or dowel rod. Add horizontal abduction to neutral and adduction across the chest with the assistance of a wand.
  - Self-assisted shoulder ROM with a wand *in sitting or standing* position by performing "gear shift" exercises (see Fig. 17.23), by sliding the arm forward on a tabletop (see Fig. 17.25), or with an overhead rope pulley system. Remind the patient to maintain an erect trunk when performing assisted shoulder motions while seated or standing.
  - Self-assisted reaching movements (to the nose, forehead, or over the head as comfort allows) to simulate functional movements.

BOX 17.4 Precautions for the Maximum Protection Phase of Rehabilitation Following Shoulder Arthroplasty

Exercise

- Short but frequent exercise sessions (four or five times per day).
- Low number of repetitions per exercise.
- Only *passive* or *assisted* shoulder ROM exercises and only within the "safe" limits of ranges noted during surgery. *Absolutely no end-range stretching.*
  - Passive external rotation to neutral after rTSA or to less than 30° after TSA to avoid excessive stress to the surgically repaired subscapularis muscle.
  - During passive or assisted shoulder rotation with the patient lying supine, position the humerus slightly anterior to the midline of the body (by placing the arm on a folded towel) to avoid excessive stress to the anterior capsule and suture line.
  - No hyperextension or horizontal abduction (beyond neutral) of the shoulder to avoid stress to the anterior capsule.
  - No combined extension, adduction, and internal rotation
  - If an overhead rope-pulley system is used for assisted elevation of the arm, initially *have the patient face the doorway and pulley apparatus,* so shoulder elevation occurs only within a limited range.
  - Maintain an erect trunk during passive or assisted elevation of the arm while sitting or standing to avoid subacromial impingement of soft tissues.
- In most instances, no active (unassisted), antigravity, dynamic shoulder exercises, particularly resisted internal rotation.
- No resistance (strengthening) exercises.
- In general, a more gradual progression of exercises following rTSA and for a patient with a severely damaged and repaired or irreparable rotator cuff mechanism who underwent TSA than for a patient with a preoperatively intact cuff.

Activities of Daily Living

- Limit activities to those that can be performed with the elbow at waist level, such as eating or writing.
- Avoid reaching behind the back to tuck in a shirt, reach into a back pocket, or following toileting.
- Avoid weight bearing on the operated extremity, such as pushing during transfers or when moving in bed, especially the first few weeks after surgery.
- Avoid lifting objects with the operated arm.
- Support the arm in a sling during extended periods of standing or walking.
- Wear the sling while sleeping or outside in crowded areas.
- No driving for 4 to 6 weeks.

- For some patients, transition to *active* (unassisted) shoulder ROM is often possible by 4 weeks.
- Functional activities with the elbow at waist level, such as hand to face and writing, are permissible.

- ***Minimize muscle inhibition, guarding, and atrophy.***
  - Gentle muscle-setting of shoulder musculature (excluding the internal rotators) with the elbow flexed and the shoulder in the plane of the scapula or neutral. Teach these exercises prior to discharge from the hospital by having the patient practice isometric contractions of the muscles of the *sound* shoulder. Postpone setting exercises (light isometrics) of the operated shoulder until about 4 to 6 weeks after surgery.
  - Scapular stabilization exercises in nonweight-bearing positions. Target the serratus anterior and trapezius muscles.

NOTE: For a patient who underwent TSA with repair of a large rotator cuff tear, it may not be permissible to begin ROM exercises immediately after surgery. When the sling or splint can be removed for exercise, perform only passive or assisted ROM throughout the first phase of rehabilitation. The range of shoulder elevation and external rotation initially permitted may be less than for shoulders that did not require cuff repair. Postpone active (unassisted), antigravity ROM and light isometrics until the second phase (approximately 6 weeks postoperatively, when repaired soft tissues are reasonably well healed).

Following rTSA, patients have a lifting limit of 1 lb or less for 6 weeks, and external rotation and elevation ROM are limited to 0° to 20° and 90° to 120°, respectively, for 3 months.[20,127] In addition, hyperextension, lifting, and supporting of body weight with the involved shoulder are all precautions following rTSA.[20] (Refer to Table 17.2 for additional precautions after rTSA.)

Criteria to progress. Criteria to advance to the second phase of rehabilitation following TSA are:

- ROM: At least 90° of passive elevation, at least 45° degrees of external rotation, and 70° of internal rotation in the plane of the scapula with minimal pain[215] or *almost* full, passive shoulder motion based on intraoperative measurements with little to no pain.[34,99]
- No pain during resisted, isometric internal rotation of the subscapularis.[34]
- Ability to perform most waist-level activities of daily living (ADLs) without pain.[99]
- For rTSA, criteria include tolerance of assisted ROM and demonstration of the ability to isometrically activate the deltoid and periscapular musculature while the joint is positioned in the scapular plane.[20]

Exercise: Moderate Protection/Controlled Motion Phase

Although suggested timelines vary from one resource to another, the moderate protection/controlled motion phase of rehabilitation, which typically begins at about 4 to 6 weeks postoperatively and extends to at least 12 to 16 weeks, focuses on gradually establishing active (unassisted) control, dynamic stability, and strength of the shoulder while continuing to increase ROM.[21,23,42,49,98,99,124,194,215]

PRECAUTIONS: During this phase of rehabilitation, although it is safe to place increasing stresses (stretching or resistance) on periarticular soft tissues, it is important to do so gradually so as not to irritate tissues that are continuing to heal. Therefore, continue with short but frequent exercise sessions and avoid vigorous stretching or resistance exercises or overuse of the involved shoulder during functional activities.

Goals and interventions. The goals and exercises for this phase of rehabilitation are as follows.

- ***Continue to increase ROM of the shoulder.***
  - Transition from passive or assisted ROM to *low-intensity, pain-free* stretching in all anatomical and diagonal planes of motion to achieve intraoperative ROM.
  - Gentle joint mobilization techniques for specific capsular restrictions.
  - In addition to therapist-assisted stretching, teach the patient how to perform gentle self-stretching exercises to increase elevation, internal/external rotation, extension, and horizontal adduction/abduction. Suggestions are pictured in the Exercise Techniques section of this chapter.
- ***Develop active control and dynamic stability and improve muscle performance (strength and endurance) of the shoulder.***
  - Continue with or gradually transition to *active* shoulder ROM exercises, initiating antigravity abduction when the patient can perform the movement without substituting scapula elevation.
  - Scapular and GH joint stabilization exercises (alternating isometrics and rhythmic stabilization) can progress from nonweight-bearing to minimal weight-bearing positions.

NOTE: For patients who have had an rTSA, maintain nonweight-bearing precautions for up to 12 weeks postoperatively.[20]

- Pain-free, low-intensity (submaximal) resisted isometrics of shoulder muscles can be incorporated, including the subscapularis and any other repaired muscle-tendon units.
- Begin dynamic resistance exercises for the scapula and shoulder musculature (between 0° and 90° of shoulder elevation) using light weights or light-grade elastic resistance. Begin in the supine position to support and stabilize the scapula and progress to the sitting position.
- Begin upper extremity endurance training with a stationary ergometer or a portable reciprocal exerciser on a table. Progress by increasing repetitions or time to increase muscular and cardiopulmonary endurance.

Criteria to progress. To advance to the final phase of rehabilitation, a patient should meet the following criteria:

- Full, passive ROM of the shoulder (based on intraoperative ranges)[34,99] or pain-free, passive or assisted shoulder flexion of at least 130° to 140° and abduction of 120°.[215]
- In the plane of the scapula, at least 60° pain-free, passive external rotation and 70° internal rotation.[215]

- Active (unassisted), antigravity elevation of the arm to at least 100° to 120° in the plane of the scapula while maintaining joint stability and using appropriate shoulder mechanics, particularly no scapula elevation during arm elevation.[215]
- 4/5 strength of rotator cuff and deltoid muscles.[49,99]
- rTSA patients should have documented improvements in function and increasing strength of the deltoid and periscapular muscles prior to progressing to the next phase.[20]

Exercise: Minimum Protection/Return to Function Phase

The minimum protection/return to functional activity phase usually begins around 12 to 16 weeks postoperatively (depending on rotator cuff tissue quality and function) and extends for several more months.[49,99,215] Pain-free strengthening of the shoulder muscles for dynamic stability and functional use of the upper extremity for progressively more demanding tasks are the primary focuses of this phase. For optimal results, the home exercise program may need to be continued for 6 months or longer, and functional and recreational activities may need to be modified.

Goals and interventions. Goals and activities for the final phase of rehabilitation include the following:[21,23,34,49,50,98,99,215]

- ***Continue to improve or maintain shoulder mobility.***
  - End-range self-stretching.
  - Grade III joint mobilization and self-mobilization, if appropriate.[21,23,34,99]
- ***Continue to improve neuromuscular control and muscle performance of the shoulder.***
  - Pain-free, low-load, high-repetition progressive resistive exercise (PRE) of shoulder musculature in anatomical and diagonal planes and in patterns of movement that replicate functional tasks throughout the available ROM. Position the patient in a variety of gravity-resisted positions.
  - Closed-chain, resisted shoulder exercises, gradually increasing the amount of weight bearing through the upper extremity.
  - Use of the involved upper extremity for lifting, carrying, pushing, or pulling activities against increasing loads.
- ***Return to most functional activities.***
  - Use of the operated upper extremity for progressively more advanced functional activities.
  - Recreational activities, such as swimming and golf are possible.
  - Modification of high-demand, high-impact work-related or recreational activities to avoid imposing excessive forces on the GH joint that could lead to loosening or premature wear of prosthetic implants.

NOTE: For the patient whose rotator cuff was irreparable or continues to be significantly deficient because of a tenuous repair and who has limited but pain-free shoulder ROM, modification of the environment and use of assistive devices may be necessary for independence in functional activities.

Outcomes

As patient selection criteria, implant design, and surgical techniques have been refined, outcomes after shoulder arthroplasty have improved. Outcomes after TSA, rTSA, or hemiarthroplasty are influenced by many factors, including the type and severity of the underlying pathology, the integrity of soft tissues, the type and quality of the surgical procedure(s) performed, and patient-related factors such as participation in a postoperative rehabilitation program.[29,33,215] The outcomes most often reported are pain relief, quality of life, passive and active shoulder ROM, and the ability to perform functional activities.

Despite an emphasis by numerous resources that a patient's participation in postoperative rehabilitation is crucial for successful outcomes, there are no studies to support this opinion, because all patients undergoing shoulder arthroplasty are given some form of postoperative exercise instruction. Furthermore, published protocols are routinely modified to meet the needs of individual patients making comparison of postoperative protocols difficult.[215]

Pain relief. A decrease in pain is the most consistent result of GH arthroplasty. Almost all patients—regardless of the underlying pathology, the type of arthroplasty, or the design of the implants—report complete or substantial relief of shoulder pain and improved functional use of the arm.[33,123,124,139,141,143,152,156,188,211]

The extent of pain relief has been shown to be associated with the underlying cause(s) of GH arthritis. Neer and associates;[141] Matsen;[123] and more recently, Norris and Iannotti[152] reported that 90% of patients with primary OA or osteonecrosis had complete or near-complete pain relief after TSA. Similar results are reported for patients with OA who underwent hemiarthroplasty.[112,124,143] Patients with RA or other synovium-based diseases also report substantial pain relief after TSA or hemiarthroplasty, although not quite to the extent reported by patients with OA or osteonecrosis.[33,176,202] However, in a sample of 191 patients after rTSA, Wall and colleagues report statistically significant improvements in pain as measured by the Constant score regardless of patient diagnosis.[211]

TSA and hemiarthroplasty have been compared to each other for pain relief effectiveness. In one prospective study of patients with OA, postoperative pain scores were similar for both groups, with patients receiving a TSA demonstrating more improvement than patients with hemiarthroplasty because of higher levels of preoperative pain.[156] In another study, patients with OA randomly assigned to either TSA or hemiarthroplasty groups were evaluated over a 24-month period and both groups reported significant pain relief and improvements in other quality-of-life parameters, with no significant differences between the groups.[112] Whether or not TSA versus hemiarthroplasty is more effective for pain relief in patients with RA has not been clearly established.[124,202]

ROM and functional use of the upper extremity. Despite the postsurgical emphasis on improving ROM and functional use of the arm during rehabilitation, improvements in these outcomes are less predictable than pain relief, with functional status improving more consistently than ROM.[59,124,152,156,179,188,215] In general, patients with primary OA or osteonecrosis demonstrate greater improvement in active flexion and rotation ROM than patients with RA, likely because of the higher incidence of cuff deficiency associated with RA or the use of more constrained prosthetic designs.[176,202,215] For example, in patients with OA or osteonecrosis, the mean active flexion changed from 105° to 161°, while in patients with RA, means range from 75° to 105°.[188,215]

Significant improvement in functional status has been reported in patients with OA or osteonecrosis following arthroplasty. Although functional improvement after arthroplasty has also been reported in patients with RA, many studies used nonstandardized measurement tools, making it difficult to compare their results with those of other studies.[215] Following rTSA, patients with primary rotator cuff arthropathy, primary OA with rotator cuff tear, or a massive rotator cuff tear had better functional and clinical outcomes than patients with post-traumatic arthritis or revision arthroplasty.[211] Regardless of the underlying pathology, resources agree that a well-functioning rotator cuff mechanism is the basis for significant postoperative gains in active ROM and functional abilities.[33,185,215]

Painful Shoulder Syndromes (Rotator Cuff Disease and Tendinopathies): Nonoperative Management

Most of the soft tissues in the suprahumeral space (see Fig. 17.7) can be a source of pain that limits movement and function and interferes with sleep. Referred to for decades as *impingement syndrome*, this common and multifactorial cause of pain was originally believed to be the result of mechanical compression and irritation of suprahumeral tissues.[80,109,117] Recent evidence suggests that noncompressive mechanisms such as tendon degenerative processes and entrapment also cause shoulder pain. For this reason, terminology such as tendinitis, tendinopathy, rotator cuff disease, and anterior shoulder pain are sometimes used instead of impingement syndrome. Various etiological factors for rotator cuff disease have been identified, leading to the classification systems summarized in Box 17.5.

Related Pathologies and Etiology of Symptoms

The cause of rotator cuff disease is often multifactorial, involving both structural and mechanical factors. The term impingement syndrome and its recent variants has traditionally described a cluster of signs and symptoms that typically includes pain with overhead reaching, a painful arc in

BOX 17.5 Categories of Painful Shoulder Syndromes

Rotator cuff disease and other painful shoulder conditions have varying etiologic factors and therefore can be categorized in several ways.

Based on Degree or Stage of Pathology of the Rotator Cuff (Neer's Classification of Rotator Cuff Disease)[140]

- *Stage I.* Edema, hemorrhage (patient usually <25 years of age)
- *Stage II.* Tendonitis/bursitis and fibrosis (patient usually 25 to 40 years of age)
- *Stage III.* Bone spurs and tendon rupture (patient usually >40 years of age)

Based on Impaired Tissue[40]

- Supraspinatus tendonitis
- Infraspinatus tendonitis
- Bicipital tendonitis
- Superior glenoid labrum and/or biceps tendon instability
- Subdeltoid (subacromial) bursitis
- Other musculotendinous strains (specific to type of injury or trauma)
- Anterior—from overuse with racket sports (pectoralis minor, subscapularis, coracobrachialis, short head of biceps strain)
- Inferior—from motor vehicle trauma (long head of triceps, serratus anterior strain)

Based on Mechanical Disruption and Direction of Instability or Subluxation

- Multidirectional instability from lax capsule with or without impingement
- Unidirectional instability (anterior, posterior, or inferior) with or without impingement
- Traumatic injury with tears of capsule and/or labrum
- Insidious (atraumatic) onset from repetitive microtrauma
- Inherent laxity

Based on Progressive Microtrauma (Jobe's Classification)[92]

- *Group 1.* Pure impingement (usually in an older recreational athlete with partial undersurface rotator cuff tear and subacromial bursitis)
- *Group 2.* Impingement associated with labral and/or capsular injury, instability, and secondary impingement
- *Group 3.* Hyperelastic soft tissues resulting in anterior or multidirectional instability and impingement (usually attenuated but intact labrum, undersurface rotator cuff tear)
- *Group 4.* Anterior instability without associated impingement (result of trauma; results in partial or complete dislocation)

Based on Degree and Frequency

- Instability → subluxation → dislocation
- Acute, recurrent, fixed

the mid-range of arm elevation, and positive provocation tests. Patients also often report waking at night with pain. Symptoms from cuff tendinopathy are usually brought on by excessive or repetitive overhead activities that place a high demand on the shoulder joint. Insight into the multifactorial nature of rotator cuff disease can be appreciated by a classification system that describes impingement as *intrinsic or extrinsic*, with extrinsic further classified as *primary, secondary, and internal.*

Additional types of musculotendinous strain in the shoulder region can occur from overuse, such as anterior pectoral region pain from playing racket sports, or from trauma such as a fall, traction on the arm, or an automobile accident.

Intrinsic Impingement: Rotator Cuff Disease

Intrinsic factors are those that compromise the structural integrity of the musculotendinous structures and include vascular changes in the rotator cuff tendons, tissue tension overload, and collagen disorientation and degeneration.[61,135] Intrinsic conditions typically involve the deep articular side of the tendons and may progress to articular-side rotator cuff tears, seen most often in those older than 40 years of age.[77]

Extrinsic Impingement: Mechanical Compression of Tissues

Extrinsic impingement is believed to occur as a result of mechanical compression of the rotator cuff against the anteroinferior one-third of the acromion in the suprahumeral space during arm elevation (Fig. 17.15). Tendon compression is believed to result from anatomical or biomechanical factors that decrease the physical dimensions of the suprahumeral space.

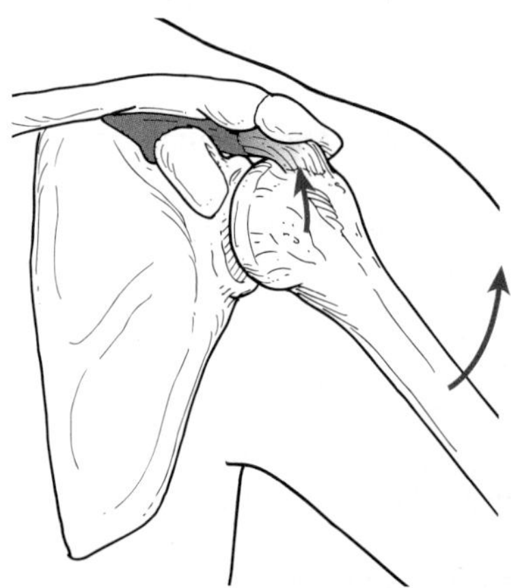

FIGURE 17.15 Decrease in the suprahumeral space during repetitive elevation activities leads to symptoms of impingement.

Primary extrinsic impingement. Primary extrinsic impingement can result from anatomical or biomechanical factors. Anatomical factors include structural variations in the acromion or humeral head, and hypertrophic degenerative changes of the AC joint and coracoacromial ligament. Neer[142] first suggested that the size and shape of the structures that make up the coracoacromial arch are related to rotator cuff impingement. In later studies, variations of the acromion were identified and classified into three shapes: type I (flat), type II (curved), and type III (hooked) (Fig. 17.16).[12] Rotator cuff pathology may be associated with types II and III—but not type I—acromial shapes.[1,133,233] Anatomical factors that decrease the suprahumeral space often have to be managed surgically.[61,168,233] Biomechanical factors include altered orientation of the clavicle or scapula during movement, or increased anterosuperior humeral head translations as may occur with a tight posterior GH capsule.[74]

Secondary extrinsic impingement. Secondary impingement describes mechanical compression of the suprahumeral tissues due to hypermobility or instability of the GH joint leading to increased translation of the humeral head. This instability may be multidirectional or unidirectional and can occur with compromised static (GH ligaments) and/or dynamic restraints (rotator cuff insufficiency).

- ***Multidirectional instability.*** Some individuals have physiologically increased connective tissue extensibility, causing excessive joint mobility. In the GH joint, this increased extensibility allows larger than normal humeral head translations in all directions.[156,181] Many individuals, particularly those involved in overhead activities, develop laxity of the capsule from continually subjecting the joint to tensile forces.[61,92] A hypermobile GH joint may be supported satisfactorily by strong rotator cuff muscles; but with muscle fatigue, poor humeral head stabilization may lead to faulty humeral mechanics, trauma, and inflammation of the suprahumeral tissues.[92,132] With multidirectional instability, the mechanical impingement of tissue in the suprahumeral space is, therefore, a secondary effect of the increased humeral head translations.[61]
- ***Unidirectional instability with or without impingement.*** Unidirectional instability (anterior, posterior, or inferior) may be the result of physiological laxity of the connective tissues, but is more often the result of trauma and usually involves rotator cuff tears. Often, there is damage to the glenoid labrum and tearing of some of the supporting ligaments associated with these traumas.

Internal extrinsic impingement. Internal impingement is a type of extrinsic impingement that occurs in a position of elevation, horizontal abduction, and maximum external rotation, primarily in throwing athletes. This position and a posterior-superior shift of the humeral head on the glenoid results in a mechanical entrapment of the posterior supraspinatus tendon between the humeral head and the labrum. Internal impingement is associated with a combination of posterior GH capsule tightness and scapula kinematic alterations.[106,138]

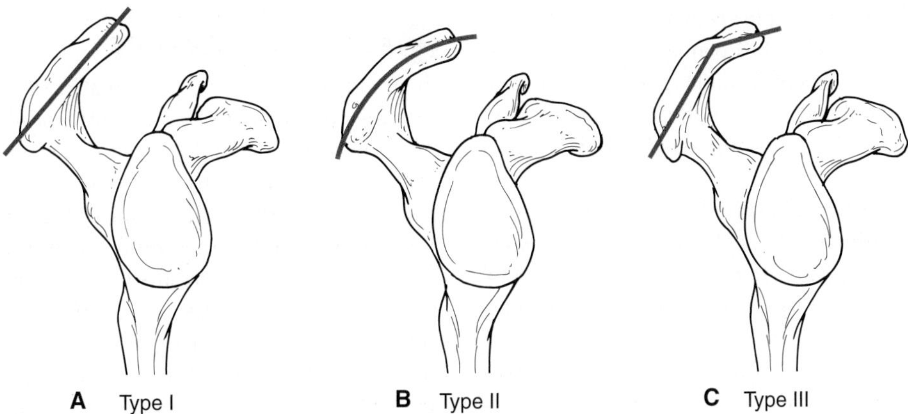

FIGURE 17.16 Classifications of the acromion by shape: **(A)** type I (flat); **(B)** type II (curved); **(C)** type III (hooked).

Tendonitis/Bursitis

Neer categorizes tendonitis/bursitis as a stage II impingement syndrome (see Box 17.5).[140] In contrast to tendinopathy, these conditions are associated with active inflammatory processes and may be localized to one or more specific tissues. The following sections describe specific pathological diagnoses and typical presenting signs and symptoms.

Supraspinatus tendonitis. With supraspinatus tendonitis, the lesion is usually near the musculotendinous junction, resulting in a painful arc with overhead reaching. There is also pain with provocation tests and pain on palpation of the tendon just inferior to the anterior aspect of the acromion when the patient's hand is placed behind the back. It is difficult to differentiate tendonitis from subdeltoid bursitis because of the anatomical proximity of these two structures.

Infraspinatus tendonitis. With infraspinatus tendonitis, the lesion is usually near the musculotendinous junction, resulting in a painful arc during overhead, forward, or cross body motions. It may present as a deceleration (eccentric) injury due to overload during repetitive or forceful throwing activities. Pain occurs with palpation of the tendon just inferior to the posterior corner of the acromion when the patient horizontally adducts and externally rotates the humerus.

Bicipital tendonitis. With bicipital tendonitis, the lesion involves the long tendon in the bicipital groove beneath or just distal to the transverse humeral ligament. Swelling in the bony groove is restrictive and compounds and perpetuates the problem. Pain occurs with Speed's test and on palpation of the bicipital groove.[119] Rupture or dislocation of the biceps tendon may compromise its role as a humeral depressor during arm elevation, promoting impingement of tissues in the suprahumeral space.[140,149]

Bursitis (subdeltoid or subacromial). When acute, the symptoms of bursitis are the same as those seen with supraspinatus tendonitis. Once the inflammation is reduced, there are no symptoms with resisted motions.

Other Impaired Musculotendinous Tissues

The following are examples of other musculotendinous problems in the shoulder region:

- The pectoralis minor, short head of the biceps, and coracobrachialis are subject to microtrauma, particularly in racquet sports requiring a controlled backward, then a rapid forward swinging of the arm. The scapular stabilizers, particularly the retractors, are also susceptible to microtrauma as they function to control forward motion of the scapula.[111]
- The long head of the triceps and scapular stabilizers may be injured in motor vehicle accidents, as the driver holds firmly to the steering wheel on impact.
- Injury, overuse, or repetitive trauma can occur in any muscle being subjected to stress.[151] Pain occurs when the involved muscle is lengthened or when contracting against resistance. Palpating the site of the lesion causes the familiar pain.

Insidious (Atraumatic) Onset

Neer has identified rotator cuff tears as a stage III impingement syndrome, a condition that typically occurs in persons over age 40 after repetitive microtrauma to the rotator cuff or long head of the biceps.[140] With aging, the distal portion of the supraspinatus tendon is particularly vulnerable to impingement or stress from overuse strain. With degenerative changes, calcification and eventual tendon rupture may occur.[61,146,154] Chronic ischemia caused from tension on the tendon and decreased healing in the elderly are possible explanations, although Neer stated that, in his experience, 95% of tears are initiated by impingement wear rather than by impaired circulation or trauma.[140]

Common Impairments of Structure and Function

Various impairments are common in rotator cuff disease; however, it is not known if they are the cause or an effect of the pathology.[28,114,117,157] A thorough examination of the cervical spine and shoulder complex is necessary to differentiate signs and symptoms related to primary and secondary impingements or other causes of shoulder pain.[19,47,119] Common impairments associated with rotator cuff disease and painful shoulder syndromes are summarized in Box 17.6.

Impaired Posture and Muscle Imbalances

Increased thoracic kyphosis, forward head, and protracted and forward-tilted scapula are often identified as related to impingement syndrome. Faulty scapular alignment may be one factor in decreasing the suprahumeral space and leading to irritation of the rotator cuff tendons with overhead activities.[114] Faulty upper quadrant posture may also lead to an imbalance in the length and strength of the scapulothoracic and GH musculature, decreasing the effectiveness of the dynamic and passive stabilizing structures of the GH joint.[221]

With increased thoracic kyphosis, the scapula is often protracted and tilted forward and the GH joint is internally rotated. With this posture, the pectoralis minor, levator scapulae, and shoulder internal rotators may become tight, and the external rotators of the shoulder and upward rotators of the scapula may test weak and have poor muscular endurance. When reaching overhead, faulty scapular and humeral mechanics may result in alterations of scapular alignment and in the muscular control of the shoulder complex.

BOX 17.6 Summary of Common Impairments With Rotator Cuff Disease and Tendinopathies

All, some, or none of the following may be present:

- Pain at the musculotendinous junction of the involved muscle with palpation, with resisted muscle contraction, and when stretched
- Positive impingement sign (forced internal rotation at 90° of flexion) and painful arc near 90° arm elevation
- Impaired posture: thoracic kyphosis, forward head, and forward (anterior) tipped scapula with decreased thoracic mobility
- Muscle imbalances: hypomobile pectoralis major and minor, levator scapulae, and internal GH joint rotators; weak serratus anterior and external GH joint rotators
- Hypomobile posterior GH joint capsule
- Hypomobile cervical and/or thoracic spine mobility, especially with secondary impingement
- Faulty kinematics during humeral elevation: decreased posterior tipping of scapula related to weak serratus anterior; scapular elevation and overuse of upper trapezius; and altered scapulohumeral rhythm during elevation or lowering of arm
- With a complete rotator cuff tear, inability to abduct the humerus against gravity
- When acute, pain referred to the C5 and C6 reference zones

 **FOCUS ON EVIDENCE**

In a study comparing the kinematics of 26 subjects without shoulder impairment and 26 with shoulder impingement, Ludewig and Cook[114] documented delayed upward rotation of the scapula during the 31° to 60° range of humeral elevation, incomplete posterior tilting of the scapula, and excessive scapular elevation in the impingement group. These motion alterations may all contribute to decreasing the available subacromial space. Decreased activation of the lower serratus anterior and increased activation of the upper trapezius were also reported. Excessive scapula elevation and upper trapezius activation were suggested as possible compensations for the reduced posterior serratus anterior function.

A study using a three-dimensional technique to compare shoulder complex kinematics between 12 asymptomatic and 10 symptomatic subjects reported that at 30° and 60° of scapular plane abduction, the symptomatic subjects had 7° and 6° more GH elevation, respectively, with less scapulothoracic upward rotation. The authors suggest the altered mechanics in the symptomatic group reflect compensatory mechanisms in the shoulder complex demonstrating regional interdependence of the joints.[107,108]

Decreased Thoracic ROM

Thoracic extension is a component motion that is needed for full overhead reaching. Incomplete thoracic extension may decrease the functional range of humeral elevation. Explanations for this regional interdependence include decreased thoracic spine mobility leading to faulty scapulothoracic mechanics and altered muscle activity.[73] Although increased thoracic kyphosis has been noted to decrease shoulder elevation,[24,60,96,121] direct evidence linking thoracic mobility to shoulder motion is not available and recent studies evaluating the effect of thoracic spine manipulation in those with rotator cuff disease have reported decreased pain without significant changes in scapula kinematics or shoulder elevation ROM.[73,137]

CLINICAL TIP

Full overhead shoulder movement is more difficult when there is increased thoracic kyphosis and forward head posture. This relationship can be used as an educational tool with a patient to demonstrate the importance of spinal posture. First, have your patient reach overhead while in a slouched posture; then, have him assume "good posture" and reach overhead again and note the difference in ROM. Reinforce the importance of spinal posture in the management and prevention of shoulder problems.

 **FOCUS ON EVIDENCE**

A study comparing the effects of thoracic manipulation on scapular mechanics and pain in 47 asymptomatic and 50 symptomatic subjects with shoulder impingement symptoms demonstrated an immediate decrease in pain and a small change in scapular mechanics in the symptomatic group relative to the asymptomatic group and those receiving a sham treatment.[73]

Rotator Cuff Overuse and Fatigue

If the rotator cuff musculature or long head of the biceps fatigue from overuse, they no longer provide the dynamic stabilizing, compressive, and translational forces that support the joint and control healthy joint mechanics. Fatigue is thought to be a precipitating factor in secondary impingement syndromes when capsular laxity is present and increased muscular effort is necessary for stability.[158] Without this dynamic stability, the tissues in the subacromial space may become impinged as a result of faulty joint mechanics. There is also a relationship between muscle fatigue and joint position sense in the shoulder that may play a role in impaired performance in repetitive overhead activities.[30]

Muscle Weakness Secondary to Neuropathy

Muscle weakness may be related to compromised nerve function. Long thoracic nerve palsy has been associated with faulty scapular mechanics due to serratus anterior muscle weakness, a movement dysfunction that may lead to rotator cuff impingement in the suprahumeral region.[181]

Hypomobile Posterior GH Joint Capsule

Loss of extensibility in the posterior GH joint capsule may negatively alter humeral head translations. Increased superior translations during arm elevation are reported in studies that have experimentally tightened the posterior capsule, an effect that would decrease the available suprahumeral space.[74]

Common Activity Limitations and Participation Restrictions

- In the acute stages, pain may interfere with sleep, particularly when rolling onto the involved shoulder.
- Pain with overhead reaching, pushing, or pulling.
- Difficulty lifting heavy loads.
- Inability to sustain repetitive shoulder activities (such as reaching, lifting, throwing, pushing, pulling, or swinging the arm).
- Difficulty with dressing, particularly putting a shirt on over the head.

Management: Painful Shoulder Syndromes

NOTE: Even though symptoms may be "chronic" in terms of long standing or recurring, the initial treatment priority is to control inflammation if present.

FOCUS ON EVIDENCE

A review of seven research articles that reported outcomes of conservative physical therapy interventions for full thickness rotator cuff tears found that the most successful treatment approaches were those that respected the stage of tissue healing and irritability of symptoms and progressed the program based on patient response (acute stage, subacute stage and reintegration to regular activities).[88]

Management: Protection Phase

Control Inflammation and Promote Healing

- Modalities and low-intensity cross-fiber massage are applied to the site of the lesion. While applying the modalities, position the extremity to maximally expose the involved region.[41,45]
- If necessary to rest the part, temporarily support the arm in a sling.

Patient Education

The environment and habits that provoke the symptoms must be modified or avoided completely during this stage. The patient should be informed about the mechanics of the irritation and the anticipated recovery, and be given guidelines regarding safe exercises at this stage of healing.

Maintain Integrity and Mobility of the Soft Tissues

- Passive, active-assistive, or self-assisted ROM is initiated in pain-free ranges.
- Multiple-angle muscle setting and protected stabilization exercises are initiated. When exercising the shoulder, it is particularly important to stimulate the stabilizing function of the rotator cuff, biceps brachii, and scapular muscles at an intensity tolerated by the patient.

PRECAUTION: Exercises during this stage must avoid the impingement positions. Often, the midrange of abduction, with internal rotation, or an end-range position when the involved muscle is on a stretch (such as putting the hand behind the back) provokes a painful response.

Control Pain and Maintain Joint Integrity

Pendulum exercises without weights can be used to cause pain-inhibiting grade II joint distraction and oscillation motions (see Fig. 17.22 in the section on exercise).

Develop Support in Related Regions

- Postural awareness and correction techniques are used. (See related information in the Interventions for Impaired Posture section in Chapter 14.)
- Supportive techniques, such as shoulder strapping or scapular taping, tactile cues, and mirrors, can be used for reinforcement. Repetitive reminders and practice of correct posture are necessary throughout the day.

FOCUS ON EVIDENCE

In a randomized placebo-controlled, crossover study[109] of 120 subjects (60 with impingement and 60 asymptomatic), postural correction with tape resulted in a significant increase in pain-free shoulder flexion and scapular plane elevation for both groups of subjects. Thoracic and scapular taping for posture correction also resulted in less forward head posture, reduced thoracic kyphosis, less lateral scapular displacement, and a less elevated and forward scapula position in both groups when compared to the effects of placebo taping.

Management: Controlled Motion Phase

After the acute symptoms are managed, the emphasis shifts to progressive movements within safe limits and using proper mechanics while the tissues heal. Individual components of desired functional movements are initiated in a controlled exercise program.[44,45,190,217,218,223] If there is functional laxity in the joint, the intervention is directed toward developing neuromuscular control and strength of both the scapula and GH joint stabilizers.[95,180,201] If there is restricted mobility that prevents normal mechanics or interferes with function, mobilization of the restricted tissue is initiated. Specific exercise techniques and progressions are described later in the chapter.

Patient Education

Patient adherence to the program and protection of healing tissues are necessary in this stage. The home exercise program is progressed as the patient learns safe and effective execution of each exercise. Continue to reinforce proper postural habits.

Develop Strong, Mobile Tissues

- Manual therapy techniques, such as cross-fiber or friction massage, can be used. The extremity is positioned so the tissue is on a stretch if it is a tendon or in the shortened position if it is in the muscle belly. The technique is applied using forces and durations that are to the tolerance of the patient.
- Following these manual techniques, the patient is instructed to perform an isometric contraction of the muscle in several positions of their available range. The intensity of contraction should not cause pain.
- The patient should be taught how to self-administer the massage and isometric techniques.

Modify Joint Tracking and Mobility

MWM may be useful to modify joint tracking and reinforce full movement when there is restriction of shoulder elevation because of a painful arc or impingement.[136] (See Chapter 5 for a description of principles.)

- *Posterolateral glide with active elevation* (Fig. 17.17 A)
  - *Patient position*: Sitting with the arm by the side and head in neutral retraction.
  - *Therapist position and procedure*: Stand on the side opposite the affected arm and reach across the patient's torso to stabilize the scapula with the palm of one hand. The other hand is placed over the anteromedial aspect of the head of the humerus. Apply a graded posterolateral glide of the humeral head on the glenoid. Request that the patient perform the previously painful elevation. Maintain the posterolateral glide mobilization throughout both elevation and return to neutral. Ensure that no pain is experienced during the procedure. Adjust the grade and direction of the glide as needed to achieve pain-free function. Add resistance in the form of elastic resistance or a cuff weight to load the muscle.
- *Self-Treatment.* A mobilization belt provides the posterolateral glide while the patient actively elevates the affected limb against progressive resistance to end-range (Fig. 17.17 B).

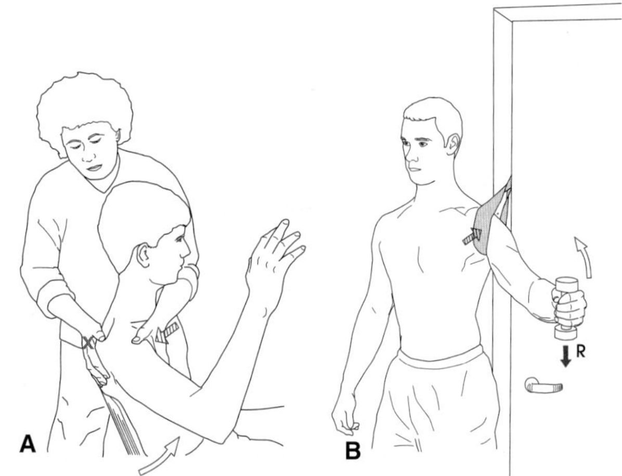

FIGURE 17.17 MWM to modify GH joint tracking and improve active elevation. A posterolateral glide is applied to the humeral head **(A)** manually or **(B)** with a belt for self-treatment, while the patient actively elevates the humerus. A weight is used to strengthen the muscles through the pain-free range.

Develop Balance in Length and Strength of Shoulder Girdle Muscles

It is important to design a program that specifically addresses the patient's impairments. Typical interventions in the shoulder girdle include but are not limited to:

- *Stretch shortened muscles.* Shortened muscles typically include the pectoralis major, pectoralis minor, latissimus dorsi, teres major, subscapularis, and levator scapulae.
- *Strengthen and train the scapulothoracic muscles.* Important scapular muscles typically include the serratus anterior and lower trapezius for posterior tilting and upward rotation of the scapula and the middle trapezius and rhomboids for scapular retraction. Because it is important that the patient avoid scapular elevation when raising the arm, emphasize maintaining scapular depression when abducting and flexing the humerus.
- *Strengthen and train the rotator cuff muscles.* Place emphasis on the shoulder external rotators.

Develop Muscular Stabilization and Endurance

- Alternating isometric resistance is applied to the scapular muscles in *open-chain positions* (side-lying, sitting, supine), including protraction/retraction, elevation/depression, and upward/downward rotation so the patient learns to stabilize the scapula against externally applied forces (see Fig. 17.37 in the exercise section).
- Scapular and GH patterns are combined using flexion, abduction, and rotation. Alternating isometric resistance is applied to the humerus while the patient holds against the changing directions of the external resistance force (see Figs. 17.38, 17.39, and 17.42 in the exercise section).
- *Closed-chain stabilization* is performed with the patient's hands fixated against a wall, a table, or the floor (quadruped position) while the therapist provides graded, alternating isometric resistance or rhythmic stabilization. If abnormal scapular winging occurs during the applied resistance, the scapular stabilizers are not strong enough for the demand and the position should be modified to reduce the challenge (see Fig. 17.43 in the exercise section). This can be accomplished by changing the patient's body position relative to gravity or modifying joint angles.
- *Muscular endurance* is progressed by increasing the amount of time the individual holds the pattern against the alternating resistance. The limit is reached when any one of the muscles in the pattern can no longer maintain the desired hold. The goal at this phase should be stabilization for approximately 3 minutes.

Progress Shoulder Function

As the patient develops strength in the weakened muscles, it becomes important to develop a balance in strength of all shoulder and scapular muscles within the range and tolerance of each muscle. To increase coordination between scapular and arm motions, dynamically load the upper extremity with submaximal resistance as the patient maintains the synergy pattern. To improve muscular endurance, increase the length of time the patient controls the correct pattern up to 3 minutes.

Management: Return to Function Phase

Specificity of training toward the desired functional outcomes begins as soon as the patient has developed control of posture and can perform the basic components of their desired activities without exacerbating the symptoms. While working with the patient, continue to teach him or her how to progress the program and prevent recurrences after discharged from therapy. Suggestions are summarized in Box 17.7.

Increase Muscular Endurance

To increase muscular endurance, repetitive loading of the defined patterns is increased from 3 minutes to 5 minutes.

Develop Quick Motor Responses to Imposed Stresses

- Apply the stabilization exercises with increased speed with shorter durations and faster transitions between the applied forces.

BOX 17.7 Patient Instructions to Prevent Recurrences of Shoulder Pain

- Prior to exercise or work, massage the involved tendon or muscle; follow with isometric resistance and then with full ROM and stretching of the muscle.
- Take breaks from activities that are repetitive in nature. If possible, alternate the stressful, provoking activity with other activities or patterns of motion.
- Maintain good postural alignment; adapt seating or workstation to minimize stress. If sport related, seek coaching in proper techniques or adapt equipment for safe mechanics.
- Prior to initiating a new activity or returning to an activity for which not conditioned, begin a strengthening and training program.

- Plyometric training in both open-chain and closed-chain patterns is initiated if power is a desired outcome (refer to Chapter 23).

Progress Functional Training

Specificity of training progresses to an emphasis on timing and sequencing of events.

- Eccentric training is progressed to maximum load.
- Desired functional activities are simulated—first under controlled conditions, then under progressively challenging conditions using acceleration/deceleration drills.
- The patient is involved in assessing performance in terms of safety, symptom provocation, postural control, and ease of execution and then practices adaptations to correct any identified problems.

Painful Shoulder Syndromes: Surgery and Postoperative Management

Surgical intervention is an option for painful shoulder syndromes when conservative management does not resolve symptoms or improve function. For an individual with primary impingement as a result of structural variations in the acromion (see descriptions and Fig. 17.16 in the previous section), subacromial decompression may be performed. An individual with a partial- or full-thickness rotator cuff tear may require surgical repair of the tissue.

Subacromial Decompression and Postoperative Management

When pain and loss of functional mobility associated with primary impingement/rotator cuff disease do not resolve sufficiently with nonoperative management, *subacromial decompression* is often warranted. This procedure is designed to restore or increase the volume of the subacromial space and provide adequate gliding room for the cuff tendons. Subacromial decompression also is referred to as *anterior acromioplasty* or *decompression acromioplasty*. Acromioplasty, which alters the shape of the acromion, is typically, but not always, one component of subacromial decompression.[126]

Indications for Surgery

The following are generally accepted indications for surgical management of impingement syndromes/rotator cuff disease.[1,56,76,81,126,142,146,168,210]

- Pain during overhead activities and loss of functional mobility of the shoulder as the result of primary impingement that persists (typically for 3 to 6 months or longer) despite a trial of nonoperative interventions.
- Stage II (Neer classification; see Box 17.5) impingement with nonreversible fibrosis or bony alterations of the subacromial compartment, calcific deposits in the cuff tendons, and symptomatic subacromial crepitus.
- Intact or minor tear of the rotator cuff.

NOTE: Patients who present with GH joint hypermobility or instability associated with a partial- or full-thickness tear of the rotator cuff are not candidates for surgical subacromial decompression alone. For these patients, subacromial decompression is combined with concomitant repair of the cuff tear; otherwise, the procedures inherent in subacromial decompression can worsen GH instability.[76,126,210]

Procedures

Surgical approach. Subacromial decompression is performed using an arthroscopic or open approach. Although an open approach has been used successfully for many years,[81,139,142,168] the preferred procedure today is an arthroscopic approach.[56,210] Unlike a traditional open approach, in which the proximal attachment of the deltoid must be detached and then repaired prior to closure,[142] the deltoid remains intact during an arthroscopic approach, which enables the patient to regain functional use of the upper extremity more rapidly after surgery. For the most part, the traditional open approach for subacromial decompression is now reserved for patients with a massive rotator cuff tear who are also undergoing an open repair. Another option preferred by some surgeons is a "mini-open" approach, which involves splitting the deltoid insertion vertically rather than detaching it.[126]

Component procedures. There are several surgical procedures that can be performed for subacromial decompression depending on the pathology observed during examination of the shoulder prior to or during surgery.[1,56,71,76,126,153,210]

- Removal of the subacromial bursa (*bursectomy*), which is typically thickened (enlarged) by chronic inflammation
- Release of the coracoacromial ligament, which is usually hypertrophied and may also be frayed, followed by complete or partial resection or recession
- Resection of the anterior acromial protuberance and contouring the undersurface of the remaining portion of the acromion (*acromioplasty*) to enlarge the subacromial space (Fig. 17.18)
- Removal of osteophytes at the AC joint and in some cases resection of the distal portion of the clavicle for advanced AC joint arthritis

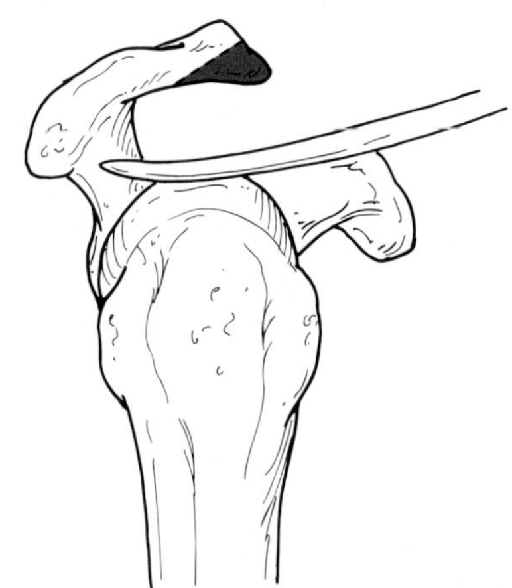

FIGURE 17.18 Arthroscopic acromioplasty showing the line of resection of the anterior acromion.

Postoperative Management

The type of surgical approach used and the integrity of the rotator cuff significantly affect rehabilitation decisions after subacromial decompression. If the rotator cuff is intact preoperatively, rehabilitation after arthroscopic decompression progresses quite rapidly because the shoulder musculature is not damaged during the procedure. In contrast, if repair of a rotator cuff tear is required in addition to decompression, or a mini-open or open approach is used, rehabilitation progresses at a slower rate to allow the repaired shoulder musculature adequate time to heal.

NOTE: The guidelines outlined in this section are for postoperative rehabilitation after *arthroscopic* subacromial decompression for a patient with primary shoulder impingement who has an *intact rotator cuff.* If subacromial decompression is combined with repair of the rotator cuff, the guidelines presented in a later section of this chapter on rehabilitation after rotator cuff repair are appropriate.

Immobilization

Following surgery the shoulder is immobilized and supported in a sling with the arm positioned at the patient's side or in slight abduction and internal rotation, with the elbow flexed to 90°. The sling is worn for comfort for 1 to 2 weeks but is removed for exercise the day after surgery.[126,210,219]

Exercise Progression

Exercises after subacromial decompression focus on many of the impairments noted for rotator cuff impingement discussed previously in this chapter. This information merits review to understand why specific exercises are included in the postoperative rehabilitation program. Because arthroscopic decompression is often performed on an outpatient basis, a patient may need to initially exercise at home with little supervision and then follow up with a series of outpatient therapy visits.

Exercise: Maximum Protection Phase

The first phase of rehabilitation after arthroscopic decompression begins on the day after surgery and extends for 3 to 4 weeks. Emphasis is placed on pain control and immediate but comfortable assisted movement of the shoulder to prevent movement restrictions as soft tissues are healing. Attaining full or nearly full passive ROM of the involved shoulder is a reasonable goal by 4 to 6 weeks postoperatively.[76]

Patient education begins immediately and is directed toward helping the patient recognize and avoid postures that contribute to symptoms during exercise and ADL. Active (unassisted) shoulder ROM is permissible as soon as motions are pain-free and proper scapulothoracic and GH control can be maintained. This may be possible as early as 2 weeks postsurgery.

Goals and interventions. The following goals and exercises are indicated for the early stage of tissue healing:[1,2,34,76,126,219]

- ***Control pain and inflammation.***
  - Use a sling when the arm is dependent.
  - Use cryotherapy and prescribed anti-inflammatory medication.
  - Shoulder relaxation exercises.
- ***Prevent loss of mobility of adjacent regions.***
  - Active ROM of the cervical spine, elbow, wrist, and hand.
- ***Develop postural awareness and control.***
  - Posture training, emphasizing cervical retraction, thoracic extension, scapula retraction, and a neutral lumbopelvic complex.
- ***Restore pain-free shoulder mobility.***
  - Assisted shoulder ROM within pain tolerance, initially guiding the involved arm with the sound upper extremity and later with a cane or wand. Start in the supine position to stabilize the scapula against the thorax and place the upper arm on a folded towel in slight abduction and flexion. Shoulder motions include elevating the arm in the plane of the scapula, forward flexion, abduction, rotation, and horizontal abduction and adduction. Progress to performing exercises in a semi-reclining position and then in a seated or standing position while maintaining thoracic extension.
  - Assisted shoulder extension in a standing position with a wand held behind the back.
  - Stretching the posterior shoulder structures in pain-free range using a cross-chest stretch into horizontal adduction. Postpone until next phase if painful.
  - Active ROM (unassisted) of the shoulder and scapula within pain-free ranges, maintaining proper scapulothoracic and GH control; begin supine and progress to sitting. Active shoulder motions may be possible by 2 weeks postoperatively.
- ***Prevent reflex inhibition and disuse atrophy of shoulder girdle musculature.***
  - *Pain-free*, low-intensity, multiple-angle isometrics of GH musculature with the arm supported and emphasis on the rotator cuff against minimal resistance. Begin submaximal isometrics a week or so postoperatively. Lightly resist with the uninvolved upper extremity. Focus on increasing repetitions more than resistance.[114,181]
  - Submaximal alternating isometric and rhythmic stabilization exercises for scapulothoracic muscles with the involved arm supported by the therapist. Target the scapular retractors and upward rotators.

Criteria to progress. Criteria to advance to the second phase include:[34,76,98,126,219]

- Minimal discomfort when the shoulder is unsupported; arm swing during ambulation is comparable to opposite arm.
- Almost full, pain-free, *passive* ROM of the shoulder (full mobility of the scapula; at least 150° of arm elevation; full internal/external rotation).
- In the supine position, pain-free *active* elevation of the arm well above the level of the shoulder.
- Pain-free, *active* external rotation of the shoulder to about 45°.
- At least fair (3/5) and preferably good (4/5) muscle testing grade of shoulder musculature.

Exercise: Moderate Protection Phase

Exercises during the second phase of rehabilitation are focused on attaining full, pain-free shoulder ROM and improving neuromuscular control and muscle performance of the rotator cuff, scapular stabilizers, and prime movers. The patient may be ready to begin this phase of rehabilitation as early as 3 to 4 weeks postoperatively but more often by 4 to 6 weeks. This phase extends over a 4- to 6-week period or until the patient meets the criteria to progress to the next phase.

Goals and interventions. The goals, exercises, and activities during the second phase of rehabilitation are:[34,76,98,219]

- ***Restore and maintain full, pain-free passive mobility of the shoulder girdle and upper trunk.***
  - Joint mobilization emphasizing posterior and caudal glides of the humerus and scapulothoracic mobility.
  - Low-intensity self-stretching of muscles that could restrict sufficient upward rotation of the scapula and rotation of the humerus, specifically the levator scapulae, rhomboids, subscapularis, latissimus dorsi, teres major, and pectoralis major and minor. Recall that tightness of these muscles may contribute to subacromial impingement during overhead movements of the arm.
  - Self-stretching of the posterior shoulder muscles and posterior capsule of the GH joint, as these structures may be tight in the presence of shoulder impingement.
  - Self-stretch the upper trunk and thoracic extension by lying supine on a rolled towel placed vertically between the scapulae.
  - Perform exercises and functional movement patterns into the acquired ROM.

- ***Reinforce posture awareness and control.***
  - Continue to emphasize cervical, thoracic, and lumbopelvic alignment during exercises and function.
- ***Develop dynamic stability, strength, endurance, and control of scapulothoracic and GH muscles.***
  - Stabilization exercises against increasing resistance and in weight-bearing positions. Emphasize isolated strengthening of the serratus anterior and trapezius muscles.
  - Upper extremity ergometry for muscular endurance. To avoid an impingement arc, initiate in a standing position rather than while seated.
  - Dynamic strengthening exercises of isolated shoulder muscles against low-loads (1- to 5-lb weight or light-grade elastic tubing), gradually increasing repetitions. Begin resisted elevation of the arm in the supine position to stabilize the scapula against the thorax; progress to sitting or standing.
  - Use the involved arm for functional activities that involve light resistance.

CLINICAL TIP

Target the upward rotators of the scapulothoracic joint (serratus anterior, upper and lower trapezius) and the rotator cuff muscles[184] as well as the latissimus dorsi, teres major, and biceps brachii, which act as humeral head depressors and therefore oppose superior translation during active elevation of the arm. Initially, perform resisted motions of the humerus below the level of the shoulder; later, progress to overhead exercises if motions remain pain free.

PRECAUTION: Be certain the patient can perform active shoulder flexion and abduction against gravity without elevating the scapula before progressing to resisted exercises above shoulder level.

Criteria to progress. The criteria to progress to the final phase of rehabilitation are:[34,98,219]

- Negative provocation tests.
- Full, pain-free, active ROM of the shoulder without evidence of substitute motions.
- At least 75% strength of the shoulder musculature compared with the sound shoulder.[219]

Exercise: Minimum Protection/Return to Function Phase

The final phase of rehabilitation usually begins 8 weeks postoperatively when soft tissues are reasonably well healed and require little to no protection. Exercises continue until about 12 to 16 weeks postoperatively or until the patient has returned to full activity. Exercises are directed toward improving strength and endurance of the shoulder girdle muscles using isolated movements and those that simulate functional activities. Patients often see continued improvement in functional use of the operated upper extremity for 6 months postoperatively.[2]

The time necessary for full recovery and unrestricted activities depends largely on the level of demand of the patient's anticipated activities. A patient wishing to return to competitive sports requires a more demanding progression of advanced exercises (e.g., plyometric training and sport-specific drills) than a sedentary individual.[34,219,222]

Goals and interventions. The goals, exercises, and activities during the final phase of rehabilitation after subacromial decompression are similar to the final phase of nonoperative management of primary impingement syndrome. Refer to the information presented in the previous section of this chapter as well as other resources.[34,45,217,219,222]

Outcomes

There appears to be no significant difference in the long-term results (pain-free ROM and return to desired functional activities) after either open or arthroscopic surgery for primary impingement syndrome with or without associated rotator cuff disease.[56,126,210] Based on the results of numerous outcome studies of open and arthroscopic procedures, 85% to 95% of patients report good to excellent results 1.0 to 2.5 years postoperatively.[1,76,126,210] In general, patients reporting the least satisfaction with their function after surgery are those who participate in high-demand athletic activities that involve overhead throwing and those with work-related injuries who are receiving workers' compensation.[126]

Several studies have documented advantages of an arthroscopic procedure rather than open surgical management of rotator cuff disease. Advantages include less postoperative pain, earlier restoration of full ROM and strength, earlier return to work (often as early as 1 week postoperatively), lower cost (shorter hospital stay or outpatient surgery), and a more favorable cosmetic result.[1,76,126,210]

Although exercises are routinely prescribed after subacromial decompression, the effectiveness of exercise has been the focus of very few studies. One prospective, randomized study compared the effectiveness of a 6-week therapist-supervised exercise program to a self-managed program after arthroscopic subacromial decompression.[2] Patients in the therapist-supervised group received exercise instruction while in the hospital and then for a 1-hour therapy session once a week for 6 weeks after discharge. Patients in the self-managed group received exercise instruction on one occasion prior to discharge from the hospital. Both groups received written instructions. At 6 weeks and at 3, 6, and 12 months, there were no significant differences in outcomes between the two groups with the exception of one variable. At 3 months postoperatively, the therapist-supervised group had a higher level of pain than the self-managed group. The authors concluded that initial, therapist-directed exercise instruction followed by a home-based, self-managed exercise program achieved rehabilitation goals as effectively as a therapist-supervised program.

Rotator Cuff Repair and Postoperative Management

Rotator cuff tears are broadly categorized as either partial-thickness or full-thickness tears. Either type may require surgical management. A *partial-thickness tear* extends inferiorly or superiorly through only a portion of the tendon from either the acromial (bursal) or humeral (articular) surface of the tendon. A *full-thickness tear* is a complete tear, extending between the superior and inferior surfaces of the tendon.[76,83,126] Both types of tears can be oriented either parallel to or perpendicular to the primary orientation of the tendon fibers.

Indications for Surgery

The primary indications for surgical management of a rotator cuff tear confirmed by imaging are pain and impaired function as the result of the following:[5,76,83,126,159,210,231]

- Partial-thickness or full-thickness tears of the rotator cuff tendons with irreversible, degenerative changes in soft tissues. Some patients with Neer stage II lesions and most with Neer stage III lesions who continue to be symptomatic and have functional limitations after a trial of nonoperative treatment are candidates for surgery.
- Acute, traumatic rupture of the rotator cuff tendons that may be combined with avulsion of the greater tuberosity, labral damage, or acute dislocation of the GH joint in individuals with no known history of prior cuff injury. Full-thickness, traumatic tears occur most often in young, active adults.

NOTE: Surgical repair is not indicated in patients who are asymptomatic despite the presence of a cuff tear confirmed by imaging.

Procedures

There are several operative options for repairing a torn rotator cuff, including arthroscopic, open, and mini-open repairs.[64,76,78,126,210] The decision about which procedure to choose depends on the severity and location of the tear, the number of tendons involved, the extent of associated lesions, the type of onset (repetitive microtrauma or traumatic injury), the quality and mobility of the torn tissues, bone quality, patient-related considerations (age, health, activity level), and the surgeon's preference and training.

Type of Repair

The type of cuff repair is typically classified by the surgical approach and techniques used. There are three categories of repair:[5,62,63,64,76,126,191,210,231]

- ***Arthroscopic approach.*** The entire procedure is performed arthroscopically and requires only a few small skin incisions for inserting surgical instruments.
- ***Mini-open (arthroscopically assisted) approach.*** There are two variations of this type of procedure, both of which involve arthroscopic subacromial decompression and a *deltoid-splitting* approach. In one variation, only the subacromial decompression is performed arthroscopically, whereas in the other variation a portion of the cuff repair itself is also performed arthroscopically.[231] In both cases, an anterolateral incision is made at the acromion and is extended distally (either 1.5 or 3.5 cm but no more than 4 cm to avoid the axillary nerve) along the fiber orientation of the deltoid. The deltoid is split longitudinally between its anterior and middle portions to allow visualization of the cuff tear without detaching the deltoid from its proximal insertion.[58,64,126,159,199]
- ***Traditional open approach.*** An anterolateral incision is made that extends obliquely from the middle one-third of the inferior aspect of the clavicle, across the coracoid process, and to the anterior aspect of the proximal humerus. The proximal insertion of the deltoid must be detached and reflected for exposure of the operative field during an open subacromial decompression and cuff repair. After the cuff repair is complete, the deltoid is reattached to the acromion.[64,83,126] As arthroscopic and arthroscopically assisted repair techniques have advanced, the use of this traditional open approach has decreased.

Components of a Rotator Cuff Repair

Regardless of the approach, subacromial decompression is performed (particularly for cuff tears associated with chronic impingement) before repair of the cuff is undertaken. After the tear is visualized, the margins of the torn tendon are débrided and released from any adherent soft tissues. The cuff tendon is then mobilized for advancement and apposition to bone that has been prepared for sutures and attached by *tendon-to-bone* fixation. Depending on whether an arthroscopic or mini-open approach is used, fixation is accomplished by sutures and suture anchors, tacks, or staples.[58,62,76,126,198,210]

In addition to subacromial decompression, other concomitant procedures may be required during the procedure. For example, capsular tightening or labral reconstruction may be performed if unidirectional or multidirectional instability of the GH joint is present. Because degenerative changes in the tendon of the long head of the biceps brachii are often "associated with chronic rotator cuff disease, a repair of this tendon also may be necessary.

Selection of Surgical Procedures

The surgeon weighs many factors when determining which type of procedure is most appropriate for each patient. One such consideration is the severity of the tear, including thickness (partial or full), size, and number of tendons torn. Although there is some variability in the literature, there are four generally accepted categories that describe the longitudinal size of rotator cuff tears: *small* (1 cm or less), *medium* (1 to 3 cm), *large* (3 to 5 cm), and *massive* (more than 5 cm or a full-thickness tear of more than one tendon).[5,58,76,212]

A small, *partial-thickness* cuff tear is usually managed surgically with a fully arthroscopic approach to débride the frayed margins of the torn tendon and includes a subacromial decompression. The torn portion of the tendon may or may not be repaired.[5,76,126,191,198,210]

Historically, small and medium *full-thickness* cuff tears only were managed with a fully arthroscopic approach.[63,76,126] With the advancement of arthroscopic techniques, however, an increasing percentage of large, full-thickness tears and some massive tears are now also managed with a fully arthroscopic approach.[210,231] Despite these surgical advances, variations of the mini-open (deltoid splitting) approach often remain the surgeon's choice for repair of medium and large tears.[58,126,199] Even some massive tears are managed with a deltoid-splitting approach.[126,212] The traditional open approach, requiring detachment and repair of the deltoid, is now primarily reserved for repairs of multiple tendon tears associated with extensive injury to the shoulder.[58,126]

The location of the cuff tear, amount of retraction and mobility of a full-thickness tear, and the quality of the remaining tendon and underlying bone also influence the surgeon's selection of the procedure expected to be most effective.[76,126,198,210] Whereas small, medium, and large tears of the supraspinatus or infraspinatus are routinely managed with arthroscopic or mini-open approaches, tears of the subscapularis are often managed with a traditional open approach.[58] Also, with poor tissue quality or significant retraction and limited mobility of the torn tendon, many surgeons believe that a stronger repair can be achieved with an open procedure instead of an arthroscopic repair.[76]

Postoperative Management

After surgical repair of a torn rotator cuff tendon, many factors influence decisions about the position and duration of immobilization, the selection and application of exercises, and the rate of progression of each patient's rehabilitation program. These factors and their potential impact are summarized in Table 17.3. These factors also will affect postoperative prognosis and outcomes.

TABLE 17.3 Factors That Influence Progression of Rehabilitation After Repair of the Rotator Cuff

Factors	Potential Impact on Rehabilitation
■ Onset of injury	■ Chronic impingement and atraumatic cuff deficiency → slower progression than after acute traumatic injury
■ Size and location of the tear	■ Larger tears with more tendons involved → slower progression
■ Associated pathologies such as GH instability or fracture	■ More involved surgeries and potential for longer period of immobilization → slower progression of exercises or the need for additional precautions
■ Preoperative strength and mobility of the shoulder	■ Preexisting weakness and atrophy of the dynamic stabilizers or limited passive and active mobility of the shoulder → slower postoperative progression
■ Patient's general health	■ Patient in poor health; history of smoking; history of inflammatory disease → slower progression
■ History of steroid injections or previous, failed cuff surgery	■ Compromised bone and tendon tissue quality, which affects the security of the repair (fixation) → slower progression
■ Pre-injury level of activity or postoperative goals	■ Higher level activities increase risk of re-injury → a more extended and advanced postoperative training program
■ Age of patient	■ Older patient → slower progression more likely
■ Type of surgical approach	■ Traditional open approach (with deltoid detachment and repair) → slightly slower progression than after an arthroscopic or arthroscopically assisted (mini-open/deltoid splitting) repair
■ Type of repair	■ Tendon to tendon → slower progression than tendon to bone
■ Mobility (no excessive tension on the repaired tendon when arm at side) and integrity of the repair	■ If mobility is inadequate → longer duration of exercise within a protected ROM during early rehabilitation
■ Patient's compliance with the program	■ Lack of compliance (doing too much or too little) can affect outcome
■ Philosophy, skill, and training of the surgeon	■ All may have an impact that could → either slower or more accelerated progression

There is little consensus in the literature or in clinical practice as to how and to what extent each of these factors, singularly or collectively, impacts the decisions made by the surgeon and the therapist about a patient's postoperative rehabilitation program. Hence, predetermined guidelines and protocols for postoperative management after rotator cuff repair are diverse and sometimes contradictory.[5,34,53,55,58,64,76,126,208] For example, some authors suggest that if deltoid detachment and repair are components of the surgery deltoid strengthening exercises should be postponed for approximately 6 to 8 weeks postoperatively until the repaired deltoid has healed.[34,55,126] In contrast, another author suggests that rehabilitation should proceed similarly regardless of whether deltoid detachment was required so long as secure fixation of the deltoid was achieved.[74]

Given the diverse characteristics of patients undergoing rotator cuff repair and the variety of surgical options available, it is not surprising that no single postoperative program can be used for all patients or yields better outcomes than other programs. Therefore, to meet each patient's needs and goals, a therapist can use published protocols or those developed at individual clinical facilities as general guidelines for postoperative management. Modifications to protocols and guidelines should be made based on ongoing examination of the patient's response to interventions and through communication with the surgeon.

Despite variations among postoperative programs, they share three common elements: (1) immediate or early postoperative motion of the GH joint; (2) control of the rotator cuff for dynamic stability; and (3) gradual restoration of strength and muscular endurance. This section will present *general* exercise guidelines that incorporate these elements into the phases of rehabilitation after arthroscopic or mini-open repair of a *full-thickness* cuff tear. Potential modifications and precautions due to a traditional open procedure or on factors such as size, location of the tear, and the quality of the repair will be noted.

NOTE: The goals, exercise interventions, and progression of rehabilitation after débridement rather than repair of a *partial-thickness* tear are comparable to postoperative management after subacromial decompression for cuff impingement presented in the previous section of this chapter.

Immobilization

The position and duration of immobilization of the operated shoulder after rotator cuff repair depends on many factors, including the size, severity, and location of the tear and the type and quality of the repair. The size of the cuff tear partially determines whether the patient's operated arm is supported in a sling (shoulder adducted, internally rotated, and elbow flexed to 90°) or in an abduction orthosis or splint (shoulder elevated in the plane of the scapula approximately 45°, shoulder internally rotated, and elbow flexed). Patients supported in an abduction splint may require assistance from a family member to support the operated arm in the 45° shoulder position when the splint is removed for exercise, dressing, or bathing.

Table 17.4 summarizes the immobilization recommendations for fully arthroscopic and mini-open/deltoid-splitting approaches. Immobilization after a traditional open procedure that involves deltoid detachment and repair is not included in Table 17.4 because of the variations in guidelines reported in the literature.[34,76,126,212]

The rationale for initially immobilizing the shoulder in abduction is based on two principles. In the abducted position, the shoulder is in a more relaxed, neutral position, reducing the possibility of reflexive muscle contractions that could disrupt the repairs. In addition, supporting the arm in abduction reduces tension on the repaired tendons and may also improve blood flow to the repair site.

Exercise Progression

Regardless of whether a patient undergoes a rotator cuff repair on an inpatient or outpatient basis, contact with a therapist for exercise instruction after surgery is usually limited to a few visits. Therefore, the emphasis of a therapist's interaction with a patient must be placed on patient education for an effective and safe home-based exercise program.

Goals and interventions for each phase of rehabilitation after arthroscopic or mini-open cuff repair follow. General guidelines for exercise and precautions after rotator cuff repair are summarized in Box 17.8. Precautions specific to a particular type of cuff tear or surgical procedure are also noted. The suggested timelines for each phase are general and must be adjusted based on factors already noted (see Table 17.3).

TABLE 17.4 Relationships between the Size of the Rotator Cuff Tear With the Type and Duration of Immobilization After Arthroscopic and Mini-Open Repair*

Size of Tear	Type and Duration of Immobilization
Small (≤ 1 cm)	Sling for 1–2 weeks; removal for exercise the day of surgery or 1 day postop
Medium to large (1 cm to 5 cm)	Sling or abduction orthosis/pillow for 3–6 weeks; removal for exercise 1–2 days postop
Massive (> 5 cm)†	Sling or abduction orthosis/pillow for 4–8 weeks; removal for exercise 1–3 days postop

*Fully arthroscopic and mini-open (arthroscopically assisted/deltoid splitting) approaches.
†A fully arthroscopic approach is not often used to repair massive cuff tears.

BOX 17.8 General Exercise Guidelines and Precautions Following Repair of a Full-Thickness Rotator Cuff Tear

Early Shoulder Motion

- Perform passive or assisted shoulder ROM within *safe and pain-free ranges* based on the surgeon's intraoperative observation of the mobility and strength of the repair, a prescribed postsurgical protocol, and the patient's comfort level during exercise.
- Only passive ROM for 6 to 8 weeks after repair of a massive cuff tear or after a traditional open approach to prevent avulsion of the repaired deltoid.
- Initially perform passive and assisted shoulder ROM in the supine position to maintain stability of the scapula on the thorax.
- Minimize anterior and superior translations of the humeral head and the potential for impingement. Position the humerus slightly anterior to the frontal plane of the body and in slight abduction.
- While at rest in the supine position, support the distal humerus on a folded towel.
- When initiating passive or assisted shoulder rotation while lying supine, position the shoulder in slight flexion and approximately 45° of abduction.
- When initiating assisted shoulder extension, perform the exercise in prone position (arm over the edge of the bed) from 90° to just short of neutral. Later progress to exercises behind the back.
- When performing assisted or active exercises in the upright position (sitting or standing), be certain that the patient maintains an erect trunk posture to minimize the possibility of impingement.
- To ensure adequate humeral depression and avoid superior translation of the head of the humerus when beginning *active* elevation of the arm, restore strength in the rotator cuff, especially the supraspinatus and infraspinatus muscles, before dynamically strengthening the shoulder flexors and abductors.
- Do not allow *active* shoulder flexion or abduction until the patient can lift the arm without hiking the shoulder.

Strengthening Exercises

- When beginning isometric resistance to scapulothoracic musculature, be sure to support the operated arm to avoid excessive tension in repaired GH musculature.
- Use low exercise loads; resisted motions should not cause pain.
- No weight-bearing (closed-chain) exercises or activities for 6 weeks.
- Delay dynamic strengthening (progressive resistive exercise) for a *minimum* of 8 weeks postoperatively for small, strong repair and for at least 3 months for larger tears.
- If the supraspinatus or infraspinatus was repaired, proceed cautiously when resisting GH joint external rotation.
- If the subscapularis was repaired, proceed cautiously with resisted GH joint internal rotation.
- After an open repair, postpone isometric resistance exercises to the repaired deltoid and cuff musculature for *at least* 6 to 8 weeks unless advised otherwise.

Stretching Exercises

- Avoid vigorous stretching, the use of contract-relax procedures, or grade III joint mobilizations for at least 6 weeks and often for 12 weeks postoperatively to give time for the repaired tendon(s) to heal and become strong.
- If the supraspinatus or infraspinatus was repaired, initially avoid end-range stretching into GH joint internal rotation.
- If the subscapularis was repaired, initially avoid end-range stretching into GH joint external rotation.
- If the deltoid was detached and repaired, initially avoid end-range shoulder extension, adduction, and horizontal adduction.

Activities of Daily Living

- Wait until about 6 weeks after a mini-open or arthroscopic repair and 12 weeks after a traditional open repair before using the operated arm for light functional activities.
- After repair of a large or massive cuff tear, avoid use of operated arm for functional activities that involve heavy resistance (pushing, pulling, lifting, carrying heavy loads) for 6 to 12 *months* postoperatively.

Exercise: Maximum Protection Phase

The priorities during the initial phase of rehabilitation are to protect the repaired tendon, which is at its weakest approximately 3 weeks after repair,[198] and to prevent the potential adverse effects of immobilization. For almost all patients, the immobilization device is removed for brief sessions of passive or assisted ROM within protected and comfortable ranges during the first few days after surgery (see Table 17.4).

The maximum protection phase extends for 3 to 4 weeks after a fully arthroscopic or mini-open repair of small or medium tears to as long as 6 to 8 weeks after repair of large or massive tears. After an arthroscopic repair of a small or medium tear, every effort is made to attain nearly full passive shoulder ROM, particularly elevation and external rotation, by 6 to 8 weeks postoperatively.[58,126,210]

Goals and interventions. The following goals and selected interventions are initiated during the maximum protection phase.[5,34,53,55,64,76,126,210,212]

- ***Control pain and inflammation.***
  - Periodic cryotherapy.
  - Arm support for comfort.

- Shoulder relaxation exercises.
- Grade I oscillations of the GH joint.
- Use of medically prescribed medications.

■ ***Prevent loss of mobility of adjacent regions.***

- Assisted ROM of the elbow.
- Active ROM of the cervical spine, wrist, and hand.
- Active scapulothoracic elevation/depression and protraction/retraction.

■ ***Prevent shoulder stiffness/restore shoulder mobility.***

- Pendulum exercises typically the first postoperative day or when the immobilizer may be removed for exercise. Emphasize using the correct technique and keeping the shoulder muscles relaxed.
- Passive ROM of the shoulder within safe and pain-free ranges. Initially perform exercises in the supine position; begin both arm elevation and external rotation in the plane of the scapula.
- Self-assisted ROM using the opposite hand or a wand by 1 to 2 weeks for patients with repairs of small to medium tears and about 2 weeks later for patients with repair of large tears.
- Active control of the shoulder with assistance as needed from the therapist or family members. With the patient lying supine, place the arm in 90° of shoulder flexion if pain free. In this position, the effect of gravity on the shoulder musculature is minimal. This position has been called the "balance point position" of the shoulder.[53] Help the patient control the shoulder while moving to and from the balance point position, making small arcs and circles with the arm.
- Active shoulder ROM by the latter part of this phase for small tears and as symptoms permit, initially supine with the elbow flexed, progressing to a semi-reclining position with the elbow less flexed.

PRECAUTION: Use only passive, non-assisted ROM for 6 to 8 weeks for a repair of a massive cuff tear or after a traditional open repair with deltoid detachment.[34,212]

■ ***Prevent or correct postural deviations.***

- Posture training and exercises to facilitate proper spinal alignment and shoulder retraction (see Chapters 14 and 16).

■ ***Develop control of scapulothoracic stabilizers.***

- Active movements of the scapula.
- Submaximal isometrics to isolated scapular muscles.[114] To avoid excessive tension in repaired GH musculature, see that the operated arm is supported but not bearing weight.
- Side-lying scapular protraction/retraction to facilitate serratus anterior function.

■ ***Prevent inhibition and atrophy of GH musculature.***

- Low-intensity, muscle-setting exercises against minimal resistance. Setting exercises should not provoke pain in a healing cuff tendon. Begin as early as 1 to 3 weeks postoperatively depending on the size of the tear and quality of the repair.[34,53,55]

PRECAUTION: Recommendations for the safest position of the shoulder in which to begin isometric training of the GH musculature after cuff repair are inconsistent. Perhaps the safest suggestion is to start in a position that creates minimal tension on the repaired cuff tendons (shoulder internally rotated and elevated in the scapular plane to about 45°, elbow flexed).[55] As the strength of the cuff muscles improves during the later phases of rehabilitation, exercises and activities can be performed with the arm positioned in more challenging and functional positions.

Criteria to progress. Criteria to advance to the second phase include:

- A well healed incision.
- Minimal pain with assisted shoulder motions.
- Progressive improvement in ROM.

Exercise: Moderate Protection Phase

The focus of the second phase of rehabilitation is to develop neuromuscular control, strength, and endurance of the shoulder while continuing to attain full or nearly full, pain-free shoulder motion. Emphasis is placed on developing control of the scapulothoracic and rotator cuff muscles.

For the patient with repair of a small or medium tear, this phase begins around 4 to 6 weeks postoperatively and extends an additional 6 weeks. For most patients, strengthening exercises typically begin around 8 weeks postoperatively. This phase may begin as late as 12 weeks for the patient with repair of a large or massive tear.

FOCUS ON EVIDENCE

Thomson et al[193] performed a systematic review of eleven RCT's comparing the effectiveness of postoperative rehabilitation protocols following rotator cuff repair. Six studies evaluated the effect of early ROM exercises and found some evidence for improved outcomes early in recovery with no detrimental long-term outcomes. With small to moderate tears and good fixation, passive ROM can begin one day following surgery, with active ROM started several days later. Patients with larger tears and additional factors such as poor tissue quality, systemic disease, or sedentary lifestyle should delay passive ROM for 4 to 6 weeks and wait to being active ROM until 6 to 8 weeks following surgery. CPM use is safe following surgery and may facilitate short-term pain relief and reduce postoperative stiffness, but does not offer any long-term benefit on outcomes.

Goals and interventions. The following goals and interventions are appropriate during this phase of rehabilitation.[5,34,53,55,58,126]

■ ***Restore nearly complete or full, pain-free, passive mobility of the shoulder.***

- Self-assisted ROM with an end-range hold by means of wand or pulley exercises, in single planes and combined

(diagonal) patterns. Add shoulder internal rotation, extension beyond neutral, and horizontal adduction.
- Mobilization of the incision site if well healed to prevent adherence of the scar.

PRECAUTION: The use of passive stretching and grade III joint mobilizations, if initiated during this phase of rehabilitation, must be done *very cautiously*. Vigorous stretching is not considered safe for 3 to 4 months, the time needed for the repaired tendons to have healed and become reasonably strong.[126]

- ***Increase strength and endurance and re-establish dynamic stability of the shoulder musculature.***
  - Active ROM of the shoulder through gradually increasing the pain-free ranges. Continue to have the patient perform active elevation of the arm in the supine position until the motion can be initiated without first elevating the scapula. When transitioning to upright positions (sitting or standing), reinforce the importance of maintaining an erect trunk during exercises.
  - Isometric and dynamic strengthening to scapulothoracic muscles. First, use alternating isometrics in non-weight-bearing positions; then progress to rhythmic stabilization during light upper extremity weight-bearing activities.
  - Submaximal multiple-angle isometrics of the rotator cuff and other GH musculature against gradually increasing resistance.
  - Dynamic strengthening and endurance training of the GH musculature within pain-free ranges against light resistance, such as light-grade elastic tubing or a 1- to 2-lb weight. Perform exercises below the level of the shoulder if pain is provoked with active movements above shoulder height.
  - Upper extremity ergometry at or just below shoulder height against light resistance to increase muscular endurance.
  - Use of the involved upper extremity for *light* (no-load or low-load) functional activities.

CLINICAL TIP

Because weakness and atrophy of the rotator cuff often are present prior to injury, strengthen and increase endurance of the cuff muscles before dynamically strengthening the shoulder abductors and flexors.

Criteria to progress. Criteria to transition to the final phase of rehabilitation and gradually return to unrestricted activities include:

- Full, pain-free passive ROM.
- Progressive improvement of shoulder strength and muscular endurance.
- A stable GH joint.

Exercise: Minimum Protection/Return to Function Phase

This final phase usually begins no earlier than 12 to 16 weeks postoperatively for patients with strong repairs or at 16 weeks or later for a more tenuous repair. This phase may continue 6 months or more depending on the patient's expected activities.

Goals and interventions. The goals and interventions during this final phase of rehabilitation are consistent with those previously discussed for late-stage nonoperative management of cuff disorders and for the final phase of rehabilitation after subacromial decompression. However, the progression of activities after a cuff repair is more gradual, and the time frame for adhering to precautions is extended.

If full ROM still has not been restored by the beginning of this phase, include passive stretching of the GH musculature and joint mobilization. Incorporate activities that move the arm into the increased ROMs, such as gently swinging a golf club or tennis racket if the motions are pain free. Advanced, task-specific strengthening activities dominate this phase of rehabilitation.

Patients are generally not allowed to return to high-demand activities for 6 months to 1 year postoperatively, depending on the patient's level of comfort, strength, and flexibility as well as the demands of the desired activities.

Outcomes

A considerable number of outcome studies of operative management of rotator cuff tears have been reported in the literature with follow-up ranging from less than 6 months to 5 years or more. Outcomes commonly measured include pain, shoulder ROM and strength, overall function, and patient satisfaction.

Long-term outcomes after fully arthroscopic, mini-open, and traditional open repairs are comparable.[76] For example, after fully arthroscopic repair of full-thickness tears (mostly small or medium but some large or massive tears), overall outcomes of several studies were reported as good to excellent in 84%[62,63] and 92%[191] of patients followed for 2 to 3 years. These results are comparable to results reported for open repairs.[76,126] However, it has been shown that regardless of the type of operative repair performed, the size of the cuff tear influences postoperative outcomes. For example, comparably favorable long-term functional outcomes and pain relief have been reported after mini-open and traditional open repairs of small to medium-sized, full-thickness tears,[7,76,126] while outcomes are less favorable after repairs of large or massive tears.[126,212]

Other factors, such as the acuity or chronicity of the tear and the patient's age also affect outcomes. Repairs of acute tears in young patients are more successful than repairs of similar size tears associated with chronic cuff impingement and insufficiency in elderly patients (>65 years).[71] The presence of fewer associated pathologies, such as a biceps tendon tear or cuff tear arthropathy, also are associated with better postoperative outcomes.[126]

Pain relief. Although the results of individual studies vary, a systematic review of the literature indicated that an average of

85% of patients who have operative repair of the rotator cuff report satisfactory relief of pain. Pain relief after arthroscopic and mini-open repairs ranges between 80% and 92%.[174] This is comparable to results of previous studies of traditional open repairs, in which satisfactory pain relief was reported by 85% to 95% of patients.[75,83] The preoperative size of the tear has an impact on pain relief with patients having small and medium tears reporting a higher percentage of satisfaction with pain relief than patients with large or massive tears.[75,126,174]

Shoulder ROM. In a prospective descriptive study of patients undergoing rotator cuff repair, the preoperative factor that most closely correlated with long-term limitation of shoulder ROM after surgery was the inability to place the hand behind the back.[203] Postoperative shoulder ROM is also associated with the size of the tear, with one study demonstrating that patients who had repairs of small to medium tears had more active flexion and abduction than patients with large tears.[83]

Strength. The rate of recovery of shoulder muscle strength also appears to be associated with the size of the tear, with faster recovery occurring with repair of small and medium tears than with repair of large or massive tears. Near-complete restoration of shoulder muscle strength occurs gradually and may take a year after repair of small and medium tears, while recovery of strength after repair of large or massive tears is inconsistent.[126,174]Although recovery of shoulder muscle strength occurs gradually throughout the first postoperative year, the most substantial gains are seen during the first 6 months.[126] In most cases, patients achieve 80% strength in the operated shoulder (compared to the noninvolved shoulder) by 6 months and 90% strength by 1 year.[171]

Functional abilities. It appears that long-term functional outcomes correlate with the size of the tear, type of repair, tissue quality, and the integrity of the repair.[126] For example, patients who have undergone a mini-open repair return to functional activities about a month earlier than those who have had an open repair.[7] However, this outcome may be skewed by the fact that mini-open repairs are performed more often in younger patients with less severe tears.

Lastly, in those patients who present with recurrence of a rotator cuff tear after repair, 80% had good to excellent short-term objective functional outcomes. This suggests that the evidence supporting a direct relationship between the integrity of the repair and functional outcomes is inconsistent.[75]

Shoulder Instabilities: Nonoperative Management

Related Pathologies and Mechanisms of Injury

GH joint hypermobility can be atraumatic or traumatic. *Atraumatic hypermobility*, often referred to as instability, can be due to generalized connective tissue laxity or from microtrauma related to repetitive activities. *Traumatic instability* is caused by a single event or a sequence of high force events that compromise the integrity of the stabilizing structures, often dislocating the GH joint. With traumatic dislocation, there is complete separation of the articular surfaces of the GH joint from direct or indirect forces applied to the shoulder.[155]Atraumatic instability may be a predisposing factor to traumatic dislocation, especially with repetitive stressful overhead activities.[85] GH joint hypermobility, regardless of whether atraumatic or traumatic, is often categorized as unidirectional or multidirectional. A secondary effect of hypermobility is a painful shoulder syndrome (described in an earlier section).

Atraumatic Hypermobility

Unidirectional instability. Unidirectional instability can be anterior, posterior, or inferior and is named for the direction in which the joint mobility is increased. It may be the result of physiological laxity of the connective tissues or repetitive non-uniform loading of the joint. With the compromise of stabilizing structures, the humeral head may continue to dislocate or sublux in the direction of the instability. This can lead to progressive degeneration and eventually tears in the supporting structures.

- *Anterior instability* usually occurs with posteriorly-directed forces applied to the arm when it is in an abducted and externally rotated position, resulting in anterior humeral head translations. If these forces occur with enough frequency and force to compromise anterior GH joint structures, instability results. Often these forces are self-generated, as in throwing athletes who repetitively position the arm such that the anterior capsule is overloaded. Positive clinical signs include apprehension, load and shift, and anterior drawer tests.[119,220]
- *Posterior instability* is much less common but can occur from repetitive posterior-directed forces applied against a forward-flexed humerus that translate the humeral head posteriorly. There is a positive posterior drawer sign with posterior instability.[119,220]
- *Inferior instability* is typically the result of rotator cuff weakness/paralysis and is frequently seen in patients with hemiplegia.[68] It is also prevalent in patients who repetitively reach overhead (workers or swimmers, for example) and those with multidirectional instability. This instability is evident with a positive sulcus sign.[119,220]

Multidirectional instability. The GH joint is considered to have multidirectional instability when stability is compromised in more than one direction. Some individuals have physiologically increased extensibility of connective tissue, causing excessive joint mobility. In the GH joint, this increased extensibility allows larger than normal humeral head translations in all directions.[155,178] Many individuals, particularly those involved in overhead activities, develop laxity of the capsule from continually subjecting the tissue to tensile forces.[61,92] Multidirectional instability is confirmed by a combination of the positive tests noted previously for unidirectional instability.

Common Impairments of Structure and Function

With atraumatic instability, symptoms are often chronic, intermittent, and activity dependent. Acute symptoms are infrequent but may occur if there is a significantly increased demand placed on the joint. Decreased endurance of the rotator cuff muscles may be a precipitating factor of repetitive trauma of the joint.

Common Activity Limitations and Participation Restrictions

- Possibility of recurrence when replicating the dislocating position or with forces applied to the arm in the dislocating position
- With anterior instability, restricted ability in sports activities such as throwing, swimming, serving, and spiking
- With posterior dislocation, restricted ability in sports activities, such as follow-through in throwing and golf; restricted ability in pushing activities, such as pushing open a heavy door or pushing one's self up out of a chair
- Discomfort or pain when sleeping on the involved side
- Inability to maintain arm positions or complete tasks requiring prolonged effort, especially overhead tasks

Traumatic Hypermobility

Traumatic anterior shoulder dislocation. Anterior dislocation most frequently occurs when there is a posteriorly directed force to the arm while the humerus is in a position of elevation, external rotation, and horizontal abduction. In that position, stability is provided by the subscapularis, GH ligaments (particularly the anterior band of the inferior ligament), and long head of the biceps.[105,170,204] A significant force to the arm may damage these structures, along with the attachment of the anterior capsule and glenoid labrum (Bankart lesion is depicted in Fig. 17.19).[43]

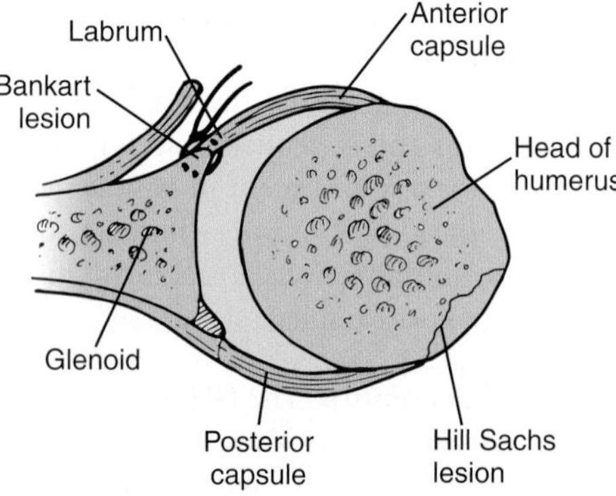

FIGURE 17.19 Lesions associated with traumatic anterior dislocation of the GH joint. A Bankart lesion is a fracture of the anterior rim of the glenoid with the attached labrum. The labrum is pulled away from the anterior glenoid along with a small piece of glenoid. A Hill-Sachs lesion, a compression fracture of the posterolateral humeral head, also may occur. *(Adapted from Tovin, BJ, and Greenfield, BH:* Evaluation and Treatment of the Shoulder—An Integration of the Guide to Physical Therapist Practice. *Philadelphia: F.A. Davis, 2001, p 295, with permission.)*

Traumatic anterior dislocation can be associated with complete rupture of the rotator cuff,[6,165] with the incidence increasing in those over 40 years of age.[43] There may also be a compression fracture (Hill-Sachs lesion, Fig. 17.19) at the posterolateral margin of the humeral head.[43] Neurological or vascular injuries may also occur during dislocations.[72] The axillary nerve is most commonly injured, but the brachial plexus or one of the peripheral nerves could be stretched or compressed.

Traumatic posterior shoulder dislocation. Traumatic posterior shoulder dislocation is less common. The mechanism of injury is usually a force applied to the arm when the humerus is positioned in flexion, adduction, and internal rotation, such as falling on an outstretched arm.[161] The injured person complains of symptoms when doing activities such as push-ups, a bench press, or follow-through on a golf swing.[72]

Recurrent Dislocations

With significant ligamentous and capsular laxity, recurrent subluxations or dislocations may occur with any movement that reproduces the humerus positions and forces that caused the original instability. These episodes result in significant pain and functional limitations. Some individuals can voluntarily dislocate the shoulder anteriorly or posteriorly without apprehension and with minimal discomfort.[155,182] The rate of recurrence after the first traumatic dislocation is highest in the younger population (< 30 years). Because they are more active and place greater demands on the shoulder, longer immobilization (> 3 weeks) is advocated after dislocation in patient's less than 30-years old. A shorter immobilization (1 to 2 weeks) is recommended for older patients.[125,128]

Common Impairments of Structure and Function

- After an acute traumatic injury, symptoms resulting from tissue damage include pain and muscle guarding due to bleeding and inflammation.
- When a dislocation is associated with a complete rotator cuff tear, there is an inability to abduct the humerus against gravity.
- Asymmetrical joint restriction/hypermobility. With anterior instability, the posterior capsule may become tight; with posterior instability, the anterior capsule may become tight. After healing from a traumatic event, there may be capsular adhesions.
- With recurrent dislocations, the individual can dislocate the shoulder at will, or the shoulder may dislocate during specific activities.

Common Activity Limitations and Participation Restrictions

- With rotator cuff rupture, inability to perform all activities requiring humeral elevation.
- Possibility of recurrence when replicating the dislocating position or with forces applied to the arm in the dislocating position.

- With anterior dislocation, restricted ability in sports activities, such as throwing, swimming, overhead serving, and spiking.
  - Restricted ability with dressing, such as putting on a shirt or jacket, and with self-grooming, such as combing the back of the hair.
  - Discomfort or pain when sleeping on the involved side.
- With posterior dislocation, restricted ability in sports activities, such as follow-through in pitching and golf; restricted ability in pushing activities, such as pushing open a heavy door or pushing one's self up from a chair.

Closed Reduction of Anterior Dislocation

NOTE: Several techniques are described in the literature utilizing either leverage or traction on the humerus to reduce an anterior dislocation.[43] Because of the risk of humeral fracture or injury to the brachial plexus or axillary blood vessels during reduction, the authors of this text recommend that these techniques should be undertaken only by someone specially trained to deal with these potential complications.

Management: Protection Phase

Protect the Healing Tissue

- Activity restriction is recommended for 6 to 8 weeks in a young patient. If a sling is used, the arm is removed from the sling only for controlled exercise. During the first week, the patient's arm may be continuously immobilized because of pain and muscle guarding.
- An older, less active patient (> 40 years of age) may require immobilization for only 2 weeks.
- The position of dislocation must be avoided when exercising, dressing, or doing other daily activities.

FOCUS ON EVIDENCE

Traditionally after acute anterior shoulder dislocation, immobilization has been instituted. However, a clinical commentary that evaluated outcomes from various studies found that the literature does not support the use of a traditional sling for immobilizing the shoulder following primary anterior shoulder dislocation.[85] It was also noted that there were significantly fewer redislocations when activity is restricted for 6 to 8 weeks in those less than 30 years of age compared to activity restriction of less than 6 weeks. The commentary also supported positioning the humerus in adduction and external rotation (rather than internal rotation) during immobilization for better approximation between the detached glenoid labrum (Bankart lesion) and the glenoid neck.

Promote Tissue Health

Protected ROM, intermittent muscle setting of the rotator cuff, deltoid, and biceps brachii muscles, and grade II joint mobilization techniques in safe directions (with the humerus at the side or in the resting position) are initiated as soon as the patient tolerates them.

PRECAUTIONS: In order not to disrupt healing of the capsule and other damaged tissues after anterior dislocation, ROM into external rotation is performed with the elbow at the patient's side, with the shoulder flexed in the sagittal plane, and with the shoulder in the resting position (in the plane of the scapula, abducted 55° and 30° to 45° anterior to the frontal plane) but not in the 90° abducted position. The forearm is moved from maximal internal rotation to 0° or possibly 10° to 15° external rotation.

CONTRAINDICATION: Extension beyond 0° is contraindicated.

Management: Controlled Motion Phase

Provide Protection

The patient continues to protect the joint and delay full return to unrestricted activity. If a sling is being used, the patient increases the time the sling is off. The sling is used when the shoulder is tired or if protection from external forces is needed.

Increase Shoulder Mobility

- Mobilization techniques are initiated using all appropriate glides except the anterior glide. The anterior glide is *contraindicated* even though external rotation is necessary for functional elevation of the humerus. For a safe stretch to increase external rotation, place the shoulder in the resting position (abducted 55° and horizontally adducted 30°); then externally rotate the humerus to the limit of its range and apply a grade III distraction force perpendicular to the treatment plane in the glenoid fossa (Fig. 17.20).
- The posterior joint structures are passively stretched with horizontal adduction self-stretching techniques.

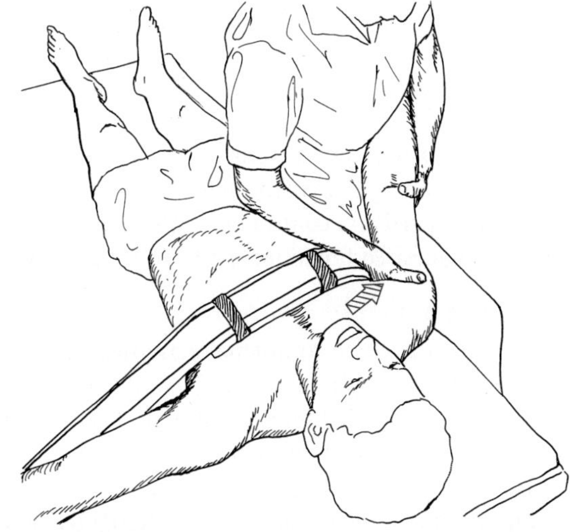

FIGURE 17.20 Mobilizing to increase GH joint external rotation when an anterior glide is contraindicated. Place the shoulder in resting position, externally rotate it, then apply a grade III distraction force.

Increase Stability and Strength of Rotator Cuff and Scapular Muscles

Both the internal and external rotators need to be strengthened as healing occurs.[22] The internal rotators and adductors must be strong to support the anterior capsule. The external rotators must be strong to stabilize the humeral head against anterior translating forces and to participate in the deltoid-rotator cuff force couple when abducting and laterally rotating the humerus. Scapulothoracic muscle strength is important for normal shoulder function and to maintain the scapula in normal alignment. The following exercises are initiated:

- *Isometric resistance* exercises with the joint positioned at the side and progressed to various pain-free positions within the available ranges.
- Partial weight-bearing and stabilization exercises.
- *Dynamic resistance,* limiting external rotation to 50° and avoiding the position of dislocation.
- At 3 weeks, supervised *isokinetic resistance* for internal rotation and adduction at speeds of 180° per second or higher may be used.[7] Position the patient standing with the arm at the side or in slight flexion and elbow flexed 90°. The patient performs internal rotation beginning at the zero position with the hand pointing anteriorly and moving across the front of the body.
- Progress to positioning the shoulder at 90° flexion. Have the patient perform the exercise from zero to full internal rotation. Do not position in 90° abduction.
- By 5 weeks, all shoulder motions are incorporated into exercises on isokinetic or other mechanical equipment except for the position of 90° abduction with external rotation.

Management: Return to Function Phase

Restore Functional Control

The following are emphasized:

- A balance in strength of all shoulder and scapular muscles
- Coordinated scapulothoracic and arm motions
- Endurance for each previously described shoulder stability exercise
- As stability improves, progress to:
  - Eccentric training to maximum load.
  - Increasing speed and control of combined motions.
  - Simulating desired functional patterns for activity.

Return to Full Activity

- The patient can return to normal activities when there is no muscle strength imbalance, good coordination is present during skilled movements, and the apprehension test is negative. Full rehabilitation takes 2.5 to 4 months.[4]
- It is important that the patient learns to recognize signs of fatigue and impingement and is educated about how to reduce the exercise load when these signs are noticed.

Closed Reduction of Posterior Dislocation

The management approach is the same as for anterior dislocation with the exception of avoiding the position of humeral flexion with adduction and internal rotation during the acute and healing phases.

CLINICAL TIP

Use of a sling following a posterior dislocation may be uncomfortable because of the adducted and internally rotated position of the humerus, particularly if the sling elevates the humerus so the head translates in a superior and posterior direction. The patient may be more comfortable with the arm hanging freely in a dependent position while kept immobile.

When mobilization is allowed, begin joint mobilization techniques using all appropriate glides except the posterior glide. Posterior glide is *contraindicated.* If adhesions develop that limit internal rotation, mobility can be regained safely by placing the shoulder in the resting position (abducted 55° and horizontally adducted 30°), internally rotating it to the limit of its range, and applying a grade III distraction force perpendicular to the treatment plane in the glenoid fossa (same as in Fig. 17.20 but with the arm internally rotated).

Shoulder Instabilities: Surgery and Postoperative Management

Surgical stabilization procedures are often necessary to repair chronic, recurrent instabilities and acute traumatic lesions in the GH, AC, and SC joints to restore function. Background information on GH joint instabilities and injuries that frequently occur with dislocations to this joint was described in the previous sections on nonoperative management. Common lesions that occur with GH instabilities are Bankart lesions, Hill-Sachs lesions, reverse Hill-Sachs lesions, and rotator cuff tears.

Glenohumeral Joint Stabilization Procedures and Postoperative Management

If a reasonable trial of nonoperative management has not prevented recurrence of GH joint instability, surgical stabilization may be considered. Recurrent instability after a traumatic event responds more favorably to surgical management than do chronic atraumatic instabilities.[11,125] Young, active patients who have sustained an acute, traumatic, anterior dislocation for the first time may elect to undergo surgery without a prior course of rehabilitation because there is a particularly high rate of recurrence of dislocation in this group after nonoperative management.[125,128]

FOCUS ON EVIDENCE

In a small randomized trial[18] of young athletes who had sustained a first-time, acute, traumatic anterior shoulder dislocation, one group (n = 14) participated in a non-operative rehabilitation program of immobilization and exercise and another group (n = 10) underwent arthroscopic repair of a Bankart lesion plus the rehabilitation program. Participants were followed for an average of 36 months. Of the 12 non-operatively managed patients who were available for follow-up, 9 (75%) experienced recurrent instability, whereas of the 9 operatively managed patients available for follow-up, only 1 (11.1%) experienced recurrent instability. Six of the 9 non-operatively treated patients who experienced recurrent instability subsequently had an open Bankart repair.

In another randomized study[102] of young patients (mean age 22 years) who sustained traumatic anterior dislocations, a trial of nonoperative management was compared to immediate arthroscopic stabilization. Over a 2-year period, 47% of the patients in the non-operative group—but only 15% of the surgical group—experienced recurrence of the dislocation. These studies demonstrate that in young patients, early surgical stabilization followed by postoperative rehabilitation significantly reduces the incidence of recurrent instability compared to non-operative management.

Indications for Surgery

The following are common indications for surgical stabilization of the GH joint.[125,128,195,210,213]

- Recurrent episodes of GH joint dislocation or subluxation that impair functional activities
- Unidirectional or multidirectional instability during active shoulder movements that causes apprehension about placing the arm in positions of potential dislocation, leading to compromised use of the arm for functional activities
- Instability-related impingement (secondary impingement syndrome) of the shoulder
- Significant inherent joint laxity resulting in recurrent involuntary dislocation
- High probability of subsequent episodes of recurrence of dislocation after an acute traumatic dislocation in young patients involved in high-risk (overhead), work-related, or sport activities
- Dislocations associated with significant cuff tears or displaced tuberosity or glenoid rim fractures
- Irreducible (chronic, fixed) dislocation
- Failure to resolve the instability and restore function with non-operative management

Procedures

Procedures designed to improve stability and prevent recurrent instability of the GH joint must balance stabilization of the joint with retention of near-normal, functional mobility. Stabilization procedures, which may involve the anterior, posterior, or inferior portions of the capsule, are performed using either an arthroscopic or open approach depending on the type of lesion(s) present and type of procedure selected by the surgeon.[125,128,161,190,210] Open stabilization procedures are highly successful (low recurrence of dislocation) and have been considered the standard for years. However, with advances in arthroscopic techniques and methods of tissue fixation, the use and success of arthroscopic stabilization procedures is much more common.[210]

Recurrent anterior (unidirectional) dislocation is by far the most common form of GH instability managed with surgical stabilization.[128] In contrast, posterior or posteroinferior instabilities are less frequently managed with surgical stabilization.[161] The surgical procedures can be organized into several categories.

Bankart repair. This repair involves an open or arthroscopic repair of a Bankart lesion, which is the detachment of the capsulolabral complex from the anterior rim of the glenoid commonly associated with traumatic anterior dislocation (see Fig. 17.19). During the repair an anterior capsulolabral reconstruction is performed to reattach the labrum to the surface of the glenoid lip.[3,65,85,90,125,1752175,210]

With an open repair, the humeral insertion of the subscapularis is detached or split longitudinally for access to the lesion and capsule.[67,125,172,175] Occasionally, access is achieved through the rotator cuff interval, which allows the subscapularis to remain intact.[125] If the subscapularis is detached, it is repaired after the labrum has been reattached. With an arthroscopic approach multiple portal sites are used, and the subscapularis is not disturbed.[3,210] Repair of a Bankart lesion is combined with an anterior capsular shift if capsular redundancy is present.

With an open procedure, the labrum is reattached with direct transglenoid sutures or suture anchors, whereas with an arthroscopic approach transglenoid sutures, suture anchors, or tacks are used.[85,210] Generally, more secure fixation is achieved with an open repair than with an arthroscopic repair, although in recent years advances in arthroscopic tissue fixation have improved.[210]

Capsulorrhaphy (capsular shift). Capsulorrhaphy, which can be performed using either an open or arthroscopic approach, involves tightening the capsule to reduce capsular redundancy and overall capsule volume by incising, overlapping in a pants-and-vest manner (imbrication), and then securing the lax or overstretched portion of the capsule (plication) with direct sutures, suture anchors, tacks, or staples.[69,90,125,128,161,210,228]

A capsular shift procedure is tailored to the direction(s) of instability: anterior, inferior, posterior, or multidirectional. For example, if a patient has recurrent anteroinferior multidirectional instability, an anterior or inferior capsular shift is performed in which this portion of the capsule is incised, tightened by imbrication (plication), and sutured. Most capsular shift procedures are performed to reduce anterior instability.[10,125,128,228]

Electrothermally assisted capsulorrhaphy. Electrothermally assisted capsulorrhaphy (ETAC) involves an arthroscopic approach that uses thermal energy (radiofrequency thermal delivery or nonablative laser) to shrink and tighten loose capsuloligamentous structures. The procedure—also referred to as a *thermal-assisted capsular shift* (TACS) or *thermocapsular shrinkage*—can be used alone but more often is used in conjunction with other arthroscopic procedures, such as repair of a glenoid tear, a capsular shift, débridement of a partial rotator cuff tear, or subacromial decompression.[54,57,125,132,197,205,210,224]

Animal and human cadaveric studies have shown that thermal energy initially makes collagen fibrils more extensible; but as the collagen tissue of the capsuloligamentous structures heals, it shortens or "shrinks," causing a decrease in capsular laxity.[84,183] If one or more of the GH ligaments is detached or if rotator cuff lesions that could be contributing to the instability are detected, they are repaired arthroscopically prior to ETAC.

Posterior capsulorrhaphy (posterior or posteroinferior capsular shift). Recurrent, involuntary posterior or posteroinferior instability can be managed with either an open or arthroscopic capsular shift to remove posterior and inferior redundancy of the capsule.[11,125,160,161,195,196,210] Additional soft tissue procedures, such as repair of a posterior labral tear (reverse Bankart lesion) or, in rare instances, plication and advancement of the infraspinatus to reinforce the posterior capsule, may be necessary. Shoulders without an effective posterior glenoid can be surgically managed with capsulolabral augmentation[210] or occasionally with a glenoid osteotomy.[125,161]

With an arthroscopic posterior stabilization, a capsular shift and repair of the posterior labrum can be accomplished without disrupting the shoulder musculature.[160] With an open stabilization, a posterolateral incision is made; the deltoid is split; and the infraspinatus, teres minor, and posterior capsule are incised.[161,196] In some instances of traumatic multidirectional instability, anterior capsulorrhaphy is used to indirectly increase the tension of the posterior capsule.[125,161,210]

Repair of a SLAP lesion. A tear of the superior labrum is classified as a SLAP lesion (*s*uperior *l*abrum extending *a*nterior to *p*osterior).[46,195,210,225] Some SLAP lesions are associated with a tear of the proximal attachment of the long head of the biceps tendon and recurrent anterior instability of the GH joint. An arthroscopic repair involves débridement of the torn portion of the superior labrum, abrasion of the bony surface of the superior glenoid, and reattachment of the labrum and biceps tendon with tacks or suture anchors. Concomitant anterior stabilization is also performed if instability is present.

Postoperative Management

General Considerations

As with rehabilitation after rotator cuff repair, guidelines for postoperative management after GH joint surgical stabilization are based on many factors. These factors, all of which can influence the composition and progression of a postoperative program, are summarized in Table 17.5. Additional factors that affect rehabilitation after GH stabilization and rotator cuff repair, such as the philosophy and training of the surgeon and a number of patient-related variables (general health, medications, preinjury functional status and postoperative goals, education, and compliance) have been addressed previously (see Table 17.3).

The content in this section identifies *general* principles of management across three broad phases of postoperative rehabilitation after a variety of GH joint surgical stabilization and reconstruction procedures. These general guidelines cannot begin to address the many variations of rehabilitation programs recommended for specific stabilization procedures. However, many detailed protocols or case-based descriptions of rehabilitation programs for use after specific procedures and for specific types of shoulder instabilities and associated lesions are available in the literature.[34,54,85,98,150,163,205,225,232]

Regardless of the type of instability, associated pathology, or type of surgical stabilization procedure, a postoperative rehabilitation program must be based on the findings of a comprehensive examination and individualized to meet the unique needs of each patient. The focus of postoperative rehabilitation is to restore pain-free shoulder mobility and muscular strength and endurance, particularly the dynamic joint stabilizers, to meet the patient's functional needs *while preventing recurrence of shoulder instability.*

Immobilization

Position. The position in which the patient's shoulder is immobilized after surgery is determined by the direction(s) of instability prior to surgery. After surgical reconstruction for recurrent anterior or anteroinferior instability, the shoulder is immobilized in a sling or splint with the arm at the side or in some amount of abduction and internal rotation, with the arm slightly anterior to the frontal plane of the body.[90,125] After surgery for posterior or posteroinferior instability, the upper extremity is supported in an orthosis with the shoulder immobilized in the "handshake" position (neutral rotation to 10° to 20° of external rotation, 20° to 30° of abduction, elbow flexed, and neutral flexion or slight extension).[125,161]

Duration. The duration of immobilization—that is, the period of time before use of the immobilizer is *completely* discontinued—is determined by many factors, including the

TABLE 17.5 Factors That Influence the Rehabilitation Program After Surgery for Recurrent Instability of the GH Joint

Factors	Potential Impact on Rehabilitation
▪ A traumatic onset of instability	▪ More conservative postoperative rehabilitation due to greater risk of recurrent dislocation[125]
▪ Severity of associated lesions	▪ Increased severity or number of associated lesions will slow the progression of rehabilitation
▪ Previous failure of a surgical Stabilization	▪ Slower progression
▪ Direction of instability	▪ Stabilization of anterior instability allows more rapid advancement than stabilization of posterior or multidirectional instabilities[161]
▪ Type of surgical approach	▪ Less postoperative pain with arthroscopic procedure but rate of progression essentially the same after open and arthroscopic stabilization procedures, because rate of healing of repaired tissues is the same in both procedures
▪ Type of procedure	▪ Electrothermally assisted capsulorrhaphy requires slower progression than arthroscopic or open capsular tightening without thermal application[54,164,205] ▪ Bony reconstruction requires slower progression than after soft tissue reconstruction
▪ Patient variables ▪ Tissue integrity ▪ Preoperative status of dynamic stabilizers ▪ Generalized joint laxity	▪ The progression of postoperative rehabilitation is more conservative for the inactive patient with multidirectional atraumatic instability who has generalized joint laxity and poor pre-operative strength of the dynamic (muscular) stabilizers

type of instability, the procedure(s) performed, and the surgeon's intraoperative assessment. This period can range from 1 to 3 weeks to as long as 6 to 8 weeks. However, the period of *continuous* immobilization of the operated shoulder (before shoulder motion can be initiated) depends on the type of procedure but is kept as short as possible. For example, after an anterior stabilization, the immobilizer may need to be worn continuously for only a day to a few days but in some cases up to 1 to 2 weeks.[128] In contrast, repairs of posterior or multidirectional instabilities, which are associated with a higher recurrence of dislocation, usually require a longer period of immobilization.[125,161,196] After a posterior stabilization procedure, the shoulder may be continuously immobilized and ROM delayed for up to 6 weeks postoperatively.[98,161]

Time frames for immobilization also vary based on the factors that influence all aspects of postoperative rehabilitation (see Table 17.4). For example, the duration of immobilization is usually shorter for an elderly patient than for a young patient, because the elderly patient is more likely to develop postoperative shoulder stiffness than the young patient. In contrast, patients with generalized hypermobility or younger patients involved in high-demand activities require longer periods of immobilization to reduce the risk of redislocation.[125]

Exercise Progression

As with the position and duration of immobilization, decisions about when the arm may be temporarily removed from the immobilizer to begin shoulder exercises and the allowable shoulder motions are based on many of the factors previously summarized (see Table 17.5).

CLINICAL TIP

During the early weeks of rehabilitation after a surgical stabilization procedure, determining what ranges fall within "safe" limits of motion is based on the extent of intraoperative ROM that was possible without placing excessive tension on the repaired, tightened, or reconstructed tissues. This information may be available in the operative report or should be communicated by the surgeon to the therapist prior to initiating postoperative exercises.

Rehabilitation after anterior stabilization (anterior capsular shift or Bankart repair) is similar after open and arthroscopic procedures. In both instances, there are precautions that must be heeded, particularly during the first 6 weeks after surgery while soft tissues are healing. During this time period after an open procedure, the anterior capsule and the detached and repaired subscapularis must be protected from excessive stresses. With an arthroscopic anterior stabilization, although the subscapularis remains intact, it is also necessary to protect the anterior capsule fixation during the initial phase of rehabilitation, because soft tissue fixation may not be as secure as the fixation used in an open procedure.

PRECAUTIONS: Precautions after arthroscopic or open anterior stabilization or reconstruction procedures are summarized in Box 17.9.[34,67,85,98,125,128,150,210] Precautions for thermally assisted capsular tightening,[54,57,164,205,224] posterior stabilization procedures,[98,160,161] and repair of a SLAP lesion[34,46,225] are noted in Box 17.10.

FOCUS ON EVIDENCE

In a study by Sachs and colleagues[175] with a 4-year follow-up of 30 patients who had sustained a traumatic anterior dislocation and undergone an open Bankart repair (that included takedown and repair of the subscapularis tendon), only postoperative subscapularis function was significantly correlated with the patients' perception of a successful outcome after surgery. Although only two patients (6.7%) reported recurrence of instability over the 4-year period, seven patients (23%) had incompetence of the subscapularis muscle. Specifically, the mean strength of the subscapularis in these patients was only 27% as strong as the non-involved shoulder, compared to the remaining patients who had mean subscapularis strength of 80%. There was no significant loss of strength in other shoulder muscles in either group of patients.

Of the patients with a reasonably strong subscapularis at the 4-year follow-up, 91% reported good to excellent results, and 100% indicated that they would have the surgery again. However, among the patients with a substantially weak subscapularis, 57% reported good to excellent results, but only 57% would undergo the surgery again. The investigators suggest that the subscapularis tendon repair and protection over the first few weeks following surgery is critical to shoulder function and patient perception of successful outcomes.

Exercise: Maximum Protection Phase

The initial phase of rehabilitation extends for about 6 weeks after surgery. Protection of the tightened capsule or repaired structures, such as the labrum or the subscapularis, is necessary during this phase while also minimizing the negative consequences of immobilization. Exercises may be initiated the day after surgery for select patients who have had an anterior stabilization procedure,[39] but more often are begun 1 to 2 weeks postoperatively.[98,150] ROM is delayed for a longer period of time after a thermally assisted stabilization,[54,57,164,205,224] a posterior stabilization procedure,[98,160,161] or repair of a SLAP lesion and torn biceps tendon[34,47,225] (see Box 17.10).

BOX 17.9 Precautions After Anterior Glenohumeral Stabilization and/or Bankart Repair*

- Limit external rotation (*ER), horizontal abduction,* and *extension* (shoulder positions that place stress on the anterior capsule) during first 6 weeks postoperatively.
  - After an arthroscopic stabilization, although the subscapularis is intact, limit ER to 5° to 10° with the arm in slight abduction or at the side for the first 2 weeks to avoid pull-out of fixation.[35] Gradually progress to 45° over the next 2 to 4 weeks with the shoulder in greater abduction. With a tenuous stabilization, may need to limit ER to only neutral for the first 4 to 6 postoperative weeks.[210]
  - After an open procedure involving subscapularis takedown and repair, limit ER to 0° (no ER past neutral), to no more than 30° to 45° or to the "safe" limits identified during the intraoperative assessment for 4 to 6 weeks.[34]
  - Postpone ER combined with full shoulder abduction for at least 6 weeks.[85]
- After an arthroscopic stabilization, progress forward flexion of the shoulder more cautiously than after an open stabilization.
- After bony procedures, delay passive or assisted ROM for 6 to 8 weeks to allow time for bone healing.[125,128]
- No vigorous passive stretching to increase end-range ER for 8 to 12 weeks after either arthroscopic or open procedure except for patients with hypoelastic tissue quality.[210]
- When stretching is permissible, avoid positioning the shoulder in abduction and external rotation during grade III joint mobilization procedures.
- After procedures with subscapularis detachment and repair, no *active* or *resisted* IR for 4 to 6 weeks; avoid lifting objects, especially if pushing the hands together is required.[34,67,85,150]
- Avoid activities involving positions that place stress on the anterior aspect of the capsule for about 4 to 6 weeks.
  - Avoid functional activities that require ER, especially if combined with horizontal abduction during early rehabilitation as when reaching to put on a coat or shirt.
  - Avoid upper extremity weight bearing particularly if the shoulder is extended, as when pushing up from the armrests of a chair.
- When dynamically strengthening the rotator cuff, maintain the shoulder in about 45°of abduction, rather than 90°.

*Precautions apply primarily to early rehabilitation during the first 6 weeks after surgery except as noted. The allowable ROM during the initial phase of rehabilitation depends on the type of pathology, surgical procedure, the patient's tissue quality (degree of hyper- or hypo-elasticity), and the intraoperative evaluation of shoulder stability.

BOX 17.10 Precautions After Selected Glenohumeral Stabilization Procedures

Thermally Assisted Capsular Tightening

- Be extremely cautious with ROM exercises for the first 4 to 6 weeks postoperatively because collagen in the thermally treated capsuloligamentous structures is initially more extensible (more vulnerable to stretch) until it heals. Some patients may begin ROM within protected ranges the day after surgery, whereas others may be required to postpone ROM exercises entirely for 2 weeks or more.
- While sleeping, complete immobilization (sling and swathe) for 2 weeks or more.
- Precautions for ROM depend on the direction of instability, patient's tissue quality (hyper- or hypoelastic), and the extent of concomitant surgical procedures necessary. For example, progress patients with congenital hyperelasticity more cautiously than those with hypoelasticity.

Posterior Stabilization Procedure and/or Reverse Bankart Repair

- Postpone all shoulder exercises or limit elevation of the arm to 90° and internal rotation (IR) to neutral or no more than 15° to 20° and horizontal adduction to neutral (up to 6 weeks postoperatively).
- Restrict upper extremity weight bearing, particularly when the shoulder is flexed, to avoid stress to the posterior aspect of the capsule, for example during closed-chain scapulothoracic and GH stabilization exercises and functional activities, for at least 6 weeks postoperatively.
- Avoid resistance exercises that direct loads and place stress on the posterior capsule, such as bench press exercises and prone push-ups until late in the rehabilitation program, if at all.

Repair of a SLAP Lesion

- For SLAP lesions where the biceps tendon is detached, progress rehabilitation more cautiously than when the biceps remain intact.
  - Limit passive or assisted elevation of arm to 60° for the first 2 weeks and to 90° at 3 to 4 weeks postoperatively.
  - Perform only passive assisted humeral rotation with the shoulder in the plane of the scapula for the first 2 weeks (ER to only neutral or up to 15° and IR to 45°); during weeks 3 to 4, progress ER to 30° and IR to 60°.
- Avoid positions that create tension in the biceps, such as combined elbow and shoulder extension (as when reaching behind the back), during the first 4 to 6 weeks postoperatively.
- Postpone active contractions of the biceps (elbow flexion with supination of the forearm) for 6 weeks and resisted biceps exercises or lifting and carrying weighted objects until 8 to 12 weeks postoperatively depending on the extent and type of biceps repair; then progress cautiously.
- If the mechanism of injury was a fall onto the outstretched hand and arm causing joint compression, progress weight-bearing exercises gradually.
- If anterior instability is also present, follow precautions in Box 17.11.
- Avoid positions of abduction combined with maximum external rotation, as this places torsion forces on the base of the biceps attachment on the glenoid.

Goals and interventions. The goals and exercises for the maximum protection phase are summarized in this section.[34,54,85,150,222,232]

- ***Control pain and inflammation.***
  - A sling for comfort when the arm is dependent or for protection when in public areas. While seated, remove the sling (if permissible) and rest the forearm on a table or wide armrest with the shoulder positioned in abduction and neutral rotation to provide support but prevent potential contracture of the subscapularis and other internal rotators of the shoulder.
  - Cryotherapy and prescribed anti-inflammatory medication
  - Shoulder relaxation exercises
- ***Prevent or correct posture impairments.***
  - Emphasis on spinal extension and scapular retraction; avoid excessive thoracic kyphosis
- ***Maintain mobility and control of adjacent regions.***
  - Active ROM of the cervical region, elbow, forearm, wrist, and fingers the day after surgery
  - Active scapulothoracic movements

PRECAUTION: Initially, strengthen the scapulothoracic muscles in open-chain positions to avoid the need for weight bearing on the operated upper extremity. When weight-bearing activities are initiated, be cautious about the position of the operated shoulder for about 6 weeks postoperatively to avoid undue stress to the vulnerable portion of the capsule.

- ***Restore shoulder mobility while protecting tightened or repaired tissues.***
  - Pendulum exercises for the first 2 weeks postoperatively.
  - Self-assisted ROM and wand exercises for the GH joint *within protected ranges* as early as 2 weeks or as late as 6 weeks postoperatively. Begin shoulder elevation in the supine position; begin humeral rotation with the shoulder in a slightly abducted and flexed position using a rolled towel under the humerus for positioning and support.
  - With an anterior stabilization, gradually progress to near-complete ROM by 6 to 8 weeks except for external rotation, extension, and horizontal abduction beyond neutral.
  - With a posterior stabilization, progress cautiously into flexion, horizontal adduction, and internal rotation.

- Progress to active shoulder ROM when motion can be performed without pain, apprehension, or use of substitute motions, such as elevating the scapula to initiate arm elevation.
- Use the operated arm for *nonweight-bearing, waist-level* functional activities with no external resistance by 2 to 4 weeks postoperatively.

- ***Prevent reflex inhibition and disuse atrophy of GH musculature.***
  - Multiple-angle, low-intensity isometric exercises of GH musculature as early as the first week or by 3 to 4 weeks postoperatively. Use caution with resisted internal rotation after subscapularis repairs.
  - *Possible* initiation of dynamic exercises against *light* resistance in protected ranges of motion at 4 to 6 weeks emphasizing the GH stabilizers.
  - Be particularly cautious when applying any type of resistance to musculature that has been torn or surgically detached, incised, or advanced and then repaired. Note that following a SLAP repair, resisted elbow flexion and resisted shoulder elevation will result in increased tensile loading of the long head of the biceps tendon.

NOTE: In some cases, dynamic exercises against light resistance are delayed until the intermediate phase of rehabilitation (about 6 to 8 weeks postoperatively), when only moderate protection is necessary.

Criteria to progress. Criteria to advance to the second phases of rehabilitation are:[34,54,85,98]

- A well healed incision.
- Reasonable improvement in ROM.
- Minimal pain.
- No sense of apprehension about instability with active motions.

Exercise: Moderate Protection Phase

The moderate protection phase of rehabilitation begins around 6 weeks postoperatively and continues until approximately 12 to 16 weeks. The focus is on maintaining joint stability while achieving nearly full active (unassisted) ROM of the shoulder; developing neuromuscular control, strength, and endurance of scapulothoracic and GH musculature; and using the upper extremity through greater ranges for functional activities.

Goals and interventions. The goals and interventions for the intermediate phase of rehabilitation are as follows.[34,54,85,98,222,232]

- ***Regain nearly full, pain-free, active ROM of the shoulder.***
  - Continue active ROM with the goal of achieving nearly full ROM by 12 weeks.
  - Incorporate ROM gains into functional activities.
  - Stretching and grade III mobilization in positions that do not provoke instability. After an anterior stabilization procedure, pay particular attention to increasing horizontal adduction, as the posterior structures may have been tight preoperatively and continue to be so postoperatively.

- ***Continue to increase strength and endurance of shoulder musculature.***
  - Alternating isometrics against increasing resistance with emphasis on the scapula and rotator cuff musculature.
  - Dynamic resistance exercises initiated or progressed using weights and elastic resistance with emphasis on scapulothoracic and GH stabilizers. Begin in midrange positions, progressing to end-range positions. Emphasize both the concentric and eccentric phases of muscle activation.
  - Dynamic strengthening in diagonal and simulated functional movement patterns.
  - Upper extremity ergometry for muscular endurance. Include forward and backward motions.
  - Progressive upper extremity weight bearing during strengthening and stabilization exercises.

PRECAUTIONS: *After anterior stabilization*, do not initiate dynamic strengthening of the internal rotators from full external rotation, particularly in the 90° abducted position. When strengthening the shoulder extensors, do not extend posterior to the frontal plane. Similarly, when strengthening the horizontal abductors, do not horizontally abduct posterior to the frontal plane. In addition, maintain the shoulder in neutral rotation during horizontal abduction and adduction. *After posterior stabilization,* do not begin dynamic strengthening of the external rotators from a position of full internal rotation initially.

Criteria to progress. Criteria to progress to the final phase of rehabilitation and the focus of exercises are similar to the criteria already identified for the final phase of rehabilitation after rotator cuff repair.

Exercise: Minimum Protection/Return to Function Phase

This phase usually begins around 12 weeks postoperatively or as late as 16 weeks, depending on individual characteristics of the patient and the surgical procedure. Stretching should continue until ROM consistent with functional needs has been attained. Gains in ROM are possible for up to 12 months as collagen tissue continues to remodel. Resistance exercises to improve strength and endurance are progressed to replicate movements involved in functional activities, including placing the joint progressively closer to positions that previously provoked instability. Plyometric training (discussed in Chapter 23) is introduced and gradually progressed, particularly in patients intending to return to high-demand sports or work-related activities. Full participation in work-related and sports activities often takes up to 6 months postoperatively.

PRECAUTIONS: Some patients may have permanent restrictions placed on functional activities that involve high-risk movements and that could potentially cause recurrence of the instability. After some anterior stabilization procedures, full external rotation in 90° of abduction may not be advisable or possible.[98]

Outcomes

A successful postoperative outcome involves regaining the ability to participate in desired functional activities without a recurrence of GH joint instability. There are many studies describing various outcomes after stabilization procedures. However, most of the studies comparing the success of one surgical intervention with that of another are not randomized—understandably so because the surgeon's examination is the basis for determining which procedure is most appropriate and will most likely lead to successful results for each patient.

Although postoperative exercise is consistently described as essential for optimal outcomes after stabilization surgery, no current evaluations of the effectiveness of postoperative exercise programs after GH stabilization are found in the literature. As with surgical decisions, most postoperative rehabilitation programs are customized to meet each patient's needs, making comparison of outcomes difficult.

Results of surgery and postoperative rehabilitation are typically reported for specific pathologies, patient populations, and surgical procedures and a variety of outcome measures are used to evaluate effectiveness. Despite this lack of consistency in reporting, some generalizations can be made.

Recurrence of instability. Recurrent instability of traumatic origin responds more favorably to surgical management than does atraumatic instability.[11,125] In addition, the rate of recurrence of instability is substantially higher in young patients (< 30 to 40 years of age) and patients who return to high-demand, work-related activities or competitive overhead sports than less active, older patients (> 30 to 40 years of age).[125,210]

The recurrence of dislocation rates after open and arthroscopic procedures have also been compared with recurrence rates after arthroscopic stabilization higher than after open stabilization.[35,125] In a review of studies on anterior stabilization procedures, the mean recurrence rate after open stabilization (Bankart lesion repair) was 11% (range 4% to 23%), but recurrence rates after arthroscopic stabilization were 18% (range 2% to 32%) with transglenoid suture fixation and 17% (range 0% to 30%) with tack fixation.[85] In a more recent review, the recurrence rates of anterior instability after an arthroscopic Bankart repair ranged from 8% to 17%.[210] Decreasing recurrence rates after arthroscopic procedures are attributed to improved surgical techniques. Today, arthroscopic stabilization has been shown in many instances to be equal to open stabilization at preventing recurrence for patients with unidirectional, anterior instability.[35,210,214] However, for multidirectional instabilities, outcomes after arthroscopic stabilization are not yet equal to outcomes after open stabilization.[210]

Outcomes after stabilization procedures for anterior and posterior instabilities also have been compared. Surgical stabilization of a recurrent, unidirectional *anterior* instability has yielded more predictable results and lower recurrence rates than stabilization of *posterior* or *multidirectional* instabilities.[11,125,161,210,228] The average recurrence rate of posterior instability after arthroscopic stabilization is particularly high. One source reported a 30% to 40% rate of redislocation,[196] and another reported rates as high as 50%.[210] In contrast, mean recurrence rates after anterior stabilization procedures have been reported at 11% and 17% to 18%, respectively, for open and arthroscopic procedures.[85]

As the preoperative diagnosis has improved and the selection of appropriate candidates for surgery has become better, the recurrence of instability after posterior stabilization has decreased. In a study[160] with a mean follow-up of 39.1 months, the recurrence rate of instability after arthroscopic posterior stabilization was only 12.1%. The patients in this study had a mean age of 25 years with a history of involuntary or voluntary dislocation of the GH joint associated with acute traumatic and chronic repetitive microtrauma.

Regarding ETAC as the primary stabilization procedure, Hawkins and colleagues[82] reported failure in 37 of 85 patients (35%). Failures were those procedures that resulted in the need for a revision stabilization, recurrent instabilities, or recalcitrant pain and stiffness. The authors noted that for their practice, ETAC is now reserved primarily for augmentation of plication or other procedures in special circumstances

Shoulder ROM. After open anterior stabilization and Bankart repair, which usually requires detachment and repair of the subscapularis, a mean loss of 12° of ER has been reported.[65] It has been suggested that there is less loss of shoulder ER after arthroscopic procedures than after open procedures.[85] However, in a nonrandomized study that compared arthroscopic and open anterior stabilization procedures, there were not statistically significant differences in ER loss between groups with mean decreases of 9° and 11°, respectively.[35]

After open GH stabilization for instability due to repetitive microtrauma, postoperative loss of shoulder ER is the most common reason athletes involved in overhead sports are unable to successfully return to competition. Loss of shoulder rotation is reported to be less after arthroscopic stabilization procedures, thus enabling a greater percentage of these athletes to return to competition.[164] Early follow-up of patients who have undergone thermally assisted capsular stabilization was encouraging,[57] but long-term outcomes do not support high rates of success. A large study of overhead athletes who underwent thermally assisted stabilization followed 130 patients for a mean of 29.3 months. Of these athletes, 113 (87%) returned to competition in a mean of 8.4 months. Although postoperative ROM was not reported, the implication was that the return of ROM after thermally assisted arthroscopic stabilization was sufficient for a high percentage of athletes being able to return to competition.[164] A recent follow-up of 101 patients with mild to moderate instability who underwent thermal capsular shrinkage for stabilization reported failure in approximately one-third of the shoulders (31%) after a mean of 39 months. The best outcomes (pain, instability, and function) were noted in those with unidirectional anterior instability or a concomitant labral repair.[200] In contrast, a comparison of outcomes at 2 years showed no statistical or clinical differences between groups of subjects who were randomized into open capsular shift ($n = 26$) or thermal shrinkage ($n = 28$) groups for MDI and failed nonoperative treatment.[134]

Acromioclavicular and Sternoclavicular Joint Stabilization Procedures and Postoperative Managemen

Acromioclavicular Joint Stabilization

A grade III separation, in which the AC and coracoclavicular ligaments are completely ruptured may be surgically stabilized with a variety of techniques.[147,167] Surgical procedures for acute dislocations include primary stabilization of the AC joint with Kirschner wires, Steinman pins, screws, or most recently bioabsorbable tacks, sutures, or fiber wires. Other procedures include a muscle-tendon transfer that moves the tip of the coracoid process with the attached tendons of the coracobrachialis and short head of the biceps to the undersurface of the clavicle[154] or the Weaver-Dunn procedure, which resects the distal clavicle and transfers the CA ligament from the acromion to the shaft of the distal clavicle.[147] Based on a small body of evidence in the literature, it appears the best results are achieved with primary AC and coracoclavicular stabilization procedures. Chronic AC dislocations, which are usually associated with degenerative changes of the AC joint, are most often managed with distal clavicle resection coupled with coracoclavicular stabilization.[153,167]

Sternoclavicular Joint Stabilization

Although most SC dislocations are managed non-operatively, an acute posterior dislocation of the SC joint that cannot be successfully reduced with a closed maneuver, or an SC joint that dislocates recurrently are both managed surgically. Surgical reduction of a traumatic anterior dislocation is not recommended.[166,229] Surgical options for posterior SC dislocations include open reduction with repair of the stabilizing ligaments or resection of a portion of the medial clavicle and fixation of the remaining clavicle to the first rib or sternum with a soft tissue graft.[166,229]

Postoperative Management

After surgical stabilization of either the AC or SC joint, the shoulder is immobilized for up to 6 weeks.[39] Exercise interventions are directed toward functional recovery as healing allows. No muscles provide dynamic stabilization of the AC and SC joints, so scapular and GH strength must be developed to provide indirect stability.

During the first few weeks of immobilization, the patient is encouraged to perform active ROM of the wrist and hand. If the elbow is supported on a table, the patient is permitted to perform active ROM of the elbow and forearm. The operated extremity, if supported, may be used for light functional activities, such as holding a utensil or typing, but weight bearing and shoulder ROM are completely prohibited during the first 6 weeks.[39]

When the immobilization can be removed, the focus of the exercise program is restoration of shoulder and elbow mobility and neuromuscular control of the shoulder complex. Shoulder ROM (passive, progressing to assisted ROM), active scapular motions, and light isometrics of the shoulder musculature are initiated at this point. Stabilization exercises, dynamic strengthening of the shoulder and scapula musculature, and stretching to restore full ROM are also introduced and progressed. Functional activities are gradually integrated into the rehabilitation program.

Exercise Interventions for the Shoulder Girdle

Exercise Techniques During Acute and Early Subacute Stages of Tissue Healing

During the *protection* and *early controlled motion* phases of management, when inflammation is present or beginning to resolve and healing tissues should not be stressed, early motion may be utilized to inhibit pain, minimize muscle guarding, and help prevent the adverse effects of complete immobilization. It is also valuable to treat associated regions, such as the cervical and thoracic spine, the scapulae, and the remainder of the upper extremity, to relieve stresses to the shoulder girdle and prevent fluid stasis in the extremity.

General guidelines for management during the acute stage are described in Chapter 10, and specific precautions for various pathologies and surgical interventions in the shoulder are identified throughout the second major section of this chapter.

Early Motion of the Glenohumeral Joint

Early motion is usually passive ROM (PROM) applied within pain-free ranges. When tolerated, active-assistive ROM (A-AROM) can be initiated. Manual PROM and A-AROM techniques are described in detail in Chapter 3. This section expands on self-assisted exercises.

Wand Exercises

- *Patient position and procedure:* Initiate A-AROM using a cane, wand, or T-bar in the supine position to provide stabilization and control of the scapula. Motions typically performed are flexion, abduction, elevation in the plane of the scapula, and internal/external rotation (Fig. 17.21 A).
- If it is necessary to relieve stress on the anterior capsule following surgical repair of the capsule or labrum, place a folded towel under the distal humerus to position the arm anterior to the frontal plane of the body when the patient performs internal or external rotation (Fig. 17.21 B).

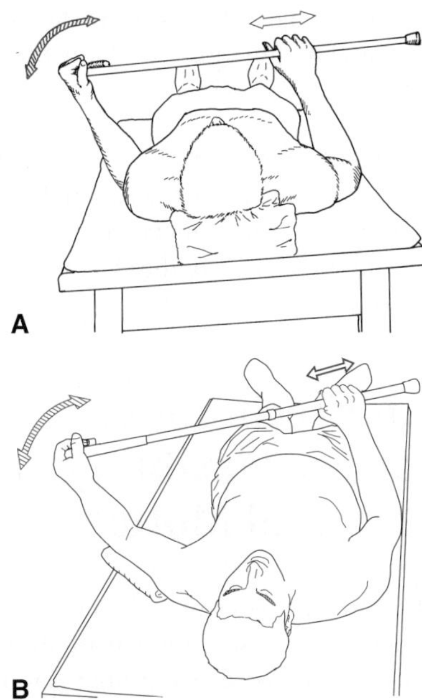

FIGURE 17.21 Self-assisted shoulder rotation using a cane **(A)** with the arm at the side and **(B)** in scaption. To relieve stress on the anterior capsule, elevate the distal humerus with a folded towel.

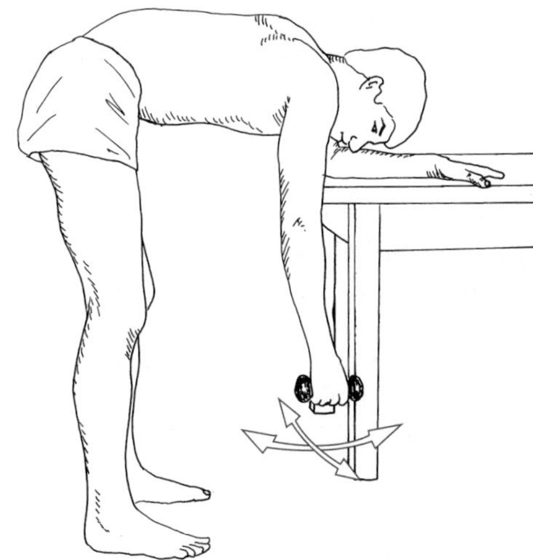

FIGURE 17.22 Pendulum exercises. For gentle distraction, no weight is used. Use of a weight causes a grade III (stretching) distraction force.

- When treating a painful shoulder syndrome (primary or secondary), grasping the wand with the forearm supinated when performing shoulder flexion and abduction may help encourage humeral external rotation.

Ball Rolling or Table Top Dusting

Patient position and procedure: Sitting with the arm resting on a table and hand placed on a 6- to 8-inch ball or towel and the humerus in the plane of the scapula. Have the patient initiate gentle circular motions of the shoulder by moving the trunk forward, backward, and to the side, allowing the hand to roll the ball or "dust the table." As pain subsides, have the patient use the shoulder muscles to actively move the ball or cloth through greater ROMs.

Wall (Window) Washing

Patient position and procedure: Standing with the hand supporting a towel or a ball against a smooth wall. Instruct the patient to perform clockwise and counterclockwise circular motions with the hand by moving the towel or rolling the ball. Progress this activity by having the patient reach upward and outward as far as tolerated without causing symptoms.

Pendulum (Codman's) Exercises

Patient position and procedure: Standing, with the trunk flexed at the hips about 90°. The arm hangs loosely downward in a position between 60° and 90° elevation (Fig. 17.22).

- A pendulum or swinging motion of the arm is initiated by having the patient move their trunk in a rhythmic rocking motion. Motions of flexion, extension, and horizontal abduction, adduction, and circumduction can be done depending on the direction the trunk rocks.[32] Increase the arc of motion as tolerated. This technique should not cause pain.
- If the patient cannot maintain balance while leaning over, have him or her hold on to a solid structure or lie prone on a table.
- If the patient experiences back pain from bending over, use the prone position.
- Adding a weight to the hand or using wrist cuffs causes a greater distraction force on the GH joint. Weights should be used only when joint stretching maneuvers are indicated late in the subacute and chronic stages—and then only if the scapula is stabilized by the therapist or a belt is placed around the thorax and scapula, so the stretch force is directed to the joint, not the soft tissue of the scapulothoracic region.

PRECAUTIONS: If a patient gets dizzy when standing upright after being bent over, have the patient sit and rest. With increased pain or decreased ROM, the technique may be an inappropriate choice. Pendulum exercises are also inappropriate for a patient with peripheral edema.

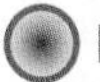

FOCUS ON EVIDENCE

An electromyographic (EMG) analysis[113] demonstrated peak percent maximum voluntary isometric contraction greater than 15% in the supraspinatus and infraspinatus muscles when asymptomatic subjects performed large diameter pendulum exercises, regardless of whether they were performed correctly (using trunk motion to create GH movement) or incorrectly (using shoulder muscles to create GH movement). These muscle activation levels may be too high for recently repaired tissues. Smaller diameter exercises kept percent activation levels below 15% for infraspinatus and below 10% for supraspinatus.

"Gear Shift" Exercises

Patient position and procedure: Sitting with the involved arm at the side, holding a cane or wand with the tip resting on the floor to support the weight of the arm. Instruct the patient to move the pole forward and back, diagonally, or laterally and medially in a motion similar to shifting gears in a car with a floor shift (Fig. 17.23).

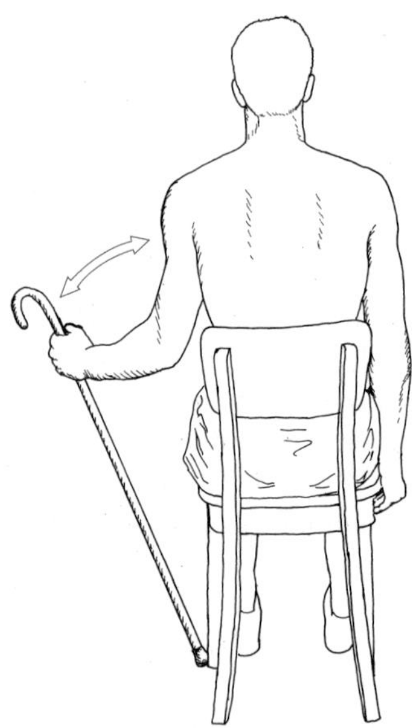

FIGURE 17.23 Gear shift exercise. Self-assisted shoulder rotation using a cane. Flexion/extension and diagonal patterns also can be done.

Early Motion of the Scapula

PROM and A-AROM of the scapula are described in Chapter 3. During the acute phase, the side-lying position is usually more comfortable than prone-lying. If the patient can perform active scapular elevation/depression and protraction/retraction, use the sitting position.

Early Neuromuscular Control

Frequently, the muscles of the rotator cuff are inhibited after trauma or surgery.[217] Initiate the following to stimulate activation and develop control in key muscles as soon as the patient tolerates it.

Multiple-Angle Muscle Setting

Begin gentle multiple-angle muscle-setting exercises of the internal and external rotators in pain-free positions of humeral flexion or scapular plane elevation. Activate the scapular and remaining GH muscles with gentle muscle-setting techniques in positions that do not exacerbate symptoms.

Protected Weight Bearing

In sitting in front of a table, have the patient lean onto his or her hands or elbows and gently move from side-to-side. This helps to seat the humeral head in the glenoid fossa and stimulate muscle action.

Exercise Techniques to Increase Flexibility and Range of Motion

To regain neuromuscular control and function in the shoulder girdle, it may be necessary to increase flexibility in restricted muscles and fascia, so proper shoulder girdle alignment and functional ranges are possible. The principles of muscle inhibition and passive stretching are presented in Chapter 4. Techniques to stretch tight joints in the shoulder girdle are discussed earlier in this chapter with reference to Chapter 5 (joint mobilization/manipulation procedures). Specific manual and self-stretching techniques are described in this section.

FOCUS ON EVIDENCE

In a randomized trial of 20 subjects with restricted GH joint mobility, the experimental group underwent a one-time intervention of soft tissue mobilization of the subscapularis, followed by contract-relax against manual resistance to the internal rotators, and then actively moved their extremity through the D_2 PNF pattern (flexion, abduction, and external rotation). The control group received no treatment; they rested for 10 minutes. The intervention group had an immediate posttreatment increase in external rotation of 16.4° ± 5.5° compared with 0.9° ± 1.5° in the control group and an increase in overhead reach of 9.6 ± 6.2 cm compared with 2.4 ± 4.5 cm in the control group. These increased motions for the intervention group were significantly greater than control group increases.[66] While this result is positive, because no long-term results were evaluated it is important to stress the need for continued self-stretching and ROM exercises as part of the patient's home exercise program.

Self-Stretching Techniques to Increase Shoulder ROM

Teach the patient a low-intensity, prolonged stretch. Emphasize the importance of not using ballistic stretches at the end of the range.

To Increase Flexion and Horizontal Adduction: Cross-Chest Stretch

- *Patient position and procedure:* Sitting or standing. Teach the patient to horizontally adduct the tight shoulder by placing the arm across the chest and then applying sustained overpressure by pulling the arm toward the chest (Fig. 17.24 A).

NOTE: The cross-chest stretch is used to increase mobility in the structures of the posterior GH joint, typically seen in shoulder impingement syndromes.[129]

- *Patient position and procedure:* Side-lying on the affected side, with the shoulder and elbow each flexed to 90° and arm internally rotated. Have the patient stretch the affected arm into horizontal adduction by reaching across the body with the opposite arm, grasping the elbow, and lifting it off the table. This side-lying position provides stabilization to the scapula (Fig 17.24 B).[226]

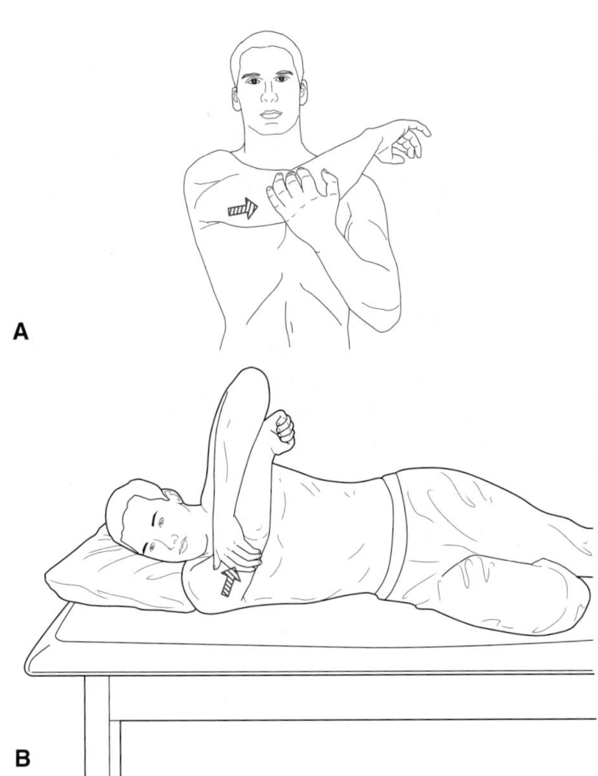

FIGURE 17.24 Self-stretching to increase horizontal adduction in standing **(A)**, and in the "sleeper position" to stabilize the scapula **(B)**.

To Increase Flexion and Elevation of the Arm

Patient position and procedure: Sitting with the involved side next to the table, forearm resting along the table edge, and elbow slightly flexed (Fig. 17.25 A). Have the patient slide the forearm forward along the table while bending from the waist. Eventually, the head should be level with the shoulder (Fig. 17.25 B).

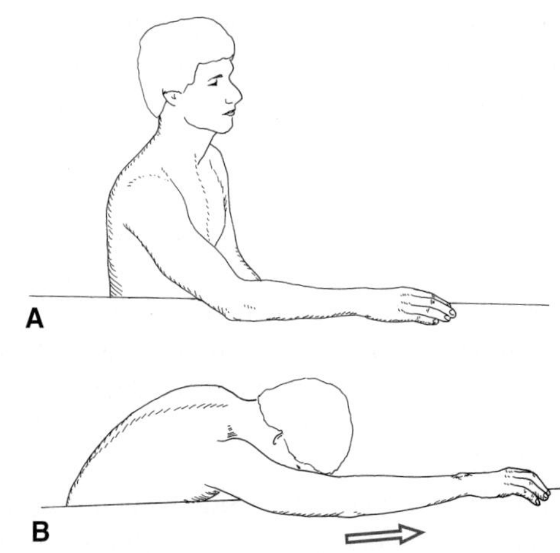

FIGURE 17.25 **(A)** Beginning and **(B)** end positions for self-stretching to increase shoulder flexion with elevation.

To Increase External (Lateral) Rotation

- *Patient position and procedure:* Standing and facing a doorframe with the palm of the hand against the edge of the frame and elbow flexed 90°. While keeping the arm against the side or in slight abduction (held in abduction with a folded towel or small pillow under the axilla), have the patient turn away from the fixed hand (Fig. 17.26 A).

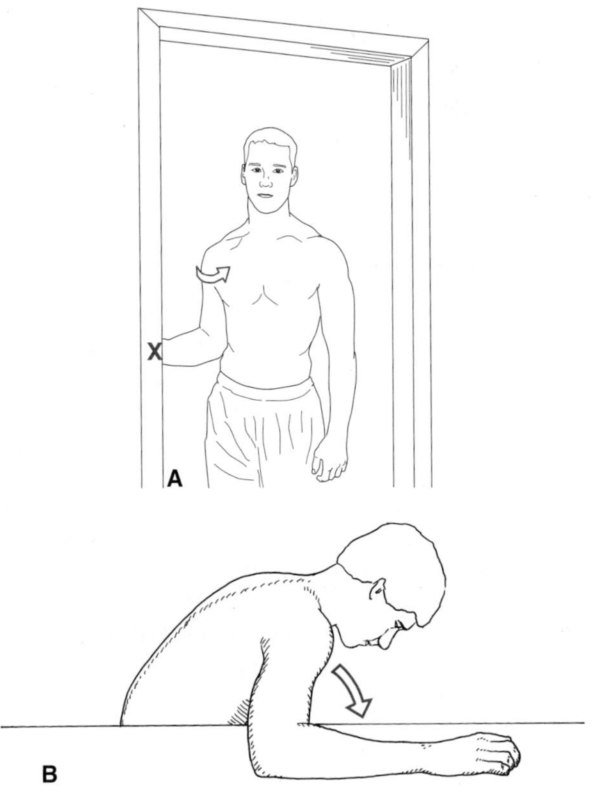

FIGURE 17.26 Self-stretching to increase external rotation of the shoulder **(A)** with the arm at the side using a doorframe and **(B)** with the arm in the plane of the scapular using a table to stabilize the forearm.

- *Patient position and procedure:* Sitting at the side of a table with the forearm resting on the table and elbow flexed to 90°. Have the patient bend from the waist, bringing the head and shoulder level with the table (Fig. 17.26 B).

PRECAUTION: Avoid the stretch position (illustrated in Figure 17.26 B) if there is anterior GH instability.

To Increase Internal Rotation

- *Patient position and procedure:* Standing facing a doorframe with the elbow flexed to 90° and the back of the hand against the frame. Have the patient turn his or her trunk toward the fixed hand.
- *Patient position and procedure:* Side-lying on the affected side, with the shoulder and elbow each flexed to 90° and arm internally rotated to end position ("sleeper" position). Have the patient then push the forearm toward the table with the opposite hand (Fig. 17.27).

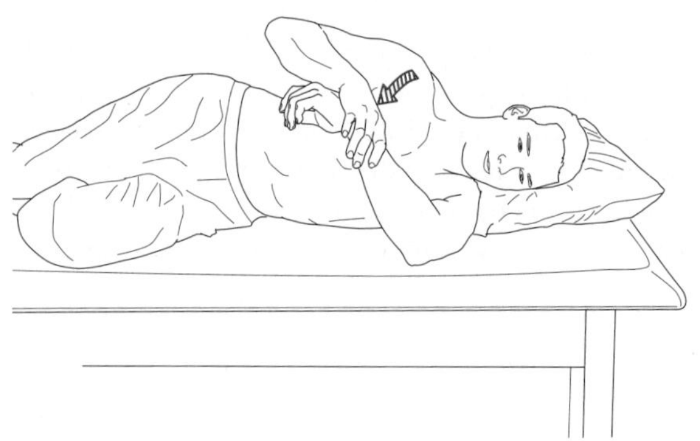

FIGURE 17.27 Self-stretching in the "sleeper position" to increase internal rotation of the shoulder using a table to stabilize the humerus.

FOCUS ON EVIDENCE

The horizontal cross-chest stretch described earlier in this section (see Fig 17.24) can also increase GH internal rotation ROM. In subjects with loss of GH internal rotation of at least 10° compared to their contralateral shoulder, performing this stretch five times daily for 30 seconds over a 4-week duration significantly increased GH internal rotation and total GH rotation compared to the opposite shoulder and to a control group.[129] Similar results were reported in another study using the horizontal adduction stretch,[122] while the side-lying "sleeper" stretch (see Fig. 17.24B) has also been shown to effectively increase GH internal rotation, total GH rotation, and reaching up the back compared to the opposite shoulder.[129]

To Increase Abduction and Elevation of the Arm

Patient position and procedure: Sitting with the side next to a table, the forearm resting with palm up (supinated) on the table and pointing toward the opposite side of the table (Fig. 17.28 A). Have the patient slide his or her arm across the table as the head is brought down toward the arm and the thorax moves away from the table (Fig. 17.28 B).

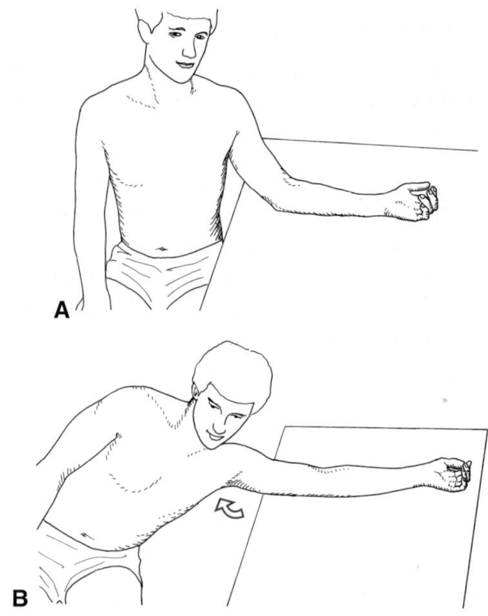

FIGURE 17.28 (A) Beginning and **(B)** end positions for self-stretching to increase shoulder abduction with elevation.

To Increase Extension of the Arm

Patient position and procedure: Standing with the back to the table, both hands grasping the edge with the fingers facing forward (Fig. 17.29 A). Have the patient begin to squat while letting the elbows flex (Fig. 17.29 B).

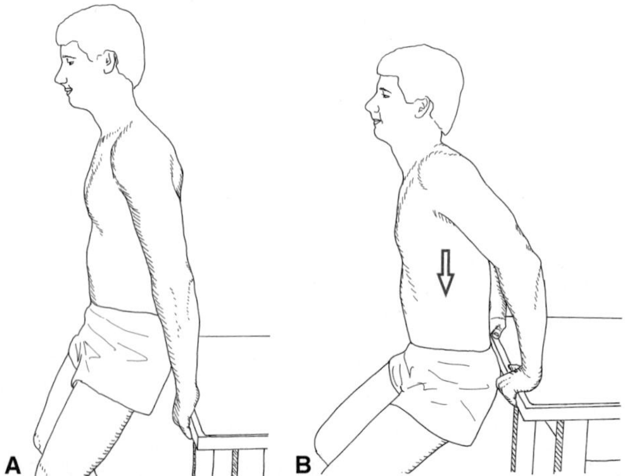

FIGURE 17.29 (A) Beginning and **(B)** end positions for self-stretching to increase shoulder extension.

PRECAUTION: If a patient is prone to anterior subluxation or dislocation, this stretching technique should not be done.

To Increase Internal Rotation, Extension, and Scapular Tilting

Patient position and procedure: Sitting or standing. Have the patient hold each end of a towel or a wand with one arm overhead and the arm to be stretched behind the lower back, and then pull up on the towel (or wand) with the overhead hand (see position in Fig. 17.13). This stretch is used to increase the ability to reach behind the back. It is a generalized stretch that does not isolate specific tight tissues. Before using it, each component of the motion should be stretched, so no one component becomes overstretched relative to the other components.

PRECAUTION: If a patient has anterior or multidirectional GH joint instability or has had recent anterior stabilization surgery to correct a dislocated shoulder, this stretch should not be done until late in the rehabilitation program when the capsule is well healed, because it forces the head of the humerus against the anterior capsule.

Manual and Self-Stretching Exercises for Specific Muscles

Manual stretching of specific multijoint muscles that affect alignment of the shoulder girdle are presented in this section along with self-stretching techniques for these muscles.

To Stretch the Latissimus Dorsi Muscle

Manual Stretch

Patient position and procedure: Supine, with hips and knees flexed so the pelvis is stabilized in a posterior pelvic tilt. If necessary, provide additional stabilization to the pelvis with one hand. With the other hand, grasp the distal humerus and flex, laterally rotate, and partially abduct the shoulder to the end of the available range. Have the patient contract into extension, adduction, and medial rotation while providing resistance for a hold–relax maneuver. During the relaxation phase, elongate the muscle (see Fig. 4.16 B).

Self-Stretch

- *Patient position and procedure:* Hook-lying with the pelvis stabilized in a posterior pelvic tilt and the arms flexed, laterally rotated, and slightly abducted overhead as far as possible (thumbs pointing toward floor). Allow gravity to provide the stretch force. Instruct the patient not to allow the back to arch.
- *Patient position and procedure:* Standing with back to a wall and feet forward enough to allow the hips and knees to partially flex and flatten the low back against the wall, with the arms in a "hold-up" position (abducted 90° and laterally rotated 90° if possible). Tell the patient to slide the back of the hands up the wall as far as possible without allowing the back to arch.

NOTE: This exercise is also used to activate the lower trapezius and serratus anterior, as they upwardly rotate and depress the scapulae during humeral abduction.

To Stretch the Pectoralis Major Muscles

Manual Stretch

Patient position and procedure: Sitting on a treatment table or mat, with the hands behind the head. Kneel behind the patient and grasp the patient's elbows (Fig. 17.30). Have the patient breathe in as he or she brings the elbows out to the side (horizontal abduction and scapular adduction). Hold the elbows at this end point as the patient breathes out. No forceful stretch is needed against the elbows, because the rib cage is elongating the proximal attachment of the pectoralis major muscles bilaterally. As the patient repeats the inhalation, again move the elbows up and out to the end of the available range and hold as the patient breathes out. Repeat only three times in succession to avoid hyperventilation.

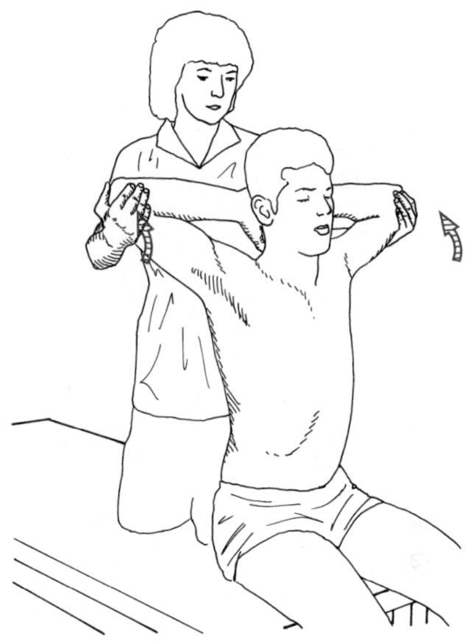

FIGURE 17.30 Active stretching of the pectoralis major muscle. The therapist gently pulls the elbows posteriorly while the patient breathes in and then holds the elbows at the end point as the patient breathes out.

PRECAUTION: Hyperventilation should not occur, because the breathing is slow and comfortable. If the patient does become dizzy, allow time to rest; then reinstruct for proper technique. Be sure the patient maintains the head and neck in the neutral position, not forward.

Self-Stretch

- *Patient position and procedure:* Standing, facing a corner or open door, with the arms in a reverse T or a V against the wall (Fig. 17.31 A & B). Have the patient lean the entire body forward from the ankles (knees slightly flexed). The degree of stretch can be adjusted by the amount of forward movement.
- *Patient position and procedure:* Sitting or standing and grasping the wand with the forearms pronated and elbows flexed 90°. Have the patient then elevate the shoulders and bring the wand behind the head and shoulders (Fig. 17.32).

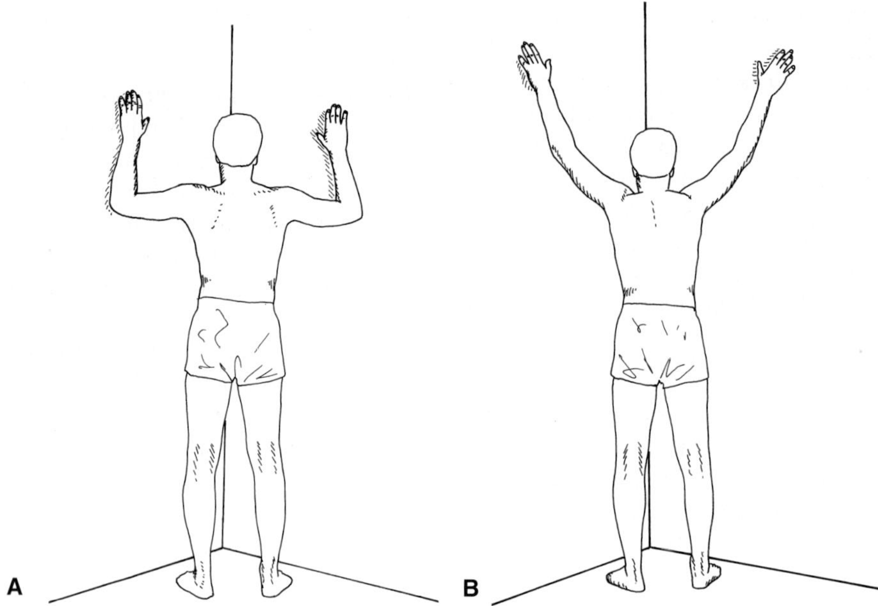

FIGURE 17.31 Self-stretching the pectoralis major muscle with the arms in a reverse-T position to stretch **(A)** the clavicular portion and in a V-position to stretch **(B)** the sternal portion.

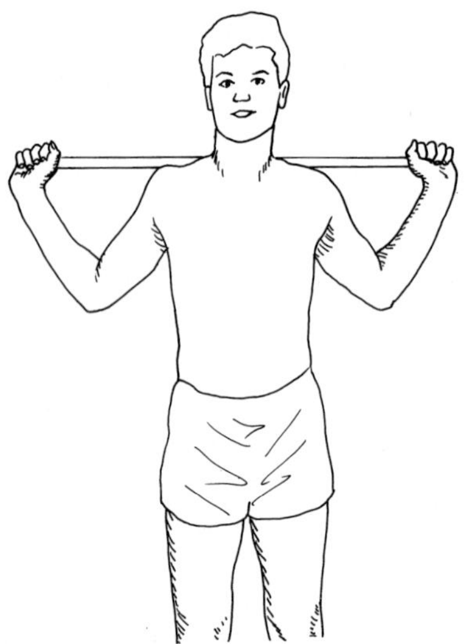

FIGURE 17.32 Wand exercises to stretch the pectoralis major muscle.

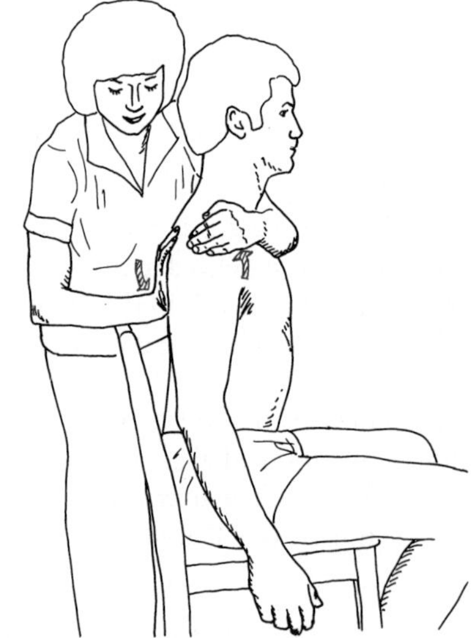

FIGURE 17.33 Active stretching of the pectoralis minor muscle. The therapist holds the scapular and coracoid process at the end point as the patient breathes out.

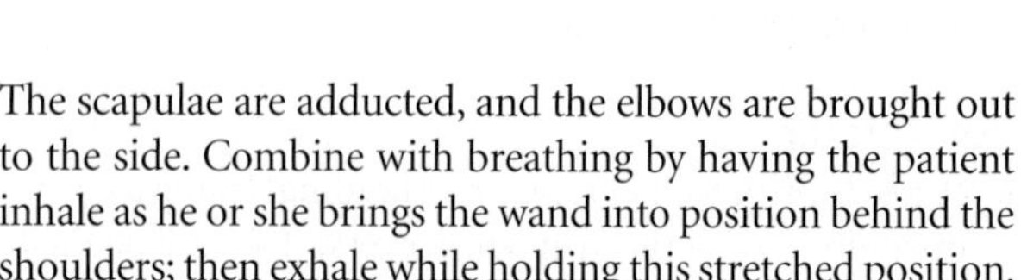

The scapulae are adducted, and the elbows are brought out to the side. Combine with breathing by having the patient inhale as he or she brings the wand into position behind the shoulders; then exhale while holding this stretched position.

To Stretch the Pectoralis Minor Muscle

Manual Stretch VIDEO 17.1

Patient position and procedure: Sitting, place one hand posterior on the scapula and the other hand anterior on the shoulder just above the coracoid process (Fig. 17.33). As the patient breathes in, tip the scapula posteriorly by pressing up and back against the coracoid process while pressing downward against the inferior angle of the scapula; then hold it at the end position while the patient breathes out. Repeat, readjusting the end position with each inhalation and stabilizing as the patient exhales.

Self-Stretch

Patient position and procedure: Standing with the involved humerus at 90° abduction and elbow at 90° flexion and the forearm stabilized against a doorway. Instruct the patient to rotate the trunk away from the involved shoulder until a stretch is felt.[17] Note that this stretch may not be appropriate for patients with anterior instability, as this is their position of apprehension and it may overly strain the anterior GH joint restraints.

To Stretch the Levator Scapulae Muscle

NOTE: The levator scapulae muscle attaches to the superior angle of the scapula and causes it to rotate downward and elevate; it also attaches to the transverse processes of the upper cervical vertebrae and causes them to backward bend and rotate to the ipsilateral side. To minimize stress to the cervical spine, it is recommended that the cervical spine and head be placed at end-range and stabilized and that the stretch force be applied against the scapula.

Manual Stretch VIDEO 17.1

Patient position and procedure: Sitting with the head rotated opposite to side of tightness (looking away from the tight side) and forward bent until a slight pull is felt in the posterolateral aspect of the neck. The arm on the side of tightness is abducted, and the hand is placed behind the head to help stabilize it in the rotated position. Stand behind the patient and stabilize with one arm; place the other hand (same side as the tight muscle) over the superior angle of the scapula (Fig. 17.34). With the muscle now in its stretched position, have the patient breathe in, then out. Hold the shoulder and scapula down to maintain the stretch as the patient breathes in again (he or she contracts the muscle against the resistance of the fixating hand). To increase the stretch, press down against the superior angle of the scapula. This is not a forceful stretch but a gentle hold-relax maneuver. Do not stretch the muscle by forcing rotation on the head and neck.

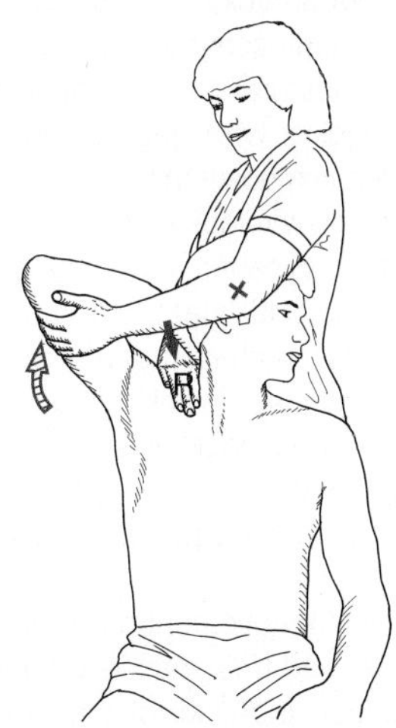

FIGURE 17.34 Stretching of the levator scapulae muscle. The therapist stabilizes the head and scapula as the patient breathes in, contracting the muscle against the resistance. As the patient relaxes, the rib cage and scapula depress, which stretches the muscle.

Self-Stretch

- *Patient position and procedure:* Standing with the head side bent and rotated away from the tight side, place the ipsilateral hand behind the head and the bent elbow against a wall. The other hand can be placed across the forehead to stabilize the rotated head. Instruct the patient to slide the elbow up the wall as he or she takes in a breath, then hold the position while exhaling (Fig. 17.35 A).
- *Patient position and procedure:* Sitting with head side bent and rotated away from the tight side. To stabilize the scapula, have the patient reach down and back with the hand on the side of the tightness and hold onto the seat of the chair. The other hand is placed on the head to gently pull it forward and to the side in an oblique direction opposite the line of pull of the tight muscle (Fig. 17.35 B).

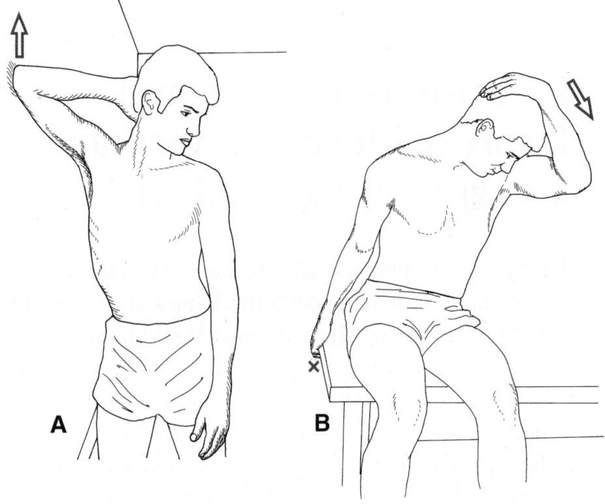

FIGURE 17.35 Self-stretching of the levator scapulae muscle **(A)** using upward rotation of the scapula and **(B)** using depression of the scapula.

To Stretch the Upper Trapezius Muscle

Manual Stretch

- *Patient position and procedure:* Sitting with the ipsilateral hand behind the back to stabilize the scapula and the head rotated to the tight side. Stand behind the patient and apply the stretch by adding a combination of cervical flexion, further rotation to the tight side, and side bending away from the tight side. A more aggressive manual stretch can be performed by using the other hand to depress the distal clavicle and the scapula.

PRECAUTION: Applying a stretch force against the head should not be done if the patient has cervical symptoms.

Self-Stretch

Patient position and procedure: Sitting or standing with the ipsilateral hand behind the back to stabilize the scapula. Instruct the patient to rotate his neck toward the tight side, then side bend away from the tight side and then add neck flexion. The patient may use the contralateral arm to grasp his or her own head to apply the stretch (Fig. 17.36).

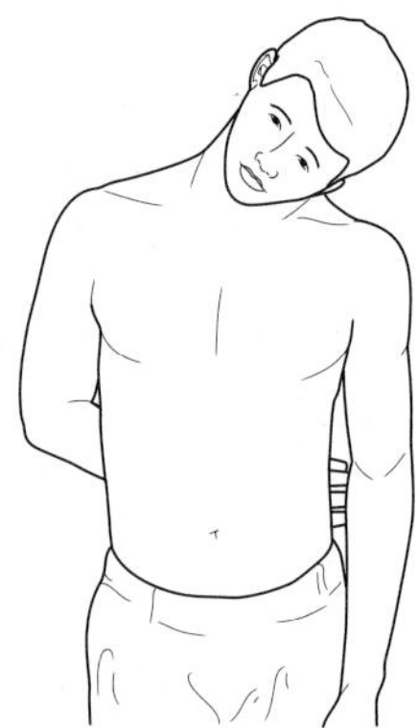

FIGURE 17.36 Self-stretching of the upper trapezius muscle.

Exercises to Develop and Improve Muscle Performance and Functional Control

Developing control of the scapulothoracic and GH musculature is fundamental to correcting pathomechanics of the shoulder girdle and for improving strength, muscle endurance, power, and performance of functional activities. During observation of scapular alignment and movement, if excessive scapular tilting, winging, or poorly coordinated scapulohumeral rhythm during humeral elevation is identified, it is important to correct these faulty mechanics with properly chosen exercises. Likewise, insufficient stabilization and control of GH rotation and translation during humeral elevation necessitate the selection of exercises that emphasize training the rotator cuff musculature.

- The exercises described in the following sections begin at the simplest or least stressful level and progress to more complex and difficult levels.
- Exercises also progress from uniplanar or isolated muscle activation to use of combined, functional patterns.
- Initially, choose exercises that help the patient focus on activating correct muscles with appropriate timing and sequencing to counteract the identified impairments.
- Then increase the challenge by emphasizing patterns of exercises that prepare the musculature to respond to functional demands.

Regardless of the level of exercise, it is important to challenge patients at intensities they can meet so they can safely progress to more intense levels. Before teaching the resistance exercises and functional training activities presented in this section, it is important that the reader understands and applies the principles of resistance exercise, open- and closed-chain training, specificity of training, aerobic conditioning, and balance training described in Chapters 6 through 8. It is also important to apply the principles of tissue healing described in Chapter 10 and integrate the precautions for exercise associated with various shoulder pathologies and surgical interventions presented in this chapter. Because posture has a direct effect on the function of the shoulder complex, refer to Chapters 14 and 16 for principles and exercises to correct postural impairments that might underlie faulty shoulder mechanics. In addition to the exercises described in this section, high-demand exercises, such as plyometric training[216] and advanced activities for balance and stability, that may be appropriate in a shoulder rehabilitation program for selected individuals are presented in Chapter 23.

Box 17.11 summarizes a sequence for progressing exercises to improve muscle performance and shoulder girdle function and move an individual toward functional recovery.

Isometric Exercises

Isometric exercises are applied along a continuum of very gentle to maximum contraction, and they are applied at varying muscle lengths by changing joint angles. Choice of the intensity, muscle length, or joint angle and the number of repetitions is based on current strength, stage of recovery after injury or surgery, and/or the pathomechanics of the region.

BOX 17.11 Summary of Exercise Progressions for Shoulder Function

- Develop awareness and control of weak or disused muscles. Place emphasis on activating scapulothoracic and trunk musculature prior to glenohumeral musculature.
- For weak or surgically repaired musculature, begin with setting exercises and multiple-angle isometrics against minimal resistance and active-assistive ROM in open- and closed-chain positions within pain-free or protected ranges.
- Provide just enough resistance and repetitions to challenge the muscles without provoking symptoms.
- Include concentric and eccentric exercises.
- Develop control in postural muscles for stability of scapular and glenohumeral joints with stabilization exercises in both open- and closed-chain positions.
- As stabilizing control develops in the scapula and GH muscles, progress to dynamic resistance exercises, emphasizing scapular and rotator cuff muscle control during open- and closed-chain motions.
- First isolate and strengthen weak motions and muscles so substitute motions and inappropriate timing of muscle actions do not dominate.
- Develop muscle endurance simultaneously with muscle strength.
- Progress to combined movement patterns that simulate functional activities and train muscle groups to function in a coordinated sequence of control and motion.
- Integrate simple functional tasks into the exercise program and progress to more complex and challenging activities, always incorporating proper body mechanics.
- Implement total body exercises to improve cardiopulmonary endurance and balance.
- As necessary, based on functional goals, incorporate high-intensity eccentric exercises and plyometric training (stretch-shortening drills)[216] and agility drills at increasing speeds of movement into the shoulder rehabilitation program.

Scapular Muscles

Patient position and procedure: Side-lying, prone-lying, or sitting, with the arm supported if necessary. Resist elevation, depression, protraction, or retraction with pressure directly on the scapula in the direction opposite the motion.

Depression (lower trapezius). Activation of the lower trapezius is indicated when there is anterior tilting and delayed upward rotation of the scapula often seen with impingement syndromes. Apply resistance against the inferior angle of the scapula (Fig. 17.37 A).

Protraction (serratus anterior). Activation of the serratus anterior is emphasized when there is scapular winging, delayed or incomplete upward rotation of the scapula with GH elevation, or with accelerated downward rotation ("dumping") of the scapula during arm lowering. Apply resistance against the axillary border of the scapula or coracoid process or indirectly against the humerus positioned in the plane of the scapula (Fig. 17.37 B).

Retraction (rhomboids and trapezius). Activation of the rhomboids and trapezius muscle groups is emphasized when the scapular posture is protracted (abducted), as typically seen with a forward head and increased kyphotic posture. Apply resistance against the medial border of the scapula.

Multiple-Angle Isometrics: GH Muscles

Patient position and procedure: Supine, sitting, or standing. If pain from joint compression occurs, a slight distractive force to the GH joint as resistance is applied may decrease patient discomfort.

External and internal rotation. Position the humerus at the patient's side in slight flexion, slight abduction, or slight scapular plane elevation and the elbow flexed 90°. Apply resistance against the dorsal surface of the forearm to resist external rotation (Fig. 17.38 A) and to the volar surface to resist internal rotation (Fig. 17.38 B).

Abduction. Maintain the humerus neutral to rotation and resist abduction at 0°, 30°, 45°, and 60°. If there are no

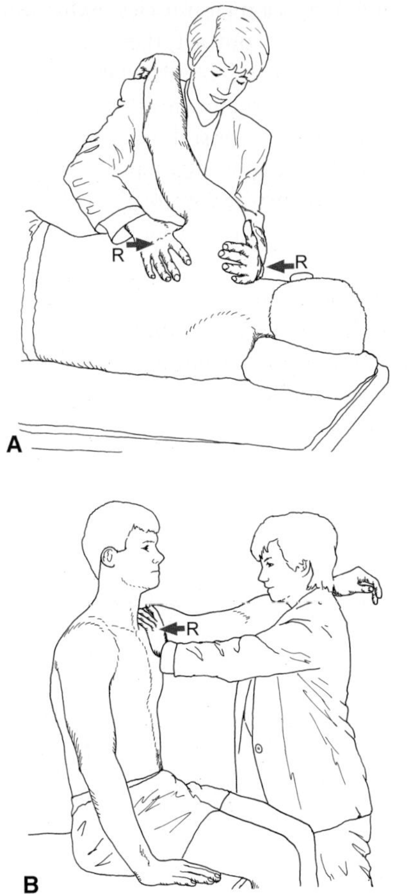

FIGURE 17.37 Isometric or dynamic manual resistance to scapular muscles. **(A)** Resistance to elevation/depression. **(B)** Resistance to protraction/retraction. Direct the patient to reach across the therapist's shoulder to protract the scapula while the therapist resists against the coracoid and acromion process. The therapist's other hand is placed behind the scapula to resist retraction.

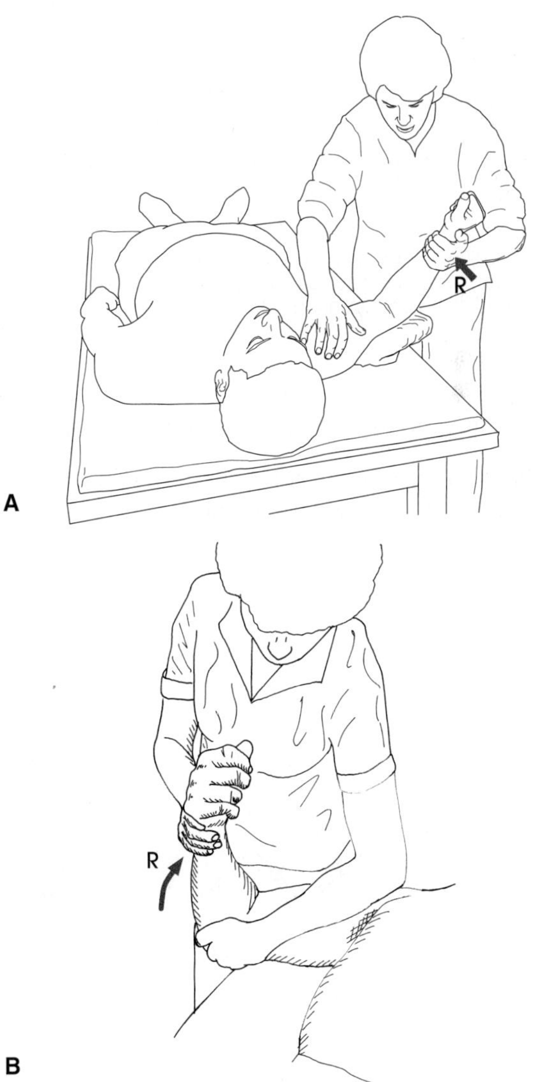

FIGURE 17.38 Isometric or dynamic resistance to shoulder rotation. **(A)** External rotation with the shoulder in the plane of the scapula. **(B)** Internal rotation with the shoulder at 90° abduction.

contraindications to motion above 90°, preposition the humerus in external rotation before elevating the humerus and resisting above 90° abduction.

Scapular plane elevation. Position midway between flexion and abduction and resist at various positions in the range, such as 30° and 60° in the plane of the scapula (Fig. 17.39).

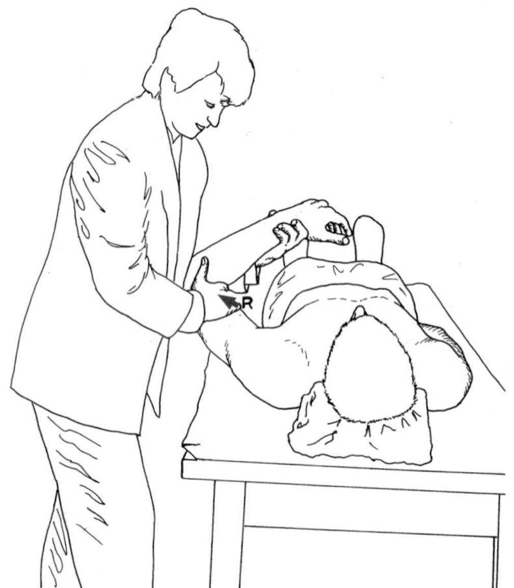

FIGURE 17.39 Isometric resistance in scapular plane elevation. The shoulder is positioned between 30° and 60° degrees of elevation, and controlled manual resistance is applied against the humerus.

Extension. Position the humerus at the side or in various positions of flexion and apply resistance against the humerus.

Adduction. Position the humerus between 15° and 30° abduction and apply resistance against the humerus.

Elbow flexion with forearm supination. Position the humerus at the side and neutral to rotation. Apply resistance to forearm flexion, causing tension in the long head of the biceps. Change the position of the shoulder into more flexion or extension and repeat the isometric resistance to elbow flexion.

Self-Applied Multiple-Angle Isometrics

Teach the patient how to independently apply isometric resistance using positions and intensities consistent with therapeutic goals. The patient can use the opposite hand (Fig. 17.40) or a stationary object, such as a wall or door frame (Fig. 17.41).

Stabilization Exercises

The application of alternating isometrics and rhythmic stabilization techniques (described in Chapter 6) is designed to develop strength and stability of proximal muscle groups in response to shifting loads. The shoulder girdle functions in both open- and closed-chain activities, and therefore, the muscles should be trained to respond to both situations.

- Begin training the scapular muscles so that when the muscles of the GH joint contract, they have a stable base on which to produce force (scapular stability).
- Initially, apply the alternating resistance slowly and instruct the patient to "hold" against the resistance.
- At the beginning of training, it also may be necessary to tell the patient which way you are going to push to help the patient focus on the contracting muscles and alternating forces.
- As the patient learns to respond by contracting the proper muscles and stabilizing the joints, increase the rapidity of the shifting resistance and decrease the verbal cues to enhance automatic responses.

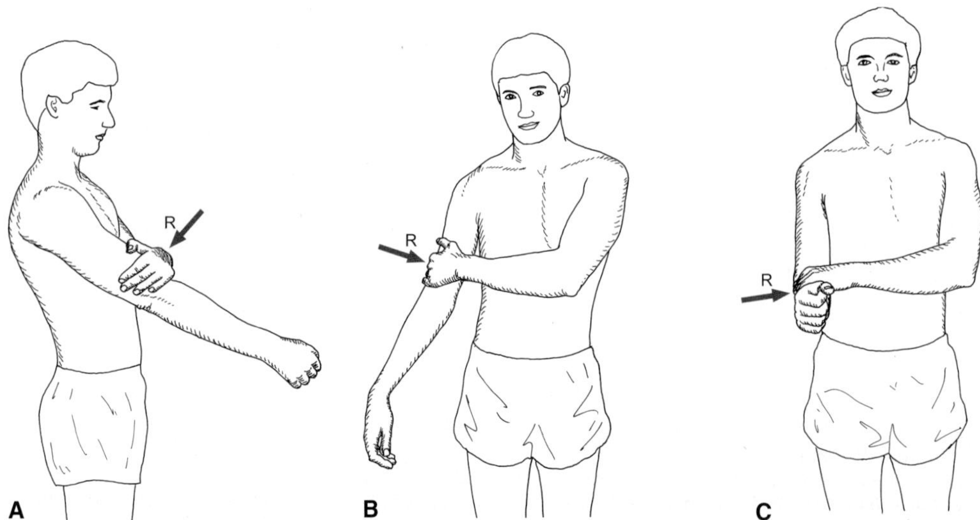

FIGURE 17.40 Self-resistance for isometric shoulder **(A)** flexion, **(B)** abduction, and **(C)** rotation.

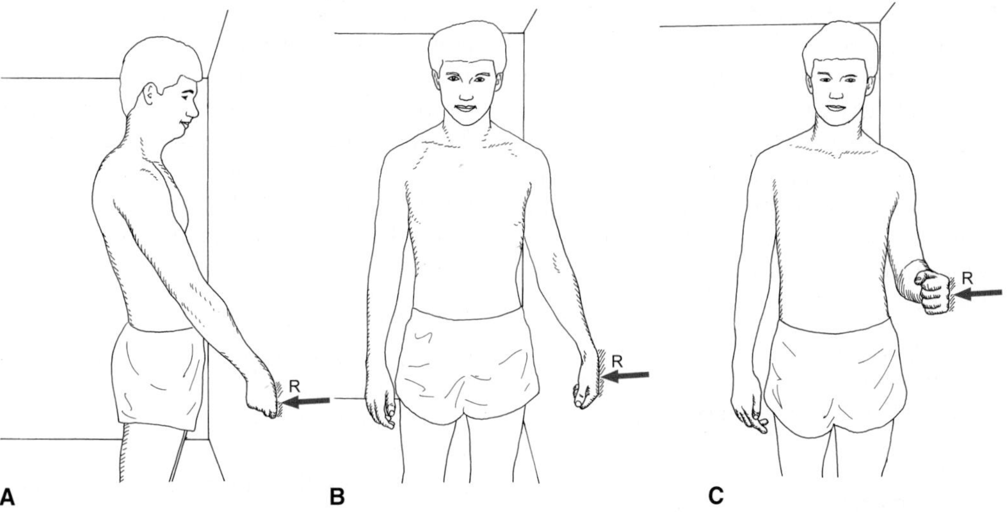

FIGURE 17.41 Using a wall to provide resistance for isometric shoulder **(A)** flexion, **(B)** abduction, and **(C)** rotation.

Open-Chain Stabilization Exercises for the Scapular Muscles VIDEO 17.2

Begin with the patient side-lying, with the affected extremity up. Drape the forearm of the involved extremity over your shoulder. The degree of shoulder flexion, scaption, or abduction can be controlled by your stance and the relative position of the patient. Progress to sitting with the patient's arm draped over your shoulder; apply resistance to all scapular motions in the same manner as described previously.

Scapular elevation/depression. Place your top hand superiorly and the other hand inferiorly around the scapula to provide manual resistance (see Fig. 17.37 A).

Scapular protraction/retraction. Place your top hand along the medial border and the other around the coracoid process to provide resistance (see Fig. 17.37 B).

Scapular upward and downward rotation. Place one hand around the inferior angle and the other hand around the acromion and coracoid process to provide resistance.

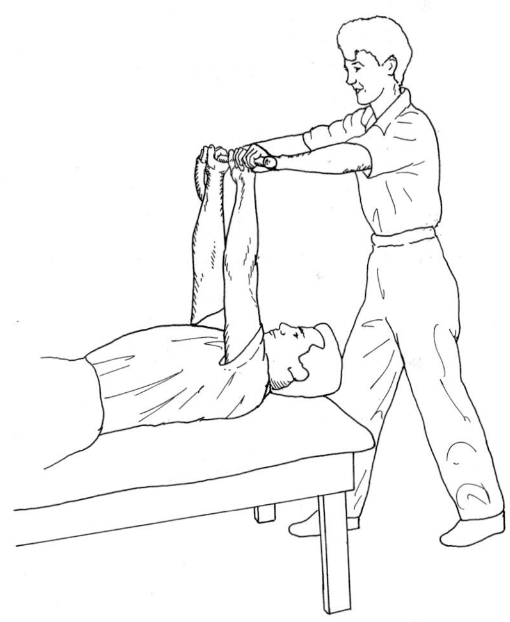

FIGURE 17.42 Stabilization exercises. The patient stabilizes with the shoulder girdle musculature (isometrically) against the resistance imposed by the therapist. Resistance to flexion/extension, abduction/adduction, and rotation is applied in a rhythmic sequence.

Open-Chain Stabilization Exercises for the Shoulder Girdle

Patient position and procedure: Supine holding a rod or ball with elbows extended and shoulders flexed to 90°. Stand at the patient's head and grasp the rod; instruct the patient to hold against or match the resistance you provide. Push, pull, and rotate the rod in various directions (Fig. 17.42). Resistance can also be applied directly against the arm or forearm.

- If too much assistance is being provided by the normal extremity, apply the stabilization technique to just the involved extremity.
- As the patient gains control, progress to sitting and then standing and have the patient hold the arm in various positions as alternating resistance is applied. Observe the scapula to be sure there is good stabilization. If not, return to the exercises described above or decrease the intensity of resistance. Progress these exercises to functional patterns as strength and control improve.

CLINICAL TIP

Studies have documented that when healthy individuals[110] or patients with shoulder instability[26] use the BodyBlade® during dynamic GH exercises (see Fig. 23.17), such as shoulder flexion and abduction, the scapulothoracic stabilizing muscles are activated to a greater extent than when the exercises are performed using weights or elastic resistance.

Static Closed-Chain (Weight-Bearing) Stabilization Exercises

Weight bearing activates the stabilizing muscles in proximal joints and may be a stimulus for improving fluid dynamics of articular cartilage as described in Chapter 5. Early during the controlled motion phase of management, it may be beneficial to initiate stabilization exercises in protected weight-bearing positions if tolerated by the healing tissues. The amount and intensity of weight bearing and resistance are progressively increased as tissues heal.

NOTE: If scapular winging occurs when the patient is weight bearing, do not progress these exercises until there is enough strength to stabilize the scapula against the rib cage.

FOCUS ON EVIDENCE

To help determine when upper extremity weight-bearing exercises could be included in an exercise program, Uhl and colleagues[206] analyzed the pectoralis major, anterior and posterior deltoid, supraspinatus, and infraspinatus with surface EMG in a progression of static exercises in 18 healthy subjects. Positions for isometric exercises included the prayer position (to simulate weight bearing against a wall), quadruped, tripod, pointer, push-up position (shoulders flexed to 90°), push-up position with feet elevated 18 inches (45 cm), and one-arm push-up position. There was a significant correlation between the increasing weight-bearing postures and increased muscular activity ($r = 0.97$, $p < 0.01$) in all the muscles. Also, the infraspinatus was the most active of the muscles tested in all positions except the prayer position (in which the pectoralis major was most active).

The authors suggest that the prayer and quadruped positions were appropriate for early rehabilitation owing to the low-activity level in all the muscles; that the tripod and pointer positions placed an intermediate demand on the infraspinatus and deltoid musculature; and that the push-up positions placed a high demand on the infraspinatus. They also conclude that the two-handed positions required less demand on the posterior deltoid but more load on the anterior deltoid and pectoralis muscles and that the one-arm push-up placed a high demand on all muscles except the supraspinatus.

■ ***Scapular stabilization.***

Patient position and procedure: Side-lying on the uninvolved side. Both the elbow and shoulder of the involved arm are flexed to 90°, with the hand placed on the table and bearing some weight. Resist the scapular motions of elevation/depression and retraction directly against the scapula; resist protraction by pushing against the elbow.

■ ***Alternating isometrics in protected weight bearing.*** VIDEO 17.3

Patient position and procedure: Sitting with forearms placed on thighs or a table or standing with hands placed on a table. Lean forward slightly to place light body weight through the extremities. Apply gentle resistance against the shoulders and ask the patient to match the resistance and "hold." Apply resistance in various directions.

■ ***Progression of closed-chain stabilization exercises.***

Patient position and procedure: Standing with shoulder at 90° and one or both hands leaning against a wall or on a ball (Fig. 17.43).

- Additional, more advanced activities include having the patient assume the quadruped (all-fours) position with hands on the floor. Apply alternating resistance against

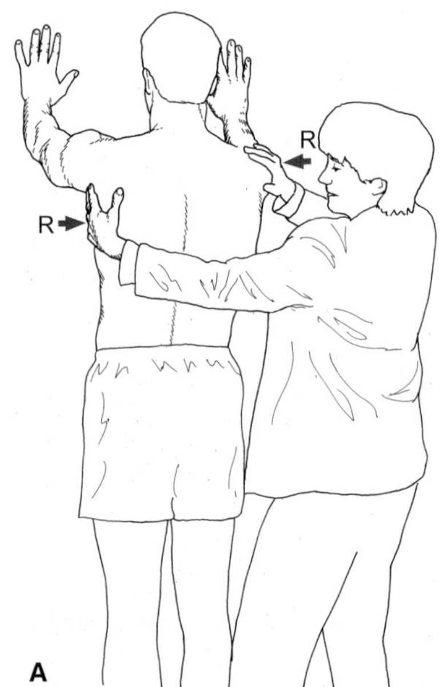

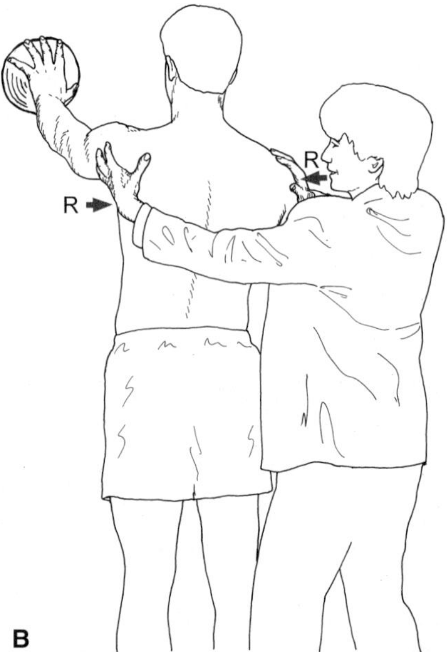

FIGURE 17.43 Closed-chain scapular and glenohumeral stabilization exercises. **(A)** Bilateral support in a minimal weight-bearing position with both hands against a wall. **(B)** Unilateral support on a less stable surface (ball). The therapist applies alternating resistance while the patient stabilizes against the resistance, or the therapist applies resistance as the patient moves from side-to-side.

the shoulders or trunk and ask the patient to "hold" against the force. Pressing forward against the trunk increases the effect of body weight through the upper extremities and requires the serratus anterior to stabilize more strongly against the additional force. As already noted, if scapular winging occurs, reduce the resistance or the degree of weight bearing.
 - Progress further by placing hands on unstable surfaces, such as a rocker or wobble board or on a ball, to require greater neuromuscular control and balance reactions. Each of these activities also can be done with weight bearing on only the involved upper extremity.

Dynamic Closed-Chain (Weight-Bearing) Stabilization Exercises

Dynamic stabilization in weight-bearing positions requires the stabilizing muscles to maintain control of the scapula and GH joint while moving the body weight over the fixed extremity or extremities.

- *Patient position and procedure:* Standing with shoulders flexed 90° and hands supported against a wall or leaning into hands on a table. Have the patient shift his or her body weight from one extremity to the other (rock back and forth). Apply resistance against the shoulders (see Fig. 17.43).
- *Progression:* Have the patient alternately lift one upper extremity and then the other, so that one extremity bears the body weight and stabilizes against the shifting load.
  - Apply manual resistance to the shoulders or strap a weight around each wrist.
  - Apply manual resistance to the shoulders or trunk that becomes more variable in direction, timing, and amount of force.
- *Patient position and procedure:* Quadruped (all-fours) position with both hands on a stable surface; have the patient raise the ipsilateral and then contralateral leg to increase serratus activity and lower trapezius activity respectively.[118]
  - *Progression:* Perform with both hands on a rocker board, wobble board, or BOSU™ or perform alternating leg raises while only one hand bears weight on a stable or unstable support surface (see Chapter 23).

Dynamic Strengthening Exercises: Scapular Muscles

It is imperative that the proximal stabilizing muscles of the thorax, neck, and scapula function properly before initiating dynamic strengthening of the muscles that move the GH joint through the ROM to avoid faulty mechanics. Strengthening exercises can be performed in both open- and closed-chain positions. Progress exercises with repetitions and resistance within the mechanical limits of the involved tissues.

Initially apply light resistance with multiple repetitions for dynamic control and muscular endurance. As control develops, progress to combined patterns of motion and training for muscle groups to function in a coordinated sequence. Begin with simple functional activities and progress to more complex and challenging activities. Both muscular endurance and strength are necessary for postural and dynamic control of activities.

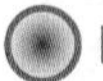

FOCUS ON EVIDENCE

A number of studies have been carried out to identify muscle activation during a variety of exercises for the shoulder girdle. Two EMG studies[51,86] analyzed exercises often used to strengthen the scapular muscles using either free weights or elastic tubing against maximum resistance. The findings of these two studies and a subsequent review of the literature[162] report the degree of trapezius and serratus anterior muscle activation during the following exercises:

- *Shoulder shrug, standing:* strongly activates the upper trapezius.
- *Full elevation of the arm above the head in the prone-lying position:* activates all three portions of the trapezius and serratus anterior when the humerus is in line with the fibers of the lower trapezius.
- *External rotation in the prone-lying position with the shoulder positioned at 90° abduction and the elbow flexed 90°:* strongly activates the lower trapezius. This position is the "best exercise" to cause maximum depression of the scapula and isolation of the lower trapezius from the middle and upper portions.[51]
- *Horizontal abduction in the prone-lying position with the shoulder in external rotation:* activates the middle and lower trapezius.
- *Rowing action, seated or prone-lying:* emphasizes the middle trapezius over the upper and lower trapezius.[162]
- *Push-up with a plus:* strong activation of serratus anterior.[162]
- *Diagonal exercises* and *shoulder abduction in the plane of the scapula above 120°*: higher activity in the serratus anterior than in the trapezius.
- *Isolated protraction exercises:* do not activate the serratus anterior to as great a degree as arm elevation exercises.[51]

In another study, based on evidence suggesting that upper trapezius activation should be minimized compared to activation of other scapulothoracic muscles during movement, Cools and associates[36] examined several exercises for the activation ratios among the muscles. Favorable exercises (those with decreased upper trapezius activation and increased lower or middle trapezius activation) included side-lying flexion, side-lying external rotation, prone horizontal abduction with humeral external rotation, and prone extension. Favorable exercises for decreased upper trapezius and increased serratus anterior activation included high rowing and arm elevation with humeral external rotation in both the sagittal and scapular planes.

Scapular Retraction (Rhomboids and Middle Trapezius)

The following exercises are designed to isolate scapular retraction. Once the patient is able to retract the scapula against resistance, combine patterns with the GH joint to progress strength and functional patterns as described in the next sections.

- *Patient position and procedure:* Prone, sitting, and standing. Instruct the patient to clasp the hands together behind the low back. This activity should cause scapular adduction. Draw attention to the adducted scapulae and have the patient hold the adducted position of the scapulae while the arms are lowered to the sides. Have the patient repeat the activity without arm motion.
- *Patient position and procedure:* Prone with the arm over the edge of the table in a dependent position and a weight in the hand. Instruct the patient to pinch the scapulae together (Fig. 17.44). Progress this exercise to prone rowing and horizontal abduction against gravity (described below).

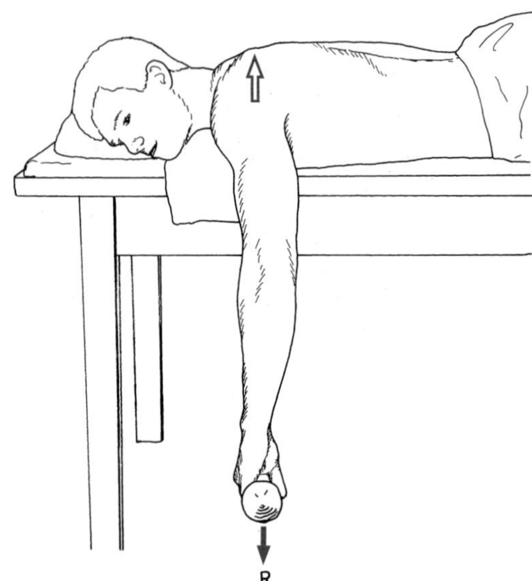

FIGURE 17.44 Scapular retraction against handheld resistance in the prone position.

- *Patient position and procedure:* Sitting or standing with the shoulder flexed to 90° and elbows extended. Have the patient grasp each end of an elastic band or tubing that has been secured at shoulder level or a two-handled pulley that is at shoulder level, and pinch the scapulae together by pulling against the resistance.

Scapular Retraction Combined With Shoulder Horizontal Abduction/Extension (Rhomboids, Middle Trapezius, Posterior Deltoid)

- *Patient position and procedure:* Prone with shoulders abducted 90°, elbows flexed, and forearms perpendicular to the floor. Instruct the patient to perform horizontal abduction with scapular retraction. This exercise can also be done with the elbows extended for greater resistance (Fig. 17.45). Progress this exercise by adding weights and then by having the patient perform the rowing motion standing or sitting in front of a length of elastic resistance that has been secured at shoulder level.

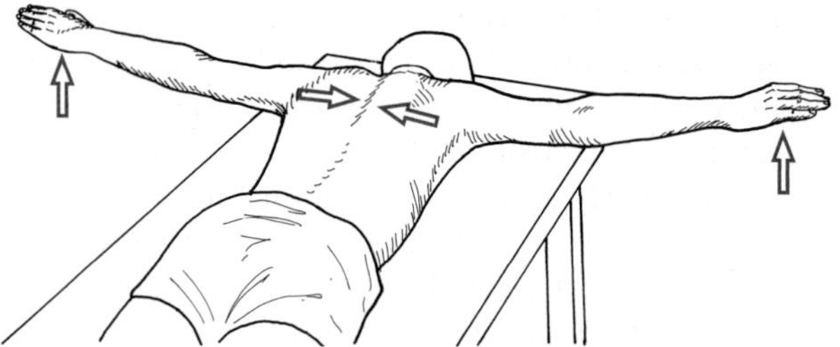

FIGURE 17.45 Horizontal abduction and scapular retraction exercises, with the arms positioned for maximal resistance from gravity. External rotation of the shoulders (thumbs pointing upward) emphasizes the middle and lower trapezius. To progress the exercise further, weights can be placed in the patient's hands.

- ***Corner press-out.***

Patient position and procedure: Standing with the back toward a corner, shoulders abducted 90°, and elbows flexed. Instruct the patient to press the elbows into the walls and push the body weight away from the corner (Fig. 17.46).

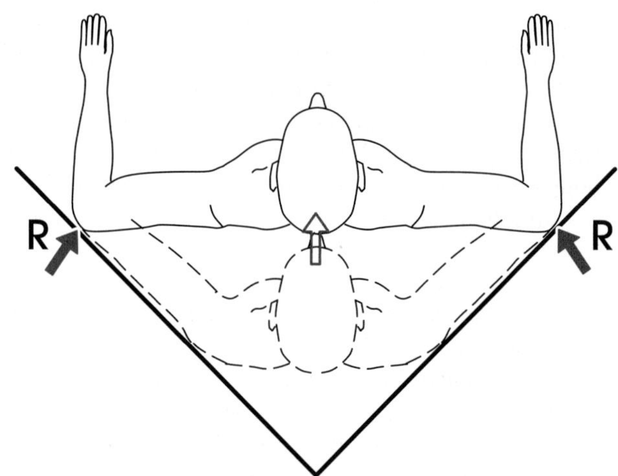

FIGURE 17.46 Corner press-out to strengthen scapular retraction and shoulder horizontal abduction (view from above).

Scapular Retraction and Shoulder Horizontal Abduction Combined With External Rotation (Rhomboids, Trapezius, Posterior Deltoid, Infraspinatus, Teres Minor)

- *Patient position and procedure:* Prone with shoulders abducted 90° and externally rotated 90° (90/90 position). The elbows can be flexed 90° (easier position) or extended (more difficult position). Instruct the patient to lift the arm a few degrees off the table. To do this correctly, the scapulae must adduct simultaneously. Greater ROM can be used if these exercises are done on a narrow bench so the arm can begin in a horizontally adducted position.
- *Patient position and procedure:* Sitting or standing with shoulders in the 90/90 position. Secure the middle of a piece of elastic resistance in front of the patient slightly above the shoulders and have the patient grasp each end of

the resistance. Then have the patient pull the hands and elbows back (moving into horizontal abduction and external rotation of the shoulder) while simultaneously adducting the scapulae (Fig. 17.47). **VIDEO 17.4**

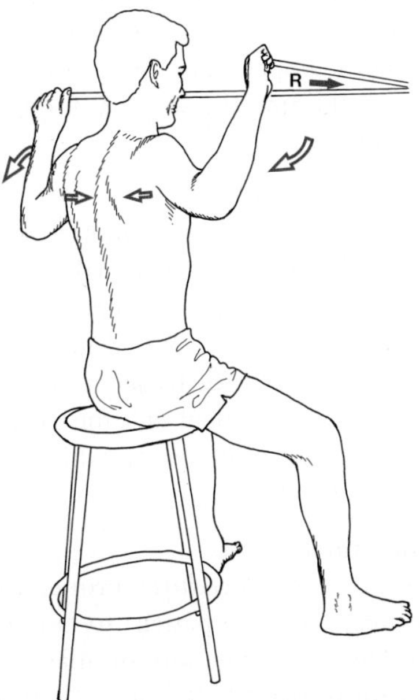

FIGURE 17.47 Combined scapular retraction with shoulder horizontal abduction and external rotation against resistance.

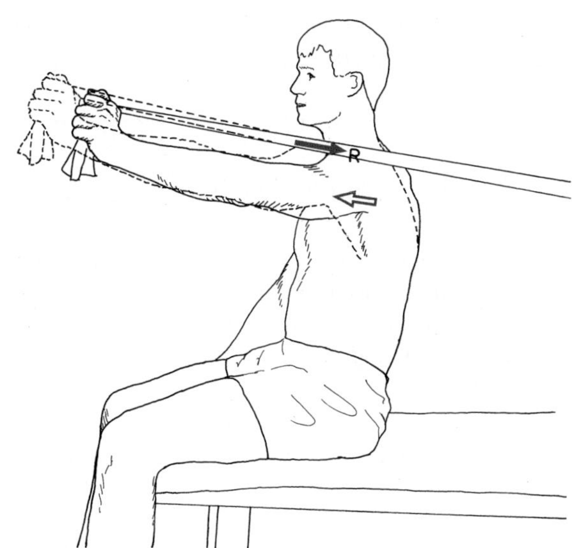

FIGURE 17.48 Scapular protraction; pushing against elastic resistance.

Scapular Protraction (Serratus Anterior)

- *Patient position and procedure:* Sitting or standing with shoulder flexed approximately 90° and elbow extended. Secure a piece of elastic resistance behind the patient at shoulder level or use a pulley system. Have the patient "push" outward against the resistance without rotating the body (Fig. 17.48).
- *Patient position and procedure:* Supine with the arm flexed 90° and slightly abducted and the elbow extended. Place a light weight in the hand if resistance is tolerated and have the patient "push" the weight upward without rotating the body.

CLINICAL TIP

According to a study by Ekstrom and colleagues,[51] isolated protraction exercises do not activate the serratus anterior as effectively as exercises that involve dynamic upward rotation of the scapula as occurs during arm elevation.

- ***Push-ups with a "plus."*** **VIDEO 17.5**

Patient position and procedure: Standing and leaning on forearms or hands against a wall. Have the patient place his or her forearms or hands directly in front or slightly to the side of the shoulders and push the trunk away from the wall. Then have the patient "give an extra push" to protract the scapulae. Progress wall push-ups to table push-ups, then to prone push-ups on the knees, and finally prone push-ups on the toes with knees extended (Fig. 17.49). Add weight around the trunk if the patient is able to tolerate greater resistance.

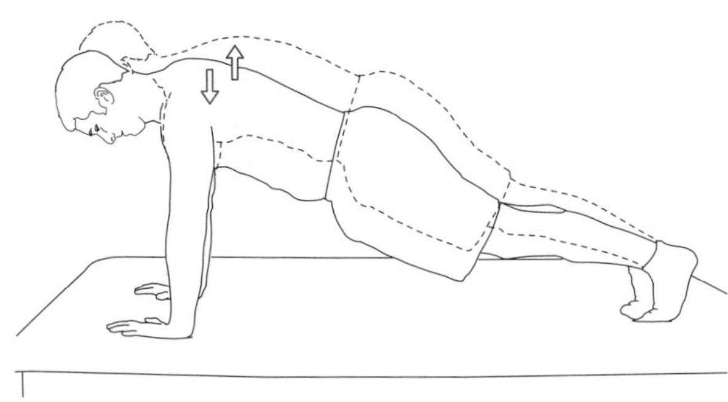

FIGURE 17.49 Push-ups with a "plus" to strengthen scapular protraction.

- ***Push-ups with a "plus" with leg lifts.***

Patient position and procedure: Quadruped (all-fours) position. Perform a push-up with a "plus" on a stable surface. Then alternately lift the lower extremities. Progress to an unstable surface (see Chapter 23 for examples).

CLINICAL TIP

A study examining scapulothoracic muscle activation compared activation during variations of the push-up with a "plus" exercise performed while in the quadruped position. The findings of this study demonstrated that raising the ipsilateral leg during the push-up with a "plus" increased serratus anterior activity, whereas raising the contralateral leg increased lower trapezius activity.[118]

Scapular Depression (Lower Trapezius, Lower Serratus Anterior)

- *Patient position and procedure:* Sitting with elbow flexed. Provide manual resistance in an upward direction under the elbow, and ask the patient to push down into your hands. Caudal gliding of the humeral head may also occur (Fig. 17.50 A).

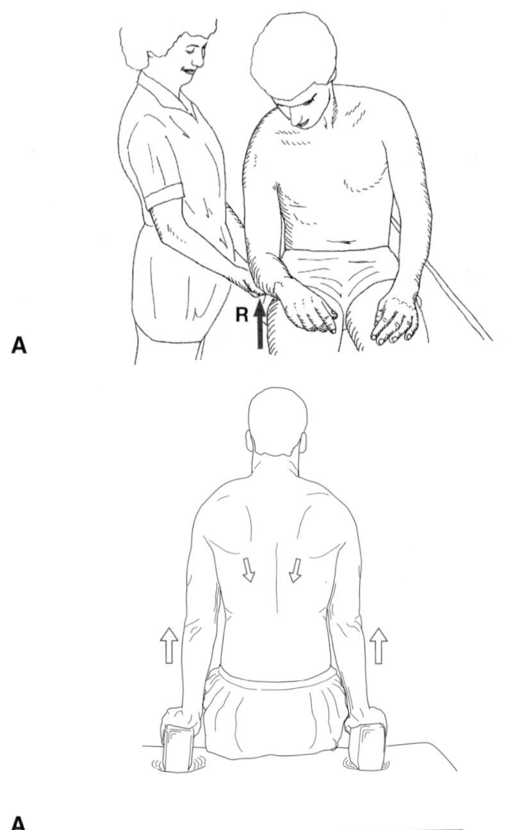

FIGURE 17.50 Exercises that emphasize the lower trapezius. (A) Shoulder girdle depression against manual resistance. (B) Closed-chain shoulder girdle depression using body weight for resistance.

- ***Upright press-up.*** VIDEO 17.5

Patient position and procedure: Sitting or standing with both hands on blocks, the armrests of a chair, or parallel bars. Have the patient push down on the hands and lift the body. After the elbows are fully extended, emphasize scapular depression. (Fig. 17.50 B).

Scapular Upward Rotation With Depression (Lower Trapezius, Serratus Anterior)

Scapular upward rotation with depression cannot be isolated from movement of the humerus. The upward rotation action of the trapezius and serratus anterior requires coordination with humeral elevation. As noted elsewhere in this chapter, a patient may substitute with scapular elevation, primarily using the upper trapezius, so this exercise draws attention to maintaining the scapula in depression while upwardly rotating.

- ***Arm slide against a wall.***

Patient position and procedure: Standing with the back to the wall, heels away from the wall enough to comfortably do a posterior pelvic tilt and maintain the back flat against the wall. Begin with arms slightly abducted and externally rotated and the elbows flexed 90°. The backs of the arms should be against the wall. Have the patient slide the hands and arms up the wall (abduction) as far as possible while maintaining the back flat against the wall.

- ***"Superman" motion prone.***

Patient position and procedure: Prone, with humerus elevated overhead. Ask the patient to barely lift the arm off the table. This end-range motion may not be possible for patients with restricted GH mobility or impingement syndrome.

- ***"Superman" motion upright.***

Patient position and procedure: Sitting or standing with arms in a comfortable overhead position. (This position can be used if the patient has a tight shoulder and cannot assume the "superman motion" while lying prone.) Secure elastic resistance overhead in front of the patient. Instruct the patient to move the shoulder into greater flexion with scapular depression. The scapular depression is most important; it may be necessary to use tactile cues on the lower trapezius to help the patient focus on scapular depression, not scapular elevation (Fig. 17.51).

Dynamic Strengthening Exercises: Glenohumeral Muscles

Dynamic strength of GH musculature coupled with strength of the scapular stabilizers is necessary for active, pain-free movement of the shoulder girdle during functional activities. Open- and closed-chain strengthening exercises should be incorporated into a shoulder rehabilitation and injury prevention program. Many of the exercises used to strengthen scapular muscles in nonweight-bearing and weight-bearing positions, described in the previous section, also dynamically strengthen some GH muscles. Additional exercises to improve dynamic strength of the shoulder girdle in anatomical and diagonal movement patterns are described in this section.

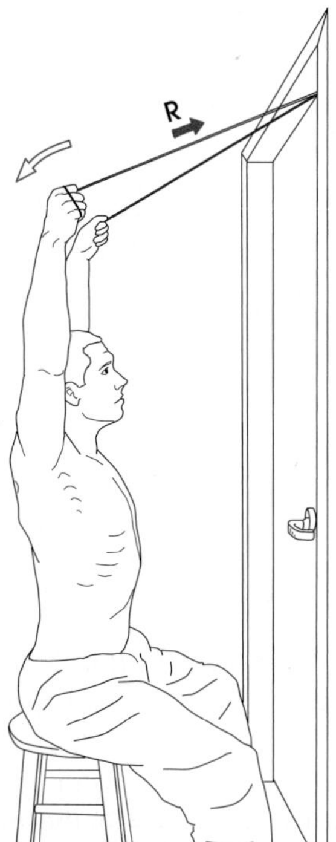

FIGURE 17.51 Scapular depression with upward rotation of the scapula against elastic resistance (also activates the upper and middle trapezius and serratus anterior).

FOCUS ON EVIDENCE

Several EMG studies have investigated exercises commonly used to activate and strengthen shoulder muscles using either free weights or elastic resistance.[8,14,86,162,163] The findings of these studies indicate the extent of activation of the rotator cuff, deltoid, pectoralis major, and latissimus dorsi muscles under maximum load conditions during the following exercises.

- *Shoulder shrug:* causes highest activation in the subscapularis, trapezius, and latissimus dorsi; also activates the supraspinatus, infraspinatus, and serratus anterior.[86]
- *Middle-grip and narrow-grip seated rowing:* activates subscapularis.[86]
- *Wide-grip seated rowing:* activates the infraspinatus and trapezius and to a lesser extent the supraspinatus.[86]
- *External rotation in prone and side-lying positions and in the plane of the scapula:* activates the infraspinatus and teres minor.[8,14,162,163]
- *Internal rotation:* movement of the forearm across the body with arm at side and elbow flexed 90° activates the subscapularis and pectoralis major.[86,162]
- *Forward punch:* causes highest activation in the supraspinatus and anterior deltoid; resistance also activates the pectoralis major and infraspinatus.[86]
- *Horizontal abduction at 100° with full external rotation:* activates the supraspinatus, middle, and posterior deltoid.[163]

Shoulder External Rotation (Infraspinatus, Teres Minor) VIDEO 17.6

Position the arm at the patient's side or in various positions of abduction, scapular plane elevation, or flexion. Flex the elbow to 90° and apply the resistive force at right angles to the forearm. Be sure the patient rotates the humerus and does not extend the elbow. When the arm is positioned at the patient's side, a folded towel placed between the elbow and side of the rib cage reminds the patient to keep the elbow at the side and ensures proper technique.[162] However, it does not significantly alter recruitment of the external rotators.[163] As indicated in the supporting evidence just presented, external rotation applied in the side-lying position (arm at side), prone-lying in the 90/90 position, and standing with the humerus in scapular plane (45° abduction, 30° horizontal adduction) produces the strongest contractions of these muscles compared with other external rotation exercises.[162,163]

- *Patient position and procedure:* Sitting or standing, using elastic resistance or a wall pulley in front of the body at elbow level. Have the patient grasp the elastic material or the pulley handle and rotate his or her arm outward (Fig. 17.52 A).
- *Patient position and procedure:* Side-lying on the uninvolved side with the involved shoulder up, the arm resting on the side of the thorax, and a rolled towel under the elbow. Have the patient use a handheld weight, cuff weight, or elastic resistance and rotate the arm through the desired ROM.
- *Patient position and procedure:* Prone on a table, upper arm resting on the table with the shoulder at 90° if possible, elbow flexed with forearm over the edge of the table. Lift the weight as far as possible by rotating the shoulder, not extending the elbow (Fig. 17.52 B).

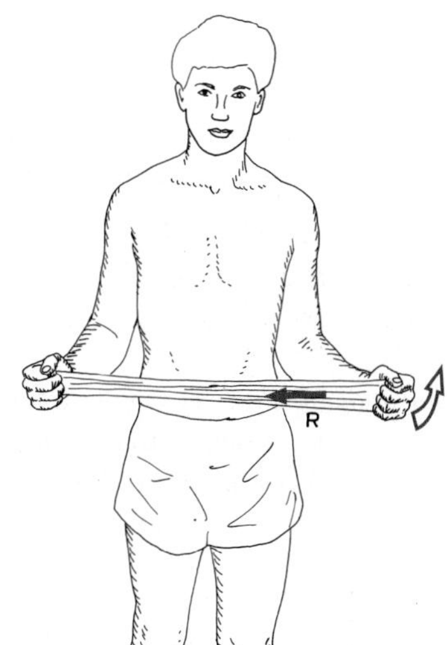

FIGURE 17.52 Resisted external rotation with **(A)** the arm at the side using elastic resistance,

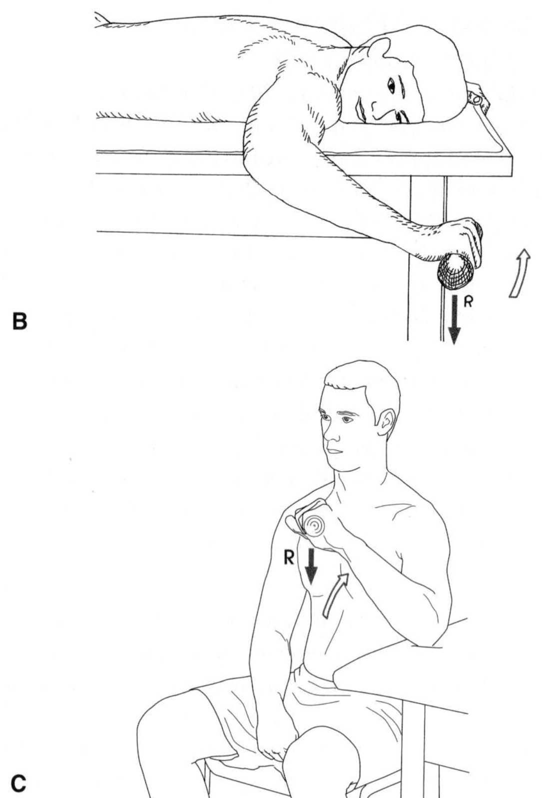

FIGURE 17.52—cont'd **(B)** the arm at 90° using a free weight and the patient lying prone, and **(C)** with the shoulder in scapular plane elevation using a free weight and the patient sitting.

- *Patient position and procedure:* Sitting with elbow flexed 90° and supported on a table so the shoulder is in the resting position (plane of the scapula). The patient lifts the weight from the table by rotating the shoulder (Fig. 17.52 C).

Shoulder Internal Rotation (Subscapularis)

Position the arm at the patient's side or in various positions of flexion, abduction, or scapular plane elevation. The elbow is flexed to 90°, and the resistive force is held in the hand.

- *Patient position and procedure:* Side-lying on the involved side with the arm forward in partial flexion. Have the patient lift the weight upward off the table into internal rotation (Fig. 17.53).
- *Patient position and procedure:* Sitting or standing using elastic resistance or a pulley system with the line of force out to the side and at the level of the elbow. Have the patient pull across the front of the trunk into internal rotation.

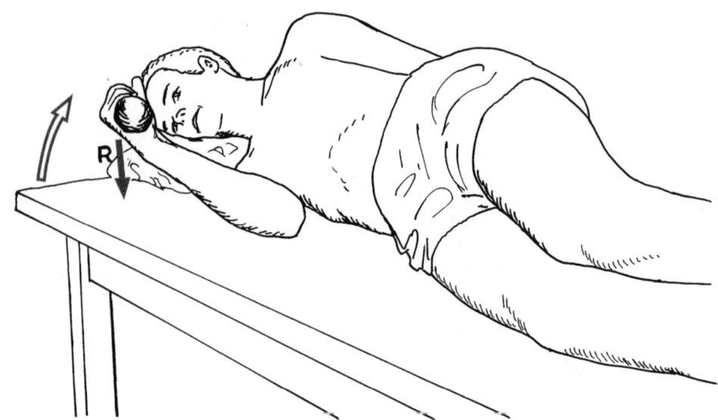

FIGURE 17.53 Resisted internal rotation of the shoulder using a handheld weight. To resist external rotation, place the weight in the patient's upper hand.

Shoulder Abduction and Elevation of the Arm in Scapular Plane (Deltoid and Supraspinatus)

Abduction exercises are classically done with the humerus moving in the frontal plane. It is commonly accepted that most functional activities occur with the humerus 30° to 45° forward to the frontal plane in which the arc of motion is more in line with the glenoid fossa of the scapula. Many abduction exercises can be adapted to be performed in the plane of the scapula.

PRECAUTION: Teach the patient that whenever the shoulder elevates beyond 90°, it must externally rotate to avoid impingement of the greater tubercle against the acromion. If the patient has impingement syndrome, limit the range to avoid the painful arc.

- *Patient position and procedure:* Sitting or standing with a weight in hand. Have the patient abduct the arm to 90° and then externally rotate and elevate the arm through the rest of the range. This same motion can be performed with elastic resistance secured under the patient's foot, but be cautious in that the greater the elastic stretch, the greater the resistance. The patient may not be able to complete the ROM because of increased resistance at the end of the range.
- *Patient position and procedure:* Side-lying with the involved arm uppermost and elbow extended. Have the patient lift a weight up to 90°. The greatest effect of the resistance is at the beginning of the range. At 90°, all of the force is through the long axis of the bone.
- *Patient position and procedure:* Standing with the humerus externally rotated (*full can position*). Have the patient raise the arm away from the side in the plane of the scapula, halfway between abduction and flexion (Fig. 17.54). Apply

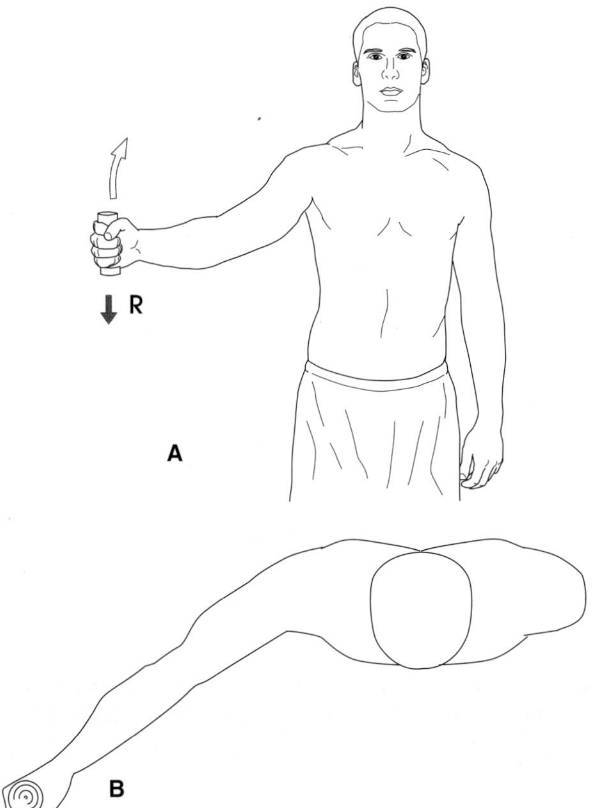

FIGURE 17.54 Abduction in the plane of the scapula. This is called the "full can" exercise because the shoulder is held in external rotation as if lifting a full can. (A) Front view. (B) Top view. If the shoulder is held in internal rotation, the exercise is called an "empty can" exercise.

resistance with a handheld weight or elastic resistance secured under the patient's foot. "Full can" elevation of the arm may also be performed in the prone position with the arm over the side of the table.

FOCUS ON EVIDENCE

EMG studies have confirmed that no one exercise isolates the action of the supraspinatus muscle from the other rotator cuff or deltoid muscles.[120,201] The supraspinatus muscle is effectively activated in both the "empty can" (humerus internally rotated)[91,217] and "full can"[89,120,201] exercises. It also contracts strongly with the military press-up[201] and horizontal abduction with external rotation exercises.[14,120,230] These findings appear to give the therapist several choices of exercises for strengthening the supraspinatus. However, several authors,[45,52,87,89,192] as well as the authors of this text, suggest that the "empty can" exercise should not be used for shoulder rehabilitation because it may cause impingement of the suprahumeral tissues, especially as the arm approaches and elevates above 90°. In support of this, when compared to the "full can" exercise, the "empty can" exercise has been demonstrated to orient the scapula in greater amounts of internal rotation and anterior tilting, positions believed to increase the risk of subacromial impingement.[192] In contrast, the "full can" position minimizes the chance of impingement.[45,89,162]

Shoulder Flexion (Anterior Deltoid, Rotator Cuff, Serratus Anterior)

Patient position and procedure: Sitting, standing, or supine and elbow extended and thumb pointing forward. Have the patient move into forward flexion of the shoulder. If a free weight is used when supine, the greatest resistance is experienced at the beginning of the range; during standing, the greatest resistive force is encountered when the shoulder is flexed to the 90° position. Elastic resistance also can be used if secured under the patient's foot or a solid object on the floor.

- ***Military press-up.***

Patient position and procedure: Sitting, arm at the side in neutral to slight external rotation with elbow flexed and forearm in mid-position (thumb pointing posterior). Have the patient lift the weight vertically to the overhead position (Fig. 17.55).

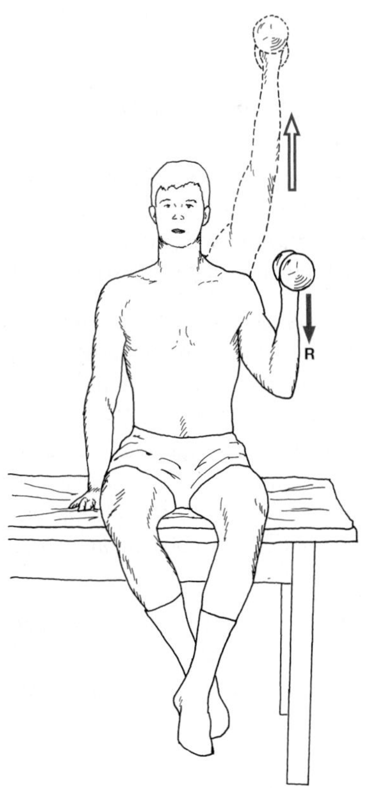

FIGURE 17.55 Military press-up. Beginning with the arm at the side in neutral to slight external rotation with elbow flexed and forearm in mid-position (thumb pointing posteriorly), the weight is lifted overhead.

Shoulder Adduction (Pectoralis Major, Teres Major, Latissimus Dorsi)

Patient position and procedure: Sitting or standing with the arm abducted. Have the patient pull down against a pulley force or elastic resistance tied overhead. The greatest resistance is when the line of the resistive force is at right angles to the patient's arm.

Shoulder Horizontal Adduction (Anterior Deltoid, Coracobrachialis, Pectoralis Major)

Patient position and procedure: Supine. Begin with one or both arms out to the side in horizontal abduction. Have the patient bring the arms forward into horizontal adduction until the arms are vertical.

Shoulder Extension (Posterior Deltoid, Latissimus Dorsi, Rhomboids)

- *Patient position and procedure:* Prone with the arm over the side of the table in 90° flexion. Have the patient lift the weight and extend the shoulder. Simultaneous elbow flexion while extending the shoulder is easier (shorter lever arm); maintaining elbow extension while extending the shoulder is more difficult (longer lever arm).
- *Patient position and procedure:* Sitting or standing with the arm flexed. A pulley or elastic resistance is secured overhead. Have the patient pull down against the resistance into extension.

Elbow Flexion (Biceps Brachii)

- ***Biceps curl.***

Patient position and procedure: Sitting or standing. Have the patient flex the elbow while holding a handheld weight and keeping the forearm supinated and the arm at the side or with the shoulder moving into slight extension (see Fig. 18.11).

NOTE: Because the biceps brachii is a two-joint muscle, the muscle not only serves to flex the elbow as its primary function, the long head assists the rotator cuff muscles by acting as an additional dynamic stabilizer of the GH joint by approximating the humeral head against the glenoid fossa and by depressing the head of the humerus as the arm elevates and the scapula upwardly rotates.[116] As such, the biceps brachii must be strengthened in a shoulder rehabilitation program.

Exercises Using Diagonal (PNF) Movement Patterns VIDEO 17.4

Proprioceptive neuromuscular facilitation (PNF) patterns involve use of the entire upper extremity or address specific regions, such as the scapula. Apply resistance manually to emphasize specific muscles in the pattern by adjusting hand placement and resistance (see Chapter 6 for complete description of patterns). As control improves, teach the patient exercises in diagonal patterns using weights or elastic resistance (Fig. 17.56).

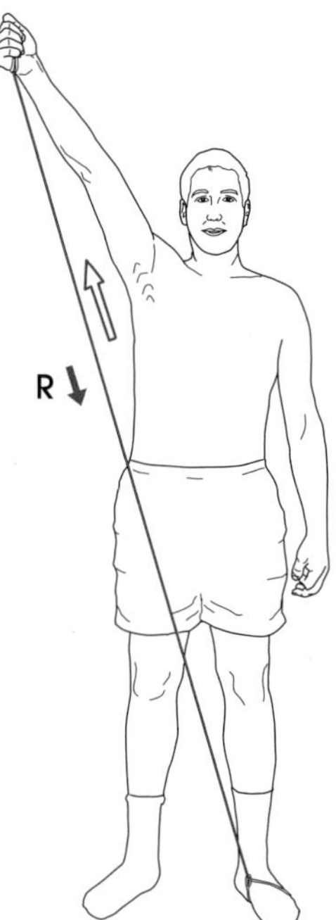

FIGURE 17.56 PNF pattern (D_2 flexion), emphasizing shoulder flexion, abduction, and external rotation against elastic resistance.

Functional Progression for the Shoulder Complex

An essential element of a shoulder rehabilitation and injury prevention program is a sequence of carefully progressed exercises and activities designed to achieve necessary and desired functional outcomes. The final section of this chapter provides a summary of key components of a functional progression for the shoulder. This progression typically includes a variety of open- and closed-chain exercises in combined movement patterns that simulate functional activities and further improve strength, power, and muscular endurance. Integrated into the functional progression are activities for balance, coordination, and skill and aerobic conditioning. A few examples of activities are presented here. Refer to Chapter 23 for further examples of activities for advanced functional training.

Exercises Using Combined Movement Patterns With Functional Activities

Exercises in combined movement patterns typically require coordination between the stabilizing and dynamic functions of the scapulothoracic and GH muscles and involve control of the entire upper extremity and trunk and sometimes of the lower extremities. Some of the strengthening exercises already presented in this chapter resist combined movements.

Component motions in functional activities, such as pulling, pushing, lifting, lowering, and carrying, involve combined movement patterns and should be practiced under progressively challenging conditions. Several examples follow:

- ***Rowing.***

Patient position and procedure: Long-sitting. Secure elastic resistance under the feet or around a solid object. Grasp both ends of the elastic material, and pull backward with the arms in a rowing action (Fig. 17.57). Vary the grip width. For a greater challenge, perform the rowing motion while seated on an unstable surface, such as a Swiss ball. As an alternative, a weight-cable system can be used for resistance.

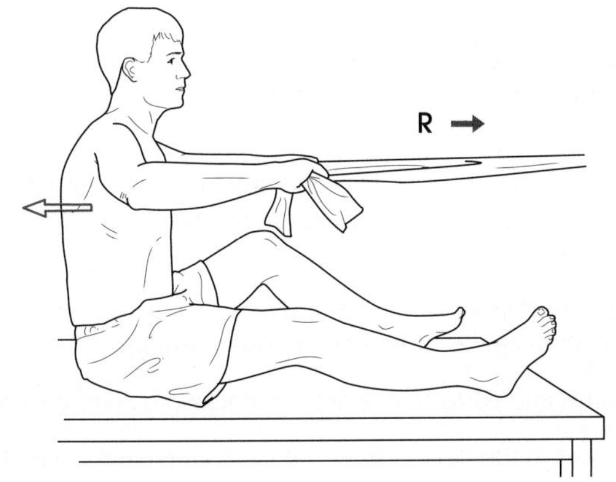

FIGURE 17.57 Simulated rowing motion against elastic resistance.

- ***"Lawnmower pull."***

Patient position and procedure: Standing with hips partially flexed and holding onto a table or chair for balance with the hand of the sound upper extremity. Have the patient reach diagonally across the midline and grasp a piece of elastic tubing that is secured under the foot of the sound side or attached to the leg of a couch or bed. Then have the patient pull diagonally and upward as if starting a lawnmower (see Fig. 18.19). This combined movement pattern may also be simulated with a free weight.

- ***Pushing a weighted cart.***

Patient position and procedure: Standing with a stable base of support. Begin by pushing the cart on a flat surface with light loads on the cart (Fig. 17.58). Emphasize proper body mechanics. Initially use both arms to push; then progress by pushing with one hand or by pushing heavier loads on uneven surfaces. Vary the activity by adjusting the width of the grip, the position of the arms, or by alternating between pushing and pulling.

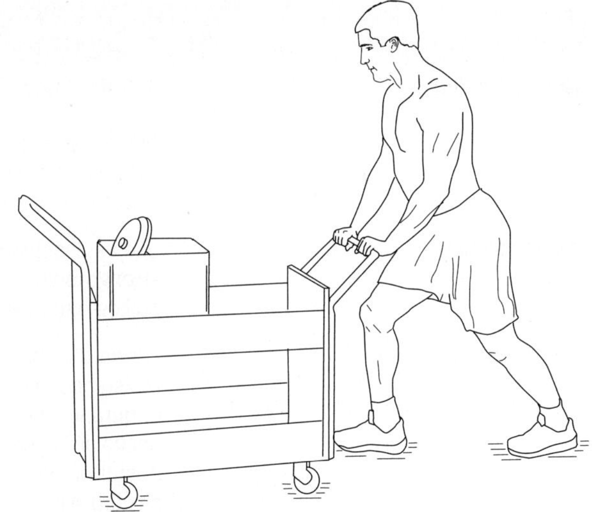

FIGURE 17.58 Pushing a weighted cart to simulate a functional activity and incorporate proper body mechanics.

Equipment

A variety of exercise devices can be used or adapted for shoulder girdle strengthening using combined movement patterns. Creativity in adapting equipment and exercises to meet progressive upper extremity challenges without exacerbating or causing recurrence of symptoms is a must. Examples of equipment and potential uses are identified in Table 17.6. Many of the activities noted are described and shown in detail in Chapter 23.

Integration of Functional Activities

Functional progression in a shoulder rehabilitation program must integrate principles of task-specific training by including a sequence of simple and easy to perform activities then progressing to complex and challenging functional activities. It is important to have the patient use the actual patterns and types of muscle contraction that will occur in their necessary and desired functional activities.

First, simulated activities should be performed with supervision and the therapist's guidance to avoid painful positions or faulty mechanics during movements of the shoulder. Then the activity can be performed independently at home or work. For example, begin by having the patient simulate the motions involved in unloading a dishwasher and placing the dishes on a low shelf or washing windows using small circular motions. If catching and throwing or swinging a bat or golf club are necessary, total body patterns are practiced.

TABLE 17.6 Exercise Devices and Potential Uses for Shoulder Girdle Rehabilitation

Exercise Device	Potential Use
BodyBlade™	Move the arm in anatomical and diagonal planes of movement, in circular (clockwise or counterclockwise) patterns, or while moving the blade away from or toward the body, as if pushing or pulling.
Rowing machine	Use as designed for endurance training and upper extremity and trunk strengthening. Emphasizes scapular retraction and trunk stabilization when pulling backward.
Upper body ergometer	Forward or backward cycling (pushing or pulling movements) against progressive resistance over an extended time period for muscular and cardiopulmonary endurance. For a patient with an impingement syndrome, place emphasis on backward cycling for scapular retraction and to target weak or underused posterior shoulder structures and minimize action of tight and overused anterior structures.
Foam roll, small ball, balance equipment (rocker or wobble board or BOSU™)	Stabilization exercises or perturbation training in prone-propping or quadruped positions on one or both hands. Emphasize upper extremity weight shifting or alternating arm or leg movements.
Stepping machine	While kneeling, perform upper extremity "climbing" motions by pushing with the hands on the steps. Emphasizes scapular protraction during pushing.
Treadmill	Kneel at the end of the treadmill and perform forward and backward hand-walking.
ProFitter™	While kneeling on the floor next to the device, place hands on the platform and slide the platform side-to-side or forward-backward using quick changes of direction.

An individual who has a sedentary lifestyle may require postural adaptations and ergonomic analysis of his or her home environment or workstation to change repetitive stress. In contrast, an athlete or industrial worker, who must perform high-demand activities over an extended time period, may require muscular and cardiopulmonary endurance or high-intensity training, such as plyometric exercises, to develop power and skill.

Independent Learning Activities

Critical Thinking and Discussion

1. Describe how the scapulothoracic and GH musculature function as dynamic stabilizers of the shoulder.
2. Which factors may alter normal upward rotation of the scapula, and how does inadequate upward rotation of the scapula adversely affect elevation of the arm?
3. Describe the relationships among cervical and thoracic posture, scapula orientation, and elevation of the arm.
4. Which mechanisms and structures could be sources of pain in extrinsic impingement syndrome?
5. How are impingement and instability related to each other in secondary impingement syndrome?
6. Describe the differences and similarities between atraumatic and traumatic instability of the GH joint.
7. A patient experienced a traumatic shoulder injury when falling down five cement steps 2 weeks ago. She now has a capsular pattern, decreased joint play, and muscle guarding with passive GH motions. She does not actively use the extremity because of pain. You observe edema in the hand. What potential complications could develop if left untreated? Design an exercise program for this patient at her present level of involvement. What would you teach the patient about her symptoms, impairments, and parameters for recovery?

8. An individual with a history of diabetes has developed a frozen shoulder. She has had shoulder discomfort for several months, but she did not seek treatment until 1 week ago when she was unable to wash or fix her hair with her left hand. Describe your intervention plan and instructions for this patient. Explain how you will determine the level of aggressiveness with which to address her ROM loss.
9. For patients with a history of recurrent anterior dislocation of the GH joint, what types of functional activities (ADL, work related, or sport related) should initially be avoided or modified during the early and intermediate stages of a rehabilitation program? What would differ with a patient with a history of recurrent posterior dislocation of the GH joint?
10. What criteria should patients with each of the following shoulder diagnoses meet before progressing to *overhead* exercises and functional activities: primary impingement syndrome, anterior GH instability, frozen shoulder, S/P rotator cuff repair?

Laboratory Practice

1. With your laboratory partner, review and practice key tests and measurements that you might need to do to determine what is causing shoulder pain and/or diminished upper extremity function. What does each of those tests indicate?
2. Mobilize the scapula with manual techniques.
3. Mobilize the GH joint capsule with manual techniques; practice the MWM techniques for the shoulder.
4. Teach your partner a series of self-mobilization techniques for the GH joint capsule.
5. Using appropriate stabilization, manually stretch all major muscle groups of the shoulder.
6. Teach your partner effective self-stretching techniques for each of these muscle groups.
7. Practice a sequence of exercises to strengthen the muscles of the scapula using manual resistance (applied by the therapist). Use open-chain and closed-chain positions.
8. Teach your partner a progressive sequence of strengthening exercises that he or she could do in a home exercise program to develop stability and dynamic control of the scapula. Apply perturbation techniques that will challenge the ability of the scapulothoracic muscles to stabilize the scapulothoracic articulation.
9. Teach your partner a progressive sequence of strengthening exercises that he or she could do in a home exercise program to develop strength, stability, and endurance of the GH muscles. Have your partner perform each exercise for a specified number of repetitions and at a specified level of resistance.
   - Describe faulty postures or motions that you will be looking for as your partner executes each exercise.
   - Describe the signs of fatigue that you may observe and the indicators of poor exercise technique.
10. Develop a series of functional activities to complement the self-stretching and self-strengthening exercises you have taught your partner.

Case Studies

1. A patient referral states: Evaluate and treat shoulder pain S/P motor vehicle accident. She was the driver of the car in a head-on collision. The patient describes shoulder pain whenever reaching overhead. She is a nurse and finds symptoms worsen when placing solutions on an IV pole, a frequent activity for her. Examination reveals painful resisted scapular protraction, elbow extension, and shoulder extension with pain on palpation of the long head of the triceps near its insertion on the inferior glenoid as well as pain in the serratus anterior in the axilla. Other impairments include weak rhomboids and lower trapezius muscles (4-/5).
   - Explain the potential mechanism of injury to these muscles from this type of accident.
   - Explain why this patient's reaching tasks would perpetuate these symptoms.
   - Outline a treatment plan that manages the acute symptoms and progresses to a therapeutic exercise program.
   - Identify a measurable functional outcome goal and interventions you would use to reach the goal.
   - As the patient's symptoms subside, how would you progress her exercise program?
2. Your patient describes pain whenever reaching overhead. He likes to play volleyball in a weekend league but otherwise has a sedentary lifestyle. On examination, you observe moderate atrophy in the infraspinous fossa, a protracted scapula, and thoracic kyphosis with forward head. You have him assume the quadruped position in anticipation of instruction in closed-chain rhythmic stabilization and scapular protraction exercises and note significant winging of the scapula.
   - Describe what muscles are likely to test weak based on these observations.
   - How would you adapt the quadruped exercise to develop control and strength in the involved muscles at a safe resistance level?
   - Based on your assumptions of muscle involvement, develop an intervention plan for this patient that includes a home exercise program. Indicate parameters (frequency, repetitions), positions, safety, and progressions.
3. You have received a referral to "evaluate and treat" a 62-year-old patient who underwent total shoulder arthroplasty for OA 2 weeks ago. The patient has been wearing a sling to support and protect the operated shoulder but has been allowed to remove the sling for daily pendulum exercises and active ROM of the elbow, wrist, and hand.
   - Prior to initiating your examination and developing an exercise program, what additional information would you like to learn from the surgeon?

- What information do you want to gather from the patient?
- What examination procedures would you wish to perform during the patient's initial visit?
- Develop, implement, teach, and then progress a series of exercises over a period of six visits with the patient.

4. Six months ago your patient underwent surgery for repair of a Bankart lesion and stabilization of the anterior capsule (capsular shift) after a traumatic anterior dislocation of the GH joint. The patient now has full ROM and 90% strength in the shoulder after a program of rehabilitation. Your patient wants to return to recreational sports, such as tennis, softball, and volleyball, but is apprehensive that the shoulder might dislocate during these activities. Design an advanced rehabilitation program to gradually return the patient to the desired recreational activities.

REFERENCES

1. Altchek, DW, et al: Arthroscopic acromioplasty: technique and results. *J Bone Joint Surg Am* 72:1198–1207, 1990.
2. Anderson, NH, et al: Self-training versus physiotherapist supervised rehabilitation of the shoulder in patients with arthroscopic subacromial decompression: a clinical randomized study. *J Shoulder Elbow Surg* 8: 99–101, 1999.
3. Arciero, RA, et al: Arthroscopic Bankart repair versus nonoperative treatment for acute, initial anterior shoulder dislocation. *Am J Sports Med* 22(5):589–594, 1994.
4. Aronen, JG, and Regan, K: Decreasing the incidence of recurrence of first-time anterior dislocations with rehabilitation. *Am J Sports Med* 12(4): 283–291, 1984.
5. Arroyo, JS, and Flatow, EL: Management of rotator cuff disease: Intact and repairable cuff. In Iannotti, JP, and Williams, GR (eds): *Disorders of the Shoulder: Diagnosis and Management.* Philadelphia: Lippincott Williams & Wilkins, 1999, p 31.
6. Atef, A, et al: Prevalence of associated injuries after anterior shoulder dislocation: a prospective study. *Int Orthop* 40(3):519–24, 2015.
7. Baker, CL, and Liu, SH: Comparison of open and arthroscopically-assisted rotator cuff repair. *Am J Sports Med* 23(1):99–104, 1995.
8. Ballantyne, BT, et al: Electromyographic activity of selected shoulder muscles in commonly used therapeutic exercises. *Phys Ther* 73(10): 668–692, 1993.
9. Bassett, RW, et al: Glenohumeral muscle force and movement mechanics in a position of shoulder instability. *J Biomech* 23:405–415, 1990.
10. Bigliani, LV, et al: Inferior capsular shift procedure for anterior-inferior shoulder instability in athletes. *Am J Sports Med* 22(5):578–584, 1994.
11. Bigliani, LV, et al: Shift of the posteroinferior aspect of the capsule for recurrent posterior glenohumeral instability. *J Bone Joint Surg Am* 77(7):1011–1020, 1995.
12. Bigliani, LJ, et al: The relationship of acromial architecture to rotator cuff disease. *Clin Sports Med* 10(4):823–838, 1991.
13. Binder, AI, et al: Frozen shoulder: a long-term prospective study. *Ann Rheum Dis* 43(3):361–364, 1984.
14. Blackburn, TA, et al: EMG analysis of posterior rotator cuff exercises. *J Athl Train* 25:40–45, 1990.
15. Borstad, JD, and Ludewig, PM: The effect of long versus short pectoralis minor resting length on scapular kinematics in healthy individuals. *J Orthop Sports Phys Ther* 35(4):227–238, 2005.
16. Borstad, JD: Resting position variables at the shoulder: evidence to support a posture-impairment association. *Phys Ther* 86(4):549–557, 2006.
17. Borstad, JD, and Ludewig, PM: Comparison of three stretches for the pectoralis minor muscle. *J Shoulder Elbow Surg* 15(3):324–330, 2006.
18. Bottoni, CR, et al: A prospective, randomized evaluation of arthroscopic stabilization versus nonoperative treatment of patients with acute traumatic, first-time shoulder dislocations. *Am J Sports Med* 30(4):576–580, 2002.
19. Boublik, M, and Hawkins, RJ: Clinical examination of the shoulder complex. *J Orthop Sports Phys Ther* 18(1):379–385, 1993.
20. Boudreau, S, et al: Rehabilitation following reverse total shoulder arthroplasty. *J Orthop Sports Phys Ther* 37(12):734–743, 2007.
21. Brems, JJ: Rehabilitation following total shoulder arthroplasty. *Clin Orthop* 307:70–85, 1994.
22. Brostrom, LA, et al: The effect of shoulder muscle training in patients with recurrent shoulder dislocations. *Scand J Rehabil Med* 24(1):11–15, 1992.
23. Brown, DD, and Friedman, RJ: Postoperative rehabilitation following total shoulder arthroplasty. *Orthop Clin North Am* 29:535, 1998.
24. Bullock, MP, Foster, NE, and Wright, CC: Shoulder impingement: the effect of sitting posture on shoulder pain and range of motion. *Man Ther* 10:28–37, 2005.
25. Burkhead, WZ, and Buark, DA: History and development of prosthetic replacement of the glenohumeral joint. In Williams, GR, et al (eds): *Shoulder and Elbow Arthroplasty.* Philadelphia: Lippincott, Williams & Wilkins, 2005, pp 3–10.
26. Buteau, JL, Eriksrud, O, and Hasson, SM: Rehabilitation of a glenohumeral instability utilizing the body blade. *Physiotherapy Theory and Practice* 23(6):333–349, 2007.
27. Cahill, JB, Cavanaugh, JT, and Craig, EV. Total shoulder arthroplasty rehabilitation. *Techniques Shld Elbow Surg* 15(1):13–17, 2014.
28. Cain, PR, et al: Anterior stability of the glenohumeral joint. *Am J Sports Med* 15(2):144–148, 1987.
29. Cameron, B, Glatz, L, and Williams, GR: Factors affecting the outcome of total shoulder arthroplasty. *Am J Orthop* 30:613–623, 2001.
30. Carpenter, JE, Blasier, RB, and Pellizzon, GG: The effects of muscle fatigue on shoulder joint position sense. *Am J Sports Med* 26(2):262–265, 1998.
31. Codman, EA: *The Shoulder.* Boston: Thomas Todd, 1934.
32. Cofield, RH, Chang, W, and Sperling, JW: Complications of shoulder arthroplasty. In Iannotti, JP, and Williams, GR (eds): *Disorders of the Shoulder: Diagnosis and Management.* Philadelphia: Lippincott Williams & Wilkins, 1999, p 571.
33. Cofield, RH, et al: Shoulder arthroplasty for arthritis. In Morrey, BF (ed): *Joint Replacement Arthroplasty,* ed. 3. Philadelphia: Churchill Livingstone, 2003, pp 438–449.
34. Cohen, BS, Romeo, AA, and Bach, BR: Shoulder injuries. In Brotzman, SB, and Wilk, KE (eds): *Clinical Orthopedic Rehabilitation,* ed. 2. Philadelphia: Mosby, 2003, pp 125–250.
35. Cole, BJ, et al: Comparison of arthroscopic and open anterior shoulder stabilization: a two- to six-year follow-up study. *J Bone Joint Surg Am* 82: 1108–1114, 2000.
36. Cools, AM, et al: Rehabilitation of scapular muscle balance. Which exercises to prescribe? *Am J Sports Med* 35(10):1744–1751, 2007.
37. Cuff, D, et al: Reverse shoulder arthroplasty for the treatment of rotator cuff deficiency. *J Bone Joint Surg Am* 90(6):1244–1251, 2008.
38. Culham, E, and Peat, M: Functional anatomy of the shoulder complex. *J Orthop Sports Phys Ther* 18(1):342–350, 1993.
39. Culp, LB, and Romani, WA: Physical therapist examination, evaluation, and intervention following the surgical reconstruction of a grade III acromioclavicular joint separation. *Phys Ther* 86(6):857–869, 2006.
40. Cyriax, J: *Textbook of Orthopaedic Medicine, Vol 1. Diagnosis of Soft Tissue Lesions,* ed. 8. London: Bailliere Tindall, 1982.
41. Cyriax, J: *Textbook of Orthopaedic Medicine, Vol 2. Treatment by Manipulation, Massage and Injection,* ed. 10. London: Bailliere Tindall, 1980.
42. Dahm, DL, and Smith, J: Rehabilitation and activities after shoulder arthroplasty. In Morrey, BF (ed): *Joint Replacement Arthroplasty,* ed. 3. Philadelphia: Churchill Livingstone, 2005, pp 502–511.
43. Dala-Ala, B, Penna, M, et al: Management of acute anterior shoulder dislocation. *Br J Sports Med* 48(16):1209–1215, 2014.

44. Davies, GJ, and Dickoff-Hoffman, S: Neuromuscular testing and rehabilitation of the shoulder complex. *J Orthop Sports Phys Ther* 18(2): 449–458, 1993.
45. Davies, GJ, and Durall, C: "Typical" rotator cuff impingement syndrome: it's not always typical. *PT Magazine* 8(5):58–71, 2000.
46. Dodson, CC, and Altchek, DW: SLAP lesions: an update on recognition and treatment. *J Orthop Sports Phys Ther* 39(2):71–80, 2009.
47. Donatelli, RA, et al: Differential soft tissue diagnosis. In Donatelli, RA (ed): *Physical Therapy of the Shoulder,* ed. 4. St. Louis: Churchill Livingstone, 2004, p 89.
48. Duan, X, et al: Total shoulder arthroplasty versus hemiarthroplasty in patients with shoulder osteoarthritis: A meta-analysis of randomized controlled trials. *Sem Arthritis Rheumatism* 43:297–302, 2013.
49. Duralde, XA: Total shoulder replacements. In Donatelli, RA (ed): *Physical Therapy of the Shoulder,* ed. 4. St. Louis: Churchill Livingstone, 2004, pp 529–545.
50. Edmonds, A: Shoulder arthroplasty. In Clark, GL, et al (eds): *Hand Rehabilitation.* New York: Churchill Livingstone, 1998, p 267.
51. Ekstrom, RA, Donatelli, RA, and Soderberg, GL: Surface electromyographic analysis of exercises for the trapezius and serratus anterior muscles. *J Orthop Sports Phys Ther* 33(5):247–258, 2003.
52. Ellenbecker, TS, and Cools, A: Rehabilitation of shoulder impingement syndrome and rotator cuff injuries: an evidence-based review. *Br J Sports Med* 44(5):319–327, 2010.
53. Ellenbecker, TS, Elmore, E, and Bailie, DS: Descriptive report of shoulder range of motion and rotational strength 6 and 12 weeks following rotator cuff repair using mini-open deltoid splitting techniques. *J Orthop Sports Phys Ther* 36(5):326–335, 2006.
54. Ellenbecker, TS, and Mattalino, AJ: Glenohumeral joint range of motion and rotator cuff strength following arthroscopic anterior stabilization with thermal capsulorrhaphy. *J Orthop Sports Phys Ther* 29(3):160–167, 1999.
55. Ellenbecker, TS: Etiology and evaluation of rotator cuff pathologic conditions and rehabilitation. In Donatelli, RA (ed): *Physical Therapy of the Shoulder,* ed. 4. St. Louis: Churchill Livingstone, 2004, p 337.
56. Ellman, H: Arthroscopic subacromial decompression. In Welsh, RP, and Shephard, RJ (eds): *Current Therapy in Sports Medicine, Vol 2.* Toronto: BC Decker, 1990.
57. Fanton, G, and Thabit, G: Orthopedic uses of arthroscopy and lasers. In Griffin (ed): *Orthopedic Knowledge. Update Sports Medicine.* Rosemont, IL: American Academy of Orthopedic Surgeons, 1994.
58. Fealy, S, Kingham, TP, and Altchek, DW: Mini-open rotator cuff repair using a two-row fixation technique outcomes analysis in patients with small, moderate and large rotator cuff tears. *Arthroscopy* 18:665–670, 2002.
59. Fenlin, JM, and Friedman, B: Shoulder arthroplasty: massive cuff deficiency. In Iannotti, JP, Williams, GR (eds): *Disorders of the Shoulder: Diagnosis and Management.* Philadelphia: Lippincott Williams & Wilkins, 1999, p 559.
60. Finley, MA, and Lee, RY: Effect of sitting posture on 3-dimensional scapular kinematics measured by skin-mounted electromagnetic tracking sensors. *Arch Phys Med Rehabil* 84(4):563–568, 2003.
61. Fu, FH, Harner, CD, and Klein, AH: Shoulder impingement syndrome: a critical review. *Clin Orthop Rel Res* 269:162–173, 1991.
62. Gartsman, GM, and Hammerman, SM: Full-thickness tears: arthroscopic repair. *Orthop Clin North Am* 28:83–98, 1997.
63. Gartsman, GM, Khan, M, and Hammerman, SM: Arthroscopic repair of full thickness tears of the rotator cuff. *J Bone Joint Surg Am* 80:832–840, 1998.
64. Ghodadra, NS, et al: Open, mini-open, and all-arthroscopic rotator cuff repair surgery: indications and implications for rehabilitation. *J Orthop Sports Phys Ther* 39(2):81–89, 2009.
65. Gill, T, et al: Bankart repair for anterior instability of the shoulder. *J Bone Joint Surg Am* 79:850–857, 1997.
66. Godges, JJ, et al: The immediate effects of soft tissue mobilization with proprioceptive neuromuscular facilitation on glenohumeral external rotation and overhead reach. *J Orthop Sports Phys Ther* 33(12):713–718, 2003.
67. Greis, PE, Dean, M, and Hawkins, RJ: Subscapularis tendon disruption after Bankart reconstruction for anterior instability. *J Shoulder Elbow Surg* 5:219–222, 1996.
68. Griffin, JW: Hemiplegic shoulder pain. *Phys Ther* 66(12):1884–1893, 1986.
69. Gross, RM: Arthroscopic shoulder capsulorrhaphy: does it work? *Am J Sports Med* 17:495–500, 1989.
70. Grubbs, N: Frozen shoulder syndrome: a review of literature. *J Orthop Sports Phys Ther* 18(3):479–487, 1993.
71. Guidotti, TL: Occupational repetitive strain injury. *Am Fam Physician* 45(2):585–592, 1992.
72. Haig, SV: *Shoulder Pathophysiology Rehabilitation and Treatment.* Gaithersbury, MD: Aspen Publishers, 1996.
73. Haik, MN, et al: Scapular kinematics pre- and post-thoracic thrust manipulation in individuals with and without shoulder impingement symptoms: a randomized controlled study. *J Orthop Sports Phys Ther* 44(7): 475–487, 2014.
74. Harryman, DT, et al: Translation of the humeral head on the glenoid with passive glenohumeral motion. *J Bone Joint Surg Am* 72(9): 1334–1343, 1990.
75. Harryman, DT II, et al: Reports of the rotator cuff: correlation of functional results with integrity of the cuff. *J Bone Joint Surg Am* 73:982–989, 1991.
76. Hartzog, CW, Savoie, FH, and Field, LD: Arthroscopic acromioplasty and arthroscopic distal clavicle resection, mini-open rotator cuff repair: Indications, techniques, and outcome. In Iannotti, JP (ed): *The Rotator Cuff: Current Concepts and Complex Problems.* Rosemont, IL: American Academy of Orthopedic Surgeons, 1998, p 25.
77. Hashimoto, T, Nobuhara, K, and Hamada, T: Pathologic evidence of degeneration as a primary cause of rotator cuff tear. *Clin Orthop Rel Res* 415:111–120, 2003.
78. Hattrup, SJ: Rotator cuff repair: relevance of patient age. *J Shoulder Elbow Surg* 4:95–100, 1995.
79. Hattrup, SJ: Complications in shoulder arthroplasty. In Morrey, BF (ed): *Joint Replacement Arthroplasty,* ed. 3. Philadelphia: Churchill Livingstone, 2003, pp 521–542.
80. Hawkins, RJ, and Abrams, JS: Impingement syndrome in the absence of rotator cuff tear (stages 1 and 2). *Orthop Clin North Am* 18(3):373–382, 1987.
81. Hawkins, RJ, et al: Acromioplasty for impingement with an intact rotator cuff. *J Bone Joint Surg Br* 70(5):795–797, 1988.
82. Hawkins, RJ, Krishnan, SG, and Karas, SG: Electrothermal arthroscopic shoulder capsulorrhaphy: a minimum 2-year follow-up. *Am J Sports Med* 35(9):1484–1488, 2007.
83. Hawkins, RJ, Misamore, GW, and Hobeika, PE: Surgery for full-thickness rotator cuff tears. *J Bone Joint Surg Am* 67:1349–1355, 1985.
84. Hayashi, K, et al: The effect of nonablative laser energy on joint capsular properties: an in vitro mechanical study using a rabbit model. *Am J Sports Med* 23(4):482–487, 1995.
85. Hayes, K, et al: Shoulder instability: management and rehabilitation. *J Orthop Sports Phys Ther* 32(10):497–509, 2002.
86. Hintermeister, RA, et al: Electromyographic activity and applied load during shoulder rehabilitation exercises using elastic resistance. *Am J Sports Med* 26(2):210–220, 1998.
87. Horrigan, JM, et al: Magnetic resonance imaging evaluation of muscle usage associated with three exercises for rotator cuff rehabilitation. *Med Sci Sports Exerc* 31(10):1361–1366, 1999.
88. Hutcherson, A and Phelan, T: Evidence-based physical therapy protocol for conservative treatment of full-thickness rotator cuff tear. *Orthop Practice* 25(4):221–230, 2013.
89. Itoi, E, et al: Which is more useful, the "full can test" or the "empty can test," in detecting the torn supraspinatus tendon? *Am J Sports Med* 27(1): 65–68, 1999.
90. Jobe, FW, et al: Anterior capsulolabral reconstruction of the shoulder in athletes in overhead sports. *Am J Sports Med* 19:428–434, 1991.
91. Jobe, FW, and Moynes, DR: Delineation of diagnostic criteria and a rehabilitation program for rotator cuff injuries. *Am J Sports Med* 10(6): 336–339, 1982.

92. Jobe, FW, and Pink, M: Classification and treatment of shoulder dysfunction in the overhead athlete. *J Orthop Sports Phys Ther* 18(2): 427–432, 1993.
93. Johnson, AJ, et al: The effect of anterior versus posterior glide joint mobilization on external rotation range of motion in patients with shoulder adhesive capsulitis. *J Orthop Sports Phys Ther* 37(3):88–99, 2007.
94. Kaltenborn, FM, et al: *Manual Mobilization of the Joints: Joint Examination and Basic Treatment, Vol 1. The Extremities*, ed. 8, Norli: Oslo, Norway, 2014.
95. Kamkar, A, Irrgang, JJ, and Whitney, SI: Nonoperative management of secondary shoulder impingement syndrome. *J Orthop Sports Phys Ther* 17(5):212–224, 1993.
96. Kanlayanaphotporn, R: Changes in sitting posture affect shoulder range of motion. *J Bodywork Movement Ther* 18:239–243, 2014.
97. Kelley, MJ, al: Shoulder pain and mobility deficit: adhesive capsulitis. Clinical practice guidelines linked to the International Classification of Functioning, Disability, and Health. *J Orthop Sports Phys Ther* 43(5): A1–A31, 2013.
98. Kelley, MJ, and Leggin, BG: Shoulder rehabilitation. In Iannotti, JP, and Williams, GR (eds): *Disorders of the Shoulder: Diagnosis and Management.* Philadelphia: Lippincott Williams & Wilkins, 1999, p 979.
99. Kelley, MJ, and Leggin, BG: Rehabilitation. In Williams, GR, et al (eds): *Shoulder and Elbow Arthroplasty.* Philadelphia: Lippincott, Williams & Wilkins, 2005, pp 251–268.
100. Kelley, MJ, McClure, PW, and Leggin, BG: Frozen shoulder: evidence and a proposed model guiding rehabilitation. *J Orthop Sports Phys Ther* 39(2):135–148, 2009.
101. Kibler, WB, et al: Scapular summit 2009: introduction. *J Orthop Sports Phys Ther* 39(11): A1–A8, 2009.
102. Kirkley, A, et al: Prospective randomized clinical trial comparing effectiveness of immediate arthroscopic stabilization versus immobilization and rehabilitation in first traumatic anterior dislocations of the shoulder. *Arthroscopy* 15:507–514, 1999.
103. Kosmahl, EM: The shoulder. In Kauffman, TL (ed): *Geriatric Rehabilitation Manual.* New York: Churchill Livingstone, 1999, p 99.
104. Kuhn, JE, Lebus, GF, and Bible, JE: Thoracic outlet syndrome. *J Am Acad Orthop Surg* 23:222–232, 2015.
105. Kumar, VP, Satku, K, and Balasubramaniam, P: The role of the long head of the biceps brachii in the stabilization in the head of the humerus. *Clin Orthop* 244:172–175, 1989.
106. Laudner, KG, et al: Scapular dysfunction in throwers with pathologic internal impingement. *J Orthop Sports Phys Ther* 36(7):485–494, 2006.
107. Lawrence, RL, et al: Comparison of 3-dimensional shoulder complex kinematics in individuals with and without shoulder pain, part 1: sternoclavicular, acromioclavicular, and scapulothoracic joints. *J Orthop Sports Phys Ther* 44(9):636–645, 2014
108. Lawrence, RL, et al: Comparison of 3-dimensional shoulder complex kinematics in individuals with and without shoulder pain, part 2: glenohumeral joint. *J Orthop Sports Phys Ther* 44(9): 646–655, 2014.
109. Lewis, JS, Wright, C, and Green, A: Subacromial impingement syndrome: the effect of changing posture on shoulder range of movement. *J Orthop Sports Phys Ther* 35(2):72–87, 2005.
110. Lister, JL, et al: Scapular stabilizer activity during bodyblade, cuff weights, and thera-band use. *J Sport Rehabil* 16:50–67, 2007.
111. Litchfield, R, et al: Rehabilitation for the overhead athlete. *J Orthop Sports Phys Ther* 18(2):433–441, 1993.
112. Lo, IK, et al: Quality-of-life outcome following hemiarthroplasty or total shoulder arthroplasty in patients with osteoarthritis: a prospective randomized trial. *J Bone Joint Surg Am* 87(10):2178–2185, 2005.
113. Long, JL, et al: Activation of the shoulder musculature during pendulum exercises and light activities. *J Orthop Sports Phys Ther* 40(4): 230–237, 2010.
114. Ludewig, PM, and Cook, TC: Alterations in shoulder kinematics and associated muscle activity in people with symptoms of shoulder impingement. *Phys Ther* 80(3):276–291, 2000.
115. Ludewig, PM, et al: Three-dimensional clavicular motion during arm elevation: reliability and descriptive data. *J Orthop Sport Phys Ther* 34(3):140–149, 2004.
116. Ludewig, PM, and Borstad, JD: The shoulder complex. In Levangie, PM, and Norkin, CC (eds): *Joint Structure and Function: A Comprehensive Analysis,* ed. 5. Philadelphia: F.A. Davis, 2011.
117. Lukasiewics, AC, et al: Comparison of 3-dimensional scapular position and orientation between subjects with and without shoulder impingement. *J Orthop Sports Phys Ther* 29(10):574–583, 1999.
118. Maenhout, A, et al: Electromyographic analysis of knee push up plus variations: what's the influence of the kinetic chain on scapular muscle activity? *Br J Sports Med* 44(14):1010–1015, 2009.
119. Magee, DJ: *Orthopedic Physical Assessment,* ed. 5. St. Louis: Saunders Elsevier, 2008.
120. Malanga, GA, et al: EMG analysis of shoulder positioning in testing and strengthening the supraspinatus. *Med Sci Sports Exerc* 28(6):661–664, 1996.
121. Malmström, EM, et al: A slouched body posture decreases arm mobility and changes muscle recruitment in the neck and shoulder region. *European J Applied Physiol* 115(12):2491–2503, 2015.
122. Manske, RC, et al: A randomized controlled single-blinded comparison of stretching versus stretching and joint mobilization for posterior shoulder tightness measured by internal rotation motion loss. *Sports Health Multidisc Approach* 2(2):94–100, 2010.
123. Matsen, FA: Early effectiveness of shoulder arthroplasty for patients who have primary degenerative disease. *J Bone Joint Surg Am* 78(2): 260–264, 1996.
124. Matsen, FA, et al: Glenohumeral arthritis and its management. In Rockwood, CA, et al (eds): *The Shoulder, Vol 2,* ed. 3. Philadelphia: Saunders, 2004, pp 879–1007.
125. Matsen, FA, et al: Glenohumeral instability. In Rockwood, CA, et al (eds): *The Shoulder, Vol 2,* ed. 3. Philadelphia: Saunders, 2004, pp 655–794.
126. Matsen, FA, et al: Rotator cuff. In Rockwood, CA, et al (eds): *The Shoulder, Vol 2,* ed. 3. Philadelphia: Saunders, 2004, pp 795–878.
127. Matsen III, FA, et al: The reverse total shoulder arthroplasty. *J Bone Jt Surg Am* 89(3):659–667, 2007.
128. Matthews, LS, and Pavlovich, LJ: Anterior and anteroinferior instability: diagnosis and management. In Iannotti, JP, and Williams, GR (eds): *Disorders of the Shoulder.* Philadelphia: Lippincott Williams & Wilkins, 1999, p 251.
129. McClure, P, et al: A randomized controlled comparison of stretching procedures for posterior shoulder tightness. *J Orthop Sports Phys Ther* 37(3):108–114, 2007.
130. McClure, PW, et al: Shoulder function and 3-dimensional kinematics in people with shoulder impingement syndrome before and after a 6-week exercise program. *Phys Ther* 84(9):832–848, 2004.
131. McClure, PW, et al: Direct 3-dimensional measurement of scapular kinematics during dynamic movements in vivo. *J Shoulder Elbow Surg* 10(3):269–277, 2001.
132. Meister, K, and Andrews, JR: Classification and treatment of rotator cuff injuries in the overhand athlete. *J Orthop Sports Phys Ther* 18(2): 413–421, 1993.
133. Miller, MD, Flatlow, EL, and Bigliani, LU: Biomechanics of the coricoacromial arch and rotator cuff: kinematics and contact of the subacromial space. In Iannotti, JP (ed): *The Rotator Cuff: Current Concepts and Complex Problems.* Rosemont, IL: American Academy of Orthopedic Surgeons, 1998, p 1.
134. Mohtadi, NG, et al: Electrothermal arthroscopic capsulorrhaphy: old technology, new evidence. A multicenter randomized clinical trial. *J Shld Elbow Surg* 23(8):1171–1180, 2014.
135. Morrison, DS, Greenbaum, BS, and Einhorn, A: Shoulder impingement. *Orthop Clin North Am* 31(2):285–293, 2000.
136. Mulligan, BR: *Manual Therapy "NAGS," "SNAGS," "MWM's" etc.,* ed. 4. Wellington, New Zealand: Plane View Press, 1999.
137. Muth, S, et al: The effects of thoracic spine manipulation in subjects with signs of rotator cuff tendinopathy. *J Orthop Sports Phys Ther* 42(12):1005–1016, 2012.
138. Myers, JB, et al: Scapular position and orientation in throwing athletes. *Am J Sports Med* 33(2):263–271, 2005.
139. Neer, CS: Surgery in the shoulder. In Kelly, WH, et al (eds): *Surgery in Arthritis.* Philadelphia: WB Saunders, 1994, p 754.

140. Neer, CS: Impingement lesions. *Clin Orthop* 173:70–77, 1983.
141. Neer, CS, Watson, KC, and Stanton, FJ: Recent experiences in total shoulder replacement. *J Bone Joint Surg Am* 64:319–337, 1982.
142. Neer, CS: Anterior acromioplasty for the chronic impingement syndrome in the shoulder: a preliminary report. *J Bone Joint Surg Am* 54(1):41–50, 1972.
143. Neer, CS: Replacement arthroplasty for glenohumeral osteoarthritis. *J Bone Joint Surg Am* 56(1):1–13, 1974.
144. Neviaser, AS, and Hannafin, JA: Adhesive capsulitis: a review of current treatment. *Am J Sports Med* 38(11):2346–2356, 2010.
145. Neviaser, RJ, and Neviaser, TJ: The frozen shoulder: diagnosis and management. *Clin Orthop* 223:59–64, 1987.
146. Neviaser, RJ: Ruptures of the rotator cuff. *Orthop Clin North Am* 18(3):387–394, 1987.
147. Neviaser, RJ: Injuries to the clavicle and acromioclavicular joint. *Orthop Clin North Am* 18(3):433–488, 1987.
148. Neviaser, TJ: Adhesive capsulitis. *Orthrop Clin North Am* 18(3): 439–443, 1987.
149. Neviaser, TJ: The role of the biceps tendon in the impingement syndrome. *Orthop Clin North Am* 18(3):383–386, 1987.
150. Nixon, RT, and Lindenfeld, TN: Early rehabilitation after a modified inferior capsular shift procedure for multidirectional instability of the shoulder. *Orthopedics* 21(4):441–445, 1998.
151. Noonan, TJ, and Garrett, WE: Injuries at the myotendinous junction. *Clin Sports Med* 11(4):783–806, 1992.
152. Norris, TR, and Iannotti, JR: Functional outcome after shoulder arthroplasty for primary osteoarthritis: a multicenter study. *J Shoulder Elbow Surg* 11(2):130–135, 2002.
153. Nuber, GW, and Bowen, MK: Disorders of the acromioclavicular joint: Pathophysiology, diagnosis, and management. In Iannotti, JP, and Williams, GR (eds): *Disorders of the Shoulder.* Philadelphia: Lippincott Williams & Wilkins, 1999, p 739.
154. O'Brien, M: Functional anatomy and physiology of tendons. *Clin Sports Med* 11(3):505–520, 1992.
155. O'Brien, SJ, Warren, RF, and Schwartz, E: Anterior shoulder instability. *Orthop Clin North Am* 18(3):395–408, 1987.
156. Orfaly, RM, et al: A prospective functional outcome study of shoulder arthroplasty for osteoarthritis with an intact rotator cuff. *J Shoulder Elbow Surg* 12:214–221, 2003.
157. Paine, RM, and Voight, M: The role of the scapula. *J Orthop Sports Phys Ther* 18:386–391, 1993.
158. Payne, LZ, et al: The combined dynamic and static contributions to subacromial impingement: a biomechanical analysis. *Am J Sports Med* 25(6):801–808, 1997.
159. Pollock, RG, and Flatow, LL: The rotator cuff. Full-thickness tears. Mini-open repair. *Orthop Clin North Am* 28(2):169–177, 1997.
160. Provencher, MT, et al: Arthroscopic treatment of posterior shoulder instability: results in 33 patients. *Am J Sports Med* 33(10):1463–1471, 2005.
161. Ramsey, ML, and Klimkiewicz, JJ: Posterior instability: diagnosis and management. In Iannotti, JP, and Williams, GR (eds): *Disorders of the Shoulder: Diagnosis and Management.* Philadelphia: Lippincott Williams & Wilkins, 1999, p 295.
162. Reinold, MM, Escamilla, T, and Wilk, KE: Current concepts in the scientific and clinical rationale behind exercises for glenohumeral and scapulothoracic musculature. *J Orthop Sports Phys Ther* 39(2):105–117, 2009.
163. Reinold, MM, et al: Electromyographic analysis of the rotator cuff and deltoid musculature during common shoulder external rotation exercises. *J Orthop Sports Phys Ther* 34(7):385–394, 2004.
164. Reinold, MM, et al: Thermal-assisted capsular shrinkage of the glenohumeral joint in overhead athletes: a 15- to 47-month follow-up. *J Orthop Sports Phys Ther* 33(8):455–467, 2003.
165. Robinson, CM, et al: Injuries associated with traumatic anterior glenohumeral dislocations. *J Bone Jt Surg* 94:18–26, 2012.
166. Rockwood, CA, and Wirth, MA: Disorders of the sternoclavicular joint. In Rockwood, CA, and Matsen, FA (eds): *The Shoulder, Vol 1,* ed. 3. Philadelphia: Saunders, 2004, p 597.
167. Rockwood, CA, Williams, GR, and Young, DC: Disorders of the acromioclavicular joint. In Rockwood, CA, and Matsen, FA (eds): *The Shoulder, Vol 1,* ed. 3. Philadelphia: Saunders, 2004, p 521.
168. Rockwood, CA, and Lyons, FR: Shoulder impingement syndrome: diagnosis, radiographic evaluation, and treatment with a modified Neer acromioplasty. *J Bone Joint Surg Am* 75(3):409–424, 1993.
169. Roddey, TS, et al: A randomized controlled trial comparing 2 instructional approaches to home exercise instruction following arthroscopic full-thickness rotator cuff repair surgery. *J Orthop Sports Phys Ther* 32(11):548–559, 2002.
170. Rodosky, MW, and Harner, CD: The role of the long head of the biceps muscle and superior glenoid labrum in anterior stability of the shoulder. *Am J Sports Med* 22:121–130, 1994.
171. Rokito, AS, et al: Strength after surgical repair of the rotator cuff. *J Shoulder Elbow Surg* 5:12–17, 1996.
172. Rowe, CR: Anterior glenohumeral subluxation/dislocation: the Bankart procedure. In Welsh, RP, and Shephard, RJ (eds): *Current Therapy in Sports Medicine, Vol 2.* Toronto, BC Decker, 1990.
173. Rundquist, PJ, and Ludewig, PM: Correlation of 3-dimensional shoulder kinematics to function in subjects with idiopathic loss of shoulder range of motion. *Phys Ther* 85(7):636–647, 2005.
174. Ruotolo, C, and Nottage, WM: Surgical and nonsurgical management of rotator cuff tears. *Arthroscopy* 18:527–531, 2002.
175. Sachs, RA, et al: Open Bankart repair: correlation of results with post-operative subscapular function. *Am J Sports Med* 33(10):1458–1462, 2005.
176. Safron, O, Seebauer, L, and Iannotti, J: Surgical management of the rotator cuff tendon-deficient arthritic shoulder. In Williams, GR, et al (eds): *Shoulder and Elbow Arthroplasty.* Philadelphia: Lippincott Williams & Wilkins, 2005, pp 105–114.
177. Salamh, PA, and Speer, KP: Post-rehabilitation exercise considerations following total shoulder arthroplasty. *Strength Conditioning J* 35(4): 56–63, 2013.
178. Schenk, T, and Brems, JJ: Multidirectional instability of the shoulder: pathophysiology, diagnosis, and management. *J Am Acad Orthop Surg* 6:65–72, 1998.
179. Schenk, T, and Iannotti, IP: Prosthetic arthroplasty for glenohumeral arthritis with an intact or repairable rotator cuff: indications, techniques, and results. In Iannotti, JP, and Williams, GR (eds): *Disorders of the Shoulder: Diagnosis and Management.* Philadelphia: Lippincott Williams & Wilkins, 1999, p 521.
180. Schieb, JS: Diagnosis and rehabilitation of the shoulder impingement syndrome in the overhand and throwing athlete. *Rheum Dis Clin North Am* 16(4):971–988, 1990.
181. Schmitt, L, and Snyder-Mackler, L: Role of scapular stabilizers in etiology and treatment of impingement syndrome. *J Orthop Sports Phys Ther* 29(1):31–38, 1999.
182. Schwartz, E, et al: Posterior shoulder instability. *Orthop Clin North Am* 18(3):409–419, 1987.
183. Selecky, MT, et al: The effects of laser-induced collagen shortening on the biomechanical properties of the inferior glenohumeral ligament complex. *Am J Sports Med* 27(2):168–172, 1999.
184. Sharkey, NA, and Marder, RA: The rotator cuff opposes superior translation of the humeral head. *Am J Sports Med* 23(3):270–275, 1995.
185. Smith, CA, and Williams, GR: Replacement arthroplasty in glenohumeral arthritis: intact or repairable rotator cuff. In Williams, GR, et al (eds): *Shoulder and Elbow Arthroplasty.* Philadelphia: Lippincott Williams & Wilkins, 2005, pp 75–103.
186. Smith, KL, and Matsen, FA: Total shoulder arthroplasty versus hemiarthroplasty—current trends. *Orthop Clin North Am* 29(3):491–506, 1998.
187. Smith, LK, Weiss, EL, and Lehmkuhl, LD: *Brunnstrom's Clinical Kinesiology,* ed. 5. Philadelphia: F.A. Davis, 1996.
188. Sperling, JW, and Cofield, RH: Results of shoulder arthroplasty. In Morrey, BF (ed): *Joint Replacement Arthroplasty,* ed. 3. Philadelphia: Churchill Livingstone, 2003, p 511–520.
189. Stokdijk, M, et al: External rotation in the glenohumeral joint during elevation of the arm. *Clin Biomech* 18(4):296–302, 2003.

190. Tate, AR, et al: Comprehensive impairment-based exercise and manual therapy intervention for patients with subacromial impingement syndrome: a case series. *J Orthop Sports Phys Ther* 40(8):474–493, 2010.
191. Tauro, JC: Arthroscopic rotator cuff repair: analysis of technique and results in 2- and 3-year follow-up. *Arthroscopy* 14:45–51, 1998.
192. Thigpen, CA, et al: Scapular kinematics during supraspinatus rehabilitation exercise: a comparison of full-can versus empty-can techniques. *Am J Sports Med* 34(4):644–652, 2006.
193. Thomson, S, Jukes, C, and Lewis J: Rehabilitation following surgical repair of the rotator cuff: a systematic review. *Physiotherapy* 102(1): 20–28, 2015.
194. Thornhill, TS, et al: Shoulder surgery and rehabilitation. In Melvin, I, and Gall, V (eds): *Rheumatologic Rehabilitation Series, Vol 5.* Surgical Rehabilitation. Bethesda, MD: American Occupational Therapy Association, 1999, p 37.
195. Tibone, JE, and McMahon, PJ: Biomechanics and pathologic lesions in the overhead athlete. In Iannotti, JP, and Williams, GR (eds): *Disorders of the Shoulder: Diagnosis and Management.* Philadelphia: Lippincott Williams & Wilkins, 1999, p 233.
196. Tibone, JE, and Bradley, JP: The treatment of posterior subluxation in athletes. *Clin Orthop* 291:124–137, 1993.
197. Tibone, JE, et al: Glenohumeral joint translation after arthroscopic, nonablative thermal capsuloplasty with a laser. *Am J Sports Med* 26(4):495–498, 1998.
198. Ticker, JB, and Warner, JP: Rotator cuff tears: principles of tendon repair. In Iannotti, JP (ed): *The Rotator Cuff: Current Concepts and Complex Problems.* Rosemont, IL: American Academy of Orthopedic Surgeons, 1998, p 17.
199. Timmerman, LA, Andrews, JR, and Wilk, KE: Mini-open repair of the rotator cuff. In Wilk, KE, and Andrews, JR (eds): *The Athlete's Shoulder.* New York: Churchill-Livingstone, 1994.
200. Toth, AP, et al: Thermal shrinkage for shoulder instability. *HSS J* 7(2): 108–14, 2011.
201. Townsend, H, et al: Electromyographic analysis of the glenohumeral muscles during a baseball rehabilitation program. *Am J Sports Med* 19:264–272, 1991.
202. Trail, IA: Replacement arthroplasty in synovial-based arthritis. In Williams, GR, et al (eds): *Shoulder and Elbow Arthroplasty.* Philadelphia: Lippincott Williams & Wilkins, 2005, pp 113–129.
203. Trenerry, K, Walton, J, and Murrrell, G: Prevention of shoulder stiffness after rotator cuff repair. *Clin Orthop* 430:94–99, 2005.
204. Turkel, SJ, et al: Stabilizing mechanisms preventing anterior dislocation of the glenohumeral joint. *J Bone Joint Surg Am* 63(8):1208–1217, 1981.
205. Tyler, TF, et al: Electrothermally-assisted capsulorrhaphy (E.T.A.C.): a new surgical method for glenohumeral instability and its rehabilitation considerations. *J Orthop Sports Phys Ther* 30(7):390–400, 2000.
206. Uhl, TL, et al: Shoulder musculature activation during upper extremity weight-bearing exercises. *J Orthop Sports Phys Ther* 33:109–117, 2003.
207. Vermeulen, HM, et al: End-range mobilization techniques in adhesive capsulitis of the shoulder joint: a multiple-subject case report. *Phys Ther* 80(12):1204–1213, 2000.
208. Vermeulen, HM, et al: Comparison of high-grade and low-grade mobilization techniques in the management of adhesive capsulitis of the shoulder: randomized controlled trial. *Phys Ther* 86(3):355–368, 2006.
209. Volpe, S, and Craig, JA: Postoperative physical therapy management of a reverse total shoulder arthroplasty. *Orthopedic Physical Therapy Practice* 21(2):11–17, 2009.
210. Wahl, CJ, Warren, RF, and Altchek, DW: Shoulder arthroscopy. In Rockwood, CA Jr, et al (eds): *The Shoulder, Vol 1,* ed. 3. Philadelphia: Saunders, 2004, pp 283–353.
211. Wall, B, et al: Reverse total shoulder arthroplasty: a review of results according to etiology. *J Bone Jt Surg Am* 89(7):1476–1485, 2007.
212. Warner, JJP, and Gerber, C: Treatment of massive rotator cuff tears: posterior-superior and anterior-superior. In Iannotti, JP (ed): *The Rotator Cuff: Current Concepts and Complex Problems.* Rosemont, IL: American Academy of Orthopedic Surgeons, 1998, p 59.
213. Warner, JP: Treatment options for anterior instability: open vs. arthroscopic. *Operative Tech Orthop* 5:233–237, 1995.
214. Weiss, KS, Savoie, FH: Recent advances in arthroscopic repair of traumatic anterior glenohumeral instability. *Clin Orthop* 400:117–122, 2002.
215. Wilcox, KB, Arslanian, LE, and Millett, PJ: Rehabilitation following total shoulder arthroplasty. *J Orthop Sports Phys Ther* 35(12):821–835, 2005.
216. Wilk, KE, et al: Stretch-shortening drills for the upper extremities: theory and clinical application. *J Orthop Sports Phys Ther* 17(5):225–239, 1993.
217. Wilk, KE, and Arrigo, C: An integrated approach to upper extremity exercises. *Orthop Phys Ther Clin North Am* 1:337–360, 1992.
218. Wilk, KE, and Arrigo, C: Current concepts in the rehabilitation of the athletic shoulder. *J Orthop Sports Phys Ther* 18(1):365–378, 1993.
219. Wilk, KE, and Andrews, JR: Rehabilitation following arthroscopic subacromial decompression. *Orthopedics* 16(3):349–358, 1993.
220. Wilk, KE, Andrews, JR, and Arrigo, CA: The physical examination of the glenohumeral joint: emphasis on the stabilizing structures. *J Orthop Sports Phys Ther* 25:380, 1997.
221. Wilk, KE, Arrigo, CA, and Andrews, JR: Current concepts: the stabilizing structures of the glenohumeral joint. *J Orthop Sports Phys Ther* 24: 364–379, 1997.
222. Wilk, KE, Meister, K, and Andrews, JR: Current concepts in the rehabilitation of the overhead throwing athlete. *Am J Sports Med* 30(1): 136–151, 2002.
223. Wilk, KE, et al: Shoulder injuries in the overhead athlete. *J Orthop Sports Phys Ther* 39(2):38–54, 2009.
224. Wilk, KE, et al: Rehabilitation following thermal-assisted capsular shrinkage of the glenohumeral joint: current concepts. *J Orthop Sports Phys Ther* 32(60):268–287, 2002.
225. Wilk, KE, et al: Current concepts in the recognition and treatment of superior labral (SLAP) lesions. *J Orthop Sports Phys Ther* 35(5): 273–291, 2005.
226. Wilk, KE, Hooks, TR, et al: The modified sleeper stretch and modified cross-body stretch to increase shoulder internal rotation range of motion in the overhead throwing athlete. *J Orthop Sports Phys Ther* 43(12): 891–894, 2013.
227. Williams, GR, and Iannotti, JP: Biomechanics of the glenohumeral joint: influence on shoulder arthroplasty. In Iannotti, JP, and Williams, GR (eds): *Disorders of the Shoulder: Diagnosis and Management.* Philadelphia: Lippincott Williams & Wilkins, 1999, p 471.
228. Wirth, MA, Blatter, G, and Rockwood, CA: The capsular imbrication procedure for recurrent anterior instability of the shoulder. *J Bone Joint Surg Am* 78(2):246–259, 1996.
229. Wirth, MA, and Rockwood, CA: Disorders of the sternoclavicular joint: pathophysiology, diagnosis, and management. In Iannotti, JP, and Williams, GR (eds): *Disorders of the Shoulder: Diagnosis and Management.* Philadelphia: Lippincott Williams & Wilkins, 1999, p 763.
230. Worrell, TW, et al: An analysis of supraspinatus EMG activity and shoulder isometric force development. *Med Sci Sports Exerc* 24(7): 744–748, 1992.
231. Yamaguchi, K, et al: Transitioning to arthroscopic rotator cuff repair: the pros and cons. *J Bone Joint Surg Am* 85:144–155, 2003.
232. Zazzali, MS, et al: Shoulder instability. In Donatelli, RA (ed): *Physical Therapy of the Shoulder,* ed. 4. St. Louis: Churchill Livingstone, 2004, pp 483–504.
233. Zuckerman, JD, et al: The influence of coracoacromial arch anatomy on rotator cuff tears. *J Shoulder Elbow Surg* 1:4–14, 1992.
234. Zuckerman, JD, Scott, AJ, and Gallagher, MA: Hemiarthroplasty for cuff tear arthropathy. *J Shoulder Elbow Surg* 9(3):169–172, 2000.

CHAPTER

18 The Elbow and Forearm Complex

CAROLYN KISNER, PT, MS ■ LYNN COLBY, PT, MS
■ CINDY JOHNSON ARMSTRONG, PT, DPT, CHT

A freely mobile but strong and stable elbow complex is required for normal upper extremity function. The design of the elbow and forearm adds to the mobility of the hand in space by shortening and lengthening the upper extremity and by rotating the forearm. The muscles provide control and stability to the region as the hand is used for various activities, from eating, dressing, and grooming to pushing, pulling, turning, lifting, throwing, catching, and reaching for objects to coordinated use of equipment, tools, and machines.[78,82,84] Most activities of daily living require a 100° arc of flexion and extension at the elbow, specifically between 30° and 130°, as well as 100° of forearm rotation, equally divided between pronation and supination.[78,82] Tasks such as drinking and eating primarily require elbow flexion, whereas a task such as reaching to tie shoelaces requires substantial elbow extension.

Injury or disease of bony, articular, or soft tissue structures of the elbow and forearm can cause pain and compromised mobility, strength, stability, and functional use of the upper extremity. Loss of active or passive elbow flexion interferes with grooming and eating, whereas loss of elbow extension restricts a person's ability to push up from a chair or reach out for objects. In general, loss of terminal flexion of the elbow contributes to greater limitation of function than loss of terminal extension.[78,82]

The anatomical and kinesiological relationships of the elbow and forearm are outlined in the first section of this chapter. Chapter 10 presents information on principles of soft tissue healing and management; the reader should be familiar with that material before establishing a therapeutic exercise program to improve function of the elbow and forearm.

Structure and Function of the Elbow and Forearm

The distal end of the humerus has two articular surfaces: the trochlea, which articulates with the ulna, and the capitulum, which articulates with the head of the radius (Fig. 18.1). Flexion and extension occur between these two joint surfaces. The radius also articulates with the radial notch on the ulna at the proximal radioulnar joint. This joint contributes to pronation and supination along with the distal radioulnar joint. The capsule of the elbow encloses the humeroulnar, humeroradial, and proximal radioulnar articulations. The distal radioulnar joint is structurally separate from the elbow complex even though its function is directly related to the proximal radioulnar joint.[82]

Joints of the Elbow and Forearm

There are four joints involved in elbow and forearm function: the humeroulnar, humeroradial, proximal radioulnar, and distal radial ulnar joints.

Elbow Joint Characteristics and Arthrokinematics

The elbow is a compound joint with a lax joint capsule, supported by two major ligaments—the medial (ulnar) and lateral (radial) collateral—which provide medial and lateral stability, respectively.[82,84]

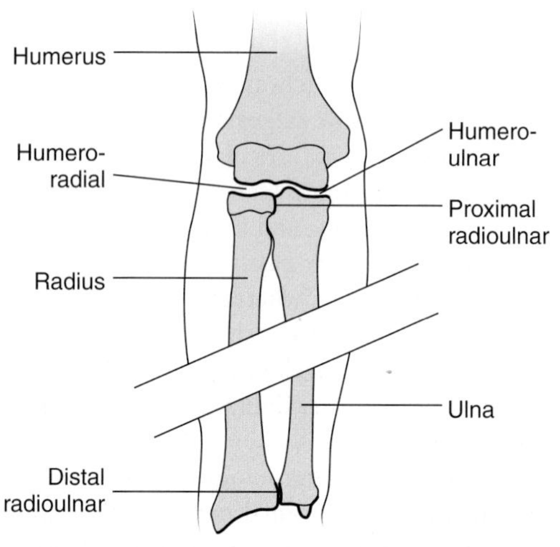

FIGURE 18.1 Bones and joints of the elbow and forearm.

Humeroulnar Articulation

Characteristics. The humeroulnar (HU) articulation is classified as a modified hinge joint. The medially placed hourglass-shaped trochlea at the distal end of the humerus is convex. The trochlear notch on the proximal ulna is concave (see Fig. 5.27). The primary motions at this articulation are flexion and extension.

Arthrokinematics. During flexion/extension the concave trochlear notch rolls and glides in the same direction in which the ulna moves, so with elbow flexion, the notch rolls and glides around the convex trochlea in an anterior direction. With elbow extension, the notch rolls and glides in a posterior direction.[82]

The axis of rotation courses slightly superior from medial to lateral due to the distal elongation of the trochlea. This asymmetry in the trochlea guides the ulna to deviate laterally relative to the humerus during extension, which is referred to as normal cubital valgus or "carrying angle." This also results in a varus angulation with elbow flexion.[82,84]

The arthrokinematics are summarized in ONLINE Box 18.1 on the FA Davis website associated with this book.

Humeroradial Articulation

Characteristics. The humeroradial (HR) articulation is classified as a modified hinge-pivot joint. The laterally placed, spherical capitulum at the distal end of the humerus is convex. The concave bony partner, the head of the radius, is located at the proximal end of the radius. Flexion/extension and pronation/supination occur at this articulation.

Arthrokinematics. As the elbow flexes and extends, the concave radial head glides in the same direction as the motion of the radius, so with elbow flexion, the concave radial head glides anteriorly, and with elbow extension, it glides posteriorly. With pronation and supination of the forearm, the radial head spins on the capitulum (see ONLINE Box 18.1).[82]

Ligaments of the Elbow

Medial (ulnar) collateral ligament. The medial (ulnar) collateral ligament complex consists of bundles of fibers that may be differentiated into anterior, posterior, and transverse portions (Fig. 18.2 A). Various portions of the ligament are taut in different ranges of motion (ROMs), providing medial support to the elbow against valgus stresses and limiting end-range elbow extension. The ligament also keeps the joint surfaces in approximation. Activities, such as throwing and golfing, impose significant stresses on the medial (ulnar) collateral ligament complex.[84]

Lateral (radial) collateral ligament. The lateral (radial) collateral ligament complex, a fan-shaped ligament on the lateral surface of the elbow, is composed of the lateral collateral ligament, the lateral ulnar collateral ligament, and the annular ligament. This complex provides stability to the lateral aspect of the elbow against varus and supination forces, stabilizes the humeroradial joint, resists longitudinal distraction, and prevents posterior translation of the radial head (Fig. 18.2 B).[84]

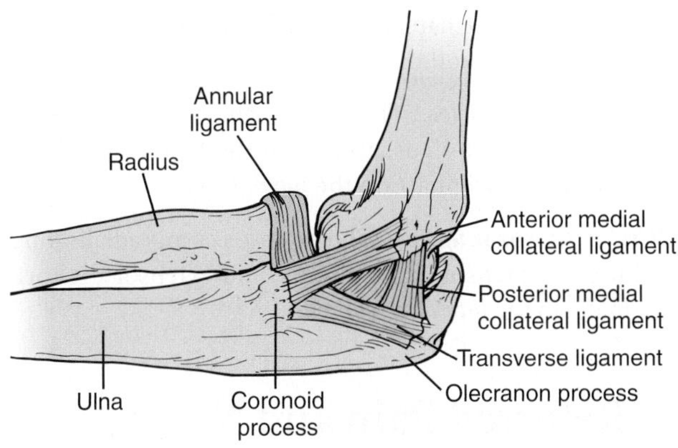

A Medial aspect

Annular ligament
Accessory collateral ligament
Lateral collateral ligament
Radius
Lateral epicondyle
Olecranon process
Ulna
Lateral ulnar collateral ligament

B Lateral aspect

FIGURE 18.2 (A) The three parts of the medial (ulnar) collateral ligament are shown on the medial aspect of the right elbow. The musculature and joint capsule have been removed to show the ligament's attachments. **(B)** The lateral collateral ligament complex includes the lateral (radial) collateral ligament, lateral ulnar collateral ligament, and annular ligament. The musculature and joint capsule have been removed to show the ligaments' attachments. *(From Norkin, CC: The elbow complex. In Levangie, PK, and Norkin, CC (eds):* Joint Structure and Function: A Comprehensive Analysis, *ed. 5. Philadelphia: F.A. Davis, 2011, p 277, with permission.)*

Forearm Joint Characteristics and Arthrokinematics

Both the proximal and distal radioulnar joints are uniaxial pivot joints that function together to produce pronation and supination (rotation) of the forearm.[84]

Proximal (Superior) Radioulnar Articulation

The proximal radioulnar (RU) articulation is within the capsule of the elbow joint but is a distinct articulation.

Characteristics. The convex rim of the radial head articulates with the relatively fixed concave radial notch on the ulna and the annular ligament. This ligament encircles the rim of the radial head and stabilizes it against the ulna (see Fig. 18.2). The primary motion of the proximal RU joint is pronation/supination.

Arthrokinematics. As the forearm rotates into pronation and supination, the convex rim of the radial head rolls and glides opposite the motion of the radius, so with pronation, the radial head rolls anteriorly (volarly) and glides posteriorly (dorsally) on the radial notch, and with supination, it rolls posteriorly (dorsally) and glides anteriorly (volarly) as the radius crosses over the relatively fixed ulna. In addition, at the humeroradial joint the radial head spins on the capitulum within the annular ligament during pronation and supination[82] (see ONLINE Box 18.1).

Distal (Inferior) Radioulnar Articulation

Characteristics. The distal RU joint is an anatomically separate joint at the distal end of the radius and ulna. The concave ulnar notch on the distal radius articulates with the convex notch on the head of the ulna. The distal RU joint, along with the proximal RU joint, participates primarily in pronation/supination.

Arthrokinematics. As the forearm rotates, the concave radius glides in the same direction as the physiological motion. It glides anterior (volar) with pronation and posterior (dorsal) with supination (see ONLINE Box 18.1).[82,84]

Muscle Function at the Elbow and Forearm

Muscles in the elbow region not only affect the function of the elbow and forearm, but also wrist and finger function.

Primary Actions at the Elbow and Forearm

Elbow Flexion

Brachialis. The brachialis is a one-joint muscle that lies deep to the biceps brachii and inserts close to the axis of motion on the ulna, so it is unaffected by the position of the forearm or the shoulder. Due to its large cross-sectional area it generates the greatest force of all the muscles that cross the elbow and its sole function is flexion of the elbow.[68,82,84]

Biceps brachii. The biceps is a two-joint muscle that crosses both the shoulder and elbow and inserts close to the axis of motion on the radius, so it also acts as a supinator of the forearm. It functions most effectively as a flexor of the elbow between 80° and 100° of flexion. For the optimal length-tension relationship, the shoulder extends to lengthen the muscle when it contracts forcefully for elbow and forearm function.[82,84]

Brachioradialis. With its insertion a great distance from the elbow on the distal radius, the brachioradialis functions to provide compression of the joint surfaces and stability to the joint. The brachioradialis is a primary elbow flexor especially during rapid movements against high resistance and acts as a pronator when the forearm is in supination and a supinator when the forearm is in pronation especially during rapid supination/pronation motions.[82,84]

Elbow Extension

Triceps brachii. The long head of the triceps brachii crosses both the shoulder and elbow; the medal and lateral heads are uniaxial and only cross the elbow joint. The long head functions most effectively as an elbow extensor if the shoulder simultaneously flexes and adducts. This maintains an optimal length-tension relationship in the muscle. Because the triceps attaches to the ulna and not the radius, it has no role in forearm rotation.[82,84]

Anconeus. The primary function of the anconeus muscle is to stabilize the elbow during extension activities as well as during active forearm supination and pronation.[68,82]

Forearm Supination

Supinator. The supinator muscle has an extensive proximal attachment and inserts distally along the proximal one third of the radius. It is capable of generating significant force regardless of the elbow position, speed, or power of the motion.[82,84]

Biceps brachii. The biceps muscle acts as a supinator if the elbow simultaneously flexes or during moderate to high powered supination activities when the elbow is flexed to 90°.[82,84]

Brachioradialis. The brachioradialis contributes to pronation and supination during short-arc, high power motions. Regardless of the position of the forearm, the brachioradialis rotates the forearm to the neutral, thumbs-up position from a fully supinated or pronated position.[82]

Forearm Pronation

Pronator teres. The pronator muscle pronates the forearm as well as stabilizes the proximal radioulnar joint by helping the radial head to maintain contact with the capitulum. The pronator teres is most active in higher-power pronation activities.[82,84]

Pronator quadratus. The pronator quadratus is the most active and consistently used pronator muscle. It also stabilizes the distal RU joint by compressing the ulnar notch of the radius against the ulnar head during pronation activities.[82,84]

Relationship of Wrist and Hand Muscles to the Elbow

Many muscles that act on the wrist and hand are attached on the medial and lateral epicondyles of the humerus. This allows for effective movement of the fingers and wrist, whether the forearm is in pronation or supination. The muscles provide stability to the elbow but contribute little to motion of the elbow. The position of the elbow affects the length-tension relationship of the muscles during their actions on the wrist and hand.[60,84] See Chapter 19 for information on the function of the wrist and hand.

Wrist flexor muscles. The flexor carpi radialis, flexor carpi ulnaris, palmaris longus, and flexor digitorum superficialis and profundus originate on the *medial epicondyle.*

Wrist extensor muscles. The extensor carpi radialis longus and brevis, extensor carpi ulnaris, and extensor digitorum originate on the *lateral epicondyle.*

Referred Pain and Nerve Injury in the Elbow Region

For a detailed description of referred pain patterns and injuries to the peripheral nerves coursing through the elbow and forearm region, see Chapter 13. ONLINE Table 13.1 summarizes the muscle involvement and functional loss that occur with each of the nerve injuries.

Common Sources of Referred Pain Into the Elbow Region

Radicular symptoms from the C5 and C6 nerve roots have been reported in patients with lateral elbow pain and from the C6 and C7 nerve roots with medial elbow pain.[2,22,96]

Nerve Disorders in the Elbow Region

Ulnar nerve. The ulnar nerve courses posteromedial to the olecranon process where it enters the cubital tunnel. After leaving the cubital tunnel, it passes between the two heads of the origin of the flexor carpi ulnaris. The most common sites for compression of the ulnar nerve in the elbow region are in the cubital tunnel and between the two heads of the flexor carpi ulnaris.[10,18]

Radial nerve. The radial nerve pierces the lateral muscular septum anterior to the lateral epicondyle and passes between the brachialis and biceps medially and the brachioradialis, extensor carpi radialis longis, and extensor carpi radialis brevis laterally. Within an area 3 cm proximal or distal to the elbow, it branches into the posterior interosseous nerve and superficial sensory nerve. The posterior interosseous nerve branch travels posterior to enter the radial/supinator tunnel (canal) between the two heads of the supinator at the arcade of Fröhse. Common sites of compression include under the extensor carpi radialis brevis, at the Arcade of Fröhse, and at the distal edge of the supinator muscle.[63,90]

Median nerve. The median nerve courses anteriorly deep in the cubital fossa, medial to the tendon of the biceps and brachial artery, where it is well protected. The nerve then progresses between the ulnar and humeral heads of the pronator teres muscle and dips under the flexor digitorum profundus muscle. Entrapment may occur between the heads of the pronator teres muscle, under the Ligament of Struthers, by the bicipital aponeurosis or deep to the flexor digitorum superficialis.[10]

Management of Elbow and Forearm Disorders and Surgeries

In order to make sound clinical decisions when treating patients with elbow and forearm disorders, it is necessary to understand the various pathologies, surgical procedures, and associated precautions and to identify presenting structural and functional impairments, activity limitations, and participation restrictions (functional limitations and possible disabilities). In this section, pathologies and surgical procedures are presented. Conservative and postoperative guidelines for managing these conditions are described in this section.

Joint Hypomobility: Nonoperative Management

Related Pathologies and Etiology of Symptoms

Pathologies, such as rheumatoid arthritis (RA), juvenile rheumatoid arthritis (JRA), and degenerative joint disease, as well as acute joint reactions after trauma, dislocations, or fractures, affect this joint complex. Postimmobilization contractures and adhesions develop in the joint capsule and surrounding tissues any time the joint is immobilized in a cast or orthosis. This typically occurs after dislocations and fractures of the humerus, radius, or ulna. The reader is referred to Chapter 11 for background information on arthritis and fractures.

Common Impairments of Structure and Function

Acute stage. When symptoms are acute, joint effusion, muscle guarding, and pain restrict elbow motion, and usually there is pain at rest. Fractures and dislocations require medical intervention; however, with proper training, therapists are capable of manipulating subluxations such as a pushed or pulled elbow (see Figs. 5.29 and 5.31, respectively).

Subacute and chronic stages. A capsular pattern usually exists in the subacute or chronic stages of tissue healing. Elbow flexion is more restricted than extension. There is a firm end-feel and decreased joint play. In long-standing arthritis of the elbow, pronation and supination also become restricted with a firm end-feel and decreased joint play in the proximal RU joint. Arthritis of the distal RU joint results in pain on overpressure.

Common Activity Limitations and Participation Restrictions

- Difficulty turning a doorknob or key in the ignition
- Difficulty or pain with pushing and pulling activities, such as opening and closing doors
- Restricted hand-to-mouth activities for eating and drinking and hand-to-head activities for personal grooming and using a telephone
- Difficulty or pain when pushing up from a chair
- Inability to carry objects with a straight arm
- Limited reach

Joint Hypomobility: Management—Protection Phase

See the Guidelines for Management Related to the Stages of Tissue Healing in Chapter 10, Box 10.1.

Educate the Patient

- Inform the patient regarding the anticipated length of acute symptoms and teach methods of joint protection and how to modify activities of daily living. For example, the patient should avoid activities that involve lifting or pushing off with the involved upper extremity.
- Instruct the patient to avoid excessive fatigue by performing exercises frequently during the day but limiting the number of repetitions during each bout (set) of exercises.

Reduce Effects of Inflammation or Synovial Effusion and Protect the Area

- Intermittent or limited immobilization in a sling or static orthosis provides rest to the elbow, but complete immobilization can lead to joint hypomobility, contractures, and limited motion; therefore, frequent periods of controlled movement within a pain-free range should be performed.

CLINICAL TIP

Posttraumatic pain and stiffness are common following both operative and nonoperative treatment of fractures and dislocations. Soft tissue structures, including muscles and ligaments, are also subject to damage with these injuries. To restore function of the elbow, good communication between the therapist and physician is critical for optimal outcomes. The key to minimizing stiffness is early motion. Minimizing immobilization by using a hinged orthosis, while limiting extension allows for early motion and provides joint protection.

- Gentle grade I or II joint distraction and oscillation techniques in the resting position may inhibit pain and move synovial fluid for nutrition in the involved joints (see Chapter 5 for principles of application and techniques).

Maintain Soft Tissue and Joint Mobility

- Passive or active-assistive ROM within limits of pain, including flexion/extension and pronation/supination
- Multiple-angle submaximal isometrics for elbow flexors, extensors, pronators, supinators, and wrist flexors and extensors in pain-free positions

Maintain Integrity and Function of Related Areas

- Shoulder, wrist, and hand ROM and activities should be encouraged within the tolerance of the individual.
- If edema develops in the hand, the arm should be elevated whenever possible. Consider retrograde massage as described in Chapter 26.

Joint Hypomobility: Management—Controlled Motion Phase

If joint hypomobility exists, ROM is increased by utilizing joint mobilization techniques as well as passive stretching and muscle inhibition techniques following the principles described in Chapters 4 and 5. Box 18.1 highlights several important precautions if joint restrictions are related to trauma.

Increase Soft Tissue and Joint Mobility

The intensity of stretching and mobilization techniques is dictated by the healing tissues, the specific pathology, and the surgical technique, as well as the amount of pain, motion, and end feel. Vigorous stretching should not be undertaken until later stages of healing. As noted in Box 18.1, high-intensity stretching of the elbow flexors is contraindicated following trauma because of the potential for development of heterotopic bone formation.

- ***Passive joint mobilization techniques.*** Because several articulations are involved with each motion at the elbow, it is important to identify which of the articulations have reduced joint play. For specific techniques to use, see Figures 5.28 through 5.33 and their descriptions in Chapter 5. Progress each technique by positioning the joint at the end of its available range before applying the mobilization technique.

BOX 18.1 Precautions Following Traumatic Injury to the Elbow

- Heterotopic ossification of the injured tissue is a potential complication and presents itself as local soft tissue swelling, warmth, and tenderness. When this occurs, stretching is ineffective and contraindicated.
- After healing of fractures in the elbow and forearm, malunion is not unusual, preventing full ROM. A bony block end-feel or an abnormal appearance of the elbow or forearm should alert the therapist to the cause of this impairment. Radiographical imaging is helpful in verifying the problem. No amount of stretching or mobilizing changes the patient's ROM. Indiscriminate stretching may lead to hypermobility of related joints, which could cause additional trauma and pain.

CLINICAL TIP

To progress joint mobility in the terminal ranges of flexion and extension, it may be necessary to emphasize the accessory motions of varus and valgus, respectively. This is accomplished with ulnar glide (for limited extension) and radial (for limited flexion) techniques.

- ***Manipulation to reduce a "pushed elbow."*** Proximal subluxation of the radius may result from falling on an outstretched hand. The radial head is pushed proximally in the annular ligament and impinges against the capitulum. This injury sometimes accompanies a fracture of the distal radius (Colles' fracture) or scaphoid and is not identified as an impairment until after the fracture has healed and the cast is removed. It is often overlooked due to the focus on the fracture site as well as soft tissue and joint restrictions caused by limited elbow motion during fracture healing. Palpation of joint space will reveal decreased space on the involved side as compared to the uninvolved side. There may be limited flexion or extension of the elbow, limited wrist flexion, and limited pronation.

CLINICAL TIP

For an acute "pushed elbow" (and no fracture), apply a distal traction to the radius to reposition the radial head. If chronic, repetitive stretching with sustained grade III distal traction to the radius is necessary (see Fig. 5.29) in addition to the soft tissue stretching and strengthening techniques needed for increasing motion.

- ***Manipulation to reduce a "pulled elbow."*** Distal subluxation of the radius is usually seen as an acute injury in children and is sometimes labeled "tennis elbow" when it occurs in adults. It occurs as a result of a forceful pull on the hand such as would occur when a child jerks away from a parent or caregiver or when an individual applies a quick force to lift a heavy object. The force causes the radius to move distally with respect to the ulna. The head of the radius is unable to glide proximally in the annular ligament when supination is attempted, resulting in the person holding the forearm in pronation. Either supination is restricted, or the patient guards against the motion.

CLINICAL TIP

With the child distracted, a quick, compressive manipulation (high-velocity thrust) of the radial head concurrently with supination is applied (see Fig. 5.31) to reposition the radial head when there is a "pulled elbow." There may be soft tissue trauma associated with the injury, which may be treated with cold and compression.

- ***Manual stretching and self-stretching.*** Use manual stretching and inhibition techniques to increase the flexibility of any periarticular tissues that are restricting mobility. Use of a light cuff weight placed around the distal forearm with the patient carefully positioned for an effective stretch provides a low-intensity, long-duration stretch and is an alternative to manual passive stretching. If elbow ROM does not steadily improve after acute symptoms have subsided, the patient may need to begin wearing a static progressive orthosis that applies a low-load, prolonged stretch force over an extended period of time. These stretching interventions are described in Chapter 4.
- ***Home instructions.*** Teach the patient self-stretching maneuvers followed by active exercise that utilizes the new range. Suggestions are provided in the last section of this chapter.

Improve Joint Tracking of the Elbow

A mobilization with movement (MWM) technique consisting of a gentle radial glide combined with the pain-free active movement of elbow flexion or extension, or pain-free gripping (depending on the patients impairment or functional limitation) with pain-free passive overpressure, may improve articular surface tracking by allowing the muscles to move the joint in a pain-free manner.[20,21,107] (Refer to the principles of MWM in Chapter 5.)

- *Patient position and maneuver*: Supine with elbow either flexed or extended to the end of the available range. Secure a mobilization belt around the patient's proximal forearm at the joint line and your hips such that the belt is horizontal. Stabilize the distal humerus by reaching inside the belt and grasping the humeral condyles. With your other hand stabilize the forearm at the wrist. Apply a gentle lateral glide to the proximal ulna with the belt by slowly moving your hips, taking care not to glide the joint too aggressively. Have the patient actively flex or extend the elbow applying a gentle passive overpressure at end range. With extension be sure to account for the carrying angle of the elbow, which may alter the treatment plane. Repeat the movement 6-10 times for up to three sets (Fig. 18.3). This is a pain-free technique.[20,21,79,107]

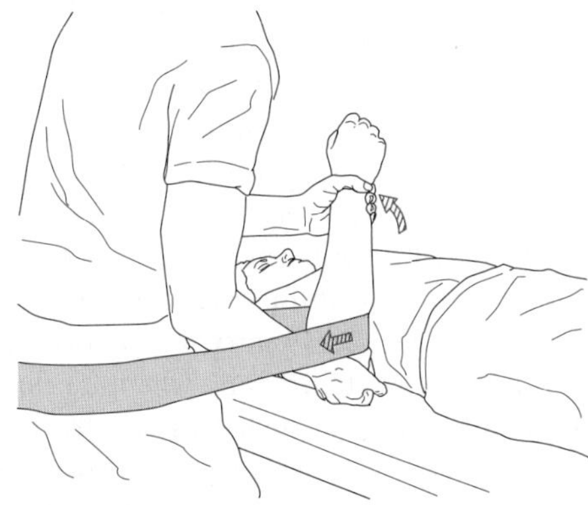

FIGURE 18.3 Mobilization with movement (MWM) to improve elbow flexion. A lateral glide is applied to the proximal ulna while the patient actively flexes their elbow, followed by a passive end-range stretch.

Improve Muscle Performance and Functional Abilities

Initiate active and low-load resistance exercises in open- and closed-chain positions to develop control, muscular endurance, and strength in the muscles of the elbow and forearm. As the patient improves, adapt the exercises to progress toward functional activities. Specific exercises are described in the exercise section of this chapter. Include the shoulder girdle, wrist, and hand in the exercise program as their flexibility and strength have an influence on the recovery of elbow function.

Joint Hypomobility: Management—Return to Function Phase

Improve Muscle Performance

Progress strengthening exercises as the joint tissue tolerates. Teach the patient safe progressions and exercise strategies that promote return to function. To prepare the joints and muscles for specific tasks, use exercises that replicate the repetitions and demands of daily activities, such as pushing, pulling, lifting, carrying, and gripping.

Restore Functional Mobility of Joints and Soft Tissues

If restrictions remain, use more vigorous manual or mechanical stretching and joint mobilization techniques.

Promote Joint Protection

Chronic arthritic conditions may require modification of high-load activities to minimize deforming stresses on the involved joints.

Joint Surgery and Postoperative Management

Intra-articular or extra-articular surgical intervention is often necessary for management of severe fractures or dislocations that affect the joints of the elbow and surrounding soft tissues. These injuries may require open reduction with internal fixation or arthroscopic or open excision of bone fragments. In adults, the most common fracture in the elbow region is a fracture of the head and neck of the radius. This type of fracture accounts for over one-third of all elbow fractures.[57,87,99,101,106,112] This injury usually occurs when a person falls on an outstretched hand when the elbow is extended and the forearm pronated, causing a fracture of the radial head with possible concurrent injuries about the elbow to include other fractures, dislocations, or ligamentous injuries.[49,57,101,106,112]

If the proximal radius is displaced and the radial head fracture is comminuted, either open reduction internal fixation, low-profile fixation, excision of the fragments of the radial head, radial head excision, or arthroplasty of the radial head are surgical options. Box 18.2 summarizes the advantages and disadvantages of surgical options for management of displaced fractures of the radial head. Radial head fractures in children, however, are relatively uncommon. When they do occur, closed reduction is preferred.[99]

Small osteochondral defects of one or more of the articular surfaces of the elbow complex occur in the skeletally mature and immature individual (often in the throwing athlete) as the result of repetitive trauma. Such defects, depending on their size, characteristics, and location, may require surgical intervention, such as removal or internal fixation of a fragment, microfracture, or autologous osteochondral or chondrocyte implantation, if nonoperative measures have been ineffective.[1,31,45,89]

Early-stage or long-standing joint disease (RA, JRA, post-traumatic arthritis) associated with synovial proliferation and destruction of articular surfaces of the elbow joints leading to pain, limitation of motion, and impaired upper extremity function may also need to be managed with extra-articular or intra-articular surgery. For example, with early-stage RA in which synovial proliferation is present but joint surfaces are still in good condition, *arthroscopic* or *open synovectomy* is the procedure of choice for relief of pain if medications have not controlled the disease.[22,26,98] Occasionally, advanced arthritis is managed surgically by *interposition arthroplasty* (only in the patient younger than 40 on a selective basis),[72,98] *resection of the radial head* with or without prosthetic implant and concomitant synovectomy, or *arthrodesis* (as a salvage procedure).[12,67] However, today, the most common surgical procedure used to manage severe destruction of the elbow joint is *total elbow arthroplasty* (TEA).[29,48,98] Table 18.1 summarizes how the severity of joint disease and the extent of soft tissue involvement influence the choice of surgical procedure for the elbow complex.[33,46,98]

The goals of surgery of the elbow joint complex and postoperative rehabilitation include (1) relief of pain, (2) restoration of bony alignment and joint stability, and (3) sufficient strength and ROM to allow functional use of the elbow and

BOX 18.2 Surgical Options for Displaced Fractures of the Radial Head

Open Reduction and Internal Fixation

- *Advantages:* Preferable technique if stable fixation can be achieved and if able to repair significant ligamentous damage; early protective postoperative motion permissible.
- *Disadvantages:* Not amenable to nonreducible fractures and less practical than radial head excision or implant for severely comminuted fractures or osteoporosis.

Low-Profile Fixation

- *Advantages:* Improved forearm rotation and flexion motion with decreased scarring as compared to other techniques. Immediate mobilization of the elbow joint is permissible.
- *Disadvantages:* Early in development including biocompatibility, which may be an issue unique to this technique.

Excision of the Radial Head

- *Advantages:* For severely comminuted, nonreducible, and unstable fractures; no potential for mechanical blockage of joint motion from malalignment of fracture fragments or internal fixation; early ROM permissible.
- *Disadvantages:* Increased valgus deformity possible with potential for early degenerative changes of the humeroulnar joint. Persistent pain and limited motion with this technique. Even with intact ligaments an alteration of the kinematics and stability of the elbow has been shown.

Excision of Fragments of the Radial Head

- *Advantages:* Not as commonly used due to improvements in fixation systems. However, technique used when small displaced fragments that block motion or loose fragments are present. Used when other fixation systems are not feasible due to small fragment size, comminution, or osteopenia.
- *Disadvantages:* Fragments that articulate with the proximal radioulnar joint should not be excised due to interference with forearm rotation.

Arthroplasty of the Radial Head

- *Advantages:* Indicated for displaced comminuted fractures of the radial head and neck where an anatomic reduction and stable internal fixation is not possible and there are associated soft tissue injuries. Radial head implants have been shown to restore the kinematics and stability of the radial head.
- *Disadvantages:* Many implants available with no studies comparing clinical outcomes or long-term results.

TABLE 18.1 Severity of Elbow Joint Disease and Selection of Surgical Procedure

Severity of Joint Disease	Selection of Surgical Procedure
■ Mild synovitis: joint surfaces normal or with minimal degeneration, osteoporosis	■ Nonoperative/medical management
■ Moderate synovitis; some loss of articular cartilage; narrowing of joint space but joint contour maintained	■ Arthroscopic synovectomy or resection of the radial head with synovectomy
■ Moderate to severe synovitis; loss of articular cartilage; loss of joint space; intact collateral ligaments	■ Resurfacing total elbow arthroplasty or, possibly in a growing child, an interpositional arthroplasty
■ Severe synovitis; destruction of articular cartilage; complete loss of joint space (bone-to-bone articulation); significant joint instability; bone loss; ankylosis	■ Semiconstrained total elbow arthroplasty

upper extremity. Surgical procedures done to relieve pain and improve elbow stability tend to be more successful than procedures done solely to increase ROM. Heterotopic bone formation, which leads to joint stiffness, is often a complication of elbow fractures, dislocations, and elbow joint surgery.[4,86] Therefore, the single goal of improving ROM is rarely an indication for surgery.

Radial Head Excision or Arthroplasty

Indications for Surgery

The following are frequently cited indications for radial head excision or arthroplasty.

- Severely comminuted fracture or fracture-dislocations of the head or neck of the radius that cannot be reconstructed and stabilized with internal fixation.[57,67,87,101,106,112]
- Chronic synovitis and mild deterioration of the articular surfaces associated with arthritis of the HR and proximal RU joints resulting in joint pain at rest or with motion, possible subluxation of the head of the radius, and significant loss of upper extremity function.[57,106]

CONTRAINDICATIONS: Radial head excision is contraindicated in the growing child. [99] Excision without replacement of the radial head is not an appropriate option in the presence of elbow instability; a displaced, comminuted fracture; and where a stable internal fixation is not achievable.[57,74,112] As with other joints, arthroplasty is also contraindicated in the presence of an active infection.

Procedure

Background

Selection of procedure. Depending on the integrity of the ligaments and stability of the elbow complex, a radial head excision may be selected or implant arthroplasty may be the better choice. Results from biomechanical studies demonstrate altered kinematics and stability after radial head excision whereas an implant restores stability and kinematics similar to the native radial head.[13,57] The use of a prosthetic implant is considered when there is more than three fracture fragments, when there is a fracture of more than 20% to 50% of the coronoid with radial head fracture, and when there is clinical instability of the elbow as the result of disruption of the supporting ligaments.[57,74,75,87]

Implant designs, materials, and fixation. There is an increasing number of prosthetic radial head implants available to surgeons. There are three major considerations for choosing the appropriate implant: (1) sizing, (2) alignment, and (3) stem fixation. Current available implants include spacer implants, press-fit and ingrowth stems, and bipolar and ceramic articulations. Silicone implants are no longer used due to significant incidence of failure producing silicone synovitis. Modular metallic (titanium) radial head implants with separate heads and stems are now used allowing for improved sizing and ease of implantation. However, the optimal radial head implant has yet to be designed and fabricated.[15,57,74,75]

Overview of Operative Procedure

The current implantation techniques vary due to the variety of implants available; however, some surgeons use an extensor digitorum splitting approach and divide the radial collateral and annular ligaments while preserving the integrity of the radial ulnar collateral ligament.[57] Others expose the joint through a posterolateral (Kocher) approach between the extensor carpi ulnaris and anconeus muscles,[87,112] while others prefer the Kaplan approach between the extensor digitorum and the extensor carpi radialis bravis.[101] Regardless of the approach, the radial head is exposed, and a radial osteotomy is performed at the level of the annular ligament to resect the head. For a severe fracture, a portion of the radial neck may also need to be excised. When exposing the operative field, effort is made not to detach intact ligaments. A concomitant synovectomy is done if proliferative synovitis is present (typically seen in RA and JRA).[57,74]

If an implant is to be inserted, the medullary canal of the radius is prepared to accept the stem of the prosthesis. If the elbow is unstable, ligamentous structures are repaired. If the radial ulnar collateral ligament is insufficient, it may be reinforced with a palmaris longus autograft or allograft.[57,74,75]

Complications

Intraoperative complications. Damage to the posterior interosseous nerve is a concern during surgical excision of the radial head regardless of whether a radial head implant is included in the procedure.[67] If an implant is inserted, malpositioning or inaccurate sizing can cause postoperative pain and humeroradial instability, compromise ROM, and eventually contribute to premature implant wear.[15,87,101,112]

Postoperative complications. Postoperatively complications of excision with or without implant may include delayed wound closure, infection, limited ROM of the elbow and/or forearm, radial tunnel syndrome, cubital laxity, persistent pain, and a sense of instability. Slight proximal migration of the radius may occur if resection does not include implantation of a prosthetic radial head.[57,74,112] This complication may or may not be associated with elbow or wrist pain. Following excision for a severe radial head fracture, osteoarthritis of the HR joint also may develop over time.[67]

As with all types of implant arthroplasty, aseptic loosing or long-term implant wear and breakage are complications that may occur, necessitating revision arthroplasty.

Postoperative Management

The goals and interventions, the rate of progression, and the length of the rehabilitation program, as well as final outcomes, are highly dependent on the extent of damage to soft tissues from injury or chronic inflammation; the integrity of repaired soft tissues, particularly the supporting ligaments of the elbow complex; the philosophy of the surgeon; and the patient's expectations of the surgery and response to treatment.

Immobilization

Depending on the extent of the surgery and the procedure performed, the elbow may be immobilized in a long arm orthosis or a hinged protective orthosis with an extension block for up to 3 weeks. The elbow is positioned at 45° to 90° with the forearm in mid pronation and the wrist in neutral. When elbow motion is permissible (often as early as 1 to 3 days after surgery or longer if significant reconstruction of ligaments was necessary), the non-hinged orthosis is removed for exercise in a protected arc of motion, but is replaced after exercise and worn at night for an extended period of time to protect healing tissues. If the stability of the elbow is in question, the patient may wear the hinged orthosis continuously to support the healing tissue, which is then adjusted to allow increased ROM as the tissue tensile strength improves.[15,35,112]

Exercise: Maximum Protection Phase

Goals and interventions. The first phase of rehabilitation (inflammatory phase) extends for the first 2 to 3 weeks after surgery and focuses on patient education that emphasizes wound care, control of pain, edema reduction, and exercises to offset the adverse effects of immobilization while protecting repaired soft tissues that maintain the stability of the elbow. The following goals and exercise-related interventions typically are included in this initial phase.[11,35]

- ***Manage edema.*** Have the patient elevate their arm above the heart (wrist above the elbow; elbow above the shoulder) and place the arm in a compressive sleeve.
- ***Maintain mobility of uninvolved joints.*** Active ROM exercises of the shoulder, wrist, and hand immediately after surgery.
- ***Maintain mobility of the elbow and forearm.*** Initiate gentle protected ROM within 2 to 3 days postoperatively. Depending on the extent of the surgical procedure or healing tissue, have the patient remove the static orthosis several times daily for self-ROM (passive or active-assisted) of the elbow and forearm within a pain-free limited arc of motion (limit extension to protect healing tissue). Active ROM is generally allowed within 1 week postoperatively and begins no longer than 3 weeks postoperatively if there was an unstable fracture or dislocation requiring immobilization. However, as noted previously, some patients must wear a hinged orthosis (with an extension block) for additional stability during ROM exercises if associated ligamentous or soft tissue reconstruction occurred.

CLINICAL TIP

Some specific motions may need to be restricted initially to prevent excessive stress on reconstructed ligaments. Restrictions vary depending on the extent of ligament disruption and the ligament (s) repaired. For example, if the radial collateral ligament complex was repaired, perform ROM exercises with the forearm in pronation to protect the healing ligament.[35]

- ***Minimize muscle atrophy.*** Submaximal, pain-free, multiple-angle isometric exercises of elbow and forearm musculature.

Exercise: Moderate and Minimum Protection Phase

Goals and interventions. The intermediate phase (fibroplastic phase) of rehabilitation begins when wound healing is satisfactory and active movements of the elbow are relatively pain free (approximately 2 to 3 weeks postoperatively) and lasts until approximately 8 weeks postoperatively. This phase of rehabilitation is characterized by continued efforts to restore nearly full or at least functional ROM for everyday activities while maintaining stability of the elbow. Exercises to improve upper extremity strength and muscular endurance and use of the involved elbow for light functional activities are introduced and progressed.

- ***Increase ROM,*** particularly if contractures were noted preoperatively.
  - Gentle (low-intensity, prolonged stretch) manual stretching, hold-relax techniques, or self-stretching

- Grade II joint mobilization techniques initially, followed by grade III mobilizations after bony and soft tissue healing has occurred

CONTRAINDICATION: When applying joint mobilization techniques, do not perform valgus/varus stretches in terminal extension/flexion, particularly if the radial head was not replaced with a prosthetic implant or if the integrity of the supporting ligaments and stability of the elbow is in question.

- Low-load, long-duration, static progressive orthotic intervention
- ***Improve functional strength and muscular endurance.***
  - Low-load (pain-free) resistance exercises (maximum 1 to 2 lb), emphasizing high repetitions
  - Initiate grip and pinch resistance exercises
  - Use of the postsurgical upper extremity for *light* activities of daily living (ADLs)

Exercise: Minimum to No Protection Phase

Goals and interventions. The final phase (remodeling phase) ranges from 2 to 6 months. The goals of this phase are to maximize ROM, increase strength and endurance, and increase function.

- ***Maximize ROM***
  - Initiate more aggressive techniques, avoiding overstretching of soft tissue and inciting an inflammatory response.
  - Progress joint mobilization techniques to grades III and IV combined with manual stretching and hold-relax techniques at end ROM.
  - Employ radial (lateral) and ulnar (medial) gapping techniques to restore end-range flexion and extension, respectively.
  - Orthotic intervention should be initiated by 8 weeks after injury or surgery if not already done so. A static progressive (more effective for extension) orthosis or a dynamic orthosis (more effective for flexion) should begin, and a wearing schedule should be determined.
- ***Restore strength and endurance***
  - Progress a resistive program using free weights, resistive bands, and/or weight machines that includes the entire upper extremity.
- ***Resumption of recreational and work-related activities.*** Patient education is a key element of helping the patient return safely to physical activities. A graded return to higher level functional activities is initiated that incorporates specific return to work and/or sport specific activities with emphasis on muscle performance.

Outcomes

The anticipated outcomes after surgical repair of the radial head following a severely displaced and comminuted fracture or due to advanced arthritis are a stable elbow and pain-free movement (flexion/extension and pronation/supination) within functional ranges. Short-term postoperative outcomes of excision arthroplasty with and without implant are similar with regard to relief of pain and functional motion. However, patients with preoperative instability necessitating an implant with ligamentous reconstruction and those with a tenuous repair of ligamentous structures have less satisfactory results than those with a stable elbow.

Some patients may develop a slight increase (about 5° to 10°) in valgus laxity of the elbow, without complaints of instability during functional activities if ligaments are intact prior to surgery or repaired at the time of surgery. Others may experience pain and instability associated with the increased laxity, thus compromising outcomes. In a study by Hall and coinvestigators, posterolateral rotary instability associated with a deficient lateral ulnar collateral ligament was identified at a mean of 44 months in only 16.6% of patients (7 of 42) who reported lateral elbow pain and a sense of instability or weakness after radial head resection (without implant).[49]

Short-term and long-term outcomes after open reduction and internal fixation for radial head fractures have been good when anatomic reduction and rigid internal fixation have been achieved and early motion has been initiated postoperatively. Outcomes for procedures using rigid metal radial head implants have also been favorable. Outcomes include pain relief, stability, and sufficient elbow and forearm ROM for functional activities, leading to relatively high patient satisfaction.[57,74]

Total Elbow Arthroplasty

Indications for Surgery

TEA is a treatment option for patients with RA; patients with debilitating, late-stage elbow arthritis; patients with a nonunion distal humerus fracture; those with bony tumors, osteonecrosis, or with dysfunctional instability; as well as for those patients who have had unsuccessful nonoperative management or unsuccessful previous surgical procedures, who are over 60 to 65 years of age and whose physical demands are relatively low.[14,27,29,51,58] However, since the first cemented TEA was introduced several decades ago, the indications for this procedure have broadened considerably as the design of prosthetic implants and surgical techniques have evolved. TEA is now considered for the younger patient depending on their postoperative demands.[25,28,46,88] A long-term follow-up of patients, who had undergone TEA at or before the age of 40 for various types of elbow arthritis, showed that 93% continued to have good to excellent outcomes at a mean duration of 91 months after surgery.[25,88]

In addition to management of advanced arthritis, TEA is now considered a preferred surgical alternative to open reduction and internal fixation for management of severely comminuted, intra-articular distal humeral fractures sustained by elderly patients.[27,29,66]

CONTRAINDICATIONS: Absolute and relative contraindications for TEA are identified in Box 18.3.[29,71] It is important to note, however, with the exception of active infection, there is lack of agreement as to which contraindications are absolute versus relative.

BOX 18.3 Contraindications to Total Elbow Arthroplasty

Absolute
- The presence of active (acute or subacute) infection in the skin, soft tissue, or bone
- Complete ankylosis of the neuropathic elbow joint
- Severely contracted, scarred, or burned skin resulting in poor-quality soft tissue at the elbow
- Inadequate muscle power of the elbow musculature

Relative
- Lack of patient compliance
- History of previous elbow infection
- Chronic instability
- Heterotopic ossification or pain-free ankylosis
- Insufficient bone stock
- Dysfunctional hand
- The younger patient with high demand

Procedure

Background

The complex structural relationships among the HU, HR, and proximal RU joints have made developing a prosthetic elbow joint a challenging task. Following introduction and use of early cemented elbow replacements,[33] incremental improvements in design, materials, fixation, and surgical technique have contributed to increasingly predictable and successful outcomes.[29,33] Elbow replacement systems include a humeral and an ulnar implant (Fig. 18.4), and some designs also include replacement of the head of the radius.[33,58,61,73,76]

Implant design and selection considerations. Early designs were *hinged (linked, articulated)* and *fully constrained* metal-to-metal humeral and ulnar implants that allowed only flexion and extension of the elbow joint.[29,33,46,93] These designs made no allowances for normal varus and valgus and rotational movements, and hence, the implants rapidly loosened at the bone-cement interface. Metal fatigue at the linkage of the prosthetic components and joint dislocation also were common complications.[9,27] As more accurate information about the biomechanical characteristics of the elbow joint became known, the design of prosthetic replacements evolved. In addition to a functional arc of flexion and extension, contemporary designs provide 5° to 10° of varus and valgus as well as rotational motion (Fig. 18.5).[27,33,56,58]

The designs of total elbow replacement can be classified into two broad categories: *linked* (articulated) and *unlinked* (nonarticulated). Rather than being fully constrained, as the early components were, linked humeral and ulnar implants are now loosely constrained and, as such, are referred to as *semiconstrained* designs.[8,58,73,76] Designs classified as unlinked favor a more anatomic and bone-preserving humeroulnar articulation with an additional radial head component in an effort to increase stability.[8,34,46,58] The most recent advance in implant design is the convertible or hybrid implant, which can be inserted as either a linked or unlinked replacement system. Use of a convertible or hybrid implant enables the surgeon to determine the more appropriate design based on intraoperative observations and evaluation.[8,58]

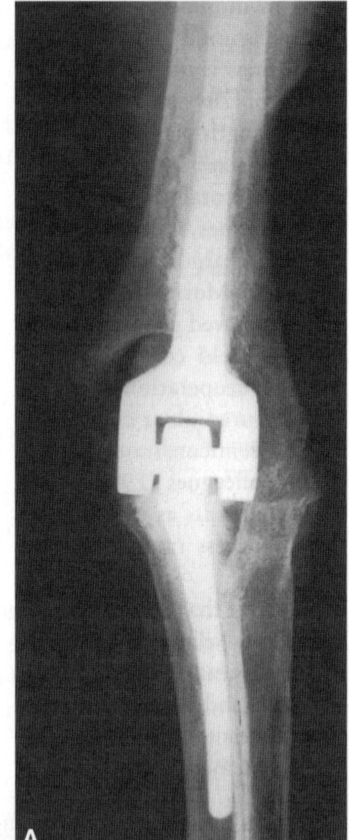

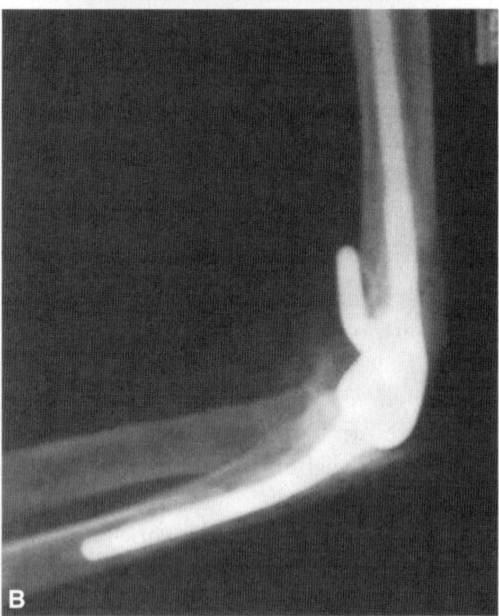

FIGURE 18.4 (A) Anteroposterior and **(B)** lateral radiographs following placement of a Conrad-Morrey (linked/semiconstrained) total elbow arthroplasty. *(From Field, LD, and Savoié, FH, III:* Master Cases: Shoulder and Elbow Surgery. *New York: Thieme, 2003, with permission.)*

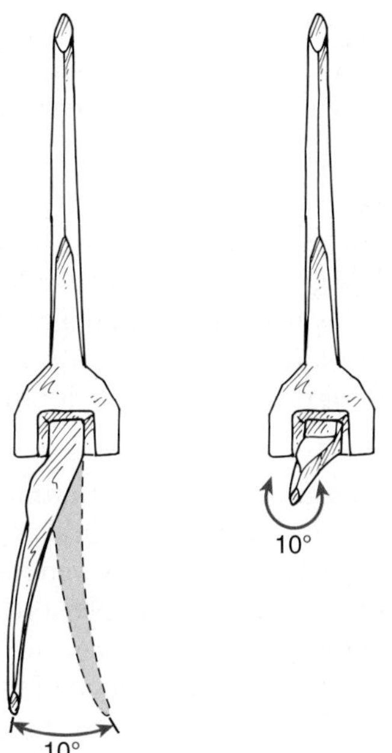

FIGURE 18.5 A linked, semiconstrained design is characterized by varus-valgus and axial rotation tolerances of several degrees at the articulation. *(From Morrey, BF [ed]:* The Elbow and Its Disorders, *ed. 4. Philadelphia: Saunders Elsevier, 2009, p 766, with permission from the Mayo Clinic Foundation.)*

The criteria for use of a linked or unlinked TEA are based in part on the characteristics of these designs with respect to stability. Linked designs derive inherent stability from one or two pins, which couple the humeral and ulnar components.[73] In addition, some semiconstrained designs have an anterior flange to enhance joint stability and decrease the risk of posterior dislocation.[33,77] Unlinked implant systems, although sometimes referred to as unconstrained, actually have varying degrees of constraint built into their designs based on the degree of congruency of the articulating surfaces.[34,58,61] The less constraining the articular surfaces of the implants, the more reliant the replacement system is on the surrounding soft tissues, particularly the collateral ligaments, for joint stability.

Semiconstrained (*linked*) implants are the most common types of elbow prostheses used in North America. Overall, linked designs, because of their inherent stability, are considered appropriate for use with a broader spectrum of patients, including those with unstable elbows, than unlinked designs.[29,33,56,58] Although both linked and unlinked designs derive some degree of stability from the supporting capsuloligamentous structures and elbow musculature, the integrity of these soft tissues is far more critical for successful use of unlinked than linked designs.[8,29,33,56,58]

In addition to considerations related to stability, the etiology and extent of joint destruction, the degree of deformity, the quality of the available bone stock, and the training and experience of the surgeon are factors that influence the type of replacement system used.[33]

Materials and fixation. A stemmed titanium humeral component that has a cobalt-chrome alloy articulating surface interfaces with a high-density polyethylene articulating surface of a stemmed ulnar component.[8,33] Currently, prosthetic components are cemented in place with polymethyl methacrylate, an acrylic cement. Some designs also have a porous-coated extramedullary flange for osseous ingrowth. To date, all-cementless fixation has not yet been developed for TEA.[29,33]

Operative Overview

The following is a brief overview of typical elements involved in a TEA.[29,3,34,46,61,73,76] A longitudinal incision is made at the posterior aspect of the elbow, either slightly lateral or medial to the olecranon process. The ulnar nerve is isolated, temporarily displaced, and protected throughout the procedure. The distal attachment of the triceps is detached and reflected laterally with a *triceps-reflecting approach* or split longitudinally and retracted along the midline with a *triceps-splitting approach*.[29,34,76] The more recently developed *triceps-sparing (triceps-preserving) approach* is also an option. It involves incisions on the medial and lateral aspects of the elbow joint. This approach preserves the attachment of the triceps tendon on the olecranon but makes insertion of the implants more technically challenging.[9,46]

As the procedure progresses, ligaments and other soft tissues are released as necessary; the posterior aspect of the capsule is incised and retracted and the joint is dislocated. In preparation for the implants, small portions of the distal humerus and proximal ulna are resected. Depending on the status of the radial head, the integrity of the collateral ligaments, and the design of the prosthesis, the head of the radius may or may not be excised. Then the intramedullary canals of the humerus and ulna and possibly the radius are prepared, and trial components are inserted. The available ROM and stability of the prosthetic joint are checked intraoperatively and x-rays are taken to confirm proper alignment of the implants. The components are then cemented in place, and the capsule and any ligaments that had ruptured prior to surgery or were released during the procedure are repaired to the extent possible or necessary based on the design of the prosthesis and the quality of the structures. If detached or split, the extensor mechanism is securely reattached or meticulously repaired. Following possible anterior transposition and careful placement of the ulnar nerve in a subcutaneous pocket, the incision is closed, and a sterile compressive dressing and posterior and/or anterior orthosis are applied to immobilize the elbow and forearm. The arm is elevated to control peripheral edema.[29]

Complications

Although the incidence of complications has declined steadily over the past few decades as selection of patients, prosthetic design, and surgical technique have improved, complications after TEA continue to occur more frequently than after total hip, knee, or shoulder arthroplasty.[56,108]

FOCUS ON EVIDENCE

In the mid-1990s, a comprehensive review of the literature indicated that the overall rates of complications following TEA ranged from 20% to 45%. A recent systematic review of the results of subsequent studies (published from 1993 to 2009), however, indicated that the mean overall rate of complications after contemporary, primary TEA (semiconstrained and nonconstrained designs) was 24.3% (± 5.8%).[108]

Complications are categorized as intraoperative and postoperative—early or late (before or after 6 weeks).[85]

Intraoperative complications. Intraoperative complications, such as fracture and component malpositioning, can significantly affect short- and long-term outcomes. Ulnar nerve damage or irritation, either transient or permanent, can also occur intraoperatively from handling or during the early weeks after surgery from compression,[9,56,85,108] typically causing paresthesia but not weakness.[97]

Postoperative complications. Deep infection, a concern after any surgery, is reported to occur in an average of 3.3% (± 2.9%) of cases following current-day TEA.[56,108] This rate is higher for TEA than large joint arthroplasties, owing to the thin layer of soft tissues covering the elbow joint and because the majority of patients undergoing TEA have inflammatory arthritis and a compromised immune system due to medication.[56,97,108]

Other postoperative complications, including joint instability, wound healing problems, and triceps insufficiency, are of particular concern during the early and intermediate phases of rehabilitation. Despite continuing improvements in implant design and fixation and surgical techniques, some complications develop several months or even years after surgery. These complications include aseptic (biomechanical) loosening of the prosthetic implants over time at the bone-cement interface (the most common long-term complication and reason for revision arthroplasty), periprosthetic fracture, and mechanical failure or premature wear of the components.[9,43,46,56,108]

It is important for a therapist to be familiar with the incidence and possible causes of complications after TEA in order to effectively structure and progress a postoperative rehabilitation program that decreases at least some of the risk factors associated with these complications. The incidence and characteristics of selected postoperative complications (joint instability, triceps insufficiency, prosthetic loosening) after TEA and factors that contribute to these complications are summarized in Box 18.4.[9,85,97,108] Precautions to reduce the risk of these and other complications are addressed in the following section on postoperative management.

Postoperative Management

The overall goal of rehabilitation after TEA is to achieve pain-free ROM of the elbow joints as well as strength of the upper extremity sufficient for functional activities while minimizing the risk of early or late postoperative complications. This goal is best achieved with an individualized rehabilitation program based on a thorough examination of each patient's postoperative status.

Immobilization

As noted previously, a soft compression dressing is applied at the close of surgery. A well-padded anterior, posterior, or hinged orthosis is used to immobilize the elbow and maintain stability and protect structures as they heal. Recommendations for the positions and duration of immobilization vary.

Position. The position of immobilization is based on a number of factors, including the surgical approach, the implant design, and which soft tissues were repaired and require protection.[7,29,34] If, for example, a triceps-reflecting approach was used for a linked TEA, full or almost full elbow extension and a neutral position of the forearm typically will be selected to protect the reattached triceps tendon.[7,29,34,51,73,77] In contrast, with an unlinked TEA, which typically requires repair of the lateral ligament complex, because of preoperative damage, or release for operative exposure of the joint, the position of immobilization is a moderate degree of flexion with limitation of full forearm supination to lessen stress on the repaired ligaments.[7,85] If a patient had a significant preoperative elbow flexion contracture that was surgically released, an anterior orthosis may be selected with the elbow placed in the available amount of extension. An extended position is also indicated if symptoms of ulnar neuropathy are present to alleviate pressure in the cubital tunnel.[9,77,85]

Duration. The period of continuous immobilization after surgery, which is kept as short as possible to avoid stiffness, also varies widely, ranging from 1 to 2 days to several weeks (in patients who are immunosuppressed or have RA with thin, friable skin).[29] This time period depends on the design of the prosthesis, the surgical approach, the integrity of ligamentous structures, intraoperative observations by the surgeon, and the integrity of the skin and subsequent wound healing. In general, unlinked/resurfacing designs, which have little inherent stability, require a longer period of immobilization than linked/semiconstrained designs.[9]

If there is increased risk of delayed wound healing because of poor skin quality or a patient's history of diabetes, smoking, or use of steroids, the elbow may be continuously maintained in extension for 10 to 14 days postoperatively to limit stress on the posterior incision.[3,77,85] Even after it is permissible to remove the orthosis for exercise or self-care, the patient is advised to continue to wear the orthosis at night for protection for up to 6 weeks.[7,29,51] If there was a preoperative flexion contracture, an adjustable orthosis that maintains the elbow in extension is worn periodically during the day for a prolonged stretch and a static (resting) orthosis is worn at night to hold the arm in a comfortably extended position. This regimen may be followed for 8 to 12 weeks postoperatively to prevent recurrence of the contracture.[29,51,73,77]

BOX 18.4 Analysis of Three Potential Complications After Total Elbow Arthroplasty

Joint Instability

- *Incidence.* One of the more common complications after TEA; predominantly a problem in unlinked arthroplasty;[9,56,108] overall rate of dislocation and symptomatic instability of contemporary TEA, an average of 3.3% (± 2.9%).[108]
  - Higher incidence with prior radial head resection.
  - Higher rate in unlinked implants (reported at 4% to 15%, mean 8%)[61] than in linked implants (reported at 0% to 14%, mean 3.5%).[55]
- *Characteristics.* Early or late onset; associated with pain and loss of function.
  - Disruption of a repaired LCL complex → posterolateral, rotary, and varus instability; disruption of a repaired MCL complex → posteromedial and valgus instability.
  - Disruption of triceps mechanism → diminished dynamic compressive forces across the joint.
- *Contributing factors.* Excessive release or inadequate or failed soft tissue repair → deficient static or dynamic stabilizers (possibly due to inadequate postoperative immobilization and excessive postoperative stresses across the elbow, particularly during the early postoperative period before soft tissue repairs have healed), malpositioning of implants, and long-term polyethylene wear of the ulnar component increase the risk of instability.[9,61,85]

Triceps Insufficiency

- *Incidence.* Primarily occurs after surgical approaches that disrupt the triceps mechanism; occurs in both linked and unlinked arthroplasty, usually during the first postoperative year.[97] Examples of rates of occurrence reported in separate retrospective studies: 1.8% of 887 elbows,[24] and 11% of 28 elbows,[55] and 2.4% (± 2.4%) of 2,938 elbows reported in a recent systematic literature review of contemporary TEA.[108]
  - Higher overall risk in patients with previous elbow surgery before TEA.[24]
- *Characteristics.* Partial or complete rupture, or avulsion, of the extensor mechanism (during the early or late postoperative period), weakness (particularly in terminal extension), often posterior elbow pain, and difficulty with pushing activities and overhead functions, such as combing one's hair.
- *Contributing factors.* Occasionally postoperative trauma but most commonly a failed surgical reattachment or repair of a poor quality tendon; premature or excessive ROM or loads on the extensor mechanism during early rehabilitation or during long-term functional use of the arm.[61]

Implant Loosening

- *Incidence.* The most common postoperative complication, occurring in linked (semiconstrained) more than unlinked (nonconstrained) implants. Overall rates are lower with contemporary TEA designs (mean, 5.1%, ± 3.4%)[56,108] than earlier designs but remain higher than after hip, knee, and shoulder arthroplasty.[85] The more constrained the design, the greater the risk of loosening.
  - Rate of clinical loosening reported in individual studies of contemporary implants up to a 6-year follow-up has been reported to range from 0% to 6%.[55,77]
  - Rates of 0% to 3% reported in patients with RA over a mean follow-up of 3.8 years[56,77] and in patients with posttraumatic arthritis with a mean follow-up of 5 years.
  - The incidence of radiological loosening is consistently higher than clinical loosening (when the patient becomes symptomatic).
- *Characteristics.* Aseptic (biomechanical) loosening, a late complication, occurs at the bone-cement interface typically of the ulnar component;[46,56] clinical loosening is associated with pain. Excludes loosening caused by infection.[9,56]
- *Contributing factors.* Inadequate cementing technique, implant malpositioning, and lack of adherence to postoperative activity modification. High-load, high-impact activities place patient at higher risk of loosening.

Exercise Progression

The progression of a postoperative exercise program after TEA varies considerably based on many factors. Key factors and their impact on postoperative rehabilitation are identified in Table 18.2.[7,34,110] The rehabilitation process proceeds most rapidly when a triceps-sparing approach is used to insert a linked replacement in a patient whose incision is healing well. On the other end of the spectrum, in which rehabilitation must progress more cautiously, is the use of a triceps-reflecting approach for an unlinked replacement, requiring release and repair of the lateral ligament complex in a patient with poor skin quality.

Just as the progression of exercise is based on the unique features of each patient's surgery, precautions are determined in a similar manner. It is particularly important for the therapist to know the status of repaired soft tissues to incorporate the necessary precautions into the exercise program. Information in the operative report and close communication with the surgeon are the best sources for these details. Specific precautions for exercise and functional use of the operated upper extremity are summarized in Box 18.5.[7,14,73,97,110] Patient education about these precautions should occur throughout the rehabilitation program. A patient's adherence to precautions ensures more positive outcomes and lessens the likelihood of short- or long-term postoperative complications related to exercise and use of the operated arm for functional activities.

Exercise: Maximum Protection Phase

The focus during the first phase of rehabilitation, which extends approximately over a 4-week period, includes control of inflammation, pain, and edema with use of medication as needed, application of cold, and regular elevation of the postsurgical arm. Emphasis is also placed on careful inspection of the wound, protection of repaired soft tissues as they begin to heal, and early ROM exercises to offset the adverse effects of immobilization without jeopardizing the stability of the

TABLE 18.2 Factors That Influence the Progression of Exercise After Total Elbow Arthroplasty

Factors	Impact on Rehabilitation
▪ Design of prosthesis: linked/semiconstrained vs. unlinked/resurfacing	▪ Earlier ROM and use of the operated upper extremity for light ADL with linked/semiconstrained replacements, which typically do not require ligament repair for joint stability ▪ More protected, controlled motion during exercise and delayed use for ADLs with unlinked/resurfacing replacements, which typically require repair of supporting ligaments for stability
▪ Surgical approach: triceps-sparing vs. triceps-splitting or triceps-reflecting	▪ Initial postoperative ROM permissible through a greater range of flexion and earlier active antigravity elbow extension, low-load resistance exercise, and light ADL with triceps-sparing approach
▪ Preoperative and postoperative status of supporting ligaments of the elbow	▪ Earlier and less protected motion during exercise, less protected use during ADs, and less time in orthosis during the day and at night if ligaments were intact preoperatively and did not undergo a release and/or repair during arthroplasty
▪ Wound healing	▪ Longer duration of immobilization of the elbow in an extension orthosis or delayed end-range flexion if posterior skin quality is poor and healing of the incision is delayed
▪ Ulnar neuropathy	▪ May require immobilization in an extension orthosis or delay of exercises to regain elbow flexion
▪ Surgical release of a preoperative elbow flexion contracture	▪ May require use of extension orthosis at night

BOX 18.5 Specific Precautions After Total Elbow Arthroplasty

ROM Exercise

- Perform ROM exercises only within the arc of motion achieved during surgery.
- To reduce postoperative stress on a repaired triceps mechanism, avoid end-range flexion during assisted ROM and active, antigravity elbow extension for 3 to 4 weeks.
- Also avoid early, end-range elbow flexion to decrease stress on the incision and reduce the risk of compromising wound healing.
- If elbow stability is questionable after an unlinked total elbow arthroplasty, limit full extension of the elbow and rotation of the forearm, particularly supination past neutral, to avoid overload on repaired lateral ligaments for 4 weeks. With an unlinked replacement, the greatest risk of instability is when the elbow is extended beyond 40° to 50°.[7]
- If symptoms of ulnar nerve compression are noted, avoid prolonged positioning or stretching into end-range flexion.

Strengthening Exercises

- Postpone resisted elbow extension for 6 weeks (or as long as 12 weeks) if a triceps-reflecting approach was used.
- When strengthening the shoulder, apply resistance above the elbow to eliminate stresses across the elbow joint.
- Weight training using moderate and high-loads is not appropriate after total elbow arthroplasty.

Functional Activities

- Avoid lifting or carrying any objects with the operated extremity for 6 weeks or objects greater than 1 lb for 3 months.
- If the triceps mechanism was detached and repaired, avoid pushing motions, including propelling a wheelchair; pushing up from a chair; and using a walker, crutches (other than forearm platform design), or a cane for at least 6 weeks or as long as 3 months.
- If an unlinked replacement was implanted, do not lift weighted objects during daily tasks with the elbow extended to avoid shear forces across the lateral ligament repair, which could contribute to posterolateral instability.
- Limit repetitive lifting to 1 lb for the first 3 months, 2 lb for the first 6 months, and no more than 5 lb thereafter. Never lift more than 10 to 15 lb in a single lift.[7,34,61]
- Do not participate in recreational activities, such as golf, volleyball, and racquet sports, that place high-loads or impact across the elbow.

prosthetic joint. Assisted ROM as tolerated and within the ranges achieved intraoperatively is typically initiated 2 to 3 days after linked TEA and a few days later after unlinked TEA if the elbow is stable.[7,29,37]

CLINICAL TIP

If there was significant preoperative instability of the elbow or if the repair of ligaments released during surgery is in question, elbow ROM typically is delayed for 7 to 10 days. When motion is initiated, the patient may need to wear a hinged orthosis for 4 to 5 weeks that allows only flexion and extension and restricts rotation of the forearm.[7,14,37]

Goals and interventions. The goals and exercise interventions during this first phase include the following:[7,14,37,51,61,73,77]

- ***Maintain mobility of the shoulder, wrist, and hand.***
  - Active ROM of these regions during the immediate postoperative period. This is particularly important for the patient with RA or JRA involving these joints.
- ***Regain motion of the elbow and forearm.***
  - After a linked TEA or if the elbow is stable after an unlinked TEA, start with gentle self-assisted elbow flexion/extension and pronation/supination with the elbow comfortably flexed and the forearm in mid-position, progressing to active ROM as tolerated. As acute symptoms subside, have the patient maintain the end-range position to apply a very low-intensity stretch.
  - If the triceps mechanism was reflected and repaired, limit assisted flexion to 90° to 100° for the first 3 to 4 weeks to avoid excessive stretch on the repaired triceps tendon. Perform active elbow flexion/extension in a seated or standing—rather than supine—position for the same time frame to avoid antigravity extension, which also could cause excessive stress to the reattached triceps mechanism and subsequent insufficiency.[7] While sitting and standing, elbow extension is a gravity-assist extension and is controlled by an eccentric contraction of the elbow flexors.
  - If a linked replacement was implanted using a triceps-sparing approach, there is little to no risk of early postoperative instability or disruption of the triceps mechanism. Therefore, active ROM in all planes of motion is permissible immediately.

NOTE: Some sources recommend after linked arthroplasty involving a triceps-reflecting approach—and if secure reattachment of the triceps tendon was achieved—that ROM exercises progress as tolerated without restriction.[14,29,77]

- ***Minimize atrophy of upper extremity musculature.***
  - Gentle, pain-free muscle-setting exercises of elbow musculature (against no resistance) while in the orthosis and later, multiple-angle setting exercises when the orthosis can be removed.
  - Low-intensity, isometric resistance exercises of the shoulder, wrist, and hand.
  - Use of the hand for light functional activities as early as 1 to 2 weeks postoperatively if a linked replacement was inserted but several weeks later after an unlinked TEA.[14,29,37,73,77]

Exercise: Moderate and Minimum Protection Phases

By about 4 to 6 weeks postoperatively, soft tissues have healed sufficiently to withstand increasing stresses. By 12 weeks, barring complications, only minimum protection is necessary; therefore, a patient typically can resume most functional activities with some imposed restrictions (see Box 18.6). However, the recommended timeline for return to a reasonably full level of activity with ongoing lifting restrictions varies from 6 weeks[34,61,73] to 3 to 4 months.[7,14,29]

Goals and interventions. The focus of rehabilitation during the intermediate and final phases is to improve ROM to the extent achieved intraoperatively, regain strength and endurance of elbow musculature, and use of the operated arm for functional activities with a permanent lifting restriction of 5 pounds.[14,29] However, these goals must be reached without disrupting repaired soft tissues or compromising the stability of the elbow prosthesis. Strength and muscular endurance usually continue to improve up to 6 to 12 months postoperatively by cautious use of the operated arm for functional activities.

Patient education, especially with regard to the resumption of functional activities, is ongoing until the patient is discharged from therapy. The following goals and interventions are added during the moderate and minimum protection phases of rehabilitation.[7]

- ***Increase ROM of the elbow.***

NOTE: It is the opinion of the authors that use of joint mobilization techniques to increase ROM of the elbow or forearm is inappropriate after TEA, particularly with linked implants and/or if the stability of the elbow is questionable. It is a more prudent choice to forego full elbow motion than to jeopardize the stability of the joint.

- Low-intensity, manual self-stretching.
- Low-load, long-duration static dynamic orthotic intervention,[104] as described and illustrated in Chapter 4 (see Fig. 4.13), or alternating use of static orthoses, fabricated in maximum but comfortable extension primarily at night.[29]

PRECAUTIONS: Emphasize end-range extension before end-range flexion to protect the posterior capsule and the triceps mechanism. If symptoms of cubital tunnel syndrome are present (aching along the ulnar forearm and hand, paresthesia, or hyperesthesia due to compression or entrapment of the ulnar nerve), avoid prolonged or repeated end-range positioning or stretching to increase elbow flexion.[3,14,18]

- ***Regain functional strength and muscular endurance of the operated extremity.***

NOTE: Some sources advocate progressive use of the postsurgical upper extremity to regain strength and muscular endurance rather than an exercise program.[61,73,77]

- Resisted, multiple-angle isometric exercises at 5 weeks if not initiated previously.
- *Light* ADLs (initially <1 lb of weight) performed with the arm positioned along the side of the trunk and the elbow flexed. If a triceps-reflecting approach was used, incorporate activities that require elbow flexion, such as eating, drinking or brushing teeth, before elbow extension. Initially modify activities to avoid those that require lifting with the elbow extended and pushing motions, such as pushing up from a chair or using a walker, axillary crutches, or a cane.
- Dynamic, open-chain resistance exercises no earlier than 6 weeks and often later using a light-weight (1 lb) or light-grade elastic resistance. Emphasize gradually increasing repetitions rather than resistance.
- Repetitive lifting during exercise and functional activities limited to 1 lb for the first 3 months and 2 lb for the next 3 months. Permanently limit repetitive lifting to no more than 5 lb and a single lift to no more than 10 to 15 lb.[7,14,29,34,61] (See Box 18.5 for additional restrictions to strengthening exercises and functional activities.)
- Low-load, closed-chain activities, such as wall push-ups, after 6 weeks or later (when the triceps mechanism and posterior capsule have healed).

CONTRAINDICATIONS: High-load progressive resistive exercise (PRE), heavy lifting during home- and work-related activities, and recreational activities that place high-loads or impact on the upper extremities (e.g., racquet and throwing sports or golf) are not allowed after TEA. These activities must be permanently avoided to reduce the risk of complications, such as elbow instability, implant loosening, and polyethylene wear.[28,37,56,59,61,108]

Outcomes

Although the results of the early use of TEA during the 1970s were unsatisfactory, improvements in prosthetic design and fixation, surgical techniques, postoperative management, and criteria for patient selection have made this procedure a reliable means for relieving pain, restoring joint stability, improving physical function and regaining patient participation.

The outcomes of TEA and postoperative rehabilitation typically are assessed by a combination of patient self-report instruments that address pain relief, function, and quality of life (e.g., the Patient Related Elbow Evaluation form or the Disabilities of the Arm, Shoulder, and Hand [DASH] questionnaire), and physician-administered tools (e.g., the American Shoulder and Elbow Surgeons Questionnaire or the Mayo Elbow Performance Score, which also include measurements of ROM, strength, and specific shoulder and elbow functions).[6,56,88,91]

Because of the variety of tools used, direct comparison among studies is often difficult.

Pain relief and patient satisfaction. Complete or nearly complete relief of pain is the most consistently positive and predictable outcome after elbow arthroplasty, occurring in more than 85% to 95% of patients.[29,91]

As noted at the beginning of this discussion on TEA, although the indications have broadened over the past four decades, elbow arthroplasty continues to be used most frequently in patients with RA followed by patients with posttraumatic arthritis. Follow-up studies of patients with these and other underlying pathologies who have undergone linked or unlinked TEA indicate an overall high rate of patient satisfaction, with 80% to 100% of patients reporting "good" or "excellent" results after linked[25,48,55,91] and unlinked[34,61,88,91] TEA.

ROM and functional use of the upper extremity. Improvements in elbow ROM after TEA have improved along with the improvements in implants and surgical techniques, although decreasing pain and maintaining stability of the prosthetic elbow postoperatively are a higher priority than gaining full ROM. Results of most studies of linked[48,55,91] and unlinked[57,91] arthroplasty indicate an increase in the arc of elbow extension/flexion and forearm rotation in patients with late-stage posttraumatic arthritis, RA, and JRA. Anecdotal evidence suggests that most gains are achieved within 6 to 12 weeks but occasionally up to 6 months postoperatively. Patients with little active movement of the elbow because of preoperative instability have exhibited marked improvement of active motion postoperatively. Examples of the arc of extension/flexion achieved after TEA are 15° to 133°,[37,50] 19° to 140°,[55] 22° to 135°,[27] and 28° to 131°, with pronation/supination of 68° and 62°, respectively.[48] Remember that arcs of 100° (from 30° to 130° of extension/flexion and 50° each of pronation/supination) are necessary for most functional activities.[78] Therefore, in all of these studies, functional ROM for extension and flexion was achieved.

It is important to note that when reviewing the literature for this summary of outcomes, there were no studies that compared outcomes after different approaches to rehabilitation.

TEA survival rates. "Survival rate" (the point at which revision arthroplasty is necessary) following current-day TEA appears to depend more on a patient's underlying pathology than on the type of prostheses implanted.[46] Relatively recent long-term studies of patients with RA, for example, have indicated that the survival rate of implants is 90% to 92% at a mean of 5 years[43,55,91] and 86% at a minimum of 10 years[43,48,91] after linked (semiconstrained) arthroplasty and after unlinked arthroplasty. Overall prosthetic survivorship rates tend to be lower and the risk of revision arthroplasty higher in patients with posttraumatic arthritis or primary osteoarthritis than in patients with RA. This may be because of generally higher activity levels—and therefore, greater loads placed across the elbow—in those with posttraumatic arthritis than in those with inflammatory disease.[43,108]

There is general consensus that for the best long-term results, a patient must be selective in the type of work-related or recreational activities performed, modifying some activities and eliminating those that impose high-loads and high impact on the elbow.

As with all types of total joint arthroplasty, TEA survival rates deteriorate over time regardless of underlying pathology, type of implant, and the extent of stress placed on the elbow.[43]

Myositis Ossificans

The terms *myositis ossificans* and *heterotopic ossification* (HO) or *ectopic bone formation* are often used interchangeably to describe the formation of bone in atypical locations of the body.[70] Some resources use the term myositis ossificans to denote only ossification of muscle. More often, the term is used generally to characterize HO or bone formation in the muscle-tendon unit, capsule, or ligamentous structures. In this text, the terms myositis ossificans and heterotopic ossification are used synonymously.

Etiology of Symptoms

The prevalence of HO following elbow fracture has been reported to be as high as 40% and is most commonly located at the posteromedial aspect of the elbow.[94] HO may develop after a comminuted fracture of the radial head, a fracture-dislocation (supracondylar or radial head fracture) of the elbow, or a tear of the brachialis tendon.[53,70,81,94] Patients with concurrent traumatic brain injury or spinal cord injury, or patients with burns to the extremities, have a much higher risk in developing this complication.[53,70,81,94] Additional risk factors for developing HO include delayed internal fixation and use of bone graft and/or bone-graft substitute. More severe HO is associated with concomitant distal humeral fracture, triad injury, and elbow fracture-dislocation. Delay in intervention increases the risk of HO.[81,94] While some believe that too much motion or aggressive stretching following injury exacerbates HO, others believe that HO occurs due to a lack of motion. There is no evidence or consensus to indicate that overstretching or participation in physical therapy contributes to HO.[94]

Clinical presentation of HO involves a restriction of joint motion after an inciting trauma. Palpation of a locking sensation at terminal extension or flexion is also an indication of HO rather than of joint contracture.[94] Heterotopic ossification begins approximately 2 weeks after the injury, and the patient often presents with swelling, warmth, and pain. As the process continues, the warmth, erythema, and swelling will gradually resolve, which may be accompanied by a gradual loss of elbow motion.[70] Palpation of the distal brachialis muscle is tender. After the acute inflammatory period, heterotopic bone formation is laid down in muscle between, not within, individual muscle fibers or around the joint capsule within a 2- to 4-week period. This makes the muscle extremely firm to touch. Although this condition can permanently restrict elbow motion, in most cases, the heterotopic bone is largely reabsorbed over several months and motion usually returns to near normal.[70]

Management

Prophylaxis use of NSAIDs should be considered for those at high risk for developing HO. If there are gastrointestinal contraindications, radiation therapy may also be considered. Surgical excision may be considered when the HO is symptomatic and/or restricts the functional arc of motion at the elbow, especially if it interferes with the patient's activities or ability to participate. When considering surgical intervention a risk-benefit ratio must be considered.[70,81] If treated operatively, the elbow is frequently managed with continuous passive motion and a hinged adjustable orthoses. Passive stretching should be introduced with extreme caution in the inflamed, posttraumatic, and/or postsurgical elbow when ROM is initiated to avoid exacerbating the inflammation, which may result in elbow contracture.[69]

Overuse Syndromes: Repetitive Trauma Syndromes

Overuse can occur in any musculotendinous structure in the elbow region, including the flexors and extensors of the elbow; however, it most commonly occurs in the muscles attached to the lateral or medial epicondyles in response to repetitive stressful forearm and wrist motions. Current evidence has shown that the traditional terms, *tendinitis* or *epicondylitis*, do not accurately reflect the true pathology of these conditions. The evidence has demonstrated that these conditions are degenerative in nature and do not reflect an inflammatory process as indicated by a lack of inflammatory cells, but rather involve dysfunctional vascular and fibrous tissue and disorganized collagen.[39,40,83] The terms *tendinosis* and *tendinopathy* refer to the degenerative changes in the tendon tissue, which includes immature fibroblastic and vascular elements, resulting in weakening of the tendinous structure.[38-40,83,105]

Related Pathologies

Lateral Elbow Tendinopathy (Tennis Elbow)

Tennis elbow is commonly referred to as lateral epicondylitis (despite current literature), lateral epicondylalgia, lateral epicondylosis, or lateral elbow tendinopathy.[100,105] Symptoms include pain over the lateral epicondyle of the humerus, primarily with gripping activities. Activities requiring firm wrist stability, such as the backhand stroke in tennis, or repetitive work tasks that require repeated wrist extension, such as computer work or pulling weeds in a garden, can stress the musculotendinous unit and cause symptoms. The primary structure involved is the origin of the extensor carpi radialis brevis muscle,[38,73,105] although the extensor digitorum is also involved in approximately 50% of patients.[83]

Positive tests of provocation include palpation tenderness on or near the lateral epicondyle, pain with resisted wrist extension performed with the elbow extended, pain with resisted middle finger extension, and pain with passive wrist flexion with the elbow extended and forearm pronated.[39,63]

NOTE: Pulled elbow, pushed elbow, radial head arthritis, radial head fracture, pinched synovial fringe, radial tunnel syndrome, cervical root compression, and periosteal bruise are also possible sources of lateral elbow pain and are sometimes inaccurately diagnosed as tennis elbow.[16,83]

Medial Elbow Tendinopathy (Golfer's Elbow)

Golfer's elbow, also known as medial epicondylitis, medial epicondylalgia, or medial epicondylosis, involves the common flexor/pronator tendon at the tenoperiosteal junction near the medial epicondyle. It is associated with repetitive movements into wrist flexion, such as swinging a golf club, pitching a ball, or work-related grasping and lifting heavy objects. Concomitant ulnar neuropathy may be an associated finding.[5,83]

Positive tests of provocation include palpation tenderness on or near the medial epicondyle, pain with resisted wrist flexion performed with the elbow extended, and pain with passive wrist extension performed with the elbow extended.

Etiology of Symptoms

The most common cause of medial or lateral epicondylalgia is excessive repetitive use or eccentric strain of the wrist or forearm muscles. The result is micro damage and partial tears, usually near the musculotendinous junction when the strain exceeds the strength of the tissues and when the demand exceeds the repair process. With repetitive trauma, fibroblastic activity and collagen weakening occurs. Recurring problems are seen because the resulting immobile or immature scar is redamaged when returning to activities before there is sufficient healing or mobility in the surrounding tissue.

Mechanical nerve pain hypersensitivity over the radial and ulnar nerves and their nerve trunks has been reported in patients with medial and lateral epicondylalgia. These findings suggest the presence of central and peripheral sensitization mechanisms in this patient population.[16,32,41,42,59,83]

Common Impairments of Structure and Function

- Gradually increasing pain in the elbow region after excessive activity of the wrist and hand
- Pain when the involved muscle is stretched or when it contracts against resistance
- Decreased muscle strength and endurance for the demand
- Decreased grip strength, limited by pain
- Proximal weakness of shoulder and scapular musculature
- Decreased mobility of the lower cervical and upper thoracic spine
- Tenderness with palpation over the lateral or medial epicondyle or tendon origin

Common Activity Limitations and Participation Restrictions

- Inability to participate in provoking activities, such as racket sports, throwing, or golf.
- Difficulty with repetitive forearm/wrist tasks, such as sorting or assembling small parts, typing on a keyboard or using a computer mouse, gripping activities, using a hammer, turning a screwdriver, shuffling papers, or playing a percussion instrument.

Nonoperative Management of Overuse Syndromes: Protection Phase

Decrease Pain

- ***Immobilization.*** Rest the muscles by immobilizing the wrist at night in an orthosis such as a wrist extension or "cock-up" orthosis.[19,20]
- ***Pain reduction.*** Use of a counterforce brace (nonarticular, proximal forearm orthosis) has demonstrated a decrease in pain and increased pain-free grip strength and function by reducing force transmission to the common tendon.[19,47,52,83,96,111]
- ***Patient instruction.*** Instruct the patient in "relative rest"—that is, to keep moving and using that arm but to avoid aggravating activities such as strong or repetitive gripping actions.[39,83]
- ***Cryotherapy.*** Use ice to help manage pain.[64]

Develop Soft Tissue and Joint Mobility

- ***Cross-friction massage.*** Apply cross-friction massage at the site of the lesion. For lateral elbow tendinopathy, find the proximal tendon of the ECRB by locating the radial head, slide dorsally around the radial head, and dive deep into the soft tissue adjacent to the radial head. Ensure you are on the correct tendon by having the patient lift the middle finger. Teach the patient cross-friction massage techniques in a home exercise program.[54,80]

- ***Neuromobilization.*** If increased symptoms occur with upper limb neurodynamic testing, use neuromobilization techniques as described in Chapter 13.
- ***Soft-tissue mobilization.*** Apply soft tissue mobilization to the wrist extensors or flexors to decrease soft tissue tightness and trigger points commonly associated with lateral and medial elbow tendinopathy.
- ***Muscle mobility techniques.*** Apply gentle hold-relax techniques to either the wrist extensor or flexor muscles (see Chapter 6). Begin with the respective muscles in the shortened position with the elbow flexed and wrist either in extension (for wrist extensor technique) or flexion (for the wrist flexor technique). Repeat the gentle resistance for five to six contractions then move the wrist toward neutral and repeat the contractions. Continue to progress the range of wrist motion without going into the painful range. Once gentle contractions in the full range of wrist motion are possible without pain, progress to lengthening the muscle across the elbow by increasing elbow extension. This progression may take several weeks. Follow the gentle hold-relax techniques with pain-free passive stretching as described in the following bullet.
- ***Passive stretching.*** Use gentle pain-free passive stretching techniques to elongate tight muscles. Hold stretches at least 20 to 30 seconds. Educate your patients that it is better to do fewer repetitions and hold them a full 20 to 30 seconds, then to perform short, quick stretches.
  - *To stretch the wrist extensors*, extend the elbow, pronate the forearm, flex and ulnarly deviate the wrist, flex the fingers, and gently press on the back of the hand until a pain-free stretch is felt in the forearm.
  - *To stretch the wrist flexors*, extend the elbow, supinate the forearm, extend and radially deviate the wrist, extend the fingers, and gently press on the palm of the hand until a pain-free stretch is felt in the forearm.

Maintain Upper Extremity Function

- ***Active ROM.*** Have the patient perform ROM to all joints to maintain the integrity of the upper extremity.
- ***Resistive exercises.*** Have the patient perform shoulder and scapular stabilization exercises with resistance applied proximal to the elbow.[17,62]

Nonoperative Management: Controlled Motion and Return to Function Phases

Utilize the following management guidelines and interventions when pain has resolved.

Increase Muscle Flexibility

- ***Manual stretching techniques.*** Continue with passive stretching as described above. In addition, use agonist contract and hold-relax techniques to elongate the tight musculature at an intensity that causes a stretching sensation but does not increase pain (principles for application of these techniques are described in Chapter 4).
- ***Self-stretching techniques.*** The patient may use a wall (see Fig. 18.10) and slide the hand along the wall until a stretch force is experienced, or the patient may use the opposite hand to apply the stretch force. These techniques are described in the self-stretching section later in the chapter.
- ***Cross-fiber (friction) massage.*** Continue with this technique as described above.

Restore Joint Tracking at the RU Joint

- ***MWM.*** These pain-free techniques are used to correct a positional fault and to bring about immediate improvement in the patient's condition.[79] Several researchers have reported decreased pain and increased grip strength during or shortly after MWM at the elbow.[20,21,107] The following techniques are used if the patient experiences pain when making a fist or with resisted wrist extension. If immediate results do not occur, either the technique is not appropriate for the patient or the technique is not being done in the correct plane, grade, or direction of mobilization.[79]
  - *Patient position and procedure:* Supine with the forearm pronated, the elbow in slight flexion, and the shoulder in internal rotation. Place the mobilization belt around the patient's proximal forearm at the joint line and over your opposite shoulder facing toward the patient's feet. Stabilize the distal humerus with the proximal hand and utilize the other hand to either stabilize the wrist during a gripping motion or to provide resistance to wrist extension depending on the patient's comparable sign. Apply a gentle lateral sustained glide to the proximal forearm with the mobilization belt while the patient slowly extends their wrist 6-10 times. Build up to 3 sets of 10 repetitions. Apply pain-free resistance to wrist extension when tolerated. The lateral glide and the muscle contraction must be pain free (A).
  - *Alternative method:* Stabilize the distal humerus with the outside hand and apply gentle lateral glide of the proximal forearm with the inside hand. Have the patient slowly extend their wrist or squeeze a foam ball 6-10 times increasing to 3 sets of 10 as tolerated (Fig. 18.6 B). Both the lateral glide and the muscle contraction must be pain free. Add a light weight to provide resistance to wrist extension when tolerated.
- ***Self-MWM.*** The patient stands with the humerus of the involved elbow stabilized against a doorframe and the forearm in the opening. The elbow is positioned at 90° with the forearm in pronation and parallel to the floor. The patient applies a gentle lateral glide to the proximal forearm with the contralateral hand and then does slow, gentle gripping of a squeezable ball (Fig. 18.6 C).

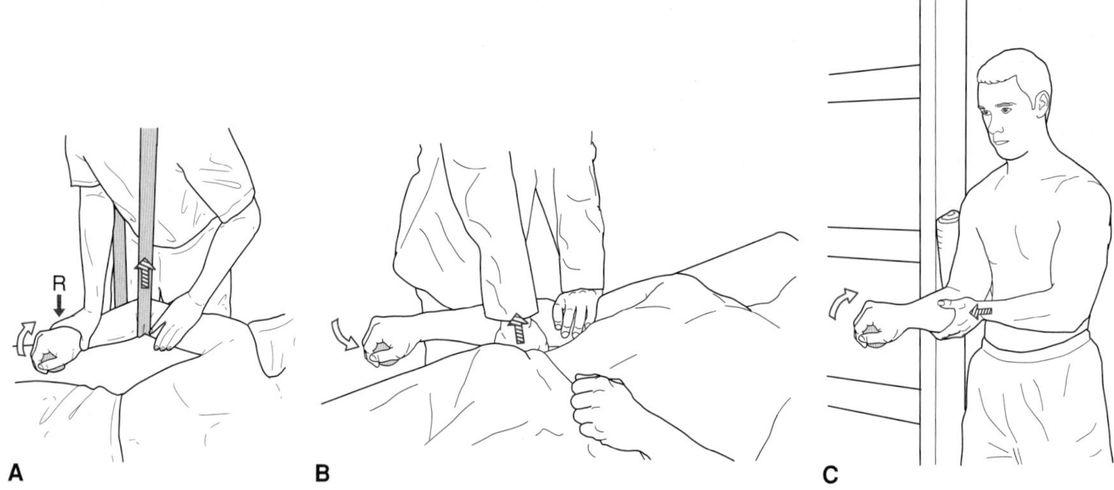

FIGURE 18.6 MWM for lateral epicondylosis. Lateral glide is applied to the proximal forearm **(A)** with active wrist extension, **(B)** with patient squeezing a ball, and **(C)** with self-mobilization.

Improve Muscle Performance and Function

- ***Counter force elbow sleeve or strap.*** Use an elbow orthosis to help reduce the load on the musculotendinous unit. This type of orthosis has been shown to have the immediate effect of improving pain-free grip strength in individuals with lateral epicondylosis.[47,52,96,111]
- ***Dynamic resistance exercise.*** Progress to dynamic exercises against manual or elastic resistance or free weights through pain-free ranges. Initially, use low-intensity resistance with multiple repetitions for muscular endurance, then progress to more intense resistance to strengthen the muscles in preparation for functional demands.
  - ***Eccentric training.*** Incorporate a progression of eccentric contractions of the involved musculotendinous unit, first within a comfortable wrist ROM against a low-intensity load, at a slow speed, and preferably with the elbow in a relatively extended position.[20,92,100,103] Use of an isokinetic dynamometer enables the patient to perform repetitive, eccentric-only contractions.[30] If elastic resistance or a free weight is used, have the patient lift the weight or lengthen the elastic band with the sound hand when returning to the starting position of wrist extension.[65]
  - ***Progressions.*** Progress to faster speeds before increasing the resistance. When resistance is increased, return to a slow speed and then again work up to a faster speed before increasing the resistance and so on. Gradually perform the eccentric contractions through a full, pain-free ROM.

FOCUS ON EVIDENCE

There is emerging evidence and moderate research support that suggests eccentric resistance training (typically combined with a program of static stretching) is effective in the treatment of lateral epicondylosis and weak evidence for the use of isokinetic and isometric exercise.[92]

Theoretical rationale suggests that progressive loading is indicated for increasing tensile strength and muscle endurance. A treatment approach that includes eccentric exercise performed in the range of 6 to 12 weeks with 3 sets of exercises consisting of 10 to 15 repetitions is effective in treating lateral epicondylosis and has the best current supporting evidence.[40,64,65,92,103]

- ***Functional patterns.*** As flexibility and strength improve and the pain is brought under control, incorporate functional training, utilizing functional patterns into the exercises. Emphasize control of the resistance through the pattern. If pain or deviation of the pattern with substitute motions occurs, have the patient rest before resuming additional repetitions. Exercises simulating the desired activity are progressed from slow, controlled motions to high speeds with low resistance to improve timing (see Fig. 18.22).
- ***General strengthening and conditioning.*** Incorporate any unused or underused part of the extremity or trunk into the training program prior to returning to the stressful activity.[38]
- ***Plyometric exercises.*** Add plyometrics to the program if the patient's goals include returning to sports or occupational activities that require elbow and forearm power. Suggestions include the following and are described and shown in Chapter 23.[38]
  - Dribbling a weighted ball against the wall or the floor
  - Flipping and catching a weighted ball
  - Bouncing a tennis ball on a short-handled racquet, progressing to a long-handled racquet
  - Rapid eccentric/concentric elbow and forearm motions against elastic resistance
  - Rapid chest passes or overhead passes using a weighted plyometric ball
- ***Activity modification.*** It may be necessary to modify the patient's activity or technique before he or she returns to the repetitive or stressful activity. For example, it may require taking tennis lessons to correct improper tennis techniques, adapting the use of a hammer or other equipment, or making ergonomic modifications of a computer workstation.[38,39,109]

NOTE: Information on ergonomic recommendations for computer workstations are described in Chapter 14.

Patient Education

- Education includes advice and techniques on prevention, recognition of provoking factors, and identification of warning symptoms.
- Teach the patient how to reduce the overload forces that caused the problem and retrain the patient in proper techniques.[38,39]
- In addition to exercises, include home instructions on the application of cross-friction massage and stretching the involved muscle prior to activity.

FOCUS ON EVIDENCE

In a descriptive study of 60 subjects with lateral epicondylalgia who were followed for 6 months after initiating physical therapy intervention, Waugh and associates[109] reported that 80% of the participants continued to improve, but only 33% had complete resolution of symptoms. The therapy intervention consisted of 8 weeks of ultrasound, deep transverse friction massage, and a stretching/strengthening program for the wrist extensor muscles; 37% of the participants also received treatment for the cervical spine or shoulder. Altogether, 50% continued with some form of therapeutic intervention after the initial 8 weeks. Those with poorer outcomes had repetitive work duties, with 92% of the repetitive duties involving computer work.

This study also reported that women who have positive cervical signs as well as repetitive job duties involving computer usage had a poorer prognosis. This was observed at both 8 weeks and 6 months. Ergonomic recommendations for postural adaptations when using a computer included having forearm support, smooth movements, and relaxed shoulders.[109]

Exercise Interventions for the Elbow and Forearm

Exercise Techniques to Increase Flexibility and Range of Motion

Prior to initiating a muscle stretching program, be sure the joint capsule is not restricting motion. Techniques to increase joint play in the elbow and forearm articulations are discussed earlier in the chapter. Principles and techniques for applying joint mobilization techniques are presented in Chapter 5.

In addition to the description of principles and techniques of stretching presented in Chapter 4, manual, mechanical, and self-stretching techniques directed to the elbow are described in this section. When teaching the patient self-stretching, emphasize the importance of maintaining a low-intensity, prolonged stretch and not applying a ballistic stretch force (bouncing at the end of the range).

Manual, Mechanical, and Self-Stretching Techniques

To Increase Elbow Extension

Mechanical Stretch: Mild Flexion Contracture

Patient position and procedure: Supine with the arm supported on the treatment table and a folded towel under the distal humerus as a fulcrum. Place a light cuff weight around the distal forearm. Position the forearm in pronation, midposition, and then supination to affect each of the three flexor muscles. Have the patient stabilize the proximal humerus with the other hand or place a sandbag or belt across the proximal humerus to stabilize it. Instruct the patient to maintain the stretch for an extended period of time.[10]

CLINICAL TIP

Of the three muscles that flex the elbow, only the biceps brachii crosses the shoulder; it also rotates the forearm. Therefore, to fully elongate the biceps brachii, the shoulder must be extended and forearm pronated in addition to extending the elbow.

Self-Stretch: Mild Flexion Contracture

Patient position and procedure: Sitting with arm supported on the treatment table and a folded towel under the distal humerus as a fulcrum. Using the opposite hand, have the patient apply the stretch force against the distal forearm positioned in pronation, midposition, and then supination to affect each of the flexor muscles.

Mechanical Stretch: Static Progressive Orthotic Intervention

Apply a low-intensity, long-duration mechanical stretch force with a static progressive orthosis to reduce a long-standing elbow flexion contracture by affecting the soft tissue properties of creep and stress-relaxation.[36,104]

FOCUS ON EVIDENCE

Ulrich and colleagues[104] carried out a prospective study to investigate the effectiveness of a patient-directed stretching program based on the principles of static progressive stretch and stress-relaxation (see Fig. 4.7 B) with 37 patients (37 elbows) with posttraumatic contractures of the elbow. Patients with any degree of heterotopic bone formation were excluded from the study. Patients performed a 30-minute stretching protocol one to three times per day in a static progressive elbow orthosis over a period of time (mean, 10 weeks; range, 2 to 25 weeks). The intensity of the stretch was controlled by the patient.

At the conclusion of the study, the mean gain in overall elbow ROM was significant (26°, range 2° to 60°), as were gains in range of elbow flexion and extension individually. Prior to the orthotic intervention program, overall elbow ROM was 81°, and it was 107° at the conclusion of the program. During the course of the study, overall patient satisfaction was good, and no patients required anti-inflammatory medication. The authors concluded that daily use of a static progressive orthosis and applying the principles of stress-relaxation over a relatively short period of time was an effective means of increasing elbow ROM.

Manual Stretch: Biceps Brachii

Patient position and procedure: Prone with the elbow in end-range but comfortable extension and forearm in pronation. Stabilize the scapula and passively extend the shoulder.

Mechanical Stretch: Biceps Brachii

Patient position and procedure: Supine with a light cuff weight around the distal forearm and the elbow in extension and forearm in pronation. Have the patient stabilize the proximal humerus with the opposite hand and then place the arm over the side of the table. Allow the elbow and shoulder to extend as far as possible and sustain the stretch position for an extended period of time (Fig. 18.7 A).

Self-Stretch: Biceps Brachii

Patient position and procedure: Standing at the side of a table. Have the patient grasp the edge of the table and walk forward, causing shoulder extension with elbow extension (Fig. 18.7 B). It is important to note that this stretching position does not include forearm pronation.

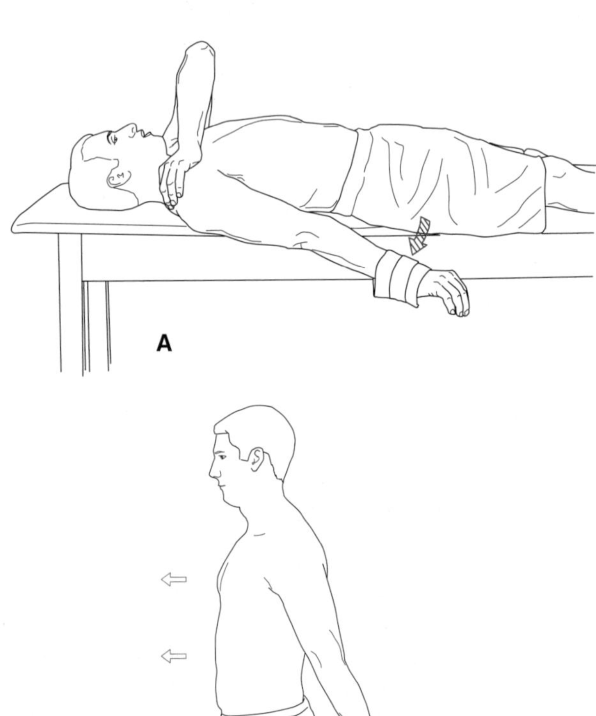

FIGURE 18.7 Self-stretching the biceps brachii musculotendinous unit includes stretching the long head across the shoulder joint **(A)** supine and **(B)** standing.

To Increase Elbow Flexion

Self-Stretch: Mild Extension Contracture

- *Patient position and procedure:* Prone-lying and propped up on elbows with forearms resting on the exercise mat. Have the patient lower the chest as far as elbow flexion allows and maintain the position as long as tolerated.
- *Patient position and procedure:* Sitting with elbow flexed as far as possible. Have the patient press against the distal forearm with the opposite hand to provide the stretch force into flexion. Alternatively, with the forearm supported on a table or arm rest of a chair, have the patient lean forward flexing the humerus against the stabilized forearm and maintaining the position as long as tolerated.

Self-Stretch: Long Head of Triceps

Patient position and procedure: Sitting or standing. Have the patient flex the elbow and shoulder as far as possible. The other hand can either push on the forearm to flex the elbow, or push the shoulder into more flexion (Fig. 18.8). Hold the stretch position as long as tolerated.

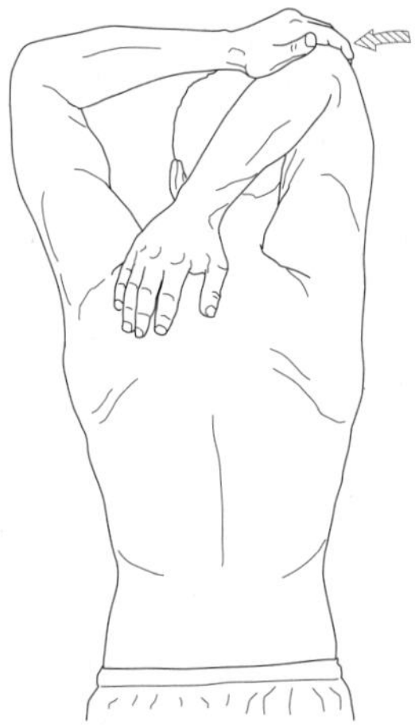

FIGURE 18.8 Self-stretching the triceps brachii musculotendinous unit includes stretching the long head across the shoulder joint.

To Increase Forearm Pronation and Supination

Patient position and procedure: Sitting with the elbow flexed to 90° stabilized against the side of the trunk or supported on a table. It is important to maintain the elbow position to prevent shoulder rotation.

Self-Stretch to Increase Pronation

Have the patient grasp the dorsal surface of the involved forearm so the heel of the uninvolved hand is against the dorsal aspect of the radius just proximal to the wrist and wrap the fingers around the ulna. Have the patient passively pronate the forearm and sustain the stretch as long as tolerated. The force is applied against the distal radius and not the carpals to avoid trauma to the wrist.

Self-Stretch to Increase Supination

Have the patient place the heel of the uninvolved hand against the volar aspect of the involved radius just proximal to the wrist, passively supinate the forearm, and sustain the stretch as long as tolerated. Be sure the force is applied against the radius, not the carpals to avoid trauma to the wrist (Fig. 18.9).

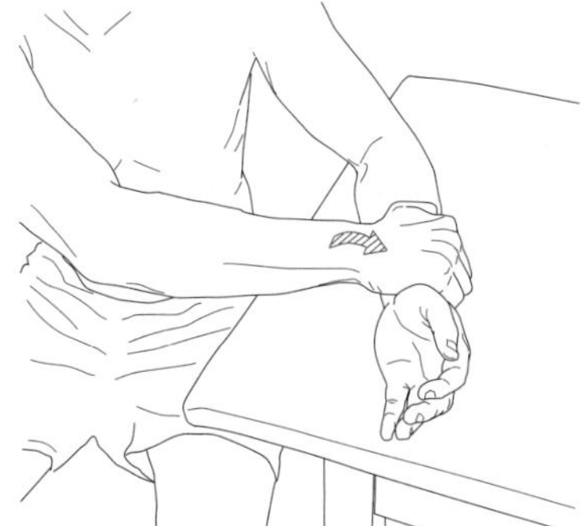

FIGURE 18.9 Self-stretching the forearm into supination. The forearm may be stabilized on a table (as pictured) or at the patient's side. It is important to maintain elbow flexion to prevent shoulder rotation and to apply the stretch force against the radius, not the hand.

Self-Stretching Techniques: Muscles of the Medial and Lateral Epicondyles

To Stretch the Wrist Extensor Muscles (From the Lateral Epicondyle)

- *Patient position and procedure:* Sitting or standing with the elbow extended and forearm pronated. While holding this position have the patient ulnarly deviate the wrist and flex the wrist and fingers; then apply a gentle stretch force against the dorsum of the hand. The patient should feel a stretching sensation along the dorsal surface of the forearm.
- *Patient position and procedure:* Standing with elbow extended, forearm pronated, and back of the hand against a wall (fingers pointing down). Have the patient then slide the back of the hand up the wall until a stretch is felt in the forearm (Fig. 18.10). For additional stretch, have the patient flex the fingers.

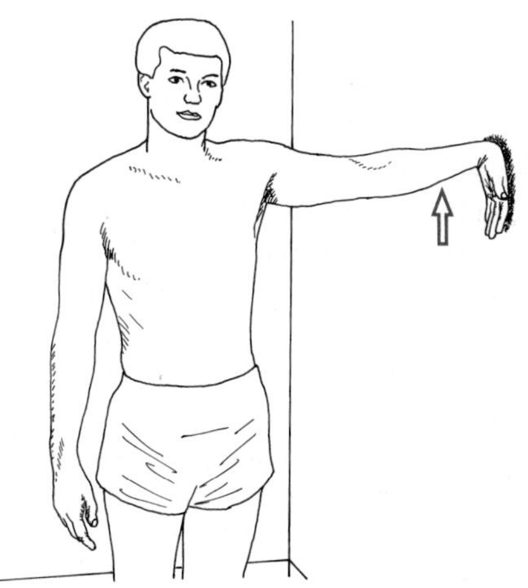

FIGURE 18.10 Self-stretching the wrist extensor muscles.

To Stretch the Wrist Flexor Muscles (From the Medial Epicondyle)

- *Patient position and procedure:* Sitting or standing with the elbow extended and forearm supinated. While holding this position, have the patient radially deviate and extend the wrist and apply a gentle stretch force with the other hand against the palm of the hand. A stretch sensation should be felt along the volar surface of the forearm.
- *Patient position and procedure:* Standing with the elbow extended and forearm supinated. Have the patient place the palm of the hand against a wall, fingers pointing down, and then move the hand up the wall until a stretch sensation is felt in the wrist flexor muscles.

Exercises to Develop and Improve Muscle Performance and Functional Control

In addition to the conditions already described in this chapter, imbalances in length and strength of muscles crossing the elbow and forearm can be the result of a variety of causes, such as nerve injury or after surgery, trauma, disuse, or immobilization. Appropriate exercises to develop neuromuscular control, increase strength, and improve muscular endurance for return to functional activities can be selected from the following exercises as well as the techniques described in Chapters 6 and 23.

For patients with elbow impairments, exercises for the regions above (shoulder girdle) and below (wrist and hand) also should be incorporated into the therapeutic exercise program to prevent complications and restore proper function of the entire upper quarter. The general principles of managing acute soft tissue lesions are discussed in Chapter 10. The exercises described in this section are for use during the controlled motion and return to function phases of intervention when tissues are in the subacute and chronic stages of healing and require only moderate to minimum protection.

Isometric Exercises

Multiple-Angle Isometric Exercises

Use manual or mechanical resistance at various positions throughout the available ROM of elbow flexion and extension and forearm rotation. Isolate the key musculature. Apply resistance at the distal forearm, not at the hand, to avoid forces across the wrist joints.

Angle-Specific Training

During isometric exercises, emphasize joint positions that simulate use of the elbow for anticipated functional activities. For example, to simulate carrying large boxes close to the chest, strengthen the elbow flexors in a 70° to 90° position with the forearm in neutral and supination. Emphasize holding objects for extended periods of time to increase muscular endurance for sustained control.

Alternating Isometrics and Rhythmic Stabilization

Open-Chain Exercises

Apply manual resistance to alternating isometric contractions of antagonists at multiple angles of elbow flexion/extension and forearm pronation/supination. Stabilize the humerus and apply the resistance against the forearm.

When the patient is able to respond to the alternating resistance at various elbow and forearm positions and at varying speeds, progress to alternating isometrics using total upper extremity patterns. To further develop stability superimposed on movement (dynamic stability), have the patient hold a vibrating BodyBlade® in various positions of the elbow, forearm, and the entire upper extremity and then during a variety of movements.

Closed-Chain Exercises

Patient positions include standing with hands against a wall or table, in the quadruped position, or in the prone push-up position (with knees or toes as a fulcrum). Have the patient hold the desired elbow position and apply alternating isometrics and rhythmic stabilization by means of manual resistance against the shoulders and trunk.

Dynamic Strengthening and Endurance Exercises

Many muscles that cross the elbow joint are multijoint muscles, such as the biceps, long head of the triceps, and wrist flexors and extensors. It is particularly important to consider the position of the shoulder and forearm during resistance training at the elbow. Dynamic strengthening and endurance activities for the *prime movers* of the elbow, forearm, and wrist using manual or mechanical resistance are noted in this section. Combined patterns of motion during open- and closed-chain activities are described in the final section describing a functional progression for the elbow and forearm.

Elbow Flexion

Muscles include the biceps brachii, brachialis, and brachioradialis.

- *Patient position and procedure:* Sitting or standing, with the humerus at the side of the chest (arm perpendicular to the floor). Have the patient hold a weight or grasp a piece of elastic band or tubing (secured under the foot or to the floor) and flex and extend the elbow. This strengthens the elbow flexors concentrically and eccentrically throughout the available ROM to simulate functional lifting and lowering. Perform this motion with the forearm supinated, pronated, and in neutral.
- *Patient position and procedure:* Supine with the humerus supported on a treatment table. When the patient is supine, the resistive force from a free weight or gravity has a greater effect on the muscles near end-range extension and has little to no effect as the elbow reaches 90°.
- *Patient position and procedure:* Standing or sitting while holding a weight with the forearm supinated. Have the patient extend the shoulder as the elbow flexes (Fig. 18.11). This combined motion elongates the biceps brachii over the shoulder as the muscle is shortening to move the elbow and thus most efficiently maintains optimal length for development of maximum tension in the *biceps*. This combined motion develops control for carrying objects at the side.

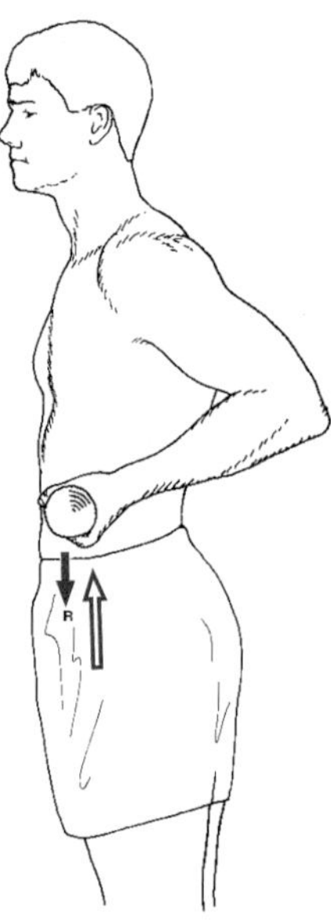

FIGURE 18.11 Resisting elbow flexion with emphasis on the biceps brachii. The shoulder extends as the elbow flexes with the forearm in supination. This combined action lengthens the proximal portion of the musculotendinous unit across the shoulder while it contracts to move the elbow, thus maintaining a more optimal length-tension relationship through a greater ROM.

Elbow Extension

Muscles include the triceps and anconeus.

- *Patient position and procedure:* Prone, humerus abducted to 90° and supported on a rolled towel on a treatment table. Have the patient extend the elbow while holding a weight. This position strengthens the elbow extensors from 90° of flexion to terminal extension.
- *Patient position and procedure:* Supine with the shoulder flexed to 90°, holding a weight in the hand. Have the patient begin with the elbow flexed and the weight either at the ipsilateral or contralateral shoulder (external or internal rotation of the shoulder); then extend and flex the elbow (lift and slowly lower the weight) to strengthen the elbow extensors concentrically and eccentrically. To help

maintain the shoulder in a stable position, have the patient stabilize the humerus in the 90° position with the opposite hand.

Long Head of Triceps With Elbow Extension

Patient position and procedure: Sitting or standing with the arm held overhead (shoulder fully flexed) and elbow flexed so the weight is near the shoulder (Fig. 18.12). Have the patient lift the weight overhead and then slowly lower the weight for concentric and eccentric strengthening. The patient may support the humerus with the opposite hand. Perform this exercise only if the patient has sufficient control of the shoulder.

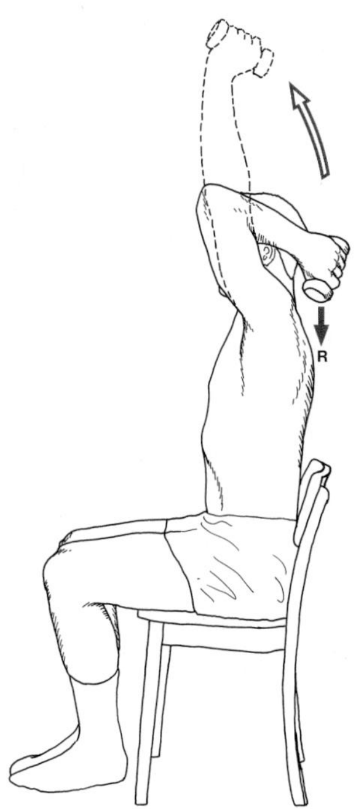

FIGURE 18.12 Resisting elbow extension, beginning with the long head of the triceps brachii on a stretch.

Pronation and Supination

Primary muscles of pronation are the pronator teres and pronator quadratus; primary muscles of supination are the supinator and biceps brachii.

Patient position: Sitting or standing with the elbow flexed to 90° and held close to the trunk. When sitting, the forearm may be on a table for support held next to the trunk.

- ***Free weights.*** When using a free weight to strengthen the pronators and supinators, the weight must be placed on one side or the other of the hand (Fig. 18.13). As the patient rotates the bar be sure that they keep the wrist in a neutral position so as not to stress the wrist especially at end ranges. The weight can also be turned through a downward arc by placing the resistance on the ulnar side of the hand.
- ***Elastic resistance.*** Have the patient grasp one end of the elastic resistance with the sound hand or by tying it to a doorknob (be sure that the elastic is secure). Have the patient grasp the other end with the involved extremity and rotate the forearm against the resistance. For greater resistance, secure the elastic resistance around the end of a short rod and have the patient pull against the resistance force.
- ***Functional activity.*** Have the patient stand, facing a doorknob with the arm kept at the side and the elbow flexed to 90° to avoid substituting with shoulder rotation. Have the patient turn the knob.

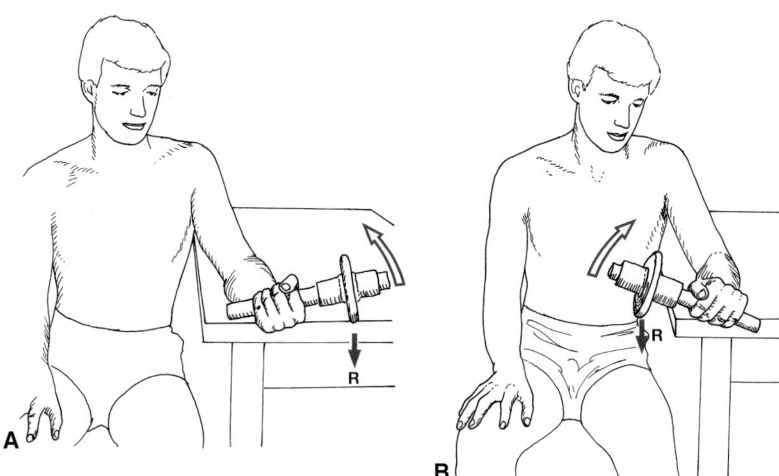

FIGURE 18.13 Mechanical resistance exercise using a small bar with an asymmetrically placed weight for strengthening **(A)** forearm pronators and **(B)** supinators. The bar also can be rotated through a downward arc to affect the other half of the range for each muscle by placing the weight on the ulnar side of the hand.

Wrist Flexion and Extension

Wrist flexion involves muscles attached to the medial epicondyle; extension involves muscles attached to the lateral epicondyle.

NOTE: In the following exercises, when the forearm is pronated, resistance is applied to the wrist extensors; when supinated, resistance is applied to the wrist flexors.

- ***Elastic resistance.*** Tie the ends of an elastic band or tubing together. While sitting, have the patient place one end of the loop under one foot. Stabilize the forearm on the thigh and place the other end of the loop across the dorsum (Fig. 18.14) or palm of the hand to resist the wrist extensors or flexors, respectively.
- ***Free weights.*** Have the patient sit, with forearm resting on a table and hand over the edge of the table holding a small weight (Fig. 18.15). Extend and flex the wrist against the resistance.
- ***Wrist roller.*** Have the patient sit or stand, with the elbows flexed or extended and the forearms pronated or supinated. Tie a 2- to 4-ft cord to the middle of a short rod and a weight to the other end of the cord. Have the patient hold each end of the rod and with an alternating wrist action, turn the rod causing the cord to wind around the rod and elevate the weight. The weight is then slowly lowered with a reverse motion (Fig. 18.16).

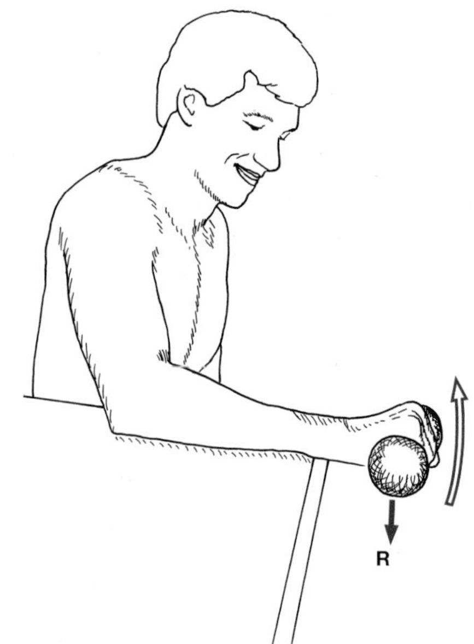

FIGURE 18.15 Strengthening the wrist extensors while grasping a handheld weight for resistance.

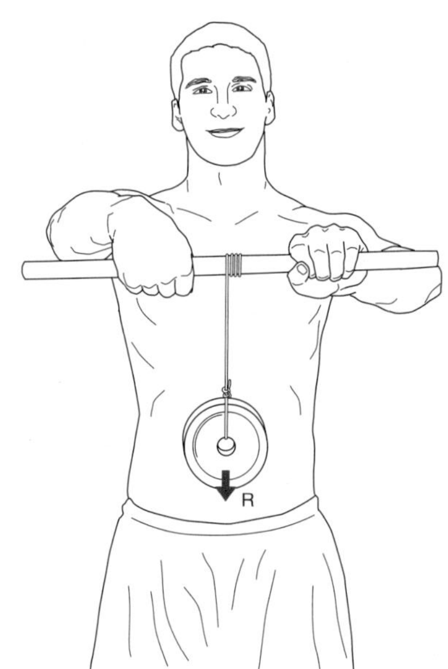

FIGURE 18.16 Wrist roller exercise to strengthen grip and develop the wrist extensors. This exercise requires stabilization in the shoulder girdle and elbow muscles. The elbows may be flexed or the forearms supinated to emphasize the elbow flexors or muscles of the medial epicondyle, respectively.

Functional Progression for the Elbow and Forearm

A comprehensive rehabilitation program for the elbow and forearm designed to achieve an individual's functional goals involves a sequence of carefully progressed exercise interventions designed to develop or restore sufficient mobility, strength, stability, muscular endurance, and power. The final section of this chapter identifies integral components and examples of exercise interventions and simulated functional activities that often are included in a functional progression for the elbow and forearm. Refer to Chapters 17 and 23 for additional exercises and activities.

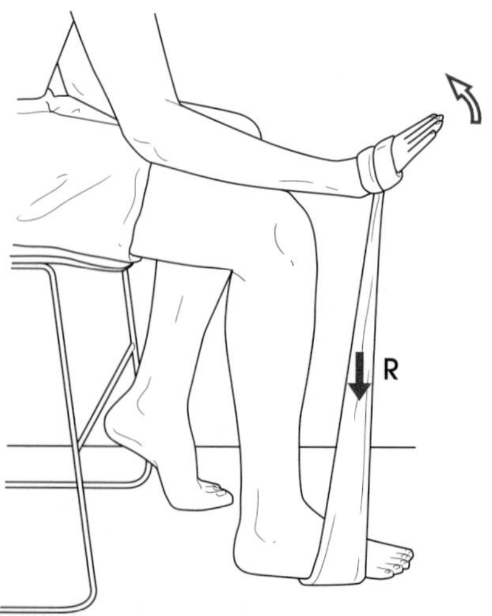

FIGURE 18.14 Strengthening the wrist extensors using elastic resistance without the use of grasp.

NOTE: Because the elbow primarily functions during activities that also involve the shoulder and hand, combined patterns of exercise that develop mobility and control the entire upper extremity should be implemented especially as it relates to proximal stabilization. Be careful that substitute motions do not occur to compensate for a weak link in the chain.

Diagonal Patterns

PNF patterns against manual or mechanical resistance. Use unilateral or bilateral diagonal patterns as described in Chapter 6. Use manual resistance, free weights, elastic resistance, a weight-pulley system, or an isokinetic dynamometer to provide the resistance as the patient moves through the diagonal patterns. Gradually increase resistance, speed (if appropriate with the choice of equipment), and repetitions.

Combined Pulling Motions

Elbow flexors are used in pulling, lifting, and carrying activities in open- and closed-chain activities. These upper extremity actions also require strength of the scapular retractors, shoulder extensors, and wrist and hand musculature. Many of the exercises that are described for the shoulder in Chapter 17 also involve resisted elbow flexion and therefore can be used to strengthen muscle groups during pulling motions. Suggestions include:

- Bilateral pull-ups against elastic resistance (Fig. 18.17).
- Closed-chain chin-ups or modified pull-ups on an overhead bar (Fig. 18.18).
- Unilateral combined pulling pattern simulating starting a lawn mower (Fig. 18.19) or bilateral or unilateral rowing motions, such as using a rowing machine.
- Pulling a variety of weighted objects with one or both arms, emphasizing elbow flexion and proper body mechanics.

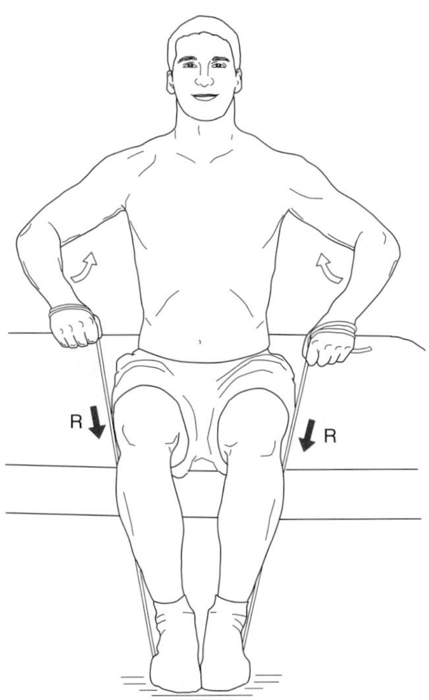

FIGURE 18.17 Bilateral pull-up against elastic resistance.

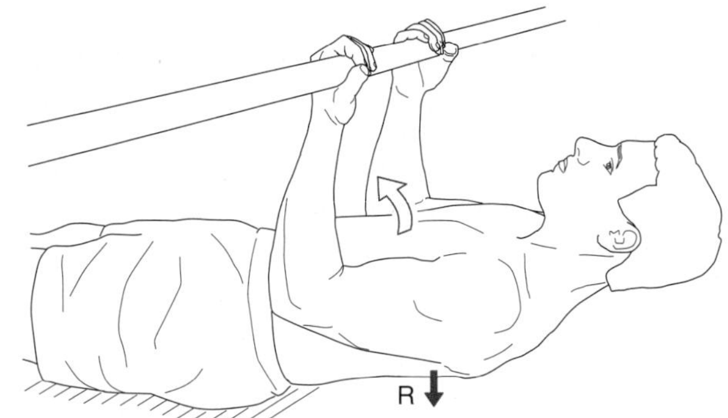

FIGURE 18.18 Closed-chain, modified chin-up using top half of body weight for resistance to strengthen the elbow flexors. This exercise may be performed in a bed with an overhead trapeze.

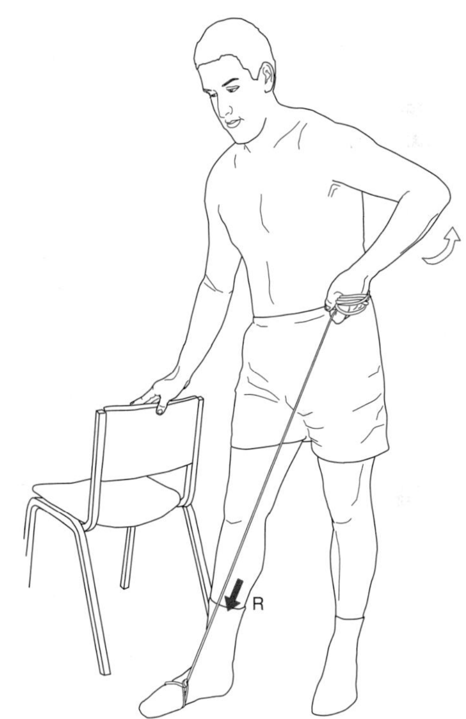

FIGURE 18.19 Simulation of a "lawn mower pull" for functional strengthening of the upper extremity.

Combined Pushing Motions

The triceps muscle is involved in pushing motions. Pushing also involves variations of shoulder flexion and scapular protraction or depression so that muscles controlling these motions are functioning with the triceps. Many of the exercises described in Chapter 17 for the shoulder and Chapter 23 also involve resisted elbow extension and may be used to strengthen muscles groups involved in pushing patterns. Suggestions include:

- Military press-up (see Fig. 17.55)
- Bench press
- Upper extremity ergometry (see Fig. 6.55)

- Wall push-ups, semi-prone or prone push-ups (Fig. 18.20 A)
- Push-ups from a chair or on parallel bars (Fig. 18.20 B)
- Stepping/stair-climbing machine with hands on the "steps" (emphasize elbow extension)
- Pushing a variety of weighted objects with one or both arms using dynamic elbow extension (Fig. 18.21)

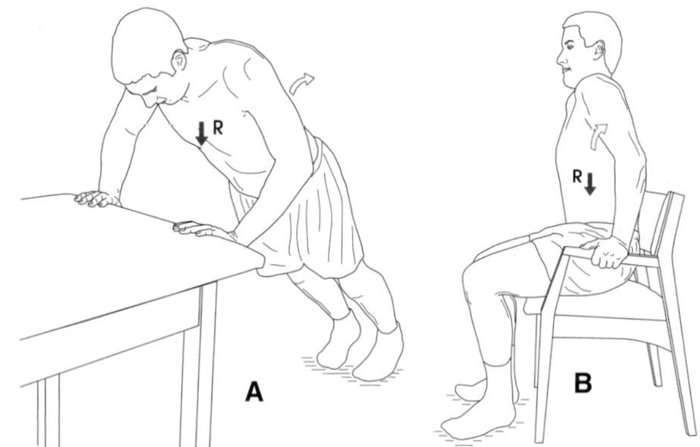

FIGURE 18.20 Closed-chain strengthening of the triceps. **(A)** Modified push-up. **(B)** Seated push-up.

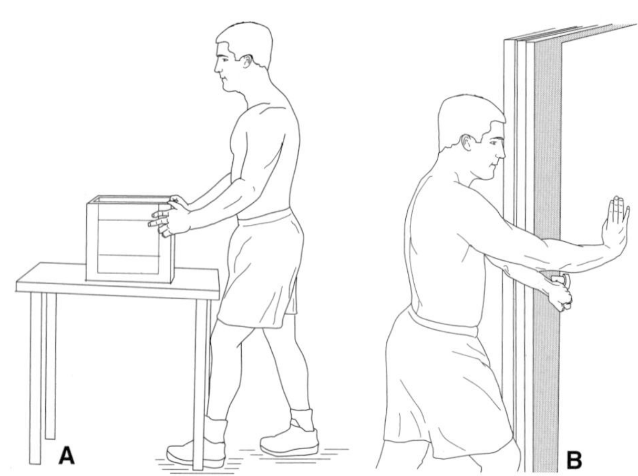

FIGURE 18.21 Strengthening the triceps with pushing activities. **(A)** Pushing weighted objects across a table. **(B)** Depressing a door handle and pushing open a door.

Plyometric Training (Stretch-Shortening Drills)

The following are suggestions for increasing power of the elbow musculature using plyometric exercises.[10,38] Advanced training activities are described in Chapter 23.

- Perform elbow flexion and extension exercises against elastic resistance, emphasizing rapid reversal between eccentric and concentric motions.
- Using a weighted ball, have the patient catch the ball and then quickly throw it back. Emphasize elbow motions with overhead passes, chest passes, and lateral passes.
- Bounce a ball against a wall or a tennis ball on a racquet with the forearm pronated and supinated.

Simulated Functional Tasks and Activities

Determine the component motions of the patient's desired functional activities as well as occupational or recreational tasks. Have the patient simulate these motions and practice the entire task. Activities could involve lifting, lowering, carrying, pushing, pulling, twisting, turning, catching, throwing, or swinging. For example, if the patient is recovering from repetitive trauma to the muscles of the lateral epicondyle when playing tennis, have the patient practice the various racquet strokes using a wall-pulley system (Fig. 18.22). Impose controlled forces to challenge the patient by increasing the time or repetitions, speed, or resistance.[38]

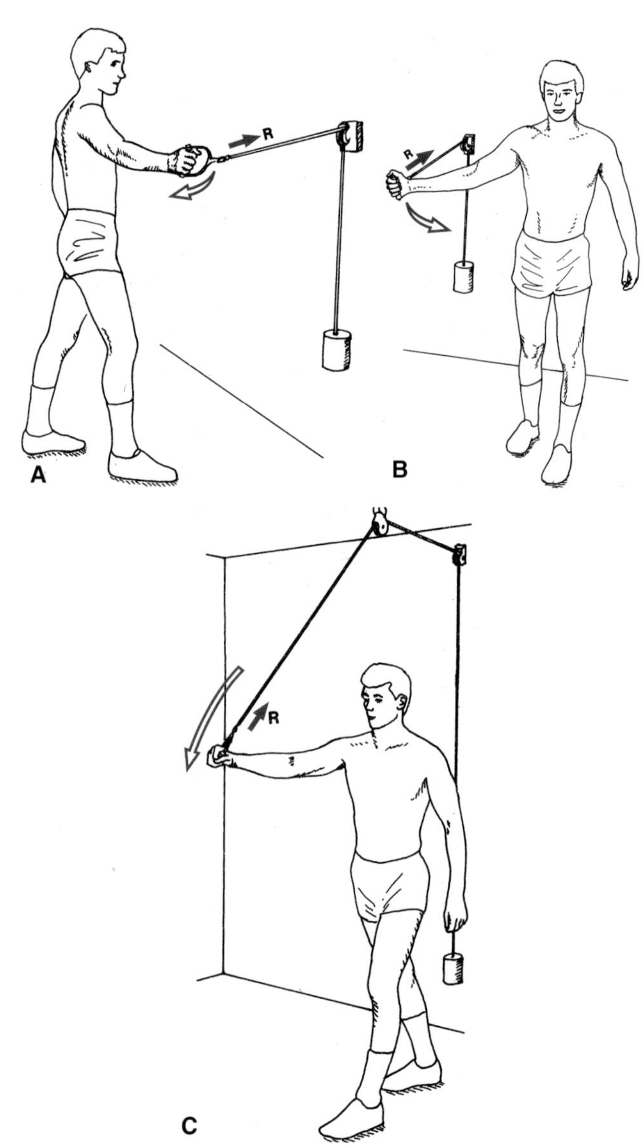

FIGURE 18.22 Mechanical resistance exercise using wall pulleys to simulate tennis swings. **(A)** Backhand stroke. **(B)** Forehand stroke. **(C)** Serve.

Independent Learning Activities

Critical Thinking and Discussion

1. Differentiate between the etiology, signs and symptoms, and management of lateral and medial epicondylalgia. Note the similarities and differences.
2. Develop, compare, and contrast the postoperative management (including an exercise progression and precautions) after two types of TEA: (1) a semiconstrained implant/triceps-reflecting approach and (2) a resurfacing implant/triceps-splitting approach.
3. The goal is to increase muscle performance and function of the elbow flexors that are currently functioning at a 3/5 strength level and endurance of four repetitions. Identify exercises that could be used at each increment of strength, including exercises for strength, endurance, power, control, stability, and function. Identify parameters for progression of each exercise and any precautions.
4. Do the same sequence of analysis and identification to increase muscle performance and function of the elbow extensors.
5. Analyze the following household, occupational, or sports-related activities. Identify the components and sequence of motions related to each of these motor tasks; pay particular attention to elbow and forearm motions during these tasks. Design a sequence of upper extremity exercises and simulated activities that could be incorporated into a late-stage rehabilitation program to prepare a patient to return to the desired task after an elbow injury.
   - Housecleaning
   - Gardening
   - Grocery store stocking
   - Carpentry
   - Volleyball
   - Tennis
   - Throwing sports

Laboratory Practice

1. Apply mobilization techniques to a laboratory partner to increase the following elbow and forearm motions: mid- and end-range elbow flexion; mid- and end-range elbow extension; and forearm pronation and supination (proximal and distal articulations).
2. Demonstrate passive stretching and hold-relax techniques to elongate the following muscles that cross the elbow: brachialis, brachioradialis, biceps, long head of the triceps, extensor digitorum, flexor carpi ulnaris, and flexor carpi radialis.
3. Using the following pieces of resistance equipment demonstrate at least two methods (set-ups) to strengthen the elbow flexors/extensors and forearm rotators: free weights, weight-pulley system, and elastic resistance. Then demonstrate a progressive sequence of resistance exercise to strengthen the same muscle groups using self-resistance (body weight or manual resistance).

Case Studies

1. Describe the mechanical problem causing impairments in the elbow and forearm in the following scenario and what techniques could be used for intervention. A patient is referred to you 4 weeks after sustaining a fracture of the distal radius with immobilization in a long arm cast following a fall on an outstretched arm and hand. She has limited elbow, forearm, and wrist motions. On palpation, you note a decreased space between the lateral aspect of the head of the radius and capitulum as well as decreased joint play at all articulations of the elbow, forearm, and wrist.
2. A 15-year-old patient with a 5-year history of polyarticular JRA just underwent open synovectomy and excision of the head of the radius with implant for late-stage joint disease of the elbow. Prior to surgery, the patient had severe pain in the elbow region, lacked full elbow flexion/extension and forearm rotation, and had limited use of the arm for functional activities. Continuous passive motion was implemented during the patient's hospitalization (3 days). A day prior to discharge, the patient was referred to physical therapy for a home program. Design an exercise program for this teenager. Prioritize and describe each exercise you want the patient to do for the first week at home. Outline a program of exercises for later use in the rehabilitation process. The patient plans to return to school within a week of discharge from the hospital. Indicate whether you recommend outpatient therapy; if so, indicate the frequency and duration; justify the need for this recommendation.

REFERENCES

1. Ahmad, CS, and El Attrache, NS: Arthroscopy in the throwing athlete. In Morrey, BF, and Sanchez-Sotelo J (ed): *The Elbow and Its Disorders,* ed. 4. Philadelphia: Saunders Elsevier, 2009, pp 587–595.
2. Anandkumar S: The effect of sustained natural apophyseal glide (SNAG) combined with neurodynamics in the management of a patient with cervical radiculopathy: a case report. *Physiother Theory Pract* 31:140–145, 2015.
3. Aiello, BJ: Median nerve compression. In Burke, SL, et al (eds): *Hand and Upper Extremity Rehabilitation,* ed. 3. Missouri: Elsevier Churchill Livingstone, 2006, pp 87–95.
4. Altman, E: Therapist's management of the stiff elbow. In Skirven, TM, et al (eds): *Rehabilitation of the Hand and Upper Extremity,* ed. 6. Philadelphia: Elsevier Mosby, 2011. 1075–1088.
5. Amin NH, Kumar NS, and Schickendantz, MS: Medical epicondylitis: evaluation and management. *J Am Acad Orthop Surg* 23:348–355, 2015.
6. Angst, F, et al: Comprehensive assessment of clinical outcomes and quality of life after total elbow arthroplasty. *Arthritis Rheum* 53:73–82, 2005.
7. Antuna, SA: Rehabilitation after elbow arthroplasty. In Williams, GR, et al (eds): *Shoulder and Elbow Arthroplasty.* Philadelphia: Lippincott Williams & Wilkins, 2005, pp 475–484.
8. Armstrong, AD, King, GJW, and Yamaguchi, K: Total elbow arthroplasty design. In Williams, GR, et al (eds): *Shoulder and Elbow Arthroplasty.* Philadelphia: Lippincott Williams & Wilkins, 2005, pp 297–312.
9. Armstrong, AD, and Galatz, LM: Complications of total elbow arthroplasty. In Williams, GR, et al (eds): *Shoulder and Elbow Arthroplasty.* Philadelphia: Lippincott Williams & Wilkins, 2005, pp 459–473.
10. Aviles, SA, Wilk, KE, and Safran, MR: Elbow. In Magee, DJ, et al (eds): *Pathology and Intervention in Musculoskeletal Rehabilitation.* Missouri: Saunders Elsevier, 2009, pp 161–212.
11. Barenholtz, A, and Wolff, A: Elbow fractures and rehabilitation. *Orthop Phys Ther North Am* 10(4):525–539, 2001.
12. Beckenbaugh, RD: Arthrodesis. In Morrey, BF, and Sanchez-Sotelo, J (eds): *The Elbow and Its Disorders,* ed. 4. Philadelphia: Saunders Elsevier, 2009, pp 949–955.
13. Beingessner, DM, et al: The effect of radial head excision and arthroplasty on elbow kinematics and stability. *J Bone Joint Surg Am* 86: 1730–1739, 2004.
14. Bennett, JB, and Mehlhoff, TL: Total elbow arthroplasty: surgical technique. *J Hand Surg (Am)* 34:933–939, 2009.
15. Beredjiklian, PK: Management of fractures and dislocations of the elbow. In Skirven, TM, et al (eds): *Rehabilitation of the Hand and Upper Extremity,* ed. 6. Philadelphia: Elsevier Mosby, 2011, pp 1049–1060.
16. Berglund, KM, Persson BH, and Denison, E: Prevalence of pain and dysfunction in the cervical and thoracic spine in persons with and without lateral elbow pain. *Man Ther* 13:295–299, 2008.
17. Bhatt, JB, and Glaser, R: Middle and lower trapezius strengthening for the management of lateral epicondylalgia: a case report. *J Orthop Sports Phys Ther* 43:841–847, 2013.
18. Bickhart, NE: Ulnar nerve compression. In Burke SL, Higgins, JP, and McClinton, MA (eds): *Hand and Upper Extremity Rehabilitation,* ed. 3. Missouri: Elsevier Churchill Livingstone, 2006, pp 96–108.
19. Bisset, LM, Collins, NJ, and Offord, SS. Immediate effects of 2 types of braces on pain and grip strength in people with lateral epicondylalgia: a randomized controlled trial. *J Orthop Sports Phys Ther* 44:120–128, 2014.
20. Bisset, LM, and Vicenzo, B: Physiotherapy management of lateral epicondylalgia. *J Physiother* 61(4):174–81, 2015.
21. Bisset, L, et al: Mobilisation with movement and exercise, corticosteroid injection, or wait and see for tennis elbow: randomised trial. *Br Med J.* e-pub 2006.
22. Buckwalter, JA, and Ballard, WT: Operative treatment of rheumatic disease. In Klippel, JH (ed): *Primer on the Rheumatic Diseases,* ed. 12. Atlanta: Arthritis Foundation, 2001, pp 613–623.
23. Caridi, J, Pumberger, M, and Hughes, A: Cervical radiculopathy: A review. *HSS Journal* 7:265–272, 2011.
24. Celli, A, et al: Triceps insufficiency following total elbow arthroplasty. *J Bone Joint Surg Am* 87(9):1957–1964, 2005.
25. Celli, A, and Morrey, BF: Total elbow arthroplasty in patients forty years of age or less. *J Bone Joint Surg (Am)* 91:1414–1418, 2009.
26. Cil A, and Morrey, BF. Synovectomy of the elbow. In Morrey, BF, and Sanchez-Sotelo, J (eds): *The Elbow and Its Disorders,* ed. 4. Philadelphia: Saunders Elsevier, 2009, pp 921–934.
27. Cil, A, Veillette, CH, Sanchez-Sotelo, J, and Morrey, BF: Linked elbow replacement: a salvage procedure for distal humeral nonunion. *J Bone Joint Surg* 90:1939–1950, 2008.
28. Clifford, PE, and Mallon, WJ: Sports after total joint replacement. *Clin Sports Med* 24:175–186, 2005.
29. Cohen, MS, and Katolik, LI: Total elbow arthroplasty. In Wolfe, SW, Hotchkiss, RN, Pederson, WC, and Kozin, SH (eds): *Green's Operative Hand Surgery, Vol 1,* ed. 6. Philadelphia, PA: Elsevier: Churchill Livingstone, 2011, pp 959–973.
30. Coisier, JL, et al: An isokinetic eccentric programme for the management of chronic lateral epicondylar tendinopathy. *Br J Sports Med* 41:269–275, 2007.
31. Coleman, SH, and Altchek, DA: Arthroscopy and the thrower's elbow. In Wolfe, SW, Hotchkiss, RN, Pederson, WC, and Kozin, SH (eds): *Green's Operative Hand Surgery, Vol 1,* ed. 6. Philadelphia, PA: Elsevier: Churchill Livingstone, 2011, pp 945–958
32. Coombes, BK, Bissett, L, and Vicenzino, B: Bilateral cervical dysfunction in patients with unilateral lateral epicondylalgia without concomitant cervical or upper limb symptoms: a cross-sectional case-control study. *J Manip Ther* 37:79–86, 2014.
33. Cooney, WP: Elbow arthroplasty: Historical perspective and current concepts. In Morrey, BF, and Sanchez-Sotelo, J (eds): *The Elbow and Its Disorders,* ed. 4. Philadelphia: Saunders Elsevier, 2009, pp 705–719.
34. Cresswell, T, and Stanley, D: Unlinked elbow arthroplasty. In Williams, GR, et al (eds): *Shoulder and Elbow Arthroplasty.* Philadelphia: Lippincott Williams & Wilkins, 2005, pp 333–345.
35. Davila, SA: Therapist's management of fractures and dislocations of the elbow. In Skirven, TM, et al (eds): *Rehabilitation of the Hand and Upper Extremity,* ed. 6. Philadelphia: Elsevier Mosby, 2011, pp 1061–1074.
36. Doornberg, JN, Ring, D, and Jupiter, JB: The effectiveness of static progressive splinting for post-traumatic elbow stiffness. *J Orthop Trauma* 20(6):400–404, 2006.
37. Edmonds, A: Elbow arthroplasty. In Burke, SL, Higgens, JP, and McClinton, MA (eds): *Hand and Upper Extremity Rehabilitation,* ed. 3. Missouri: Elsevier Churchill Livingstone 2006, pp 431–437.
38. Ellenbecker, TS, Pieczynski, TE, and Davies, GJ: Rehabilitation of the elbow following sports injury. *Clin Sports Med* 29:33–60, 2010.
39. Fedorczyk, JM: Tendinopathies of the elbow, wrist, and hand: histopathology and clinical considerations. *J Hand Ther* 25:191–201, 2012.
40. Fedorczyk, JM: Tennis elbow: blending basic science with clinical practice. *J Hand Ther* 19:146–153, 2006.
41. Fernandez-Carnero, J, et al: Widespread mechanical pain hypersensitivity as sign of central sensitization in unilateral epicondylalgia: A blinded, controlled study. *Clin J Pain* 25:555–561, 2009.
42. Fernádez-de-las-Peñas, C, et al: Specific mechanical pain hypersensitivity over peripheral nerve trunks in women with either unilateral epicondylalgia or carpal tunnel syndrome. *J Orthop Sports Phys Ther* 40(11):751–760, 2010.
43. Fevang, B-TS, et al: Results after 562 total elbow replacements: a report from the Norwegian arthroplasty register. *J Shoulder Elbow Surg* 18:449–456, 2009.
44. Field, LD, and Savoié, FH, III: *Master Cases: Shoulder and Elbow Surgery.* New York: Thieme, 2003.
45. Field, LD, and Savoié, FH, III: Management of loose bodies and other limited procedures. In Morrey, BF, and Sanchez-Sotelo, J (eds): *The Elbow and Its Disorders,* ed. 4. Philadelphia: Saunders Elsevier, 2009, pp 579–586.
46. Gallo, RA, Payatakes, A, and Sotereanos, DG: Surgical options for the arthritic elbow. *J Hand Surg* 33(5):746–759, 2008.

47. Garg, R, et al: A prospective randomized study comparing a forearm strap brace versus a wrist splint for the treatment of lateral epicondylitis. *J Should Elbow Surg* 19:508–512, 2010.
48. Gill, DRJ, Morrey, BF, and Adams, RA: Linked total elbow arthroplasty in patients with rheumatoid arthritis. In Morrey, BF, and Sanchez-Sotelo, J (eds): *The Elbow and Its Disorders,* ed. 4. Philadelphia: Saunders Elsevier, 2009, pp 782–791.
49. Hall, JA, and McKee, MA: Posterolateral rotary instability of the elbow following radial head resection. *J Bone Joint Surg Am* 87(7):1571–1579, 2005.
50. Hastings, H, and Theng, CS: Total elbow replacement for distal humerus fractures and traumatic deformity: results and complications of semiconstrained implants and design rationale for the Discovery Elbow System. *Am J Orthop* 32:20–28, 2003.
51. Hughes, JS, Morrey, BF, and King, GJW: Unlinked arthroplasty: In Morrey, BF, and Sanchez-Sotelo, J (eds): *The Elbow and Its Disorders,* ed. 4. Philadelphia: Saunders Elsevier, 2009, pp 720–753.
52. Jafarian, FS, Demneh, ES, and Tyson, SF: The immediate effect of orthotic management on grip strength for patients with lateral epicondylosis. *J Orthop Sports Phys Ther* 39(6):484–489, 2009.
53. Jawa, A, Jupiter, JB, and Hotchkiss, RN: Complex traumatic elbow dislocation. In Wolfe SW, Hotchkiss, RN, Pederson, WC, and Kozin, SH (eds): *Green's Operative Hand Surgery, Vol 1,* ed. 6. Philadelphia, PA: Elsevier: Churchill Livingstone, 2011, pp 869–885.
54. Joseph, MF, Taft, K, Moskawa, M , and Denegar, CR: Deep friction massage to treat tendinopathy: a systematic review of a classic treatment in the face of a new paradigm of understanding. *J Sports Rehab* 21(4):343–353, 2012.
55. Kelly, EV, Coghlan, J, and Bell, S: Five- to thirteen-year follow-up of the GBS III total elbow arthroplasty. *J Shoulder Elbow Surg* 13:434–440, 2004.
56. Kim, JM, Mudgal, CS, Konopka, JF, and Jupiter, JB: Complications of total elbow arthroplasty. *J Am Acad Orthop Surg* 19:328–330, 2011.
57. King, JGW: Total elbow arthroplasty. In Wolfe SW, Hotchkiss, RN, Pederson, WC, and Kozin, SH (eds): *Green's Operative Hand Surgery, Vol 1,* ed. 6. Philadelphia, PA: Elsevier: Churchill Livingstone, 2011, pp 783–819.
58. Kokkalis, ZT, Schmidt, CC, and Sotereanos, DG: Elbow arthritis: Current concepts. *J Hand Surg* 34A:761–768, 2009.
59. Lee, BP, Adams, RA, and Morrey, BF: Wear and elbow replacement. In Morrey, BF, and Sanchez-Sotelo, J (eds): *The Elbow and Its Disorders,* ed. 4. Philadelphia: Saunders Elsevier, 2009, pp 880–884.
60. Lin, F, et al: Muscle contribution to elbow joint valgus stability. *J Shoulder Elbow Surg* 16:795–802, 2007.
61. Linscheid, RL, and Morrey, BF: Resurfacing elbow replacement arthroplasty. In Morrey, BF (ed): *Joint Replacement Arthroplasty,* ed. 3. Philadelphia: Churchill Livingstone, 2003, pp 303–315.
62. Lucado, AM, Kolber, MJ, and Cheng, MS. Upper extremity strength characteristics in female recreational tennis players with and without lateral epicondylalgia. *J Orthop Sports Phys Ther* 42:1025–1031, 2012.
63. Magee, DJ: *Orthopedic Physical Assessment,* ed. 6. St. Louis: Saunders, 2014.
64. Manias, P, and Stasinopoulos, D: A controlled clinical pilot trial to study the effectiveness of ice as a supplement to the exercise programme for the management of lateral elbow tendinopathy. *Br J Sports Med* 40:81–85, 2006.
65. Martinez-Sivestrini, JA, et al: Chronic lateral epicondylitis: comparative effectiveness of a home exercise program including stretching alone versus stretching supplemented with eccentric or concentric strengthening. *J Hand Ther* 18(4):411–419, 2005.
66. McKee, MD, et al: A multicenter, prospective randomized, controlled trial of open reduction—internal fixation versus total elbow arthroplasty for displaced intra-articular distal humeral fractures in elderly patients. *J Shoulder Elbow Surg* 18(1):3–12, 2009.
67. Monica, JT, and Mudogal, CS: Radial head arthroplasty. *Hand Clin* 26:403–410, 2010.
68. Morrey, BF: Anatomy of the elbow joint. In Morrey, BF, and Sanchez-Sotelo, J (eds): *The Elbow and Its Disorders,* ed. 4. Philadelphia: Saunders Elsevier, 2009, pp 11–38.
69. Morrey, BF: Splints and bracing at the elbow. In Morrey, BF, and Sanchez-Sotelo, J (eds): *The Elbow and Its Disorders,* ed. 4. Philadelphia: Saunders Elsevier, 2009, pp 164–169.
70. Morrey, BF: Ectopic ossificans about the elbow. In Morrey, BF, and Sanchez-Sotelo, J (eds): *The Elbow and Its Disorders,* ed. 4. Philadelphia: Saunders Elsevier, 2009, pp 472–486.
71. Morrey, BF: Linked arthroplasty: rationale, indications and surgical technique. In Morrey, BF, and Sanchez-Sotelo, J (eds): *The Elbow and Its Disorders,* ed. 4. Philadelphia: Saunders Elsevier, 2009, pp 765–781.
72. Morrey, BF, and Larson, AN: Interposition arthroplasty of the elbow. In Morrey, BF, and Sanchez-Sotelo, J (eds): *The Elbow and Its Disorders,* ed. 4. Philadelphia: Saunders Elsevier, 2009, pp 935–948.
73. Morrey, BF: Linked arthroplasty. In Williams, GR, et al (eds): *Shoulder and Elbow Arthroplasty.* Philadelphia: Lippincott Williams & Wilkins, 2005, pp 475–484.
74. Morrey, BF: Radial head fracture. In Morrey, BF, and Sanchez-Sotelo, J (eds): *The Elbow and Its Disorders,* ed. 4. Philadelphia: Saunders Elsevier, 2009, pp 359–388.
75. Morrey, BF: Radial head prosthetic replacement. In Morrey, BF (ed): *Joint Replacement Arthroplasty,* ed. 3. Philadelphia: Churchill Livingstone, 2003, pp 294–302.
76. Morrey, BF: Semiconstrained total elbow replacement: indications and surgical technique. In Morrey, BF (ed): *Joint Replacement Arthroplasty,* ed. 3. Philadelphia: Churchill Livingstone, 2003, pp 316–328.
77. Morrey, BF, and Adams, RA: Results of semiconstrained replacement for rheumatoid arthritis. In Morrey, BF (ed): *Joint Replacement Arthroplasty,* ed. 3. Philadelphia: Churchill Livingstone, 2003, pp 329–337.
78. Morrey, BF, and An, K: Functional evaluation of the elbow. In Morrey, BF, and Sanchez-Santolo, J (eds): *The Elbow and Its Disorders,* ed. 4. Philadelphia: Saunders Elsevier, 2009, pp 80–89.
79. Mulligan, BR: *Manual Therapy "NAGS," "SNAGS," "MWM'S" etc.,* ed. 6. Wellington: Plane View Press, 2010.
80. Nagrale, AV, Herd, CR, Ganvir, S, and Ramteke, G: Cyriax physiotherapy versus phonophoresis with supervised exercise in subjects with lateral epicondylalgia: a randomized clinical trial. *J Man Manip Ther* 17(3):171–178, 2009.
81. Nauth, A, et al: Heterotopic ossification in orthopaedic trauma. *J Orthop Trauma* 26:684–688, 2012.
82. Neumann, DA: Elbow and forearm. In Neumann, DA: *Kinesiology of the Musculoskeletal System: Foundations for Rehabilitation,* ed. 2. St. Louis: Mosby/Elsevier, 2010, pp 173–215.
83. Nirschl, RP, and Alvarado, GJ: Tennis elbow tendinosis. In Morrey, BF, and Sanchez-Sotelo, J (eds): *The Elbow and Its Disorders,* ed. 4. Philadelphia: Saunders Elsevier, 2009, pp 626–642.
84. Norkin, CC: The elbow complex. In Levangie, PK, and Norkin, CC (eds): *Joint Structure and Function: A Comprehensive Analysis,* ed. 5. Philadelphia: F.A. Davis, 2011, pp 271–304.
85. O'Driscoll, SW: Complications of total elbow arthroplasty. In Morrey, BF, and Sanchez-Santolo, J (eds): *Joint Replacement Arthroplasty,* ed. 3. Philadelphia: Churchill Livingstone, 2003, pp 352–378.
86. O'Driscoll, SW: Elbow dislocation. In Morrey, BF, and Sanchez-Santolo, J (eds): *The Elbow and Its Disorders,* ed. 4. Philadelphia: Saunders Elsevier, 2009, pp 436–449.
87. Pappas, N, and Bernstein, J: Fractures in brief: radial head fractures. *Clin Orthop Relat Res* 468:914–916, 2010.
88. Park, JG, Cho, NS, Song, JH, Lee, DS, and Rhee, YG: Clinical outcomes of semiconstrained total elbow arthroplasty in patients who were forty years of age or younger. *J Bone Joint Surg* 97:1781–1791, 2015.
89. Petrie, RS, and Bradley, JP: Osteochondral defects in the elbow. In Mirzayan, R (ed): *Cartilage Injury in the Athlete.* New York: Thieme, 2006, pp 201–216.
90. Pitts, G, and Umansky, SC: Radial nerve compression. In Burke SL, Higgins, JP, and McClinton, MA (eds): *Hand and Upper Extremity Rehabilitation,* ed. 3. Missouri: Elsevier Churchill Livingstone 2006, pp 109–120.

91. Plaschke, HC, Thillemann, TM, Brorson, S, and Olsen, BS: Outcome after total elbow arthroplasty: a retrospective study of 167 procedures performed from 1981 to 2008. *J Should Elbow Surg* 24(12):1982–1990, 2015.
92. Raman, J, MacDermid, JC, and Grewal, R: Effectiveness of different methods of resistance exercises in lateral epicondylosis—a systematic review. *J Hand Ther* 25:5–26, 2012.
93. Ramsey, ML: The history and development of total elbow arthroplasty. In Williams, GR, et al (eds): *Shoulder and Elbow Arthroplasty.* Philadelphia: Lippincott Williams & Wilkins, 2005, pp 271–278.
94. Ranganathan, K, et al: Heterotopic ossification: basic-science principles and clinical correlates. *J Bone Joint Surg* 97:1101–1111, 2015.
95. Regan, WD, and Morrey, BF: Physical examination of the elbow. In Morrey, BF, and Sanchez Sotelo, J (eds): *The Elbow and Its Disorders,* ed. 4. Philadelphia: Saunders Elsevier, 2009, pp 67–79.
96. Sadeghi-Demneh, E, and Jafarian, F. The immediate effects of orthoses on pain in people with lateral epicondylalgia. *Pain Res Treat* 2013:1–6, 2013.
97. Sanchez-Sotelo, J, and Morrey, BF: Total elbow arthroplasty. *J Am Academy Orthop Surgeons* 19(2):121–125, 2011.
98. Stanley, D: Surgical and postoperative management of elbow arthritis. In Skirven et al (eds): *Rehabilitation of the Hand and Upper Extremity,* ed. 6. Philadelphia: Elsevier Mosby, 2011. pp 1420–1426.
99. Stans, AA: Fractures of the neck of the radius in children. In Morrey, BF, and Sanchez-Sotelo, J (eds): *The Elbow and Its Disorders,* ed. 4. Philadelphia: Saunders Elsevier, 2009, pp 268–282.
100. Stasinopoulos, D, Stasinopoulos, K, and Johnson, MI: An exercise programme for the management of lateral elbow tendinopathy. *Br J Sports Med* 39:944–947, 2005.
101. Stevens, CG, and Wright, TW: Radial head fractures. *Oper Tech Orthop* 23:188–197, 2013.
102. Tanaka, N, et al: Kudo total elbow arthroplasty in patients with rheumatoid arthritis. *J Bone Joint Surg Am* 83:1506–1513, 2001.
103. Tyler, TF, Thomas, GC, Nickolas, SJ, and McHugh, MP: Addition of isolated wrist extensor eccentric exercise to standard treatment for chronic lateral epicondylosis: a prospective randomized trial. *J Shoulder Elbow Surg* 19:917–922, 2010.
104. Ulrich, SD, et al: Restoring range of motion via stress relaxation and static progressive stretch in posttraumatic elbow contractures. *J Shoulder Elbow Surg* 19:196–201, 2010.
105. van Hofwegen, C, Baker III, CL, and Baker Jr, CL: Epicondylitis in the athlete's elbow. *Clin Sports Med* 29:577–597, 2010.
106. Van Riet, RP, Van Glabbeek, F, and Morrey, BF: Radial head fracture. In Morrey, BF, and Sanchez-Sotelo, J (eds): *The Elbow and Its Disorders,* ed. 4. Philadelphia: Saunders Elsevier, 2009, pp 359–381.
107. Vicenzino, B, Cleland, JA, and Bisset, L: Joint manipulation in the management of lateral epicondylalgia: a clinical commentary. *J Man Manip Ther* 15(1):50–56, 2007.
108. Voloshin, I, et al: Complications of total elbow replacement: a systematic review. *J Shoulder Elbow Surg* 20:158–168, 2011.
109. Waugh, EJ, Jaglal, SB, and Davis, AM: Computer use associated with poor long-term prognosis of conservatively managed lateral epicondylalgia. *J Orthop Sports Phys Ther* 34(12):770–780, 2004.
110. Wilk, KE, and Andrews, JR: Elbow injuries. In Brotzman, SB, and Wilk, KE (eds): *Clinical Orthopedic Rehabilitation,* ed. 2. Philadelphia: Mosby, 2003, pp 85–123.
111. Yoon, JJ, and Bae, H: Change in electromyographic activity of wrist extensor by cylindrical brace. *Yonsei Med J* 54:220–224, 2013.
112. Yoon, AM, et al: Radial head fractures. *J Hand Surg* 37A:2626–2634, 2012.

CHAPTER

19

The Wrist and Hand

■ CAROLYN KISNER, PT, MS ■ LYNN COLBY, PT, MS
■ CINDY JOHNSON ARMSTRONG, PT, DPT, CHT

The wrist is the final link of joints that positions the hand for functional activities. It functions to control the length-tension relationship of the multiarticular muscles of the hand as they adjust to various activities. The wrist is often considered the most complex joint of the body, both from an anatomical and physiological perspective. However, there are two points of consensus regarding the wrist: (1) the structure and biomechanics of the wrist as well as the hand vary significantly from person to person and (2) even subtle variations can produce differences in the way a particular functional activity occurs.[9] The hand is a valuable tool through which we control and manipulate our environment and express ideas and talents. It also has an important function of providing sensory feedback to the central nervous system.

This chapter is divided into three major sections. The first section briefly reviews the rather complex structure and function of the wrist and hand—information that is important to know in order to effectively treat patients with wrist and hand pathology. The second section describes common disorders and guidelines for conservative and postoperative management. The last section describes exercise techniques commonly used to meet the goals of treatment during the stages of tissue healing and phases of rehabilitation.

Structure and Function of the Wrist and Hand

The bones of the wrist include the distal radius and ulna. The scaphoid (S), lunate (L), triquetrum (Tri), and pisiform (P) make up the proximal carpal row; the trapezium (Tm), trapezoid (Tz), capitate (C), and hamate (H) make up the distal carpal row. Five metacarpals and 14 phalanges make up the hand and the five digits (Fig. 19.1).

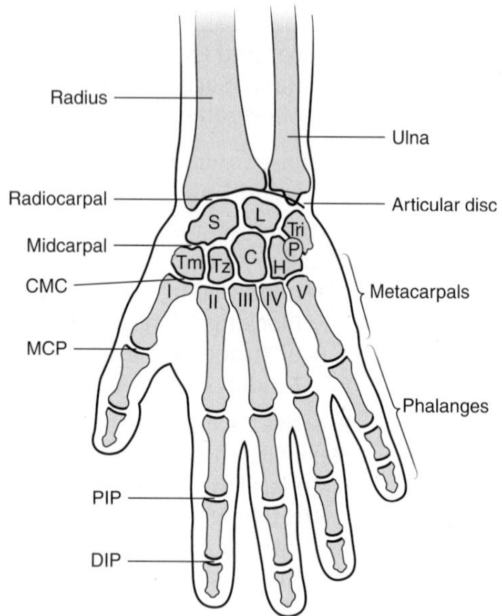

FIGURE 19.1 Bones of the wrist and hand complex.

Joints of the Wrist and Hand

Wrist Joint: Characteristics and Arthrokinematics

The distal radioulnar (RU) joint is not considered part of the wrist joint, although pain and impairments in this forearm articulation are often described by the patient as wrist pain. Structure and function of the RU joints are described in Chapter 18.

The wrist joint is multiarticular and is made up of two compound joints, the radiocarpal/ulnocarpal and midcarpal joints. It is biaxial, allowing flexion, extension, radial deviation, and ulnar deviation. However, due to an oblique axis of rotation, most activities are carried out with an oblique wrist motion from extension with radial deviation to flexion with ulnar deviation. This oblique plane of motions is referred to as the "dart thrower's motion" (DRT) and is an important concept when developing treatment plans for individuals with wrist pathology.[24,53] Stability is provided by numerous extrinsic ligaments: the ulnar and radial collateral, the dorsal and volar (palmar) radiocarpal, the ulnocarpal and the triangular fibrocartilage complex, as well as a multitude of intrinsic intercarpal ligaments.[9,102]

The pisiform is categorized as a carpal bone and aligned volar to the triquetrum in the proximal carpal row. It is not part of the wrist joint per se but functions as a sesamoid bone in the flexor carpi ulnaris tendon.

Radiocarpal Joint

Characteristics. The radiocarpal (RC) and ulnocarpal (UC) joints are enclosed in a loose but strong capsule that is reinforced by the ligaments shared with the midcarpal joint. The biconcave articulating surface is made up of the distal end of the radius and articular disc (an integral part of the triangular fibrocartilage complex) and is angled slightly volarly and ulnarly.[9,102] The biconvex articulating surface of the proximal carpal row includes the scaphoid, lunate, and triquetrum. The triquetrum primarily articulates with the disc. These three carpals are bound together with numerous interosseous ligaments.

Arthrokinematics. With motions of the wrist, the convex proximal row of carpals slides on the concave distal radius and articular disc in the direction opposite the physiological motion of the hand. The arthrokinematics are summarized in ONLINE Box 19.1 available on the FA Davis website related to this textbook.

Midcarpal Joint

Characteristics. The midcarpal joint is a compound joint between the proximal and distal carpal rows. It has a capsule that is also continuous with the intercarpal articulations. The combined distal surfaces of the distal carpal row (scaphoid, lunate, and triquetrum) articulate with the proximal carpal row (trapezium, trapezoid, capitate, and hamate).

Arthrokinematics. The midcarpal joint is divided into radial and ulnar compartments.

- The *ulnar compartment* consists of the articulating surfaces of the capitate and hamate and is, in essence, convex, which slides on the concave articulating surfaces of a portion of the scaphoid, lunate, and triquetrum. Therefore, with flexion and extension, as well as radial and ulnar deviation, the distal component of the ulnar compartment (capitate and hamate) slides opposite the physiological motion.
- The *radial compartment* of the midcarpal joint consists of the articulating concave surfaces of the trapezium and trapezoid, which slide on the convex distal surface of the scaphoid. With flexion and extension, the distal component of the radial compartment (trapezium and trapezoid) slides in the same direction as the physiological motion. However, during radial and ulnar deviation, it has been shown through cineradiography (three-dimensional CT scan) that the proximal row of carpal bones "rock" slightly either volarly or dorsally and, to a lesser extent, "twist." The

rocking motion is most pronounced in the scaphoid, which moves volarly (flexes) during radial deviation and slightly dorsally (extends) during ulnar deviation.

 **FOCUS ON EVIDENCE**

According to Moojen, at 20° of ulnar deviation, the scaphoid rotates dorsally about 20° relative to the radius, and at 20° of radial deviation, the scaphoid moves volarly about 15°, which allows for a few more degrees of radial deviation.[9,96,97,102] The exact mechanism that produces this motion is not well understood; however, it is theorized that it occurs because of the passive forces of the ligaments and compression between the adjacent carpals.[102]

Hand Joints: Characteristics and Arthrokinematics

Carpometacarpal Joints of Digits 2 through 5

Characteristics. The carpometacarpal (CMC) joints are enclosed in a common joint cavity and include the articulations of each metacarpal with the distal row of carpals and the articulations between the bases of each metacarpal.

The joints of digits 2 and 3 are difficult to classify due to their jagged interlocking articular surfaces; however, they are most often considered to be planar joints. These interlocking surfaces, combined with strong ligaments, allow for very little motion as stability at these joints is paramount to the overall stability of the hand and forms the central pillar. The slightly convex bases of the fourth and fifth metacarpals articulate with the slightly concave surface of the hamate and allow for important mobility to the hand. The fourth and fifth metacarpal joints are able to "fold" or rotate toward the center of the hand, deepening the palmar concavity. This motion occurs by flexion and internal rotation of the fourth and fifth metacarpals moving toward the third digit and is often referred to as "cupping" of the hand.[9,103] This motion improves the ability of the hand to grasp objects of various sizes. Extension of the metacarpals contributes to flattening of the hand, which improves the ability to release objects.

Arthrokinematics. The slightly concave proximal surfaces of the metacarpals slide in a volar direction on the relatively convex surfaces of the distal carpal row with flexion and in a dorsal direction with extension motions in the hand (see ONLINE Box 19.1).

Carpometacarpal Joint of the Thumb (Digit 1)

Characteristics. The CMC joint of the thumb is a saddle-shaped (sellar) joint between the trapezium and base of the first metacarpal. The longitudinal diameter of the articular surface of the trapezium is concave in the dorsal to volar direction, while the transverse diameter of the articular surface is convex in the radial to ulnar direction. The proximal articular surface of the thumb metacarpal joint is convex in the dorsal to volar direction and concave in the radial to ulnar direction, thus opposite to the surface of the trapezium. The thumb CMC joint has a lax capsule and wide range of motion (ROM) that allows the thumb to fully oppose the other digits, which greatly enhances prehension activities.[9,103]

Arthrokinematics. A change in terminology relative to thumb CMC joint motion was adopted by the American Academy of Orthopaedic Surgeons (AAOS), the American Society for Surgery of the Hand (ASSH), the International Federation of Societies for Surgery of the Hand (IFSSH), and the American Society of Hand Therapists (ASHT) in the early 1990s. Many publications in the United States and internationally have since incorporated this terminology when discussing the thumb CMC joint.[13,72,84,100,114]

- The motions previously known as CMC abduction and adduction are termed *palmar abduction* and *adduction* (moving away from or toward the palm); in this plane the distal surface of the metacarpal is convex and the proximal surface of the trapezium is concave. Since the distal segment moves on the proximal segment, the motion is convex on concave; therefore, the metacarpal slides in the opposite direction of the physiological motion.
- The motions previously known as CMC flexion and extension are termed *radial abduction* and *adduction* (moving away or toward the radius). In this plane, the distal surface of the metacarpal is concave, and the proximal surface of the trapezium is convex; therefore, the motion is concave on convex and the metacarpal slides in the same direction as the physiological motion (see ONLINE Box 19.1).

Metacarpophalangeal Joints of Digits 2–5

Characteristics. The metacarpophalangeal (MP) joints are condyloid joints, which allows for flexion/extension and abduction/adduction. The MP joints of the fingers are surrounded by a relatively lax articular capsule, allowing for significant accessory motion and axial rotation of the proximal phalanx. This mobility enables the fingers to better conform to the shapes of objects and increases the control of grasp. Each joint is supported by a volar plate and two collateral ligaments. The collaterals become taut in full flexion and prevent abduction and adduction in this position.[9,103]

Arthrokinematics. The distal end of each metacarpal is convex, and the proximal phalanx is concave. The proximal surface of the proximal phalanx rolls and slides in the same direction as the physiological motion (see ONLINE Box 19.1).

Interphalangeal Joints and MP Joint of the Thumb

Characteristics. There is a proximal interphalangeal (PIP) joint and a distal interphalangeal (DIP) joint for each digit, 2 through 5. The thumb has only one IP joint, although the MP joint of the thumb is uniaxial and therefore functions similarly to the IP joints. The MP joint of the thumb differs in that it is reinforced by two sesamoid bones on the volar surface, which improves the leverage of the flexor pollicis brevis muscle. Each of these joints is a uniaxial hinge joint.

The capsule of each joint is reinforced with collateral ligaments. Unlike the MP joints, the collateral ligaments of the IP joints remains relatively constant throughout the ROM. There is increasing flexion/extension ROM in the MP joints as you move from radial to ulnar digits of 2 through 5. This allows for greater opposition of the ulnar fingers to the thumb and also causes a potentially tighter grip on the ulnar side of the hand.

Arthrokinematics. The articulating surface at the distal end of each phalanx is convex; the articulating surface at the proximal end of each phalanx is concave. Therefore, the proximal surface of each phalanx rolls and slides in the same direction as the physiological motion (see ONLINE Box 19.1).

Hand Function

Muscles of the Wrist and Hand

The complex function of the hand occurs as a result of an intricate balance and control of forces between the extrinsic and intrinsic muscles of the wrist and hand. The primary and secondary actions of the wrist and hand muscles are summarized in Table 19.1 and depicted in Figure 19.2.

TABLE 19.1 Muscles of the Wrist and Hand

Action	Prime Movers	Secondary Movers
Wrist		
Flexion	Flexor carpi radialis Flexor carpi ulnaris Palmaris longus	Flexor digitorum superficialis Flexor digitorum profundus Flexor pollicis longus
Extension	Extensor carpi radialis longus Extensor carpi radialis brevis Extensor carpi ulnaris Extensor digitorum	Extensor indicis Extensor digiti minimi Extensor pollicis brevis Abductor pollicis longus
Radial deviation	Flexor carpi radialis longus Extensor carpi radialis longus Extensor carpi radialis brevis	Flexor pollicis longus Extensor pollicis brevis Abductor pollicis longus
Ulnar deviation	Flexor carpi ulnaris Extensor carpi ulnaris	
Thumb (Digit 1)		
CMC opposition	Opponens pollicis	
CMC radial adduction	Opponens pollicis	
CMC radial abduction	Abductor pollicis longus	Extensor pollicis longus
CMC palmar abduction	Opponens pollicis Abductor pollicis longus Abductor pollicis brevis Extensor pollicis brevis	Flexor pollicis brevis (superficial head)
CMC palmar adduction	Adductor pollicis (first volar interossei)	Flexor pollicis brevis (deep head) Extensor pollicis longus
MP flexion	Flexor pollicis brevis	Flexor pollicis longus
MP extension	Extensor pollicis brevis Extensor pollicis longus	Extensor pollicis longus
IP flexion	Flexor pollicis longus	
IP extension	Extensor pollicis longus	

TABLE 19.1 Muscles of the Wrist and Hand—cont'd

Action	Prime Movers	Secondary Movers
Digits 2 through 5 (function of these muscles varies with joint positions/motions)		
MP flexion	Lumbricals Volar and dorsal interossei Flexor digitorum superficialis Flexor digitorum profundus	
MP extension	Extensor digitorum Extensor digiti minimi Extensor indices	
MP abduction	Dorsal interossei Abductor digiti minimi	(Note: Proximal wing tendons of the interossei have more influence on the MP joint)[9]
MP adduction	Volar interossei	
IP flexion	Flexor digitorum superficialis (PIP only) Flexor digitorum profundus (PIP and DIP)	
IP extension	Lumbricals, dorsal and volar interossei, and extensor digitorum via extensor mechanism	(Note: Distal wing tendons of the interossei have more influence on the IP joints)[9]

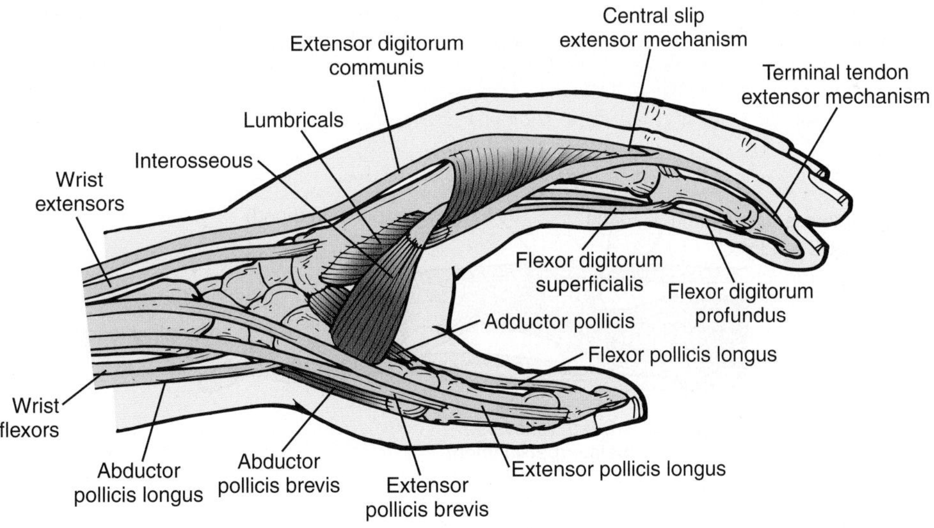

FIGURE 19.2 The extrinsic and intrinsic muscles of the wrist and hand create a balance of forces that affect hand function.

Length-Tension Relationships

The position of the wrist controls the length of the extrinsic muscles of the digits. As the fingers or thumb flex, the wrist extensor muscles must stabilize the wrist to prevent the flexor digitorum profundus and flexor digitorum superficialis or the flexor pollicis longus from simultaneously flexing the wrist. As the grip becomes stronger, synchronous wrist extension lengthens the extrinsic flexor tendons across the wrist and maintains a more favorable overall length of the musculotendinous unit for a stronger contraction.

For strong finger or thumb extension, the wrist flexor muscles stabilize the wrist so the extensor digitorum, extensor indicis, extensor digiti minimi, or extensor pollicis longus muscles can function more efficiently.

Extensor Mechanism

Structurally, the foundation of the extensor mechanism is made up of the extensor digitorum tendon (with the extensor indicis and extensor digiti minimi), the extensor hood, the central tendon, and the lateral bands (stabilized by the triangular ligament) that merge into the terminal tendon. The passive components of the extensor mechanism include the triangular ligament and the sagittal bands (which prevent bowstringing of the extensor mechanism and centralize the extensor tendons at the MP joints). The active components of the extensor mechanism include the dorsal interossei, the volar interossei, and the lumbrical muscles (collectively referred to as the intrinsic muscles) (Fig. 19.3).[9,103]

- The extensor digitorum tendon passes dorsal to the MP joint axis, and an active contraction of the extensor digitorum creates tension in the sagittal bands, pulling the bands proximally resulting in extension of the proximal phalanx.
- An isolated contraction of the extensor digitorum produces MP joint hyperextension with IP joint flexion. The IP joint flexion is produced from passive pull of the extrinsic flexor tendons. This position is called clawing or the hook position.
- PIP and DIP extension is interdependent, meaning when the PIP joint extends, the DIP joint will extend as well and is produced by the interossei and lumbrical muscles through their pull on the extensor hood.
- There must also be tension in the extensor digitorum tendon for there to be IP extension. This occurs either by active contraction of the muscle, causing MP extension concurrently as the intrinsic muscles contract, or by passive tension of the extensor digitorum tendon, which occurs with MP flexion.[9]
- The dorsal interossei, the volar interossei, and the lumbricals pass volar to the joint axis of the MP joint and insert into the extensor mechanism proximal to the PIP joint. Therefore, when the extensor digitorum, the interossei, and the lumbricals all contract simultaneously, the MP joint and the IP joints will all extend. Although when the interossei and the lumbricals contract in the absence of active contraction of the extensor digitorum, the MP joints will flex and the IP joints will extend.

Control of the Unloaded (Free) Hand

Anatomical factors, muscular contraction, and viscoelastic properties of the muscles influence finger motion.[9,103]

- When only the extrinsic extensor and flexor muscles contract, clawing motions occur in the digits.
- Closing motions occur with extrinsic flexor muscle contractions but also require the viscoelastic force of the interossei and, to a lesser extent, the lumbricals. In addition, the extensor digitorum muscle acts as a "brake" at the MP joints, allowing for more refined and controlled motion at the IP joints.
- Opening motions require synergistic contraction of the extrinsic extensor, as well as the intrinsic muscles accompanied by viscoelastic resistance of the flexor digitorum profundus.
- Reciprocal motion of MP flexion and IP extension is caused by the intrinsic muscles. The lumbrical removes the viscoelastic tension from the profundus tendon and, along with the interossei, acts as a strong IP extensor.

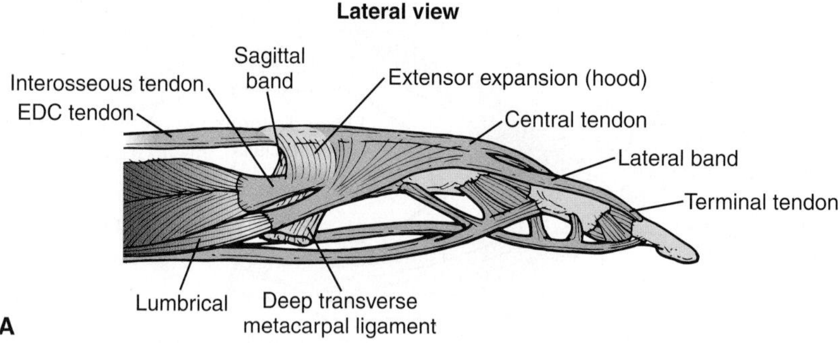

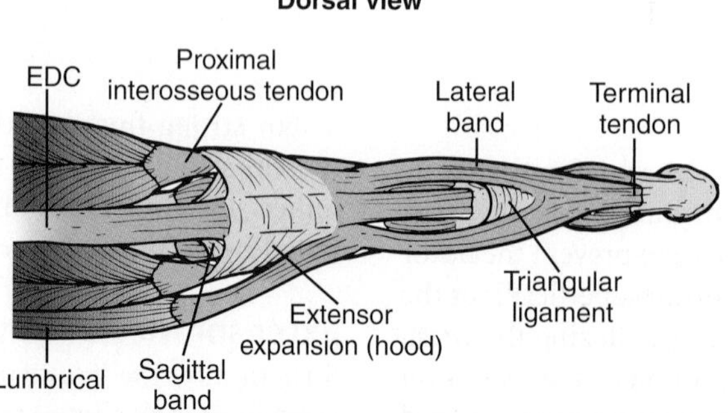

FIGURE 19.3 Anatomical structures of the extensor mechanism: **(A)** lateral view and **(B)** dorsal view. See text for description of functional relationships.

Grips and Prehension Patterns

The nature of the intended activity dictates the type of grip used.[6,9,103]

Power Grips (Full Hand Prehension)

Description. Power grips involve clamping an object with partially flexed fingers against the palm of the hand and with counter pressure from the palmarly adducted thumb. Power grips are primarily isometric functions. The fingers assume a position of sustained flexion, which varies in degree with the size, shape, and weight of an object. The thumb reinforces the fingers and helps make small adjustments to control the direction of the force. Varieties include cylindrical grip, spherical grip, hook grip, and lateral prehension.[9,102]

Muscle control. The muscles primarily function with isometric contractions.[6,9,101,102]

- Maximum grip force occurs with the wrist positioned in slight extension and slight ulnar deviation stabilized by the extrinsic wrist extensors.
- Extrinsic finger flexors, especially the flexor digitorum profundus muscles of the fourth and fifth digits, provide the major gripping force.
- The extensor digitorum provides a compressive force to the MP joints, which increases stability and also provides a balancing force for the flexors.
- Interossei rotate and radially abduct the first phalanx for positioning to compress the external object and flex the MP joint.
- With the exception of the fourth lumbrical, lumbricals do not participate in the power grip.
- The thenar muscles and adductor pollicis provide compressive forces against the object being gripped.

Precision Patterns

Description. Prehension patterns involve manipulating an object that is not in contact with the palm of the hand between the opposing thumb and fingers. The muscles primarily function isotonically. The sensory surfaces of the digits are used for maximum sensory input to influence delicate adjustments. With small objects, precise handling occurs primarily between the thumb and index finger. Varieties include pad-to-pad, tip-to-tip, and pad-to-side prehension.

Muscle control. The primary dynamic function of the muscles includes the following:[9,85,103]

- Extrinsic muscles provide the compressive force to hold the objects between the fingers and thumb.
- For manipulation of an object, the interossei abduct and adduct the fingers; the thenar muscles control movement of the thumb; and the lumbricals help move the object away from the palm of the hand. The amount of participation of each muscle varies with the amount and direction of motion.

Combined Grips

Description. Combined grips involve digits 1 and 2 (and sometimes 3) performing precision activities, whereas digits 3 through 5 supplement with power.

Pinch. Pinch requires holding an object between the thumb and index or middle finger, as in precision handling, but may require primarily an isometric hold. The thenar eminence muscles, the adductor pollicis, the interossei, and the extrinsic flexors provide compression between the thumb and fingers. The lumbricals also participate.

Major Nerves Subject to Pressure and Trauma at the Wrist and Hand

For a detailed description of peripheral nerve injuries and entrapments in the wrist and hand region, as well as complex regional pain syndromes and their management, see Chapter 13.

Nerve Disorders in the Wrist

Median nerve. The most common site for compression of the median nerve is in the carpal tunnel.

Ulnar nerve. The most common site for compression of the ulnar nerve is in the ulnar tunnel (also called Guyon's canal).

Referred Pain and Sensory Patterns

The hand is the terminal point for the C6, C7, C8, and T1 nerve roots coursing through the median, ulnar, and radial nerves (see Figs. 13.5, 13.6, and 13.7). Injury or entrapment of these nerves may occur anywhere along their course, from the cervical spine to their termination. What the patient perceives as pain or a sensory disturbance in the hand may be from injury of the nerve anywhere along its course, or the pain may derive from irritation of tissue of common segmental origin, such as the zygapophyseal facet joints of the spine. For treatment to be effective, it must be directed to the source of the problem, not to the site where the patient perceives the pain or sensory changes. Therefore, a thorough history is taken and examination of the entire upper quarter must be done, including the cervical spine when referred pain patterns or sensory changes are reported by the patient.[86,92]

Management of Wrist and Hand Disorders and Surgeries

To make sound clinical decisions when treating patients with wrist and hand disorders, it is necessary to understand the various pathologies, surgical procedures, and associated precautions and to identify presenting structural impairments, activity limitations, and participation restrictions. In this section, common pathologies and surgeries and conservative and postoperative management are presented.

Joint Hypomobility: Nonoperative Management

Pathologies, such as rheumatoid arthritis (RA) and degenerative joint disease (DJD), affect the joints of the wrist and hand and may have a significant effect on participation and functional abilities of an individual as a result of pain, impaired mobility, and potential joint deformities. Impaired joint, tendon, and muscle mobility also occurs any time joints are immobilized due to fractures, trauma, or surgery. Chapter 11 describes the etiology and general guidelines for management of impairments due to these joint pathologies. This section focuses on specific interventions for the wrist and hand.

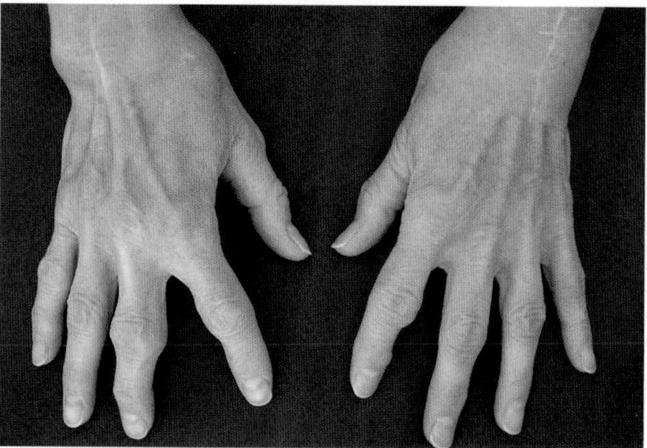

FIGURE 19.4 Joint deformities seen in the hand of a patient with rheumatoid arthritis. Note the hypertrophy of the IP joints, rheumatoid nodules, and volar subluxation of the triquetrum. This patient had fusion of the wrist joints due to pain and complete destruction of the joints, which has helped prevent the deforming, bowstringing effect of the extrinsic tendons on the MP joints. *(Courtesy of Turtle Services Limited, www.turtleserviceslimited.org/.)*

Common Joint Pathologies and Associated Impairments

Rheumatoid Arthritis

The following is a summary of signs, symptoms, and resulting impairments typically seen in the wrist and hand with RA.[2,18,104,134]

Acute stage. There is pain, swelling, warmth, and limited motion from synovial inflammation (synovitis) and tissue proliferation, most commonly in the MP, PIP, and wrist joints bilaterally. There is also inflammation (tenosynovitis) and synovial proliferation in the extrinsic tendons and tendon sheaths. In addition, an individual with RA may experience:

- Progressive muscle weakness and imbalances in length and strength between agonists and antagonists and between intrinsic and extrinsic muscles.
- Carpal tunnel syndrome in conjunction with tenosynovitis due to compression of the median nerve from the swollen tissue.
- General systemic as well as muscular fatigue.

Advanced stages. Joint capsule weakening, cartilage destruction, bone erosion, and tendon rupture, as well as imbalances in musculotendinous forces leading to joint instabilities, subluxations, and deformities (Fig. 19.4). Typical deformities and the pathomechanics in the hand include:[2,18]

- *Volar subluxation of the triquetrum on the articular disk and ulna.* The extensor carpi ulnaris tendon displaces volarly and causes a flexor force at the wrist joint.
- *Ulnar subluxation of the carpals.* This causes radial deviation of the wrist.
- *Ulnar drift of the fingers and volar subluxation of the proximal phalanx.* There is stretching or rupture of the collateral ligaments at the MP joints and a bowstringing effect from the extrinsic tendons.[2,18]
- *Swan-neck deformity.* Laxity of the PIP joint with an overstretched volar (palmar) plate and bowstringing of the lateral bands of the extensor hood result in hyperextension of the PIP and flexion of the DIP joints (Fig. 19.5A). Tight or overactive interossei muscles pulling on the extensor tendon reinforces the hyperextension of the hypermobile PIP joints, and increased passive tension in the flexor digitorum profundus tendon causes flexion of the DIP joint.
- *Boutonnière deformity.* Stretching or rupture of the central band (central slip) of the extensor hood results in the lateral bands of the extensor mechanism migrating volarly to the PIP joint, causing PIP flexion and DIP extension (Fig. 19.5B).

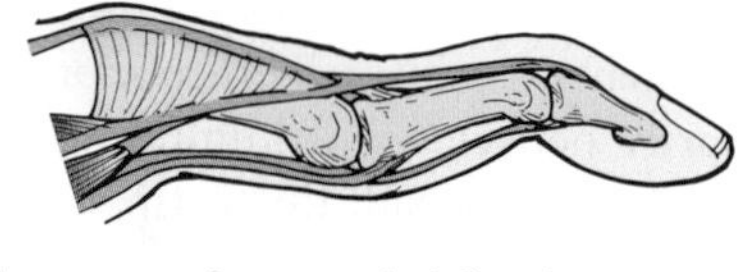

A Swan-neck deformity

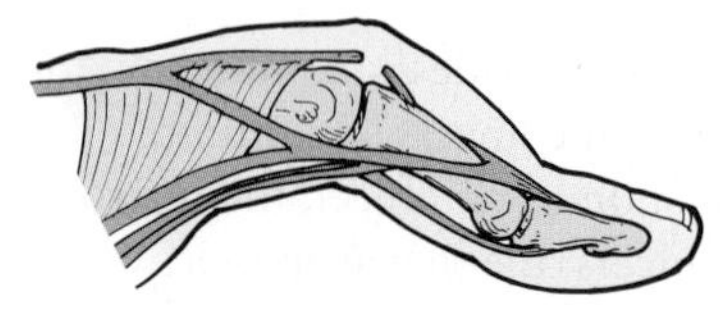

B Boutonnière deformity

FIGURE 19.5 (A) Swan-neck and **(B)** boutonnière deformities. See text for description of the pathomechanics.

- *Zigzag deformity of the thumb.* Muscle imbalances and ligamentous laxity lead to metacarpal dislocation of the thumb and deformities similar to a swan-neck or boutonnière deformity. Tightness in the adductor pollicis contributes to deformities in the thumb.[2,104]

Degenerative Joint Disease/Osteoarthritis and Posttraumatic Arthrosis

Age and repetitive joint trauma lead to degenerative cartilaginous and bony changes in susceptible joints. DJD, or osteoarthritis (OA), most commonly involves the CMC joint of the thumb, and DIP joints of the digits, although the effects of trauma can occur in any joint.

Posttraumatic arthrosis can develop in any joint of the wrist or hand as the result of a severe intra-articular fracture or fracture-dislocation. For example, at the wrist, deficiency of the scapholunate interosseous ligament as the result of a severe wrist sprain can alter joint alignment, which can cause articular degeneration over time. In the fingers, the PIP joint is a common site of articular fracture and subsequent joint degeneration.

The following is a summary of signs, symptoms, and resulting impairments commonly seen in DJD or posttraumatic arthrosis.[15]

Acute stage. During the early stages of DJD, symptoms include achiness and feelings of stiffness, which abate with movement. Following stressful activities or trauma, joint swelling, warmth, and restricted and painful motion occur.

Advanced stages. With degeneration, there is capsular laxity resulting in hypermobility or instability; with progression, contractures and limited motion develop. Affected joints may become enlarged or sublux (Fig. 19.6). Limitation of both flexion and extension with a firm capsular end-feel develops in the affected joints. There is general muscle weakness, weak grip strength, and poor muscular endurance. Pain may also be a limiting factor in pinch and gripping activities.

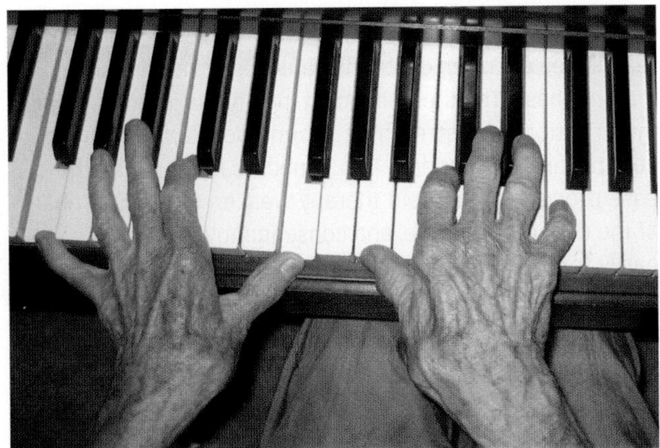

FIGURE 19.6 Advanced-stage osteoarthritis of the hands of an 86-year-old pianist. Note the carpometacarpal (CMC) joint subluxation at the base of each thumb. Atrophy of the first dorsal interossei, nodules, and joint enlargements are apparent, but the individual is still functional.

PRECAUTION: After trauma, the therapist must be alert to signs of a fracture in the wrist or hand because small bone fractures may not show on radiographs for as many as 2 weeks. Signs include swelling, muscle spasm when passive motion is attempted, increased pain when the involved bone is stressed (e.g., deviation toward the involved bone), and tenderness on palpation over the fracture site.[64]

Postimmobilization Hypomobility

Immobilization may be necessary following a fracture, surgery, or trauma, or it may be used to rest a part when an individual sustains repetitive stress. Structural impairments may occur from the lack of motion and muscle contraction, including:

- Decreased ROM and decreased joint play with firm end-feel and pain on overpressure.
- Tendon adhesions as the result of inflammation in a tendon or its sheath.
- Decreased muscle performance including muscle weakness, weak grip strength, decreased flexibility, and decreased muscle endurance.

Common Impairments of Function, Activity Limitations, and Participation Restrictions

When joint pathology is acute, many prehension activities are painful, interfering with activities of daily living (ADLs and IADLs), such as dressing, eating, grooming, and toileting, or almost any functional activity that requires pinching, gripping, and fine-finger dexterity, including writing and typing.

Functional loss may be minor or significant depending on which joints are involved; the amount of restricted movement and residual weakness, fatigue, or dexterity loss; and the type of grip or amount of precision handling required.

Joint Hypomobility: Management—Protection Phase

General guidelines for managing acute joint lesions are described in Chapter 11, with special concerns for patients with RA and OA summarized in Boxes 11.2 and 11.4, respectively.

Control Pain and Protect Joints[15,111]

Patient education. Teach the patient how to protect involved joints and control pain with activity modification, ROM exercises, and appropriate use of an orthosis.[15,108,111]

Pain management. In addition to physician-prescribed medications or nonsteroidal anti-inflammatory medications and modalities, gentle grade I or II distraction and oscillation techniques may inhibit pain and move synovial fluid for nutrition in the involved joints.

Orthoses. Use an orthosis to rest and protect the involved joints. Instruct the patient to remove the orthosis for brief periods of nonstressful motion throughout the day.

Activity modification. Analyze the patient's daily activities and recommend adaptations or assistive devices to minimize repetitive or excessive stresses on the joints. This is particularly important for patients with chronic arthritic disorders to prevent repetitive trauma and to minimize joint-deforming forces.[15,108] Examples are summarized in Box 19.1.

Maintain Joint and Tendon Mobility and Muscle Integrity

Passive, assistive, or active ROM. It is important to move the joints as tolerated, because immobility of the hand quickly leads to muscle imbalance and contracture formation or further articular deterioration. Warm water aquatic therapy is an effective method of combining nonstressful, nonweight-bearing exercises with therapeutic heat.

Tendon-gliding exercises. Have the patient perform full motion in the uninvolved joints and as much motion as possible in the involved joints to prevent adhesions between the long tendons or between the tendons and their synovial sheaths.[59] Tendon-gliding exercises are described in the exercise section of this chapter.

Multiple-angle muscle setting exercises. Perform gentle, pain-free, isometrics of all wrist and hand musculature. Resistive ROM exercises usually are not tolerated if there is joint effusion or inflammation; therefore, isometric resistance within the tolerance of pain is performed.

BOX 19.1 Joint Protection in the Wrist and Hand

Purpose. Performance of daily activities with minimal pain, stress to joints, and energy expenditure. Most of these principles are applicable to any arthritic problem in the hand but are especially important in the hand affected by rheumatoid arthritis.[15]

Respect pain. Monitor activities; stop when fatigue or discomfort begins to develop. Modify or discontinue any activity or exercise that causes pain that lasts longer than 1 hour after stopping the activity.

Maintain strength and ROM. Integrate exercises into daily activities.

- Look for early signs of muscle tightness in the intrinsic muscles. If tight, initiate stretching. One cause of swan-neck deformity is tight interossei muscles pulling on the extensor tendon, leading to hyperextension of hypermobile PIP joints.
- Strengthen radial deviation of the MP joints of the fingers to counter the ulnar drifting of the fingers that occurs in many functional activities.

Balance activity level and rest. More rest than normal is required during the active phases of RA. Conserve energy and perform activities in the most economical way or do the most important activities first.

Avoid deforming positions or one position for prolonged periods.

Avoid using strong grasping activities that facilitate the deforming force. Typical joint deformities with RA include radial deviation and extension of the wrist and ulnar deviation and volar subluxation of the MP joints. Adaptive suggestions include:

- Open jars with the left hand or with an assistive device.
- Cut food with the blade of the knife protruding from the ulnar side of the hand.
- Stir food with spoon on the ulnar side of the hand.
- Build up the handles of eating utensils.
- Use stronger, larger joints whenever feasible. For example, carry items in a shoulder bag or over the forearm or with two hands rather than with one hand.
- Avoid twisting or wringing motions with the fingers. Press water out of a rag by opposing the palms of both hands together.

Joint Hypomobility: Management—Controlled Motion and Return to Function Phases

With joint pathology, increase ROM by utilizing joint mobilization techniques to stretch the capsule as well as passive stretching and muscle inhibition techniques to elongate the periarticular connective tissue and musculotendinous units following the principles described in Chapters 4 and 5. It is also critical to determine if scar tissue has formed in the long tendon sheaths in the hand and, if so, to attempt to re-establish smooth tendon gliding.

Increase Joint Play and Accessory Motions

Joint mobilization techniques. Determine which of the articulations of the distal RU, wrist, hand, or digits are restricted because of decreased joint play and apply grade III sustained or grade IV oscillation techniques to stretch the capsules. See Figures 5.33 through 5.43 for mobilizing restricted joints of the distal forearm, wrist, hand, and digits.

PRECAUTIONS: For patients with RA, joint mobilization techniques are often contraindicated, especially in the inflammatory phase. The therapist must modify the intensity of joint mobilization and stretching techniques that are used to counter any restrictions. This is necessary because the disease process and steroid therapy weaken the tensile quality of the connective tissue, and consequently the tissue is more easily torn.

Improve Joint Tracking and Pain-Free Motion

Mobilization with movement (MWM) techniques may be applied to increase ROM and/or decrease the pain associated with movement.[99] (The principles of MWM are described in Chapter 5.)

MWM of the wrist. Have the patient seated with the elbow flexed and forearm supinated (patient's palm facing toward his or her face); stabilize the distal radius and ulna with one hand, and place the other hand on the ulnar aspect of the proximal carpal row.

- Apply a gentle pain-free radial glide to the proximal row of carpals, utilizing the web space of your hand. Have the patient then perform active wrist extension or flexion to the end of the available range and, with his or her free hand, apply gentle overpressure at the end of the pain-free range (Fig. 19.7).

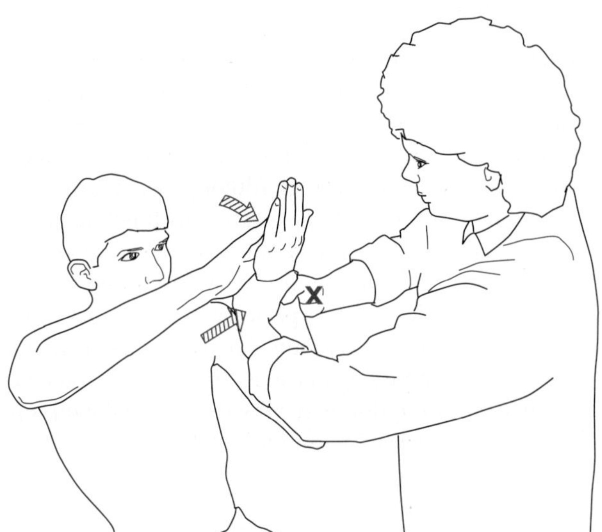

FIGURE 19.7 Mobilization with movement (MWM) to increase wrist flexion or extension. Apply a very gentle lateral glide while the patient actively flexes or extends the wrist and then applies a passive stretch force with his other hand at the end of the range.

- Rotation of the carpals, either dorsally or volarly, may need to be combined with the glide to achieve pain-free, end-range loading.

MWM can also be used with patients who experience pain over an individual carpal bone. In these cases, the MWM is really used to "reposition" a carpal bone in relation to an adjacent carpal (either proximal or distal). Provide a sustained gentle dorsal or volar glide to a specific carpal bone while the patient either performs pain-free wrist flexion, extension, radial or ulnar deviation 6-10 times or performs a pain-free gripping force. Repeat for 3 sets of 6-10 repetitions, ensuring that the technique remains pain free.[99]

MWM of the MP and IP joints of the digits. Gently radially or ulnarly glide the involved phalanx in a painless direction, then have the patient actively flex or extend the finger and apply a pain-free, end-range stretch. Rotation of the more distal phalanx may be required in conjunction with the medial or lateral glide to achieve painless end-range overpressure.[99]

Improve Mobility, Strength, and Function

Carefully examine the multijoint and intrinsic muscles for restricted motion due to contractures or adhesions and poor movement patterns due to weakness or imbalances in strength. Stretching, tendon gliding, and strengthening exercises are described in the exercise sections of this chapter. Utilize techniques that specifically address the impairments the patient demonstrates. Once range is gained, it is critical that the patient uses the new range with active ROM and functional activities.

CLINICAL TIP

Strong muscles help protect the joints, but in the hand, imbalanced muscle forces lead to deformities. Teach isometric exercises in pain-free positions by showing the patient how to use one hand to resist the other in carefully controlled positions and directions. These exercises can be done throughout the day whenever the patient feels discomfort in his or her joints.

Neuromuscular control and strength. Progress exercises with controlled and nondestructive force to increase strength and muscle balance between antagonists and to progress endurance training. With pathological joints, use caution when applying weights so as not to stress the joints beyond the capability of the stabilizing tissues.

Functional activities. Develop exercises that prepare the patient for functional activities. Consider prehension patterns that are required for the patient's job, recreational, and daily activities. Include exercises that require coordination and fine finger dexterity.

Conditioning exercises. Initiate physical conditioning exercises using activities that do not provoke joint symptoms, such as aquatic exercises or cycling.

Joint protection. Reinforce use of joint protection techniques as summarized in Box 19.1.

FOCUS ON EVIDENCE

In a systematic literature review of randomized, controlled trials of adult patients with RA, the reviewers concluded that there is evidence to support the idea that low-intensity therapeutic exercise is beneficial for reducing pain and improving functional status (including hand grip strength) in patients with RA, whereas high-intensity exercise programs may exacerbate symptoms.[109]

Joint Surgery and Postoperative Management

Long-standing RA, OA, or posttraumatic arthritis affecting the joints and soft tissues of the wrist and hand can lead to chronic pain, instability and deformity of joints, restricted ROM, loss of strength in the hand, and impaired function of the upper extremity. When nonoperative management is not sufficient, surgical intervention coupled with individually designed and carefully supervised postoperative rehabilitation is indicated to improve and restore function.

Some of the more common surgical options for management of arthritis of the wrist and hand are listed in ONLINE Box 19.2 on the FA Davis website.

Soft tissue procedures, such as synovectomy, tenosynovectomy for chronic tenosynovitis of the extensor and flexor tendons of the wrist, repair of ruptured tendons, capsulotomy or release of other soft tissues for correcting a deformity, or muscle balancing of the wrist or finger joints, are employed independently or concomitantly when articular surfaces of the involved joints remain reasonably intact.[21,35,59,7687,139] If joint deterioration is significant, resection arthroplasty, such as resection of the distal ulna (Darrach procedure) or proximal row carpectomy; arthrodesis; or implant arthroplasty, performed in conjunction with soft tissue repair or reconstruction, is a surgical option for advanced joint deterioration.[21,76,80,139]

Some procedures are selected to relieve pain and others to minimize or delay further deformity. For example, if medical management of RA of the wrist does not adequately control synovitis, tenosynovectomy is performed to remove proliferated synovium from tendon sheaths and to prevent erosion or rupture of tendons before significant deformity and loss of active control of the wrist and fingers occur.[32,35,76,139] If rupture occurs, tendon repair or transfer can improve function of the hand and delay or prevent subluxation and dislocation of joints or fixed deformities.[32,35,59,61]

Partial or complete arthrodesis of the wrist and arthrodesis of an individual joint of a digit, such as the CMC joint of the thumb, yields predictable and durable results. Fusion corrects deformity and gives the patient stability and relief of pain with only some compromise of function despite the loss of joint motion.[76,80] If fusion is inappropriate and pain-free functional mobility is necessary, implant arthroplasty—either interposition arthroplasty or total joint replacement—is an option. In many instances, a combination of joint and soft tissue procedures is indicated.[17,21,35,80] For the most part, however, arthroplasty is reserved for the patient who requires only low-demand use of the hand.

General goals. The goals of surgery and postoperative management of advanced arthritis and associated deformities of the wrist and hand include[17,21,32,59,80] (1) relief of pain, (2) restoration of normal or sufficient function of the wrist and hand, (3) correction of instability or deformity, (4) restoration of ROM, and (5) improved strength of the wrist and fingers for functional grips and pinch.

A discussion of several types of arthroplasty and general guidelines for postoperative management follow. Information on surgical management and postoperative rehabilitation of tendon repairs and transfers associated with RA is then outlined. Given the complexity of hand rehabilitation, suggested phase-specific guidelines for exercise, founded on principles of tissue healing, must be individualized for each patient and determined by the patient's level of participation in the rehabilitation process and response to exercise.

Successful outcomes are contingent upon close communication among the surgeon, therapist, and patient or patient's family. An effective postoperative rehabilitation program combines early, supervised therapy with patient education and progresses to long-term self-management by the patient.[59,81] Although rehabilitation is deemed essential after each of the surgical interventions covered in this section, postoperative protocols vary and have not been compared for each type of procedure, making it difficult to suggest that there is one best approach to postoperative management.

Wrist Arthroplasty

Although arthrodesis of the wrist continues to be the most common surgical intervention for late-stage arthritis of the wrist, arthroplasty has become an acceptable alternative, particularly for patients with arthritis and impaired mobility of other joints of the extremities. Although wrist arthrodesis has not been shown to limit upper extremity function in daily living activities in patients with only posttraumatic arthritis of the wrist, it is thought that loss of wrist motion may adversely affect function, such as personal care, in patients with RA who also have impaired mobility of other upper extremity joints.[32,80,130] For these patients, wrist arthroplasty (total joint replacement) is an option that provides relief of symptoms while retaining some wrist mobility.[32,35,130]

Indications for Surgery

The following are common indications for arthroplasty of the wrist:[1,17,21,35,107,130]

- Severe pain in the wrist region as the result of deterioration of the articular surfaces of the distal radius, carpals, and distal ulna from chronic arthritis (usually RA, but also OA and posttraumatic arthritis) that compromises hand and upper extremity function
- Deformity and marked limitation of wrist motion that cause muscle-tendon imbalances of the digits
- Subluxation or dislocation of the RC joint
- Appropriate procedure for *low-demand* upper extremity functional needs
- Appropriate procedure for patients with bilateral wrist involvement in which arthrodesis of both wrists would limit rather than improve overall function
- Also appropriate procedure for patients with significant stiffness of the ipsilateral shoulder, elbow, or finger joints in whom unilateral wrist arthrodesis would further limit, rather than improve, functional use of the upper extremity

CONTRAINDICATIONS: Box 19.2 identifies some absolute and relative contraindications to wrist arthroplasty and arthroplasty of the joints of the fingers and thumb.[1,17,21,107]

Procedures

Implant Design, Materials, and Fixation

Numerous designs of total wrist replacement arthroplasty have been developed and consistently refined over the past few decades, making arthroplasty available not only to patients with late-stage joint disease, but also those with severe deformity and collapse of the wrist joint.[17,32,107,130]

BOX 19.2 Contraindications to Arthroplasty of the Wrist or Digits

Absolute
- Active infection
- Expected high-demand use of the hand (e.g., manual labor) or high-impact sport activities (e.g., tennis and volleyball)
- Inadequate motor control of the wrist or hand as the result of neurological damage
- Rupture of the radial wrist extensors
- Limited ROM without pain

Relative
- Severe and irreparable deformity of the wrist or digits
- Rupture of multiple extensor tendons of the digits
- Inadequate, poor quality bone stock
- Need for ambulation aids (e.g., crutches or a walker) that place significant forces across the wrist and hand
- Compromised immune system

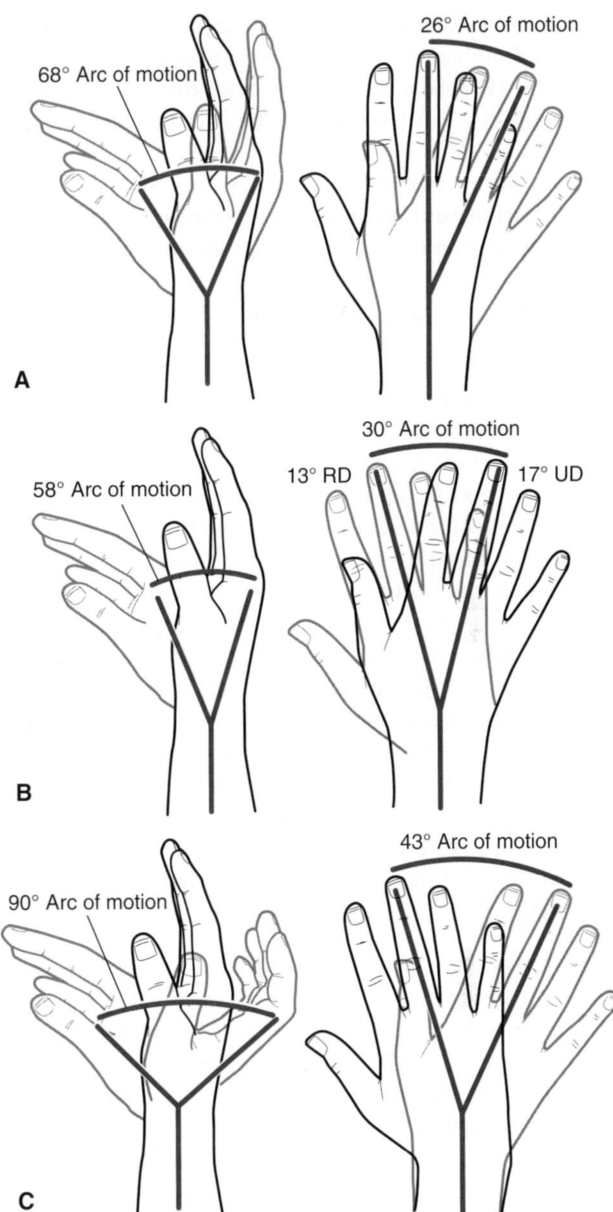

FIGURE 19.8 Arc of motion achieved with **(A)** the Universal 2, **(B)** the ReMotion, and **(C)** the Maestro joint implants.

However, a total wrist arthroplasty is still contraindicated for individuals with a nonfunctional hand due to neurological dysfunction as well as in high-demand patients, laborers, and those with previous history of sepsis or deep local infection. It is also contraindicated for those patients who require the use of assistive devices for support during ambulation or transfers.

Implants used in total wrist arthroplasty have undergone considerable changes aimed at increasing implant survivorship. Currently there are three implant designs approved by the US Food and Drug Administration: the Universal 2 (which uses an ellipsoidal articulation with a beaded porous coating and radial and ulnar variable-angle screws), the ReMotion (designed to allow some degree of intercarpal rotation—the polyethylene ellipse snaps on a ball on the proximal side of the carpal plate), and the Maestro (which mimics a proximal row carpectomy and depends on replacement of the capitate head. The articulation is achieved with a polyethylene proximal component seated into the radius. Follow-up studies have demonstrated that the Universal 2 produces an average total arc of motion of 68° (42° of flexion and 26° of extension and an average of 1° of radial deviation and 26° of ulnar deviation) (Fig. 19.8A). The ReMotion produces a flexion-extension arc of 58°, and radial deviation/ulnar deviation of 30° (13° of radial deviation and 17° of ulnar deviation) (Fig. 19.8B). The Maestro, the newest of the implants, produces an average flexion-extension arc of 90° (43° of flexion and 47° of extension) and a radial/ulnar deviation arc of 43° (14° of radial deviation and 29° of ulnar deviation) (Fig. 19.8C) and is the only implant currently on the market that has achieved functional ROM.[107,130,153,]

Operative Overview

Total wrist arthroplasty requires a longitudinal incision along the dorsal aspect of the wrist in line with the third metacarpal.[17,21,80,130] Concomitant *dorsal clearance* (synovectomy of the wrist and tenosynovectomy of the extensor tendons) is often necessary. The retinaculum is incised and reflected, and the digital extensor tendons are retracted for access to the joint capsule.

The distal portions of the radius, the proximal row (scaphoid, lunate, and triquetrum), and the proximal half of the capitate are resected. The axis of rotation for the wrist lies at the proximal third of the capitate; therefore, the closer the center of the implant to the original, normal center, the better the balance of the implant and ultimately the better the functional outcome of the arthroplasty. An intercarpal fusion of the distal carpal row is performed to support the distal component of the implant, which is subsequently secured to the distal carpal row. With instability and subluxation of the radiocarpal joint, capsule and ligament reconstruction typically is performed to improve wrist stability. Soft tissue balancing is critical for satisfactory results.[80,130]

After closure of the dorsal incision, the hand is placed in a long-arm or short-arm bulky compression dressing and elevated for several days postoperatively to control edema.

Postoperative Management

Immobilization

At 2 to 5 days' following surgery, the bulky dressing is removed and the wrist and forearm are placed in a short-arm volar wrist orthosis with the wrist positioned in 10° to 15° extension. The orthosis allows full, unrestricted finger ROM and opposition of the thumb. At this stage it is important to encourage finger and thumb mobility while in the orthosis. Early on, the patient may have difficulty with activation and glide of the finger extensor muscles because of the surgical approach; therefore, it is beneficial to have the patient perform place and hold exercises for the digital extensors to assist with tendon glide and muscle activation.[26,80]

Depending on the stability of the prosthesis, gentle active ROM of the wrist may begin as early as 2 weeks progressing to passive range stretching begun at approximately 4 weeks. During the first 4 to 6 weeks, the patient will wear the orthosis most of the time, only removing for bathing and exercises.[26,80,130]

Exercise Progression

As with arthroplasty of other large or small joints, the goals and progression of exercise during each successive phase of rehabilitation after wrist arthroplasty are based on the stages of soft tissue healing. If concomitant extensor tendon repairs were also done, the guidelines and time frame for exercise are adjusted and special precautions are taken, as discussed in a later section of the chapter on repair of extensor tendon ruptures in RA.

CLINICAL TIP

When implementing a postoperative exercise program after any type of wrist arthroplasty, stability of the wrist always takes precedence over restoration of wrist mobility. As a point of interest with regard to wrist ROM, the results of biomechanical studies of normal individuals performing a variety of functional activities have revealed that no more than 40° of wrist flexion or extension and a combined 40° of radial and ulnar deviation is used during most activities.[102]

For protection of the wrist after arthroplasty, precautions, identified in Box 19.3, must be incorporated into postoperative exercises and functional activities during and after rehabilitation.[26,80,130,134]

BOX 19.3 Precautions After Wrist Arthroplasty

- Avoid weight bearing on the operated hand during transfers, ambulation with assistive devices, or other daily living activities.
- If ambulation aids are required because of lower extremity joint involvement, use forearm-support crutches or walker.
- Avoid functional activities that place more than 5- to 10-lb loads on the wrist.
- Wear a wrist orthosis for additional protection during functional activities.
- Permanently refrain from high-impact vocational or recreational activities, such as heavy labor or racquet sports.

Exercise: Maximum and Moderate Protection Phases

The focus of rehabilitation during the maximum protection phase is to control pain and peripheral edema, protect the wrist, and prevent stiffness of the rest of the upper extremity. When the orthosis can be removed for wrist exercises, protection of the wrist is still essential.

The emphasis during the moderate protection (controlled motion) phase, which typically begins about 4 weeks postoperatively, is to gradually restore active control and mobility of the digits, wrist, and forearm motion without jeopardizing wrist stability.

Goals and interventions. The following goals and interventions should be considered before and after the wrist orthosis can be removed for exercise.[26,80,130]

- ***Maintain and later improve mobility of uninvolved joints.***
  - Begin active ROM exercises of the digits, elbow, and shoulder while the wrist is immobilized and the use of the hand is restricted.
  - At 6 weeks postoperatively, if there was limited finger mobility preoperatively, initiate gentle passive stretching of the fingers with the wrist in a neutral position and selectively use a low-load, dynamic or static progressive finger orthosis during the day to increase mobility for a sufficient level of hand function.
  - Grade II and possibly grade III joint mobilization techniques are appropriate if the joints of the digits are not inflamed.
- ***Restore control and mobility of the wrist.***
  - Edema control and scar management are an essential part of the program.
  - Include active ROM and tendon-gliding exercises with the wrist in neutral (see Fig. 19.16 A through E in the exercise section of this chapter).
- ***Regain use of wrist, finger, and thumb musculature.***
  - Start with gentle setting (place and hold) exercises and progress to low-intensity, isometric resistance exercises of the wrist and finger musculature.
  - Begin to use the hand for light (minimum-load) functional activities around 6 to 8 weeks.[118]

Exercise: Minimum Protection/Return to Function Phase

During the final phase of rehabilitation, which usually does not begin until 8 to 10 weeks postoperatively, regaining sufficient strength and muscular endurance of the entire upper extremity for functional activities is the priority.[26,80] Patient education focuses on incorporating joint protection during functional activities (refer to Box 19.1). Use of a resting orthosis is advisable at night, particularly if a wrist flexion contracture persists.

Goals and interventions. The following goals and interventions can be progressed as the extent of protection decreases:

- ***Regain functional strength of the hand and wrist.***
  - Transition to low-intensity, dynamic resistance (about 1 lb) exercises of the hand and wrist.[26,81]
  - Emphasize simulated functional movement patterns, such as various types of grasping activities, being certain to reinforce principles of joint protection. If not previously initiated, begin to use the hand for light functional activities.[130]
  - Advise patients regarding avoidance of repetitive forceful activities (i.e., hammering), heavy manual labor, and contact sports.[130]

Outcomes

A successful outcome after wrist arthroplasty gives the patient a stable, pain-free wrist with functional ROM. Postoperative outcomes typically measured are pain relief, use of the hand for functional activities, wrist and forearm ROM, and grip strength. Instruments, such as the Disabilities of the Arm, Shoulder, and Hand (DASH) questionnaire and the Patient-Rated Wrist Evaluation, are used to assess pain, function, and satisfaction.[107]

For the patient with late-stage arthritis in multiple joints, the sequencing of joint surgeries is critical for successful outcomes. For example, a hip or knee replacement should be done before wrist arthroplasty to avoid the need to place weight on the wrist replacement when using an assistive device for ambulation.[1]

Pain relief. Barring complications, short- and long-term relief of pain after total wrist arthroplasty[17,21] is a consistent finding.[107,130] For example, Ferreres and associates[62] reviewed midterm results using the Universal 2 implant in 22 wrists (22 patients) with an average follow up of 5.5 years (range 3 to 9 years). Fifteen of the 22 patients had RA, 2 had wrist destruction from advanced Keinbocks disease, and the remaining 5 patients had nonrheumatoid inflammatory arthritis. Following the procedure, 10 patients reported being very satisfied and 10 patients were satisfied. Pain during ADLs was absent or slight in 17 patients, and when discomfort was present, it was attributed to neighboring diseased joints. Similar results have been found with the ReMotion and Maestro implants.[107]

Wrist and forearm ROM, strength, and function. Improvement in ROM is less predictable than pain relief. ROM of the wrist achieved postoperatively is usually about 25° to 35° of extension and 30° to 40° of flexion; 10° of radial deviation and 15° of ulnar deviation, however, these ranges can be highly variable.[130] A functional level of active wrist ROM appears to be retained over an extended number of years.

Grip strength and use of the operated hand for functional activities routinely improve after wrist arthroplasty. Relief of pain has an obvious impact on hand function. Concomitant soft tissue repair, such as repair of ruptured tendons, also contributes to improved function.[107] Furthermore, arthroplasty provides some additional length to the wrist, which in turn improves the length-tension relationship of the muscle-tendon units that cross the wrist.[17]

Complications. Potential complications, any of which can compromise outcomes following wrist arthroplasty, fall into two broad categories: intraoperative and postoperative.[1,63]

During surgery, there is a risk of fracture of the radius or carpal bone during component implantation, particularly if there is weakening of the cortical bone from long-standing synovitis. This complication requires use of a bone graft and an extended period of immobilization, which can result in postoperative tendon adhesions and stiffness of the wrist. There is also risk of intraoperative damage to an extensor tendon when exposing the joint, requiring repair of the tendon and modification of postoperative exercises so as not to place excessive stress on the repaired tendon.[63]

Postoperative complications include wound infection, dislocation or component loosening, and component wear and eventual breakage.[1] However, results of recent modifications to implant designs that rely on the distal component fixed to the carpus with concomitant intercarpal fusion have significantly reduced the incidence of loosening when compared to older models fixed into the metacarpal shafts.[63,130] Complications may require an alternative procedure or revision arthroplasty. If a silicone implant arthroplasty fails, total wrist arthroplasty is still possible; if a total wrist arthroplasty fails because of mechanical loosening or component failure, revision arthroplasty and wrist arthrodesis are still viable alternatives.[1,17,63,130]

Metacarpophalangeal Implant Arthroplasty

Arthroplasty of the MP joints of fingers (digits 2 to 5), combined with necessary reconstruction of soft tissues, is the most common surgical procedure performed to manage impaired function and progressive deformity as the result of late-stage RA of the hand.[32,40,128]In patients with RA, hand function has been shown to improve over a 1-year period following MP arthroplasty when combined with ongoing medical management. In contrast, the level of hand function does not deteriorate but does not improve over the same time period with ongoing medical management alone.[33] Arthroplasty is also an option for patients with idiopathic OA and posttraumatic arthritis of the MP joints.[40,89,115,130,132]

For MP arthroplasty to be successful, a patient must have intact extensor digitorum tendons, or repair of these tendons must be performed. The two procedures may be staged, one prior to the other, or performed simultaneously as determined by the surgeon. Other procedures to balance soft tissues must accompany MP arthroplasty for improved hand function postoperatively.[33,88,132]

If joints other than the MP joints are involved, which is often the case in RA, surgeries are carefully sequenced. For example, if the wrist is involved, a radiolunate or total wrist arthrodesis for pain-free wrist stability in a functional position may be necessary prior to MP arthroplasty. In contrast, a swan-neck deformity of a finger is managed with PIP fusion in 30° to 40° of flexion, but typically it is done after—not before—MP arthroplasty.[32,33,134]

Similar to wrist arthroplasty, the overall goals of this surgery and postoperative management are to relieve pain, correct alignment of the fingers, improve active hand opening and grasp, and improve the cosmetic appearance of the hand.[32,88,130]

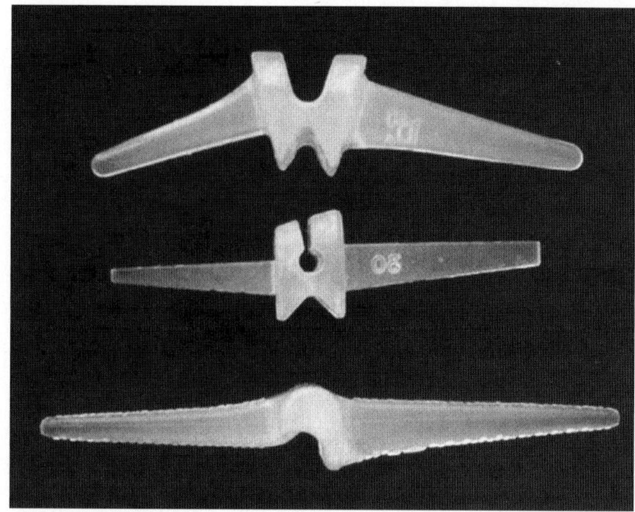

FIGURE 19.9 Lateral view of the three most common silicone-based implants: Neuflex (*top*), Avanta (*middle*), Swanson (*bottom*). Note that the Avanta and Swanson implants are of a 0° bend type. *(From Manuel, JLM, and Weiss, APC: Silicone metacarpophalangeal joint arthroplasty. In Strickland, JW, and Graham, TJ [eds]:* Master Techniques in Orthopedic Surgery—The Hand, *ed. 2. Philadelphia: Lippincott Williams & Wilkins, 2005, p 393, with permission.)*

Indications for Surgery

The following are common indications for arthroplasty of the MP joint(s):[32,33,80,88,130]

- Pain at the MP joint(s) of the hand and diminished hand function as the result of deterioration of the articular surfaces, usually because of RA but sometimes as the result of OA or posttraumatic arthritis
- Instability, often coupled with volar subluxation, and deformity (flexion and ulnar drift) of the MP joint(s) that cannot be corrected with soft tissue releases and reconstruction alone
- Stiffness and decreased active ROM of the MP joints, often associated with a deficient extensor mechanism, causing inability to open the hand to grasp large objects
- Poor appearance of the hand as the result of deformity

Procedures

Implant Design, Materials, and Fixation

MP joint arthroplasty is designed to provide a balance of stability and mobility to the MP joints for patients with late-stage arthritis. Several designs using different materials and methods of fixation have been developed over the past few decades. Currently there are three types of implants available in the United States for MP arthroplasty: pyrolytic carbon (pyrocarbon) MP joint implants, silicone elastomer implants, and surface replacement implants. Both the pyrolytic carbon implant as well as the surface replacement implant attempt to recreate more normal anatomy and may offer patients improved function in the long term.[5,49,80,128] The silicone elastomer implant (Fig. 19.9) has been used since the 1960s and with its known material and long track record, is predictable and dependable in low-demand patients.[5,32,80,130] Silicone elastomer implants have traditionally been used for patients with RA and less commonly in traumatic or isolated degenerative arthritis.

FOCUS ON EVIDENCE

Kevin Chung and colleagues[37] performed the largest collaborative multicenter prospective cohort study to date, comparing the silicone elastomer implant to a nonsurgical group. A total of 67 surgical patients and 95 nonsurgical patients with severe subluxation and/or ulnar drift of the fingers at the MP joints were recruited. Outcomes included the Michigan Hand Outcomes Questionnaire (MHQ), the Arthritis Impact Measurement Scales 2 (AIMS2), grip/pinch strength, the Jebsen-Taylor Test, ulnar deviation, extensor lag, and arc of motion at the MP joints. At 3 years, data was available on 42 surgical and 73 nonsurgical patients and demonstrated significant improvement in mean overall MHQ score and the MHQ function, ADLs, aesthetics, and satisfaction scores in the surgical group as compared to the nonsurgical group. Ulnar deviation (20°), extensor lag (30°), and arc of motion (99°) in the MP joints also improved significantly in the surgical group. The AIMS2 scores and grip/pinch did not show improvement. Complications were reported as minimal with a fracture rate of 9.5%.

As an alternative to silicone elastomer implants, two-component, convex-concave implants have been developed. The surface replacement (SRA) implant provides a medial–lateral stability in flexion, and the radius of the curvature of the articular surfaces allows for the potential of a near normal arc of motion. The components are designed to be cemented; however, noncemented components are being considered for the future.[80,128] The indications for SRA are the same for silicone implants; however, the need for functional collateral ligaments is critical in both the surface replacement and pyrolytic designs.[49,128] The pyrolytic carbon implant has demonstrated properties similar to cortical bone, and wear models have demonstrated no evidence of wear or wear debris, no evidence of inflammation, and excellent bone-implant incorporation. The material properties of the pyrolytic carbon implant provide a good alternative for patients with degenerative or traumatic arthritis of the MP joint. For those patients with RA, where there are signs of instability, dislocation, and cortical bone loss, traditional silicone implants remain the most favorable option.[32,37,49,80,128]

FOCUS ON EVIDENCE

Wagner and colleagues[146] performed a prospective study over 14 years (1998 to 2012) of 254 MP arthroplasties in 110 patients using the pyrocarbon implant design. Of those, 164 patients had inflammatory arthritis (51 required prednisone and 93 required methotrexate), 37 had posttraumatic arthritis, and 53 had osteoarthritis. Of the 254 arthroplasties over 14 years, 26 required revision surgery. The 2-, 5-, and 10-year survival rates were 96%, 89%, and 77%, respectively. The risk for revision surgery was greatest in smokers and those with inflammatory arthritis requiring either prednisone or methotrexate. The 5-year survival rate was not significantly different for inflammatory arthritis (90%), osteoarthritis (85%), and posttraumatic arthritis (85%). The authors concluded that patients overall experience provided predictable pain relief and improvements in ROM and pinch strength and that MP arthroplasties using a pyrocarbon implant demonstrated a nearly 90% 5-year survival rate with a relatively low rate of complications regardless of the diagnosis.

Operative Overview

MP arthroplasty and related soft tissue balancing involve the following procedures.[5,40,88,115,128] The involved MP joints are approached by either a single, transverse incision over the dorsal aspect of the metacarpal heads or by double, longitudinal incisions made between the index and middle fingers and the ring and little fingers. The joint capsule is exposed by carefully separating the extensor tendons, which are often ulnarly displaced from the underlying capsule, and longitudinally incising the extensor hood. The tendons are retracted; the ulnar and possibly the radial collateral ligaments, if intact, are reflected from the head of each metacarpal; and the dorsal aspect of the capsule is incised (capsulotomy). Every effort is made to preserve the radial collateral ligaments. A synovectomy is performed if necessary. If a significant flexion contracture exists, the volar aspect of each capsule may also be incised to allow greater extension of the MP joints.

The heads (distal aspect) of the metacarpals and proximal aspect of the first phalanges of the involved joints are excised, and the intramedullary canals of the metacarpals and proximal phalanges are widened to accept the prosthetic implants. After insertion of the implants, the ROM of the replaced joints is checked. The joint capsule, radial collateral ligament (if preserved), and extensor mechanism of each digit are repaired. The wound is then closed, and a bulky compression dressing and volar hand and forearm orthosis are placed on the hand. The hand is elevated to control edema.[5,80,128]

Postoperative Management

As with arthroplasty of the wrist or other joints of the digits, the postoperative rehabilitation program is founded on the principles of soft tissue healing and includes phase-specific goals and interventions, including the use of dynamic and/or static orthoses and a supervised home exercise program.

General postoperative guidelines from a number of resources for a progression of exercises combined with the use of orthoses to maintain alignment and protect soft tissues as they heal are summarized in this section.[28,40,80] These guidelines must be individualized based on the type of arthroplasty and soft tissue procedures performed and each patient's response. Ongoing patient education and close communication with the surgeon are essential for effective outcomes. Postoperative rehabilitation continues for 3 to 6 months.

Immobilization

Initially, the wrist and hand are continuously immobilized in the bulky compression dressing and volar orthosis applied at the end of surgery, with the wrist positioned in neutral, the MP joints in full extension and either neutral or slight radial deviation (opposite the position of deformity), and the distal joints (PIP and DIP) are free.[5,32,40,80,115]

Continuous immobilization is not lengthy but varies with the type of arthroplasty, the type and quality of the soft tissue repairs, and the stability of the reconstructed joints. If only an MP implant was performed, the hand remains immobilized for only a few days. If, in addition to the MP arthroplasty, ruptured extensor tendons were repaired or transferred, the hand remains immobilized longer to protect the tendons.[61]

Dynamic orthoses. When the compression dressing is removed, the hand is placed in a dynamic MP extension orthosis with an outrigger (Fig. 19.10). The orthosis is worn to protect

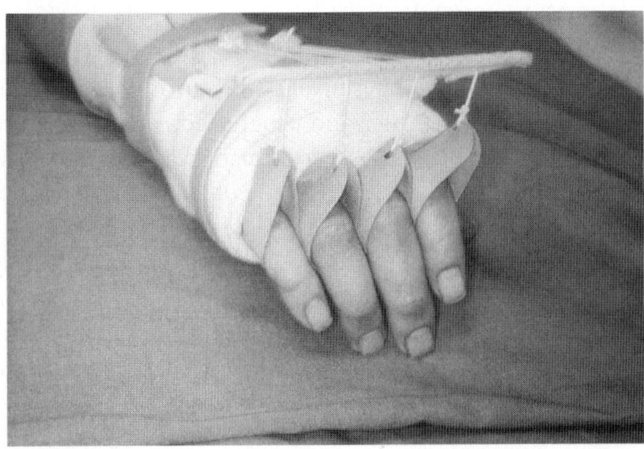

FIGURE 19.10 A dynamic extension orthosis with rubber bands attached to a dorsal outrigger used after MP arthroplasty; permits active MP flexion; and, at rest, maintains the MP joints in extension and sometimes slight radial deviation. *(Courtesy of Janet Bailey, OTR/L, CHT.)*

healing structures, maintain alignment (to prevent recurrent flexion and ulnar drift deformities at the MP joints), and control and guide the range and plane of motion during exercises as soft tissues heal.[20,33,80]

The dynamic orthosis holds the wrist in about 10° to 15° of extension and the MP joints in neutral (at 0°) and slight radial deviation, but it does not control motion in the IP joints. Slings under the proximal phalanx of each finger with spring and fishing line, rubber bands, or elastic cord attached to the outrigger of the orthosis hold the MP joints in a neutral (0°) position when the hand is at rest but still allow active flexion of the MP joints within a functional range. The finger slings are placed around the proximal phalanges with a 90° angle of pull from the proximal phalanx to the outrigger. It is critical to maintain the MP joints in a neutral position of extension when at rest. The pull must also be in the radial direction to prevent recurrence of the ulnar drift and also to prevent radial and ulnar instability by decreasing stress on the radial aspect of the capsule. The patient wears the dynamic orthosis throughout the day for about 6 weeks.[33,80,130]

Static orthoses. A static orthosis is provided for the patient to wear while sleeping. The night orthosis is made with the wrist and MP joints in neutral extension with control of the alignment of the fingers. The night orthosis is worn for 3 to 6 months after surgery or longer as determined by joint alignment and/or the presence of an extensor lag.[32,80]

Exercise Progression

Protected motion in a dynamic orthosis is initiated as early as 3 to 5 days or as late as 10 to 14 days postoperatively when the bulky compression dressing is removed and orthoses have been fabricated.[20,32,40,80,128] Within the first week, emphasis is placed on edema management and gentle active ROM and passive ROM for MP joint flexion and extension within the orthosis with careful monitoring of alignment and rotation.[32,80] Time frames may vary with the type of procedures performed, the underlying pathology, and the stability of the joint. Even after the bulky dressing is removed, exercise may be delayed for a patient with poor soft tissue quality and potential joint instability or delayed wound healing.

With OA or posttraumatic arthritis, the involved MP joints are usually stable postoperatively. Therefore, MP exercises typically are begun earlier and progressed more rapidly in these patients than is permissible for patients with RA, whose joints tend to be less stable as the result of long-standing tissue inflammation and deformities.[115]

Lubahn and associates[80] proposed general goals following MP joint arthroplasty: optimal wound healing, prevention of scar adhesion, management of postoperative edema, neutral alignment with a 35° to 45° arc of motion at the MP joints, and optimal performance of ADLs and vocation/avocational activities. Amadio and Shin[5] reported an expected outcome of a 30° to 40° arc of motion; however, Chung[34] and colleagues studied 162 patients with 180 arthroplasties, and their results demonstrated a 28° arc of motion for the index finger, 28° for the long finger, 32° for the ring finger, and 35° for the small finger, which is slightly less than others have reported. Regardless, appropriate treatment leads to improved motion. The most effective treatment is one based on the individual's tissue response to the exercises and the orthotic positioning program. The most important outcome is for the patient to achieve functional motion in the fingers and satisfaction that their pain has been relieved and their deformity has been improved.[33,37,80,128]

CLINICAL TIP

During the course of rehabilitation, active MP flexion usually plateaus before active MP extension, with flexion levelling off at about 3 to 4 months; however, extension often continues to improve for up to a year.[46]

Exercise: Maximum Protection Phase

For the first 3 weeks, the emphasis is on edema management with active ROM and gentle passive stretching performed within the orthosis. The MP joint is flexed, with the shelf position (MP flexion with IP extension) emphasized, followed by the fingers slowly flexing into the palm. The focus is on the range of the MP joint. During the second week after surgery, collagen formation increases around the capsule and the implant and the joint become more stable. This may appear as increased stiffness of the MP joints; therefore, it is important to monitor the ROM to ensure that the motion is maintained during this time of scar production and maturation.[80]

CLINICAL TIP

Extra attention must be given to the small finger, because the small finger may demonstrate weak flexor power due to chronic subluxation at the MP joint. Buddy taping the small finger to the ring finger at the proximal phalanx may assist with small finger MP joint flexion.[80]

Goals and interventions. The following goals and exercises are emphasized during the maximum protection phase:[20,80,147]

- ***Maintain mobility of the shoulder, elbow, and forearm.***
  - Perform active shoulder, elbow, and forearm ROM. This is particularly important for patients whose RA is affecting multiple joints of the body.
- ***Improve functional ROM of the fingers and maintain gliding of tendons within their sheaths.***
  - To facilitate ROM, edema management techniques including compression sleeves or compression wrapping is initiated.
  - Begin active and gentle passive stretching of the MP, PIP, and DIP joints into flexion and extension within the dynamic orthosis. Emphasize the shelf position of the MP joints followed by flexion of the PIP and DIP joints into the palm of the hand closely monitoring alignment and rotation.

PRECAUTIONS: Carefully observe the incision during MP flexion, being certain to avoid excessive tension on the skin and delay wound closure.

- ***Prevent adhesions along the healed incision.***
  - Perform gentle mobilization of the scar when sutures have been removed.

Exercise: Moderate and Minimum Protection Phases

The *moderate protection phase* begins at about 3 weeks when the implant is clinically stable. The emphasis at this time is to achieve full *active* extension of the MP joints to neutral (no extensor lag) and continue to increase active MP flexion for functional use of the hand. If MP joint flexion is not at the desired range, passive flexion cuffs or rubber band traction may be initiated at this time. The frequency and duration of orthotic positioning is determined by the patient's active and passive motion at this time.

At 4 weeks, in the late fibroblastic stage, coordination and muscle balancing exercises to maintain flexion and extension begin. Light strengthening exercises may also be initiated. It is important to review the joint protection principles and modify the behaviors as needed. At 5 weeks, light ADLs and functional activities are initiated utilizing the joint protection principles. The dynamic orthosis may be continued as needed to assist with alignment and to provide an extension assist if an extensor lag is present. By 6 weeks, the daytime dynamic extension orthosis is gradually discontinued; however, it may be helpful for some patients to use a hand-based dynamic orthosis to maintain the MP joints in extension, yet allow for flexion during functional activities.[80,128] Or, if additional support for alignment is needed, a soft hand-based or forearm-based ulnar drift orthosis may be beneficial. The static night orthosis is continued for an additional 3 to 6 months. During the *minimum protection phase*, which begins around 8 weeks postoperatively, scar maturation is underway; progressive strengthening of the wrist and hand musculature and increasing use of the hand for functional activities while reinforcing principles of joint protection are emphasized. In most instances, a patient is allowed full use of the hand for light to moderate functional tasks by 12 weeks postoperatively.

Goals and interventions. During the moderate and minimum protection phases, goals include the following:[20,40,80]

- ***Continue to increase ROM and active control of the MP joints.***
  - Have the patient continue active flexion exercises in the dynamic orthosis until the daytime orthosis is discontinued. Continue passive stretching, one finger at a time, to increase flexion.
  - Emphasize active MP extension with the wrist in neutral and the IP joints flexed (the hook fist position of the hand) to reinforce the action of the extensor digitorum (ED) muscle and minimize influence of the intrinsic finger extensors. This movement also promotes gliding of the extrinsic extensors in the tendon sheaths.
  - Reinforce MP extension by maintaining the extended position briefly with each repetition.
  - Teach the patient to perform active radial deviation of the MP joints by placing the open hand palm-down on a table, stabilizing the dorsum of the hand with the opposite hand, and sliding ("walking") the fingers toward the thumb.
  - Include active composite finger flexion and opposition of the thumb to each digit, emphasizing pad-to-pad pinch rather than lateral pinch.
- ***Restore ROM of the wrist.***
  - When the dynamic orthosis can be removed during exercise, initiate active ROM of the wrist, emphasizing wrist extension. Be sure the fingers are relaxed during wrist motions.
- ***Improve functional strength of the hand and wrist.***
  - Have the patient begin isometric flexion and extension against submaximal manual resistance or a solid object at 4 weeks postoperatively. Then transition to resisted dynamic finger flexion and extension using a variety of exercise devices, such as a small spring-loaded hand exerciser or exercise putty beginning around 6 weeks.[80]
  - Include resisted radial deviation of the digits. For example, have the patient place the hand on a table palm-down and stabilize the dorsum of the involved hand with the opposite hand. Abduct the index finger against the resistance of a rubber band or push against a coffee cup and slide it across the table.[20]
- ***Regain use of the hand for functional activities while protecting the operated joints to prevent recurrence of deformity.***
  - Reinforce principles of joint protection and energy conservation through patient education (see Box 19.1). Emphasize avoidance of stresses on the fingers in an ulnar direction.
  - Perform simulated functional grasping activities, beginning with light prehension activities. Use the hand for light to moderate functional activities by 5 to 6 weeks postoperatively.
  - Modify ADLs that could contribute to deforming stresses on the MP or other involved joints.[80] Consider use of a commercially fabricated, hand-based, digital alignment orthosis made of neoprene during heavier, more stressful activities.

Outcomes

A successful outcome provides the patient with pain-free, stable, and properly aligned MP joints combined with improved active extension of the digits while retaining or improving MP flexion sufficient for functional grasp. Of these outcomes, pain relief and improved deformity is the primary value of MP arthroplasty.[37]

Pain relief and patient satisfaction. Pain relief is excellent or good for most patients, and correction of a flexion/ulnar drift deformity is consistently sufficient after MP arthroplasty. Both of these outcomes contribute to patient satisfaction because they improve hand function and the cosmetic appearance of the hand.[33,80,128]

ROM and hand function. As previously noted, approximately 70° of active flexion of the MP joints with full active extension to neutral and correction of ulnar drift of the fingers are considered an ideal overall result.[80]

This degree of mobility enables a patient to open the hand far enough to grasp large objects, touch the fingertips of the ulnar digits to the palm (which is necessary for grasping small objects), and touch the tips of the index finger and thumb for pinch. Less MP flexion in the index and middle fingers is acceptable because limited motion of the MP joints enhances stability and allows dexterity and pinch without compromising functional grasp. In a review of a number of short- and long-term studies of patients with various types of arthritis undergoing MP arthroplasty, the postoperative range of MP flexion/extension varied considerably from study to study, with the mean arc of active motion for all fingers reported to be 40° to 45° and a mean extensor lag of 15°. When comparing pre- and postoperative mobility, the total range of flexion/extension may increase only to a small or moderate extent, but the arc of active motion postoperatively often is elevated and becomes more functional. Few studies have directly compared one type of prosthetic implant to another. However, Delaney and colleagues[47] performed a prospective, double-blind study of patients with RA, which followed patients for 2 years postoperatively, and compared the results of two types of silicone implants, the Swanson and the Neuflex® designs (see Fig. 19.9). The findings indicated a significantly greater improvement in MP flexion in patients who received the Neuflex® design than in patients who received the Swanson implant, but there was no significant difference in active MP extension, ulnar deviation, or grip strength between the two groups. Of interest in this study is that the Neuflex® implant, which is performed in 30° of flexion, did not adversely affect active MP extension, which had been a concern of the investigators.

Although satisfactory improvement of MP mobility and a significant correction of deformity (decreased ulnar drift of the fingers) are predictable outcomes after joint arthroplasty, grip and pinch strength do not seem to increase significantly or consistently or they improve only modestly. For example, results of a study by Chung and associates [33] demonstrated that grip and pinch strength had decreased at 6 months after surgery (compared to preoperative measurements) and then gradually increased to preoperative levels by 1 year.

Complications. As the result of a number of complications, approximately 70% of MP silicone implants survive 10 years before revision is necessary.[40,80,123] However, some postoperative complications affect outcomes but do not necessitate additional surgery. Delayed wound healing is a short-term complication that may have an adverse effect on re-establishing adequate MP flexion for functional grasp.[134]

As with the wrist, the most common long-term complication after silicone implant arthroplasty is breakage of the implant,[32,49,123] whereas subluxation or dislocation, mechanical loosening, and implant fracture are common reasons for failure of the two-component metal-plastic and pyrocarbon designs.[32,40,123] It is believed that these long-term complications can be minimized if the patient adheres to joint protection principles by consistently avoiding heavy loads, high-impact activities and deforming forces on the reconstructed joints.

Proximal Interphalangeal Implant Arthroplasty

There are a number of joint and soft tissue procedures for managing arthritis and associated deformities of the PIP joints. They include soft tissue release and reconstruction for swan-neck and boutonnière deformities[32,134] and implant arthroplasty or arthrodesis when there is significant destruction of the articular surfaces.[1,136] PIP arthroplasty is used more frequently for late-stage OA or posttraumatic arthritis than for RA but may or may not be preferable to arthrodesis to improve functional use of the hand.

In the ulnar digits, where mobility of the PIP joints is particularly important for functional grasp, arthroplasty may be the procedure of choice.[136] However, in the index finger, where stability of the PIP joint is a necessity for many functional tasks, arthrodesis is often preferable.[4,73,128,145] If the MP and PIP joints are involved, as is often the case in patients with RA, the MP joint is usually replaced, but the PIP joint deformity (usually a swan-neck deformity) is corrected by soft tissue reconstruction or fusion.[4,59]

Indications for Surgery

In general, PIP implant arthroplasty is indicated for patients with isolated PIP involvement, particularly those who are free of MP joint disease. Implant arthroplasty of contiguous joints (both the MP and PIP joints) is not recommended.[59] The following are commonly accepted indications for PIP joint arthroplasty.[4,59,60]

- PIP joint pain and destruction of the articular surfaces (with or without joint subluxation) secondary to OA or posttraumatic arthritis (less frequently indicated for RA) when nonoperative management has been unsuccessful
- Loss of hand function as the result of joint stiffness, deformity, and decreased ROM that cannot be corrected with soft tissue reconstruction and/or nonoperative treatment
- Only occasionally for isolated boutonnière deformity or swan-neck deformity if fusion is not a viable option

NOTE: Necessary prerequisites for PIP arthroplasty include adequate bone stock, intact neurovascular system, and functioning flexor/extensor mechanisms.[128]

Procedure

Implant Design, Materials, and Fixation

The type of arthroplasty of the PIP joint selected by the surgeon depends on the underlying pathology, the extent of associated impairments and deformities, and the experience of the surgeon. The selection of PIP joint implants available for use today for patients without RA include the silicone elastomer one-piece flexible implant, such as the Swanson, Neuflex, or SBI devices, and surface replacement implants, including titanium-polyethylene (TI) and pyrocarbon (PY).[5,23,44,80,136]

The silicone implant, originally designed by Swanson during the 1960s, remains in use today.[5,44,71,136] A surface replacement design affords greater joint mobility than the one-piece silicone design but provides no inherent stability. Therefore, when PIP arthroplasty is deemed appropriate for patients with RA, who typically have compromised joint stability as the result of damage to periarticular soft tissues secondary to chronic synovitis, a one-piece silicone implant tends to be used to provide some stability to the joint. In contrast, surface replacement arthroplasty is used almost exclusively in patients with OA or posttraumatic arthritis because the collateral ligaments usually are intact or repairable.[5,44,59,71]

Operative Overview

A curved, longitudinal incision is made along the dorsal aspect of the PIP joint. Occasionally, a volar (palmar) or lateral approach is used.[23,59,80] With a dorsal approach, either a *central slip-sparing technique* (which leaves the central tendon intact) or a *central slip-splitting technique* (where the central tendon is incised longitudinally) is used. The latter approach is selected when there is significant joint deformity. Table 19.2 provides an overview of which soft tissues are released, repaired, and require protection during the postoperative program and which structures remain intact during the operative procedure.[4,5,16,59,60,80]

CLINICAL TIP

Although published resources provide descriptions of the various surgical approaches, it is important to review the operative report in a patient's medical record to learn what type of surgical approach was used and which soft tissue structures were incised or released, repaired prior to closure, and will require protection during rehabilitation.

Portions of the head of the proximal phalanx and the base of the middle phalanx are resected. The intramedullary canals of the proximal and middle phalanges are reamed and prepared for the prosthetic implant(s), which is then inserted.

If necessary, the volar plate is released for a flexion contracture, and the extensor tendon mechanism (if split during the approach) is repaired followed by repair of the joint capsule. The wound is closed and a supportive bulky compression dressing is applied holding the PIP joint in extension.

Postoperative Management

Immobilization

At approximately 3 to 5 days postoperatively the surgical dressing is removed and a custom forearm-based dynamic PIP extension orthosis is fabricated with the wrist in 15° of extension and the MP joints in 20° of flexion. This daytime orthosis allows for a passive PIP extension assist and active PIP flexion. A static forearm-based night orthosis is also fabricated with the wrist in 15° of extension, the MP joints in slight flexion, and the IP joints in near full extension.[4,5,59,80,116]

The duration of immobilization varies with the type of arthroplasty, whether extensor tendon or collateral ligament reconstruction of the fingers was part of the procedure, and the surgeon's philosophy; however, it is generally accepted that the dynamic orthosis is discontinued at around 4 weeks if the patient demonstrates full PIP extension and buddy taping is initiated during the day. The protective night orthosis may be continued for up to 3 months postoperatively for those patients having difficulty maintaining their extension and to protect the repaired joints.[5,59,60,80,116]

Exercise Progression

The sequence of exercises after PIP arthroplasty emphasizes early but protected motion of the operated and adjacent joints. PIP exercises in the dynamic orthosis are initiated 3 to 5 days postoperatively with a limited arc of motion starting with 0° to 30°. At 2 weeks, PIP joint motion is increased to 45° if there is no extension lag. At 4 weeks, if the patient demonstrates full active extension, the arc of flexion is increased to 60°. By 6 weeks, a 0° to 75° arc of motion should be achieved and gentle stretching is initiated. By 3 months, the goal is 0° to 75° and activity as tolerated.[5,80,116]

TABLE 19.2 Comparison of Surgical Approaches for PIP Joint Arthroplasty

Type of Approach	Structures Released, Repaired, and Protected Postoperatively	Structures Left Intact
Dorsal approach—central slip-sparing technique	Collateral ligaments incised/repaired; Volar plate disrupted	Central tendon/extensor mechanism intact; allows AROM immediately after surgery
Dorsal approach—central slip-splitting technique	Central tendon incised longitudinally and detached; delays AROM after surgery Volar plate may or may not be disrupted	Collateral ligaments intact; provides joint stability

The goals of exercise during each of the following phases of rehabilitation after PIP arthroplasty are similar to those already detailed in this chapter for rehabilitation after MP arthroplasty. Only guidelines and precautions unique to PIP arthroplasty or procedures for associated correction of specific soft tissue deformities of the PIP joints are addressed in this section.

Exercise: Maximum and Moderate Protection Phases

The primary goals of the maximum and moderate protection phases of rehabilitation after PIP arthroplasty are to control peripheral edema and restore functional mobility of the operated joint(s) without compromising the repair or reconstruction of soft tissues.

In most instances, the emphasis is to regain full or nearly full active PIP extension while gradually increasing PIP flexion by 10° to 15° per week.[5,60,80,116]

CLINICAL TIP

A balance of ROM exercises to regain flexion and extension must occur. Regaining PIP flexion should not be at the expense of attaining full or nearly full active PIP extension, so there is little to no extensor lag.[80]

Goals and interventions. The following goals and interventions are recommended as general guidelines during the first 6 to 8 weeks after surgery. Detailed protocols describing use of orthoses and progression of exercises following different types of PIP arthroplasty are described in several resources:[5,60,80,116,148]

- ***Maintain mobility of the wrist, MP, and DIP joints.***
  - Immediately after surgery, initiate active ROM of all joints not restricted by the bulky dressing.
- ***Restore ROM of the operated joints.***
  - Begin active PIP flexion in the dynamic orthosis 0° to 30° of each involved PIP joint for 2 weeks. At 2 weeks if there is no extension lag, increase the motion to 45°. At 4 weeks, if the PIP joint has full active extension, the arc of flexion is increased to 60°. By 6 weeks postoperatively, the goal is to achieve 0° to 75° of active PIP joint motion.[5,60,80,116] Stabilize the MP and DIP joints in neutral to direct motion to the PIP joint (promotes joint mobility and tendon gliding).
  - If a *boutonnière deformity* was corrected (which requires reconstruction of the extensor mechanism), follow the guidelines and precautions described in Box 19.4.[134]
  - If a *swan-neck deformity* was corrected, follow the guidelines and precautions noted in Box 19.5.[59] A central, slip-splitting approach is necessary for correcting a swan-neck deformity to allow the tension on the extensor mechanism to be adjusted and greater excursion of the PIP joint into flexion.

BOX 19.4 Postoperative Guidelines and Precautions After Correction of a Boutonnière Deformity

Exercise

- Maintain as much extension as possible of the PIP joint through the use of an extension orthosis and exercise for 3 to 6 weeks postoperatively. Remove the orthosis only for exercise and wound care.
- Initiate early DIP flexion exercises with the PIP joint stabilized in extension to maintain the length of the oblique retinacular ligament.
- Begin active or assisted PIP flexion/extension exercises by 10 to 14 days or sooner postoperatively. Stabilize the MP joint in neutral (on a book or at the edge of a table) during PIP movements.
- Emphasize PIP extension and DIP flexion during exercise.

Precautions

- Avoid hyperextension of the DIP joint.
- Because correction of a boutonnière deformity requires a central slip-splitting approach and repair of the extensor mechanism, avoid resisted exercises and stretching of the extensor mechanism of the PIP joint for 6 to 8 weeks or as long as 12 weeks postoperatively.

BOX 19.5 Postoperative Guidelines and Precautions after Correction of a Swan-Neck Deformity

Exercise

- Maintain the PIP joint(s) in 20° to 30° of flexion and the DIP joint(s) in full extension with the use of a static digital orthosis.[59]
- Initiate active ROM exercises at the PIP and DIP joints several days postoperatively.[59]
- Perform DIP extension exercises with the PIP joint stabilized in slight flexion.
- Stabilize the DIP joint in neutral during PIP ROM exercises.
- Emphasize PIP flexion and DIP extension.

Precautions

- Limit PIP extension to 10° of flexion during exercise to avoid excessive stretch to the volar aspect of the capsule.
- Avoid extreme flexion of the DIP joint.

PRECAUTION: During ROM exercises, it is essential to avoid lateral and rotational stresses to the operated joints that could compromise the integrity of the collateral ligaments and joint stability.

Exercise: Minimum Protection/Return to Function Phase

The primary goal of the minimum protection phase shifts from restoration of functional ROM to improving strength in the hand and wrist and gradually incorporating safe but progressive use of the hand into functional ADLs. This transition occurs around 6 to 8 weeks postoperatively. The status of the soft tissue repairs, particularly the extensor tendons, determines how early resisted exercises are initiated. For optimal results, rehabilitation may need to continue (through adherence to a home program) for 3 to 6 months or longer postoperatively.

As with MP arthroplasty, low-intensity strengthening exercises can be performed with equipment specifically designed for hand rehabilitation, such as exercise putty, or through graded functional activities that involve resisted movements. Principles of joint protection (see Box 19.2) are integrated into daily living through patient education, with attention to continued avoidance of lateral stresses to the PIP joints.

Outcomes

After PIP joint arthroplasty, an optimal result provides the patient with a pain-free, mobile, but stable and well-aligned joint for functional use of the hand.[16,59,80,128] Pain relief is the most consistent outcome after PIP arthroplasty. Although patients typically report improvement in use of the hand for functional activities, improvements in ROM and grip strength tend to be marginal at best.[49,148]

Successful outcomes are dependent on proper balancing and repair of the collateral ligaments, adequate soft tissue coverage, and lack of infection following surgery. Outcomes usually are better in patients with OA than in those with posttraumatic arthritis or RA and in fingers without preoperative deformity,[128] but there is no conclusive evidence that one surgical approach or type of current-day arthroplasty is superior to another.[49]

Optimal ROM for functional use of the hand after arthroplasty of the PIP joint is 45° to 70° of active flexion and full or almost full active extension (no extensor lag). However, postoperative ROM reported in most studies is substantially less than optimal.[5]

If the extensor tendon mechanism is intact and a central slip-sparing approach is used, which allows early initiation of mobility exercises, approximately 10° more PIP flexion can be expected than if a central slip-splitting approach is used or repair of extensor tendons is required. If a swan-neck deformity was corrected, a slight (up to 10°) flexion contracture at the PIP joint is acceptable to protect the volar aspect of the joint capsule and possibly avoid recurrence of the deformity.

Complications. The potential complications that can arise following PIP arthroplasty are similar to those associated with MP arthroplasty. Sclerosis around the implant and eventual implant loosening or breakage are long-term complications seen with one-piece silicone implant arthroplasty; however, silicone synovitis is rare.[49,123] Joint instability, subluxation, and dislocation are complications seen with the two-component metal-plastic or pyrocarbon surface replacements because these designs have no inherent stability. Loosening is a long-term complication that may occur regardless of whether cemented or noncemented fixation was used. A unique complication reported only in pyrocarbon designs is an audible squeaking of the implant during joint motion.[49,123]

Patients must continue to avoid forceful grasping and high-impact activities and must practice principles of joint protection for a lifetime to prevent common long-term complications, such as fracture of the implant.[60]

Carpometacarpal Arthroplasty of the Thumb

The CMC joint of the thumb, also called the trapeziometacarpal or basal joint, is one of the most common sites for arthritis in the body. The constant multiplanar forces to which this joint is subjected to over the course of daily activities, work, and recreation can lead to arthritis in one of every three women and one of every eight men.[12,14,19] Pain is the primary reason for patients seeking treatment. Patients with CMC arthritis often describe a constant ache that becomes sharp in nature with activities such as gripping, pinching, or twisting motions. Difficulty and pain with writing is a common complaint. Additional difficulties with participation or activity limitations are specific to an individual's work or recreational pursuits.[14,43]

Indications for Surgery

The following are common indications for CMC arthroplasty of the thumb:[12,14,19,110,132]

- Failure of conservative care including activity modification, hand therapy, orthosis support, anti-inflammatory medication, and intra-articular corticosteroid injections.
- Ongoing disabling pain at the base of the thumb, specifically the CMC joint, as the result of OA, posttraumatic arthritis, or RA. However, most CMC arthroplasties are performed for degenerative joint diseases and less often for synovium-based diseases.
- Dorsal-radial instability (subluxation or dislocation) of the first metacarpal on the trapezium, leading to a hyperextension deformity at the MP joint of the thumb.
- Stiffness and limited ROM (often an adduction contracture) of the thumb.
- Decreased pinch and grip strength because of CMC pain or subluxation.
- Arthrodesis of the CMC joint is inappropriate.

Procedures

Background and Surgical Options

There are a myriad of surgical options from which to choose. The type of procedure selected depends on the degree of ligament laxity, the extent of destruction of the articular surfaces, the underlying pathology, the expected demands that will be placed on the hands postoperatively, and most frequently the surgeons' background and training during residency or fellowship.[11,12,14,41,70] Badia[11] described a classification and treatment system based on arthroscopic findings to assist surgeons in determining the most appropriate course of treatment relative to the stage of arthritis. He defines arthroscopic stage I osteoarthritis as synovitis with intact articular cartilage, and the treatment of choice would by synovectomy. He defines arthroscopic stage II as loss of articular cartilage on the ulnar third of the thumb metacarpal and the central third of the trapezium with disruption of the dorsal radial ligament and attenuation of the anterior oblique ligament. For these patients, he recommends synovectomy, removal of loose bodies and arthroscopic thermal shrinkage (capsulorraphy), and metacarpal extension osteotomy when necessary. He defines arthroscopy stage III as loss of articular cartilage on the trapezium and metacarpal, for which he recommends hemitrapeziectomy with interposition arthroplasty.[11,110] Arthrodesis, rather than arthroplasty, is an option for patients who use the hand for high-demand occupational activities. However, for the patient whose activities place less stress on the hand, there are a number of soft tissue and bony procedures that relieve pain and restore joint stability but preserve functional mobility at the base of the thumb.[12,19,41,70,104] Retaining some CMC joint mobility is particularly important for the patient with RA, who typically has loss of mobility of other joints of the hand and wrist.[138]

Currently there are eight commonly used surgical procedures to treat CMC OA that have been presented in the literature: (1) volar ligament reconstruction, (2) metacarpal osteotomy, (3) CMC arthrodesis, (4) total joint replacement, (5) trapeziectomy, (6) trapeziectomy with tendon interposition, (7) trapeziectomy with ligament reconstruction, and (8) trapeziectomy with ligament reconstruction and tendon interposition (LRTI).[12,14,143] Among these procedures, ligament reconstruction alone is used when there is pain and instability but little to no loss of articular cartilage.[41] Trapezial resection with tendon interposition is by far the most widely used approach to treatment when there is joint subluxation and loss of the joint space due to deterioration of articular cartilage.[14,19,22,59,70,110,132,138,143] Trapezial resection, combined with ligament reconstruction but without tendon interposition, also has been shown to be an effective surgical approach to treatment.[19,22,110,143]

Surface replacement arthroplasty is an alternative to trapezial resection/tendon interposition arthroplasty for a select few patients with CMC OA. Surface replacement arthroplasty involves either resurfacing one articular surface or replacing the surfaces of the trapezium and metacarpal (also known as a total joint surface replacement) with a two-component, saddle-shaped rigid implant that is cemented in place.[14,41,70,144] A patient must have good quality bone stock to be a candidate for surface replacement arthroplasty. In the past decade, total joint arthroplasty using a semiconstrained cemented implant that allows freedom of motion while providing good stability has gained popularity. The main advantage of using a total joint arthroplasty is that if the implant fails or the patient is symptomatic, the implant can be removed and the trapezium resected, allowing for the standard LRTI procedure to be performed. However, the current indications for a total joint arthroplasty is for older women with limited hand use due to reports of heterotopic ossification and implant loosening.[12,14] On the other hand, preliminary studies of the newer implants are showing promise by allowing for a minimally invasive procedure with minimal bone resection and providing sufficient stability while allowing for biologic ingrowth at the new joint location.[12,69,143,144]

Operative Overview

LRTI arthroplasty. For an LRTI, a dorsal incision is made at the base of the thumb, with careful attention paid to protecting the branches of the superficial radial nerve. The trapezium is resected (trapeziectomy), the EPB tendon is reflected, and a hole is created in the base of the metacarpal perpendicular to the nail plate. A portion of the FCR tendon is harvested through a proximal transverse incision. The tendon is passed through the base of the metacarpal and between the thumb and index metacarpal. The remainder of the tendon is rolled into a ball and inserted into the trapezial space. The capsule is repaired, being sure to include the tendon reconstruction in the repair. Before wound closure, the MP joint is evaluated as indicated and treated with a capsulodesis or arthrodesis, along with possible transfer of the EBP tendon to the first metacarpal base. The capsule and adjacent soft tissues are then repaired, and the wound is subsequently closed.[8,12,14,16,22,59,70]

Surface replacement arthroplasty. For a partial trapeziectomy with interposition of a biologic implant, a dorsal approach is used. Approximately 2 mm of the distal trapezial articular surface is removed, and a shallow trough is made in the dorsal surfaces of the metacarpal base and the trapezium. The trough allows for the implant to lie flush to the bone. The implant is inserted into the space and secured to the bone. The capsule is closed over the implant, and the wound is closed.[14,110,144] With a two-component design, after the capsule has been split longitudinally, the distal portion of the trapezium and the base of the first metacarpal are resected. The trapezium and the intramedullary canal of the metacarpal are prepared, and the prosthetic components are inserted and cemented in place. The capsule is repaired, and as with soft tissue interposition arthroplasty, the abductor pollicis longus may be advanced to enhance joint stability. Joint stability and ROM are assessed prior to closure and application of a bulky compression dressing.

Postoperative Management

The overall goal of rehabilitation following CMC arthroplasty is to attain sufficient pain-free mobility of the thumb for functional activities while maintaining joint stability for strong pinch and grasp. It may take up to a year after surgery for a patient to achieve optimal results.

Immobilization

With all procedures, the thumb and hand are immobilized postoperatively in a bulky compression dressing and elevated for several days to a week to control edema.

After the postoperative dressing is removed, the hand is placed in a static, forearm-based thumb spica cast for the first 4 to 6 weeks. The cast is later replaced with a custom removable orthosis, with the CMC joint immobilized in palmar abduction (40° to 60°), the MP joint in slight flexion, and the wrist in neutral to slight extension.[8,14,19,43,70] The IP joint of the thumb and the fingers are left free.

The length of time the CMC joint is *continuously* immobilized depends on the surgery. The time frame varies from just 1 to 2 weeks after total surface replacement arthroplasty[43] to 3 to 5 weeks after ligament reconstruction/tendon interposition arthroplasty or resurfacing arthroplasty with prosthetic implants.[19,41,43,59,104]

After surgery, when ROM exercises are permitted, the orthosis is removed during the day for frequent exercise sessions. From 8 to 12 weeks, as the patient uses the hand for functional activities, the use of a daytime orthosis is gradually discontinued. Use of a night orthosis to stabilize the thumb continues for 8 to 12 weeks or until the joint is stable and essentially pain free.[19]

Exercise Progression

Progression of exercises varies with the type of arthroplasty. Guidelines presented in this section are for *ligament reconstruction/tendon interposition arthroplasty*, still the most common form of CMC arthroplasty. Management guidelines unique to total surface replacement arthroplasty also are noted. Precautions after CMC arthroplasty are summarized in Box 19.6.[8,14,19]

Exercise: Maximum Protection Phase

The focus of the first 6 weeks of rehabilitation is to control pain and edema, maintain ROM in nonimmobilized joints, and initiate protected motion of the CMC joint when it is permissible to remove the thumb spica orthosis for exercise.[8,14,19,70]

BOX 19.6 Precautions After CMC Arthroplasty of the Thumb

- Initially refrain from full CMC radial adduction (sliding the thumb across the palm to the base of the fifth finger) as this motion places excessive stress on the dorsal aspect of the capsule and ligament reconstruction. Be certain it is possible to oppose the thumb to each fingertip before attempting to touch the base of the fifth finger.
- When stretching to increase CMC palmar abduction, apply the stretch force to the metacarpal, not the first phalanx, to avoid hyperextension or compromising stability of the MP joint. Follow the same precaution during light resistance exercises.
- Avoid forceful pinch and grasp for at least 3 months after surgery.
- Modify ADLs to limit heavy lifting. If occasionally heavy lifting is necessary, advise the patient to wear a protective orthosis.

Goals and interventions. The following are suggested goals and exercise interventions for the first 6 weeks after surgery:

- ***Maintain mobility of the fingers and IP joint of the thumb.***
  - During the period of continuous immobilization of the wrist and CMC and MP joints of the thumb, have the patient perform active ROM of the fingers, IP joint of the thumb, elbow, and shoulder.
- ***Initiate protected mobility of the thumb and wrist.***
  - When permissible, begin active ROM of the wrist and controlled ROM of the thumb within protected ranges.
  - After *tendon interposition arthroplasty*, protected ROM is not initiated until about 4 to 6 weeks after surgery to allow time for the reconstructed soft tissues to adequately heal .[8,41,43,70,110,138,147]
  - After *total surface replacement arthroplasty*, ROM may be initiated at about 1 week postoperatively because of the inherent stability of the cemented implants.[41] When it is permissible to remove the orthosis for exercise, begin active wrist ROM in all directions and CMC ROM with active radial and palmar abduction, opposition, and circumduction. Also include active MP flexion and extension, being certain to stabilize the CMC joint.

Exercise: Moderate and Minimum Protection Phases

While continuing to regain ROM, the focus of rehabilitation during the intermediate and final phases of rehabilitation gradually shifts to developing grip and pinch strength for functional tasks.

Goals and interventions. Consider the following goals and interventions:

- ***Re-establish functional mobility of the hand and wrist.***
  - Continue active ROM exercises, gradually increasing the range.
  - At about 8 weeks, begin gentle self-stretching exercises.
- ***Regain strength and functional use of the hand and wrist.***[8,19,43,138,147]
  - At about 8 weeks postoperatively, initiate isometric exercises against light resistance, emphasizing palmar abduction, radial abduction, opposition, and circumduction.
  - If the CMC joint is stable and pain free, progress to dynamic resistance exercises to regain pinch and grip strength.
  - Between 8 and 12 weeks, remove the orthosis when using the hand for light ADLs, such as buttoning and unbuttoning.
  - Incorporate principles of joint protection during strengthening exercises and ADLs.
  - Continue to increase use of the hand for light to moderate ADLs over the next 4 to 6 weeks. A patient typically can return to light-duty work by 3 to 4 months and can resume most functional activities by 4 to 6 months.

Outcomes

Most of the studies reported in the literature have investigated outcomes of trapezial resection/tendon interposition arthroplasty with limited evidence reported on the results of surface replacement arthroplasty. Based on data from a variety of instruments that measure pain, ROM, hand function, patient satisfaction, and quality of life, pain-free ROM of the basal joint of the thumb and improved hand function, measured by patient's dexterity, pinch, and grasp, are considered successful overall outcomes following CMC arthroplasty.[12,14,19,41,69] The time required to achieve maximum benefit from the surgery is typically 6 to 12 months.[14]

Among the procedures available, trapezial resection/tendon interposition arthroplasty with or without ligament reconstruction yields the most predictable and successful outcomes.[14,41,70] In a review of tendon interposition arthroplasty, outcomes appear better when the procedure includes reconstruction of ligaments, possibly because the CMC joint is more stable with reconstruction.[41]

Pain relief and patient satisfaction. Regardless of the type of CMC arthroplasty, the most consistent and predictable benefit of these procedures is relief of pain.[12,14,19,41,59,,77,143] For example, in a review of outcomes of a number of studies for patients with OA who had undergone tendon interposition arthroplasty with or without ligament reconstruction, 94% of patients reported long-term relief of pain.[132] Although tendon interposition is designed to resurface the deteriorated joint to make motion more comfortable, in a prospective, randomized study of patients with OA, investigators compared the results of trapezial resection and ligament reconstruction with and without the use of tendon interposition. They found that at a mean of 48 months after surgery, both groups had equally satisfactory pain relief.[77]

A patient's quality of life also improves after CMC arthroplasty. In a follow-up study of 103 patients with OA who had primary tendon interposition arthroplasty, participants completed several standardized self-assessment questionnaires at a mean of 6.2 years after surgery.[7] In an overall rating, 79 of 103 reported their quality of life had improved greatly, and an additional 15 reported slight improvement.

ROM and hand function. Active ROM of the thumb, particularly opposition, and dexterity usually improve after CMC arthroplasty. Increased radial and palmar abduction widen the web space, making it easier to open the hand to grasp large objects. However, the results of some studies of ligament reconstruction/tendon interposition arthroplasty indicate that preoperative and postoperative ROM is essentially unchanged. Although evidence is limited, surface replacement arthroplasty is thought to produce greater improvement in ROM compared with soft tissue procedures, especially in the short term.[41,69,143,144] However, results of a recent study of total surface replacement arthroplasty (two-component, metal-plastic design) demonstrated that although significant pain relief and improvement of bilateral hand function occurred in some tests, there was no significant improvement in range of opposition or grip and pinch strength at a mean follow-up of 3 years after surgery.[69,142]

In contrast, other studies that follow patients for several years after surgery indicate that measurements of pinch and grip strength as well as performance of functional tasks improve significantly.[41] The most successful long-term functional outcomes have been reported for patients who use the hand primarily for low-demand activities.[12,14,69]

Complications. Complications vary with the type of CMC arthroplasty. Overall, the rate of complications is low, with inadequate pain relief and recurrence of joint instability the most common complications that necessitate revision arthroplasty. In a retrospective study of 606 primary tendon interposition-ligament reconstruction arthroplasties performed over a 16-year period, only 3.8% were known to have required a revision procedure for mechanically based pain.[42] Neuropathic pain also can develop after CMC arthroplasty. The pain may be caused by damage to or impingement of the radial nerve (radial sensory neuritis), carpal tunnel syndrome, or complex regional pain syndrome.[14]

For arthroplasties that include implantation of prosthetic components, loosening and dislocation are the most common complications. Overall, implant loosening is more likely to occur with uncemented fixation but has been reported to occur in cemented procedures as well.[69,142]

Tendon Rupture Associated With RA: Surgical and Postoperative Management

Background and Indications for Surgery

Tendon ruptures in the hand are common in patients with chronic tenosynovitis associated with RA. The site of the rupture may be in the wrist or the hand. When a tendon ruptures, there is a sudden loss of active control of one or more of the digits. Rupture of a single or multiple tendons is usually painless and occurs during unremarkable use of the hand.[16,59,61,124] Such ruptures are evidence of severely diseased tendons.

The extensor tendons are affected far more frequently than the flexor tendons. In order of frequency, extensor tendons that most often rupture are the common extensor tendons to the small and ring fingers and the extensor pollicis longus (EPL). The most common flexor tendon to rupture is the flexor pollicis longus (FPL).[2,59,61,81,124,125]

The causes of rupture include infiltration of proliferative synovium in the tendon sheaths and into tendons, which subsequently weakens the affected tendon; abrasion and fraying of a tendon as it moves over a bony prominence roughened or eroded by synovitis; periodic use of local steroid injections over time; or ischemic necrosis caused by direct pressure from hypertrophic synovium, particularly at the dorsal retinaculum, that compromises blood supply to a tendon. Common sites of abrasion that affect the extensors are the distal ulna, Lister's (Radial) tubercle, and the volar aspect of the scaphoid where it contacts the flexor tendons.[2,59,61,81,124,125]

The indication for surgery is loss of function of the hand. Rupture of a single tendon, such as the extensor digiti minimi, may not impair a patient's function, whereas rupture of multiple tendons simultaneously or over a period of time may cause significant limitations of function and disability.

Procedures

The surgical procedures available for treatment of tendon ruptures in RA vary depending on which tendon(s) has ruptured, the number of ruptured tendons, the location of the rupture, the condition of the tendon at the site of rupture, and the quality of the remaining intact tendons of the hand. Options include:[16,38,59,81,124]

- ***Tendon transfer.*** A tendon is removed from its normal distal attachment and attached at another site. For example, the extensor indicis (EI) can be transferred if the EPL has ruptured. A flexor tendon can also be transferred to the dorsal surface of the hand to act as an extensor if multiple extensor tendons have ruptured.[38,59,81,124,125]
- ***Tendon graft reconstruction.*** A portion of another tendon that acts as a "bridge" is inserted between and sutured to the two ends of the ruptured tendon. The palmaris longus tendon is often selected as the donor tendon. A wrist extensor tendon may be selected if a wrist arthrodesis is performed at the time of the tendon reconstruction.[38,59,81]
- ***Tendon anastomosis (side-to-side tenorrhaphy).*** The ruptured tendon is sutured to an adjacent intact tendon. This is a common option at the wrist for the finger extensor tendons.[81,124,125]
- ***Direct end-to-end repair.*** The two ends of the ruptured tendon are re-opposed and sutured together. This option is used only occasionally because the ends of the ruptured tendons in patients with RA are usually frayed. Therefore, a considerable portion of the frayed tendon(s) must be resected, which shortens the tendon, making it difficult to suture end to end.[59,124]

Concomitant procedures in the rheumatoid hand include tenosynovectomy, removal of osteophytes from bony prominences, and ligament reconstruction or arthrodesis for instability. If late-stage MP joint disease also is present and passive extension of the MP joints is significantly limited, arthroplasty of the involved joints may be indicated as well, either simultaneously with the tendon procedure or during two separate operations as determined by the surgeon. Without adequate joint mobility, the transferred or reconstructed extensor tendons become adherent, resulting in a poor outcome.[124,125]

Postoperative Management

The guidelines described in this section apply only to management of tendon transfer, reconstruction, or repair of extensor tendons in the rheumatoid hand. As mentioned previously, rupture of extensor tendons occurs far more frequently than flexor tendon rupture. As with postoperative management for other surgeries described in this chapter, pain and edema control and exercises for the uninvolved joints are always essential components of rehabilitation.

Tendon transfers and reconstruction are delicate procedures requiring ongoing communication between the therapist and surgeon and active involvement of the patient in the postoperative program. The goal of any tendon transfer is to redistribute power in the hand in order to improve function. Communication with the patient and establishing realistic goals and expectations is important, as the tendon transfer does not return normal joint motion but rather improves current function. Therefore, patient education is woven into every phase of rehabilitation.[81]

Immobilization

A bulky compression dressing is applied to the hand and wrist at the close of extensor tendon surgery to control edema. The surgical compression dressing is removed after several days, and the wrist and hand are then immobilized in a forearm-based volar resting orthosis, which holds the wrist in 30° to 40° extension and the MP joints in 10° to 20° of flexion with the IP joints free to minimize any possible tension on the transfer.[81,125]

For example, after side-to-side finger extensor transfer or extensor tendon reconstruction, the wrist and all fingers are immobilized in extension in the orthosis, but the thumb is free to move. After reconstruction of a ruptured EPL tendon or transfer of the EI tendon to restore thumb extension, the wrist is immobilized in extension, the thumb in palmar abduction, and the MP and IP joints in neutral to slight extension with the fingers free to move.[81]

Continuous immobilization of the wrist and digits is maintained for approximately 3 to 4 weeks to protect the healing tendons.[59,81,124,125] Use of a daytime orthosis is discontinued at about 12 weeks; however, use of a night orthosis typically continues for 6 months or longer.

CLINICAL TIP

Use of dynamic orthosis and early mobilization (a few days after surgery) is not typically recommended for tendon reconstruction or transfers in the rheumatoid hand. Tissue healing is slower and the risk of re-rupture higher postoperatively for patients with long-standing, systemic disease (who likely have been treated periodically with corticosteroids) than in otherwise healthy patients who have sustained an acute laceration or rupture of a tendon in the hand.[59,124,125]

Exercise Progression

During each phase of postoperative rehabilitation after extensor tendon transfer or reconstruction, exercises are progressed very slowly and very gradually. Precautions during exercise and functional use of the hand are summarized in Box 19.7.

Exercise: Maximum Protection Phase

During the first 6 weeks after surgery, the priorities of rehabilitation are edema control and protection of the transferred or reconstructed tendon(s), followed by carefully controlled mobility of the operated areas to prevent adherence of healing tissues. It is usually permissible to remove the protective orthosis for exercise at around 3 to 4 weeks. If tendon quality is poor and the security of the sutured tissues is in question, exercise may be delayed until about 6 weeks postoperatively.[81]

BOX 19.7 Precautions After Extensor Tendon Transfers or Reconstruction in the Rheumatoid Hand

- During the early phase of rehabilitation, do not initiate MP extension from full, available MP flexion to avoid excessive stretch on the operated tendon(s).
- Postpone stretching to increase MP flexion if there is a deficit in active extension.
- Avoid activities or hand postures that combine finger flexion or thumb radial abduction and radial adduction with wrist flexion, as this places extreme stress on the reconstructed or transferred extensor tendons. If a patient must use the hands for transfer activities, avoid weight bearing on the dorsum of the hand.
- Avoid vigorous gripping activities that could potentially overstretch or rupture the reconstructed or transferred extensor tendon(s).

Goals and interventions. The goals and intervention during the first phase of rehabilitation include the following:[61,81]

- ***Maintain mobility of the elbow and forearm, uninvolved digits, and other uninvolved joints.***
  - While the operated hand is immobilized, perform active ROM of all necessary joints.
- ***Re-establish mobility and control of the repaired or transferred extensor muscle-tendon units.***
  - When the orthosis may be removed for exercise, initiate active wrist motions with the fingers relaxed.
  - Begin assisted MP extension of each of the fingers or thumb with the wrist and IP joints of each digit stabilized in neutral.
  - Perform *place and hold* exercises by passively positioning the operated MP joint first in a neutral and later in a slightly extended position. Have the patient briefly hold the position. This emphasizes end-range extension to prevent an extensor lag.
  - Progress to active MP extension with the wrist in neutral, initially from slight MP flexion with the palm of the hand on a table and the fingers relaxed over the edge.

CLINICAL TIP

To help a patient learn the new action of a transferred tendon, initially have the patient focus on the original action (function) of the muscle-tendon unit. For example, if the EI was transferred to replace the action of the EPL of the thumb, have the patient think about extending the index finger when trying to actively extend the thumb. Use biofeedback or functional electrical stimulation (FES) to assist with the motor learning.[81]

- ***Regain active flexion of the digits.***
  - Initiate MP flexion of the fingers by having the patient relax the ED after active extension rather than actively flexing the fingers.
  - Progress to active MP flexion within a protected range with the wrist and PIP joints stabilized in neutral. With the wrist and MP joints stabilized in extension, actively flex (hook fist/intrinsic minus position) and extend (straight hand position) the PIP joints. Performing PIP flexion while in wrist and MP extension prevents stiffness of the IP joints without placing a stretch on the repaired ED tendon(s). It is important to attain full fist closure with the wrist in extension in the first 4 weeks because an inability to achieve a full fist, particularly of the ring and small fingers, indicates a functional restriction as opposed to a slight extensor lag.[124]

Exercise: Moderate and Minimum Protection Phases

By 6 to 8 weeks postoperatively, the transferred or reconstructed tendon can withstand greater stresses. Use of the hand for light functional activities usually begins at this time. At about 8 weeks, use of a daytime orthosis is gradually decreased and typically discontinued by 12 weeks postoperatively; however, use of an orthosis at night may continue for up to 6 months depending on the function of the transfer.[81]

Goals and interventions. Consider the following goals and interventions to progress the rehabilitation program:

- ***Continue to increase active mobility of the operated digits.***
  - Add gentle passive stretching to increase MP extension or flexion if one or both motions are restricted.
  - Continue active MP extension exercises to prevent an extensor lag. If MP extension to neutral is possible (no extensor lag), perform active MP extension with the palm of the hand on a flat surface, and extend each finger beyond neutral.
  - With the wrist in neutral or slight extension, gradually increase MP flexion by touching each fingertip to the palm of the hand (first straight and then full-fist positions) or the thumb to each fingertip and gradually to the base of the fifth finger.
- ***Regain strength, control, and functional use of the hand.***
  - Incorporate active movements of the digits into manual dexterity and coordination activities that simulate functional activities. Remove the orthosis for functional activities that involve light grasp, such as picking up or holding light objects or folding clothing.
  - Around 8 to 12 weeks add isometric and dynamic, *submaximal* resistance exercises to improve functional strength and endurance of the hand.
  - Through ongoing patient education, reinforce principles of joint protection during functional use of the hand.

Outcomes

The results of surgical intervention and postoperative management of ruptured tendons in the hands of patients with RA is highly dependent on the extent of involvement in the joints and soft tissues of the hand and wrist preoperatively. It is often difficult to differentiate postoperative functional improvement strictly as the result of a tendon transfer or reconstruction from procedures performed concurrently, such as joint arthroplasty or arthrodesis.

Barring complications, the most common of which is tendon re-rupture, a few generalizations can be made.[59,61] Patients with a recent rupture of a single tendon, who have full passive ROM of the affected joint, realize an optimal postoperative outcome: full functional grasp and no extensor lag in the involved digit. The greater the number of tendon ruptures or associated impairments, such as joint contractures, fixed deformities, or joint instabilities, the more complicated the surgical treatment and the poorer the results.[59]

Repetitive Trauma Syndromes/Overuse Syndromes

Disorders from cumulative or repetitive trauma in the wrist and hand lead to significant loss of hand function and lost work time.[58] The causes are related to repeated movements over an extended period of time. The resulting inflammation can affect muscles, tendons, synovial sheaths, and nerves. Diagnoses include carpal tunnel syndrome, trigger finger, de Quervain's disease, and tendinopathy (tendonitis/tenosynovitis). Management of carpal tunnel syndrome and nerve compression in the tunnel of Guyon is described in Chapter 13.

Tendinopathy

Etiology of Symptoms

Pathological breakdown of the tendon structure results from continued or repetitive use of the involved muscle beyond its ability to adapt, the effects of RA, a stress overload to the contracting muscle (such as strongly gripping the steering wheel during a motor vehicle accident), or roughening of the surface of the tendon or its sheath.[45,58,117,149]

Common Impairments of Structure and Function

- Pain whenever the related muscle contracts or whenever there is movement that causes gliding of the tendon through the sheath.
- Warmth and tenderness with palpation in the region of inflammation.
- In RA, synovial proliferation and swelling in affected tendon sheaths, such as over the dorsum of the wrist or in the flexor tendons in the carpal tunnel.
- Frequently, an imbalance in muscle length and strength or poor endurance in the stabilizing muscles. The fault may be more proximal in the elbow or shoulder girdle, causing excessive load and substitute motions at the distal end of the chain.

Common Activity Limitations and Participation Restrictions

A common limitation of tendinopathy is the inability to perform repetitive or sustained work, recreational, or leisure gripping activities or hand motions that require contraction of the involved musculotendinous unit due to pain that worsens with the provoking activity.[57]

Management: Protection Phase

Follow the guidelines for acute lesions described in Chapter 10, with special emphasis on education, relieving the stress in the involved musculotendinous unit, and maintaining a healthy environment for healing with nondestructive forces.

- ***Patient education.*** Inform the patient how the mechanism of injury and repetitive activity is provoking the symptoms. Explain the necessity to modify the activity to allow healing. Engage the patient in the rehabilitation program.
- ***Rest the part.*** Rest the involved joints and involved tendon with the use of an orthosis.[78]
- ***Tendon mobility.*** If the tendon is in a sheath, apply transverse friction massage while the tendon is in an elongated position, so mobility develops between the tendon and sheath.[78]
  - Teach the patient gentle stretching and tendon-gliding exercises to improve mobility and prevent adhesions. (These are described in the exercise section of this chapter.)
- ***Muscle integrity.*** Teach the patient how to perform multi-angle muscle setting isometrics in pain-free positions followed by pain-free ROM.

Management: Controlled Motion and Return to Function Phases

- ***Exercise progression.*** Progress to dynamic exercises, adding resistance within the tolerance of the healing musculotendinous structure.
- ***Biomechanical assessment.*** Assess the biomechanics of the functional activity provoking the symptoms and design a program to regain a balance in the length, strength, and endurance of the muscles. Frequently, problems arise in the wrist and hand because of poor stabilization or endurance in the shoulder or elbow.
- ***Prevention.*** Continue to emphasize the importance of self-monitoring the symptoms, maintaining a safe exercise program, and unloading the wrist/hand when symptoms occur.[45]

FOCUS ON EVIDENCE

Backstrom[10] reported a case study of a patient diagnosed with de Quervain's disease of 2 months' duration in which MWM was used in addition to physical agents, exercise, and transverse friction massage. Pain was markedly reduced from 6/10 to 3/10 (50%) by the third intervention, and by the completion of 12 sessions, it was 0 to 1/10. The author proposed that the subtle malalignment in the wrist joints associated with the overuse syndrome perpetuated the symptoms and that the MWM helped restore normal arthrokinematics. The MWM techniques used included active movements of the thumb and wrist while a passive radial glide of the proximal row of carpals was applied (similar to Fig. 19.7). The principles of MWM are described in Chapter 5.

Traumatic Lesions of the Wrist and Hand

Simple Sprain: Nonoperative Management

After trauma from a blow or a fall, an excessive stretch force may strain the supporting ligamentous tissue. There may be a related fracture, subluxation, or dislocation.

Common Impairments of Structure

- Pain at the involved site whenever a stretch force is placed on the ligament
- Possible hypermobility or instability in the related joint if supporting ligaments are torn

Common Impairments of Function, Activity Limitations, and Participation Restrictions

- With a simple sprain, pain may interfere with functional use of the hand for a couple of weeks whenever the joint is stressed. Consider the use of an orthosis or tape to protect the ligament without a limitation of function provided the orthosis does not interfere with the task.
- With significant tears, there is instability, and the joint may sublux or dislocate with provoking activities, requiring surgical intervention.

Management

Follow the guidelines in Chapter 10 for treating acute lesions with emphasis on maintaining mobility while minimizing stress to the healing tissue. If immobilization is necessary to protect the part, only the involved joint should be immobilized. Joints above and below should be free to move. This maintains mobility of the long tendons in their sheaths that cross the involved joint. Avoid positions of stress and activities that provoke the symptoms while healing.

Lacerated Flexor Tendons of the Hand: Surgical and Postoperative Management

Background and Indications for Surgery

Lacerations of flexor tendons can occur in various areas (zones) along the volar surface of the fingers, palm, wrist, and distal forearm and cause an immediate loss of hand function, consistent with the tendons severed. The musculotendinous structures damaged depend on the location and depth of the wound. Damage to one or more tendons may be accompanied by vascular, nerve, and skeletal injuries, which can cause additional loss of function and complicate management. An acute rupture of a flexor tendon may also occur as the result of a closed traumatic injury to the hand.[3,12,101,129,137]

The volar surfaces of the forearm, wrist, palm, and fingers are divided into five zones; the thumb is divided into three zones. These zones are illustrated in Figure 19.11. The anatomical landmarks for each of the zones are described in Box 19.8.[65,82,90,127,129,134,137] Use of this system of classifying lacerations improves consistency of communication and can provide a basis for predicting outcomes.[137]

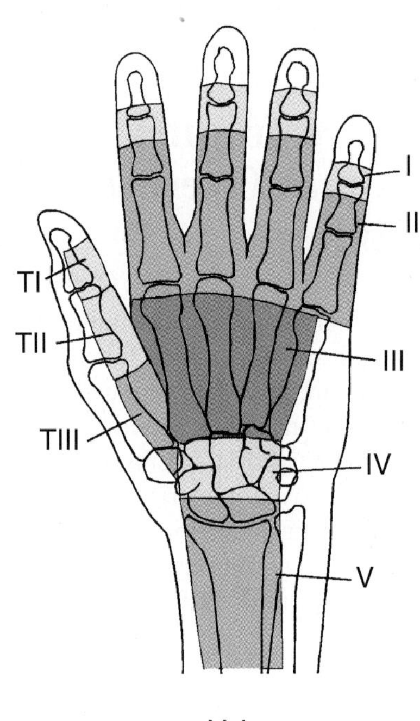

FIGURE 19.11 Flexor tendon zones; volar aspect of the hand and wrist.

Knowledge of the complex anatomy, kinesiology of the hand, and tendon healing properties is essential to understand the impairments and functional implications caused by damage to the flexor tendons in each of these zones. Box 19.9 identifies common impairments associated with damage in each of the zones.[90,112]

When severed or ruptured, flexor tendons readily retract, thus requiring surgical intervention in most instances to restore function to the hand and prevent deformity. Repair and rehabilitation of lacerations in zone II, traditionally referred to as "no-man's land," pose a particular challenge to hand surgeons and therapists.[82,95,122,127,129,137,153] Because of the confined space in which the extrinsic flexors of the fingers lie and the limited vascular supply to the tendons in zone II, healing tissues in this area are prone to excursion-restricting adhesions. Scar tissue formation during the healing process can interrupt tendon-gliding in the synovial sheath and subsequently restrict ROM of the involved fingers.[122,137]

BOX 19.8 Flexor Tendon Zones: Anatomical Landmarks

Zones of the Fingers, Palm, Wrist, and Forearm

- I—from the insertion of the FDP on the distal phalanx to just distal of the FDS insertion on the middle phalanx
- II—from the distal insertion of the FDS tendon to the level of the distal palmar crease (just proximal to the neck of the metacarpals)
- III—from the neck of the metacarpals, proximally along the metacarpals to the distal border of the carpal tunnel
- IV—the carpal tunnel (area under the transverse carpal ligament)
- V—area just proximal to the wrist (proximal edge of the carpal ligament) to the musculotendinous junction of the extrinsic flexors in the distal forearm

Zones of the Thumb

- T-I—from the distal insertion of the FPL on the distal phalanx of the thumb to the neck of the proximal phalanx.
- T-II—from the proximal phalanx, across the MP joint to the neck of the first metacarpal.
- T-III—from the first metacarpal to the proximal margin of the carpal ligament.

In zone IV (the carpal tunnel), the extrinsic flexor tendons of the digits (FDS, FDP, and FPL) lie in close proximity to each other. An injury in this zone may lead to adherence of adjacent tendons to each other in the carpal tunnel and impairment of differential gliding between the tendons.[68]

Procedures

Types and Timing of Operative Procedures

Many factors influence the type of surgical repair selected to manage a flexor tendon injury.[65,90,127,134] Injury-related factors include the mechanism of injury; the type and location (zone) of the laceration; the extent of associated skin, vascular, nerve, and skeletal damage; the degree of wound contamination; and the time elapsed since the injury. Surgery-related factors include timing of the repair, if there is a need to stage surgeries, and the hand surgeon's background and experience. Patient-related influences are the patient's age, health, and lifestyle (especially nutrition and smoking). These factors also have a significant impact on postoperative rehabilitation and outcomes of a tendon repair.[82,95,137,153]

Types of repair or reconstruction. Surgical options for repair of lacerations or a closed rupture of flexor tendons can be classified by the *type* of procedure.[65,90,98,137]

- ***Direct repair.*** An end-to-end repair in which the tendon ends are re-opposed and sutured together.
- ***Tendon graft.*** An autogenous donor tendon (autograft), such as the palmaris longus, is sutured in place to replace the damaged tendon. This is necessary when the ends of the severed tendon(s) cannot be brought together without undue tension. Tendon grafts are performed in one or more stages depending on the severity, type, and location of injury.

A straight laceration usually lends itself well to a direct (end-to-end) repair, whereas a jagged laceration that frays the tendon may require a tendon graft.[150]

Timing of a repair. Another method of classifying and describing tendon repairs is the *timing* of the repair, as related to the elapsed time since the injury. The timing of a repair after an acute tendon injury is critical because the severed ends of the tendon begin to soften and deteriorate quickly and the proximal portion of the tendon retracts. These factors make it difficult to reattach the tendon with a strong repair at its normal length. However, only a tendon laceration associated with major damage to the vascular system is considered an emergency situation.[90,122,127] Although better outcomes are thought to occur if the repair is done within the first few days,

BOX 19.9 Consequences of Injury to the Volar Surface of the Hand, Wrist, and Forearm

- *Zone I.* Only one tendon, the FDP, can be severed as can the A-4 and A-5 retinacular pulleys, which are important for maintaining the mechanical advantage of the FDP for complete finger flexion (full fist).
- *Zone II.* FDS and FDP tendons, a double-layered synovial sheath and multiple annular pulleys (including A-1) of the flexor retinaculum (the fibrous sheath that approximates the tendons to the underlying bones and maintains them relatively close to the joints for full tendon excursion) can all be damaged. Inability to flex the PIP and DIP joints occurs if both tendons are severed. Potential damage to the vincula, the vascular structures that provide blood, and supplement nutrition derived from synovial diffusion can compromise tendon healing.
- *Zone III.* In addition to loss of the FDP and FDS, damage to lumbricals can disrupt MP flexion.
- *Zone IV.* Damage in this zone (in the carpel tunnel) can affect all three extrinsic flexors of the digits—FDP, FDS, and FPL—which disrupts finger and thumb flexion. Synovial sheath also sustains damage. Nerve injury frequently accompanies laceration in this zone.
- *Zone V.* Laceration in the forearm can cause major damage to flexor tendons of the digits and wrist, resulting in loss of wrist and digital flexion. The median and ulnar nerves and the radial and ulnar arteries also lie superficial in this zone.
- *Zones T-I and T-II.* Damage to the retinacular pulley system of the thumb, synovial sheath in addition to the FPL, and possibly the distal insertion of the FPB can occur; IP and MP flexion are disrupted.
- *Zone T-III.* Potential damage to the thenar muscles.

a delay of up to 10 days yields results equal to those of an immediate repair. Delays beyond 2 weeks are associated with poorer outcomes.[127,137,150] If a repair must be delayed for more than 3 to 4 weeks, a direct repair is no longer possible, which necessitates a tendon graft.[127]

Categories of surgeries based on elapsed time include:[65,90,127,134]

- ***Immediate primary repair:*** A repair done within the first 24 hours after injury.
- ***Delayed primary repair:*** A repair performed up to 10 days after injury.
- ***Secondary repair:*** A repair done 10 days to 3 weeks after injury.
- ***Late reconstruction:*** Surgery performed well beyond 3 to 4 weeks, sometimes months after the injury.
- ***Staged reconstruction:*** Multiple separate surgeries performed over a period of weeks or months.[98,121,122] A staged reconstruction enables a surgeon to prepare an extensively damaged or scarred tendon bed months prior to a tendon graft, so adhesions are less likely to develop.

A simple, clean, acute laceration of a tendon without associated injuries of the hand is most often managed with a *direct primary repair*, either immediate or delayed a few days.[82,127,134] However, if the wound is not clean, a *delayed primary repair* allows time for medical intervention to reduce the risk of infection. Lengthy delays that necessitate a *secondary repair* or *late reconstruction* are often associated with multiple injuries, such as extensive skin loss, fractures that cannot be stabilized immediately, or long-standing scarring and contractures. If there is damage to one or more of the tendon pulleys, these must be repaired before the lacerated tendon can be repaired effectively.[121,122,127,137]

Of the multiple-stage reconstructions for extensive and complex flexor tendon injuries of the hand, the *Hunter two-stage reconstruction passive or active implant* is most widely known. During the first stage of this procedure, the scarred and adherent portions of the damaged flexor tendon are resected. An implant (rod) made of silicone is then secured in place to act as a *tendon spacer* around which a new sheath develops over a period of 3 months. In addition, a damaged retinacular pulley system is reconstructed, and any contractures are released during the first surgery. During the second phase, the implant is removed, and a donor tendon (graft) is drawn through the new sheath and sutured in place.[98,121,127,137,153]

Operative Overview

Some general aspects of the many variations of operative procedures for primary flexor tendon injuries are described in this section.[65,90,98,122,127,134,137] However, careful review of a patient's operative report and close communication with the hand surgeon are necessary sources of specific details of each patient's surgery.

Surgical approach. For example, for repair of lacerated finger tendons in zone II, a volar, zigzag approach, designed to avoid the lines of stress or a lateral incision, may be elected by the surgeon although the zig-zag approach is more common. When surgically repairing a lacerated tendon, the incision is made between the annular pulleys to ensure optimal excursion. This approach preserves the function of these fibrous sheaths, which encircle the finger flexors and keep the tendons close to the joints, preventing bowstringing of the tendon.

Suturing technique. For a direct repair after the tendon ends are located, prepared, and re-opposed, there are a number of delicate suturing techniques that can be employed.[65,82,90,127,129,134,137,150] Core sutures and epitendinous sutures are used to hold the tendon ends together. A larger number of suture strands across the repair site (e.g., four or six strands instead of two) produces a proportionally stronger repair. Running, locked epitendinous sutures used in addition to core sutures appear to further increase the initial strength of the repair.[65,127,129,149]

CLINICAL TIP

Suturing technique and the number of suture strands influence the initial strength of the repair and consequently the type and timing of motion allowable postoperatively.

Suturing technique must also address the vascular supply to the repaired tendon. Nonreactive sutures are placed in the nonvascular volar aspect of the tendon so as not to disturb the vincula, which lies in the dorsal aspect of the tendon and provides its blood supply.[129,134,137] When present, as in zones II and IV, the synovial sheath is also repaired to re-establish circulation of synovial fluid, an important source of nutrition to the healing tendons.[65,129]

Closure. After all repairs have been completed, the incision(s) is closed, and the hand and wrist are immobilized in a bulky compression dressing and elevated to control edema. The compression dressing remains in place for 1 to 3 days. When the bulky surgical dressing is removed, it is replaced with a light compressive dressing and an orthosis.

Postoperative Management

General considerations. After surgical intervention for a flexor tendon injury, a strong, well-healed tendon that glides freely is the cornerstone for restoring functional mobility and strength in the hand.[3,55,68,112] Every effort is made to prevent excursion-restricting adhesions from forming while simultaneously protecting the repaired tendon as it heals. Box 19.10 summarizes the factors that contribute to adhesion formation after tendon repair.[55,68,112,127]

Many of the same patient and injury-related factors—already noted—that a surgeon weighs when determining the most appropriate approach to surgical management for a patient's hand injury also influence the complex components and progression of postoperative rehabilitation. In addition,

BOX 19.10 Factors That Contribute to Adhesion Formation After Tendon Injury and Repair

- Location of the injury and repair: higher risk in flexor zone II and extensor zone III; tendons glide in a closely confined area
- Extent of trauma: higher risk with extensive trauma and damage to associated structures
- Reduced blood supply, subsequent ischemia, and reduced nutrition to healing tendons
- Excessive handling of damaged tissues during surgery
- Ineffective suturing technique
- Damage or resection of components of the tendon sheath
- Prolonged immobilization after injury or repair, which prevents tendon-gliding
- Gapping of the repaired tendon ends associated with *excessive* stress to the healing tendon

surgery-related factors, including the type and timing of the repair, suturing technique, strength of the tendon repair, and the need for concomitant operative procedures, affect rehabilitation and eventual outcomes. Furthermore, therapy-related factors—in particular the time at which therapy is initiated, the use of early or delayed mobilization procedures, the quality of the orthosis, the expertise of the therapist, and ultimately the quality and consistency of the patient's involvement in the rehabilitation process—influence outcomes.

Extensive research has been done on the process of tendon healing, the tensile strength of tendon repairs, adhesion formation, and tendon excursion and imposed stresses (loading) on a repaired tendon during digital motion. A number of sources provide an in-depth analysis and summary of basic and clinical studies, typically animal and cadaveric, but some are *in vivo* human studies, as they apply to rehabilitation.[3,29,55,66,127,129,134]

The purpose of this section is to examine and summarize current concepts and approaches to immobilization and exercise used in rehabilitation after flexor tendon injury and repair. Therapists treating patients after tendon repair must be familiar with the various postoperative protocols or guidelines used by referring hand surgeons and those described in the literature.

A therapist's knowledge of the underlying concepts in any protocol is essential for effective communication with the surgeon. A therapist's skill in applying and teaching exercise procedures is equally necessary for effective patient education and helping a patient achieve optimal functional outcomes. This knowledge enables a therapist to make sound clinical judgments to determine when the progression of activities in a protocol preferred by a referring surgeon is safe or when activities must be adjusted based on each patient's responses. Remember, a regimented protocol is only safe and effective when there are no postoperative variables, a situation that certainly does not occur in the clinical setting.[39,112]

Approaches to postoperative management. There are two basic approaches to management after flexor tendon repair characterized by the timing and type of exercises in the program. They are categorized as *early controlled motion*, either passive or active, and *delayed motion*.

Numerous published protocols with considerable variability fall within these categories. Most current-day programs emphasize early controlled (protected) motion after surgery and include both passive and active exercises of the operated digit(s). Advances in surgical management (in particular, improved suturing techniques) that establish a relatively strong initial tendon repair allow the use of early motion.

FOCUS ON EVIDENCE

Trumble and colleagues[140] studied 103 patients with zone II flexor tendon repair who were randomized to either early active motion with place and hold or a passive motion protocol. ROM was measured at 6, 12, 26, and 52 weeks following the repair. Outcome measures also included dexterity tests, the DASH outcome questionnaire, and a satisfaction score. Ninety-three patients completed the study. At all points in the study, patients treated with the active motion protocol had greater ROM. At 52 weeks, the total active motion (TAM) for the active place and hold group was a mean of 156° +/- 25°, compared with 128° +/- 22° ($p < 0.05$) in the passive group. The authors also report that the active motion group had significantly smaller flexion contractures and greater satisfaction scores ($p < 0.05$). There was no difference between groups in either the DASH score or dexterity tests. They concluded that active motion therapy provides greater active finger motion than passive motion therapy after zone II flexor tendon repair without risk of tendon rupture (3%). In addition, they reported that concomitant nerve injuries, multiple digit injuries, and a history of smoking negatively impact the final outcome of tendon repairs.

Box 19.11 summarizes the rationale for early protected motion as soon as a day or two after tendon repair based on four decades of evidence derived from scientific studies.[29,55,65,66,68,82,112,127,131,132] However, there are instances when a traditional, delayed motion approach must be used. Indications for prolonged (3 to 4 weeks) immobilization after tendon repair (and therefore delayed motion) are noted in Box 19.12.[48,112,122,127]

Key elements of early passive and active motion approaches and the delayed motion approach with regard to immobilization and selection and progression of exercises are presented in the following sections. More detailed descriptions of these approaches, as well as specific protocols advocated by various practitioners and researchers, are available in many sources.[29,39,55,66,68,112,131,134,147,150]

With all approaches, the postoperative goals and interventions for pain reduction, edema control, and maintenance of function in uninvolved regions (e.g., the elbow and shoulder) are consistent with management following other operative procedures previously discussed in this chapter. Patient

BOX 19.11 Rationale for Early Controlled Motion After Tendon Repair

- Decreases postoperative edema.
- Maintains tendon-gliding and decreases the formation of adhesions that can limit tendon excursion and that consequently limit functional ROM. Gliding deteriorates by 10 days after repair when a tendon is immobilized.
- Increases synovial fluid diffusion for tissue nutrition, which increases the rate of tendon healing.
- Increases wound maturation and the tensile strength of the repaired tendon more rapidly than continuous immobilization by means of *appropriate-level* stresses achieved with early tendon motion. The repair site loses strength during the first 2 weeks after surgery.
- Decreases gap formation at the repair site, which in turn increases the tensile strength of the repair.

BOX 19.12 Indications for Use of Prolonged Immobilization and Delayed Motion After Flexor Tendon Repair

- Patients who are unable to comprehend and actively participate in an early controlled motion exercise program. This includes:
  - Children less than 5 years of age
  - Patients with diminished cognitive capacity associated with head injury, developmental disability, or psychological impairment
- Patients who have the cognitive ability to understand and follow an early controlled motion program but who are unlikely to adhere to the program. This includes:
  - The unmotivated patient
  - The overzealous, impatient individual with a history of a previously failed repair
  - Patients in whom repair of other hand injuries or surgeries necessitates extended immobilization of the hand

education is of the utmost importance for effective outcomes after hand surgery.

NOTE: Unless otherwise noted, the guidelines described in this section for immobilization and exercise are for injury and primary repair or one-stage tendon grafts of the FDS and/or FDP muscle-tendon units in zones I, II, and III. The guidelines are similar but not addressed for zones T-I and T-II of the thumb. Postoperative guidelines for multistage or late reconstructions are progressed in a similar but more cautious manner. Refer to other resources for this information.[48,55,66,68,112,131]

Immobilization

The duration, type, and position of immobilization must be considered.

Duration of immobilization. With some exceptions previously noted (see Box 19.12), when prolonged immobilization (3 to 4 weeks) is necessary, the repaired tendon is continuously immobilized after surgery for up to 5 days while the bulky compression dressing is kept in place. This allows some time for postoperative edema to decrease.

Type or method of immobilization. This usually depends on the preference of the hand surgeon and therapist, the approach to postoperative exercise, and the stage of tissue healing. If motion of the operated digit is to be delayed for 3 to 4 weeks, a cast or static orthosis provides the immobilization. Early controlled motion approaches require the fabrication of different types of customized orthoses.

There are three general types of orthoses used after flexor tendon repair: a static dorsal blocking orthosis;[50,55,68,112,127] a dorsal blocking orthosis with dynamic traction, originally proposed by Kleinert[75,79] and subsequently modified and improved by clinicians and researchers;[55,112,122] and a dorsal tenodesis orthosis with a wrist hinge.[29,112,127,134] Descriptions of these static and dynamic orthosis techniques for immobilization and/or exercise are noted in Box 19.13. Figure 19.12 shows an example of a dorsal blocking orthosis with dynamic traction. The orthosis allows active extension of the involved finger, and the elastic band passively returns the finger to a flexed position. (See Fig. 19.13A for a depiction of a dorsal tenodesis orthosis.)

Position of immobilization. The typical position of immobilization for repairs of flexor tendons in zones I, II, and III is

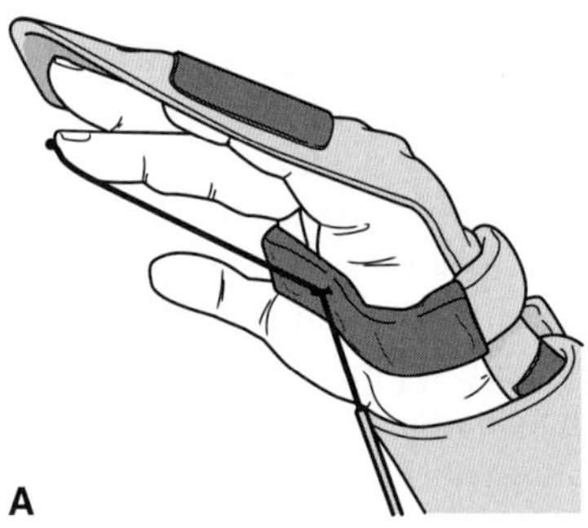

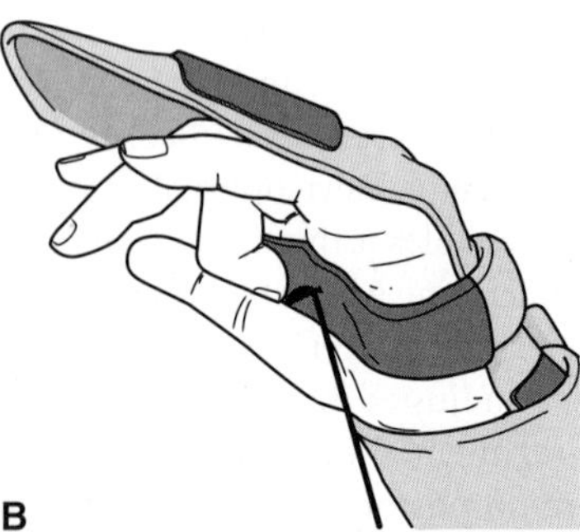

FIGURE 19.12 A dorsal-blocking orthosis with dynamic traction for early controlled motion after flexor tendon repair; **(A)** showing active extension and **(B)** passive flexion.

BOX 19.13 Static and Dynamic Dorsal Blocking Orthoses: Position and Use

Static Dorsal Blocking Orthosis

- Covers the dorsal surface of the entire hand and two-thirds of the forearm (the thumb is free).
- Positioned in wrist and MP flexion and IP extension to avoid excessive tension on the repaired flexor tendon. The degrees of flexion may vary with the philosophy of the surgeon or therapist and the approach (protocol) implemented.
- Fabricated with straps placed across the volar aspect of the hand and forearm to hold the wrist and fingers in the correct position.
- Restricts wrist and MP extension.
- Worn during early phases of rehabilitation. Distal straps of the orthosis are loosened or removed for early exercises.
- Also worn as a protective night orthosis.

Dorsal Blocking Orthosis With Dynamic Traction

- Allows early motion of the operated joint while the hand is in the orthosis.
- Fabricated with an elastic band (or nylon cord), which is attached to the nail of the operated finger (or all four fingers), passes under a palmar bar that acts as a pulley, and then is attached proximally at the wrist.
- At rest, the elastic band provides dynamic traction that holds the operated finger in flexion.
- Allows *active extension* of the IP joints to the surface of the dorsal orthosis.
- When PIP and DIP extensors relax, tension from the elastic band pulls on the finger, causing *passive flexion*.

Dorsal Tenodesis Orthosis With Wrist Hinge

- Worn *exclusively* for exercise sessions.
- No dynamic traction with elastic bands.
- Allows full wrist flexion and limited (approximately 30°) wrist extension but maintains the MP joints in at least 60° of flexion and the IP joints in full extension when the straps are secured.
- Loosening of straps across the fingers allows active wrist extension during initial passive IP flexion and later when finger flexion is maintained for several seconds by a static contraction of the IP flexors.

wrist and MP flexion coupled with PIP and DIP extension. This position prevents full lengthening and undue stress on the repaired FDS and/or FDP tendons while minimizing the risk of IP flexion contractures. The recommended degrees of wrist and MP flexion differ somewhat from one source to another. Recommended positions range from 10° to 45° of wrist flexion and from 30° to 70° of MP flexion with the IP joints in full but comfortable extension depending on the zone.[29,50,55,68,112,127,134] The wrist typically is positioned in less flexion than the MP joints. The trend over the years has been to fabricate orthoses that allow less wrist and MP flexion than early protocols increasing patient comfort and reducing the risk of carpal tunnel syndrome.[55,112]

The wrist is typically positioned at neutral with 60° to 70° MP flexion following a zone IV repair.[68]

Exercise: Early Controlled Motion Approaches

There are two basic approaches to the application of early, controlled motion to maintain tendon-gliding and prevent tendon adhesions after flexor tendon repair: early passive motion and early active motion. The way in which passive or active motion of the repaired tendon is achieved, however, varies among protocols.

Early controlled passive motion. Historically, the use of early passive motion has been based on the work of Duran and Houser[50] and of Kleinert and associates.[75,79] Both groups proposed early passive flexion of the IP joints within a protected range postoperatively, but they used different approaches to the use of orthoses and exercise. Duran advocated use of a static dorsal blocking orthosis and early removal of the orthosis or loosening of the stabilization straps for passive ROM exercise of the IP joints of the operated finger(s). Kleinert and colleagues advanced use of a dorsal blocking orthosis with dynamic traction for early exercise (see Fig. 19.12). Within the confines of the orthosis, the patient performs *active extension* of the operated finger with the elastic bands producing passive flexion allowing excursion of the repaired tendon without active tension in the finger flexors. A gentle manual push into full composite flexion using the uninvolved hand may be added to increase passive flexion.

NOTE: When a dynamic traction orthosis is used during the day, a static dorsal blocking orthosis is worn at night. The night orthosis holds the IP joints in extension, the wrist in 10° to 30° of flexion, and the MP joints in 50° to 70° flexion to prevent IP flexion contractures.

These original passive motion protocols have been modified over the past 3 decades. Today, some surgeons and therapists use selected elements (use of an orthosis and/or exercise) of these passive motion approaches.[29,31,113,122,140] However, use of early *active* motion that imposes controlled stresses on the repaired tendon is gradually replacing passive motion approaches.[31,68,113,140]

Early controlled active motion. The primary feature that distinguishes an early active motion from an early passive motion approach is the use of *minimum-tension, active contractions* of the repaired muscle-tendon units initiated during the acute stage of tissue healing, often by the first 24 to 72 hours but no later than 5 days postoperatively.[29,55,68,112,127,134,140] Some passive exercises are also incorporated into active regimens.

Based primarily on experimental studies using animal models, it is hypothesized that gentle stresses placed on a repaired tendon by means of a very low-intensity static or dynamic muscle contraction, which "pulls" the repaired tendon through its sheath, is a more effective method of creating tendon excursion (gliding) than "pushing" the tendon with passive motion.[3,39,55,57,66] Early active motion has become more widely accepted because stronger suturing techniques produce a repair that can withstand early, controlled stresses.

PRECAUTION: Proponents of early, active tendon mobilization caution that this approach is recommended only for primary tendon repairs, using the stronger four- and six-strand core and epitendinous suture techniques (in contrast to two-strand suturing) in carefully selected patients who have access to rehabilitation with an experienced hand therapist and are most likely to adhere to the prescribed exercise and orthosis regimen.[29,31,55,66,127,131,134,137]

There are two ways in which early active motion can be implemented. Both methods are founded on an analysis and application of evidence in the scientific literature on tendon repair and healing, tendon excursion, and imposed loading on repaired tendons.[31,39,55,134]

- ***Place-and-hold approach.*** One approach uses "place-and-hold" exercises by means of *static* muscle contractions to generate active tension of the finger flexors and impose controlled stress on the repaired tendon. (Place-and-hold exercises are described in the phase-specific exercises that follow.) This approach to early active motion is used in the Indiana protocol.[29,31,134,151]
- ***Dynamic approach.*** The other approach to early active motion, developed by Evans,[55,57] uses *dynamic*, short-arc, minimum muscle tension exercises to impose initially low-intensity stresses on the healing tendon.
- ***Combined approach.*** Groth[66] proposed a conceptual model for the use of early active motion and application of progressive forces to the healing tendon after flexor tendon repair that combines elements of both the place-and-hold and dynamic approaches. In addition, in the rationale for this model, Groth discusses the effects of each level of exercise on internal tendon loads and tendon excursion supported by key evidence from the literature when available.
  - A unique feature of Groth's model is that it is criterion based rather than time based. By providing criteria for progressing exercises based on optimal tendon loading, this program provides a mechanism for an individualized sequence of exercises adjusted for each patient rather than using predetermined timelines for progression.
  - The model contains eight progressive levels of active exercises, from the least to the greatest levels of loading on the tendon. The sequence is preceded by warm-up exercises (slow, repetitive passive finger motions in protected ranges). As with other early active motion approaches, exercises are begun during the first few days after surgery and are progressed until conclusion of postoperative rehabilitation. Box 19.14 describes the eight-level sequence of exercises in Groth's conceptual model.[66,112,137]

BOX 19.14 A Sequence of Exercises for Early Active Motion With Progressive Tendon Loading After Flexor Tendon Repair[66]

Warm-Up

Warm-up exercises (passive finger motions within protected ranges precede each exercise session).

Progressive Levels of Exercise*

- Level 1—place-and-hold finger flexion
- Level 2—active composite finger flexion
- Level 3—hook and straight fist finger flexion
- Level 4—isolated finger joint motion
- Level 5—continuation of levels 1–4 of exercise and discontinuation of protective orthosis with introduction of gradually increasing use of the hand for functional activities
- Level 6—resisted composite finger flexion
- Level 7—resisted hook and straight fist exercises
- Level 8—resisted isolated joint motion.

* *Note:* Exercise sequence is from least to greatest tendon loading. Repetitions are highest at the lowest level of loading and least at the highest level of loading. Progression to the next level occurs when specific criteria are met.

A number of retrospective studies and prospective, non-randomized case series have been published describing the effectiveness of early active motion or early passive motion approaches to postoperative rehabilitation following flexor tendon repair.

FOCUS ON EVIDENCE

Chesney and colleagues[31] performed a systematic review of flexor tendon rehabilitation protocols in zone II of the hand. The authors looked at all rehabilitation protocols published with the exception of immobilization. The protocols were broadly classified as either passive flexion and active extension protocols (Kleinert-type), controlled passive motion protocols (Duran-type), combined "controlled passive motion" protocols (combined Kleinert and Duran with elements from both), and early active motion protocols (protocols utilizing place and hold). The primary outcomes they considered were the rate of tendon rupture, the ROM of the injured digit, as well as quality of life and patient satisfaction. Results of their review demonstrated that both early active motion protocols and combined protocols result in low rates of tendon rupture and acceptable ROM; however, there isn't a protocol that is superior to another. The takeaway is that the literature does not support any one protocol and that more research is needed including randomized controlled trials comparing the different protocols side by side to not only determine the most effective protocol, but also to determine which protocol is most cost effective.

Exercise: Maximum Protection Phase

NOTE: The guidelines for exercises described in this section focus on the application of early active motion after *zone I, II, or III primary flexor tendon repairs* and are drawn from several resources.

The maximum protection phase of rehabilitation begins within the first few days after surgery and continues for 3 to 5 weeks. This is the period of time when the tendon repair is weakest. The goals of this phase of rehabilitation are pain and edema control and protection of the newly repaired tendon while imposing very low-level, controlled stresses on the tendon to maintain adequate tendon gliding and prevent adhesions that can restrict tendon excursion. Interventions in this phase include elevating the hand, orthosis use and care, wound management and skin care, and passive and active exercises.

During the first phase of rehabilitation, exercises are performed in a static dorsal blocking orthosis or in a wrist tenodesis orthosis (Fig. 19.13 A) specifically designed for exercise. With both methods, the stabilization straps are loosened to allow finger flexion. The following exercises are performed frequently (hourly) during the day and continue for about the first 4 weeks.

- ***Passive ROM exercises.*** On an hourly basis perform passive MP, PIP, and DIP flexion and extension of each individual joint to the extent the dorsal orthosis allows, followed by composite passive flexion in the confines of the orthosis. Composite flexion can include passive movements into full fist and straight fist positions.
- ***Independent motions of the PIP and DIP joints for differential gliding of the FDP and FDS tendons.*** For example, the DIP joint must be flexed and extended separately while each PIP joint is stabilized in flexion. In this way, as the DIP joint is passively extended, the FDP repair site glides distally, away from the FDS repair.[68,112]

PRECAUTION: It is essential to maintain the MP joints in flexion during passive ROM of the IP joints to avoid excessive stretch of the repair site, which could cause gapping of the reopposed tendon ends during IP extension.

- ***Place-and-hold exercises.*** Many programs initiate place-and-hold exercises of the repaired digit with the patient wearing either a dorsal blocking orthosis[55,151] or a tenodesis orthosis.[29,39,66,112] With the MP joints in flexion, passively place the IP joints in a partially flexed position and have the patient hold the position independently for 5 seconds with a minimum static contraction of the finger flexors. If the patient is wearing a tenodesis orthosis, combine place-and-hold finger flexion with active wrist extension (Fig. 19.13 B and C). Have the patient relax and allow the wrist to passively flex and the digits to passively extend. Initially, have the patient practice this with the uninjured hand or use biofeedback to learn how to hold the position with a minimum of force production in the FDP and FDS.

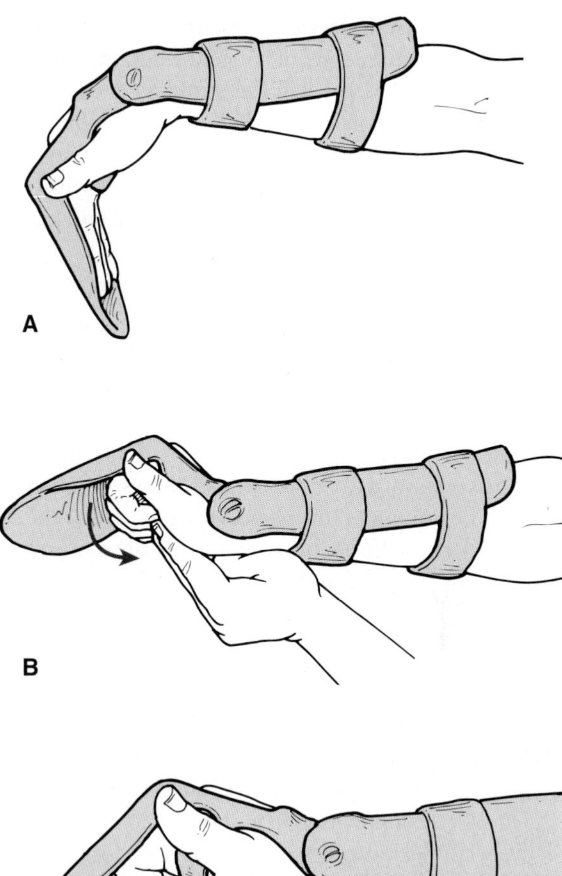

FIGURE 19.13 Orthosis and exercise for early active motion post-flexor tendon repair. **(A)** Following removal of the surgical compression dressing and fabrication of a static dorsal-blocking splint, a tenodesis splint with a wrist hinge is fabricated. **(B)** The tenodesis orthosis allows full wrist flexion but limits wrist extension to 30°. During early movement of the fingers, the MP joints are maintained in at least 60° of flexion, as the IP joints are passively moved and placed in composite flexion. **(C)** Then the patient actively extends the wrist while maintaining the flexed finger position with a static muscle contraction and the least amount of tension possible in the finger flexors. *(From Strickland, JW: Flexor tendon injuries. In Strickland, JW, and Graham, TJ [eds]:* Master Techniques in Orthopedic Surgery—The Hand, *ed. 2. Philadelphia: Lippincott Williams & Wilkins, 2005, p 262, with permission.)*

FOCUS ON EVIDENCE

Research has shown that it is preferable to perform place-and-hold exercises with the wrist extended and the MP joints placed in flexion because wrist extension is the position in which the IP joints can be moved by contraction of the FDS and FDP with the *least* amount of contraction force and, therefore, a very low-level load on the repaired tendon.[29,39]

- ***Minimum-tension, short-arc motion (SAM).*** Some programs begin active, dynamic finger flexion during the first few days after surgery if the suturing technique and strength of the repair allow.[39,55,112] Active contractions that generate minimum tension—just enough tension to overcome the resistance of the extensors and cause flexor tendon excursion—are performed with the wrist in slight extension and the MP joints flexed.

Exercise: Moderate Protection Phase

The moderate protection phase begins at about 4 weeks and continues until 8 weeks postoperatively. The focus during this phase is on safely increasing stresses on the repaired tendon and achieving full active flexion and extension of the wrist and digits and differential gliding of the tendons. If a tenodesis orthosis was worn for early active exercises, it is discontinued at the beginning of this phase. However, use of the static dorsal blocking orthosis continues during the day except for exercise until at least 6 to 8 weeks. Use of a night orthosis continues for protection or to decrease or prevent a flexion contracture. Exercises include:

- ***Place-and-hold exercises.*** Continuation of place-and-hold exercises but with gradually increasing tension.
- ***Active ROM.*** Continuation or initiation of active composite flexion and extension of the IP joints with the MP joints flexed, MP flexion/extension with the IP joints relaxed and active wrist flexion and extension with the fingers relaxed.
- ***Tendon-gliding and blocking exercises.*** These exercises are initiated at about 5 to 6 weeks (see Figs. 19.16 and 19.17 and the descriptions in the final section of this chapter).

PRECAUTION: Avoid finger extension combined with wrist extension for about 6 to 8 weeks, as this position places extreme tension on the repaired flexor tendon.

Exercise: Minimum Protection/Return to Function Phase

The minimum protection/return to function phase begins at approximately 8 weeks postoperatively and is characterized by gradually progressed resistance exercises to improve strength and endurance, dexterity exercises, and use of the hand for light (1 to 2 lb) functional activities. (Refer to the final section of this chapter for suggested exercises and activities.)

Use of a protective orthosis is discontinued; however, intermittent use of an orthosis may be necessary if the patient has a persistent extensor lag or flexion contracture. After primary flexor tendon repairs, most patients return to full activity by 12 weeks after surgery.

Exercise: Delayed Motion Approach

In instances where continuous immobilization of a repaired flexor tendon extends for 3 to 4 weeks (see Box 19.12 for indications), some degree of tendon healing and adhesion formation already has occurred by the time exercises can be initiated.

PRECAUTION: Despite the extended period of immobilization, at 3 to 4 weeks, the tendon repair must still be protected in a dorsal blocking orthosis and exercises must be performed in protected positions and progressed gradually.

Exercises such as passive ROM, tendon-blocking and tendon-gliding, and active ROM can be initiated when the cast is removed. Exercises used in early motion approaches are appropriate. The reader is also referred to additional resources that provide detailed exercise programs when delayed mobilization is necessary.[48,112]

Outcomes

Functional outcomes. There is a substantial body of evidence on flexor tendon repairs, some of which is based on longitudinal clinical outcome studies.[137] A literature review[129] indicated that with the advances made in flexor tendon surgery and rehabilitation techniques over the past few decades, recovery of good or excellent function can be expected in 80% or more of patients after flexor tendon injury and repair. Two factors that have contributed considerably to a high rate of favorable outcomes are the use of improved suturing techniques that produce a strong repair site and implementation of early motion in rehabilitation programs.

There are several quantitative assessment tools used in outcome studies of tendon repair.[112] It is helpful to become familiar with the more frequently used assessments in order to understand the findings of studies. With some of these tools, results are reported as excellent, good, fair, and poor. For the most part, these terms are not simply subjective descriptors but rather are associated with objective measurement tools. For example, in the Strickland system,[31] the terms refer to a percentage of "normal" TAM (total active flexion minus deficits in active extension) of the PIP and DIP joints achieved after zone I, II, or III repairs and rehabilitation.

Some generalizations can be made about outcomes after flexor tendon repair. Findings in the literature indicate that immediate primary and delayed primary repairs (up to 10 days after injury) yield equally positive outcomes.[122] However, late reconstructions and multistage reconstructions, not surprisingly, result in poorer outcomes (less active and passive ROM, greater functional limitations) than primary repairs.[48,98,127] This is consistent with the findings that the greater the severity and number of associated injuries, the less favorable the outcomes.[112]

Studies dating back to the 1980s have documented that the use of 4 weeks of uninterrupted immobilization leads to a slower return of tensile strength in the repaired tendon and greater adhesion formation than the use of early mobilization.[112] Although extended immobilization continues to be the treatment of choice for children less than 7 to 10 years of age,[54] there is emerging evidence demonstrating positive results using both early active and early passive motion protocols depending on the child's developmental maturity and caregiver support.[94,106141]

Studies of various approaches to early motion (passive or active) after flexor tendon repair demonstrate superior outcomes when compared with outcomes after extended immobilization. Although the use of early motion in rehabilitation after flexor tendon repair has been well documented in the literature and is now the "norm" for treatment, there continues to be limited evidence to definitively indicate any one protocol as superior over the others.[31]

The prospective randomized study by Trumble and coinvestigators[140] highlighted previously in this section lends further support for the use of early active motion for the management of repaired flexor tendons; however, additional research including randomized controlled trials is still needed.[31]

Complications. The most frequent early complication after surgery is rupture of the repaired tendon, and the most frequent late complication is flexion contracture or a deficit in active extension of the repaired DIP and/or PIP joints, typically as the result of tendon adhesions.[51,134] Overall, the rate of postoperative complications is higher in zone II repairs than in other zones.[95] Most ruptures usually occur around 10 days postoperatively when the repaired tendon is in its most weakened state.[95] A rupture may occur during strong gripping activities or as the result of encountering an unexpected high load, but it also may occur while the patient is asleep if the hand is unprotected during the first few months after surgery.

Although there is general agreement that early motion after tendon repair reduces adhesion formation, there have been concerns that initiating early active contractions (static or dynamic) of the PIP or DIP flexors, which place active tension on the newly repaired tendon, may increase the risk of tendon rupture. Overall, however, rupture rates are low and appear to be relatively equal to those seen with early passive flexion/active extension programs.[51] In the systematic review by Chesney[31] and colleagues, rupture rate was lowest in the combined Kleinert and Duran protocols (2.3%) and highest in the Kleinert protocols (7.1%); however, no statistical difference was found. Equal rupture rates (4%) have occurred in zone II tendon repairs when early passive motion and early active motion (place-and-hold) approaches to therapy were implemented.[140]

Lacerated Extensor Tendons of the Hand: Surgical and Postoperative Management

Background and Indications for Surgery

Laceration and traumatic rupture of the extensor tendons of the fingers, thumb, or wrist are often considered as being less serious than flexor tendon injury. Treatment and rehabilitation are often believed to be less intricate, less time-consuming, and associated with a more favorable prognosis than flexor tendon injuries. Experience, however, demonstrates that extensor tendon injuries can be just as complex, time-consuming, frustrating, and disappointing.[39,91,119] Their superficial location makes the extensor tendons vulnerable to damage when trauma occurs to the dorsum of the hand. Furthermore, extensor tendons in the digits are substantially thinner than flexor tendons, making them more prone to traumatic rupture and difficult to repair.[52,105,119,130]

As with the flexor surface, the extensor surface of the hand, wrist, and forearm is divided into zones (Fig. 19.14). The dorsal surface of the fingers and wrist are divided into seven zones, and the thumb into four zones. Each of these zones is identified by specific anatomical landmarks, as noted in Box 19.15.[52,56,91,105,119] The odd-number zones correspond to the location of the DIP, PIP, MP, and wrist joint regions, while the even-number zones correspond to the bones. Although not depicted in Figure 19.14, the dorsal surface of the distal and middle forearm is often identified as zones VIII and IX,

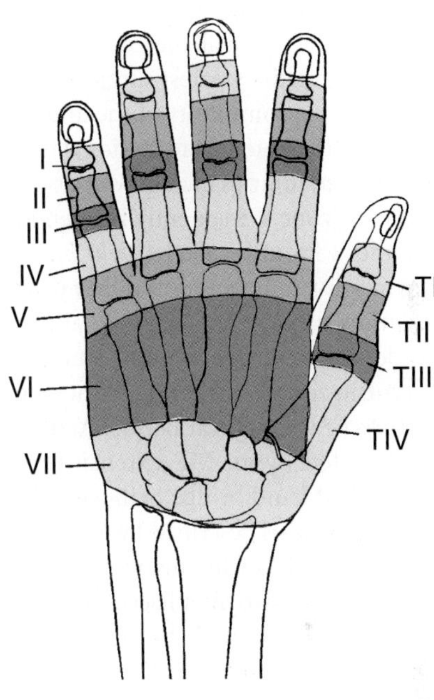

FIGURE 19.14 Extensor tendon zones; dorsal aspect of the hand and wrist.

BOX 19.15 Extensor Tendon Zones: Anatomic Landmarks

Zones of the Dorsal Surfaces of the Fingers, Hand, Wrist, and Forearm

- I—DIP joint region
- II—middle phalanx
- III—PIP joint region
- IV—proximal phalanx
- V—apex of the MP joint region
- VI—dorsum of the hand
- VII—wrist region/dorsal retinaculum
- VIII and IX—distal and middle forearm

Zones of the Thumb

- T-I—IP joint region
- T-II—proximal phalanx
- T-III—MP joint region
- T-IV—metacarpal
- T-V—carpometacarpal joint region

respectively. The area at the CMC joint of the thumb is often identified as zone T-V.[52,56,105]

The extensor mechanism of the hand and wrist is complex. The structural characteristics of these mechanisms vary in each zone. Damage in one zone produces compensatory imbalances in adjacent zones. Knowledge of the anatomy and kinesiology of the extensor mechanism is basic to an understanding of how a patient's physical impairments and functional limitations occur according to the structures damaged in each zone. Box 19.16 identifies key structures and characteristic impairments associated with tendon rupture or laceration by zone.[52,91,119,126,130] Of all the extensor zones, injuries in zones III and VII pose the greatest surgical and rehabilitative challenges due to the complexity of the underlying structures in that area and the potential for residual functional loss or deformity. However, injuries in zone V are by far the most common. Injuries to zone V frequently happen as a result of a punch to another's mouth, called a *fight bite.* With these cases, there is a high risk of infection and they usually become septic. This requires surgical debridement and intravenous antibiotics, in addition to the repair of the tendon.[91,130] Other injuries also occur in zone V, including blunt trauma, which can cause rupture to the sagittal bands. Acute injuries in zone V can be treated by an MP extension orthosis for 6 weeks or the sagittal band bridge orthosis (similar to the "relative extension" orthosis described by Howell and associates), which places the MP of the involved finger in relative hyperextension as compared to the adjacent fingers (25° to 35°) and is worn for 8 weeks. However, chronic injuries in zone V are treated with primary repair rather than sagittal band reconstruction.[56,67,68,91,130,]

Depending on the type and location of injury to the extensor mechanism and the extent of associated skeletal, joint, vascular, or nerve damage, surgery may or may not be indicated. The tendons of the extensor system distal to the dorsum of the hand have many soft tissue attachments along various structures, making extensor tendons far less likely to retract when lacerated or ruptured than flexor tendons.[105] Consequently, with a rupture (closed injury) or a simple laceration in zones I to III, the tendon is re-opposed and managed by uninterrupted immobilization in an orthosis for 6 to 8 weeks as it heals.[39,52,119,126,130] For example, this is a common course of treatment for a *mallet finger* (or thumb) deformity, which is a closed rupture of the terminal extensor tendon in zone I, usually from forceful hyperflexion.[39,52,105,119,126,130]

Nevertheless, surgical intervention, even for a simple distal tendon injury, may be necessary to restore active ROM, muscular balance, strength, and function to the hand and prevent contractures and deformity. Although the extensor muscles of the digits are substantially weaker than the flexors, an intact extensor mechanism is essential for functional grasp and release.[119]

Procedures

Types of Repairs and Reconstruction

Surgical options for extensor tendon repair include a direct (end-to-end) repair or a reconstruction. As with flexor tendon repair or reconstruction, surgeries are classified as primary (immediate repair or delayed up to 10 days), secondary repair, or reconstruction, which may involve a tendon lengthening, tendon grafts (for larger defects that cannot be addressed by tendon lengthening procedures), or tendon transfers.[119,126,130] These terms already have been defined in the previous section of this chapter on flexor tendon repair and rehabilitation. Operative procedures, such as tendon transfers, for ruptured, diseased extensor tendons associated with RA also were described earlier in the chapter.

BOX 19.16 Consequences of Injury to the Dorsal Structures of the Hand and Wrist

- ***Zones I and II.*** Damage to the terminal extensor leads to inability to actively extend the DIP joint (extensor lag) and eventual DIP flexion contracture and deformity (mallet finger). A swan-neck deformity secondary to an unopposed central slip and migration of the extensor mechanisms proximally may also develop. Damage in those zones is usually the result of a closed rupture rather than a laceration.
- ***Zones III and IV.*** Damage to the central slip and possibly the lateral bands results in an inability to actively extend the PIP joint from a 90° flexed position. Flexion contracture of the PIP joint and eventually a boutonnière deformity develop as the lateral bands slip volarly and cause hyperextension of the DIP joint.
- ***Zone V.*** Damage to the common extensor tendons (ED), extensor indicis (EI), extensor digiti minimi (EDM), and sagittal bands that surround the MP joints causes inability to actively extend the MP joints, eventually resulting in MP flexion contractures.
- ***Zones VI and VII.*** The juncturae tendium along the dorsum of the hand (VI) and the dorsal retinaculum (VII) under which multiple extensor tendons of the wrist and digits pass in close proximity can be damaged. A bowstring effect occurs in the extensor tendons if the retinaculum, which acts as a pulley, is lacerated. The synovial sheath through which the tendons glide in zone VII can also be damaged, subsequently compromising synovial diffusion and nutrition to the tendons. Injuries in zones VI and VII can result in loss of extension of the digits and wrist.
- ***T-I and T-II.*** Damage to the EPL and possibly the EPB (if laceration is in the proximal region of the proximal phalanx) leads to loss of hyperextension of the IP joint (mallet thumb deformity) and weakened MP extension.
- ***T-III and T-IV.*** Damage to EPB leads to weakened MP extension and transfers extension forces to IP joint, leading to a flexion deformity of the MP joint and a hyperextension deformity of the IP joint if the EPL is intact.

Operative Overview

Although similar definitions exist for extensor and flexor tendon procedures, there are substantial differences in operative techniques used to repair extensor versus flexor tendons. These differences are based largely on the fact that extensor tendons are morphologically thinner and flatter than flexor tendons. This fact led to the belief that extensor tendon repairs are more prone to gapping, have less tensile strength, and are more likely to rupture than flexor tendons after repair. However, stronger suturing techniques, specifically designed for extensor tendon repair and reconstruction, are used more frequently today, allowing early postoperative mobilization of the repaired tendon while lessening concerns of gapping and rupture.[52,91,119,126]

Zone III primary repair. Operative procedures for repair of lacerated or ruptured extensor tendons vary significantly in the distal versus the proximal zones. In this overview, only repair of a zone III laceration is described, simply as an example. Detailed descriptions of operative techniques for primary repair and late reconstruction of extensor tendons in all zones of the hand, wrist, and forearm can be found in several sources.[16,52,91,105,126,130]

Closed or open injury to the extensor mechanism over the PIP joint in zone III may injure the central slip, the lateral bands, or both. This can result in a PIP joint extensor lag and DIP joint hyperextension, called a boutonniere deformity. The cause of a closed boutonnière deformity involves blunt trauma to the dorsum of the PIP joint and volar dislocation that results in an avulsion of the central slip, with or without a piece of bone. Treatment for acute central slip injuries in zone III, includes using an orthosis in full PIP extension for 6 weeks in order to allow the central slip to heal, during which time active DIP flexion exercises are done hourly in order to draw the lateral bands dorsally. After the initial 6 weeks, a night orthosis is used for an additional 4 to 6 weeks.[52,133] For open injuries to zone III, the central slip is repaired, and if the central slip is not robust enough for a direct repair, a suture anchor can be used to the middle phalanx to facilitate tendon-to-bone fixation.[52,133]

If damaged, the lateral bands are repaired. If a boutonnière deformity is evident or likely to develop, a K-wire may be inserted to immobilize the PIP joint in extension for about 3 weeks and then removed. After closure of the area, a bulky compression dressing immobilizes the repaired tissues and controls edema.[52,57,133]

Postoperative Management

General considerations. The overall goal of postoperative rehabilitation after extensor tendon injury and repair is the same as after flexor tendon repair—that is, to restore mobility and strength to the hand and wrist for functional activities. Adhesion formation is a concern in the extensor tendons after repair, just as it is after repair of the flexor tendons. As noted previously, extensor tendons of the fingers are less likely to retract after laceration or rupture because of the extensor mechanism's multiple soft tissue linkages to surrounding structures. However, these attachments make extensor tendons prone to adhesion formation and loss of excursion during the healing process.[91,105,119] As with management after flexor tendon repair, emphasis after extensor tendon repair is placed on preventing adhesions that restrict tendon gliding, limit joint ROM, and functional use of the hand. (Refer to Box 19.10 to review factors that contribute to adhesion formation.)

The components and progression of postoperative rehabilitation and eventual outcomes after extensor tendon repair are influenced by many of the same factors that influence rehabilitation and outcomes of flexor tendon repair, including the location (level) and severity of the injury; the specifics of the surgical procedure(s), particularly the type of suturing technique and strength of the repair; and the timing of and the patient's access and commitment to a supervised rehabilitation program with an experienced hand therapist.[39,56,57,91,119]

Approaches to postoperative management. Two general approaches to rehabilitation after surgical repair of extensor tendon injuries are described in the literature: prolonged, uninterrupted immobilization with motion of the injured region(s) delayed for 3 to 6 weeks or, in carefully selected patients, early controlled passive or active motion initiated during the first few postoperative days. The latter is based on the same rationale as for early mobilization of flexor tendon repairs (see Box 19.11).

There are situations when an extended immobilization/delayed motion approach is the only appropriate method of management (see Box 19.12). Some studies continue to show that in many instances this traditional approach yields acceptable results in certain cases.[39,56] However, some studies have shown that extensor tendon repairs, managed with prolonged immobilization, are more likely to develop adhesions, resulting in only marginal outcomes (increased incidence of extensor lag, joint contracture, and boutonnière deformity). In addition, these and other studies have demonstrated that early motion programs after *primary* repair of acute extensor tendon injuries in zones III and VII are effective and safe[25,56,57,130] and produce superior outcomes compared with prolonged immobilization/delayed motion programs.[39,56] Consequently, early motion approaches have become more widely used in recent years.

It should be noted, however, that prolonged immobilization continues to be the most frequently selected method of treating zone I and II extensor tendon injuries.[39,56,57,119,126,130] Late reconstruction, which is more complex and usually involves tendon grafts, also is managed in most cases with continuous, extended immobilization and delayed motion.[126]

Immobilization

Immobilization typically is maintained with a volar (palmar) orthosis after the bulky surgical dressing is removed a few days postoperatively. The duration of immobilization, the type(s) of immobilization selected, the joints immobilized, and the position of immobilization are based on the location (zone) of the injury and repair and the structures involved.

Duration of immobilization. If a patient is a good candidate for an early motion program, the duration of uninterrupted immobilization often is just a few days. If delayed motion is a more appropriate course of action, uninterrupted immobilization ranges from 3 to 6 weeks. In early motion programs, some type of a protective orthosis is used during exercise for about 6 weeks after surgery.

Types of immobilization. Either static or dynamic orthoses or a combination of both is used. Depending on the joints immobilized, a forearm and wrist-based or a hand-based orthosis is indicated to block excessive flexion at the region of the repair and prevent stretching of the repaired tendon(s). A static orthosis is considered a low-profile orthosis, whereas a dynamic orthosis (see Fig. 19.10) with its outrigger secured to the dorsal surface of the orthosis for the elastic band and sling attachments is a high-profile orthosis. The slings and elastic band attachments hold the digits in extension at rest but allow active flexion.

For a delayed motion program, a static volar or a removable circumferential orthosis is fabricated and worn on a continuous basis (other than daily skin care). A dynamic orthosis, worn during the day for frequent exercise sessions, is an integral component of many early motion programs, but a static orthosis must be worn at night to protect the repair. Some early active motion programs use only static orthoses that allow active motion when the straps are loosened but otherwise prevent excessive motion of joints. Special static orthoses for the repaired digits are fabricated and used only during short-arc exercises to limit the range of allowable motion (see Fig. 19.15).[56,83]

The joints are immobilized in an extended position or a position that places only minimal tension on the tendon to protect the repair from excessive stretch and potential gapping. As examples, for a zone I or II repair, the DIP is placed in hyperextension, for a zone III/IV repair, the PIP and sometimes the DIP joints are placed in extension, but for a zone V/VI repair, the wrist is held in 30° of extension and the MP joints in 30° to 45° of flexion. Recommended positions of the joints proximal or distal to the injured zone vary considerably. Several resources provide detailed information on immobilization and use of orthoses after extensor tendon repairs.[30,39,56,83]

Exercise: Early Controlled Active Motion Approach

As interest in the application of early active motion after tendon repair has grown, so have the number of studies describing details of exercise programs and outcomes. In addition to one example of an early active motion program for zone III/IV repairs presented in this section, guidelines for early mobilization of zones V, VI, and VII also have been proposed and detailed in the literature.[27,30,56,57,67,83,93]

CLINICAL TIP

The distinguishing feature common to all early active motion programs following extensor tendon repair is that low-intensity and controlled active contractions of the repaired muscle-tendon units are initiated during the first few postoperative days, albeit in the confines of some type of static volar orthosis.

As noted previously, extensor tendon repairs in zones III and IV are especially prone to adhesion formation because of multiple soft tissue attachments of the extensor mechanism to surrounding structures and the broad bone-tendon interface of the proximal phalanx along which the extensor mechanism must glide.[56,57,105,119] Evans[56,57] proposed an early motion program of using orthoses and exercise for repairs of the central slip that involves minimal active tension of the repaired extensors for controlled SAM of the PIP and DIP joints.

FOCUS ON EVIDENCE

Evans[56] compared the results of a prolonged immobilization/delayed motion program and an early SAM program in 55 patients who had undergone primary repair of 64 fingers for injury of the central slip. Patients in one group (36 digits) were managed with 3 to 6 weeks (mean 32.9 days) of continuous immobilization, whereas patients in the early motion group (28 digits) began active motion in a protected range at 2 to 11 days (mean 4.59 days) after surgery. After 6 weeks of treatment, patients in the delayed motion group had significantly less PIP flexion (44°) than the early motion group (88°). At discharge, the delayed motion group continued to have significantly less PIP flexion (72° after 76 days) than the early motion group (88° at 51 days). In addition, at discharge, the delayed motion group had significantly less DIP flexion than the early motion group (37.6° and 45.0°, respectively). It also is interesting to note that at discharge, the delayed motion group compared to the early motion group had significantly greater PIP extensor lag (8.1° and 2.9°, respectively). However, at the initiation of treatment, the delayed motion group had a 13° PIP extensor lag, whereas the early motion group had only a 3° lag.

Key elements of the early, short-arc, active motion program for central slip repairs include the following orthosis and exercise procedures:[30,56,57,83]

Use of customized static volar orthoses. Several types of customized orthoses are used with this approach. A static, hand-based volar orthosis is fabricated and applied as soon as the surgical dressing is removed. It holds only the PIP and DIP joints in 0° extension; the wrist and MP joints are free. This orthosis is removed for exercise on an hourly basis during the day but replaced between exercise sessions.

- A forearm-based resting orthosis is worn at night for protection for at least 6 weeks postoperatively.
- Two static, volar, finger-based, template orthoses are fabricated and worn only during exercise to limit joint motion,

extensor tendon excursion, and the level of stress on the repaired central slip. One orthosis is molded to limit PIP flexion to 30° and DIP flexion to 20° or 25° during exercise. A second template orthosis is fabricated to hold the PIP joint in full extension during isolated DIP flexion limited to 30° to 35° (Fig. 19.15).

- The PIP exercise orthosis is revised during the second week of exercise to allow 40° of flexion if no extensor lag is present. The PIP flexion allowed by the orthosis is increased incrementally by 10° each week thereafter.

Exercise progression. The patient is taught the concept of minimum active tension (MAT) to protect healing tissues during tendon excursion. MAT is just enough tension generated during an active muscle contraction to overcome the elastic resistance of an antagonist.[56]

- Exercises are initiated within the first few postoperative days and performed hourly during the day. While actively holding the wrist in 30° of flexion and manually stabilizing the MP joint in neutral to slight flexion, the patient performs active PIP and DIP flexion within the limits allowed by the PIP exercise orthosis (Fig. 19.15 A), followed by full active extension held for several seconds (Fig. 19.15 B).
- The patient also performs active, isolated DIP flexion/extension in the second volar template orthosis that stabilizes the PIP joint in full extension.
- Exercises continue regularly during the day for several weeks using revised exercise orthoses. Ideally, by the end of 4 weeks, the patient achieves 70° to 80° of active flexion and full extension of the PIP joint.
- Composite MP, PIP, and DIP flexion (full fist) is postponed for at least 4 weeks or when the exercise orthoses have been discontinued.
- By 6 to 8 weeks, low-intensity resisted exercises are initiated along with gradual use of the hand for functional activities.

Exercise: Delayed Mobilization Approach

If a traditional approach to postoperative management of extensor tendon repairs is used, exercises are delayed for at least several weeks after surgery. Special considerations and precautions for exercise using a delayed motion approach are summarized by zones in Box 19.17.[30,56]

Guidelines for resistance exercises to strengthen the hand and continuation or modification of an orthosis for protection are not addressed in this summary. In general, an orthosis is continued during the day if an extensor lag persists and at night for protection for about 12 weeks. If grasp is limited because of insufficient finger flexion, passive stretching is initiated, or a dynamic flexor orthosis may be incorporated into the program by alternating the flexion and extension orthoses.

Resistance to the repaired muscle-tendon unit is not initiated until 8 to 12 weeks postoperatively regardless of the site of the repair. First, emphasis is placed on gradually strengthening the extensors to prevent or minimize an extensor lag. After 10 to 12 weeks, *low-intensity* resisted grasp and pinch activities are initiated to gradually strengthen the flexors if no extensor lag is present.

Outcomes

Outcomes, including complications, after extensor tendon repair and postoperative rehabilitation are well documented in the literature. Early and late complications are similar to those occurring after flexor tendon repair, including rupture, adhesion formation, and limited motion. Outcomes typically measured and reported after extensor tendon repair are ROM of the wrist and/or digits and grip strength with only limited information reported on use of the hand for functional activities.

Digital motion often is expressed in terms of "pad-to-palm" distances or TAM (active flexion minus extensor lag). These figures are then compared to the contralateral hand or to the "normal" population and are typically expressed as excellent, good, fair, or poor. For example, if ROM is only 75% of that found in normal individuals or if there is < 15° of extensor lag in a digit and sufficient digital flexion to touch the pad of the distal phalanx to the mid-palm, the result is described as "good." To understand the results of studies on tendon repair, it is necessary to have some understanding of the various assessment tools.

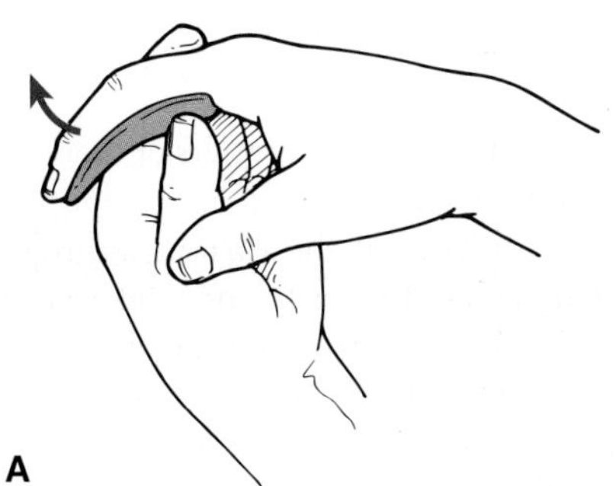

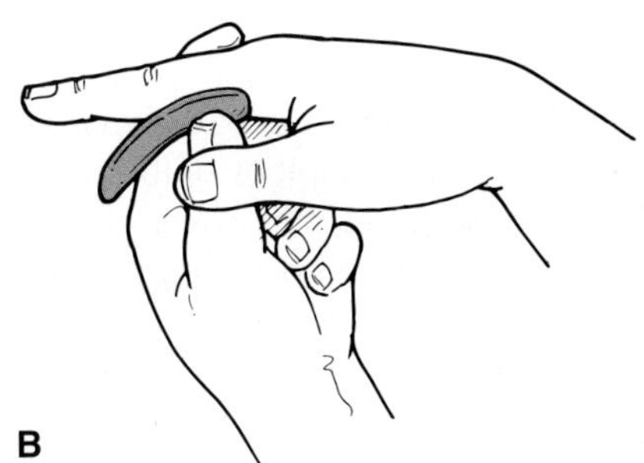

FIGURE 19.15 One of two static volar template orthoses used during early short-arc exercises of the PIP and DIP joints after repair of the extensor mechanism in zones III/IV. During exercise, the patient actively holds the wrist in approximately 30° of flexion and manually holds the MP joint in neutral to slight flexion. **(A)** Using minimal active tension during combined active PIP and DIP flexion, the orthosis initially limits PIP and DIP flexion to 30° and 20° to 25°, respectively, to prevent excessive stretch of the repair site. **(B)** The patient actively and slowly extends the PIP and DIP joints to full extension and briefly holds the extended position.

BOX 19.17 Special Considerations for Exercise After Extensor Tendon Repair and Extended Immobilization

Zones I and II

- Tendon injuries in these zones are typically managed nonoperatively.
- PIP and MP AROM while the DIP is continuously immobilized in extension for at least 4 weeks but more often 6 to 8 weeks.
- When orthosis can be removed for exercise, perform active DIP extension and very gentle active flexion with the MP and PIP joints stabilized in neutral. Briefly hold the extended position with each repetition.
- Emphasize active extension more than flexion to avoid an extensor lag.
- After initiating exercises, use an orthosis between exercise sessions an additional 2 weeks or longer if an extensor lag develops.

PRECAUTION: Increase active flexion of the DIP joint *very gradually,* initially limiting flexion to 20° to 25° during the first week of exercise. The strong FDP can easily place excessive stress on the terminal extensor tendon and cause gapping or rupture of the repair. Progress active flexion by about 10° per week. Do not attempt full DIP flexion for about 3 months.

Zones III and IV

- If the lateral bands were intact, begin DIP AROM 1 week postoperatively while the PIP joint is immobilized in extension in a volar orthosis or cylinder cast. Early DIP motion prevents adherence and loss of extensibility of the lateral bands and oblique retinacular ligaments and loss of mobility of the DIP joint.
- If the lateral bands were damaged and repaired, postpone DIP ROM until 4 to 6 weeks postoperatively.
- At a minimum of 3 to 4 weeks but more often at 6 weeks, the volar orthosis is removed for active ROM of the PIP joints with the MP joints stabilized. Emphasize active extension more than flexion.

PRECAUTIONS: Progress PIP flexion in *very gradual* increments; limit PIP flexion to 30° the first week of PIP ROM exercises. Increase an additional 10° per week if no extensor lag.

- If the wrist and MP joints have been immobilized postoperatively, include active ROM of the wrist with the MP and PIP joints stabilized and active MP ROM with the wrist and PIP joints stabilized in extension.

Zones V and VI

- When the volar orthosis can be removed for exercise (between 3 and 4 weeks or as late as 6 weeks postoperatively), begin active or assisted MP extension and passive flexion with the wrist and IP joints stabilized in neutral and the forearm *pronated.* Actively hold the extended position for a few seconds with each repetition. Let the extensors relax to flex the MP joints.
- Add carefully controlled active MP flexion within a protected range with the wrist stabilized in extension.
- Emphasize active MP extension more than flexion to prevent an extensor lag.

PRECAUTION: Initially limit active MP flexion to 30° in the index and middle fingers and 35° to 40° in the ring and small fingers.

- During active IP flexion and extension exercises, stabilize the MP joints in neutral and the wrist in slight extension. Encourage full-range DIP motion.
- Combine active MP extension with active PIP flexion (hook fist position) and PIP extension (straight hand position).
- Incrementally progress to full fist position over several weeks if no extensor lag develops.

Zone VII

- If the wrist extensors are intact and only extrinsic finger extensors have been repaired follow the guidelines for zone V/VI repairs.
- If the wrist extensors were repaired, begin active wrist extension from neutral to full extension in a gravity-eliminated position (forearm in mid-position) at 3 to 4 weeks.
- Incrementally increase wrist flexion beyond neutral between 5 and 8 weeks postoperatively.
- Perform radial and ulnar deviation with the wrist in neutral.

Some generalizations about outcomes can be drawn from the literature regarding the severity and location of the injury. As with flexor tendon injuries, the greater the extent of associated skeletal, joint, vascular, or nerve injuries, the poorer are the results of the repair with respect to extensor lag and digital flexion for grasp. For example, in a study of outcomes after extended immobilization following extensor tendon repair, 64% of patients with simple tendon injuries had good results, whereas only 47% of patients with associated skeletal or joint injuries had good results.[105] In the same study, investigators found that repairs of distal injuries (zones I to IV) had less favorable results than repairs of more proximal injuries (zones V to VIII).

Outcomes of the various approaches to postoperative management of extensor tendon injuries are reported in the literature on an ongoing basis. With regard to the timing of the surgical intervention, for example, primary repairs of acute injuries (rupture or laceration), whether repaired immediately or delayed for up to 10 days, yield equally good results.[119] As noted throughout this section on extensor tendon injury and repair, numerous studies have been published describing outcomes of the various approaches to postoperative management. Although some studies support the use and effectiveness of prolonged immobilization of extensor tendon repairs, there is growing use and ongoing modification and refinement of early controlled motion approaches to help patients achieve the best possible outcomes.

For example, a dynamic extension orthosis, a mainstay of early passive mobilization protocols for more than 20 years, now is being re-evaluated. Although some studies [25,120] have demonstrated that high-profile, dynamic orthoses continue to be used and are effective, other studies reflect a return to the use of low-profile, static orthoses if coupled with early active motion.[56,93]

In a prospective, randomized, controlled trial, Kitis[74] and associates compared static and dynamic orthosis management of extensor tendon repairs in zones V to VII. Between January 2009 and June 2011, they compared the results of patients randomized into a static group (n = 25) or a dynamic group (n = 27). All patients underwent extensor tendon repair within 24 hours using Kessler's method using a two-strand core suture of 4.0 nylon and a circumferential running suture of 6.0 nylon. Following surgery, the patients were seen in the clinic 3 to 5 days postoperatively. Twenty-five patients with 39 fingers were treated with controlled movement with a volar static orthosis (wrist in 30°-35° extension and MP joints in 45° of flexion with the orthosis extending distally to the middle of the proximal phalanx), and 27 patients with 44 fingers were treated with a dynamic orthosis. Those in the static group were allowed to actively flex and extend their IP joints within the limits of the orthosis. Active motion of the wrist was initiated after 3 weeks with gravity eliminated, followed by extension of the MPs, followed by full extension of the IPs. Exercises were performed 10 times each waking hour. At 4 weeks, the orthosis was removed and wrist AROM was initiated against gravity. At 6 weeks, the patients were allowed to use the involved hand for light ADLs, and at 8 weeks, gradual resistance was initiated. The dynamic group was placed in an extension orthosis positioned dorsally, which allowed full IP motion and 30° of active MP flexion with passive rubber band extension. The patients were instructed to actively flex the MP joints to 30° as permitted by the orthosis 10 times every waking hour. At 4 weeks, the dynamic group was allowed active MP and IP extension, and the dynamic orthosis was discontinued except at night. At 5 weeks, active wrist flexion and extension was allowed, as well as a full active fist. Between 8 to 12 weeks, the dynamic group progressed to resistive exercises and was allowed to perform normal hand activities. Outcome measures included the measurement of TAM, grip strength, and the DASH questionnaire, which were measured in both groups at 4 weeks, 12 weeks, and 6 months postoperatively. The authors reported no ruptures in either group and concluded that the use of dynamic orthoses for extensor tendon lacerations in zones V to VII provides improved functional outcomes when compared with the use of static orthoses.

Exercise Interventions for the Wrist and Hand

Techniques for Musculotendinous Mobility

Active muscle contraction and specific motions of the digits and wrist are used to maintain or develop mobility between the multijoint musculotendinous units and other connective tissue structures in the wrist and hand. Because adhesions between the various structures can become restrictive or incapacitating, *tendon-gliding exercises* and *tendon-blocking exercises* are used whenever possible to develop or maintain mobility. This is particularly important when there has been immobilization after trauma, surgery, or fracture and scar tissue adhesions have developed. If restrictions occur as a result of scar tissue adherence between tendons or between tendons and surrounding tissues, mobilization techniques described in this section may be necessary. General stretching techniques also may be necessary; they are described in the next section. The tendon-gliding and tendon-blocking exercises described here may also be used to develop neuromuscular control and coordinated movement.

Tendon-Gliding and Tendon-Blocking Exercises

Place-and-Hold Exercises

Place-and-hold exercises are a form of gentle muscle setting (static/isometric) exercises that are used during the early postoperative period following tendon repair before active ROM is initiated but when a minimal level of stress on the repaired tendon and passive joint movement are beneficial for maintaining joint mobility and tendon excursion.

- Following flexor tendon repair, the patient usually wears a dorsal blocking orthosis[39,55,56,57] or a tenodesis orthosis.[29,112,134] With the MP joints in flexion, passively place the IP joints in a partially flexed position and have the patient hold the position independently for 5 seconds with a minimum static contraction of the finger flexors.
- If the patient is wearing a tenodesis orthosis, combine place-and-hold finger flexion with active wrist extension (see Fig. 19.13 B and C). Have the patient relax and allow the wrist to passively flex and the digits to passively extend.
- Following extensor tendon repair, when the volar blocking orthosis may be removed for exercise, passively position the joint in the zone of the repair first in a neutral and later in a slightly extended position utilizing the sagittal band bridge or relative extension orthoses. Have the patient hold the position for 5 to 10 seconds. This emphasizes end-range extension to prevent an extensor lag.

- Have the patient practice the exercise with the uninjured hand or use biofeedback to learn how to hold the position with a minimum of force production.

Flexor Tendon-Gliding Exercises

Flexor tendon-gliding exercises are designed to maintain or develop free gliding between the FDP and FDS tendons and between the tendons and bones in the wrist, hand, and fingers.[112] There are five positions in which the fingers move during tendon-gliding exercises: straight hand (all the joints are extended); hook fist (MP joints are extended, IP joints are flexed); full fist (all the joints are flexed); table-top position, also known as the intrinsic plus hand (MP joints are flexed, IP joints are extended); and straight fist (MP and PIP joints are flexed, DIP joints are extended) (Fig. 19.16). The following progression is suggested:

- Initiate the exercises with the wrist in neutral position.
- Once full range of the finger motions is achieved, progress to doing the gliding\exercises with the wrist in flexion and in extension to establish combined finger and wrist mobility.
- Full excursion and tendon-gliding of all the extrinsic muscles are accomplished by starting with the wrist and fingers in full extension, then moving to full wrist and finger flexion, and then reversing the motion.

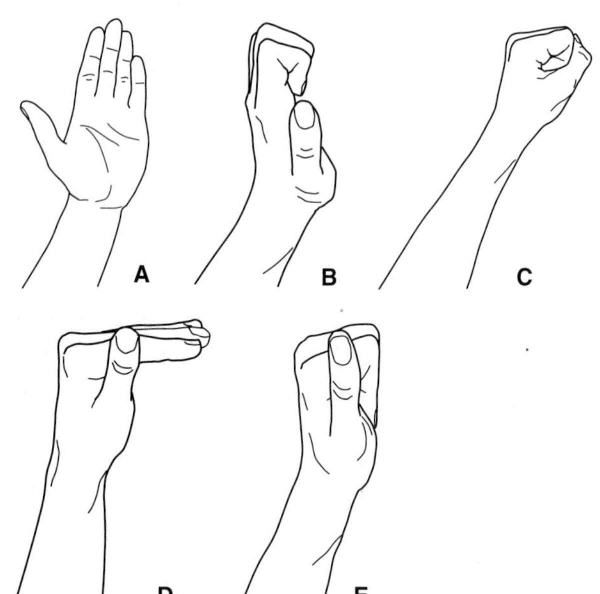

FIGURE 19.16 The five finger positions used for flexor tendon-gliding exercises: **(A)** straight hand, **(B)** hook fist, **(C)** full fist, **(D)** table top (intrinsic plus), and **(E)** straight fist.

Hook-fist position. Have the patient move from the straight hand to the hook-fist position by flexing the DIP and PIP joints while maintaining MP extension (Fig. 19.16 A and B). Maximum gliding occurs between the profundus and superficialis tendons and between the profundus tendon and the bone. (There is also gliding of the extensor digitorum tendons; this motion is used with the extensor gliding exercises.)

Full fist. Have the patient move to the full fist position by flexing all the MP and IP joints simultaneously (Fig. 19.16 C). Maximum gliding of the profundus tendon with respect to the sheath and bone as well as over the superficialis tendon occurs.

Straight fist. Have the patient move from the table-top position (Fig. 19.16 D) to the straight fist position by flexing the PIP joints while maintaining the DIP joints in extension (Fig. 19.16 E). Maximum gliding of the superficialis tendon occurs with respect to the flexor sheath and bone.

Thumb flexion. Have the patient flex the MP and IP joints of the thumb full range. This promotes maximum gliding of the flexor pollicis longus.

Flexor Tendon-Blocking Exercises

Blocking exercises for the flexor tendons (Fig. 19.17) not only develop gliding of the tendons with respect to the sheaths and related bones; they also require neuromuscular control of individual joint motions. Therefore, they use the mobility gained by the flexor tendon-gliding exercises and are a progression of the flexor tendon-gliding exercises. Progress to manual resistance as the tissues heal and can tolerate resistance.

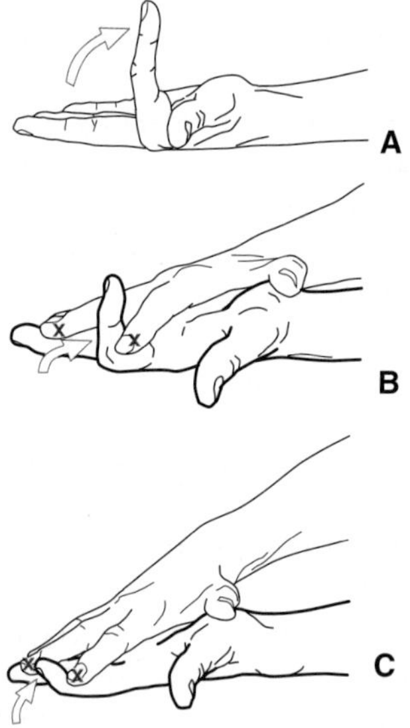

FIGURE 19.17 Flexor tendon blocking exercises: **(A)** isolated MP flexion of one digit, **(B)** isolated PIP flexion (flexor digitorum superficialis) of one digit, and **(C)** isolated DIP flexion (flexor digitorum profundus) of one digit.

PRECAUTION: These exercises should not be used in the early stages of flexor tendon healing after repair because of the stress placed on the tendons.

Patient position and stabilization: Sitting with the forearm supinated and the back of the hand resting on a table. The opposite hand provides stabilization and "blocking" against unwanted movement. Each finger performs the exercise separately.

Isolated MP flexion (lumbricals and palmar interossei). With the patient's hand stabilized, have the patient flex only the MP joint of one digit (Fig. 19.17 A). If necessary, stabilize the rest of the fingers in extension against the table with the other hand. With improved control, the hand does not have to be stabilized against the table.

PIP flexion (flexor digitorum superficialis). Have the patient stabilize the proximal phalanx of one digit with the opposite hand and, if possible, flex just the PIP joint of the one digit while keeping the DIP joint extended and the rest of fingers on the table (Fig. 19.17 B).

If the patient has difficulty doing this, stabilize the other digits in extension with the opposite hand.

DIP flexion (flexor digitorum profundus). Have the patient attempt to flex just the distal phalanx (Fig. 19.17 C). Stabilize the middle phalanx of one digit with the other hand. Vary this exercise by increasing the range of MP and PIP flexion to the point at which the patient just begins to lose DIP motion; stabilize in this position and have the patient attempt DIP flexion.

Full fist. When full independent tendon-gliding is available, the patient should be able to make a full fist. Progress the exercises described by adding resistance.

Exercises to Reduce an Extensor Lag

The extrinsic finger extensors (extensor digitorum , extensor indicis, and extensor digiti minimi) are more superficial than the flexor tendons and therefore more easily damaged. Their prime function is to extend the MP joints. Extension of the IP joints requires active interaction with the intrinsic muscles of the hand via the extensor mechanism. Adhesions within their sheaths at the wrist or between tendon and bone restrict tendon-gliding both proximally (restricting active finger extension) and distally (restricting active and passive finger flexion).

When full passive range of extension is available but the person cannot actively move the joint through the full range of extension, it is called an *extensor lag*. An extensor lag can occur as the result of weakness but is frequently caused by adhesions that prevent gliding of the tendons when the muscles contract.

One purpose of the following exercises is to maintain mobility and thus prevent adhesions. The exercises also are used to regain control of finger extension. Mobilization of adhesions is described immediately following the differential gliding of extensor tendon exercises. Stretching techniques are described in the next section.

Isolated MP extension. Have the patient move from the full fist position (see Fig. 19.16C) to the hook-fist position (see Fig. 19.16 B).

- If the patient has difficulty maintaining the IP joints in flexion, have him or her hook the fingers around a pencil while extending the MP joints.
- Begin with the wrist in neutral and progress to positioning the wrist in flexion and extension while performing MP extension.

Isolated PIP and DIP extension. Extension of the IP joints requires intrinsic and extrinsic muscle (extensor digitorum) control.

- For strongest participation of the lumbricals, stabilize the MP joint in flexion while the patient attempts IP extension, moving from the full fist position (see Fig. 19.16 C) to the table-top position (see Fig. 19.16 D).
- Progress to stabilizing the palm of the hand on the edge of a table (or block) with the PIP or DIP joint partially flexed over the edge.
- Have the patient extend the involved phalanx through the ROM.

Terminal-range extension of IP joints. Progress to the terminal range by stabilizing the entire hand, palm side down on a flat surface, and have the patient extend the involved phalanx into hyperextension. If there is not enough range available, place a pencil or block under the proximal phalanx or middle phalanx so the PIP or DIP joint can go through a greater range (Fig. 19.18).

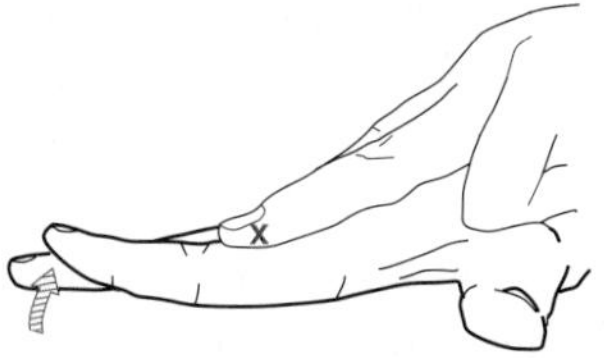

FIGURE 19.18 Terminal extension of the PIP joint. The MP joint is stabilized in extension, and the patient lifts the middle and distal phalanges off the table.

Extensor Tendon-Gliding Exercises

Differential gliding of the extensor digitorum tendons to each of the fingers can be achieved by the following progression.

- Teach the patient to passively flex the MP and IP joints of one finger with the opposite hand while actively maintaining the other fingers in extension.
- If the patient has difficulty doing this, begin with the involved hand resting on a table with the palm up. Stabilize three of the four fingers against the table while passively flexing one of the digits (Fig. 19.19). Then instruct the patient to attempt to actively keep the fingers against the table while one of the digits is passively flexed.
- Progress by having the patient actively maintain the fingers in extension with the fingers spread out and then actively flex each finger in turn while the other fingers remain extended.
- Have the patient flex the middle and ring fingers while maintaining extension of the index and little fingers (long horn sign). This promotes isolated control of the extensor indicis and extensor digiti minimi tendons and promotes their gliding on the extensor digitorum tendons.

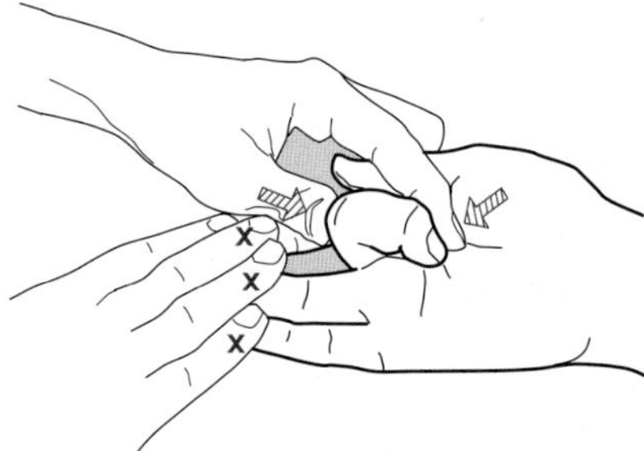

FIGURE 19.19 Differential gliding of the extensor digitorum tendons. Move each digit into flexion while stabilizing the other digits in extension.

Scar Tissue Mobilization for Tendon Adhesions

Ideally, the tendon-gliding exercises described previously in this section maintain or develop mobility between the long tendons and surrounding connective tissues or within their sheaths. However, when there has been inflammation and immobilization during the healing process following trauma or surgery, scar tissue adhesions may form and prevent gliding of the tendons. Contraction of the muscle does not result in movement of the joint or joints distal to the site of the immobile scar.

Techniques to mobilize the adhesive scar tissue include the application of friction massage directly to the adhesion. This is superimposed on active and passive stretching techniques (described in the next section) and the tendon-gliding techniques already described. To apply friction massage, hold the tendon in its lengthened position; apply pressure with your thumb, index, or middle finger and massage perpendicular to the tendon and longitudinally in proximal and distal directions. A sustained force against the adhesion allows for creep and eventual movement of the scar. Techniques to mobilize the flexor and extensor tendons follow.

To Mobilize the Long Finger Flexor Tendons

Adhesions between the flexor tendons and their sheaths or between tendons and underlying bones restrict tendon-gliding in both a proximal and distal direction so the joints distal to the scar do not flex when the muscle contracts. Passive movement into flexion of the joints distal to the adherent scar is possible if there are no capsular restrictions. Full range of extension of the joints distal to the scar is not possible actively or passively owing to the inability of the tendon to glide distally.

The following is a suggested progression in intensity of scar tissue mobilization:

- Begin the stretching routine by passively moving the tendon in a distal direction by extending the finger joints as far as possible and applying a sustained hold to allow for creep. Follow this with active contraction of the flexor muscle to create a stretch force against the adhesion in a proximal direction using the patterns of movement described for tendon-gliding exercises (see Fig. 19.16).
- If active and passive stretching, described in the above technique, does not release the adhesion, extend the MP and IP joints as far as allowed, stabilize them, and apply friction massage with your thumb or finger at the site of the adhesion while the tendon is held in its stretched position. Apply the massaging stretch force across the tendon and in a longitudinal direction, both proximally and distally. When applying friction massage in a proximal direction, ask the patient to simultaneously contract the flexor muscle in order to superimpose an active stretch force.
- After friction massage, have the patient repeat the flexor tendon-gliding exercises to utilize any gained mobility.

To Mobilize the Extensor Tendons and the Extensor Mechanism

If the extensor tendons or extensor mechanism has restricted mobility because of adhesions, muscle action is not transmitted through the mechanism to extend the joint or joints distal to the restriction. Without free gliding, an extensor lag may result. As defined earlier, an extensor lag is the loss of active extension when there is full passive extension. The following is a progression in intensity of scar tissue mobilization:

- Stretch the adhesion in a distal direction by passively flexing the joint distal to the site. Follow this by having the patient attempt to actively extend the joint and put tension on the scar in a proximal direction.

PRECAUTION: If the extensor lag increases (i.e., flexion increases, but there is no active extension through the increased range), the tendon distal to the adhesion, rather than the adhesion, may be stretching. Do not continue with passive stretching into flexion, but rather emphasize friction massage applied to the scar tissue.

- Apply friction massage at the site of the adhesion with the tendon kept taut by holding the joint at the end of its range of flexion. Apply friction massage across the fibers and in a distal and proximal direction. When applying friction massage in a proximal direction, have the patient actively contract the extensors to assist with the mobilization effort.
- Follow these mobilization techniques with extensor tendon-gliding exercises, as described in the previous section.

Exercise Techniques to Increase Flexibility and Range of Motion

Stretching the muscles and connective tissue structures of the wrist and hand requires knowledge of the unique anatomical relationships of the multijoint musculotendinous units and the extensor mechanism of the digits. These are described in the first section of this chapter. The principles and techniques of stretching are presented in Chapter 4, and special note is made of the importance of stabilization when stretching the multijoint muscles of the hand and fingers. This is re-emphasized here. In addition, because scarring and adhesions can restrict tendon-gliding and therefore motion of the digits, it is important to recognize these restrictions and utilize specific techniques that address the adhesions as presented in the previous section. Before stretching muscle or connective tissue, there should be normal gliding of the joint surfaces to avoid joint damage. Use joint mobilization techniques to stretch the joint capsule and restore gliding (see Chapter 5).

NOTE: The patient position for most wrist and hand exercises is sitting with the forearm supported on a treatment table unless otherwise noted.

General Stretching Techniques

When stretching to increase wrist flexion or extension, it is important that the fingers are free to move so the extrinsic finger flexor and extensor musculotendinous units do not restrict motion at the wrist. Similarly, when stretching ligaments and other periarticular connective tissues across individual finger joints, it is important that there is no tension on the multijoint tendons. The following techniques are initially applied by the therapist and then are taught to the patient as self-stretching techniques for a home exercise program when he or she understands how to safely apply the stretch force and stabilization.

To Increase Wrist Extension

- Have the patient place the palm of the hand on a table with the fingers flexed over the edge. Use the other hand to stabilize the dorsal surface of the hand to maintain the palm against the table. Then have the patient move the forearm up over the stabilized hand (similar to Fig. 19.21 except the fingers are over the edge of the table so they are free to flex and the stretch occurs only at the wrist).
- Have the patient place the palms of the hands together at right angles to each other and allow the fingers to intertwine and flex. Instruct the patient to press the restricted hand in a dorsal direction with the palm of the other hand and sustain the stretch.

To Increase Wrist Flexion

- Have the patient place the dorsal surface of the hand on a table. Use the other hand to provide stabilization against the palm of the hand. Have the patient move the forearm up over the stabilized hand.
- Have the patient sit with the forearm pronated and resting on a table and the wrist at the edge of the table. Press against the dorsal surface of the hand with the opposite hand to flex the wrist.
- Have the patient place the dorsum of both hands together. Then, with the fingers relaxed, move the forearms so the wrists flex toward 90°.

To Increase Flexion or Extension of Individual Joints of the Fingers or Thumb

To increase extension at any one joint, begin by positioning the patient's forearm on a table in supination; to increase flexion, position the forearm in pronation. Place the phalanx to be stretched at the edge of the table. Show the patient how to apply the stretch force against the distal bone while stabilizing the proximal bone against the table.

Stretching Techniques for the Intrinsic and Multijoint Muscles

Self-Stretching the Lumbricals and Interossei Muscles

Have the patient actively extend the MP joints, flex the IP joints, and apply a passive stretch force at the end of the range with the opposite hand (Fig. 19.20A).

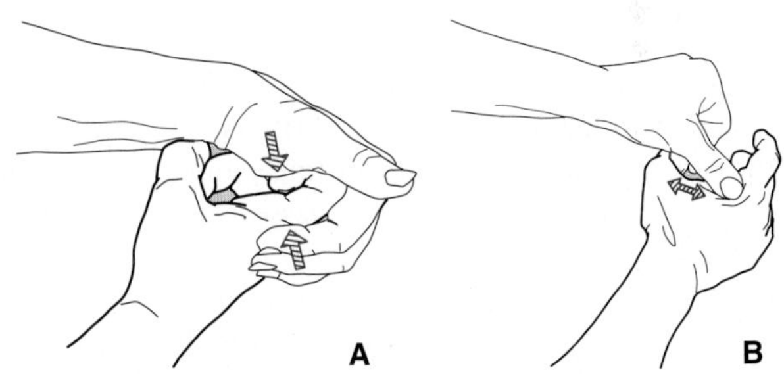

FIGURE 19.20 Self-stretching **(A)** the lumbricals with MP extension and IP flexion and **(B)** the adductor pollicis with CMC abduction of the thumb. To increase thumb abduction, it is critical that the stretch force is applied against the metacarpal head, not the proximal or distal phalanges.

Self-Stretching the Interossei Muscles

Have the patient place the hand flat on a table with the palm down and the MP joints extended. Instruct the patient to abduct or adduct the appropriate digit and apply the stretch force to the distal end of the proximal phalanx. Holding the adjacent digit provides stabilization.

Self-Stretching the Adductor Pollicis

Have the patient rest the ulnar border of the hand on the table and palmarly abduct the thumb.Instruct the patient to apply the stretch force with the crossed thumb and index or long finger of the other hand against the metacarpal head of the thumb and index finger and attempt to increase the web space (Fig. 19.20 B).

PRECAUTION: It is critical that the patient does not apply the stretch force against the proximal or distal phalanx. This places stress on the ulnar collateral ligament of the MP joint of the thumb and can lead to instability at that joint and poor functional use of the thumb. Palmar and radial abduction occur at the CMC joint at the articulation between the metacarpal and the trapezium.

Manual Stretching of the Extrinsic Muscles

Because they are multijoint muscles, the final step in a stretching progression is to elongate each tendon of the extrinsic muscles over all the joints simultaneously. However, do not initiate stretching procedures in this manner because joint compression and damage can occur to the smaller or less stable joints. Begin by allowing the wrist and more proximal finger joints to relax; stretch the tendon unit over the most distal joint first. Stabilize the distal joint at the end of the range, and then stretch the tendon unit over the next joint. Next, stabilize the two joints and stretch the tendon over the next joint. Progress in this manner until the desired length is reached.

PRECAUTION: Do not let the PIP and MP joints hyperextend as the tendons are stretched over the wrist.

Self-Stretching the Flexor Digitorum Profundus and Superficialis

Have the patient begin by resting the palm of the involved hand on a table; then extend the DIP joint, using the other hand to straighten the joint. While keeping it extended, have the patient straighten the PIP and MP joints in succession. If the patient can actively extend the finger joints to this point, the motion should be performed unassisted. With the hand stabilized on the table, have the patient then begin to extend the wrist by bringing the arm up over the hand. The patient moves just to the point of feeling discomfort, holds the position, and then progresses as the length increases (Fig. 19.21).

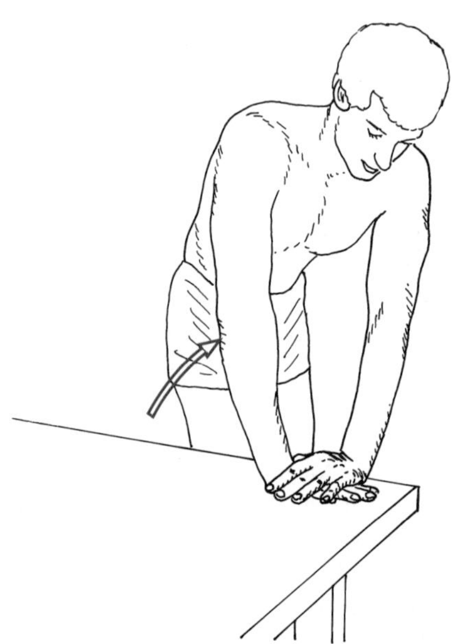

FIGURE 19.21 Self-stretching of the extrinsic finger flexor muscles, showing stabilization of the small distal joints. To isolate stretch to the wrist flexors, allow the fingers to flex over the edge of the table.

Self-Stretching the Extensor Digitorum

The fingers are flexed to the maximum range, beginning with the most distal joint first and progressing until the wrist is simultaneously flexed. The opposite hand applies the stretch force.

Exercises to Develop and Improve Muscle Performance, Neuromuscular Control, and Coordinated Movement

Exercises described in this section are for use during the controlled motion and return to function phases of rehabilitation when the tissues are in the subacute and chronic stages of healing and require only moderate or minimum protection. In addition to the conditions already described in this chapter, imbalances in the length and strength of the wrist and hand muscles may be caused by nerve injury, trauma, disuse, or immobilization.

Appropriate exercises to develop fine finger dexterity or strength and muscular endurance for strong or repetitive gripping can be selected from the following exercises or their adaptations. The flexor tendon-blocking exercises and extensor tendon-gliding exercises described previously in this section may be used to strengthen the musculature by adding resistance manually or mechanically. Exercises for shoulder, elbow, and forearm strength and muscular endurance also should be included to restore proper function in the upper extremity.

Techniques to Strengthen Muscles of the Wrist and Hand

If the musculature is weak, use progressive strengthening exercises, beginning at the level of the patient's ability. Use active-assistive, active, or manual resistance exercises as described in Chapters 3 and 6 of this text. Use mechanical resistance to progress strengthening exercises.

To Strengthen Wrist Musculature

Allow the fingers to relax. Exercise the wrist muscles in groups if their strength is similar. If one muscle is weaker, the wrist should be guided through the range desired to minimize the action of the stronger muscles. For example, with wrist flexion, if the flexor carpi radialis is stronger than the flexor carpi ulnaris, have the patient attempt to flex the wrist toward the ulnar side as you guide the wrist into flexion and ulnar deviation. If the muscle is strong enough to tolerate resistance, apply manual resistance over the fourth and fifth metacarpals.

Wrist flexion (flexor carpi ulnaris and radialis) and extension (extensor carpi radialis longus and brevis and extensor carpi ulnaris). Have the patient sit with the forearm supported on a table, grasping a weight or elastic resistance that is secured on the floor. The forearm is supinated to resist flexion or pronated to resist extension (Fig. 19.22).

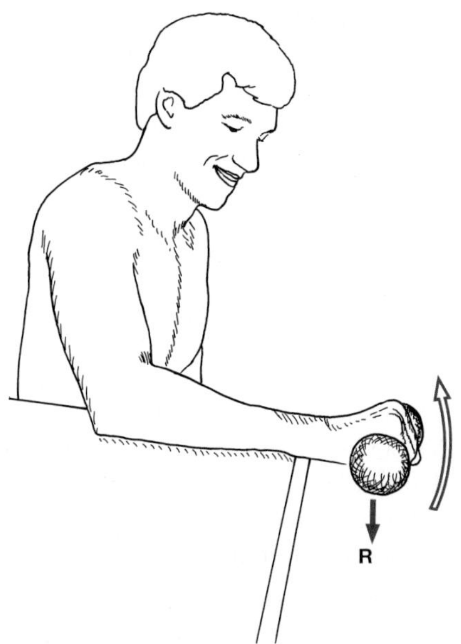

FIGURE 19.22 Mechanical resistance to strengthen wrist extension. Note that the forearm is pronated. To resist wrist flexion, the forearm is supinated.

Wrist radial deviation (flexor and extensor carpi radialis muscles and abductor pollicis longus) and ulnar deviation (flexor and extensor carpi ulnaris muscles). While standing, have the patient hold a bar with a weight on one end. To resist radial deviation, the weight is on the radial side of the wrist (Fig. 19.23A); to resist ulnar deviation, the weight is on the ulnar side of the wrist (Fig. 19.23 B).

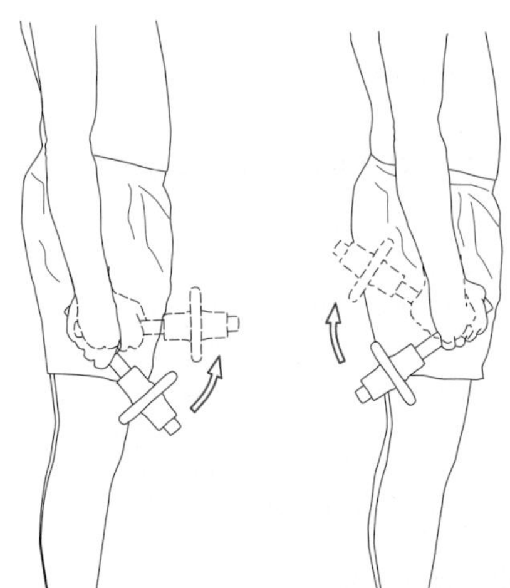

FIGURE 19.23 Mechanical resistance to strengthen **(A)** radial deviation and **(B)** ulnar deviation of the wrist using a weighted bar.

Functional progression for the wrist. Progress to controlled patterns of motion requiring stabilization of the wrist for functional hand activities such as repetitive gripping, picking up and releasing objects of various sizes and weights, and opening and closing the screw lid on a jar. Develop muscular endurance and progress to the desired functional pattern by loading the upper extremity to the tolerance of the wrist stabilizers. When the stabilizers begin to fatigue, stop the activity.

CLINICAL TIP

Functional progression of exercises for the wrist and hand should incorporate the entire upper extremity. When performing shoulder, elbow, or forearm exercises, emphasize safe wrist patterns of motion or wrist stabilization (i.e., do not let the wrist collapse into end-range flexion or extension).

To Strengthen Weak Intrinsic Musculature

NOTE: Imbalance from weak intrinsic muscles leads to a claw hand.

MP joint flexion with IP joint extension (lumbricals). Begin with the MP joints stabilized in flexion. Have the patient actively extend the PIP joint against resistance along the middle phalanx (the final position is table top). Increase the resistance by resisting the distal phalanx. Resistance may be applied manually or with rubber bands.

- Have the patient start with the MP joints extended and the PIP joints flexed; then actively push the fingertips outward, performing the desired combined motion (Fig. 19.24A and B). For resistance, have the patient push the fingers into the palm of the other hand (Fig. 19.24C), or push the fingers into exercise putty with the desired motion.

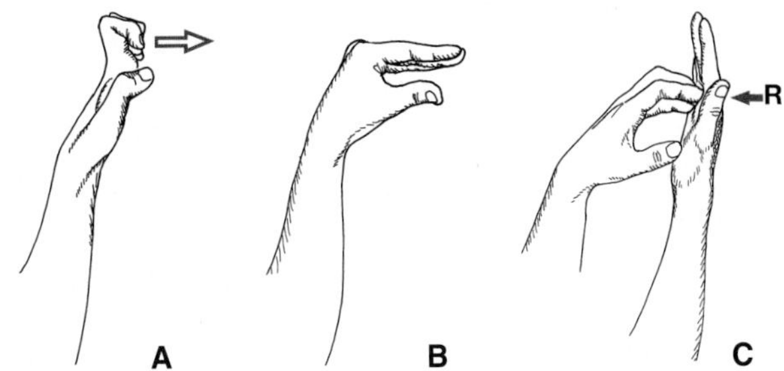

FIGURE 19.24 To strengthen intrinsic muscle function for combined MP flexion and IP extension, the patient begins with **(A)** MP extension and IP flexion and **(B)** pushes his fingertips outward. The same motion is resisted by **(C)** pushing the fingertips against the palm of the other hand.

- Begin with all the finger joints extended. Have the patient maintain the IP joints in extension and flex the MP joints to the table-top position. Apply resistance against the proximal phalanx.

Isolated or combined abduction/adduction of each finger (dorsal and volar interossei). Have the patient rest the palm of the hand on a table. Apply resistance at the distal end of the proximal phalanx, one finger at a time, for either abduction or adduction.

- For self-resisted adduction, have the patient interlace the fingers of both hands (or intertwine with your fingers) and squeeze the fingers together or squeeze exercise putty between two adjacent fingers.

- For self-resisted abduction, place a rubber band around two digits and have the patient spread them apart.

Palmar abduction of the thumb (abductor pollicis brevis and longus). Have the patient rest the dorsum of the hand on a table. Apply resistance at the base of the first phalanx of the thumb as the patient lifts the thumb away from the palm of the hand.

- Place a rubber band or band of exercise putty around the thumb and base of the index finger and have the patient abduct the thumb against the resistance.

Opposition of the thumb (opponens policis). Have the patient use various prehension patterns such as tip-to-tip and tip-to pad, with the thumb opposing each digit in succession, and pad-to-side, with the thumb approximating the lateral side of the index finger.

- Have the patient pinch exercise putty, a pliable ball, or a spring-loaded clothespin.

To Strengthen Weak Extrinsic Muscles of the Fingers

NOTE: The wrist must be stabilized for the action of the extrinsic hand musculature to be effective. If wrist strength is inadequate for stabilization, manually stabilize it during exercises and use an orthosis for functional activities.

Metacarpophalangeal extension (extensor digitorum, indicis, and digiti minimi). Place the hand on a table with the palm down and digits over the edge. Place a small strap over the distal end of the proximal phalanx with a small weight hanging from it or secure an elastic band or tubing around the proximal phalanx and have the patient extend the MP joint.

IP flexion (flexor digitorum profundus and superficialis). Have the patient apply self-resistance by starting with the hands pointing in opposite directions and placing the pads of each finger of one hand against the pads of each finger of the other hand (or against your hand) and then curl the fingers against the resistance provided by the other hand (Fig. 19.25).

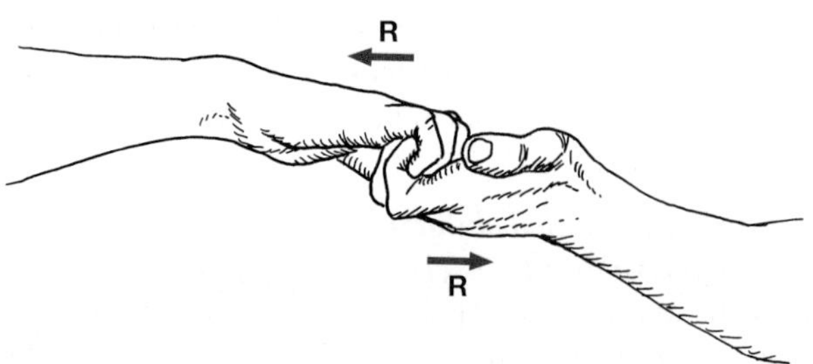

FIGURE 19.25 Self-resistance to strengthen extrinsic finger flexor muscles.

Mechanical Resistance Techniques for Combined Intrinsic and Extrinsic Muscle Function

NOTE: Proper stabilization is important; either the patient's stabilizing muscles must be strong enough or the weakened areas must be supported manually. If a weight causes stress because the patient cannot control it, the exercise is detrimental rather than beneficial.

Towel or newspaper crumple. Spread a towel out on a table. Have the patient place the palm of the hand down at one end of the towel and crumple the towel into the hand while maintaining contact with the heel of the hand. The same exercise can be carried out by placing a stack of newspapers under the hand. The patient crumples the top sheet into a ball, tosses it into a basket for coordination and skill practice, and repeats the exercise with each sheet in succession.

Disk weight resistance. Have the patient grasp a disk weight in the manner described in each of the following exercises:

- With the forearm pronated (palm down), pick up the disk with the tips of all five digits spread around the outer edge. Have the patient hold the position for isometric resistance. To increase the effect of the resistance to the flexors, have the patient extend one digit at a time.
- Pick up the side of the disk with either tip-to-tip or pad-to-pad prehension of thumb and fingers.
- With the hand palm down on a table, place the disk on the dorsum of the fingers; then lift the disk by hyperextending the fingers.

Other resistance aids. Resistive devices, such as putty, spring-loaded hand exercisers, and various grades and sizes of soft balls, can be used for specific muscles or general strengthening. Observe the pattern used by the patient and be sure he or she does not substitute or develop damaging forces.

Dexterity and Functional Activities

Fine-Finger Dexterity

Functional use of the hand for manipulating small objects or skillfully controlling delicate devices requires use of the thumb in opposition to the index and middle fingers. Have the patient perform activities such as picking up small objects of various sizes, twisting nuts on and off bolts, drawing, writing, tying a string or ribbon, opening and closing small bottles or boxes, and typing on a keyboard.

Functional Activities

Progress to specific activities needed for ADLs, work, hobbies, or recreational function. For the patient to return to independent function using the hand, he or she must not only have neuromuscular control and strength, but must also have muscular endurance, coordination, and fine finger dexterity for the desired activity. This requires careful questioning and analysis of the patient's desired outcomes. Consider each of the power grips and prehension patterns and adapt the exercises to meet the goals.

Independent Learning Activities

Critical Thinking and Discussion

1. Review all of the power grips and prehension patterns and identify the primary muscles that function when performing each action.
2. Summarize the sensory and motor impairments, deformities, and associated activity limitations and/or participation restrictions that may occur in the wrist and hand as the result of a lesion of (1) the median nerve, (2) the radial nerve, and (3) the ulnar nerve.
3. Differentiate between a boutonnière deformity and a swan-neck deformity of the fingers. What are the underlying factors that contribute to these deformities? After surgical repair of each of these deformities, how should an exercise program be designed to increase hand function but prevent recurrence of these deformities?
4. Identify key structures by the zone in the hand and wrist that could be damaged as the result of a laceration at each zone of the dorsal and volar aspects of the hand and wrist. What functional impairments occur as the result of damage in each zone?
5. Make a case for the use of early controlled motion after surgical repair of a flexor or extensor tendon injury. Explain the key features of different approaches to the use of early motion in an exercise program. Also identify circumstances in which the use of early controlled motion would be inadvisable or not possible.
6. Analyze and summarize the similarities and differences in the components and progression of exercise programs after flexor or extensor tendon repairs using early controlled mobilization versus delayed mobilization approaches.

Laboratory Practice

1. Mobilize each forearm, wrist, and finger joint with joint mobilization and passive stretching techniques (refer to Chapters 4 and 5).
2. Practice each tendon-gliding exercise and identify the purpose for each one.
3. Teach your partner strengthening exercises for each muscle or muscle group in the hand using resistance putty.
4. Identify three alternative resistance devices that can be used to strengthen each muscle and pattern of motion in the hand.
5. Observe someone tying laces on a shoe, identify the muscles functioning, and design an exercise program that could be used to develop neuromuscular control or strengthen each of the muscles.

Case Studies

1. A patient is referred to you early in the development of symptoms that stem from RA. He currently is in remission after his first serious flare of the disease and desires a home exercise program to safely improve the use of his hands. He is a sales associate who travels frequently. He keeps his records on a computer. His grip strength is reduced 50%; he has 25% loss of joint ROM and decreased joint play in the wrist, MP, and IP joints. Detectable synovial hypertrophy is minimal, and there are no joint subluxations. Consider what precautions should be followed with this disease to prevent the deforming forces of improperly applied exercises and daily forces. Establish a program of intervention for this patient.
2. A patient is referred to you 2 months after a distal radius fracture. Her hand is swollen and sensitive to touch, and she currently is developing contractures and weakness in the hand related to complex regional pain syndrome (CRPS) (see Chapter 13). Joint contractures exist in the forearm, wrist, and hand. You determine that the patient is in the second stage of the disease. Establish a plan for intervention.
3. A patient with RA who has just undergone MP implant arthroplasties of the ring and small fingers has been referred to you for an exercise program. For the past 4 weeks, the patient has been wearing a dynamic extension orthosis that allows active MP flexion and assists MP extension. The patient is now allowed to remove the orthosis for active ROM of the wrist and hand. Your examination reveals that the patient has an extensor lag and also has restricted flexion of the fingers. Design and progress an exercise program for this patient. What precautions should be incorporated into each phase of the program?
4. A patient who underwent a ligament reconstruction tendon interposition arthroplasty for posttraumatic arthritis of the CMC joint of the thumb 4 weeks ago has been referred to you. The thumb spica cast was removed at 3½ weeks postoperatively, and the patient is now wearing a thumb spica orthosis that may be removed for exercise. Develop and progress an exercise program for the patient. The patient has already returned to his or her position in an office. The patient would like to be able to resume golf on a recreational basis.
5. An 8-year-old child who sustained a zone III laceration of the volar aspect of the index and middle fingers of the nondominant hand while carving a pumpkin has been referred to you after surgical repair of the FDP and FDS tendons. The child's hand has been immobilized in a cast for 3 weeks after the repair in a position of wrist and finger flexion. The child is now wearing a dorsal blocking orthosis that may be removed for exercise. The child's active and passive extension is significantly limited. Design and progress an exercise program for this child. Identify activities that the child must do under direct supervision and those that he or she may do independently.

REFERENCES

1. Adams, BD: Complications of wrist arthroplasty. *Hand Clin* 26: 213–220, 2010.
2. Alter S, Feldon, P, and Terrono, AL: Pathomechanics of deformities in the arthritic hand and wrist. In Skirven, TM, Osterman, AL, Fedorczyk, JM, and Amadio, PC (eds): *Rehabilitation of the Hand and Upper Extremity, Vol II,* ed. 6. Philadelphia, PA: Elsevier Mosby, 2011, pp 1321–1329.
3. Amadio, PC: Advances in understanding of tendon healing and repairs and effect on postoperative management. In Skirven, TM, Osterman, AL, Fedorczyk, JM, and Amadio, PC (eds): *Rehabilitation of the Hand and Upper Extremity, Vol I,* ed. 6. Philadelphia, PA: Elsevier Mosby, 2011, pp 439–444.
4. Amadio, PC, Murray, PM, and Linscheid, RL: Arthroplasty of the proximal interphalangeal joint. In Morrey, BF (ed): *Joint Replacement Arthroplasty,* ed. 3. Philadelphia: Churchill Livingstone, 2003, pp 163–174.
5. Amadio, PC, and Shin, AY: Arthrodesis and arthroplasty of small joints of the hand. In Wolfe SW, Hotchkiss, RN, Pederson, WC, and Kozin, SH (eds): *Green's Operative Hand Surgery, Vol I,* ed. 6. Philadelphia, PA: Elsevier: Churchill Livingstone, 2011, pp 389–406.
6. Anson, JG, et al: EMG discharge patterns during human grip movement are task-dependent and not modulated by muscle contraction modes: a transcranial magnetic stimulation (TMS) study. *Brain Research* 934: 162–166, 2002.
7. Angst, F, et al: Comprehensive assessment of clinical outcome and quality of life after resection interposition arthroplasty of the thumb saddle joint. *Arthritis Rheum* 53(2):205–213, 2005.
8. Ataker, Y, Gudemez, E, Ece, SC, Canbulat, N, and Gulgonen, A: Rehabilitation protocol after suspension arthroplasty of thumb carpometacarpal joint arthritis. *J Hand Ther* 25:374–383, 2012.
9. Austin, NM: The wrist and hand complex. In Levange, PK, and Norkin, CC (eds): *Joint Structure and Function: A Comprehensive Analysis,* ed. 5. Philadelphia: F.A. Davis, 2011, pp 305–353.
10. Backstrom, KM: Mobilization with movement as an adjunct intervention in a patient with complicated de Quervain's tenosynovitis: a case report. *J Orthop Sports Phys Ther* 32(3):86–97, 2002.
11. Badia, A: Trapeziometacarpal arthroscopy: A classification and treatment algorithm. *Hand Clinics* 22: 153–163, 2006.
12. Badia, A: Management of the osteoarthritic thumb carpometacarpal joint. In Skirven, TM, Osterman, AL, Fedorczyk, JM, and Amadio, PC (eds): *Rehabilitation of the Hand and Upper Extremity, Vol II,* ed. 6. Philadelphia, PA: Elsevier Mosby, 2011, pp 1356–1366.
13. Barakat, MJ, Field, J, and Taylor, J: The range of movement of the thumb. *Hand* 8:179–182, 2013.
14. Barron, OA, and Catalano, LW: Thumb basal joint arthritis. In Wolfe SW, Hotchkiss, RN, Pederson, WC, and Kozin, SH (eds): *Green's Operative Hand Surgery, Vol I,* ed. 6. Philadelphia, PA: Elsevier: Churchill Livingstone, 2011, pp 407–426.
15. Beasley J: Therapist's examination and conservative management of arthritis of the upper extremity. In Skirven, TM, Osterman, AL, Fedorczyk, JM, and Amadio, PC (eds): *Rehabilitation of the Hand and Upper Extremity, Vol II,* ed. 6. Philadelphia, PA: Elsevier Mosby, 2011, pp 1330–1343.
16. Beasley, RW: *Surgery of the Hand.* New York: Thieme, 2003.
17. Beckenbaugh, RD: Arthroplasty of the wrist. In Morrey, BF (ed): *Joint Replacement Arthroplasty,* ed. 3. Philadelphia: Churchill Livingstone, 2003, pp 244–265.
18. Bielefeld, T, and Neumann, DA: The unstable metacarpophalangeal joint in rheumatoid arthritis: anatomy, pathomechanics, and physical rehabilitation considerations. *J Orthop Sports Phys Ther* 35(8):502–520, 2005.
19. Bielefeld, TM, and Neumann, DA: Therapist's management of the thumb carpometacarpal joint with osteoarthritis. In Skirven, TM, Osterman, AL, Fedorczyk, JM, and Amadio, PC (eds): *Rehabilitation of the Hand and Upper Extremity, Vol II,* ed. 6. Philadelphia, PA: Elsevier Mosby, 2011, pp 1366–1375.
20. Biese, J, and Goudzward, P: Postoperative management of metacarpophalangeal implant resection arthroplasty. *Orthop Phys Ther Clin North Am* 10(4):595–616, 2001.
21. Bodell, LS, and Leonard, L: Wrist arthroplasty. In Berger, RA, and Weiss, A (eds): *Hand Surgery, Vol II.* Philadelphia: Lippincott Williams & Wilkins, 2004, pp 1340–1394.
22. Bodin, ND, Spangler, R, and Thoder, JJ: Interposition arthroplasty options for carpometacarpal arthritis of the thumb. *Hand Clin* 26: 339–350, 2010.
23. Bouacida, S, Lazerges, C, Coulet, B, and Chammas, M: Proximal interphalangeal joint arthroplasty with Neuflex implants: relevance of the volar approach and early rehabilitation. *Chirurgie de la main, Elsevier Masson* 33:350–355, 2014.
24. Brigstocke, GHO, Hearnden, A, Holt, C, and Whatling, G: In-vivo confirmation of the use of the dart thrower's motion during activities of daily living. *J Hand Surg Eur* 39:373–378, 2014.
25. Brüner, S, et al: Dynamic splinting after extensor tendon repair in zones V to VII. *J Hand Surg Br* 28(3):224–227, 2003.
26. Burke, SL: Wrist arthroplasty. In Burke, SL, Higgins, JP, McClinton, MA, Saunders, RJ, and Valdata, L (eds): *Hand and Upper Extremity Rehabilitation,* ed. 3. St Louis, MO, Elsevier Churchill Livingstone, 2007, pp 522–527.
27. Burns, MC, Berby, B, and Neumeister, MW. Wyndell Merritt immediate controlled active motion (ICAM) protocol following extensor tendon repairs in zone IV-VII: review of literature, orthosis design and case study—a multimedia article. *Hand* 8:17–22, 2013.
28. Burr, N, Pratt, AL, and Smith, PJ: An alternative splinting and rehabilitation protocol for metacarpophalangeal arthroplasty in patients with rheumatoid arthritis. *J Hand Ther* 15(1):41–47, 2002.
29. Cannon, NM: *Diagnosis and Treatment Manual for Physicians and Therapists,* ed. 4. Indianapolis: Hand Rehabilitation Center of Indiana, 2001.
30. Carney, KL, and Griffin-Reed, N: Rehabilitation after extensor injury and repair. In Berger, RA, and Weiss, APC (eds): *Hand Surgery, Vol I.* Philadelphia: Lippincott Williams & Wilkins, 2004, pp 767–778.
31. Chesney, A, et al: Systematic review of flexor tendon rehabilitation protocols in zone II of the hand. *Plast Reconstr Surg* 127:1583–1592, 2011.
32. Chim HW, Reese, SK, Toomey, SN, and Moran, SL: Update on the surgical treatment for rheumatoid arthritis of the wrist and hand. *J Hand Ther* 27:134–142, 2014.
33. Chung, KC, et al: A multicenter clinical trial in rheumatoid arthritis comparing silicone metacarpophalangeal joint arthroplasty with medical treatment. *J Hand Surg Am* 34(5):815–823, 2009.
34. Chung, KC, et al: Outcomes of silicone arthroplasty for rheumatoid metacarpophalangeal joints stratified by fingers. *J Hand Surg* 34A: 1647–1652, 2009.
35. Chung, KC, and Kotsis, SV: Outcomes of hand surgery in the patient with rheumatoid arthritis. *Curr Opin Rheumatol* 22:336–341, 2010.
36. Chung, KC, and Pushman, AG: Current concepts in the management of the rheumatoid hand. *J Hand Surg* 36A:736–747, 2011.
37. Chung, KC, et al: Long-term follow up for rheumatoid arthritis patients in a multicenter outcomes study of silicone metacarpophalangeal joint arthroplasty. *Arthritis Care Res* 64:1292–1300, 2012.
38. Chung, US, Kim, JH, Seo, WS, and Lee, KH: Tendon transfer or tendon graft for ruptured finger extensor tendons in rheumatoid hands. *J Hand Surg Eur* 35E:279–282, 2010.
39. Clancy, SP, and Mass, DP: Current flexor and extensor tendon motion regimens: a summary. *Hand Clin* 29:295–309, 2013.
40. Cooney, WP III, Linscheid, RL, and Beckenbaugh, RD: Arthroplasty of the metacarpophalangeal joint. In Morrey, BF (ed): *Joint Replacement Arthroplasty,* ed. 3. Philadelphia: Churchill Livingstone, 2003, pp 175–203.
41. Cooney, WP III: Arthroplasty of the thumb axis. In Morrey, BF (ed): *Joint Replacement Arthroplasty,* ed. 3. Philadelphia: Churchill Livingstone, 2003, pp 204–225.
42. Cooney, WP, III, Leddy, TP, and Larson, DR: Revision of thumb trapeziometacarpal arthroplasty. *J Hand Surg Am* 31(2):219–227, 2006.
43. Crosby, CA, et al: Rehabilitation following thumb CMC, radiocarpal and DRUJ arthroplasty. *Hand Clin* 29:123–142, 2013.
44. Daecke, W, et al: A prospective, randomized comparison of 3 types of proximal interphalangeal joint arthroplasty. *J Hand Surg* 37A: 1770–1779, 2012.

45. Davenport, TE, et al: The EdUReP model for nonsurgical management of tendinopathy. *Phys Ther* 85(10):1093–1103, 2005.
46. Delaney, R, and Stanley, J: A postoperative study of the range of movement following metacarpophalangeal joint replacement: optimum time of recovery. *Br J Hand Ther* 5(3):85–87, 2000.
47. Delaney, R, Trail, IA, and Nutall, D: A comparative study of outcome between the Neuflex and Swanson Silastic metacarpophalangeal joint replacements. *J Hand Surg Br* 30(1):3–7, 2005.
48. Diao, E, and Chee, N: Staged/delayed tendon reconstruction. In Skirven, TM, Osterman, AL, Fedorczyk, JM, and Amadio, PC (eds): *Rehabilitation of the Hand and Upper Extremity, Vol I,* ed. 6. Philadelphia, PA: Elsevier Mosby, 2011, pp 479–486.
49. Drake, ML, and Segalman, KA: Complications of small joint arthroplasty. *Hand Clin* 26:205–212, 2010.
50. Duran, RJ, and Houser, RC: Controlled passive motion following flexor tendon repair in zones II and III. In AAOS (ed): *Symposium on Tendon Surgery in the Hand.* St. Louis: CV Mosby, 1975.
51. Dy, CJ, et al: Complications after flexor tendon repair: A systematic review and meta-analysis. *J Hand Surg* 37A:543–551, 2012.
52. Dy, CJ, Rosenblatt, L, and Lee, SK: Current methods and biomechanics of extensor tendon repairs. *Hand Clin* 29, 261–268, 2013.
53. Edirisinghe, Y, et al: dynamic motion analysis of dart throwers motion visualized through computerized tomography and calculation of the axis of rotation. *J Hand Surg Eur* 39:364–372, 2014.
54. Elhassan, B, et al: Factors that influence the outcome of zone I and zone II flexor tendon repairs in children. *J Hand Surg Am* 31:1661–1666, 2006.
55. Evans, RB: Early active motion after flexor tendon repairs. In Berger, RA, and Weiss, APC (eds): *Hand Surgery, Vol I.* Philadelphia: Lippincott Williams & Wilkins, 2004, pp 709–735.
56. Evans, RB: Clinical management of extensor tendon injuries: the therapist's perspective. In Skirven, TM, Osterman, AL, Fedorczyk, JM, and Amadio, PC (eds): *Rehabilitation of the Hand and Upper Extremity, Vol I,* ed. 6. Philadelphia, PA: Elsevier Mosby, 2011, pp 521–554.
57. Evans, RB: Managing the injured tendon: Current concepts. *J Hand Ther* 25:173–190, 2012.
58. Fedorczyk, JM: Tendinopathies of the elbow, wrist and hand: Histopathology and clinical considerations. *J Hand Ther* 25:191–201, 2012.
59. Feldon, P, Terrono, AL, Nalebuff, EA, and Millender, LH: Rheumatoid arthritis and other connective tissue disorders. In Wolfe SW, Hotchkiss, RN, Pederson, WC, and Kozin, SH (eds): *Green's Operative Hand Surgery, Vol II,* ed. 6. Philadelphia, PA: Elsevier: Churchill Livingstone, 2011, pp 1993–2065.
60. Feldscher, SB: Postoperative management for PIP joint pyrocarbon arthroplasty. *J Hand Ther* 23(3):315–322, 2010.
61. Ferlic, DC: Repair of ruptured finger extensors in rheumatoid arthritis. In Strickland, JW, and Graham, TJ (eds): *The Hand,* ed. 2. Philadelphia: Lippincott Williams & Wilkins, 2005, pp 457–462.
62. Ferreres, A, Lluch, A, and del Valle, M: Universal total wrist arthroplasty: midterm follow-up study. *J Hand Surg Am* 36:967–973, 2011.
63. Gaspar, MP, Kane, PM, and Shin, EK: Management of complications of wrist arthroplasty and wrist fusion. *Hand Clinics* 31:277–292, 2015.
64. Green, JB, et al: Hand, wrist and digit injuries. In Magee, DJ, Zachazewski, JE, and Quillen, WS (eds): Pathology and intervention in musculoskeletal rehabilitation. St Louis, MO:Saunders Elsevier 2009, pp 213–305.
65. Griffin, M, et al: An overview of the management of flexor tendon injuries. *The Open Orthop J* 6:28–35, 2012.
66. Groth, GN: Pyramid of progressive force exercises to the injured flexor-tendon. *J Hand Ther* 17(1):31–42, 2004.
67. Howell, JW, Merritt, WH, and Robinson, SJ: Immediate controlled active motion following zone 4-7 extensor tendon repair. *J Hand Ther* 18: 182–190, 2005.
68. Howell, JW, and Peck, F: Rehabilitation of flexor and extensor tendon injuries in the hand: Current updates. *Injury, Int J Care Injured* 44: 397–402, 2013.
69. Huang, K, Hollevoet, N, and Giddins, G: Thumb carpometacarpal joint total arthroplasty: a systematic review. *J Hand Surg Eur* 40E: 338–350, 2015.
70. Igoe, D, Middleton, C, and Hammert W: Evolution of basal joint arthroplasty and technology in hand surgery. *J Hand Ther* 27:115–121, 2014.
71. Jacobs, BJ, Verbruggen, G, and Kaufmann, RA: Proximal interphalangeal joint arthritis. *J Hand Surg Am* 35A:2107–2116, 2010.
72. Jacobs, MA, and Austin, NM: *Orthotic Intervention for the Hand and Upper Extremity: Splinting Principles and Process,* ed. 2. Baltimore, MD: Lippincott Williams & Wilkins, 2014, pp 26–46.
73. Jennings, CD, and Livingstone, DP: Surface replacement arthroplasty of the proximal interphalangeal joint using the SR PIP implant: long-term results. *J Hand Surg Am* 40 (3):469–473, 2015.
74. Kitis, A, et al: Comparison of static and dynamic splinting regimens for extensor tendon repairs in zones V to VII. *J Plast Surg Hand Surg* 46:267–271, 2012.
75. Kleinert, HE, Kutz, JE, and Cohen, MJ: Primary repair of zone 2 flexor tendon lacerations. In AAOS (ed): *Symposium on Tendon Surgery in the Hand.* St. Louis: CV Mosby, 1975, 91–104.
76. Kozlow, JH, and Chung, KC: Current concepts in the surgical management of rheumatoid and osteoarthritic hands and wrists. *Hand Clinics* 27:31–41, 2011.
77. Kriegs-AU, G, et al: Ligament reconstruction with or without tendon interposition to treat primary thumb carpometacarpal osteoarthritis: a prospective randomized study. *J Bone Joint Surg Am* 86(2):209–218, 2004.
78. Lee, MP, Biafora, SJ, and Zelouf, DS: Management of hand and wrist tendinopathies. In Skirven, TM, Osterman, AL, Fedorczyk, JM, and Amadio, PC (eds): *Rehabilitation of the Hand and Upper Extremity, Vol I,* ed. 6. Philadelphia, PA: Elsevier Mosby, 2011, pp 569–588.
79. Lister, GD, et al: Primary flexor tendon repair followed by immediate controlled mobilization. *J Hand Surg* 2(6):441–451, 1977.
80. Lubahn J, Wolfe, TL, and Feldscher, SB: Joint replacement in the hand and wrist: surgery and therapy. In Skirven, TM, Osterman, AL, Fedorczyk, JM, and Amadio, PC (eds): *Rehabilitation of the Hand and Upper Extremity, Vol II,* ed. 6. Philadelphia, PA: Elsevier Mosby, 2011, pp 1376–1398.
81. Lubahn J, and Wolfe, TL: Surgical treatment and rehabilitation of tendon ruptures and imbalances in the rheumatoid hand. In Skirven, TM, Osterman, AL, Fedorczyk, JM, and Amadio, PC (eds): *Rehabilitation of the Hand and Upper Extremity, Vol I,* ed. 6. Philadelphia, PA: Elsevier Mosby, 2011, pp 1399–1407.
82. Lutsky, KF, Giang, EL, and Matzon, JL: Flexor tendon injury, repair and rehabilitation. *Orthop Clin N Am* 46:67–76, 2015.
83. Lutz, K, Pipicelli, J, and Grewal, R. Complications of extensor tendon injuries. *Hand Clin* 31:301–310, 2015.
84. MacDermid, J (ed): *Clinical Assessment Recommendations: Impairment-Based Conditions,* ed. 3. Mt. Laurel, NJ: American Society of Hand Therapists, 2015.
85. Magee, DJ: *Orthopedic Physical Assessment,* ed. 5. St Louis, MO: Saunders, Elsevier, 2008.
86. Magee, DJ, Zachazewski, JE, and Quillen, WS: *Pathology and Intervention in Musculoskeletal Rehabilitation.* St Louis, MO: Saunders, Elsevier, 2009.
87. Malahias, M, et al: The future of rheumatoid arthritis and hand surgery – combining evolutionary pharmacology and surgical technique. *The Open Orthop J* 6:88–94, 2012.
88. Manuel, JL, and Weiss, AC: Silicone metacarpal phalangeal joint arthroplasty. In Strickland, JW, and Graham, TJ (eds): *Master Techniques in Orthopedic Surgery: The Hand,* ed. 2. Philadelphia, Lippincott Williams and Wilkins, 2005, pp 391–403.
89. Martin, AS, and Awan, HM: Metacarpophalangeal arthroplasty for osteoarthritis. *J Hand Surg Am* 40:1871–1872, 2015.
90. Mass, DP: Early repairs of flexor tendon injuries. In Berger, RA, and Weiss, APC (eds): *Hand Surgery, Vol 1.* Philadelphia: Lippincott Williams & Wilkins, 2004, pp 679–698.
91. Matzon, JL, and Bozentka, DJ: Extensor tendon injuries. *J Hand Surg* 35A:854–861, 2010.
92. McClure, P: Upper quarter screen. In Skirven, TM, Osterman, AL, Fedorczyk, JM, and Amadio, PC (eds): *Rehabilitation of the Hand and Upper Extremity, Vol I,* ed. 6. Philadelphia, PA: Elsevier Mosby, 2011, pp 124–131.

93. Merritt, WH: Relative motion splint: active motion after extensor tendon injury and repair. *J Hand Surg Am* 39:1187–1194, 2014.
94. Moehrlen, U, Mazzone, L, Bieli, C, and Weber, DM: Early mobilization after flexor tendon repair in children. *Eur, J Pediatr Surg* 19:83–86, 2009.
95. Moment, A, Grauel, E, and Chang, J: Complications after flexor tendon injuries. *Hand Clin* 26:179–189, 2009.
96. Moojen, TM, et al: Three-dimensional carpal kinematics in vivo. *Clin Biomech* 17:506–514, 2002.
97. Moojen, TM, et al: In vivo analysis of carpal kinematics and comparative review of the literature. *J Hand Surg* 28:81–872, 2003.
98. Moore, T, Anderson, B, and Seiler II, JG: Flexor tendon reconstruction. *J Hand Surg* 35(6):1025–1030, 2010.
99. Mulligan, BR: *Manual Therapy "NAGS," "SNAGS," MWM, etc.*, ed. 6. Wellington: Plane View Press, 2010.
100. Nallakaruppan, V, et al: The effect of blocking radial abduction on palmar abduction strength of the thumb. *J Hand Surg Eur* 37E: 269–274, 2011.
101. Netscher, DT, and Badal, JJ: Closed flexor tendon ruptures. *J Hand Surg Am* 39 (11):2315–2323, 2014.
102. Neumann, DA: Wrist. In Neumann, DA (ed): *Kinesiology of the Musculoskeletal System: Foundations for Rehabilitation,* ed. 2. St Louis: Mosby/Elsevier, 2010, pp 216–243.
103. Neumann, DA: Hand. In Neumann, DA (ed): *Kinesiology of the Musculoskeletal System: Foundations for Rehabilitation,* ed. 2. St Louis: Mosby/Elsevier, 2010, pp 244–297.
104. Neumann, DA, and Bielefeld, T: The carpometacarpal joint of the thumb: stability, deformity, and therapeutic intervention. *J Orthop Sports Phys Ther* 33(7):386–399, 2003.
105. Newport, ML: Early repair of extensor tendon injuries. In Berger, RA, and Weiss, APC (eds): *Hand Surgery, Vol I.* Philadelphia: Lippincott Williams & Wilkins, 2004, pp 737–752.
106. Nietosvaara, Y, et al: Flexor tendon injuries in pediatric patients. *J Hand Surg Am* 32:1549–1557, 2007.
107. Ogunro, S, Ahmed, I, and Tan, V: Current indications and outcomes of total wrist arthroplasty. *Orthop Clin N Am* 44:371–379, 2013.
108. Ottawa Panel: Ottawa Panel evidence-based clinical practice guidelines for patient education in the management of rheumatoid arthritis. *Health Ed J* 71:397–451, 2012.
109. Ottawa Panel: Ottawa Panel evidence-based clinical practice guidelines for therapeutic exercises in the management of rheumatoid arthritis in adults. *Phys Ther* 84(10):934–972, 2004.
110. Park, MJ, Lee, AT, and Yao, J: Treatment of thumb carpometacarpal arthritis with arthroscopic hemitrapeziectomy and interposition arthroplasty. *Orthop* 35(12):1759–1763, 2012.
111. Park, Y, and Chang, M: Effects of rehabilitation for pain relief in patients with rheumatoid arthritis: a systematic review. *J Phys Ther Sci* 28: 304–308, 2016.
112. Pettengill, K, and Van Strien, G: Postoperative management of flexor tendon injuries. In Skirven, TM, Osterman, AL, Fedorczyk, JM, and Amadio, PC (eds): *Rehabilitation of the Hand and Upper Extremity, Vol I,* ed. 6. Philadelphia, PA: Elsevier Mosby, 2011, pp 457–478.
113. Quadlbauer, S, et al: Early passive movement in flexor tendon injuries of the hand. *Arch Orthop Trauma Surg* 136:285–293, 2016.
114. Rayan, G, and Akelman, E (eds): *The Hand: Anatomy, Examination and Diagnosis,* ed. 4. Lippincott Williams & Wilkins, Philadelphia, PA: American Society for Surgery of the Hand, 2011.
115. Rettig, LA, Luca, L, and Murphy, MS: Silicone implant arthroplasty in patients with idiopathic osteoarthritis of the metacarpophalangeal joint. *J Hand Surg Am* 30:667–672, 2005.
116. Riggs, JM, Lyden, AK, Chung, KC, and Murphy, SL: Static versus dynamic splinting for proximal interphalangeal joint pyrocarbon implant arthroplasty: a comparison of current and historical cohorts. *J Hand Ther* 24:231–239, 2011.
117. Riley, G: Tendinopathy—from basic science to treatment. *Nat Clin Pract Rheumatol* 4(2):82–89, 2008.
118. Rizzo, M, and Beckenbaugh, RD: Results of biaxial total wrist arthroplasty with a modified (long) metacarpal stem. *J Hand Surg Am* 28: 577–584, 2003.
119. Rosenthal, EA, and Elhassan, BT: The extensor tendons: evaluation and surgical management. In Skirven, TM, Osterman, AL, Fedorczyk, JM, and Amadio, PC (eds): *Rehabilitation of the Hand and Upper Extremity, Vol I,* ed. 6. Philadelphia, PA: Elsevier Mosby, 2011, pp 487–520.
120. Sameem, M, et al: A systematic review of rehabilitation protocols after surgical repair of the extensor tendons in zones V-VIII of the hand. *J Hand Ther* 24:365–373, 2011.
121. Samora, JB, and Klinefelter, RD: Flexor tendon reconstruction. *J Am Acad Orthop Surg* 24:28–36, 2016.
122. Sandvall, BK, Kuhlman-Wood K, Recor, C, and Friedrich, JB: Flexor tendon repair, rehabilitation and reconstruction. *Plast Reconstr Surg* 132:1493–1503, 2013.
123. Satteson, ES, Langford, MA, and Li, Z: The management of complications of small joint arthrodesis and arthroplasty. *Hand Clin* 31: 243–266, 2015.
124. Schindele, S, Kloss, D, and Herren, D: Options in extensor tendon reconstruction in rheumatoid arthritis. *Elsevier, International Congress Series* 1295:94–106, 2006.
125. Schindele, SF, Herren, DB, and Simmen, BR: Tendon reconstruction for the rheumatoid hand. *Hand Clin* 27:105–116, 2011.
126. Schubert, CD, and Guinta, RE: Extensor tendon repair and reconstruction. *Clin Plastic Surg* 41:525–531, 2014.
127. Seiler, JG: Flexor tendon injury. In Wolfe SW, Hotchkiss, RN, Pederson, WC, and Kozin, SH (eds): *Green's Operative Hand Surgery, Vol I,* ed. 6. Philadelphia, PA: Elsevier: Churchill Livingstone, 2011, pp 189–238.
128. Shin, AY, and Amadio, PC: The stiff finger. In Wolfe, SW, Hotchkiss, RN, Pederson, WC, and Kozin, SH (eds): *Green's Operative Hand Surgery, Vol I,* ed. 6. Philadelphia, PA: Elsevier: Churchill Livingstone, 2011, pp 355–406.
129. Singh, R, Rymer, B, Theobald, P, and Thomas, PBM: A review of current concepts in flexor tendon repair: physiology biomechanics, surgical technique and rehabilitation. *Orthop Reviews* 7:101–105, 2015.
130. Stanley, J: Arthoplasty and arthrodesis of the wrist. In Wolfe SW, Hotchkiss, RN, Pederson, WC, and Kozin, SH (eds): *Green's Operative Hand Surgery, Vol I,* ed. 6. Philadelphia, PA: Elsevier: Churchill Livingstone, 2011, pp 429–463.
131. Starr, HM, Snoddy, M, Hammond, KE, and Seiler, JG: Flexor tendon repair rehabilitation protocols: a systematic review. *J Hand Surg* 38A: 1712–1717, 2013.
132. Steinberg, DR: Osteoarthritis of the hand and digits: metacarpophalangeal and carpometacarpal joints. In Berger, RA, and Weiss, APC (eds): *Hand Surgery, Vol II.* Philadelphia: Lippincott Williams & Wilkins, 2004, pp 1269–1278.
133. Straugh RJ: Extensor tendon injury. In Wolfe SW, Hotchkiss, RN, Pederson, WC, and Kozin, SH (eds): *Green's Operative Hand Surgery, Vol I,* ed. 6. Philadelphia, PA: Elsevier: Churchill Livingstone, 2011, pp 159–188.
134. Strickland, JW: Flexor tendon injuries. In Strickland, JW, and Graham, TJ (eds): *Master Techniques in Orthopedic Surgery: The Hand,* ed. 2. Philadelphia: Lippincott Williams & Wilkins, 2005, pp 251–266.
135. Strickland, JW, and Dellacqua, D: Rheumatoid arthritis in the hand and digits. In Berger, RA, and Weiss, APC (eds): *Hand Surgery, Vol II.* Philadelphia: Lippincott Williams & Wilkins, 2004, pp 1179–211.
136. Sweets, TM, and Stern, PJ: Proximal interphalangeal joint arthroplasty. *J Hand Surg Am* 35:1190–1193, 2010.
137. Taras JS, Martyak, GG, and Steelman, PJ: Primary care of flexor tendon injuries. In Skirven, TM, Osterman, AL, Fedorczyk, JM, and Amadio, PC (eds): *Rehabilitation of the Hand and Upper Extremity, Vol I,* ed. 6. Philadelphia, PA: Elsevier Mosby, 2011, pp 445–456.
138. Terrono, AL, Nalebuff, EA, and Philips, CA: The rheumatoid thumb. In Skirven, TM, Osterman, AL, Fedorczyk, JM, and Amadio, PC (eds): *Rehabilitation of the Hand and Upper Extremity, Vol I,* ed. 6. Philadelphia, PA: Elsevier Mosby, 2011, pp 1344–1355.
139. Trieb K: Treatment of the wrist in rheumatoid arthritis. *J Hand Surg* 33A:113–123, 2008.
140. Trumble, TE, et al: Zone-II flexor tendon repair: a randomized prospective trial of active place-and-hold therapy compared with passive motion therapy. *J Bone Joint Surg Am* 92:1381–1389, 2010.

141. von der Heyde, R: Flexor tendon injuries in children: rehabilitative options and confounding factors. *J Hand Ther* 28:195–200, 2015.
142. van Rijn, J, and Gosens, T: A cemented surface replacement prosthesis in the basal thumb joint. *J Hand Sur* 35(4):572–579, 2010.
143. Vermeulen, GM, et al: Surgical management of primary thumb carpometacarpal osteoarthritis: a systematic review. *J Hand Surg* 36A: 157–169, 2011.
144. Vitale, MA, Taylor, F, Ross, M, and Moran, SL: Trapezium prosthetic arthroplasty (silicone, Artelon, metal and pyrocarbon). *Hand Clin* 29:37–55, 2013.
145. Vitale, MA, et al: Prosthetic arthroplasty versus arthrodesis for osteoarthritis and posttraumatic arthritis of the index finger proximal interphalangeal joint. *J Hand Surg Am* 40(10):1937–1948, 2015.
146. Wagner, ER, Weston, J, Houdek, MT, Moran, SL, and Rizzo, M: Pyrocarbon in metacarpophalangeal arthroplasty: a longitudinal analysis of 253 cases: level 4 evidence. *J Hand Surg Am* 40:e54, 2015.
147. Weiss, S, and Falkenstein, N: *Hand Rehabilitation: A Quick Reference Guide and Review,* ed. 2. St Louis: Mosby, 2004.
148. Wijk, I, et al: Outcomes of proximal interphalangeal joint pyrocarbon implant. *J Hand Surg* 35(1):A38–A43, 2010.
149. Wolfe, SW: Tendinopathy. In Wolfe SW, Hotchkiss, RN, Pederson, WC, and Kozin, SH (eds): *Green's Operative Hand Surgery, Vol II,* ed. 6. Philadelphia, PA: Elsevier: Churchill Livingstone, 2011, pp 2067–2088.
150. Wong, JKF, and Peck, F: Improving results of flexor tendon repair and rehabilitation: *Plast Reconstr Surg* 134:913e–925e, 2014.
151. Yen, CH, Chan, WL, Wong, WC, and Mak, KH: Clinical results of early active mobilization after flexor tendon repair. *Hand Surg* 13: 45–50, 2008.
152. Yeoh, D, and Tourret, L: Total wrist arthroplasty: a systematic review of the evidence from the last 5 years. *J Hand Surg* 40E:458–468, 2015.
153. Yuste, V, et al: Influence of patient and injury-related factors in the outcomes of primary flexor tendon repair. *Eur J Plast Surg* 38:49–54, 2015.

CHAPTER

20

The Hip

CAROLYN KISNER, PT, MS ■ LYNN COLBY, PT, MS ■ JOHN BORSTAD, PT, PHD

The hip is similar to the glenohumeral joint in that it is a triaxial joint, functions in all three planes, and is the proximal link to its extremity. In contrast to the highly mobile shoulder, however, the hip is a stable joint that is adapted for upright standing and weight bearing activities. At the same time, at least 120° of hip flexion and 20° each of abduction and external rotation are necessary to carry out activities of daily living (ADLs) in what is considered a "normal" manner.[120] Because forces from the lower extremities are transmitted upward through the hips to the pelvis and trunk during gait and other lower extremity activities, and because the hips support the weight of the head, trunk, and upper extremities, the health of the hip joint is vital for most functional activities.

This chapter is divided into three major sections. The first section briefly reviews the anatomy and function of the hip and its relation to the pelvis, lumbar spine, and knee. The second section describes common disorders of the hip and provides guidelines for conservative and postoperative management, expanding on the information and principles of management presented in Chapters 10 through 13. The reader should be familiar with that material as well as the components of a comprehensive examination of the hip and pelvis before determining a diagnosis and establishing a therapeutic exercise program. The third section describes exercise interventions commonly used to meet the treatment goals for the hip region.

Structure and Function of the Hip

The pelvic girdle links the lower extremity to the trunk and plays a significant role in the function of the hip as well as the spinal joints. The proximal femur and the pelvis comprise the hip joint (Fig. 20.1). The unique characteristics of the pelvis and femur that affect hip function are reviewed in this section. The function of the pelvis with respect to spinal mechanics is described in greater detail in Chapter 14.

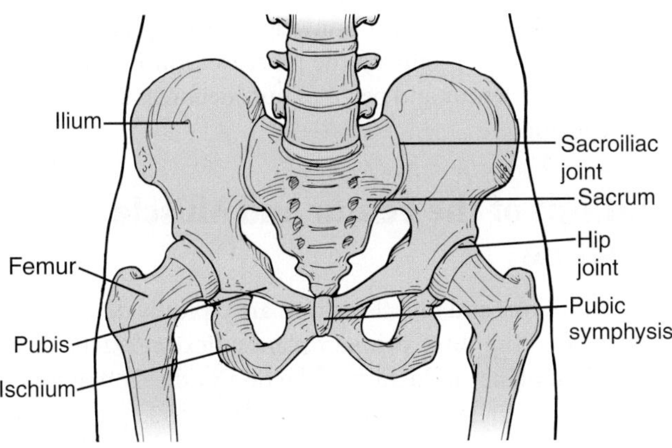

FIGURE 20.1 Bones and joints of the pelvis and hip.

Anatomical Characteristics of the Hip Region

Bony Structures

The structure of the pelvis and femur are designed for weight bearing and transmitting proximally and distally generated forces through the hip joint.

The Pelvis

Each innominate bone of the pelvis is formed by the union of the ilium, ischium, and pubic bones and therefore is a structural unit. The right and left innominate bones articulate anteriorly with each other at the pubic symphysis and posteriorly with the sacrum at the two sacroiliac joints.[93] Slight motion occurs at these three joints to help attenuate forces transmitted through the pelvic region, but the pelvis basically functions as a unit in a closed chain.

The Femur

The shape of the femur is designed to manage the effect of gravity on the head, arms, and trunk and to transmit ground reaction forces to the acetabulum of the pelvis. In the frontal plane, the angle of inclination (normally 125°) between the axis of the femoral neck and the shaft of the femur allows a bending moment to attenuate these forces, and there is a slight anterior bowing of the shaft in the sagittal plane that also helps absorb and transmit force.[93] Similar to the humerus, there is an angle of torsion of the femur formed by the transverse axis of the femoral condyles and the axis of the neck of the femur. This angle ranges from 8° to 25°, with an average angle of 12°.

Hip Joint Characteristics and Arthrokinematics

Characteristics

The hip is a ball-and-socket (spheroidal) triaxial joint made up of the head of the femur and acetabulum of the pelvis. It is supported by a strong articular capsule that is reinforced by the iliofemoral, pubofemoral, and ischiofemoral ligaments. The two hip joints are linked to each other through the bony pelvis, which is integrated with the vertebral column through the sacroiliac and lumbosacral joints.[93]

Articular Surfaces

The concave bony surface of the hip joint, the acetabulum, is located in the lateral aspect of the pelvis and is oriented laterally, anteriorly, and inferiorly (see Fig. 20.1). The concavity is deepened by a ring of fibrocartilage, the acetabular labrum. The articular cartilage of the acetabulum is horseshoe shaped and thicker in the lateral region, where the major weight-bearing forces are transmitted. The central portion of the acetabular surface is nonarticular.

The convex bony surface is the spherical head of the femur, which is attached to the femoral neck. The neck and head of the femur project anteriorly, medially, and superiorly.

Ligaments

Three ligaments reinforce the joint capsule: the iliofemoral and pubofemoral ligaments are located anteriorly (Fig. 20.2 A), and the ischiofemoral ligament is located posteriorly (Fig. 20.2 B).[93,117,121]

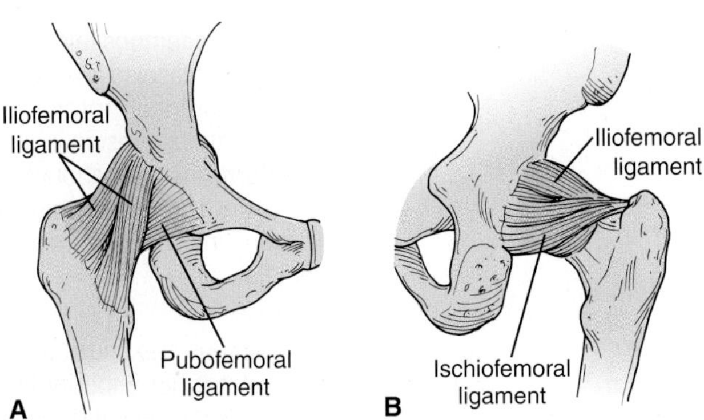

FIGURE 20.2 Ligaments supporting the hip joint. **(A)** Anterior view. **(B)** Posterior view.

There is general agreement in the literature that all three capsular ligaments limit excessive extension of the hip, and the iliofemoral ligament, also known as the Y ligament of Bigelow, is the strongest of the three.[64,93,117,121] In addition to their ability to limit extension, additional motions are limited by each individual ligament. The iliofemoral ligament, which reinforces the anterior portion of the capsule, is also thought to limit external rotation of the hip.[117,121] The pubofemoral ligament, which supports the inferior as well as anterior portion of the capsule, is believed to limit abduction.[117,121] Lastly, the ischiofemoral ligament, reinforcing the posterior aspect of the capsule, may also limit internal rotation and may limit adduction when the hip is flexed.[64,117,121]

Arthrokinematics of the Hip Joint

During many activities, such as squatting, walking, or doing leg-press exercises, both the pelvis and femurs are moving. Therefore, joint mechanics can be described by the movement of the femur in the acetabulum or by the pelvis on the femur.

Motions of the femur. The convex femoral head slides in the direction opposite the physiological motion of the femur. Thus, with hip flexion and internal rotation, the articulating surface slides posteriorly; with extension and external rotation, it slides anteriorly; with abduction, it slides inferiorly; and with adduction, it slides superiorly.The arthrokinematics are summarized in ONLINE Box 20.1 available on the FA Davis website.

Motions of the pelvis. When the lower extremity is stabilized distally, as when standing or during the stance phase of gait, the concave acetabulum moves on the convex femoral head in the same direction as the pelvic motion. The pelvis is a link in a closed chain; therefore, when the pelvis moves, there is motion at both hip joints as well as at the lumbar spine.

Influence of the Hip Joint on Balance and Posture Control

The joint capsule is richly supplied with mechanoreceptors that respond to variations in position, stress, and movement to control posture, balance, and movement. Reflex muscle contractions of the entire kinematic chain, known as balance strategies, occur in a predictable sequence when standing balance is disturbed and regained. Joint pathologies, restricted motion, or muscle weakness can impair balance and postural control. Refer to Chapter 8 for an in-depth discussion of these concepts.

Functional Relationships in the Hip Region

The hip functions in both nonweight-bearing and weight-bearing activities, requiring the muscles to move the femur or control the femur and pelvis as outside forces are imposed on the region.

Motions of the Femur and Muscle Function

Femur motions and muscle actions are typically described as occurring in the three primary planes: flexion/extension in the sagittal plane, abduction/adduction in the frontal plane, and internal/external rotation in the transverse plane. Most of the muscles at the hip can produce motion in several planes. The primary and secondary actions of the hip muscles are summarized in Table 20.1.[63,93,118]

TABLE 20.1 Muscles of the Hip: Open-Chain (Nonweight-Bearing) Function

Action	Prime Movers	Secondary Movers (action depends on hip joint position)
Flexion		
	▪ Iliopsoas ▪ Rectus femoris (also extends knee) ▪ Tensor fasciae latae (also abducts and internally rotates hip and maintains tension in iliotibial band) ▪ Sartorius (also abducts and externally rotates hip and flexes and internally rotates knee)	Pectineus Adductor longus Adductor magnus Gracilis
Extension		
	▪ Gluteus maximus (also externally rotates hip; superior fibers insert into iliotibial band) ▪ Hamstrings: long head of biceps femoris, semitendinosus, semimembranosus (also flex knee)	Gluteus medius (posterior fibers) Adductor magnus Piriformis

TABLE 20.1 Muscles of the Hip: Open-Chain (Nonweight-Bearing) Function—cont'd

Action	Prime Movers	Secondary Movers (action depends on hip joint position)
Abduction		
	■ Gluteus medius ■ Gluteus minimus ■ Tensor fasciae latae (also flexes hip)	Piriformis Sartorius Rectus femoris
Adduction		
	■ Adductor magnus ■ Adductor longus ■ Adductor brevis ■ Gracilis ■ Pectineus	Biceps femoris (long head) Gluteus maximus (posterior fibers) Quadratus femoris Obturator externus
External (Lateral) Rotation		
	■ Obturator internus and externus ■ Gemellus superior and inferior ■ Quadratus femoris ■ Piriformis ■ Gluteus maximus	Gluteus medius (posterior fibers) Gluteus minimus (posterior fibers) Sartorius Biceps femoris (long head)
Internal (Medial) Rotation		
	No prime movers	Gluteus medius (anterior fibers) Gluteus minimus (anterior fibers) Tensor fasciae latae Adductor longus and brevis Adductor magnus (posterior fibers) Pectineus

Note: Prime motions are described from the anatomic position; actions of some muscles change as the hip position changes.

Motions of the Pelvis and Muscle Function

The pelvis is the connecting link between the spine and lower extremities (Fig. 20.3A). A consequence of pelvis movement, therefore, is motion at the hip joints and lumbar spine articulations. Another consequence of this linked system is that contraction of the hip musculature will cause pelvic motion through reverse action. In this case, if pelvic movement is not desired during femur motion at the hip joint, the pelvis must be stabilized using the trunk musculature.

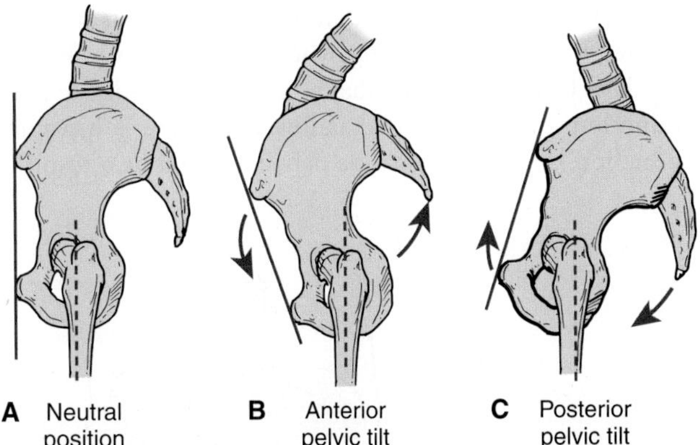

FIGURE 20.3 (A) Neutral position of the pelvis. **(B)** Anterior pelvic tilt. **(C)** Posterior pelvic tilt. With anterior pelvic tilt, the decreased angle between the pelvis and femur results in hip flexion, and with posterior pelvic tilt, the increased angle results in hip extension.

Anterior Pelvic Tilt

The anterior superior iliac spines of the pelvis move anteriorly and inferiorly and thus closer to the anterior aspect of the femur as the pelvis rotates forward around the transverse axis of the hip joints (Fig. 20.3 B). This pelvic motion results in hip flexion and increased lumbar spine extension.[93]

- Muscles causing this motion are the hip flexors and back extensors.
- If hip flexion through femur movement is the desired motion, the pelvis must be stabilized by the abdominals to prevent anterior pelvic tilting.
- During standing, if the line of gravity of the trunk shifts anterior to the axis of the hip joints, the effect is an anterior pelvic tilt moment. Stability is provided by the abdominal muscles and hip extensor muscles.

Posterior Pelvic Tilt

The posterior superior iliac spines of the pelvis move posteriorly and inferiorly, thus closer to the posterior aspect of the femur as the pelvis rotates backward around the axis of the hip joints (Fig. 20.3 C). This results in hip extension and lumbar spine flexion.[93]

- Muscles causing this motion are the hip extensors and trunk flexors (abdominals).
- If hip extension through femur movement is the desired motion, the lumbar extensors contract to stabilize the pelvis.
- During standing the line of gravity of the trunk normally falls posterior to the axis of the hip joints, creating a posterior pelvic tilt moment. Dynamic stability is provided by the hip flexors and back extensors and passive stability by the iliofemoral ligament.

Pelvic Shifting

During standing, a forward translatory shift of the pelvis results in extension of the hip and extension of the lower lumbar spinal segments. There is a compensatory posterior shifting of the thorax on the upper lumbar spine with increased flexion of these spinal segments. This is often seen with slouched or relaxed postures (see Fig. 14.18 B in Chapter 14). Little muscle action is required; the posture is maintained by the iliofemoral ligament at the hip, anterior longitudinal ligament of the lower lumbar spine, and posterior ligaments of the upper lumbar and thoracic spine.

Lateral Pelvic Tilt

Frontal plane pelvic motion results in opposite motions at each hip joint. Pelvic motion is defined by what is occurring to the iliac crest that is opposite the weight-bearing extremity (that is, the side of the pelvis that is moving). When one crest elevates, it is called hip hiking; when it lowers, it is called hip or pelvic drop. On the side that is elevated, there is hip joint adduction; on the side that is lowered, there is hip joint abduction (Fig. 20.4 A). These pelvic motions also result in lumbar spine motion, with lateral flexion occurring toward the elevated crest (convexity of the lateral curve is toward the lowered side).[93]

- Muscles causing lateral pelvic tilting include the quadratus lumborum on the side of the elevated crest and reverse muscle pull of the gluteus medius on the stance side hip.
- When hip abduction through femur movement is the desired motion, the pelvis must be stabilized by the lateral abdominals (internal and external obliques) on the side of the moving femur. When standing, the stance side gluteus medius prevents the pelvis from tilting downward.
- With an asymmetrical slouched posture, the person shifts the trunk weight onto one lower extremity and allows the pelvis to drop on the other side. Passive support comes from the iliofemoral ligament and iliotibial band on the stance leg side.
- When standing on one leg, gravity creates an adduction moment at the hip, tending to cause the pelvis to drop on the unsupported side (hip or pelvic drop). This is prevented by the gluteus medius stabilizing the pelvis on the stance side.

Pelvic Rotation

Pelvic rotation occurs around one lower extremity that is fixed on the ground. The unsupported lower extremity swings forward or backward along with the pelvis. When the unsupported side of the pelvis moves forward, it is called forward rotation of the pelvis.[93] The trunk concurrently rotates in the opposite direction, and the hip joint on the stabilized side rotates internally. When the unsupported side of the pelvis moves backward, it is called posterior rotation; the hip joint on the stabilized side concurrently rotates externally, and the trunk rotates opposite (Fig. 20.4 B).

- Muscles causing pelvic rotation are the hip rotators working in synergy with the oblique abdominal muscles, the transversus abdominis, and the multifidus.
- When hip rotation through femur movement is the desired motion, the pelvis must be stabilized by the trunk musculature.

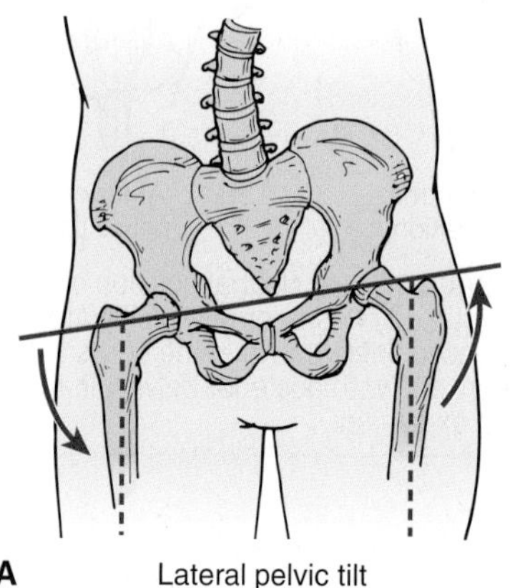

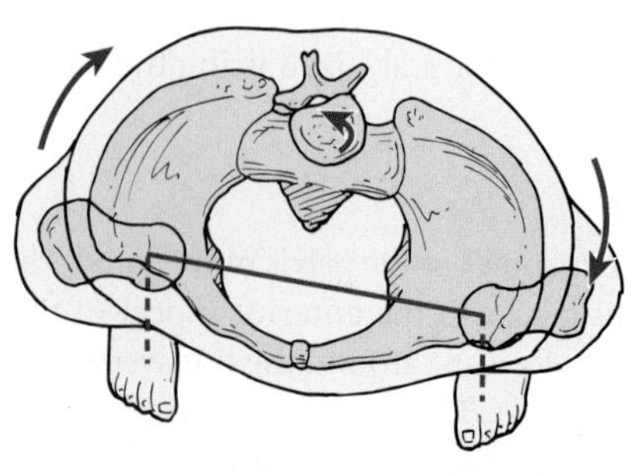

FIGURE 20.4 (A) Lateral pelvic tilt. Elevation of the iliac crest (hip hiking) causes relative adduction of the hip on the elevated side, and lowering of the iliac crest (hip drop) causes relative abduction of the hip on the lower side. **(B)** Pelvic rotation. Forward motion (forward rotation) of the pelvis causes relative external rotation of the hip; and backward motion (posterior rotation) of the pelvis causes relative internal rotation of the hip.

Pelvifemoral Motion

A combined movement occurs between the lumbar spine and pelvis during maximum forward bending of the trunk as when reaching toward the floor or the toes.[93] This motion is also known as lumbopelvic rhythm.[26] Although there is considerable variability in the participation of each of the joints, the motion typically is described as beginning with forward bending of the head.

- As the head and upper trunk initiate flexion, the pelvis shifts posteriorly to maintain the center of gravity over the base of support.
- The trunk continues to forward-bend, controlled by the extensor muscles of the spine, until approximately 45°. At this point for an individual with relatively normal flexibility, the posterior ligaments become taut, and the superior facets of the zygapophyseal joints slide upward, resulting in passive tension in the facet capsules.
- Once all of the vertebral segments are at the end of the range and stabilized by the posterior ligaments and facets, the pelvis begins to rotate forward (anterior pelvic tilt), controlled by the gluteus maximus and hamstring muscles.
- The pelvis continues to rotate forward until full muscle length is reached. Final range of motion (ROM) in forward bending is dictated by the flexibility of the various back extensor muscles and fasciae as well as hip extensor muscles (including the hamstrings).

The return to the upright position begins with the hip extensor muscles rotating the pelvis posteriorly through reverse muscle action (posterior pelvic tilt), then with the back extensor muscles extending the spine from the lumbar region upward. Variations in the normal synchronization of this activity occur because of training (as with dancers and gymnasts), faulty habits, restricted muscle or fascia length, or injury and faulty proprioception.

Hip, Knee, and Ankle Functional Relationships in Weight Bearing

During weight bearing, control of hip positions and motions affects the alignment and function of the entire lower extremity.

Hip flexion/extension. Hip flexion in weight bearing is typically accompanied by knee flexion and ankle dorsiflexion. These actions are controlled by the hip extensor (gluteus maximus and hamstrings), knee extensor (quadriceps femoris), and ankle plantarflexor (gastrocnemius and soleus) muscles. Hip extension in weight bearing causes knee extension by pulling the femur posteriorly and contributes to the locking mechanism at the knee.

Hip abduction/adduction. With unilateral weight bearing, gravity creates an adductor moment at the hip that is stabilized by the gluteus medius (preventing pelvic drop). Typically, this results in a varus moment at the knee, approximating the medial knee compartment. However, if the gluteus medius is weak, there is increased adduction of the femur and increased valgus moment at the knee, imposing greater stress on the medial collateral ligament, medial patellofemoral ligament, and anterior cruciate ligament.[133]

Hip rotation. Internal rotation of the hip results in the femur rotating medially on a fixed tibia at the knee. The force through the tibia causes eversion of the calcaneus and pronation of the foot when weight bearing. The reverse occurs with hip external rotation. This total chain response occurs repeatedly during the loading and terminal stance phases of gait as the ground reaction forces are absorbed and the body is moved forward. A total chain response also occurs during loading of the extremities when descending stairs or landing a jump.

Pathomechanics in the Hip Region

Abnormal structure or impaired function of the hip—such as a leg-length discrepancy, decreased flexibility, or muscle timing and strength imbalances—can contribute to stress through the spine or other joints of the lower extremities.

Decreased Flexibility

Decreased flexibility of the structures around the hip joint may have the effect of weight-bearing forces and movement being transmitted to the spine rather than being absorbed by the pelvis. For example, tight hip flexors will cause increased lumbar extension (lordosis) as the thigh extends. Hip flexion contractures with incomplete hip extension during weight bearing also place added stresses on the knee because the knee cannot lock while the hip is in flexion unless the trunk is bent forward. During weight bearing, tight adductors cause pelvic drop opposite to the side of tightness and compensatory side-bending of the trunk toward the side of tightness. The opposite occurs with tight abductors.

Muscle Weakness

Decreased hip abductor, extensor, and external rotator muscle strength is associated with valgus collapse at the knee (increased valgus and internal rotation of the femur) during weight-acceptance activities and may contribute to impairments throughout the lower extremity as described in the following examples.[133]

Patellofemoral impairment. Higher valgus moments at the knee as a result of weak hip abductors have been associated with patellofemoral impairments, which occur more often in women than in men (see Chapter 21).[133,134]

Anterior cruciate ligament strain. Valgus collapse and decreased hip extensor activation are more common in women than in men who have sustained an anterior cruciate ligament injury. It is suggested that this pattern increases anterior shear of the tibia and strain of the anterior cruciate ligament during loading (hip-knee flexion when landing following a jump).[133]

Piriformis syndrome. Hip extensor and abductor weakness resulting in hip adduction and internal rotation (valgus collapse) during functional activities has been identified as the possible cause of sciatic nerve compression secondary to piriformis muscle overuse. Strengthening and functional retraining of the gluteus maximus and gluteus medius along with correction of the faulty movement patterns were reported to alleviate the symptoms and functional improvement.[159]

Hip Muscle Imbalances and Their Effects

It is important to recognize that imbalances in muscle function (dominance of one muscle over another when performing an activity) that cause faulty movement patterns may be due to muscle strength and length deficits as well as altered proprioception and neuromuscular control.[63] Faulty mechanics from any of these factors may cause hip, knee, or back impairments and pain.[142] Overuse syndromes, soft tissue pain, and joint pain may all develop in response to continued abnormal stresses. The following are common hip muscle imbalances that may result in lower extremity impairments.

Shortened tensor fasciae latae (TFL) and/or gluteus maximus. The TFL and approximately one-third of the gluteus maximus insert into the iliotibial (IT) band. Decreased flexibility in either of these muscles has an effect on the tension transmitted through the IT band. Postural impairments often associated with a shortened TFL or gluteus maximus include an anterior pelvic tilt posture, slouched posture, or flat back posture (see Fig. 14.18 and related discussion in Chapter 14).[142] Overuse syndromes associated with greater tension of the IT band include trochanteric bursitis in the hip region and IT band friction syndrome in the knee (see description of this in the patellofemoral impairment section in Chapter 21).

Dominance of the TFL over the gluteus medius. The imbalance resulting from an apparent weakness of the gluteus medius with compensatory dominance of the TFL functioning as a hip abductor results in increased tension on the IT band,[142] valgus collapse of the knee during weight bearing with hip/knee flexion (see Fig. 21.9), and increased dynamic Q-angle.[63] This may lead to lateral knee pain (IT band syndrome) or patellofemoral pain syndrome from increased bowstring effect on the extensor mechanism (see the description of the bowstring effect and Fig. 21.3 in Chapter 21).

Dominance of the two-joint hip flexor muscles over the iliopsoas. Dominance of the TFL, rectus femoris, and/or sartorius muscles may contribute to faulty hip mechanics or knee pain from overuse of these muscles as they cross the knee.

Dominance of hamstring muscles over the gluteus maximus. Faulty posture and decreased functional activation of the gluteus maximus may decrease the flexibility of this muscle and limit the range of hip flexion.[142] Excessive lumbar spine flexion may result whenever full range of hip flexion is attempted. Limited mobility of the gluteus maximus also causes increased tension on the IT band, an alteration associated with trochanteric or lateral knee pain.

With decreased activation of the gluteus maximus, the hamstrings dominate as hip extensors.[142] Overuse of the hamstring muscles may result in cramping of the muscle with high-intensity exercise[165] or may result in decreased hamstring flexibility and muscle imbalances with the quadriceps femoris muscles at the knee.[142] In this muscle imbalance, the hamstrings dominate the knee stabilizing function by increased posterior pulling on the tibia to extend the knee in closed-chain activities. This alters the mechanics at the knee and may lead to overuse syndromes in the hamstring tendons or in anterior knee pain from modified quadriceps forces.[142]

Use of lateral trunk muscles for hip abductors. Relying on the lateral trunk muscles to perform the task of controlling the pelvis normally accomplished by the hip abductors results in excessive trunk motion and increased stress on the lumbar spine.

Asymmetrical Leg Length

Functional and structural asymmetries of the lower extremities affect the orientation and position of the pelvis.

Unilateral short leg. A unilateral short leg causes lateral pelvic tilting (drop on the short side) and side-bending of the trunk away from the short side (convexity of the lateral lumbar curve toward the side of short leg). This may lead to a functional—or eventually a structural—scoliosis. Causes of a short leg could be unilateral lower extremity faults, such as flat foot, genu valgum, coxa vara, tight hip muscles, anteriorly rotated innominate bone, poor standing posture, or asymmetrical bone growth.

Coxa valga and coxa vara. A pathologically large angle of inclination between the femoral neck and shaft of the femur is called *coxa valga*, and a pathologically smaller angle is called *coxa vara*. Unilateral coxa valga results in a relatively longer leg on that side and associated genu varum. Unilateral coxa vara leads to a relatively shorter leg with associated genu valgum.

Anteversion and retroversion. An increase in the torsion of the femoral neck is called *anteversion* and causes the shaft of the femur to be rotated medially. A decrease in the torsion is called *retroversion* and causes the shaft of the femur to be rotated laterally. Anteversion often results in genu valgum and pes planus. Unilateral anteversion results in a relatively shorter leg on that side; retroversion causes the opposite effect.

The Hip and Gait

During the normal gait cycle, the hip goes through 40° of flexion and extension ROM (10° extension at terminal stance to 30° flexion at midswing and initial contact). There is also lateral pelvic tilt and hip abduction/adduction of 15° (10° adduction at initial contact, 5° abduction at initial swing) and hip internal/external rotation along with pelvic rotation totaling 15° transverse plane motion (peak internal rotation at the end of loading, peak external rotation at the end of preswing). Loss of any of these motions affects the smoothness of the gait pattern.[130]

Hip Muscle Function and Gait

Hip Flexors

The hip flexors control hip extension at the end of stance and then contract concentrically to initiate swing.[130] With loss of flexor function, a posterior lurch of the trunk to initiate swing may be seen. Contractures of the hip flexors prevent complete extension during the second half of stance, thus shortening the stride. To compensate for a flexor contracture, a person increases the lumbar lordosis or walks with the trunk bent forward.

Hip Extensors

The hip extensors control the flexor moment during the loading response, and the gluteus maximus initiates hip extension.[124,130] With loss of extensor function, a posterior lurch of the trunk occurs at foot contact to shift the center of gravity of the trunk posterior to the hip. With contractures of the gluteus maximus, some decreased range occurs in the terminal swing as the femur comes forward, or the person may compensate by rotating the pelvis increasingly forward. The lower extremity may rotate outward because of the external rotation component of the muscle, or the gluteus maximus may place greater tension on the iliotibial band through its attachment, leading to irritation along the lateral aspect of the knee with repetitive activity.

Hip Abductors

The hip abductors control the lateral pelvic tilt during swinging of the opposite leg.[124,130] With loss of gluteus medius function, the trunk shifts laterally over the weak hip during stance when the opposite leg swings. This lateral shift also occurs with a painful hip to minimize the torque produced by gravity on the head, arms, and trunk and to subsequently decrease the abductor muscle force required. The tensor fasciae latae also functions as an abductor and can affect gait if it becomes tight.

Effect of Musculoskeletal Impairments on Gait

Bone and joint deformities change alignment of the lower extremity and therefore the mechanics of gait. Painful conditions cause antalgic gait patterns, which are characterized by decreased stance time on the painful side to avoid the stress of weight bearing.

Referred Pain and Nerve Injury

The hip is innervated primarily from the L3 spinal level; hip joint irritation is usually felt along the L3 dermatome reference from the groin, down the front of the thigh to the knee.[38,90] For a detailed description of referred pain patterns and peripheral nerve injuries in the hip and buttock region, see Chapter 13.

Major Nerves Subject to Injury or Entrapment

Sciatic nerve. Entrapment may occur when the sciatic nerve passes deep to the piriformis muscle (occasionally it passes over or through the piriformis).

Obturator nerve. Isolated injury is rare, although prolonged fetal head pressure during labor or damage from forceps delivery may occur.

Femoral nerve. Injury may result from fractures of the upper femur or pelvis, reduction of congenital dislocation of the hip, or pressure during a forceps labor and delivery.

Common Sources of Referred Pain in the Hip Region

If painful symptoms are referred to the hip region from other sources, primary treatment must be directed to the source of the irritation. Common sources of referred pain in the hip region include:

- Nerve roots or tissues derived from spinal segments L1, L2, L3, S1, and S2.
- Lumbar intervertebral and sacroiliac joints.

Management of Hip Disorders and Surgeries

To make sound clinical decisions when treating patients with hip disorders, it is necessary to understand the various pathologies, surgical procedures, and associated precautions and to identify each patient's presenting structural and functional impairments, activity limitations, and participation restrictions. In this section, common pathologies and surgeries of the hip region are described. Conservative and postoperative management of these conditions is also discussed in this section.

Joint Hypomobility: Nonoperative Management

Related Pathologies and Etiology of Symptoms

Osteoarthritis (OA), rheumatoid arthritis (RA), aseptic necrosis, slipped epiphyses, dislocations, and congenital deformities can lead to degenerative changes in the hip joint (see Fig. 11.2).

Osteoarthritis (Degenerative Joint Disease)

OA is the most common arthritic disease of the hip joint. Etiological factors include the aging process, joint trauma, repetitive abnormal stresses, obesity, hip developmental disorders, or disease.[32] The degenerative changes include articular cartilage breakdown and loss, capsular fibrosis, and osteophyte formation at the joint margins.[47] These effects usually occur in regions undergoing the greatest loading forces, such as the superior weight-bearing surface of the acetabulum (see Fig. 11.6).

Postimmobilization Hypomobility

Restricted capsular and surrounding periarticular tissue mobility may occur any time the joint is immobilized after a fracture or surgery.

Common Impairments of Structure and Function

- Pain experienced in the groin and referred along the anterior thigh and knee in the L3 dermatome.
- Stiffness after rest.
- Limited motion with a firm capsular end-feel.[153] Initially, limitation is only in internal rotation; in advanced stages, the hip is fixed in adduction, has no internal rotation or extension past neutral, and is limited to 90° flexion.[38]
- Asymmetry in lower extremity weight bearing and an antalgic gait usually with a compensated gluteus medius (abductor) limp and slower speed (related to shorter step length and stance duration).[36]
- Limited hip extension leading to increased extension forces on the lumbar spine and possible back pain.
- Limited hip extension preventing full knee extension when standing or during gait, leading to altered knee stresses.
- Impaired balance and postural control.

A clinical prediction rule (CPR) recently developed by Sutlive and associates[153] (summarized in Box 20.1) identifies five examination variables that can be used for the diagnosis of hip OA. The diagnostic variables are based on a preliminary study of 72 subjects over the age of 40 with unilateral buttock, groin, or anterior thigh pain. Patients with radiographic changes had an increased likelihood of having clinically relevant symptoms. Neither a validation study nor an impact analysis of this CPR have been reported.

Other functional impairments, such as decreased muscle strength and limited functional abilities, have been identified in individuals with hip OA.

BOX 20.1 Clinical Prediction Rule for the Diagnosis of Osteoarthritis of the Hip[153]

Variables*

- Squatting aggravates symptoms per self-report.
- Active hip flexion causes lateral hip pain.**
- The scour test with adduction causes lateral hip or groin pain.
- Active hip extension causes pain.
- Passive internal rotation is less than or equal to 25°.**

*Results of the study indicated that if three of the five variables were present, the likelihood of having hip OA increased from a 29% to 68% probability; if four of the five variables were identified, the likelihood increased to 91%.

**Interrater reliability for identifying the end feels of flexion and internal rotation was 0.85 and 0.88, respectively.

FOCUS ON EVIDENCE

A cross-sectional study compared 26 patients with hip OA who were not surgical candidates with a matched control group without OA for function and disability. Significant differences between the groups included mild to moderate pain level, decreased knee extension strength, and decreased hip ROM in the hip OA group. Functionally, those with OA walked a shorter distance in 6 minutes, but there were no significant differences in strength of the hip flexors/extensors, knee flexors, or ankle dorsiflexors/plantarflexors.[141]

Common Activity Limitations and Participation Restrictions

Hip joint impairments interfere with many weight-bearing activities and ADLs.[31,141]

Early stages. There is progressive pain with continued weight bearing and walking or at the end of the day after repetitive lower extremity activities. The pain may interfere with work or routine household activities that involve prolonged weight bearing.

Progressive degeneration. The individual experiences increased difficulty rising from a chair, walking long distances or on uneven surfaces, climbing stairs, squatting, and other weight-bearing activities and begins to have limitations in routine ADLs, such as bathing, toileting, and dressing (putting on pants, hose, socks).

CLINICAL TIP

To measure the extent of impairments (e.g., pain, ROM, strength) and activity and participation restrictions (walking distance or speed, ability to climb/descend stairs, ADLs, and quality of life) use tools such as the Western Ontario and McMaster Universities Osteoarthritis Index (WOMAC), the Arthritis Impact Measurement Scale (AIMS), Lower Extremity Functional Scale (LEFS), the Hip disability and Osteoarthritis Outcome Score (HOOS), the Harris Hip Score, and others as identified in the ***Clinical Practice Guidelines.***[32,45]

Management: Protection Phase

Chapter 11 describes the general principles and plan of care in the treatment of OA and RA, and Chapter 10 describes general management of joints during acute, subacute, and chronic stages of tissue injury and repair. In conjunction with medical management of inflammation and pain, correcting faulty mechanics is an integral part of decreasing hip pain. Faulty hip mechanics may be caused by conditions such as obesity, leg-length differences, muscle length and strength imbalances, sacroiliac dysfunction,[31,32] poor posture, or injury to other joints linked to hip motion.[25] The following goals and interventions are emphasized when the symptoms are acute and during the protection phase of nonoperative management.

Provide Patient Education

- Explain how the stresses of weight bearing and other activities impact symptoms and joint health and describe how interventions may minimize symptoms.
- Teach safe ambulatory patterns and a home exercise program that emphasizes nonimpact activities and frequent ROM.

Decrease Pain at Rest

- Apply grade I or II oscillation techniques with the joint in the resting position.
- Have the patient rock in a rocking chair to provide gentle oscillations to the lower extremity joints and possibly a stimulus to the joint mechanoreceptors.

Decrease Pain During Weight-Bearing Activities

- Provide assistive devices for ambulation to help reduce stress on the hip joint. If the pain is unilateral, teach the patient to walk with a single cane or crutch on the side opposite the painful joint.
- If leg-length asymmetry is causing hip joint stress, gradually elevate the short leg with lifts in the shoe.
- Modify chairs to provide an elevated and firm surface and adapt commodes with an elevated seat to make sitting down and standing up easier.

Decrease Effects of Stiffness and Maintain Available Motion

- Teach the patient the importance of moving the hips through their ROM frequently throughout the day. When the acute symptoms are medically controlled, have the patient perform active or assisted ROM as they are able.
- If a pool is available, have the patient perform ROM in the buoyant environment.
- Initiate nonimpact activities such as swimming, gentle water aerobics, or stationary cycling.

Management: Controlled Motion and Return to Function Phases

As symptoms subside, the emphasis of management includes the following goals and interventions.

Progressively Increase Joint Accessory Motion and Soft Tissue Mobility

Joint mobilization techniques.[32] Progress joint mobilization to stretch grades (grade III sustained or grade III and IV oscillation) using glide directions that stretch restricting capsular tissue at the end of the available ROM (see Figs. 5.45 through 5.47 in Chapter 5). Vigorous stretching should not be undertaken until the chronic stage.

Stretching techniques. Stretch any range-limiting tissues. Suggested manual stretching techniques are described in Chapter 4, and self-stretching techniques are described in the exercise section later in this chapter.

Improve Joint Tracking and Pain-Free Motion

Mobilization with movement (MWM) techniques[110] may be applied through the use of a mobilization belt to produce a pain-free inferolateral glide and then superimposing motion to the end of the available range. As with all MWM techniques, no pain should be experienced during application of the technique. Principles of MWM are described in Chapter 5; specific MWM techniques for the hip are described here.

Increase Internal Rotation

Patient position: Supine with the involved hip flexed and a mobilization belt secured around the proximal anterior-medial thigh and your pelvis.

Procedure: Stabilize the patient's pelvis with the palm of the hand closest to the patient's head. Use the mobilization belt to produce a pain-free inferolateral glide while the caudal hand grips around the flexed thigh and shin to create pain-free, end-range internal rotation (Fig. 20.5 A).

Increase Flexion

Patient position: Supine with the involved hip flexed and a mobilization belt secured around the proximal anterior-medial thigh and the pelvis.

Procedure: Stabilize the patient's pelvis with the palm of the hand closest to the patient's head. Use the mobilization belt to produce a pain-free inferolateral glide while the caudal hand grips around the flexed thigh and shin to create pain-free, end-range flexion (Fig. 20.5 B).

Increase Extension

Patient position: Supine with the pelvis near the end of the treatment table in the Thomas test position (opposite thigh held against the chest) and a mobilization belt secured around the proximal medial thigh and your pelvis.

Procedure: Stabilize the patient's pelvis with the palm of the hand closest to the patient's head. Use the mobilization belt to produce a pain-free, inferolateral glide, while the caudal hand presses against the extended thigh to create pain-free, end-range extension (Fig. 20.5 C).

Increase Extension During Weight Bearing

Patient position: Standing with the unaffected foot up on a stool and a mobilization belt secured around the proximal medial thigh and your pelvis.

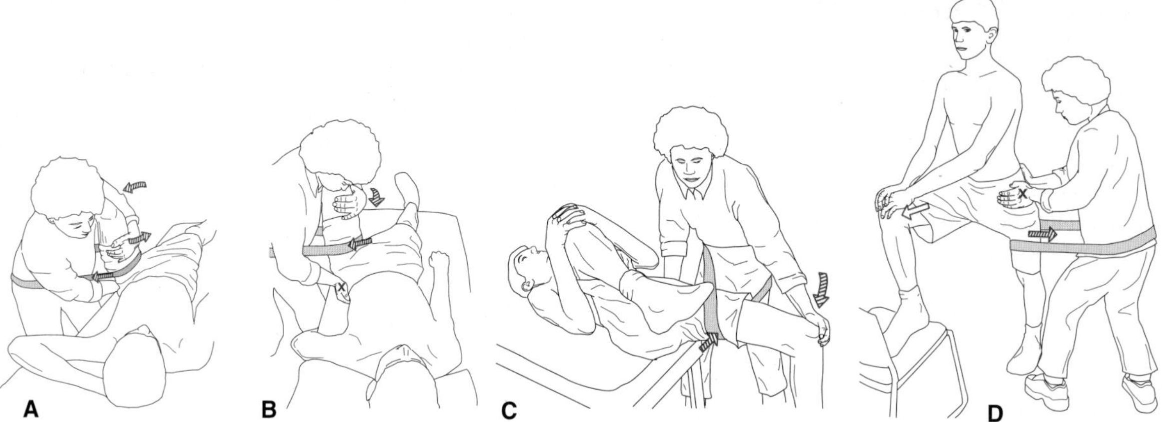

FIGURE 20.5 Mobilization with movement using an inferolateral glide increasing **(A)** pain-free internal rotation, **(B)** pain-free flexion, **(C)** pain-free extension, and **(D)** a lateral glide increasing extension during weight bearing.

Procedure: Stabilize the pelvis with both hands and apply a pain-free, lateral glide with the mobilization belt, while the patient lunges forward to produce painless extension of the affected hip (Fig. 20.5 D).

Improve Muscle Performance in Supporting Muscles, Balance, and Aerobic Capacity

- Initiate exercises that develop strength and control of the hip musculature, especially the gluteus maximus, gluteus medius, and rotators, and that improve stability and balance when performing weight-bearing activities. Begin with submaximal isometric resistance; progress to dynamic resistance as the patient tolerates movement. If any exercises exacerbate the joint symptoms, reduce the intensity. Also reassess the patient's functional activities and adapt them to reduce the stress.
- Progress to functional exercises as tolerated using closed-chain and weight-bearing activities. The patient may require assistive devices while weight bearing. Use a pool or tank to reduce the effects of gravity to allow partial weight-bearing exercises without stress.
- Develop postural awareness and balance.
- Progress the low-impact aerobic exercise program (swimming, cycling, or walking within tolerance).

Provide Patient Education

Help the patient establish a balance between activity and rest and teach them the importance of minimizing stressful, deforming forces by maintaining muscle strength and flexibility in the hip region.

FOCUS ON EVIDENCE

Two systematic reviews of studies examining the effects of exercise in the management of hip and knee OA describe support for aerobic exercise and strengthening exercises to reduce pain and disability.[138,139] The consensus of the studies is that there are few contraindications and that exercise is relatively safe in patients with OA.[138] However, exercise should be individualized and patient centered, with consideration for age, comorbidity, and general mobility.

An outcome review[39] summarized that moderate- or high-intensity exercises in patients with RA have minimal effect on the disease activity, but there is insufficient radiological evidence on the effect in large joints. Long-term moderate- or high-intensity exercises that are individualized to protect radiologically damaged joints improve aerobic capacity, muscle strength, functional ability, and psychological well-being in patients with RA.

A committee appointed by the Osteoarthritis Research International performed an extensive systematic review and developed a consensus recommendation for the management of hip and knee OA.[172] Suggested interventions included referral to a physical therapist for evaluation and instruction in exercises to "reduce pain and improve functional capacity" as well as use of assistive devices when appropriate. The report also supported the importance of regular aerobic exercise, muscle strengthening, and ROM.

Clinical Practice Guidelines (CPGs) for Hip OA developed by the Orthopaedic Section of the American Physical Therapy Association[32] recommend patient education; functional, gait, and balance training; manual therapy; and flexibility, strengthening, and endurance exercises.

Joint Surgery and Postoperative Management

A number of surgical options are available to manage early- and late-stage hip joint injury or disease and fractures that compromise the vascular supply to the head of the femur. As a result of advances in arthroscopy of the hip, small- to medium-size, full-thickness lesions of the articular cartilage of the acetabulum and head of the femur as well as other joint pathologies, such as acetabular labral tears, femoroacetabular impingement (FAI), and capsular laxity, are now managed arthroscopically.[44,45, 175,177] *Microfracture*, a type of *chondroplasty*, is a procedure designed to repair small lesions of the articular cartilage.[44] Other arthroscopic procedures for the hip include *debridement* for removal of a loose body within the joint, *labral resection* or *repair* for acetabular-labral fraying or a tear, *osteoplasty* and *rim trimming* for FAI, and *capsulorrhaphy* or capsular *plication* for capsular laxity.[44] In-depth information on FAI can be found in a later section on Painful Hip Syndromes in this chapter and in other resources.[45, 175,176,177]

Surgical procedures to manage late-stage deterioration of the hip joint include *osteotomy* (an extra-articular procedure) and arthroplasty, specifically *hip resurfacing arthroplasty (surface replacement)*,[55,69] *hemiarthroplasty*,[99] and *total hip arthroplasty (THA)*.[37,76,94] *Arthrodesis* and *resection arthroplasty* of the hip are considered salvage procedures after failure of arthroplasty and when revision arthroplasty is contraindicated or not feasible.[94]

The goals of joint surgery and postoperative management are to provide the patient with (1) a pain-free hip, (2) a stable joint for lower extremity weight bearing and functional ambulation, and (3) adequate ROM and strength of the lower extremity for functional activities.

For an effective, safe postoperative rehabilitation program, it is important for the therapist to have a basic understanding of the more common surgical procedures for hip joint disease and deformity, plus a thorough knowledge of appropriate therapeutic exercise interventions and their progression. An overview of two of the more common procedures—THA and hemiarthroplasty—and guidelines for postoperative management are described in the following sections.

Arthroscopic Procedures for the Hip

Indications for Surgery

The following are common indications for arthroscopic interventions from injuries and disorders affecting the hip joint:[44,45,175,176,177]

- Anterior hip/groin pain as the result of focal lesions of the articular cartilage acetabulum or femoral head and often found in conjunction with FAI and/or an acetabular labral tear or fraying that is not relieved by a course of conservative (nonoperative) treatment
- Intra-articular loose bodies leading to clicking, catching, or locking of the hip joint
- Laxity of the hip capsule typically leading to anterior instability of the hip
- Intra-articular examination of the hip

Procedures

A surgeon's selection of one or more arthroscopic procedures for the hip to relieve or reduce a patient's structural or functional impairments is based on a number of criteria including the type, size, and location of the defect or lesion and patient-related factors, such as age, desired activity level, and an ability to participate in a postoperative rehabilitation.[44,45,175,176]

Chondroplasty/microfracture. One of several arthroscopic procedures can be performed for repair of small to medium articular cartilage lesions. Microfracture involves creating small fractures of subchondral bone in the area of the chondral lesion to stimulate growth of fibrocartilage to replace the damaged hyaline cartilage.[44]

Resection or repair of a labral tear of the acetabulum. Arthroscopic resection and removal (debridement) of the unstable portion of a torn or frayed labrum, while preserving as much stable tissue as possible, is performed to reduce hip pain or the catching sensation a patient may have been experiencing over a period of time. Repair of a labral tear typically is selected for management of an acute tear, usually caused by trauma and to preserve the congruity of the hip joint.

Osteoplasty and rim trimming. These bony procedures are designed to reduce the structural abnormalities of the femoral head, acetabulum, or both and subsequent abutment of bony structures, which often lead to FAI and the development of labral fraying or tears and articular cartilage lesions.[44,176]

Capsular modification: plication or thermal-assisted capsulorrhaphy. These procedures are designed to surgically decrease or shrink the size of the joint capsule to reduce capsular laxity, joint instability, and the risk of labral tears and articular cartilage injury.[44]

Postoperative Management

Rehabilitation following any of the arthroscopic procedures for the hip is criterion based and time based, is geared to the type and number of procedures carried out, and is individualized to each patient.

Interventions in the postoperative program include patient education emphasizing avoidance of symptom-provoking positions of the lower extremities; weight bearing with some degree of protection; and therapeutic exercises to improve ROM and flexibility, strength and endurance, and neuromuscular control and balance. Postoperative rehabilitation guidelines for the arthroscopic hip procedures described in this section are based on several resources in the literature and summarized in Table 20.2.[44,45,175,176,177]

Additional postoperative interventions. There are a number of interventions common to the arthroscopic surgical procedures for the hip addressed in Table 20.2. They include the use of a modified Bledsoe orthosis for 10 to 14 postoperative days to limit hip motion. Another range-limiting device is an antirotation bolster to limit external rotation for 10 to 14 days following labral resection or repair, microfracture, and osteoplasty and for up to 4 weeks after capsular plication or thermal-assisted capsulorrhaphy. However, active internal rotation from neutral while lying supine is initiated during the early postoperative days to reduce the risk of capsular adhesions. Sometimes a CPM unit for hip flexion and extension within a limited range

TABLE 20.2 Guidelines for Postoperative Management Following Arthroscopic Procedures for the Hip

Type of Arthroscopic Procedure	Weight-Bearing Restrictions*	Exercise Guidelines and Progression*
Microfracture/Chondroplasty		
	▪ Restrict weight bearing to protect early fibrocartilage formation and for pain control ▪ Minimal (touch-down) weight bearing for 4–6 weeks[44] or up to 8 weeks[176] postop, progressing to weight bearing as tolerated ▪ Use of ambulation aids for joint protection	▪ Hip ROM ▪ Active-assistive ROM on first postop day within protected ranges ▪ Full ROM permitted after 2 weeks ▪ Strengthening and balance exercises ▪ Active ROM at 2 weeks; avoid supine SLRs for 3–4 weeks to minimize compressive forces on the hip ▪ Low-load PRE at 4–6 weeks ▪ Resistance and balance exercises in weight bearing after 6 weeks
Resection or Repair of an Acetabular Labral Tear		
	▪ *After resection and debridement:* partial weight bearing for up to 2 weeks postop ▪ *After repair:* partial weight-bearing for up to 4 weeks postop ▪ Gradual progression of weight bearing based on joint irritability and pain ▪ Use of ambulation aids for joint protection	▪ Hip ROM ▪ Active-assistive ROM on first postop day, gradually progressing to active ROM ▪ Stationary cycling with seat raised (to limit hip flexion) within first postop week ▪ Limit hip flexion to 80°-90° ▪ Full ROM (abduction and external rotation) permitted by 2 weeks postop ▪ Strengthening and balance exercises ▪ Active ROM by 2 weeks, progressing with low-load resistance ▪ Progressive weight bearing and balance exercises incorporating weight-bearing restrictions
Osteoplasty and Rim Trimming		
	▪ Minimal (touch-down) weight bearing for 4–6 weeks to allow bony healing, gradually progressing to weight bearing as tolerated ▪ Use of ambulation aids for joint protection	▪ Hip ROM ▪ Active-assistive ROM within protected ranges on postop day 1 ▪ Full ROM permitted by 2 weeks ▪ Strengthening and balance exercises ▪ Active ROM permitted after 2 weeks; progress by adding light resistance. ▪ Avoid supine SLRs for 3–4 weeks postop to minimize compressive forces on the hip. ▪ When weight bearing is permitted as tolerated, begin weight-bearing exercises and balance progression.
Capsular Modification: Plication or Thermal-Assisted Capsulorrhaphy		
	▪ Partial weight bearing for 10–14 days;[44] up to 4 weeks[176] ▪ Use of ambulation aids for protection of joint capsule	▪ Hip ROM ▪ Active-assistive ROM on first postop day, gradually progressing to active ROM. After anterior capsular modification, limit external rotation beyond 10° for 3–4 weeks,[44,176] ▪ Stationary cycling within first postop week ▪ Full ROM permitted after 4 weeks postop ▪ Strengthening and balance exercises ▪ Resistance exercises in weight-bearing and balance exercises when full weight bearing allowed SLRs = straight-leg raises

*NOTE: Weight-bearing and ROM restrictions vary based on the underlying diagnoses that necessitated the arthroscopic procedure(s)

is used postoperatively. Ankle pumping exercises to reduce the risk of a deep vein thrombosis (DVT) and setting exercises (quadriceps and gluteal muscles) are routinely begun on postoperative day 1 and 2, respectively. Typically, if full, passive hip ROM is not achieved by 4 to 6 weeks after surgery, stretching exercises are initiated to increase hip muscle flexibility. Stabilization exercises, targeting lumbopelvic musculature, also are an integral component of the rehabilitation program.

Standing and ambulation with crutches or a walker while partial-weight bearing on the operated side can begin on the day of or after surgery. Before full-weight bearing is permitted, aquatic activities and ambulation can also begin after the incision is well healed. Resumption of functional activities occurs gradually, but typically sooner after labral resection, labral repair, or capsular modification than after microfracture, osteoplasty, or rim trimming.

Sport-specific rehabilitation. As postoperative rehabilitation for management of arthroscopic procedures for the hip has evolved during the past decade, guidelines for sport-specific training for the intermediate and advanced phases of recovery are being developed in clinical settings and published in the literature.[175,176]

Total Hip Arthroplasty

One of the most widely performed surgical interventions for advanced arthritis of the hip joint is THA (Fig. 20.6). OA is the underlying pathology that accounts for most primary total hip procedures.[37]

Indications for Surgery

The following are common indications for THA, sometimes referred to as total hip replacement:[37,46,50,101]

- Severe hip pain with motion and weight bearing with significant motion limitation as the result of joint deterioration and loss of articular cartilage associated with OA, RA or traumatic arthritis, ankylosing spondylitis, or osteonecrosis (avascular necrosis)
- Nonunion fracture, instability or deformity of the hip
- Bone tumors
- Failure of conservative management or of previous joint reconstruction procedures (osteotomy, resurfacing arthroplasty, femoral stem hemiarthroplasty, and primary THA)

Because the projected life span of primary THA procedures is about 20 years, they were historically used for patients older than 60 to 65 years of age or for the very inactive younger patient with multijoint involvement, such as RA.[37,50] However, with advances in component design, materials, and fixation, plus improvements in surgical techniques, THA is now an option for some younger (< 60 years of age), moderately active individuals.[8,51] These individuals are counseled by the surgeon to anticipate the need for revision arthroplasty later in life.

There are a number of instances in which THA is contraindicated. Absolute and relative contraindications are noted in Box 20.2.[8,14,37]

Preoperative Management

Preoperative contact with a patient prior to elective surgery typically occurs on an outpatient basis individually or in

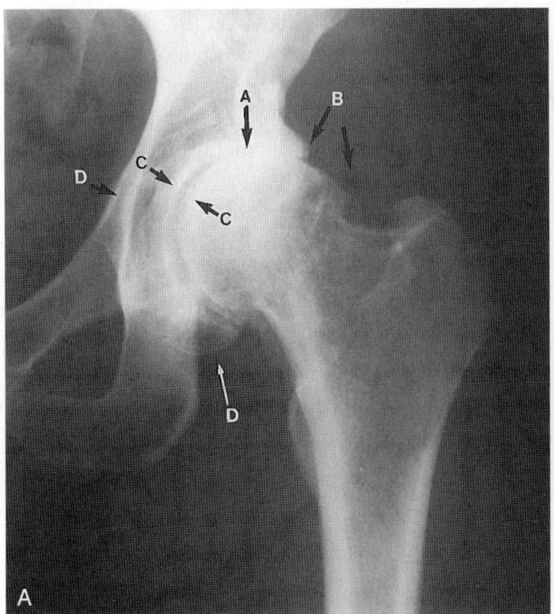

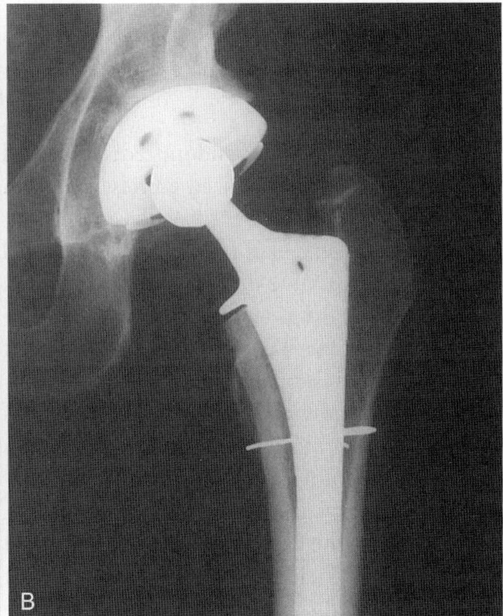

FIGURE 20.6 Total hip arthroplasty. **(A)** The preoperative film of a severely degenerative hip joint demonstrates the classic signs of degenerative joint disease. Arrow A shows a narrowed joint space with superior migration of the femoral head; B shows osteophyte formation at the joint margins of both the acetabulum and femoral head; C shows sclerosis of subchondral bone on both sides of the joint surface; and D shows acetabular protrusion (a bony outpouching of the acetabular cup in response to the progressive superior and medial migration of the femoral head). **(B)** Postoperative film shows a total hip arthroplasty. Both the acetabular and femoral portions of the joint have been resected and replaced with prosthetic components. *(From McKinnis, LN: Fundamentals of Musculoskeletal Imaging, ed. 4. Philadelphia: F.A. Davis, 2014, p 354, with permission.)*

BOX 20.2 Contraindications to Total Hip Arthroplasty

Absolute
- Active joint infection
- Systemic infection or sepsis
- Chronic osteomyelitis
- Significant loss of bone after resection of a malignant tumor or inadequate bone stock that prevents sufficient implant fixation
- Neuropathic hip joint
- Severe paralysis of the muscles surrounding the joint

Relative
- Localized infection, such as bladder or skin
- Insufficient function of the gluteus medius muscle
- Progressive neurological disorder
- Highly compromised/insufficient femoral or acetabular bone stock associated with progressive bone disease
- Patients requiring extensive dental work—dental surgery should be completed before arthroplasty
- Young patients who must or are most likely to participate in high-demand (high-load, high-impact) activities

BOX 20.3 Components of Therapy-Related Preoperative Management: Preparation for Total Hip Arthroplasty

- Examination and evaluation of pain, ROM, muscle strength, balance, ambulatory status, leg lengths, gait characteristics, use of assistive devices, general level of function, and perceived level of disability. Consider gathering pre-operative information using a valid outcome measure, such as the Harris Hip Score, Hip Outcome Score, or Lower Extremity Functional Scale.
- Information for patients and their families about joint disease and the operative procedure in nonmedical terms.
- Postoperative precautions and their rationale including positioning and weight bearing.
- Functional training for early postoperative days including bed mobility, transfers, and gait training with assistive devices.
- Early postoperative exercises.
- Criteria for discharge from the hospital.

a group several days before surgery. Patient information sessions often are coordinated and conducted by a team of professionals from multiple disciplines who are likely to be involved with a patient's postoperative care. These sessions typically include a combination of patient education, assessment and documentation of the patient's preoperative status, and instruction regarding a pre-surgical exercise program.[13,94,112,126] Box 20.3 summarizes possible components of preoperative management.[13,66,94,112,126]

FOCUS ON EVIDENCE

Wang and colleagues[166] conducted a randomized, controlled investigation to determine if a customized exercise program initiated before scheduled THA had an effect on the ambulatory abilities of patients after surgery. Gait function was evaluated with the 25-Meter Walk Test and the 6-Minute Walk Test. Participants in the exercise group (n = 15) took part in two facility-based and two home-based exercise sessions of stationary bicycling and resistance training each week for 8 weeks prior to surgery. Individualized exercise programs resumed at 3 weeks postoperatively and continued through 12 weeks. Control group subjects (n = 13) received only advice routinely provided by a hospital physical therapist. At 3 weeks postoperatively, the exercise group demonstrated significantly greater gait velocity and stride length, and at 12 weeks, they demonstrated significantly greater 6-minute walking distance than the control group. The investigators concluded that a customized strength and endurance training program prior to and after THA improved the rate of recovery of ambulatory function.

Procedures

Background

Prosthetic designs and materials. THA has been performed successfully since the early 1960s.[37,50] Sir John Charnley,[29] a surgeon from England, is credited with the initial research and clinical application of total hip replacement, which has evolved into contemporary hip arthroplasty. A variety of implant designs, materials, and surgical approaches have been developed and modified over the years.[37,50,69] Today, total hip implant systems are typically composed of an inert metal (cobalt-chrome and titanium) modular femoral component and a high-density polyethylene acetabular component. Occasionally, metal-on-metal[69,149] and ceramic surfaces are used in the design.[37,69]

Cemented versus cementless fixation. The revolutionary aspect of the early THA procedures was the use of acrylic cement (methyl methacrylate) for prosthetic fixation. Cement fixation allowed very early postoperative weight bearing, which shortened the period of rehabilitation, whereas prior to the use of cement fixation patients were subjected to months of restricted weight bearing and limited mobility.[37] Although cement fixation has its drawbacks, it continues to be used regularly today, particularly in THA for elderly and physically inactive younger patients.[15,69,125,135]

A significant postoperative complication associated with cement fixation is aseptic (mechanical) loosening of the prosthetic components at the bone-cement interface. This loosening subsequently leads to a gradual recurrence of hip pain and the need for surgical revision.[15,37,135] Patients who most often develop implant loosening are the younger, physically active patients. In contrast, loosening has not been shown to be a particularly prevalent problem in elderly patients or in young patients with multijoint involvement and limited physical activity.[50,135]

The problem of mechanical loosening gave rise to the development and use of cementless (biological) fixation.[37,50] Cementless fixation is achieved by using implants that allow osseous ingrowth into a porous beaded or textured surface or by a precise press-fit technique.[17,85,160] Smooth (nonporous) femoral components also are being used with cementless arthroplasty. Some components are manufactured with a coating of a bioactive compound called hydroxyapatite, designed to promote initial osseous ingrowth.[28] Ingrowth of bony tissue occurs over a 3- to 6-month period with continued bone remodeling beyond that time period. Initial long-term studies of cementless fixation have demonstrated better fixation durability of the acetabular component than of the femoral stem component.[69]

Improvements in both cemented and cementless fixation continue, as does debate over the indications, benefits, and disadvantages of both forms of fixation. Cementless fixation is more often the choice for the patient under 60 years of age who is physically active and has good bone quality.[17,85,160] Its use continues to grow as the average age of the patient undergoing THA decreases and improvements in femoral stem fixation evolve.[69] However, cement fixation continues to be used routinely for elderly patients and those with osteoporosis and poor bone stock.[15,125,135] In some cases a combination of fixation procedures, known as a hybrid procedure, involving a cementless acetabular component and a cemented femoral stem component is used.[113]

Operative Overview

The operative approaches used to gain access to the involved joint and to implant the prosthetic components during THA can be divided into two broad categories: *traditional (conventional or standard)* and *minimally invasive* approaches. Original hip arthroplasty procedures used long surgical incisions (15 to 25 cm) to expose the joint. Although long-term outcomes have been successful, *traditional* surgical approaches impose substantial trauma to soft tissues that may increase the postoperative recovery period.

A recent advance in primary hip arthroplasty—the use of minimally invasive approaches through "mini-incisions"—allows adequate exposure of the joint for insertion of the prosthetic components while decreasing soft tissue trauma. Brief overviews of the various types of *traditional* and minimally invasive surgical approaches follow, focusing on which muscles are incised or left intact during the procedure.[3,42,59,69,71,88] The integrity of the muscles and other soft tissues surrounding the prosthetic hip influences its postoperative stability and the extent of restrictions placed on the patient, most notably during the early phase of postoperative recovery.

Traditional surgical approaches. There are several approaches that may be used during traditional THA procedures: posterior (or posterolateral), lateral, anterolateral, anterior, and transtrochanteric. Each has its advantages and disadvantages.[3,42,59] In addition to the following information, ONLINE Table 20.1(available on the FA Davis website) summarizes the key features of each approach and their potential impact on function.

- ***Posterior or posterolateral approaches.*** These are the most frequently used approaches for primary THA. To access the joint through a posterior approach, the gluteus maximus is split in line with the muscle fibers. With a posterolateral approach, the interval between the gluteus maximus and medius is split. The piriformis and short external rotator tendons are transected near their insertion. The capsule is incised, and the gluteus maximus tendon may be released from its insertion on the femur in preparation for posterior dislocation of the hip and insertion of the components. Although an intact gluteus medius may result in earlier recovery of a normal gait pattern after surgery, the primary disadvantage of this approach is that it is associated with the highest incidence of postoperative joint instability and resulting subluxation or dislocation of the hip.[71,81,106,107] To reduce the risk of postoperative dislocation, repair of the posterior capsule and muscles is advocated to improve the soft tissue constraint to the posterior aspect of the joint.[30]
- ***Direct lateral approach.*** This approach requires longitudinal division of the tensor fasciae latae (TFL), release of up to one-half of the proximal insertion of the gluteus medius, and longitudinal splitting of the vastus lateralis.[3,59] The gluteus minimus also is partially detached from the trochanter. A lateral approach may also involve a trochanteric osteotomy. Disruption of the abductor mechanism is associated with postoperative weakness of this muscle group, leading to gait abnormalities such as a positive Trendelenburg sign.
- ***Anterolateral approach.*** With this approach, an incision is centered over the greater trochanter, lateral to the TFL. The IT band is split, and the anterior one-third of the gluteus medius and minimus are detached from their insertion on the greater trochanter to be reattached at closure.[71,88,96] In some instances, the anterior one-third of the vastus lateralis is detached as well.[96] Unlike the posterior/posterolateral approach, the external rotators usually remain intact in the anterolateral approach. A capsulotomy is performed and the hip dislocated anteriorly for adequate exposure of the joint. Although this approach allows for precise implant positioning, leg length correction, and excellent postoperative stability, it is associated with delayed recovery of the abductor muscles. Consequently, postoperative gait asymmetries persist for a longer period of time than with an anterior approach.[88] Compared with the posterior approach, the incidence of postoperative dislocation is lower in the anterolateral approach.[37,59] Therefore, it is also indicated for patients with muscle imbalances associated with stroke or cerebral palsy whose standing posture is characterized by hip flexion and internal rotation joint positions that place them at high risk of dislocation with a posterior approach.[3,59]

- ***Anterior approach.*** An incision is made lateral and distal to the anterior superior iliac spine, slightly anterior to the greater trochanter, and medial to the TFL. Although no muscles are detached with this approach, the rectus femoris and sartorius are retracted medially for exposure of the joint. The capsule is incised, and the hip is dislocated anteriorly in preparation for insertion of the components.[88] A key advantage of the direct anterior approach is that weight bearing as tolerated is permitted immediately after surgery. However, this approach is used infrequently for primary THA because visualization of the surgical field is more challenging.
- ***Transtrochanteric approach.*** This approach was first used with very early primary THA[29] but is now used primarily in complex revision arthroplasty. The transtrochanteric approach involves an osteotomy of the greater trochanter at the insertion of the gluteus medius and minimus and affords excellent exposure for insertion of the prosthetic components.[71] Following component placement, the trochanter is reattached and wired in place to stabilize the osteotomy site. The trochanter is often reattached in a position to improve the mechanical efficiency of the gluteus medius muscle.[3,59] An extended period of nonweight bearing and adherence to abduction precautions are required until bony healing has occurred. Complications associated with trochanteric osteotomy include nonunion and greater than usual soft tissue irritation and pain from a considerable amount of internal fixation.

Minimally invasive approaches. As with traditional THA, minimally invasive THA is an open procedure. With minimally invasive procedures, however, the joint is approached through one or two small incisions, usually less than or equal to 10 cm in length.[14] The characteristics of minimally invasive approaches for THA are summarized in Box 20.4.

The rationale for choosing minimally invasive THA over traditional THA is that the smaller incisions and muscle-sparing techniques reduce soft tissue trauma during surgery, potentially improving and accelerating a patient's postoperative recovery.[9,14]

Benefits cited by advocates of minimally invasive THA are:[3,9,13,14,71,140]

- Decreased blood loss.
- Reduced postoperative pain.
- Shorter length of hospital stay and lower cost of hospitalization.
- More rapid recovery of functional mobility.
- Better cosmetic appearance of the surgical scar.

Proponents of minimally invasive THA note that the procedures are more technically challenging, specifically with regard to insertion and alignment of the prosthetic components.[4,10,170] Depending on the surgeon's experience with the new approach and selection of patients, there is speculation that rates of postoperative complications will be higher.[4,10] In general, the results of studies have supported the in-hospital benefits of minimally invasive THA, such as less blood loss, less postoperative pain, and shorter hospital stay, when compared with traditional THA.[122,137,170] However, the claim of rapid recovery of functional mobility, typically measured by gait analysis following minimally invasive versus traditional THA, has yet to be determined.[42,96,131,137]

Numerous studies have compared MI and traditional procedures for in-hospital and postsurgical outcomes for THA. The most recent systematic reviews and meta-analyses of these studies report some small but minor benefit to using minimally invasive surgery.[18,151,171] When a posterior approach is used in patients with degenerative hip disease, MI results in statistically significant improvement in operating time, length of hospital stay, blood loss, and the Harris Hip Score for function.[18] The authors of this analysis note that the higher Harris Hip Scores for patients who have had the MI procedure do not reach the threshold for a clinically important difference. When analyzing studies using all surgical approaches for a variety of diagnoses, MI results in reduced length of hospital stay and reduced blood loss, but no other surgical, functional, or radiological benefits.[171] Details of studies that have compared these procedures are summarized in the outcomes section on THA.

Implantation of components and closure. After dislocation of the joint, an osteotomy is performed at the femoral neck, and the head is removed. Another option used by some

BOX 20.4 Features of Minimally Invasive Total Hip Arthroplasty

- Length of incision: < 10 cm, depending on the location of the approach and the size of the patient[14,71]
- Most, if not all, muscles and tendons left intact
- Single-incision or two-incision surgical approach
  - *Single incision*: posterior,[52] anterior,[95,96,131] or occasionally lateral.[10,68]
  - *Two-incision*: two 4- to 5-cm incisions, one anterior for insertion of acetabular component and one posterior for placement of femoral component.[5,13,140,154]
- Incision location and muscles disturbed
  - *Posterior approach*: an incision extending mostly distal to the greater trochanter between the gluteus medius and piriformis muscles; short external rotators may or may not be incised (later repaired); abductor mechanism consistently is left intact.[52,170]
  - *Anterior approach*: an incision beginning just lateral and distal of the anterior superior iliac spine extending in a distal and slightly posterior direction along the belly of the tensor fasciae latae (TFL); sartorius and rectus femoris retracted medially and the TFL laterally; leaves all muscles intact; no postoperative precautions.[13,95,96,131]
  - *Lateral approach*: least commonly used; splits the middle-third of the gluteus medius; anterolateral incision into the capsule leaves the posterior capsule intact, eliminating the need to observe postoperative precautions for prevention of posterior dislocation.[10,68]

surgeons for minimally invasive procedures is to cut the femoral neck *in situ* without dislocating the hip.[13,95,154] The acetabulum is reamed and remodeled, and a high-density polyethylene cup is inserted into the prepared surface.[125] The intramedullary canal of the femoral shaft may be broadened if necessary, and the stemmed, metal prosthesis is inserted into the shaft of the femur.[15,135] With both components in place, the alignment is checked radiographically and stability and ROM are assessed.

After the prosthetic hip is reduced, the capsule typically is repaired. The remaining layers of soft tissues that were incised or detached are securely repaired and appropriately balanced for length and mobility prior to closure.

CLINICAL TIP

Although published resources contain a wealth of information about implant design, methods of fixation, and soft tissues incised or detached in the various conventional and minimally invasive surgical approaches for THA, the best resource a therapist can use to understand the unique features of a patient's surgery and then plan an individualized postoperative rehabilitation program is the operative report found in the patient's medical record.

Complications

The incidence of intraoperative and early and late postoperative complications after primary, traditional THA is relatively low. However, some surgeons are concerned that minimally invasive procedures will result in a higher incidence of complications due to decreased visual exposure of the hip joint during surgery and the more technically demanding nature of the approaches.[4,10] To date, this concern has not been consistently supported by evidence-based studies.[69,71] Although only a small percentage of complications require revision arthroplasty, any complication can hamper rehabilitation and diminish functional mobility.

Intraoperative complications. Intraoperative complications associated with THA include malpositioning of the prosthetic components, femoral fracture, insufficient equalization of leg lengths, and nerve injury.

Early postoperative complications. In addition to the medical complications, such as infection, DVT, or pneumonia that can occur after any surgery, postoperative complications that may occur during the early period of recovery (before 6 weeks or up to 2 to 3 months) include infection or delayed wound healing, dislocation of the prosthetic joint, disruption of a bone graft site before sufficient bone healing has occurred, and a persistent functional leg-length discrepancy.[106]

Late complications. Late complications include mechanical loosening of either implant at the bone-cement or bone-implant interface; polyethylene wear; atraumatic or traumatic periprosthetic fracture; and, in rare instances, heterotopic ossification.[71] Of these late complications, mechanical loosening of the components is by far the most common and typically requires revision arthroplasty.

Dislocation: a closer look. Dislocation of the operated hip is a complication that occurs most frequently during the first 2 to 3 months postoperatively when soft tissues around the hip joint are healing. The frequency of early dislocation after primary THA is reported to be less than 1% to slightly more than 10%, with a mean of just less than 2%.[100] During the first postoperative year, revision arthroplasty rates (5.1%) are higher than rates for primary THA (1.7%).[73] Most dislocations are nontraumatic, occur in a posterior direction,[81,107] and are usually associated with a posterior surgical approach.[3,59] Although less common, dislocation can also occur after anterior, anterolateral, and direct lateral approaches.[81,107,129] Patient-related and surgery/prosthesis-related risk factors that may contribute to dislocation are noted in Table 20.3.[73,100] Precautions to reduce the risk of dislocation after THA are addressed in the following section on postoperative management (see Box 20.6). Although a first-time dislocation usually can be managed with closed reduction and conservative treatment, recurrent dislocation after THA typically requires additional surgery.

Leg length inequality: a closer look. Leg length inequality is one of the more common complaints during the early

TABLE 20.3 Risk Factors Contributing to Joint Dislocation After Total Hip Arthroplasty

Patient-Related Factors	Surgery/Prosthesis-Related Factors
▪ Age > 80 to 85 years[100,107] ▪ THA for femoral neck fracture	▪ Surgical approach: higher risk with posterior than anterior, anterolateral, or lateral approaches
▪ Medical diagnosis: higher risk in patients with inflammatory arthritis (mostly RA) than patients with OA[73,174]	▪ Design of femoral component: higher risk with smaller-sized femoral head[73] ▪ Malpositioning of the acetabular component
▪ Poor quality soft tissue from chronic inflammatory disease ▪ History of prior hip surgery ▪ Preoperative and postoperative muscle weakness (particularly the abductor mechanism)[69] and contractures ▪ Cognitive dysfunction, dementia	▪ Inadequate soft tissue balancing during surgery or poor quality soft tissue repair ▪ Experience of the surgeon

recovery period after THA and is associated with pain and a sense of instability and exertion while walking.[33,128] Quite often a functional leg length discrepancy and pelvic obliquity that is evident during standing and walking is the result of muscle spasm, muscle weakness (particularly the gluteus medius), and residual contracture of hip muscles. This type of leg length discrepancy usually resolves with conservative management during the first postoperative year.[33] However, a true leg length discrepancy may be the result of over-lengthening the limb during surgery, malpositioning of the prosthetic implants (usually the acetabular component), or recurrent postoperative dislocation. If significant, it may necessitate further surgery or revision arthroplasty.[128] Leg length differences of greater than 20 mm are associated with significant gait abnormalities and protracted low back pain.[173]

Postoperative Management

Early Mobilization

After THA, there is no need for immobilization of the operated hip. To the contrary, postoperative rehabilitation emphasizes early movement and patients are encouraged to regularly move the hip through allowed ROM. An exception to this postoperative strategy may be required when the patient is lying supine in bed, depending on the surgical approach used and the stability of the prosthetic hip. In such cases, the operated limb is positioned in slight abduction and neutral rotation using an abduction pillow or wedge.[94]

Weight-Bearing Considerations

After cemented THA, patients are usually permitted to bear as much weight as tolerated almost immediately after surgery.[15,125,135] In contrast, with cementless or hybrid THA, weight bearing on the operated limb is often restricted for the first few weeks or more. A number of factors affect the extent and duration of postoperative weight-bearing restrictions. Box 20.5 summarizes these factors.

Although it has been customary to limit weight bearing after cementless and hybrid THA,[17,160] this practice deserves a closer look. The rationale for restricted weight bearing is based on the assumption that early, excessive loading of the operated limb could cause micromovement at the bone-implant interface, thereby jeopardizing the initial stability of the implant(s), interfering with osseous ingrowth, and contributing to eventual loosening of the prosthetic implants. There is little evidence, however, to support these concerns.[65]

Moreover, there are potential benefits to safe levels of early weight bearing after THA, specifically the reduction of bone demineralization from decreased weight bearing and earlier recovery of functional mobility.[20,22] Gradually progressed weight bearing also promotes activation of the weakened hip abductor muscles for stabilization of the pelvis and a more symmetrical gait pattern.[65]

To further strengthen the case for early weight bearing as tolerated, it has been established that many patients have difficulty learning and integrating prescribed weight-bearing limitations into daily functional activities and consequently place greater loads than recommended on the operated extremity, particularly once postoperative pain has subsided.[162] For example, a recent analysis of walking on level surfaces and stairs showed that THA patients had foot loads of between 41% and 88% of their peak presurgical loading, even after being trained with a scale to use only 10% loading.[143] It is also known that some resisted movements of the lower extremity performed in the supine position impose loads on the hip considerably greater than body weight.[120]

In light of these considerations, the need for weight-bearing restrictions after cementless THA is being re-examined.

BOX 20.5 Early Postoperative Weight-Bearing Restrictions After Total Hip Arthroplasty

Method of Fixation

- *Cemented.* Immediate postoperative weight bearing as tolerated.[15,94,125]
- *Cementless and hybrid.* Recommendations vary from partial weight bearing (toe-touch or touch-down) for at least 6 weeks[17,76,81,97] to weight bearing as tolerated (no restrictions) immediately after surgery.[13,20,22]

Surgical Approach

- *Traditional versus minimally invasive.* Weight bearing usually more restricted after standard (traditional) approach because of more extensive surgical disturbance and repair than minimally invasive approach.[14] Weight bearing as tolerated may be permissible immediately after minimally invasive procedure.[13]
- *Trochanteric osteotomy.* Although used infrequently, restricted weight bearing at least 6 to 8 weeks or possibly 12 to 16 weeks for bone healing.

Other Factors

- *Use of bone grafts.* Nonweight bearing or restricted weight bearing during bone healing.
- *Poor quality of patient's bone.* Extended restrictions so as not to jeopardize the stability of the prosthetic implants.

FOCUS ON EVIDENCE

Several randomized, controlled investigations have demonstrated that immediate weight bearing as tolerated after cementless or hybrid hip arthroplasty does not result in higher rates of adverse effects.[20,22,74] Bottner et al[22] compared patients who were allowed immediate weight bearing with no restrictions to a group restricted to toe-touch weight bearing with the use of two crutches for 6 weeks. Boden et al[20] evaluated an immediate weight-bearing group that initially used one crutch to a group using two crutches and limited to 10% body weight for 3 months. Kishida et al[74] compared a group that was allowed full weight bearing on the second day after surgery to a group limited to touchdown weight bearing for 3 weeks, partial weight bearing for the next 6 weeks, and full weight bearing at 6 weeks. None of the studies found significant between group differences in adverse effects, including implant fixation integrity, for up to 5 years after surgery. The authors suggest that early weight bearing as tolerated after cementless or hybrid primary THA can be safe in younger patients (< 60 to 65 years of age) with excellent bone quality. It is important to note that patients in these studies were relatively young compared with most patients undergoing hip arthroplasty.

A systematic review of the literature comparing unrestricted to restricted weight bearing notes moderate to strong evidence in support of immediate weight bearing to tolerance for a young, healthy population following cementless primary THA.[65] However, in the clinical setting, the responsibility of determining the need for protected weight bearing during the early phase of postoperative rehabilitation after THA remains with the surgeon.

Exercise Progression and Functional Training

Therapeutic exercise has been part of postoperative rehabilitation for patients after THA for many years. Despite this, the optimal exercises and their doses are not fully established, perhaps because surgical procedures and approaches continue to evolve and interventions are still adapting to these changes. A consensus survey on physical therapy-related intervention for early inpatient total hip rehabilitation was a step forward in the development of consistent guidelines for postoperative THA management,[43] although many of the exercises and functional activities identified in this document have not been evaluated for effectiveness or efficacy.[104] The goals, guidelines, and precautions for exercise and functional activities after primary THA discussed in this section represent not only those interventions identified in the aforementioned consensus survey, but also exercises and activities selected from current literature.[24,40,62,94,112,123,166]

FOCUS ON EVIDENCE

Several single-subject studies have measured *in vivo* hip forces acting and acetabular contact pressures during exercise and gait.[53,79,80,152] Although these studies analyzed only two patients after insertion of a femoral endoprosthesis, not a total joint replacement, the results raise questions about assumptions made by clinicians regarding the selection and progression of exercises and functional activities during THA rehabilitation. The results suggest that some active or resistive exercises—such as maximal effort gluteal setting, unassisted heel slides, and manually resisted isometric abduction—may generate acetabular contact pressures that are greater than weight-bearing contact pressures.[53,152]

Accelerated Rehabilitation

One change in postoperative management is the trend toward accelerated rehabilitation, particularly for patients under 60 to 65 years of age who have undergone minimally invasive THA and wish to resume an active lifestyle as quickly as possible following surgery.[13,41] Although "accelerated rehabilitation" following minimally invasive THA has not been clearly defined, two characteristics stand out—a rapid progression to full weight bearing during ambulation and discontinuing crutch and cane use as soon as possible.

There is concern, however, that progressing ambulation at this rate in the presence of postoperative strength and balance deficits could result in persistent gait asymmetries, increase the risk of injury, or jeopardize short- and long-term outcomes.[42] In addition, during functional activities that require endurance, persistent muscular weakness and fatigue may increase the stresses placed on the prosthetic hip, thereby contributing to biomechanical loosening of the components over time.[147]

Therefore, before discontinuing use of an ambulation aid, it is important to regain sufficient strength of the hip abductors and extensors to maintain stability and symmetry during ambulation. With this in mind, it is clear that an individualized program of strengthening exercises must be an integral component of accelerated rehabilitation.[65]

Exercise: Maximum Protection Phase After Traditional THA

Common impairments exhibited by patients during the acute and subacute stages of soft tissue healing and the initial phase of rehabilitation after THA are pain secondary to the surgical procedure, decreased ROM, muscle guarding and weakness, impaired postural stability and balance, and decreased functional mobility (transfers and ambulation activities). Depending on the type of component fixation used and the surgeon's preference, weight-bearing restrictions may also interfere with some functional activities.

The emphasis of this phase of rehabilitation after a conventional surgical approach is on patient education to reduce the risk of early postoperative complications, in particular dislocation of the operated hip. (Risk factors for dislocation after THA are noted in Table 20.3.) Precautions during functional activities are determined by the surgical approach used and input from the surgeon about the intraoperative stability of the hip replacement (Box 20.6).[81,94,106,107,129]

Selected exercises and functional training begin as soon as the patient is medically stable, typically the day of surgery when possible. The frequency of treatment by a therapist is often twice a day until the patient is discharged from the hospital.[43,123] The average length of hospitalization after a THA is age dependent, with younger patients averaging 3 days and older patients 4 days.[169]

Goals and interventions. The following goals and interventions apply to the initial postoperative days while the patient is hospitalized and continue through the first few weeks after

BOX 20.6 Early Postoperative Motion Precautions After Total Hip Arthroplasty*

Posterior/Posterolateral Approaches

ROM
- Avoid hip flexion > 90° and adduction and internal rotation beyond neutral.

ADL
- Transfer to the sound side from bed to chair or chair to bed.
- Do not cross the legs.
- Keep the knees slightly lower than the hips when sitting.
- Avoid sitting in low, soft chairs.
- If the bed at home is low, raise it on blocks.
- Use a raised toilet seat.
- Avoid bending the trunk over the legs when rising from or sitting down in a chair or dressing or undressing.
- When bathing, take showers, or use a shower chair in the bathtub.
- When ascending stairs, lead with the sound leg; when descending, lead with the operated leg.
- Pivot on the sound lower extremity.
- Avoid standing activities that involve rotating the body toward the operated extremity.
- Sleep in supine position with an abduction pillow; avoid sleeping or resting in a side-lying position.

Anterior/Anterolateral and Direct Lateral Approaches

ROM
- Avoid hip flexion > 90°.**
- Avoid hip extension, adduction, and external rotation past neutral.
- Avoid the combined motion of hip flexion, abduction, and external rotation.
- If the gluteus medius was incised and repaired or a trochanteric osteotomy was done, do not perform active, antigravity hip abduction for at least 6 to 8 weeks or until approved by the surgeon.

ADL
- Do not cross the legs.
- During early ambulation, step to, rather than past, the operated hip to avoid hyperextension.
- Avoid activities that involve standing on the operated extremity and rotating away from the involved side.

Transgluteal Approach (Trochanteric Osteotomy)***

ROM
- Avoid hip adduction past neutral
- No active, antigravity hip abduction for at least 6 to 8 weeks or until approved by the surgeon
- No exercises that involve weight bearing on the operated leg

ADL
- Sleep in supine position with abduction pillow
- Do not cross legs
- Maintain weight-bearing restrictions during all ADLs

*Precautions apply to traditional total hip arthroplasty and may or may not be necessary after minimally invasive procedures, depending on the surgeon's guidelines.

**Although a posterior surgical approach is associated with the highest risk of dislocation, all patients routinely are asked to limit hip flexion to < 90° and rotation to < 45° for about 6 weeks regardless of the surgical approach used.[129]

***Follow weight-bearing restrictions for 6 to 8 weeks or up to 12 weeks for bone healing to occur.

surgery when the patient is at home or in a subacute healthcare or skilled nursing facility.

- ***Prevent vascular and pulmonary complications.***
  - Ankle pumping exercise to prevent venous stasis, thrombus formation, and the potential for pulmonary embolism.
  - Deep breathing exercise and bronchial hygiene until the patient is regularly mobile to prevent postoperative atelectasis or pneumonia.
- ***Prevent postoperative dislocation or subluxation of the operated hip.***
  - Patient and caregiver education about motion restrictions, safe bed mobility, transfers, and precautions during ADLs (see Box 20.6).
  - Monitor the patient for signs and symptoms of joint dislocation, such as shortening of the operated lower extremity.
- ***Achieve independent functional mobility prior to discharge.***
  - Bed mobility, rising from and sitting down in a chair, and transfer training, emphasizing proper trunk and lower extremity alignment and integrating weight-bearing and motion restrictions.

CLINICAL TIP

Rising from a low chair imposes particularly high-loads across the hip joint, producing loads approximately eight times the patient's body weight.[120] If the posterior capsule was incised during surgery, this places the involved hip at a high risk of posterior dislocation until soft tissues around the hip joint have healed sufficiently (at least 6 weeks) or until the surgeon indicates that unrestricted functional activities are permissible. Therefore, teach the patient the importance of sitting only on a chair with an elevated seat and to avoid sitting on soft, low furniture.

- Ambulation with an assistive device (initially a walker or two crutches) immediately after surgery, adhering to weight-bearing restrictions and gait-related ADL precautions. Emphasize a stable, symmetrical gait pattern. Progress to one crutch or a cane depending on pain, strength of hip abductors, and gait symmetry.
- Stair training with an assistive device, both ascending and descending, initially one step at a time.

PRECAUTION: Even if a patient is permitted to bear full weight on the operated extremity and discontinue crutch or cane use as tolerated, have the patient continue to use an ambulation aid when ascending and descending stairs during the first few weeks after surgery to reduce the risk of placing excessive torsional forces on the prosthetic hip joint.[65]

- ***Maintain a functional level of strength and muscular endurance in the upper extremities and nonoperated lower extremity.***
  - Active-resistive exercises in functional movement patterns, targeting muscle groups used during transfers and ambulation with assistive devices.
- ***Prevent reflex inhibition and atrophy of musculature in the operated limb.***
  - *Submaximal* muscle-setting exercises of the quadriceps, hip extensor, and hip abductor muscles—just enough to elicit a muscle contraction.

PRECAUTION: If a trochanteric osteotomy was performed, avoid even low-intensity isometric contractions of the hip abductors during the early postoperative phase unless initially approved by the surgeon and performed strictly at a minimum intensity. (See Box 20.6 for additional precautions after trochanteric osteotomy.)

- ***Regain active mobility and control of the operated extremity.***
  - While in bed, active-assistive ROM exercises of the hip within protected ranges.
  - Active knee flexion and extension exercises while seated in a chair, emphasizing terminal knee extension.
  - Active hip rotation, maintaining motion limitations based on the surgical approach.
  - If the status of the abductor muscles permits, active, gravity-eliminated hip abduction in the supine position by sliding the leg on a low-friction surface or active antigravity abduction combined with external rotation (clam exercise) in the side-lying position (with a pillow between the thighs to prevent hip adduction past neutral).
  - Active hip ROM (forward and backward pendular motions) in the standing position with the hands on a stable surface to maintain balance.
  - Bilateral, closed-chain, weight-shifting activities, heel raises, and mini-squats, while maintaining symmetrical alignment and weight-bearing limitations on the operated extremity.
- ***Prevent a flexion contracture of the operated hip.***
  - Avoid use of a pillow under the knee of the operated extremity while in supine.

Criteria to progress. The criteria to advance to the next phase of rehabilitation is highly dependent on weight-bearing and ROM restrictions; however, the following criteria typically must be met:

- Well-healed incision; no signs of wound drainage or infection
- Independent level-ground ambulation with one crutch or a cane or no assistive device if weight-bearing restrictions permit
- Ability to bear full weight on the operated extremity without pain and with a fully extended knee
- Functional ROM of the hip
- Muscle strength of operated hip: at least 3/5

Exercise: Moderate Protection Phase After Traditional THA

After traditional THA, the intermediate phase of rehabilitation begins at about 4 to 6 weeks postoperatively. Full weight bearing may be permitted for some patients, but some degree of protection may be necessary for 12 weeks postoperatively for others. The extent of protection of the operated hip varies substantially based on the surgical approach, the type of fixation used, and the surgeon's preference. Full healing of soft tissue and bone continues for up to a year after surgery.

The exercises described for this phase may be carried out under therapist supervision or as part of a home program. Exercises and functional training focus on restoring muscle strength (particularly the hip abductors and extensors), postural stability and balance, a symmetrical gait pattern, muscular and cardiopulmonary endurance, and functional ROM. Exercises that target impairments in other body regions can also be included to improve overall function.

Postoperative precautions during ADL may continue for at least 12 weeks and sometimes considerably longer.[94,112] Patient education should focus on the return to anticipated activities in the home, workplace, or recreational setting.

Goals and interventions. The following are the goals and interventions for the intermediate (moderate protection) phase of rehabilitation:

- ***Regain strength and muscular endurance, emphasizing strength of hip abductors and extensors.***

PRECAUTION: The initiation and progression of resistance training to strengthen hip abductor muscles depends on the integrity of the abductor mechanism, which can be compromised during some surgical approaches. Likewise, progressing from bilateral to unilateral closed-chain training depends on when full weight bearing on the operated extremity is permitted.

  - While standing on the sound lower extremity, open-chain exercises within the permissible ranges in the operated leg against light resistance. Initially, emphasize increasing the number of repetitions rather than the resistance to improve muscular endurance.
  - Bilateral, closed-chain exercises to strengthen hip and knee extensors, such as mini-squats against light-grade elastic resistance or while holding light weights in both hands when unsupported standing, are permitted. Reinforce symmetrical alignment of the lower extremities during standing exercises.
  - Unilateral, closed-chain exercises, such as hip hiking or forward and lateral step-ups (to a low step) while standing on the operated extremity and partial lunges

with the involved foot forward when full weight bearing, are permitted on the operated lower extremity. During step-ups and lunges, apply elastic resistance around the lateral thigh of the operated extremity to simultaneously strengthen the hip abductors and hip extensors.

- ***Improve cardiopulmonary endurance.***
  - Nonimpact aerobic conditioning program, such as progressive stationary cycling, swimming, or water aerobics.
- ***Restore ROM while adhering to precautions.***
  - Gravity-assisted supine stretch to neutral in the Thomas test position. Pull the uninvolved knee to the chest while relaxing the operated hip. (At least 10° of hip extension beyond neutral is needed for a normal gait pattern.)
  - Resting in a prone position for a prolonged passive stretch of the hip flexor muscles.
  - Integrate gained ROM into functional activities.

PRECAUTION: Check with the surgeon before initiating a stretch of the hip flexors to neutral or into hyperextension, particularly if an anterior or anterolateral approach was used during surgery. In addition, prone lying may not be permissible or comfortable for the patient at this time.

- ***Improve postural stability, balance, and gait.***
  - Progressive balance activities in standing (see Chapters 8 and 23.)
  - Gait training, emphasizing an erect trunk, vertical alignment, equal step lengths, and a neutral symmetrical alignment of the pelvis and extremities.
  - If full weight bearing is not yet permitted, continue or progress to use of a cane (in the hand *contralateral* to the operated hip) and progress weight bearing on the operated limb. Practice walking on uneven and soft surfaces to challenge the balance system.
  - Continue cane use until weight-bearing restrictions are discontinued or if the patient exhibits gait deviations, such as a positive Trendelenburg sign on the operated lower extremity, indicating hip abductor weakness. Cane use is also recommended during extended periods of ambulation to decrease muscle fatigue.
  - For selected patients, consider treadmill walking to practice a symmetrical gait pattern.

FOCUS ON EVIDENCE

Use of a cane in the contralateral hand by patients after a hip replacement has been shown to decrease electromyographic (EMG) activity in the hip abductor muscles to a significant degree regardless of whether moderate or near-maximum force is applied on the cane.[116] In the same study, ipsilateral cane use produced no significant decrease in EMG activity in the hip abductor muscles. The degree to which the decreases in EMG activity reflected a reduction in forces imposed on the prosthetic hip joint was not determined in this study. However, in single-subject studies of two patients with femoral endoprostheses, acetabular contact pressures were reduced by using a cane in the contralateral hand.[53,79,80]

Criteria to progress. The criteria to progress to advanced training during a final phase of rehabilitation include the following:

- Pain-free ambulation with or without a cane
- Functional ROM and strength of the operated hip
- Independence in ADL

Exercise: Minimum Protection Phase and Resumption of Full Activity

After traditional THA, the final phase of rehabilitation begins when the patient has met the criteria to progress. This usually occurs around 12 weeks postoperatively. Continued training for restoration of strength, muscular and cardiopulmonary endurance, balance, and a symmetrical gait pattern should be the focus of this phase, coupled with a gradual resumption or modification of functional activities. Return to a full level of functional activities may take at least a year.[132]

Extended rehabilitation and modification of activities. Weakness of the hip abductors leading to pelvic obliquity and an asymmetrical gait pattern often presents preoperatively in patients with hip OA and has been shown to persist in some patients for months following THA.[147] With this in mind, patients, especially those wishing to return to an active lifestyle, may benefit from an extended strength training program that targets the hip musculature.

If ongoing rehabilitation services are available to a patient, the following activities should be considered:

- Integrate strength, endurance, and balance training into simulated functional activities to prepare for independence.
- To improve muscular and cardiopulmonary endurance, progressively increase the length of time and distance of a low-intensity walking program. Aim for a target frequency of 2 to 4 days a week for 30 minutes each session for the walking program.
- Through patient education, reinforce the importance of selecting or modifying activities to reduce or minimize the forces and demands placed on the prosthetic hip. When a patient's employment involves heavy labor, vocational retraining or an adjustment in work-related activities is advised.

CLINICAL TIP

When walking and carrying a heavy object in one hand, suggest that the patient hold it on the same side as the operated hip. EMG studies have shown that under these circumstances the forces imposed on the abductor muscles of the operated hip are significantly lower than when the load is carried on the contralateral arm. This was found to hold true with and without cane usage.[114,115] Theoretically, this reduces the amount of stress imposed on the hip replacement over time.

Return to sport activities. The younger, active patient who has undergone THA usually has a desire to resume sport-related or fitness activities at some point following surgery.

Several factors, including the level of demand or degree of impact or twisting movements involved in the activity, the frequency of repetitive motions, and the potential for falls or contact, influence a surgeon's recommendation or approval for a patient to participate in various athletic activities. A patient's body weight, overall level of fitness, and his or her experience with the activity prior to surgery also affect whether or not an activity is allowable.[34,61,75,97]

To prolong the life of the hip replacement, a patient is routinely advised to refrain from high-impact sports and recreational activities. Activities that impose heavy rotational forces on the operated hip are of particular concern and could contribute to long-term loosening and wear of the prosthetic implants and eventual failure of the hip replacement. However, with a foundation of sufficient strength, endurance, balance, and use of proper biomechanics during functional activities, a patient can gradually and safely return to low- and moderate-impact sports and fitness activities following THA.

Table 20.4 lists the sports-related, recreational, and fitness activities highly recommended, recommended with caution, or not recommended based on a 2007 survey and the consensus of arthroplasty surgeons' opinions.[75] Ninety percent of the surgeons responding agreed that patients could return to selected activities by 6 months after undergoing THA.

Outcomes

Pain relief, patient satisfaction, and quality of life. Most studies evaluating patient satisfaction, perceived levels of pain, function, and quality of life after THA reflect a marked decrease in pain and improvement in function.[84,132] However, patient's and surgeon's perceptions of satisfaction do not always agree. Lieberman and associates[87] demonstrated that when a patient reported little or no pain following THA, the patient's and surgeon's assessments of pain and level of satisfaction were similar. However, when patient's reported continuing pain after THA, there was less agreement between the patient's and surgeon's assessments of the level of patient satisfaction. This result explains why there is a need for outcome assessments from both the patient and the health-care professional.

Several factors may contribute to unsatisfactory outcomes following THA. Fortin and colleagues[48] investigated the timing of THA and subsequent outcomes and determined that, not surprisingly, patients who had the worst physical function and pain before surgery had the poorest outcomes 2 years after surgery. Another long-term, prospective study (mean 3.6 years) of patients who had undergone unilateral THA for OA also confirmed that a higher preoperative level of pain predicted poorer outcomes.[119] This study also revealed that an older age at the time of surgery and the presence of postoperative low back pain were predictors of poor self-assessed outcomes.[119]

Physical functioning. Improvements in ROM, postural stability, strength, and functional mobility occur gradually after THA. Patients typically achieve 90% of their expected level of overall functional improvement by the end of the first postsurgical year. Over the next 1 to 2 years, patients report additional gains in strength and improved function, reaching a plateau at approximately 2 to 3 years after surgery.[132]

Trudelle-Jackson and colleagues[161] evaluated ROM, static muscle strength, and single-leg balance in a group of 15 patients with a mean age of 62 years (range, 51 to 77 years) 1 year after unilateral, primary THA. They found no significant differences in ROM between the operated and uninvolved hips and small—but not statistically significant—differences in the strength of hip and knee musculature. However, they did find substantial differences between the operated leg and the uninvolved leg for all parameters of balance measured during a one-leg stance. In addition, patients' self-assessed levels of physical function were moderately associated with muscle strength but only weakly with postural stability.

Implant design, fixation, and surgical approach. Several decades of studies indicate that both cemented and cementless THA result in equally positive postoperative outcomes in all

TABLE 20.4 Guidelines for Participation in Sport, Recreational, and Fitness Activities Following THA[75]

Allowed	Allowed With Caution and Prior Experience	Not Allowed*
▪ Golf ▪ Swimming ▪ Walking (outdoor/treadmill) ▪ Stationary cycling or use of elliptical trainer ▪ Cross-country ski unit ▪ Bowling ▪ Low-impact aerobics ▪ Speed walking ▪ Hiking ▪ Stair-climbing or rowing units ▪ Doubles tennis ▪ Use of weight machines	▪ Pilates ▪ Cross-country skiing ▪ Rollerblading ▪ Ice skating ▪ Downhill skiing	▪ Jogging/running ▪ Baseball/softball ▪ Racquetball/squash ▪ Snow boarding ▪ High-impact aerobics ▪ Contact sports (football, basketball, soccer)

Note: Whether singles tennis or martial arts was allowable was not determined in the survey.

areas of assessment, with the most consistent being pain reduction.[85,135] In-depth analyses and current information on outcomes of specific prosthetic designs, as well as outcome assessments of cemented, cementless, and hybrid procedures, can be found in the references previously cited in the operative overview of THA presented earlier in this chapter.

Woolson and colleagues[170] conducted a retrospective comparative study of 135 patients who had undergone primary, unilateral THA with either a standard posterior approach or a minimally invasive posterior approach. The participating surgeons determined which patients met the criteria for the minimally invasive procedure with regard to health history and body mass index. Consequently, the minimally invasive group was thinner and healthier than the conventional THA group. Despite this, there were no significant differences between the groups with respect to surgical outcomes (operating time, blood loss, need for transfusion) or in length of hospital stay or the percentage of patients discharged directly home. However, there was a higher rate of complications in the minimally invasive group, including wound complications, component malpositioning, and leg-length discrepancy. More recently, Goosen and colleagues reported no significant differences in perioperative blood loss or complications between subjects randomized to minimally invasive (n = 60) and traditional (n = 60) THA groups,[56] although mean operation times were shorter in the minimally invasive group. Similarly, Repantis and colleagues[137] noted no perioperative or immediate postoperative benefit to the minimally invasive approach over the traditional approach for THA. In this comparison, the same experienced surgeon performed either an anterior minimally invasive procedure (n = 45) or an anterior traditional procedure (n = 45). Although the minimally invasive group had lower pain intensity at 2 weeks postoperatively, there were no differences between groups for function or walking endurance.[137]

Ogonda and colleagues[122] conducted a randomized controlled trial comparing minimally invasive and traditional THA in 219 patients undergoing primary, unilateral, hybrid THA performed by the same surgeon. In both groups, a single incision, posterior approach was used, with the only differences being a shorter skin incision and less TFL disturbance during the minimally invasive approach. All patients participated in exercise and functional training after surgery. The only statistically significant group difference identified was less blood loss in the minimally invasive group, with no significant differences in postoperative pain and use of pain medication, ability to transfer and ambulate with an assistive device, length of hospital stay, or discharge to home or transitional facility. At 6 weeks postsurgery, there continued to be no significant differences between groups related to function or complications. Dorr and colleagues[42] reported similar in-hospital findings, with less pain on each postoperative day and a shorter hospital stay for a minimally invasive group compared with a traditional THA group.

A number of prospective, randomized studies have been conducted to compare improvements in gait following minimally invasive versus traditional, unilateral THA. Results of a study by Mayr and coinvestigators[96] demonstrated significant improvement in several gait parameters at 6 weeks in the group that underwent minimally invasive THA but not in the traditional THA group. At 12 weeks, however, both groups showed significant improvements in gait, but the minimally invasive group improved in a larger number of the parameters measured. In contrast, another gait study reported no significant differences in gait characteristics between the minimally invasive and traditional THA groups at 10 days and 12 weeks after surgery.[131] Recently published analyses reported similar results, with no differences in walking speed, step length, cadence, or pelvic and thoracic motion between minimally invasive groups and traditional approach groups.[109,136] It is important to note that postoperative rehabilitation in these studies was uniform between groups, which may have contributed to the similarity of outcomes in the minimally invasive and traditional THA groups.

Lastly, Dorr and colleagues[42] also investigated improvements in functional mobility following THA and found that 87% of patients in the minimally invasive group used just one assistive device (crutch or cane) for ambulation at the time of discharge compared to 53% of the traditional THA group. However, there was no significant difference in walking distance at the time of discharge between the two groups. With the mixed findings from studies such as these, it is difficult to draw evidence-based conclusions about the impact of minimally invasive procedures versus traditional THA on early postoperative ambulation.

Impact of rehabilitation. Despite the number of sources in the literature that emphasize the importance of rehabilitation programs or, more specifically, a postoperative exercise and ambulation program after THA, the impact of postoperative interventions following THA has not been clearly established. Studies have demonstrated that access to inpatient physical therapy services does[49,111] and does not[82] decrease a patient's length of stay in an acute care facility after THA. It has also been shown that the use of physical therapy services after THA increases the probability of discharge to the home setting rather than to another healthcare facility.[49] The inclusion of exercise and gait training interventions provided by a physical therapist in addition to instruction given by a multidisciplinary hip group immediately after surgery resulted in greater hip ROM and strength and improved mobility than instruction alone at 15 days postsurgery.[163]

In a nonrandomized study of the effectiveness of a 6-week home exercise program with patients who were 6 to 48 months post THA, the two exercise groups (one performing ROM and hip muscle isometrics and the other performing ROM, isometric, and eccentric exercises) increased their walking speed, whereas a control group (no exercise program) did not. Interestingly, strength improvements were noted in all three groups.[132]

A randomized trial that enrolled subjects 3 months after posterolateral THA showed that participants who completed

12 sessions of training that was led by a physical therapist and emphasizing walking skills had significantly greater improvements on several performance-based and self-report outcome measures. When compared to a control group that did not have supervised therapy, greater improvements were noted at 5 months postsurgery in the intervention group for the 6-minute walk test, stair climbing time, figure-of-eight test, the Index of Muscle Function, hip extension ROM, the Harris Hip Score, and self-efficacy in the training group. Group differences in walking distance and stair climbing persisted at 12 months postsurgery, and there were fewer fall events reported in the walking skill training group.[62]

Mikkelsen and colleagues evaluated the effect of a twice-weekly progressive resistance training intervention following THA, comparing it to a home program of standard hip and knee resistance exercises. The intervention group (n = 32) performed 30 to 40 minutes of unilateral hip strengthening exercises on strength-training machines, using both concentric and eccentric contraction and loads that increased based on the repetition maximum, while the control group (n = 30) performed 10 repetitions of unloaded hip and knee movements twice a day for 4 weeks, followed by the same movements against elastic resistance for an additional 6 weeks. After 10 weeks of training, there were statistically significant group differences for maximal walking speed and stair climbing time in favor of the intervention group, but no other significant differences, including measures of hip strength and power.[102]

Hemiarthroplasty of the Hip

Indications for Surgery

The following are some of the main indications for prosthetic replacement of the proximal femur:[54,76,78]

- Acute, displaced intracapsular (subcapital, transcervical) fractures of the proximal femur in an elderly patient with poor bone quality and an anticipated low-demand level of activity after surgery[54,76,101,126,127,155]
- Failed internal fixation of intracapsular fractures associated with osteonecrosis of the head of the femur[76,101,126]
- Severe degeneration of the head of the femur associated with long-standing hip disease or deformity, resulting in disabling pain and loss of function that cannot be managed with nonoperative procedures[76,101,127]

NOTE: Patients with preexisting degenerative hip disease who sustain a femoral fracture are candidates for primary THA rather than hemiarthroplasty.[46,101] Acute, severely comminuted intertrochanteric fractures are *infrequently* managed by primary hemiarthroplasty.[101,156]

FOCUS ON EVIDENCE

A recent assessment of the American Board of Orthopaedic Surgery database regarding femoral neck fractures showed that between 1999 and 2011, the use of THA increased 7% while the use of hemiarthroplasty decreased 4%. Patients younger than 65 years old were even more likely to have THA than arthroplasty.[103]

Procedures

Background. Historically, acute displaced proximal femur fractures were treated with unipolar (fixed head), uncemented metal-stemmed endoprostheses. The primary complication associated with these single-component implants, regardless of design or fixation, was progressive erosion of the acetabular cartilage and subsequent pain.

To decrease acetabular wear, the bipolar hemiarthroplasty was developed. The bipolar design is composed of multiple components: a metal femoral ball-and-stem prosthesis that moves within a free-riding polyethylene shell, which in turn inserts into a metal cup that moves within the acetabulum. The purpose of the multiple-surface, load-bearing design is to dissipate the forces that previously acted directly on the acetabulum through the interposed components.[70,101,126] Contemporary versions of both unipolar and bipolar prostheses are in use today, with debate among surgeons regarding the advantages and disadvantages of one design versus the other.[70,101,126]

Operative procedure. A posterolateral approach is most commonly used for hemiarthroplasty. After visualizing the joint and removing the head of the femur, the metal-stemmed prosthesis is inserted into the shaft of the proximal femur. The femoral stem usually is cemented in place, although bio-ingrowth fixation is also used. Procedures for closure are consistent with THA.

Postoperative Management

For the most part, the postoperative care and rehabilitation for hemiarthroplasty are similar to that described for THA. This includes the considerations and precautions for positioning and ADL, as well as the components and progression of the exercise and ambulation program. As with postoperative management after THA, the selection and progression of exercises and functional activities after hemiarthroplasty tend to reflect the opinions of surgeons and therapists and are based on the potential of specific exercises to remediate impairments and improve function. As a result, the effectiveness of exercise after hemiarthroplasty remains largely unreported. Only limited information on the impact of specific exercises and gait-related activities on the hip joint, per se, after hemiarthroplasty is available in the literature. Some findings from several single-subject studies of two patients with femoral endoprostheses have already been discussed in the previous section of this chapter on THA.[53,79,80,152]

PRECAUTION: Given the significant concerns for long-term erosion of acetabular cartilage after hemiarthroplasty, avoiding exercises that impose the greatest compressive or shearing forces across the hip joint is of critical importance. Exercises should be performed initially at a *submaximal* level and then progressed gradually. *Unassisted* heel slides and *maximum* effort gluteal setting exercises may need to be avoided during the acute phase of postoperative rehabilitation.[152] In the post-acute rehabilitation period, manually resisted hip abduction should be progressed gradually because maximum-effort hip abduction is thought to generate greater forces across the hip joint than protected weight-bearing activities.[53]

Outcomes

Present-day modular, unipolar, and bipolar hemiarthroplasty procedures appear to yield similar results in pain relief, functional outcomes, and type and rate of complications.[76,101,126] Although acetabular wear was identified as the primary concern after the unipolar replacement used several decades ago, the mechanical effectiveness of the bipolar prosthesis in preventing acetabular erosion has yet to be firmly established.[76] In a study of community-dwelling patients age 65 years or older (mean age 80 years) who had undergone hemiarthroplasty with either a bipolar implant or a modular unipolar implant, there were no significant differences between the two groups at 1 year and 4 to 5 years of follow-up with regard to functioning in daily activities or rates of dislocation, infection, or mortality.[167] Results of another study suggest that joint ROM may decrease over time after bipolar hemiarthroplasty, possibly due to the design of the implants. This decreased range was not associated with diminished functional abilities.[70]

Lastly, the use of hemiarthroplasty versus screw fixation for displaced femoral neck fractures in elderly patients was examined in a large (over 4,000 patients), retrospective study conducted in Norway.[54] Results of the study showed that the patients who had undergone hemiarthroplasty had significantly less postoperative pain, fewer secondary surgeries, and were more satisfied with the outcome of the surgery than the group who had undergone internal fixation (screw fixation) of the fracture site.

Hip Fractures: Surgical and Postoperative Management

Hip Fracture: Incidence, Risk Factors, and Impact on Function

A prevalent musculoskeletal occurrence in the elderly is fracture of the hip or, more correctly, fracture of the most proximal portion of the femur in the hip region. The acute signs and symptoms of hip fracture are pain in the groin or hip region, pain with active or passive motion of the hip, or pain with lower extremity weight bearing. The fractured lower extremity appears to be shorter by several centimeters and assumes a position of external rotation.[76,127]

In the United States, the vast majority of hip fractures occur in individuals between the ages of 75 to 85 years, with women accounting for 77.2% of the fractures in this age group.[23] Worldwide, the incidence of hip fracture has stabilized and appears to have decreased slightly in the United States between 1985 and 2005.[23] The total number of hip fractures per year is expected to increase, however, mainly because of the higher proportion of elderly in the population.[76,127] Fewer than 3% of hip fractures are sustained by persons less than 50 years of age[76,127] and are usually associated with high-force, high-impact trauma or with repetitive microtrauma, such as from distance running.

Multiple risk factors, including those related to fall risk, contribute to the increased incidence of hip fracture with age.[27] Risk factors for falls and the potential for hip fractures in the elderly include age-related loss of muscle strength and flexibility, balance and gait deficits associated with musculoskeletal or neurological disorders, low vision, cognitive decline, and medication effects. Loss of bone density and strength associated with osteoporosis typically occurs in the proximal femur, distal radius, and spine, making these sites more susceptible to fracture.[76,127] A forceful rotational motion between the pelvis and lower extremity or the impact from a fall can both cause a fracture of the fragile proximal femur. Although 90% of all hip fractures in the elderly are associated with a fall,[76] it is not yet known if trauma from the fall caused the hip fracture or if a pathological fracture of the hip resulted in the fall.

In addition to the potential fracture mechanisms noted, the inability to absorb the impact of a fall also contributes to the risk of sustaining a fracture.[127] In addition, the characteristics of falling also change with age. As walking speed decreases with age, an older person usually drops and falls to the side, rather than falling forward on outstretched hands as occurs with faster walking speeds.[76,127]

Hip fracture in the elderly is associated with significant functional impairments and loss of independence. Many patients who survive for more than 1 year following hip fracture have limitations in ADLs and functional mobility and require assistance to transfer, dress, walk, and climb stairs.[89,148] The combination of limitations attributable to the hip fracture (not simply age), reduced activity and subsequent deconditioning during the recuperative period, and activity avoidance for fear of falling make it difficult to return to prefracture activity and functional levels.[89,91] Consequently, long-term nursing care or permanent placement in skilled nursing or assisted living facilities is often required.

Postfracture mortality rates in the United States declined from 1985 to 2005.[23] This decline may be the result of improved surgical techniques, which have reduced the need for prolonged immobilization or restricted weight bearing, thus decreasing postoperative complications such as pneumonia and thromboemboli.

Sites and Types of Hip Fracture

Fractures of the proximal femur are broadly classified as *intracapsular* or *extracapsular* and then further subdivided by specific location (Fig. 20.7). Sites and specific types of hip fracture are noted in Box 20.7.[76,98,101,155–157] Of these sites, fractures in the intertrochanteric region are most common, accounting for approximately 50% of all proximal femur fractures.[98] Intracapsular fractures may compromise the vascular

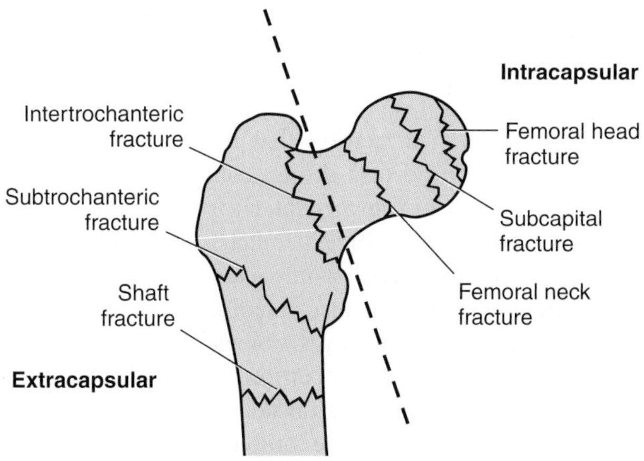

FIGURE 20.7 Fractures of the proximal femur are broadly divided into *intracapsular* and *extracapsular* sites. *(From McKinnis, LN: Fundamentals of Musculoskeletal Imaging, ed. 4. Philadelphia: F.A. Davis, 2014, p 350, with permission.)*

BOX 20.7 Common Sites and Types of Hip Fracture

Intracapsular

- Fracture site proximal to the attachment of the hip joint capsule
- Further subdivided into *femoral head, subcapital* and *femoral neck* (*transcervical* or *basicervical* fractures)
- May be displaced, nondisplaced, or impacted
- May disturb the blood supply to the head of the femur resulting in avascular necrosis or nonunion

Extracapsular

- Fracture site distal to the capsule to a line 5 cm distal to the lesser trochanter
- Further subdivided into *intertrochanteric* (between the greater and lesser trochanters) or *subtrochanteric* and *stable* or *unstable* (comminuted)
- Does not disturb the blood supply to the head of the femur, but nonunion may occur as the result of fixation failure

supply to the head of the femur, which increases the risk of delayed healing, nonunion, or osteonecrosis (avascular necrosis) of the head of the femur. These complications occur far more frequently with displaced versus nondisplaced intracapsular fractures.[76,101] Intracapsular fractures are most often sustained by elderly women.[76,101]

In contrast, fracture-dislocation and acetabular trauma are most common in the young, active individual.[76] Most fracture-dislocations occur in a posterior direction, often causing traumatic disruption of the vascular supply to the head of the femur and damage to joint cartilage. Over time, osteonecrosis and posttraumatic arthritis may result from this type of trauma, necessitating prosthetic replacement of the hip joint.

Nonoperative Management

In some situations, nonoperative management is the only treatment option after hip fracture. Traction is one appropriate alternative treatment for nonambulatory individuals or for medically unstable patients who cannot undergo a surgical procedure.[76,127] The patient remains in bed and the leg in traction just long enough for early healing to occur, followed by bed-to-chair mobilization. If weight bearing or ambulation is feasible, it is delayed until bone healing is sufficient, usually by 10 to 12 weeks or as long as 16 weeks after fracture.

Open Reduction and Internal Fixation of Hip Fracture

Indications for Surgery

Surgical intervention by means of open (or possibly closed) reduction followed by stabilization with internal fixation (Figs. 20.8 and 20.9) is indicated for the following types of proximal femur fracture:[76,127,155–157]

- Displaced or nondisplaced intracapsular femoral neck fractures
- Fracture-dislocations of the head of the femur
- Stable or unstable intertrochanteric fractures
- Subtrochanteric fractures

In the elderly patient, displaced intracapsular fractures often are managed with prosthetic replacement of the femoral

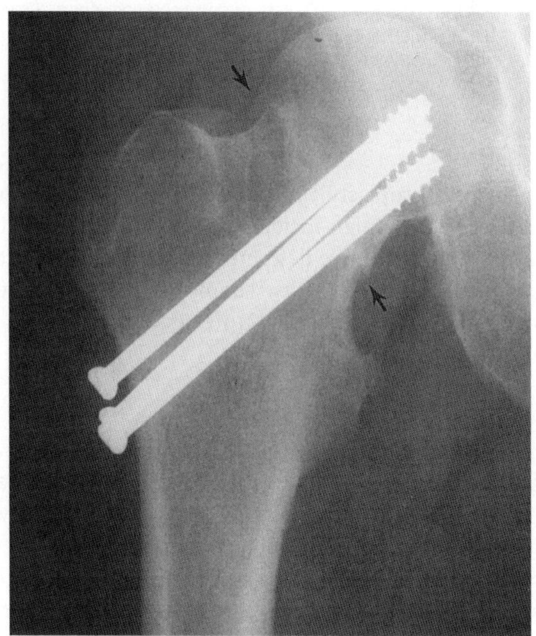

FIGURE 20.8 Reduction and internal fixation of a complete fracture of the femoral neck. Restoration of alignment and good compression is obtained via fixation with three compression screws. The black arrows mark the extent of the fracture line. *(From McKinnis, LN: Fundamentals of Musculoskeletal Imaging, ed. 4. Philadelphia: F.A. Davis, 2014, p 351, with permission.)*

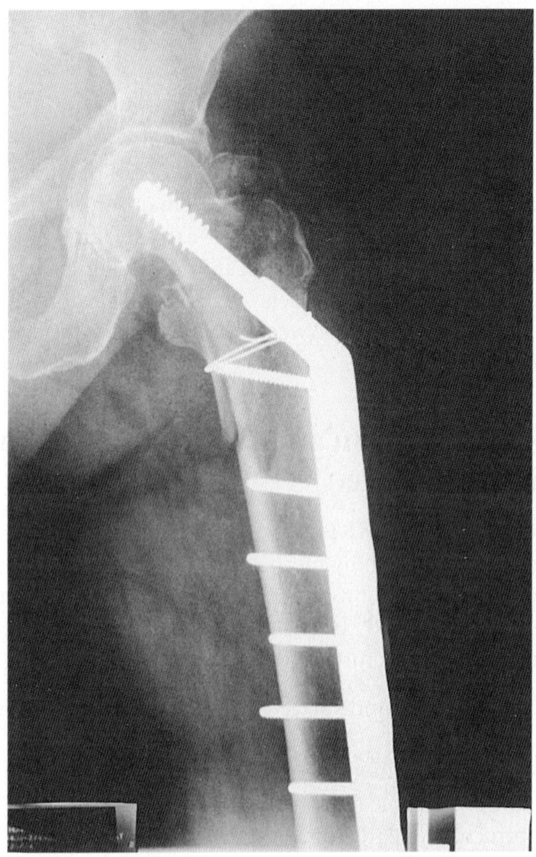

FIGURE 20.9 Intertrochanteric fracture of the hip. This postoperative image shows fracture fixation via a side plate and screw combination device. The fracture line is evident, extending through the intertrochanteric region to the proximal femoral shaft. Some comminution is evident, and a large fragment on the medial shaft is noted. The imposed added densities of soft tissue are seen. *(From McKinnis, LN: Fundamentals of Musculoskeletal Imaging, ed. 4. Philadelphia: F.A. Davis, 2014, p 353, with permission.)*

head (hemiarthroplasty), rather than internal fixation, to avoid the relatively high incidence of nonunion.[54,126] There is, however, no definitive determination as to which procedure provides superior results.[54] Some severely comminuted (unstable) intertrochanteric fractures may also be managed with hemiarthroplasty.[76,101,156]

Procedures

The goal of surgery is to achieve maximum stability and restore the bony alignment of the hip. Surgery is indicated during the first 24 to 48 hours after injury, particularly with intracapsular femoral neck fractures because the risk of disrupted vascular supply to the head of the femur is high. A variety of internal fixation devices are used to stabilize the many types of proximal femur fracture. The type and severity of the fracture, the associated injuries, and the patient's age and physical and cognitive status all influence the surgeon's choice of procedure.[76,127] The type of procedure performed, in turn, affects the progression of postoperative rehabilitation.

Types of fixation and surgical approach. The most common modern, internal fixation devices used include the following:[2,76,127,155–157]

- Intramedullary nail fixation that interlocks proximally in the femoral head or a sliding compression screw for intertrochanteric or subtrochanteric fractures.
- *In situ* fixation with multiple parallel cancellous lag screws or pins for nondisplaced or impacted femoral neck fractures and possibly for displaced femoral neck fractures in active patients less than 65 years of age.
- Dynamic extramedullary fixation with a sliding (compression) hip screw and lateral side plate for stable intertrochanteric fractures; may be combined with an osteotomy for unstable (comminuted) fractures. The dynamic hip screw allows sliding between the screw and plate and creates compression across the fracture site during early weight bearing.

An open surgical approach along the lateral aspect of the hip is used in these fixation procedures, although some aspects of the procedures may be performed percutaneously. The degree of soft tissue disruption differs with each procedure. The tensor fasciae latae, vastus lateralis, or gluteus medius may need to be incised parallel to the fibers and a capsulotomy is generally performed with femoral neck fractures.

Postoperative Management

The ultimate goal of surgical intervention and postoperative care after hip fracture is to return the patient to their preferred living environment[108] at their pre-injury level of function.[76,127] It is generally agreed that rehabilitation services during recovery, including postoperative exercise and functional training across the continuum of care, are recommended and contribute to optimal outcomes.[35,108]

During the initial phase of postoperative rehabilitation in the acute care setting, the emphasis is on mobilization (getting the patient up and moving as quickly as possible) while protecting the stabilized fracture site. This prevents or minimizes the adverse effects of prolonged bed rest. In addition to helping the patient learn to move safely in bed, transfer, and ambulate independently with an assistive device, early postoperative rehabilitation typically includes patient or caregiver education, deep breathing and coughing exercises, lower extremity edema control (use of compressive stockings), proper positioning in bed to avoid contractures, and an exercise program.

After discharge from the hospital, postoperative functional training and a progression of exercises typically continue in a transitional, subacute rehabilitation or skilled nursing facility or at home. Despite consensus that rehabilitation after hospital discharge is an essential aspect of postoperative care,[108] there is little evidence that suggests one rehabilitation setting is superior to another for functional outcomes, and there is insufficient evidence to inform decisions about the optimal components of subacute rehabilitation.[35]

What is known, however, is that most patients are discharged from subacute rehabilitation services after achieving independence in ambulation and necessary ADLs. On average, 85% to 95% of patients receiving physical therapy in the home setting are discharged from services by 7 to 9 weeks after hip fracture.[92] Often, services are discontinued despite persistent impairments and functional deficits and well before patients have attained a pre-injury level of function, which in turn increases the risk of future injury.[19]

Weight-Bearing Considerations

The amount of weight bearing permissible during early ambulation and transfers is always determined by the surgeon for each patient on an individual basis. Factors that influence the decision are the patient's age and bone quality, the fracture location and pattern, the type of fixation used to stabilize the fracture site, and the degree of intraoperative stability achieved.[76,78,127] Recommendations range from nonweight bearing, toe-touch or touch-down weight bearing (< 10 lb), to weight bearing as tolerated. Current internal fixation methods have decreased the need for extended nonweight-bearing or toe-touch status after surgery.

Many fixation procedures used make early weight bearing possible. Some examples of fractures and fixation procedures in which weight bearing as tolerated is permissible immediately after surgery are:

- Nondisplaced, rigidly fixed, or impacted femoral neck fractures managed with *in situ* fixation.[76,78,127,155]
- Stable (noncomminuted) intertrochanteric fractures managed with a dynamic (sliding) compression screw and lateral side plate fixation.[76,127,156]
- Stable intertrochanteric and subtrochanteric fractures managed with interlocking intramedullary nailing and bone-to-bone fixation.[2,76,127,157]

Even when weight bearing is limited during ambulation and transfers, the fracture site is still subjected to significant forces through hip muscle activation. For example, moving in bed, sitting up at the edge of the bed, and active and resisted ROM exercises all generate forces across the hip that approach or even exceed those incurred during full weight-bearing ambulation.[120] Based on this, studies are investigating the risks associated with early weight bearing after open reduction and internal fixation of hip fractures.

FOCUS ON EVIDENCE

In one study, elderly patients with stable as well as comminuted intertrochanteric fractures treated with dynamic compression screw and plate fixation were all allowed to bear weight as tolerated during ambulation with an assistive device immediately after surgery. One year postoperatively, there was no significant difference between the rate of implant failure and revision surgery in the patients with stable fractures and those with comminuted fractures. The investigators concluded that, at least in elderly patients with comminuted and noncomminuted intertrochanteric fractures that were stabilized intraoperatively, there was little biomechanical justification for nonweight-bearing restrictions postoperatively.[78]

Excluded from this generalization were patients with complex fractures in whom satisfactory intraoperative stabilization could not be achieved, young patients with displaced femoral neck fractures with *in situ* fixation, and patients with severe bone disease (e.g., as the result of malignancy).

Despite the findings of this study and the recognized benefits of early ambulation and exercise, there is always a risk, albeit small, of failure of the internal fixation in some patients. Therefore, it is important to recognize the signs of possible displacement or loosening of the fracture stabilization device as summarized in Box 20.8. The presence of any of these signs or symptoms should be reported immediately to the surgeon.[76,127]

Exercise and Functional Training

Decreased joint mobility, ROM, muscle performance, balance, and loss of functional mobility are the most common physical impairments after open reduction and internal fixation of hip fracture. Exercise and functional training continue to be the interventions routinely included throughout current-day postoperative rehabilitation to reduce impairments and improve functional outcomes.[92]

During the initial postoperative period, hip and even knee motions are quite painful, affecting ROM and strength of the involved lower extremity. In addition, some degree of tissue protection is necessary over the course of soft tissue healing (approximately 6 weeks) and bone healing (10 to 16 weeks).[155–157] These factors affect the progression of exercise and functional training, as do the location and stability of the fracture site, type of internal fixation used, and the soft tissues traumatized at the time of the injury and during surgery. Special considerations for exercise and ambulation after various types of hip fracture and with specific surgeries are noted in Box 20.9.[76,127,155–157]

The following sections outline a progression of exercises and functional training after open reduction and internal fixation of hip fractures.

BOX 20.8 Signs and Symptoms of Possible Failure of the Internal Fixation Mechanism

- Severe, persistent groin, thigh, or knee pain that increases with limb movement or weight bearing
- Progressive limb length inequality (shortening of the involved lower extremity) that was not present immediately after surgery
- Persistent external rotation of the operated limb
- A positive Trendelenburg sign during weight bearing on the involved limb that does not resolve with strengthening exercises

BOX 20.9 Special Considerations for Exercise and Gait After Internal Fixation of Fractures of the Proximal Femur

- Multiple hip muscles are traumatized by fracture of the hip, leading to postoperative pain, reflex inhibition, and weakness. Fractures at these sites may cause damage to the following muscles.
  - Greater trochanter: gluteus medius
  - Lesser trochanter: iliopsoas
  - Subtrochanteric region: gluteus maximus
- The tensor fasciae latae (TFL) and vastus lateralis (VL) are usually incised during surgery, causing postoperative pain, inhibition, and weakness during hip abduction and knee flexion.
- Adhesion formation between the incised TFL and VL may develop and restrict motion. Hip adduction and internal rotation and knee flexion place a stretch on the TFL and VL, respectively, during ROM exercises and therefore are often painful.
- If there is shortening of the involved limb after fracture and internal fixation, the distance between the distal insertion of the gluteus medius on the greater trochanter and the center of axis of hip motion is often decreased, thus diminishing the mechanical advantage of the muscle and causing weakness and a positive Trendelenburg sign during ambulation.
- Intracapsular fractures typically traumatize the capsule, and internal fixation requires an incision into the capsule (capsulotomy). Both predispose the capsule to postoperative restriction.

Exercise: Maximum Protection Phase

Exercises begin on the first postoperative day to prevent complications and to restore a patient's control of the involved hip during functional activities. Initially, exercises are directed toward restoring ROM of the involved hip and developing balance and strength in the upper extremities and uninvolved lower extremity to facilitate ambulation with an assistive device. It is reasonable to expect to achieve 80° to 90° of active hip flexion (with the knee flexed) by 2 to 4 weeks postoperatively.[76]

There is lack of consensus about the appropriate time to begin resistance exercises with the involved lower extremity. Low-intensity resistance exercises *of the operated hip* may be delayed until 4 to 6 weeks postoperatively to allow time for any surgically incised hip muscles to heal. However, resistance exercises of knee and ankle musculature may be initiated as soon as tolerable.

FOCUS ON EVIDENCE

Mitchell and colleagues[105] conducted a randomized, controlled trial to determine the effects of 6 weeks of quadriceps resistance exercises during the early phase of postoperative rehabilitation after hip fracture. The study included 80 patients described as "frail elderly" (all > 65 years of age, mean 80 years). All subjects performed a standard therapy program of ROM exercises and functional training after surgery. Half of the patients also performed bilateral resisted knee extension exercises at 16 days postoperatively, beginning with 3 sets of 12 repetitions at the 50% 1-RM intensity twice a week, and progressing to 80% intensity by the fifth week.

After 6 weeks of resistance training, the bilateral quadriceps strength of the intervention group increased to a significantly greater extent than that of the control group. Based on a functional mobility test, the intervention group also demonstrated a significantly greater reduction in functional impairments and activity limitations than the control group. However, there were no significant differences in improvement between groups regarding gait velocity or test scores measuring independence in ADL. There were no training-related adverse events during the study.

The authors concluded that moderate- to high-intensity postoperative quadriceps resistance training during early recovery after hip fracture was functionally beneficial and well tolerated by the participants despite their age and frailty.

Goals and interventions. The following are goals, exercises, and functional training interventions typically initiated in the hospital setting and continued following discharge from the hospital.[11,12,72,92] Patient education occurs throughout this phase of rehabilitation emphasizing progressive use of the operated extremity, safety, the prevention of postoperative complications, and reducing the risk of a future fall.

- ***Prevent vascular and pulmonary complications.***
  - Ankle pumping exercises performed regularly throughout the day to maintain circulation and reduce the risk of DVTs and thromboemboli.
  - Deep breathing exercises and airway clearance to prevent pulmonary complications.
- ***Improve strength in the upper and sound lower extremities.***
  - Exercises against progressive levels of resistance targeting key muscle groups used to lift body weight during bed mobility, standing transfers, and ambulation with assistive devices.
  - Emphasis on closed-chain training with most weight on the sound extremity, such as bridging exercises, to simulate the movement patterns used during these activities.
- ***Re-establish balance, postural stability, and safe and independent functional mobility within weight-bearing restrictions.***
  - Weight-shifting activities in bilateral stance.
  - Heel and toes raises in bilateral stance.
  - Stabilization exercises in bilateral stance (alternating isometrics/rhythmic stabilization).

- Balance activities with self-initiated perturbations by reaching in various directions.
- Bed mobility, transfers, and gait training with an assistive device.

■ ***Prevent postoperative reflex inhibition of hip and knee musculature.***

- Low-intensity isometric (setting) exercises of the hip and knee musculature of the operated extremity. Depending on the fracture site and its stability, perform submaximal gluteal, abductor, adductor, and quadriceps and hamstring setting exercises.

■ ***Restore mobility and control of the operated hip and adjacent joints.***

- Assisted, progressing to active ROM of the involved hip and knee in progressively more challenging positions as pain and fracture healing permit. For example, in the supine position, perform heel slides before straight leg raises (SLRs). When the knee is flexed, the shorter moment arm places lower rotational loads on the fracture site than a long moment arm.
- Pelvic tilts and knee-to-chest movements with the *uninvolved* leg to prevent stiffness in the low back region.
- Unassisted hip flexion, abduction, and extension while standing on the sound leg and holding onto a stable surface for balance before progressing to SLRs in a horizontal position.
- Low-intensity, dynamic resistance exercises in weight-bearing and nonweight-bearing positions as the stability of the fracture site allows.

PRECAUTION: When initiating setting and dynamic exercises of the involved hip after comminuted subtrochanteric fractures that required medial cortex reconstruction, postpone contractions of the abductor and adductor muscles for 4 to 6 weeks to avoid stresses across the fracture site.[157]

Exercise: Moderate and Minimum Protection Phases

By 6 weeks, soft tissues are healed; by 8 to 12 weeks, depending on the age and health of the patient, some degree of bone healing has occurred. By 6 weeks of rehabilitation, except in unusual situations, at least partial weight bearing or full weight bearing as tolerated is now permissible. By 8 to 12 weeks, although a patient gradually can be weaned from use of an assistive device during ambulation, most continue to use at least a cane well beyond this time frame.

During the intermediate and final phases of rehabilitation, the emphasis is on increasing strength and functional control of the involved lower extremity and gradually increasing the patient's level of functional activities. However, patients often are discharged from supervised therapy by 7 to 9 weeks or no later than 12 weeks postoperatively.

Extended exercise programs after surgery for hip fracture. Several studies have demonstrated that after a standard course of postoperative rehabilitation and with clearance from the patient's surgeon, an extended program of properly supervised, carefully progressed resistance exercises for strength training, begun as early as 6 weeks or as late as 5 to 7 months postoperatively (depending on the intensity of the exercise program), is safe and effective.[19,60,67,91,145,146]

The intensity, frequency, and duration of the extended exercise program varied in these studies, and the equipment used for resistance training ranged from elastic resistance products to weight machines. Features of the exercise programs implemented in three of the studies are summarized in Table 20.5. Additional details and outcomes of these studies are addressed at the conclusion of this section on postoperative management after hip fracture.

CLINICAL TIP

After hip fracture surgery, mildly to moderately frail elderly individuals who complete a standard course of postoperative therapy followed by 6 months of an extended exercise program that includes progressive resistance exercise training can expect that their fractured extremity will achieve a level of strength at least equivalent to that of their nonfractured extremity.[67]

TABLE 20.5 Summary of Studies of Extended Exercise Programs Following Surgery for Hip Fracture

First Author and Type of Study	Subjects: (n) and Mean Age	Setting, Format, and Timing of Intervention	Frequency, Duration, and Types of Exercise	Features of PRE Training
Binder[19] RCT with two groups	$N = 90$ Intervention group: $n = 46$; 80 years Control group: $n = 44$; 81 years	Facility based; group format for intervention group and home-based program for control group Begun no more than 16 weeks postsurgery	*Intervention group*: Two 3-month phases, three weekly sessions Phase 1: total of 22 exercises (flexibility, balance, aerobic training, low-intensity resistance exercises)	One or two sets, six to eight reps at 65% of initial 1-RM progressing to three sets, 8 to 12 reps at 85%–100% initial 1-RM Weight machines Exercises: bilateral knee flexion and extension,

Continued

TABLE 20.5 Summary of Studies of Extended Exercise Programs Following Surgery for Hip Fracture—cont'd

First Author and Type of Study	Subjects: (n) and Mean Age	Setting, Format, and Timing of Intervention	Frequency, Duration, and Types of Exercise	Features of PRE Training
			Phase 2: Moderate- to high-intensity PRE added to shortened phase 1 program *Control group*: A portion of phase 1 exercises, no PRE	leg press, seated bench press, biceps curl, seated rowing
Hauer[60] RCT with two groups Mangione[91] RCT with three groups	N = 28; all at least 75 years Intervention group: n = 15; 81.7 years Control group: n = 13; 80.8 years	Facility based; group format; begun 6–8 weeks postfracture	*Intervention group*: Three weekly sessions for 3 months; PRE, balance, and functional training *Control group*: Stretching, seated calisthenics, memory tasks.	Two sets at 70%–90% of 1-RM intensity Weight machines and body weight resistance Exercises: leg press, hip/knee extension, plantarflexion
Mangione[91] RCT with three groups	N = 33 Resistance group: n = 11; 77.9 years Aerobic group: n = 12; 79.8 years Control group: n = 10; 77.8 years	Home based; individual format; begun 19.4, 19.7, and 12.6 weeks after surgery, respectively, for resistance, aerobic, and control groups	Total of 3 months: two sessions weekly for 2 months, followed by 1 session weekly for 1 month	Three sets of eight reps at the 8-RM intensity Portable resistance unit or body weight resistance Exercises: supine hip and knee extension, hip abduction, standing hip extension; standing plantarflexion (heel raises)
Latham[83] RCT with two groups	N = 232; Intervention: n = 120 (Age 77.2) Control: n = 112 (Age 78.9)	Home based; individual format after traditional rehab; time since fracture 9.5 months for intervention group, 8.6 months for control group	6-month program: Three sessions per week *Intervention Group:* Functional tasks and standing exercises. *Control Group:* Nutrition education for cardiovascular health.	Functional tasks with elastic resistance; Standing exercises with weighted vests and varying step heights
Singh[150] RCT with two groups	N = 124; Intervention: n = 62 (Age 80.1) Control: n = 62 (Age 78.4)	Clinic based, individually prescribed; training began 6 to 8 weeks after fracture	12-month program: Twice per week *Intervention Group:* High-intensity PRE *Control Group*: Usual multidisciplinary care	Whole-body PRE (80% of peak upper and lower body strength); Progressive balance training

Goals and interventions. The following goals and exercises are appropriate during the intermediate and advanced phases of rehabilitation.

- ***Increase flexibility of any chronically shortened muscles.*** Muscles typically involved include the ankle plantarflexors, hip flexors, and hamstrings. Suggested stretching techniques include:
  - Heel cord stretching with a towel or with the assistance of a caregiver while sitting on a bed with the knee extended and later while standing.

- Hip flexor stretching in the supine (Thomas test) position.
- Hamstring stretching by sitting on the edge of a table with one leg supported in hip flexion and knee extension and the other in extension over the side of the support surface (see Fig. 20.18).

- ***Improve strength and muscular endurance in the lower extremities for functional activities.*** Refer to the section on exercise interventions later in the chapter for descriptions of the following exercises.
  - Bilateral, closed-chain active exercises, such as mini-squats and heel raises using body weight as the source of resistance and a table or walker for support and balance as soon as partial weight bearing on the operated lower extremity is permissible.
  - Lunges and forward and lateral step-ups when weight bearing to tolerance is allowable.
  - Open-chain hip and knee exercises initially against light to moderate resistance (up to 5 lb) with elastic resistance or cuff weights. Emphasize hip extension and abduction for a positive impact on ambulation.
  - Task-specific training, such as stair-climbing or carrying small loads while ambulating.
- ***Improve postural stability, neuromuscular responses, standing balance, and functional mobility.***
  - A progression of balance activities appropriate for the patient's age and desired activity level (refer to Chapters 8 and 23).
  - Progressive ambulation on various surfaces and at varying speeds.
- ***Increase aerobic capacity/cardiopulmonary endurance.***
  - Stationary bicycling, upper body ergometry, or treadmill walking.
  - Aerobic conditioning activities, possibly in an age-appropriate, community-based exercise class, to increase walking distance and velocity.

FOCUS ON EVIDENCE

A ***CPG for hip fracture management in the elderly***[1] notes moderate support that supervised occupational and physical therapy across the continuum of care improves functional outcomes and prevents falls and strong support for intensive physical therapy after discharge following a femur fracture.

Outcomes

General outcomes. The true measure of success of surgical intervention and postoperative rehabilitation after hip fracture is the extent to which a patient can return to his or her prefracture level of function. The level of pre-injury functional mobility in patients with femoral neck fractures has been shown to be a critical factor in postoperative survival.[66] In one follow-up study of patients after hip fracture, only 33% had regained their pre-injury level of function in basic ADL and instrumental ADL (IADL) 1 year postoperatively.[72] Given the advanced age and health status of the typical patient who sustains a hip fracture, it is not surprising that 1 year postoperative mortality rates are high, ranging from 12% to 36% depending on the mean age, general health status, and severity of the fracture.[76] Beyond 1 year of recovery, mortality rates are equal to age-matched subjects who have not sustained a hip fracture.[76]

Among patients who survive 1 year postoperatively, 83% demonstrated the ability to ambulate independently (50 feet on an uncarpeted surface) in one study.[11] In another study, 92% of patients returned to independent ambulation, but only 41% regained their prefracture level of ambulation.[77] In a study of community-dwelling older adults (mean age 83.4 years) 6 months after discharge from the hospital following a fall-related hip fracture, 53.3% (48/90) had experienced one or more falls.[148] The need for an assistive device during ambulation after hip fracture and the patient's prefracture fall history were predictors of a fall after hospital discharge.

Impact of rehabilitation. According to a report of the National Center for Medical Rehabilitation Research, the use of therapeutic exercise is one of the least examined factors affecting outcomes after hip fracture.[168] The minimal evidence that does exist indicates that rehabilitation is associated with positive outcomes. For example, in one study, the number of visits to physical therapy has been positively associated with the ability to ambulate independently.[11] Another study indicated that the frequency of physical therapy visits increased the likelihood of regaining functional independence and going directly home from an acute care setting after hip fracture surgery.[58]

In a randomized, controlled study, subjects who participated in a 1-month home exercise program increased their knee extensor strength and increased their walking velocity to a greater extent than the control group.[145] Another randomized, controlled study that evaluated a 6-month home exercise program of functional tasks and strengthening exercises demonstrated significant improvements in performance-based and subjective outcome measures for the intervention group relative to the control group.[83] Another study compared the effects of a 2-week program of weight-bearing versus non-weight-bearing exercises initiated during inpatient rehabilitation and found that both groups demonstrated substantial improvements in lower extremity muscle strength, balance, gait, and other functional tasks. However, there were no significant differences between groups.[146] This study supports the value of both types of exercise during early rehabilitation.

In the studies summarized in this section (see Table 20.6), muscle strength and performance on a variety of functional mobility and ADL tests improved to a significantly greater extent in the groups who participated in resistance training than in the groups who participated in low-intensity or no resistance training.[19,60,91] The resistance training group in the study by Binder and colleagues[19] also reported a significant decrease in the perceived levels of disability, whereas the control group, who performed only low-intensity exercises, did not. The resistance training group in the investigation by Hauer and associates[60] noted improved perception of walking steadiness but no change in fear of falling.

Moderate- to high-intensity resistance training after discharge from a "standard" postoperative program appears to be not only feasible, but also safe. Other than reports of mild muscle soreness during the early weeks of resistance exercise programs, training-related adverse events were reported in only one study, and these events were not specific to the involved hip.[19] A more recent study evaluating a multidisciplinary intervention that included high-intensity exercises showed reductions in risk of death and nursing home admissions, plus lower reliance on assistive devices.[150] However, not all extended rehabilitation programs after hip fracture have been shown to be effective. The results of a study of individuals enrolled in a long-term, home-based, multifaceted rehabilitation program (including extensive ADL and IADL training) in comparison to a traditional postoperative exercise and ambulation program for 6 months postoperatively demonstrated no significant between group differences.[158]

Painful Hip Syndromes: Nonoperative Management

Related Pathologies and Etiology of Symptoms

Painful symptoms in the hip region other than arthritis may be caused by pathologies involving the muscles, tendons, bursae, or the acetabular labrum. Often, symptoms occur as a result of overuse or repetitive trauma to the tissues and may have underlying structural or faulty mechanical predisposing factors.

FOCUS ON EVIDENCE

The ***CPG for Nonarthritic Hip Joint Pain linked to the International Classification of Functioning, Disability and Health***[45] identifies intra-articular structures as potential sources of nonarthritic hip pain, including femoroacetabular impingement, structural instability, labral tears, chondral lesions, loose bodies, and ligamentous teres tears, as well as acknowledging extra-articular structural impairments in the musculoskeletal system.

Musculotendinous Factors

Overuse or trauma to any of the musculotendinous units in the hip region can result from excessive strain during a muscle contraction or from repetitive use with inadequate time allowed for the injured tissue to heal between activities.

Tendinopathies and muscle strains. Commonly strained muscles include the hip flexors, adductors, and hamstrings. Decreased flexibility and muscle fatigue may predispose an individual to strains and/or injury during an activity or sporting event; sudden falls, such as slipping on ice, may also cause a muscle strain.

Repetitive trauma. Strength and flexibility imbalances among agonist/antagonist muscle pairs or among synergistic muscles may result in overuse injuries related to repetitive or high-intensity activities. Common overuse syndromes at the hip may reflect dominance of the tensor fasciae latae and rectus femoris as hip flexors, abductors, and internal rotators with apparent weak gluteus medius and gluteus minimus muscles or dominance of the hamstrings over the gluteus maximus.[142] Overuse of the piriformis muscle with apparent weakness of the gluteus maximus and medius muscles has also been reported.[159] Because of the relationship of these muscles with the pelvis and knee as well as the effect of faulty mechanics on weight-bearing function, patients with these muscle imbalances may also present with low back or knee symptoms.

Bursitis

Trochanteric bursitis. With inflammation of the trochanteric bursa, pain is experienced over the lateral hip and possibly down the lateral thigh to the knee when the iliotibial band rubs over the greater trochanter. Discomfort may be experienced after standing asymmetrically for long periods with the affected hip elevated and adducted and the pelvis dropped on the opposite side. Ambulation and climbing stairs aggravate the condition. Muscle flexibility, strength imbalances, and the resulting faulty pelvic motion may be the predisposing factors leading to bursal irritation.

Psoas bursitis. Pain is experienced in the groin or anterior thigh and possibly into the patellar area when there is inflammation of the psoas bursa. Activities requiring excessive, repetitive hip flexion aggravate the condition.

Ischiogluteal bursitis (Tailor's or Weaver's Bottom). When there is inflammation of the ischiogluteal bursa, pain is experienced around the ischial tuberosity, especially when sitting. If the adjacent sciatic nerve is irritated from the swelling, symptoms of sciatica may occur.

Femoroacetabular Impingement

Trauma, acetabular labral impingement, capsular laxity, dysplasia, and degeneration are causative factors for tears in the acetabular labrum leading to anterior hip or groin pain.[6,57,86,164] There may be associated structural abnormalities in the acetabulum or femur.[6] Acetabular labral pathology is associated with hip OA in older patients.[57] Patients usually present with pain that is activity dependent and describe mechanical symptoms such as clicking, locking, catching, or giving way.[86] Groin pain is most often related to an anterior tear, and buttock pain is most often related to a posterior tear. With an anterior lesion, positive tests typically include pain with the impingement test (combined flexion, adduction, and internal rotation) and with the scour test.[6] The log roll test may elicit pain or clicking when rolling the femur into internal rotation, and there may be restricted mobility and groin pain with the FABER (flexion, abduction, external rotation) test. Muscle flexibility and strength imbalances have been reported, including tightness of hip flexors and lumbar extensors and weak, inhibited gluteal and abdominal muscles.[57] Radiographic imaging and MRI (using gadolinium contrast) are usually performed to diagnose labral pathology.

CLINICAL TIP

Although FAI is often treated surgically, a period of conservative management is advocated that addresses any biomechanical impairment. Emphasize alignment of the hip joint, reduce anteriorly directed forces on the joint, and develop a length/strength balance in the muscles of the hip. Strengthen the hip abductors, gluteus maximus, iliopsoas, and external rotators and develop flexibility in the hamstring muscles. Avoid hip rotation under loads (pivoting) and correct faulty gait, such as knee hyperextension, which causes hip hyperextension during stance.[86] No exercise should cause pain.

Common Impairments of Structure and Function

Pain. With musculotendinous strains, symptoms occur when the involved muscle is contracted or stretched or when the provoking activity is repeated, often restricting participation in daily activities, community mobility, or sports activities. With impingement (bursa or labral tears), symptoms typically occur when the involved tissue is pinched between opposing structures.

Gait deviations. Slightly shorter stance occurs on the painful side. There may be a slight lurch or shift in the gait to minimize forces on the impaired structures.

Imbalance in muscle flexibility and neuromuscular control. Flexibility or altered patterns of activation in synergistic muscles may be precipitating factors in many painful hip syndromes. Imbalances are described in the introductory section of this chapter and summarized in the descriptions of painful hip syndromes.

Decreased muscular endurance. Muscle fatigue may lead to altered joint posture, stress, and imbalanced muscle use as described previously.

Management: Protection Phase

Patient Education

Advise the patient on the importance of modifying activities. Tailor the modifications to the patient's impairments, such as avoiding the impinged position; altering the sitting, standing, or sleeping positions that provoke symptoms; using an assistive device temporarily to reduce stress; or avoiding exercises that aggravate the patient.[45]

Control Inflammation and Promote Healing

When there is chronic irritation or inflammation from an acute injury, follow the guidelines as described in Chapter 10, with emphasis on resting the involved tissue by not stressing or putting pressure on it.

Develop Support in Related Areas

Initiate exercises to maximize neuromuscular control and alignment of the pelvis and hip and to develop strength in weak muscles. Avoid stressing the inflamed tissue during exercise. Patient education and cooperation are necessary to reduce repetitive trauma.

Management: Controlled Motion Phase

When acute symptoms have decreased, initiate a progressive exercise program within the tolerance of the involved tissues to improve muscle performance. The program should emphasize regaining a balance in length; neuromuscular control; strength; and endurance in the muscles of the hip, trunk, and the rest of the lower extremity.

Develop a Strong Mobile Scar and Regain Flexibility

Remodel the scar in muscle or tendon, if suspected, by applying cross-fiber massage to the site of the lesion (if accessible) followed by multiple-angle submaximal isometrics in pain-free positions.

Develop a Balance in Hip Muscle Length and Strength

Specific exercises are described in the exercise sections of this chapter.

- Stretch any muscles that are restricting motion with gentle, progressive techniques. Instruct the patient to do self-stretching with proper stabilization to ensure that the stretches are performed safely and effectively.
- Begin developing neuromuscular control to train muscles to optimally align the femur with emphasis on hip external rotation, external rotation combined with abduction, and hip extension with emphasis on the gluteus maximus.
- When the patient is aware of proper muscle control and is able to maintain segment alignment, progress to strengthening the weakened muscles through the range of joint motion.
- Initiate controlled weight-bearing exercises when tolerated. Because the individual is probably standing and walking during daily activities, they may not tolerate additional closed-chain activities than those initiated during the healing stage, so proceed with caution. Carefully observe the exercises so proper movement patterns are used.

CLINICAL TIP

With the common faulty pattern of increased hip adduction and internal rotation when bearing weight, valgus collapse at the knee is also likely. Increase the patient's awareness of knee alignment by having them focus on maintaining the knee in line vertically over the foot when descending stairs or sitting down.

- Muscles not directly involved in the pathology should be stretched and strengthened if they are contributing to asymmetrical forces. The patient may not have sufficient trunk coordination or strength, which may also contribute to the underlying problem if hip muscles must overcompensate. (See Chapter 16 for suggestions for developing control and stabilizing function in the trunk muscles.)
- Use exercises that encourage symmetrical muscle activation, such as biking or partial weight-bearing and weight-shifting activities in the parallel bars. Observe the coordination and movement patterns between the trunk, hip, knee, and ankle.
- Stop exercise with the onset of fatigue, when substitute motions appear, or if pain develops in the weakest segment in the chain.

Develop Muscle and Cardiopulmonary Endurance

- For muscle endurance, have the patient perform each exercise safely for 1 to 3 minutes before progressing to the next level of difficulty.
- Determine aerobic activities that do not exacerbate the patient's symptoms. It may be that the patient simply needs to modify the intensity of the activities used in their current aerobic program.

Patient Education

Initiate a home exercise program as soon as the patient has demonstrated correct neuromuscular control and safety and independence with stretching, strengthening, and aerobic activities. Provide regular follow-up instruction for modification and progression of the program.

Management: Return to Function Phase

- Progress closed-chain and functional training to include balance, neuromuscular control, and muscular endurance.
- Use specificity principles; increase eccentric resistance and demand for controlled speed if necessary for return to work, activities, or sporting events.
- Progress to patterns of motion consistent with the desired outcome. Use acceleration/deceleration drills and plyometric training.
- Assess total body functioning while the patient performs the desired activity. Facilitate the proper timing and sequencing of events during functional movements.
- Prior to returning to the desired function, have the patient practice the activity in a controlled environment and for an abbreviated time period. As tolerated, introduce variability in the environment and increase the intensity and duration of activities.

FOCUS ON EVIDENCE

The CPGs for Nonarthritic Hip Joint Pain[45] support interventions that include patient education and counseling that minimize aggravating factors and manage pain; joint and soft tissue mobilization procedures for hip joint capsular and fascial restrictions; therapeutic exercise for flexibility, strengthening, and conditioning; and neuromuscular reeducation for coordination.

Exercise Interventions for the Hip Region

No matter what the cause, muscle strength or flexibility imbalance in the hip can lead to abnormal lumbopelvic and hip mechanics, which can contribute to low back, sacroiliac, or hip pain (see Chapters 14 through 16). Abnormal hip mechanics from muscle flexibility and strength imbalances may also affect the knee and ankle during weight-bearing activities, potentially causing overuse syndromes or increased stress in these regions (see Chapters 21 and 22).

Exercise Techniques to Increase Flexibility and Range of Motion

The exercise techniques in this section are suggestions for correcting limited flexibility of the musculature and periarticular tissues crossing the hip. Principles and techniques of passive stretching and neuromuscular inhibition are presented in Chapter 4 and those of joint mobilization/manipulation in Chapter 5. Specific manual and self-stretching techniques are described in this section.

Flexibility (self-stretching) exercises, chosen according to the degree of limitation and ability of the patient to participate, can be valuable for reinforcing therapeutic interventions performed by the therapist. Not all of the following exercises are appropriate for every patient. Consequently, the therapist should select exercises and their intensity appropriate for each patient's level of function and progress each exercise as indicated. Recall that when the patient is able to contract the muscle opposite the range-limiting muscle, not only is the agonist being trained, but there is the added benefit of reciprocal inhibition of the shortened (antagonist) muscles. This principle is key to achieving effective joint control in the newly gained ROM.

Techniques to Stretch Range-Limiting Hip Structures

NOTE: Two-joint muscles can restrict full ROM of the hip when simultaneously lengthened at the knee joint. This first section describes stretches to increase hip motions only. Therefore, the two-joint muscles must be kept on slack across the knee during these stretches. Techniques to stretch specific two-joint muscles are described in the second section.

To Increase Hip Extension

Prone Press-Up

Patient position and procedure: Prone with hands on a table at shoulder level. Have the patient press the thorax upward and allow the pelvis to sag (see Fig. 15.4B).

PRECAUTION: This exercise also moves the lumbar spine into extension; if it causes pain to radiate into the patient's leg rather than providing just a stretch sensation in the anterior trunk, hip, and thigh, it must not be performed.

"Thomas Test" Stretch

Patient position and procedure: Supine with the hips near the end of the treatment table, both hips and knees flexed, and the contralateral thigh held against the chest with the arms. Have the patient slowly lower the thigh to be stretched toward the table in a controlled manner and allow the knee to extend, so the two-joint rectus femoris does not limit the range. Do not allow the thigh to externally rotate or abduct. Direct the patient to let the weight of the leg produce the stretch force and to relax the tight muscles at the end of the range (Fig. 20.10). The therapist may apply a passive stretch force manually, or a hold-relax technique may be used by applying a force to the distal thigh (see Fig. 4.26).

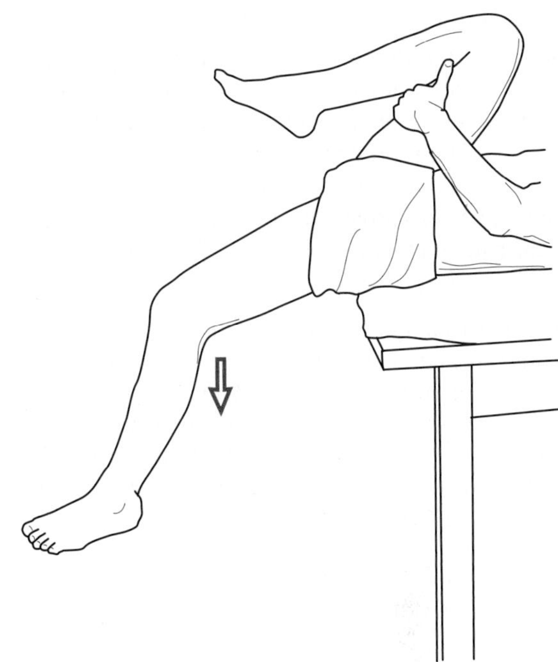

FIGURE 20.10 Self-stretching to increase hip extension. The pelvis is stabilized by holding the opposite hip in flexion. The weight of the thigh provides a stretch force as the patient relaxes. Allowing the knee to extend emphasizes the one-joint hip flexors (iliopsoas), whereas maintaining the knee in flexion and hip neutral to rotation as the thigh is lowered emphasizes the two joint rectus femoris and tensor fasciae latae muscles.

Modified Fencer Stretch

Patient position and procedure: Stand in a fencer's lunge-like posture with the involved leg in back (extended) and uninvolved leg forward. Position the back leg in the same plane as the front leg and the foot pointing forward. Have the patient first do a posterior pelvic tilt and then shift the body weight onto the anterior leg until a stretch sensation is felt in the anterior hip region of the back leg (Fig. 20.11). If the heel of the back foot is kept on the floor, this exercise may also stretch the gastrocnemius muscle.

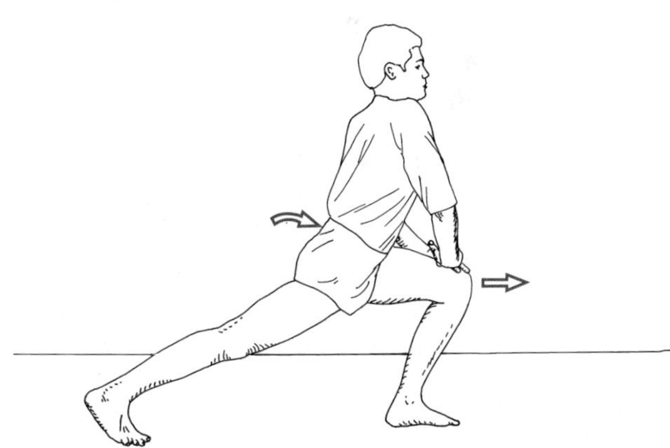

FIGURE 20.11 Self-stretching of the hip flexor muscles and soft tissue anterior to the hip using a modified fencer's squat posture.

Kneeling Fencer Stretch

Patient position and procedure: Kneel on the side to be stretched, with the uninvolved leg forward in hip/knee flexion and the foot on the ground. Have the patient first do a posterior pelvic tilt and then shift the body weight onto the anterior leg until a stretch sensation is felt in the anterior hip region of the back leg. Positioning the involved hip in internal rotation may enhance this stretch.

To Increase Hip Flexion

Bilateral Knee to Chest Stretch

Patient position and procedure: Supine. Have the patient bring both knees toward the chest and grasp the thighs firmly until a stretch sensation is felt in the posterior hip region. Monitor the position carefully, because if the pelvis lifts up off the mat, the lumbar spine flexes and the stretch force is transmitted there instead of to the hips.

Unilateral Knee to Chest Stretch

Patient position and procedure: Supine. Have the patient bring one knee to the chest and grasp the thigh firmly against the chest while keeping the other lower extremity extended on the mat. This position isolates the stretch force to the hip being flexed and helps stabilize the pelvis.

To emphasize a stretch of the gluteus maximus muscle, have the patient pull the knee toward the opposite shoulder.

Quadruped (All Fours) Stretch

Patient position and procedure: On hands and knees. Have the patient rock the pelvis into an anterior tilt, causing lumbar extension (Fig. 20.12 A); then maintain the lumbar extension and shift the buttocks back in an attempt to sit on the heels. The hands remain forward (Fig. 20.12 B). It is important not to let the lumbar spine flex while holding the stretch position, so the stretch affects the hip.

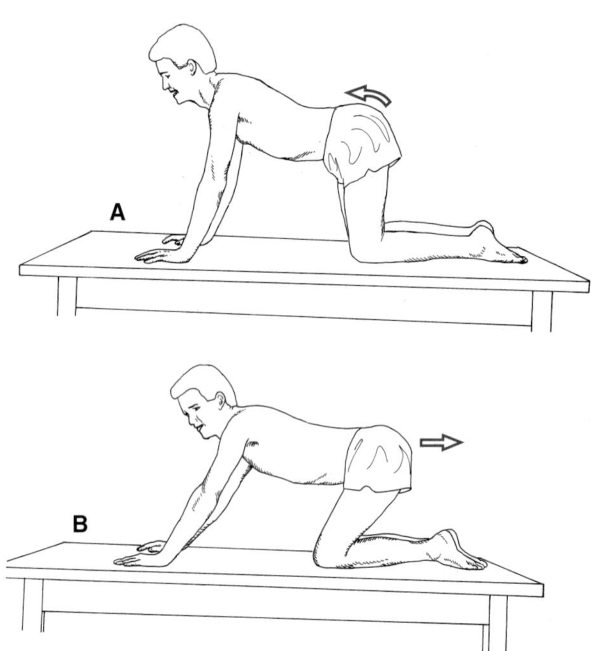

FIGURE 20.12 Gluteus maximus self-stretch with lumbar spine stabilization. **(A)** The patient on all fours rocks into an anterior pelvic tilt, causing lumbar extension. **(B)** While maintaining lumbar extension, the patient shifts the buttocks back, attempting to sit on the heels. When lordosis can no longer be maintained, the end-range of hip flexion is reached; this position is held for the stretch.

Short-Sitting Stretch

Patient position and procedure: Sitting in a chair or at edge of elevated exercise mat (so that the hips are positioned in 90° of flexion) with the pelvis rotated anteriorly and the low back extended to stabilize the spine. Have the patient grasp the front of the chair seat (or mat) and lean or pull the trunk forward, keeping the back arched, so the motion occurs only at the hips.

To Increase Hip Abduction

Patient position and procedure: Supine with both hips flexed 90°, knees extended, and legs and buttocks against the wall. Have the patient abduct both hips as far as possible with gravity causing the stretch force (Fig. 20.13).

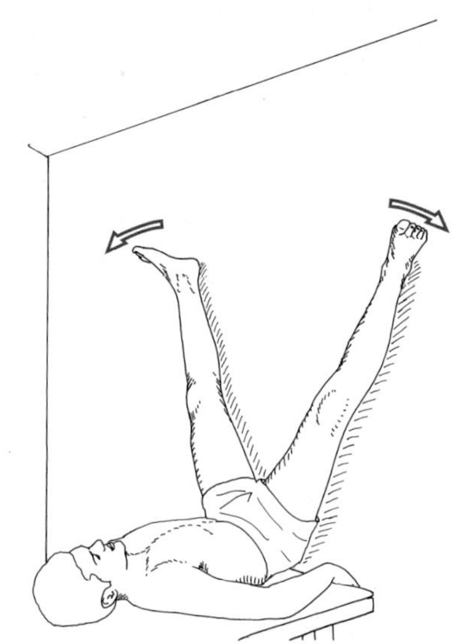

FIGURE 20.13 Self-stretching of the adductor muscles with the hips at 90° of flexion.

To Increase Hip Abduction and External Rotation Simultaneously

- *Patient position and procedure:* Sitting or supine with soles of feet together and hands on the inner surface of the knees. Have the patient push the knees down toward the floor with a sustained stretch. The stretch can be increased by pulling the feet closer to the trunk.

NOTE: When this stretch is performed supine, teach the patient to stabilize the pelvis and lumbar spine by actively contracting the abdominal muscles and maintaining a neutral spinal position.

- *Patient position and procedure:* Sitting or supine hook-lying, with ankle of extremity to be stretched placed on the opposite thigh (FABER or figure-4 position) (Fig. 20.14).

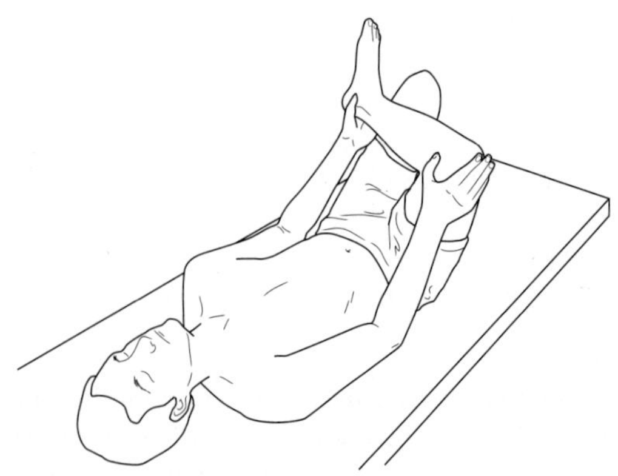

FIGURE 20.14 Self-stretching to increase hip abduction and external rotation using the figure-4 position.

Have the patient push the knee down with one hand while stabilizing the ankle on the thigh with the other hand.

To increase the stretch on the posterior hip musculature, have the patient bend forward at the hips (or bring the flexed knee toward the chest if in hook-lying) while maintaining the lumbar spine in extension and pelvis in midline (not tipping to one side).

- *Patient position and procedure:* Standing in a fencer's position but with the back leg externally rotated. Have the patient shift the weight onto the front leg until a stretch sensation is felt along the medial thigh in the hind leg.

To Increase Hip Internal Rotation

Patient position and procedure: Long-sitting position on a mat with the leg of the hip to be stretched flexed and crossed over the opposite leg (Fig. 20.15). Keep the foot planted and adduct and internally rotate the hip by moving the knee medially.

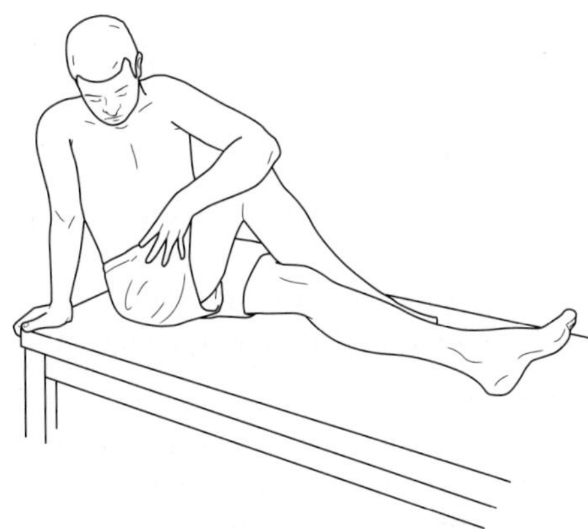

FIGURE 20.15 Self-stretching to increase internal rotation of the hip.

Techniques to Stretch Range-Limiting, Two-Joint Muscles

Rectus Femoris Stretches

NOTE: The rectus femoris is the only 2-joint component of the quadriceps femoris muscle group. It is elongated using hip extension while maintaining the knee in flexion.

"Thomas Test" Stretch

Patient position and procedure: Supine with the hips near the end of the treatment table, both hips and knees flexed, and the thigh on the side opposite the tight hip held against the chest with the arms. While keeping the knee flexed, have the patient lower the thigh to be stretched toward the table in a controlled manner. Do not allow the thigh to externally rotate or abduct. Direct the patient to let the weight of the leg produce the stretch force and to relax the tight muscles at the end of the range. The patient can attempt to further extend the hip by contracting the extensor muscles (see Fig. 20.10 but with the knee flexed).

NOTE: This is the same stretch used to increase hip extension—except to stretch the rectus femoris, the knee is kept flexed so the range for hip extension is less.

Prone Stretch

Patient position and procedure: Prone with the knee flexed on the side to be stretched. Have the patient grasp the ankle on that side (or place a towel or strap around the ankle to pull on) and flex the knee. As the muscle increases in flexibility, place a small folded towel under the distal thigh to further extend the hip.

NOTE: Do not allow the hip to abduct or externally rotate or allow the spine to hyperextend.

Standing Stretch

Patient position and procedure: Standing with the hip extended and knee flexed and grasping the ankle. Instruct the patient to maintain a posterior pelvic tilt and neutral hip abduction/adduction and not allow the back to arch or side bend during this stretch (Fig. 20.16).

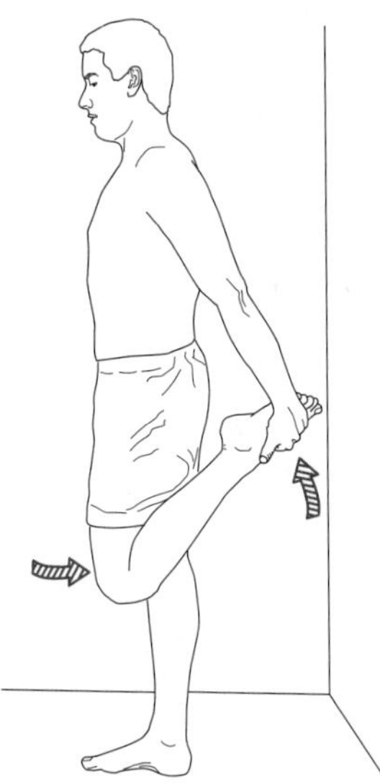

FIGURE 20.16 Self-stretching of the rectus femoris while standing. The femur is kept in line with the trunk. Care must be taken to maintain a posterior PT and not arch or twist the back.

NOTE: If the rectus femoris is too tight to stretch safely in this manner, the patient may place his or her foot on a chair or bench located behind the body rather than grasping the ankle.

Hamstrings Stretches

NOTE: The two-joint hamstring muscle group is stretched by flexing the hip while maintaining the knee in extension.

Straight Leg Raising

Patient position and procedure: Supine with a towel behind the thigh. Have the patient perform an SLR of the restricted extremity by maintaining the knee in extension and flexing the hip, and pulling on the towel to move the hip into more flexion.

Hamstrings Stretch in Doorway

Patient position and procedure: Supine, on the floor, with one leg through a doorway and the other leg (the one to be stretched) propped up against the door frame. For an effective stretch, the pelvis and opposite leg must remain on the floor with the knee extended.

- To increase the stretch when the patient is able, have the patient move the buttock closer to the doorframe, keeping the knee extended (Fig. 20.17 A).
- Teach the patient to perform the hold-relax/agonist contraction technique by pressing the heel of the leg being stretched against the doorframe, causing an isometric contraction, relaxing it, then lifting the leg away from the frame (Fig. 20.17 B).

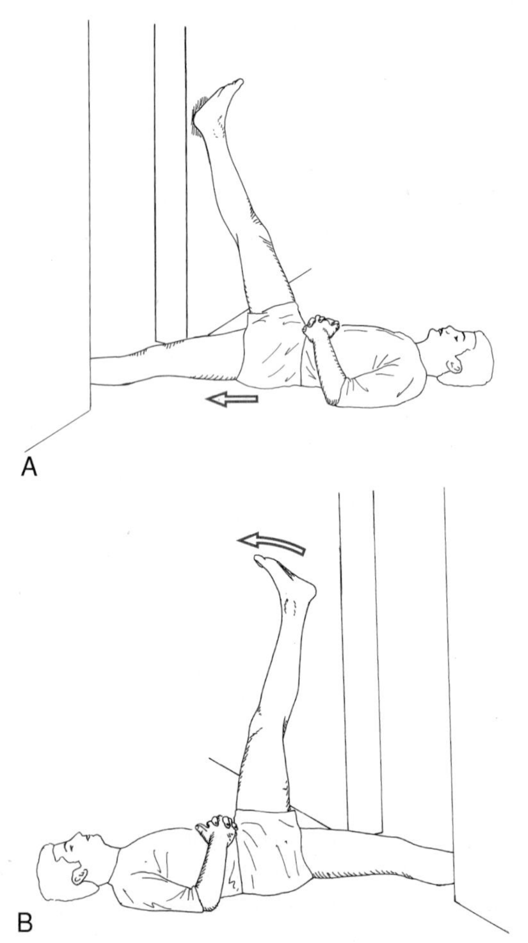

FIGURE 20.17 Self-stretching of the hamstring muscles. Additional stretch can occur if the person either **(A)** moves the buttock closer to the door frame or **(B)** lifts the leg away from the doorframe.

Hamstrings Stretch on Chair or Table

- *Patient position and procedure:* Sitting with the leg to be stretched extended to another chair, or sitting at the edge of a treatment table, with the leg to be stretched on the table and the opposite foot on the floor. Have the patient lean the trunk forward toward the thigh, maintaining the back in neutral so there is motion only at the hip joint (Fig. 20.18).

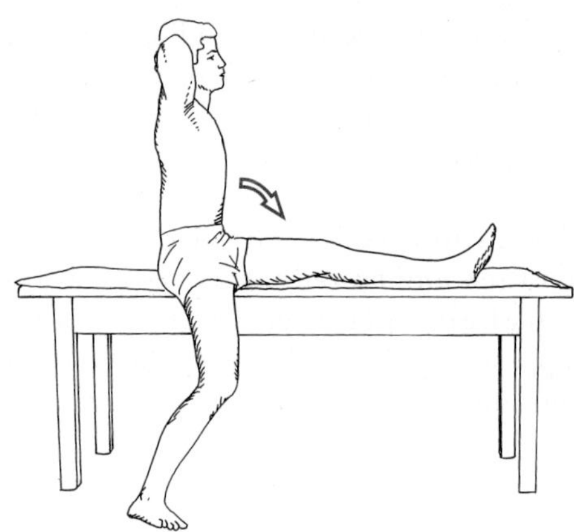

FIGURE 20.18 Self-stretching the hamstring muscles by leaning the trunk toward the extended knee, flexing at the hips.

- *Alternate position:* Standing with the extremity to be stretched on a stool or the seat of a chair. Have the patient lean the trunk forward toward the thigh, keeping the back stabilized in neutral so that motion is only at the hip joint.

Bilateral Toe Touching

NOTE: Bilateral toe touching exercises are often used to stretch the hamstring muscles in exercise classes. It is important to recognize that having the patient reach for the toes does not selectively stretch the hamstrings but stretches the low back and mid-back as well. Toe touching is considered a general flexibility exercise and tends to mask shortening of soft tissues in one region and overstretch areas already flexible. Whether a person can touch the toes depends on many factors (e.g., body type; arm, trunk, and leg length; flexibility in the thoracic and lumbar regions; and hamstring and gastrocnemius length).

Patient position and procedure: Standing. To discourage the "toe touch" idea, teach the patient to place the hands on the hips when bending forward. To specifically stretch the hamstrings using the forward-bend method while standing, teach the patient to first do an anterior pelvic tilt to extend the lumbar spine; then maintain the back position and bend only at the hips ("hinge at the hips") moving only through the range of forward bending in which the spine can be maintained in extension. The stretch sensation should be felt in the hamstring region.

PRECAUTION: This stretching technique should not be used when the patient has low-back impairments because forward bending greatly increases muscle activation and mechanical stress to the tissues of the low back.

Tensor Fasciae Latae and Iliotibial Band Stretches

NOTE: The tensor fasciae latae (TFL) inserts into the iliotibial (IT) band, which inserts into the extensor mechanism and lateral fascia of the knee. The TFL is a hip flexor, abductor, and internal rotator; for an effective stretch, all *three* components must be addressed. In addition, for an effective stretch of the muscle, the IT band must be positioned across the greater trochanter and the knee must be flexed. Adding knee flexion at later stages is a more aggressive technique that may also enhance the effectiveness of TFL stretches.

Supine Stretch

Patient position and procedure: Supine with two pillows under the hips and back to position the hips in extension. Instruct the patient to cross the uninvolved extremity over the top of the involved extremity, so the involved thigh has room to move into adduction and internal rotation. The foot of the uninvolved extremity is placed lateral to the knee of the adducted thigh and assists in holding the stretch position (Fig. 20.19).

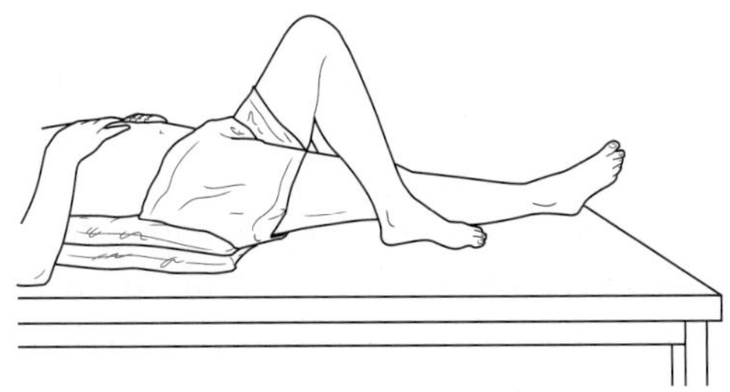

FIGURE 20.19 Self-stretching of the tensor fascia latae: supine. Pillows support the spine and pelvis, allowing the hips to extend. The crossed-over foot stabilizes the femur in adduction and external rotation.

Side-Lying Stretch

- *Patient position and procedure:* Side-lying, with the leg to be stretched uppermost. The bottom extremity is flexed for support, and the pelvis is tilted laterally, so the waist is against the mat or floor. Abduct the top leg and align it in the plane of the body (in extension). While maintaining this position, have the patient externally rotate the hip and then gradually lower (adduct) the thigh to the point of stretch (Fig. 20.20 A).

NOTE: It is critical to keep the trunk aligned and not allow it to roll backward. If the trunk rolled backward, the hip would then flex, and the iliotibial tract would slip in front of the greater trochanter, preventing an effective stretch.

- *Progression:* Secure a belt or sheet around the ankle of the involved leg and have the patient hold onto the other end placed over the shoulder (Fig. 20.20 B). Instruct the patient to first flex the knee and abduct the hip and then extend the hip. (This ensures that the IT band is positioned over the greater trochanter.) Then have the patient adduct the hip in slight external rotation until tension is felt along the lateral aspect of the knee. If tolerated, a 2- to 5-lb weight is placed distally over the lateral thigh for added stretch, and the position maintained for 20 to 30 minutes (also see manual stretching Fig. 4.29).

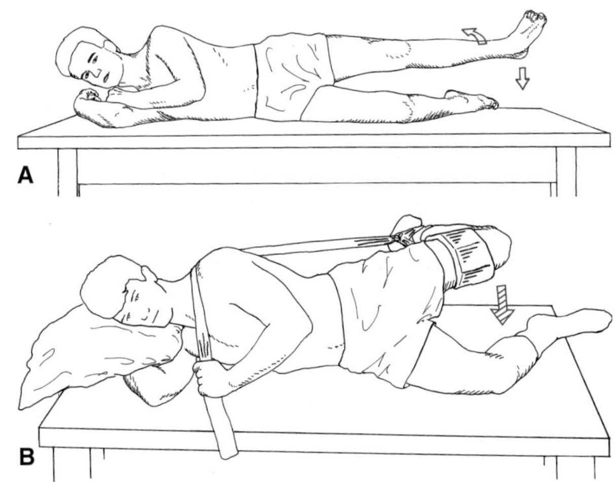

FIGURE 20.20 Self-stretching of the tensor fascia latae: side-lying. **(A)** The thigh is abducted in the plane of the body; then it is extended and externally rotated, then slowly lowered. Additional stretch occurs by flexing the knee. **(B)** Progress the intensity of a sustained stretch by pulling the hip into extension with a strap and adding a weight.

- ***Fascial release procedure for the IT band in side-lying.*** Refer to the description and illustration of the foam roller release in Chapter 21 (see Fig. 21.22).

Standing Stretch

Patient position and procedure: Standing with the side to be stretched toward a wall and the hand on that side placed on the wall. Have the patient extend, adduct, and externally rotate the extremity to be stretched and cross it behind the other extremity. With both feet on the floor, have the patient shift his or her pelvis toward the wall and allow the normal knee to bend slightly (Fig. 20.21). There is a slight side-bending of the trunk away from the side being stretched.

Exercises to Develop and Improve Muscle Performance and Functional Control

During the controlled motion and return to function phases of intervention, when only moderate or minimum protection of healing tissues is necessary, the patient must learn to develop control of hip movement while using good trunk stability. For a muscle that has not been functioning normally

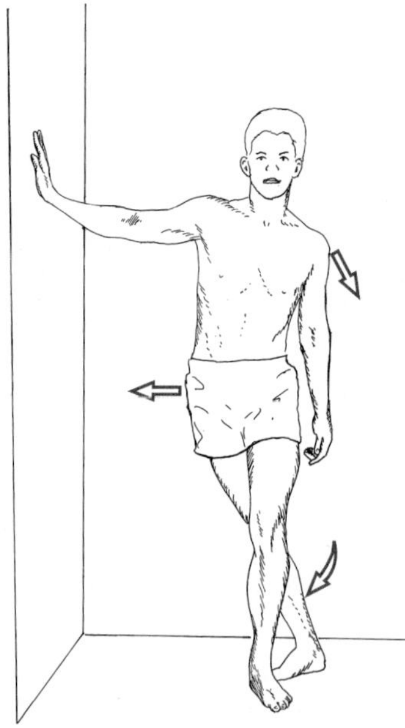

FIGURE 20.21 Self-stretching of the tensor fasciae latae: standing. The pelvis shifts toward the tight side with a slight side bend of the trunk away from the tight side. Increased stretch occurs when the extremity is positioned in external rotation prior to the stretch.

because other muscles are more active, exercises begin with developing patient awareness of muscle contractions and movements through graded isometrics and controlled ROM exercises. If muscle shortening has prevented full ROM, development of muscle control in any newly gained range must immediately follow stretching activities. Principles for improving muscle performance as well as techniques for manual resistance exercise and methods of mechanical resistance are described in Chapter 6. Manually applied resistance should be used when muscles are weak or when helping the patient focus on activating specific muscles.

Exercises described in the following sections may be adapted for home exercise programs and progressed by integrating advanced function training exercises described in Chapter 23. Choose exercises that challenge the patient to progress toward the functional goals established in the plan of care.

Open-Chain (Nonweight-Bearing) Exercises

Even though weight-bearing activities dominate lower extremity function, when a patient is weak or has poor control of specific muscles or movement patterns, it is advantageous to begin exercises in nonweight-bearing positions, so the individual can learn to isolate muscle activity and control specific motions. In addition, many functional activities have a nonweight-bearing component, such as the swing phase in gait, lifting the leg up to a step when going upstairs, and lifting the lower extremity into a car or onto a bed.

To Develop Control and Strength of Hip Abduction (Gluteus Medius, Gluteus Minimus, and Tensor Fasciae Latae)

NOTE: When a patient is observed to flex and internally rotate the thigh when abducting the hip, there may be a muscle activation imbalance between the TFL and gluteus medius. Most often, the TFL is dominant and the stabilizing forces from the gluteus medius are poorly controlled with this movement pattern.[142] To manage this, the posterior fibers of the gluteus medius and minimus must be trained to contract and control external rotation while the TFL relaxes. If there is sufficient control of rotation, abduction is performed utilizing the optimum synergy between these muscles. Techniques to address this imbalance are described in the following sections.

Supine Abduction

Patient position and procedure: Supine with the hips and knees extended. Have the patient concentrate on isolated hip abduction while keeping the trunk still. Do not let the femur roll outward into external rotation. Supine abduction is the easiest position in which to initiate motion, because the influence of gravity on the abductors is eliminated.

- For very weak abductors (< 3/5 manual muscle test grade), provide assistance or place a skate or towel under the leg to minimize the effects of friction.
- If the abductors are not strong enough to progress to antigravity training in the side-lying position, place a weight, such as a sandbag, along the lateral aspect of the thigh or ankle and have the patient push the weight outward.

Side-Lying Abduction

NOTE: If the TFL is tight, the range into extension or adduction may be limited. It is important to stretch this muscle (see Figs. 20.19, 20.20, and 20.21) prior to performing hip abduction to strengthen the gluteus medius. Be certain that the patient does not let the hip flex or internally rotate during these exercises to minimize action of the TFL. If the patient has difficulty controlling hip rotation while abducting in the side-lying position, first develop strength in the external rotators as described later in this section.

Patient position and procedure: Side-lying with the bottom hip and knee flexed for stability. Have the patient lift the top leg into abduction, keeping the hip neutral to rotation and in slight extension. Do not allow the hip to flex or the trunk to roll backward.

- Add ankle weights to provide resistance as the patient's strength improves.

Standing Abduction

Patient position and procedure: In single-leg stance, have the patient move the nonweight-bearing lower extremity out to the side. Instruct the patient to maintain the trunk upright in neutral alignment and avoid hiking the pelvis and flexing or rotating the abducting hip.

- Add resistance by applying an ankle weight on the moving leg or by using pulleys or elastic resistance applied at right angles to the moving extremity.
- The abductors on the weight-bearing lower extremity contract isometrically to stabilize the pelvis (see Fig. 20.26 B).

To Develop Control and Strength of Hip Extension (Gluteus Maximus)

Gluteal Muscle Setting

Patient position and procedure: Supine or prone. Use gluteal setting exercises to increase awareness of the contracting muscle; teach the patient to "squeeze" (contract) the buttocks.

Standing Leg Lifts With Trunk Support

Patient position and procedure: Standing at the edge of a treatment table with the trunk flexed and supported on the table. Have the patient alternately extend one hip, then the other. This is done with the knee flexed to train the gluteus maximus while relaxing the hamstrings. To progress, add weights or elastic resistance to the distal thigh.

CLINICAL TIP

When attempting hip extension with the knee flexed, if the hamstrings cramp from active insufficiency, the patient is using the hamstrings rather than the gluteus maximus and should learn to alter this contraction pattern. Help them refocus on the maximus by using isometrics in various positions before progressing with this exercise.

Quadruped Leg Lifts

Patient position and procedure: In the quadruped position or lying prone over a large gym ball, have the patient alternately extend each hip while keeping the knee flexed (Fig. 20.22). Combine this exercise with trunk stabilization by first having the patient find the neutral pelvic position, drawing in the abdominal muscles, then extending the hip (see Chapter 16).

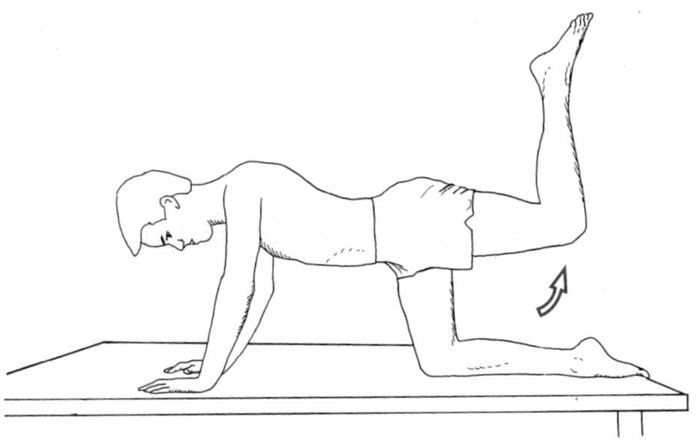

FIGURE 20.22 Isolated training and strengthening of the gluteus maximus. Starting in the quadruped position, extend the hip while keeping the knee flexed to rule out use of the hamstring muscles. Do not to extend the hip beyond the available ROM to avoid causing stress to the sacroiliac or lumbar spinal joints.

CLINICAL TIP

When instructing a patient in hip extension exercises, care is taken not to extend the hip beyond the available range of hip extension; otherwise, the motion causes stress in the sacroiliac joint or lumbar spine. Emphasize spinal stabilization when performing hip extension.

Standing Extension

Patient position and procedure: In single-leg stance, have the patient extend the opposite hip (see Fig. 20.26 A). Instruct the patient to maintain the trunk upright in neutral alignment and not allow the moving hip to extend beyond the normal range.

- To add resistance, apply an ankle weight on the moving leg or by using pulleys or elastic resistance applied at right angles to the moving extremity.
- The hip musculature on the weight-bearing lower extremity must contract isometrically to stabilize the pelvis.

To Develop Control and Strength of Hip External Rotation

Prone Isometrics

Patient position and procedure: Prone with knees flexed and about 10 inches apart. Have the patient press the medial aspect of the heels together, causing an isometric contraction of the external rotators. This also may be done with the knees extended; emphasize the sensation of the thighs rolling outward, not adducting.

Clam Shell Exercise

NOTE: Clam shell exercises combine hip external rotation with abduction.

Patient position and procedure: With the patient side-lying, lower extremities partially flexed at the hips and knees, and the heel of the top leg resting on the heel of the bottom leg, have the patient lift the knee of the top leg, keeping the heels together. Add resistance by tying an elastic band around the thighs or by placing a cuff weight around the distal thigh of the top leg (Fig. 20.23).

- Variations of the clam shell exercise include beginning with the patient supine in the hook-lying position with an elastic band around the distal thigh for resistance and progressing to a modified bridge position or side plank position using the elastic band around the knee for resistance. These last two positions require good trunk stabilization while moving the hips through the abduction/external rotation motion.

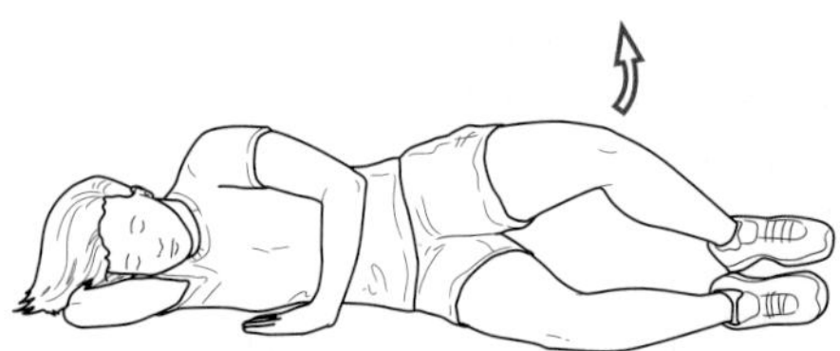

FIGURE 20.23 Clam exercises to develop control and initiate antigravity strengthening of the external rotators. Wrap an exercise band around the thighs or add a weight to top leg to increase resistance.

Side-Lying External Rotation: Progression

Patient position and procedure: Hip and knee of top leg extended and aligned with the trunk. First, have the patient roll the leg outward. Then progress to lifting the lower extremity into abduction with the hip externally rotated. Apply elastic resistance or a cuff weight around the thigh when resistance is tolerated.

NOTE: Do not allow the patient to roll the trunk backward or flex the hip, as this exercise is done to minimize substitution with the tensor fasciae latae.

Sitting: External Rotation

Patient position and procedure: Sitting with knees flexed over the edge of a treatment table. Secure an elastic band or tubing around the patient's ankle and the table leg on the same side. For resisted external rotation have the patient move the foot toward the opposite leg, pulling against the resistance (Fig. 20.24).

NOTE: Do not allow substitution with knee flexion or extension or hip abduction.

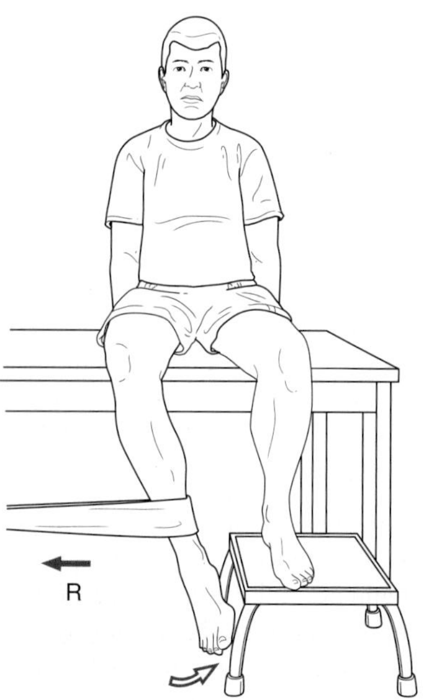

FIGURE 20.24 Strengthening the external rotators in a sitting position with elastic resistance.

To Develop Control and Strength of Hip Flexion (Iliopsoas and Rectus Femoris)

Supine Heel Slides

Patient position and procedure: Begin in hip and knee extension and have the patient flex the hip and knee by sliding the heel toward the buttock.

Hip and Knee Flexion

Patient position and procedure: Standing in front of a step or stool and holding onto a stable object for balance if necessary. Have the patient lift the leg (flex the hip and knee) and place the foot on the step and then return the foot to the floor. Alternate with the other leg for bilateral strengthening.

- To progress resistance add an ankle weight and/or the height of the step.
- Variations include having the patient perform alternating hip/knee flexion (high-step marching) or climbing a flight of stairs.

Straight-Leg Hip Flexion

Patient position and procedure: Supine, or standing and holding on to a stable structure for balance if necessary. Have the patient flex the hip while maintaining the knee in extension. For resistance when supine, add cuff weights; when standing, secure elastic resistance around the patient's distal thigh or leg.

To Develop Control and Strength of Hip Adduction

Side-Lying Adduction

Patient position and procedure: With the bottom leg aligned in the plane of the trunk (hip extension) and the top leg flexed forward with the foot on the floor or with the thigh resting on a pillow, have the patient lift the bottom leg upward into adduction. Weights can be added to the ankle to progress strengthening (Fig. 20.25 A). A more difficult position is to have the patient hold the top leg in abduction and adduct the bottom leg upward to meet it (Fig. 20.25 B).

Standing Adduction

Patient position and procedure: Have the patient adduct the leg across the front of the weight-bearing leg. Add ankle weights to provide resistance, or fasten elastic resistance or a pulley at right angles to the moving leg.

Closed-Chain (Weight-Bearing) Exercises

Weight-bearing exercises in the lower extremity involve all of the joints in the chain and are therefore not limited to hip muscles. Most activities bring into play antagonistic, two-joint muscles in which each muscle is being lengthened across one joint while it is shortening across another, thus maintaining an optimal length-tension relationship. In addition to causing motion, a prime function of the muscles in weight bearing is to control the forces of gravity and momentum for balance

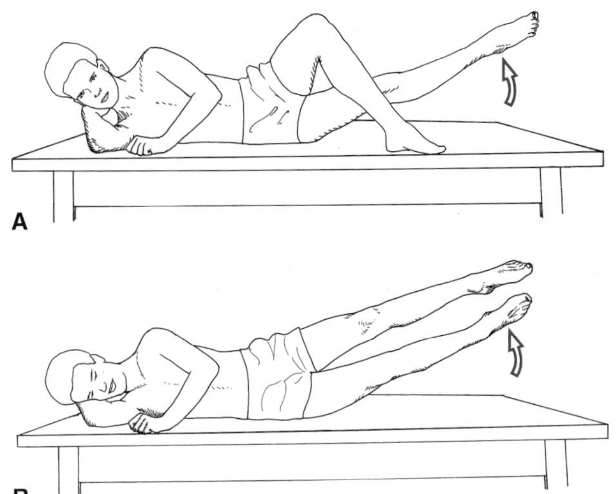

FIGURE 20.25 Training and strengthening the hip adductors. **(A)** The top leg is stabilized by flexing the hip and resting the foot on the mat while the bottom leg is adducted against gravity. **(B)** The top leg is isometrically held in abduction while the bottom leg is adducted against gravity.

and stability. Therefore, the exercises for the hip described in this section include balance and stabilization training as well as strengthening and functional exercises. More advanced balance and functional exercises are described in Chapter 23.

A number of EMG studies have analyzed lower extremity exercises used to strengthen hip musculature in both non-weight-bearing and weight-bearing positions. Two such studies, primarily of weight-bearing exercises, are summarized in Box 20.10.[7,41]

Exercises performed in weight-bearing postures described in the following section are closely related and are progressed concurrently as the patient is able. If the patient does not tolerate or is not permitted to be full weight bearing, begin exercises with upper extremity assistance, such as parallel bars, or utilize a therapeutic pool if one is available and the patient has no open wounds (see Chapter 9).

Closed-Chain Isometric Exercises

Alternating Isometrics and Rhythmic Stabilization

Patient position and procedure: Standing; begin with bilateral standing and progress the patient to unilateral standing. Alternating isometrics and rhythmic stabilization develop postural adjustments to applied forces.

- Apply manual resistance against the pelvis in alternating directions and ask the patient to hold (with isometric contractions). There should be little or no movement.
- Vary the force and direction of resistance; also vary where the force is applied by shifting the resistance from the pelvis to the shoulders and eventually against outstretched arms (see Fig. 22.15).
- At first, use verbal cueing. Then, as the patient learns control, apply the varying forces without warning.

Stabilization in Single-Leg Stance

Patient position and procedure: Standing on the involved leg with elastic resistance placed around the thigh of the opposite extremity and secured to a stable upright structure. If the uninvolved knee is stable, the resistance can be applied around the ankle. Have the patient maintain alignment and stability of the trunk and the weight-bearing extremity while moving the opposite extremity forward, backward, and to the side.

- To resist *hip flexion of the moving thigh*, have the patient face away from where the resistance is secured. This requires stabilization by the posterior muscles on the stance side.
- To resist *extension of the moving thigh*, have the patient face toward where the resistance is secured (Fig. 20.26 A). This requires stabilization by the anterior muscles on the stance side.

BOX 20.10 EMG Analysis of Selected Weight-Bearing Exercises Used to Strengthen Lower Extremity Musculature*

Gluteus maximus: > 40% MVC (strong contraction)

- Single-limb wall slide,[7] single-limb squat, and single-limb deadlift[41]
- Single-limb mini-squat[7]
- Step-ups (forward, lateral, retro)[7]
- Lunges (transverse, forward, sideways)[41]

Gluteus maximus: < 40% MVC

- Side-lying hip abduction, clam with 60° hip flexion[41]
- Transverse hop, forward hop, and clam with 30° hip flexion[41]

Gluteus medius: > 40% MVC (strong contraction)

- Side-lying hip abduction[41]
- Single-limb wall slide[7]
- Lateral band walk, single-limb deadlift, sideways hop[41]
- Forward step up[7]
- Sideways hop, transverse hop, transverse lunge, forward hop, forward lunge, clam with 30° hip flexion[41]

Gluteus medius: < 40% MVC

- Sideways lunges and clam exercise (in the side-lying position) with 60° hip flexion[41]

Biceps femoris: < 40% MVC

- Single-leg wall squat, mini-squat, and forward step-up[7]
- Retro step-up and lateral step-up are 10% and 9% MVC, respectively[7]

*The clam exercise was performed in a nonweight-bearing position. The exercises are listed from most effective to least effective for activating each muscle as normalized to its own maximum voluntary contractions (MVC).

- To resist *abduction* and *adduction,* have the patient face so the band is directed toward one side and then the other (Fig. 20.26 B).

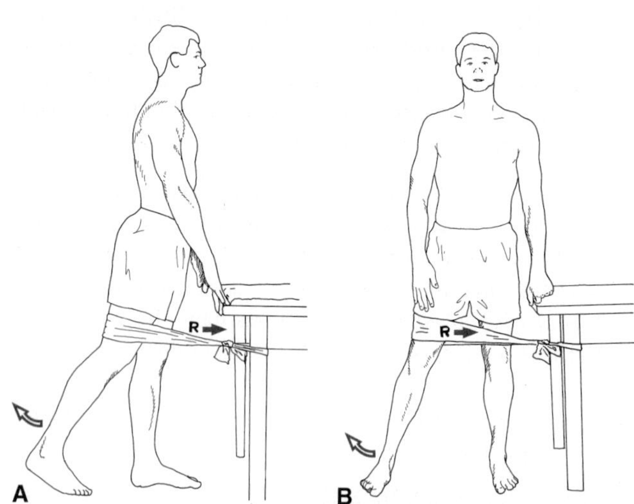

FIGURE 20.26 Closed-chain stabilization and strengthening exercises with elastic resistance around the opposite leg. **(A)** Resisting extension on the right requires stabilization of the anterior muscles of the left side. **(B)** Resisting abduction on the right requires stabilization by the left frontal plane muscles. To increase difficulty, the resistance is moved distally onto the leg.

NOTE: Although the nonweight-bearing extremity is moving against resistance, the emphasis of the exercise is to develop stability and strengthen the weight-bearing side. Therefore, fatigue is determined when the patient can no longer hold the weight-bearing extremity or pelvis stable.

These stabilization exercises can be used for balance training by having the patient vary the speed of the moving leg.

Closed-Chain Dynamic Exercises

Hip Hiking/Pelvic Drop

Patient position and procedure: Standing with one leg on a 2- to 4-inch block and using a wall or stable surface for balance if necessary. Alternately lower and elevate the pelvis on the side of the unsupported leg (Fig. 20.27). This develops control of the abductors of the stance leg and hip hikers on the unsupported side.

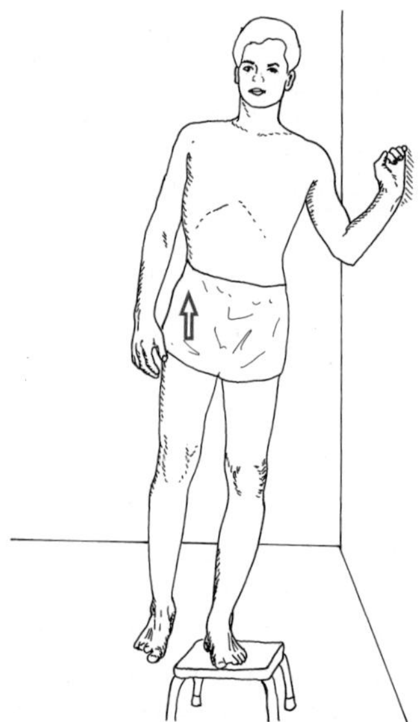

FIGURE 20.27 Training the hip abductor and hiker muscles for frontal plane strengthening and stability.

FOCUS ON EVIDENCE

In an EMG study by Bolgla and Uhl,[21] a series of 16 healthy subjects performed 6 different abductor exercises using a constant weight. The authors documented significantly greater maximum voluntary contraction of the gluteus medius in the stance leg (weight-bearing leg) during the pelvic drop exercise than during other hip abduction exercises. In addition, standing hip abduction showed significantly greater hip abductor activity on the weight-bearing side than on the moving (open-chain) side; the activity on the weight-bearing side had a comparable maximum voluntary contraction as side-lying hip abduction.

Bridging

Patient position and procedure: Begin in the hook-lying position. Have the patient press the upper back and feet into the mat, elevate the pelvis, and extend the hips. This strengthens the hip extensors in coordination with the trunk stabilizers (Fig. 20.28).

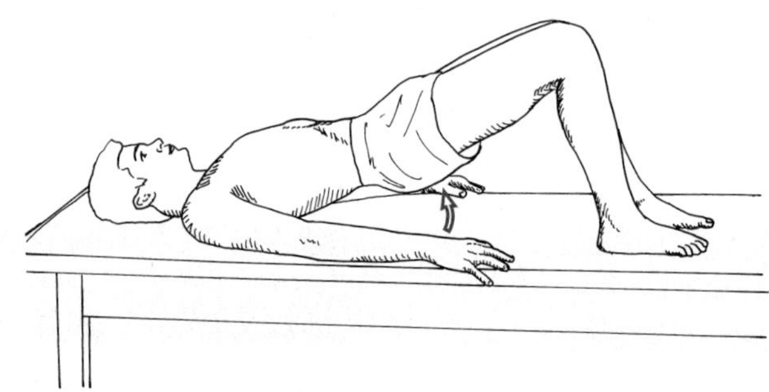

FIGURE 20.28 Training and strengthening the hip extensor muscles using bridging exercises. Resistance can be added against the pelvis.

- *Progressions:* Apply resistance against the anterior pelvis manually or by strapping a weighted belt around the pelvis. Have the patient hold the bridge position and alternately extend the knees. To challenge proprioception and balance, perform bridging exercises using a large gym ball positioned either under the back with feet on the floor or under the feet while lying on the floor.
- *Variation:* Apply elastic resistance around the thighs. While maintaining the bridge position, have the patient abduct and externally rotate the thighs to coordinate strengthening of the gluteus maximus, medius, and external rotators.

Wall Slides

Patient position and procedure: Standing and resting the back against a wall with feet forward and a shoulder-width apart. Have the patient slide the back down the wall by flexing the hips and knees, then slide up the wall by extending the hips and knees (Fig. 20.29 A). This strengthens the hip and knee extensors eccentrically and concentrically. If sliding the back directly against the wall causes excessive friction, place a towel behind the patient's back.

- *Progressions:* Place a large exercise ball behind the back. This requires additional control because the surface is less stable (Fig. 20.29 B). Add arm motions and weights to develop coordination and increase strength. To develop isometric strength, have the patient hold the flexed position and superimpose arm motions with weights. Tie these exercises in with the functional activity of sit-to-stand (with arm assistance if necessary) to and from various chair heights.

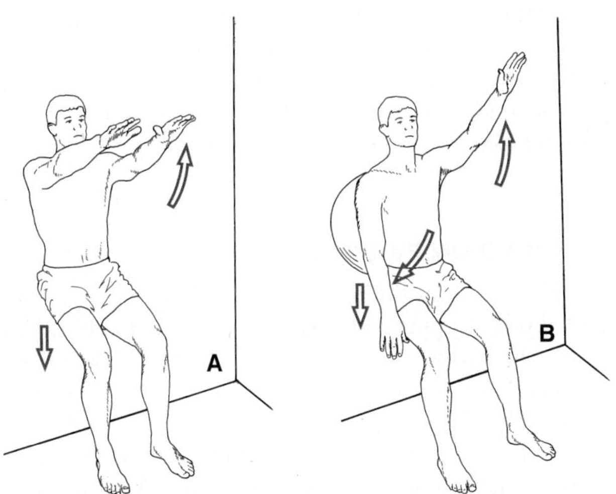

FIGURE 20.29 Wall slides/partial squats to develop eccentric control of body weight. **(A)** The back sliding down a wall, superimposing bilateral arm motion for added resistance. **(B)** The back rolling a gym ball down the wall, superimposing antagonistic arm motion to develop coordination.

Partial Squats/Mini-Squats VIDEO 20.1

Patient position and procedure: In bilateral stance, have the patient lower the body by flexing the hips and knees as if sitting on a chair. Add resistance by having the patient hold weights in the hands, or use elastic resistance secured under the feet (see Fig. 21.27). Progress to safe lifting techniques that involve squatting.

NOTE: If there is need to protect the ACL following ACL reconstruction, limit knee flexion range from 0° to 60° (see Box 21.10 in Chapter 21). Have the patient lower the hips as if preparing to sit on a chair so the knees do not move anterior to the toes. To reduce patellofemoral compression, instruct the patient to squat only through pain-free ranges and avoid deep knee bends.

- *Variations:* Apply elastic resistance around the thighs. While abducting and externally rotating the thighs against the resistance, have the patient perform partial squats (Fig. 20.30) or side-step in one direction and then the other (hips slightly flexed) to coordinate strengthening of the gluteus maximus, medius, and external rotators.

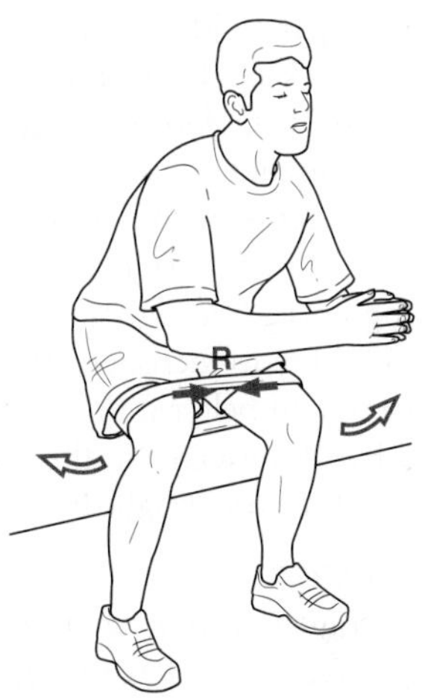

FIGURE 20.30 Elastic resistance around thighs is used to activate the hip external rotators and abductors while performing partial squats to develop strength of the hip and knee extensors.

Single-Limb Deadlift VIDEO 20.1

Patient position and procedure: In unilateral stance with the weight-bearing hip and knee in 30° flexion. Have the patient bend forward at the hips and reach for the toes of the stance leg with the contralateral hand while extending the hip and knee of the nonweight-bearing leg behind (Fig. 20.31). Then return to the upright starting position. This strengthens the hip extensors of the weight-bearing extremity eccentrically and concentrically.

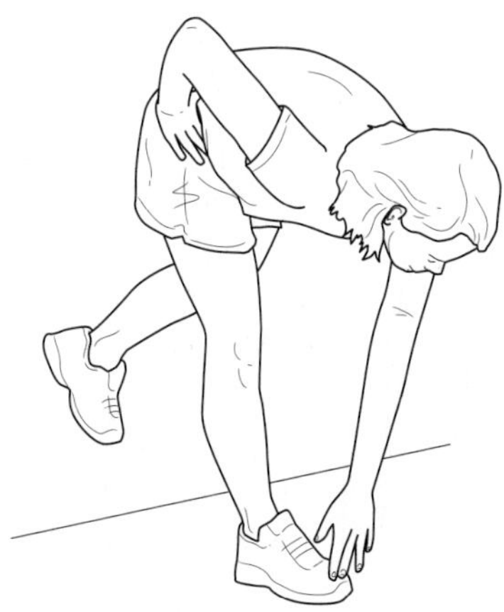

FIGURE 20.31 Single-limb deadlift to strengthen the hip extensors and develop control in the knee.

Step-Ups and Step-Downs

Patient position and procedure: Begin with a low step, 2 to 3 inches in height; increase the height as the patient is able. Have the patient step up and down, forward, laterally, or backward.

- Be sure the patient places the entire foot on the step and lifts and lowers the body with smooth motion. When stepping up, be certain the patient avoids a lurching motion of the trunk or pushing off with the trailing extremity.
- Make sure the patient keeps the trunk upright and the knee aligned vertically over the foot to prevent hip adduction and internal rotation and subsequent valgus collapse. If valgus positioning occurs, reinforce activation of the gluteus medius with manual resistance applied to the lateral thigh of the stepping leg (see Fig. 21.28 A).
- *Progression:* In addition to increasing the step height, add resistance with a weight belt, elastic resistance around the waist (see Fig. 21.28 B), weights in the hands, or a weight around the ankle of the nonweight-bearing leg.

Partial and Full Lunges

Patient position and procedure: After assuming a forward stride position, have the patient flex the hip and knee of the forward extremity and then return upright. Repeat with the same leg or alternate legs. Begin by flexing the knee within a small range, progressing to 90° knee flexion. Instruct the patient to keep the knee in alignment with the forward foot and not bend the knee forward of the foot.

- Use a cane or rod for balance, or hold on to a stable surface for support (parallel bars, treatment table, countertop) if the patient has difficulty controlling the movement (Fig. 20.32).
- It is important to keep the toes pointing forward, bend the knee in the same plane as the feet, and keep the back upright.

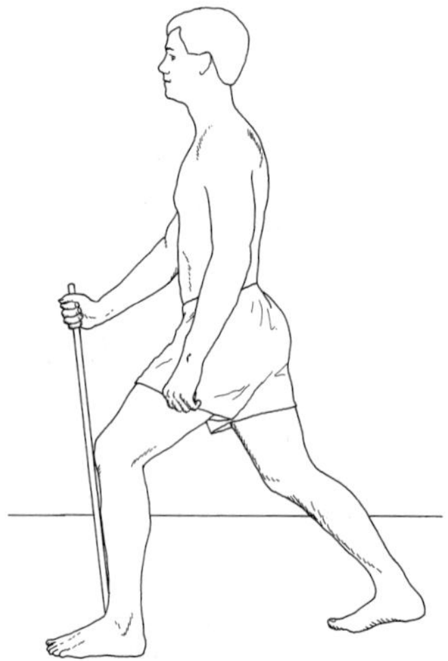

FIGURE 20.32 Partial lunge with cane assistance to develop balance and control for lowering body weight.

- *Progressions:* Hold weights in the hands for additional resistance, take a longer stride, or lunge forward onto a small step. Integrate a function into this exercise by lunging and picking up objects from the floor.

NOTE: A patient with an ACL-deficient knee or a surgically repaired ACL should not flex the knee forward beyond the toes when performing lunges, because this increases the shear force and stress to the ACL. An individual with patellofemoral pain typically experiences increased pain under these circumstances because the external torque generated by the force of gravity acting on the body is greater when the mass is posterior to the knee flexion/extension axis. Adapt the position of the knee or body based on the patient's symptoms and presenting pathology.

Resisted Side Stepping

Patient position and procedure: Patient standing upright or in a partial squat position with an elastic band secured around the knees or distal legs (or the two ends of the band can be held in each hand with the band under both feet). Have the patient step sideways and return, or walk sideways with additional side steps 8 to 10 times then return by leading with the other leg.

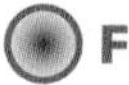 **FOCUS ON EVIDENCE**

In an EMG study by Berry et al,[16] 24 healthy adults performed resisted side stepping with an elastic band around the ankles in both the upright and partial squat positions. The authors consistently recorded significantly greater muscle activation levels in the gluteus maximus, gluteus medius, and tensor fascia latae of the stationary limb compared to the moving limb in both positions. The gluteus medius and maximus had greater activation in the squat position, whereas the tensor had higher values in the upright position.

Resisted Side Sliding

Patient position and procedure: Standing upright or in a partial squat position with an elastic band secured around the ankles. Place a towel under the moving foot and have the patient slide that foot along the floor into hip abduction and return with hip adduction while maintaining stability in the stationary leg (Fig. 20.33).

Functional Progression for the Hip

For a patient to return to full function, the level of challenge from the exercise program must meet the demands that will be imposed during ADL, IADL, work, or sports-related

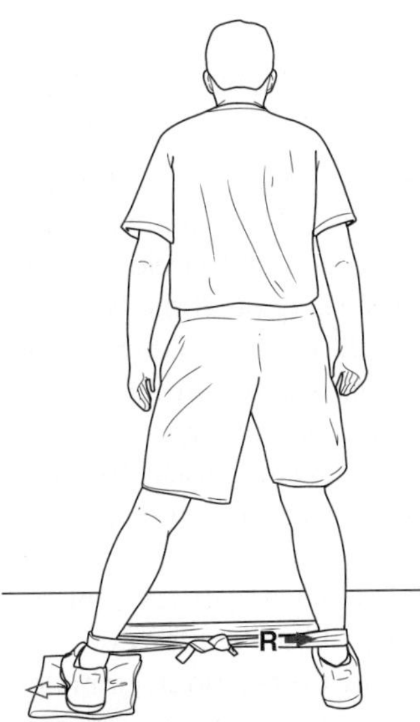

FIGURE 20.33 Standing side slides with elastic resistance; the stationary leg provides stability and control of the body weight while the moving leg slides along the floor into abduction and adduction.

tasks. An outcome may be simply learning how to ambulate forward, backward, and around obstacles safely, or it may involve developing a high level of strength, endurance, coordination, balance, and skill.

The progression of exercises typically begins with isolated activation, control, endurance, and strengthening of the impaired muscles and advances to a variety of open- and closed-chain exercises in combined movement patterns that simulate functional activities to further improve strength, power, and muscular endurance. Balance, coordination, skill, and aerobic conditioning are also integrated into the exercise program as weight-bearing tolerance improves.

Key components of functional exercise progressions for the hip incorporate the entire lower extremity as well as the trunk and upper extremities. Suggestions are summarized in Box 20.11. Details of progressions of exercises for advanced training are described in Chapter 23. Also, refer to Chapter 16 for progressions of spinal exercises and safe body mechanics, Chapter 7 for principles of aerobic exercise, and Chapter 8 for principles of balance training.

BOX 20.11 Summary of Functional Progressions for the Hip

For each activity, adapt the exercise to challenge the patient, but avoid unsafe stresses to the tissues.

- *Balance activities.* Initiate balance activities at the level of weight bearing allowed and progress from bilateral to unilateral activities. Add sagittal and frontal plane arm movements; progress to transverse and diagonal planes. Advance balance/perturbation training activities from stable to unstable surfaces.
- *Ambulation activities.* Increase challenges for ambulation, such as having the patient walk on uneven surfaces, turn, maneuver backward, and walk up and down ramps first under supervision and then unassisted. As soon as the patient is able, have him or her practice rising up and sitting down from chairs of various heights and climbing and descending flights of stairs. Add resistance and speed as tolerated.
- *Safe body mechanics.* Incorporate exercises that prepare the patient for use of safe body mechanics, such as repetitive squats and lunges. Progress the exercises by having the patient lift and carry or push and pull various loads as part of the exercise routine. Utilize safe patterns of motion that replicate functional requirements.
- *Aerobic training.* Cardiopulmonary endurance exercises that replicate functional demands are introduced early in the rehabilitation program and progressed as the patient tolerates.
- *Agility drills.* Use agility drills such as maneuvering around and stepping over obstacles. Incorporate running, jumping, hopping, skipping, and side-shuffle drills.
- *Advanced strength training.* Incorporate maximum eccentric loading into a weight training progression. Any of the previously described exercises can be adapted, but it is critical to assist the patient through the concentric phase of the exercise and guard him or her through the eccentric phase as the resistance is greater than what the muscle can control concentrically. Also include isokinetic training, particularly at medium and fast speeds (velocity spectrum training), if equipment is available.
- *Plyometric training.* If the patient is returning to activities that require strength and power, incorporate plyometric drills. For example, have the patient jump from a box or step; flex the hips, knees, and ankles to absorb the impact of landing; and immediately jump back up to the box or step.

Independent Learning Activities

Critical Thinking and Discussion

1. Describe the function of the primary muscle groups of the hip joint in open- and closed-chain situations. Include their role in stabilizing the pelvis during single-leg stance and the effects on the spine when the pelvis is moved by the hip musculature.
2. Describe the role of the hip during the gait cycle. Include hip muscle activity, hip and pelvic motions needed, and pathological gait patterns that may be related to muscle weakness or restricted motion.
3. Analyze the type of gait deviations a patient might exhibit after internal fixation of a fracture of the proximal femur, THA, or hip hemiarthroplasty.
4. After THA or internal fixation of a hip fracture, what are the signs that dislocation of the hip or loss of fracture stabilization has occurred?

Laboratory Practice

1. Identify and practice the techniques you would use to treat a mobility impairment if the results of your examination included decreased joint play versus restricted flexibility in the hip musculature. Include exercises that could be used in a home exercise program.
2. Demonstrate a progression of exercises to develop control and strength in the gluteus medius muscle after total hip replacement.
3. Develop an exercise routine and progression for an individual with hip muscle weakness who wants to return to work that requires walking, lifting objects that weigh up to 45 lb, and climbing ladders with 45-lb weights.

Case Studies

1. Mr. C, 57 years of age, is a mail carrier; he has walked his mail route for 32 years. Over the past year, he has noticed that his hip hurts after sitting for more than 1 hour and that there is a marked increase in pain when first getting up out of a chair and walking. He also has noticed that there is increased discomfort in his hip and knees near the end of each workday. The medical diagnosis is OA. Strength testing reveals generally 4/5 on manual muscle tests except the gluteus medius, which is 3+/5. There is mild tightness in the hip flexors, including the rectus femoris and tensor fasciae latae. Mr C wants to avoid being a "candidate for total hip replacement surgery."
   - Explain why the patient's job would perpetuate these symptoms.
   - Outline a plan to manage the symptoms; identify measurable goals and interventions you would use to reach the goals.
   - What can the patient do to protect his hip joints?
2. Ms. J, a 31-year-old mother, recreational tennis player, and bowler, is recovering from multiple femoral fractures she sustained in an automobile accident 3 months ago. There is radiological healing of all the fracture sites, and she is now allowed full weight bearing and no restrictions in activities. She has significant hip mobility impairments from joint restrictions and muscle weakness.
   - What joint ranges and muscle strength levels are needed for her to return to her functional and recreational activities?
   - Outline a plan to manage the symptoms; identify measurable goals and interventions you would use to reach the goals. Using the taxonomy or motor skills described in Chapter 1, develop a series of progressively more challenging motor tasks under varying environmental conditions.
3. Mr. P is a 32-year-old firefighter who strained his right hamstring muscles near the ischial tuberosity while pulling a heavy individual out of a burning building 4 days ago. Currently, he is experiencing considerable pain, especially when rising from or lowering himself into a chair and climbing or descending stairs, and is unable to sit on hard surfaces (because of pressure as well as flexing the hip). Hip flexion is limited to 90° and SLR to 45°. He tolerates minimal resistance to hip extension or knee flexion. This individual must be able to climb a ladder while wearing his gear (40 lb) and air pack (40 lb) and carrying a 20-lb hand tool; in addition, he must be able to carry a 175-lb individual across his shoulder, drag a heavy body across the floor, climb five flights of stairs while wearing full gear, and run a half mile in 5 minutes to be able to return to work.
   - Explain why this patient has impaired function in biomechanical terms.
   - Establish goals that reflect treatment of the impairments and desired functional outcomes.
   - Design a program of intervention at each stage of tissue healing.
   - Design a series of exercises that can be used to prepare Mr. P for return to function once the muscle has healed.
4. A 78-year-old woman who lives at home with her husband has been referred to you for home-based physical therapy. Ten days ago she underwent cemented THA with a posterolateral approach for late-stage posttraumatic arthritis associated with injuries sustained in a horseback riding accident 30 years ago. She has been home from the hospital for 5 days. She is ambulating with a walker on level surfaces, and weight bearing is tolerated. The patient's long-term goals are to be able to participate in a community-based fitness program for older adults and resume travel with her husband.
   - Continue progressing her exercise program that was initiated in the hospital.

- Review the precautions she must take for the next 6 to 12 weeks during ADLs.
- Make suggestions on how she or her husband might adapt the home environment to help her adhere to the precautions.
- To help her meet her long-term goals, design a sequence of progressively more demanding functional activities, integrating the taxonomy of motor tasks (addressed in Chapter 1) and the principles of aerobic conditioning (discussed in Chapter 5).

REFERENCES

1. American Academy of Orthopaedic Surgeons (AAOS): *American Academy of Orthopaedic Surgeons Clinical Practice Guideline on Management of Hip Fracture in the Elderly*. Rosemont, IL: AAOS, 2014.
2. Anglen, JO, and Weinstein, JN: Nail or plate fixation of intertrochanteric hip fractures: changing pattern of practice: a review of the American Board of Orthopedic Surgery database. *J Bone Joint Surg Am* 90(4): 700–707, 2008.
3. Antoniou, J, Greidanus, NV, and Proprosky, WG: Surgical approaches and anatomic considerations. In Pellicci, PM, Tria, AJ, and Garvin, KL (eds): *Orthopedic Knowledge Update, 2. Hip and Knee Reconstruction*. Rosemont, IL: American Academy of Orthopedic Surgeons, 2000, p 91.
4. Archibeck, MJ, et al: Second-generation cementless total hip arthroplasty: eight to eleven year results. *J Bone Joint Surg Am* 83:1666–1673, 2001.
5. Archibeck, MJ, and White, RE: Learning curve for the two-incision total hip replacement. *Clin Orthop* 429:232–238, 2004.
6. Austin, AB, et al: Identification of abnormal hip motion associated with acetabular labral pathology. *J Orthop Sports Phys Ther* 38(9):558–564, 2008.
7. Ayotte, NW, et al: Electromyographical analysis of selected lower extremity muscles during 5 unilateral weight-bearing exercises. *J Orthop Sports Phys Ther* 37(2):48–55, 2007.
8. Babis, GC, Morrey, BF, and Berry, DJ: The young patient: indications and results. In Morrey, BF, and Berry, DJ (eds): *Joint Replacement Arthroplasty*, ed. 3. Philadelphia: Churchill-Livingstone, 2003, pp 696–707.
9. Baerga-Varela, L, and Malanga, GA: Rehabilitation and minimally invasive surgery. In Hozack, WJ, et al (eds): *Minimally Invasive Total Joint Arthroplasty*. Heidelberg: Springer Verlag, 2004, pp 2–5.
10. Bal, BS, et al: Early complications of primary total hip replacement performed with a two-incision minimally invasive technique. *J Bone Joint Surg Am* 87(11):2432–2438, 2005.
11. Barnes, B, and Dunovan, K: Functional outcomes after hip fracture. *Phys Ther* 67:1675–1679, 1987.
12. Beaupre, LA, et al: Best practices for elderly hip fracture patients: a systematic overview of the evidence. *J Gen Intern Med* 20(11): 1019–1025, 2005.
13. Berger, RA, et al: Rapid rehabilitation and recovery with minimally invasive total hip arthroplasty. *Clin Orthop* 429:239–247, 2004.
14. Berry, DJ, et al: Minimally invasive total hip arthroplasty: development, early results, and critical analysis. *J Bone Joint Surg Am* 85:2235–2246, 2003.
15. Berry, DJ, and Duffy, GP: Cemented femoral components. In Morrey, BF, and Berry, DJ (eds): *Joint Replacement Arthroplasty*, ed. 3. Philadelphia: Churchill Livingstone, 2003, 617–636.
16. Berry, JW, et al: Resisted side stepping: the effect of posture on hip abductor muscle activation. *J Orthop Sports Phys Ther* 45(9):675–682, 2015.
17. Berry, DJ, Morrey, BF, and Cabanela, MG: Uncemented femoral components. In Morrey, BF, and Berry, DJ (eds): *Joint Replacement Arthroplasty*, ed. 3. Philadelphia: Churchill Livingstone, 2003, 637–656.
18. Berstock, JR, Blom, AW, and Beswick, AD: A systematic review and meta-analysis of the standard versus mini-incision posterior approach to total hip arthroplasty. *J Arthroplasty* 29:1970–1982, 2014.
19. Binder, EF, et al: Effects of extended outpatient rehabilitation after hip fracture: a randomized controlled trial. *JAMA* 292(7):837–846, 2004.
20. Bodén, H, and Adolphson, P: No adverse effects of early weight bearing after uncemented total hip arthroplasty. *Acta Orthop Scand* 75(1):21–29, 2004.
21. Bolgla, LA, and Uhl, TL: Electromyographic analysis of hip rehabilitation exercises in a group of healthy subjects. *J Orthop Sports Phys Ther* 35(8):487–494, 2005.
22. Bottner, F, et al: Implant migration after early weight bearing in cementless hip replacement. *Clin Orthop* 436:132–137, 2005.
23. Brauer, CA, et al: Incidence and mortality of hip fractures in the United States. *JAMA* 302(14):1573–1579, 2009.
24. Bukowski, EL: Practice guidelines: acute care management following total hip arthroplasty (postoperative days 1–4). *Orthop Phys Ther Pract* 17(3):10–14, 2005.
25. Bullock-Saxton, JE: Local sensation changes and altered hip muscle function following severe ankle sprain. *Phys Ther* 74(1):17–28, 1994.
26. Cailliet, R: *Low Back Pain Syndrome*, ed. 5. Philadelphia: F.A. Davis, 1995.
27. Campbell, AJ, and Robertson, MC: Implementation of multifactorial interventions for fall and fracture prevention. *Age Aging* 35(Suppl 2): ii60–ii64, 2006.
28. Capello, WN, et al: Arc-deposited hydroxyapatite-coated cups. *Clin Orthop* 41:305–312, 2005.
29. Charnley, J: Total hip replacement by low friction arthroplasty. *Clin Orthop* 72:7–21, 1974.
30. Chu, FY, et al: The effect of posterior capsulorrhaphy in primary total hip arthroplasty. *J Arthroplasty* 15(2):194–199, 2000.
31. Cibulka, MT, and Delitto, A: A comparison of two different methods to treat hip pain in runners. *J Orthop Sports Phys Ther* 17(4):172–176, 1993.
32. Cibulka, MT, et al: Hip pain and mobility deficits—hip osteoarthritis: clinical practice guidelines linked to the international classification of functioning, disability, and health from the Orthopaedic Section of the American Physical Therapy Association. *J Orthop Sports Phys Ther* 39(4):A1–A25, 2009.
33. Clark, CR, et al: Leg-length discrepancy after total hip arthroplasty. *J Am Acad Orthop Surg* 14(1):38–45, 2006.
34. Clifford, PE, and Mallon, WJ: Sports after total joint replacement. *Clin Sports Med* 24:175–186, 2005.
35. Colon-Emeric, CS: Postoperative management of hip fractures: interventions associated with improved outcomes. *BoneKEy Reports* 1:Article Number 241, 2012. doi:10.1038/bonekey.2012.241
36. Constantinou, M, et al: Spatial-temporal gait characteristics in individuals with hip osteoarthritis: a systematic literature review and meta-analysis. *J Orthop Sports Phys Ther* 44(4):291–303, 2014.
37. Coventry, MB, and Morrey, BF: Historical perspective of hip arthroplasty. In Morrey, BF and Berry, DJ (eds): *Joint Replacement Arthroplasty*, ed. 4. Philadelphia: Churchill Livingstone, 2003, pp 557–565.
38. Cyriax, J: *Textbook of Orthopaedic Medicine, Vol 1. Diagnosis of Soft Tissue Lesions*, ed. 8. London: Bailliere Tindall, 1982.
39. De Jong, Z, and Vlieland, TP: Safety of exercise in patients with rheumatoid arthritis. *Curr Opin Rheumatol* 17(2):177–182, 2005.
40. Di Monaco, M, and Castiglioni, C: Which type of exercise therapy is effective after hip arthroplasty? A systematic review of randomized controlled trials. *Eur J Phys Rehabil Med* 49:893–907, 2013.
41. Distefano, LJ, et al: Gluteal muscle activation during common therapeutic exercises. *J Orthop Sports Phys Ther* 39(7):532–540, 2009.
42. Dorr, LD, et al: Early pain relief and function after posterior minimally invasive and conventional total hip arthroplasty: a prospective, randomized blinded study. *J Bone Joint Surg Am* 89:1153–1160, 2007.
43. Enloe, J, et al: Total hip and knee replacement treatment: a report using consensus. *J Orthop Sports Phys Ther* 23(1):3–11, 1996.
44. Enseki, KR, et al: The hip joint: arthroscopic procedures and postoperative rehabilitation. *J Orthop Sports Phys Ther* 36(7):516–525, 2006.

45. Enseki, K, et al: Nonarthritic hip joint pain: clinical practice guidelines linked to the international classification of functioning, disability and health from the orthopaedic section of the American Physical Therapy Association. *J Orthop Sports Phys Ther* 44(106):A1–A32, 2014.
46. Fehring, TK, and Rosenberg, AG: Primary total hip arthroplasty: indications and contraindications. In Callaghan, JJ, Rosenberg, AG, and Rubash, HE (eds): *The Adult Hip, Vol II*. Philadelphia: Lippincott-Raven, 1998, p 893.
47. Fife, RS: Osteoarthritis, epidemiology, pathology, and pathogenesis. In Klippel, JF (ed): *Primer on Rheumatic Diseases,* ed. 13. Atlanta: Arthritis Foundation, 2007.
48. Fortin, PR, et al: Timing of total joint replacement affects clinical outcomes among patient with osteoarthritis of the hip or knee. *Arthritis Rheum* 46(12):3327–3330, 2002.
49. Freburger, JK: An analysis of the relationship between utilization of physical therapy services and outcomes of care for patients after total hip arthroplasty. *Phys Ther* 80(5):448–458, 2000.
50. Galante, JO: An overview of total joint arthroplasty. In Clohisy, J, et al (eds): *The Adult Hip, Vol II*. Philadelphia: Lippincott Williams & Wilkins, 2014.
51. Garvin, KL, et al: Low wear rates seen in THAs with highly crosslinked polyethylene at 9 to 14 years in patients younger than age 50 years. *Clin Orthop Rel Res* doi 10.1007/s11999-015-4422-7, 2015.
52. Gerlinger, TL, Ghate, RS, and Paprosky, WG: Posterior approach: backdoor in. *Orthopedics* 28(9):931–933, 2005.
53. Givens-Heiss, DL, et al: In vivo acetabular contact pressures during rehabilitation. Part II. Post acute phase. *Phys Ther* 72(10):700–705, 1992.
54. Gjertsen, JE, et al: Internal screw fixation compared with bipolar hemiarthroplasty for treatment of displaced femoral neck fractures in elderly patients. *J Bone Joint Surg Am* 92:619–628, 2010.
55. Goldberg, VM: Surface replacement solutions for the arthritic hip. *Orthopedics* 28(9):943–944, 2005.
56. Goosen, JHM, et al: Minimally invasive versus classic procedures in total hip arthroplasty. A double-blind randomized controlled trial. *Clin Orthop Rel Res* 469:200–208, 2011.
57. Groh, MM, and Herrera, J: A comprehensive review of hip labral tears. *Burr Rev Musculoskelet Med* 2:105–117, 2009.
58. Gucione, AA, Fogerson, TL, and Anderson, JJ: Regaining functional independence in the acute care setting following hip fracture. *Phys Ther* 76(8):818–826, 1996.
59. Hanssen, AD: Anatomy and surgical approaches. In Morrey, BF, and Berry, DJ (eds): *Joint Replacement Arthroplasty,* ed. 3. Philadelphia: Churchill Livingstone, 2003, pp 566–593.
60. Hauer, K, et al: Intensive physical training in geriatric patients after severe falls and hip surgery. *Age Aging* 31:49–57, 2002.
61. Healy, WL, Iorio, R, and Lemos, MJ: Athletic activity after joint replacement. *Am J Sports Med* 29(3):377–387, 2001.
62. Heiberg, KE, et al: Effect of a walking skill training program in patients who have undergone total hip arthroplasty: Followup one year after surgery. *Arthritis Care Res* 64(3):415–423, 2012.
63. Heiderscheit, BC: Lower extremity injuries: is it just about hip strength? *J Orthop Sports Phys Ther* 40(2):39–41, 2010.
64. Hewitt, J, et al: The mechanical properties of the human hip capsule ligaments. *J Arthroplasty* 17:82–89, 2002.
65. Hol, AM, et al: Partial versus unrestricted weight bearing after an uncemented femoral stem in total hip arthroplasty: recommendation of a concise rehabilitation protocol from a systematic review of the literature. *Arch Orthop Trauma Surg* 130:547–555, 2010.
66. Holt, EM, et al: 1000 femoral neck fractures: the effect of pre-injury mobility and surgical experience on outcome. *Injury* 25(2):91–95, 1994.
67. Host, HH, et al: Training-induced strength and functional adaptations after hip fracture. *Phys Ther* 87(3):292–303, 2007.
68. Hozack, WJ: Direct lateral approach: splitting the difference. *Orthopedics* 28(9):937–938, 2005.
69. Huo, MH, Gilbert, NF, and Parvizi, J: What's new in total hip arthroplasty? *J Bone Joint Surg Am* 89:1874–1885, 2007.
70. Izumi, H, et al: Joint motion of bipolar femoral prostheses. *J Arthroplasty* 10(2):237–243, 1995.
71. Jacobs, CA, Christensen, CP, and Berend, ME: Sport activity after total hip arthroplasty: changes in surgical technique, implant design, and rehabilitation. *J Sport Rehabil* 18:47–59, 2009.
72. Jette, AM, Harris, BA, and Clearly, PD: Functional recovery after hip fracture. *Arch Phys Med Rehabil* 68(10):735–740, 1987.
73. Khatod, M, et al: An analysis of the risk of hip dislocation with a contemporary total hip registry. *Clin Orthop Rel Res* 447:19–23, 2006.
74. Kishida, Y, et al: Full weight-bearing after cementless total hip arthroplasty. *Internat Orthop* 25:25–28, 2001.
75. Klein, GR, et al: Return to athletic activity after total hip arthroplasty: consensus guidelines based on a survey of the Hip Society and American Association of Hip and Knee Surgeons. *J Arthroplasty* 22(2):171–175, 2007.
76. Koval, KJ, and Zuckerman, JD: *Hip Fractures: A Practical Guide to Management.* New York: Springer-Verlag, 2000.
77. Koval, KJ, et al: Ambulatory ability after hip fracture: a prospective study in geriatric patients. *Clin Orthop* 310:150–159, 1995.
78. Koval, K, et al: Weight bearing after hip fracture: a prospective series of 596 geriatric hip fracture patients. *J Orthop Trauma* 10(8):526–530, 1996.
79. Krebs, DE, et al: Exercise and gait effects on in vivo hip contact pressures. *Phys Ther* 71(4):301–309, 1991.
80. Krebs, DE, et al: Hip biomechanics during gait. *J Orthop Sports Phys Ther* 28(1):51–59, 1998.
81. Lachiewicz, PF: Dislocation. In Pellicci, PM, Tria, AJ, and Garvin, KL (eds): *Orthopedic Knowledge Update, 2. Hip and Knee Reconstruction.* Rosemont, IL: American Academy of Orthopedic Surgeons, 2000, p 149.
82. Lang, KE: Comparison of 6- and 7-day physical therapy coverage on length of stay and discharge outcome for individuals with total hip and knee arthroplasty. *J Orthop Sports Phys Ther* 28(1):15–22, 1998.
83. Latham, NK, et al: Effect of a home-based exercise program on functional recovery following rehabilitation after hip fracture. A randomized clinical trial. *JAMA* 311(7):700–708, 2014.
84. Laupacis, A, et al: The effect of elective total hip replacement on health-related quality of life. *J Bone Joint Surg Am* 75(11):1619–1626, 1993.
85. Lewallen, DG: Cementless primary total hip arthroplasty. In Pellicci, PM, Tria, AJ, and Garvin, KL (eds): *Orthopedic Knowledge Update, 2. Hip and Knee Reconstruction.* Rosemont, IL: American Academy of Orthopedic Surgeons, 2000, p 195.
86. Lewis, CL, and Sahrmann, SA: Acetabular labral tears. *Phys Ther* 86: 110–121, 2006.
87. Lieberman, JR, et al: Differences between patients' and physicians' evaluation of outcome after total hip arthroplasty. *J Bone Joint Surg Am* 78(6):835–838, 1996.
88. Lugade, V, et al: Gait asymmetry following an anterior and anterolateral approach to total hip arthroplasty. *Clin Biomech* 25(7):675–680, 2010.
89. Magaziner, J, et al: Changes in functional status attributable to hip fracture: a comparison of hip fracture patients to community-dwelling aged. *Am J Epidemiol* 157(11):1023–1031, 2003.
90. Magee, DJ: *Orthopedic Physical Assessment,* ed. 6. St. Louis: Saunders, Elsevier, 2014.
91. Mangione, KK, et al: Can elderly patients who have had a hip fracture perform moderate- to high-intensity exercise at home? *Phys Ther* 85(8):727–739, 2005.
92. Mangione, KK, et al: Interventions used by physical therapists in home care for people after hip fracture. *Phys Ther* 88(2):199–210, 2008.
93. Martin, RI, and Kivlan, B: The hip complex. In Levangie, PK, and Norkin, CC (eds): *Joint Structure and Function: A Comprehensive Analysis,* ed. 5. Philadelphia: F.A. Davis, 2011, pp 358–398.
94. Martin, SD, et al: Hip surgery and rehabilitation. In Melvin, JL, and Gall, V (eds): *Rheumatologic Rehabilitation Series, Vol 5. Surgical Rehabilitation.* Bethesda, MD: American Occupational Therapy Association, 1999, p 81.
95. Matta, JM, and Ferguson, TA: The anterior approach for hip replacement. *Orthopedics* 28(9):927–928, 2005.
96. Mayr, E, et al: A prospective randomized assessment of earlier functional recovery in THA patients treated by minimally invasive direct anterior approach: a gait analysis study. *Clin Biomech* 24:812–818, 2009.

97. McGrorey, BJ, Stewart, MJ, and Sim, FH: Participation in sports after total hip and knee arthroplasty: a review of the literature and survey of surgical preferences. *Mayo Clin Proc* 70(4):342–348, 1995.
98. McKinnis, LN: *Fundamentals of Musculoskeletal Imaging,* ed. 4. Philadelphia: F.A. Davis, 2014.
99. McMinn, DJW: Avascular necrosis in the young patient: a trilogy of arthroplasty options. *Orthopedics* 28(9):945–947, 2005.
100. Meek, RMD, et al: Epidemiology of dislocation after total hip arthroplasty. *Clin Orthop* 447:9–18, 2006.
101. Meere, PA, DiCesare, PE, and Zuckerman, JD: Hip fractures treated by hip arthroplasty. In Callaghan, JJ, Rosenberg, AG, and Rubash, HE (eds): *The Adult Hip, Vol II.* Philadelphia: Lippincott-Raven, 1998, p 1221.
102. Mikkelsen, LR, et al: Effect of early supervised progressive resistance training compared to unsupervised home-based exercise after fast-track total hip replacement applied to patients with preoperative functional limitations. A single-blinded randomized controlled trial. *Osteoarthr Cartil* 22:2051–2058, 2014.
103. Miller, BJ, et al: Changing trends in the treatment of femoral neck fractures. *J Bone Joint Surg Am* 96:e149(1–6), 2014.
104. Minns Lowe, CJ, et al: Effectiveness of land-based physiotherapy exercise following hospital discharge following hip arthroplasty for osteoarthritis: an updated systematic review. *Physiother* 101:252–265, 2015.
105. Mitchell, SL, et al: Randomized controlled trial of quadriceps training after proximal femoral fracture. *Clin Rehabil* 15(3):282–290, 2001.
106. Mohler, CG, and Collis, DK: Early complications and their management. In Callaghan, JJ, Rosenberg, AF, and Rubash, HE (eds): *The Adult Hip, Vol II.* Philadelphia: Lippincott-Raven, 1998, p 1125.
107. Morrey, BF: Dislocation. In Morrey, BF, and Berry, DJ (eds): *Joint Replacement Arthroplasty,* ed. 3. Philadelphia: Churchill Livingstone, 2003, pp 875–890.
108. Morris, AH, and Zuckerman, JD: National consensus conference on improving the continuum of care for patients with hip fracture. *J Bone Joint Surg Am* 84:670–674, 2002.
109. Muller, M, et al: The direct lateral approach: impact on gait patterns, foot progression angle and pain in comparison with a minimally invasive anterolateral approach. *Arch Orthop Trauma Surg* 132:725–731, 2012.
110. Mulligan, BR: *Manual Therapy "NAGS", "SNAGS", "MWM'S" etc.,* ed. 6. Wellington: Plane View Services Limited, 2010.
111. Munin, ME, et al: Early inpatient rehabilitation after elective hip and knee arthroplasty. *JAMA* 279(11):847–862, 1998.
112. Munin, MC, et al: Rehabilitation. In Callaghan, JJ, Rosenberg, AG, and Rubash, HE (eds): *The Adult Hip, Vol II.* Philadelphia: Lippincott-Raven, 1998, p 1571.
113. Nelson, C, Lombardi, PM, and Pellicci, PM: Hybrid total hip replacement. In Pellicci, PM, Tria, AJ, and Garvin, KL (eds): *Orthopedic Knowledge Update, 2. Hip and Knee Reconstruction.* Rosemont, IL: American Academy of Orthopedic Surgeons, 2000, p 207.
114. Neumann, DA: An electromyographic study of the hip abductor muscles as subjects with hip prostheses walked with different methods of using a cane and carrying a load. *Phys Ther* 79(12):1163–1173, 1999.
115. Neumann, DA: Hip abductor muscle activity in patients with a hip prosthesis while carrying loads in one hand. *Phys Ther* 76(12): 1320–1330, 1996.
116. Neumann, DA: Hip abductor muscle activity as subjects with hip prostheses walk with different methods of using a cane. *Phys Ther* 78(5): 490–501, 1998.
117. Neumann, DA: Hip. In Neumann, DA: *Kinesiology of the Musculoskeletal System: Foundations for Rehabilitation,* ed. 2. St. Louis: Mosby/Elsevier, 2010, pp 465–519.
118. Neumann, DA: Kinesiology of the hip: a focus on muscular actions. *J Orthop Sports Phys Ther* 40(2):82–94, 2010.
119. Nilsdotter, AK, et al: Predictors of patient relevant outcomes after total hip replacement for osteoarthritis: a prospective study. *Ann Rheum Dis* 62(10):923–930, 2003.
120. Nordin, M, and Frankel, VH: Biomechanics of the hip. In Nordin, M, and Frankel, VH (eds): *Basic Biomechanics of the Musculoskeletal System,* ed. 3. Philadelphia: Lippincott Williams & Wilkins, 2001, p 202.
121. Oatis, CA: *Kinesiology: The Mechanics and Pathomechanics of Human Movement,* ed. 3. Philadelphia: Lippincott Williams & Wilkins, 2016.
122. Ogonda, L, et al: A minimal-incision technique in total hip arthroplasty does not improve early postoperative outcomes: a prospective, randomized, controlled trial. *J Bone Joint Surg Am* 87(4):701–710, 2005.
123. Okoro, T, et al: What does standard rehabilitation practice after total hip replacement in the UK entail? Results of a mixed methods study. *BMC Musculoskelet Disorders* 14:91–98, 2013.
124. Olney, SJ, and Eng, J: Gait. In Levangie, PK, and Norkin, CC (eds): *Joint Structure and Function: A Comprehensive Analysis,* ed. 5. Philadelphia: F.A. Davis, 2011, pp 528–571.
125. Papagelopoulos, PJ, and Morrey, BF: Cemented acetabular components. In Morrey, BF, and Berry, DJ (eds): *Joint Replacement Arthroplasty,* ed. 3. Philadelphia: Churchill Livingstone, 2003, pp 602–608.
126. Papagelopoulos, PJ, and Sim, FH: Proximal femoral fracture: Femoral neck fracture. In Morrey, BF and Berry, DJ (eds): *Joint Replacement Arthroplasty,* ed. 3. Philadelphia: Churchill Livingstone, 2003, pp 722–732.
127. Parker, MJ, Pryor, GA, and Thorngren, K: *Handbook of Hip Fracture Surgery.* Oxford: Butterworth-Heinemann, 1997.
128. Parvizi, J, et al: Surgical treatment of limb-length discrepancy following total hip arthroplasty. *J Bone Joint Surg Am* 85(12):2310–2317, 2003.
129. Peak, EL, et al: The role of patient restrictions in reducing the prevalence of early dislocation following total hip arthroplasty. *J Bone Joint Surg Am* 87(2):247–253, 2005.
130. Perry, J: *Gait Analysis: Normal and Pathological Function.* Thorofare, NJ: Slack, 1992.
131. Pospischill, M, et al: Minimally invasive compared with traditional transgluteal approach for total hip arthroplasty. *J Bone Joint Surg Am* 92:328–337, 2010.
132. Poss, R: Total joint replacement: optimizing patient expectations. *J Am Acad Orthop Surg* 1(1):18–23, 1993.
133. Powers, CM: The influence of abnormal hip mechanics on knee injury: a biomechanical perspective. *J Orthop Sports Phys Ther* 40(2):42–51, 2010.
134. Prins, MR, and van der Wurff, P: Females with patellofemoral pain syndrome have weak hip muscles: a systematic review. *Aust J Physiother* 55:9–15, 2009.
135. Ranawat, CS, Rasquinna, VJ, and Rodriguez, JA: Results of cemented total hip replacement. In Pellicci, PM, Tria, AJ, and Garvin, KL (eds): *Orthopedic Knowledge Update, 2. Hip and Knee Reconstruction.* Rosemont, IL: American Academy of Orthopedic Surgeons, 2000, p 181.
136. Reininga, IHF, et al: Comparison of gait in patients following a computer-navigated minimally invasive anterior approach and a conventional posterolateral approach for total hip arthroplasty: A randomized controlled trial. *Orthop Res* 31:288–294, 2013.
137. Repantis, R, Bouris, T, and Korovessis, P: Comparison of minimally invasive approach versus conventional anterolateral approach for total hip arthroplasty: a randomized controlled trial. *Eur J Orthop Surg Traumatol* 25:111–116, 2015.
138. Roddy, E, et al: Evidence-based recommendations for the role of exercise in the management of osteoarthritis of the hip or knee—the MOVE consensus. *Rheumatology* 44(1):67–73, 2005.
139. Roddy, E, Zhang, W, and Doherty, M: Aerobic walking or strengthening exercise for osteoarthritis of the knee? A systematic review. *Ann Rheum Dis* 64(4):544–548, 2005.
140. Rosenberg, AG: A two-incision approach: promises and pitfalls. *Orthopedics* 28(9):935–937, 2005.
141. Rydevik, K, et al: Functioning and disability in patients with hip osteoarthritis with mild to moderate pain. *J Orthop Sports Phys Ther* 40(10):616–624, 2010.
142. Sahrmann, SA: *Diagnosis and Treatment of Movement Impairment Syndromes.* St. Louis: CV Mosby, 2002.
143. Schaefer, A, et al: Incompliance of total hip arthroplasty (THA) patients to limited weight bearing. *Arch Orthop Trauma Surg* 135:265–269, 2015.
144. Shashika, H, Matsuba, Y, and Watanabe, Y: Home program of physical therapy: effect on disabilities of patients with total hip arthroplasty. *Arch Phys Med Rehabil* 77(3):273–277, 1996.

145. Sherrington, C, and Lord, SR: Home exercise to improve strength and walking velocity after hip fracture: a randomized, controlled trial. *Arch Phys Med Rehabil* 78:208–212, 1997.
146. Sherrington, C, Lord, SR, and Herbert, RD: A randomised trial of weight-bearing versus nonweight-bearing exercise for improving physical abilities in inpatients after hip fracture. *Aust J Physiother* 49:15–22, 2003.
147. Shih, CH, et al: Muscular recovery around the hip joint after total hip arthroplasty. *Clin Orthop* 302:115–120, 1994.
148. Shumway-Cook, A, et al: Incidence of and risk factors for falls following hip fracture in community-dwelling older adults. *Phys Ther* 85(7): 648–655, 2005.
149. Silva, M, Heisel, C, and Schmalzried, TP: Metal-on-metal total hip replacement. *Clin Orthop* 430:53–61, 2005.
150. Singh, NA, et al: Effects of high-intensity progressive resistance training and targeted multidisciplinary treatment of frailty on mortality and nursing home admissions after hip fracture: A randomized controlled trial. *J Am Med Directors Assoc* 13:24–30, 2012.
151. Smith, TO, Blake, V, and Hing, CB: Minimally invasive versus conventional exposure for total hip arthroplasty: A systematic review and meta-analysis of clinical and radiological outcomes. *Internat Orthop* 35:173–184, 2011.
152. Strickland, EM, et al: In vivo acetabular contact pressures during rehabilitation. Part I. Acute phase. *Phys Ther* 72(10):691–699, 1992.
153. Sutlive, TG, Lopez, HP, and Schnitker, D: Development of a clinical prediction rule for diagnosing hip osteoarthritis in individuals with unilateral hip pain. *J Orthop Sports Phys Ther* 38(9):542–550, 2008.
154. Tanzer, M: Two-incision total hip arthroplasty. *Clin Orthop* 441:71–79, 2005.
155. Taylor, KW, and Murthy, VL: Femoral neck fractures. In Hoppenfeld, S, and Murthy, VL (eds): *Treatment and Rehabilitation of Fractures.* Philadelphia: Lippincott Williams & Wilkins, 2000, p 258.
156. Taylor, KW, and Hoppenfeld, S: Intertrochanteric fractures. In Hoppenfeld, S, and Murthy, VL (eds): *Treatment and Rehabilitation of Fractures.* Philadelphia: Lippincott Williams & Wilkins, 2000, p 274.
157. Taylor, KW, and Murthy, VL: Subtrochanteric femur fractures. In Hoppenfeld, S, and Murthy, VL (eds): *Treatment and Rehabilitation of Fractures.* Philadelphia: Lippincott Williams & Wilkins, 2000, p 288.
158. Tinetti, ME, et al: Home-based multicomponent rehabilitation program for older persons after hip fracture: a randomized trial. *Arch Phys Med Rehabil* 80:916–922, 1999.
159. Tonley, JC, et al: Treatment of an individual with piriformis syndrome focusing on hip muscle strengthening and movement reeducation: a case report. *J Orthop Sports Phys Ther* 40(2):103–111, 2010.
160. Trousdale, TR, and Cabahela, ME: Uncemented acetabular components. In Morrey, BF and Berry, DJ (eds): *Joint Replacement Arthroplasty,* ed. 3. Philadelphia: Churchill Livingstone, 2003, pp 609–616.
161. Trudelle-Jackson, E, Emerson, R, and Smith, S: Outcomes of total hip arthroplasty: a study of patients one year postsurgery. *J Orthop Sports Phys Ther* 32(6):260–267, 2002.
162. Tveit, M, and Kärrholm, J: Low effectiveness of partial weight bearing: continuous recording of vertical loads using a new pressure-sensitive insole. *J Rehabil Med* 33:42–46, 2001.
163. Umpierres, CS, et al: Rehabilitation following total hip arthroplasty evaluation over short follow-up time: randomized clinical trial. *J Rehabil Res Develop* 51(10):1567–1578, 2014.
164. Valenzuela, F, et al: A retrospective study to determine the effectiveness of nonoperative treatment of hip labral tears. *Orthop Practice* 22(3): 147–152, 2010.
165. Wagner, T, et al: Strengthening and neuromuscular reeducation of the gluteus maximus in a triathlete with exercise-associated cramping of the hamstrings. *J Orthop Sports Phys Ther* 40(2):112–119, 2010.
166. Wang, AW, Gilbey, HJ, and Ackland, TR: Perioperative exercise programs improve early return of ambulation function after total hip arthroplasty: a randomized, controlled trial. *Am J Phys Med Rehabil* 81(11):801–806, 2002.
167. Wathe, RA, et al: Modular unipolar versus bipolar prosthesis: a prospective evaluation of functional outcomes after femoral neck fracture. *J Orthop Trauma* 9(4):298–302, 1995.
168. Weinrich, M, et al: Timing, intensity, and duration of rehabilitation for hip fracture and stroke: report of a workshop at the National Center for Medical Rehabilitation Research. *Neurorehabil Neural Repair* 18(1):12–28, 2004.
169. Wolford, ML, Palso, K, and Bercovitz, A: Hospitalization for total hip replacement among inpatients aged 45 and over: United States, 2000-2010. *Centers for Disease Control and Prevention, National Center for Health Statistics,* Data Brief Number 186, 2015.
170. Woolson, ST, et al: Comparison of primary total hip replacement performed with a standard incision or a mini-incision. *J Bone Joint Surg Am* 86:1353–1358, 2004.
171. Xu, C-P, et al: Mini-incision versus standard incision total hip arthroplasty regarding surgical outcomes: A systematic review and meta-analysis of randomized controlled trials. *PLoS ONE* 8(11): e80021, 2013.
172. Zhang, W, et al: OARSI recommendations for the management of hip and knee osteoarthritis, Part II: OARSI evidence-based, expert consensus guidelines. *Osteoarthritis and Cartilage* 16:137–162, 2008.
173. Zhang, Y, et al: Total hip arthroplasty: Leg length discrepancy affects functional outcomes and patient gait. *Cell Biochem Biophys* 72:215–219, 2015.
174. Zwartelé, RE, Brand, R, and Doets, HC: Increased risk of dislocation after primary total hip arthroplasty in inflammatory arthritis. *Acta Orthop Scand* 75(6):684–690, 2004.
175. Philippon, MJ, Weiss, DR, Cuppersmith, DA, Briggs, KK, and Hay, CJ: Arthroscopic labral repair and treatment of femoroacetabular in professional hockey players. *Am J Sports Med* 38: 99–104, 2010.
176. Pierce, CM, et al: Ice hockey goaltender rehabilitation, including on-ice progression, after arthroscopic hip surgery for femoroacetabular impingement. *J Orthop Sports Phys Ther* 43(3): 129–141, 2013.
177. Wahoff, M, and Ryan, M Rehabilitation after hip femoroacetabular impingement arthroscopy. *Clin Sports Med* 30:463–482, 2011.

CHAPTER

21

The Knee

■ LYNN COLBY, PT, MS ■ CAROLYN KISNER, PT, M
■ JOHN BORSTAD, PT, PHD

The knee joint is designed for mobility and stability; it functionally lengthens and shortens the lower extremity to raise and lower the body or to move the foot in space. Along with the hip and ankle, it supports the body when standing, and it is a primary functional unit in walking, climbing, running, and sitting activities.

As in the other regional chapters of the text, this chapter is divided into three primary sections. Highlights of the anatomy and function of the knee complex are reviewed in the first section of the chapter, followed by material on the management of knee disorders and surgeries. The third section includes exercise interventions for the knee region. Chapters 10 through 13 present general information on principles of management. The reader should be familiar with the material in these chapters as well as have a background in examination and evaluation in order to effectively design a therapeutic exercise program to improve knee function in patients with impairments due to injury or pathology or following surgery.

Structure and Function of the Knee

The bones of the knee joint consist of the distal femur with its two condyles, the proximal tibia with its two tibial plateaus, and the large sesamoid bone in the quadriceps tendon, the patella. It is a complex joint both anatomically and biomechanically (Fig. 21.1).[108] The proximal tibiofibular joint is anatomically close to the knee but is enclosed in a separate joint capsule and functions with the ankle. Therefore, the proximal tibiofibular joint is discussed in Chapter 22.

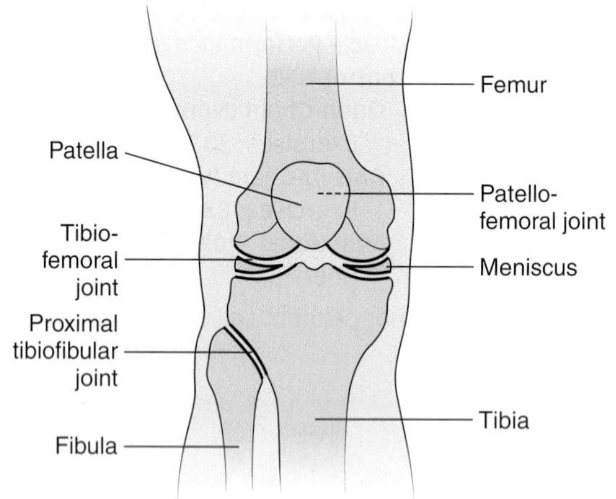

FIGURE 21.1 Bones and joints of the knee and leg.

Joints of the Knee Complex

A lax joint capsule encloses two articulations: the tibiofemoral and the patellofemoral joints. Recesses from the capsule form the suprapatellar, subpopliteal, and gastrocnemius bursae. Folds or thickenings in the synovium persist from embryologic tissue in as many as 60% of individuals and may become symptomatic with microtrauma or macrotrauma.[24,136]

Tibiofemoral Joint

Characteristics. The knee joint is a biaxial, modified hinge joint with two interposed menisci supported by ligaments and muscles. Anteroposterior stability is provided by the cruciate ligaments; mediolateral stability is provided by the medial (tibial) and lateral (fibular) collateral ligaments (MCL and LCL), respectively (Fig. 21.2).[37,108]

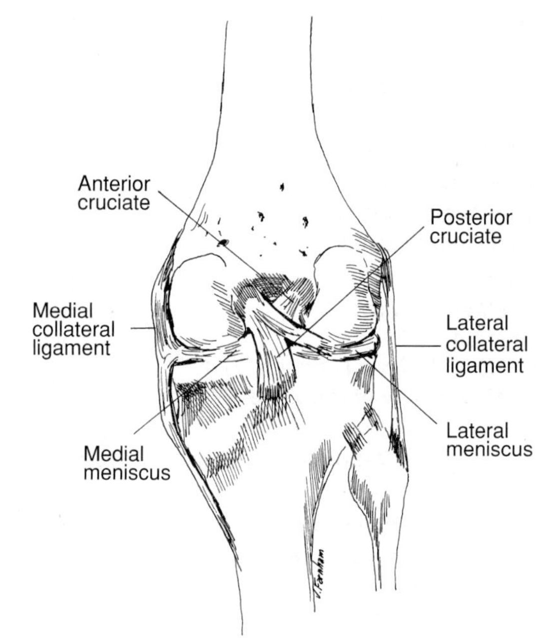

FIGURE 21.2 The medial meniscus is attached to the medial collateral, anterior cruciate, and posterior cruciate ligaments. The lateral meniscus is also attached to the posterior cruciate ligament. (Joint capsule removed for visualization). *(From Hartigan, E, Lewek, M, and Snyder-Mackler, L: The knee. In Levangie, PK, and Norkin, CC (eds):* Joint Structure and Function: A Comprehensive Analysis, *ed. 5. Philadelphia: F.A. Davis, 2011, with permission.)*

- The convex bony partner is composed of two asymmetrical condyles on the distal end of the femur. The medial condyle has a longer surface than the lateral condyle, which contributes to the locking mechanism at the knee.
- The concave bony partner is composed of two tibial plateaus on the proximal tibia with their respective fibrocartilaginous menisci. The medial plateau is larger than the lateral plateau.
- The menisci improve the congruency of the articulating surfaces. They are connected to the tibial condyles and capsule by the coronary ligaments, to each other by the transverse ligament, and to the patella via the patellomeniscal ligaments.[108] Anterior and posterior meniscofemoral ligaments connecting the lateral meniscus to the femur may also be present.[104] The medial meniscus is firmly attached to the joint capsule as well

as to the MCL, anterior and posterior cruciate ligaments (ACL and PCL), and semimembranosus muscle. The lateral meniscus attaches to the PCL and the tendon of the popliteus muscle through capsular connections.[108] Because the medial meniscus has more extensive attachments than the lateral meniscus (see Fig. 21.2), it has a greater chance of sustaining a tear when there is trauma to the knee.

Arthrokinematics. Joint mechanics are affected by open- and closed-chain positions of the extremity. and are summarized in ONLINE Box 21.1 available on the FA Davis web site.

- With motions of the tibia while in a nonweight-bearing, open kinematic chain, the concave plateaus slide in the same direction as the bone motion.
- With motions of the femur on a fixed tibia while in a weight-bearing, closed kinematic chain, the convex condyles slide in the direction opposite to the bone motion.
- Axial rotation occurs between the tibia and femur as the knee flexes and extends due to the asymmetrical condyles. In nonweight bearing extension the tibia rotates laterally on the femur, and with flexion it rotates medially.

Screw-home mechanism. The axial rotation that occurs between the femoral condyles and the tibia during the final degrees of extension is called the locking, or screw-home, mechanism. When the tibia is fixed with the foot weight bearing on the ground, terminal extension results in the femur rotating internally (the medial condyle slides farther posteriorly than the lateral condyle). Concurrently, the hip moves into extension. Tension in the iliofemoral ligament, which occurs with hip extension, reinforces the medial rotation of the femur to lock the knee. As the knee is unlocked, the femur rotates laterally. Unlocking of the knee occurs indirectly with hip flexion and directly from action of the popliteus muscle. Individuals who cannot lock their knee into extension because they lack full hip extension (hip flexion contracture) are unable to benefit from this passive stabilizing function during standing.

Patellofemoral Joint

Characteristics. The patella is a sesamoid bone in the quadriceps tendon. It articulates with the intercondylar (trochlear) groove on the anterior aspect of the distal femur. Its articulating surface is covered with smooth hyaline cartilage. The patella is embedded in the anterior portion of the joint capsule and is connected to the tibia by the ligamentum patellae. Many bursae surround the patella.[108]

Mechanics. As the knee flexes, the patella first contacts the intercondylar groove with its inferior margin and maintains contact with the groove as flexion increases. With extension, the patella remains seated in the groove until near full knee extension, when there is a small amount of superior patellar translation in the proximal intercondylar groove.[154] If patellar movement is restricted, it interferes with the range of knee flexion and may contribute to an extensor lag with active knee extension.[289]

Patellar Function

The primary function of the patella is to increase the moment arm of the quadriceps muscle in its function to extend the knee. The cartilaginous surface of the patella also reduces friction and dissipates forces between the patella and the femoral condyles.[108]

Patellar Alignment

The alignment of the patella in the frontal plane is influenced by the direction of the quadriceps muscle group composite force vector and by its attachment to the tibial tubercle via the patellar tendon. The result of these opposing forces is a bowstring effect on the patella that produces a lateral pull. The bowstring effect can be estimated by measuring the Q-angle. The *Q-angle* is the angle formed by two intersecting lines: one from the anterior superior iliac spine to the midpatella and the other from the tibial tubercle through the midpatella (Fig. 21.3).[108,178] A normal Q-angle, which tends to be greater in women than men, is 10° to 15°. A higher Q-angle suggests greater lateral bowstring forces on the patella.

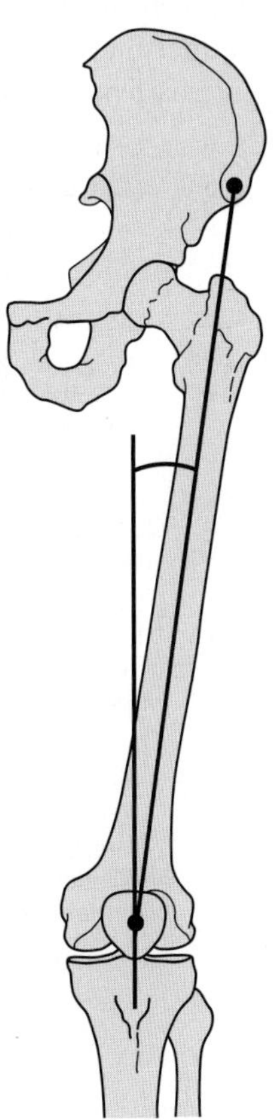

FIGURE 21.3 The Q-angle is the angle formed by the intersection of a line drawn from the center of the patella to the anterosuperior iliac spine and a line drawn from the center of the patella to the tibial tuberosity. These two lines represent forces that create a bowstring effect on the patella. An increased Q-angle is a factor contributing to excessive lateral tracking of the patella. *(From McKinnis, LN: Fundamentals of Musculoskeletal Imaging, ed. 4. Philadelphia: F.A. Davis, 2014, p 375, with permission.)*

Forces Maintaining Alignment

In addition to the bony restraints of the trochlear groove (femoral sulcus), the patella is stabilized by passive and dynamic restraints. The superficial portion of the extensor retinaculum, to which the vastus medialis (VM) and vastus lateralis (VL) muscles attach, provides dynamic stability to the patella in the transverse plane. The medial and lateral patellofemoral ligaments, which attach to the adductor tubercle medially and iliotibial (IT) band laterally, provide passive restraints to the patella in the transverse plane.[108] The medial and lateral patellotibial ligaments and patellar tendon combine to stabilize the patella against the superiorly directed pull of the quadriceps muscle group (Fig. 21.4).

Patellar Malalignment and Tracking Problems

Malalignment and tracking problems of the patella may be caused by several factors that may or may not be interrelated.[99]

Increased Q-angle. With an increased Q-angle, there may be increased force between the lateral patellar facet and lateral femoral condyle when the knee flexes during weight bearing. Structurally, an increased Q-angle may occur with a wide pelvis, femoral anteversion, coxa vara, genu valgum, and/or laterally displaced tibial tuberosity. Lower extremity motions in the transverse plane that may increase the Q-angle are external tibial rotation, internal femoral rotation, and a pronated subtalar joint. Dynamic knee valgus (see Fig. 21.9), where the knee joint center moves medially relative to the foot during weight-bearing activities, also increases the Q-angle.[233,234]

FOCUS ON EVIDENCE

A recent MRI study[277] comparing femoral and patellar orientation at multiple knee angles during weight bearing in females with ($n = 15$) and without ($n = 15$) patellofemoral pain showed significant group-by-angle interactions for three of four outcome variables (femoral medial rotation, lateral patellar displacement, and patellar tilt, but not patellar rotation). Subjects in the patellofemoral pain group demonstrated significantly altered joint kinematics compared to the control group, with the greatest differences between groups at 0° knee flexion. The authors propose that increased femoral medial rotation is the main mechanism responsible for these kinematic differences.

Muscle and fascial tightness. A tight IT band and lateral retinaculum prevent medial translation of the patella. Tight ankle plantarflexors result in pronation of the foot when the ankle dorsiflexes, causing lateral torsion of the tibia and functional lateral displacement of the tibial tuberosity promoting an increased lateral force on the patella.[166] Tight rectus

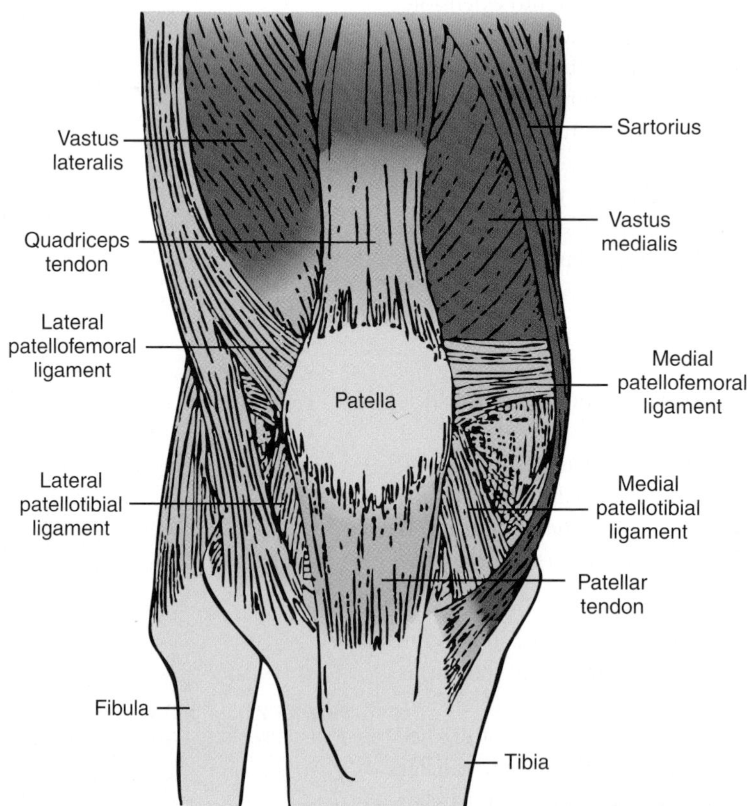

FIGURE 21.4 The extensor retinaculum is reinforced medially by the transversely oriented medial patellofemoral ligament and the longitudinally oriented medial patellotibial ligament. The lateral patellofemoral ligament and lateral patellotibial ligament help resist an excessive medial glide of the patella. *(From Hartigan, E, Lewek, M, and Snyder-Mackler, L: The knee. In Levangie, PK, and Norkin, CC (eds):* Joint Structure and Function: A Comprehensive Analysis, *ed. 5. Philadelphia: F.A. Davis, 2011, p 403, with permission.)*

femoris and hamstring muscles may affect knee mechanics and lead to compensations.[172]

Hip muscle weakness. Hip abductor and external rotator weakness may result in femur adduction and knee valgus and contribute to increased medial rotation of the femur observed under weight bearing in subjects with patellofemoral pain syndrome.[125,194]

Patellar Compression

Patellar contact. The posterior surface of the patella has several facets and is not completely congruent with the trochlear groove on the femur. When the knee is in complete extension (0°), the patella is superior to the trochlear groove. By 15° of flexion, the inferior border of the patella begins to articulate with the superior aspect of the groove. As knee flexion increases, the patella slides distally in the groove, and surface contact area increases. Beyond 60° of flexion the contact area either continues to increase, levels off, or decreases, depending on the source.[98,99] As the knee flexes past 90°, the quadriceps tendon comes in contact with the trochlear groove as the patella slides inferiorly.

Compression forces. In full extension, because there is minimal to no contact of the patella with the trochlear groove, there is no compression of the articular surfaces. Furthermore, the nearly parallel alignment of the femur and tibia creates minimal compressive loading through a small sagittal plane bowstring effect. The resultant force from this quadriceps and patellar tendon bowstring effect causes increased compressive forces as the knee flexes, but there is also greater joint surface contact area to dissipate these higher forces. Patellofemoral joint reaction forces rise rapidly between 30° and 60°, but there is controversy regarding the extent of joint reaction forces at higher flexion angles.

- During squatting, the joint reaction force continues to rise until 90° and then levels off or decreases because the quadriceps tendon begins making contact with the trochlear groove and dissipates some of the force.[98]
- In an open-chain, nonweight-bearing exercise with a free weight on the distal leg, the greatest joint reaction force in the patellofemoral articulation occurs at around 30° of flexion.[98] This is more likely due to the changing moment arm of the weight rather than the resultant force of the quadriceps and patellar tendons.
- An increased Q-angle causes increased lateral facet compression as the knee flexes.[234]

Muscle Function

Knee Extensor Muscle Function

The quadriceps femoris muscle group is the only muscle crossing anterior to the flexion/extension axis of the knee and is the prime mover (agonist) for knee extension. Other muscles that can act to extend the knee require the foot to be fixed, creating a closed chain. In this situation, the hamstrings and the soleus muscles can cause or control knee extension by pulling the proximal tibia posteriorly.

Closed-chain function. During standing and the stance phase of gait, the knee is an intermediate joint in a closed chain. The quadriceps muscle controls the amount of knee flexion and also extends the knee through reverse muscle pull on the femur. In the erect standing posture when the knee is locked in extension, the quadriceps need not function when the gravity line falls anterior to the flexion/extension axis. In this case, tension in the hamstring and gastrocnemius tendons support the posterior capsule of the knee.

Patella. The patella improves the mechanical advantage of the knee extensors by increasing the moment arm between the extensor force vector and the knee joint flexion/extension axis. Its greatest effect on the leverage of the quadriceps is during knee extension from 60° to 30° and the effect rapidly diminishes from 15° to 0° of extension.[101,108]

Torque. The peak extension torque produced by the quadriceps muscle occurs between 70° and 50°.[34] The physiological advantage of the quadriceps rapidly decreases during the last 15° of knee extension because of its shortened length. This, combined with its decreased mechanical advantage in the last 15°, requires the muscle to significantly increase its contractile force when large demands are placed on the muscle during terminal extension.[101]

- During standing closed-chain activities, assistance for knee extension is provided by the hamstring and soleus muscles. In addition, the ACL and the hamstring muscle group contractile force counter the anterior translation force produced by quadriceps muscle contractions.[75,171]
- During open-chain knee extension exercises in the sitting or supine position, when the resistive torque is maximum in terminal extension because of the resistance moment arm, a relatively strong contraction of the quadriceps muscle is required to overcome the physiological and mechanical disadvantages of the muscle to complete the final 15° of motion.[101] However, recall that the compressive loads on the patella also decrease in terminal extension because of its superior location with respect to the trochlear groove and the relatively small sagittal plane bowstring effect of the quadriceps and patellar tendon.

CLINICAL TIP

Be aware of the effect of the external resistance and how the muscle is challenged differently through the range of motion. During open-chain exercises with fixed resistance such as an ankle weight, the resistance torque is most challenging for the quadriceps in terminal extension, while there is minimal challenge midrange where the muscle is capable of generating greater tension. This paradox will impact the effectiveness of the exercises performed by the patient, their comfort during the exercise, and the joint loading that occurs across the range of motion.

Knee Flexor Muscle Function

The hamstring muscles are the primary knee flexors and also influence rotation of the tibia on the femur. Because the hamstrings are two-joint muscles, they contract more efficiently when the decrease in length during knee flexion is offset by increased length through hip flexion. During closed-chain weight-bearing activities, the hamstring muscles can assist with knee extension by pulling the tibia posteriorly.

- The gastrocnemius muscle also can function as a knee flexor, but its prime function at the knee during weight bearing is to support the posterior capsule against hyperextension forces.
- The popliteus muscle supports the posterior capsule and acts to unlock the extended knee.
- The pes anserinus muscle group (sartorius, gracilis, and semitendinosus) provides medial stability to the knee and affects rotation of the tibia in a closed chain.

Dynamic Stability of the Knee

Because of the incongruity between the rounded femoral condyles and nearly flat tibial plateaus, there is minimal knee stability provided by the bony architecture. The cruciate and collateral ligaments provide significant passive stability to the knee throughout joint motion. Dynamic stability is the ability of a joint to remain stable in the presence of rapidly shifting loads during motion.[122] Dynamic stability requires motor control of the neuromuscular system to coordinate muscle activity around the joint. The complex feedforward and feedback responses mediated by the central nervous system modulate muscle stiffness and are important for providing dynamic knee stability under varying loads and stresses imposed on the joint structures.[309] As summarized in a clinical commentary by Williams,[309] clinical and scientific evidence is accumulating to substantiate exercise programs designed for the purpose of developing dynamic stability of the knee—that is, to improve dynamic control of the knee via neuromuscular responses in order to reduce knee ligament stress and minimize the risk of injury during high-intensity activities.

The Knee and Gait

During the normal gait cycle, the knee goes through a range of 60° (0° extension at initial contact or heel strike to 60° at the end of initial swing). There is also some medial rotation of the femur as the knee extends at initial contact and just prior to heel-off.[108,212,228]

Muscle Control of the Knee During Gait

Stability during the gait cycle is efficiently controlled by the normal function of the muscles that cross the knee joint.[212,228]

Quadriceps. The quadriceps muscle controls the amount of knee flexion during initial contact and loading response and then extends the knee toward midstance. It again controls the amount of flexion during preswing (heel-off to toe-off) and prevents excessive knee flexion (heel rise) during initial swing. With loss of quadriceps function, the patient lurches the trunk anteriorly during initial contact to stabilize the joint by moving the trunk center of gravity anterior to the knee flexion/extension axis.[283]

Hamstrings. The hamstring muscles primarily decelerate and control knee extension during terminal swing. Loss of function may result in the knee snapping into extension prior to initial contact. The hamstrings also provide posterior support to the knee capsule when the knee is extended during stance, and loss of this function results in progressive genu recurvatum.[283]

Soleus. The single joint ankle plantarflexor muscles (primarily the soleus) help limit the amount of knee flexion during preswing by controlling the forward movement of the tibia over the fixed foot. Loss of function results in compensatory hyperextension of the knee during preswing. Loss of heel rise during the preswing phase resulting in a lag or slight dropping of the pelvis on that side may also occur with soleus dysfunction.

Gastrocnemius. The gastrocnemius muscle provides posterior support to the extended knee at the end of loading response or foot flat and just prior to preswing or heel-off. Loss of gastrocnemius function results in hyperextension of the knee during these periods as well as loss of propulsion from plantarflexion during preswing or push-off.

Hip and Ankle Impairments

Because the knee is the intermediate joint between the hip and foot, problems in these two areas can interfere with knee function during gait. Examples include the following.

Hip flexion contractures. Inability to extend the hip prevents the knee from extending just before terminal stance (heel-off).

Length/strength imbalances. With asymmetry of length, strength, or neuromuscular control of hip and knee muscles, unbalanced forces may stress structures of the knee, giving rise to pain during walking or running. For example, a tight tensor fasciae latae or gluteus maximus muscle may increase stress on the IT band and lead to lateral knee pain, or it could affect patellofemoral joint kinematics and lead to anterior knee pain. Weak hip external rotators and abductors result in femoral internal rotation, which can create a relative lateral displacement of the patella and subsequent patellofemoral pain.[277] Overuse of the hamstring muscle group may result in compensatory increases in quadriceps femoris muscle activation and result in anterior knee pain (see Chapter 20 for discussion of muscle imbalances in hip).

Foot impairments. The position and function of the foot and ankle affect the stresses transmitted to the knee. For example, with pes planus or pes valgus, there is an overall medial rotation of the lower extremity, with increased Q-angle and an increased bowstring effect on the patella.[166]

Referred Pain and Nerve Injuries

For a detailed description of referred pain patterns and peripheral nerve injuries in the knee region, see Chapter 13.

Major Nerves Subject to Injury at the Knee

The sciatic nerve divides into the tibial and common peroneal nerves just proximal to the popliteal fossa. These nerves are relatively well protected deep in the fossa.

- The *common fibular (peroneal) nerve* (L2–L4) becomes superficial where it winds around the fibula just below the fibular head, a common site for injury. Symptoms of sensory loss and muscle weakness are distal to that site.
- The *saphenous nerve* (L2–L4) is a sensory nerve that innervates the skin along the medial side of the knee and leg. It may be injured with trauma or surgery in that region, resulting in chronic pain syndromes.

Common Sources of Referred Pain

Nerve roots and tissues derived from spinal segments L3 refer to the anterior aspect, and those from S1 and S2 refer to the posterior aspect of the knee.[50] The hip joint, which is primarily innervated by L3, may refer symptoms to the anterior thigh and knee. In cases of referred pain, therapeutic exercise for the knee is beneficial only for preventing disuse of the knee musculature; primary treatment must be directed to the source of the nerve irritation.

Management of Knee Disorders and Surgeries

To make sound clinical decisions when treating patients with knee disorders, it is necessary to understand the various pathologies, surgical procedures, and associated precautions and to identify the structural and functional impairments, activity limitations, and participation restrictions. In this section, common pathologies and surgical procedures are presented and conservative and postoperative management of these conditions is described.

Joint Hypomobility: Nonoperative Management

Common Joint Pathologies and Associated Impairments

Osteoarthritis (OA) and rheumatoid arthritis (RA), as well as acute trauma, can all affect the knee joints. In addition, decreased flexibility and adhesions can develop in the joints and surrounding tissues any time the knee joint is immobilized following an injury, surgery, or fracture. The etiology of arthritic and joint symptoms and general management guidelines are described in Chapter 11; this section applies that information to management of the knee joint.

Osteoarthritis (Degenerative Joint Disease)

OA, often referred to as degenerative joint disease, is the most common disease affecting weight-bearing joints. In the knee, articular cartilage destruction is more often apparent on the medial joint compartment than the lateral compartment (Fig. 21.5).

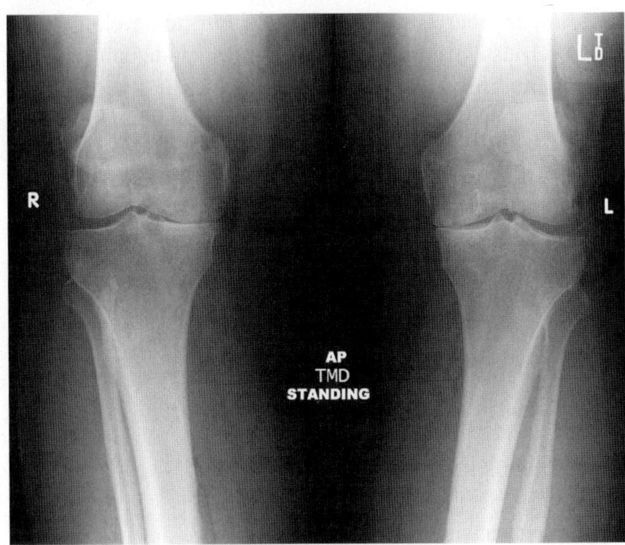

FIGURE 21.5 Advanced bilateral, medial compartment degenerative joint disease in the knees of a 52-year-old computer programmer/analyst who subsequently underwent right total knee arthroplasty.

One-third of individuals older than age 65 have radiographic evidence of knee OA.[16] Pain, muscle weakness, medial compartment laxity, and motion limitations affect function and lead to disability. Deformity such as genu varum commonly develops in the knees in the presence of OA, although genu valgum may occur in some individuals. Knee instability (the sensation of knee buckling or shifting) is frequently reported by individuals with knee OA and significantly contributes to impaired physical function.[77] Factors such as excess weight, joint trauma, developmental deformities, quadriceps weakness, and abnormal tibial rotation are risk factors for developing OA of the knee.[6,16]

FOCUS ON EVIDENCE

An investigation of 52 patients with medial compartment knee OA by Schmitt and associates[255] found that self-reported knee instability contributed to limited function during daily living. However, the study showed no direct relationship between the severity of reported knee instability and the amount of medial joint laxity, varus alignment of the knee, or quadriceps muscle strength.

In a study of 220 patients with OA, 95% of the subjects reported lack of knee confidence during gait; pain during gait and fear of movement being high correlates with lack of confidence.[272]

Posttraumatic Arthritis

Posttraumatic arthritis of the knee occurs in response to any injury that affects the joint structures, particularly following traumatic ligament and meniscal tears. With these injuries, joint swelling may be immediate, indicating bleeding within the joint, or progressive (more than 4 hours to develop), indicating serous effusion. Acute symptoms include pain, limited motion, and muscle guarding. Trauma, including repetitive microtrauma, is a common cause of degenerative changes in the knee joint.

Rheumatoid Arthritis

Early-stage RA usually manifests first in the hands and feet but with progression of the disease process, the knees may also become involved. With RA, the joints become warm and swollen and limited motion develops. In addition, a genu valgum deformity commonly develops during the advanced stages of the disease.

Postimmobilization Hypomobility

When the knee has been immobilized for several weeks or longer, such as during healing of a fracture or after surgery, the capsule, muscles, and soft tissue develop contractures and motion becomes restricted. Tissue adhesions may restrict caudal gliding of the patella, which limits knee flexion, and may cause pain if the tissue tightness results in increased patellofemoral joint compression forces. If proximal gliding of the patella is restricted when the quadriceps muscle contracts, an extensor lag may occur with active knee extension.[281] This usually occurs after operative repairs of some knee ligaments, when the knee is immobilized in flexion for a prolonged period.

Common Structural Impairments

- With joint involvement, the pattern of restriction at the knee is usually more loss of flexion than extension.
- When there is effusion (swelling within the joint), a joint position near 25° of flexion is often most comfortable for the patient because this position has the greatest capsule distensibility. Minimal joint motion is possible in the presence of effusion.
- Reflex inhibition and resulting weakness of the quadriceps femoris muscle occurs because of joint distention.[279] Symptoms such as joint distention from effusion, stiffness, pain, and reflex quadriceps inhibition may cause an extensor (quadriceps) lag in which the active range of knee extension is less than the passive range available.[281]
- Impaired balance responses such as increased body sway under both static and dynamic conditions have been reported in patients with knee arthritis.[300]

Common Impairments, Activity Limitations, and Participation Restrictions

- With acute symptoms and in advanced stages of joint degeneration, there is pain during motion, weight bearing, and gait that may interfere with work or routine household and community activities.
- There is limitation of, or difficulty controlling, weight-bearing activities that involve knee flexion, such as sitting down and rising from a chair or a commode, descending or ascending stairs, stooping, squatting, or rising from the floor.[74]
- With end-stage arthritis, physical activity is markedly curtailed with less participation in leisure and household activities.[291]

Joint Hypomobility: Management—Protection Phase

See Chapter 11 for general guidelines for the management of acute joint lesions and specific guidelines for OA and RA.

Control Pain and Protect the Joint

Patient education. It is important to teach the patient methods to protect the joint including bed positioning, use of orthotics to avoid deforming contractures, range of motion (ROM) and muscle-setting exercises to maintain mobility and promote blood flow, and safe functional activities that reduce stresses on the knee.

Functional adaptations. Instruct the patient to minimize stair-climbing, use elevated seats on commodes, and avoid deep-seated or low chairs in order to minimize the high muscle forces required in these knee flexion ranges while bearing weight. If necessary during an acute flare of arthritis, have the patient use crutches, canes, or a walker to distribute forces through the upper extremities while walking.

Maintain Soft Tissue and Joint Mobility

Passive, active-assistive, or active ROM. Use ROM techniques within the limits of pain and available motion. The patient may be able to perform active ROM in the gravity-eliminated, side-lying position, or self-assisted ROM.

Grade I or II joint distraction and anterior/posterior glides. Apply gentle manual techniques, if tolerated, with the joint in or near resting position (25° flexion). These techniques are used to inhibit pain as well as maintain joint mobility. Stretching is contraindicated at this stage.

Maintain Muscle Function and Prevent Patellar Adhesions

Setting exercises. Perform pain-free quadriceps ("quad sets") and hamstring muscle-setting exercises with the knee in pain-free positions, quad sets with leg raises, and submaximal closed-chain muscle setting exercises. Muscle-setting exercises are described in detail in the last section of this chapter. Quad sets may help maintain mobility of the patella when the tibiofemoral joint is immobilized and therefore are routinely taught following surgery or when the joint is immobilized.

Joint Hypomobility: Management—Controlled Motion and Return to Function Phases

As joint effusion decreases and tissues are able to tolerate increased stresses, the goals of treatment change to deal with the impairments interfering with function. The patient is progressed through controlled motion exercises and activities that focus on safely returning to desired functional activities.

Educate the Patient

- Inform the patient about his or her condition, what to expect regarding recovery, and how to protect the joints.
- Teach the patient safe exercises to do at home, how to progress them, and how to modify them if symptoms are exacerbated by the disease, overuse, or the exercises. Exercises that include specifically designed strengthening, stretching, ROM, and use of a stationary bicycle have been shown to improve functional outcomes in patients with OA in a home exercise program.[59] It is important to emphasize that maintaining strength in the supporting muscles helps protect and stabilize the joint and that balance exercises help reduce the incidence of falls.
- Instruct the patient to perform active ROM and muscle-setting techniques frequently during the day, especially prior to bearing weight, in order to reduce the painful symptoms that occur with initial weight bearing.[74]
- The patient with OA or RA should be cautioned to alternate activity with rest.

FOCUS ON EVIDENCE

In a randomized, controlled study[59] of 134 patients with knee OA, a clinic treatment group ($n = 66$) received supervised exercise, manual therapy, and home exercises for 4 weeks. A home exercise group ($n = 68$) performed home exercises only. Outcomes consisted of the distance walked in 6 minutes and the Western Ontario and McMaster Universities Osteoarthritis Index (WOMAC). Both groups improved at 4 weeks; the clinic treatment group improved 52% on the WOMAC, whereas the home exercise group improved 26%. Both groups improved 10% on the 6-minute walk distances. At 1 year, there was no difference between the groups, and both groups demonstrated improvement over baseline measurements. However, the clinic treatment group was less likely to be taking medication for the arthritis and was more satisfied with the outcome of their rehabilitation. The lack of long-term maintenance highlights the importance of patient education and adherence to a prescriptive long-term home exercise program.

Decrease Pain From Mechanical Stress

Continue use of assistive devices for ambulation if necessary. The patient may progress by using less assistance or may ambulate for periods without assistance. Continue use of elevated seats on commodes and chairs, if needed, to reduce the mechanical stresses imposed when attempting to stand.[74]

Increase Joint Play and Range of Motion

PRECAUTION: Do not increase ROM unless the patient has sufficient strength to control the motion already available. A mobile weight-bearing joint with inadequate muscle control causes impaired stability and makes lower extremity weight-bearing function difficult.

Joint mobilization. When there is loss of joint play and decreased mobility, joint mobilization techniques should be used. Apply grade III or IV sustained or oscillatory techniques to the tibiofemoral and patellofemoral articulations with the joint positioned at the end of its available range. (See Figs. 5.49 through 5.54 and their descriptions in Chapter 5.) As ROM increases, integrate the rotational accessory motions that accompany flexion and extension.[134]

- To increase *flexion*, position the tibia in medial rotation and apply the posterior glide against the anterior aspect of the medial tibial plateau.
- To increase *extension*, position the tibia in lateral rotation and apply the anterior glide against the posterior aspect of the lateral tibial plateau.
- Medial and lateral gliding of the tibia on the femur may also be done to regain mobility for flexion and extension.

Stretching techniques. Passive and proprioceptive neuromuscular facilitation (PNF) stretching techniques are used to increase extensibility of the muscles and extracapsular noncontractile soft tissues that are restricting knee motion. Specific techniques are described in the last section of this chapter.

PRECAUTIONS: Techniques that force the knee into flexion by using the tibia as a lever or by using strong quadriceps contractions (during a hold-relax maneuver) may exacerbate joint symptoms.

Incorporate the following to minimize joint trauma from stretching.

- Mobilize the patellofemoral and tibiofemoral joints before stretching in order to facilitate the natural joint arthrokinematics during the stretch maneuvers.

- Apply soft tissue or friction massage to loosen adhesions or contractures prior to stretching. Include deep massage around the patellar borders.
- Modify the intensity of the contractions used during PNF stretching techniques to decrease the effects of joint compression. If activating the quadriceps for a hold-relax technique to increase knee flexion aggravates anterior knee pain, an agonist contraction technique with the hamstring muscles can be used instead.
- Use low-intensity, long-duration stretches within the patient's tolerance.

Mobilization with movement. Mobilization with movement (MWM) may be applied to increase ROM and/or decrease the pain associated with movement by facilitating joint arthrokinematics. Mulligan[195] states that MWM is more effective with loss of knee flexion than extension. The principles of MWM are described in Chapter 5.

MWM: Lateral or Medial Glides

Patient position and procedure: Supine for extension or prone for flexion. Apply a pain-free medial or lateral glide to the tibial plateau manually or with a mobilization belt. The direction of glide is often in the direction of the pain (i.e., lateral knee pain responds best to a lateral glide of the tibia and medial knee pain to a medial glide).[195]

- While sustaining the mobilization, ask the patient to actively move to the end of the available pain-free range of flexion or extension.
- Add pain-free overpressure to achieve the benefit of end-range loading.

MWM: Internal Tibial Rotation for Flexion—Manual Technique

Patient position and procedure: Supine with the knee flexed to the end of its available pain-free range. Apply internal rotation mobilization to the tibia with manual pressure from one hand on the anteromedial tibial plateau simultaneously with pressure from the other hand on the posterolateral tibial plateau, posterior to the fibular head.

- Sustain the internal rotation mobilization and ask the patient to flex the knee using a mobilization belt looped around the foot. Hold the position at the end of the available pain-free range for several seconds (Fig. 21.6).

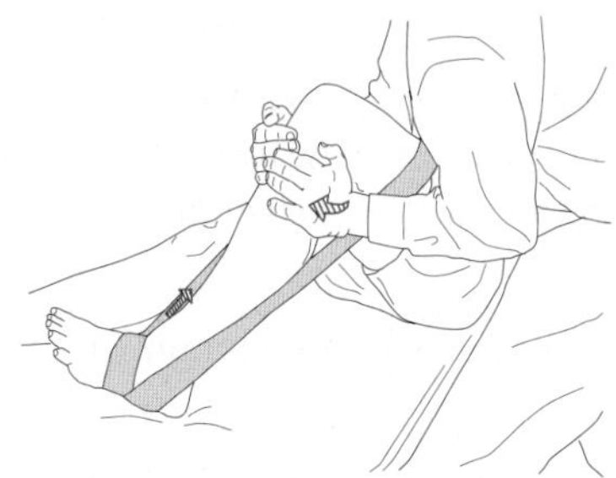

FIGURE 21.6 MWM with internal tibial rotation to increase knee flexion.

MWM: Internal Rotation for Flexion—Self-Treatment

Patient position and procedure: Standing with the foot of the involved leg on a chair and knee flexed. Position the foot such that the tibia is internally rotated. Have the patient apply internal rotation pressure against the anteromedial and posterolateral tibial plateaus and shift the weight forward to flex the knee to the end of the available pain-free range (Fig. 21.7).

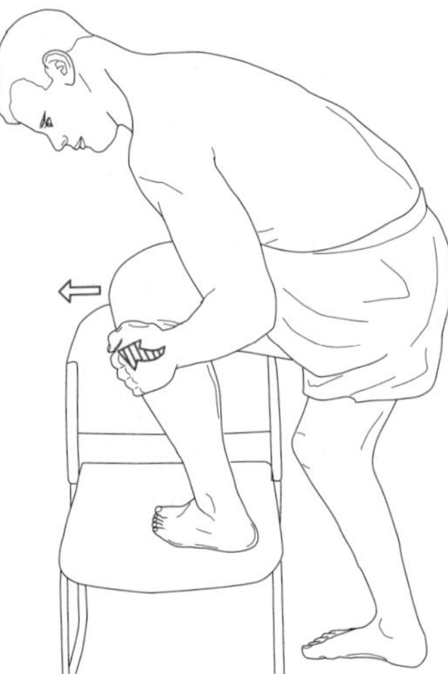

FIGURE 21.7 Self-treatment using MWM with internal tibial rotation to increase knee flexion.

Improve Muscle Performance in Supporting Muscles

Exercises identified in this section are described in detail in the last section of this chapter.

Progressive strengthening. Begin with multiple-angle isometrics to both knee flexors and extensors and active ROM exercises in open- and closed-chain positions using a moderate progression of repetitions and resistance through arcs of pain-free motion. Exercise intensity should be within the tolerance of the joint and should not exacerbate symptoms.

- When performing open-chain exercises, patients experience less pain with faster speeds and light resistance compared to slow speeds with heavy resistance.
- Resistance to knee extension through the mid-ROM (45° to 90°) tends to exacerbate patellofemoral pain because of the increased joint compressive forces on the patella. Apply resistance in arcs of motion that are pain free on either side of the symptomatic range. This can be done using manual or mechanical resistance.
- Strengthen both hip and ankle musculature using open- and closed-chain exercises to balance forces throughout the lower extremities and progress the patient toward functional independence. (See Chapters 20 and 22 for hip and ankle exercises.)

Muscular endurance training. Increase repetitions at each resistance level before increasing resistance.

Functional training. Climbing steps, sitting down and rising up from chairs and commodes, and using safe body mechanics to lift objects from the floor are often difficult in individuals with knee arthritis. It is imperative to strengthen the knee musculature using modifications of functional activities, gradually removing the modifications and progressing the difficulty as strength improves.

- ***Step-up and step-down exercises (forward, backward, lateral).*** Begin with a low step height, and progress to the step height the patient requires for home and community mobility. Progress to functional activities, such as climbing stairs or ladders, depending on the desired outcomes.
- ***Wall slides and minisquats to 90°, if tolerated.*** Stay within a range that does not exacerbate symptoms. Tie these exercises in with the functional activities of sitting down and sit-to-stand (with arm assistance if necessary) to and from various chair heights. Determine if chair adaptation is needed for safe function. Teach proper lower extremity alignment and posterior weight shift to activate and strengthen the gluteus maximus.
- ***Partial lunges.*** Concentrate on trunk control and keeping the knee over the stance foot during the motion. Have the patient activate the lumbopelvic musculature to stabilize the pelvis during the lunge activity. Progress by gradually increasing the depth of the lunge and by picking up small objects from the floor to simulate effective body mechanics.
- ***Balance activities.*** Balance activities are initiated at the level the patient can control. Detailed suggestions are outlined in Chapters 8 and 23.
- ***Ambulation.*** Decrease use of assistive devices as quadriceps strength improves to a manual muscle test level of 4/5 and as joint motion during gait becomes normalized and symmetrical. Practice walking on a variety of terrains and inclines, and include changes of direction, first with assistance and then independently.

Improve Cardiopulmonary Endurance

Select and adapt activities to minimize irritating stresses on the knee.

- ***Swimming, water aerobics, and aquatic exercises*** provide an environment for improving muscular and cardiopulmonary function with minimal joint loading.
- ***Bicycling*** is a low-impact form of exercise. Adjust the seat height so the knee goes into complete extension (but not hyperextension) when the pedal is at the lowest point of its arc. If using a stationary bike, begin with low resistance and progress as tolerated.
- ***High impact activities—with caution.*** For some patients, progression to running or jumping rope and other high-impact, faster-paced, or more intense activities can be undertaken so long as the joint remains asymptomatic. If joint deformity is present and proper biomechanics cannot be restored, the patient should be discouraged from progressing to these activities to prevent further joint damage.

Outcomes

Two systematic reviews of studies designed to examine the effects of exercise in the management of hip and knee OA support aerobic exercise and strengthening exercises to reduce pain and disability.[248,249] The consensus of expert opinion cited by Roddy[248] is that (1) there are few contraindications and (2) exercise is relatively safe in patients with OA but should be individualized and patient-centered with consideration for age, comorbidity, and general mobility. Similarly, the Cochrane Database of Systematic Reviews;[80] the Philadelphia Panel Evidence-Based Clinical Practice Guidelines;[229] and, more recently, a summary of systematic reviews of studies on physical therapy interventions for patients with knee OA[127] indicated that there is evidence to support strengthening, stretching, and functional exercises as interventions for the management of knee pain as the result of OA and to improve physical function.

Another study followed 285 patients with knee OA for 3 years and found that factors that protected the individuals from poor functional outcomes included strength and activity level, as well as mental health, self-efficacy, and social support.[264]

An outcome review[57] summarized that moderate- or high-intensity exercises for patients with RA have minimal effect on the disease activity but that there is insufficient radiological evidence regarding the effect of exercise on large joints. The review also indicated that long-term moderate- or high-intensity exercises that are individualized to protect radiologically damaged joints improve aerobic capacity, muscle strength, functional ability, and psychological well-being of patients with RA. Subjects with RA who participated in a combined aerobic, strength, and functional activity program and continued that program through an 18-month follow-up maintained knee extensor muscle strength while those who did not continue exercising lost strength. Aerobic fitness declined and functional ability was maintained from baseline in both groups at the 18-month follow-up.[56]

Finally, a recent systematic review by the Osteoarthritis Research Society International recommended referral to physical therapy services as a nonpharmacological intervention to improve functional capacity of patients with symptomatic OA.[318]

Joint Surgery and Postoperative Management

A range of surgical options for management of knee arthritis is available when joint pain and synovitis cannot be controlled with conservative therapy and appropriate medical management, or when destruction of articular surfaces, deformity, or motion restriction have progressed to the point that functional abilities are significantly impaired.

The surgical procedure selected depends on the patient's signs and symptoms, activity level and age, type of disease, severity of articular damage or joint deformity, and involvement of other joints. *Arthroscopic débridement* and *lavage* are used to remove loose bodies that may cause symptoms such as swelling and intermittent locking of the knee.[17,260] Several procedures to repair damaged articular cartilage have been developed, with mixed results. *Abrasion arthroplasty*, a procedure designed to smooth worn articular surfaces and stimulate growth of replacement cartilage has had only limited success. [17,260] More recently developed procedures to repair small, localized articular cartilage defects of the knee, such as *microfracture*,[94,262] *osteochondral autograft transplantation (mosaicplasty)*,[13,106,143] and *autologous chondrocyte implantation*,[44,95,303] appear to hold promise.

Synovectomy had been the procedure of choice for the young patient with unremitting joint effusion, synovial proliferation, and/or pain as the result of RA or juvenile RA and minimal articular surface destruction, but it is now used infrequently.[35,223,260] *Osteotomy* of the distal femur or proximal tibia (an extra-articular procedure) redistributes weight-bearing forces between the tibia and femur in an attempt to reduce joint pain during activities and delay the need for knee arthroplasty.[17,35,260] In the past, high tibial osteotomy was considered a surgical option for the active patient younger than age 50 to 55 years without active systemic disease, significant motion limitations, or joint deformity. However, advancements in arthroplasty have meant that joint replacement is now performed more frequently in younger patients, making osteotomy a less common surgical option.[39]

When erosion of articular surfaces becomes severe and pain is unremitting, *total knee arthroplasty (total knee replacement)* is the surgical procedure of choice to reduce pain, correct deformity, and improve functional movement.[123,167,258] Only in highly selective situations is *arthrodesis* (fusion) of the knee used as a salvage procedure to provide a patient with a stable and pain-free knee.

Regardless of the type of surgery, the goals of surgery and postoperative management are to (1) reduce pain, (2) correct deformity or instability, and (3) restore lower extremity function. Carefully progressed postoperative rehabilitation is essential for optimal functional outcomes.

Repair of Articular Cartilage Defects

Injuries of the ligaments or menisci of the knee and acute or chronic patellofemoral dysfunction are often associated with articular surface damage. Surgical management of chondral defects has proved challenging because of the limited capacity of articular cartilage to heal.[44,153] However, several surgical procedures are available to repair cartilage lesions when nonoperative management or palliative arthroscopic débridement and lavage have been unsuccessful. The strategies for these surgical procedures focus on either repair or restoration.[242]

Cartilage repair procedures include microfracture or bone drilling,[94,153,242,262,282] while restoration procedures range from osteochondral autograft transfer (OAT), osteochondral allograft transplant,[13,18,106,143] and autologous chondrocyte implantation.[95,153,242,303] These procedures are designed to stimulate growth of hyaline cartilage within focal articular cartilage defects and to prevent progressive deterioration of joint cartilage leading to OA.[44,153]

Descriptions of procedures specific to the knee are presented in this section. Regardless of the cartilage procedure selected, each requires the patient's ability and willingness to adhere to a lengthy rehabilitation process.

Indications for Surgery

The primary indication for repair or restoration of an articular cartilage defect is a symptomatic knee caused by a small to relatively large focal lesion of the tibiofemoral or patellofemoral joint surfaces. Lesions are most commonly located on the weight-bearing portions of the medial or lateral femoral condyles, the trochlear groove, and the patellar facets.

Selection criteria when choosing the procedure include the size of the chondral lesion, the depth and location of the lesion, the elapsed time since the occurrence of the defect, and the patient's age and intended activity level. In general, defects greater than 1 to 2 cm^2 but no more than 4 cm^2 are considered suitable for repair. Defects larger than 4 cm^2 are more appropriate for restoration techniques.[242] Most patients who undergo articular cartilage repair are young and active. [44,153]

CLINICAL TIP

A system for classification of cartilage lesions developed by the International Cartilage Repair Society is based on a five-point grading scale. Lesions range from grade 0 (normal cartilage without notable defects) to grade 4 (severely abnormal, full-thickness osteochondral defects).[32]

Procedures

Microfracture. Microfracture is indicated for repair of small defects, usually of the medial or lateral femoral condyle or the patella. The procedure is performed arthroscopically and uses a nonmotorized awl to systematically penetrate the subchondral bone and expose the bone marrow. This first-option treatment is designed to stimulate a marrow-based repair response leading to local ingrowth of cartilaginous repair tissue (fibrocartilage) to mend the lesion.[44,94,153,262,282] Autologous matrix-induced chondrogenesis is a newer technique that combines microfracture with the application of a bilayer collagen membrane to stabilize the ingrowth and guide the repair.[242]

Osteochondral autograft transfer. For focal lesions involving chondral or subchondral tissue of the weight-bearing surfaces of the knee, osteochondral graft transplantation may be selected. This is an arthroscopic or mini open procedure that transplants intact mature articular cartilage along with some underlying bone, resulting in a bone-to-bone graft.[13,18,106,143] *Mosaicplasty* is a similar technique that uses multiple small-diameter osteochondral plugs that are harvested and press-fit into the chondral defect, instead of the single piece of tissue that is used in the OAT procedure.[13,18,106,143]

Donor sites are most often nonweight-bearing, nonarticulating portions of the supracondylar ridge of the lateral femoral articulating surfaces.[13]

Autologous chondrocyte implantation. This procedure, also referred to as chondrocyte transplantation, is used in younger patients with a single, larger (2- to 4-cm^2) full-thickness chondral and osteochondral defect of the femoral condyle or patella.[44,95,303] The procedure occurs in two stages. First, healthy articular cartilage is harvested arthroscopically from the patient. Then chondrocytes are extracted from the articular cartilage, cultured for several weeks, and processed in a laboratory to increase the volume of healthy tissue. The second stage involves the implantation of the chondrocytes during an arthrotomy (open procedure). After debriding the chondral defect sites, they are covered with a periosteal patch harvested from the proximal medial tibia, and the patch is secured with fibrin glue. Millions of autologous chondrocytes are then injected under the patch into the articular defects.

Patient positioning during the first 4 hours after surgery is critical. Patients are positioned so the effect of gravity distributes the chondrocytes evenly along the base of the defect.[240] For example, after a patellar surface repair, the patient is positioned in prone.

Maturation of the implanted chondrocytes is a lengthy process. It may take as long 6 months for the graft site to become firm and as long as 9 months for the graft to become as durable as the healthy tissue surrounding the graft.[95]

Osteochondral allograft transplant. For defects larger than 4 cm^2, the only option for repair—although used infrequently—is an osteochondral allograft of intact articular cartilage from a cadaveric donor. Intact grafts are harvested and stored for up to 4 weeks before implantation in the defect.[55] Frozen allografts have also been used in some patients with good long-term results,[22,226] although freezing the graft material may kill articular chondrocytes and lead to graft failure.[44,153]

Other procedures. If coexisting ligament or meniscus pathology or tibiofemoral or patellofemoral malalignment is identified prior to or concomitant with surgical repair, reconstruction or realignment must be carried out for the articular cartilage repair to be successful. The most common procedures are ACL reconstruction and meniscus repair for tibiofemoral articular defects and lateral retinacular release for patellar defects.[13,95]

Postoperative Management

A cautiously progressed and closely monitored rehabilitation program is critical for a successful outcome after articular cartilage repair procedures. The components and progression of a rehabilitation program, including exercise, ambulation, and functional activities, must be carefully graded to protect the repair or graft and prevent further articular damage while applying controlled stresses to stimulate the healing process.

There are many common elements to the progression of postoperative exercises and functional activities after microfracture, osteochondral autologous transplantation, and autologous chondrocyte implantation, yet they also vary to some degree. Detailed postoperative protocols, as well as comprehensive clinical practice guidelines for each of these procedures, have been published.[13,95,143,142,240] In addition to the type of repair, the rehabilitation progression is based on the size, depth, and location of the articular defect, the concomitant surgical procedures, and patient-related factors such as age, body mass index, health history, and preoperative activity level.

The goals during rehabilitation after articular cartilage repair are similar to those for most knee rehabilitation programs presented in this chapter. Protected weight bearing over an extended period of time and early motion are essential after articular cartilage repair to promote maturation and maintain the health of the repaired or implanted cartilage. Special considerations for exercise and weight bearing associated with the various articular cartilage procedures are summarized in Box 21.1.[13,95,143,142,240,303]

Total Knee Arthroplasty

Total knee arthroplasty (TKA), also called total knee replacement, is a widely performed procedure for advanced arthritis of the knee. TKA is primarily performed in older patients (≥70 years of age), but over the past few decades the proportion of younger patients undergoing TKA has increased significantly.[146] The overarching goals of TKA are to relieve pain and improve a patient's physical function and quality of life.[189,258]

Indications for Surgery

The following are common indications for TKA:[123,167,258]

- Severe joint pain with weight bearing or motion that compromises functional abilities
- Extensive destruction of knee articular cartilage secondary to advanced arthritis
- Marked deformity of the knee such as genu varum or valgum
- Gross instability or motion limitation
- Failure of nonoperative management or a previous surgical procedure

Procedure

Background

Prosthetic replacement of one or more surfaces of the knee joint was developed during the 1960s. To address problems with early prosthetic designs, semiconstrained, two-component designs were created, and design innovations continue to this day. For the patient with severe anterior knee pain resulting from advanced patellofemoral deterioration, a three-component, total condylar design that includes patellofemoral joint resurfacing was developed. For advanced arthritis of only the medial or lateral aspect of the knee, the unicompartmental (unicondylar) knee arthroplasty (UKA) was developed as an alternative to TKA.[197,217,252,290]

A therapist's knowledge of the different types of TKA and UKA used today enhances communication between the therapist and surgeon and provides a foundation for rehabilitation decisions.

BOX 21.1 Special Considerations and Precautions for Rehabilitation After Articular Cartilage Repair*

- The larger the lesion, the slower and more cautious the rehabilitation progression.
- Early but controlled ROM is advocated to facilitate the healing process and begins immediately or within a day or two after surgery (CPM, passive or assisted exercise).
- Controlled (protected) weight bearing initiated as early as possible is beneficial to the healing process, but adherence to weight-bearing restrictions is critical.
- Duration and degree of weight-bearing restrictions vary with the defect size and the type and location of the repair.*
  - Longer period of protected weight bearing for osteochondral transplantation/mosaicplasty and autologous chondrocyte implantation than after microfracture
  - Longer period of protected weight bearing for a femoral condyle repair (up to 8 to 12 weeks) than for a patellar defect (up to 4 weeks)
  - Full weight bearing is delayed for as long as 8 to 12 weeks
- Protective bracing may be used postoperatively.
  - Typically locked in extension, except during exercise
  - Worn during weight-bearing activities 4 to 6 weeks
  - Worn during sleep for as many as 4 weeks
  - An unloading brace may be used after repair of a femoral condyle defect during the period of protected weight bearing to shift the weight away from the repair
- Return to functional activity.[142]
  - In general, low-impact sports such as swimming, skating, rollerblading, and cycling are permitted at about 6 months
- High-impact sports, such as jogging, running, and aerobics are usually permitted at:
  - 8–9 months for small lesions
  - 9–12 months for larger lesions
- Higher-impact sports such as tennis, basketball, football, and baseball are usually permitted by 12–18 months.

*Considerations and precautions vary with the size, depth, and location of the articular defect, type of surgical repair and concomitant procedures, and patient-related factors (e.g., age, body mass index, health history, and preoperative activity level).

Types of knee arthroplasty. Contemporary knee replacement procedures can be divided into several categories based on component design, surgical approach, and type of fixation (Box 21.2).[124,167,194,197,258,290] One category is based on the number of components implanted or articulating surfaces replaced. Another is based on the degree of constraint or amount of inherent congruency/stability built into the design. Most TKA procedures today involve a two-component (bicompartmental), semiconstrained prosthetic system that replaces the proximal tibia and distal femur (Fig. 21.8). These systems are typically composed of a modular or nonmodular femoral component with a metal articulating surface paired with a single all-polyethylene or metal-backed modular or nonmodular tibial component with a polyethylene articulating surface.[124,167,258]

Occasionally, a tricompartmental design, which also resurfaces the posterior aspect of the patella with a polyethylene component, is selected if the patellofemoral joint is symptomatic.[123,167,258] For the younger patient (< 55 years of age) with advanced disease of only the medial or lateral compartment of the knee joint, a unicompartmental design is often selected to replace just one tibial plateau and one femoral condyle.[197,217,252,258,290]

Intact MCL and LCL are necessary prerequisites for semiconstrained and unconstrained TKA.[123,167,258] Fully constrained

BOX 21.2 Total Knee Arthroplasty: Design, Surgical Approach, and Fixation

Number of Compartments Replaced

- Unicompartmental: only the medial or lateral joint surface is replaced
- Bicompartmental: entire femoral and tibial surfaces are replaced
- Tricompartmental: femoral, tibial, and patellar surfaces are replaced

Implant Design

- Degree of constraint
  - Unconstrained: no inherent stability in the implant design; used primarily with unicompartmental arthroplasty
  - Semiconstrained: provides some degree of stability with little compromise of mobility; most common design used for total knee arthroplasty
  - Fully constrained: significant congruency of components; most inherent stability but motion is considerably limited
- Fixed-bearing or mobile-bearing design
- Cruciate-retaining or cruciate-excising/substituting

Surgical Approach

- Standard/traditional versus minimally invasive
- Quadriceps-splitting versus quadriceps-sparing

Implant Fixation

- Cemented
- Uncemented
- Hybrid

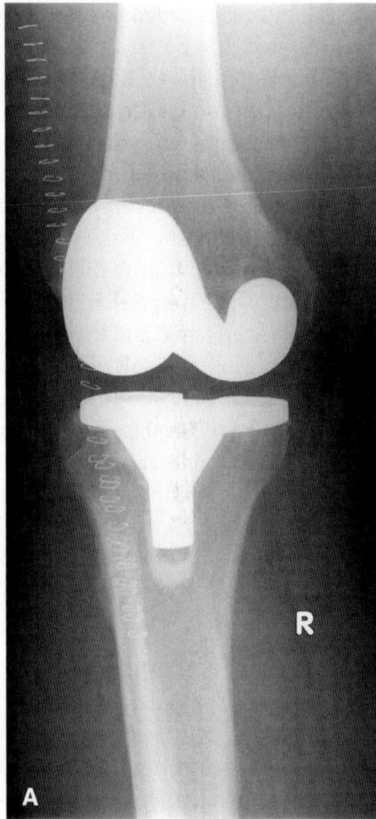

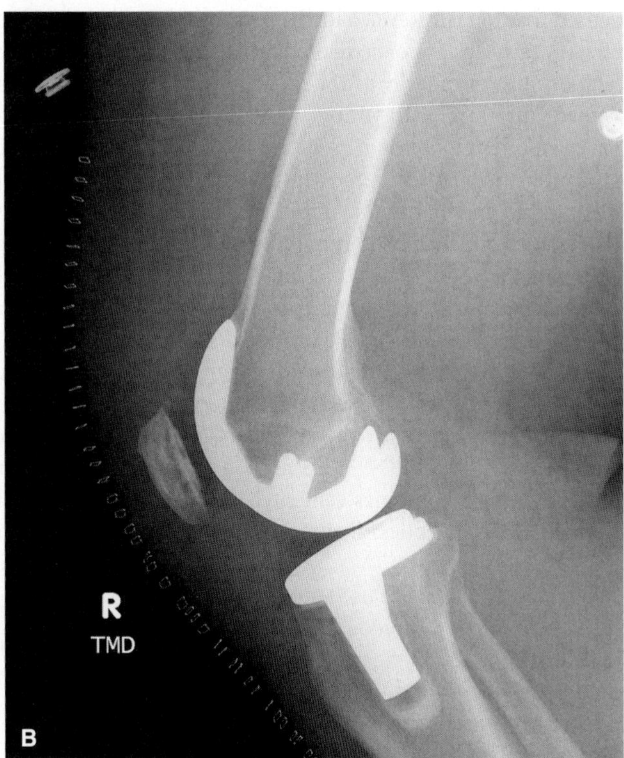

FIGURE 21.8 Posterior cruciate-retaining total knee arthroplasty of the right knee with cemented fixation. **(A)** Anteroposterior view. **(B)** Lateral view.

designs, now used infrequently, are reserved for the low-demand patient who has marked instability of the knee, extensive bone loss, severe deformity, or who has had previous TKA revisions.[123,167] Contemporary fully constrained designs are not hinged but have inherent medial-lateral (ML) and anterior-posterior (AP) stability, with some degree of rotation of the tibia on the femur allowed to lessen the problem of progressive loosening of the prosthetic components over time.[123,167]

TKA designs are also classified as mobile-bearing or fixed-bearing. The most recent development in the evolution of TKA is the introduction of the mobile-bearing, bicompartmental prosthetic knee. A mobile-bearing knee has a rotating platform inserted between the femoral and tibial components whose top surface is congruent with the femoral implant (round-on-round articulation) but whose undersurface is flat for rotation and sliding of the tibial component (flat-on-flat articulation).[38,194,258] A fixed-bearing knee does not have such an insert.[60,258] The purpose of the mobile-bearing insert is to decrease long-term wear of the polyethylene tibial component. A mobile-bearing knee design is recommended for the active patient, younger than 55 to 65 years of age.[258]

Another way to classify TKA design is based on the status of the PCL. Designs are described as cruciate-retaining or cruciate-excising/substituting.[123,167,213,216,258] Although the ACL is routinely excised during knee replacement—except with UKA—the PCL can be preserved or sacrificed. If the PCL is intact to provide posterior stability to the knee, one of several cruciate-retaining designs that require less congruency and allow some degree of AP glide can be used. If the PCL is irreparably deficient, a cruciate-excising/substituting prosthesis is selected. This type of design has inherent posterior stability from the congruency of the components, a posterior prominence in the tibial component, or a cam-post mechanism built into the design. Cruciate-retaining and cruciate-excising designs can be either fixed-bearing or mobile-bearing.[258]

Surgical approach. TKA and UKA procedures are also described in terms of the surgical approach employed.[28,41,197,258] Since the inception of knee arthroplasty, an open approach requiring a relatively long anterior incision has been employed to provide sufficient exposure of the knee joint during the procedure. A recent advance is the development of *minimally invasive* knee arthroplasty.[28,197] As with traditional joint arthroplasty, minimally invasive arthroplasty is an open procedure. However, minimally invasive TKA involves a smaller incision and less soft tissue disruption to reduce postoperative pain and increase the rate of postoperative recovery. Standard (traditional) and minimally invasive surgical approaches are described later in this section.

Fixation. The method of fixation—cemented, uncemented, or "hybrid"—is another way to classify TKA procedures—that is, implants are held in place with acrylic cement, bone ingrowth (uncemented), or a combination of these two methods.[167,215,239,302] Initially, almost all total knee replacements relied on cemented fixation. However, a long-term complication associated with early designs of cemented prostheses was biomechanical loosening, primarily of the tibial component at the bone-cement interface, with young, active patients at highest risk for component loosening.[302]

To address the problem of loosening, cementless (biological) fixation relying on rapid growth of bone into the surfaces of a porous-coated or beaded prosthesis was introduced and recommended primarily for the young, active patient.[123,167,215,258,302] In addition, a hydroxyapatite coating on the prosthesis can be used to enhance the ingrowth of bone.[260] However, long-term follow-up demonstrated that although the femoral component reliably achieved fixation to bone, tibial component loosening occurred at an even higher rate with all-cementless fixation compared with cemented fixation.[215,302] This finding gave rise to the "hybrid" TKA, which combines cemented fixation of the tibial component and cementless fixation of the femoral component.

Currently, all-cemented fixation is used most often, and all-cementless is used least often. A surgeon's decision whether to employ hybrid fixation is based on the patient's age, bone quality, and expected activity level and the tightness of fit of the femoral component achieved during surgery.[258] Design modifications to augment fixation of the tibial component (e.g., with pegs or screws) continue, although the long-term value of these designs has yet to be determined.[123,316]

In summary, research and development continue on TKA biomechanics, prosthetic designs, fixation methods, materials with better wear qualities, and surgical techniques using sophisticated instrumentation for alignment and placement of the components.

Operative Overview

An incision along the midline or anteromedial aspect of the knee can be used with either the standard or minimally invasive approach. Key features of these two types of approaches are compared in Table 21.1.[28,41,197,258] A quadriceps-splitting or a quadriceps-sparing approach is used to reach the capsule for an arthrotomy. The knee is flexed, and osteophytes, menisci, and the ACL are resected. If a posterior cruciate-substituting prosthesis is to be implanted, the PCL is also excised.

A series of surgical techniques are performed prior to inserting the implants.[124,258] Contemporary TKA usually employs either computer-assisted navigation during surgery or custom-made cutting blocks based on presurgical images to ensure precise placement and alignment of the components. Small portions of the distal femur and proximal tibia are removed and prepared for the implants. If a patellar implant is indicated, the patellar surface also is prepared and the prosthesis inserted. After trial components are inserted, soft tissue tension, collateral ligament balance, ROM, and patellar tracking are assessed. The lateral retinaculum may be released to improve patellar tracking.[144,258] Permanent components are inserted, and the capsule and other soft tissues are repaired. The area is thoroughly irrigated, and the wound is closed with a small suction drain in place and the knee positioned in extension. A sterile dressing is placed over the incision, and the area is covered from foot to thigh with a compression wrap.

Complications

The incidence of complications after TKA is low. Intraoperative complications, such as an intercondylar fracture or damage to a peripheral nerve, are uncommon. Because minimally invasive TKA is considered more technically challenging than conventional TKA,the rate of intraoperative complications, such as fracture or malpositioning of an implant, is higher with a minimally invasive than a standard approach.[28,87] An increased incidence of intraoperative technical errors is associated with patient obesity.[129]

Early and late postoperative complications include infection, joint instability, polyethylene wear, and component loosening. As with arthroplasty of other joints, there is a risk of wound-healing problems and deep vein thrombosis (DVT) during the first few months after surgery. Although the incidence of deep periprosthetic infection is low, it is the most common reason for early failure and the need for revision arthroplasty. In contrast, polyethylene wear of the patellar and tibial components is the most common late complication

TABLE 21.1 Features of Standard and Minimally Invasive Surgical Approaches for Total Knee Arthroplasty

Standard Traditional Approach	Minimally Invasive Approach
▪ Anteromedial parapatellar vertical or curved incision from the distal aspect of the femoral shaft, running medial of the patella to just medial of the tibial tubercle, ranging from 8–12 cm[28] or 13–15 cm[258] in length ▪ Necessary soft tissue releases prior to eversion of the patella ▪ Anterior capsule release ▪ Dislocation of the tibiofemoral joint prior to bone cuts and implantation of components	▪ Reduced length of anteromedial skin incision 6–9 cm in length[28] ▪ No patellar eversion ▪ Anterior capsule release ▪ No tibiofemoral dislocation ▪ *In situ* bone cuts ▪ *In situ* implantation of components

requiring revision.[52,196] The incidence of biomechanical loosening has been reduced significantly with the newer prosthetic designs and improved surgical techniques.[196,259] If mechanical loosening develops over time, it occurs most often at the tibial component and with cementless or hybrid TKAs rather than fully cemented replacements.[215]

Other postoperative complications that can compromise a patient's functional recovery include limited knee flexion, joint instability leading to subluxation,[52,258] and patellar instability or tracking problems leading to impaired function of the extensor mechanism (most often an extensor lag).[144,258] Additionally, obesity has been shown to limit mobility outcomes after TKA compared to nonobese patients.[129]

Postoperative Management

Goals and interventions during progressive phases of postoperative rehabilitation after TKA are summarized in Table 21.2. Guidelines are similar for management after UKA. Interventions also may include preoperative patient education on an individual or group basis.[260] Following surgery, patients routinely receive gait training and exercise instruction while hospitalized and in a subacute rehabilitation facility. Many patients also

TABLE 21.2 Total Knee Arthroplasty: Interventions for Each Phase of Rehabilitation

Phase and General Time Frame	Maximum Protection Phase: Weeks 1–4	Moderate Protection Phases: Weeks 4–8	Minimum Protection/Return to Function Phases: Beyond Week 8
Patient presentation			
	■ Patient enters rehabilitation 1–2 days postoperatively ■ Postoperative compression dressing ■ Postop pain controlled ■ ROM 10°–60° ■ Weight bearing as tolerated with cemented prosthesis, delayed with uncemented or hybrid	■ Minimum pain ■ Full weight bearing except with uncemented or hybrid ■ ROM 0°–90° ■ Joint effusion controlled ■ Impaired balance and functional mobility ■ Diminished muscle function and cardiopulmonary endurance	■ Muscle function: 70% of noninvolved extremity ■ No symptoms of pain or swelling during previous phase ■ Impaired balance and functional mobility
Key examination procedures			
	■ Pain (0–10 scale) ■ Monitor for hemarthrosis ■ ROM ■ Patellar mobility ■ Muscle control ■ Soft tissue palpation	■ Pain assessment ■ Joint effusion—girth ■ ROM ■ Patellar mobility ■ Gait analysis	■ Pain assessment ■ Muscular strength testing ■ Patellar alignment/stability ■ Gait analysis ■ Functional status
Goals			
	■ Control postoperative swelling ■ Minimize pain ■ ROM 0°–90° ■ 3/5 to 4/5 strength of quadriceps ■ Ambulate with or without assistive device ■ Establish home exercise program	■ Reduce swelling ■ ROM 0°–110° or greater ■ Full weight bearing ■ 4/5 to 5/5 strength ■ Unrestricted ADL function ■ Improved balance, neuromuscular control, and functional mobility ■ Adherence to home exercise program	■ Develop maintenance program and educate patient on importance of adherence including methods of joint protection ■ Community ambulation ■ Improve cardiopulmonary endurance/aerobic fitness

Continued

TABLE 21.2 Total Knee Arthroplasty: Interventions for Each Phase of Rehabilitation—cont'd

Phase and General Time Frame	Maximum Protection Phase: Weeks 1–4	Moderate Protection Phases: Weeks 4–8	Minimum Protection/Return to Function Phases: Beyond Week 8
Interventions			
	■ Pain modulation modalities ■ Compression wrap to control effusion ■ Ankle pumps to minimize risk of DVT ■ A-AROM and AROM ■ Muscle setting quadriceps, hamstrings, and adductors (may augment with E-stim) ■ Patellar mobilization (grades I and II) ■ Gait training ■ Flexibility program hamstrings, calf, IT band ■ Trunk/pelvis stabilization exercises	■ Patellar mobilization ■ LE stretching program ■ Closed-chain strengthening ■ Limited range PRE ■ Tibiofemoral joint mobilization, if appropriate and needed ■ Proprioceptive training ■ Stabilization and balance exercises ■ Protected aerobic exercise—swimming, cycling or walking	■ Continue as previous phase; advance as appropriate ■ Progression of balance and advanced functional activities ■ Implement exercise specific to identified deficits and expected functional tasks

receive home-based or outpatient therapy after discharge from inpatient care.

A patient is advanced from one phase of rehabilitation to the next based on an evaluation of their signs and symptoms and responses to selected interventions rather than solely at designated time periods. Accordingly, the timelines noted in Table 21.2 and described in the following sections are intended to serve only as general guidelines.

NOTE: The postoperative guidelines in Table 21.2 and the following sections reflect recommendations for patients who have undergone *primary* TKA in which a *standard* surgical approach was used. The suggested timelines for the progression of exercises and weight bearing tend to be more rapid after UKA than TKA and after minimally invasive compared with traditional arthroplasty, but slower after complex revision arthroplasty versus primary arthroplasty.

Immobilization and Early Motion

After primary TKA, the knee is either immobilized in a bulky compression dressing for a day, or subjected to mechanical continuous passive motion (CPM). The position of immobilization after primary TKA is usually extension.[258] Although uncommon, an alternative approach is to immobilize the knee in a 90° flexion splint immediately after surgery and for brief intervals during the next day or two to achieve knee flexion as soon as possible while maintaining knee extension with exercises.[117] With a complicated revision arthroplasty, an extended period of immobilization may be required.

During the initial postoperative period, it may be advisable for the patient to wear a posterior extension orthosis during ambulation until quadriceps control is reestablished. An extension orthosis is also indicated at night for the patient who is having difficulty achieving full knee extension or who had a significant preoperative knee flexion contracture.[39,258]

After first being introduced, CPM was used routinely following TKA during the patient's hospitalization.[97] Early studies demonstrated benefits of CPM, including decreased need for postoperative pain medication, decreased incidence of deep vein thrombosis, and increased or more rapid recovery of ROM.[131,161,176] Over time, however, this practice has decreased as early mobility has been shown to be equally effective in realizing these benefits.[109]

Customary practice for the past 2 decades has been to initiate early postoperative exercise following TKA except in some instances of complex revision arthroplasty.[66] Chapter 3 includes a section on the history and current guidelines for using CPM.

Weight-Bearing Considerations

The extent to which weight bearing is allowable after primary TKA depends on the type of prosthesis implanted; the type of fixation used; the patient's age, size, and bone quality; and whether a knee immobilizer is worn during ambulation or transfers. With *cemented fixation*, weight bearing as tolerated using crutches or a walker is usually permitted immediately after surgery. The patient progresses to full weight bearing over a 6-week period.[239]

With *biological/cementless fixation*, recommendations for weight bearing vary from permitting only touch-down weight bearing for 4 to 8 weeks while using crutches or a walker[215] to weight bearing as tolerated within a few days after surgery while using crutches or a walker.[39,258,260]

A cane can be used during the progression from partial to full weight bearing. Ambulation without an assistive device, particularly during outdoor walking, is not advisable until the patient has attained full or nearly full, active knee extension ROM, and adequate strength of the quadriceps and hip musculature to control the operated lower extremity.[39,167,215,260]

Exercise Progression

Goals and exercises for progressive phases of postoperative rehabilitation after current-day TKA, noted in Table 21.2, are discussed in the following sections.[11,39,66,180,185,231,260,317] Precautions for exercise during rehabilitation are summarized in Box 21.3.

Many of the exercises described for the early phase of rehabilitation were reported in a consensus document developed by physical therapists on the management of hospitalized patients after TKA.[66] Prior to discharge from inpatient rehabilitation, a home exercise program serves as the foundation for the remainder of the rehabilitation process, with some patients also undergoing home-based or outpatient rehabilitation for a limited number of visits.

BOX 21.3 Exercise Precautions Following TKA

- Monitor the integrity of the surgical incision during knee flexion exercises. Watch for signs of excessive tension on the wound, such as drainage or skin blanching.
- Postpone SLRs in side-lying positions for 2 weeks after cemented arthroplasty and for 4 to 6 weeks after cementless/hybrid arthroplasty to avoid varus and valgus stresses to the operated knee.
- Confer with the surgeon to determine when it is permissible to initiate exercises against low-level resistance. It may be as early as 2 weeks or as late as 3 months postoperatively.
- If a posterior cruciate-sacrificing (posterior-stabilized) prosthesis was implanted, avoid hamstring strengthening in a sitting position to reduce the risk of posterior dislocation of the knee.[39]
- Tibiofemoral joint mobilization techniques to increase knee flexion or extension may or may not be appropriate, depending on the design of the prosthetic components. It is advisable to discuss the use of these techniques with the surgeon before initiating them.
- Postpone unsupported or unassisted weight-bearing activities until strength in the quadriceps and hamstrings is sufficient to stabilize the knee.

Exercise: Maximum Protection Phase

The focus of management during the first phase of rehabilitation and the acute/inflammatory and early subacute stage of tissue healing, which extends for about 4 weeks, is to control pain and swelling, achieve independent ambulation and transfers using an assistive device, prevent early postoperative medical complications such as pneumonia and DVT, and minimize the adverse effects of postoperative immobilization. The ROM goal is to attain 90° of knee flexion and full knee extension by the end of this first phase of rehabilitation. However, full knee extension may not be possible until joint swelling has subsided.

It is well established that pain and joint swelling limit the function of the quadriceps muscle. In addition, there is a high correlation between quadriceps muscle weakness and impaired functional abilities during the initial period of recovery after TKA.[187] Regaining quadriceps muscle strength, particularly in terminal extension, as early as possible after TKA is essential for functional control of the knee during ambulation and stair climbing. In addition to early postoperative exercise, neuromuscular electrical stimulation or biofeedback of the quadriceps may be beneficial as it has been shown to be safe when initiated as early as 2 days following surgery.[8,185]

FOCUS ON EVIDENCE

Mizner and coinvestigators[188] compared the voluntary activation and force-producing capacity of the quadriceps femoris muscle group in 52 patients (mean age 64.9 years, range 49 to 78 years) 3 to 4 weeks after unilateral, cemented primary TKA for OA to 52 healthy individuals (mean age 72.2 years, range 64 to 85 years) without knee pathology. All patients in the TKA group had participated in a standard exercise program following surgery. Quadriceps force production and volitional activation of the operated limb were 64% and 26% less in the TKA group than in the healthy group, respectively, but there were no significant differences of the noninvolved knees in the TKA group compared with the healthy group. Based on the results of their study, the investigators recommended the use of neuromuscular electrical muscle stimulation or biofeedback as an adjunct to an individualized postoperative exercise program to augment quadriceps muscle force production after TKA.

Results of a prospective, randomized, controlled study conducted by Avramidis and colleagues[9] support the recommended use of neuromuscular electrical stimulation in addition to a postoperative exercise program after TKA. Thirty patients scheduled to undergo primary TKA were randomly assigned to either a treatment group or a control group (15 patients per group). Both groups underwent an individualized program of exercise and gait training following surgery, while the treatment group also received electrical stimulation to the vastus medialis muscle 4 hours a day for 6 weeks beginning on postoperative day 2. Patients in the treatment group demonstrated a significantly faster walking speed than those in the control group at 6 weeks and 12 weeks postoperatively.

Goals and interventions. The following goals and exercise interventions are included in the initial phase of rehabilitation after TKA.[11,39,66,180,185,260,317]

- ***Prevent vascular and pulmonary complications.***
  - Ankle pumping exercises with the leg elevated immediately after surgery to prevent venous stasis and reduce the risk of a DVT or pulmonary embolism
  - Deep breathing exercises
- ***Control pain and swelling.***
  - Cold, compression, and elevation
- ***Minimize reflex inhibition or loss of knee and hip musculature strength.***
  - Muscle-setting exercises of the quadriceps (preferably coupled with neuromuscular electrical stimulation), hamstrings, and hip extensors and abductors
  - Active-assisted and active straight leg raise (SLR) exercises in supine and prone positions the first day or two after surgery, postponing SLRs in side-lying positions for as long as 2 weeks after cemented TKA and for as long as 4 to 6 weeks after cementless/hybrid replacement to avoid varus or valgus stresses to the operated knee
  - Active-assisted ROM progressing to active ROM of the knee while seated and standing for antigravity knee extension and flexion, respectively
  - As weight bearing on the operated lower extremity permits, terminal knee extension in standing, wall slides in a standing position, minisquats, and partial lunges to develop control of the knee extensors and reduce the risk of an extensor lag
- ***Maintain or improve strength of the contralateral lower extremity.***
  - PRE of nonoperated lower extremity, particularly the quadriceps and hip extensors and abductors[317]
- ***Regain knee ROM.***
  - Heel-slides in a supine position or while seated with the foot on the floor to increase knee flexion
  - Neuromuscular facilitation and inhibition techniques, such as the agonist-contraction technique (described in Chapter 4), to decrease muscle guarding and increase knee flexion
  - Gravity-assisted knee flexion by having the patient sit and dangle the lower leg over the side of a bed
  - Gravity-assisted or self-assisted knee extension in the supine or long-sitting position by periodically placing a rolled towel under the heel and leaving the knee unsupported, or by gently pressing downward on the distal femur with both hands
  - Gentle inferior and superior patellar gliding techniques

PRECAUTION: Avoid placing a pillow or rolled towel under the knee while lying supine or while seated with the operated leg elevated to reduce the risk of developing a knee flexion contracture.

- ***Improve trunk stability and balance.***
  - Trunk stabilization exercises
  - Balance activities in sitting and weight shifting in bilateral stance while adhering to weight-bearing restrictions
- ***Reestablish functional mobility.***
  - Gait training with an appropriate assistive device to maintain weight-bearing restrictions
  - Functional training (bed mobility, sit-to stand transfers, basic ADLs)

Criteria to progress. The criteria to progress to the intermediate phase of rehabilitation include the following:

- Minimal swelling and pain
- Well-healed incision with no signs of infection
- Independent basic ADLs and ambulation with appropriate assistive device
- Full or nearly full active knee extension and 90° knee flexion

Exercise: Moderate Protection/Controlled Motion Phase

The emphasis of the intermediate phase of rehabilitation, which begins at about 4 weeks and extends to 8 to 12 weeks postoperatively, is to achieve approximately 110° knee flexion and active knee extension to 0° and to regain lower extremity strength and muscular endurance, balance, cardiopulmonary endurance, and additional functional mobility.

By 4 to 6 weeks postoperatively, if nearly full knee extension has been achieved and the strength of the quadriceps is sufficient, most patients transition to using a cane during ambulation. This makes it possible to focus on normalizing the patient's gait, sit-to-stand, and stair ascent and descent patterns and on improving the speed and duration of walking. In general, most improvements in a patient's functional abilities and quality of life tend to occur by 3 months postoperatively.[132]

Goals and interventions. The goals and exercise interventions for the intermediate phase of rehabilitation are the following:[11,39,66,180,187,231,260,317]

- ***Increase strength and endurance of knee and hip musculature.***
  - Multiple-angle isometrics and low-intensity dynamic resistance exercises of the quadriceps, hamstrings, and hip musculature (extensors, abductors, external rotators) against a light grade of elastic resistance or a cuff weight around the ankle
  - Resisted SLRs in various positions to increase the strength of hip and knee musculature
  - As weight bearing allows, continue or begin closed-chain exercises including resisted terminal knee extension in standing, standing wall slides, minisquats, partial lunges, and the sit-to-stand task emphasizing proper lower extremity alignment. Include scooting forward and backward on a wheeled stool to improve functional control of the knee.
  - Add forward and backward step-ups/downs, progressing to lateral. Reinforce proper lower extremity alignment. To progress, increase the step height or perform against elastic resistance.
  - Stationary cycling with the seat positioned as high as possible to emphasize knee extension
  - Include strengthening exercises for the noninvolved lower extremity

- ***Continue to increase knee ROM.***
  - Low-intensity self-stretching using a prolonged stretch or hold-relax technique to increase knee flexion and extension if limitation persists. Flexibility of the hip flexors, hamstrings, and calf muscles also may need to be improved for standing and ambulation activities.
  - Stationary cycling with seat lowered to increase knee flexion
  - Grade III inferior or superior patellar mobilization techniques to increase knee flexion or extension, respectively, if insufficient patellar mobility is restricting ROM
- ***Improve standing balance and trunk stability.***
  - Trunk stabilization exercises
  - Proprioceptive and balance training progressing from bilateral to unilateral stance on stable surface, then to balance activities on an unstable surface
  - Functional reaching activities while standing or stooping
  - Tandem walking, grapevine walking initially in parallel bars for safety (see Chapter 23 for additional activities)

PRECAUTION: A progression of balance activities for patients with TKA is typically safe to begin about 8 weeks postoperatively but must be based on the ability to control the knee during stance, weight-bearing restrictions, and the absence of pain.[231]

- ***Continue to improve functional mobility.***
  - Symmetrical heel-toe walking, ambulation on a variety of surfaces and inclines, kneeling and getting up to a standing position, and ascending and descending stairs
  - Functional exercises: backward walking, side-stepping, marching, stepping over small objects

FOCUS ON EVIDENCE

Following TKA or UKA, patients often report difficulty kneeling or the inability to kneel even a year after surgery. Although many functional activities, such as housework and gardening, involve kneeling, patient education about this skill is not always included in postoperative rehabilitation. Jenkins and associates[130] conducted a single-blind, prospective, randomized, controlled study to investigate the impact of kneeling instruction following partial knee replacement. All patients participated in postoperative rehabilitation, but at 6 weeks after surgery, only half received a single physical therapy intervention of advice and instruction on kneeling. At 1 year following surgery, patient-reported kneeling ability was significantly better in the group who received kneeling advice and instruction than in the group that did not. As such, the investigators suggested that kneeling advice and instruction should be included in postoperative rehabilitation after partial knee replacement. Although the findings of this study may have implications for patients who have undergone TKA, the investigators pointed out that the results of the study can be applied to patients following only partial knee replacement.

- ***Improve cardiopulmonary endurance.***
  - Aerobic conditioning on a stationary cycle or upper body ergometer, emphasizing increased duration

Criteria to progress. The following criteria typically must be met to progress to the final phase of rehabilitation following TKA:

- AROM: full knee extension (no extensor lag), 110° knee flexion
- Quadriceps/hamstring and hip muscle strength: at least 70% (or 4/5 muscle testing grade) compared to uninvolved leg
- Minimal to no pain during exercises and ambulation with or without a cane

Exercise: Minimum Protection/Return to Function Phase

Beginning at approximately 8 to 12 weeks after surgery, the emphasis of the final phase of rehabilitation is on task-specific strengthening exercises, proprioceptive and balance training, advanced functional training (see Chapter 23), and continued cardiopulmonary conditioning so that the patient develops the strength, power, balance, and endurance needed to return to a full level of functional activities in the community. (Refer to Table 21.2 for a summary of goals and interventions during the final phase of rehabilitation.)

Despite persistent strength and power deficits, altered movement patterns, and insufficient speed and endurance during functional activities, patients often are discharged from supervised therapy 2 to 3 months postoperatively after attaining functional ROM of the knee and the ability to ambulate independently with an assistive device. However, deficits in physical function have been shown to persist for an average of 10 months[297] to a year or more after surgery.[187]

It is likely that some patients, especially those living in the community, could benefit from an intensive exercise program during the late phases of rehabilitation to perform demanding physical activities more efficiently, such as ascending and descending stairs and returning to selected recreational activities.

FOCUS ON EVIDENCE

Moffet and associates[189] conducted a single-blind, randomized, controlled study to determine the effectiveness of an intensive, supervised functional training program initiated 2 months after primary TKA for OA. Patients in the experimental group (n =38) participated in facility-based, twice-weekly, 60- to 90-minute exercise sessions consisting of hip and knee strengthening exercises, task-specific functional exercises, and aerobic conditioning. Patients also received a home program to be followed on the days they did not participate in the supervised program. Patients in the control group (n =39) participated in a home exercise program for 6 weeks with periodic home visits by a therapist. No exercise-related adverse events occurred during the study.

Patients were evaluated by means of the 6-minute walk test and two functional outcome and quality-of-life (QOL) measures prior to beginning the exercise program (baseline measurement at 2 months after surgery), at the conclusion of the 6-week exercise program, and at 6 and 12 months postoperatively. The two groups were comparable at baseline. At the conclusion of the intervention and at the 6- and 12-month follow-ups, patients in the intensive exercise group walked significantly longer distances (walked at a faster speed) during the 6-minute walk test than did those in the control group. Functional abilities and QOL were significantly better for the intensive exercise group than the control group immediately after the 6-week program and at 6 months postoperatively. At 1 year after surgery there were no significant differences in function or QOL measures between the two groups.

The investigators concluded that an intensive, functionally oriented exercise program initiated 2 months after primary TKA was safe and effective for improving physical function and QOL.

With the trend toward an increasing number of young (< 60 years of age) and active patients undergoing TKA,[126] patient education is essential to help patients understand the detrimental effects of repetitive, high-impact activities (work related, fitness related, and recreational) on the prosthetic implants and to learn how to select activities that promote fitness but are least likely to reduce the longevity of the prosthetic knee.[110,147,174] Accordingly, patients are advised to participate in low-impact physical activities after TKA to reduce the risk of component wear and mechanical loosening over time and the premature need for revision arthroplasty.

For the patient who wishes to participate in athletic activities after TKA, there are a number of considerations. Factors that influence participation include the level of demand (intensity and load) of an athletic activity, a patient's body weight, overall level of fitness, and preoperative experience with the activity and the technical quality of the knee replacement and related soft tissue balancing or reconstruction.[110,147]

Physical activities for fitness and recreation that are highly recommended, recommended with caution, or not recommended after TKA are noted in Box 21.4.[110,147,174]

BOX 21.4 Recommendations for Participation in Physical Activities Following TKA

Highly Recommended*
- Stationary cycling
- Swimming, water aerobics
- Walking
- Golf (preferably with golf cart)
- Ballroom or square dancing
- Table tennis

Recommended if Participated Prior to TKA**
- Road cycling
- Speed/power walking
- Low-impact aerobics
- Cross-country skiing (machine or outdoor)
- Table tennis
- Doubles tennis
- Rowing, canoeing
- Bowling

Not Recommended***
- Jogging, running
- Basketball
- Volleyball
- Singles tennis
- Baseball, softball
- High-impact aerobics
- Stair-climbing machine
- Handball, racquetball, squash
- Football, soccer
- Gymnastics, tumbling
- Water-skiing

*Low impact, low load; appropriate at a moderate or high intensity on a regular basis for aerobic fitness.
**Moderate impact; appropriate on a recreational basis if performed at low or moderate intensity.
***High impact, high load; peak load occurs during knee flexion.

Outcomes

Although the ideal knee replacement that replicates the normal biomechanics of the native knee joint has yet to be developed, knee arthroplasty has been shown to be a successful procedure for patients with advanced joint disease. Extensive research has been published on patient-related outcomes and the survivorship associated with a wide variety of prosthetic designs, surgical techniques, methods of fixation, and types of materials.[123,124,163,258,316] Because of the variability of procedures and the fact that outcomes are often based on nonrandomized, retrospective studies, it has been difficult to draw general conclusions.[259] However, a recent large-scale (2,352 patients), multicenter, randomized study comparing patient-related outcomes following three variations of total knee component designs demonstrated no significant differences in clinical, functional, and QOL improvements between the randomized groups at 2 years following surgery.[132]

Patient-related outcomes after knee arthroplasty that have the most influence on patient satisfaction are relief of pain and an improved ability to perform necessary and desired functional activities for an extended number of years. Approximately 90% of patients who undergo primary TKA can expect 10 to 20 years of satisfactory function before revision arthroplasty may need to be considered.[258] For example, Dixon and colleagues[60] reported a 92.6% survival rate of modular, fixed-bearing TKA in patients followed for a minimum of 15 years.

Parameters typically measured by means of self-report and performance-based instruments to determine the success of knee replacement surgery are the level of pain, overall QOL, knee ROM, strength of the knee musculature, and a patient's ability to perform functional activities safely and with ease.

An understanding of evidence-based outcomes following TKA can assist a therapist in developing realistic goals with a patient and better determining a patient's prognosis.

Pain relief. Almost all patients who undergo knee arthroplasty report a significant reduction of pain during knee motion and weight bearing, with most patients reporting good to excellent pain relief.[85,258,259,298]

ROM. Improvements in knee ROM are not as predictable as relief of pain. Stiffness often persists after the initial recovery from surgery has occurred.[85] However, it also has been reported that ROM may continue to improve up to 12 to 24 months postoperatively.[273] Factors that influence postoperative ROM include preoperative ROM, the underlying disease, obesity, postoperative pain, and whether a primary or a revision arthroplasty was performed. Complications such as component malpositioning, inadequate soft tissue balancing or reconstruction, infection, and mechanical loosening of an implant can adversely affect postoperative ROM.[220,269]

Patients with restricted ROM preoperatively often continue to have limited postoperative knee flexion, extension, or both despite an aggressive exercise program.[269,273] In fact, the most important predictor of long-term postoperative knee ROM is preoperative ROM.[155,257,269] For example, in a study of 358 patients who underwent primary TKA for OA, total ROM of the knee was 110° preoperatively and 113° postoperatively due to a reduction in the average knee flexion contracture from 12° to 9°.[257] The results of several other studies found that despite patients' participation in an outpatient or home-based postoperative rehabilitation program, there was no significant change in preoperative versus postoperative knee ROM at 6 months[11,187] or at 12 months after surgery.[238]

Differences in prosthetic design, such as mobile-bearing versus fixed-bearing[38,258] or PCL-retaining versus PCL-substituting (posterior stabilized) designs,[213,216,258] and in the method of fixation[215,258] do not appear to affect ROM outcomes after primary TKA. A comparison of five designs of posterior cruciate-substituting implants, for example, showed no significant differences in the extent of improvement of knee ROM among designs.[257]

Limited knee ROM has a substantial impact on postoperative function, particularly if knee flexion is less than 90° and knee extension is limited by more than 10° to 15°.[258] With less than 90° to 100° of knee flexion, it is difficult to negotiate stairs, and having less than 105° makes it difficult to stand up from a standard height chair without using arm support.[258] In a retrospective study of more than 5,000 total knee arthroplasties, Ritter and associates[246] determined that greater than 105° of knee flexion was necessary for optimal postoperative function. Results of their study indicated that functional outcomes were highest when at least 128° of knee flexion was achieved following surgery but were substantially compromised if < 118° was achieved. In contrast, lack of full knee extension because of contracture or an extensor lag is thought to be a source of a patient's perception of knee pain or instability during ambulation activities, particularly when ascending and descending stairs.[144,258]

Strength and endurance. It takes a minimum of 3 to 6 months after surgery for a patient to regain preoperative strength levels in the quadriceps and hamstrings of the operated knee.[144,187,273] Quadriceps weakness tends to persist longer after knee arthroplasty than does knee flexor weakness.[273] Furthermore, quadriceps weakness of the contralateral (nonoperated) side is a predictor of impaired functional outcomes at 1 and 2 years following unilateral TKA.[317]

Studies of patients after unilateral TKA with a conventional surgical approach have demonstrated that quadriceps strength in the operated leg correlates highly with performance on tests of functional abilities during the first 6 months after surgery.[187] For example, a study by Farquhar and associates[70] demonstrated that at 3 months post-TKA, patients had quadriceps weakness and an altered sit-to-stand movement pattern reflected by the use of increased hip flexion and greater reliance on hip extensor strength, thus reducing the demand on the knee extensors. Of additional interest was the finding that at 1 year after surgery, despite improved symmetry of quadriceps strength, the altered sit-to-stand pattern persisted, perhaps as the result of habit.[70]

Quadriceps strength is also significantly less than in similarly aged healthy individuals 6 months to a year after surgery[67,85,187,298] and the noninvolved leg 1 to 2 years postoperatively.[251,270] It has been suggested that eversion of the patella during a conventional surgical approach may contribute to impaired function of the quadriceps mechanism after surgery.[163,270]

A recent systematic review of lower limb isometric strength following TKA concluded that there were strength deficits in the quadriceps, hamstring, and calf of the involved leg at multiple time-points postoperatively when compared to unimpaired control groups. Quadriceps and calf strength deficits persisted for up to 3 years following surgery.[254]

Given the number of studies that have identified significant quadriceps weakness after TKA and the high correlation between quadriceps strength and functional performance, there is substantial evidence to support the importance of quadriceps-strengthening exercises in postoperative rehabilitation programs to optimize function after TKA.

Physical function and activity level. The greatest and most rapid improvements in physical performance following TKA occur during the first 12 weeks with an additional but small amount of improvement occurring beyond 12 weeks.[137] Relief of pain appears to significantly improve a patient's QOL and ability to perform functional activities. However, just 1 month after TKA, functional performance is dramatically worse than the preoperative level of function, despite a patient's participation in a rehabilitation program beginning the day after surgery.[11]

A systematic review of the literature by Ethgen and colleagues[69] revealed that a patient's postoperative level of function and QOL, as measured by self-report questionnaires, typically begins to surpass the preoperative level at approximately 3 months, with most improvement in function occurring by 6 months. However, results of some studies have shown that additional improvements may occur for a year or more postoperatively.[273,298]

Overall, when comparing preoperative with postoperative function, patients with high preoperative scores on functional measures achieved a higher level of function postoperatively than patients with low preoperative functional scores.[79]

A survey of 176 patients (mean age, 70.5 years) by Weiss and colleagues[301] 1 year or more after TKA identified patients' level of participation in activities of graduated difficulty and determined which activities were most important to patients. The survey also identified activities that were difficult after TKA. The results of the survey indicated that in addition to basic ADLs—walking, stair-climbing, and personal care—patients performed a wide range of therapeutic and recreational activities after TKA. The activities in which the highest percentage of patients participated were stretching exercises (73%), leg-strengthening exercises (70%), gardening (57%), and stationary cycling (51%). These same activities were rated as important by patients. Functions that were the most difficult and most often caused knee pain were squatting (75%) and kneeling (70%).

Bradbury and colleagues[30] studied the pre- and postoperative sports participation of 160 patients who had undergone TKA 5 years earlier. Preoperatively, there were no significant differences in knee ROM, walking abilities, and radiographs in the patients who did and did not participate in sports activities. Postoperatively, the investigators found that 51 (65%) of the 79 patients (mean age 73 years at the 5-year follow-up) who had regularly (at least twice a week) participated in sports activities during the year prior to surgery were participating in some type of sport at the 5-year follow-up. Patients were more likely to return to low-impact rather than high-impact activities. Of the patients who did not regularly participate in a sport before surgery, none took up a sport postoperatively.

Despite an overall positive impact of TKA on physical function, long-term studies indicate that functional abilities typically remain below norms for age-matched, healthy populations.[11,67,79,] A follow-up study of 276 community-dwelling patients 6 months after primary TKA revealed that overall physical function improved significantly for all patients, although 60% reported moderate to extreme difficulty descending stairs and 64% continued to have a similar degree of difficulty with heavy household tasks.[133]

Results of another study indicated that 1 year after TKA, despite a relative absence of pain and some improvement in functional abilities, significant deficits in strength and function were apparent when compared with the abilities of age-matched, healthy individuals.[298] The post-TKA patients had less strength of the knee musculature, slower walking and stair-climbing speeds, and a higher perceived level of exertion during activities than healthy individuals. The authors pointed out that the post-TKA patients as a group were heavier than the control group and suggested that general physical deconditioning may have contributed to the postoperative group's functional limitations. This study emphasized the need for inclusion of a low-impact aerobic conditioning program during rehabilitation after TKA.

Patellofemoral Dysfunction: Nonoperative Management

Related Patellofemoral Pathologies and Etiology of Symptoms

Patellofemoral pain syndrome (PFPS) is a clinical diagnosis that encompasses multiple features, most commonly involving a general description of anterior knee pain, provoked by physical activities such as running and by increased PF joint compressive forces during activities such as squatting, sitting with flexed knees, and ascending and descending stairs.[46,151,313] The cause of anterior knee pain may be direct trauma; overuse; faulty patellar tracking; joint degeneration; soft tissue length and strength imbalances in the hip, knee, or ankle/foot; or a combination of factors.[33,56,151,172,233,234,236,251,282,299,298] For effective treatment, an attempt should be made to determine the causative factors based on the patient's history and a comprehensive examination. To encompass this variety of potential causes, several classification systems have been proposed and are summarized in this section.[120,307] In addition, consensus papers from several research retreats[46,54,235] have organized the condition into three primary categories—local, distal, and proximal—in order to identify etiologic factors. Because interventions should be directed to the underlying problem, it is helpful to look at the various diagnoses within the context of these three categories.

Local Factors

Local factors include structures around the knee joint itself, such as the infrapatellar fat pad, ligaments, quadriceps tendon, retinaculum, and subchondral bone. Symptoms may be provoked by faulty mechanics or activities that directly influence local factors such as those identified in the following diagnoses.

PF Instability

Instability includes subluxation or dislocation related to a single episode or recurrent episodes. Instability may be related to an abnormal Q-angle, dysplastic trochlea (shallow groove or flat lateral femoral condyle), patella alta, tight lateral retinaculum, or inadequate medial stabilizers (vastus medialis oblique muscle and medial patellofemoral ligament). Patellar instability is most often in a lateral direction. Dislocation may derive from direct trauma to the patella or from a forceful quadriceps contraction while the foot is planted and the femur is externally rotating while the knee is flexed. Recurrent dislocation is usually an indication for surgery to reorient the stabilizing forces across the PF joint.

PF Pain With Malalignment or Biomechanical Dysfunction

Patella alta or baja and lateral patellar tilt are specific alignment alterations possible at the patellofemoral joint. Impairments that may contribute to biomechanical dysfunction include a tight lateral retinaculum, weak vastus medialis obliquus (VMO) muscle, neuromuscular deficits in the hip musculature, and generalized joint hypermobility. These impairments usually result in clinical evidence of abnormal patellar tracking, and there may be discordant firing of the quadriceps muscle.[120]

FOCUS ON EVIDENCE

Although it is widely reported that PF malalignment is seen in patients with PFPS and may be associated with symptoms, the evidence to support the existence of abnormal alignment in PFPS is lacking. Specifically, because there is little evidence to support the validity and reliability of various testing procedures currently used to measure patellar position and tracking, only assumptions can be made as to the relationship between malalignment and PFPS.[311]

PF Pain Without Malalignment

Patellofemoral pain without malalignment includes many subcategories of lesions that cause anterior knee pain.

Soft tissue lesions. Soft tissue lesions include plica syndrome, fat pad syndrome, tendonitis, IT band friction syndrome, and bursitis.

- *Plica syndrome* describes a condition where embryological synovial tissue remnants or bands around the patella cause joint irritation during motion. With chronic irritation, the tissue remnant becomes an inelastic, fibrotic band that is tender during palpation. When symptoms are acute, the tissue is painful during palpation. Bands may be palpable medial to the patella, although there are variations in location.[24,136]
- *Fat pad syndrome* involves irritation of the infrapatellar fat pad from trauma or overuse.
- *Tendonitis* of the patellar or quadriceps tendons, sometimes called *jumper's knee*, typically occurs from overuse as the result of repetitive explosive jumping activities. Tenderness occurs at the attachment of the tendons on the patella. Symptoms may be related to or exacerbated by quadriceps tightness.[299]
- *IT band friction syndrome* is irritation of the IT band as it passes over the lateral femoral condyle during activities. Irritation may be the result of tight tensor fasciae latae or gluteus maximus muscles (see discussion in Chapter 20). Because the IT band attaches to the patella and lateral retinaculum, anterior knee pain may also be noted with IT band friction syndrome.
- *Prepatellar bursitis*, also known as housemaid's knee, can result from prolonged kneeling or recurrent minor trauma to the anterior knee. When inflamed, there may be restricted motion due to swelling and direct pressure or pressure from the patellar tendon will be painful.

Tight medial and lateral retinacula or patellar pressure syndrome. There is increased contact force between the patella and distal femur in the trochlear groove.

Osteochondritis dissecans of the patella or femoral trochlea. Osteochondral lesions result in pain on the posterior patellar surface that increases during squatting, stooping, ambulating, and descending steps. There may be loose bodies within the joint that cause the knee to give way or lock.

Traumatic patellar chondromalacia. Chondromalacia is softening and fissuring of the cartilaginous posterior patellar surface, diagnosed with arthroscopy or arthrography.[120] It may eventually predispose the joint to degenerative arthritis or basal degeneration of the middle and deep zones of the cartilage.[96] Causes include trauma, surgery, prolonged or repeated stress, or lack of normal stress such as during periods of immobilization.[214]

PF OA. OA may be idiopathic or posttraumatic and is diagnosed by radiographic changes consistent with degeneration.

Apophysitis. Osgood-Schlatter disease (traction apophysitis of the tibial tuberosity) and Sinding-Larsen Johansson syndrome (traction apophysitis on the inferior pole of the patella) occur during adolescence as a result of overuse during rapid growth. They are self-limiting conditions.

Symptomatic bipartite patella. Most bipartite patellae (split due to patellar ossification variants) are asymptomatic, but trauma may disrupt the chondro-osseous junction, leading to symptoms.[120]

Trauma. Trauma includes tendon rupture, patella fracture, contusion, and articular cartilage damage that results in inflammation, swelling, limited motion, and pain when contracting the quadriceps, such as during stair climbing, squatting, and resisted knee extension.

Proximal Factors

Factors arising from the hip and pelvis region include increased hip adduction and internal rotation during specific tasks such as running and single-limb activities of squatting, jumping, and drop landing. These hip kinematic alterations may be associated with hip abductor, extensor, and eternal rotator muscle weakness.

FOCUS ON EVIDENCE

The summary statement of the 3rd International Patellofemoral Pain Research Retreat[313] summarized studies that show evidence of greater hip adduction in women who develop PFP and conflicting results regarding contralateral pelvic drop. Studies also identified reduced hip extension moments during running, weaker isometric hip extension, and delayed activation in gluteus medius in those with PFP.

Distal Factors

Factors arising from the foot include an externally rotated foot during relaxed stance, rearfoot eversion at heel strike, delayed or prolonged rearfoot eversion during walking and running, and increased midfoot mobility.[54] The extent to how these factors are related to the development of PF joint symptoms remains unclear.[313]

FOCUS ON EVIDENCE

A systematic review of 7 prospective studies[151] identified the female gender and low peak torque in the quadriceps muscles as risk factors for developing PFPS. There was contradictory evidence for onset timing of VMO before VL and lack of evidence supporting the magnitude of the Q-angle as risk factors. Because of limitations in the studies reviewed, no additional risk factors were identified.

Common Impairments

Impairments of Structure and Function. Impairments that may be associated with PF dysfunction include the following:[33,56,136,151,172,230,233-236,251,296,299,313]

- Pain in the retropatellar region
- Pain along the patellar tendon or at the subpatellar fat pads
- Patellar crepitus; swelling or locking of the knee
- Altered lower extremity alignment (Fig. 21.9), specifically increased hip adduction and internal rotation and dynamic knee valgus that occurs during weight-bearing activities, such as ascending and descending stairs, squatting, or landing after a jump[125,177,233,234,236,247,278]
- Weakness of the hip abductor, external rotator, and/or extensor muscles[25,125,177,230,233,234,247,278]
- Weakness, and atrophy in the quadriceps muscles[93,94,151]
- Decreased flexibility of the tensor fasciae latae, hamstrings, quadriceps, or gastrocnemius and soleus muscles[230,233,237]
- Overstretched medial retinaculum
- Restricted lateral retinaculum, IT band, or fascial structures around the patella
- Decreased medial gliding or medial tipping of the patella
- Pronated foot

FOCUS ON EVIDENCE

There are a substantial number of studies that have reported altered lower extremity kinematics and/or hip musculature strength and activation deficits in individuals with PF pain versus those without.[25,125,177,230,233-236,247,278] Overall, the findings of most of these studies have revealed greater hip adduction and/or internal rotation during weight-bearing activities that involve knee flexion, such as squatting, ascending or descending stairs, or landing from a jump, in individuals with PF pain. Decreased strength of hip extensors, external rotators, and/or abductors, typically measured during a maximum voluntary isometric contraction, has also been identified in those with PF pain.

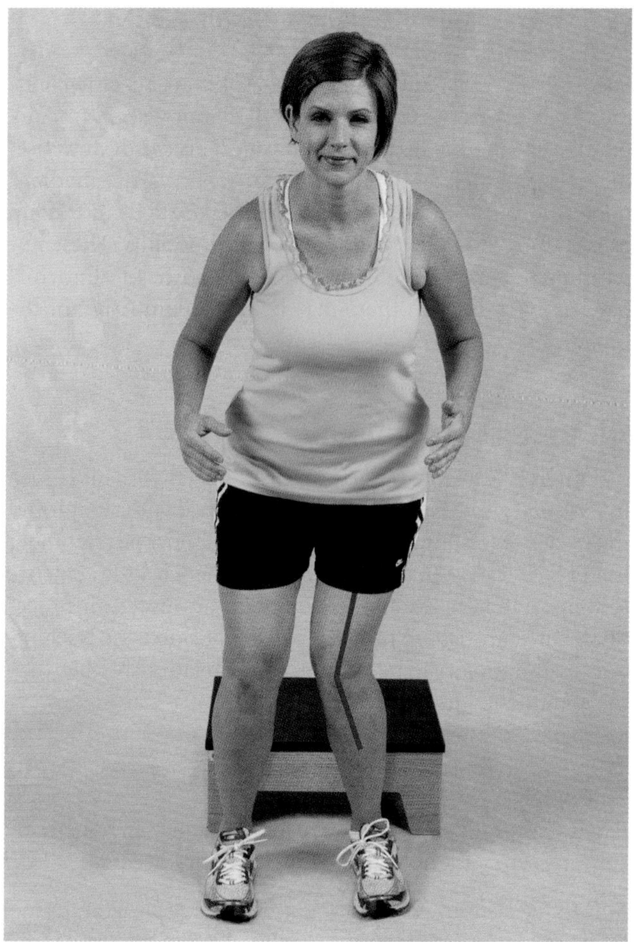

FIGURE 21.9 Excessive hip adduction and internal rotation with valgus collapse at the knee during descent from a step.

McKenzie and colleagues[177] reported diminished strength of hip extensors, abductors, and external rotators, as well as excessive hip adduction and internal rotation during stair descent and ascent in subjects with PFPS. Souza and colleagues[278] reported that females with PFPS had significantly decreased strength of the hip extensors and abductors with increased hip internal rotation during step-down movements, a drop-jump, and running, but no increase in hip adduction. In contrast, Bolgla and colleagues[25] identified weakness of the hip abductors and external rotators but no evidence of abnormal hip kinematics during stair descent in females with PFPS. The inconsistent findings may be attributed to a number of factors including differences in weight-bearing tasks and measurement techniques.

Although these studies suggest that an interdependence exists between the knee and more proximal regions of the body, specifically the hip, pelvis, and trunk, it is also important to recognize that the retrospective nature of these studies demonstrate associations—not cause-and-effect relationships—among altered hip mechanics, deficits in hip muscle performance, and signs and symptoms of PF dysfunction.[113,233,236]

Activity limitations and participation restrictions. Limitations and restrictions associated with the impairments include the following:

- Limited performance of basic ADLs as the result of pain or poor knee control (valgus collapse)
- Pain-related limitations of functional activities that are necessary to carry out ADLs and IADLs; work; and community, recreational, or sport activities, such as getting in or out of a chair or car, ascending and descending stairs, walking, jumping, or running.
- Inability to maintain prolonged flexed knee postures, such as sitting or squatting, as the result of pain and stiffness in the knee

Patellofemoral Symptoms: Management—Protection Phase

When symptoms are acute, treat them as any acute joint problem—with modalities, rest, gentle motion, and muscle-setting exercises in pain-free positions. Quadriceps inhibition is common with pain and joint effusion,[286] making it imperative to minimize these impairments in this management phase. Supporting the patella with a brace or tape may unload the joint and relieve the irritating stress. Foot orthoses may relieve pain and stress in patients with identified foot impairments.[235]

Patellofemoral Symptoms: Management—Controlled Motion and Return to Function Phases

When signs of acute pain and inflammation are no longer present, management is directed toward correcting or modifying the biomechanical or alignment factors that may be contributing to the impairment. Because no one factor or combination of factors has been identified as the direct cause or effect of PF pain symptoms, it is imperative to develop interventions that address the scope of impairments identified during the examination.[234] It is also important to integrate the concept of regional interdependence in the application of exercise interventions by addressing the local, distal, and proximal factors that may place excessive stress through the PF joint.[113,233]

Management during the controlled motion and return to function phases of rehabilitation typically emphasizes increasing strength, dynamic control, and pain-free mobility of the knee and hip, and foot; modifying abnormal movement strategies that may contribute to impairments; improving stability of the lower extremity, pelvis and trunk; and on improving balance, and functional abilities.

Patient Education

Instructions. Because end-range stress and prolonged postures tend to exacerbate symptoms, instruct the patient to avoid positions and activities that provoke the symptoms.

- Minimize or avoid stair climbing and descending until the hip and knee muscles are strengthened to a level at which they can control knee function without symptoms.
- Avoid sitting with the knees flexed for prolonged periods because increased knee flexion magnifies PF joint compressive forces. Periodically perform ROM of the knee while sitting to relieve stasis.

Home exercise program. Implement a home exercise program to reinforce the supervised training. Prior to discharge, provide instructions for a safe progression of exercises and functional activities.

Increase Flexibility of Restricting Tissues

Identify all structures that may contribute to faulty mechanics and establish a stretching program to increase mobility. The gastrocnemius, soleus, quadriceps, hamstring, and tensor fasciae latae (TFL) muscles have been identified as specific muscles with reduced flexibility in some individuals with patellofemoral dysfunction.[230,233,296] Self-stretching techniques are described in the exercise section of this chapter. Techniques to stretch the two-joint muscles that cross the hip and knee are described in Chapter 20, and those that cross the knee and ankle are described in Chapter 22.

Because restrictions related to insertion of the IT band and the lateral retinaculum may contribute to decreased patellar mobility and faulty patellar tracking in some patients with PFPS, specific techniques to address these impairments are described in this section.

Patellar mobilization: medial glide. Position the patient side-lying. Stabilize the femoral condyles with one hand under the femur, and glide the patella medially with the base of the other hand (Fig. 21.10).[99] There is usually greater mobility with the knee near extension; progress by positioning the knee in greater flexion prior to performing the medial glide.

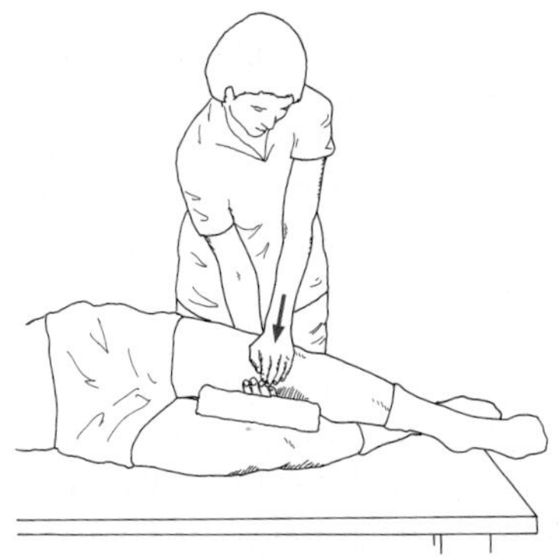

FIGURE 21.10 Medial glide of the patella.

Medial tipping of the patella. Position the patient supine. Place the thenar eminence at the base of the hand over the medial aspect of the patella. Apply a posterior force to tip the patella medially. While the patella is held in this position, apply friction massage with the other hand along the lateral border (Fig. 21.11). Teach the patient to self-stretch in this manner.

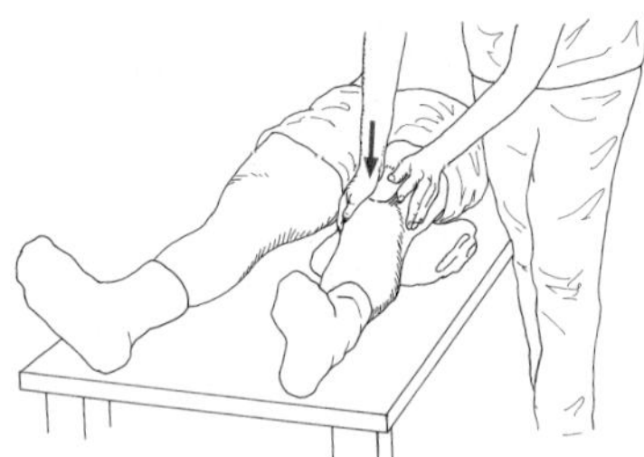

FIGURE 21.11 Medial tipping of the patella with friction massage along the lateral border.

Patellar taping. Although taping to realign the patella and provide a prolonged stretch may have merit,[99,172] the primary benefit of taping appears to be reduced anterior knee pain during provoking activities after being taped.[23,49] The mechanism behind pain relief from tape is not known but may be due to patellar realignment or improved neuromuscular function.

FOCUS ON EVIDENCE

A multicenter, single-blind study demonstrated little to no change in patellar alignment from the application of three different patellar taping techniques. Decreased symptoms occurred in 71 subjects with PFPS, regardless of the direction in which the tape was applied.[310] The investigators suggested that taping may alter proprioceptive input and increase tolerance to functional training and recommended its use while focusing treatment on proximal muscle weakness.

Improve Muscle Performance and Neuromuscular Control

Because many possible diagnoses fall under the category of PFPS, various influences may precipitate or perpetuate the symptoms. Importantly, not all patients with PF symptoms benefit from the same exercises, making it imperative that the therapist design a progression of exercises that addresses each patient's specific impairments. In addition, it is now well accepted that exercise programs for patients with PFPS should target proximal regions, specifically the hip extensors and abductors in order to affect alignment and control of the knee.[84,168,200,296] Impaired strength, endurance, and neuromotor control of the knee and hip musculature, as well as impaired stability of the trunk and pelvis, must be addressed.[233-236]

In addition to the knee exercises described later in this chapter, exercises to improve muscle performance and functional control in regions proximal and distal to the knee are described in Chapters 16, 20, and 22, respectively. Advanced functional exercises for the lower extremity are described in Chapter 23.

Nonweight-Bearing (Open-Chain) Exercises

There is controversy regarding compressive forces and stress on the PF joint with open-chain exercises.[67,98] The type of resistance (constant, variable, or isokinetic) places different demands on the quadriceps muscle in terms of the required effort through the ROM. The resultant force from the quadriceps and patellar tendon vary through the ROM, as does the patellar contact area, which subsequently varies the pressure and stress on the PF articulating surfaces. With little or no contact of the patella with the trochlear groove from 0° to 15° of flexion,[67] pain felt in that range could derive from irritation of the patellar fat pads or synovial tissue. Greatest patellar stress is at 60° and compression loads at 75°, so when maximum torque from the resistance force is applied in these ranges, pain may be provoked.[67] The location of the joint pathology also affects where in the range the pain is noted.[98] It is recommended to identify where in the ROM pain is felt and avoid resistance loads in that range.

Quadriceps setting (quad sets) in pain-free positions. Have the patient set the quads with the knee in various positions. Because the location of irritation in the ROM varies among patients with PF dysfunction, identify pain-free positions to ensure nondestructive loading.[67,98]

Quad sets with straight-leg raise. Have the patient perform SLR exercises in supine or long-sitting positions to target quadriceps control.

Progression of resisted isometrics. Initiate multiple-angle isometrics against resistance to knee extension in pain-free positions as tolerated by the patient.

Short-arc terminal extension. Begin with the patient supine and knee flexed around 20° (see Fig. 21.23). If tolerated and the motion is not painful, apply light resistance at the ankle. Strengthening in terminal extension trains the muscle to function where it is least efficient because of its shortened position and where there is minimal joint compression because the patella is superior to the femoral groove. End-range knee extension is needed for activities such as lifting the leg into bed or a car.

PRECAUTION: If there is irritation of the suprapatellar pouch or bursa, terminal knee extension may be painful and should be avoided until the pain subsides.

Weight-Bearing (Closed-Chain) Exercises

A progression of closed-chain/axial-loading exercises, typically performed in weight-bearing positions, should be a major component of an exercise program for PFPS to reduce PF symptoms; increase muscle performance and dynamic control of knee, hip, and trunk; and to improve neuromuscular control/response time and balance.[12,26,115,168,200,296] When excessive knee valgus occurs during weight-bearing activities involving dynamic knee flexion (e.g., squats, lunges, stair ascent or descent, or landing from a jump), it may indicate hip abductor, extensor, and/or external rotator weakness. Strengthening these muscle groups in weight-bearing positions and practicing movement strategies in proper alignment should be a priority.[115,168,233,234,296]

PRECAUTION: Because there are higher patellar compressive loads when the knee is flexed beyond 60° during weight bearing, exercises and activities with the knee flexed beyond this angle may provoke symptoms. Use caution when the patient is ready to progress beyond 60°. Have the patient carefully monitor symptoms and stop the exercise if symptoms develop.

- If full weight bearing is painful, begin with partial weight-bearing exercises. Progress exercises in standing as tolerated.
- To improve strength and muscular endurance, have the patient perform multiple repetitions of appropriate exercises until PF symptoms or loss of control just begins to occur. Do not push beyond that point in order to avoid faulty mechanics or loss of control.
- Initiate terminal knee extension against light resistance in standing for end-range knee control (see Fig. 21.26).
- Introduce bilateral minisquats and progress to unilateral early in the exercise program when weight bearing and partial squatting are tolerated and do not provoke symptoms (see Fig. 21.27). Be sure that the knees remain aligned over the toes during squatting.
- Progress dynamic exercises by adding double-leg, then single-leg standing wall slides, short-step, then long-step lunges, and forward, backward, and lateral step-ups and step-downs to the exercise program. Add elastic resistance for further challenge.
- Select resistance equipment for progressive strengthening and muscular endurance training that incorporates weight bearing, such as the seated leg press, the Total Gym® unit, and the stepping machine.
- Combine balance and agility training with strengthening exercises in weight-bearing positions.
- Include plyometric training for individuals wishing to return to high-demand activities if symptoms do not recur (see Chapter 23).

Functional Activities

Practice simulated functional activities and activity-specific drills without provoking symptoms to prepare the patient to return to the desired activities (see Chapter 23). If abnormal lower extremity alignment occurs during weight-bearing activities despite improvements in muscle strength and endurance, integrate movement reeducation into activity-specific drills to reinforce proper movement strategies.

Modify Biomechanical Stresses

Assess lower extremity mechanics, and modify any faulty alignment. If the patient exhibits excessive foot pronation, a medial wedge foot orthosis may reduce the stresses at the knee and decrease PF pain.[65,102]

Outcomes

Several systematic reviews of the literature focusing on quality randomized, controlled studies for PFPS have revealed that interventions most effective for reducing pain and improving function were quadriceps strengthening, acupuncture, and combinations of interventions that include quadriceps strengthening with patellar taping and use of biofeedback.[14,23,49] The effectiveness of a patellar brace was neither refuted nor supported, nor was the use of manual therapy techniques, such as stretching and manipulation. One systematic review looking specifically at the effect of exercise for PFPS concluded that exercise therapy is important to relieve pain and improve measures of patient reported activity limitations and participation restrictions.[46]

No particular exercise approach has been found to be superior to another for reducing symptoms and improving function. A recent systematic review of studies that utilized therapist-guided quadriceps muscle–strengthening exercises provided strong evidence that there was no difference in effectiveness based on the type of exercises used.[145]

There is a substantial body of evidence indicating that decreased strength and flexibility of regions proximal to the knee are associated with PFPS, and randomized controlled studies are now documenting the effectiveness of treatment programs that target the hip, pelvis, and trunk. A systematic review and meta-analysis of studies on the effectiveness of exercise programs that emphasize proximal musculature concluded that there is strong evidence supporting proximal rehabilitation, with or without quadriceps rehabilitation, utilizing both open- and closed-kinetic-chain exercises for pain reduction and improved function in subjects with PFPS.[149]

Fukuda[84] conducted a randomized, controlled study of 70 sedentary females with anterior knee pain: 22 received knee exercises that emphasized stretching and strengthening the knee musculature, 23 received the same program with the addition of hip strengthening and stretching, and 25 served as controls. After intervention (3 times a week for 4 weeks) both exercise groups showed significant improvement in function and reduced pain compared to the controls. The group that performed the combined hip and knee exercise program showed greater improvement than the knee exercise group in all measures, although only pain reduction during stair descent reached statistical significance. Using only hip-strengthening exercises for 8 weeks,[139] Khayambashi et al documented improved pain and health status in females compared to those not receiving exercises; the improvement was maintained at a 6-month follow-up for those in the exercise group.

Dolak et al[61] conducted a randomized controlled study of 33 females with PFPS who either received hip strengthening or quadriceps strengthening for 4 weeks; both groups then received the same functional weight-bearing exercises for an additional 4 weeks. After the initial 4 weeks, those in the hip strengthening group had significant decrease in pain compared with the quad strengthening group. By emphasizing hip strength and not stressing the patella with quadriceps exercises during the initial 4 weeks, the authors suggest the PF pain was allowed time to heal while preparing the hip for the functional exercise phase of the program. Both groups improved function (measured by the lateral step-down test) and decreased pain by 8 weeks.[61]

Baldon et al[12] measured multiple parameters, including pain, function, kinematics, trunk endurance, and eccentric hip and knee muscle strength, in a randomized study of 31 recreational female athletes. The experimental group received exercises that emphasized hip muscle strengthening, limb and trunk movement control, and functional stabilization training; the control group received stretching and traditional exercises emphasizing quadriceps strengthening. Measurements were collected after 8 weeks of interventions with a follow up at 3 months. Both groups had decreased pain at 8 weeks; those in the experimental group demonstrated greater improvement and function, including improved trunk and extremity alignment during a single-leg squat at 8 weeks and less pain at 3 months.[12]

Patellar Instability: Surgical and Postoperative Management

Following conservative management of a primary (first-time) patellar dislocation, the of dislocation recurrence rate is between 15% to 44% and as high as 50% after subsequent episodes.[47] When nonoperative interventions fail to control instability and related symptoms such as recurrent dislocation or chronic subluxation, pain, crepitus, or PF joint degeneration, surgery is usually indicated.

Surgical interventions can be used to alter patellar alignment, correct tension imbalances of the static stabilizers (see Fig. 21.4), modify the Q-angle (see Fig. 21.3 for depiction of Q-angle measurement), improve patellar tracking, and débride or repair PF joint articular surfaces. The correct surgical procedure is selected following a thorough physical examination coupled with radiographic and arthroscopic evaluations to determine the etiology of symptoms and identify the factors contributing to patellar instability.

Overview of Surgical Options

Surgical options for lateral patellar instability are noted in Box 21.5.[40,45,47,85,86,88,89,119,183,184,199,221,232,241] Numerous variations of operative procedures fall under each of these options. Procedures may be arthroscopic, open, or a combination of these approaches.

When soft tissue factors contribute to lateral patellar instability, a proximal realignment procedure, such as MPFL repair or reconstruction or VMO imbrication, is often selected. When an osseous factor is the underlying cause, a distal realignment procedure that involves a tibial tubercle osteotomy with patellar tendon transfer is performed. Repair of chondral lesions associated with acute or recurrent patellar dislocation or trauma may also be necessary.[184] In contrast, TKA or patellectomy (a salvage procedure) is performed only for end-stage PF arthritis and collapse of the joint space.[86,184,221]

The two broad categories of surgery for patellofemoral instability—proximal and distal realignment of the extensor mechanism—may be performed with or without a lateral retinacular release (LRR). As an independent procedure, LRR can alleviate or reduce patellofemoral pain if the cause of the pain is compression of lateral knee structures (lateral compression syndrome) related to excessive lateral tilt of the patella, but it is not recommended for management of lateral patellar instability.[47,78,86,184,232]

BOX 21.5 Surgical Options for Management of Lateral Patellar Instability and Associated Structural Impairments

Soft Tissue and Osseous Procedures for Patellar Instability
- Medial patellofemoral ligament repair or reconstruction with autograft or allograft
- Medial retinacular imbrication (advancement)
- Lateral retinacular release, including release of the lateral patellofemoral and patellotibial ligaments
- Imbrication and medialization of the VMO
- Distal realignment of the extensor mechanism (anteromedialization of the tibial tubercle and insertion of the patellar tendon)
- Trochleoplasty (to improve the size/shape of the trochlear groove) for trochlear dysplasia

Articular Cartilage Procedures
- Arthroscopic débridement
- Repair of patellofemoral articular cartilage lesions (microfracture, osteochondral autograft transfer/mosaicplasty, autologous chondrocyte implantation)
- Abrasion arthroplasty/chondroplasty of the posterior surface of the patella (used less frequently with the advent of surgeries to repair articular cartilage)

Procedures for End-Stage Patellofemoral Arthritis
- TKA or replacement arthroplasty of the posterior surface of the patella
- Patellectomy (salvage procedure)

FOCUS ON EVIDENCE

Several current literature reviews[45,47,241] report that the use of LRR *in isolation* for recurrent or acute lateral patellar instability yields poor long-term outcomes (high recurrence rates for dislocation). According to another review,[86] LRR failed to realign the patella more medially. All reviews concluded that LRR in isolation is not effective for treatment of lateral patellar instability.

Operative procedures other than proximal or distal realignment are also used for recurrent patellar instability. Trochleoplasty, which involves deepening of the trochlear sulcus, may be indicated if trochlear dysplasia is contributing to patellar instability.[47] When excessive rotational deformity of the lower extremity is the underlying cause of severe patellar malalignment and recurrent instability, a supratubercle, derotational, high tibial osteotomy may be indicated as an alternative to proximal or distal realignment procedures.[224]

Following proximal or distal extensor mechanism realignment, a number of factors influence the rate of progression of rehabilitation. Factors include the type of surgical procedure performed; the patient's age, general health, and severity of patellofemoral symptoms prior to surgery; the presence of other pathologies; the desired functional outcomes; and the patient's adherence to the prescribed home exercise program and motivation to return to functional activities.

Proximal Extensor Mechanism Realignment: Medial Patellofemoral Ligament Repair or Reconstruction and Related Procedures

Repair, realignment, or reconstruction of the static and dynamic medial patellar support structures are surgical options for the patient with recurrent lateral patellar instability causing pain and compromised function.[4,40,47,201] MPFL repair or reconstruction, with or without LRR, is the primary surgical option when conservative management is unsuccessful. MPFL repair or reconstruction may also be indicated following an acute, first-time lateral patellar dislocation as the result of trauma. Other proximal realignment procedures include VMO imbrication (advancement) and medial retinacular reefing/tightening. These soft tissue procedures are appropriate for the skeletally immature patient with patellar instability and may be used in conjunction with a distal realignment involving an osteotomy in the skeletally mature patient.[86,119]

Indications for Surgery

Although opinions vary among surgeons, the following are cited as indications for MPFL repair or reconstruction and other proximal realignment procedures with or without LRR.[4,40,47,86,88,119,199,201,221,232]

- Deficiency (acute tear, chronic laxity) of the medial patellar support structures, in particular the MPFL, leading to patellar malalignment and recurrent instability
- Excessive (or abnormal) lateral patellar tracking and VMO insufficiency
- Painful, lateral compressive forces at the PF joint and persistent lateral patellar tilt despite a previous LRR
- The skeletally immature patient with patellar instability for the purpose of realignment.[119]

CONTRAINDICATIONS: Proximal realignment procedures are not appropriate for patients with medial patella articular degeneration, patella alta, or trochlear dysplasia because surgery may exacerbate or have no impact on symptoms.[86,119]

Procedures

Background and Operative Overview

Proximal realignment procedures combine an open surgical approach through a medial parapatellar incision with an arthroscopic examination of the knee; LRR; débridement of any loose osteochondral fragments or partial-thickness lesions; and, if necessary, microfracture for full-thickness chondral lesions.[184]

MPFL repair or tightening. An acute lateral patellar dislocation usually results in disruption of the MPFL and is managed with a direct repair.[40,119] Repair is also an option if the ligament is lax as the result of recurrent dislocations. To expose the MPFL, the medial retinaculum must be opened. Depending on the location of the tear(s), the ligament is reattached to the femoral condyle, the patella, or both bony surfaces using suture anchors. If the midsubstance of the ligament is disrupted, fragments are repaired with nonabsorbable locking sutures in a pants-over-vest fashion.

MPFL reconstruction. This procedure is used if the MPFL is incompetent as the result of recurrent lateral dislocation or subluxation or if a previous repair or reefing of the ligament has failed. Reconstruction involves reinforcement of the MPFL with an autogenous hamstring, TFL, or quadriceps tendon graft or allograft.[4,62,201] Depending on the type of reconstruction and graft selected, the patellar and femoral ends of the graft are secured in drill holes with sutures, suture anchors, or screw fixation. Some procedures do not use drill holes which eliminates the risk of patellar fracture.

VMO imbrication (advancement). This procedure improves the resting length-tension relationship of the VMO by moving the muscle to a more central and distal location.[86,199,221,232]

Lateral retinacular release and other concomitant procedures. If a lateral patellar tilt is identified, LRR is indicated to reduce the tilt and restore patellar alignment in the trochlea.[45,86,232,241] LRR is performed arthroscopically through several lateral parapatellar portals by "releasing" the lateral structures supporting the patellofemoral joint. Specifically, the superficial and deep portions of the lateral retinaculum and the lateral patellofemoral and patellotibial ligaments are released with an incision that extends from the superior lateral pole of the patella to just lateral and inferior to the patellar tendon.[184] The location of the incision is such that the superior lateral and inferior lateral geniculate arteries are cut and must be cauterized immediately and tied. The release leaves the tendinous portion of the VL muscle intact so as not to compromise quadriceps function. Electrocautery[199] and, most recently, radiofrequency ablation[89] are alternatives to surgically incising the retinaculum. The advantages of these methods for releasing the lateral structures are less bleeding and subsequent hemarthrosis.

In addition to repair or reconstruction of the MPFL, the medial patellotibial and medial patellomeniscal ligaments may be tightened or repaired.[86,88] A bony distal realignment procedure may also be combined with a medial soft tissue repair or reconstruction.[86,88,199]

Complications

Postoperative complications that can occur with any of the patellofemoral surgeries include a superficial infection, an intra-articular infection, or a DVT. Patellar adhesions and arthrofibrosis can compromise postoperative ROM. In rare instances, complex regional pain syndrome can develop (see Chapter 13).[48]

Complications following proximal realignment. Several complications can increase medial articular surface loading and exacerbate pain, including "overtensioning" the native MPFL or graft tissue during repair or reconstruction, overtightening other medial soft tissues, inaccurate graft placement, and/or excessive imbrication of the VMO.[4,40,47] Significant scarring or overtightening of medial tissues may also cause increased patellar rotation and excessive medial tracking leading to retropatellar erosion and/or increased risk of *medial* instability of the patella.[40,86] In contrast, inadequate medial tightening or VMO realignment may result in no change in patellar position and tracking, or in the patient's symptoms. Although the risk of patellar fracture is low, it is a complication that can occur during MPFL reconstruction procedures that require patellar drill holes for graft placement and fixation.[47]

Entrapment, irritation, or a neuroma of the saphenous nerve as it passes the adductor tubercle and splits at the pes anserine tendon can also occur with any procedure involving structures on the medial side of the knee.[86]

Complications following LRR. Because of the location of the geniculate artery, hemarthrosis can occur if it is not adequately cauterized during surgery. Thermal injury to overlying skin can occur with radiofrequency ablation or electrocautery.[89] Another complication, postoperative medial patellar subluxation, can develop if the lateral release extends too far proximally and causes weakness of the VL muscle. In rare instances, rupture of the quadriceps tendon occurs following VMO advancement.

Postoperative Management

Postoperative rehabilitation after MPFL repair or reconstruction or other proximal realignment procedures follows a course summarized in Table 21.3.[4,40,88,164,201] The patient is progressed through each phase of rehabilitation based on signs and symptoms and the attainment of phase-specific goals.[209]

TABLE 21.3 MPFL Repair or Reconstruction: Intervention for Each Phase of Postoperative Rehabilitation

Phase and General Time Frame	Maximum Protection Phase: Weeks 1–4	Moderate Protection Phase: Weeks 4–8	Minimum Protection Phase: Weeks 8–12 and Beyond
Patient presentation			
	▪ Rehab begins within 1–2 days after surgery ▪ Postoperative pain ▪ ROM limited ▪ Weight bearing as tolerated in locked extension orthosis	▪ Minimum pain ▪ Joint effusion controlled ▪ Full weight bearing with orthosis locked until full, active knee extension achieved ▪ Functional ROM of knee ▪ Able to perform SLR (no extensor lag) by 6 weeks	▪ No pain, swelling, or tenderness ▪ No signs or symptoms of patellar subluxation, during the previous phase ▪ Muscle function: at least 75% (4/5 MMT) of noninvolved extremity ▪ Unrestricted ADL and IADL
Key examination procedures			
	▪ Pain (0–10 scale) ▪ Monitor for hemarthrosis ▪ ROM ▪ Muscle control—ability to perform quad set ▪ MMT: hip muscle strength ▪ Soft tissue palpation	▪ Pain assessment ▪ Joint effusion—girth ▪ ROM ▪ Muscle control ▪ Gait analysis	▪ Pain assessment ▪ Muscle strength ▪ Neuromuscular balance ▪ Patellar alignment and stability ▪ Functional status

TABLE 21.3 MPFL Repair or Reconstruction: Intervention for Each Phase of Postoperative Rehabilitation—cont'd

Phase and General Time Frame	Maximum Protection Phase: Weeks 1–4	Moderate Protection Phase: Weeks 4–8	Minimum Protection Phase: Weeks 8–12 and Beyond
Goals			
	▪ Control postoperative ▪ swelling ▪ Minimize pain ▪ Knee ROM: 0°–90° (end of week 4) ▪ 3/5 muscle strength ▪ Ambulate full weight bearing on operated side without assistive device but in locked brace ▪ Establish home exercise program	▪ Control swelling ▪ Knee ROM: 0°–120° (end of week 6) ▪ 0°–135° (end of week 8) ▪ 4/5 to 5/5 strength ▪ Improve neuromuscular control ▪ Normalize the gait pattern ▪ Adherence to home program	▪ Functional knee ROM ▪ 75% muscle strength compared to nonoperated lower extremity ▪ Gradual return to ADL and IADL ▪ Educate patient on resuming activity slowly, monitoring signs and symptoms ▪ Develop maintenance program and educate patient on importance of adherence
Interventions			
	▪ Compression wrap to control effusion ▪ Pain modulation modalities ▪ Gait training with crutches in locked brace, weight bearing as tolerated ▪ Ankle pumps ▪ Knee: A-AROM→AROM in range-limiting brace ▪ Superior and inferior patellar mobilization (grades I and II) ▪ Setting exercises: quadriceps, hamstrings, and gluteal muscles (may augment with pain-free NMES over VMO) ▪ Four-position SLRs in locked brace for hip strength ▪ Flexibility program hamstring, calf, IT band	▪ LE flexibility program ▪ Continued open-chain (SLR without lag) and closed-chain strengthening ▪ Limited-range PRE ▪ Proprioceptive training ▪ Stabilization and balance exercises ▪ Gait training ▪ Low-intensity stationary cycling in range-limiting brace for aerobic conditioning	▪ Continue stretching for LE flexibility ▪ Progress PRE for strengthening ▪ Advanced closed-chain exercise ▪ Aerobic conditioning program: cycling, swimming, or walking program ▪ Walk-jog progression at week 10 ▪ Agility drills by week 10–12 ▪ Implement drills specific to occupation or sport ▪ Consider bracing for high-demand activity occupation ▪ Task-specific training. Simulated functional tasks based on signs and symptoms

Immobilization and Weight-Bearing Considerations

A compression dressing is applied following surgery, and the knee is immobilized in a range-limiting, hinged orthosis locked in extension or in a posterior orthosis to prevent excessive knee flexion and protect the soft tissues. Some surgeons allow early ROM in a protected range within a few days after surgery,[4,40,164,201] whereas others advocate continuous immobilization for a week postoperatively.[119,232] Depending on the surgeon's preference, protected ROM is performed with the patient wearing the range-limiting orthosis or with it removed for therapy.

During ambulation with crutches in the early postoperative period, the knee orthosis is locked in extension. Weight-bearing status on the operated extremity ranges from 25% of body weight to weight bearing as tolerated. Full weight bearing with the immobilizer locked is permitted by about 4 weeks after surgery.[201] Full weight bearing with the orthosis unlocked and without an assistive device is permitted only when the patient can control the knee and has achieved full, pain-free passive and active knee extension (no evidence of an extensor lag/quadriceps lag).[164,232]

Exercise Progression

Exercise goals following proximal realignment are directed toward restoring and improving the function of the entire lower extremity and trunk, not just the knee.[78,164,168,234] As with nonoperative management of patellofemoral dysfunction, many of the rehabilitation exercises focus on regaining pain-free knee ROM, maintaining patellar mobility, and recruiting the quadriceps mechanism as a unit and the VMO in particular. These interventions are designed to prevent or remediate patellar motion restrictions and an extensor lag.[56,135,164,281,289] A more recent but equally important postoperative focus is remediating strength deficits in the trunk; pelvis; and hip abductor, external rotator, and extensor muscles and improving flexibility of the hip and ankle musculature.[125,168,230,233,234]

Exercise goals, a progression of exercise interventions, and criteria to progress from one phase of rehabilitation to the next after proximal realignment procedures are summarized in the following sections.[88,164,201] Exercise precautions after proximal and distal extensor realignment procedures are noted in Box 21.6.[119,164,201]

Exercise: Maximum Protection Phase

Goals and interventions. During the first 4 weeks after surgery, the repaired or reconstructed medial patellar tissues are in the acute and subacute stages of healing and vulnerable to excessive stresses. The goals and interventions during this period are directed toward achieving independent ambulation with crutches; controlling pain and swelling; preventing complications, such as a DVT or adhesions; regaining quadriceps control; and restoring ROM of the knee while protecting the reconstructed soft tissues (see Table 21.4).

- ***Achieve independent ambulation.*** Gait training with crutches for protected weight bearing and knee orthosis locked in extension
- ***Control pain and swelling.*** Apply cold and compression regularly throughout the day.
- ***Patient education.*** Review weight-bearing and exercise precautions with the patient to protect the repaired ligament or graft tissue while it is most vulnerable to excessive stresses (see Box 21.6). Establish and teach a home exercise program.
- ***Restore ROM.*** Perform knee flexion/extension exercises (PROM, A-AROM, and AROM) within a day or two after surgery. Follow the surgeon's preference regarding removing the orthosis for ROM. Depending on the type of repair or reconstruction performed, the goal is to attain full passive and active knee extension and *at least* 90° flexion by the end of week 4.[88,164,201] Stretch hip and ankle musculature, if restricted.
- ***Maintain patellar mobility.*** Apply gentle (grades I and II) patellar mobilization (superior and inferior) to reduce pain and prevent tissue adhesions.
- ***Reestablish neuromuscular control and improve muscle performance.*** Begin gentle quadriceps setting for knee control augmented with pain-free neuromuscular electrical muscle stimulation or biofeedback. While wearing the orthosis locked in extension, initiate SLRs in supine, prone, and side-lying positions for hip control. With the orthosis unlocked, begin partial-range heel-slides in the supine position and bilateral minisquats and heel raises when 50% pain-free weight bearing on the operated side is allowed.

BOX 21.6 Exercise Precautions After Proximal or Distal Realignment of the Extensor Mechanism

- Initiate PROM or A-AROM_AROM exercises in a hinged, range-limiting orthosis to prevent excessive knee flexion or a valgus stress to the knee.
- Progress knee flexion gradually so as not to disrupt sutures after MPFL repair or reconstruction, advancement of the VMO, or tibial tubercle osteotomy with medial transfer of the patellar tendon.
- When assisting with supine-lying hip and knee flexion/extension ROM, stand on the contralateral side of the operated extremity to avoid placing a valgus stress on the knee and stretching repaired medial structures.
- Perform SLR on the operated side with the orthosis locked in extension.
- Begin weight-bearing exercises, such as weight shifting, in bilateral stance with the knee orthosis locked in extension.
- Begin bilateral closed-chain exercises, such as minisquats, in the unlocked, range-limiting knee orthosis when 50% weight bearing on the operated side is permissible.
- Continue to keep the orthosis locked in extension during closed-chain exercises or ambulation in full weight bearing until quadriceps control has been established (full, active knee extension/no extensor lag).
- Postpone unilateral weight-bearing exercises that involve full weight on the operated side and without the orthosis:
  - For at least 4 to 6 weeks after soft tissue reconstruction
  - For at least 8 weeks or until radiographic healing has occurred after a distal realignment involving a tibial tubercle osteotomy
- Do not perform a maximum voluntary contraction of the quadriceps for at least 12 weeks after VMO advancement or tibial tubercle osteotomy.

Criteria to progress. Criteria to progress to the intermediate phase of rehabilitation include:[164,201]

- Minimal pain and swelling
- Incision healing well; no signs of infection
- Full, active knee extension (no evidence of extensor lag) and at least 90° of knee flexion

Exercise: Moderate Protection/Controlled Motion Phase

Goals and interventions. During the intermediate phase of rehabilitation, from approximately 4 to 8 weeks postoperatively, soft tissues are in the repair and remodeling stage of healing. Full weight bearing without an assistive device but with the orthosis locked is usually permitted by 4 to 6 weeks after surgery. The patient should be able to achieve functional knee ROM by the end of this phase of rehabilitation.

As symptoms subside and quadriceps activation improves, the focus of this phase is to establish a normal gait pattern with the orthosis unlocked, increase knee ROM, and restore hip and ankle flexibility and function. It is also important to develop strength and endurance of the hip and trunk muscles, improve neuromuscular control/response times, ensure sufficient balance and proprioception, regain cardiopulmonary endurance, and progress and reinforce the home exercise program.

- ***Normalize the gait pattern.*** If full weight bearing is pain free and quadriceps control is sufficient, practice walking with crutches or a cane with the orthosis unlocked.
- ***Restore ROM and joint mobility.*** Begin low-intensity, prolonged stretching and grade III joint mobilization to increase ROM of restricted areas. Achieve 0° to 120° knee ROM by the end of week 6 and 0° to 135° by the end of week 8.[4,88,164] Stretch all tight lower extremity musculature, specifically the gastrocnemius, soleus, hamstring muscles, and IT band, because they have been shown to be tight in patients with PF dysfunction.[230]
- ***Improve muscle performance.*** Progress pain-free, closed-chain, and open-chain resistance training to increase strength and muscular endurance of the entire lower extremity. Emphasize knee extensor and hip extensor, abductor, and external rotator strengthening exercises. (Suggestions for a progression of nonweight-bearing and weight-bearing exercises are noted in the previous section on nonoperative management and described in the final section of this chapter and Chapter 20.)

PRECAUTION: The patient must only perform resisted exercises in pain-free ranges and in positions consistent with weight-bearing precautions. During weight-bearing exercises, reinforce proper lower extremity alignment to avoid knee valgus during flexion.

- ***Improve neuromuscular control and response time, proprioception, and balance.*** While wearing the orthosis locked in extension, begin neuromuscular/proprioceptive training and stabilization and balance activities on a stable surface and progress to unstable surfaces. Emphasize maintaining proper lower extremity alignment. Progress from bilateral to unilateral stance and by adding first uniplanar and then multiplanar movements of the nonaffected extremities or trunk. As knee control improves, unlock the orthosis during training.
- ***Improve cardiopulmonary endurance.*** Begin a stationary cycling program while wearing the range-limiting orthosis. Begin with a high seat and low resistance. If wound healing is adequate, pool exercise such as walking, marching, or jogging can begin.

Criteria to progress. The following criteria should be achieved to advance to the final phase of rehabilitation.[164]

- No swelling or extensor lag
- Knee ROM: 0° to 135°
- Sufficient strength of knee and hip musculature (at least 75% compared to nonoperated side) to initiate lower extremity functional activities

Exercise: Minimum Protection/Return To Function Phase

Goals and interventions. During the final phase of rehabilitation, which extends from 8 to 12 weeks and beyond, the patient gradually participates in more demanding functional activities. By 12 weeks postoperatively, the patient should be able to begin land-based jogging, and by 16 to 20 weeks, they should be able to return to a full level of activity without symptoms. It may be necessary to modify or limit some activities to minimize the risk of provoking symptoms or the recurrence of instability.[4]

Emphasize activity-specific training, always maintaining proper lower extremity alignment. The patient's lifestyle may need to be modified temporarily to avoid symptom-provoking activities. Develop and implement a self-managed program to continue to improve and maintain strength, flexibility, and balance and devise a plan for adherence to this program.

NOTE: Continued use of patellar taping or a patellar tracking orthosis during exercise may be useful during the progression of exercises and transition to high-demand functional activities.

Refer to the exercise progression previously discussed for advanced nonoperative management and selected exercises described in the final sections of this chapter and Chapter 20. More advanced exercises, including plyometric training and agility drills, are described in Chapter 23.

Outcomes

Outcomes reported after MPFL repair or reconstruction vary considerably among studies because the procedures used differ widely, with some performed in isolation and others combined with lateral release or distal realignment. For the patient with a first-time lateral dislocation, rates of subsequent patellar dislocation were similar for nonoperative management and surgical repair, suggesting there is no advantage of undergoing surgery prior to a course of nonoperative exercises.[219]

Camp and colleagues[40] carried out a retrospective review of 27 patients (29 knees) who underwent MPFL repair at an average of 19 years of age for recurrent patellar instability. The success rate for the prevention of recurrence of patellar dislocation for an average of 4 years following MPFL repair was 72% (21 of 29 knees), which the investigators considered a relatively high rate of recurrence. The patients who reported a postoperative dislocation subsequently underwent additional procedures, including MPFL reconstruction and/or distal realignment (tibial tubercle osteotomy). Recurrent instability following MPFL reconstruction has been associated with malpositioning of the MPFL graft during surgery.[27]

In contrast, MPFL reconstruction procedures have resulted in high patient satisfaction and low redislocation rates. For example, in a retrospective case series, Drez and coinvestigators[62] reported the use of MPFL reconstruction with a soft tissue graft (and no distal realignment) in 15 patients with recurrent lateral instability after first-time patellar dislocation. At a mean follow-up of 31.5 months (minimum of 2 years), 93% of patients had excellent results (10 patients) or good results (3 patients) on an objective functional outcome and patient satisfaction scale. Only 1 of the 15 patients reported one episode of subluxation during the follow-up period.

There is general agreement that LRR performed in isolation is not an effective procedure for management of acute or chronic patellar instability.[45,47,232,241] The poor results can be attributed to the inability of LRR to align the patella in a more medial position.[86]

Poor outcomes, overall, following the many proximal realignment procedures described in the literature appear to be due more to retropatellar pain than to recurrent instability.[119] Patients with generalized joint hypermobility or uncorrected trochlear dysplasia tend to have a high rate of redislocation and typically require a distal realignment procedure.[88]

Distal Realignment Procedures: Patellar Tendon With Tibial Tubercle Transfer and Related Procedures

For a patient with recurrent subluxation/dislocation of the patella, a distal realignment of the extensor mechanism may be the surgical intervention of choice. A medial transfer of the tibial tubercle is performed to decrease laterally directed forces on the patella by improving patellar tracking and shifting contact stresses away from chondral lesions of the distal and lateral articular surface of the patella.[47,85] Anterior tubercle transfers are done to increase the patellar lever arm, which decreases quadriceps forces and in turn, patellofemoral contact forces.[105] Combined medial and anterior transfers are used when realignment and reduced forces are both deemed necessary.[105] Distal realignment procedures may be used in isolation or coupled with LRR or a proximal soft tissue procedure, such as MPFL repair or reconstruction or medial capsular reefing.[47,88,199]

Indications for Surgery

The following are indications for distal realignment procedures:[47,85,86,184,199,221,232]

- Recurrent episodes of lateral patellar instability and a sense of the knee "giving way" because of patellar malalignment due to lateralization of the tibial tubercle and patellar tendon insertion
- Painful lateral tracking of the patella with no instability
- Anterior knee pain associated with patellar maltracking and patellofemoral arthrosis (chondral or osteochondral defects) of the lateral and distal retropatellar surfaces
- Abnormally increased Q-angle
- Excessive tibial tubercle-trochlear groove distance (> 15 mm)

CONTRAINDICATION: Bony procedures are not recommended for the skeletally immature patient whose tibial tubercle growth plate is open. Recurvatum of the knee can develop with premature closure of this epiphyseal plate.[85,119]

Procedures

Background and Operative Overview

The purpose of distal realignment procedures is to reduce patellar instability and anterior knee pain by reducing laterally directed forces on the patella, reducing the magnitude of patellofemoral contact forces and improving patellar tracking.[47,85,86,221,232] Distal realignment procedures are performed using an open surgical approach. However, arthroscopic examination of the knee joint, débridement of the articular surface of the patella, and sometimes an LRR may precede the distal realignment procedure.

A number of surgical techniques for distal realignment have been reported.

Tibial tubercle transfer (Elmslie-Trillat procedure). An osteotomy of the tibial tubercle is performed; the bony prominence is then transferred medially and secured with screw fixation.[47,85,88]

Anteriorization (elevation) of the tibial tubercle. Often combined with a medial tibial tubercle transfer, this procedure involves displacing the tubercle anteriorly by means of a bone graft.[232] This serves to reduce contact forces on the patella and offloads the distal patellar articular surfaces.[47,85,232]

Distal medialization of the patellar tendon. This procedure involves only a soft tissues transfer for the skeletally immature patient.

Complications

Uncommon but serious complications associated with distal realignment procedures include tibial fracture during placement of fixation screws, neurovascular injury during surgery, inadequate skin closure or sloughing over the osteotomy site, soft tissue infection or osteomyelitis, and nonunion of the transposed bone.[85,232] Redislocation can occur laterally because of undercorrection or medially with overcorrection, particularly in patients who return to high-demand activities.[85,199]

Pain at the anterior tibial tubercle from the fixation screws is not unusual. Therefore, screws are routinely removed 6 to 12 months after surgery.[85] As with all patellofemoral surgeries, patellar adhesions can occur, restricting knee motion. Because distal realignment shifts retropatellar loads medially and proximally, excessive medialization of the tibial tubercle and patellar tendon can cause excessive contact pressure on the medial patellar facet and medial compartment, contributing to arthrosis of these areas over time.[47]

Postoperative Management

Immobilization and Weight-Bearing Considerations

Depending on the type of fixation used, rehabilitation after distal realignment involving bony procedures must progress more gradually than rehabilitation following proximal realignment of soft tissues. Ambulation with crutches while wearing a knee orthosis locked in extension is permissible the day after surgery. Weight bearing is limited to touch-down/toe-touch for the first 4 weeks or until radiographic verification of bone callus formation has occurred at the osteotomy site.[85,164] Weight bearing is progressed gradually, with full weight bearing permissible without the immobilizer at 8 weeks if quadriceps control is sufficient.[164]

Exercise Progression

ROM also is progressed more gradually than after soft tissue procedures (refer to exercise precautions noted in Box 21.6). A range-limiting orthosis is worn that allows motion from only 0° to 30°[164] or 0° to 60°[88] of flexion during the first week; to 90° of flexion by the end of week 4; and to 135° by the end of week 8.[164] Closed-chain exercises are initiated in the range-limiting knee orthosis as increased weight bearing is permitted. Otherwise, exercises are similar to those for nonoperative management, LRR, and proximal realignment procedures. The return to full activity generally takes about 5 to 6 months and is based on bone healing and lower extremity strength.

Outcomes

Patients without degeneration of the retropatellar surface or those with lateral and distal lesions tend to have better results than those with medial articular lesions or advanced PF arthritis.[47,184] Outcomes following medial tibial tubercle transfer were shown to be better for patients with painful lateral patellar tracking without instability than for patients with at least a 1-year history of recurrent instability.[142] However, because improvement occurred in both groups of patients tibial tubercle transfer appears beneficial for painful maltracking and recurrent instability.

Distal realignment procedures are often coupled with a proximal repair and/or lateral release to correct malalignment and relieve symptoms. Results of studies of combined procedures reflect good to excellent outcomes for most patients. Garth and colleagues[88] studied a group of young adults (mean age, 18 years) with recurrent patellar instability after an acute, traumatic, lateral dislocation of the patella. After undergoing distal realignment coupled with MPFL repair and advancement of the patellomeniscal ligament, 90% (18 of 20) of the patients reported good to excellent results in knee function and patient satisfaction and no recurrence of instability at a minimum follow-up of 24 months. In another study[199] evaluating the combination of three procedures (lateral release, repair of medial supporting structures, and distal realignment), 32 of 42 knees (76%) in 37 patients had good or excellent outcomes at follow-up (mean, 44 months; range, 25 to 85 months), with only four knees experiencing redislocations.

Ligament Injuries: Nonoperative Management

Mechanisms of Injury

Ligament injuries occur most frequently in individuals between 20 and 40 years of age during sport participation (e.g., skiing, soccer, football) but can occur in individuals of all ages. The ACL is the most commonly injured knee ligament. Often, more than one knee ligament is damaged during a single injury episode.

FOCUS ON EVIDENCE

Sprain and strain injuries are classified as knee instability and movement coordination impairments in the **Clinical Practice Guidelines** linked to the International Classification of Functioning, Disability, and Health.[159]

Anterior Cruciate Ligament

ACL injuries can occur from both contact and noncontact mechanisms (Fig. 21.12). The most common contact mechanism is a force applied to the lateral side of the knee that results in a large valgus moment. This mechanism can injure not only the ACL, but also the MCL and the medial meniscus. Such an injury is termed the "unholy triad" or "terrible triad" injury because of the frequency with which these three structures are injured in a single trauma (Fig. 21.13).

The most common noncontact injury occurs through a rotational mechanism in which the tibia is externally rotated on the planted foot. Literature supports that this mechanism accounts for as many as 78% of all ACL injuries.[208] The second most common noncontact mechanism is forceful hyperextension of the knee.

With prolonged ambulation on a knee that has a deficient ACL, the secondary restraints (LCL and posterolateral joint capsule) are stressed and become lax, and a "quadriceps avoidance gait" may develop.[116] The quadriceps avoidance gait in ACL-deficient knees was originally documented and described by Berchuck and colleagues[15] as a reduction in the magnitude of the flexion moment about the knee during the limb loading phase of gait due to the patient's effort to reduce contraction of the quadriceps.

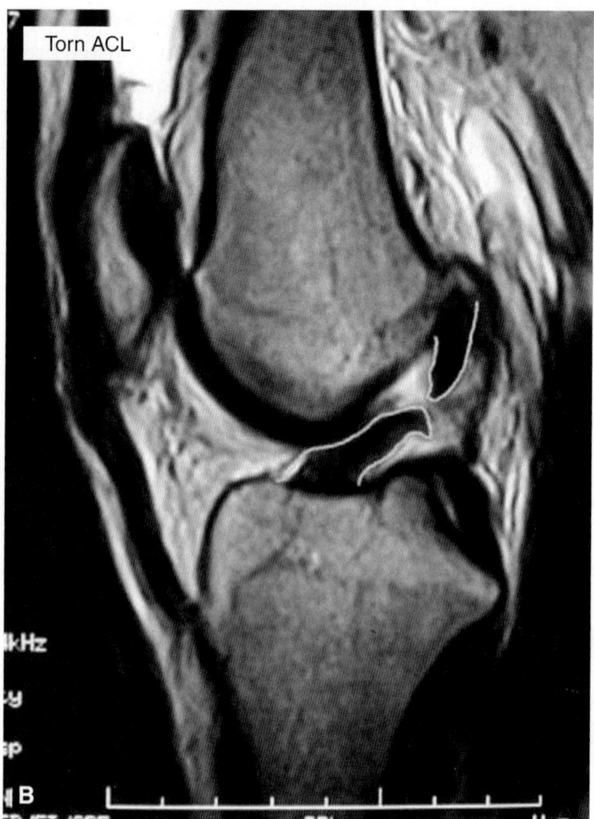

FIGURE 21.12 Sagittal MRI demonstrating a complete midstructure tear of the anterior cruciate ligament (outlined). *(From McKinnis, LN:* Fundamentals of Musculoskeletal Imaging, *ed. 4. Philadelphia: F.A. Davis, 2014, p 396, Fig. 13.48 B, with permission.)*

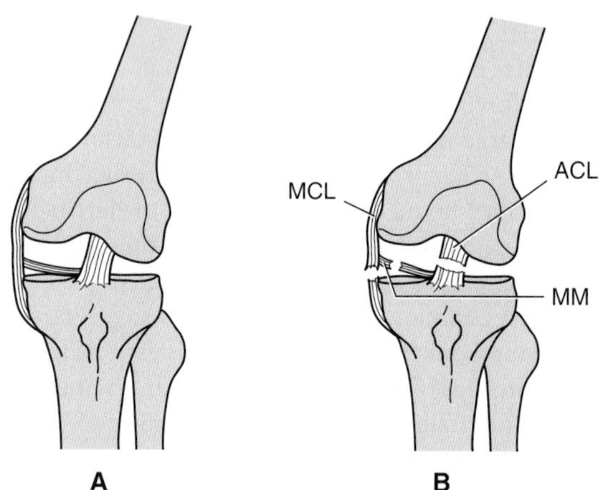

FIGURE 21.13 The "terrible triad," a combination of injuries to the medial meniscus (MM), medial collateral ligament (MCL), and anterior cruciate ligament (ACL). **(A)** Intact ligaments stretched by valgus force. **(B)** Rupture of the MCL, ACL, and MM. *(From McKinnis, LN:* Fundamentals of Musculoskeletal Imaging, *ed. 4. Philadelphia: F.A. Davis, 2014, p 395, Fig. 13.45 A and B, with permission.)*

Posterior Cruciate Ligament

PCL (Fig. 21.14) injuries occur most commonly from a forceful trauma to the anterior tibia while the knee is flexed, such as contact with the car dashboard in a motor vehicle accident or falling onto a flexed knee. A study by Schulz[256] evaluating 587 acute and chronic PCL-deficient knees reported that the three most common mechanisms of injury were a "dashboard"/anterior injury mechanism (38.5%); followed by a fall on the flexed knee with the foot in plantarflexion (24.6%); and lastly, a sudden, violent hyperflexion of the knee joint (11.9%).

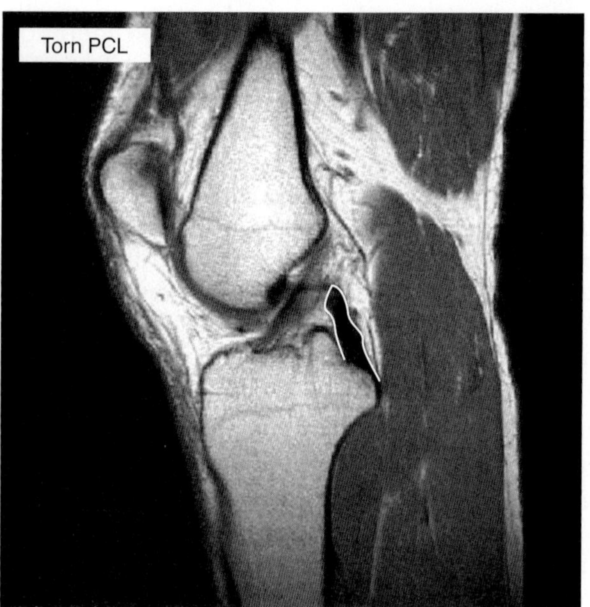

FIGURE 21.14 Sagittal MRI demonstrating a rupture of the posterior cruciate ligament seen as an interruption in the cordlike structure (outlined). *(From McKinnis, LN:* Fundamentals of Musculoskeletal Imaging, *ed. 4. Philadelphia: F.A. Davis, 2014, p 396, Fig. 13.47 B, with permission.)*

Medial Collateral Ligament

Isolated injuries to the MCL can occur from valgus moments that create high tensile loads across the medial joint line of the knee. Injuries to the MCL can be partial or incomplete and are graded utilizing a I, II, III grading classification of ligament injuries described in Chapter 10 (see Fig. 21.13).

Lateral Collateral Ligament

Injuries to the LCL are infrequent and are usually the result of a traumatic varus moment at the knee that loads the ligament. With this mechanism, it is not uncommon for additional ligaments, the joint capsule, and sometimes the menisci to also be damaged and result in posterolateral knee instability.

Ligament Injuries in the Female Athlete

The increased number of females participating in organized sports since the passage of Title IX in 1972 has also resulted in a concurrent increase in the number of injuries to female athletes. A significant percentage of these injuries are ACL tears, specifically from noncontact mechanisms. In fact, when injury to the ACL is sustained in a noncontact manner, a woman is three times more likely to tear the ACL than is a man.[8] This phenomenon has led the American Academy of Orthopaedic Surgeons to publish a consensus paper examining the risk factors and prevention strategies of noncontact ACL injuries.[100] In addition, clinicians and scientists interested in ACL injury gender bias have met regularly to present research, develop consensus, and suggest future investigations on gender bias in ACL injuries.[53]

Risk factors identified in the consensus papers generated by these groups fall into four major categories: biomechanical, neuromuscular, structural, and hormonal, and they are summarized here.[53,100]

- ***Biomechanical risk factors*** include the effect of the total chain (trunk, hip, knee, and ankle) on ACL injuries, including awkward or improper dynamic body movements during activities such as deceleration and changes of direction. For example, increased hip adduction is related to increased knee valgus, which is associated with ACL injury risk in the female. Also, decreased hip and knee flexion angles have been demonstrated during cutting activities in the female athlete.
- ***Neuromuscular risk factors*** have an influence on biomechanical factors in that neuromuscular control influences joint position and movement. Valgus collapse at the knee and decreased use of the hip extensors have been reported to be more common in women who have sustained an ACL injury than in men with an ACL injury. It is suggested that this is related to increased anterior shear of the tibia and strain of the ACL during deceleration such as landing with hip-knee flexion following a jump.[233] Not only are females weaker in hip and knee strength compared to males (normalized to body weight), but muscle timing and activation patterns of the quadriceps, hamstrings, and gastrocnemius muscles also differ between males and females.
- ***Structural risk factors*** include femoral notch size, ACL size, and lower extremity alignment. The femoral notch height is smaller and notch angle larger in the male compared to the female, which may affect ACL size. The female ACL is smaller than the male ACL even when adjusted for body size. The ACL in the female has a lower modulus of elasticity (i.e., less stiff) and lower failure strength (i.e., fails at a lower load), leading to greater joint mobility than in the male.
- ***Hormonal differences*** between males and females may also be a factor related to the increased incidence of female ACL injuries. There are hormone receptor sites for estrogen, progesterone, and testosterone in the ACL of humans. The sex hormones have a time-dependency effect that influences ACL tissue characteristics, such as increasing risk of injury during the pre-ovulatory phase of the menstrual cycle in females.[159]

Common Impairments, Activity Limitations, and Participation Restrictions

- Following trauma, the joint usually does not swell for several hours. If blood vessels are torn, swelling is usually immediate.
- If tested when the joint is not swollen, the patient feels pain when the injured ligament is stressed.
- If there is a complete tear, instability is detected when the torn ligament is tested.
- When effused, motion is restricted, the joint assumes a position of minimum stress (usually flexed 25°), and the quadriceps muscles are inhibited.[279]
- When acute, the knee cannot bear weight, and the person cannot ambulate without an assistive device.
- With a complete tear, there is instability, and the knee may give way during weight bearing, preventing the return to specific work, sport, and recreational activities requiring dynamic knee stability.

Conservative Management of Ligament Injuries

Acute sprains, partial ligament tears, and sometimes complete rupture of a single knee ligament can be treated conservatively with rest, joint protection, and exercise. After the acute stage of healing, exercises should focus on ROM, balance, normalizing the gait pattern , and developing strength and endurance of muscles that support and dynamically stabilize the joint during functional activities.[59,76,121] The degree of instability following a ligament tear affects the demands the patient can place on the knee when returning to full activity.

A patient's preinjury activity level and the postinjury level of activity to which he or she expects to return both influence the success of a nonoperative treatment program. Relatively sedentary individuals can usually function with some loss of knee stability and can expect to return to preinjury activities following a course of nonoperative management. For select athletes who wish to return to high-demand activities following ACL injury, an intensive rehabilitation program, including balance/perturbation training to stimulate neuromuscular control and develop dynamic knee stability, can be effective.[75,76] In contrast, for patients with extensive ligament damage or concomitant injuries (such as meniscus damage) and poor dynamic knee stability after a period of nonoperative treatment, surgical reconstruction is typically recommended for return to high-level work or sports and preinjury level of function.

FOCUS ON EVIDENCE

The descriptive terms "potential coper" and "potential noncoper" have been used in the literature[64,76,121,190] to identify and classify those individuals early after ACL injury who are good versus poor candidates for nonoperative rehabilitation. Potential copers are described as having sufficient dynamic knee stability; the ability to compensate following injury; and good potential to return to preinjury, high-level activities following a course of nonoperative treatment. In contrast, potential noncopers are thought to have poor potential to return to preinjury activities following nonoperative treatment; these individuals typically have poor dynamic knee stability and are advised to consider surgical management. A study by Moksnes and associates[190] evaluated both copers and noncopers after 1 year of intensive rehabilitation. For those not undergoing surgery, 19 of the 27 noncopers (70%) showed excellent knee function and were reclassified as true copers. In the coper group, 15 of 25 (60%) were true copers. (The term "true coper" applies to individuals able to return to preinjury activity level 1 year after ACL injury with no episodes of the knee giving way during activities.)

The results suggest limited prognostic accuracy of the screening examination and therefore support the importance of including all patients with ACL injury in intensive rehabilitation, not just those who initially meet the definition of coper.

If the collateral or coronary ligaments are involved, because of their superficial location, they may benefit from cross-fiber massage to align the healing fibers and maintain their mobility. Because of the structural characteristics of the MCL (a broad, flat ligament with deep and superficial portions, parallel alignment of collagen fibers, and fan-shaped attachments proximally and distally), injuries to this ligament are typically managed with a conservative (nonsurgical) approach.[306] Conservative management of knee ligament injuries is described in Table 21.4; progression is based on presenting signs and symptoms.[209]

Nonoperative Management: Maximum Protection Phase

Follow the principles described for an acute joint lesion earlier in this chapter.

- If possible, examine before effusion sets in.
- Utilize cold and compression with rest and elevation.
- Teach protected weight bearing with use of crutches and partial weight bearing as tolerated.
- Teach safe transfer activities to avoid pivoting on the involved extremity.
- Initiate quadriceps-setting exercises. The knee may not fully extend for end-range muscle-setting exercises, so begin the exercises in the range most comfortable for the patient. As the swelling decreases, initiate ROM within tolerance.

TABLE 21.4 Nonoperative Management of Knee Ligament Injuries: Intervention for Each Phase of Rehabilitation*

Phase and General Time Frame	Maximum Protection Phase: Weeks 1–3	Moderate Protection Phase: Weeks 3–6	Minimum Protection Phase: Weeks 5–8 and Beyond
Patient presentation			
	■ Joint effusion ■ Pinpoint tenderness ■ Decreased ROM	■ Minimal tenderness ■ Joint effusion controlled ■ No increased instability ■ Full or nearly full ROM	■ No instability ■ No effusion of tenderness ■ 4/5 to 5/5 strength (MMT) ■ Unrestricted ADL function ■ Muscle function 70% of noninvolved extremity
Key examination procedures			
	■ Pain scale ■ Joint effusion ■ Ligament stability ■ ROM ■ Muscle control ■ Functional status ■ Patellar mobility	■ Pain scale ■ Joint effusion ■ Ligament stability ■ ROM ■ Muscle control/ strength ■ Functional status	■ Ligament stability ■ Muscle control ■ Functional status
Goals			
	■ Protect healing tissues ■ Prevent reflex inhibition of muscle ■ Decrease joint effusion ■ Decrease pain ■ Establish home exercise program	■ Full, pain-free ROM ■ Restore muscular strength ■ Normalize gait without assistive device ■ Normalize ADL function ■ Adherence to home program	■ Increase strength ■ Increase power ■ Increase endurance ■ Improve neuromuscular control ■ Improve dynamic stability ■ Regain ability to function at highest desired level ■ Transition to maintenance program

TABLE 21.4 Nonoperative Management of Knee Ligament Injuries: Intervention for Each Phase of Rehabilitation*—cont'd

Phase and General Time Frame	Maximum Protection Phase: Weeks 1–3	Moderate Protection Phase: Weeks 3–6	Minimum Protection Phase: Weeks 5–8 and Beyond
Interventions			
	▪ PRICE (protective bracing, rest, ice, compression elevation) ▪ Ambulation training with crutches; weight bearing as tolerated ▪ PROM/A-AROM ▪ Patellar mobilization (grades I and II) ▪ Muscle setting quadriceps, hamstrings, and adductors (may augment with E-stim) ▪ SLRs ▪ Aerobic conditioning	▪ Continue multiple-angle isometrics ▪ Initiate PRE ▪ Closed-chain strengthening ▪ LE flexibility exercises ▪ Endurance training (e.g., bike, pool, ski machine) ▪ Perturbation/balance training ▪ Stabilization exercises ▪ Initiate a walk/jog program at the end of this phase ▪ Initiate skill-specific drills at the end of this phase	▪ Continue LE flexibility ▪ Advance PRE strengthening ▪ Advance closed-chain exercises ▪ Advance perturbation training ▪ Advance endurance training ▪ Isokinetic training (if available) ▪ Progress running program; full speed jog, sprints, figure-eight running, and cutting ▪ Implement drills specific to sport or occupation ▪ Determine need for protective bracing prior to return to sport or work

*Note: This is based on grade II ligament injury but may be accelerated for grade I or decelerated for grade III injuries.

Adapted from Wilk, KE, and Clancy, WG: Medial collateral ligament injuries: Diagnosis, treatment, and rehabilitation in knee ligament injuries. In Engle, RP (ed): *Knee Ligament Rehabilitation.* New York: Churchill Livingstone, 1991, with permission.

Nonoperative Management: Moderate Protection (Controlled Motion) Through Return to Activity Phases

As swelling decreases, examine the patient for impairments and functional losses. Initiate joint movement and exercises to improve muscle performance, functional status, and cardiopulmonary conditioning.[64,159]

Improve Joint Mobility and Protection

Joint mobility. Use supine wall slides (see Fig. 21.19), patellar mobilizations, and stationary cycling; encourage as much movement as possible. Unless there has been an extended period of immobilization, there should be minimal need to stretch contractures.

Protective bracing. Bracing may be necessary for weight-bearing activities to decrease stress to the healing ligament or to provide stability when ligament integrity has been compromised. Bracing can be one of two types: (1) range-limiting post-operative type braces that are used to protect healing tissues and discontinued during later phases of rehabilitation or (2) functional braces that are used during advanced rehabilitation and upon return to functional activities. The patient must be advised to modify activities until appropriate stability is obtained.

Improve Muscle Performance

Strength and endurance. Initiate isometric quadriceps and hamstring exercises, and progress to dynamic strength and muscular endurance training. Quadriceps strength is important for knee stability.[159]

- Utilize both open-chain and closed-chain resistance.
  - Open-chain resistance has been shown to be more effective for increasing quadriceps strength than closed-chain single-leg squat in patients with an ACL injury.[288]
  - Progress closed-chain exercises using partial squats, step-ups, leg press, and heel raises.
- Reinforce quadriceps contractions with high-intensity electrical stimulation if there is an extensor lag.[275]

FOCUS ON EVIDENCE

Eitzen and associates[64] reported results of a progressive 5-week exercise program with patients (n =100) who had a recent ACL injury (within 3 months) prior to deciding on whether or not to have reconstructive surgery. Pre- and post-tests included isokinetic quadriceps and hamstring strength, four single-leg hop tests, two self-assessment questionnaires, and a global rating of knee function. Both potential copers and noncopers without additional symptomatic injuries were included in the study. The program utilized progressive strength training (heavy resistance open and closed chain); plyometric, balance, and stability exercises; and perturbation training. A standardized response mean for each variable was calculated and demonstrated clinically relevant improvements in both groups. Adverse events (swelling, pain, or knee giving way) occurred in only 5 subjects.

Neuromuscular control. Neuromuscular control is compromised when stabilizing muscles fatigue.[118] Emphasize neuromuscular reeducation (proprioceptive training) with stabilization, acceleration, deceleration, and perturbation training in weight-bearing positions.[159] Begin with low-intensity, single-plane movements and progress to high-intensity, multiplane movements. These exercises are described in Chapter 8 and summarized in the last section of this chapter.

 **FOCUS ON EVIDENCE**

In a randomized, controlled study, 26 athletes with an acute ACL injury or rupture of ACL grafts participated in a standard rehabilitation program or a standard rehabilitation program with perturbation training.[75] Of those in the perturbation group (n =12), only one had unsuccessful rehabilitation, with the knee giving way while playing football prior to completing the program. In the control group (no perturbation training; n =14), one-half of the subjects had unsuccessful outcomes and were considered at high risk for re-injury at the 6-month follow-up examination. The authors stated that although both groups returned to high-level physical activities, those in the perturbation-training group demonstrated greater long-term success.

Improve Cardiopulmonary Conditioning

Utilize a program that is consistent with the patient's goals, such as biking (begin with a stationary bike), jogging (begin with walking on a treadmill), using a ski machine, or swimming.

Progress to Functional Training

Develop activity-specific exercises and drills that replicate the demands of the individual's outcome goals.[294] Suggestions for functional training are described in the exercise section of this chapter and Chapter 23.

Ligament Injuries: Surgical and Postoperative Management

Background

Knee ligaments are the key static stabilizing structures for accessory and rotational motions of the tibiofemoral joint (see Fig. 21.2). The main accessory motions of the joint are anterior and posterior translation and medial and lateral translation, while the primary rotational motions are varus and valgus moments and long-axis rotation. Strong ligamentous support is necessary because the shallow concave tibial articulating surface allows significant translatory motions if unrestrained. Acute traumatic disruption or chronic laxity of the ligaments results in increased accessory and/or rotational joint motions, which can impair functional abilities and accelerate joint degeneration. Although injuries to each of the four primary knee ligaments (ACL, PCL, MCL, and LCL) are discussed extensively in the literature, the ACL is, by far, the most frequently injured and surgically repaired. [19,208]

General considerations and indications for ligament surgery. Factors influencing the decision for surgical reconstruction include the specific ligament injured, the location and extent of the lesion, the degree of instability experienced by the patient, the presence of concomitant pathology such as a meniscal or articular cartilage damage, and the potential for achieving the patient's desired level of function.[1,2,72,138,186,271] The risk of re-injury and prevention of future impairment are also considerations because if not managed adequately, acute ligament injury can lead to chronic joint instability.[19] In turn, chronic instability is thought to contribute to degeneration of articular cartilage and early-onset OA.[160]

Surgical intervention for ligament injury is indicated when the patient has failed to achieve functional goals established in a conservative rehabilitation program or has early joint degeneration. Many authors[19,33,82,186,267,271] recommend surgical intervention for acute, isolated ACL and LCL injuries after a brief period of acute symptom management in recreationally active individuals. Surgical management of chronic ligament deficiency is rcommended when a patient's function has become compromised or when secondary joint pathology has developed. However, there is no evidence to suggest that ACL reconstruction prevents or reduces the rate of progression of early-onset joint degeneration.[160]

Types of ligament surgery. Ligament surgeries are classified as *intra-articular*, *extra-articular*, or combined procedures and can be performed using an open, arthroscopically assisted, or all-arthroscopic approach.[33,150,186] Initially, intra-articular procedures were performed through an open approach and involved a direct repair of the ligament. The repair was accomplished by re-opposing and suturing the torn ligament. Postoperatively, a long period (usually 6 weeks) of immobilization and restricted weight bearing were required because of extensive tissue disruption associated with the open approach and the poor healing qualities of ligamentous tissue.[150] Surgical outcomes were unacceptable due to postimmobilization contractures, patellofemoral dysfunction, muscle weakness, and an unacceptably high incidence of rerupture. Consequently, direct ligament repairs were abandoned and reconstruction procedures were developed.

Intra-articular reconstruction of ligament injuries is the primary means by which ACL and PCL injuries are managed surgically. In general terms, reconstruction involves using a tissue graft to replicate the function of the damaged ligament and act as an inert restraint of the knee.[20,33,150,165,186,205,271] Initially, intra-articular reconstructions were performed through an open approach, and the need for lengthy postoperative immobilization continued.[150] Today, intra-articular ligament reconstructions are performed through an arthroscopically assisted or all-arthroscopic approach, causing far less tissue damage and resulting in a more rapid postoperative recovery.

NOTE: Overviews of intra-articular ACL and PCL reconstruction procedures are described later in this chapter.

Extra-articular reconstructions involve transposing either dynamic musculotendinous or static tissue restraints to locations that provide external stability to the knee joint. Extra-articular procedures are used rarely today as primary procedures because they do not restore normal kinematics to the knee as effectively as intra-articular procedures. Extra-articular procedures used to augment intra-articular reconstructions have shown little additional benefit.[150]

Grafts: Types, healing characteristics, and fixation. The tissue used for intra-articular reconstructions is most often an *autograft* (the patient's own tissue), but is occasionally an *allograft* (donor tissue) or a *synthetic graft* (Fig. 21.15).[140,182,205,267] An allograft or synthetic graft is used only when a suitable autograft is not available—for example, when a patient's own tissue is not suitable for graft harvesting.[150,205] Autografts are preferred for intra-articular reconstruction because remodeling and incorporating both allografts and synthetic grafts after implantation may be slower than with the patient's native tissue.[182] (Refer to Chapter 12 and Box 12.9 for additional information about tissue grafts.)

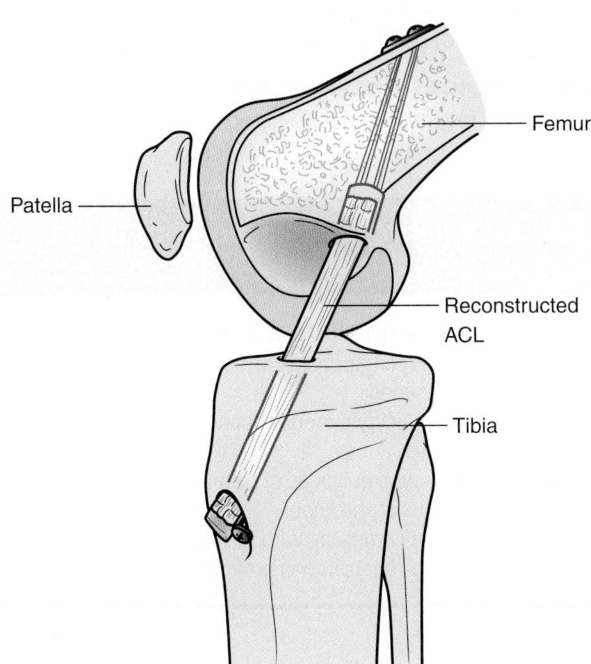

FIGURE 21.15 Lateral view of the knee depicting graft placement for ACL reconstruction.

Although several types of tissues are harvested for knee ligament reconstruction,[140,152,165, 182,191,205] the bone-patellar tendon-bone autograft has the longest history of successful and continued use as a replacement ligament, has been the gold standard for ACL reconstruction for several decades,[33,71,150,152,194] and remains the most frequently selected graft for the procedure.[20,72,81,140,152,165,186] An alternative graft that has also become widely used for ACL reconstruction is a semitendinosus-gracilis tendon graft.[71,150,152,191,263,287] Research has shown that the material strength and stiffness of both of these grafts are greater than that of the native ACL.[263]

An extensive body of knowledge exists on graft healing, placement, and fixation, as well as the strength and stiffness of the tissues used as grafts and their responses to imposed loads. Most of this research has focused on grafts for ACL reconstruction because of the much higher incidence rates and subsequent reconstructions for this injury.[20,31,81,138,152,271]

CLINICAL TIP

Because graft type and graft fixation characteristics affect rehabilitation and surgical outcomes, it is important to understand that an implanted graft undergoes a series of changes as it heals. Initially, there is a period of avascular necrosis during which the graft loses substantial strength. This period is followed by a period of revascularization, then remodeling, and finally maturation, which typically takes at least 1 year. During the first 6 to 8 weeks postoperatively, graft integrity is most vulnerable to excessive loads because the strength of the graft is derived solely from the fixation, not the graft itself.[20,31,138,140]

With advances in graft selection, preparation, placement, and fixation and with the evolution of arthroscopic techniques, the need for a long postoperative period of immobilization and protected weight bearing following primary ACL reconstruction has been eliminated.[20,31,271] Nevertheless, there is still a need to carefully limit and progress the stresses imposed on the healing graft during early rehabilitation.

General considerations for rehabilitation. The expected outcomes following ligament reconstruction and postoperative rehabilitation are (1) restoration of joint stability and motion, (2) pain-free and stable weight bearing, (3) sufficient postoperative strength and endurance to meet functional demands, and (4) the ability to return to preinjury activities.

Whenever possible, successful postoperative outcomes start with a *preoperative* program that includes edema control, exercise to minimize atrophy and maintain ROM, protected ambulation, and patient education.[59,190,225,265] Preoperative intervention is often possible because ligament reconstruction is usually delayed until acute symptoms subside. Exercises used for preoperative therapy are similar to those used for the early phase of nonoperative management of ligament injuries discussed in the previous section of this chapter. Depending on the location and extent of injury, a preoperative exercise program may be carried out for several weeks or months before a surgical decision is made.[190] Regardless of the duration of the preoperative exercise program, exercises should not cause additional swelling or pain.

The progression and duration of postoperative rehabilitation programs published in the literature vary and no single program has been shown to be optimal. Throughout rehabilitation, open communication with the surgeon enables the therapist to discuss any precautions or concerns specific to the individual patient and their procedure.

Regardless of the ligament injured or specific surgical procedure, the emphasis of rehabilitation is on restoring the patient's functional abilities while protecting the healing graft and preventing postoperative complications and re-injury. Early controlled motion and weight bearing decrease the incidence of postoperative complications such as contracture, patellofemoral pain, and muscle atrophy[225,265,250,308] and allow patients to return to activity as quickly as possible without compromising the integrity of the reconstructed ligament.[198,250]

To progress patients through rehabilitation after ligament reconstruction, contemporary practice follows guidelines that are based on the attainment of specific criteria and measurable goals or performance on functional tests rather than time-based protocols.[112,155,157,198,209,308] For example, exercises and activities are advanced only after the patient achieves full, active knee extension or a specific benchmark on a single-leg balance test. This transition to criterion-based progression is advocated to ensure a safe return to high-level sporting activities and to prevent re-injury.[198,308]

FOCUS ON EVIDENCE

Clinical practice guidelines (CPGs) have been published that summarize available evidence and provide recommendations to support evidence-based decision-making during rehabilitation following ligament injury and surgery.[159] One published CPG reports that there is moderate evidence to support immediate postoperative bracing, immediate mobilization (motion), and neuromuscular electrical stimulation for patients following ACL reconstruction and for in-clinic and home exercises for patients with knee stability impairments. The same CPG notes strong evidence for both nonweight-bearing and weight-bearing exercises for those with stability and movement coordination impairments.[159]

Another CPG reports moderate evidence supporting early, accelerated, and nonaccelerated postoperative rehabilitation protocols following ACL reconstruction, as all three have similar outcomes.[3]

Anterior Cruciate Ligament Reconstruction

Because the healing capacity of a torn ACL is poor, surgical reconstruction is frequently recommended to restore knee stability, particularly in the young, active individual.[19,138] Although the incidence of re-injury of the knee is lower after ACL reconstruction than with nonoperative management, particularly in patients younger than 25 years of age,[63] many individuals who have sustained an acute, primary ACL injury participate in a conservative course of treatment before choosing between surgical reconstruction or further nonoperative treatment.[64,190]

Indications for Surgery

Although there are no rigid criteria for patient selection, the most frequently cited indications for ACL reconstruction include the following:[19,33,165,186,190,191]

- Disabling instability of the knee due caused by a complete or partial acute ACL tear or chronic ACL laxity
- Frequent episodes of the knee giving way during routine ADLs as the result of significantly impaired dynamic knee stability despite a course of nonoperative management
- A positive pivot-shift test indicating rotational instability associated with concomitant injury to other knee structures such as the MCL
- Injury of the MCL at the time of ACL injury to prevent lax healing of the MCL
- Increased risk of re-injury because of participation in high-demand work, sports, or recreational activities

NOTE: Increased anterior translation of the tibia on the femur compared with the contralateral, noninvolved knee, as measured by an arthrometer, is not considered a reliable indication for ACL reconstruction because a strong correlation among these measurements of stability and a patient's symptoms of instability has not been established.[19]

CONTRAINDICATIONS: Relative, not absolute, contraindications for ACL reconstruction are noted in Box 21.7.[19,33,165,191]

BOX 21.7 Relative Contraindications to ACL Reconstruction

- Relatively inactive individual with little to no exposure to work, sport, and recreational activities that place high demands on the knee
- Inability to make lifestyle modifications that eliminate high-risk activities
- Inability to cope with episodes of instability
- Advanced arthritis of the knee
- Poor likelihood of complying with postoperative restrictions and adhering to a rehabilitation program

Procedures

Operative Overview

Surgical approach, graft selection, and harvesting. To reduce tissue damage and reduce recovery time, the current standard practice for most reconstruction procedures is the use of arthroscopically assisted or endoscopic techniques.[19,20,71,150] In an arthroscopically assisted approach, only the intra-articular portions of the procedure, such as meniscus débridement or repair, enlargement of the intercondylar notch of the femur, or drilling the femoral and tibial bone tunnels, are performed arthroscopically.[150]

The most common ACL reconstruction procedure today is an arthroscopically assisted or endoscopic procedure using an autograft. If a bone-patellar tendon-bone graft is selected, it is harvested through a small, longitudinal incision over the patellar tendon from the patient's involved knee[20,33,72,165,186] or occasionally from the contralateral knee.[267] The central one-third of the patellar tendon with small bone fragments from the patella and tibial tubercle attached is harvested. These fragments serve as bone plugs for graft fixation. When a semitendinosus-gracilis tendon autograft (hamstring tendon graft) is used, it is harvested through an incision over the tibial insertion of the semitendinosus and gracilis tendons.[71,191,263,268,271,280,287] Hamstring tendon grafts harvested with bony attachment to allow faster ligament incorporation are becoming more common.[169]

Although systematic reviews indicate no significant difference in outcomes based on the use of bone-patellar tendon-bone versus hamstring tendon grafts,[159] there are advantages, disadvantages, and potential complications associated with each type of autograft. For example, the transition from mechanical fixation to biological fixation is thought to occur more rapidly with a patellar tendon graft, which involves bone-to-bone healing, than with a hamstring tendon graft, which requires tendon-to-bone healing (6 to 8 weeks versus 12 weeks, respectively).[271] Other reported advantages and disadvantages of these two types of autografts are summarized in Boxes 21.8 and 21.9.[1,71,150,152,169,250,263,268,280,287] Recently, the use of a bone-hamstring tendon-bone autograft for ACL reconstruction was reported, allowing bone-to-bone healing and affording some of the same advantages associated with a bone-patellar tendon-bone autograft.[169]

Graft placement and fixation. After the graft is harvested and prepared for implantation, the arthroscopic instrumentation is reinserted and femoral and tibial bone tunnels are drilled.[20,82,150,165] Graft placement (see Fig. 21.15) is achieved by passing the graft through the tunnels to its final position in the tibia and femur. Precise anatomical graft placement is crucial for restoration of joint stability and mobility; improper placement can lead to loss of postoperative ROM.[1] A graft placed too far posteriorly may result in failure to regain full flexion, and a graft placed too far anteriorly may limit extension.[31]

NOTE: Limited ROM into extension also may be caused by graft impingement due to an inadequate femoral notch size or buildup of scar tissue in the notch.[1] A *femoral notchplasty* (enlargement of the intercondylar notch) is often performed during the reconstruction to ensure adequate graft clearance during knee extension.

Graft fixation is vital to the success of ACL reconstruction. With a bone-patellar tendon-bone graft, both bone plugs are secured in the prepared tunnels (bone-to-bone fixation) by means of screw fixation (metal or bioabsorbable interference screws).[31,33,82,152,165,271] Several types of soft tissue fixation devices are used to secure a hamstring tendon graft, including endobuttons, washers, and staples, while interference and transfixation screws may also be used.[31,71,138,191,263] Despite fixation advances, strong tendon-bone integration remains a challenge, particularly at the tibial site.

BOX 21.8 Advantages and Disadvantages/Complications of the Bone-Patellar Tendon-Bone Autograft

Advantages

- High tensile strength/stiffness, similar or greater than the ACL
- Secure and reliable bone-to-bone graft fixation with interference screws
- Rapid revascularization/biological fixation (6 weeks) at the bone-to-bone interface permitting safe, accelerated rehabilitation
- Ability to return to preinjury, high-demand activities safely

Disadvantages/Potential Complications

- Anterior knee pain in area of graft harvest site
- Pain during kneeling
- Extensor mechanism/patellofemoral dysfunction
- Long-term quadriceps muscle weakness
- Patellar fracture during graft harvest (rare, but significant adverse effects)
- Patellar tendon rupture (rare)

BOX 21.9 Advantages and Disadvantages/Complications of the Semitendinosus-Gracilis Autograft

Advantages

- High tensile strength/stiffness greater than ACL with quadrupled graft
- No disturbance of epiphyseal plate in skeletally immature patient
- Evidence of hamstring tendon regeneration at donor site
- Loss of knee flexor muscle strength remediated by 2 years postoperatively

Disadvantages/Potential Complications

- Tendon-to-bone fixation devices (particularly tibial fixation) not as reliable as bone-to-bone fixation
- Longer healing time (12 weeks) at tendon-bone interface
- Hamstring muscle strain during early rehabilitation
- Short- and long-term knee flexor muscle weakness (not associated with functional limitation)
- Possible increased anterior knee translation (not associated with functional limitations)

An advantage of current-day fixation devices is that they can withstand early but controlled tensile forces on the graft so that with proper placement and fit of these fixation devices there is a low risk of compromising the security of the graft itself.[20,31,71] This, in turn, permits early weight bearing and ROM of the knee, both of which are typical elements of contemporary, accelerated rehabilitation programs.[21,90,112,157,198,263,250,308]

After graft fixation and prior to closure, the knee is moved through the ROM to check the graft's integrity and the tension on the graft during movement. As with graft placement, proper graft tension at the time of fixation has a direct effect on postoperative joint mobility and stability. Too little tension can result in excessive knee laxity and potential instability, and too much tension can limit knee ROM.[20] After the incision is closed, a small compression dressing is immediately placed on the knee, and the knee may be immobilized for protection.

Complications

There are a number of intraoperative and postoperative complications that can compromise outcomes after ACL reconstruction (see Boxes 21.8 and 21.9). Even minor technical errors during reconstruction can adversely affect function. As discussed in the previous section, inappropriate placement of the graft or bone tunnels, problems with graft harvesting such as inadequate graft length, and improper graft tension can adversely affect joint stability and mobility.[1,261] Insufficient graft length occurs more frequently during hamstring than patellar tendon graft harvesting. If graft fixation is insufficient, graft slippage and early failure can occur.[261,263] With a bone-patellar tendon-bone graft, a bone plug can fracture during harvesting or implantation, necessitating an alternative autograft or an allograft.[261]

Potential postoperative complications are knee pain, loss of motion, persistent strength deficits, and inadequate joint stability.[1,191,261] Anterior knee pain at the patellar tendon graft donor site or at the patellofemoral joint is common and may affect functional activities. A neuroma of the infrapatellar branch of the saphenous nerve can cause significant knee pain during kneeling.

Loss of full knee extension and persistent quadriceps weakness are recognized as significant complications after ACL reconstruction, particularly if full extension is not achieved preoperatively.[170] Permanent damage to the extensor mechanism is possible after patellar tendon graft harvesting, leading to quadriceps weakness or even patellar tendon rupture in rare instances. Limited ROM of the knee may have been present prior to surgery or may develop after surgery possibly from scar tissue in the intercondylar notch that will then require arthroscopic notchplasty. Loss of patellar mobility may also be a source of limited knee ROM.

FOCUS ON EVIDENCE

McHugh and associates[175] evaluated 102 patients (age 31 ± 1 year) within 2 weeks and 6 months after primary ACL reconstruction to determine preoperative indicators of postoperative knee extension motion loss and quadriceps weakness. They found that patients with loss of knee extension preoperatively were more likely to have limited knee extension postoperatively. However, a preoperative quadriceps muscle strength deficit did not predict postoperative quadriceps weakness 6 months after surgery.

Lastly, graft failure and the need for revision reconstruction may occur even in the absence of risk factors related to surgical technique. Graft failure is most likely to occur during the early months after surgery,[83] and the most common cause of graft failure is poor adherence to postoperative rehabilitation, in particular prematurely returning to high-risk, high joint-load activities.[1,83,261]

Postoperative Management

Advances in surgical techniques and a better understanding of graft healing and the impact of stress on the healing graft, early postoperative motion and weight bearing—often referred to as "accelerated rehabilitation"—has become the standard of care after primary ACL reconstruction with an autogenous graft for the active, typically young patient.[21,36,90,112,157,198,222,225,265,266,308] Accelerated rehabilitation is based on the premise that a precisely placed and appropriately tensioned graft not only is strong enough to withstand the stresses of early motion and weight bearing, but is subjected to favorable healing conditions in response to these stresses.[20,36,265,266,250,308]

Table 21.5 outlines a contemporary, accelerated program following primary ACL reconstruction. The sequence of goals and interventions identified in Table 21.5 and described in the phases of rehabilitation that follow reflects guidelines common to a number of published programs.[21,36,90,112,159,181,198,222,225,243,245,250,265,288,308]

NOTE: It is important to recognize that although the descriptor "accelerated" is used frequently in the literature to characterize current-day rehabilitation after primary ACL reconstruction, there is no consensus on the initiation, progression, or duration of postoperative exercise, weight bearing, and other interventions.

Immobilization and Bracing

The rationale for a brief period of immobilization and using a brace in the early phase of rehabilitation after ACL reconstruction is to protect the graft from excessive strain and prevent the loss of full knee extension.[20,244,314] However, with advances in graft fixation, the use of immobilization and protective bracing are no longer universally recommended.[20,21,222,265,308]

Decisions about immobilization and postoperative bracing are based on many factors. These include the surgeon's philosophy, the type of graft used, intraoperative observations about the quality of fixation, comorbidities and concomitant surgical procedures, and an assessment of the patient's expected level of adherence to a postoperative rehabilitation program.[112,225]

Types of postoperative bracing. Bracing the knee after ACL reconstruction falls into two broad categories: *rehabilitative*

TABLE 21.5 ACL Reconstruction: Interventions for Postoperative Rehabilitation

Phase and General Time Frame	Maximum Protection Phase: Day 1–Week 4	Moderate Protection Phase: Weeks 4–10	Minimum Protection Phase: Weeks 11–24
Patient presentation			
	■ Pain and hemarthrosis ■ Decreased ROM ■ Diminished voluntary quadriceps activation ■ Ambulation with crutches ■ Use of protective bracing (if prescribed)	■ Pain controlled ■ Joint effusion controlled ■ Full or near full knee ROM ■ Fair plus to good muscle strength (3+/5 to 4/5) ■ Muscular control of joint ■ Independent ambulation	■ No joint instability ■ No pain or swelling ■ Full knee ROM ■ Muscle function: 75% of noninvolved extremity ■ Symmetrical gait ■ Unrestricted ADL ■ Possible use of functional brace or sleeve
Key examination procedures			
	■ Pain scale ■ Joint effusion—girth ■ Ligament stability—joint arthrometer (days 7–14) ■ ROM ■ Patellar mobility ■ Muscle control ■ Functional status	■ Pain scale ■ Effusion—girth ■ Ligament stability—joint arthrometer ■ ROM ■ Patellar mobility ■ Muscle strength testing ■ Functional testing	■ Ligament stability—joint arthrometer ■ Muscle strength testing ■ Functional testing ■ Full clinical examination
Goals			
	■ Protect healing tissues ■ Prevent reflex inhibition of muscle ■ Decrease joint effusion ■ ROM 0°–110° ■ Active control of ROM ■ Weight bearing: 75% to weight bearing as tolerated ■ Establish home exercise program	■ Full, pain-free ROM ■ 4/5 muscular strength (MMT) ■ Dynamic control of knee ■ Improved kinesthetic awareness ■ Normalize gait pattern and ADL function ■ Adherence to home program	■ Increase muscle strength, endurance, and power ■ Improve neuromuscular control, dynamic stability, and balance ■ Regain cardiopulmonary endurance ■ Transition to maintenance program ■ Regain ability to function at highest desired level ■ Reduce risk of re-injury
Interventions			
	Weeks 0–2 ■ PRICE: (protective bracing, rest, ice, compression, elevation) ■ Gait training: crutches, partial weight bearing to WBAT ■ PROM/A-AROM (range-limiting brace, if prescribed ■ Patellar mobilization (grades I/II) ■ Muscle setting, isometrics: quadriceps, hamstrings, adductors at multiple angles (may augment with E-stim)	Weeks 5–6 ■ Multiple-angle isometrics ■ Closed-chain strengthening and PRE ■ LE stretching program ■ Endurance training (bike, pool, elliptical trainer) ■ Proprioceptive training in single-leg stance: balance board, BOSU ■ Stabilization exercises, elastic bands, band walking Weeks 7–10 ■ Advance strengthening (include PNF), endurance, and flexibility exercises	Weeks 11–24 ■ Continue LE stretching ■ Advance PRE/initiate isokinetic training (if desired) ■ Advance closed-chain exercise ■ Initiate plyometric drills: bounding, jumping ■ Initiate plyometric drills (bouncing, jumping rope, box jumps: double-/single-leg) ■ Advance proprioceptive and balance training

Continued

TABLE 21.5 ACL Reconstruction: Interventions for Postoperative Rehabilitation—cont'd

Phase and General Time Frame	Maximum Protection Phase: Day 1–Week 4	Moderate Protection Phase: Weeks 4–10	Minimum Protection Phase: Weeks 11–24
	■ Assisted SLRs—supine ■ Ankle pumps Weeks 2–4 ■ Continue as above ■ Progress to full weight bearing; begin closed-chain squats; heel/toe raises ■ SLRs in four planes ■ Low-load PRE: hamstrings ■ Open-chain knee extension (range 90°–40°) ■ Trunk/pelvis stabilization ■ Aerobic conditioning: stationary cycle	■ Proprioceptive training: high speed stepping drills, unstable surface challenge drills, balance beam ■ Initiate a walk/jog program at the end of this phase	■ Progress agility drills (figure-eight, skill-specific patterns) ■ Simulated work or sport-specific training ■ Transition to full-speed jogging, sprints, running, and cutting

bracing and *functional bracing*.[20,244,314] Rehabilitative bracing uses a hinged orthosis with a locking mechanism that can restrict the allowable ROM. It is typically only worn for the first 6 weeks following surgery. In contrast, a functional brace is worn when returning to high-demand sports or work-related activities to potentially reduce the risk of re-injury.

Brace use and initiation and progression of knee ROM. If a rehabilitative brace is prescribed after surgery, it may be locked initially to maintain the knee in full extension. If locked in full extension for a short period of time, the brace is unlocked for exercise as soon as ROM is permitted. It is worn throughout the day for a few weeks to 6 weeks[20] and is sometimes worn during sleep for protection during the first postoperative week.[225] The brace is also locked in full extension during ambulation with crutches to prevent graft injury in the event of a fall.[112,157,225,265,308] When ROM is initiated, the rehabilitative brace can be set to incrementally progress the range of knee flexion that is allowed during exercise and functional activities.

CLINICAL TIP

Guidelines for the duration of immobilization in extension and the initiation and progression of knee ROM vary somewhat.[7,20,21,112,191,198,222,225,265,308] The literature supports the initiation of immediate or at least early knee motion (within the first week after primary, isolated ACL reconstruction) to reduce pain and adverse effects on articular cartilage and soft tissues surrounding the joint and improve ROM outcomes.[20,36,159]

Full, active knee extension and 90° to 110° of flexion ROM is expected by 4 to 6 weeks postoperatively. The patient is weaned from brace use at about 6 weeks postoperatively if full extension has been achieved. Depending on the stability of the knee, the protective brace may need to be worn longer in some cases. These timelines are progressed more slowly when ACL reconstruction is combined with another procedure, such as a collateral ligament, meniscus, or articular cartilage repair.[222]

Some patients are advised to wear a functional brace during the advanced phases of rehabilitation and when participating in high-demand sports or heavy manual labor after rehabilitation is completed. However, the effectiveness of functional bracing after ACL reconstruction is unclear because the literature contains conflicting evidence.[159]

Despite the widespread use of protective bracing following ACL reconstruction, the literature provides a critical analysis of its efficacy during early rehabilitation and when returning to high-risk activities.

FOCUS ON EVIDENCE

The literature reflects a common belief that protective bracing during early recovery and when returning to activities following ACL reconstruction leads to improved outcomes by decreasing pain, joint swelling, and wound drainage by improving knee extension and by protecting the graft from excessive strain and the risk of re-injury. However, a recent systematic review by Wright and Fetzer[314] of 12 level I randomized, controlled trials determined that there is insufficient evidence to support the effectiveness of bracing. All but one of these studies evaluated bracing during early rehabilitation. The review indicated no significant differences between groups who did and did not use protective bracing during early recovery in outcomes such as postoperative pain, anterior-posterior knee stability, ROM, and functional testing. No conclusions could be drawn about the effectiveness of functional bracing to prevent re-injury during high-demand activities because of low re-injury rates in the study that evaluated this outcome. The overall conclusion of the review was that the available evidence does not support the routine use of protective bracing after ACL reconstruction.

Weight-Bearing Considerations

Early weight bearing is possible after primary ACL reconstruction with a bone-patellar tendon-bone or hamstring tendon autograft because of advances in graft fixation. Recommendations for the period of protected weight bearing immediately after surgery range from some degree of restricted weight bearing the first 2 weeks to weight bearing as tolerated with use of two crutches immediately after surgery.[21,71,157,198,222,250,265,294,308] Weight bearing is increased during the next 2 to 3 weeks based on the patient's symptoms. A longer duration of protected weight bearing will be required when other structures in the knee have been injured and/or repaired.[308]

Full weight bearing and ambulation without crutches, with or without an unlocked protective brace, is usually permitted by 4 weeks if weight bearing is pain free and the patient has achieved full, *active* knee extension and sufficient strength of the quadriceps to control the knee.[21,112,191,198,225]

Weight-bearing recommendations do not appear to be based on the type of graft or graft fixation used or whether protective bracing is worn but rather are determined on an empirical basis. The few randomized studies that have evaluated the effects of immediate and delayed weight bearing during the first few weeks after surgery indicate that both produce similar outcomes.[20]

FOCUS ON EVIDENCE

Tyler and colleagues[295] compared the effects of immediate versus delayed weight bearing during the first 2 weeks after ACL reconstruction with a bone-patellar tendon-bone graft in 49 patients. An immediate weight-bearing group was advised to bear weight as tolerated and discontinue crutch use as soon as they felt comfortable doing so while the delayed weight-bearing group was advised not to wear a shoe on the operated side and remain nonweight bearing during ambulation with crutches for the first 2 weeks. After that, there were no restrictions placed on the progression of weight bearing. Neither group wore protective bracing. With the exception of weight-bearing status, the rehabilitation program for all patients was the same.

At a mean of 7.3 months postsurgery, there were no significant differences between groups with respect to knee ROM, knee stability, VMO activation, or overall function. However, patients in the immediate weight-bearing group had a lower incidence of anterior knee pain than the patients in the delayed weight-bearing group (8% and 35%, respectively). The investigators concluded that immediate weight bearing did not compromise knee joint stability or function and was beneficial in that it resulted in a lower incidence of postoperative anterior knee pain.

Exercise Progression

A progression of carefully selected exercises and functional activities coupled with patient education is a foundation of rehabilitation following ACL injury and reconstruction.

Preoperative exercise. Because surgery is typically delayed until acute symptoms have subsided, there is ample time to implement a *preoperative* exercise program to restore full knee ROM, particularly extension; prevent atrophy and weakness of leg musculature; and address the strength and flexibility of hip and ankle muscles.[59,107,190,225,265,308]

Postoperative exercise progression. After ACL reconstruction, exercise begins immediately on the first postoperative day. Use of strong grafts, such as bone-patellar tendon-bone and quadrupled hamstring autografts, and reliable graft fixation make early motion possible.[21,112,198,222,225,265,308]

Sometimes CPM is used while a patient is hospitalized or when at home after discharge. Although a valid mechanism for controlling postoperative pain and initiating early motion,[171,265] it is being used infrequently for postoperative care.[112] Two recent systematic reviews indicate no additional long-term benefit of CPM after ACL reconstruction.[274,315]

CLINICAL TIP

Be mindful that a tendon graft goes through a necrotizing process the first 2 to 3 weeks postoperatively before revascularization commences and maturation gradually occurs.[20,81,138,140] Exercises must be progressed cautiously during each phase of rehabilitation, even during accelerated programs. If protective bracing has been prescribed, exercises are carried out while wearing the brace.

The rate of progression of exercise and functional training after ACL reconstruction depends on many factors. Patient-related factors such as age and preinjury health status affect the healing process, enabling younger, healthier patients to progress more rapidly. The type of graft and graft fixation also may influence the exercise progression. Some resources advocate more rapid progression of exercise for bone-to-bone fixation with a patellar tendon graft than for tendon-to-bone fixation with a quadrupled hamstring graft, suggesting that bone-to-bone healing may be faster than soft tissue-to-bone healing.[112,225,308] In contrast, others advocate the same accelerated program for both procedures.[71,250,263] If concomitant injuries are present or were managed surgically, the progression of exercises is more gradual than after isolated ACL injury and reconstruction.[222]

Exercises for progressive phases of rehabilitation after ACL reconstruction, summarized in Table 21.5, are described in the following sections. Exercise precautions are noted in Box 21.10.[21,90,112,175,198,222,245,265,275,304,308]

BOX 21.10 Exercise Precautions After ACL Reconstruction

Resistance Training—General Precautions
- Progress exercises more gradually for reconstruction with hamstring tendon graft than bone-patellar tendon-bone graft.
- Progress knee flexor strengthening exercises cautiously if a hamstring tendon graft was harvested and knee extensor strengthening if a patellar tendon graft was harvested.

Closed-Chain Training
- When squatting in an upright position, be sure that the knees do not move anterior to the toes as the hips descend because this increases shear forces on the tibia and could potentially place excess stress on the autograft.
- Avoid closed-chain strengthening of the quadriceps between 60° to 90° of knee flexion.*

Open-Chain Training
- During PRE to strengthen hip musculature, initially place the resistance above the knee until knee stability and control is established.
- Avoid resisted, open-chain knee extension (short-arc quadriceps training) between 45° or 30° to full extension for at least 6 weeks or as long as 12 weeks.*
- Avoid applying resistance to the distal tibia during quadriceps strengthening.*

*Contraction of the quadriceps in these positions and ranges causes the greatest anterior tibial translation and can create potentially excessive stress to the graft during the early stage of healing.[67,101,304,308]

Exercise: Maximum Protection Phase

During the early postoperative period, a delicate balance exists between adequate protection of the healing graft and the donor site with the prevention of adhesions, contractures, articular degeneration, muscle weakness, and atrophy associated with immobilization. Early motion generates stresses that benefit the graft but must be carefully controlled to avoid excessive tension on the graft during the first 6 to 8 weeks after implantation.

The following goals and exercise interventions are emphasized during the first 4 weeks after surgery when considerable protection of knee structures is warranted.[21,112,157,159,175,198,222,225,265,308]

Goals. Immediately after surgery through the first few postoperative weeks, in addition to controlling pain and swelling and initiating ambulation with crutches, exercise goals are to prevent reflex inhibition of knee musculature, prevent adhesions, restore knee mobility, regain kinesthetic awareness and neuromuscular control of the lower extremity, and improve strength and flexibility of hip and ankle musculature.

The goal for knee ROM is to achieve 90° of flexion and full passive extension by the end of the first 1 to 2 weeks as joint swelling subsides and to reach 110° to 125° of flexion by 3 to 4 weeks.

Interventions. Pain, joint swelling, and peripheral edema are controlled in a standard manner. Exercises begin the day of or the day after surgery with an emphasis on (1) preventing vascular complications (DVTs), (2) activating knee musculature, and (3) reestablishing knee mobility. Patient education during the first phase of rehabilitation supports these interventions through the home exercise program.

CLINICAL TIP

It is important to activate and strengthen the quadriceps early in the rehabilitation process to reestablish dynamic knee extension control, particularly for safe weight-bearing activities. However, it is equally important to activate and strengthen the hamstrings as they provide a dynamic restraint to limit anterior translation of the tibia on the femur.

When a protective brace has been prescribed, weight-bearing exercises are performed while in the brace. Low-intensity closed-chain exercises and proprioceptive/neuromuscular control training are initiated as soon as weight bearing is permissible. The value of early closed-chain/weight-bearing exercises and proprioceptive/neuromuscular control training for quadriceps control after ACL reconstruction is supported by many studies and is discussed in the exercise section of this chapter.[11,36,59,112,121,157,181,198,243,245,265,250,308]

The following exercises are advocated for the maximum protection phase:[21,90,112,157,157,175,181,198,222,225,243,245,265,304,308]

- ***Ankle pumping exercises.*** Perform ankle pumping frequently throughout the day to reduce DVT risk.
- ***Voluntary isometric and dynamic activation of knee musculature.***
  - Begin muscle setting of quadriceps, hamstrings, and hip abductors, adductors, and extensors within the patient's comfort level. An isometric quadriceps contraction with the knee in full extension generates little to no anterior translation of the tibia on the femur because the knee is in a closed-pack position.
  - Use electrical stimulation or biofeedback to augment quadriceps activation. A recent literature review concluded that neuromuscular electric stimulation may be more effective in improving quadriceps strength than exercise alone. However, there were no differences found in long-term functional performance.[141]
  - Perform four-position SLRs, first with assistance, then progress to active hip motions with the knee maintained in extension. Add external resistance when the patient is able to maintain knee extension control during hip movements.
  - When knee movement is permissible, initiate low-intensity, multiple-angle isometrics of the knee musculature with emphasis on quadriceps control and co-contraction of the quadriceps and hamstrings.

- Consider *low-intensity*, eccentric quadriceps training between 20° and 60° on a motorized, eccentric ergometer, if available. Negative work training, if progressed gradually, has been shown to be safe when initiated as early as 3 weeks after ACL reconstruction.[90]
- To activate the hamstrings dynamically, include supine heel-slides to a comfortable level of hip and knee flexion, standing knee flexion (hamstring curls without resistance added), and scooting *forward* while seated on a rolling stool.

PRECAUTION: Postpone dynamic activation of the knee flexors if a hamstring graft was used for reconstruction (see Box 21.10).

- ***ROM and patellar mobility.***
  - Begin ROM in a protected range. Include therapist-controlled PROM or A-AROM within the patient's comfort level.
  - Include patellar mobilization to prevent adhesions.
  - To increase passive knee extension, have the patient assume a supine or long-sitting position and prop the heel on a rolled towel or bolster with the knee unsupported (see Fig. 21.18).
  - To increase knee flexion, include supine, gravity-assisted wall slides (see Fig. 21.19) or dangle the leg while sitting on the side of a bed.
  - Stretch hip and ankle musculature if flexibility is limited.
- ***Neuromuscular control/responses, proprioception, stability, and balance.***
  - Begin neuromuscular training with trunk and lower extremity stabilization exercises in bilateral stance. Have the patient wear a protective brace locked in extension, if prescribed. Distribute weight equally on both lower extremities, and support some weight through the upper extremities. Have the patient maintain a stable, well-aligned position and apply alternating resistance with varying directions and speeds to the pelvis.
  - Progress training with weight-shifting activities and bilateral minisquats in the 0° to 30° range and with stepping and marching movements. Gradually decrease upper extremity support. When the knee is pain free and full weight bearing is possible, progress to unilateral stabilization activities.
  - Perform *nonresisted*, multijoint movements, such as stationary cycling and exercise on a seated leg press machine or in a semireclining position on a Total Gym® unit, at 3 to 4 weeks. If incision healing allows, begin exercises in a pool.

Criteria to progress to next phase. Criteria include:

- Minimal pain and swelling
- Full, *active* knee extension (no extensor lag)
- At least 110° knee flexion
- Quadriceps strength at least 50% to 60% of contralateral side (measured isometrically at 60°)
- No evidence of excessive joint laxity (determined by arthrometric measurements)

Exercise: Moderate Protection/Controlled Motion Phase

The moderate protection phase begins about 4 to 5 weeks postoperatively or when identified criteria have been met and extends to about 10 to 12 weeks postoperatively. The emphasis of this phase is to achieve full knee ROM; increase strength, dynamic stability, and endurance; and to normalize gait and neuromuscular control/response time and balance in preparation for a transition to functional activities. A protective brace may be worn for gait and most exercises until about 6 weeks when brace use is gradually discontinued.

CLINICAL TIP

By 8 to 10 weeks graft revascularization is becoming well established and exercises can be performed more vigorously while continuing to closely monitor the patient's response.[81,138,140]

Goals. Rehabilitation goals during the intermediate phase are to attain full ROM (full knee extension and 125° to 135° flexion); improve lower extremity strength and muscular endurance; ambulate without assistive device or protective brace using a normal gait pattern; continue to improve neuromuscular control/response time, proprioception, and balance; and regain cardiopulmonary fitness.

Interventions. Include and progress the following interventions during the moderate protection phase:[21,90,112,157,157,175,181,198,225,243,245,265,308]

- ***ROM and joint mobility.***
  - Continue low-intensity, end-range self-stretching to gain full knee ROM.
  - Use grade III joint mobilization techniques to restore full knee flexion.
  - Continue flexibility exercises for hip and ankle musculature, especially the hamstrings, IT band, and plantarflexors.
- ***Strength and muscle endurance.***
  - Continue closed-chain exercises against body weight resistance (bridging, wall slides, partial squats, straight-line lunges, step-ups/step-downs, heel raises).
  - Progress from double-leg to single-leg exercises.
  - Initiate open-chain hip extension and abduction and knee extension/flexion against light-grade elastic resistance in appropriate portions of knee ROM (see Box 21.10). The literature supports both closed-chain and open-chain training for ACL deficiency[64,288] or following ACL reconstruction.[159]

FOCUS ON EVIDENCE

Although an emphasis has been placed on closed-chain strengthening during the past few decades,[36] recent studies also demonstrate the value in including both open- and closed-chain exercises in an ACL rehabilitation program.[181] Bynum and colleagues[36] compared open- and closed-chain rehabilitation after primary ACL reconstruction with a bone-patellar tendon-bone autograft. When strengthening exercises were initiated, one group followed an open-chain regimen and the other a closed-chain regimen. One year after surgery, patients in the closed-chain exercise group had significantly less anterior knee pain, closer to normal knee stability as measured by an arthrometer, earlier return to functional activities, and greater overall satisfaction with the outcome of the surgery compared with the open-chain group.

A subsequent study by Mikkelsen and associates[181] demonstrated that the addition of open-chain quadriceps strengthening at 6 weeks postoperatively resulted in no significant differences in anterior knee laxity between a group that performed closed- and open-chain strengthening and a group that performed only closed-chain strengthening. A significantly higher proportion of participants who performed the additional open-chain training returned to sports at their pre-injury level, and did so on average 2 months sooner, than those who trained with closed-chain exercises only.

- ***Neuromuscular control/responses, proprioception, and balance.***
  - Progress neuromuscular training with stabilization and static and dynamic balance activities in bilateral stance, progressing to unilateral stance on stable and then unstable surfaces. Focus on developing quick responses to alternating resistance and unexpected perturbations in varying directions.
  - Emphasis on hip and lumbopelvic stability as well as awareness of proper lower extremity alignment and knee control is crucial to correct pathomechanical alignment or movements.[233]
- ***Gait training.*** Practice ambulation in a controlled environment without bracing or with the protective brace unlocked and without crutches. Emphasize symmetrical alignment, step length, and timing to reestablish a normal gait pattern.
- ***Aerobic conditioning.*** Continue stationary cycling, increasing the duration and speed, or initiate a swimming or pool walking/running program, treadmill walking, or use of an elliptical trainer or stepping machine.
- ***Activity-specific training.*** Integrate simulated functional activities or components of activities into the exercise program.

Criteria to progress to next phase. Criteria to progress to the advanced phases of rehabilitation include:

- Absence of pain and joint effusion
- Full, active knee ROM
- At least 75% strength of knee musculature compared to the contralateral side
- Hamstrings/quadriceps ratio > 65%
- Functional hop test > 70% of contralateral side
- No evidence of knee instability on arthrometer readings or clinical examination

Exercise: Minimum Protection/Return to Function Phase

The advanced phase of rehabilitation and preparation for a return to a preinjury level of activity begins at about 10 to 12 weeks postoperatively or when the patient has met specified criteria. Most post-ACL reconstruction rehabilitation programs described in the literature continue until about 6 months postoperatively.[20,21,112,198,222,225,308] The intensity and duration of training are typically based on the patient's goals and the level of activity to which the patient wishes to return. Individuals involved in high joint-loading, work-related activities, or competitive sports are advised to participate in a maintenance exercise program.

Goals. From 12 to 24 weeks postoperatively, the aims are to further increase strength, endurance, and power; further enhance neuromuscular control and agility; and participate in progressively demanding functional activities.

Interventions. Exercise interventions during the final phase of rehabilitation include PRE with an emphasis on eccentric training, advanced closed-chain strengthening (lunges, step-ups, step-downs against elastic resistance); advanced neuromuscular, balance, and agility training with directional changes, acceleration, and deceleration; plyometrics; and activity-specific drills coupled with a gradual return to progressively demanding activities. Patient education emphasizing prevention of re-injury continues throughout the advanced phases of rehabilitation and as the patient returns to full activity. (Refer to the exercise section of this chapter and to Chapter 23 for examples of exercises and activities.)

A functional knee brace may be worn to reduce the risk of re-injury during high-demand activities, particularly those that involve turning, twisting, cutting, or jumping motions. As noted previously in this section, conflicting evidence exists for the use of functional bracing following ACL reconstruction.[159] For additional information on efficacy of functional bracing, refer to the section on Outcomes.

Return to activity. Recommended timelines for returning to vigorous activities, including competitive sports, range from 6 months to a year after surgery.[21,250,263] Criteria to return to a preinjury level of activity must be individualized for each patient and are contingent on clinical examination findings, particularly quadriceps strength, knee stability, and the expected work, recreational, or sports-related demands. Box 21.11 identifies criteria, suggested by several sources,[107,148,157,198,250,304,308] that should be met prior to a return to high-risk, high joint-loading activities.

Outcomes

ACL reconstruction followed by a carefully progressed postoperative rehabilitation program is a reliable means of reestablishing knee stability. Long-term success rates following ACL

BOX 21.11 Criteria Used to Inform Decisions About Return to High-Demand Activities After ACL Reconstruction

- No knee pain or joint effusion during final phase of rehabilitation
- Full, active knee ROM
- Quadriceps strength > 85% to 90% of contralateral side or peak torque/body mass 40% and 60% for men and 30% and 50% for women (tested at 300°/sec and 180°/sec, respectively).
- Hamstring strength 100% of contralateral side
- Hamstring/quadriceps ratio > 70%
- No postoperative history of knee instability/giving way
- Negative pivot shift test
- Knee stability measured by arthrometer: < 3 mm difference between reconstructed and uninjured side
- Proprioceptive testing: 100%
- Functional testing (a series of hop, jump, and/or squat tests): > 85% or > 90% of contralateral side or normative values
- Acceptable patient-reported score on comprehensive, quantitative knee function measurement tool, such as the International Knee Documentation Committee Subjective Knee Form
- Acceptable confidence and motivation based on standardized outcome measures for psychological variables such as kinesiophobia or emotional preparedness for return to activities

reconstruction range from 82% to 95%, and graft failure leading to recurrent instability occurs in approximately 8% of patients.[2] However, outcomes are predicated on numerous factors, including the patient's age, sex, overall health status, and preinjury activity level; the presence or absence of injuries associated with the ACL injury; the surgical procedure; postoperative complications; and the patient's adherence to the rehabilitation program. The effects of several of these variables are addressed in this section.

Graft selection and outcomes. Numerous prospective and retrospective studies have been conducted comparing the effects of graft selection on outcomes. Bone-patellar tendon-bone and hamstring tendon autografts are studied most often. An extensive review and analysis of the literature revealed that although both types of grafts have their merits and limitations (summarized in Boxes 21.9 and 21.10), long-term (2 years or more) functional outcomes are essentially the same.[268]

Approaches to rehabilitation. There are few studies that have evaluated the effects of postoperative exercise program variables such as the components and rate of progression of rehabilitation and the degree of supervision. Neuromuscular training is one ACL postoperative rehabilitation component that has been studied. Risberg and colleagues[243] compared a program of neuromuscular training to a traditional strength-training program over a 6-month period after ACL reconstruction and showed that the neuromuscular training group had significantly better scores on selected functional tests than the traditional strength-training group. There were no significant between group differences in knee pain, joint laxity, proprioception, or knee muscle strength. Although the study did not include a long-term follow-up, the investigators concluded that neuromuscular training is an important component of rehabilitation following ACL reconstruction.

Beynnon and coinvestigators[21] compared outcomes between accelerated (19 weeks) and nonaccelerated (32 weeks) rehabilitation programs following ACL reconstruction with bone-patellar tendon-bone autografts. The two programs contained the same rehabilitation components but were implemented over two different timelines. At 24 months postoperatively, there were no significant between group differences in knee laxity, functional testing, patient satisfaction, or activity level.

The effect of supervision during rehabilitation has also been studied. Specifically, home-based rehabilitation with limited therapist supervision has been compared with clinic-based rehabilitation with therapist supervision throughout the program. Two literature reviews report that, for the most part, these two approaches produced similar outcomes.[20,315] Importantly, all participants in these studies had some direct instruction and supervision from a therapist. The reviewers emphasized the importance of therapist-directed assessments and initial instruction in an exercise program and recommended periodic, rather than continuous, supervision over the course of rehabilitation.

Functional bracing. The effect of functional bracing during the intermediate and advanced phases of rehabilitation and its use during high-risk sports after completion of rehabilitation is unclear. Risberg and colleagues[244] prospectively investigated 60 patients randomly assigned to a braced or a nonbraced group. After ACL reconstruction with a patellar tendon autograft, patients in the braced group wore a protective brace for 2 weeks and then wore a functional brace for an additional 10 weeks. At the conclusion of rehabilitation, the braced group was advised to wear the functional brace for all high joint-loading activities. The nonbraced group had no brace at any time during or after rehabilitation. Both groups underwent the same rehabilitation program and patient education. At a 2-year follow-up, there were no significant differences between groups for knee ROM, knee joint laxity, muscle strength, functional testing, or ACL re-injury rates. These results are similar to those of a more recent study by McDevitt and associates,[173] who found that wearing an "off-the-shelf" functional brace for 1 year after ACL reconstruction during all high-demand activities (jumping, pivoting, and cutting) had no significant impact on knee function or re-injury.

Sterret and colleagues[284] also investigated the role of functional bracing in preventing re-injury in patients returning to downhill skiing after ACL reconstruction. Investigators prospectively evaluated 820 skiers who had undergone ACL reconstruction with a patellar tendon autograft at least 2 years previously. Of the 820 post-ACL reconstruction skier/employees, 257 were considered at significant risk for re-injury of the ACL based on the results of preseason screening. These individuals were given and advised to wear a functional knee brace during skiing. The remaining 563 skier/employees were not determined to be at significant risk for re-injury and were not issued a functional brace. There were a total of 61 ACL re-injuries: 51 in the nonbraced skiers and 10 in the braced skiers. The nonbraced group was 2.74 times more likely to sustain re-injury to the ACL than the braced group. The authors recommend functional knee bracing after recovery from ACL reconstruction for patients returning to the high-risk sport of skiing regardless of their assessed risk of re-injury.

Posterior Cruciate Ligament Reconstruction

In contrast to ACL injury, injury of the PCL is relatively infrequent.[312] When a PCL injury does occur, it usually is accompanied by damage to other structures of the knee. There is general agreement that a PCL injury combined with an injury to another ligament or knee structure usually warrants early surgical intervention.[73,210,211]

When an isolated PCL injury occurs, most patients respond well to nonoperative management and are able to return to a preinjury level of activity. However, an increased incidence of OA in the medial compartment of the knee over time has been observed following a PCL injury.[312] Motion analysis of the PCL-deficient knee has detected altered kinematics of the medial compartment of the knee, specifically anterior subluxation of the medial femoral condyle.[156] These kinematic changes may explain the degenerative changes observed in the PCL-deficient knee and lend support for managing the injury with surgical intervention.

Indications for Surgery

Although there is limited consensus, the most frequently cited indications for surgical reconstruction of the PCL include the following.[5,43,73,211,271,312]

- Complete tear or avulsion of the PCL with posterolateral, posteromedial, or rotary instability of the knee combined with damage to another ligament and often the menisci or articular cartilage
- Isolated, symptomatic, grade 3 PCL tear with greater than 8- to 10-mm posterior tibial displacement compared with the contralateral knee, resulting in instability during functional activities
- Persistent pain and instability after an unsuccessful course of nonoperative treatment following an isolated PCL injury
- Chronic PCL insufficiency associated with posterolateral instability, pain, limitations in functional activities, and articular surface degeneration

Procedures

Operative Overview

There are a number of arthroscopic, arthroscopically assisted, or open procedures used for management of a torn or ruptured PCL. Although a tear mechanism that includes a bony avulsion is occasionally managed with primary repair, reconstruction is the much more frequent procedure.[73] As with ACL reconstruction, PCL reconstruction involves implantation of a graft to replace the damaged ligament. Graft options using single-bundle or double-bundle reconstruction include a bone-patellar tendon-bone autograft, a hamstring or quadriceps tendon autograft, an Achilles tendon or anterior tibialis tendon allograft, or occasionally a synthetic graft.[5,43,73,211,271,312]

The operative procedure begins with diagnostic arthroscopy followed by graft harvest. There are two methods of graft placement—transtibial tunnel and tibial inlay.[43] With the arthroscopic transtibial technique, femoral and tibial tunnels are drilled and prepared, and the graft is drawn through and secured in the tunnels with bony or soft tissue fixation devices. The tibial inlay technique can be performed as an open procedure through a posteromedial incision or less frequently as an arthroscopic procedure. No significant differences in outcomes have been identified following the transtibial versus the open tibial inlay procedures.[43]

Graft placement must be precise to mimic the function of the native PCL regardless of the method used. Prior to closure, the knee is flexed and extended to ensure that graft placement and tension allow full ROM. After wound closure, a sterile compression dressing is applied, and the knee is immobilized in full extension.

Complications

Because PCL reconstruction involves the posterior aspect of the knee, there is risk of damage to the popliteal neurovascular bundle, particularly while drilling the tibial bone tunnel. Postoperative bleeding can lead to compartment syndrome. If a patellar tendon autograft was used, the patient may experience anterior knee pain and pain during kneeling. Knee flexion motion can become limited postoperatively. As with any ligament reconstruction, graft failure can occur, leading to joint instability and the need for revision reconstruction.[43,73]

Postoperative Management

Immobilization, Protective Bracing, and Weight Bearing

The knee is immobilized in a hinged, range-limiting protective brace locked in full extension following surgery. The immobilizer is worn during the day and even during sleep for the first 4 to 8 weeks to prevent posterior displacement of the tibia as the result of gravity or sudden contraction of the knee flexors. It may be unlocked or removed for therapy 1 day to a week after surgery and removed after the first postoperative week for bathing.[5,43,73,210,211,312] The protective brace remains locked in extension during weight bearing and ambulation for an extended period of time.

FOCUS ON EVIDENCE

In theory, protective bracing is prescribed following PCL reconstruction to prevent posterior tibial translation that could disrupt the graft in the early stage of healing. However, a recent literature review indicates that there is no evidence to support this assumption.[159]

In contrast to weight bearing after ACL reconstruction, weight bearing is progressed more gradually after PCL surgery.[43,73,210,211,312] The time frames for initiating and progressing weight bearing range from partial weight bearing (about 30%[43]) immediately after surgery using two crutches and wearing the protective brace locked in extension[51,210,211] to nonweight bearing for a week to 5 weeks postoperatively.[73,312] Weight bearing is increased over several weeks while keeping the brace locked in extension. As quadriceps control of full knee extension improves and pain and joint effusion are well controlled, the brace is unlocked, allowing movement in a protected range during ambulation with crutches and weight-bearing exercises.

Crutches are discontinued and full weight bearing with the brace unlocked is permitted when the patient has met specified criteria (Box 21.12), typically by 8 to 10 weeks postoperatively.[43,51,210,211] Brace use is discontinued gradually after meeting these criteria.

Exercise Progression

Postoperative exercises during rehabilitation following PCL reconstruction are similar to those performed after ACL reconstruction (see Table 21.5).[43,51,73,210,211] The key differences are that exercises are progressed more gradually, and those that place posterior shear forces on the tibia are postponed during the initial and intermediate phases of rehabilitation when the graft is most vulnerable.

Strengthening the quadriceps is emphasized for knee control after PCL reconstruction because it acts as a dynamic restraint to posterior tibial translation. When resistance exercises for hamstring strengthening are initiated during advanced rehabilitation, they are adjusted based on the stability of the knee. Box 21.13 summarizes precautions for exercise and functional activities after PCL reconstruction.[43,51,210,211]

Exercise: Maximum Protection Phase

The emphasis during the first, maximum protection phase of rehabilitation, which extends for 4 to 6 weeks, is to protect the integrity of the graft while simultaneously beginning to regain function, mobility, and quadriceps control.[43,51,73,210,211]

Goals. The goals during this phase of rehabilitation are to control or reduce acute symptoms, prevent vascular complications, reestablish quadriceps control, maintain patellar mobility, regain approximately 90° of knee flexion by 2 to 4 weeks after initiating knee motion, begin to reestablish neuromuscular control and balance, improve strength and flexibility of the hip and ankle musculature if limited, and improve cardiopulmonary fitness.[43,51,210,211]

Interventions. Control pain and swelling using effective methods such as cold, compression, and elevation. Immediately

BOX 21.12 Suggested Criteria for Ambulation Without Crutches After PCL Reconstruction

- Minimal to no pain or joint effusion
- Full, active knee extension (no extensor lag) with a straight-leg raise in the supine position
- Passive and active knee flexion from 0° to at least 90°
- Quadriceps strength: approximately 70% compared with the contralateral side or at least 4/5 manual muscle test grade
- No gait deviations

BOX 21.13 Exercise Precautions After PCL Reconstruction

General Precautions
- Avoid exercises and activities that place excessive posterior shear forces and cause posterior displacement of the tibia on the femur, thus disrupting the healing graft.
- Throughout the rehabilitation process, limit the numbers of repetitions of knee flexion to minimize potential abrasion to the PCL graft.

Early and Intermediate Rehabilitation
- Begin exercise to restore knee flexion while in a seated position, allowing gravity to passively flex the knee and the hamstrings to remain essentially inactive.
- During squatting exercises to increase quadriceps strength:
  - Avoid excessive trunk flexion, because it causes increased activity in the hamstrings.
  - Avoid knee flexion past 60° to 70°, because it tends to cause posterior translation of the tibia.
- When performing open-chain exercises to strengthen hip musculature, such as resisted SLRs in standing, place resistance above the knee.
- Postpone open-chain, active knee flexion against the resistance of gravity (prone or standing) for 6 to 12 weeks.

Advanced Rehabilitation
- Postpone resistance training for the knee flexors, such as use of a hamstring curl machine, for 5 to 6 months.
- When performing resisted hamstring curls, use low-loads.
- Avoid downhill inclines during walking, jogging, or hiking.
- Avoid activities that involve knee flexion combined with rapid deceleration when one or both feet are planted.
- Postpone returning to vigorous functional activities for at least 9 to 12 months.
- Consider wearing a functional knee brace during high-demand activities.

after surgery, begin ankle-pumping exercises, patellar-gliding techniques, quadriceps-setting exercises augmented by neuromuscular electrical stimulation, and four-position SLRs while wearing the protective brace locked in full extension. Use an upper extremity ergometer for aerobic conditioning. Establish a home exercise program.

When knee motion is permitted, follow the exercise precautions for early rehabilitation previously noted (see Box 21.13). Begin multiple-angle isometrics of the quadriceps from full extension to 25° to 30° of flexion. Perform assisted knee extension, progressing to active knee extension while seated. To regain knee flexion, begin with *gravity-assisted* flexion in a seated position. Hold the patient's leg in full knee extension and have the patient control leg lowering as gravity induces knee flexion.

Begin trunk and lower extremity stabilization exercises and heel raises in a supported standing position while following weight-bearing restrictions and wearing the locked brace. When it is permissible to unlock the protective brace, begin closed-chain quadriceps strengthening in bilateral stance while holding on to a stable surface for support. As with ACL reconstruction, hip and lumbopelvic stabilization is critical to controlling knee movements.[233] Stretch the hip and ankle musculature, in particular the hamstrings, IT band, and plantarflexors.

Criteria to progress to next phase. Criteria to advance to the intermediate phase of treatment include:[43,51,210,211]

- Minimal joint swelling
- Full, active knee extension (no extensor lag)
- At least 100° of knee flexion
- A grade of 3/5 quadriceps strength on manual muscle test
- Knowledge of home program and exercise and activity precautions

Exercise: Moderate and Minimum Protection Phases

Goals and interventions. As with early rehabilitation, the goals and interventions during the intermediate and advanced phases of rehabilitation following PCL reconstruction are similar to those following ACL reconstruction (see Table 21.5). However, the suggested timelines continue to be more extended, particularly for hamstring strengthening.

The exercises and activities during the intermediate phase of rehabilitation are essentially an extension of those initiated during the first phase. By 9 to 12 weeks postoperatively, the patient should have achieved full knee ROM (0° to 135°), making it possible to discontinue use of the protective brace if quadriceps control is sufficient.[43,51,210,211]

During the intermediate and advanced phases of rehabilitation, precautions to prevent excessive posterior translational forces on the tibia during exercises and functional activities continue (see Box 21.13). Strengthening continues to focus on the quadriceps to reestablish full, active knee extension, while also emphasizing the quadriceps, hip, and ankle musculature for the return to functional weight-bearing activities.

Initiating resistance training to improve strength and muscular endurance of the hamstrings depends on the posterior stability of the knee. Strengthening of the knee flexors is typically delayed until 2 to 3 months postoperatively and then progressed cautiously. Begin hamstring strengthening with closed-chain exercises, such as bilateral bridging that progresses to unilateral. A recent literature review supports an eccentric squat program following PCL reconstruction.[159] Add open-chain hamstring strengthening (hamstring curls) when posterior knee stability allows.

Advanced neuromuscular training with plyometrics, balance activities, and agility drills, plus progressive aerobic conditioning and activity-specific training, are critical for a safe transition to a full level of functional activities. A full return to vigorous activities after PCL reconstruction may take 9 months to a year.[43,51,73,210,211]

Meniscus Tears: Nonoperative Management

Mechanisms of Injury

The medial meniscus is injured more frequently than the lateral meniscus. Meniscal injuries may occur during femur on tibia rotation during weight bearing when the foot is firmly fixed on the ground, as when pivoting, getting out of a car, or in many sport- or work-related activities. Medial meniscus injuries often accompany ACL tears. Simple squatting or high-force trauma may also cause a meniscus tear.

Common Impairments and Activity Limitations

A meniscus tear can cause acute locking of the knee or chronic symptoms with intermittent catching/locking. There is joint swelling and some degree of quadriceps atrophy, with pain along the joint line during forced hyperextension or maximum flexion due to stress to the coronary ligament.[142] When there is joint catching/locking, the knee does not fully extend and there is a springy end feel with passive extension. When the joint is swollen, there is usually end-range flexion or extension motion limitation. The McMurray test or Apley's compression/distraction test may be positive.[162]

With an acute meniscus tear the patient may be unable to bear weight on the involved side. Unexpected locking or giving way during ambulation often occurs, causing safety problems.

Management

- Often the patient can actively move the leg to "unlock" the knee, or the unlocking happens spontaneously.
- Passive manipulative reduction of the medial meniscus may unlock the knee (Fig. 21.16).
  - *Patient position and procedure:* Supine. Passively flex the involved knee and hip, and simultaneously rotate the

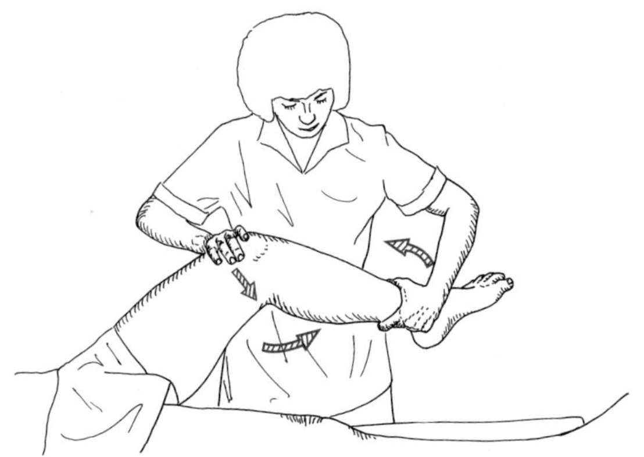

FIGURE 21.16 Manipulative reduction of a medial meniscus. Internally and externally rotate the tibia during hip and knee flexion (not shown); then laterally rotate the tibia and apply a valgus stress to the knee during knee extension. The meniscus may click into place.

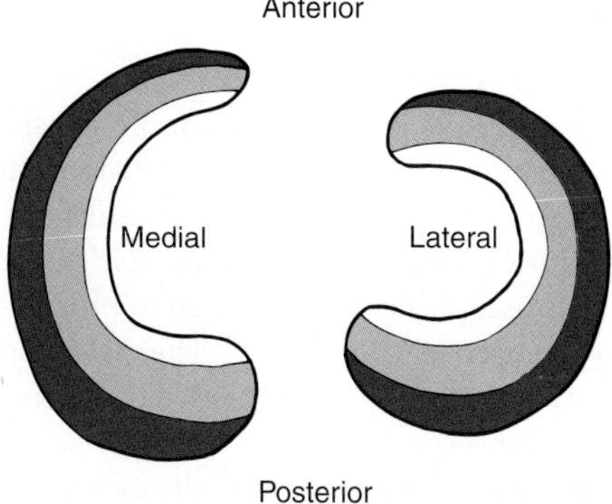

FIGURE 21.17 Vascularity of the medial and lateral menisci. The peripheral zone (outer one-third) is highly vascular; the central one-third is relatively avascular; and the inner one-third is avascular.

tibia internally and externally. When the knee is fully flexed, externally rotate the tibia and apply a valgus stress at the knee. Hold the tibia in this position and extend the knee. The meniscus may click into place.
  - Once reduced, the knee may react as an acute joint lesion. If this occurs, treat as described earlier in the chapter in the section on nonoperative management of joint hypomobility.
- After acute symptoms have subsided, exercises should be performed in open- and closed-chain positions to improve strength, endurance, and functional stability and to prepare the patient for functional activities.

Meniscus Tears: Surgical and Postoperative Management

With a significant meniscus tear or rupture or if nonoperative management of a partial tear is unsuccessful, surgical intervention may be necessary. Surgical procedures aim to retain as much of the meniscus as possible to preserve the load transmission and shock-absorbing functions of the tissue and reduce tibiofemoral articular surface stresses.

Primary surgical options are *partial meniscectomy* and *meniscal repair*, both of which are preferable to total meniscectomy.[285,292] The surgical approach used is influenced by the location and nature of the tear, as well as the patient's age and level of activity. Tears located toward the vascularized perimeter heal well, while tears extending into the less vascularized central portion have marginal healing properties (Fig. 21.17).[293] Age and the patient's activity level factor into the decision-making process because it has been shown that removing even a portion of a meniscus increases the long-term risk of articular degeneration.[293]

Partial meniscectomy is often used to manage complex, fragmented tears and tears involving the central (middle third), relatively avascular zone of a meniscus.[292] In contrast, peripheral tears are usually repaired rather than excised.[293] However, the young or physically active older patient with a central zone tear may also be good candidates for a repair.[111,203,204] If there is extensive damage to a major portion of the meniscus and it is determined to be unsalvageable, total meniscectomy remains the only surgical option.[292]

For the relatively young and/or active patient who previously underwent total meniscectomy and now is symptomatic as the result of early osteoarthritic changes in the tibiofemoral joint, a recently developed option—*meniscal transplantation*—using human allograft tissue has become available.[111,206,227] Although this procedure is expected to fail in the long term with only a 40% survival rate reported after 15 years, the short-term benefits of symptom resolution and improved function is justified for this population.[202]

The progression of postoperative rehabilitation and the time required to return to full activity after each of these procedures depends on the extent and location of the tear and the type of surgical approach and procedure performed. Rehabilitation proceeds more conservatively after meniscus repair or transplantation and after total meniscectomy than after a partial meniscectomy. Any damage and repair or reconstruction of other soft tissues of the knee will also affect the course and progression of rehabilitation after surgery.

Meniscus Repair

Indications for Surgery

Repair of a torn meniscus is indicated in the following situations:[111,203,292]

- A lesion in the vascular outer third of the medial or lateral meniscus
- A tear extending into the central, relatively avascular third of the meniscus of a young (younger than age 40) or physically active older (older than age 50) individual

CONTRAINDICATIONS: Contraindications include the presence of a tear localized to the innermost, avascular third of the meniscus, a tear with considerable tissue fragmentation, or a tear that cannot be completely re-opposed during surgery.[111]

Procedure

Operative Overview

Prior to the operative procedure, a comprehensive arthroscopic examination of the joint is performed to determine if a meniscus tear is suitable for repair and to identify any concomitant injuries. The meniscus repair itself is performed using an arthroscopically assisted open approach or a fully arthroscopic approach.[111,192,193,203] The determination of which approach is used is primarily based on the location and nature of the tear.[292]

There are several surgical procedures—referred to as inside-out, outside-in, or all-inside techniques—for meniscus repair. The inside-out and outside-in techniques are arthroscopically assisted, with a portion of the procedure being performed through an incision at the posteromedial or posterolateral aspect of the knee.[192,203] The all-inside technique is fully arthroscopic.[193,293]

Variations in fixation include suturing with nonabsorbable or bioabsorbable sutures or the use of other devices such as darts or staples. Of the many repair variations, the arthroscopically assisted, inside-out suture repair is most common and considered by some in the orthopedic community to be the "gold standard."[111,192,203,293]

At the beginning of the procedure, small incision portals are made and saline is arthroscopically introduced into the joint to distend the capsule. After the joint is examined, arthroscopic débridement is performed to remove all unstable tissue fragments and prepare the torn meniscus for repair. The repair procedure is performed endoscopically or through a posteromedial or posterolateral incision. During the repair the edges of the tear are closely approximated and sutured every 3 to 4 mm to ensure complete closure with no gapping. All sutures are tied with the knee fully extended or in 10° of flexion to allow full extension postoperatively without causing undue stress on the repaired meniscus.

Several methods to improve healing by introducing growth factors or endogenous blood to the tear site are also used with meniscal repairs. Trephination (creating several burr holes) or rasping of the tear surface to cause local bleeding are two such methods. Similarly, a fibrin clot from the patients' venous blood may be created and used to augment healing.[128] These clots are applied to the tibial joint surface at the tear site prior to tightening the sutures and reduced failure rates from 64% to 8% in one early study.[114]

After closure, a compression dressing is applied to control postoperative joint effusion and the knee is immobilized.

NOTE: Detailed descriptions of medial and lateral meniscal allograft transplantation techniques are published in several resources.[91,111,206,207,227]

Complications

Complications specific to meniscus surgery include intraoperative damage to the neurovascular bundle at the posterior aspect of the knee during the suturing process. With a medial meniscus repair, there is a risk of damage to the saphenous nerve; with a lateral meniscus repair, there is risk of damage to the peroneal nerve. Postoperatively, these same nerves can become entrapped by adherent scar tissue.[192,292,293]

A postoperative flexion contracture or extensor lag compromises knee alignment and stability during gait and functional activities. The risk of failure of the repair is greatest during activities that involve joint loading and knee flexion beyond 45° and highest during the first few postoperative months.[179,285]

Postoperative Management

Factors that influence the components and progression of postoperative rehabilitation after meniscus repair are noted in Box 21.14.[51,111,179,203] Some variables permit relatively rapid rehabilitation, whereas others necessitate a more cautious progression. For example, exercise and weight bearing are progressed more rapidly after repair of a peripheral zone tear than after a central tear and after a single tear than after a complex pattern tear.

Malalignment of the knee affects compressive forces on a repaired meniscus and thus influences the progression of weight bearing during ambulation and exercise. With varus alignment, a repaired medial meniscus is subjected to increased stress and increased risk of displacement during healing. In such a case, weight bearing must be progressed more slowly than when there is normal knee alignment.[51]

NOTE: Although timelines vary somewhat in published postoperative guidelines, the progression of exercises presented in the following rehabilitation program is appropriate after *isolated* meniscus repair in a stable knee. These same guidelines are appropriate after meniscal transplantation, although the duration of rehabilitation and protection of the transplanted meniscus is extended.[111,227] If a concomitant procedure such as ligament reconstruction is performed, adjustments to protect the affected structure will be necessary.

Immobilization, Protective Bracing, and Weight Bearing

Immobilization and protective bracing. The knee is maintained in full extension in the postoperative immobilizer and then in a long-leg brace after the compression dressing is

BOX 21.14 Factors Influencing the Progression of Rehabilitation After Meniscus Repair

- Location and size of the tear (i.e., the zone[s] affected and their vascularity)
- Type of tear (tear pattern and complexity)
- Type of surgical fixation device used
- Alignment of the knee joint (normal, varus, valgus)
- Concomitant injuries (ligament, chondral defect) with or without reconstruction or repair

removed a few days after surgery.[51,111,292] Occasionally, for carefully selected patients with a peripheral zone repair, no protective bracing is used after the postoperative dressing is removed.[192] Thigh-high compression stockings to control swelling may be worn.

To protect the repaired meniscus during the first few postoperative weeks, the range-limiting long-leg brace is worn continuously (day and night) and locked in full extension. The brace can be unlocked periodically during the day to initiate early ROM exercises and for bathing. Depending on the site of the lesion and repair, flexion motion is kept between 0° to no more than 90° for 2 weeks or longer. Thereafter, weekly 10° increases in flexion ROM are allowed until full flexion has been achieved.[111] The brace is unlocked throughout the day as early as 2 weeks postoperatively if the patient has achieved full knee extension.

After a central zone repair, the patient typically wears the brace for about 6 weeks or until adequate quadriceps control has been reestablished. After a meniscal transplant, the brace may be worn even a few weeks longer.

Weight bearing. Following a peripheral zone repair, partial weight bearing (ranging from 25% to 50%) during ambulation with crutches and with the brace locked in full extension is allowed during the immediate postoperative period (first 2 weeks).[111] The percent of body weight permitted during weight bearing is lower and progressed more cautiously after a central zone repair or meniscus transplantation. If quadriceps control is sufficient, full weight bearing may be permitted by 4 weeks after a peripheral repair[111] and by 6 to 8 weeks after a central repair or transplantation.[51,111,179,206,227]

FOCUS ON EVIDENCE

A recent literature review compared outcomes of "standard" with "accelerated" rehabilitation programs following meniscus repairs.[142] In the standard programs, knee ROM and weight bearing were delayed for a period of time after surgery, whereas in the accelerated programs, ROM and weight bearing as tolerated were permitted immediately after surgery. The review found no deleterious effects from accelerated rehabilitation and no significant differences in patient outcomes between the standard versus accelerated groups. Importantly, there were conflicting timeframes for the rate of progression of knee motion and weight bearing across studies. Therefore, ROM and weight bearing must be progressed gradually, regardless of the procedure, and must be based on the patient's signs and symptoms.

Exercise: Maximum Protection Phase

Exercises and gait training with crutches begin the first postoperative day. A standard approach to control pain, joint effusion, and vascular complications is used. Patient education focuses on establishing a home exercise program and reinforcing weight-bearing precautions. Exercise precautions are noted in Box 21.15.[51,111,179,292,293]

BOX 21.15 Exercise Precautions After Meniscus Repair*

General Precautions

- Progress exercises and weight bearing more gradually after central zone meniscus repairs or meniscus transplantations than after peripheral zone repairs.
- If the patient experiences a clicking sensation in the knee during exercise or weight-bearing activities, report it immediately to the surgeon.

Early and Intermediate Rehabilitation

- Increase knee flexion gradually, especially after a central zone repair.
- If a stationary bicycle is used for cardiopulmonary conditioning, set the seat height as high as possible to limit the range of knee flexion.
- During weight-bearing exercises, such as lunges and squats, do not perform knee flexion beyond 45° for 4 weeks or beyond 60° to 70° for 8 weeks. Flexion beyond 60° to 70° places posterior translation forces on a repaired meniscus, increasing the risk of displacement during early healing.
- Postpone use of a leg press machine until about 8 weeks. Limit motion from 0° to 60°.
- Avoid twisting motions during weight-bearing activities.
- Postpone hamstring curls until about 8 weeks.

Advanced Rehabilitation

- Do not perform exercises that involve deep squatting, deep lunges, twisting, or pivoting for at least 4 to 6 months. (The greater the flexion angle, the greater the stress on the meniscus.)
- Do not begin jogging or running program until 5 to 6 months.

Return to Activity

- Refrain from recreational and sports activities that involve repetitive, high joint compressions and shear forces.
- Avoid prolonged squatting in full flexion.

*These precautions also are applicable after meniscus transplantation, but time frames for the precautions are extended.

Goals. During the first 4 weeks after surgery, exercise goals are to regain functional ROM, prevent patellar restrictions, reestablish control of knee musculature, restore postural stability, improve strength and flexibility of the hip and ankle, and maintain cardiopulmonary fitness. By 4 weeks, the patient should achieve full, active knee extension. Recommendations for maximum flexion during the first 2 weeks vary from 60° to 90°.[29,51,111,179,292] After 4 weeks, the patient should attain 120° of knee flexion.[111]

Interventions. During the first 4 weeks after meniscus repair, the following interventions are included:[29,51,111,179]

- ***Knee ROM.*** CPM may be prescribed at the surgeon's discretion. The day after surgery, begin A-AROM and AROM exercises of the knee within a protected range. Knee flexion may be restricted by a hinged, range-limiting brace. Include exercises such as gravity-assisted knee flexion in a sitting position and with assistance, then progress to active heel slides in a supine position.

- ***Patellar mobility.*** Teach the patient grade I and II patellar gliding exercises.
- ***Activation of knee musculature.***
  - Emphasize quadriceps control in full extension with quadriceps-setting exercises, assisted SLRs in the supine position, and assisted progression to active open-chain knee extension/flexion in a sitting position for concentric/eccentric quadriceps control. Augment quadriceps activation with neuromuscular electrical stimulation or biofeedback.
  - Perform hamstring-setting exercises and multiple-angle isometrics.
- ***Neuromuscular control/responses, proprioception, and balance.***
  - Begin balance training in a standing position within the limits of weight-bearing restrictions and with the brace locked in extension.
  - Emphasize trunk and lower extremity stabilization exercises.
  - When it is permissible to unlock the brace during carefully controlled weight bearing, initiate bilateral closed-chain exercises, such as minisquats and standing wall slides, initially limiting flexion to no more than 45°.
- ***Flexibility and strength of the hip and ankle musculature.***
  - Stretch the hamstrings and plantarflexors, if restricted.
  - Begin gluteal and adductor setting exercises the first postoperative day. Perform four-position SLRs with the brace locked or with the brace unlocked when the patient can perform an SLR in supine position without an extensor lag.
  - Perform bilateral heel raises when 50% weight bearing on the operated extremity is permitted.
- ***Cardiopulmonary function.*** Use an upper body ergometer for aerobic conditioning exercises.

Criteria to progress to next phase. The following criteria should be met:

- Minimal joint effusion and pain
- Evidence of superior gliding of the patella with quadriceps setting
- Full, active knee extension (no extensor lag)
- Approximately 120° of knee flexion

FOCUS ON EVIDENCE

A ***CPG*** for meniscal and articular cartilage lesions reports moderate evidence supporting the use of therapeutic exercise for strengthening, endurance, and functional performance for patients who have undergone a surgical meniscectomy and for the application of neuromuscular electrical stimulation to increase muscle strength in patients with meniscal or chondral injuries. All other recommendations regarding interventions for patients with meniscus or cartilage lesions were weak or conflicting.[158]

Exercise: Moderate Protection/Controlled Motion Phase

The moderate protection phase extends from 4 to 6 weeks to about 12 weeks postoperatively. The knee brace is discontinued at about 6 to 8 weeks if there is adequate control of the knee and no extensor lag. Use of a cane or single crutch is advisable to provide some degree of protection during ambulation.

Goals. Restoring full knee ROM; improving lower extremity flexibility, strength, and muscular endurance; continuing to reestablish neuromuscular control and balance; and improving overall aerobic fitness are emphasized during the moderate protection phase of rehabilitation.

Interventions. Include and progress the following exercises and activities during the intermediate phase of rehabilitation:[29,51,111,179]

- ***ROM.*** Progress low-load, long-duration stretching exercises if the patient is having difficulty achieving full knee ROM.
- ***Muscle performance (strength and muscular endurance).***
  - Initiate stationary cycling against light resistance.
  - Use elastic resistance for low-intensity, open-chain, and closed-chain exercises.
  - Progress hip- and ankle-strengthening exercises. Emphasize strengthening of the hip abductors and extensors.
- ***Neuromuscular control/responses, proprioception, and balance.*** With each of these activities, emphasize maintaining proper lower extremity alignment.
  - Continue or—if not initiated previously—begin closed-chain exercises. Add disturbed balance activities (perturbation training) standing on an unstable surface, such as a minitrampoline or BOSU.
  - When full weight bearing is permissible, begin unilateral balance activities, partial lunges, step-ups, and step-downs. Practice walking on an unstable surface, such as high-density foam rubber.
  - Initiate low-intensity agility drills.
- ***Flexibility of the hip and ankle.*** Stretch the IT band and rectus femoris after the patient has achieved full knee flexion with hip flexion.
- ***Cardiopulmonary fitness.*** Begin stationary cycling or a pool-walking program at the beginning of this phase. Initiate treadmill training, land walking, a cross-country ski machine or elliptical trainer at around 9 to 12 weeks.
- ***Functional activities.*** Gradually resume light functional activities during this phase.

Criteria to progress to next phase. By 12 to 16 weeks postoperatively, the following criteria should be met:

- No pain or joint effusion
- Full, active knee ROM
- Lower extremity strength (maximum isometric contraction): 60% to 80% compared to the contralateral side

Exercise: Minimum Protection/Return to Function Phase

Some degree of protection is still warranted at the beginning of the final phase of rehabilitation, which typically begins at around 12 to 16 weeks and may continue until 6 to 9 months. The return to a high level of physical activity depends on achieving adequate strength, full, nonpainful ROM, and an acceptable clinical examination.[51,111,179]

Goals. The primary goal of this phase is to prepare the patient to resume a full level of functional activities using normal movement patterns while continuing patient education to reinforce the importance of selecting activities that do not overstress the repaired meniscus (see Box 21.15).

Interventions. During advanced resistance training, focus on movement patterns that simulate functional activities. Begin and gradually progress drills, such as plyometric training and agility drills, to improve power, coordination, and rapid response times. Continue to stress the importance of proper trunk and lower extremity alignment. Increase the duration or intensity of the aerobic conditioning program. Transition from a walking program to a jogging/running program, if desired, at about 4 to 6 months. A detailed progression of aerobic conditioning activities after meniscus repair is available in published resources.[111,179]

Outcomes

Medial or lateral meniscus repair is a well-tested procedure that results in predictably successful outcomes, particularly for suture repair of a peripheral zone tear.[111,192,293] Although repairing tears that extend into the central zone has less predictable results, there is increasing evidence that these repairs heal well and provide long-term relief of symptoms.[203,204]

Although the various surgical techniques used and the frequency of concomitant pathologies and surgeries make it difficult to compare across studies, several generalizations can be made. One of the most important factors influencing outcomes of meniscus repair is the status of the ACL. When an ACL injury occurs in combination with a meniscus tear, patients who undergo ACL reconstruction have better outcomes than patients with ACL deficiency. Recurrent tears of a repaired meniscus occur more frequently in an ACL-deficient knee than in an ACL-stable knee.[204,293]

Although the patient's age is cited as a factor influencing surgical decisions regarding meniscal repairs, a study by Noyes and colleagues[203] demonstrated high success rates following repair of central zone tears in a group of patients 40 years of age or older. With regard to postoperative rehabilitation, no single protocol has been shown to result in superior outcomes.[293]

Lastly, short-term results of meniscus transplantation with an allograft appear to be promising but are challenging to summarize because of evolving surgical techniques. Long-term effectiveness of current-day procedures has yet to be determined.[91,206,227]

Partial Meniscectomy

Indications for Surgery

The following are indications for partial meniscectomy as a surgical option for a meniscus tear:[292]

- A displaced tear of the meniscus that is associated with pain and locking of the knee sustained by an older, inactive individual
- A tear extending into the central, less vascular third of the meniscus that is not determined repairable when arthroscopically visualized and probed
- A tear localized to the avascular inner third of the meniscus

Procedure

Arthroscopic meniscectomy is usually performed under local anesthesia on an outpatient basis. Small portal incisions are made and saline is injected through one of the portals to distend the knee. The torn portion of the meniscus is identified, grasped, and divided endoscopically by knife or scissors and removed by vacuum. Intra-articular debris or loose bodies are also removed. After the knee is irrigated and drained, skin incisions at the portal sites are closed, and a compression dressing is applied.[285,292]

Postoperative Management

The overall goal of rehabilitation after partial meniscectomy is to restore ROM of the knee and develop strength in the lower extremity to reduce stresses on the knee and protect its articular surfaces. The progression of exercises and functional activities depends on the patient's presenting signs and symptoms.

Immobilization and Weight Bearing

A compression dressing is placed on the knee, but it is not necessary to immobilize the knee postoperatively. For the first few postoperative days, cryotherapy, compression, and elevation of the operated leg are used to control edema and pain. Weight bearing is progressed as tolerated.[51,292]

Exercise: Maximum and Moderate Protection Phases

Although the ideal situation is to begin exercise instruction on the day of or after surgery, most patients do not see a therapist for supervised exercise immediately after an outpatient procedure. When a patient is referred for supervised therapy, the emphasis is often placed on establishing a home exercise program. Under these circumstances, it is preferable to teach the patient initial exercises to reduce atrophy and prevent contracture *preoperatively*, so he or she can initiate the exercises at home immediately after surgery.

There is no need for an extended period of maximum protection following arthroscopic partial meniscectomy because there is little soft tissue trauma during surgery. Moderate protection is warranted for approximately 3 to 4 weeks. All exercises and weight-bearing activities should be pain free and progressed gradually during the first few postoperative weeks.[29]

Goals. During the early phase of rehabilitation, the emphasis of treatment is to control inflammation and pain, reestablish independent ambulation, and restore knee control and ROM.

Interventions. Immediately after surgery, begin muscle-setting exercises, SLRs, active knee ROM, and weight bearing as tolerated. Full weight bearing is usually achieved by 4 to 7 days, and at least 90° of knee flexion and full extension are attained by 10 days. Initiate closed-chain exercises and stationary cycling a few days after surgery, or as pain and weight bearing status allow, with the goal of regaining dynamic strength and endurance.

PRECAUTION: Patients who have undergone partial meniscectomy must be cautioned not to progress themselves too quickly. An accelerated progression of exercise can cause recurrent joint effusion and may damage articular cartilage.

Exercise: Minimum Protection/Return to Function Phase

By 3 or 4 weeks postoperatively, minimum protection of the knee is necessary, but full, pain-free, active knee ROM and a normal gait pattern should be achieved before progressing to high-demand exercises. Resistance training, endurance activities, bilateral and unilateral closed-chain exercises, and proprioceptive/balance training to develop neuromuscular control can all be progressed rapidly. Advanced activities such as plyometrics, maximum effort isokinetic training, and simulated high-demand functional activities can be initiated as early as 4 to 6 weeks or 6 to 8 weeks postoperatively with emphasis on reestablishing normal mechanics in movement.

PRECAUTION: High-impact weight-bearing activities such as jogging or jumping, if included in the program, should be added and progressed cautiously to prevent articular damage. Improper lower extremity alignment during weight bearing, such as valgus collapse and/or pelvic drop should be corrected prior to advancing with plyometric and high-impact activities.

Exercise Interventions for the Knee

Strength and flexibility imbalances between muscle groups can be caused by several factors such as disuse, faulty joint mechanics, joint swelling, immobilization (due to fracture, surgery, or trauma), and nerve injury. In addition to the hamstrings and rectus femoris, most of the two-joint muscles that cross the knee function primarily at the hip or the ankle, yet have an effect on the knee. If there is an imbalance in length or strength in the hip or ankle muscles, altered mechanics may manifest throughout the lower extremity.[113,253] Refer to the chapters on the hip and the ankle and foot for a complete picture of these interrelationships.

Exercise Techniques to Increase Flexibility and Range of Motion

When attempting to increase ROM, the mechanics of the tibiofemoral and patellofemoral joints and their importance in lower extremity function must be respected. Because the knee is a weight-bearing joint, mobility coupled with adequate strength and stability is necessary for normal function.

Principles of passive stretching and PNF stretching are presented in Chapter 4, joint mobilization/manipulation of the extremities is described in Chapter 5, and techniques directed toward specific tibiofemoral joint and patella restrictions are presented earlier in this chapter. Additional manual and self-stretching techniques to increase knee ROM are described in this section.

To Increase Knee Extension

Decreased extensibility of the hamstring musculature and periarticular tissue posterior to the knee can restrict full knee extension. Increasing knee extension is a two-step process. First, full extension of the knee is obtained without placing tension on the hamstrings at the hip by maintaining the hip at or near 0° extension. After full knee extension has been attained, a stretch is applied to the two-joint hamstring muscle group by progressively flexing the hip while maintaining the knee in extension (SLR position). Techniques to stretch the hamstrings using SLRs are described in Chapter 4 and the exercise section of Chapter 20.

PNF Stretching Techniques

- *Patient position and procedure:* Supine, with the hip and knee extended as much as possible. Have the patient perform an isometric contraction of the knee flexors as you resist with your hand placed proximal to the heel. Then ask the patient to relax as you passively extend the knee into the newly gained range, or have the patient actively extend the knee as far as possible (hold-relax and hold-relax/agonist-contraction techniques, respectively).
- *Patient position and procedure:* Prone, with the hip and knee extended as much as possible. Place a small pad or folded hand towel under the femur proximal to the patella to protect the patellofemoral joint from compressive forces. Stabilize the pelvis to prevent hip flexion, and then apply the hold-relax technique to increase knee extension.

Gravity-Assisted Passive Stretching Techniques

Use a low-intensity, long-duration stretch to ensure that the patient stays as relaxed as possible.

Prone Hang

Patient position and procedure: Prone, hips extended with the patient's foot off the edge of the treatment table. Place a rolled towel under the patient's femur just proximal to the patella and a cuff weight around the ankle. As the muscle relaxes, the weight places a sustained passive stretch on the hamstrings, which increases knee extension.

Supine Heel Prop

Patient position and procedure: Supine, with the knee extended as far as possible. Place a rolled towel or padding under the distal leg and heel to elevate the calf and knee off **the table** (Fig. 21.18). For a sustained stretch, secure a cuff weight across the distal femur but proximal to the patella to avoid patellar compression.

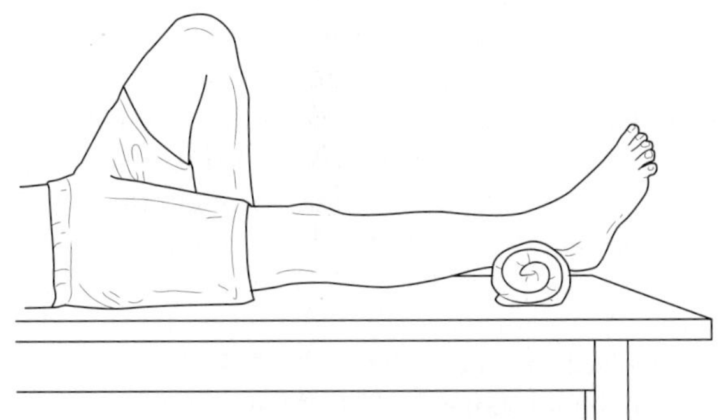

FIGURE 21.18 Heel prop in supine to increase knee extension. A cuff weight or sandbag placed across the distal femur increases the stretch force.

NOTE: This position is not effective for severe knee flexion contractures. Use it only for restrictions that are near the end of the range of knee extension.

Self-Stretching Technique

Patient position and procedure: Long-sitting, with the distal leg supported on a rolled towel. Have the patient press down with the hands against the femur just above (not on) the patella to cause a sustained force to increase knee extension.

To Increase Knee Flexion

Before stretching to increase knee flexion, be sure the patella is mobile and is able to glide distally in the trochlear groove as the knee flexes; otherwise, it restricts knee flexion. Patellar mobilization techniques to increase patellar gliding are described in Chapter 5 (see Figs. 5.53 and 5.54). Techniques to increase mobility of the IT band at the knee to improve patellar tracking are described later in this section. Once full range of knee flexion is restored, the two-joint rectus femoris and TFL muscles should be stretched across the hip joint while maintaining the knee in flexion. These techniques are described in Chapter 20.

PNF Stretching Techniques

Patient position and procedure: Sitting, with the knee at the edge of the treatment table and flexed as far as possible. Place your hand just proximal to the ankle and manually resist an isometric contraction of the knee extensors. Have the patient relax as you passively flex the knee to the end of the range, or have the patient actively flex as far as possible.

Gravity-Assisted Passive Stretching Technique

Patient position and procedure: Sitting with the lower legs dangling and knee flexed to the end of the available range. Instruct the patient to relax the thigh muscles and let the weight of the leg create a low-intensity, long-duration stretch. Place a light cuff weight around the distal leg to increase the stretch force.

Self-Stretching Techniques

Gravity-Assisted Supine Wall Slides

Patient position and procedure: Supine, with buttocks close to the wall and lower extremities resting vertically against the wall (hips flexed, knees extended). Have the patient slowly flex the involved knee by sliding the foot down the wall until a gentle stretch sensation is felt. Hold the position for a period of time, then slide the foot back up the wall (Fig. 21.19).

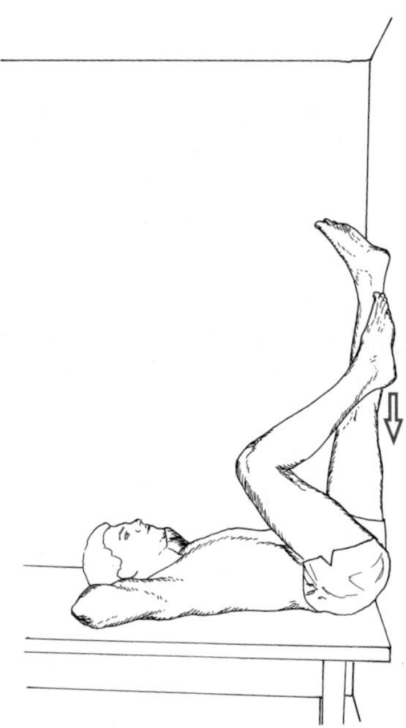

FIGURE 21.19 Gravity-assisted supine wall slide. The patient flexes the knee to the limit of its range and holds it there for a sustained stretch.

Self-Stretch With Uninvolved Leg

Patient position and procedure: Sitting with legs dangling over the edge of a bed and ankles crossed. Using the uninvolved leg, have the patient apply sustained pressure to the involved leg just above the ankle to increase knee flexion.

Rocking Forward on a Step

Patient position and procedure: Standing, with the foot of the involved knee on a step. Have the patient rock forward over the stabilized foot, flexing the knee to the limit of its range, then rock back and forth in a slow, rhythmic manner, or sustain the stretched position (Fig. 21.20). Begin with a low step or stool; increase the height as more range is obtained.

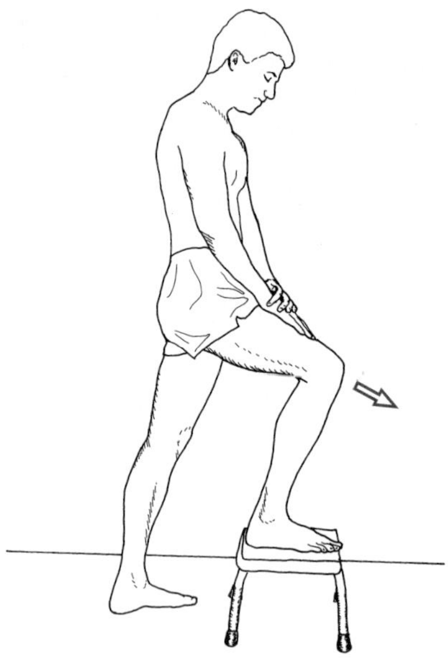

FIGURE 21.20 Self-stretching on a step to increase knee flexion. The patient places the foot of the involved side on a step, then rocks forward over the stabilized foot to the limit of knee flexion to stretch the quadriceps femoris muscle. A higher step is used for greater flexion.

PRECAUTION: Do not allow the patient to move into a position that causes pinching at the anterior aspect of the ankle.

Sitting

Patient position and procedure: Sitting in a chair, with the involved knee flexed to the end of its available range and the foot firmly planted on the floor. Have the patient move forward in the chair, not allowing the foot to slide. Hold the position for a comfortable, sustained stretch of the knee extensors (Fig. 21.21).

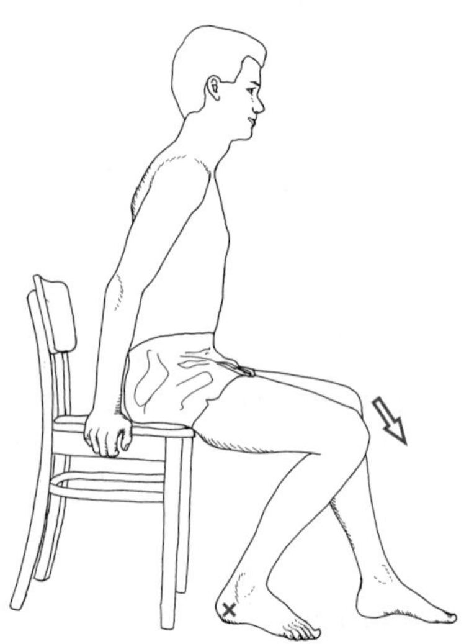

FIGURE 21.21 Self-stretching in a chair to increase knee flexion. The patient fixates the foot of the involved leg on the floor and then moves forward in the chair over the stabilized foot to place a sustained stretch on the quadriceps femoris muscle and increase knee flexion.

To Increase Mobility of the IT Band at the Knee

The IT band is a strong fibrous band of connective tissue that is not easily stretched. Mobility of the IT band distal attachment at the knee is necessary for proper patellar tracking and knee flexion and, if restricted, may contribute to patellofemoral pain or patellar maltracking. The distal attachment of the TFL and approximately one-third of the gluteus maximus insert into the proximal IT band and also affect its mobility. Stretching of these muscles is described in Chapter 20. The "foam roller fascial release" that follows is used to increase the mobility of the IT band and its effect at the knee.

Foam Roller Fascial Release

Patient position and procedure: Side-lying with the involved thigh on a foam roller (dense foam cylinder) positioned perpendicular to the femur. Maintain the hip of the involved side in extension, flex the top hip and knee, and plant the foot on the floor (Fig. 21.22). Have the patient prop on the forearm or hands to lift the trunk and adduct the hip of the involved leg. Then roll the lateral thigh proximally and distally on the roll along the IT band or maintain a sustained pressure against the IT band.

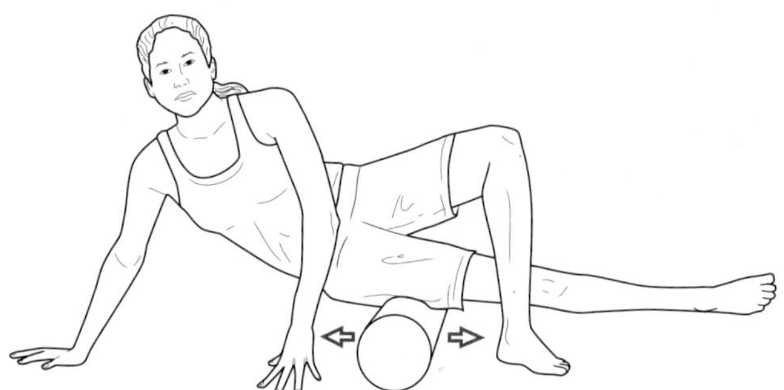

FIGURE 21.22 Foam roller fascial release for a tight IT band.

NOTE: The planted foot, along with the hands, serve to guide the rolling motion and can partially reduce the pressure on the lateral thigh, making the release technique more tolerable.

Exercises to Develop and Improve Muscle Performance and Functional Control

The primary emphasis of strengthening exercises for the knee muscles are to develop stability and sound patellofemoral and extensor mechanism biomechanics. After stability and patellar mechanics are well established, the emphasis shifts to the coordination and timing of muscle contractions, as well as the endurance needed to perform functional activities. To accomplish this, closed-chain exercises using low-intensity (low resistance) and a high number of repetitions are more effective than open-chain exercises for improving dynamic functional stability and muscular endurance of the knee.

Although closed-chain control of the knee is essential, remember that the knee functions in both an open- and closed-chain fashion during most daily activities. Not only do the quadriceps and hamstrings function using co-contractions during closed-chain activities, but they also contract independently using concentric and eccentric contractions during functional activities. To be most effective, exercises under all these conditions should be incorporated into a comprehensive knee rehabilitation program. It is also important to change the position of the hip during quadriceps- and hamstring-strengthening exercises to affect the length-tension relationship of the rectus femoris and hamstrings.[74]

- In the exercises that follow, open-chain exercises are described before closed-chain exercises simply because weight bearing after knee injury or surgery is often restricted for a period of time.
- Isolated activation of knee musculature also is necessary for functional activities that involve open-chain movements, such as lifting the leg to get in and out of bed or a car or flexing and extending the knee during dressing.
- The quadriceps has been shown to develop greater strength using resisted open-chain than closed-chain exercises.[288]
- Closed-chain strengthening should be initiated first in partial weight bearing and later in full weight bearing as healing allows and then integrated with balance and proprioceptive training and functional weight-bearing activities.

Considerable research has been done comparing joint reaction forces and muscle function during open- and closed-chain exercises. Comparisons of outcomes are difficult because of differing research designs and exercise variables.[67] Table 21.6 summarizes results from a study comparing two dynamic exercises, with recommendations for exercise modification with specific knee impairments. Special adaptations also have been highlighted in the conservative management and surgical management sections of this chapter.

Open-Chain (Nonweight-Bearing) Exercises

To Develop Control and Strength of Knee Extension (Quadriceps Femoris)

A wide variety of static and dynamic exercises can be used to improve the function of the quadriceps femoris muscles in open-chain positions. Because of variations in muscle fiber orientation and attachments of the knee extensor muscles, individual components of the quadriceps femoris muscle group place different biomechanical stresses on the patella.

Although it is not possible to isolate contraction of the different parts of the quadriceps femoris muscle because of the common innervation, emphasis is often placed on activation of the VMO and vastus medialis muscles to prevent potentially harmful lateral patellar tracking. Tactile cues, biofeedback, and electrical muscle stimulation over the VMO may reinforce awareness of the muscle contracting for patellar control.

TABLE 21.6 Comparison of Forces and Muscle Action at the Knee During Dynamic Open-Chain and Closed-Chain Exercises[67,304]

Parameter	Open-Chain Exercise—Variable Resistance: Sitting, Knee Extension Machine	Closed-Chain Exercise—Variable Resistance: Squatting, Leg-Press Machine (Body Moving Away from Fixed Feet)
Rectus femoris development	More effective	Less effective
VMO development	Less effective	More effective for VMO (and VL)
Other muscle development	None	Effective for hamstrings
ACL tensile forces*	ACL under tension at < 25°	
PCL tensile forces*	PCL under tension from 25°–95° (peak at 1.0 × body weight)	PCL under tension throughout range (1.5–2.0 × body weight)
Patellofemoral compression	Peak stress at 60°, peak compression at 75°‡	Compression increases with knee flexion, peaking at 90°†
Tibiofemoral compression	Higher compression (more stability) < 30°	Higher compression (more stability) > 70°

*The 0°–25° range should be excluded in open-chain exercises following ACL injury but may be included after PCL injury.
†Squat exercises: exercise only from 0°–50° with patellofemoral dysfunctions.
‡Open-chain exercise from 0°–30° and 75°–90° with patellofemoral dysfunctions. (Note: there is controversy in the literature regarding compressive forces in the patellofemoral joint from 0° to 30°.)

Quadriceps Setting (Quad Sets)

Patient position and procedure: Supine, sitting in a chair (with the heel on the floor) or long-sitting with the knee extended (or flexed a few degrees) but not hyperextended. Have the patient contract the quadriceps isometrically, causing the patella to glide proximally; then hold for a count of 10, and repeat.

- Use verbal cues such as, "Try to push your knee back and tighten your thigh muscle" or "Try to tighten your thigh muscle and pull your kneecap up." When the patient sets the muscle properly, offer verbal reinforcement immediately and then have the patient repeat the activity.
- Have the patient dorsiflex the ankle and then hold an isometric contraction of the quadriceps.[7]
- Monitor the gluteus maximus to make sure that the patient is not compensating with hip extension as a result of an inhibited quadriceps.

Straight-Leg Raise

CLINICAL TIP

A supine SLR combines dynamic hip flexion with an isometric contraction of the quadriceps. The effective resistance of gravity (or any additional weight added at the ankle) decreases as the lower extremity elevates because of the decreasing moment arm of the resistance force. Consequently, the greatest resistance is encountered during the first few degrees of the SLR and resistance progressively decreases with greater hip flexion. The rectus femoris (which is also a hip flexor) is the primary muscle in the quadriceps group that is active during the SLR exercise.[276]

Patient position and procedure: Supine, with the knee extended. To stabilize the pelvis and low back, the opposite hip and knee are flexed, and the foot is placed flat on the exercise table. First, have the patient set the quadriceps muscle, and then lift the leg to about 45° of hip flexion while keeping the knee extended. Have the patient hold the leg in that position for a count of 10 and then lower it.

- To progress, have the patient lift to only 30° and then to only 15° of hip flexion, and hold the position.
- To increase resistance, place a cuff weight around the patient's ankle.

FOCUS ON EVIDENCE

It has been proposed that if an SLR in the supine position is coupled with external rotation or isometric adduction of the hip, the VMO or VM muscles are preferentially activated and strengthened.[7,34,56,172] The rationale for advocating these exercises is that many fibers of the VMO muscle originate from the adductor magnus tendon.[7,135] Although a number of authors[6] have advocated these SLR adaptations to increase the medially directed forces on the patella, there is lack of evidence to substantiate the effect.

Straight-Leg Lowering

Patient position and procedure: Supine. If the patient cannot perform an SLR because of a quadriceps lag or weakness, begin by passively placing the leg in 90° of SLR position (or as far as the flexibility of the hamstrings allows), and have the patient gradually lower the extremity while keeping the knee fully extended.

- Be prepared to control the descent of the leg with your hand under the heel as the torque created by gravity increases.
- If the knee begins to flex as the extremity is lowered, have the patient stop at that point, then raise the extremity upward to 90°.
- Have the patient repeat the motion and attempt to lower the extremity a little farther each time while keeping the knee extended.
- When the patient can keep the knee extended while lowering the leg through the full ROM, SLRs can be initiated.

Multiple-Angle Isometric Exercises

- *Patient position and procedure:* Supine or long-sitting. Have the patient perform bent leg raises with the knee in multiple angles of flexion.
- *Patient position and procedure:* Seated at the edge of a treatment table. When tolerated, apply resistance just above the ankle to strengthen the quadriceps isometrically in varying degrees of knee flexion. Co-contraction of the quadriceps and hamstrings can be activated (except in the last 10° to 15° of knee extension) by having the patient push the thigh into the table while holding the knee in extension against resistance.[103]

Short-Arc Terminal Knee Extension

CLINICAL TIP

Although in the past it was thought that the VMO was responsible for the terminal phase of knee extension, it is now well documented that all components of the quadriceps femoris muscle group are active throughout active knee extension and that the VMO primarily affects patellar alignment.[276]

Patient position and procedure: Supine or long-sitting. Place a rolled towel or bolster under the knee to support it in flexion (Fig. 21.23). The patient can also assume a short-sitting position at the edge of a table with the seat of a chair or a stool placed under the heel to stop knee flexion at the desired angle. Begin with the knee in a few degrees of flexion. Increase the degrees of flexion as tolerated by the patient or dictated by the condition.

- Initially, have the patient extend the knee only against the resistance of gravity. Later, add a cuff weight around the

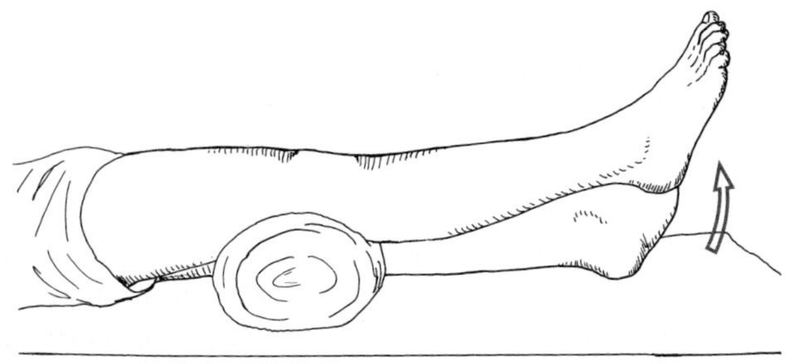

FIGURE 21.23 Short-arc terminal extension exercise to strengthen the quadriceps femoris muscle. When tolerated, resistance is added proximal to the ankle.

ankle to increase the resistance if the patient does not experience pain or crepitation.

- Combine short-arc terminal knee extension with an isometric hold and/or a SLR when the knee is in full extension.
- To reduce lateral shear forces at the knee, have the patient invert the foot as he or she extends the knee.[7,101]

PRECAUTION: When adding resistance to the distal leg, the amount of force generated by the quadriceps muscle increases significantly in the terminal ranges of knee extension. In this portion of the range, the quadriceps has a poor mechanical advantage and poor physiological length while having to contract against an external resistance force that has a long lever arm. The amount of muscle force generated causes an anterior translation force on the tibia, which is restrained by the ACL. This exercise is not appropriate for a patient during the early phase of postoperative rehabilitation when the reconstructed ligament is most vulnerable to imposed loads.

Full-Arc Extension

Patient position and procedure: Sitting or supine. Have the patient extend the knee from 90° to full extension. Apply resistance to the motion as tolerated.

CLINICAL TIP

Resistance applied from 90° to 60° in a nonweight-bearing position causes less anterior tibial translation than squatting (a closed-chain activity) in this range. Resistance applied in open-chain extension from 30° to 0°, however, increases anterior translation more than does performing minisquats in the same range.[304]

- Apply resistance through the full arc of motion only during the later phases of rehabilitation if the knee is pain free, stable, and asymptomatic. If there is pain, resistance should be applied only through those portions of the range with no symptoms.
- Various forms of resistance equipment discussed in Chapter 6 can be used to strengthen the knee extensors. Emphasize high-repetition, low-resistance training with weight-training equipment and medium- to high-velocity training with isokinetic equipment to minimize compressive and shear forces on knee joint structures during exercise. When using equipment, the tibial pad against which the patient pushes while extending the knee can be placed proximally on the lower leg to decrease excessive stress on supporting structures of the knee.[305]
- If a cuff weight is applied to the tibia to provide resistance, it causes a distraction to the joint and stress on the ligaments when the patient sits or lies supine with the knee flexed to 90° and the tibia over the edge of the treatment table. To avoid this stress on ligaments, place a stool under the foot so it is supported when the leg is in the dependent position.[37]

To Develop Control and Strength of Knee Flexion (Hamstrings)

Hamstring Setting (Hamstring Sets)

Patient position and procedure: Supine or long-sitting, with the knee in extension or slight flexion with a towel roll under the knee. Have the patient isometrically contract the knee flexors by gently pushing the heel into the treatment table just enough to feel tension develop in the muscle group. Have the patient relax and then repeat the contraction.

Multiple-Angle Isometric Exercises

Patient position and procedure: Supine or long-sitting. Apply either manual or mechanical resistance to a static hamstring muscle contraction with the knee flexed to several positions in the ROM.

- Place the tibia in internal or external rotation prior to resisting knee flexion to emphasize the medial or lateral hamstring muscles, respectively.
- Teach the patient to apply self-resistance at multiple points in the ROM by placing the opposite foot behind the ankle of the leg to be resisted.

Hamstring Curls

- *Patient position and procedure:* Standing, holding onto a solid object for balance. Have the patient lift the foot and flex the knee (Fig. 21.24). Maximum resistance from gravity occurs when the knee is at 90° flexion. Apply resistance with ankle weights or a weighted boot. If the patient flexes the hip, stabilize it by having the patient place the anterior thigh against a wall or solid object.
- *Patient position and procedure:* Prone. Place a small folded towel or piece of foam rubber under the femur just proximal to the patella to avoid compression of the patella between the treatment table and the femur. With a cuff weight around the ankle, have the patient flex the knee to only 90°. Maximum resistance from gravity occurs when the knee first starts to flex at 0°. If hamstring curls are performed in the prone position using manual resistance, a weight-pulley system or isokinetic equipment resistance to the knee flexors can be applied throughout the full range of knee flexion.

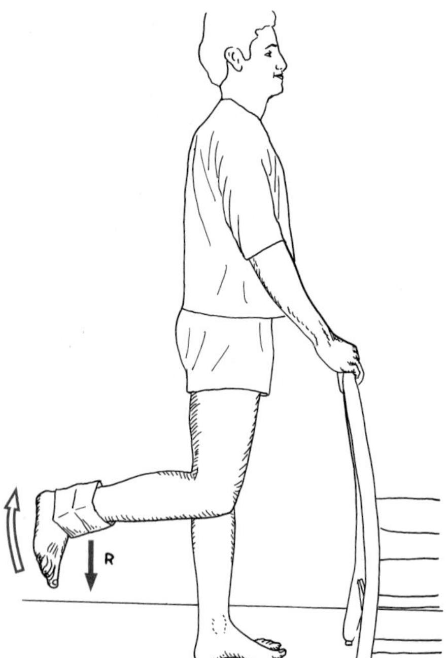

FIGURE 21.24 Hamstring curls; resistance exercises to the knee flexors with the patient standing. Maximal resistance occurs when the knee is at 90°.

PRECAUTION: Open-chain hamstring curls performed against resistance placed on the distal tibia cause posterior tibial translation. A patient with a PCL injury or reconstruction should avoid this exercise during the early stages of rehabilitation.

Closed-Chain (Weight-Bearing) Exercises

Progressive closed-chain exercises are beneficial for activating and training the muscles of the lower extremity to respond to specific functional demands. As the quadriceps contract eccentrically to control knee flexion or concentrically to extend the knee, the hamstrings and soleus function to stabilize the tibia against the anterior translating force of the quadriceps at the knee joint. This synergy, along with the compressive loading on the joints, provides support to the cruciate ligaments.[67,218] In addition, because the hip extends and the ankle plantarflexes as the knee extends (and vice versa) during closed-chain activities, the two-joint hamstrings and gastrocnemius and the one-joint soleus are maintaining favorable length-tension relationships through action at the hip and ankle, respectively.

Initiation of closed-chain exercises. During rehabilitation, closed-chain exercises can be incorporated into an exercise regimen as soon as partial or full weight bearing is safe. In certain portions of the ROM, closed-chain strengthening exercises generate less shear force on the knee joint than open-chain quadriceps-strengthening activities. Therefore, resistance can be added to closed-chain activities sooner after injury or surgery than can be added to open-chain exercises while still protecting healing structures such as the ACL. Clinically, closed-chain exercises enable the patient to develop strength, endurance, and stability of the lower extremity in functional patterns sooner after knee injury or surgery than do open-chain exercises. The progression of closed-chain exercises described in Chapter 20 is also appropriate for knee rehabilitation programs.

Partial weight-bearing and support techniques. If the patient does not tolerate or is not permitted to bear full weight on the involved extremity, begin exercises with upper extremity assistance, such as in the parallel bars or in a pool, to partially unload body weight and avoid excessive biomechanical stress. Also consider use of supportive taping techniques or bracing to ensure proper alignment during weight bearing. Begin exercises at a level tolerated by the patient and at which there is complete control and no exacerbation of symptoms.

CLINICAL TIP

Because the knee is the intermediate link in the lower extremity chain, it is significantly influenced by hip and trunk function, as well as foot and ankle function, during weight bearing.[113,234] Therefore, exercises for these regions should be included in the rehabilitation of the knee if impairments are detected during the examination. Specifically, look for:

- Tightness of the TFL, gluteus maximus, rectus femoris, hamstrings, or gastrocnemius-soleus muscle group
- Weakness of the gluteus medius, external rotators, or gluteus maximus

Closed-Chain Isometric Exercises

Closed-chain isometric exercises are done to facilitate co-contraction of the quadriceps and hamstrings.

Setting Exercises for Co-Contraction

Patient position and procedure: Sitting on a chair, with the knee extended or slightly flexed and the heel on the floor. Have the patient press the heel against the floor and the thigh against the seat of the chair and concentrate on contracting the quadriceps and hamstrings simultaneously to facilitate co-contraction around the knee joint. Hold the muscle contraction, relax, and repeat. Use biofeedback to enhance learning of the co-contraction.

Alternating Isometrics and Rhythmic Stabilization

Patient position and procedure: Standing, with weight equally distributed through both lower extremities. Apply manual resistance to the pelvis in alternating directions as the patient holds the position. This facilitates isometric contractions of muscles in the ankles, knees, and hips.

- Increase the speed of application of the resistive forces to train the muscles to respond to sudden shifts in forces.
- Progress the stabilization activity by applying the alternating resistance against the shoulders to develop trunk stabilization and then by having the patient bear weight only on the involved lower extremity while resistance is applied.

- Progress to weight bearing on unstable surfaces as balance and stability improve.

Closed-Chain Isometrics Against Elastic Resistance

Patient position and procedure: Standing on the involved extremity, loop elastic resistance around the thigh of the opposite extremity and secure it to a stable object (see Fig. 20.26 in Chapter 20). Have the patient flex and extend the hip of the nonweight-bearing lower extremity at varying speeds to facilitate co-contraction of muscles and stability of the weight-bearing leg. This closed-chain exercise also facilitates proprioceptive input and balance on the weight-bearing (involved) lower extremity.

Closed-Chain Dynamic Exercises

Scooting on a Wheeled Stool

Patient position and procedure: Sitting on a rolling stool or chair. Have the patient "walk" the feet forward to use the hamstrings or "walk" backward to use the quadriceps (Fig. 21.25). Be certain the knee is aligned vertically over the foot to avoid hip adduction, internal rotation, and subsequent valgus alignment of the lower leg.

- Increase the challenge of the exercise by having the patient steer around an obstacle course, roll the stool across carpeting, or pull against a resistance, such as pulling another person who is also on a rolling stool.

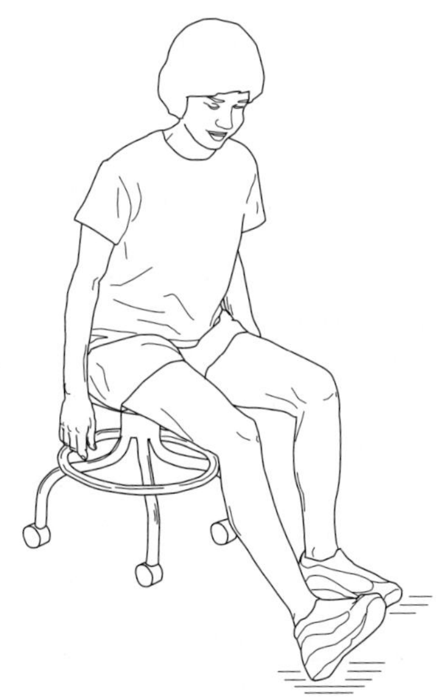

FIGURE 21.25 Forward scooting on a wheeled stool to strengthen knee flexors and backward scooting to strengthen knee extensors.

NOTE: Patient position is standing in all of the following exercises.

Unilateral Closed-Chain Terminal Knee Extension

Patient position and procedure: Standing, elastic resistance looped around the distal thigh of the involved extremity and secured to a stationary structure (Fig. 21.26). Have the patient actively perform terminal knee extension while bearing partial to full weight on the involved extremity.

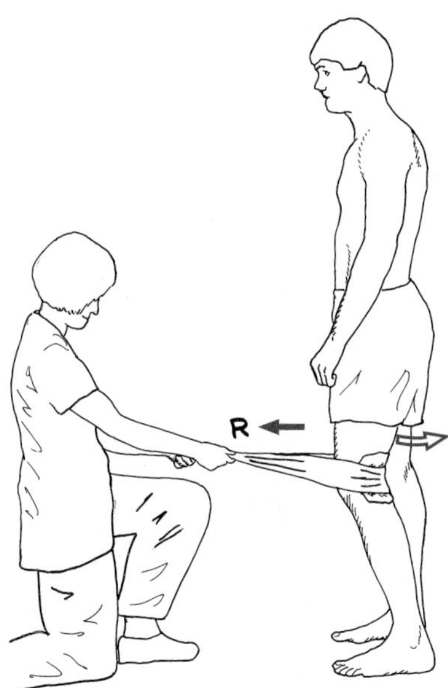

FIGURE 21.26 Unilateral closed-chain terminal knee extension.

Partial Squats, Minisquats, and Short-Arc Training

Patient position and procedure: Begin by having the patient flex both knees up to 30° to 45° and then return to full extension. Progress by holding elastic resistance that is secured under both feet (Fig. 21.27 A) or by holding weights in the hands. The patient should maintain the trunk upright, concentrate on maintaining a posterior weight shift, and lower the hips as though sitting down before moving the knees. The knees should maintain alignment with the toes to prevent valgus collapse and should not move forward beyond the toes to ensure gluteal activation and decreased patellofemoral joint forces.

- Progress squats to greater ranges of knee flexion during the advanced phases of treatment if necessary.
- Increase the difficulty of the exercise by performing unilateral resisted minisquats (Fig. 21.27 B) or squatting on unstable surfaces. Advanced activities are described and illustrated in Chapter 23.

Standing Wall Slides

Patient position and procedure: Standing, with back against the wall (see Fig. 20.29 A in Chapter 20). Flex the hips and knees and slide the back down and then up the wall, lowering and lifting the body weight.

- Apply elastic resistance around both thighs just proximal to the knees to provide added resistance to the hip abductors. This encourages the patient to maintain knee alignment over the toes to prevent or correct a valgus collapse.
- As control improves, have the patient move into greater knee flexion, up to a maximum of 60°. Knee flexion beyond 60° is not recommended to avoid excessive tibiofemoral joint shear forces and patellofemoral joint compressive forces.

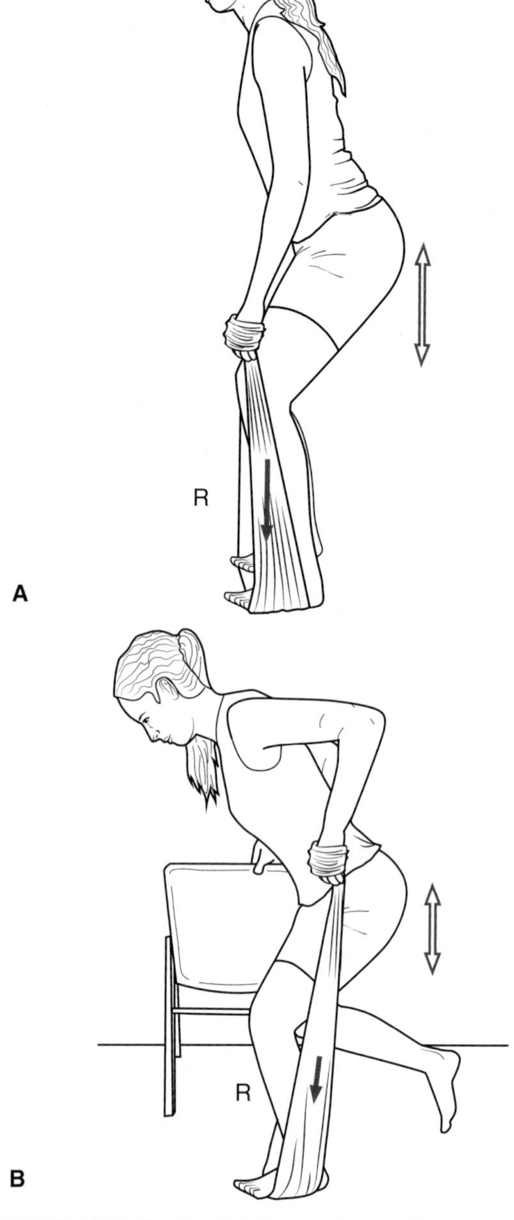

FIGURE 21.27 Resisted minisquats using elastic resistance; closed-chain short-arc training in **(A)** bilateral stance and **(B)** unilateral stance.

- Add isometric training by having the patient stay in the partial-squat position. If the patient is able, he or she maintains the partial squat and alternately extends one leg and then the other.
- Wall slides performed with a gym ball behind the back decrease stability and require greater control (see Fig. 20.29 B in Chapter 20).
- Increase the difficulty of the exercise by performing wall slides in unilateral stance (see Fig. 23.29 in Chapter 23).

Forward, Backward, and Lateral Step-Ups and Step-Downs VIDEO 21.1

Patient position and procedure: Begin with a low step, 2 to 3 inches in height, and increase the height as the patient is able. Make sure the patient keeps the trunk upright and the knee aligned vertically over the foot to avoid valgus collapse.

- To reinforce proper lower extremity alignment and stimulate firing of the gluteus medius during forward step-ups, apply a graded manual resistive force to the lateral aspect of the forward thigh (Fig. 21.28 A).
- Emphasize control of body weight during concentric (step-up) and eccentric (step-down) quadriceps activities. To emphasize the quadriceps and minimize pushing off with the plantarflexors of the trailing extremity, teach the patient that the trailing heel must be the last to leave the floor and the first to return.
- Add resistance with a weight belt or handheld weights, or place elastic resistance (Fig. 21.28 B) or a belt attached to a pulley system around the patient's hips.
- Progress to stepping up to or down from higher surfaces, and add rotational movements.

FOCUS ON EVIDENCE

An EMG study[9] of five weight-bearing exercises in single-leg stance demonstrated the following quadriceps recruitment from greatest activation to least (66% to 55% MVIC): wall squat (wall slide), forward step-up, minisquat, reverse step-up, and lateral step-up.

A kinematic study evaluating patellar joint forces and stress during forward step-up, lateral step-up and forward step-down activities showed the peak PF joint stress was greatest during the eccentric phase (by 7%) in the forward step-down due to a higher knee extensor moment when compared to the two step-up activities.[42]

Partial and Full Lunges

Lunges may be performed by varying the length of the stride, by stepping into a lunge and bringing the trailing leg forward, or by stepping into a lunge and pushing back to the starting position. In addition, maintaining the lunge position and raising and lowering the body with the trunk erect will progress the exercise.

Patient position and procedure: Begin with the feet together, and then have the patient lunge forward with the involved extremity using a small stride and a small amount of knee flexion (see Fig. 20.32). Then return to the upright position by extending the knee and bringing the foot back beside the other foot. As the patient gains control, increase the stride length and knee flexion accordingly.

- Maintain the knee in alignment with the toes (to avoid hip adduction and internal rotation), and do not flex the forward leg beyond a vertical line coming up from the toes.[68]

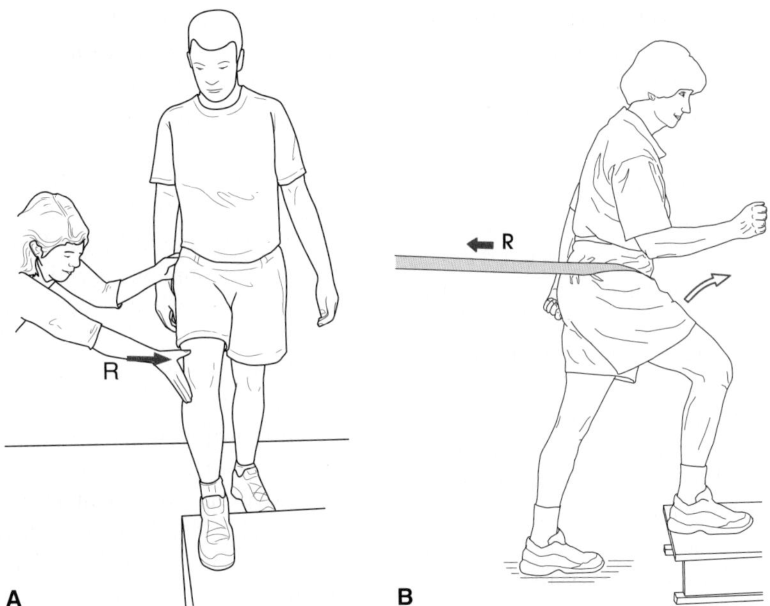

FIGURE 21.28 (A) A forward step-up with manual pressure applied to the lateral thigh to reinforce proper lower extremity alignment and stimulate the gluteus medius. (B) Resisted step-ups against elastic resistance or a pulley to strengthen knee extensors.

- To increase the challenge, add weights around the trunk or in the patient's hands, and increase the speed of the activity as control improves.
- Progress by having the patient lunge forward in a diagonal direction, then out to the side, then diagonally backward, and then directly backward. (See Chapter 23 for descriptions and illustrations of advanced progressions.)

Functional Progression for the Knee

To prepare for functional activities, it is important to develop adequate strength, stability, power, muscular and cardiopulmonary endurance, coordination and timing of movements, and the ability to control balance and to respond to expected or unexpected perturbations. Each of these elements is necessary for skill acquisition. The principle of specificity of training is applied to progress the patient's activities toward the desired functional outcomes. A brief summary of the key components of a functional progression for knee rehabilitation follows, with references to other chapters for additional information.

Strength and Muscle Endurance Training

Strength. Advanced strengthening often involves high-load eccentric exercises or velocity-spectrum training. Resistance equipment, such as a leg press unit, a Total Gym® unit, or an isokinetic dynamometer, provide progressive loading of knee musculature beyond that of elastic resistance and cuff weights. During high-load, open-chain knee extension exercises, placing the tibial pad of the dynamometer close to the knee joint reduces anterior shear forces on the knee.[305]

Muscular endurance. To improve muscular endurance, exercises previously described in this chapter are progressed by increasing the number of repetitions or the time spent at each resistance level. Equipment typically used for cardiopulmonary training, such as a treadmill, stationary bicycle, or stair-stepping unit, also can be used to develop lower extremity muscular endurance. Characteristics of exercise regimens designed to progressively develop strength and muscular endurance and features of various types of equipment are addressed in Chapters 6 and 7.

Cardiopulmonary Endurance Training

A progression of aerobic activities, such as swimming, cycling, walking, running and using an upper extremity ergometer, elliptical trainer, stair-stepper, or cross-country ski machine are graded to the patient's tolerance and integrated into a rehabilitation program for cardiopulmonary endurance. These activities also increase muscular endurance in multiple muscle groups. If the patient is planning on returning to a sport activity, choose a conditioning activity that best replicates the muscle activity used. Refer to Chapter 7 for training guidelines.

Balance and Proprioceptive Activities (Perturbation Training)

A progression of balance activities requiring trunk and lower extremity control is an essential component of a rehabilitation program to improve or restore a patient's functional capabilities.[75,76,294,309] As soon as partial to full weight bearing is permitted, balance training can progress from basic activities in bilateral stance on a stable surface to more challenging activities in unilateral stance on unstable surfaces. Examples include stabilization exercises against alternating resistive forces; maintaining balance during multidirectional arm movements; and controlled weight shifting, stepping, and marching movements, to more challenging activities in unilateral stance on unstable surfaces. A sequence of activities for postural control and progressive balance training is described and illustrated in Chapters 8, 16, and 23.

Plyometric Training and Agility Drills

Plyometrics. Plyometric training, also referred to as stretch-shortening drills, is designed to improve power and develop quick neuromuscular responses. This form of training is appropriate during the advanced phase of rehabilitation for selected patients intending to return to high-demand work- or sport-related activities. Training involves high-speed movements and quick changes of direction. Examples of lower extremity plyometric training include forward-backward and side-to-side shuffles, use of a Pro-Fitter®, and jumping on and off surfaces of varying heights and landing using proper mechanics to reduce the risk of injury. Refer to Chapter 23 for a progression of lower extremity plyometric activities.

Agility. Agility drills are designed to develop coordination, balance, and quick neuromuscular responses. Drills involve practicing activities that include directional changes at varying speeds of movement. Activities include maneuvering around or stepping over obstacles in the environment first while walking and then while running, pivoting, cutting, or hopping. Examples of agility drills are in Chapter 23.

Simulated Work-Related Activities and Sport-Specific Drills

A final component of an individualized rehabilitation program involves practicing activities that simulate the physical demands of a patient's work or desired recreational or sport activity. Simulated activities and drills enable a patient to practice under supervised conditions to receive feedback on correct mechanics. For example, the patient returning to a repetitive lifting job should practice activities that develop strength and endurance in the trunk stabilizers and hip and knee extensors while maintaining safe body mechanics.

Examples of early balance activities for the lower extremity are described in the exercise section of Chapter 20. A progression of lifting tasks and application of proper body mechanics are described in Chapters 8 and 16. Descriptions of sport-specific drills are beyond the scope of this textbook but can be found in a number of resources.

Independent Learning Activities

Critical Thinking and Discussion

1. Consider each of these functional activities: Putting on socks and shoes, rising from a chair, climbing on to a city bus.
   - What ROM is needed in the knee joint for each activity?
   - If motion is restricted in either flexion or extension, what muscles may also have decreased mobility? What arthrokinematic motions may also be limited?
   - What muscles are functioning during the activities, and what level of strength is needed?
2. Describe an intervention program to address loss of strength and/or ROM that is limiting these activities. What is the logical progression of the intervention?
3. For all the two-joint muscles that cross the knee, describe their function at both the knee and the adjacent joint. How can each muscle function most efficiently at the knee in terms of its length-tension relationship?
4. Describe the function of the knee during the gait cycle.
   - How much ROM is needed, and when during the gait cycle does the maximum degree of flexion and extension occur?
   - When during the gait cycle is each of the muscles active at the knee, and what are their functions?
   - What gait deviations occur when there is muscle shortening, muscle weakness, and joint pain? Explain why each deviation occurs.
5. Two patients, both in their seventies, underwent TKA 10 days ago because of joint degeneration from OA of the right knee and have been referred to you in your home health practice. One patient had a cemented TKA, and the other had a "hybrid" TKA. How does their postoperative management differ, or how is it similar?
6. Describe the structures involved with a lateral retinacular release, a proximal realignment of the extensor mechanism, and a distal realignment procedure. How do these differences impact postoperative rehabilitation?
7. What muscles could be weak or tight when a patient demonstrates pelvic drop and valgus collapse at the knee during a single-leg knee bend 6 months following ACL reconstruction? Describe interventions that can be used to correct these problems.

Laboratory Practice

1. Design, set up, and perform a circuit-training course to improve hamstring and quadriceps muscle activation, strengthening, and balance. Sequence the activities from basic to advanced. Observe the accuracy and safety with each exercise, and consider the stresses involved.
2. Using mechanical resistance (pulleys, elastic resistance, and free weights), perform exercises to meet each of these objectives:
   - Strengthening the quadriceps with the greatest mechanical torque occurring when the knee is at 90°, at 45°, and at 25°.

- Strengthening the hamstrings with the greatest mechanical torque occurring when the knee is at 90°, at 45°, and at 0°.

3. Review the joint mobilization techniques for the knee; include basic glides, accessory motions, patellar mobilizations, and mobilization with movement techniques.
   - Identify and practice techniques that increase knee extension, beginning with the knee at 45° and progressing by 15° increments until full extension is reached.
   - Do the same for knee flexion, beginning at 25° and progressing by 15° increments until full range is achieved. What accessory motions are necessary?
   - What knee motions may be restricted if the patella does not glide distally?
   - What knee function may be lost if the patella does not glide proximally?
4. Review and practice soft tissue and patellar mobilization techniques that are used to increase the mobility of the lateral retinaculum and IT band. How does mobilizing this tissue improve patellar tracking? What proximal muscles help to support normal patellar alignment during dynamic activities?
5. Review and practice self-stretching techniques with and without equipment for all of the two-joint muscles at the knee.

Case Studies

1. Mrs. James is a 49-year-old mother of three children. She is in good health but is recently experiencing considerable right knee pain, especially when standing after prolonged sitting, when descending stairs, and when on her feet for longer than 2 hours. She reports a right proximal tibial fracture 15 years ago that took approximately a year to return to normal mobility. On examination there is no obvious deformity or joint swelling. Knee flexion is 125° with a firm end feel and pain on overpressure; extension is 0° with firm end feel and pain on overpressure. There is a slight decrease in posterior glide accessory motion of the tibia and decreased mobility of the patella on the right compared to the left. Strength of the knee flexors and extensors is 4/5 bilaterally. She complains of pain in the right knee when squatting; pain begins at 45° flexion. She stops when the knees are at 75°, saying it hurts too much. She bends forward from the waist to pick up objects from the floor. She has difficulty lowering herself down to a low chair in a controlled manner.
   - List her impairments and functional limitations and state appropriate goals.
   - Develop an exercise program to meet the goals. Describe the exercises you will begin with and why they are appropriate. Explain how you will progress each exercise and the program.
   - List the possible manual techniques that would be beneficial to her and describe the rationale for each one.
   - Discuss the home exercises you would suggest and describe how you would teach them to her.
2. Mr. Ray, who is 25 years of age, was in a serious automobile accident and sustained femur and patella fractures of his left leg. His leg was immobilized in a long-leg cast for 3 months, followed by a short-leg cast for an additional month. He was allowed to perform partial weight bearing when in the short-leg cast. The cast was removed this morning, and he is to begin rehabilitation, although he will not be allowed full weight bearing for an additional month. He describes significant stiffness and discomfort when flexing his knee. Observation reveals significant atrophy in his left thigh and leg. There are no open sores or joint swelling. Range is limited to 25° flexion and 20° extension, with no joint play in the tibiofemoral or patellofemoral joints. He has the ability to do quadriceps and hamstring sets, but strength could not be tested.
   - Answer the same questions as in the previous case.
   - Even though patients in this and the previous case have restricted motion and demonstrate weakness, what are the differences in intervention strategies? Are there different precautions that you will follow during treatment? If so, what are they?

REFERENCES

1. Allum, R: Aspects of current management: complications of arthroscopic reconstruction of the anterior cruciate ligament. *J Bone Joint Surg Br* 85:12–16, 2003.
2. American Academy of Orthopedic Surgeons: ACL injury: does it require surgery? Available at www.orthoinfo.aaos.org; Accessed February 15, 2016.
3. American Academy of Orthopaedic Surgeons (AAOS): American Academy of Orthopaedic Surgeons clinical practice guideline on management of anterior cruciate ligament injuries. *AAOS* Sept 5:619, 2014.
4. Anbari, A, and Cole, BJ: Medial patellofemoral ligament reconstruction: a novel approach. *J Knee Surg* 21(3):241–245, 2008.
5. Anderson, JK, and Noyes, FR: Principles of posterior cruciate ligament reconstruction. *Orthopedics* 18(5):493–500, 1995.
6. Andriacchi, TP, and Numdermann, A: The role of ambulatory mechanics in the initiation and progression of knee osteoarthritis. *Curr Opin Rheumatol* 18:514–518. 2006.
7. Antich, TJ, and Brewster, CE: Modification of quadriceps femoris muscle exercises during knee rehabilitation. *Phys Ther* 66(8):1246–1251, 1986.
8. Arendt, E, and Dick, R: Knee injury patterns among men and women in collegiate basketball and soccer. *Am J Sports Med* 23(6):694–701, 1995.
9. Avramidis, K, et al: Effectiveness of electrical stimulation of the vastus medialis muscle in the rehabilitation of patients after total knee arthroplasty. *Arch Phys Med Rehabil* 84(12):1850–1853, 2003.
10. Ayotte, NW, et al: Electromyographical analysis of selected lower extremity muscles during 5 unilateral weight-bearing exercises. *J Orthop Sports Phys Ther* 37(2):48–55, 2007.
11. Bade, MJ, Kohrt, WM, and Stevens-Lapsley, JE: Outcomes before and after total knee arthroplasty compared to healthy adults. *J Orthop Sports Phys Ther* 40(9):559–567, 2010.
12. Baldon, R, et al: Effects of functional stabilization training on pain, function, and lower extremity biomechanics in women with patellofemoral pain: a randomized clinical trial. *J Ortho Sports Phys Ther* 44(4):240–251, 2014.

13. Bartha, L, et al: Autologous osteochondral mosaicplasty grafting. *J Orthop Sports Phys Ther* 36(10):739–750, 2006.
14. Barton, CJ, Webster, KE, and Menz, HB: Evaluation of the scope and quality of systematic reviews on nonpharmacological conservative treatment for patellofemoral pain syndrome. *J Orthop Sports Phys Ther* 38: 529–541, 2008.
15. Berchuck, M, et al: Gait adaptations by patients who have a deficient anterior cruciate ligament. *J Bone Joint Surg Am* 72(6):871–877, 1990.
16. Berenbaum, F: Osteoarthritis, epidemiology, pathology, and pathogenesis. In Klippel, JH, et al (eds): *Primer on the Rheumatic Diseases,* ed. 12. Atlanta: Arthritis Foundation, 2001, pp 285–293.
17. Bert, JM: Arthroscopic treatment of degenerative arthritis of the knee. In Insall, JN, and Scott, WN (eds): *Surgery of the Knee,* ed. 5. New York: Churchill Livingstone, 2012, pp 229–234.
18. Bertlet, GC, Mascia, A, and Miniaci, A: Treatment of unstable osteochondritis dessicans lesions of the knee using autogenous osteochondral grafts (mosaicplasty). *Arthroscopy* 15:312–316, 1999.
19. Beynnon, BD, et al: Treatment of anterior cruciate ligament injuries. Part 1. *Am J Sports Med* 33(10):1579–1602, 2005.
20. Beynnon, BD, et al: Treatment of anterior cruciate ligament injuries. Part 2. *Am J Sports Med* 33(11):1751–1767, 2005.
21. Beynnon, BD, et al: Rehabilitation after anterior cruciate ligament reconstruction: a prospective, randomized, double-blind comparison of programs administered over 2 different time intervals. *Am J Sports Med* 33(3):347–355, 2005.
22. Bianchi, G, et al: The use of unicondylar osteoarticular allografts in reconstructions around the knee. *Knee* 16:1–5. 2009.
23. Bizzini, M, et al: Systematic review of the quality of randomized, controlled trials for patellofemoral pain syndrome. *J Orthop Sports Phys Ther* 33(1):4–20, 2003.
24. Blackburn, TA, Eiland, WG, and Bandy, WG: An introduction to the plica. *J Orthop Sports Phys Ther* 3(4):171–177, 1982.
25. Bolgla, LA, et al: Hip strength and hip and knee kinematics during stair descent in females with and without patellofemoral pain syndrome. *J Orthop Sports Phys Ther* 38(1):12–18, 2008.
26. Boling, NC, et al: Outcomes of a weight-bearing rehabilitation program for patients diagnosed with patellofemoral pain syndrome. *Arch Phys Med Rehabil* 87:1428–1435, 2006.
27. Bollier, M, et al: Technical failure of medial patellofemoral ligament reconstruction. *Arthroscopy* 27(8):1153–1159. 2011.
28. Bonutti, PM: Minimally invasive total knee arthroplasty—Midvastus approach. In Hozack, WJ, et al (eds): *Minimally Invasive Total Joint Arthroplasty.* Heidelberg: Springer, 2004, pp 139–145.
29. Boyce, DA, and Hanley, ST: Functional based rehabilitation of the knee after partial meniscectomy or meniscal repair. *Orthop Phys Ther Clin North Am* 3:555, 1994.
30. Bradbury, N, et al: Participation in sports after total knee replacement. *Am J Sports Med* 26(4):530–535, 1998.
31. Brand, J, Jr, et al: Graft fixation in cruciate ligament reconstruction. *Am J Sports Med* 28:761–774, 2000.
32. Brittberg, M, and Winalski, CS: Evaluation of cartilage injuries and repair. *J Bone Joint Surg Am* 85-A(Suppl 2):58–69, 2003.
33. Brodersen, MP: Anterior cruciate ligament reconstruction. In Morrey, BF (ed): *Reconstructive Surgery of the Joints,* ed. 2. New York: Churchill Livingstone, 1996, p 1639.
34. Brownstein, BA, Lamb, RL, and Mangine, RE: Quadriceps, torque, and integrated electromyography. *J Orthop Sports Phys Ther* 6(6):309–314, 1985.
35. Buckwalter, JA, and Ballard, WT: Operative treatment of arthritis. In Klippel, JH (ed): *Primer on the Rheumatic Diseases,* ed. 12. Atlanta: Arthritis Foundation, 2001, pp 613–623.
36. Bynum, EB, Barrick, RL, and Alexander, AH: Open versus closed kinetic chain exercises after anterior cruciate ligament reconstruction: a prospective study. *Am J Sports Med* 23(4):401–406, 1995.
37. Cailliet, R: *Knee Pain and Disability,* ed. 3. Philadelphia: F.A. Davis, 1992.
38. Callaghan, JJ, et al: Mobile-bearing knee replacement: concepts and results. *Instr Course Lect* 50:431–449, 2001.
39. Cameron, H, and Brotzman, SB: The arthritic lower extremity. In Brotzman, SB, and Wilk, KE (eds): *Clinical Orthopedic Rehabilitation,* ed. 2. Philadelphia: Mosby, 2003, pp 441–474.
40. Camp, CL, et al: Medial patellofemoral ligament repair for recurrent patellar dislocation. *Am J Sports Med* 38(11):2248–2254, 2010.
41. Carrey, CT, and Tria, AJ: Surgical principles of total knee replacement: incisions, extensor mechanism, ligament balancing. In Pellicci, PM, Tria, AJ, and Garvin, KL (eds): *Orthopedic Knowledge Update, 2. Hip and Knee Reconstruction.* Rosemont, IL: American Academy of Orthopedic Surgeons, 2000, p 281.
42. Chinkulprasert, C, Vachalathiti, R, and Powers, CM: Patellofemoral joint forces and stress during forward step-up, lateral step-up, and forward step-down exercises. *J Orthop Sports Phys Ther* (41(4):241–248, 2011.
43. Chu, BI, et al: Surgical techniques and postoperative rehabilitation for isolated posterior cruciate ligament injury. *Orthop Phys Ther Prac* 19(3):185–189, 2007.
44. Chu, C: Cartilage therapies: Chondrocyte transplantation, osteochondral allografts, and autographs. In Pedowitz, RA, O'Conor, JJ, and Akeson, WH (eds): *Daniel's Knee Injuries: Ligament and Cartilage Structure, Function, Injury, and Repair,* ed. 2. Philadelphia: Lippincott Williams & Wilkins, 2003, pp 227–237.
45. Clifton, R, Ng, CY, and Nutton, RW: What is the role of lateral retinacular release? *J Bone Joint Surg Br* 92(1):1–6, 2010.
46. Clijsen, R, Suchs, J, and Taeymans, J: Effectiveness of exercise therapy in treatment of patients with patellofemoral pain syndrome: systematic review and meta-analysis. *Phys Ther,* 94:1697–1708, 2014.
47. Colvin, AC, and West, RV: Patellar instability. *J Bone Joint Surg Am* 90: 2751–2762, 2008.
48. Cooper, DE, DeLee, MD, and Ramamurthy, S: Reflex sympathetic dystrophy of the knee. *J Bone Joint Surg Am* 71(3):365–369, 1989.
49. Crossley, K, et al: A systematic review of physical interventions for patellofemoral pain syndrome. *Clin J Sport Med* 11(2):103–110, 2001.
50. Cyriax, J: *Textbook of Orthopaedic Medicine, Vol 1. Diagnosis of Soft Tissue Lesions,* ed. 8. London: Bailliere Tindall, 1982.
51. D'Amato, M, and Bach, BR: Knee injuries. In Brotzman, SB, and Wilk, KE (eds): *Clinical Orthopedic Rehabilitation,* ed. 2. Philadelphia: Mosby, 2003, pp 251–370.
52. D'Antonio, JA: Complications of total hip and knee arthroplasty: lessons learned. In Hozack, WJ, et al (eds): *Minimally Invasive Total Joint Arthroplasty.* Heidelberg: Springer, 2004, pp 304–308.
53. Davis, I, Ireland, ML, and Hanaki, S: ACL injuries—the gender bias. *J Orthop Sports Phys Ther* 37(2):A1–A7, 2007.
54. Davis, IS, and Powers, C: Patellofemoral pain syndrome: proximal, distal, and local factors. *J Orthop Sports Phys Ther* 40(3):A3–A9, 2010.
55. De Caro, F, et al: Large fresh osteochondral allografts of the knee: A systematic clinical and basic science review of the literature. *Arthroscopy* 31(4):757–765. 2015.
56. de Jong Z, et al: Long-term follow-up of a high-intensity exercise program in patients with rheumatoid arthritis. *Clin Rheumatol* 28(6): 663–671, 2009.
57. de Jong, Z, and Vlieland, TP: Safety of exercise in patients with rheumatoid arthritis. *Curr Opin Rheumatol* 17(2):177–182, 2005.
58. Dewan, AK, et al: Evolution of autologous chondrocyte repair and comparison to other cartilage repair techniques. *Biomed Research International* Article ID 272481:11 pages, 2014.
59. Deyle, GD, et al: Physical therapy treatment effectiveness for osteoarthritis of the knee: a randomized comparison of supervised clinical exercise and manual therapy procedures versus a home exercise program. *Phys Ther* 85:1301–1317, 2005.
60. Dixon, MC, et al: Modular fixed-bearing total knee arthroplasty with retention of the posterior cruciate ligament: a study of patients followed for a minimum of fifteen years. *J Bone Joint Surg Am* 87(3):598–603, 2005.
61. Dolak, KL, et al: Hip strengthening prior to functional exercises reduces pain sooner than quadriceps strengthening in females with patellofemoral pain syndrome: a randomized clinical trial. *J Orthop Sports Phys Ther* 41(8):560–570, 2011.

62. Drez, D, Edwards, TB, and Williams, CS: Results of medial patellofemoral ligament reconstruction in the treatment of patellar dislocations. *Arthroscopy* 17(3):298–306, 2001.
63. Dunn, WR, et al: The effect of anterior cruciate ligament reconstruction on the risk of knee re-injury. *Am J Sports Med* 32(8):1906–1914, 2004.
64. Eitzen, I, et al: A progressive 5-week exercise therapy program leads to significant improvement in knee function early after anterior cruciate ligament reconstruction. *J Orthop Sports Phys Ther* 40(11):705–721, 2010.
65. Eng, JJ, and Peirrynowski, MR: Evaluation of soft foot orthotics in the treatment of patellofemoral pain syndrome. *Phys Ther* 73(2):62–68, 1993.
66. Enloe, J, et al: Total hip and knee replacement programs: a report using consensus. *J Orthop Sports Phys Ther* 23(1):3–11, 1996.
67. Escamilla, RF, et al: Biomechanics of the knee during closed kinetic chain and open kinetic chain exercises. *Med Sci Sports Exerc* 30(4):556–569, 1998.
68. Escamilla, RF, et al: Patellofemoral joint force and stress between a short- and long-step forward lunge. *J Orthop Sports Phys Ther* 38(11):681–690, 2008.
69. Ethgen, O, et al: Health-related quality of life in total hip and total knee arthroplasty: a qualitative and systematic review of the literature. *J Bone Joint Surg Am* 86:963–974, 2004.
70. Farquhar, SJ, Reisman, DS, and Snyder-Mackler, L: Persistence of altered movement patterns during a sit-to-stand task 1 year following unilateral total knee arthroplasty. *Phys Ther* 88(5):567–579, 2008.
71. Feller, JA, and Webster, KE: A randomized comparison of patellar tendon and hamstring tendon anterior cruciate ligament reconstruction. *Am J Sports Med* 31(4):564–573, 2003.
72. Fineberg, MS, Zarins, B, and Sherman, OH: Practical considerations in anterior cruciate ligament replacement surgery. *Arthroscopy* 16(7): 715–724, 2000.
73. Finger, S, and Paulos, LE: Arthroscopic-assisted posterior cruciate ligament repair/reconstruction. In Jackson, DW (ed): *Master Techniques in Orthopedic Surgery: Reconstructive Knee Surgery,* ed. 2. Philadelphia: Lippincott Williams & Wilkins, 2003, pp 159–177.
74. Fisher, NM, et al: Quantitative effects of physical therapy on muscular and functional performance in subjects with osteoarthritis of the knees. *Arch Phys Med Rehabil* 74(8):840–847, 1993.
75. Fitzgerald, GK, et al: The efficacy of perturbation training in nonoperative anterior cruciate ligament rehabilitation programs for physically active individuals. *Phys Ther* 80(2):128–140, 2000.
76. Fitzgerald, GK, Axe, MJ, and Snyder-Mackler, L: Proposed practice guidelines for nonoperative anterior cruciate ligament rehabilitation of physically active individuals. *J Orthop Sports Phys Ther* 30:194–203, 2000.
77. Fitzgerald, GK, Piva, SR, and Irrgang, JJ: Reports of knee instability in knee osteoarthritis: prevalence and relationship to physical function. *Arthritis Rheum* 51:941–946, 2004.
78. Ford, DH, and Post, WR: Open or arthroscopic lateral release: indications, techniques, and rehabilitation. *Clin Sports Med* 16:29–49, 1997.
79. Fortin, PR, et al: Outcomes of total hip and knee replacement: preoperative functional status predicts outcomes at six months after surgery. *Arthritis Rheum* 42:1722–1728, 1999.
80. Fransen, M, McConnell, S, and Bell, M: Exercise for osteoarthritis of the hip or knee. *The Cochrane Database of Systematic Reviews* 2003, Issue 2. Art. No.: CD004376. doi:10.1002/14561858.CD004376.
81. Fu, FH, et al: Current trends in anterior cruciate ligament reconstruction. Part I. Biology and biomechanics of reconstruction. *Am J Sports Med* 27(6):821–830, 1999.
82. Fu, FH, et al: Current trends in anterior cruciate ligament reconstruction. Part II. Operative procedures and clinical correlations. *Am J Sports Med* 28(1):124–130, 2000.
83. Fujimoto, E, et al: An early return to vigorous activity may destabilize anterior cruciate ligaments reconstructed with hamstring grafts. *Arch Phys Med Rehabil* 85:298–302, 2004.
84. Fukuda, TY, et al: Short-term effects of hip abductors and lateral rotators strengthening in females with patellofemoral pain syndrome: a randomized, controlled clinical trial. *J Orthop Sports Phys Ther* 40(11):736–742, 2010.
85. Fulkerson, JP: Anteromedial tibial tubercle transfer. In Jackson, DW (ed): *Master Techniques in Orthopedic Surgery: Reconstructive Knee Surgery,* ed. 2. Philadelphia: Lippincott Williams & Wilkins, 2006, pp 13–25.
86. Fulkerson, JP: Diagnosis and treatment of patients with patellofemoral pain (Review). *Am J Sports Med* 30:447–456, 2002.
87. Gandhi, R, et al. Complications after minimally invasive total knee arthroplasty as compared with traditional incision techniques: a meta-analysis. *J Arthroplasty.* 26:29–35, 2011.
88. Garth, WP, DiChristina, DG, and Holt, G: Delayed proximal repair and distal realignment after patellar dislocation. *Clin Orthop* 377:132–144, 2000.
89. Gasser, SI, and Jackson, DW: Arthroscopic lateral release of the patella with radiofrequency ablation. In Jackson, DW (ed): *Master Techniques in Orthopedic Surgery: Reconstructive Knee Surgery,* ed. 2. Philadelphia: Lippincott Williams & Wilkins, 2006, pp 3–13.
90. Gerber, JP, et al: Safety, feasibility, and efficacy of negative work exercise via eccentric muscle activity following anterior cruciate ligament reconstruction. *J Orthop Sports Phys Ther* 37(1):10–18, 2007.
91. Gersoff, WK: Meniscal transplantation. In Mirzayan, P (ed): *Cartilage Injury in the Athlete.* New York: Thieme, 2006, pp 263–271.
92. Giles, LS, et al: Does quadriceps atrophy exist in individuals with patellofemoral pain? A systematic literature review with meta-analysis. *J Orthop Sports Phys Ther* 43(11):766–776, 2013.
93. Giles, LS, et al: Atrophy of the quadriceps is not isolated to the vastus medialis oblique in individuals with patellofemoral pain. *J Orthop Sports Phys Ther* 45(8):613–619, 2015.
94. Gill, TJ, Asnis, PD, and Berkson, EM: The treatment of articular cartilage defects using the microfracture technique. *J Orthop Sports Phys Ther* 36(10):728–738, 2006.
95. Gillogly, SD, Myers, TH, and Reinold, MM: Treatment of full-thickness chondral defects in the knee with autologous chondrocyte implantation. *J Orthop Sports Phys Ther* 36(10):751–764, 2006.
96. Goodfellow, J, Hungerford, D, and Woods, C: Patello-femoral joint mechanics and pathology of chondromalacia patellae. *J Bone Joint Surg Br* 58(3):291–299, 1976.
97. Gose, JC: CPM in the postoperative treatment of patients with total knee replacements. *Phys Ther* 67(1):39–42, 1987.
98. Grelsamer, RP, and Klein, JR: The biomechanics of the patellofemoral joint. *J Orthop Sports Phys Ther* 28(5):286–298, 1998.
99. Grelsamer, RP, and McConnell, J: *The Patella: A Team Approach.* Gaithersburg, MD: Aspen, 1998.
100. Griffin, LY, et al: Noncontact anterior cruciate ligament injuries: risk factors and prevention strategies. *J Am Acad Orthop Surg* 8(3):141–150, 2000.
101. Grood, ES, et al: Biomechanics of the knee: extension exercise. *J Bone Joint Surg Am* 66(5):725–734, 1984.
102. Gross, MT, and Foxworth, JL: The role of foot orthoses as an intervention for patellofemoral pain. *J Orthop Sports Phys Ther* 33(11):661–670, 2003.
103. Gryzlo, SM, et al: Electromyographic analysis of knee rehabilitation exercises. *J Orthop Sports Phys Ther* 20(1):36–43, 1994.
104. Gupte, CM, et al: A review of the function and biomechanics of the meniscofemoral ligaments. *Arthroscopy* 19(2):161–171, 2003.
105. Hall, MJ, and Mandalia, VI: Tibial tubercle osteotomy for patella-femoral joint disorders. *Knee Surg Sports Traumatol Arthroscopy* Oct 2014, doi:10.1007/s00167-014-3388-4.
106. Hangood, L: Mosaicplasty. In Insall, JN, and Scott, WN (eds): *Surgery of the Knee, Vol 1,* ed. 3. New York: Churchill Livingstone, 2001, p 357.
107. Hartigan, EH, Axe, MJ, and Snyder-Mackler, L: Timeline for noncopers to return-to-sports criteria after anterior cruciate ligament reconstruction. *J Orthop Sports Phys Ther* 40(3):141–154, 2010.
108. Hartigan, E, Lewek, M, and Snyder-Mackler, L: The knee. In Levangie, PK, and Norkin, CC (ed): *Joint Structure and Function: A Comprehensive Analysis,* ed. 5. Philadelphia: F.A. Davis, 2011, pp 396–439.
109. Harvey, LA, Brosseau, L, and Herbert, RD: continuous passive motion following total knee arthroplasty in people with arthritis. *Cochrane Database of Systematic Reviews* Issue 2:Article number CD004260, 2014. doi: 10.1002/14651858.CD004260.pub3.

110. Healy, WL, Iorio, R, and Lemos, MJ: Athletic activity after total knee arthroplasty. *Clin Orthop* 390:65–71, 2000.
111. Heckman, TP, Barber-Westin, SD, and Noyes, FR: Meniscal repair and transplantation: indications, techniques, rehabilitation, and clinical outcomes. *J Orthop Sports Phys Ther* 36(10):795–815, 2006.
112. Heckman, TP, Noyes, FR, and Barber-Westin, SD: Autogenic and allogenic anterior cruciate ligament rehabilitation. In Ellenbecker, TS (ed): *Knee Ligament Rehabilitation.* New York: Churchill Livingstone, 2000, p 132.
113. Heiderscheidt, B: Lower extremity hip injuries: is it just about strength? (Editorial) *J Orthop Sports Phys Ther* 40(2):39–41. 2010.
114. Henning, CE, et al: Arthroscopic meniscal repair using an exogenous fibrin clot. *Clin Orthop Relat Res* 252:64–72. 1990.
115. Herrington, L, and Al-Sherhi, A: A controlled trial of weight-bearing versus nonweight-bearing exercises for patellofemoral pain. *J Orthop Sports Phys Ther* 37(4):155–160, 2007.
116. Hewett, TE, Blum, KR, and Noyes, FR: Gait characteristics of the anterior cruciate ligament-deficient varus knee. *Am J Knee Surg* 10(4): 246–254, 1997.
117. Hewitt, B, and Shakespeare, D: Flexion versus extension: a comparison of postoperative total knee arthroplasty mobilization regimes. *Knee* 8:305–309, 2001.
118. Hiemstra, LA, Lo, I, and Fowler, PJ: Effect of fatigue on knee proprioception: implications for dynamic stabilization. *J Orthop Sports Phys Ther* 31(10):598–605, 2001.
119. Hinton, RY, and Sharma, KM: Acute and recurrent patellar instability in the young athlete. *Orthop Clin North Am* 34:385–396, 2003.
120. Holmes, SW, and Clancy, WG: Clinical classification of patellofemoral pain and dysfunction. *J Orthop Sports Phys Ther* 28(5):299–306, 1998.
121. Hurd, WJ, Axe, MJ, and Snyder-Mackler, L: A 10-year prospective trial of a patient management algorithm and screening examination for highly active individuals with anterior cruciate ligament injury. Part 1. Outcomes. *Am J Sports Med* 36:40–47, 2008.
122. Hurd, WJ, Axe, MJ, and Snyder-Mackler, L: A 10-year prospective trial of a patient management algorithm and screening examination for highly active individuals with anterior cruciate ligament injury. Part 2. Determinants of dynamic knee stability. *Am J Sports Med* 36:48–56, 2008.
123. Insall, JN, and Clark, HD: Historic development, classification and characteristics of total knee prostheses. In Insall, JN, and Scott, WN (eds): *Surgery of the Knee, Vol 2,* ed. 3. New York: Churchill Livingstone, 2001, p 1516.
124. Insall, JN, and Easley, ME: Surgical techniques and instrumentation in total knee arthroplasty. In Insall, JN, and Scott, WN (eds): *Surgery of the Knee, Vol 2,* ed. 3. New York: Churchill Livingstone, 2001, p 1553.
125. Ireland, ML, et al: Hip strength in females with and without patellofemoral pain. *J Orthop Sports Phys Ther* 33(11):671–676, 2003.
126. Jain, NB, et al: Trends in epidemiology of knee arthroplasty in the United States 1990–2000. *Arthritis Rheum* 52(12):3928–3933, 2005.
127. Jamtvedt, G, et al: Physical therapy interventions for patients with osteoarthritis of the knee: an overview of systematic reviews. *Phys Ther* 88(1):123–136, 2008.
128. Jarit, GJ, and Bosco, JA: Meniscal repair and reconstruction. *Bull NYU Hosp Joint Diseases* 68(2):84–90. 2010.
129. Jarvenpaa, J, et al: Obesity may impair the early outcome of total knee arthroplasty. *Scand J Surg* 99(1):45–49, 2010.
130. Jenkins, C, et al: After partial knee replacement patients can kneel, but they need to be taught to do so: a single-blind, randomized, controlled trial. *Phys Ther* 88(9):1012–1021, 2008.
131. Johnson, DP: The effect of continuous passive motion on wound healing and joint mobility after knee arthroplasty. *J Bone Joint Surg Am* 72(3):421–426, 1990.
132. Johnston, L, et al: The knee arthroplasty trial (KAT) design features, baseline characteristics, and two-year functional outcomes after alternative approaches to knee replacement. *J Bone Joint Surg Am* 91(1): 134–141, 2009.
133. Jones, CA, Voaklander, DL, and Suarez-Almazor, ME: Determinants of function after total knee arthroplasty. *Phys Ther* 83(8):696–706, 2003.
134. Kaltenborn, FM, et al: *Manual Mobilization of the Joints: Joint Examination and Basic Treatment, Vol I. The Extremities,* ed. 8. Oslo, Norway: Morli, 2014.
135. Karst, GM, and Jewett, PD: Electromyographic analysis of exercises proposed for differential activation of medial and lateral quadriceps femoris muscle components. *Phys Ther* 73(5):286–295, 1993.
136. Kegerreis, S, Malone, T, and Ohnson, F: The diagonal medial plica: an underestimated clinical entity. *J Orthop Sports Phys Ther* 9(9):305–309, 1988.
137. Kennedy, DM, et al: Assessing recovery and establishing prognosis following total knee arthroplasty. *Phys Ther* 88(1):22–32, 2008.
138. Khatod, M, and Akeson, WH: Ligament injury and repair. In Pedowitz, RA, O'Connor, JJ, and Akeson, WH (eds): *Daniel's Knee Injuries: Ligament and Cartilage Structure, Function, Injury, and Repair,* ed. 2. Philadelphia: Lippincott Williams & Wilkins, 2003, pp 185–201.
139. Khayambashi, K, et al: The effects of isolated hip abductor and external rotator muscle strengthening on pain, health status, and hip strength in females with patellofemoral pain: a randomized controlled trial. *J Orthop Sports Phys Ther* 42(1):22–29, 2011.
140. Kim, CW, and Pedowitz, RA: Principles of surgery. Part A. Graft choice and the biology of graft healing. In Pedowitz, RA, O'Connor, JJ, and Akeson, WH (eds): *Daniel's Knee Injuries: Ligament and Cartilage Structure, Function, Injury, and Repair,* ed. 2. Philadelphia: Lippincott Williams & Wilkins, 2003, pp 435–455.
141. Kim, K, et al: Effects of neuromuscular electrical stimulation after anterior curciate ligament reconstruction on quadriceps strength, function, and patient-oriented outcomes: a systematic review. *J Orthop Sports Phys Ther* 40(7):383–391, 2010.
142. Koeter, S, Diks, MJ, and Anderson PG: A modified tibial tubercle osteotomy for patellar maltracking: results at two years. *J Bone Joint Surg Br* 89:180–185, 2007.
143. Koh, JL, Hangody, L, and Rathonyi, GK: Osteochondral autograft transfer (OATS/mosaicplasty). In Mirzayan, R (ed): *Cartilage Injury in the Athlete.* New York: Thieme Medical Publishing, 2006, pp 124–140.
144. Kolessar, DJ, and Rand, JA: Extensor mechanism problems following total knee arthroplasty. In Morrey, BF (ed): *Reconstructive Surgery of the Joints,* ed. 2. New York: Churchill Livingstone, 1996, p 1533.
145. Kooiker, L, et al: Effects of physical therapist-guided quadriceps-strengthening exercises for the treatment of patellofemoral pain syndrome: a systematic review. *J Orthop Sports Phys Ther* 44(6):391–402, 2014.
146. Kremers, HM, et al: Prevalence of total hip and knee replacement in the United States. *J Bone Joint Surg Am* 97:1386–1397. 2015.
147. Kuster, MS: Exercise recommendations after total joint replacement: a review of the current literature and proposal of scientifically based guidelines. *Sports Med* 32(7):433–445, 2002.
148. Kvist, J: Rehabilitation following anterior cruciate ligament injury: current recommendations for sports participation. *Sports Med* 34:269–280, 2004.
149. Lack, S, et al: Proximal muscle rehabilitation is effective for patellofemoral pain: A systematic review with meta-analysis. *Br J Sports Med* 49(21): 1365–1376, 2015.
150. Laimins, PD, and Powell, SE: Principles of surgery. Part C. Anterior cruciate ligament reconstruction: Techniques past and present. In Pedowitz, RA, O'Connor, JJ, and Akeson, WH (eds): *Daniel's Knee Injuries: Ligament and Cartilage Structure, Function, Injury, and Repair,* ed. 2. Philadelphia: Lippincott Williams & Wilkins, 2003, pp 472–491.
151. Lankhorst, NE, Bierma-Zeinstra, SMA, Van Middlekpoop, M: Risk factors for patellofemoral pain syndrome: a systematic review. *J Orthop Sports Phys Ther* 42(2):81–93, 2012.
152. Lee, S, et al: Outcome of anterior cruciate ligament reconstruction using quadriceps tendon autograft. *Arthroplasty* 20:795–802, 2004.
153. Lewis, PB, et al: Basic science and treatment options for articular cartilage injuries. *J Orthop Sports Phys Ther* 36(10):717–728, 2006.

154. Lin, F, et al: In vivo and noninvasive six degrees of freedom patellar tracking during voluntary knee movement. *Clin Biomech* 18:401–409, 2003.
155. Lizaur, A, Marco, L, and Cebrian, R: Preoperative factors influencing the range of movement after total knee arthroplasty for severe osteoarthritis. *J Bone Joint Surg Br* 79(4):626–629, 1997.
156. Logan, M, et al: The effect of posterior cruciate ligament deficiency on knee kinematics. *Am J Sports Med* 32(8):1915–1922, 2004.
157. Logerstedt, D, and Sennett, BJ: Case series utilizing drop-out casting for the treatment of knee joint extension motion loss following anterior cruciate ligament reconstruction. *J Orthop Sports Phys Ther* 37(7): 404–411, 2007.
158. Logerstedt, DS, et al: Knee pain and mobility impairments: meniscal and articular cartilage lesions. *J Orthop Sports Phys Ther* 40(6):A1–A35. 2010.
159. Logerstedt DS, et al: Knee stability and movement coordination impairments: knee ligament sprain. *J Orthop Sports Phys Ther* 40(4): A1–A37, 2010.
160. Lohmander, LS, et al: The long-term consequences of anterior cruciate ligament and meniscus injuries: osteoarthritis. *Am J Sports Med* 35: 1756–1769, 2007.
161. Lynch, PA, et al: Deep venous thrombosis and continued passive motion after total knee arthroplasty. *J Bone Joint Surg Am* 70(1):11–14, 1988.
162. Magee, DJ: *Orthopedic Physical Assessment,* ed. 6. Philadelphia: Saunders (Elsevier), 2014.
163. Mahoney, OM, et al: The effect of total knee arthroplasty design on extensor mechanism function. *J Arthroplasty* 17:416–421, 2002.
164. Mangine, RE, et al: Postoperative management of the patellofemoral patient. *J Ortho Sports Phys Ther* 28(5):323–335, 1998.
165. Manifold, SG, Cushner, FD, and Scott, WN: Anterior cruciate ligament reconstruction with bone-patellar tendon-bone autograft: Indications, technique, complications, and management. In Insall, JN, and Scott, WN (eds): *Surgery of the Knee, Vol 1,* ed. 3. New York: Churchill Livingstone, 2001, p 665.
166. Martin, RL, and Kivlan, B: The ankle and foot complex. In Levangie, PK, and Norkin, CC (eds): *Joint Structure and Function. A Comprehensive Analysis,* ed. 5. Philadelphia: F.A. Davis, 2011, pp 444–485.
167. Martin, SD, Scott, RD, and Thornhill, TS: Current concepts of total knee arthroplasty. *J Orthop Sports Phys Ther* 28(4):252–261, 1998.
168. Mascal, CL, Landel, R, and Powers, C: Management of patellofemoral pain targeting hip, pelvis, and trunk muscle function: 2 case reports. *J Orthop Sports Phys Ther* 33(11):642–660, 2003.
169. Matsumoto, A, et al: A comparison of bone-patellar tendon-bone and bone-hamstring tendon-bone autografts for anterior cruciate ligament reconstruction. *Am J Sports Med* 34(2):213–219, 2006.
170. Mauro, CS, et al: Loss of extension following anterior cruciate ligament reconstruction: analysis of incidence and etiology using IKDC criteria. *Arthroscopy* 24:146–153, 2008.
171. McCarthy, MR, et al: The effects of immediate continuous passive motion on pain during the inflammatory phase of soft tissue healing following anterior cruciate ligament reconstruction. *J Orthop Sports Phys Ther* 17(2):96–101, 1993.
172. McConnell, J: The management of chondromalacia patellae: a long-term solution. *Aust J Physiother* 32:215–233, 1986.
173. McDevitt, ER, et al: Functional bracing after anterior cruciate ligament reconstruction: a prospective, randomized, multicenter study. *Am J Sports Med* 32(8):1887–1892, 2004.
174. McGrory, BJ, Stuart, MJ, and Sim, FH: Participation in sports after hip and knee arthroplasty: review of literature and survey of surgeon preferences. *Mayo Clin Proc* 70:342–348, 1995.
175. McHugh, MP, et al: Preoperative indicators of motion loss and weakness following anterior cruciate ligament reconstruction. *J Orthop Sports Phys Ther* 27(6):407–411, 1998.
176. McInnes, J, et al: A controlled evaluation of continuous passive motion in patients undergoing total knee arthroplasty. *JAMA* 268(11): 1423–1428, 1992.
177. McKenzie, K, et al: Lower extremity kinematics of females with patellofemoral pain syndrome with stair stepping. *J Orthop Sports Phys Ther* 40(10):625–632, 2010.
178. McKinnis, LN: *Fundamentals of Musculoskeletal Imaging,* ed. 4. Philadelphia: F.A. Davis, 2014.
179. McLaughin, J, et al: Rehabilitation after meniscus repair. *Orthopedics* 17(5):463–471, 1994.
180. Meier, W, et al: Total knee arthroplasty: muscle impairments, functional limitations, and recommended rehabilitation approaches. *J Orthop Sports Phys Ther* 38(5):246–256, 2008.
181. Mikkelsen, C, Werner, S, and Eriksson, E: Closed kinetic chain alone compared to combined open and closed kinetic chain quadriceps strengthening with respect to return to sports: a prospective, matched, follow-up study. *Knee Surg Sports Traumatol Arthrosc* 8:337–342, 2000.
182. Miller, SL, and Gladstone, JN: Graft selection in anterior cruciate ligament reconstruction. *Orthop Clin North Am* 33:675–638, 2002.
183. Minas, T, and Bryant, T: The role of autologous chondrocyte implantation in the patellofemoral joint. *Clin Orthop* 436:30–39, 2005.
184. Minas, T: Surgical management of patellofemoral disease. In Mizrayan, R (ed): *Cartilage Injury in the Athlete.* New York: Thieme, 2006, pp 273–285.
185. Mintken, PE, et al: Early neuromuscular electrical stimulation to optimize quadriceps muscle function following total knee arthroplasty: a case report. *J Orthop Sports Phys Ther* 37(7):364–371, 2007.
186. Mirza, F, et al: Management of injuries to the anterior cruciate ligament: results of a survey of orthopaedic surgeons in Canada. *Clin J Sport Med* 10(2):85–88, 2000.
187. Mizner, RL, Petterson, SC, and Snyder-Mackler, L: Quadriceps strength and time course of functional recovery after total knee arthroplasty. *J Orthop Sports Phys Ther* 35(7):424–436, 2005.
188. Mizner, RL, Stevens, JE, and Snyder-Mackler, L: Voluntary activation and decreased force production of the quadriceps femoris muscle after total knee arthroplasty. *Phys Ther* 83(4):359–365, 2003.
189. Moffet, H, et al: Effectiveness of intensive rehabilitation on functional ability and quality of life after first total knee arthroplasty: a single-blind, randomized trial. *Arch Phys Med Rehabil* 85:546–555, 2004.
190. Moksnes, H, Snyder-Mackler, L, and Risberg, MA: Individuals with an anterior cruciate ligament-deficient knee classified as noncopers may be candidates for nonsurgical rehabilitation. *J Orthop Sports Phys Ther* 38(10):586–595, 2008.
191. Mologne, TS, and Friedman, MJ: Arthroscopic anterior cruciate reconstruction with hamstring tendons: Indications, surgical technique, complications, and their treatment. In Insall, JN, and Scott, WN (eds): *Surgery of the Knee, Vol 1,* ed. 3. New York: Churchill Livingstone, 2001, p 681.
192. Mooney, MF, and Rosenberg, TD: Meniscus repair: The inside-out technique. In Jackson, DW (ed): *Master Techniques in Orthopedic Surgery: Reconstructive Knee Surgery,* ed. 2. Philadelphia: Lippincott Williams & Wilkins, 2003, pp 57–71.
193. Morgan, CD, and Leitman, EH: Meniscus repair: the all-inside arthroscopic technique. In Jackson, DW (ed): *Master Techniques in Orthopedic Surgery: Reconstructive Knee Surgery,* ed. 2. Philadelphia: Lippincott Williams & Wilkins, 2003, pp 73–91.
194. Morrey, BF, and Pagnano, MW: Mobile-bearing knee. In Morrey, BF (ed): *Joint Replacement Arthroplasty,* ed. 3. Philadelphia: Churchill Livingstone, 2003, pp 1013–1022.
195. Mulligan, BR: *Manual Therapy "NAGS", "SNAGS", "MWM's": etc.,* ed. 6. Wellington: Plane View Services Limited, 2010.
196. Mulvey, TJ, et al: Complications associated with total knee arthroplasty. In Pellicci, PM, Tria, AJ, and Garvin, KL (eds): *Orthopedic Knowledge Update 2. Hip and Knee Reconstruction.* Rosemont, IL: American Academy of Orthopedic Surgeons, 2000, p 323.
197. Murray, DW: Mobile bearing unicompartmental knee replacement. *Orthopedics* 28(9):985–987, 2005.
198. Myer, GD, et al: Rehabilitation after anterior cruciate ligament reconstruction: criterion-based progression through the return-to-sport phase. *J Orthop Sports Phys Ther* 36(6):385–402, 2006.

199. Myers, P, et al: The three-in-one proximal and distal soft tissue patellar realignment procedure: results and its place in the management of patellofemoral instability. *Am J Sports Med* 27:575–579, 1999.
200. Nakagawa, TH, Muniz, TB, and Baldon, R: The effect of additional strengthening of hip abductor and lateral rotator muscles in patellofemoral pain syndrome: a randomized, controlled pilot study. *Clin Rehabil* 22:1051–1056, 2008.
201. Noyes, FR, and Albright, JC: Reconstruction of the medial patellofemoral ligament with autologous quadriceps tendon. *Arthroscopy* 22(8):904, e1–e7, 2006.
202. Noyes, FR, and Barber-Westin, SD: Meniscal transplantation in symptomatic patients under fifty years of age. Survivorship analysis. *J Bone Joint Surg Am* 97:1209–1219. 2015.
203. Noyes, FR, and Barber-Westin, SD: Arthroscopic repair of meniscus tears extending into the avascular zone with or without anterior cruciate ligament reconstruction in patients 40 years of age and older. *Arthroscopy* 16(8):882–829, 2000.
204. Noyes, FR, and Barber-Westin, SD: Arthroscopic repair of meniscal tears extending into the avascular zone in patients younger than twenty years of age. *Am J Sports Med* 30(4):589–600, 2002.
205. Noyes, FR, Barber, SD, and Mangine, RE: Bone-patellar ligament-bone and fascia lata allografts for reconstruction of the anterior cruciate ligament. *J Bone Joint Surg Am* 72(8):1125–1136, 1990.
206. Noyes, FR, Barber-Westin, SD, and Rankin, M: Meniscal transplantation in symptomatic patients less than fifty years old. *J Bone Joint Surg Am* 86(7):1392–1404, 2004.
207. Noyes, FR, Barber-Westin, SD, and Rankin, M: Meniscal transplantation in symptomatic patients less than fifty years old: surgical technique. *J Bone Joint Surg Am* 87(Suppl 1, Part 2):149–165, 2005.
208. Noyes, FR, et al: Arthroscopy in acute traumatic hemarthrosis of the knee: incidence of anterior cruciate tears and other injuries. *J Bone Joint Surg Am* 62:687–695, 1980.
209. Noyes, FR, DeMaio, M, and Mangine, RE: Evaluation-based protocol: a new approach to rehabilitation. *J Orthop Sports Phys Ther* 14(12): 1383–1385, 1991.
210. Noyes, FR, Heckman, TP, and Barber-Westin, SD: Posterior cruciate ligament and posterolateral reconstruction. In Ellenbecker, TS (ed): *Knee Ligament Rehabilitation.* New York: Churchill Livingstone, 2000, pp 167–185.
211. Noyes, FR, Barber-Westin, SD, and Grood, ES: New concepts in the treatment of posterior cruciate ligament ruptures. In Insall, JN, and Scott, WN (eds): *Surgery of the Knee, Vol 1,* ed. 3. New York: Churchill Livingstone, 2001, p 841.
212. Olney, SJ, and Eng, J: Gait. In Levangie, PK, and Norkin, CC (eds): *Joint Structure and Function: A Comprehensive Analysis,* ed. 5. Philadelphia: F.A. Davis, 2011, pp 528–571.
213. Ortiguera, CJ, Hanssen, AD, and Stuart, MJ: Posterior cruciate-substituting and sacrificing total knee arthroplasty. In Morrey, BF (ed): *Joint Replacement Arthroplasty,* ed. 3. Philadelphia: Churchill Livingstone, 2003, pp 982–992.
214. Outerbridge, RE, and Dunlop, J: The problem of chondromalacia patellae. *Clin Orthop* 110:177–196, 1975.
215. Pagnano, MW, Papagelopoulas, PJ, and Rand, JA: Uncemented total knee arthroplasty. In Morrey, BF (ed): *Joint Replacement Arthroplasty,* ed. 3. Philadelphia: Churchill Livingstone, 2003, pp 993–1001.
216. Pagnano, MW, and Rand, JA: Posterior cruciate ligament retaining total knee arthroplasty. In Morrey, BF (ed): *Joint Replacement Arthroplasty,* ed. 3. Philadelphia: Churchill Livingstone, 2003, pp 976–981.
217. Pagnano, MW, and Rand, JA: Unicompartmental total knee arthroplasty. In Morrey, BF (ed): *Joint Replacement Arthroplasty,* ed. 3. Philadelphia: Churchill Livingstone, 2003, pp 1002–1012.
218. Palmitier, RA, et al: Kinetic chain exercises in knee rehabilitation. *Sports Med* 11(6):402–413, 1991.
219. Palmu, S, et al: Acute patellar dislocation in children and adolescents: a randomized, clinical trial. *J Bone Joint Surg Am* 90:463–470, 2008.
220. Papagelopoulos, PJ, and Sim, FH: Limited range of motion after total knee arthroplasty: etiology, treatment, and prognosis. *Orthopedics* 20:1061–1065, 1997.
221. Papagelopoulos, PJ, Sim, FH, and Morrey, BF: Patellectomy and reconstructive surgery for disorders of the patellofemoral joint. In Morrey, BF (ed): *Reconstructive Surgery of the Joints,* ed. 2. New York: Churchill Livingstone, 1996, p 1671.
222. Paris, MJ, Wilcon, RB, III, and Millett, PJ: Anterior cruciate ligament reconstruction: surgical management and postoperative rehabilitation considerations. *Orthop Phys Ther Pract* 17(4):14–24, 2005.
223. Patel, D: Arthroscopic synovectomy. In Jackson, DW (ed): *Master Techniques in Orthopedic Surgery: Knee Surgery,* ed. 2. Philadelphia: Lippincott Williams & Wilkins, 2003, pp 417–425.
224. Paulos, L, et al: Surgical correction of limb malalignment for instability of the patella: a comparison of 2 techniques. *Am J Sports Med* 37(7):1288–1300, 2009.
225. Paulos, LE, Walther, CE, and Walker, JA: Rehabilitation of the surgically reconstructed and nonsurgical anterior cruciate ligament. In Insall, JN, and Scott, WN (eds): *Surgery of the Knee, Vol 1,* ed. 3. New York: Churchill Livingstone, 2001, p 789.
226. Pearsall, AW, et al: The evaluation of refrigerated and frozen osteochondral allografts in the knee. *Surg Sci* 2:232–241. 2011.
227. Pepe, MD, Giffin, JR, and Haner, CD: Meniscal transplantation. In Jackson, DW (ed): *Master Techniques in Orthopedic Surgery: Reconstructive Knee Surgery,* ed. 2. Philadelphia: Lippincott Williams & Wilkins, Philadelphia, 2003, pp 93–101.
228. Perry, J: *Gait Analysis: Normal and Pathological Function.* Thorofare, NJ: Slack, 1992.
229. Philadelphia Panel: Evidence-Based Clinical Practice Guidelines on Selected Rehabilitation Interventions for Knee Pain. *Phys Ther* 81(10): 1675–1700, 2001.
230. Piva, SR, Coodnight, EA, and Childs, JD: Strength around the hip and flexibility of soft tissues in individuals with and without patellofemoral pain syndrome. *J Orthop Sports Phys Ther* 35(12):793–801, 2005.
231. Piva, SR, et al: A balance exercise program appears to improve function for patients with total knee arthroplasty: a randomized, clinical trial. *Phys Ther* 90(6):880–894, 2010.
232. Post, WR, and Fulkerson, JP: Surgery of the patellofemoral joint: Indications, effects, results, and recommendations. In Insall, JN, and Scott, WN (eds): *Surgery of the Knee, Vol 1,* ed. 3. New York: Churchill Livingstone, 2001, p 1045.
233. Powers, CM: The influence of abnormal hip mechanics on knee injury: a biomechanical perspective. *J Orthop Sports Phys Ther* 40(2):42–51, 2010.
234. Powers, CM: The influence of altered lower-extremity kinematics on patellofemoral joint dysfunction: a theoretical perspective. *J Orthop Sports Phys Ther* 33(11):639–646, 2003.
235. Powers, CM, et al: Patellofemoral pain: proximal, distal, and local factors—2nd international research retreat. *J Orthop Sports Phys Ther* 42(6):A1–A54, 2012.
236. Prims, MR, and van der Wurff, P: Females with patellofemoral pain syndrome have weak hip muscles: a systemic review. *Austral J Physiother* 55(1):9–15, 2009.
237. Rabin, A, et al: Factors associated with visually assessed quality of movement during a lateral step-down test among individuals with patellofemoral pain. *J Orthop Sports Phys Ther* 44(12):937–946, 2014.
238. Rajan, RA, et al: No need for outpatient physiotherapy following total knee arthroplasty. *Acta Orthop Scand* 75(1):71–73, 2004.
239. Rand, JA: Cemented total knee arthroplasty: Techniques. In Morrey, BF (ed): *Reconstructive Surgery of the Joints,* ed. 2. New York: Churchill Livingstone, 1996, p 1389.
240. Reinold, MM, et al: Current concepts in rehabilitation following articular cartilage repair procedures in the knee. *J Orthop Sports Phys Ther* 38(10):774–795, 2006.
241. Ricchetti, ET, et al: Comparison of lateral release versus lateral release with medial soft-tissue realignment for the treatment of recurrent patellar instability: a systematic review. *Arthroscopy* 23:463–468, 2007.
242. Richter, DL, et al: Knee articular cartilage repair and restoration techniques: A review of the literature. *Sports Health* doi:10.1177/1941738115611350. 2015.

243. Risberg, MA, et al: Neuromuscular training versus strength training first 6 months after anterior cruciate ligament reconstruction: a randomized, clinical trial. *Phys Ther* 87:737–750, 2007.
244. Risberg, MA, et al: The effect of knee bracing after anterior cruciate ligament reconstruction: a prospective, randomized study with two years' follow-up. *Am J Sports Med* 27:76–83, 1999.
245. Risberg, MA, et al: Design and implementation of a neuromuscular training program following anterior cruciate ligament reconstruction. *J Orthop Sports Phys Ther* 31(11):620–631, 2001.
246. Ritter, MA, et al: The effect of postoperative range of motion on functional outcomes after posterior-cruciate retaining total knee arthroplasty. *J Bone Joint Surg Am* 90(4):777–784, 2008.
247. Robinson, RL, and Nee, RJ: Analysis of hip strength in females seeking physical therapy for unilateral patellofemoral pain syndrome. *J Orthop Sports Phys Ther* 37(5):232–238, 2007.
248. Roddy, E, et al: Evidence-based recommendations for the role of exercise in the management of osteoarthritis of the hip or knee—The MOVE consensus. *Rheumatology* 44(1):67–73, 2005.
249. Roddy, E, Zhang, W, and Doherty, M: Aerobic walking or strengthening exercise for osteoarthritis of the knee? A systematic review. *Ann Rheum Dis* 64(4):544–548, 2005.
250. Roe, J, et al: A 7-year follow-up of patellar tendon and hamstring grafts for arthroscopic anterior cruciate ligament reconstruction: differences and similarities. *Am J Sports Med* 33(9):1337–1345, 2005.
251. Rossi, MD, and Hassan, S: Lower-limb force production in individuals after unilateral total knee arthroplasty. *Arch Phys Med Rehabil* 85: 1279–1284, 2003.
252. Saccomanni, B: Unicompartmental knee arthroplasty: a review of literature. *Clin Rheumatol* 29:339–346, 2010.
253. Sahrmann, S: *Diagnosis and Treatment of Movement Impairment Syndromes.* St. Louis: Mosby, 2002.
254. Schache, MB, McClelland, JA, and Webster, KE: Lower limb strength following total knee arthroplasty: A systematic review. *Knee* 21:12–20. 2014.
255. Schmitt, LC, et al: Instability, laxity, and physical function in patients with medial knee osteoarthritis. *Phys Ther* 88(12):1506–1516, 2008.
256. Schulz, MS, et al: Epidemiology of posterior cruciate ligament injuries. *Arch Orthop Trauma Surg* 123:186–191, 2003.
257. Schurman, DJ, and Rojer, DE: Total knee arthroplasty: range of motion across five systems. *Clin Orthop* 430:132–137, 2005.
258. Scott, RD: *Total Knee Arthroplasty.* Philadelphia: Saunders, 2006.
259. Scott, RD, et al: Long-term results of total knee replacement. In Pellicci, JM, Tria, AJ, and Garvin, KL (eds): *Orthopedic Knowledge Update, 2. Hip and Knee Reconstruction.* Rosemont, IL: American Academy of Orthopedic Surgeons, 2000, p 301.
260. Sculco, T, et al: Knee surgery and rehabilitation. In Melvin, JL, and Gall, V (eds): *Rheumatologic Rehabilitation Series, Vol 5. Surgical Rehabilitation.* Bethesda, MD: American Occupational Therapy Association, 1999, p 121.
261. Sekiya, JK, Ong, BC, and Bradley, JP: Complications in anterior cruciate ligament surgery. *Orthop Clin North Am* 34:99–105, 2003.
262. Sethi, P, Mirzayan, R, and Kharrazi, D: Microfracture technique. In Mirzayan, R (ed): *Cartilage Injury in the Athlete.* New York: Thieme Medical Publishers, 2006, pp 116–123.
263. Shaieb, MD, et al: A prospective, randomized comparison of patellar tendon versus semitendinosus and gracilis tendon autografts for anterior cruciate ligament reconstruction. *Am J Sports Med* 30(2):214–220, 2002.
264. Sharma, L, et al: Physical functioning over three years in knee osteoarthritis: role of psychosocial, local mechanical, and neuromuscular factors. *Arthritis Rheum* 48(12):3359–3370, 2003.
265. Shelbourne, KD, and Kloutwyk, TE: Rehabilitation after anterior cruciate ligament reconstruction. In Pedowitz, RA, O'Connor, JJ, and Akeson, WH (eds): *Daniel's Knee Injuries: Ligament and Cartilage Structure, Function, Injury, and Repair,* ed. 2. Philadelphia: Lippincott Williams & Wilkins, 2003, pp 493–500.
266. Shelbourne, KD, and Trumper, RV: Anterior cruciate ligament reconstruction: Evolution of rehabilitation. In Ellenbecker, TS (ed): *Knee Ligament Rehabilitation.* New York: Churchill Livingstone, 2000, pp 106–117.
267. Shelbourne, KD, and Urch, SE: Primary anterior cruciate ligament reconstruction using the contralateral autogenous patellar tendon. *Am J Sports Med* 28(5):651–658, 2000.
268. Sherman, OH, and Banffy, MB: Anterior cruciate ligament reconstruction: which graft is best? *Arthroscopy* 20(9):974–980, 2004.
269. Shoji, H, and Solomonov, M: Factors affecting postoperative flexion in total knee arthroplasty. *Clin Orthop* 13(6):643–649, 1990.
270. Silva, M, and Schmalzried, T: Knee strength after total knee arthroplasty. *J Arthroplasty* 18:605–611, 2003.
271. Singhal, MC, Fites, BS, and Johnson, DL: Fixation devices in ACL surgery: what do I need to know? *Orthopedics* 28(9):920–924, 2005.
272. Skou, ST, Rasmussen, S, et al: Knee confidence as it relates to self-reported and objective correlates of knee osteoarthritis: a cross-sectional study of 220 patients. *J Orthop Sports Phys Ther* 45(10):765–771, 2015.
273. Smidt, GL, Albright, JP, and Deusinger, RH: Pre- and postoperative functional changes in total knee patients. *J Orthop Sports Phys Ther* 6(1):25–29, 1984.
274. Smith, T, and Davies, L: The efficacy of continuous passive motion after anterior cruciate ligament reconstruction: a systematic review. *Phys Ther Sport* 8:141–152, 2007.
275. Snyder-Mackler, L, et al: Strength of the quadriceps femoris muscle and functional recovery after reconstruction of the anterior cruciate ligament. *J Bone Joint Surg Am* 77(8):1166–1173, 1995.
276. Soderberg, GL, and Cook, TM: An electromyographic analysis of quadriceps femoris muscle setting and straight leg raising. *Phys Ther* 63:1434–1438, 1983.
277. Souza, RB, et al: Femur rotation and patellofemoral joint kinematics: a weight-bearing magnetic resonance imaging analysis. *J Orthop Sports Phys Ther* 40(5):277–285, 2010.
278. Souza, RB, and Powers, CM: Differences in hip kinematics, muscle strength, and muscle activation between subjects with and without patellofemoral pain. *J Orthop Sports Phys Ther* 39(1):12–19, 2009.
279. Spencer, JD, Hayes, KC, and Alexander, IJ: Knee joint effusion and quadriceps reflex inhibition in man. *Arch Phys Med Rehabil* 65(4): 171–177, 1984.
280. Spindler, KP, et al: Anterior cruciate ligament reconstruction autograft choice: bone-tendon-bone versus hamstring. Does it really matter? A systematic review. *Am J Sports Med* 32(8):1986–1995, 2004.
281. Sprague, R: Factors related to extension lag at the knee joint. *J Orthop Sports Phys Ther* 3(4):178–182, 1982.
282. Steadman, JR, et al: Outcomes of microfracture for traumatic chondral defects of the knee: average 11-year follow-up. *Arthroscopy* 19:477–484, 2003.
283. Steindler, A: *Kinesiology of the Human Body Under Normal and Pathological Conditions.* Springfield, IL: Charles C Thomas, 1955.
284. Sterett, WI, et al: Effect of functional bracing on knee injury in skiers with anterior cruciate ligament reconstruction: a prospective cohort study. *Am J Sports Med* 34(10):1581–1585, 2006.
285. Stone, RC, Frewin, PR, and Gonzales, S: Long-term assessment of arthroscopic meniscus repair: a two to six year follow-up study. *Arthroscopy* 6(2):73–78, 1990.
286. Stratford, P: Electromyography of the quadriceps femoris muscles in subjects with normal and acutely effused knees. *Phys Ther* 62(3): 279–283, 1982.
287. Tadokoro, K, et al: Evaluation of hamstring strength and tendon regrowth after harvesting for anterior cruciate ligament reconstruction. *Am J Sports Med* 32(7):1644–1650, 2004.
288. Tagesson, S, et al: A comprehensive rehabilitation program with quadriceps strengthening in closed versus open kinetic chain exercise in patients with anterior cruciate ligament deficiency: a randomized, clinical trial evaluating dynamic tibial translation and muscle function. *Am J Sports Med* 36(2):298–307, 2008.
289. Tamburello, T, et al: *Patella hypomobility as a cause of extensor lag.* Research presentation. Overland Park, KS, May 1985.
290. Tanavalee, A, Choi, YJ, and Tria, AJ: Unicondylar knee arthroplasty: past and present. *Orthopedics* 28(12):1423–1433, 2005.
291. Thomas, SG, Pagura, SM, and Kennedy, D: Physical activity and its relationship to physical performance in patients with end stage knee osteoarthritis. *J Orthop Sports Phys Ther* 33(12):745–754, 2003.

292. Torchia, ME: Meniscal tears. In Morrey, BF (ed): *Reconstructive Surgery of the Joints,* ed. 2. New York: Churchill Livingstone, 1996, p 1607.
293. Tsai, AMH, and Pedowitz, RA: Meniscus injury and repair. In Pedowitz, RA, O'Connor, JJ, and Akeson, WH (eds): *Daniel's Knee Injuries: Ligament and Cartilage Structure, Function, Injury, and Repair,* ed. 2. Philadelphia: Lippincott Williams & Wilkins, 2003, pp 239–251.
294. Tyler, TF, and McHugh, MP: Neuromuscular rehabilitation of a female Olympic ice hockey player following anterior cruciate ligament reconstruction. *J Orthop Sports Phys Ther* 31(10):577–587, 2001.
295. Tyler, TF, et al: The effect of immediate weight bearing after anterior cruciate ligament reconstruction. *Clin Orthop* 357:141–148, 1998.
296. Tyler, TF, et al: The role of hip muscle function in the treatment of patellofemoral pain syndrome. *Am J Sports Med* 34:630–636, 2006.
297. Valtonen, A, et al: Muscle deficits persist after unilateral knee replacement and have implications for rehabilitation. *Phys Ther* 89(10): 1072–1079, 2009.
298. Walsh, M, et al: Physical impairments and functional limitations: a comparison of individuals 1 year after total knee arthroplasty with control subjects. *Phys Ther* 78:248–258, 1998.
299. Waryasz, GR, and McDermott, AY: Patellofemoral pain syndrome (PFPS): a systematic review of anatomy and potential risk factors. *Dyn Med* 26:7–9, 2008.
300. Wegener, L, Kisner, C, and Nichols, D: Static and dynamic balance responses in persons with bilateral knee osteoarthritis. *J Orthop Sports Phys Ther* 25(1):13–18, 1997.
301. Weiss, JM, et al: What functional activities are important to patients with knee replacements? *Clin Orthop* 404:172–188, 2002.
302. Whiteside, LA: Fixation in total knee replacement: Bone ingrowth. In Pellicci, PM, Tria, AJ, and Garvin, KL (eds): *Orthopedic Knowledge Update, 2. Hip and Knee Reconstruction.* Rosemont, IL: American Academy of Orthopedic Surgeons, 2000, p 275.
303. Wiley, JW, Bryant, T, and Minas, T: Autologous chondrocyte implantation. In Mirzayan, R (ed): *Cartilage Injury in the Athlete.* New York: Thieme Medical Publishers, 2006, pp 141–157.
304. Wilk, KE, and Andrews, JR: Current concepts in the treatment of anterior cruciate ligament disruption. *J Orthop Sports Phys Ther* 15(6): 279–293, 1992.
305. Wilk, KE, and Andrews, JR: The effects of pad placement and angular velocity on tibial displacement during isokinetic exercise. *J Orthop Sports Phys Ther* 17(1):24–30, 1993.
306. Wilk, KE, and Clancy, WG: Medial collateral ligament injuries: Diagnosis, treatment, and rehabilitation in knee ligament injuries. In Engle, RP (ed): *Knee Ligament Rehabilitation.* New York: Churchill Livingstone, 1991, p 71.
307. Wilk, KE, et al: Patellofemoral disorders: a classification system and clinical guidelines for nonoperative rehabilitation. *J Orthop Sports Phys Ther* 28(5):307–322, 1998.
308. Wilk, KE, Reinold, MM, and Hooks, TR: Recent advances in the rehabilitation of isolated and combined anterior cruciate ligament injuries. *Orthop Clin North Am* 34:107–137, 2003.
309. Williams, GN, et al: Dynamic knee stability: current theory and implications for clinicians and scientists. *J Orthop Sports Phys Ther* 31(10): 546–566, 2001.
310. Wilson, T, Carter, N, and Gareth, T: A multicenter, single-masked study of medial, neutral, and lateral patellar taping in individuals with patellofemoral pain syndrome. *J Orthop Sports Phys Ther* 33(8): 437–448, 2003.
311. Wilson, T: The measurement of patellar alignment in patellofemoral pain syndrome. Are we confusing assumptions with evidence? *J Orthop Sports Phys Ther* 37(6):330–341, 2007.
312. Wind, WM, Bergfeld, JA, and Parker, RD: Evaluation and treatment of posterior cruciate ligament injuries: revisited. *Am J Sports Med* 32(7):1765–1775, 2004.
313. Witvrouw, E, et al: Patellofemoral pain: consensus statement from the 3rd International Patellofemoral Pain Research Retreat held in Vancouver, September 2013. *Br J Sports Med* 48:411–414. 2014.
314. Wright, RW, and Fetzer, GB: Bracing after ACL reconstruction: a systematic review. *Clin Orthop Relat Res* 455:162–168, 2007.
315. Wright, RW, et al: A systematic review of anterior cruciate ligament reconstruction rehabilitation, part I: continuous passive motion, early weight bearing, postoperative bracing, and home-based rehabilitation. *J Knee Surg* 21:217–224, 2008.
316. Wright, TM: Biomechanics of total knee design. In Pellicci, PM, Tria, AJ, and Garvin, KL (eds): *Orthopedic Knowledge Update, 2. Hip and Knee Reconstruction.* Rosemont, IL: American Academy of Orthopedic Surgeons, 2000, p 265.
317. Zeni, JA, and Snyder-Mackler, L: Early postoperative measures predict 1- and 2-year outcomes after unilateral total knee arthroplasty: importance of contralateral limb strengthening. *Phys Ther* 90(1):43–55, 2010.
318. Zhang W, et al: OARSI recommendations for the management of hip and knee arthritis, Part II: OARSI evidence-based, expert consensus guidelines. *Osteoarthritis and Cartilage* 16:137–162, 2008.

CHAPTER

22

The Ankle and Foot

LYNN COLBY, PT, MS ■ CAROLYN KISNER, PT, MS
■ JONATHAN ROSE, PT, MS, SCS, ATC ■ JOHN BORSTAD, PT, PHD

The joints, ligaments, and muscles of the ankle and foot provide stability and mobility in the terminal structures of the lower extremity. During standing, the foot bears the weight of the body with minimum muscle energy expenditure. The foot must also be both pliable and relatively rigid depending on various functional demands. This versatility allows the foot to absorb forces, accommodate to uneven surfaces, and serve as a structural lever to propel the body forward during walking and running.

A clear understanding of the complex anatomy and kinesiology of the ankle and foot is important when treating impairment in this region of the body. The first section of this chapter reviews highlights of these areas the reader should know and understand. The second section contains guidelines for the management of disorders and surgeries in the foot and ankle region, and the third section describes exercise interventions for this region. Chapters 10 through 13 present general information on principles of management; the reader should be familiar with the material in these chapters and should have a background in examination and evaluation in order to effectively design a therapeutic exercise program to improve ankle and foot function in patients with impairments from injury, pathology, or recovery following surgery.

Structure and Function of the Ankle and Foot

The bones of the ankle and foot consist of the distal tibia and fibula, 7 tarsals, 5 metatarsals, and 14 phalanges (Fig. 22.1).

Structural Relationships and Motions

Anatomical Characteristics

The leg is structurally adapted to transmit ground reaction forces from the foot upward to the knee joint and femur during upright activities. Depending on the activity, the foot and ankle provide a foundation of either stability or motion to the distal extremity that assists the leg in managing forces and demands. The motions in the ankle and foot are defined using primary plane and triplanar descriptors.

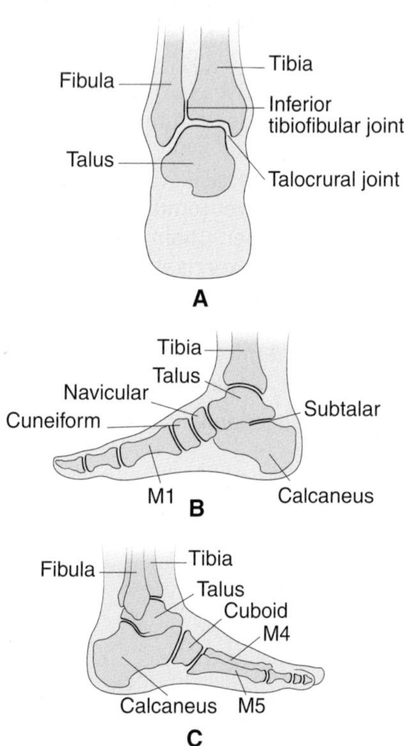

FIGURE 22.1 Bones of the ankle and foot. **(A)** Anterior view of the lower leg and ankle, **(B)** medial and **(C)** lateral views of the ankle and foot.

Leg

The tibia and fibula make up the leg. These two bones are bound together by an interosseous membrane between the bones, strong anterior and posterior inferior tibiofibular ligaments that hold the distal tibiofibular articulation together, and a strong capsule that encloses the proximal tibiofibular articulation. Unlike the radius and ulna in the upper extremity, the tibia and fibula do not rotate around each other, but there is slight movement between the two bones that allows greater ankle joint motion.

Foot

The foot is divided into three segments: hindfoot, midfoot, and forefoot.

Hindfoot. The talus and calcaneus make up the posterior foot segment.

Midfoot. The navicular, cuboid, and three cuneiforms make up the middle foot segment.

Forefoot. Five metatarsals and 14 phalanges make up the anterior foot segment. Each toe has 3 phalanges except for the large toe, which has 2.

Motions of the Foot and Ankle Defined

Primary Plane Motions

Although motions in the foot and ankle do not occur purely in the cardinal planes, they are still defined as follows:[71,211,293]

Sagittal plane motion around a frontal (coronal axis). *Dorsiflexion* is movement in a dorsal direction, which decreases the angle between the leg and dorsum of the foot, and *plantarflexion* is movement in a plantar direction. Motion occurring at the toes may also be called dorsiflexion, or extension, and plantarflexion, or flexion.

Frontal plane motion around a sagittal (anteroposterior) axis. *Inversion* is inward turning of the foot, and *eversion* is outward turning. Normally, an inward and outward motion is described by the terms abduction and adduction, but because the foot is at a right angle to the leg, the terms abduction and adduction are not used for this frontal plane motion.

Transverse plane motion around a vertical axis. *Abduction* is movement away from the midline, and *adduction* is movement toward the midline.

Triplanar Motion

Triplanar motion occurs around an oblique axis at each articulation of the ankle and foot. The definitions are descriptive of the movement of the distal bone on the proximal bone. When the proximal bone moves on the stabilized distal bone, as occurs in weight bearing, the motion of the proximal bone is opposite, although the relative joint motion is the same as defined.

Pronation. Pronation is a combination of dorsiflexion, eversion, and abduction. During weight bearing, pronation of the subtalar and transverse tarsal joints causes the arch of the foot to lower, and there is a relative supination of the forefoot with dorsiflexion of the first metatarsal and plantarflexion of the fifth metatarsal. This is the loose-packed or mobile position of the foot and is assumed when the foot absorbs the impact of weight bearing and rotational forces of the rest of the lower extremity and when the foot conforms to the ground.[71]

Supination. Supination is a combination of plantarflexion, inversion, and adduction. In the closed-chain, weight-bearing foot, supination of the subtalar and transverse tarsal joints with a pronation twist of the forefoot (plantarflexion of the first metatarsal and dorsiflexion of the fifth metatarsal) increases the arch of the foot and is the close-packed or stable position of the joints of the foot. This is the position the foot assumes when a rigid lever is needed to propel the body forward during the push-off phase of ambulation.[211,293]

NOTE: The terms *inversion* and *supination*, as well as *eversion* and *pronation*, are often used interchangeably.[252] This text uses the discrete terms defined above.

Joint Characteristics and Arthrokinematics: Leg, Ankle, and Foot

The characteristics of each joint in the leg, ankle, and foot dictate how they contribute to the function of the ankle and foot complex.[211,293]

Tibiofibular Joints

Anatomically, the superior and inferior tibiofibular joints are separate from the ankle, but they provide accessory motions that allow greater movement at the ankle. Fusion or immobility in these joints impairs ankle function. The strong mortise formed by the distal ends of the tibia and fibula makes up the proximal surface of the ankle (talocrural) joint.

Superior tibiofibular joint characteristics. The superior tibiofibular joint is a plane synovial joint made up of the fibular head and a facet on the posterolateral aspect of the rim of the tibial condyle. The facet faces posteriorly, inferiorly, and laterally. Although near the knee joint, it has its own capsule that is reinforced by the anterior and posterior tibiofibular ligaments.

Inferior tibiofibular joint characteristics. The inferior tibiofibular joint is a syndesmosis with fibroadipose tissue between the two bony surfaces. This strong articulation is supported by the crural tibiofibular interosseous ligament and the anterior and posterior tibiofibular ligaments.

Accessory motions. With dorsiflexion and plantarflexion of the ankle, there are slight accessory movements of the fibula. The direction of movement is variable depending on facet orientation of the proximal tibiofibular joint and elasticity in the tibiofibular ligaments. However, movement is necessary to allow full range of the talus in the mortise during ankle dorsiflexion.

Ankle (Talocrural) Joint

Characteristics. The ankle (talocrural) joint is a synovial hinge joint formed by the mortise (distal end of the tibia and the tibial and fibular malleoli) and trochlea (dome) of the talus. It is enclosed by a relatively thin and weak capsule. It, along with the subtalar joint, is supported medially by the medial collateral (deltoid) ligament and laterally by the lateral collateral (anterior and posterior talofibular and calcaneofibular) ligaments (Fig. 22.2).

The fibular malleolus extends farther distally and posteriorly than the tibial malleolus, so the mortise angles outward and downward. This causes the axis of motion to be rotated laterally 20° to 30° and inclined downward 10°. The surface of the mortise is congruent with the articulating surface of the body of the talus.

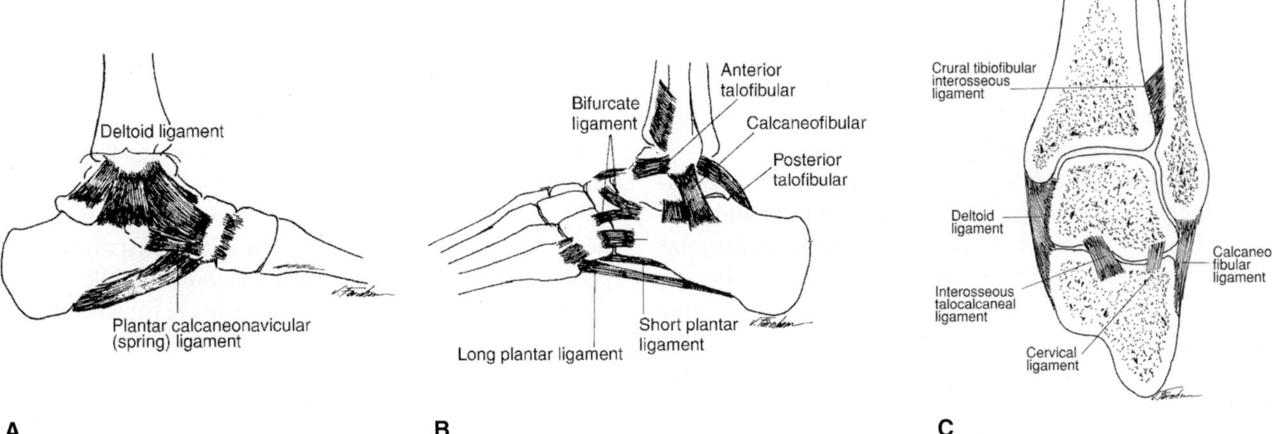

FIGURE 22.2 Ligaments of the ankle and foot. **(A)** Medial view, **(B)** lateral view, and **(C)** posterior (cross-sectional) view. *(From Martin, RL, and Kivlan, B: The ankle and foot complex. In Levangie, PK, and Norkin, CC (eds):* Joint Structure and Function, *ed. 5. Philadelphia: F.A. Davis, A and B, p 445; C, p 449, with permission.)*

The surface of the talus is wedge-shaped, wider anteriorly, and also cone-shaped, with the apex pointing medially. As a result of the orientation of the axis and the shape of the talus when the foot dorsiflexes, the talus also abducts and slightly everts (pronation). When the foot plantarflexes, the talus also adducts and slightly inverts (supination). Dorsiflexion is the close-packed, stable position of the talocrural joint; plantarflexion is the loose-packed position.

CLINICAL TIP

It is important to recognize that the stable positions of the ankle and the foot do not always coincide. For example, when a person walks in high heels, the ankle joint is more vulnerable to injury, because the talocrural joint is in a less stable, plantarflexed position while the subtalar and transverse tarsal joints are in a close-packed (rigid) position.

Arthrokinematics. The concave articulating surface is the mortise; the convex articulating surface is the body of the talus. With physiological motions of the foot, the articulating surface of the talus slides in the opposite direction. The arthrokinematics are summarized in ONLINE Box 22.1 and available on the FA Davis web site related to this textbook.

Subtalar (Talocalcaneal) Joint

Characteristics. The subtalar (talocalcaneal) joint is a complex joint with three articulations between the talus and calcaneus. It has an oblique axis of motion that lies approximately 42° from the transverse plane and 16° from the sagittal plane, allowing the calcaneus to pronate and supinate in a triplanar motion on the talus.

Frontal plane inversion (turning heel inward) and eversion (turning heel outward) can be isolated only with passive motion. The subtalar joint is supported by the medial and lateral collateral ligaments, which also support the talocrural joint; the interosseous talocalcaneal ligament in the tarsal canal; and the posterior and lateral talocalcaneal ligaments (see Fig. 22.2). In closed-chain activities, the joint attenuates the rotatory forces between the leg and foot so that, normally, excessive inward or outward turning of the foot does not occur as the foot maintains contact with the supporting surface.

Of the three articulations between the talus and calcaneus, the posterior is separated from the anterior and middle by the tarsal canal. The canal divides the subtalar joint into two joint cavities. The posterior articulation has its own capsule. The anterior articulations are enclosed in the same capsule as the talonavicular articulation, forming the talocalcaneonavicular joint. Functionally, these articulations work together.

Arthrokinematics. The facet on the bottom of the talus in the posterior compartment is concave, and the opposing facet on the calcaneus is convex. The facets of the anterior and middle articulations on the talus are convex, whereas the opposing facets on the calcaneus are concave. With open-chain physiological motions of the subtalar joint, the convex posterior portion of the calcaneus slides opposite to the motion; the concave anterior and middle facets on the calcaneus slide in the same direction, similar to turning a doorknob. With the component motion of eversion, as the calcaneus swings laterally, the posterior articulating surface slides medially, and with inversion, the posterior articulating surface slides laterally.

Talonavicular Joint

Characteristics. Anatomically and functionally, the talonavicular joint is part of a complex articulation between the talus and navicular as well as the anterior and medial facets of the subtalar joint. It is supported by the spring, the deltoid, the bifurcate, and the dorsal talonavicular ligaments. The triplanar motions of the navicular on the talus function with the subtalar joint, resulting in pronation and supination.

During pronation, in the weight-bearing foot, the head of the talus drops plantarward and medially, resulting in a pliable foot and decreased medial longitudinal arch. In essence, as the calcaneus everts, it cannot also dorsiflex and abduct with the foot on the ground, so the talus plantarflexes and inverts on the calcaneus. This downward and inward motion of the talar head results in an upward and outward motion of the navicular and a flattening of the arch. During supination, the opposite occurs, resulting in a structurally stable foot and an increased medial longitudinal arch. The calcaneus inverts, and the talus dorsiflexes and everts, resulting in the navicular plantarflexing, inverting, and adducting.

Arthrokinematics. The head of the talus is convex; the proximal articulating surface of the navicular is concave. With physiological motions of the foot, the navicular slides in the same direction as the motion of the forefoot. In the open-chain motion of pronation, the navicular slides dorsally and laterally (abduction and eversion), resulting in a flattening of the medial longitudinal arch. With supination, the navicular slides in a plantar and medial direction (adduction and inversion) (see ONLINE Box 22.1).

Transverse Tarsal Joint

Characteristics. The transverse tarsal joint is a functionally compound joint between the hindfoot and midfoot that includes the anatomically separate talonavicular and calcaneocuboid joints. The talonavicular joint is described in the previous section. The calcaneocuboid joint is saddle-shaped. The transverse tarsal joint participates in the triplanar pronation/supination motions of the foot and makes compensatory movements to accommodate variations in the ground. Passive accessory motions include abduction/adduction, inversion/eversion, and dorsal/plantar gliding.

Arthrokinematics. The articulating surface of the calcaneus is convex in a dorsal-to-plantar direction and concave in a medial-to-lateral direction. The articulating surface of the cuboid is reciprocally concave and convex.

Remaining Intertarsal and Tarsometatarsal Joints

The remaining intertarsal and tarsometatarsal joints are plane joints that reinforce the function of transverse tarsal joints and, during weight bearing, help regulate the position of the forefoot on the ground.

Metatarsophalangeal and Interphalangeal Joints of the Toes

The metatarsophalangeal (MTP) and interphalangeal (IP) joints of the toes are the same as the metacarpophalangeal and IP joints of the hand except that, in the toes, extension range of motion (ROM) is more important than flexion. Extension of the MTP joints is necessary for normal walking. Also, unlike the thumb, the large toe does not function separately from the other digits.

Function of the Ankle and Foot

Structural Relationships

Interdependence of leg and foot motions. In the weight-bearing foot, subtalar motion and tibial rotation are interdependent. Supination of the subtalar joint results in or is caused by lateral rotation of the tibia, and conversely, pronation of the subtalar joint results in or is caused by medial rotation of the tibia.[211,293]

Arches. The arches of the foot are visualized as a twisted osteoligamentous plate, with the metatarsal heads being the horizontally placed anterior edge of the plate, and the calcaneus being the vertically placed posterior edge. The twist causes the longitudinal and transverse arches. When the foot is bearing weight, the plate tends to untwist and flatten the arches slightly.[211]

- Primary support of the arches comes from the spring ligament, with additional support from the long plantar ligament, the plantar aponeurosis, and short plantar ligament (see Fig. 22.2). During push-off in gait, as the foot plantarflexes and supinates and the MTP joints go into extension, increased tension is placed on the plantar aponeurosis, which helps increase the arch. This is called the windlass effect.
- In the normal static foot, muscles do little to support the arches, yet without muscle tension, the passive supports stretch and foot pronation increases under weight-bearing loads. In this respect, muscles contribute to arch support during ambulation.

Effect on posture. During standing with weight equally distributed in both lower extremities, if one foot/ankle complex is more pronated than the other, the overall effect is a frontal plane asymmetry with a "short leg" on that side. All typical landmarks (crest of the ilium, greater trochanter, popliteal crease, head of the fibula, and medial malleolus) on the side of the pronated foot are slightly lower.

Abnormal foot postures. A person with a varus deformity of the calcaneus (observed nonweight bearing) may compensate by standing with a pronated (or everted) calcaneus posture.[72] Internal rotation of the leg, valgus at the knee, and internal rotation of the femur may also be seen with the pronated foot posture. The terms *pes planus*, *pronated foot*, and *flat foot* are often used interchangeably to mean a pronated posture of the hindfoot and decreased medial longitudinal arch. Pes cavus and supinated foot describe a high-arched foot.[252]

Muscle Function in the Ankle and Foot

Plantarflexors. Plantarflexion is caused primarily by the two-joint gastrocnemius muscle and the one-joint soleus muscle; these muscles attach to the calcaneus via the Achilles tendon.

Secondary plantarflexors. Other muscles passing posteriorly to the axis of motion of plantarflexion contribute minimally to that motion, but they have other functions.

- Tibialis posterior is a strong *supinator* and *invertor* that supports the medial longitudinal arch during weight bearing[247] and controls and reverses pronation during the loading response of gait.
- The flexor hallucis longus and flexor digitorum longus muscles flex the toes and help support the medial longitudinal arch. To prevent clawing of the toes (MTP extension with IP flexion), intrinsic muscles must also function at the MTP joints.
- The fibularis longus and brevis muscles primarily *pronate* the foot at the subtalar joint, and the longus gives support to the transverse and lateral longitudinal arches during weight-bearing activities.

Dorsiflexors. Dorsiflexion of the ankle is caused by the tibialis anterior muscle (which also inverts the ankle), the extensor hallucis longus and extensor digitorum longus (which also extend the toes), and the fibularis tertius muscles.

Intrinsic muscles. Intrinsic muscles of the foot function similarly to those of the hand (except there is no thumb-like function in the foot). In addition, they provide support to the arches during gait.

Stability in standing. During normal standing, the gravitational line is anterior to the axis of the ankle joint, creating a dorsiflexion moment. The soleus muscle contracts to counter the gravitational moment through its pull on the tibia. Other extrinsic foot muscles help stabilize the foot during postural sway.

The Ankle/Foot Complex and Gait

During the normal gait cycle, the ankle goes through a ROM of 32° to 35°. Approximately 7° of dorsiflexion occurs at the end of midstance, as the heel begins to rise, and 25° of plantarflexion occurs at the end of stance (toe off).[254]

Function of the Ankle and Foot Joints During Gait

The shock-absorbing, terrain-conforming, and propulsion functions of the ankle and foot include the following:[211,254,267]

- During the *loading response* (heel strike to foot flat), the heel strikes the ground in neutral or slight supination. As the foot lowers to the ground, it begins to pronate to its loose-packed position. The entire lower extremity rotates inward, reinforcing the loose-packed position of the foot. With the foot in a lax position, it can conform to variations in the ground contour and absorb some of the impact forces as the foot is lowered.
- Once the foot is fixed on the ground, dorsiflexion begins as the tibia advances over the foot. The tibia also rotates internally, which reinforces pronation of the subtalar joint and loose-packed position of the foot.
- During *midstance* and continuing through *terminal stance*, the tibia begins to rotate externally, initiating supination of the hindfoot and locking of the transverse tarsal joint. This brings the foot into its close-packed position, which is reinforced as the heel rises and the foot rocks up onto the toes, causing toe extension and tightening of the plantar aponeurosis (windlass effect). This stable position converts the foot into a rigid lever, ready to propel the body forward as the ankle plantarflexes from the pull of the gastrocnemius-soleus muscle group.

Muscle Control of the Ankle and Foot During Gait

Muscles of the ankle and foot function in the following manner during the gait cycle.[211,254,267]

Ankle dorsiflexors. The ankle dorsiflexors function during the initial foot contact and loading response (heel strike to foot flat) to counter the plantarflexion torque and to control the lowering of the foot to the ground. They also function during the swing phase to keep the foot from plantarflexing and dragging on the ground. With loss of the dorsiflexors, foot slap occurs at initial foot contact, and the hip and knee flex excessively during swing to prevent the toes from catching on the ground.

Ankle plantarflexors. Early in stance, the ankle plantarflexors function eccentrically to control the rate of forward movement of the tibia. Then, at around 40% of the cycle (midstance), there is a burst of concentric activity to initiate plantarflexion of the ankle for push off. Loss of function results in a slight lag of the lower extremity during terminal stance with no push-off.

Ankle evertors. Contraction of the peroneus longus muscle late in the stance phase facilitates transfer of weight from the lateral to the medial side of the foot. It also stabilizes the first ray and facilitates the pronation twist of the tarsometatarsal joints, as increased supination occurs in the hindfoot.

Ankle inverters. The tibialis anterior helps control the pronation force on the hindfoot, and the tibialis posterior helps control the pronation force on the medial longitudinal arch during the loading response of gait.

Intrinsic muscles. The intrinsic muscles support the transverse and longitudinal arches during gait.

Referred Pain and Nerve Injury

Several major nerves terminate in the foot. Injury or entrapment of the nerves may occur anywhere along their course—from the lumbosacral spine to near the nerves' termination. For treatment to be effective, it must be directed at the source of the problem. Therefore, a thorough history is obtained, and an examination is performed when the patient reports referred pain patterns, sensory changes, or muscle weakness. For a detailed description and illustrations of referred pain patterns and peripheral nerve innervations in the foot and ankle region, see Chapter 13 and related figures.

Major Nerves Subject to Pressure and Trauma

Common fibular nerve. Pressure on the common fibular (formerly common peroneal) nerve may occur as it courses laterally around the fibular neck and passes through an opening in the fibularis longus muscle.

Posterior tibial nerve. Entrapment in the tarsal tunnel, causing tarsal tunnel syndrome, may occur from a space-occupying lesion posterior to the medial malleolus.

Plantar and calcaneal nerves. These branches of the posterior tibial nerve may become entrapped as they turn under the medial aspect of the foot and pass through openings in the abductor hallucis muscle. Overpronation presses the nerves against these openings. Irritation of the nerves may elicit symptoms similar to those of acute foot strain (tenderness at the posteromedial plantar aspect of the foot), painful heel (inflamed calcaneal nerve), and pain in a pes cavus foot.

Common Sources of Segmental Sensory Reference in the Foot

The foot is the terminal point for the L4, L5, and S1 nerve roots coursing through the terminal branches of the fibular and tibial nerves. Referred pain may occur with irritation to tissues derived from the same spinal segments, or sensory changes from irritation or damage to these nerve roots (see Fig. 13.2).

Management of Foot and Ankle Disorders and Surgeries

To make sound clinical decisions when managing patients with foot and ankle disorders, it is necessary to understand the various pathologies, surgical procedures, and associated precautions, and to correctly identify impairments, activity limitations, and participation restrictions. In this section, common pathologies and surgeries are presented and the conservative and postoperative management of these conditions are described using principles of tissue healing and exercise intervention.

Joint Hypomobility: Nonoperative Management

Common Joint Pathologies and Etiology of Symptoms

Pathologies such as rheumatoid arthritis (RA), juvenile rheumatoid arthritis (JRA), and degenerative joint disease (DJD) will affect the foot and ankle complex, as will acute joint reactions after trauma, dislocation, or fracture. Postimmobilization contractures and adhesions can develop in the joint capsules and surrounding tissues when a joint is immobilized in a cast or orthosis for a period of time. The reader is referred to Chapter 11 for background information on arthritis, postimmobilization stiffness, and etiology of symptoms. The following section is specific to joint conditions of the ankle and foot.

RA. Pathology of the foot and ankle as the result of RA commonly affects the forefoot early in the disease process; the hindfoot later; and, least frequently, the ankle.[146,214] RA in the MTP, subtalar, and talocrural joints of the foot can lead to progressive instabilities and painful deformities such as hallux valgus and subluxation of the metatarsal heads. Tendon rupture within the foot and ankle may also result from chronic inflammation and can contribute to deformity.[146]

DJD and joint trauma. Degenerative symptoms occur in joints that are repetitively traumatized, and acute joint symptoms are often seen in conjunction with ankle sprains, chronic instability, or fracture. Posttraumatic arthritis leading to DJD is by far the most common type of arthritis affecting the ankle, accounting for approximately 70% to 80% of all ankle arthritis. In contrast, primary osteoarthritis, common in the hip and knee, is rare in the ankle, even in the older adult population.[214,346]

Postimmobilization stiffness. Contractures and adhesions in the capsule and surrounding periarticular soft tissues may occur any time the joint is immobilized after a fracture or surgery.

Gout. Symptoms commonly affect the MTP joint of the great toe, causing pain during terminal stance, resulting in decreased stance time and lack of smooth push-off.

Common Impairments of Structure and Function, Activity Limitations, and Participation Restrictions

In RA, many of the impairments and deformities listed here occur with progression of the disease.[146,308] With DJD and postimmobilization stiffness, only the affected joint(s) is limited.[44] Activity limitations and participation restrictions occur primarily as a result of loss of weight-bearing abilities.

- ***Restricted motion.*** When symptoms are acute, the patient experiences swelling and restricted, painful motion, particularly during weight-bearing activities. When symptoms are chronic, there is restricted motion, decreased joint play, and a firm capsular end-feel in the affected joint.
  - ***Proximal and distal tibiofibular joints.*** Restricted accessory motion in these joints can occur with periods of immobilization and limit ankle and subtalar joint motion.
  - ***Talocrural joint.*** Passive plantarflexion is more limited than dorsiflexion (unless the gastrocnemius-soleus muscle group also is shortened, in which case dorsiflexion is limited accordingly).[57]
  - ***Subtalar, transverse tarsal, and tarsometatarsal joints.*** Progressive limitation of supination develops until eventually the joint fixes in pronation with flattening of the medial longitudinal arch.[57] The close-packed position of the tarsals (supination) becomes more and more difficult to assume during the terminal stance (push-off) phase of gait. Moderate to severe foot pain is experienced with midfoot arthritis, especially during weight bearing.[277]
  - ***MTP joint of the large toe.*** Gross limitation of extension and some limitation of flexion develop; the rest of the MTP joints are variable. Lack of extension restricts the terminal stance phase of gait with an inability to rock up onto the metatarsal heads. This exacerbates the pronation posture and inability to supinate the foot during push-off in gait.
- ***Alignment deformities.*** Deformities occur due to a variety of factors including but not limited to muscle imbalances,

tendon rupture, faulty footwear, trauma, and heredity. Common deformities of the forefoot are described in Box 22.1.[205,308]

- ***Muscle weakness and decreased muscular endurance.*** Inhibition resulting from pain and relatively limited use of the extremities leads to impaired muscle function.
- ***Impaired balance and postural control.*** The sensory receptors in the ankle joints and ligaments, as well as in the muscle spindles, provide important information for using the *ankle strategy* for maintaining balance. The ankle strategy is used in balance control during perturbations (See Chapter 8). Faulty feedback and balance deficits occur when there is instability, muscle impairments, or arthritis.
- ***Increased frequency of falling.*** Impaired balance or a sense of instability (giving way) of the ankle may lead to frequent falling or fear of falling, thus restricting community outings.[214]
- ***Painful weight bearing.*** When symptoms are acute, weight-bearing activities are painful, preventing independent ambulation and causing difficulty in rising from a chair and ascending and descending stairs.
- ***Gait deviations.*** With pain during weight bearing, there is a short stance phase, reduced single limb support, and decreased stride length on the side of involvement. Because of the restricting motion and loss of effective plantarflexion and supination in the arthritic foot as well as pain in the forefoot area under the metatarsal heads, push-off is ineffective during terminal stance. Little or no heel rise occurs; instead, the person lifts up the involved foot to initiate the swing phase.
- ***Decreased ambulation.*** Because of decreased ankle and foot mobility and resulting decreased length of stride, distance and speed of ambulation are decreased; assistive devices may be necessary for ambulation. If pain, balance, or restricted motion is severe, a wheelchair may be required for mobility.

BOX 22.1 Common Arthritis-Related Forefoot Deformities

- ***Hallux valgus.*** This deformity in the great (large) toe develops as the proximal phalanx shifts laterally toward the second toe. Eventually the flexor and extensor muscles of the great toe shift laterally and further accentuate the deformity. The bursa over the medial aspect of the metatarsal head may become inflamed and the bone may hypertrophy, causing a painful bunion.
- ***Hallux limitus/hallux rigidus.*** Narrowing and eventual obliteration of the first MTP joint space occur with progressive loss of extension. This affects terminal stance by not allowing the foot to roll over the metatarsal heads and great toe for normal push-off. Instead, the individual turns the foot outward and rolls over the medial aspect of the large toe. This faulty pattern accentuates hallux valgus and foot pronation, and usually the MTP joint is quite painful.
- ***Dorsal subluxation/dislocation of the proximal phalanges on the metatarsal heads.*** If this occurs, the fat pad, which normally is under the metatarsal heads, migrates dorsally with the phalanges, and the protective cushion during weight bearing is lost, leading to pain, callus formation, and potential ulceration.
- ***Claw toe (MTP hyperextension and IP flexion) and hammer toe (MTP hyperextension, PIP flexion, and DIP hyperextension).*** These deformities result from muscle imbalances between the intrinsic and extrinsic muscles of the toes. Friction from shoes may cause calluses to form where the toes rub.

Joint Hypomobility: Management—Protection Phase

The interventions selected for management depend on the signs and symptoms present. For acute problems, follow the general outline presented in Chapter 10 and summarized in Box 10.1. Suggested interventions for the various goals are described in this section.[158,214,308] Box 22.2 lists the general non-operative intervention options for individuals with arthritis.

Educate the Patient and Provide Joint Protection

- Teach a home exercise program at the level of the patient's abilities.
- Teach the patient signs of systemic fatigue (especially in RA), local muscle fatigue, and joint stress and ways to modify exercises and activities to remain active within safe levels.
- Emphasize the importance of daily ROM and endurance activities.
- Educate on joint protection, specifically the need to avoid faulty foot and ankle postures and to protect the feet from the deforming, weight-bearing forces and trauma imposed by improperly fitting footwear.
- If necessary, instruct the patient in safe use of assistive devices to decrease the effects of weight bearing and pain.

Decrease Pain

In addition to physician-prescribed medication, intra-articular injections of corticosteroids or nonsteroidal anti-inflammatory

BOX 22.2 Nonoperative Interventions for Ankle Arthritis[108,242]

- Nonsteroidal anti-inflammatory agents
- Corticosteroid injections
- Viscosupplementation
- Physical therapy
- Activity modification
- Orthotics

medications and therapeutic use of modalities, the following are used to manage painful symptoms:

- ***Manual therapy techniques.*** Gentle grade I or II distraction and oscillation techniques may inhibit pain and move synovial fluid for nutrition within the involved joints.
- ***Orthotic devices.*** Orthotic shoe inserts and well-constructed shoes help protect the joints by providing support and realigning forces.[158,277] Such support has been shown to decrease pain and improve functional mobility. An orthosis or bracing may also be used to stabilize an arthritic joint.

FOCUS ON EVIDENCE

Kavlak and colleagues[158] reported the effects of prescribed orthotic devices in 18 patients with RA (no control group) and a variety of bilateral foot deformities, including pes planus, hallux valgus, hammer toe, subluxation of the metatarsal heads, and others. All patients in the study were community walkers with no history of foot or ankle surgery. All patients were prescribed custom-made orthotic inserts and shoe modifications, such as a medial longitudinal arch support, metatarsal pad, or heel and forefoot wedge, to meet their individual needs. Pain, temporal-distance characteristics of gait, and energy expenditure during walking were measured before and after the patients had been wearing the custom orthoses for 3 months. There was a significant reduction in pain and energy cost during ambulation and increases in step and stride length after use of the orthotic devices for 3 months. There were no significant changes in foot angle or the width of the base of support. The authors concluded that appropriately prescribed orthoses and shoe modifications were important elements of nonoperative treatment of foot pain and impaired gait in patients with RA.

Maintain Joint and Soft Tissue Mobility and Muscle Integrity

- ***Passive, active-assistive, or active ROM.*** It is important to move the joints as tolerated. If active exercises are tolerated, the benefits of the muscle action make them preferable to passive motion.
- ***Aquatic therapy.*** Aquatic therapy is an effective method of combining therapeutic heat with low-impact buoyancy-assisted exercises.
- ***Muscle setting.*** Apply resistance to generate gentle, multi-angle, muscle-setting exercises in pain-free positions at intensities that do not exacerbate symptoms.

Joint Hypomobility: Management—Controlled Motion and Return to Function Phases

Examine the patient for signs of decreased muscle flexibility, joint restrictions, muscle weakness, and balance impairments. Initiate exercises and mobilization procedures at a level appropriate for the condition of the patient.

PRECAUTIONS WITH RA: Because the disease process and use of steroid therapy weaken the tensile quality of the connective tissue, modify the intensity of joint mobilization and stretching techniques used to manage motion restrictions. It may be necessary to continue joint protection with orthotics, proper fitting shoes, and assistive devices for ambulation.[308] Encourage the patient to be active, but to also be aware of pain and fatigue.

Increase Joint Play and Accessory Motions

Joint mobilization techniques. Determine which articulations are restricted owing to decreased joint play and apply grade III sustained or grade III and IV oscillation techniques to stretch the limitations. (See Figures 5.55 through 5.64 and their descriptions in Chapter 5 for techniques to mobilize the leg, ankle, and foot articulations.) Mobilizing the toes is the same as the fingers (see Figs. 5.42 through 5.43).

Because weight-bearing forces and arthritic joint changes accentuate pronation, mobilizing to increase pronation should be undertaken cautiously in an arthritic foot. Perform these techniques only in the stiff foot after immobilization when the foot does not pronate sufficiently during the loading response in gait.

CLINICAL TIP

Extension of the toes at the MTP joints is important during terminal stance for normal push-off and development of the windlass effect in gait. The great toe requires from 40° to 50° extension to function effectively during this phase of gait.[254,267]

Improve Joint Tracking of the Talocrural Joint

Apply mobilization with movement (MWM) techniques to increase ROM and/or decrease pain associated with movement.[241] The principles of MWM are described in Chapter 5.

MWM: Plantarflexion

Patient position and procedure: Supine with hip and knee flexed and heel on the table (Fig. 22.3). Stand at the foot of the table facing the patient and contact the patient's anterior tibia with the palm of your hand (for the right foot use the left hand). Produce a pain-free graded posterior glide of the tibia on the talus. The patient should now be unable to plantarflex. While maintaining the posterior tibial glide grip the talus with your other hand (for the right foot, use the right hand) and create a passive end-range plantarflexion movement, causing the talus to roll anteriorly.

The sustained plantarflexion must be painless. Repeat 6 to 10 repetitions for 3 to 4 sets and reassess range.

MWM: Dorsiflexion

Patient position and procedure: Standing with the affected foot placed on a chair or stool (Fig. 22.4). Kneel on the floor facing the patient with a mobilization belt around your

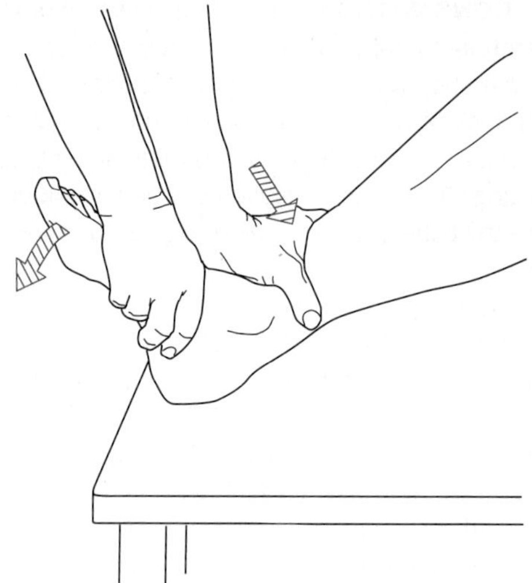

FIGURE 22.3 Mobilization with movement to increase ankle plantarflexion. Maintain a posterior glide of the tibia while moving the talus into plantarflexion. This should not cause pain.

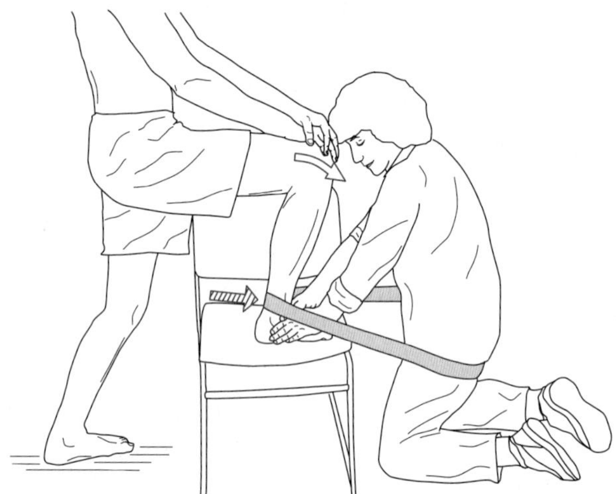

FIGURE 22.4 MWM to increase ankle dorsiflexion. Maintain an anterior glide of the tibia with the mobilization belt while the patient lunges forward into ankle dorsiflexion. This should not cause pain.

buttocks and the patient's Achilles tendon (padded with a towel). Place the web space of both hands around the neck of the talus with the palms on the dorsum of the foot. Hold the foot down and back and the subtalar joint in neutral pronation/supination. Use the belt to produce a pain-free graded anterior gliding force to the ankle joint. While maintaining this mobilization, have the patient lunge forward, bringing the affected ankle into dorsiflexion and causing painless end-range loading. Repeat 6 to 10 repetitions for 3 to 4 sets and reassess.

Increase Mobility of Soft Tissues and Muscles

Perform stretching techniques as described in Chapter 4. Self-stretching techniques are described later in this chapter.

Regain Balance in Muscle Strength and Prepare for Functional Activities

Initiate resistive exercises at a level appropriate for the weakened muscles. Begin with isometric resistance in pain-free positions and progress to dynamic resistance exercises through pain-free ranges using open- and closed-chain exercises. Resistive exercises are described later in this chapter.

CLINICAL TIP

Use a pool or tank to reduce stress on the foot and ankle joints for low-load, weight-bearing exercises; ambulatory activities; and for low-impact aerobic exercises.

Improve Balance and Proprioception

Initiate protected balance exercises, and progress the intensity as tolerated. Determine the level of stability and safety during ambulation and continue use of assistive devices if necessary to help prevent falls.

Develop Cardiopulmonary Fitness

Low-impact aerobic exercises should be initiated early in the treatment program and progressed as the patient is able. Water aerobics, swimming, treadmill walking, and bicycling may be within the patient's tolerance. A person with OA or RA should not perform high-impact (jumping, hopping, and jogging) aerobic exercises.

Joint Surgery and Postoperative Management

Advanced arthritis of the ankle or the joints of the foot can cause severe pain, motion limitations, gross instability or deformity, and significant loss of function during weight-bearing activities (Fig. 22.5). Unlike the hip and knee joints, the ankle is rarely affected by primary idiopathic arthritis, even in the elderly.[108,242,346] Instead, trauma is the most common cause of ankle and foot arthritis. When nonoperative management fails to alleviate symptoms, surgical options for early and advanced disease may be necessary[20,78,108,113,167,214,242,273,291,346,349,364] Selecting a specific surgical procedure depends upon the joint(s) involved, the extent of articular damage, the severity of instability or deformity, bone quality, and the postoperative functional goals of the patient.

The goals of surgery for arthritis are pain relief with maximum function. Arthroscopic repair of small osteochondral lesions, debridement of a symptomatic joint, and distraction arthroplasty are used for management of early joint changes, particularly in an individual younger than 50 years old whose symptoms are unsuccessfully managed conservatively and who is unwilling to consider arthrodesis or arthroplasty.[108,214,243] These procedures, however, offer little symptomatic relief or functional improvement when there is

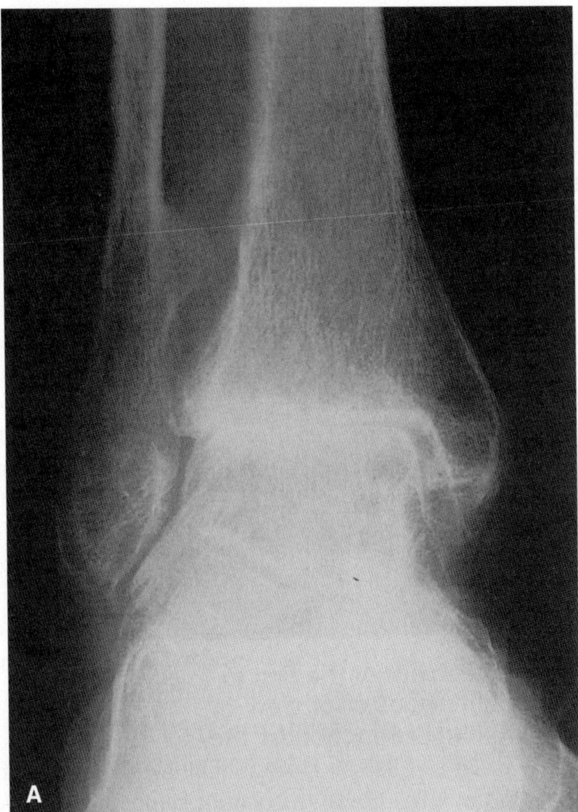

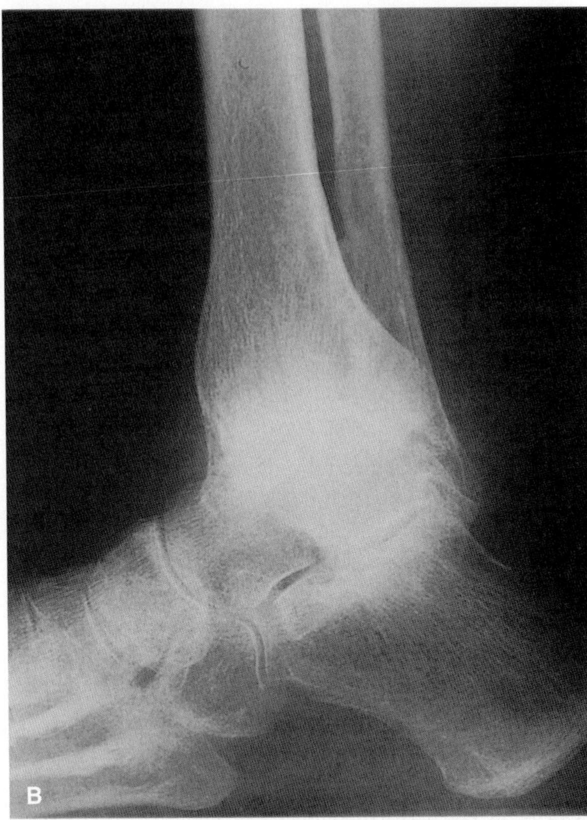

FIGURE 22.5 Late-stage arthritis of the ankle. **(A)** Mortise view of the ankle shows severe loss of the normal joint space and partial erosion of the lateral tibia. **(B)** Lateral view shows tibial erosion with mild joint space loss in the subtalar region and significant osteophyte formation in the anterior ankle. *(From Hasselman, CT, Wong, YS, and Conti, SF: Total ankle replacement. In Kitaoka, HB (ed):* Master Techniques in Orthopedic Surgery: The Foot and Ankle, *ed. 2. Philadelphia: Lippincott Williams & Wilkins, 2002, Fig. 39.1, p 583, with permission.)*

significant destruction of articular cartilage.[78,108,214,243,346,364] For symptomatic stage 3 ankle arthritis, ankle arthrodesis and ankle arthroplasty become the most viable surgical options.[103,108,113,242] Arthrodesis is typically performed in younger patients with high functional demands[45,108,130,214,242,346] and has the advantage of pain relief during weight bearing but the disadvantage of limited motion with functional activities. Following ankle arthrodesis, pain-free compensatory motion must be available in adjacent joints to absorb weight-bearing forces during ambulation. Although ankle arthrodesis is performed 6 times more frequently than total ankle arthroplasty,[276] replacement arthroplasty is becoming a more common procedure in the United States.[20,108,273] Replacement arthroplasty of the ankle[108,113,130,167,170,172,243,283,291] or toes[349] has the advantage of motion preservation and predictable pain relief, with the disadvantage of more frequent complications.

Following joint surgery and postoperative rehabilitation for the ankle and foot, anticipated benefits include:[108,214,242,243,346,349]

- Pain relief with weight bearing and joint motion
- Deformity correction
- Restored stability or mobility to affected joints
- Improved muscle strength and endurance
- Improved ambulation and lower extremity function

Rehabilitation includes postoperative exercise; gait training with assistive devices; fabrication of foot orthoses; joint and soft tissue mobilization; neuromuscular reeducation; and patient education including information about activity modification (activities of daily living [ADLs] and recreational activities) and shoe fit and selection.

Total Ankle Arthroplasty

Individuals with pain and disability from advanced, symptomatic ankle arthritis have two potential surgical procedures, total ankle arthroplasty (TAA) and ankle arthrodesis. TAA is an option for carefully selected patients who have pain and impaired functional mobility from advanced, symptomatic arthritis of the talocrural joint. TAA provides pain relief while preserving functional ankle joint motion, reducing stress on adjacent joints more effectively than arthrodesis.[108,243,318] Until recently, the ideal candidate for TAA was the thinner individual older than age 50 with low physical demands, minimal joint deformity, and near full ROM.[113] Recent reports indicate that although obesity remains a risk factor for postoperative complications, improvement in pain and function is similarly beneficial for active individuals younger than 50 years old.[167,283,371] Therefore, TAA is becoming a management option for younger, more active individuals (typically those with either posttraumatic arthritis or RA) who wish to continue to participate in moderately demanding activities. Improvements in implant design, instrumentation for implant alignment, and the use of bio-ingrowth fixation have broadened the selection criteria for TAA,[66,108,113,130,131,243,283,291] resulting in an increased number of TAA procedures.[273,276]

Indications for Surgery

Although end-stage ankle arthritis is the primary indication for TAA, there is little clinical guidance on which to base more specific indications for this surgery.[66,108,113,130,243,283,291] Commonly cited indications describe the adult patient with end-stage ankle arthritis who has failed conservative management and has persistent pain that compromises functional mobility. Conditions include advanced degenerative or inflammatory joint disease, including posttraumatic arthritis; primary OA, RA, or JRA; or avascular necrosis of the dome of the talus. This patient should have:[108,243]

- Low to moderate physical demands
- Sufficient integrity of ligaments for ankle stability
- A flexible deformity that can be passively corrected to neutral or less than 5° of hindfoot valgus
- Adequate vascular flow and soft tissue envelope to allow for wound healing.

TAA can also be performed following ankle arthrodesis as a salvage procedure for an individual with persistent pain during weight bearing and long-term, unsatisfactory functional results.

Contraindications

There are a number of absolute and relative contraindications to current-day TAA.[108,113,243] Absolute contraindications include active or chronic ankle infection; severe osteoporosis or poor bone stock; avascular necrosis of a significant portion of the body of the talus; peripheral neuropathy leading to decreased sensation or paralysis; impaired lower extremity vascular supply; and long-term corticosteroid use. As with replacement of other joints, TAA is contraindicated for the skeletally immature individual.

Relative contraindications include a remote history of infection; severe malalignment (hindfoot varus or valgus deformity > 20°); presence of marked instability; restricted total arc of sagittal plane motion (combined dorsiflexion and plantarflexion) less than 20°; positive tobacco use; obesity; and the need to return to high demand, high-impact physical activity.

Procedure

Implant Design, Materials, and Fixation

Current total ankle systems consist of three components: a metallic baseplate that is fixed to the tibia, a domed or condylar-shaped metal component that resurfaces the talus, and a polyethylene bearing surface interposed between the tibial and talar components.[108,113,243] Because contemporary prosthetic designs more closely mimic the characteristics of a normal ankle joint, ROM available in several of these systems is nearly equivalent to that of a normal ankle.[353] Contemporary TAA also requires far less bony resection and typically utilizes cementless (bio-ingrowth) fixation with hydroxyapatite coated metal implants.[243]

Contemporary implants are divided into two basic categories: fixed-bearing and mobile- bearing. A system is considered fixed-bearing if the polyethylene bearing surface is fixed to the tibial baseplate and mobile-bearing if the polyethylene component is not fixed. The mobile-bearing design allows for joint surface sliding (anterior-posterior and medial-lateral directions) and rotation of the free polyethylene component.[243,383] Polyethylene component movement in a mobile-bearing design should, in theory, maintain a congruent articulation between the talar and polyethylene components, decreasing mechanical wear.[243,292] Valderrabano et al,[355] however, found very little anterior-posterior movement of the talar polyethylene component, noting that the mobile-bearing design functioned largely like a fixed-bearing design. Aside from the mobile-bearing Scandinavian Total Ankle Replacement (STAR) system, the implants approved for use in the United States are fixed-bearing designs (Fig. 22.6).[243]

Operative Overview

General TAA procedure. Although there are numerous variations of TAA operative techniques, the following steps represent the key components.[17,34,108,130,167,209,243,307] Any significant deformity above or below the ankle joint is corrected before placement of the system implants.[243] An

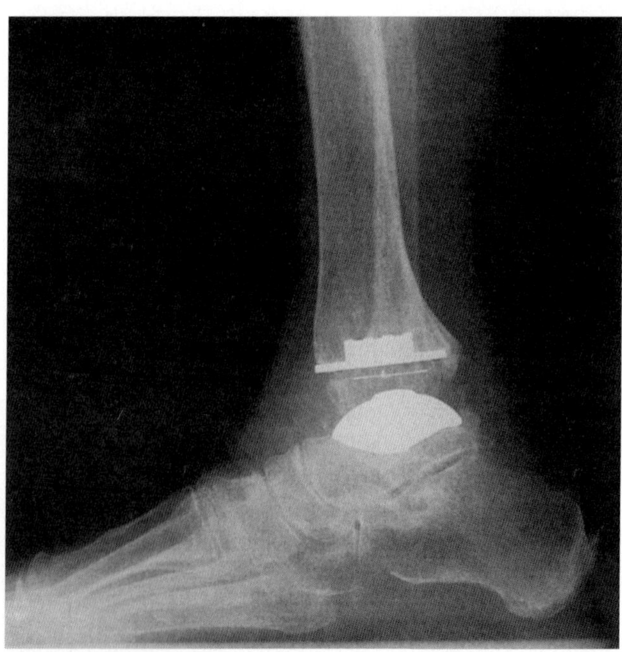

FIGURE 22.6 Total ankle arthroplasty. Lateral view of a total ankle replacement in a 78-year-old woman 1 year after surgery for posttraumatic arthritis. *(From Kitaoka, HB, and Claridge, RJ: Ankle replacement arthroplasty. In Morrey, BF (ed):* Joint Replacement Arthroplasty, *ed. 3, 2003, p 1148, with permission from The Mayo Clinic Foundation.)*

anterior longitudinal incision between the tibialis anterior and extensor hallucis tendon is the most widely used approach. The extensor retinaculum and capsule are incised to expose the dorsal ankle and talonavicular joints. The joint is debrided and osteophytes are removed from the dorsal talonavicular joint. An external distraction device is used to separate the joint surfaces and facilitate bone resection. Small portions of the distal tibia and talar dome are excised, followed by preparation of the joint surfaces. In some cases, the medial and lateral malleolar recesses are also resurfaced. Trial implants are inserted to evaluate their alignment and the range of dorsiflexion available. Permanent implants are selected and inserted. Any necessary soft tissue balancing or repair is performed. After the wound is closed, a bulky compression dressing and well-padded, posterior orthosis or short-leg cast is applied to control swelling and limit ROM.

Adjunctive procedures. If there is less than 5° of dorsiflexion because of a gastrocnemius-soleus contracture, a percutaneous lengthening of the Achilles tendon is performed. When a larger surface for fixation of the tibial prosthesis is needed, fusion of the tibiofibular syndesmosis with screw fixation is performed through a lateral incision.[113,170,243] In the case of a significant varus or valgus hindfoot deformity, a subtalar arthrodesis is performed.[130,243,307] Ligamentous stability is imperative for optimal outcome, so if instability persists intraoperatively after placement of the permanent implants, a lateral ligament reconstruction is performed.[243]

Complications

The current rate of complications after contemporary TAA appears to have decreased compared to rates with early implant designs and surgical techniques.[114,123,167,243,371] However, insufficient evidence is available to draw a firm conclusion regarding true complication rates, with reports varying widely.[176,180,182,360] Krause et al[176] pooled data from 20 studies published between 1999 and 2009 and reported an average 5-year complication rate of 29.5% (range 4.4% to 98.1%). Despite improvements in implant design, surgical technique, and patient selection, complication rates of >50% have been reported at intermediate and long-term follow-up evaluations.[176,180,182,302,321] Complication rates are higher in obese individuals, individuals with diabetes, and individuals who use tobacco.[250,299,300,371]

Complications can occur intraoperatively, in the early postoperative period, and in the long term. Fracture of the medial or lateral malleolus is the most frequent intraoperative complication, reported to occur in approximately 10% of procedures, with one report citing a 38% incidence rate.[11,108,176,243,290,302] Other intraoperative complications include implant malpositioning, tendon laceration, and nerve injury. As with all types of joint arthroplasty, postoperative infection is a potential complication. Deep infection rates range from 1% to 5%.[176,263] Postoperative edema in the ankle and foot also increases the risk of delayed wound healing by prolonging the immobilization period, delaying early ankle motion, and potentially leading to poor ROM outcomes.[108,167,209,243,245] Tarsal tunnel syndrome, soft tissue impingement, or complex regional pain syndrome occasionally develop, causing foot and ankle pain. (Complex regional pain syndromes and interventions are described in Chapter 13.) Box 22.3 summarizes common early postoperative and long-term complications associated with TAA.[17,108,113,130,176,180,182,243,263,291,302] Any of these complications can adversely affect the progression of rehabilitation and the short-term and long-term outcomes of TAA. Persistent or severe complications may necessitate revision arthroplasty or ankle arthrodesis.

Postoperative Management

There are few published guidelines in the literature for postoperative management of patients who have undergone TAA. Those that are available vary considerably regarding the duration of immobilization, weight-bearing restrictions, and the initiation and progression of exercise. There is a lack of evidence to support whether ROM exercises should be initiated a few days postoperatively or delayed several weeks until there is evidence of bone ingrowth into the implants. It is also unclear whether protected motion has a positive impact on ROM outcomes or if it is detrimental to implant fixation or wound healing.[243,292] Due to the higher rate of complications, postoperative management typically is less aggressive (longer periods of restricted weight bearing and longer periods of immobilization) for TAA when compared to total hip and knee arthroplasty.

The guidelines and precautions in the following sections for postoperative management summarize the recommendations of several authors based on their experience and training.[6,17,34,130,150,209,214,291]

BOX 22.3 Potential Postoperative Complications of Total Ankle Arthroplasty

Early Postoperative Complications → Potential Consequence(s)

- Delayed wound healing → an extended period of restricted ankle motion
- Delayed union or nonunion of a tibiofibular syndesmosis fusion → an extended immobilization and restricted weight-bearing period
- Tarsal tunnel syndrome or complex regional pain syndrome

Late Postoperative Complications → Potential Consequence(s)

- Component migration or impaction → malalignment and premature component wear
- Mechanical (aseptic) loosening (most often the talar component) → pain and impaired functional mobility
- Hindfoot arthritis (most often the subtalar joint) → pain and impaired weight-bearing abilities
- Heterotopic bone formation → restricted motion

Immobilization and Weight-Bearing Considerations

Immobilization. After the wound is closed following surgery, the ankle is placed in a compression dressing and immobilized in a neutral position in a well-padded short leg cast or posterior orthosis. This is left in place for 10 to 21 days, after which time it is replaced with a short-leg walking cast, controlled ankle motion (CAM) walker boot, or ankle foot orthosis. The duration of continuous immobilization and initiation of ROM exercises varies depending on the type of implant fixation used, the types of concomitant surgical procedures performed during the arthroplasty, and the surgeon's recommendations. Length of immobilization depends on the most restrictive tissue healing consideration. For example, if a tibiofibular syndesmosis or subtalar fusion was performed, no motion is allowed for 6 weeks or until there is evidence of bony union.[170,150] If a soft tissue procedure is required (e.g., ligamentous reconstruction), the period of immobilization may be extended. Without adjunctive procedures, immobilization following cementless fixation ranges from 2 to 6 weeks.[17,150,214,291]

Weight bearing. Recommendations for the initiation and extent of weight bearing after TAA vary significantly and can be affected by many factors including the causative pathology, the type of fixation, adjunctive procedures, patient characteristics, and physician preference. Guidelines range from non-weight bearing for 3 to 6 weeks[6,150,214,291] to minimal immediate postoperative weight bearing that progresses to weight bearing as tolerated within the first 2 weeks.[6,17,34,130,150,176] Adjunctive procedures can delay weight bearing. If a tibiofibular syndesmosis or hindfoot fusion is performed, or if an intraoperative malleolar fracture requires fixation, weight bearing is delayed for at least 6 weeks.[167,170,176]

In most cases, full weight bearing is generally achieved by 6 weeks following surgery.[6,130,150,214] Weight bearing is initiated with the leg in an ankle immobilizer.[6,150,176] After the initial period of restricted weight bearing, a patient gradually progresses to full weight bearing over several weeks while remaining in the immobilizer. This gradual progression to full weight bearing in the immobilizer is followed by a gradual return to full weight bearing without the immobilizer after 6 weeks.[150]

Exercise: Maximum Protection Phase

The first phase of postoperative rehabilitation, which extends for about 6 weeks, focuses on the patient becoming functionally mobile while protecting the operative ankle. Postoperative edema management and deep vein thrombosis prevention are critical in this period of restricted mobility and weightbearing.[18] During this phase, ankle ROM exercises are usually initiated. [6,150,214]

Goals and interventions. In addition to elevation and compression for edema management, maintenance of mobility to joints distal and proximal to the ankle, and strength and endurance training of the upper extremities and contralateral lower extremity, goals and interventions include the following:[17,150,214,290]

- ***Prevent postoperative complications***
  - Patient education related to signs/symptoms associated with deep vein thrombosis and infection.
- ***Re-establish independent ambulation and functional mobility***
  - Gait training with assistive devices
  - Transfers and mobility
  - Patient education regarding weight-bearing restrictions
- ***Minimize atrophy of the ankle and foot muscles of the operative limb***
  - Low-intensity, isometric (muscle-setting) exercises of the ankle musculature within the immobilizer.
- ***Prevent stiffness of the operated ankle and foot and loss of tissue extensibility of surrounding soft tissues.***
  - Active ROM of the toes
  - Gentle ankle active ROM exercises if removal of the immobilizer is permitted and the wound demonstrates sufficient healing. Initially include active ROM dorsiflexion/plantarflexion. Inversion, eversion and circumduction may be postponed until after 6 weeks after surgery.[6,150]

NOTE: ROM of the operative ankle may be permitted as early as 2 weeks after surgery or delayed as long as postoperative week 6.[150]

Exercise: Moderate and Minimum Protection Phases

Except in cases of poor soft tissue healing or delayed bony ingrowth, use of the immobilizer is generally discontinued and weight bearing restrictions are removed about 6 weeks after surgery. During the moderate and minimum protection phases of postoperative rehabilitation after TAA, emphasis is placed on increasing the range of functional ankle dorsiflexion and plantarflexion and increasing the strength of the plantarflexors.[6,150,214] Improving standing balance and ankle proprioception are also important for a gradual return to functional activities. Formal rehabilitation is generally completed 3 to 6 months after surgery.[150]

CLINICAL TIP

The level of physical activity possible after TAA depends on many factors, including patient characteristics (obesity, general health), the underlying pathology (DJD, OA, or RA), other joint involvement, prior level of activity, and the patient's goals for recovery. These factors should be considered and discussed when setting patient-centered goals.

Goals and interventions. During the moderate and minimum protection phases, the goals and interventions include:[6,150,292]

- ***Achieve 100% of the ROM obtained intraoperatively.***
  - Active, pain-free ROM exercises in nonweight-bearing positions, followed by active pain-free ROM in weight

positions. Include dorsiflexion, plantarflexion, inversion, eversion, and circumduction.
- Stretching of the gastrocnemius-soleus muscle group is indicated if dorsiflexion is limited. Begin with a towel stretch in a long-sitting position; progress to standing on a wedge for an extended period of time.

CLINICAL TIP

An arc of motion that ranges from 20° plantarflexion to 10° of dorsiflexion is necessary for normal gait over level surfaces.[267] Achievement of 20° of dorsiflexion is needed for descending stairs.[205] The amount of ankle dorsiflexion achieved while pedaling a bicycle can be adjusted by raising or lowering the seat height. A lower seat height requires greater dorsiflexion.

- ***Restore strength, muscular endurance, and balance in the lower extremities for functional activities.***
  - Low-intensity, high-repetition, open-chain, resisted exercise using elastic resistance initially, progressing to closed-chain exercises including squats, lunges, heel raises, and arch raises.
  - A progression of bilateral and unilateral balance activities beginning on stable surface and introducing progressive surface instability (refer to Chapters 8 and 23 for examples).
- ***Improve aerobic capacity and cardiopulmonary endurance.***
  - Swimming, stationary cycling, and treadmill walking.
- ***Resume a safe level of work-related and recreational activities.***
  - Integration of strength and balance training into simulated functional activities.
  - Activity modification for joint protection.
  - Patient education to help the patient return to safe and appropriate activities.

PRECAUTION: No clinical studies have demonstrated that participation in high-level athletic activities are associated with increased TAA failure.[133] However, plyometric training and other activities that involve high-impact and quick stop-and-go motions are generally considered inappropriate following TAA.[197,354]

Return to fitness and sports activities. With advances in TAA design and surgical techniques, plus expanding knowledge of long-term outcomes, it is now possible for selected patients to participate in low to moderately demanding fitness and sport activities.[133,197,354] These patients typically are younger (<60 years of age), were physically active prior to surgery, and underwent TAA for posttraumatic arthritis. A consensus of recommendations has recently been published, indicating activities that surgeons routinely recommend or prohibit following TAA (Table 22.1 summarizes these activity recommendations). Low-impact activities that do not require quick stop-and-go motions are routinely recommended; moderate-impact activities and activities performed in a motion limiting boot are allowed in patients with previous experience. High-impact activities, activities with risk of contact or collision, or activities that require cutting or jumping are not recommended.[133,354] Participation in fitness and sport activities is recommended only after completion of an individualized rehabilitation program in patients who are free from complications.[197,250,354]

Outcomes

Although early TAA afforded pain relief for a period of time,[113] unacceptable complication rates led to poor functional outcomes and patient dissatisfaction.[113,291,292] Modern

TABLE 22.1 Suggested Activity Recommendations Following TAA[197]

Allow All Patients	Allow Patients With Previous Experience	Not Recommended
Aquatic Fitness/Swimming	Doubles tennis	Court Sports
Biking	Hiking	▪ Badminton
▪ Road	Skating	▪ Basketball
▪ Stationary	▪ Rollerblading	▪ Racquetball/Squash
Bowling	▪ Ice skating	▪ Singles tennis
Dancing	Skiing	▪ Volleyball
Elliptical and stairclimber	▪ Cross country	Field Sports
Golf	▪ Downhill	▪ American football
Low-impact aerobics	Lower extremity resistance training	▪ Soccer
Pilates/Yoga	▪ Free weights	▪ Lacrosse
Walking/Speed walking	▪ Machines	▪ Baseball/Softball
	Mountain biking	Gymnastics
		High-impact aerobics
		Jogging/Running
		Snowboarding
		Waterskiing

surgical techniques and more judicious patient selection have resulted in more encouraging outcomes, although long-term success rates remain unknown.[17,113,122,291,292] It is important to note that although prospective and retrospective studies have compared implant designs, no studies to date have compared rehabilitation factors, such as early vs. delayed weight bearing or ROM exercises following TAA.

Pain, ROM, general level of function, patient satisfaction, and postoperative complications are the outcomes most often reported in follow-up studies. A variety of quantitative assessment instruments are used to measure pain relief, postoperative function, and patient satisfaction. Two examples of validated assessment instruments are the Ankle Osteoarthritis Scale (AOS) and the American Orthopedic Foot and Ankle Society Questionnaire (AOFAS). Survival rates, the percentage of prostheses not requiring removal at given time points after surgery, are also frequently reported.

Prosthesis survival rates. Arthroplasty survival rates reported in the literature vary, but they appear to be trending upward.[113,182,251,318] Labek et al[182] reported 5-year survival rates just below 90% in most data sets, and limited data sets demonstrate 10-year survival rates of approximately 75%. Evidence from prospective studies suggest similar TAA survival rates for patients with OA (primary or posttraumatic arthritis) and RA at mid-term (5 years)[265] and long-term (14 years)[173] follow-up. Relative to patient age, prospective studies indicate no difference in implant survival rates for patients older or younger than 50 years of age at short-term (3 years)[66] or mid-term (median follow up of 6 years)[170] follow-up. Retrospective studies indicate that obesity negatively impacts long-term survival rates and results in increased postoperative complications.[30,250,299,371]

When considering reports of TAA outcomes, note that many of the published reports represent studies conducted by implant developers.[165] Labek et al[180,181] noted a significant difference in the revision rates in published sample series compared with those taken from national joint registries. Revision rates collected in national joint registries are approximately twice as high as those reported in published sample series studies. Labek et al[180,182] suggest that because implant developers represent 50% of the published sample series content, their data may be proportionately overrepresented and thus influence outcomes reported in systematic reviews.

Pain relief, functional improvement, and patient satisfaction in different populations. Bai et al[17] prospectively compared outcomes following mobile-bearing TAA in patients with posttraumatic arthritis versus primary OA. At a mean follow-up of 38 months, no significant between-group differences were found in ankle ROM, radiographic findings, and an ankle-hindfoot assessment scale. Survival rates of the implants were comparable between the posttraumatic and primary OA groups (97% and 100%, respectively) at the conclusion of the study. However, complication rates were significantly higher (38% vs. 27%) in the posttraumatic arthritis group than in the primary OA group.

Gaudot et al[101] retrospectively compared outcomes of statistically paired individuals with mobile-bearing versus fixed-bearing TAA implants. The authors found no statistical difference for postoperative complications between the two groups at a mean follow-up of 24 months. While postoperative AOFAS scores were significantly higher than preoperative scores for both groups, the fixed-bearing group postoperative scores were significantly higher than those in the mobile-bearing group. No between-group postoperative differences were reported for ankle ROM or radiographic imaging. The authors concluded that fixed-bearing TAA had results equivalent to, if not better than, mobile-bearing.

In a multicenter study, Daniels et al[58] prospectively followed 281 individuals who underwent TAA for an average of 5.5 years. Seventeen percent of the patients required a subsequent revision surgery, and the major complication rate was 19%. Final AOS total, pain, disability scores, and SF-36 physical component summary score all significantly improved when compared to baseline measures. When compared to 107 individuals who underwent ankle arthrodesis, no significant postoperative group differences were found for any outcome variables.

Although several studies report no difference in pre- and postoperative ROM, Ajis et al[6] reported significant improvement in dorsiflexion at 6 weeks and 6 months following TAA. Dorsiflexion increased from a preoperative mean of 6.6° to a 12-month postoperative mean of 12.0°, while total arc of sagittal plane motion (terminal plantarflexion to terminal dorsiflexion) increased from 22.7° preoperatively to 24.3° postoperatively, a change that was not statistically significant.

Outcomes for a frequently used second generation, two-component system and more recently developed third generation, three-component (mobile-bearing) designs have been reported but not directly compared. Knecht[170] reported positive outcomes (reduced pain and increased function) in 66 patients who had undergone a two-component ankle replacement a mean of 9 years earlier. The mean total arc of dorsi- and plantarflexion measured in 33 patients was 18°.

Buechel and colleagues[34] followed 50 patients (mean age 49 years), who had received a mobile-bearing replacement with cementless fixation. They reported 48% excellent and 40% good results at a mean follow-up of 5 years (range 2 to 10 years). Of the 50 patients who participated in the study, 26% reported no pain after TAA, 60% reported slight or mild pain, and 14% reported moderate or severe pain that interfered with functional activities. The mean total arc of dorsi- and plantarflexion was 28°. In a short-term follow-up study of 116 patients who had a different mobile-bearing prosthesis implanted in 122 ankles, 84% of patients were satisfied, with 82% reporting good or excellent results at an average of 19.9 months.[131] The mean total arc of ankle dorsi- and plantarflexion was 39°. Although postoperative gains in ROM reported in these studies were small (often as little as 5° to 10°), gains of even a few degrees have been reported to improve functional mobility.[292]

Participation in physical activities. Although most TAA outcome studies evaluate prosthetic survival rates or clinical variables, the ability to return to a physically active lifestyle is also of interest. Naal et al[246] compared the preoperative and postoperative activity levels of 101 patients who had undergone TAA secondary to posttraumatic arthritis (46.5%), primary OA (34.7%), or RA (18.8%). One year prior to surgery, 62.4% were active in sport and fitness activities, while 66.3% were active at an average of 3.7 years after surgery. The types of activities and the frequency of participation before and after surgery were essentially unchanged; however, 65% of those surveyed indicated that performance during their preferred activities had improved following TAA. Swimming, cycling, and weight training for fitness were the most frequently reported activities before and after surgery. Although some patients participated in high-impact sports (i.e., jogging, soccer, and tennis) before surgery, few or none participated in these activities at follow-up, perhaps because of postoperative patient education. Of the three diagnostic groups, the individuals in the posttraumatic arthritis group reported decreased sport and fitness participation and were the least satisfied with their ability to participate in sport.

Schuh et al[303] prospectively collected sport and recreational activity participation rates in 21 patients scheduled for TAA. Following TAA, participation rates declined from 86% to 76%, but this change was not statistically significant. The most common activities reported post-TAA were cycling (45%), swimming (45%), hiking (25%), Nordic walking (20%), and skiing (15%). A recent systematic review of post-TAA activity indicated that sport and recreation participation remains relatively unchanged following TAA, and there is no evidence identifying sport activity as a risk factor for TAA failure.[133] In general, surgeons are comfortable recommending low-impact sports and aerobic activities to most TAA recipients.[197]

Valderrabano and coinvestigators[354] studied 147 patients (mean age 59.6 years, range 28 to 86 years) who participated in sports and recreational activities before and after TAA. Of these patients, 89% had a preoperative diagnosis of posttraumatic arthritis or primary OA, and only 11% had a diagnosis of RA. A combined total of 83% of all patients in the study reported excellent or good results and 69% were pain-free postoperatively. Just prior to surgery, 36% of patients were active in sports/recreational activities, and 56% were active at a mean of 2.8 years after surgery. This change reflected an increase in the activity level of the patients with posttraumatic arthritis and primary OA, not of the patients with RA. The most frequently reported preoperative activities (in descending order) were cycling, swimming, hiking, and low-impact aerobics. After surgery, hiking was most frequently reported followed by cycling, swimming, and aerobics. The only significant change in activity before and after surgery was an increase in hiking (participation spiked from 25.5% to 52.8%). The authors recommended that before initiating any sport activity after ankle replacement, a patient should complete postoperative rehabilitation and be free of complications.

Arthrodesis of the Ankle and Foot

Ankle arthrodesis (fusion) is the most frequently used surgery for late-stage arthritis of the ankle or foot and toe joints.[20,273,276] Although the rate of TAA has been increasing, ankle arthrodesis is still performed over six times more frequently than replacement.[276] Ankle fusion (AF) is the procedure of choice for relatively young, active patients with posttraumatic arthritis and gross instability of the ankle and hindfoot.[315,346] Arthrodesis also is an option for patients with hindfoot or forefoot involvement as the result of RA or JRA.[84,242,244] Deformities of the forefoot such as hallux valgus or hallux rigidus and severe deterioration of the MTP joint of the first toe are also managed with arthrodesis.[7,108,242,244]

Indications for Surgery

The following are frequently cited indications for surgical fusion of selected joints of the ankle and foot:[2,7,84,113,242,244,294,346]

- Debilitating pain, particularly during weight bearing, and severe articular degeneration secondary to posttraumatic or postinfectious arthritis, OA, RA, or other inflammatory arthropathies
- Marked instability or stiffness of one or more joints that is unresponsive to conservative management
- Deformity of the ankle, foot, or toes associated with chronic joint malalignment as the result of congenital anomalies, neuromuscular disorders, or arthritis
- Osteonecrosis of the talus
- A salvage procedure after failed total ankle arthroplasty

Generally, indications for arthrodesis and arthroplasty are very similar. Arthrodesis has been the "gold standard" option for younger patients with high functional demands and pain-free compensatory movements.[214,242,346] However, as ankle arthroplasty implants and techniques have improved, patients under the age of 50 with the above conditions can determine the most appropriate procedure based on the risks and benefits of the respective procedures.[243,283]

Contraindications to Surgery

Absolute contraindications include vascular impairment or infection of the limb. Relative contraindications include uncontrolled diabetes, active tobacco use, and severe ipsilateral subtalar arthrosis or contralateral ankle arthrosis.[242]

NOTE: For patients with RA or primary RA of both ankles, bilateral arthrodesis is rarely performed because loss of dorsiflexion bilaterally limits an individual's ability to rise from a chair or ascend and descend stairs.

Procedures

There are many types of arthrodesis; however, all involve the use of bone grafts coupled with internal fixation devices (see Fig. 12.2) or occasionally external skeletal fixation for bony ankylosis.[84,242] Common to all techniques is appropriate positioning of the ankle to maximize function: neutral dorsiflexion/plantarflexion, approximately 5° of external rotation, 5° of valgus, and slight posterior translation of the talus under the tibia.[108,242] Internal fixation is considered the best fusion technique and can be achieved via multiple compression screws, pins, an intramedullary nail, or a plate. The type of fixation selected depends on the joints involved and extent of deformity. For correction of severe deformity or tendon rupture, concomitant soft tissue procedures are required.[108,145,242]

Arthrodesis at the ankle or foot has traditionally been performed through an open approach. Over the past decade, however, mini-open, arthroscopically-assisted and fully arthroscopic arthrodesis of the ankle have become viable surgical options.[84,102,108,145,242,260,305,341] Although previously reserved for ankles with minimal deformity, arthroscopic fixation has recently been shown to be a viable option for ankles with deformity greater than 15°.[59,104,289] The benefit of an arthroscopic approach is the reduced rate of wound healing complications secondary to less soft tissue disruption during surgery.[145,242,328,346] There have also been reports of shorter hospital stays, decreased blood loss, lower morbidity, and reduced time to union with an arthroscopic approach. However, these potential benefits are based largely on data from nonrandomized, retrospective studies rather than controlled comparisons to an open approach.[59,84,104,248,348,379]

Common Types of Arthrodesis

Arthrodesis of the ankle. This procedure fuses the talus to the tibia in a position that maximizes function: 0° dorsiflexion and 5° to 10° external rotation of the foot to match the contralateral Fick angle.[108,242,294,346] Slight plantarflexion may be tolerated, but a talocrural joint fixed in dorsiflexion may result in intractable heel pain.[242] Once osteophytes are removed and the tibial and talar articular surfaces are prepared, internal fixation is achieved with two or three screws connecting the tibia and talus. Fixation of the fibula to the talus and tibia with a plate and transmalleolar screws can provide an added measure of stability. Bone graft is often used to augment bone healing.[242] Although ankle arthrodesis provides pain relief and ankle stability, dorsiflexion and plantarflexion are lost, thus altering the biomechanics and speed of gait and increasing energy expenditure during ambulation.[346] The hindfoot and forefoot compensate to a great extent for the loss of motion at the ankle. Despite this, an asymmetrical gait pattern is detectable in most patients after ankle arthrodesis.[45]

FOCUS ON EVIDENCE

Thomas et al[347] reported significant between-group differences in gait between 27 patients who had undergone tibiotalar arthrodesis and 27 age-matched control subjects. Cadence and stride length were significantly decreased in the arthrodesis group as were motions of the hindfoot and midfoot during the swing and stance phases of gait. In addition, radiographic evaluation demonstrated evidence of severe hindfoot arthritis in 15% of the arthrodesis group. The arthrodesis group was analyzed at a mean duration of 44 months' postsurgery.[347]

Arthrodesis of the hindfoot. Hindfoot arthrodesis is indicated when conservative management (including arch supports, appropriate footwear, ankle and hindfoot bracing, and oral or injected anti-inflammatory medication) has failed. Severe pain, instability, or chronic hindfoot deformity (pes valgus or pes planus) as the result of advanced hindfoot arthritis may require a triple arthrodesis or a single-joint fusion.[232,280,325] Procedures include talonavicular, talocalcaneal (subtalar), or triple arthrodesis. A triple arthrodesis—often indicated for a rigid hindfoot deformity—involves fusion of the talocalcaneal, talonavicular, and calcaneocuboid joints.[5,231,280,325] A talocalcaneal arthrodesis is indicated to correct heel valgus if the midtarsal joint has been spared. A single-joint fusion, such as a talonavicular arthrodesis, may be sufficient to correct a chronic but flexible hindfoot deformity.[280] In most instances, the hindfoot is positioned in 5° of valgus in each of these fusions.

Talonavicular, subtalar, or triple arthrodesis provides permanent medial-lateral stability and pain relief in the hindfoot, but pronation and supination of the ankle are eliminated or substantially diminished.[343] It is interesting to note that fusion of the talonavicular joint alone indirectly reduces motion at the subtalar and calcaneocuboid joints, providing frontal plane stability without fusing additional joints.[331,343]

Arthrodesis of the first toe. Arthrodesis of the first MTP joint for hallux rigidus and hallux valgus provides pain relief at rest and with ambulation in 80% to 90% of patients.[7,60,86,97,280] The position of fusion is neutral rotation, 10° to 20° of valgus and 15° to 30° of dorsiflexion. Although the toe may not contact the ground during quiet stance, this position allows adequate push-off during ambulation and does not necessarily require customized footwear.[60,97,280] If the lateral MTP joints are involved, fusion of the great toe is performed after excision arthroplasty of the lateral joints.[97,280,349]

Comparisons of first MTP arthrodesis to arthroplasty have generally favored arthrodesis for pain relief, balance, ambulation, and cosmesis.[280] Recent studies report mixed results, noting higher patient satisfaction with arthroplasty but better functional results with arthrodesis.[86,286] Long-term outcomes of the newer generation first MTP prostheses have not yet been determined.[280]

Arthrodesis of the IP joints of the toes. Fusion of the IP joints of the toes in a neutral position for hammer toes (typically toes 2 to 3) provides relief of pain with ambulation and improved shoe fit.[146,280,334]

Complications

The overall complication rate associated with arthrodesis is relatively low but can vary by patient population, the joint involved, and the surgical technique.[242,346,379] The most common complication is nonunion, occurring in up to 10% of arthrodesis procedures.[114,242,248,280,379] The smaller the area of the bony surfaces and the poorer their vascular supply, the higher the rate of nonunion. Factors that contribute to nonunion include postoperative infection, malalignment of the fused joint, and a patient's use of tobacco before and after surgery.[168,231] Table 22.2 summarizes risk factors for nonunion in foot and ankle arthrodesis.[242,344] Arthrodesis nonunion typically requires revision arthrodesis.[242,379]

In addition to pain and decreased function associated with nonunion, nerve damage can occur due to the surgical procedure; and neuromas can develop postoperatively.[242] These conditions can lead to postoperative pain and limited function. Occasionally postoperative stress fracture of a fused bone or an adjacent bone occurs. Subsequent arthritis in adjacent joints requires arthrodesis in up to 5% of individuals.[379] Delayed wound healing is a particular problem in patients with poor vascularity of the foot and ankle.

Postoperative Management

Immobilization. The method and duration of immobilization of the fused joint(s) are determined by the surgeon and are based on the fusion site, the type of fixation used, the quality of fixation achieved, the patient's bone quality, and the presence of factors that affect bone healing.

After surgical fixation and wound closure, a compression dressing and orthosis are applied and worn for 48 to 72 hours for edema control.[84,242,280] For ankle or hindfoot arthrodesis, a short-leg, nonweight-bearing cast is applied following removal of the postoperative dressing. This is typically worn for 4 to 8 weeks and is changed as needed to accommodate limb-swelling changes. A short-leg walking cast or rigid boot is applied at 4 to 8 weeks, and immobilization continues for an additional 6 to 8 weeks.[84,168,231,242,280,290,294] After arthrodesis of the first MTP joint, a short-leg cast or surgical shoe with a flat, rigid sole is worn to protect the joint as it heals.[86,97,280,286]

TABLE 22.2 Risk Factors Associated With Arthrodesis Nonunion[344]

Patient Factors		Surgical Factors
Systemic	**Local**	
Diabetes Tobacco/Alcohol Use Osteoporosis NSAID/Corticosteroid use Weight bearing compliance	Infection Vascularity Avascular necrosis Soft tissue injury	Open/Arthroscopic Construct stability Surgeon experience Revision arthrodesis

When radiographs show evidence of fusion, the patient is weaned from the immobilizer over several weeks.[84,242,280] After orthosis use is discontinued, the patient should be advised of proper shoe selection, modification, and fit. The use of a custom-made foot orthosis may be necessary for support, relief of pressure or shock absorption.[285,314] Rocker bottom shoes have been recommended following ankle arthrodesis, but a recent biomechanical study determined that running shoes provided similar—or better—beneficial effects in gait parameters including speed and forefoot maximal force.[14]

Weight-bearing considerations. As with postoperative immobilization, the timing and extent of weight bearing permissible following arthrodesis varies widely in published guidelines.[36,84,112,183,242] The same considerations that influence decisions about immobilization also influence the progression of postoperative weight bearing on the operated extremity. The most prevalent practice is to substantially restrict weight bearing for a minimum of 6 weeks after ankle and hindfoot arthrodesis. Mobility is accomplished with a wheelchair, a standard walker, crutches, or rolling knee walker. When radiographs show evidence of bony union, partial weight bearing is initiated in a rigid short-leg boot or shoe. Most individuals progress to full weight bearing in typical footwear by 12 to 16 weeks postoperatively. With midfoot and forefoot arthrodesis, partial to full weight bearing is initiated earlier, either immediately or within the first 4 weeks.[28,112,183]

FOCUS ON EVIDENCE

In an effort to reduce recovery time and improve quality of life following arthrodesis, early weight bearing has been explored. Cannon et al[36] conducted a nonrandomized, retrospective study of two groups of patients following arthroscopic ankle arthrodesis. One group (n = 15) was immobilized and instructed in either non-weight bearing or touch weight bearing for 8 weeks. A second group (n = 21) was immobilized in a removable orthosis and encouraged to begin weight bearing as tolerated immediately following surgery. No difference in time to union was found when comparing the two groups. Additional trials using randomization and controls are still needed to fully assess the effects of early weight bearing.

Postoperative exercises. Prior to bony fusion, care is needed to avoid stressing the fixation. Initially, postoperative exercises focus on active ROM of the nonoperated joints proximal or distal to the joints that are immobilized. If the patient is wearing a removable orthosis, active ROM exercises of the nonoperated joints confined by the immobilizer may be permissible early in the rehabilitation program as well.[36,385] For example, after ankle or hindfoot arthrodesis, exercises to maintain toe mobility are indicated in addition to knee

ROM.[385] For a patient with RA, active ROM is essential in all involved joints not restricted by the immobilization device.

When bony fusion has occurred and use of the immobilizer has been discontinued, postimmobilization muscle weakness, balance deficiencies, and adjacent joint hypomobilities should be addressed. The type of fixation should be considered in exercise prescription. For example, a subtalar fusion will limit inversion and eversion of the foot, reducing the capacity for isotonic posterior tibialis strengthening.

Return to physical activities. Studies with relatively small samples have investigated the ability of individuals to return to physical activities following arthrodesis. Romeo et al[285] compared the rate and type of recreational sport activities in 33 patients (22 males, 11 females) after calcaneal fractures treated with subtalar joint arthrodesis. The percentage of individuals reporting sports participation did not change following arthrodesis. The authors noted a shift from high- to low-impact activities and from longer to shorter duration exercise sessions. Shuh et al[303] reported that 18 out of 20 patients (90%) reported sport activity prior to ankle arthrodesis and 15 out of 20 reported similar activity after arthrodesis. Although specific activity rates varied in these studies, the most common postoperative activities included cycling, swimming, hiking, skiing, and exercise walking.[285,303] A survey of surgeons and athletic trainers concluded that participation in low-impact sports is recommended and participation in high-impact sports is discouraged.[365] Low-impact sport participation that requires dorsiflexion beyond neutral, such as cycling, can be difficult following ankle arthrodesis because of the restricted dorsiflexion inherent in the procedure.

Outcomes

Short- and intermediate-term outcomes. Following arthrodesis, fusion rates of greater than 90% should be expected in uncomplicated cases.[84,114,176,242,348] Factors contributing to nonunion include multiple fusion sites, open technique, greater preoperative deformity, and underlying inflammatory arthropathy. When healing is complete after arthrodesis, pain relief and joint stability are predictable outcomes, generally resulting in improved functional mobility. Following ankle arthrodesis, postoperative walking speed is significantly improved when compared to baseline measures; however, speed remains significantly reduced when compared to controls.[19,313,340] Because dorsiflexion and plantarflexion are lost, the speed and biomechanics of gait are altered, resulting in an asymmetrical gait pattern in most individuals. These alterations result in increased energy expenditure and compensation from the hindfoot and midfoot.[32,96,288,313,340] After ankle arthrodesis, patients face functional challenges such as difficulty walking on uneven surfaces or inclines and ascending and descending stairs.

Long-term outcomes. Although arthrodesis provides pain relief in the fused joint(s), biomechanical studies show that the procedure increases stress on neighboring joints.[142,368] Several clinical studies demonstrate accelerated degenerative changes in the subtalar and tarsometatarsal joints following ankle arthrodesis.[19,77,79,96,313] Given that traditional arthrodesis indications include age < 50 years, long-term adverse functional outcomes are a concern. Coester et al[45] carried out a long-term follow-up study of 23 patients who had undergone isolated talocrural arthrodesis for posttraumatic arthritis a mean duration of 22 years earlier and found a significantly higher rate of arthritis in the ipsilateral hindfoot and midfoot joints compared to the same joints in the contralateral limb. In addition, based on information from standardized, self-report functional assessment instruments, ipsilateral foot pain interfered with the functional mobility of almost all patients. For this reason, the long-term cost-effectiveness of arthrodesis compared to arthroplasty has been questioned. Two recent studies concluded that although direct costs associated with arthrodesis are significantly lower than with ankle arthroplasty, arthroplasty results in approximately 2 additional quality-adjusted life years.[54,179]

Leg, Heel, and Foot Pain: Nonoperative Management

The cause of pain in the leg, heel, or foot is often multifactorial, but it most commonly occurs from biomechanical stress or overload. Pain is typically described as an overuse syndrome from repetitive microtrauma, but is also described as non-inflammatory degeneration.[345] The increased biomechanical stress may be from obesity, work habits, faulty alignment of the lower extremity, muscle imbalances or fatigue, changes in exercise or functional routines, training errors, improper footwear for the ground, functional demands placed on the feet, or a combination of several of these factors[226,345] (see Table 22.3).[213,226,345] Symptoms persist because continued overload is placed on the tissue before it is adequately healed. A common cause predisposing this region to painful syndromes is excessive pronation of the subtalar joint during weight-bearing activities. Increased pronation could be related to a variety of causes including excessive joint mobility, inadequate neuromuscular control,

TABLE 22.3 Intrinsic and Extrinsic Factors Associated With Heel Pain

Intrinsic Factors	Extrinsic Factors
Pes cavus foot type	Running
High BMI	Increase in exercise routine
Decreased ankle dorsiflexion	Work demands
Weak foot intrinsic musculature	Assembly line work
Faulty lower extremity alignment	Work requiring in/out of vehicles
Female gender	Improper footwear

leg length discrepancy, femoral anteversion, external tibial torsion, genu valgum, or muscle flexibility and strength imbalances in the lower extremity. Often there is a hypomobile gastrocnemius-soleus complex related to the abnormal foot pronation.

Related Pathologies and Etiology of Symptoms

The extrinsic foot musculature symptoms can develop at or near proximal attachments in the leg (shin splints); at the ankle where the tendons course around bony prominences; or at distal attachments in the foot (tendinopathy). Symptoms may also develop in the intrinsic foot muscles as well as in the plantar fascia (plantar fasciitis). Several common syndromes are described in this section.

Heel Pain

Heel pain is most often experienced on either the plantar surface of the heel or near the postero-superior calcaneus. Plantar surface pain at the insertion of the plantar fascia is common and may be related to overstretch of this tissue. Plantar pain may also result from calcaneal heel spurs or tissue bruising after high-impact forces related to jumping or falling. Posterior pain is most often located near the insertion of the Achilles tendon due to insertional tendinopathy or inflammation of one of the Achilles bursa.[345]

FOCUS ON EVIDENCE

The Heel Pain Committee of the American College of Foot and Ankle Surgeons (ACFAS) published a revised ***Clinical Practice Guideline (CPG)***[345] that categorizes mechanical heel pain as plantar heel pain (including plantar fasciitis, plantar fasciosis, and heel spurs) and posterior heel pain (including insertional Achilles tendinopathy and bursitis). The Orthopaedic Section of the American Physical Therapy Association has published two separate ***CPGs,*** one for Achilles pain, stiffness, and muscle power deficits (Achilles tendinitis), and one for heel pain (plantar fasciitis).[39,213,226] Recommendations from these ***CPGs*** are included in the following sections.

Plantar fasciitis. Pain is usually experienced along the plantar aspect of the heel, where the plantar fascia inserts on the medial tubercle of the calcaneus. The site is typically very tender to palpation. Pain occurs on initial weight bearing after periods of rest (start-up pain), then decreases, but returns as weight-bearing activity increases.[213,226,345] Associated impairments include hypomobile gastrocnemius-soleus muscles and plantar fascia pain or restriction when extending the toes (windlass effect).[98,213] Martin et al[213] suggest research to explore the role of decreased intrinsic muscle strength as a causative factor in plantar fascia pain. A high body mass index, inappropriate footwear, and either a flexible flat foot (pes planus) or a high arch foot (pes cavus) may be predisposing factors. Pressure transmitted to the irritated site with weight bearing or stretch forces to the fascia, as when extending the toes during push-off, causes pain. Gait mechanics may be impaired, with avoidance of heel strike during loading response and decreased push-off during terminal stance. Although an infracalcaneal spur (heel spur) is frequently found in individuals with plantar fasciitis, its presence or absence does not necessarily correlate with symptoms.[345]

Insertional Achilles tendinopathy and bursitis. Pain is experienced at the calcaneal insertion of the Achilles tendon.[39,345] Associated impairments include decreased ankle dorsiflexion[206,317,373] abnormal subtalar ROM, decreased ankle plantarflexion strength,[206,310,311] and increased foot pronation with walking or running.[376] Reported risk factors include obesity, hypertension, diabetes, and use of certain medications including fluoroquinolone (antibiotic) and statin medications.[39,40,210] Ultrasound imaging may be able to identify tendinopathy prior to onset of pain and dysfunction.[93,94] Once symptomatic, pain and stiffness follow a typical tendinopathy pattern: symptoms in the tendon begin following a period of inactivity, decrease with a return to activity, but eventually increase as activity continues. Changes in shoe heel height can provoke symptoms, particularly for individuals walking long distances in a low-heeled shoe when they are accustomed to high heels.

Tendinosis, Tendonitis, and Tenosynovitis

Tendinopathy is an umbrella term that indicates a disorder of the tendon. Tendinosis describes a long-standing, chronic, degenerative tendon that is absent of inflammatory mediators or cells. Tendinitis indicates an acute inflammatory process in the tendon. Differentiation between tendinitis and tendinosis is critical to successful physical therapy intervention. Tenosynovitis is inflammation of the tendon synovial sheath, which may occur in the sheath of the posterior tibialis tendon as it passes posterior to the medial malleolus.

Any tendon of the extrinsic foot muscles may become irritated as it approaches and crosses behind or over the ankle or at the insertion on the foot. Pain occurs during or after repetitive activity. When the foot and ankle are evaluated, pain is experienced at the site of the lesion during resistance to the muscle action and when the involved tendon is placed on stretch or palpated.[39,345]

A common site for Achilles tendinopathy symptoms is 2 to 6 cm proximal to the calcaneal insertion in the midsubstance of the tendon.[39] With Achilles tendinopathy, the affected leg will demonstrate decreased plantar flexor strength and endurance, as demonstrated by a limited ability to perform repetitive unilateral heel raises when compared to the unaffected side.[310] Tendon degeneration in the posterior tibialis tendon is also a common source of pain that can lead to impaired walking or acquired pes planus.[178] Symptoms in the anterior or posterior tibialis tendons or fibularis tendons are often associated with athletic activities such as running and court sports.

 **FOCUS ON EVIDENCE**

Volume 45, No. 11 of the *Journal of Orthopaedic & Sports Physical Therapy* (November 2015) is a special journal issue encompassing current basic and applied science as it relates to the pathophysiology, examination, evaluation, and treatment of tendinopathy. Relative to the foot and ankle, Michener and Kulig[233] compare and contrast the pathophysiologic changes and treatment strategies for management of supraspinatus and Achilles tendinopathy. Couppe et al[53] review literature related to eccentric Achilles tendon loading as a treatment for tendinosis, concluding that tendon loading is generally beneficial but that current literature does not support one optimal loading strategy. Silbernagel and Crossley[309] describe an evidence-based decision-making process used to return an athlete with midportion Achilles tendinopathy back to full sport participation while minimizing the chance of recurrence.

Shin Splints

This term is used to describe activity-induced leg pain along the posterior medial or anterior lateral aspects of the proximal two-thirds of the tibia. It may include different pathological conditions such as musculotendinopathy, stress fractures of the tibia, periosteitis, compartment syndrome, or irritation of the interosseous membrane. Muscle fatigue with vigorous weight-bearing exercise, often associated with a significant increase in intensity or duration, may precipitate the condition.

Anterior shin splints. Overuse of the anterior tibialis muscle is the most common type of shin splint. Impairments associated with shin splints include hypomobile gastrocnemius-soleus complex, weak anterior tibialis muscle, and excessive pronation with walking or running[306,350] Pain increases with active dorsiflexion and when the muscle is stretched into plantarflexion.

Posterior shin splints. A tight gastrocnemius-soleus complex and a weak or inflamed posterior tibialis muscle, along with increased foot pronation, are associated with posteromedial shin splints. Pain is experienced when the foot is passively pronated to end range with overpressure and/or actively supinated against resistance.

Common Impairments of Structure and Function, Activity Limitations, and Participation Restrictions

- Pain with repetitive activity, on palpation of the involved site, with stretch of the involved musculotendinous unit, and with resistance to the involved muscle
- Pain on initial weight bearing and with repetitive weight-bearing activities and gait
- Muscle length-strength imbalances, especially tight gastrocnemius-soleus muscle group
- Abnormal foot posture, including that created by faulty footwear
- Decreased length of time the individual can tolerate standing
- Decreased distance or speed of ambulation, which may limit associated community and work activities and recreational and sport activities

Leg, Heel, Foot Pain: Management—Protection Phase

If signs of local inflammation are present (erythema, edema, warmth), treat as an acute condition with rest and appropriate modalities (See Chapter 10 for general principles and guidelines). Stress relief can be achieved with immobilization in a cast or orthosis with the foot slightly plantarflexed; or with a temporary heel lift, a shoe orthotic, or calcaneal taping.[39,76,134,144,213] Interventions in the protection phase include:

- Cross-friction massage to the site of the lesion
- Submaximal muscle-setting contractions
- Passive stretch of the plantarflexors
- Active ROM within pain-free range
- Activity modification or avoidance
- Supportive taping or orthotic prescription[39,144,178,213,226,247,345]

Leg, Heel, Foot Pain: Management—Controlled Motion and Return to Function Phases

When symptoms become subacute, the entire lower extremity as well as the foot should be examined for impaired alignment or muscle flexibility and strength imbalances. Eliminating or modifying causative factors in the lower extremity kinetic chain is important to improve outcomes and to correct alignment.[44,381] Orthotic devices may be necessary to correct alignment.[39,144,178,213,345] A comprehensive movement screen such as described by Cook et al[46] can also be useful in determining aberrant movement patterns, asymmetries, weakness, or tightness remote to the painful area that may be contributing to the problem. Detailed descriptions of stretching and strengthening exercises for the ankle and foot are found in the last section of this chapter.

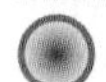 **FOCUS ON EVIDENCE**

A multicenter, randomized study of 60 subjects with plantar heel pain compared two treatment groups, one receiving electrophysical agents and exercise and the other treated with manual interventions (vigorous soft tissue techniques and joint mobilization directed at the hip, knee and ankle/foot as needed) and exercise. Both groups demonstrated significant improvement in functional measures and pain, with those receiving the specific manual interventions and exercise showing greater increases at 4-week (function and pain) and 6-week (function only) follow-ups.[44] Individuals with plantar heel pain symptoms less than 7 months' duration were more likely to respond positively to treatment, while age and BMI were not related to the treatment response.[218]

Educate the Patient and Provide Home Exercises

- Help the patient incorporate home exercises and soft tissue and joint mobilization into his or her daily routine.
- If the patient experiences pain when first bearing weight, especially in the morning and after prolonged sitting, teach the patient to do ROM exercises with the foot for several minutes before standing. Emphasize full dorsiflexion active ROM.
- Teach prevention, including the following principles.
  - Before intense exercise, use gentle repetitive warm-up activities followed by stretching of tight muscles.
  - Use proper foot support for the ground conditions.
  - Allow time for recovery from microtrauma after high-intensity exercise bouts.

Increase Mobility of Range-Limiting Structures

- The gastrocnemius-soleus muscle complex is frequently hypomobile in cases of foot problems and should be stretched if limiting dorsiflexion. Restricted mobility causes the foot to pronate when the ankle dorsiflexes.

CLINICAL TIP

Instruct patients with pes planus to wear supportive shoes with medial arch support when performing gastrocnemius-soleus stretches to protect the foot.[153]

- With heel pain, apply joint and soft tissue mobilization techniques.
  - Deep massage to the insertion of the plantar fascia at the medial calcaneal tubercle and the gastrocnemius-soleus tendon.
  - Joint mobilization directed to specific limitations such as lateral glide to the subtalar joint to improve rear foot inversion and posterior glide to the talus to improve ankle dorsiflexion.
  - Joint mobilization at the knee or hip as needed.[44]
- Stretching exercises to the plantar fascia that includes toe extension with ankle dorsiflexion and eversion.[67]
- Stretching exercises to any lower extremity region that may affect alignment and function of the foot and ankle.

Improve Muscle Performance

- Begin with resistive isometric and progress to resistive dynamic exercises to the foot and ankle in open- and closed-chain activities.
- For medial and lateral support, develop a balance in strength between the muscle groups, especially the invertors and evertors.[39,178]
- Emphasize muscular endurance and train the muscles to respond to eccentric loading.
- With plantar fasciitis, the intrinsic muscles need to be strengthened. Include exercises that require toe control such as gathering a towel or picking up small objects.

FOCUS ON EVIDENCE

Barefoot running is a recent trend among recreational runners. It is proposed that barefoot running facilitates mid-foot strike during the contact phase of the running cycle, reducing ground reaction force and decreasing injuries.[189,194,322] Limited evidence supports an association between barefoot running and reduced ground reaction force at impact.[117] It is also theorized that barefoot running strengthens the muscles of the foot and lower leg and improves proprioception.[190] A recent prospective study randomly assigned 29 experienced runners to an 8-week running program completed in either running shoes or while barefoot. Although both groups demonstrated significant improvement in some performance outcome measures, there were no between group differences noted. The authors suggest that 8 weeks may be an insufficient amount of time to observe changes related to footwear.[240]

Ligamentous Injuries: Nonoperative Management

Ankle sprain is one of the most common musculoskeletal injuries with physically active individuals who are at higher risk than the general population.[90,91,370] First-, second-, and third-degree (grades I-III) sprains are usually managed conservatively.[154,220] The most common type of ankle sprain is caused by inversion stress and can result in a partial or complete tear of the anterior talofibular (ATF) ligament and often the calcaneofibular (CF) ligament (see Fig. 22.2).[69,90,154,281,370] The posterior talofibular (PTF) ligament, the strongest of the lateral ligaments, is rarely torn in isolation; significant inversion stress is required to tear the PTF ligament.[278] If the inferior tibiofibular ligaments are torn after torsional stress to the ankle, the mortise becomes unstable.[21,140] Rarely do the components of the deltoid ligament become strained; rather, there is greater likelihood of an avulsion from or fracture of the medial malleolus with significant eversion stress. Depending on the severity of injury, the joint capsule also may be involved, and intra-articular pathology, including cartilage lesions, may occur.[327]

Prospective cohort studies note that a history of a previous ankle sprain is a risk factor for future sprain,[13,62,85,129,174,175,324,351] as is participation in organized or recreational athletic activities.[69,90,370] Using an external support (lace-up ankle brace or athletic ankle taping) has been shown to decrease the incidence of ankle sprains.[68,147,188] Conflicting evidence exists related to age, gender, physical characteristics, postural control, general ligamentous laxity, and foot type as risk factors for ankle sprain.[212] Table 22.4 details evidence-based risk factors associated with acute lateral ankle sprains.[212]

Common Impairments of Structure and Function, Activity Limitations, and Participation Restrictions

- Pain when the injured tissue is stressed in mild to moderate injuries.
- Excessive motion or instability of the related joint in the case of complete tears.
- Proprioceptive deficit manifested as decreased ability to perceive passive motion and development of balance impairments.[374]
- Related joint symptoms and reflex muscle inhibition.[259]
- Possible decreased ROM of the talocrural joint in recurrent lateral ankle sprains due to anterior subluxation and impaired tracking of the talus in the mortise.[366]
- Postural control deficits following an acute lateral ankle sprain in both the injured and uninjured limb.[192,225]
- Restricted ambulation (requiring an assistive device) during the acute and subacute phases. With chronic instability, the individual may have difficulty walking or running on uneven surfaces or making quick changes in direction. He or she may be unable to land safely when jumping or hopping.

FOCUS ON EVIDENCE

A randomized controlled trial (N = 40) incorporated a repeated measures design to demonstrate the efficacy of a balance-training program using elastic tubing as a perturbation force. Individuals with chronic ankle instability (CAI) (n = 20) were matched with healthy normal subjects (n = 20). Subjects in each group were randomly assigned to either an elastic tubing balance exercise group or to a control. Total travel distance of the center of pressure was measured at baseline, after 4 weeks of training, and at a 4-week follow-up session. The 4-week elastic resistance balance-training program caused a significant improvement in balance for the exercise group when compared to the control; and significant improvement in the CAI group compared to the healthy normal group. Improvements in balance persisted 4 weeks following the intervention. The authors concluded that elastic resistance for balance perturbation should be considered for both home and clinic use in individuals with CAI.[120]

Ankle Sprain: Management—Protection Phase

See Chapter 10 for principles of treatment during the stages of inflammation and repair.

FOCUS ON EVIDENCE

The Orthopaedic Section of the American Physical Therapy Association published a ***CPG*** to guide evidence-based management of ankle ligament sprains.[212] The National Athletic Trainer's Association published a position statement guiding the conservative management of ankle sprains in athletes.[154] Recommendations from both of these papers are incorporated into the following section.

- Use compression, elevation, and repeated intermittent applications of ice to minimize swelling.[25,26,105,358] Randomized controlled trials have failed to demonstrate consistent support for electrical or acoustic modalities.
  - Electrotherapy: There is moderate evidence both for and against the use of electrotherapy to manage acute pain and swelling, with a trend toward no benefit.[88,208,227,316]
  - Ultrasound: Clinicians should not use ultrasound for the management of acute ankle sprains.[363]
- Provide external support (brace, semi-rigid ankle orthotic, or walking boot) in conjunction with progressive, functional weight bearing.[31,47,151]
- Use gentle joint mobilization techniques to maintain mobility and inhibit pain.[195]
- Perform gentle sagittal plane active ROM in a pain-free range.
- Educate the patient.
  - Teach the patient the importance of RICE (rest, ice, compression, and elevation), and instruct the patient to apply ice every 2 waking hours during the first 24 to 48 hours.
  - Teach partial weight bearing with crutches and instruct in progressive weight bearing.
  - Teach muscle-setting (isometric) exercises and active toe curls to help maintain muscle integrity and assist with circulation.

TABLE 22.4 Intrinsic and Extrinsic Factors Associated With Acute Lateral Ankle Sprain

Intrinsic Risk Factors	Extrinsic Risk Factors
Previous ankle sprain[13,62,85,129,174,175,324,351]	Athletic participation without external support[68,147,188]
Decreased ankle dorsiflexion ROM[62]	Failure to warm-up prior to activity[124]
	Failure to participate in balance/proprioceptive training[141,223,224,236,282,297,356,362]

FOCUS ON EVIDENCE

Bleakley et al[27] randomly assigned individuals (N = 101) to either accelerated rehabilitation (AR) or standard protection (SP) groups after acute grade I and II lateral ankle sprains (average 2 days' postinjury). Individuals in the AR group (n = 50) received early therapeutic exercise as well as cryotherapy and advice for early progressive weight bearing. The SP group (n = 51) initially received only cryotherapy and advice for progressive weight bearing; therapeutic exercise was initiated after 1 week. After the first week, both groups completed a progressive therapeutic exercise regime that consisted of muscle strengthening, neuromuscular training, and sport-specific functional exercise. The AR group demonstrated significant improvement in ankle function at weeks 1 and 2 and significantly greater physical activity during the first week. At 16 weeks, both groups reported good ankle function with just four re-injuries (two in each group). This finding supports early initiation of therapeutic exercise following acute ankle sprain.

Ankle Sprain: Management—Controlled Motion Phase

- As the acute symptoms subside, continue to provide protection for the involved ligament with an orthosis during weight bearing. Commercial orthoses, such as an air splint, provide medial-lateral stability while allowing dorsiflexion and plantarflexion.[22,118,159]
- Provide gait training to normalize walking over level ground and on stairs.
- Apply cross-friction massage to the ligaments as tolerated.
- Use grade II joint mobilization techniques to maintain mobility of the joint, particularly posterior glide of the talus.
- Advance therapeutic exercise resistance or intensity. Avoid end-range inversion. Exercises should be completed frequently throughout the day.
  - Nonweight-bearing active ROM into dorsiflexion, plantarflexion, inversion, and eversion; toe curls; and ankle alphabet.
  - Sitting with the heel on the floor and performing foot intrinsic exercises: towel gathering or picking up objects with the toes.
- Stretch the gastrocnemius-soleus muscle group to restore full ankle dorsiflexion. Begin with towel stretch in long sitting, then progress to weight bearing stretches.
- As swelling decreases and weight bearing tolerance increases, progress to progressive resistive exercise (strength and endurance) and neuromuscular re-education (balance and proprioception).[141] Include isometric and isotonic exercise, bicycle ergometry, and partial to full weight-bearing balance board exercises. Initially, have the patient wear a range-limiting brace or orthosis to prevent excessive stress on the healing ligament.

Ankle Sprain: Management—Return to Function Phase

- Progress strengthening exercises by adding elastic resistance to foot movements in long-sitting (open-chain) and sitting with the heel on the floor for partial weight bearing.
- Progress neuromuscular reeducation training to improve balance, coordination, stability, and neuromuscular response in full weight bearing. Progressively challenge dynamic lower extremity stabilizers by introducing varying degrees of surface instability and external perturbation.
- Incorporate movement patterns, such as forward/backward walking and cross-over side stepping with elastic resistance secured around the unaffected lower extremity.[120]
- Utilize an unstable surface, such as a BOSU®, BAPS® board, or mini-trampoline, or an ankle destabilization shoe or boot.[73,74]
- Depending on the final goals of rehabilitation, train the ankle with weight-bearing activities, such as walking on uneven ground, jogging, running, jumping, hopping, and sprinting. Incorporate agility activities such as controlled twisting, turning, and lateral weight shifting. Provide distracting activities such as ball toss to increase automaticity of postural control.[274,287]
- When the patient is involved in sports activities, the ankle should be splinted or taped and appropriate shoes should be worn to protect the ligament from re-injury.[68,147,188]

CLINICAL TIP

Use of external support during neuromuscular training has been shown to decrease muscle activation in the lower extremity.[88,261] To maximize the neuromuscular benefit of training, select balance and proprioception exercises that can be completed safely without external support.

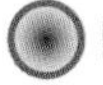

FOCUS ON EVIDENCE

McKeon and Hertel[224] performed a systematic literature review to determine the effectiveness of balance and coordination training for individuals with lateral ankle instability. Prophylactic balance training substantially reduced the risk of sustaining ankle sprains, with a greater effect seen in those with a history of a previous sprain. There was inadequate evidence to show that training prevented sprains for those without previous injury. The review also demonstrated that balance and coordination training substantially improved treatment outcomes after acute ankle sprains. A recent randomized controlled trial (N = 522), not included in this systematic review, found a 35% reduction in ankle sprain recurrence in individuals who completed an unsupervised proprioceptive training program following usual care for lateral ankle sprain.[141] Neuromuscular reeducation for balance and proprioceptive training should be performed following lateral ankle sprain to reduce re-injury rates.[154,212]

In a prospective study, 384 individuals with subacute ankle sprain (< 2 months from injury) were randomly assigned to one of three treatment arms: training group (n = 120), brace group (n = 126), or combination group (n = 138). The training group completed an 8-week independent neuromuscular training program; the brace group received a semi-rigid brace to be worn during all sporting activities for 12 months; and the combination group received both the neuromuscular training program and a semi-rigid brace to be worn during all sporting activities for 8 weeks. Re-injury was tracked for 1 year. During the 1-year follow up, 69 participants (20%) reported a subsequent ankle sprain: 29 (27%) in the training group, 17 (15%) in the brace group, and 23 (19%) in the combination group. The brace group re-injury rate was significantly lower than the training group, but not significantly different than the combination group. There was no between-group difference in the severity of subsequent ankle sprains. An extended period of brace wear following lateral ankle sprain is indicated to reduce re-injury rates.[147]

Traumatic Soft Tissue Injuries: Surgical and Postoperative Management

Repair of Complete Lateral Ankle Ligament Tears

A third-degree (grade 3) sprain of the lateral ankle, which usually occurs as the result of a severe inversion injury, causes a complete tear of the ATF ligament, often the CF ligament, and infrequently the PTF ligament (Fig. 22.7).[281]

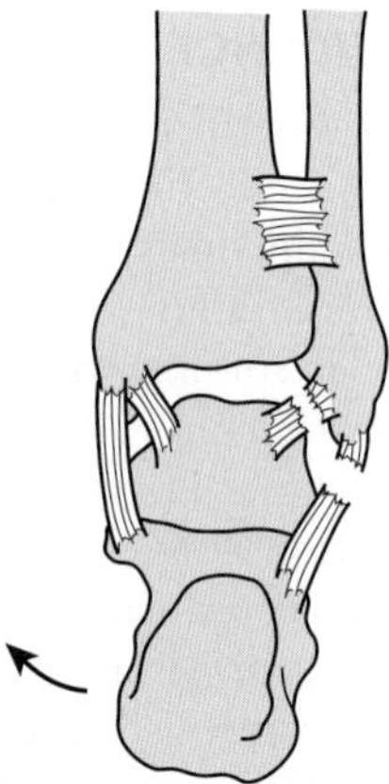

FIGURE 22.7 A complete tear of the lateral collateral ligament complex as the result of a severe (grade 3) inversion injury of the ankle. *(From McKinnis, LN:* Fundamentals of Musculoskeletal Imaging, *ed. 3. Philadelphia: F.A. Davis, 2010, p 432, with permission.)*

Tearing of both the ATF and CF ligaments leads to combined instability of the tibiotalar and subtalar joints. The ATF ligament is most likely to tear when forceful inversion occurs while the ankle is plantarflexed.[164,304,357,384] Injuries associated with lateral ankle sprain include articular cartilage (talar dome) lesions, fibularis tendon tearing or subluxation, a transverse fracture of the lateral malleolus, syndesmosis sprain, or an avulsion fracture of the base of the fifth metatarsal.[70,89,281,284,364]

In addition to significant swelling, tenderness, and pain, a complete tear of one or more lateral ligaments causes marked mechanical instability and functional instability of the ankle during weight-bearing activities.[125,128,132] Mechanical instability is defined as ankle mobility beyond the physiologic ROM, increased talar tilt, and an anterior drawer sign indicative of join laxity. Functional instability is characterized by the patient's sensation of the ankle "giving way."[125,132,329] The severity of functional ankle instability does not appear to be directly related to the magnitude of anterior joint displacement or talar tilt.[56,132] It has been hypothesized that functional ankle instability results from both peripheral and central sensorimotor deficits.[121,126] This may account for the feeling of "giving way" experienced by many patients who have no evidence of mechanical instability with physical examination after a lateral ankle sprain. Despite normal joint motion and no apparent laxity, these individuals report significant functional limitations. Hiller et al[128] proposed multiple subgroupings of individuals with ankle instability symptoms, positing that ankle instability results from an interaction between mechanical, functional, and perceived instability.

After an acute, grade 3 inversion injury, nonoperative treatment is successful for most individuals. However, some patients develop chronic ankle instability with continued pain, recurrent sprains, and a consistent feeling of the ankle "giving way." For patients with demonstrated instability who do not respond to conservative management and for select patients with acute lateral ankle injuries who regularly engage in high-impact activities, surgical repair or reconstruction may be required to manage the instability and return the patient to the desired level of function.[3,171,281] The overall goal of surgery and postoperative management is to restore joint stability while retaining pain-free, functional ROM of the ankle and subtalar joints.[3,171,281,296]

Indications for Surgery

The following have been frequently cited indications for surgical reconstruction or repair of the lateral ankle soft tissue structures:[3,89,109,171,281,296]

- Chronic mechanical and functional instability of the ankle during activity that is not resolved with several months of conservative management.
- Acute, radiographically or arthroscopically confirmed third-degree lateral ankle sprain resulting in complete tear of the ATF and/or CF ligaments.

Procedures

Types of Stabilization Procedures

There are numerous surgical procedures that may be used for reconstruction or repair of the lateral ankle ligaments and soft tissue structures (Fig. 22.8).[37,52,89,109,143,171,266,281,296,320,338] Procedures are dichotomized into two broad categories: repair and reconstruction.[215,281] Surgical repair techniques involve a direct end-to-end anatomic suturing of the torn or attenuated (overstretched) ATF or CF ligaments; surgical reconstruction uses tenodesis (tendon graft) to reconstruct the lateral ankle complex. Either procedure can be performed via arthroscopy or open procedure.[3,109,336]

The type of procedure selected depends on the severity and chronicity of the instability, the presence of comorbidities, the patient's age and anticipated postoperative activity level, and the surgeon's preferred method. Repair is typically the preferred procedure for patients with chronic lateral ankle instability who have normal body mass and ADL requirements. Reconstruction is reserved for individuals who may stress the ankle to a greater degree than normal.[109,215]

Direct repair. The surgery most commonly performed for a primary repair is the *modified Broström procedure,* also known as the *Broström-Gould procedure.*[89,109,215,281] This procedure involves an anatomic repair of the ATF and/or CF ligament(s) with one or more of the following techniques:

- Direct, end-to-end repair of midsubstance tear
- Imbrication (overlap/suture with pants-and-vest technique) of stretched ligament
- Anchoring of avulsed ligament to bone

The anatomic repair is augmented by suturing the lateral portion of the extensor retinaculum to the fibula, reinforcing the repaired structures. Retinacular reinforcement is regarded as a critical element to the success of the procedure.[109]

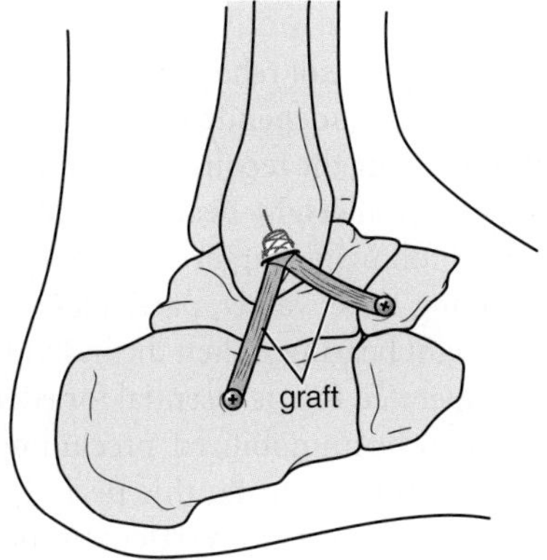

FIGURE 22.8 Lateral view of the ankle depicting reconstruction of torn ATF and CF ligaments using a tendon graft to augment stability. Proximal advancement of the extensor retinaculum (not shown) over the reconstructed ligaments and suture attachment to the distal fibula provides additional stability.

Reconstruction with augmentation. Reconstruction procedures, in general, are employed when direct repair is not an option because of poor ATF and/or CF ligament tissue quality or when a patient's weight (more than 200 to 250 lb) will overly stress a direct repair. Reconstruction with augmentation is also used as a revision procedure when previous direct repair has failed to prevent a recurrence of instability. Current lateral ankle reconstruction procedures utilize anatomic reconstruction of the ATF and CF ligaments with tendon autograft or allograft. These procedures route the transferred tendon graft in such a way as to replicate the anatomic positions of the ATF and CF ligament origin and insertion sites.[109] The transferred tendon can be secured to the bone with anchors, interference screws, or endobutton devices.[109,171,281,336]

The ipsilateral fibularis brevis tendon is the most commonly used autologous graft. The tendon can be completely excised with the distal muscle fixed to the fibularis longus; or the tendon can be split, sparing the stabilizing action of the muscle. [281,296] To preserve the integrity of the fibularis brevis tendon, reconstruction procedures using a gracilis[52,336] or semitendinosis[137] tendon autograft, or an anterior tibialis[83] or bone-patellar tendon[332] allograft, have been developed.

Surgical Approach

Repair and reconstruction have historically been performed as open procedures. Arthroscopy, previously reserved for perioperative examination to guide open reconstruction, has recently demonstrated promising short-term clinical results.[3,48,51,110,166,217,336,337,361] Arthroscopic direct repair and reconstruction have been described with early promising results in nonrandomized, case series reports. Techniques vary, but both procedures follow the general tenets for repair and reconstruction described above. In a recent systematic review that included published reports of arthroscopic repair (21 studies) and arthroscopic reconstruction (6 studies), Matsui et al[216] concluded there is insufficient evidence to support a high grade of recommendation for minimally invasive surgery.

Operative Overview

Prior to an open repair or reconstruction for lateral ankle instability, arthroscopy is performed to assess the extent of intra-articular pathology. A high percentage (77% to 95%) of chronically unstable ankles exhibit associated intra-articular pathology, specifically small articular cartilage lesions, which are thought to be a precursor to osteoarthritis of the ankle.[89,138,333] If a chondral lesion is identified, arthroscopic subchondral drilling (microfracture) is typically performed.[138,339]

After arthroscopy an oblique or curvilinear incision is made beginning at the anterior aspect of the distal fibula and extending distally along the lateral aspect of the ankle and foot. If a direct repair (Broström-Gould) procedure[119] is used, torn or avulsed structures are repaired with permanent sutures by excision and end-to-end repair, a vest-over-pants (imbrication) technique, or through drill holes in the bone.

The repair is augmented by suturing the lateral portion of the extensor retinaculum to the distal fibula.[281] If an autologous fibularis brevis tendon graft is to be used to provide additional reinforcement (Chrisman-Snook procedure),[43] the tendon is split longitudinally. One half of the tendon is transected from the musculotendinous junction, leaving the distal insertion intact. Bone tunnels are drilled in the fibula and calcaneus. The graft is passed through bone tunnels and, after appropriate tensioning, is secured either to the base of the fifth metatarsal or to the distal fibula with permanent sutures. If a semitendinosis or gracilis graft is used, a third bone tunnel is drilled in the lateral neck of the talus and the free graft is secured in the tunnel with a biotenodesis screw.[52,83,281,338] With either a fibularis graft or a free graft, the extensor retinaculum is advanced proximally and sutured over the ligament repair to the distal fibula for additional reinforcement.

Prior to wound closure, ankle stability and ROM are checked. The foot and ankle are placed in a compression dressing in a nonwalking bivalve cast or posterior orthosis with the ankle in 0° of dorsiflexion and slight eversion. The leg is elevated for edema management.

Postoperative Management

Postoperative care varies by procedure and surgeon. Direct repair procedures rely on biomechanically weaker suture repair when compared to the strong fixation of allograft tissue reconstruction.[215,281] Because of this, post-operative progression of direct repair has traditionally been more conservative than for reconstruction, despite scant evidence to support this approach.[217,270]

Initial management generally consists of a period (2 to 6 weeks) of nonweight-bearing immobilization followed by 2 to 4 weeks of weight bearing to tolerance in a walking boot.[264,281] Protected ROM exercise is initiated after the initial immobilization period; terminal inversion is avoided. The exercise progression after surgery is similar to that used for nonoperative management of lateral ankle sprains. Postoperative management attempts to restore normal ROM and neuromuscular control while preventing re-injury.[264]

Immobilization and Weight-Bearing Considerations

Immobilization. After some degree of swelling has subsided, usually within 3 to 5 postoperative days, the compression dressing and protective cast or orthosis is removed and a short leg cast is reapplied. Depending on the type and strength of the repair, the cast is removed at 2 to 6 weeks and replaced with an air-stirrup-type orthosis, a removable cast boot, or a CAM walking brace, which is worn for several additional weeks.[52,89,264,281,372] Once in a removable boot or orthosis, patients are encouraged to perform active ROM dorsiflexion/plantarflexion and restricted active ROM inversion/eversion (10°-15° arc of motion).[264]

By 6 to 12 weeks, the patient gradually discontinues use of the immobilizer during ambulation. However, patients returning to athletic activities that involve jumping, running, and quick changes of direction are advised to wear a protective orthotic device or to tape the ankle for at least 3 to 6 months to prevent re-injury.

Weight bearing. Although recent reports indicate that immediate weight bearing to tolerance is safe and beneficial,[235,270] a period of nonweight bearing in the protective orthosis or cast is still frequently recommended.[264,281] Following removal of the compression dressing, the return to weight bearing schedule can vary. Although Pearce et al[264] recommend weight bearing as tolerated 10 to 14 days following surgery, other authors recommend nonweight bearing for 6 weeks.[52,281,332,338] Full weight bearing without the immobilizer is typically permitted 6 to 12 weeks following surgery.

FOCUS ON EVIDENCE

Individuals who underwent reconstruction of the ATF ligament with a gracilis autograft using interference screw fixation were randomly assigned to a typical rehabilitation (TR) group (immobilization/restricted weight bearing; n = 15) or an accelerated rehabilitation (AR) group (no immobilization/weight bear to tolerance; n = 18). All patients were followed for 2 years and outcome measures included stress radiography, self-reported functional scores (Karlsson and Peterson scoring system), and time between surgery and full return to activity. Two years postoperatively, both groups (TR and AR) demonstrated significantly improved stability and functional scores when compared to preoperative measures. There were no between group differences at 2 years in either of these measures. All patients were able to return to their previous athletic activity, with the AR group returning to activity significantly faster than the IR group (13.4 ± 2.2 weeks vs. 18.5 ± 3.5 weeks, respectively). No differences in performance ability were observed between group, and no cases of re-injury were reported in either group. The authors concluded that immediate mobility and weight bearing following reconstruction with interference screw fixation is safe and preferable.[235]

Exercise: Maximum Protection Phase

The focus of the first phase of rehabilitation, which lasts from 4 to 6 weeks, is to regain independent mobility for functional activities while protecting the repaired or reconstructed lateral ankle structures. Nonweight-bearing ambulation with crutches is typical following surgery. Some individuals may elect to use a rolling knee walker, particularly for extended periods of nonweight bearing. When the individual is seated, elevation of the operated foot is essential for edema management. The ankle may be immobilized, precluding ROM exercise. If ROM is permitted during this period, active ROM dorsiflexion/plantarflexion and restricted range inversion/eversion (10°-15° arc of motion) should be initiated.[264] Muscle-setting exercises in a neutral ankle position can be performed in or out of the immobilizer.[235,264]

Goals and interventions. Limited evidence guides exercise prescription during the immediate postoperative phase. The following exercise-related goals and interventions are appropriate during the first postoperative phase.[215,235,264,329,372]

- ***Prevent reflex inhibition of immobilized muscle groups.***
  - Submaximal muscle-setting (isometric) exercises in neutral ankle position, including the fibularis muscles.
- ***Prevent stiffness of the operated ankle and foot and loss of extensibility of surrounding soft tissue.***
  - Active ROM in pain-free range for ankle plantarflexion and dorsiflexion. Active ROM in pain-free, restricted arc ROM for inversion and eversion (10°-15° arc of motion).[264]
  - Active ROM of the toes.
- ***Maximize independent mobility.***
  - Gait and transfer training with appropriate assistive device. Adherence to weight-bearing restrictions.
- ***Maintain strength of nonimmobilized muscle groups.***
  - Perform active and resistive exercises of the hip and knee of the operated lower extremity and resistance exercises of the upper extremities and non-operative lower extremity.
  - Perform mini-squats in bilateral stance with appropriate weight bearing.

Exercise: Moderate and Minimum Protection Phases

Interventions in the moderate protection phase are initiated 4 to 6 weeks after surgery. At this time, healing structures are able to sustain controlled and progressive stress. Ankle ROM typically is limited and may be painful with end-range overpressure. Lower extremity balance and strength are impaired.

This phase is characterized by a gradual weaning from the immobilizer or brace accompanied by restoration of full, pain-free ankle joint mobility. Neuromuscular control, strength, and balance deficits are addressed while minimizing risk of re-injury. Gait training restores normal walking gait.

The minimum protection phase typically begins 8 to 12 weeks following surgery. The focus of the final rehabilitation phase is to restore full muscle strength and endurance of the operated extremity equal to that of the sound side; re-establish a normal, pain-free running gait pattern; and prepare for return to desired work-, sport-, or recreation-related activities. Interventions should emphasize restoring sensorimotor acuity, reducing functional deficits, improving postural control, and preventing re-injury.[264]

CLINICAL TIP

With proper precautions, a return to functional activities, including sport, may be possible 3 to 4 months postoperatively.[235,264,372] Fibularis muscle strength, assessed with handheld dynamometry, should test normal compared to the contralateral ankle.[264] No instability should be noted with anterior drawer or medial talar tilt tests. The following functional tests help determine readiness for return to sport progression:

- Single-leg hop tests (for horizontal distance; for vertical distance; triple hop test; figure-of-8 hop test; and 6-meter timed hop test)[192,298]
- Star Excursion Balance test[106,126,192]
- Foot and Ankle Ability Measure functional questionnaire[38,81]
- Finally, a patient's perceived readiness for return to sport should be considered[12]

Goals and interventions. The following exercise-related goals and interventions are appropriate during the intermediate and final phases of rehabilitation:

- ***Restore pain-free ROM of the operated ankle.*** If strict immobilization was performed during the maximum protection phase, dorsiflexion will likely be limited to just a few degrees beyond neutral. To increase ankle ROM:
  - Progress AROM, achieving full ankle ROM by 8 weeks.
  - Initiate active multiplanar movements, such as figure-of-eight or ankle alphabet active ROM
  - Perform grade II or III joint mobilization techniques to the tibiotalar and tibiofibular joint if joint restriction limits dorsi- or plantarflexion.
  - Add self-stretching exercises to improve muscle flexibility, particularly for the gastrocnemius-soleus complex. Begin with a towel stretch; progress to standing on a wedge for an extended duration.
- ***Increase strength of ankle and foot musculature in both lower extremities.***

CLINICAL TIP

Functional ankle instability has been shown to be associated with decreased strength (peak torque) of the ankle evertors of the involved ankle when compared to the contralateral ankle in individuals who have not undergone a surgical stabilization procedure.[295] In addition, the extent of strength loss in the ankle musculature has been shown to be associated with the chronicity of the instability.[1] Therefore, after surgical repair or reconstruction of the lateral ligaments, improving eversion strength is particularly important for developing dynamic stability.

  - Perform progressive resistance exercises of all ankle muscles. Begin in nonweight-bearing and progress to weight-bearing positions.
  - Unilateral calf raises should initially be performed with upper extremity support to minimize chance of re-injury due to balance loss.
  - Emphasize strengthening of the ankle evertors. For dynamic strengthening, perform eversion against elastic or manual resistance in cardinal or diagonal planes.[116]

- Include bilateral hip and knee strengthening in weight-bearing positions, emphasizing proximal control (see Chapters 20 and 21).
- Progress to plyometric training when weight bearing is pain free, ankle is stable with stress testing, and 25 unilateral heel raises can be performed.[264,311] Begin with bilateral jumping, progress to unilateral hopping forward, backward, diagonally, and side-to-side. Plyometrics initially should be performed with external ankle support (bracing or taping).[147,281] Refer to Chapter 23 for a full description of plyometric activities.

■ ***Improve muscular endurance and cardiopulmonary fitness.***
- Begin with pool walking, swimming, stationary bicycling, treadmill walking, or using a cross-country ski machine. Progress to deep-water running and outdoor walking, jogging, or running. Land-based activities should initially be performed with external ankle support (bracing or taping).[147,281]

■ ***Improve neuromuscular control, balance reactions, dynamic stability, and agility.***
- Initiate progression of bilateral and unilateral balance activities beginning on stable surface and introducing progressive surface instability (refer to Chapters 8 and 23 for examples).
- Initiate unilateral balance training at about 6 weeks postoperatively or when full weight bearing on the involved extremity is tolerated.
  - Progress from firm surface to soft surface (mini-trampoline or dense foam) to unstable surface (balance board or BOSU®)
  - Ankle proprioception may also be targeted on specific destabilization tools (ankle destabilization boot, ankle destabilization sandal, air bladder) with moderate inversion ROM (10°-15°) localized only under the rearfoot.[74,92]
- Progress to activities to improve agility, such as grapevine walking (carioca), lateral shuffles, use of a slide board, and pivoting and cutting activities.
- Refer to Chapter 23 for a sequence of balance and agility activities.

FOCUS ON EVIDENCE

For patients with a functionally unstable ankle, proprioceptive/balance training using rocker or wobble boards has been shown to be an effective method of improving joint proprioception (joint position sense) and single-leg standing ability and muscle reaction times during balance activities.[73,74,82] Evidence is mixed regarding effect of balance training on postural sway, although this form of neuromuscular training is thought to demonstrate short-term effectiveness.[63,212,224]

In a prospective study by Verhagen et al,[362] 1,127 male and female professional volleyball players were randomly assigned by team to a training group or a control group. Throughout the 36-week volleyball season, the training groups participated in a proprioceptive training program consisting of a variety of balance activities, some on balance boards. The control groups were not given any training program. Injuries were tracked for both groups over the course of the season. Among players who had a history of ankle sprains prior to the beginning of the study, those who participated in the balance training program had a significantly lower incidence of acute lateral ankle sprains during the season than those in the control group. Among training and control group players who did not have a history of lateral ankle sprains, there was no significant difference in the incidence of ankle injury during the season. The authors concluded that proprioceptive training was effective in preventing recurrence of lateral ankle injury in adult volleyball players.

Although this and other studies have not involved patients undergoing rehabilitation after repair or reconstruction of the lateral ankle ligaments, proprioceptive training programs such as these may be beneficial for the postoperative patient.

■ ***Re-establish pain-free, symmetrical weight bearing during gait and related activities.***
- Begin gait training in a pool or land-based training on level surfaces as soon as ambulation in a controlled ankle motion brace (which allows dorsi- and plantarflexion) is permitted.
- Emphasize symmetrical weight bearing during sit-to-stand movements and eventually ascending and descending stairs
- Progress to ambulation and functional activities without the brace.

■ ***Safely return to functional activities and prevent re-injury.*** The late rehabilitation phase typically occurs between 8 to 12 weeks postoperatively. Patients should demonstrate normal gait over level and uneven ground, and with ascending/descending stairs. Ankle strength should be ≥ 90% of the contralateral side.[342] Functional hop test performance (figure-of-eight, side-to-side) should demonstrate appropriate weight-bearing neuromuscular control and performance ≥ 90% compared to the contralateral side.[141,270] Precautions to reduce the risk of re-injury when returning to sports or high-demand activities after repair or reconstruction of lateral ankle ligaments are summarized in Box 22.4.

Outcomes

An optimal postoperative outcome after lateral ankle repair or reconstruction is an ankle that has full mobility but remains stable and pain free during functional activities. Systematic reviews demonstrate that both repair and reconstruction procedures can predictably restore stability and return individuals to sport.[63,160,268] Published trials can be divided into those that treated individuals with acute lateral ankle sprain, and those that treated individuals with chronic ankle instability (characterized by recurrent ankle sprains and a feeling of "giving way").

BOX 22.4 Activity-Related Precautions to Reduce the Risk of Re-injury After Lateral Ligament Reconstruction of the Ankle

- Modify activities, if possible, by participating in low-impact sports, such as swimming, cycling, low-impact aerobics, or cross country skiing.
- Minimize or avoid participation in activities that involve high-impact (basketball, volleyball), rapid stopping and starting and changes of direction (tennis, soccer), or traversing uneven surfaces.
- If involved in activities associated with high risk of ankle injury:
  - Participate in a preseason injury prevention program that includes progressive proprioceptive and plyometric training and continue the program throughout a sport season.[82,362]
  - Wear a prescribed orthotic device, such as a functional stirrup brace or orthosis, to provide medial-lateral stability of the ankle.[68,147,159,221,222,326] Ankle taping has been shown to have prophylactic benefit in individuals with history of ankle sprain; however, both higher cost and higher incidence of integumentary problems favors the use of brace.[186,234,253]

Surgical management of acute lateral ankle sprain. Kerkoffs et al,[160] in a Cochrane Review, compared surgical to conservative management of acute lateral ankle sprain. No difference in return to previous level of sport participation was found, but surgical intervention resulted in a significant decrease in the number of individuals with recurrent ankle sprains compared to the conservative treatment group. A recent review had similar findings, noting that surgical intervention results in improved objective stability and decreased recurrence rates.[268] It is important to note that many of the studies included in these reviews are more than 20 years old and that only one of the included studies was published in the last 10 years. A recent randomized controlled trial of male military conscripts compared long-term outcomes for individuals with acute lateral ankle sprain treated with either direct repair (n = 25) or functional treatment (n = 26).[271] Functional treatment included immediate weight bearing to tolerance in a semi-rigid ankle orthotic for 3 weeks and therapeutic exercise guided by a physiotherapist. Individuals in the surgical group followed a similar postoperative weight-bearing, bracing, and exercise regimen. All patients in both groups recovered their preinjury activity level and completed military service. Fifteen (60%) of the surgical group and 18 (69%) of the functional treatment group returned for long-term follow-up (mean duration 14 years). Prevalence of re-injury was 1 out of 15 in the repair group and 7 out of 18 in the functional treatment group. Stress radiographs showed no difference between groups for anterior drawer or medial talar tilt. Evidence of osteoarthritis on MRI was observed in 4 out of 15 individuals in the repair group and 1 out of 18 in the functional treatment group. The authors concluded that both methods of management are appropriate for return to preinjury activity level and that although surgical repair decreases risk of subsequent ankle sprain, there may be an increased risk of subsequent osteoarthritis. There is insufficient evidence from high quality randomized controlled trials to strongly recommend surgical management of acute lateral ankle sprains.[160,268,271]

Surgical management of chronic ankle instability. Relatively few studies compare surgical to conservative management for chronic ankle instability. A recent review by de Vries et al[63] included four studies using several different surgical procedures including direct repair and reconstruction. All studies were judged at high risk for bias, generally related to blinding and selective reporting. The authors concluded that there was insufficient evidence to support any one surgical technique over others for chronic ankle instability. Individual should fail conservative management, specifically neuromuscular training, prior to surgical stabilization. Following surgery, postoperative management should include early mobility and weight bearing vs. 6 weeks of nonweight-bearing immobilization.

Direct repair vs. allograft reconstruction. Both direct repair and allograft reconstruction result in predictable stability and good to excellent patient satisfaction.[89,110,187,215,216,337] Although not an optimal result, a slight loss of ankle motion (5°-10° of inversion) occurs most often after surgical reconstruction procedures.[135,338] Krips et al[177] evaluated two groups of athletes (n = 77) who had undergone either direct repair (DR) or an allograft reconstruction (AR) procedure for chronic lateral ankle instability 2 to 10 years (mean 5.4 years) earlier. There were no between group differences in preoperative age, activity level, or gender. All DR and AR participants had failed 6 months of conservative management. The AR group had significantly more patients with decreased ankle dorsiflexion than DR group (15/36 vs. 3/41). Patients did not have limited plantarflexion, eversion, or inversion in either group. Individuals in the DR group reported functional abilities as "excellent" or "good" at a significantly higher rate than those in the AR group (88% DR vs. 58% AR). AR group participants reported lower activity level, lower push-off power on the operated extremity during running, and lesser perceived ankle stability than those in the DR group. The authors concluded that direct repair was a better choice than tenodesis for primary repair of chronic ankle instability in an athletic population.

This difference in outcomes is becoming less of a concern with improved anatomic reconstruction techniques.[137,301,336,338] Improved allograft anatomical reconstruction surgical techniques, which more closely restores ankle kinematics, do not appear to be associated with restricted postoperative ROM or increased incidence of arthritis.[272] A nonrandomized cohort study compared outcomes in individuals after lateral ankle repair (n = 61) or anatomic reconstruction (n = 25). At a minimum of 2-year follow-up, there were no significant differences in satisfaction, function (Foot and Ankle Disability Index), or activity levels (Tegner Activity Scale). ROM was not assessed.[215]

A recent review concluded there was insufficient high quality evidence to strongly support any specific surgical procedure for treating ankle instability.[63] Although direct repair is currently considered the preferred procedure for primary ankle stabilization, further research comparing allograft reconstruction techniques to direct repair are needed to draw a firm conclusion.[109,135,177,187,215,216] Regardless of procedure, it is unlikely that rearfoot motion mechanics are completely restored by either procedure.[272]

Participation in sporting activities. Most individuals return to previous level of sport following lateral ankle stabilization surgery.[109,199,215] A consecutive series of 42 professional athletes with acute grade III lateral ankle ligament injury were treated with direct repair stabilization (Broström procedure). All athletes returned to training at a median of 63 days and to full sport participation at a median of 77 days. Forty patients reported being very satisfied and two partly satisfied. There were no serious complications related to the surgery.[372] Long-term sport participation demonstrates increased attrition. Maffulli et al[198] reported sport participation rates of 38 individuals 9 years (range 5 to 13 years) after Broström repair for management of chronic lateral ankle instability. Twenty-two (58%) individuals practiced sport at preinjury levels; 6 (16%) individuals were still active but in less demanding sports (cycling and tennis); and 10 (26%) were no longer active in sport. Of the 10 patients who had abandoned sport, 6 had experienced a subsequent traumatic inversion injury on the repaired ankle and did not feel sport participation was a viable option. Comparing baseline to follow-up plain film radiographs, degenerative changes were found in 15 patients (39%); degenerative changes did not correlate with return to sport activity. Overall, 76% of individuals reported good to excellent outcomes; 68% of individuals did not experience a subsequent ankle inversion injury; and 74% of individuals continued sport participation.

Repair of a Ruptured Achilles Tendon

Acute rupture of the Achilles tendon is a common soft tissue injury, occurring in the fourth to sixth decade of life for individuals who participate in exercise or athletic activities, with males affected about three times more than females.[99,163,275] The rupture usually is associated with a forceful contraction of the gastrocnemius-soleus muscles (triceps surae) during sudden acceleration or abrupt deceleration, such as jumping or landing.[16,35] Degenerative and mechanical factors appear to increase the risk of acute rupture.[35] The combination of a relatively hypovascular tendon, increased stiffness with aging, and repetitive microtrauma is thought to result in an inadequate reparative response and attrition of viable tissue. A concentric or eccentric mechanical overload completes the rupture.[16,41,275,352] Other factors thought to contribute to Achilles rupture include diabetes, cigarette smoking, preinjury use of quinolone antibiotics, and preinjury steroid injections in the tendon or paratendon.[127,275]

The tendon most frequently ruptures 3 to 4 cm proximal to the calcaneal insertion.[352] At the time of injury, a complete rupture leads to pain, swelling, a palpable defect, and significant weakness in plantarflexion. On clinical examination, the concordant presence of the following three findings are highly suggestive of a complete Achilles rupture:[100]

- Abnormal Thompson Squeeze Test (squeezing the calf muscle while the patient is prone to elicit ankle plantar flexion)
- Decreased ankle resting compared with the contralateral side (normal resting tension is approximately 20°-30° plantarflexion)
- Palpable defect in the Achilles tendon

An acute rupture of the Achilles tendon can be managed nonoperatively or surgically. Both options have advantages and disadvantages. With surgical repair followed by rehabilitation there is a lower risk of re-rupture of the tendon than with conservative management.[23,148,162,163,375] However, there is also a risk of postoperative wound closure problems, infection, and nerve injury (typically sural) that is not present with nonoperative management. With either management strategy, there is a relatively long recovery period and persistent weakness compared to the contralateral limb. There is general agreement that surgical intervention is preferable for younger, active individuals and athletes who desire to return to sport[64,193,200,323] and that conservative management is preferable for the older, relatively sedentary individual.[42,87,163,378] However, recent studies employing early functional mobilization rehabilitation protocols have demonstrated similar outcomes for operative and conservative management.[249,258,377,382] Presently, there is insufficient evidence to clearly support conservative versus surgical management. Re-rupture rates are relatively low following either strategy as long as early mobilization is utilized.[377,382] Both patient and surgeon must weigh the advantages and disadvantages of surgery and nonoperative treatment and arrive at an individualized treatment strategy.

FOCUS ON EVIDENCE

In the last decade, nonoperative management has evolved from 6 to 8 weeks of immobilization and restricted weight bearing to a more accelerated and functional rehabilitation approach.[80,229,249,377] Controlled and progressive loading of the tendon during the proliferative inflammatory phase (days to weeks following injury) has been shown to be beneficial to recovery.[95] Olsson et al[258] randomly assigned 100 individuals with acute Achilles tendon rupture into either a surgical repair group (surgery; n = 49) or conservative management group (nonsurgical; n = 51). Both groups completed an accelerated rehabilitation protocol that included immediate weight bearing to tolerance in a walker boot with three heel wedges holding the foot in an equinus (roughly 20° plantarflexion) position. Over the course of 8 weeks, heel wedges were sequentially removed, allowing progressively increased dorsiflexion to neutral. Both groups were weaned from the boot and into shoes with heel lifts (surgical group at 6 weeks, nonsurgical group at 8 weeks) and then weaned from heel lifts (surgical group at 10 weeks, nonsurgical group at 14 weeks). During the first 8 weeks, both groups completed exercise, but the nonsurgical group was limited to toe flexion/extension active ROM. The surgical group completed progressive, range-limited active ROM and light resistance gastrocnemius/soleus exercises. After the initial protective phase, both groups completed a standardized rehabilitation program that included therapeutic and functional exercises; the surgical group exercise progression was progressed more quickly than the nonsurgical group. There were no between-group significant differences in self-reported symptoms, physical activity level, or quality of life. Both groups returned to preinjury physical activity level at 12 months. At 12 months, the surgical group showed significantly better performance on hop tests. Although not statistically significant, five patients in the nonsurgical group sustained a re-rupture, whereas no re-ruptures occurred in the surgical group. The authors concluded that although stable surgical repair with accelerated tendon loading could be performed without major soft tissue complications, the treatment was not superior to nonsurgical management in terms of functional results, physical activity, or quality of life.

Indications for Surgery

The following are frequently cited indications for surgical repair or reconstruction of an acute or chronic rupture of the Achilles tendon:

- Acute, complete rupture of the Achilles tendon[16,42,352]
- The individual wishes to return to high-demand functional activities[10,16,42,258,382]
- Chronic, previously undiagnosed or untreated complete rupture in which end-to-end apposition cannot be achieved by conservative means[239,369]

Procedures

Primary Versus Delayed Repair

A considerable number of surgical procedures and techniques have been described for repair or reconstruction of a ruptured Achilles tendon.[16,24,55,249,258,369,377] An open, minimally invasive, or percutaneous surgical approach can be used for a primary repair.[16,42,191,352] Although minimally invasive techniques have been described,[199,201,196] an open approach typically is used for a delayed repair requiring reconstruction of the neglected Achilles tendon rupture (>1 month postrupture).[4,269,369]

Primary repair of an acute rupture generally is performed within the first few days after the injury. It is usually accomplished with a direct, end-to-end repair in which the ends of the torn tendon are re-opposed and sutured together.[16,352] The repair can be augmented with autograft or allograft, and this is more commonly performed with delayed repair.[16,199,269,352] Structures that may serve as a donor graft are the flexor hallucis longus, plantaris, fibularis brevis, semitendinosis, or a flap of fascia from the gastrocnemius.[199,269,352]

Operative Overview

Primary repair. In an open primary repair, an approximately 10-cm posterior incision is made at the distal leg medial to the Achilles tendon. A postero-medial incision avoids damage to the sural nerve. The tendon ends are identified, debrided, and sutured in re-opposition.[16,352] Core tendon sutures can be supplemented with epitendinous sutures to reinforce the repair.[258] Augmentation for primary repair is sometimes utilized, with inconclusive evidence.[42,352] With a percutaneous repair, the tendon ends are located and sutured together through several small puncture wounds that are made along the medial and lateral aspects of the Achilles tendon or through several small transverse incisions made directly over the tendon.[16,115,200,201,352] Mini-open repair uses a less lengthy skin incision than an open approach (approximately 5 cm). The tendon end is identified, sutured, and anchored to a bony drill hole for the repair.[24,228] In each of these approaches, the tendon is repaired while the ankle is maintained in a slightly plantarflexed or neutral position.

Delayed repair/reconstruction. With a tendon autograft reconstruction, a second incision is made to harvest the graft. For example, a fibularis brevis autograft requires release through a 2-cm incision at the base of the fifth metatarsal. The autograft is passed through, tensioned, and sutured to the opposed Achilles tendon stumps.[202]

Before closure, the ankle is moved into passive dorsiflexion to assess the integrity of the repair or reconstruction. After closure, a compression dressing and below knee posterior orthosis are applied with the ankle positioned in approximately 20° of equinus.[16] If immediate or very early weight bearing is to be allowed by the surgeon, a walking boot with heel wedges (approximately 20°) is applied.[258]

NOTE: An above-knee cast is applied (and later replaced with a below-knee cast) if the quality of the repair is tenuous.[16]

Complications

Complications associated with surgical repair or reconstruction of a ruptured Achilles tendon are summarized in Box 22.5.[9,16,148,163,228,238,249,258,319,378,382] Reports of complications typically separate re-rupture from other complications. Postoperative re-rupture is relatively uncommon with an incidence rate of approximately 3% to 5%.[16,152] Infection, adhesions, and sural nerve sensory disturbance are the most commonly reported complications.[152] A recent meta-analysis revealed a risk ratio of 3.9 in favor of nonoperative treatment for complications other than re-rupture; this translates to one additional complication (other than re-rupture) expected for every seven patients treated surgically.[319] The risk of complications associated with operative management decreases with

BOX 22.5 Complications Following Primary Repair of a Ruptured Achilles Tendon

- Tendon re-rupture or failure of the tendon to heal (palpable gap)
- Wound complications: infection, delayed healing of the incision
- Sural nerve injury leading to altered sensitivity of the lateral border of the foot
- Adherent or hypertrophic scarring
- Deep vein thrombosis or pulmonary embolism
- Restricted ankle ROM as the result of joint hypomobility or soft tissue adhesions or contractures, leading to impaired function, such as difficulty ascending or descending stairs due to limited dorsiflexion
- Strength and muscular endurance deficits, typically of the plantarflexors
- Pain at the site of a suture knot
- Complex regional pain syndrome (rare)

minimally invasive and percutaneous procedures when compared with an open approach for repair.[163,228,238]

Postoperative Management

Guidelines for postoperative rehabilitation after a primary open repair of an acute Achilles tendon rupture vary considerably in the literature and clinical practice. Historically, the surgery was followed by approximately 6 weeks of immobilization and nonweight bearing to avoid stress on the repair site. However, studies have demonstrated that the tendon benefits from early loading and motion during the healing process.[15,155,169] Translating basic science research into clinical practice, recent research has employed early weight bearing and mobilization following Achilles tendon repair.[184,203,204,249,258,377] Individuals with Achilles tendon repair following early weight bearing and mobilization protocols have demonstrated improved outcomes, including earlier return to walking, work, and pre-injury activity level; higher patient satisfaction; and no increased rate of re-rupture.[33,139,359] This has led to an AAOS ***CPG*** recommendation of no more than 2 weeks of protected weight bearing (strength of recommendation: moderate) and the use of a protective device that allows mobilization by 2 to 4 weeks postoperatively (strength of recommendation: moderate).[42]

NOTE: In the context of postoperative Achilles tendon repair literature, "early mobilization" implies that the patient is becoming more mobile; mobilization or loading of the tendon is controlled with slow, progressive ankle ROM. Early end-range ankle dorsiflexion is avoided during the protected phase of rehabilitation. Box 22.6 provides guidelines for early treatment following Achilles tendon repair.

Guidelines for management after percutaneous repair vary as well and are often quite similar to postoperative guidelines following open repair or reconstruction. Early weight bearing and mobilization following percutaneous repair have demonstrated positive outcomes similar to open repair.[8,61] Therefore, specific guidelines for percutaneous repair are not addressed in the following sections but can be found in other resources.[8,55,61,115,200]

BOX 22.6 Features of Early Weight-Bearing and Remobilization Programs After Repair of Acute Achilles Tendon Rupture*

Weight-Bearing Guidelines

- Initiated as tolerated while using crutches immediately after surgery[156,203] or after 1 or 2 weeks[229,237,279,330,377] in a below-knee orthosis with the ankle immobilized most often in plantarflexion or possibly neutral
- Progress gradually to full weight-bearing status between 3 to 6 weeks postoperatively[156,279,330,377]
- Orthosis worn during all weight-bearing activities for 6 to 8 weeks after surgery[279,330]
- Full weight bearing without the functional orthosis but wearing regular shoes with bilateral heel lifts when orthosis discontinued beginning at about 6 to 8 weeks postoperatively[156,326,330]

ROM Exercises

- Immediately[58,79,81,126] or by 1 to 2 weeks[237,279,326,330,377] after surgery, active plantarflexion and dorsiflexion of the operated ankle initiated while wearing a functional brace or orthosis to prevent dorsiflexion beyond 15° to 20° of equinus or to no more than a neutral position
- During the first 4 to 6 weeks and with the orthosis removed, ankle inversion and eversion while maintaining the ankle in plantarflexion[377]
  - By 6 to 8 weeks, dorsiflexion to 10° beyond neutral permitted in the orthosis and inversion/eversion out of the orthosis[156,237]

* During the first 6 postoperative weeks, all ankle ROM exercises are performed while seated or supine. Beyond 6 to 8 weeks postoperatively, guidelines are similar for early remobilization and conventional (traditional) programs.

Immobilization and Weight-Bearing Considerations

Immobilization with restricted weight-bearing approach. This approach may be utilized for a tenuous repair or repair/reconstruction of a failed primary repair.[367] The ankle is immobilized in approximately 20° of plantarflexion for approximately 6 weeks. The patient remains nonweight bearing during all or most of this time.[16,230,367] Following the period of strict immobilization, a CAM orthosis is applied, generally allowing plantarflexion, but limiting dorsiflexion to 0°. Although this approach is safe and associated with a low risk of re-rupture, it has been shown in some studies to lead to deficits in ankle strength (gastrocnemius/soleus) and ROM (dorsiflexion).[33,139,230,352,359]

Early remobilization and weight-bearing approach. After primary direct repair of the Achilles tendon, early motion and weight bearing are now recommended because of advances in surgical procedures and a better understanding of the benefits of early loading and motion during the tendon healing process.[42,229,249,330,377] Postoperatively, the ankle is immobilized in equinus for a short period (less than 2 weeks) to minimize wound complications. Individuals are encouraged to use crutches and bear weight to tolerance in a protective boot or walking cast that maintains the ankle in approximately 20° of plantarflexion.[42,258,352,377] If a boot is used, it is typically a hinged CAM orthosis that can be locked in various positions to limit end range dorsiflexion.[42,279]

After the initial period of immobilization (1 to 2 weeks), the CAM brace is opened to allow movement in a protected range, generally limiting dorsiflexion beyond neutral.[237,249,258,377] As an alternative, a rigid dorsal orthosis that allows plantarflexion but limits dorsiflexion to 0° may be used.[155,203] During the first 6 weeks of rehabilitation, the protective orthosis is worn during ambulation with progressive weight bearing and at all other times (including sleep) except when removed for wound care or for therapeutic exercises.

When the patient is able to ambulate on level surfaces without pain while fully weight bearing on the operated extremity, the protective boot or orthosis is gradually discontinued (usually 6 to 8 weeks postoperatively).[249,258] After discontinuing the functional brace or orthosis, a 1- or 1.5-cm bilateral heel lift is used initially to prevent tendon lengthening and to reduce tendon strain during functional activities.[249,258]

Although published guidelines for initiating and progressing weight bearing and allowing ankle mobility have differed from study to study, it has become apparent that allowing individuals to bear weight in a range-limiting orthosis during the initial protective phase leads to higher patient satisfaction, earlier return to functional activities, and no difference in re-rupture rates.[33,139] Common to all protocols is the use of safe levels of applied stress while protecting the healing tendon. Close communication among the surgeon, therapist, and patient is essential for success. Table 22.5 summarizes immobilization and weight-bearing guidelines associated with postoperative Achilles tendon repair management.[33,42,139,258,377]

Active plantarflexion and dorsiflexion of the operated lower extremity in the CAM orthosis can be initiated immediately[155,203] or by 1 to 2 weeks postoperatively.[201,237,249,258,330,377] The CAM

TABLE 22.5 Conventional Postoperative Management After Achilles Tendon Repair or Reconstruction With Graft*

Postoperative Time Period	Type and Position of Ankle Immobilization**	Weight-Bearing Guidelines
From 0–2 weeks		
	▪ Compression dressing and posterior orthosis, *OR* ▪ Walking boot set at 20° equinus, *OR* ▪ CAM orthosis that allows free plantarflexion but restricts dorsiflexion to -20°	▪ Partial weight bearing with bilateral axillary crutches
From 2 to 4 weeks		
	▪ CAM orthosis that allows free plantarflexion but restricts dorsiflexion to -20°	▪ Weight bearing as tolerated in walking boot or CAM orthosis; crutches as needed
From 4 to 6 weeks		
	▪ CAM orthosis that allows free plantarflexion but restricts dorsiflexion to -10° (week 4) and 0° (week 5)	▪ Full weight bearing in walking boot or brace, wean from crutches
From 6 to 8 weeks		
	▪ CAM orthosis that allows free plantarflexion but restricts dorsiflexion to 10° (week 6) ▪ Wean from CAM orthosis to shoes with 1- to 1.5-cm bilateral heel lift (week 7)	▪ Full weight bearing in functional brace or shoe with heel lift
Beyond 8 weeks		
	▪ Wean from heel lifts by 10 weeks	▪ Full weight bearing in regular shoe without lifts by 10 weeks

*All time periods are approximately 2 weeks longer after reconstruction with tendon graft.

** Immobilizer may be worn during ambulation for a longer period of time if wound healing is delayed or the quality of the repair is tenuous.

orthosis initially should restrict dorsiflexion beyond 20° of equinus. Active ROM dorsiflexion is allowed to increase as the CAM orthosis allows more motion. During the first 2 to 4 weeks, and with the orthosis removed, ankle inversion and eversion are initiated with the ankle in plantarflexion. [258,377] Initially, all ROM is completed actively while seated or supine. After 6 weeks postoperatively, bilateral standing exercises are introduced to improve active and passive ROM.[249,258,377]

FOCUS ON EVIDENCE

Until the late 1980s, 6 weeks of cast immobilization was standard postoperative management following Achilles tendon repair. As stated above, subsequent research has demonstrated the positive effects of early functional rehabilitation.[155,203,229,249,258,330,377,382] However, early functional rehabilitation regimens primarily involved either early weight bearing[49,50,330] or early ankle motion exercises,[155,156] but not necessarily both in combination. High quality, randomized controlled trials have combined these approaches.[8,107,161,203,204] Huang et al[139] recently completed a systematic review with meta-analysis that compared the following approaches:

- Comparison 1 (Early WBing + ROM): Early weight bearing with an ankle motion exercise regimen versus immobilization
- Comparison 2 (Early ROM only): Isolated early ankle motion exercises without early weight bearing versus immobilization

For the Early WBing + ROM vs. immobilization comparison, a total of 279 individuals were included.[203,204,50,49,161] The average time to weight bearing allowance was 4.1 days. Individuals who completed early weight-bearing and ROM exercises performed significantly better on 11 of 15 outcome measures when compared to individuals who received cast immobilization. Significantly better outcomes included:

- Higher satisfaction rate (93.6% vs. 77.5%)
- Time to return to sport
- Number of individuals returning to sport
- Normal ankle ROM
- Decreased tendon elongation
- Higher percentage of heel raise ability

There was no difference in the rates of re-rupture or major complications when comparing the two groups; but the rigid cast immobilization group had a higher rate of minor complications.

For the Early ROM vs. immobilization comparison, 171 individuals were included.[155,156] The average time to weight bearing allowance was 3.3 weeks. When compared to the immobilization group, individuals who completed early ROM had significantly superior outcomes in time to return to sport and decreased tendon elongation. No difference was observed between the 2 groups for rates of re-rupture, major, or minor complications.

Based on these results, the authors concluded that protocols employing early weight-bearing and early ROM exercise achieve superior results when compared to cast immobilization or early ankle ROM exercise with delayed weight bearing. Relatively few advantages are demonstrated when comparing early ROM exercise without weight bearing to rigid immobilization.

Two published case series have described outcomes following early weight bearing and ROM without postoperative bracing.[75,380] One day following endoscopic Achilles tendon repair, Doral permitted 28 males to bear weight as tolerated with axillary crutches and no brace/orthosis/cast. At an average of 28 months after surgery, individuals demonstrated no between ankle difference in plantarflexion strength, ankle ROM, or hop test performance. No re-ruptures were reported and all patients returned to same pre-injury sports and/or ADL level. Yotsumoto et al[380] investigated the effectiveness of a new Achilles tendon repair technique for allowing early mobilization without a postoperative immobilization orthosis in 20 patients (14 male, 6 female). Following surgery, individuals completed active and passive ankle ROM exercise. Partial weight bearing was initiated at 1 week after confirmation of 0° dorsiflexion, and full weight-bearing ambulation was allowed at 4 weeks. Heel lifts were used in individuals with strong tension of the gastrocnemius/soleus. The authors reported the following average times to achieve outcomes:

- Symmetrical ROM: 3.2 ± 0.7 weeks
- Normal walking without pain or fear: 4.5 ± 0.7 weeks
- 20 continuous single-leg heel raises of the operative foot: 9.9 ± 1.7 weeks.
- Resumption of sport activity: 15.4 weeks
- Resumption of labor: 12 weeks

No postoperative complications were found, and subjects achieved an average Achilles Tendon Rupture Score of 98.3 ± 2.4 at 24 weeks following surgery. Both studies concluded that early mobilization without immobilization is an option in select patients following Achilles tendon repair.

Exercise Progression

Although timing and progression of exercise may differ depending on the surgery (primary direct repair or reconstruction of a neglected rupture), the types of exercise included in a postoperative rehabilitation program are similar. In the phases of rehabilitation that follow, a progression of exercises is presented that is designed to help an individual achieve treatment goals that allow return to pre-injury function. The time frame for the initiation of weight bearing on the operated extremity, initiation of ankle ROM (particularly dorsiflexion), and resumption of pre-injury work-related and sports activities should be determined through consultation with the surgeon.

Exercise: Maximum Protection Phase

Achilles tendon repair frequently is performed on an outpatient basis. Therefore, patient education is essential before surgery or prior to discharge. It focuses on wound care (if the immobilizer is removable), controlling peripheral edema by elevating the operated leg, gait training with appropriate assistive device, and a home exercise program.

Goals and interventions. The following treatment goals are appropriate during the first 2 to 6 weeks after surgery.

- ***Re-establish independent ambulation and functional mobility.*** Instruct in gait and transfer training in protective orthosis with assistive devices, emphasizing weight-bearing restrictions.
- ***Maintain ROM of nonimmobilized joints.*** In a seated, supine or prone position, perform active ROM of the hip, knee, and toes of the operated side while wearing the immobilizer.
- ***Prevent reflex inhibition of immobilized muscle groups.*** Begin submaximal, pain-free muscle-setting exercises of the ankle in the immobilizer within the first few days after surgery. Start with setting exercises of the dorsiflexors, invertors, and evertors. Submaximal gastrocnemius/soleus muscle setting is typically initiated after 2 weeks, although a recent study included this exercise immediately postoperatively.[258] With a stable repair, it is possible to initiate nonweight-bearing isotonic strengthening against low loads (light grade elastic resistance) for the dorsiflexors, invertors, evertors, and plantarflexors after 2 weeks.[258]
- ***Prevent joint stiffness and soft tissue adhesions in the operated ankle and foot.*** Initiate ROM exercises in protected ranges. Active dorsiflexion should not exceed 0° for the first 4 weeks;[33] active ROM dorsiflexion can be completed in the CAM orthosis to prevent overstretching the repaired tendon. Active inversion and eversion should be performed in a plantarflexed position. Active ROM plantarflexion can be completed without restriction.
- ***Begin to restore balance reactions in standing.*** Perform weight-shifting activities in bilateral stance while wearing the protective orthosis. Use the parallel bars or another stable surface for upper extremity support as needed.
- ***Maintain cardiopulmonary fitness.*** Use an upper extremity ergometer for endurance training if available. After 2 weeks, initiate exercise bike in protective orthosis with minimal resistance.

Exercise: Moderate Protection Phase

At the end of the maximum protection phase (typically 4 to 6 weeks after surgery), the patient is advanced to full weight bearing in a CAM orthosis or walking boot that is progressed to 0° dorsiflexion. Weaning from the orthosis and into a shoe with heel lifts begins 6 to 8 weeks postoperatively.[33,184,203,258,377] As the patient is weaned from the orthosis, it may be necessary to resume using a cane or crutch for a period of time to normalize gait mechanics.

During the moderate protection phase of rehabilitation, which begins at 4 to 6 weeks and extends to 12 weeks postoperatively, the stress placed on the operated tendon is gradually increased. Patients continue supervised as well as independent exercise. Initially, exercise may be completed in the protective orthosis; as the patient weans from the orthosis, exercises are completed without the device. Precautions for progressing exercises and functional activities are noted in Box 22.7.[33,139,258,330,377]

Goals and interventions. The following goals and exercises are implemented during the intermediate phase of rehabilitation:

- ***Increase ROM of the operated ankle with joint mobilization and stretching techniques.***
  - Grade III joint mobilization techniques if ankle or foot joints are restricted.
  - Gentle self-stretching exercises, such as a towel stretch in a sitting position, to increase ankle dorsiflexion with the knee slightly flexed. Progress to stretch with knee fully extended.
  - Gentle manual self-stretching to regain full inversion/eversion and dorsiflexion/plantarflexion and toe extension.
  - Active ankle ROM with patient seated and foot on a wobble or rocker board.
  - Self-stretching to increase dorsiflexion by standing on a wedge in bilateral stance with knees slightly flexed. Progress to stretch with knees fully extended. Initiate unilateral standing stretches of plantarflexors at the end of this phase of rehabilitation (approximately 12 weeks after surgery).
- ***Improve strength and muscular endurance of the operated lower extremity.*** Initiate or progress low-load, high repetition resistance exercises at 6 to 8 weeks. Begin with open-chain exercises, and progress to seated then standing closed-chain exercises. Emphasize controlled, eccentric loading of the plantarflexors. Perform closed-chain exercises without the orthosis as its use is gradually discontinued. Examples of resistance exercises include:
  - Open-chain resistance exercises for the hip, knee, and ankle musculature against a light grade of elastic resistance.
  - Closed chain exercises such as unilateral heel raising and lowering while seated; add light resistance as tolerated, typically by 8 weeks.
  - Standing bilateral heel raising/lowering with body weight resistance. Postpone unilateral heel raising/lowering until 10 to 12 weeks after surgery.[258,330]
  - Partial lunges with involved leg forward, bilateral mini-squats, and toe raises.
  - As strength progresses, add external resistance (handheld weights, weight belt, or weighted backpack) to supplement body weight with standing exercises.

CLINICAL TIP

A resistance training program should focus on improving muscular endurance as well as strength. Substantial deficits in muscular endurance of the gastrocnemius-soleus muscles of the operated leg compared with the contralateral limb (as determined by number of unilateral heel raises performed in standing) have been shown to persist for at least a year after

BOX 22.7 Precautions and Guidelines for Exercise and Functional Activities Following Achilles Tendon Repair*

General Precautions

- Progress all exercises very cautiously that place resistance or a stretch on the gastrocnemius-soleus muscle group intentionally, following postoperative guidelines.
- Postpone all unilateral weight-bearing exercises on the operated side until full weight bearing without pain is possible.

Stretching to Increase Ankle Dorsiflexion

- Initiate active ROM dorsiflexion within the protected range by week 3 following surgery.[33,258,377]
- Begin stretching program in nonweight-bearing exercises (such as a towel stretch with slight knee flexion).
- Limit dorsiflexion to no more than 10° beyond neutral until 8 weeks after surgery. Progress to full ankle dorsiflexion (bilateral symmetry) by 12 weeks.
- Initiate weight-bearing stretches in *sitting* with feet on the floor, a low incline wedge (<10°), or a rocker board.
- Begin standing stretches in *bilateral* stance with knees bent only if pain free. This can be accomplished with a modified runner's wall stretch or a low incline (≤ 10°) wedge.
- Postpone *unilateral* standing stretches or bilateral standing stretches with heels over the edge of a step until advanced postoperative activities are permitted (approximately 12 weeks).

Resistance Exercises

- Begin strengthening exercises for ankle and foot musculature in nonweight-bearing positions against low loads (light-grade elastic resistance) before progressing to closed-chain exercises against body weight.
- Initiate heel raises in a seated position with gradual addition of external resistance before progressing to bilateral heel raises in standing.
- Progress heel raising/lowering exercises from bilateral to unilateral only if performed pain free (see suggested sequence in Box 22.11). Unilateral heel raising/lowering should be postponed until approximately 10 to 12 weeks postoperatively.

Advanced Training (Plyometric, Agility, Sport-Specific Training)

- Begin plyometric training in a pool (chest-deep progressing to waist deep immersion).
- Initiate advanced land-based training program (running, plyometrics, etc.) after 12 weeks if the individual meets the following criteria:
  - Ambulates pain free with normal gait and no assistive device
  - Normal dorsiflexion ROM (excessive dorsiflexion compared to contralateral limb indicates elongated tendon; advanced training may be delayed).
  - Completes 5 unilateral heel raises at ≥ 90% of the limb's maximum heel-rise height
- Begin with bilateral land-based plyometric activity, teaching the individual correct landing techniques. Advance to unilateral activities when proper joint alignment and controlled deceleration on the operative limb is achieved.
- Initiate return to running progression on level treadmill.
- Teach the patient correct landing technique for proper alignment during jumping and hopping exercises
- Wear a prescribed functional ankle-foot orthosis or tape the ankle during high-impact, high-velocity activities to minimize the risk of tendon re-rupture

* Precautions are applicable to conventional and early ROM/weight-bearing approaches to rehabilitation.

surgical repair of Achilles tendon ruptures.[29] The gastrocnemius-soleus complex also has been shown to produce significantly less work, calculated using force times distance with the heel-rise work test, than the contralateral limb at 1 year following repair.[311]

- ***Improve balance reactions.*** While wearing the functional orthosis, initiate or progress proprioceptive/balance training in bilateral stance on a firm surface. Progress to pliant surfaces (foam, air bladder, or mini-trampoline) and narrow the base of support (tandem stance, unilateral stance).
  - While continuing to wear the orthosis, progress to balance training in unilateral stance when full weight bearing is tolerated on the operated limb.
  - Transition to a sequence of more advanced balance exercises in supportive shoes (usually with a heel lift) after use of the functional brace has been discontinued.
- ***Re-establish a symmetrical gait pattern.*** When full weight bearing is comfortable and as the patient is weaned from the orthosis, progress gait training. Emphasize symmetrical alignment and weight shifting as well as equal step lengths and timing, paying particular attention to push-off on the operated side.
- ***Improve cardiopulmonary endurance.*** Begin or progress level-surface treadmill walking or stationary cycling (recumbent or upright) while wearing the functional brace or a regular shoe with a heel lift. If necessary, raise the seat height of the upright bicycle to accommodate for limited dorsiflexion. Progress to treadmill walking on an incline.

Exercise: Minimum Protection/Return to Function Phase

The final phase of rehabilitation, which begins around 12 to 16 weeks postoperatively, is directed toward returning a patient to a preinjury level of function for expected work-related demands and desired recreational/athletic activities. Stretching exercises continue if full ROM has not been achieved. During this phase, interventions should emphasize transition to independent maintenance.

Strength and muscular endurance training continues, emphasizing eccentric loading of the gastrocnemius-soleus muscle group with heel-lowering exercises in unilateral stance (see Fig. 22.17) and with resistance equipment. Descending stairs step over step also emphasizes eccentric loading. Depending on the patient's preinjury activity level, plyometric training can be initiated in a pool (see Chapter 23).

Having achieved functional criteria, individuals begin land-based plyometric training and treadmill walking on an incline at 12 to 16 weeks.[229,258,377] Advance to jogging, running, agility drills (cutting, pivoting), and sport-specific training. Patient education is a priority and focuses on ways to reduce the risk of re-rupture of the repaired tendon. Emphasize appropriate active warm-up and stretching prior to strenuous activity. If the strength of the operated extremity is relatively comparable to that of the contralateral extremity (dynamometry and/or heel-rise test),[335] the individuals progress from bilateral to unilateral plyometrics.[258] Individuals are permitted to gradually return to sporting activity 4 to 6 months after surgery.[249,258,352,377] Clinical criteria for return to sport activity include strength and ROM within normal limits. Functional criteria include pain-free walking and running and functional hop testing with limb symmetry indexes > 90% of the contralateral limb.

Outcomes

The ideal outcome is for a patient to return to a preinjury level of physical activity without pain or re-rupture of the repaired Achilles tendon. Patients undergoing primary repair of an acute rupture have consistently better outcomes than those who undergo a delayed repair for a chronic or neglected rupture. A surgical delay of up to 30 days following rupture has no negative impact; however, longer delays result in less satisfactory outcomes.[16,352] Active individuals 30 years or younger are at the highest risk of re-rupture following primary repair of an acute rupture.[279] The overall risk of re-rupture is approximately 3%.[16,184,230,319]

Numerous studies have compared methods of managing acute Achilles tendon ruptures. Operative management has been compared to nonoperative management, open procedures have been compared to minimally invasive procedures, and conservative management (strict immobilization/restricted weight) has been compared to "accelerated rehabilitation" (early motion/early weight bearing) in both operative and nonoperative management. Outcomes typically reported include re-rupture rate, ROM, strength, functional or sport-related activity level, and patient satisfaction. The following sections reflect conclusions drawn from systematic reviews of the literature as well as individual studies.

Nonoperative versus operative management. Despite a plethora of randomized controlled trials, it is unclear whether surgical or nonsurgical management provides superior results. Early systematic reviews concluded that operative management resulted in fewer re-ruptures when compared to nonoperative management.[23,163,378] However, the postoperative and nonoperative management generally included restricted weight bearing and delayed ROM for 6 weeks, a management strategy that is no longer in alignment with the current ***CPG***.[42]

A recent meta-analysis included results from 10 randomized controlled trials comparing operative and nonoperative outcomes in individuals with acute Achilles tendon rupture.[319] Postoperative management (conservative vs. functional rehabilitation) was determined to be a significant cause of heterogeneity among the studies. When considering only the results from five studies that employed functional rehabilitation (early weight bearing and ROM), surgical treatment and nonsurgical treatment were equivalent with regard to the re-rupture rate. Other findings included:

- Complications other than re-rupture favor nonoperative management (relative risk: 3.9)
- Time to return to work favors operative management (19 days earlier return to work)
- ROM results did not show a clinically important difference
- Strength results did not show a clinically important difference
- Functional outcomes did not show a clinically important difference

The authors concluded that nonoperative management with functional rehabilitation should be considered as a viable management option. This conclusion is echoed by the meta-analysis conducted by van der Eng et al, who found no difference in the re-rupture rates or the occurrence of major or minor complications between surgically and conservatively managed individuals.[359] Despite the equivocal results of these meta-analyses, surgeons generally consider surgical management the best option for high level athletes who desire a full return to sport activity.[16]

Regardless of operative or nonoperative management, over 30% of individuals are reported to have some degree of impairment including pain, decreased strength, and/or decreased ROM at 1 to 5 years after injury.[16,255,256,311,312] Studies of National Football League (NFL) and National Basketball Association (NBA) players with an Achilles tendon rupture have demonstrated that only 61% to 78% of professional athletes are able to return to previous level of play following surgical repair.[10,207,219,262] NBA basketball athletes who did return to previous level of play demonstrated significantly decreased playing time and player efficiency rating when compared to matched controls.[10] In the season following repair, NFL athletes who underwent Achilles tendon repair played in fewer games and at a lower performance level when compared to the season prior to injury.[207,262]

Olsson et al[257] investigated predictors of clinical outcome in 93 individuals following acute Achilles tendon repair. All participants completed an accelerated rehabilitation protocol consisting of early weight bearing and ROM. Independent (predictor) variables included treatment (surgical versus nonsurgical), age, sex, BMI, and patient-reported measures at time of inclusion (Physical Activity Scale and European Quality of Life Scale). Although surgical treatment resulted in lower degree of symptoms at 6 months, no difference in function was found between surgically and nonsurgically managed individuals at 6 and 12 months. Increasing age was a strong predictor of decreased function at both 6 and 12 months. Individuals with higher BMI experienced greater symptoms, but no effect on function was found.

Open versus minimally invasive repair. Traditionally, open repair has been considered the "gold standard" for Achilles tendon repair due to a low rate of re-rupture.[16] Percutaneous or minimally invasive techniques have been associated with a lower overall complication rate but increased risk of sural nerve injury.[16,162,163] Recent studies have challenged these assumptions.

A study of 211 individuals treated with minimally invasive surgical repair of an Achilles tendon rupture, sural nerve injury occurred in 41 (19%) and re-ruptures in 17 (8%).[228] A retrospective cohort study of 270 individuals treated with open (n = 169) or percutaneous Achilles repair demonstrated no difference in the major or minor complication rates. Most patients in both groups returned to baseline activities by 5 months following surgery.[136] A systematic review of compared open and minimally invasive repairs found comparable outcomes in ROM and ankle function in most of the included studies.[65] Open repair resulted in a higher percentage of complications when compared to minimally invasive procedures (14% vs. 6%, respectively), including a higher rate of re-rupture (3.4% vs. 2.2%, respectively). Minimally invasive repair resulted in more nerve injuries than open repair (2.9% vs. 1.8%, respectively). Individuals returned to work more quickly following minimally invasive procedures. The authors concluded that minimally invasive and open surgery are grossly equivalent procedures in terms of outcomes but that the cost and risk profile favors minimally invasive procedures.

Summary. In summary, there continues to be controversy as to whether surgical or nonoperative treatment is the better option for management of acute Achilles tendon rupture.[111,185,352] It is increasingly clear that postoperative and nonoperative management strategies previously considered "accelerated" have become the standard of care. Early weight bearing and ROM are now the recommended rehabilitation approach for primary Achilles tendon repair.[33,80,139,157,184,230,249,258,319,352]

Exercise Interventions for the Ankle and Foot

Exercise Techniques to Increase Flexibility and Range of Motion

Loss of flexibility in the ankle and foot can result from a variety of causes. Restoration of motion may be necessary to correct alignment or for normal biomechanics during walking and running. Joint mobilization techniques are used to increase accessory motion of the joint surfaces. These techniques are described in detail in Chapter 5. Manual passive stretching and PNF stretching techniques are described in Chapter 4. Self-stretching techniques to improve flexibility and ROM are the emphasis of this section.

Flexibility Exercises for the Ankle Region

Increase Ankle Dorsiflexion

The muscles that restrict dorsiflexion of the ankle are the one-joint soleus and the two-joint gastrocnemius. To effectively stretch the gastrocnemius, the knee must be extended while dorsiflexing the ankle. To isolate stretch to the soleus, the knee must be flexed during dorsiflexion to take tension off the gastrocnemius. Most of the following stretching exercises can be adapted with the knee in flexion or extension, so both of the plantarflexor muscles can be stretched.

PRECAUTION: When a patient uses weight-bearing exercises to stretch the plantarflexor muscles, shoes with arch supports should be worn or a folded washcloth placed under the medial border of the foot to minimize the stress to the arches of the foot.

FOCUS ON EVIDENCE

In a study of 30 subjects (15 with pes planus and 15 with neutral foot alignment), the effects of weight-bearing dorsiflexion stretches on the displacement of the myotendinous junction of the medial gastrocnemius, rearfoot angle, and navicular height were measured. Results showed a significantly greater displacement (elongation) at the myotendinous junction when the arch was supported in both groups, with a greater displacement occurring in subjects with pes planus. When the subjects with pes planus stretched without arch support, there was a significant increased rearfoot angle and drop in navicular height.[153]

- *Patient position and procedure:* Long-sitting (knees extended) or with the knees partially flexed. Have the patient strongly dorsiflex the feet, attempting to keep the toes relaxed.
- *Patient position and procedure:* Long-sitting or with the knee partially flexed and with a towel or belt looped under the forefoot. Have the patient pull with equal force on both ends of the towel to move the foot into dorsiflexion.
- *Patient position and procedure:* Sitting with the foot flat on the floor. Have the patient slide the foot backward, keeping the heel on the floor.
- *Patient position and procedure:* Standing. Have the patient stride forward with one foot, keeping the heel of the back foot flat on the floor (the back foot is the one being stretched). If necessary, have the patient brace his or her

hands against a wall. To provide stability to the foot, the patient partially rotates the back leg inward so the foot assumes a supinated position and locks the joints of the foot. The patient then shifts body weight forward onto the front foot. To stretch the gastrocnemius muscle, the knee of the back leg is kept extended; to stretch the soleus, the knee of the back leg is partially flexed.

- *Patient position and procedure:* Standing on an inclined board with feet pointing upward and heels downward (Fig. 22.9). Greater stretch occurs if the patient leans forward. Because the body weight is on the heels, there is little stretch on the long arches of the feet. Little effort is required to maintain this position for extended periods.
- *Patient position and procedure:* Standing, with the forefoot on the edge of a step or stool and heel over the edge. Have the patient slowly lower the heel over the edge (heel drop).

PRECAUTION: This stretch may create muscle soreness because it requires that the patient control an eccentric contraction of the plantarflexors.

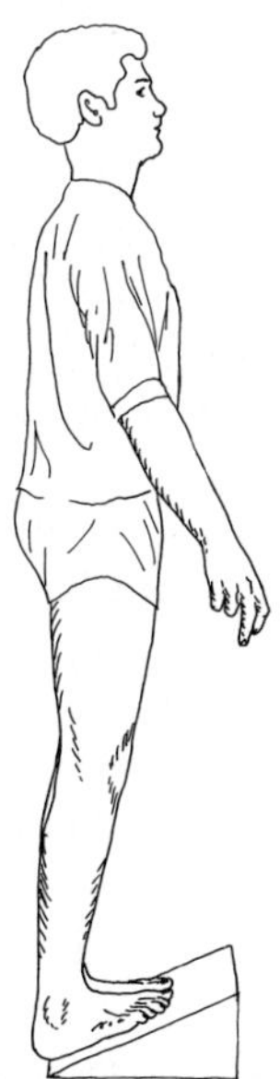

FIGURE 22.9 Self-stretching the gastrocnemius muscle to increase ankle dorsiflexion.

Increase Ankle Inversion

- *Patient position and procedure:* Sitting, with the foot to be stretched placed across the opposite knee. Have the patient grasp the midfoot and hindfoot with the opposite hand and lift the foot into inversion. Emphasize turning the heel inward, not just twisting the forefoot.
- *Patient position and procedure:* Long-sitting with a towel or belt looped under the foot. Have the patient pull on the medial side of the towel to cause the heel and foot to turn inward (Fig. 22.10). This technique also can be used to turn the foot outward by pulling on the lateral side of the towel. It is important that the motion includes the heel, not just the forefoot.

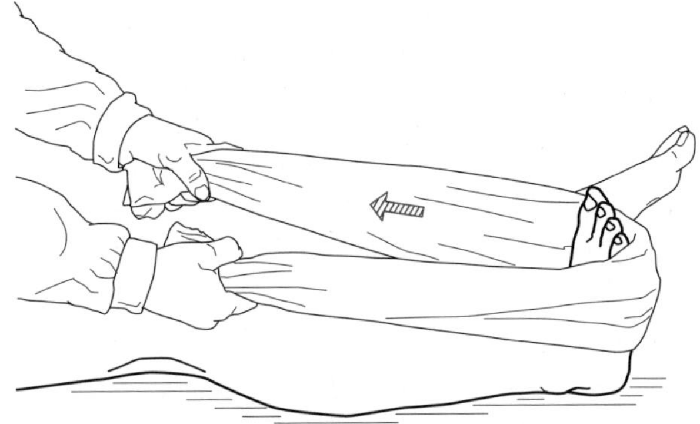

FIGURE 22.10 Self-stretching the ankle and foot into inversion by pulling with the medial side of the towel.

- *Patient position and procedure:* Sitting or standing, with feet pointing forward. Have the patient roll to the lateral border of each foot so the soles are turned inward.
- *Patient position and procedure:* Standing or walking, with the involved foot on a slanted board, placing the lateral aspect of the foot to be stretched on the lower side of the board. Bilateral stretching can be accomplished if hinged planks are placed in an inverted-V position and the patient stands or walks on them.

Increase Ankle Plantarflexion and Eversion

It is uncommon for plantarflexion and eversion to be restricted because gravity plantarflexes the foot in the supine position and the body's weight everts the foot in the standing position. Eversion, which is a component of pronation, is the loose-packed position of the foot and is perpetuated with weight bearing. The exception for restricted talocrural plantarflexion is when there is a capsular pattern at the joint as a result of arthritis. If the restriction is from joint hypomobility, it is treated with joint mobilization techniques.

Increase Ankle Dorsiflexion and Eversion

Patient position and procedure: Long-sitting with a towel or belt looped under the foot. Have the patient pull on the lateral side of the towel to cause the heel and foot to turn outward.

Flexibility Exercises for Limited Mobility of the Toes

Tight extrinsic muscles of the toes occur with claw toes and hammer toes, causing the MTP joints to extend and the IP joints to flex. There is often weakness of the intrinsic muscles. To stretch the intrinsic muscles, emphasize *MTP flexion* and *IP extension.*

Passive MTP Flexion

Patient position and procedure: Sitting with the foot crossed onto the opposite knee. Show the patient how to stabilize the foot under the metatarsal heads (MTP joints) with the thumbs and passively flex the MTP joints by applying pressure against the proximal phalanges. Or, have the patient attempt active flexion of the MTP joints, assisting the motion if necessary.

Passive IP Extension

Patient position and procedure: Sitting with the foot crossed onto the opposite knee. Teach the patient to stabilize the proximal phalanx of the involved toe and passively stretch the long flexors across each joint by moving the middle and/or distal phalanx into extension.

Active MTP Flexion

Patient position and procedure: Standing with the toes over the edge of a stool or book and the MTP joints at the edge. Have the patient attempt to flex the MTP joints over the edge of the stool. Ideally, the patient should try to keep the IP joints of the toes extended, but many individuals cannot do this.

Great Toe Extension

Extension of the great toe at the MTP joint is critical during the push-off phase of gait. In addition to joint mobilization techniques, passive stretching and self-stretching techniques should be used.

- *Patient position and procedure:* Sitting with the foot resting on the opposite knee. Show the patient how to stabilize the foot around the head of the first metatarsal with one hand and passively *extend* the MTP joint by applying pressure against the proximal phalanx.
- *Patient position and procedure:* Sitting with the feet placed on the floor. Have the patient slide the foot to be stretched backward by flexing the knee while keeping the toes on the floor and raising the heel off the floor.
- *Patient position and procedure:* Standing with the involved foot in a backward stride position. The patient may lean his or her hands against a wall for support. Have the patient keep the toes on the floor and rock forward lifting the heel until a stretch is felt under the first toe. A sustained stretch or a gentle rocking stretch can be used.

Stretching the Plantar Fascia of the Foot

- *Patient position and procedure:* Sitting with the foot placed across the opposite knee. Teach the patient to use his or her thumbs to apply deep massage horizontally and longitudinally across the plantar surface of the foot.
- *Patient position and procedure:* Sitting with a ball, small roller, or plastic bottle under the foot. Have the patient roll the foot forward and backward across the curved surface, using as much pressure as is comfortable. Pressing down on the knee with one or both hands can exert additional force.

Exercises to Develop and Improve Muscle Performance and Functional Control

Causes of strength and flexibility imbalances of the ankle and foot include disuse, immobilization, nerve injury, and progressive joint degeneration. In addition, imbalances occur from the weight-bearing stresses that are imposed on the feet. Imbalances can be the cause or the effect of faulty lower extremity mechanics. Because the lower extremities bear weight, realignment by strengthening exercises alone is of limited value. Strengthening exercises undertaken in conjunction with conscious correction, appropriate stretching, balance training, and other necessary measures (such as using orthotic inserts or adaptations for shoes, bracing, orthoses, or surgery) improve alignment, so structurally safe weight bearing is possible. In addition, knowledge of the types of shoes used or surfaces encountered during walking or sports activities may be a lead to the source of faulty mechanics, which then can be adjusted. (Techniques of orthopaedic adaptations for shoes, bracing, and orthoses are beyond the scope of this text.)

Most functional demands on the ankle and foot occur during weight-bearing activities. Kinesthetic input from skin, joint, and muscle receptors and the resulting joint and muscle responses are different in open- and closed-chain activities.[261] Therefore, whenever possible, use of progressive weight-bearing exercises is important to simulate functional activities. In addition to the exercises described in this section, refer to Chapter 23 for total lower extremity functional exercises performed in the standing position that influence muscle control at the hip, knee, and ankle.

Exercises to Develop Dynamic Neuromuscular Control

- *Patient position and procedure:* Long-sitting or with the knees partially flexed. Have the patient practice contracting each of the major muscles while concentrating on his or her actions—for example, dorsiflexion with inversion (anterior tibialis), plantarflexion with inversion (posterior tibialis), and eversion (fibularis muscles).
- *Patient position and procedure:* Long-sitting or with the knee partially flexed. Instruct the patient to "draw" the alphabet in space, leading with the toes but moving at the ankle. For variety, have the patient "print" using capital letters, then with lower case letters, or "write" words such as his or her name or address.

- *Patient position and procedure:* Sitting on a chair or low mat table with feet on the floor. Place a number of small objects, such as marbles or dice, to one side of the involved foot. Have the patient pick up one object at a time by curling the toes around it and then place the object in a container on the other side of the foot. This exercise emphasizes the plantar muscles as well as inversion and eversion.
- *Patient position and procedure:* Sitting with feet on the floor or standing. Have the patient curl the toes against the resistance of the floor. Place a towel or tissue paper under the feet, and have the patient attempt to wrinkle it up by keeping the heel on the floor and flexing the toes.
- *Patient position and procedure:* Sitting, with the feet on the floor. Have the patient attempt to raise the medial longitudinal arch while keeping the forefoot and hindfoot on the floor. External rotation of the tibia—but not abduction of the hips—should occur. The activity is repeated until the patient has consistent control; then it is performed while standing as a progression.
- *Patient position and procedure:* Sitting with a tennis ball placed between the soles of the feet. Instruct the patient to roll the tennis ball back and forth from heel to forefoot.
- *Patient position and procedure:* Sitting, with both feet or the involved foot only on a rocker or balance board. Have patient perform controlled ankle and foot motions (with or without the assistance of the normal foot) into dorsiflexion and plantarflexion and inversion and eversion (Fig. 22.11). If the equipment permits, the patient also can perform circumduction in each direction. Progress this activity to the standing position to further develop control and balance.

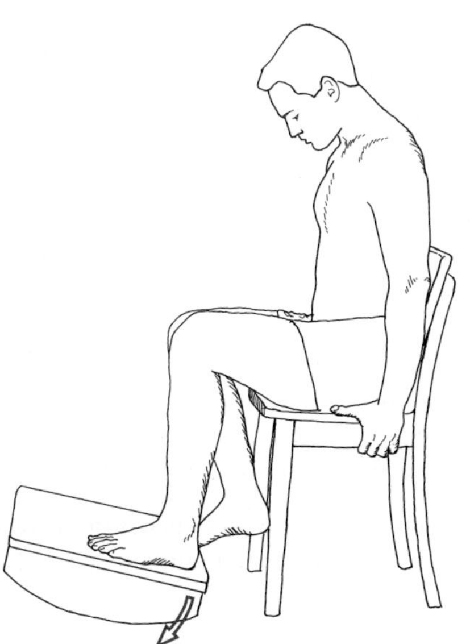

FIGURE 22.11 Using a rocker board to develop control of ankle motions with the patient sitting. The normal foot can assist the involved side in the early phases of rehabilitation. This activity can be progressed by using only the involved foot and then performing the motions in standing.

- *Patient position and procedure:* Standing. Have the patient practice walking while concentrating on placement of the feet and shifting body weight with each step. The patient begins by accepting body weight on the heel, then shifting the weight along the lateral border of the foot to the fifth metatarsal head and across to the first metatarsal head and great toe for push-off.

Open-Chain (Nonweight-Bearing) Exercises

Plantarflexion

Patient position and procedure: Long-sitting with the leg resting on a rolled towel to slightly elevate the heel off the treatment table. Have the patient hold both ends of an elastic band that is looped under the forefoot, then plantarflex the foot against the resistance (Fig. 22.12).

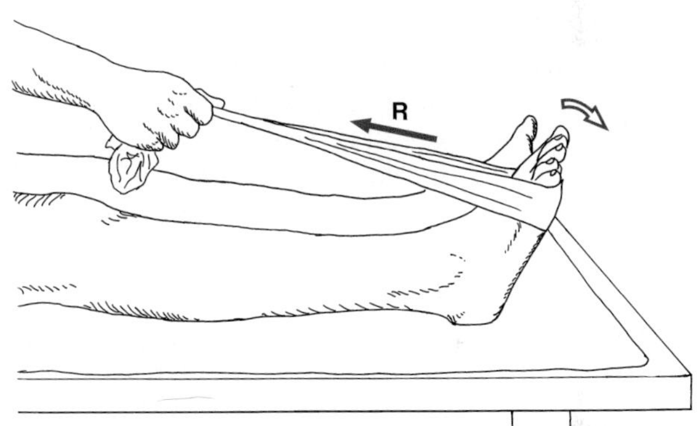

FIGURE 22.12 Resisting the ankle plantarflexor muscles with an elasticized material.

Isometric Eversion and Inversion

Patient position and procedure: Long-sitting or sitting in a chair with knees flexed.

- To resist *eversion*, the ankles are crossed; instruct the patient to press the lateral borders of both feet together against each other.
- To resist *inversion*, the medial borders of the feet are placed beside each other; instruct the patient to press the medial borders of the feet against each other.

Eversion and Inversion With Elastic Resistance

Patient position and procedure: Long-sitting, supine, or sitting with the feet resting on the floor.

- To strengthen *evertors*, place a loop of elastic tubing around both feet and have the patient evert one or both feet against the resistance (Fig. 22.13). Instruct the patient to keep the knees still and turn the foot outward, not allowing the thigh and leg to abduct or externally rotate.
- To strengthen *invertors*, tie the elastic band or tubing to a structure on the lateral side of the foot. Again, have the

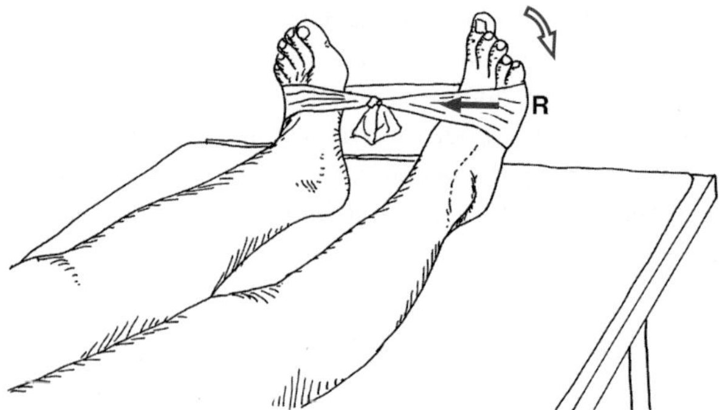

FIGURE 22.13 Resisting the ankle evertor muscles with an elasticized material.

patient keep the legs stationary and only turn the foot inward without allowing the hip to adduct and internally rotate.

Adduction With Inversion and Abduction With Eversion Using Weights

Patient position and procedure: Sitting with the foot on the floor. Place a towel under the forefoot and a weight on the end of the towel (Fig. 22.14). Have the patient pull the weighted towel along the floor with the forefoot by keeping the heel fixed on the floor and swinging the foot either inward or outward.

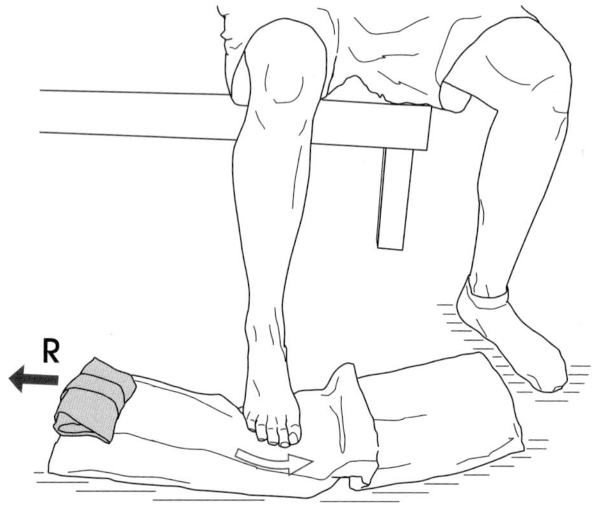

FIGURE 22.14 Resisting ankle adduction and inversion with a weight on the end of the towel. The heel is kept stationary while a windshield wiper motion of the foot is used to pull the towel along the floor. Abduction with eversion can be resisted by placing the weight on the towel on the medial side of the foot.

Dorsiflexion

Patient position and procedure: Long-sitting or supine with a rolled towel under the distal leg to elevate the heel slightly. Tie both ends of an elastic band or tubing to the foot board of a bed (or other object), and loop the elastic over the dorsum of the foot. Have the patient dorsiflex the ankle against the resistance (Fig. 22.15).

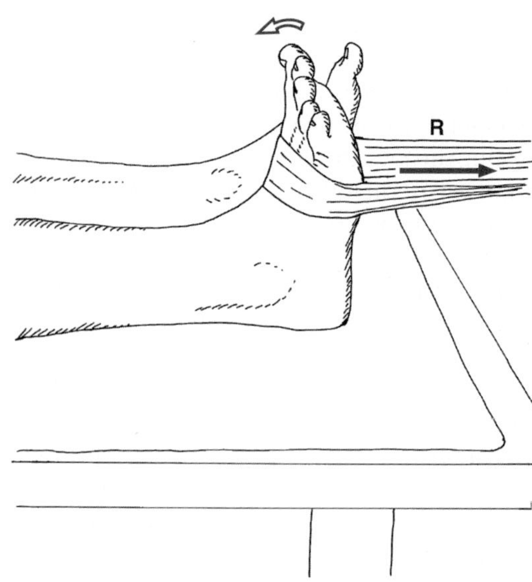

FIGURE 22.15 Resisting the ankle dorsiflexor muscles with an elasticized material.

All Ankle Motions

Patient position and procedure: Sitting in a chair or standing with one or both feet in a box filled with sand, foam, dry peas, dry beans, or other similar type material to offer resistance to various foot motions. Have the patient plantarflex, dorsiflex, invert, and evert the foot and ankle, and curl the toes with the foot on top or with the foot dug into the medium.

Closed-Chain (Weight-Bearing) Exercises

For these exercises, the patient position is standing. If the patient does not initially tolerate full weight bearing without reproduction of symptoms, begin with the patient standing in parallel bars using both hands for support, holding onto a stable object, harnessed into a body weight support system, or exercising in a pool to reduce weight-bearing forces. Progress from bilateral to unilateral stance. Refer to Table 6.9 for general guidelines for progression of closed-chain exercises.

Stabilization Exercises

Begin stabilization exercises for the ankle and foot in bilateral stance, progressing to unilateral stance and by standing on a flat, stable surface and later on less stable surfaces.

- Apply resistance to the patient's pelvis in various directions while he or she attempts to maintain control. At first, use verbal cues, then resist without warning. Also, increase the speed and intensity of the perturbation forces.
- Have the patient hold onto a wooden dowel rod or cane with both hands. Apply the resistance through the rod in various directions and with varying intensities and speeds as the patient attempts to remain stable (Fig. 22.16).
- Progress to standing only on the involved foot.

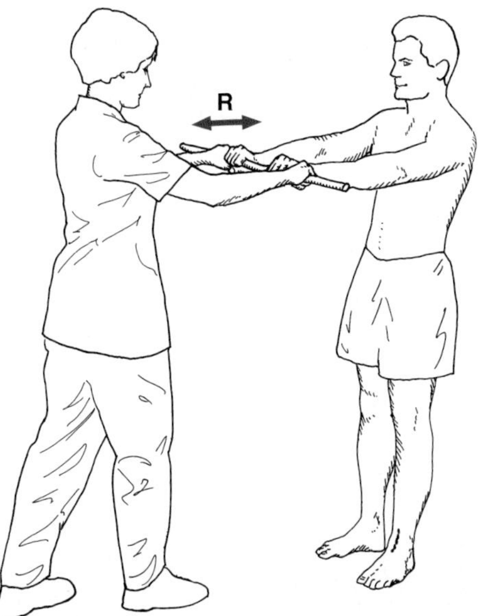

FIGURE 22.16 Stabilization exercises with the patient standing and maintaining balance against the alternating resistance forces from the therapist. The therapist applies force through the rod in backward/forward, side-to-side, and rotational directions. This can be progressed by standing on only the involved foot and by removing visual input.

- Have the patient stand on the involved leg and maintain a stable position of the ankle and foot while moving the opposite leg forward, backward, and to the side against the resistance of an elastic band or tubing secured around the ankle of the moving limb and a table leg (similar to Fig. 20.22).

Dynamic Strength Training

- Have the patient perform bilateral toe and heel raises and rock outward to the lateral borders of the feet. Progress to performing these exercises unilaterally. When tolerated, add resistance with a weighted backpack, weight belt, or handheld weights. Progress to jumping, then hopping on level surfaces and then on and off a platform for explosive concentric and eccentric loading.
- For *eccentric loading* of the gastrocnemius-soleus muscle group without concentric loading of the affected ankle, have the patient perform the following sequence.[149] While positioned next to a stable surface (wall, countertop) using one hand for balance, have the patient stand on a low platform on the *sound* lower extremity and the *affected* foot in maximum plantarflexion with the ball of the foot on the floor. Transfer body weight onto the ball of the foot of the *affected* side while lifting the sound lower extremity off the step; and then slowly lower the heel to the floor (Fig. 22.17) using a lengthening contraction of the gastrocnemius-soleus muscle group. Repeat the sequence by stepping back onto the platform with the sound limb.

CLINICAL TIP

Resistance training that emphasizes eccentric contractions of the ankle plantarflexors has been shown to decrease pain and increase physical functioning in patients with midposition Achilles tendinopathy.[38] Eccentric loading, emphasizing heel-lowering exercises, has also been investigated for management of insertional Achilles tendinopathy with promising results.[149]

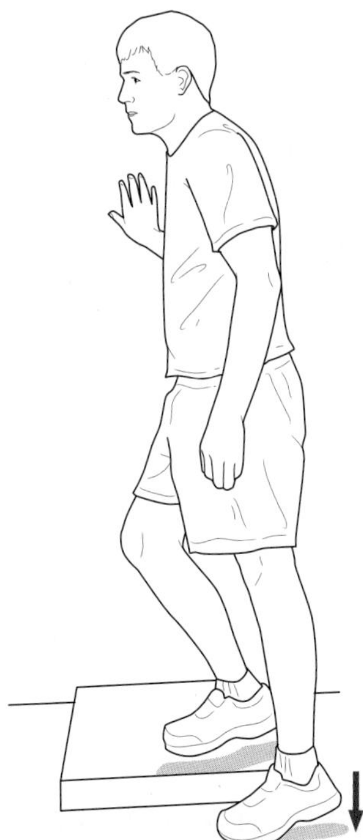

FIGURE 22.17 Eccentric loading of the gastrocnemius-soleus muscle group is accomplished by shifting weight from the foot on the step to the ball of the plantar flexed foot then lowering the heel of the involved ankle.

Resisted Walking

- Have the patient walk on heels and on toes against resistance. Apply manual resistance against the patient's pelvis, or have the patient walk against a weight-pulley system or elastic resistance secured around the pelvis.
- Apply an elastic band around the ankle of the sound lower extremity and secure the band to a stable object.[120] While bearing weight on the involved lower extremity:
  - Bring the sound leg one step forward against the resistance of the elastic band to strengthen the ankle dorsiflexors of the weight-bearing limb (Fig. 22.18 A and B).
  - Move the sound leg one step backward against the resistance of the elastic band to strengthen the ankle plantarflexors of the weight-bearing limb (Fig. 22.19 A and B).

Functional Progression for the Ankle and Foot

As with functional training for the hip and knee, implement a progression of exercises that prepares a patient recovering from structural or functional impairments of the ankle to return safely to their desired occupational and recreational activities. To meet these challenges, a patient must develop

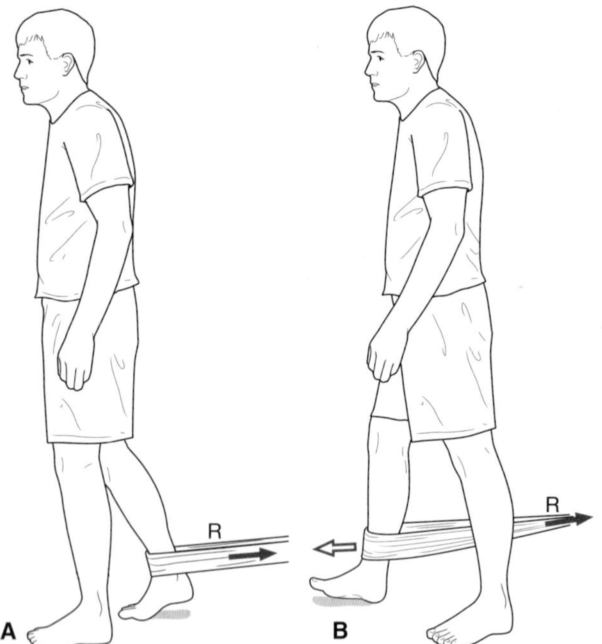

FIGURE 22.18 **(A)** Starting position for activation of the ankle dorsiflexors of the *weight-bearing limb* by advancing the opposite limb forward against resistance of an elastic band; **(B)** ending position.

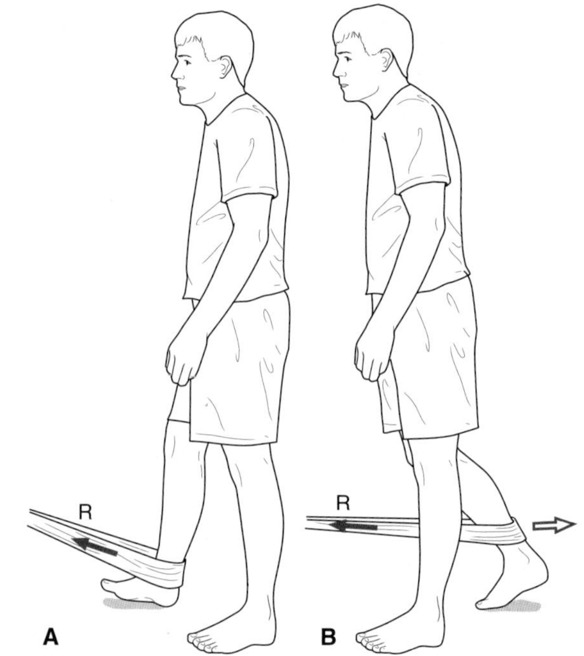

FIGURE 22.19 **(A)** Starting position for activation of the ankle plantarflexors of the *weight-bearing limb* by advancing the opposite limb backward against resistance of an elastic band; **(B)** ending position.

sufficient strength, endurance, and flexibility, as well as power, balance, coordination, agility, aerobic fitness, and task-specific skills. (Refer to Chapters 7 and 8 respectively for principles of aerobic conditioning and balance training.)

A functional progression of exercises for the ankle and foot must involve the entire body—lower extremities, trunk, and upper extremities. A variety of advanced stability, balance, strengthening, plyometric, and agility exercises that could be used for the patient with dysfunction of the ankle and/or foot are described and illustrated in Chapter 23. Some of the closed-chain strengthening exercises and functional progressions described in Chapters 20 and 21 are applicable as well (see Box 20.11).

Selected equipment also is valuable for improving function of the ankle and foot. Training on a stationary bicycle, treadmill, cross-country ski machine, or mini-trampoline is useful for developing endurance of ankle musculature. A slide board can be used to develop coordination, control, and dynamic ankle stability. Use of balance equipment, such as a rocker or wobble board or BOSU®, imposes a significant challenge on dynamic stabilizers of the ankle as does walking or running on uneven surfaces.

Independent Learning Activities

Critical Thinking and Discussion

1. Observe how the foot and ankle function as a unit in several activities, such as walking up steps, walking on uneven surfaces, and walking in high-heeled shoes versus low-heeled shoes.
   - What motions do you observe in the talocrural, subtalar, transverse tarsal, and MTP joints? Describe how the mechanics change across activities.
   - What muscles are functioning to move or control each joint? Describe how muscle function and demand changes across activities.
2. Describe the role of the ankle and foot during the gait cycle.
   - How much ROM is needed at the ankle, and which muscles are acting to cause or control the motion? What other forces are causing or controlling motion at the ankle?
   - What gait deviations occur if there is muscle shortening or weakness at the ankle? Describe potential deviations with involvement of the plantarflexors, inverters, evertors, and dorsiflexors.
   - After a unilateral arthrodesis of the talocrural joint (ankle fused in neutral), what deviations will occur in

the gait cycle? How will such a procedure affect the proximal joints of the lower extremity and/or the pelvis and trunk?
- Describe the mechanics and function of pronation and supination in the foot during the gait cycle. Explain how the gait cycle would be affected if a patient had flexible flat feet versus rigid supinated feet.

3. Compare and contrast an exercise program for a patient who has had a repair or reconstruction of torn lateral ligaments of the ankle versus a patient who has had a repair of a ruptured Achilles tendon. How will precautions and selection of exercises differ after these two types of surgical repairs?
4. Discuss the benefits and limitations of total ankle arthroplasty versus arthrodesis of the ankle.

Laboratory Practice

1. Review all the joint mobilization techniques for the leg, ankle, and foot; include basic glides, accessory motions, and mobilization with movement techniques.
   - Identify and practice techniques that you could use to increase ankle plantarflexion; begin with the ankle at zero, and progress at 15° increments until full plantarflexion is reached.
   - Do the same for ankle dorsiflexion, subtalar inversion and subtalar eversion, and MTP extension.
2. Set up a circuit-training course for the foot and ankle musculature to increase strength, muscular endurance, stability, balance, and neuromuscular reactions. Sequence the activities from basic to advanced, and observe accuracy and safety with each exercise. Identify other muscles in the lower extremity, trunk, or arms that are also being affected by the exercises.

Case Studies

1. Carl has a 10-year history of RA. His acute symptoms are managed with medication, so he is able to walk with a cane. He complains of increased pain after walking 15 minutes, considerable stiffness, and generalized weakness. He walks with short step lengths and has minimal push-off. Ankle ROM: dorsiflexion 10°, plantarflexion 15°, inversion 0°, eversion 8°. He stands with pronated feet and has dorsal migration of the first phalanges and moderate hammer toes. He tolerates moderate resistance in his lower leg/ankle musculature, but he is unable to demonstrate toe walking or do bilateral toe raises even one time.
   - List his impairments and activity limitations.
   - Develop a list of short- and long-term goals
   - Develop a program of intervention to meet the goals. How will you initiate the intervention? How will you sequence the interventions? What techniques will you use and how will you progress them?
   - Describe your rationale for the manual techniques and exercises you select, for those deemed not appropriate, and for the home interventions you would teach the patient.
   - Identify any precautions that are present for your interventions, as well as those that you must teach the patient.
2. Sandy sustained a boot-top fracture of the tibia and fibula as the result of a fall while downhill skiing. She was immobilized in a long-leg cast for 6 weeks, followed by a short-leg cast for 4 weeks. She was allowed partial weight bearing while wearing the short-leg cast. The cast was removed this morning. She now reports significant stiffness and discomfort when attempting to move her ankle and foot. Observation reveals lower leg atrophy, but no edema or joint swelling. ROM in the ankle and foot is minimal, and there is no accessory gliding of the fibula at the proximal or distal tibiofibular joints. Strength was not tested, although the patient can activate all muscles.
   - Answer the same questions posed in Case 1.
   - What are the key differences between Sandy and Carl regarding the intervention strategies and precautions?
   - How will you determine the progression of weight-bearing activities?
3. Ron is a 35-year-old computer programmer who plays recreational basketball. He sustained a severe inversion strain of his right ankle when landing on the foot of an opponent during a recent game. He wrapped the ankle with a compression wrap and applied ice to it for 2 days. On the third day, a radiograph determined that there was no fracture but he was diagnosed with a grade II instability of the ATF ligament. Observation reveals significant swelling and discoloration of the anterior and lateral ankle region. He experiences a marked increase in pain with inversion and plantarflexion motions, anterior gliding of the talus, and palpation over the ATF ligament. Because of muscle guarding, strength was not tested.
   - Identify structural and functional impairments, activity limitations, and participation restrictions.
   - Determine goals and an intervention strategy for this patient.
   - Describe how the intervention will be progressed.
   - Ron wants to know how soon he can return to playing basketball. What criteria will you use to make this judgment, and how will you protect his ankle when he does return?
4. Jamaal is an active 43-year-old dentist who ruptured his (L) Achilles tendon during a weekend tennis match. At the time of the injury, he experienced acute pain above his heel that persisted for a brief period of time. He was able to return home, where he rested for the remainder of the day while applying ice to the posterior aspect of the lower leg. Jamaal went to an urgent care facility the next day because he was having some difficulty walking and ascending and descending stairs. Physical examination suggested a ruptured Achilles tendon, which was confirmed by an MRI. An open primary repair of the tendon was performed two days later on an outpatient basis. Following surgery, the

involved ankle was immobilized in a short-leg cast with the ankle positioned in plantarflexion for 2 weeks. He has been ambulating nonweight bearing with crutches since surgery. At the 2-week postoperative visit to the surgeon, the cast was removed and replaced with an ankle-foot orthosis, which was set in slight plantarflexion. He is now permitted to bear partial weight on the involved foot within pain tolerance while wearing the orthosis. Jamaal has been referred to physical therapy to begin rehabilitation, using an early remobilization and weight-bearing approach. He is allowed to remove the orthosis for ankle ROM exercises.

- Describe a sequence of exercises and criteria for progression that you would teach Jamaal that is consistent with this accelerated functional approach to Achilles repair management.
- What precautions are included in your treatment plan?
- Describe the additional intervention strategies that will be used to prepare Jamaal to return to playing tennis.

REFERENCES

1. Abdel-Aziem, AA, and Draz, AH: Chronic ankle instability alters eccentric eversion/inversion and dorsiflexion/plantarflexion ratio. *J Back Musculoskelet Rehabil* 27(1):47–53, 2014.
2. Abidi, NA, Gruen, GS, and Conti, SF: Ankle arthrodesis: indications and techniques. *J Am Acad Orthop Surg* 8(3):200–209, 2000.
3. Acevedo, JI, and Mangone, P: Ankle instability and arthroscopic lateral ligament repair. *Foot Ankle Clin* 20(1):59–69, 2015.
4. Ahmad, J, Jones, K, and Raikin, SM: Treatment of chronic Achilles tendon ruptures with large defects. *Foot Ankle Spec* 20(10):1–9, 2016
5. Ahmad, J, and Pedowitz, D: Management of the rigid arthritic flatfoot in adults: triple arthrodesis. *Foot Ankle Clin* 17(2):309–22, 2012.
6. Ajis, A, Henriquez, H, and Myerson, M: Postoperative range of motion trends following total ankle arthroplasty. *Foot Ankle Int* 34(5):645–656, 2013.
7. Alexander, IJ: Hallux metatarsophalangeal arthrodesis. In Kitaoka, HB (ed): *Master Techniques in Orthopedic Surgery: The Foot and Ankle*, ed. 2, Philadelphia: Lippincott Williams & Wilkins, 2002, pp 45–60.
8. Al-Mouazzen, L, et al: Percutaneous repair followed by accelerated rehabilitation for acute Achilles tendon ruptures. *J Orthop Surg Hong Kong* 23(3):352–356, 2015.
9. Amendola A: Outcomes of open surgery versus nonoperative management of acute Achilles tendon rupture. *Clin J Sport Med* 24(1):90–91, 2014.
10. Amin, NH, et al: Performance outcomes after repair of complete Achilles tendon ruptures in national basketball association players. *Am J Sports Med* 41(8):1864–1868, 2013.
11. Anderson, T, Montgomery, F, and Carlsson, A: Uncemented STAR total ankle prostheses. Three to eight-year follow-up of fifty-one consecutive ankles. *J Bone Joint Surg Am* 85–A(7):1321–1329, 2003.
12. Ardern, CL, et al: Psychological responses matter in returning to preinjury level of sport after anterior cruciate ligament reconstruction surgery. *Am J Sports Med* 41(7):1549–1558, 2003.
13. Arnason, A, et al: Risk factors for injuries in football. *Am J Sports Med* 32:5S–16S, 2004.
14. Arno, F, and Roman, F: The influence of footwear on functional outcome after total ankle replacement, ankle arthrodesis, and tibiotalocalcaneal arthrodesis. *Clin Biomech* 32:34–39, 2016.
15. Aspenberg, P: Stimulation of tendon repair: mechanical loading, GDFs and platelets. A mini-review. *Int Orthop* 31(6):783–789, 2007.
16. Azar, F: Traumatic disorders. In Canale ST and Beaty JH (eds) *Campbell's Operative Orthopaedics,* ed. 12. Philadelphia: Elsevier/Mosby; 2013, p. 2311–2362, 2013.
17. Bai, L-B, et al: Total ankle arthroplasty outcome comparison for post-traumatic and primary osteoarthritis. *Foot Ankle Int* 31(12):1048–1056, 2010.
18. Barg, A, Henninger, HB, and Hintermann, B: Risk factors for symptomatic deep-vein thrombosis in patients after total ankle replacement who received routine chemical thromboprophylaxis. *J Bone Joint Surg Br* 93(7):921–927, 2011.
19. Barton, T, Lintz, F, and Winson, I: Biomechanical changes associated with the osteoarthritic, arthrodesed, and prosthetic ankle joint. *Foot Ankle Surg* 17(2):52–57, 2011.
20. Best, MJ, Buller, LT, and Miranda, A: National trends in foot and ankle arthrodesis: 17-year analysis of the National Survey of Ambulatory Surgery and National Hospital Discharge Survey. *J Foot Ankle Surg* 54(6):1037–1041, 2015.
21. Beumer, A, et al: Effects of ligament sectioning on the kinematics of the distal tibiofibular syndesmosis: a radiostereometric study of 10 cadaveric specimens based on presumed trauma mechanisms with suggestions for treatment. *Acta Orthop* 77(3):531–540, 2006.
22. Beynnon, BD, et al: A prospective, randomized clinical investigation of the treatment of first-time ankle sprains. *Am J Sports Med* 34(9): 1401–1412, 2006.
23. Bhandari, M, et al: Treatment of acute Achilles tendon ruptures: a systematic overview and metaanalysis. *Clin Orthop* 400:190–200, 2002.
24. Bijlsma, T, and van der Werken, C: Operative treatment of Achilles tendon rupture: a minimally invasive technique allowing functional after-treatment. *Orthop Traumatol* 8(4):285–290, 2000.
25. Bleakley, C, McDonough, S, and MacAuley, D: The use of ice in the treatment of acute soft-tissue injury: a systematic review of randomized controlled trials. *Am J Sports Med* 32(1):251–261, 2004.
26. Bleakley, CM, et al: Cryotherapy for acute ankle sprains: a randomised controlled study of two different icing protocols. *Br J Sports Med* 40(8):700–705, 2006.
27. Bleakley, CM, et al: Effect of accelerated rehabilitation on function after ankle sprain: randomised controlled trial. *BMJ* 340:c1964, 2010.
28. Blitz, NM, et al: Early weight bearing after modified lapidus arthrodesis: a multicenter review of 80 cases. *J Foot Ankle Surg* 49(4):357–362, 2010.
29. Bostick, GP, et al: Factors associated with calf muscle endurance recovery 1 year after Achilles tendon rupture repair. *J Orthop Sports Phys Ther* 40(6):345–351, 2010.
30. Bouchard, M, et al: The impact of obesity on the outcome of total ankle replacement. *J Bone Joint Surg Am* 97(11):904–910, 2015.
31. Boyce, SH, Quigley, MA, and Campbell, S: Management of ankle sprains: a randomised controlled trial of the treatment of inversion injuries using an elastic support bandage or an Aircast ankle brace. *Br J Sports Med* 39(2):91–96, 2005.
32. Braito, M, et al: Are our expectations bigger than the results we achieve? A comparative study analysing potential advantages of ankle arthroplasty over arthrodesis. *Int Orthop* 38(8):1647–1653, 2014.
33. Brumann, M, et al: Accelerated rehabilitation following Achilles tendon repair after acute rupture—Development of an evidence-based treatment protocol. *Injury* 45(11):1782–1790, 2014.
34. Buechel, FFS, Buechel, FFJ, and Pappas, MJ: Ten-year evaluation of cementless Buechel-Pappas meniscal bearing total ankle replacement. *Foot Ankle Int* 24(6):462–472, 2003.
35. Calhoun, JH: Acute repair of the Achilles tendon. In Kitaoka, HB (ed): *Master Techniques in Orthopedic Surgery: The Foot and Ankle,* ed. 2. Philadelphia: Lippincott Williams & Wilkins, 2002, pp 311–332.

36. Cannon, LB, Brown, J, and Cooke, PH: Early weight bearing is safe following arthroscopic ankle arthrodesis. *Foot Ankle Surg* 10(3):135–139, 2004.
37. Cannon, LB, and Slater, HK: The role of ankle arthroscopy and surgical approach in lateral ankle ligament repair. *Foot Ankle Surg* 11(1):1–4, 2005.
38. Carcia, CR, Martin, RL, and Drouin, JM: Validity of the Foot and Ankle Ability Measure in athletes with chronic ankle instability. *J Athl Train* 43(2):179–183, 2008.
39. Carcia, CR, et al: Achilles pain, stiffness, and muscle power deficits: Achilles tendinitis. *J Orthop Sports Phys Ther* 40(9):A1–A26, 2010.
40. Carmont, MR, et al: Simultaneous bilateral Achilles tendon ruptures associated with statin medication despite regular rock climbing exercise. *Phys Ther Sport* 10(4):150–152, 2009.
41. Chen, TM, et al: The arterial anatomy of the Achilles tendon: anatomical study and clinical implications. *Clin Anat* 22(3):377–385, 2009.
42. Chiodo, CP, et al: American Academy of Orthopaedic Surgeons clinical practice guideline on treatment of Achilles tendon rupture. *J Bone Joint Surg Am* 92(14):2466–2468, 2010.
43. Chrisman, OD, and Snook, GA: Reconstruction of lateral ligament tears of the ankle. An experimental study and clinical evaluation of seven patients treated by a new modification of the Elmslie procedure. *J Bone Joint Surg Am* 51(5):904–912, 1969.
44. Cleland, JA, et al: Manual physical therapy and exercise versus electrophysical agents and exercise in the management of plantar heel pain: a multicenter randomized clinical trial. *J Orthop Sports Phys Ther* 39(8):573–585, 2009.
45. Coester, LM, et al: Long-term results following ankle arthrodesis for post-traumatic arthritis. *J Bone Joint Surg Am* 83–A(2):219–228, 2001.
46. Cook, G: *Movement: Functional Movement Systems: Screening, Assessment, Corrective Strategies.* Aptos, CA, USA: On Target Publications, 2010.
47. Cooke, MW, et al: Treatment of severe ankle sprain: a pragmatic randomised controlled trial comparing the clinical effectiveness and cost-effctiveness of three types of mechanical ankle support with tubular bandage. The CAST trial. *Health Technol Assess Winch Engl* 13(13):1–121, 2009.
48. Corte-Real, NM, and Moreira, RM: Arthroscopic repair of chronic lateral ankle instability. *Foot Ankle Int* 30(3):213–217, 2009.
49. Costa, ML, et al: Randomised controlled trials of immediate weight-bearing mobilisation for rupture of the tendo Achilles. *J Bone Joint Surg Br* 88(1): 69–77, 2006.
50. Costa, ML, et al: Immediate full-weight-bearing mobilisation for repaired Achilles tendon ruptures: a pilot study. *Injury* 34(11):874–876, 2003.
51. Cottom, JM, and Rigby, RB: The "all inside" arthroscopic Broström procedure: a prospective study of 40 consecutive patients. *J Foot Ankle Surg* 52(5):568–574, 2013.
52. Coughlin, MJ, et al: Comprehensive reconstruction of the lateral ankle for chronic instability using a free gracilis graft. *Foot Ankle Int* 25(4): 231–241, 2004.
53. Couppé, C, et al: Eccentric or concentric exercises for the treatment of tendinopathies? *J Orthop Sports Phys Ther* 45(11):853–863, 2015.
54. Courville, XF, Hecht, PJ, and Tosteson, ANA: Is total ankle arthroplasty a cost-effective alternative to ankle fusion? *Clin Orthop* 469(6): 1721–1727, 2011.
55. Cretnik, A, Kosanovic, M, and Smrkolj, V: Percutaneous suturing of the ruptured Achilles tendon under local anesthesia. *J Foot Ankle Surg* 43(2):72–81,2004.
56. Croy, T, et al: Anterior talocrural joint laxity: diagnostic accuracy of the anterior drawer test of the ankle. *J Orthop Sports Phys Ther* 43(12): 911–919, 2013.
57. Cyriax, J: *Textbook of Orthopaedic Medicine, Vol 1. Diagnosis of Soft Tissue Lesions*, ed. 8. London: Bailliére Tindall, 1982.
58. Daniels, TR, et al: Intermediate-term results of total ankle replacement and ankle arthrodesis: a COFAS multicenter study. *J Bone Joint Surg Am* 96(2):135–142, 2014.
59. Dannawi, Z, et al: Arthroscopic ankle arthrodesis: are results reproducible irrespective of pre-operative deformity? *Foot Ankle Surg* 17(4):294–299, 2011.
60. Dayton, P, and McCall, A: Early weightbearing after first metatarsophalangeal joint arthrodesis: a retrospective observational case analysis. *J Foot Ankle Surg* 43(3):156–159, 2004.
61. De la Fuente, C, et al: Prospective randomized clinical trial of aggressive rehabilitation after acute Achilles tendon ruptures repaired with Dresden technique. *Foot* 26:15–22, 2016.
62. de Noronha, M, et al: Intrinsic predictive factors for ankle sprain in active university students: a prospective study. *Scand J Med Sci Sports* 23(5): 541–547, 2013.
63. de Vries, JS, et al: Interventions for treating chronic ankle instability. *Cochrane Database Syst Rev* (8):CD004124, 2011.
64. Deangelis, JP, et al: Achilles tendon rupture in athletes. *J Surg Orthop Adv* 18(3):115–121, 2009.
65. Del Buono, A, Volpin, A, and Maffulli, N: Minimally invasive versus open surgery for acute Achilles tendon rupture: a systematic review. *Br Med Bull* 109:45–54, 2014.
66. Demetracopoulos, CA, et al: Effect of age on outcomes in total ankle arthroplasty. *Foot Ankle Int* 36(8):871–880, 2015.
67. Digiovanni, BF, et al: Plantar fascia-specific stretching exercise improves outcomes in patients with chronic plantar fasciitis. A prospective clinical trial with two-year follow-up. *J Bone Joint Surg Am* 88(8):1775–1781, 2006.
68. Dizon, JMR, and Reyes, JJB: A systematic review on the effectiveness of external ankle supports in the prevention of inversion ankle sprains among elite and recreational players. *J Sci Med Sport* 13(3):309–317, 2010.
69. Doherty, C, et al: The incidence and prevalence of ankle sprain injury: a systematic review and meta-analysis of prospective epidemiological studies. *Sports Med* 44(1):123–140, 2014.
70. Dombek, MF, et al: Peroneal tendon tears: a retrospective review. *J Foot Ankle Surg* 42(5):250–258, 2003.
71. Donatelli, RA: Normal anatomy and biomechanics. In Donatelli, RA (ed): *The Biomechanics of the Foot and Ankle*, ed. 2. Philadelphia: F.A. Davis, 1996, p 3.
72. Donatelli, RA: Abnormal biomechanics. In Donatelli, RA (ed): *The Biomechanics of the Foot and Ankle*, ed. 2. Philadelphia: F.A. Davis, 1996, p 34.
73. Donovan, L, Hart, JM, and Hertel, J: Effects of 2 ankle destabilization devices on electromyography measures during functional exercises in individuals with chronic ankle instability. *J Orthop Sports Phys Ther* 45(3):220–232, 2015.
74. Donovan, L, et al: Rehabilitation for chronic ankle instability with or without destabilization devices: A randomized controlled trial. *J Athl Train* 51(3):233–251, 2016.
75. Doral, MN: What is the effect of the early weight-bearing mobilisation without using any support after endoscopy-assisted Achilles tendon repair? *Knee Surg Sports Traumatol Arthrosc* 21(6):1378–1384, 2013.
76. Drake, M, Bittenbender, C, and Royles, RE: The short-term effects of treating plantar fasciitis with a temporary custom foot orthosis and stretching. *J Orthop Sports Phys Ther* 41(4):221–231, 2011.
77. Dubois-Ferrière, V, et al: Clinical outcomes and development of symptomatic osteoarthritis 2 to 24 years after surgical treatment of tarsometatarsal joint complex injuries. *J Bone Jt Surg Am* 98(9):713–720, 2016.
78. Easley, ME, Sides, SD, and Toth, AP: Osteochondral lesions of the talus. In Mirzayan, R (ed): *Cartilage Injury in the Athlete.* New York: Thieme Medical Publications, 2006, pp 171–186.
79. Ebalard, M, et al: Risk of osteoarthritis secondary to partial or total arthrodesis of the subtalar and midtarsal joints after a minimum follow-up of 10 years. *Orthop Traumatol Surg Res* 100(4):S231–S237, 2014.
80. Ecker, TM, et al: Prospective use of a standardized nonoperative early weightbearing protocol for Achilles tendon rupture: 17 years of experience. *Am J Sports Med* 44(4):1004–1010, 2016.

81. Eechaute, C, et al: The clinimetric qualities of patient-assessed instruments for measuring chronic ankle instability: a systematic review. *BMC Musculoskelet Disord* 8:6, 2007.
82. Eils, E, and Rosenbaum, D: A multi-station proprioceptive exercise program in patients with ankle instability. *Med Sci Sports Exerc* 33(12):1991–1998, 2001.
83. Ellis, SJ, et al: Results of anatomic lateral ankle ligament reconstruction with tendon allograft. *HSS J* 7(2):134–140, 2011.
84. Elmlund, AO, and Winson, IG: Arthroscopic ankle arthrodesis. *Foot Ankle Clin* 20(1):71–80, 2015.
85. Engebretsen, AH, et al: Intrinsic risk factors for acute ankle injuries among male soccer players: a prospective cohort study. *Scand J Med Sci Sports* 20(3):403–410, 2010.
86. Erdil, M, et al: Comparison of arthrodesis, resurfacing hemiarthroplasty, and total joint replacement in the treatment of advanced hallux rigidus. *J Foot Ankle Surg* 52(5):588–593, 2013.
87. Erickson, BJ, et al: Trends in the Management of Achilles Tendon Ruptures in the United States Medicare Population, 2005-2011. *Orthop J Sports Med* doi:10.1177/2325967114549948, 2014.
88. Feger, MA, et al: Electrical stimulation as a treatment intervention to improve function, edema or pain following acute lateral ankle sprains: A systematic review. *Phys Ther Sport* 16(4):361–369, 2015.
89. Ferke, RD, and Chams, RN: Chronic lateral instability: arthroscopic findings and long-term results. *Foot Ankle Int* 28(1):24–31, 2007.
90. Ferran, NA, and Maffulli, N: Epidemiology of sprains of the lateral ankle ligament complex. *Foot Ankle Clin* 11(3):659–662, 2006.
91. Fong, DT-P, et al: A systematic review on ankle injury and ankle sprain in sports. *Sports Med* 37(1):73–94, 2007.
92. Forestier, N, Terrier, R, and Teasdale, N: Ankle muscular proprioceptive signals' relevance for balance control on various support surfaces: an exploratory study. *Am J Phys Med Rehabil* 94(1):20–27, 2015.
93. Fredberg, U, Bolvig, L, and Andersen, NT: Prophylactic training in asymptomatic soccer players with ultrasonographic abnormalities in Achilles and patellar tendons: the Danish Super League Study. *Am J Sports Med* 36(3):451–460, 2008.
94. Fredberg, U, and Bolvig, L: Significance of ultrasonographically detected asymptomatic tendinosis in the patellar and Achilles tendons of elite soccer players: a longitudinal study. *Am J Sports Med* 30(4): 488–491, 2002.
95. Freedman, BR, et al: Nonsurgical treatment and early return to activity leads to improved Achilles tendon fatigue mechanics and functional outcomes during early healing in an animal model. *J Orthop Res* doi:10.1002/jor.23253, 2016.
96. Fuentes-Sanz, A, et al: Clinical outcome and gait analysis of ankle arthrodesis. *Foot Ankle Int* 33(10):819–827, 2012.
97. Fuhrmann, RA, and Pillukat, T: Arthrodesis of the first metatarsophalangeal joint. *Oper Orthop Traumatol* 24(6):513–526, 2012.
98. Fuller, EA: The windlass mechanism of the foot. A mechanical model to explain pathology. *J Am Podiatr Med Assoc* 90(1):35–46, 2000.
99. Ganestam, A, et al: Increasing incidence of acute Achilles tendon rupture and a noticeable decline in surgical treatment from 1994 to 2013. A nationwide registry study of 33,160 patients. *Knee Surg Sports Traumatol Arthrosc* 24(12):3730–3737, 2016.
100. Garras, DN, et al: MRI is unnecessary for diagnosing acute Achilles tendon ruptures: clinical diagnostic criteria. *Clin Orthop* 470(8):2268–2273, 2012.
101. Gaudot, F, et al: A controlled, comparative study of a fixed-bearing versus mobile-bearing ankle arthroplasty. *Foot Ankle Int* 35(2):131–140, 2014.
102. Gharehdaghi, M, Rahimi, H, and Mousavian, A: Anterior ankle arthrodesis with molded plate: technique and outcomes. *Arch Bone Jt Surg* 2(3):203–209, 2014.
103. Giannini, S, et al: The treatment of severe posttraumatic arthritis of the ankle joint. *J Bone Joint Surg Am* 89(3):15–28, 2007.
104. Gougoulias, NE, Agathangelidis, FG, and Parsons, SW: Arthroscopic ankle arthrodesis. *Foot Ankle Int* 28(6):695–706, 2007.
105. Green, T, et al: A randomized controlled trial of a passive accessory joint mobilization on acute ankle inversion sprains. *Phys Ther* 81(4): 984–994, 2001.
106. Gribble, PA, Hertel, J, and Plisky, P: Using the Star Excursion Balance Test to assess dynamic postural-control deficits and outcomes in lower extremity injury: a literature and systematic review. *J Athl Train* 47(3):339–357, 2012.
107. Groetelaers, RPTGC, et al: Functional treatment or cast immobilization after minimally invasive repair of an acute Achilles tendon rupture: prospective, randomized trial. *Foot Ankle Int* 35(8):771–778, 2014.
108. Grunfeld, R, Aydogan, U, and Juliano, P: Ankle arthritis: review of diagnosis and operative management. *Med Clin North Am* 98(2): 267–289, 2014.
109. Guillo, S, et al: Consensus in chronic ankle instability: aetiology, assessment, surgical indications and place for arthroscopy. *Orthop Traumatol Surg Res* 99(8):S411–S419, 2013.
110. Guillo, S, et al: Arthroscopic anatomical reconstruction of the lateral ankle ligaments. *Knee Surg Sports Traumatol Arthrosc* 24(4):998–1002, 2016.
111. Gulati, V, et al: Management of Achilles tendon injury: A current concepts systematic review. *World J Orthop* 6(4):380–386, 2015.
112. Gutteck, N, et al: Immediate fullweightbearing after tarsometatarsal arthrodesis for hallux valgus correction—does it increase the complication rate? *Foot Ankle Surg* 21(3):198–201, 2015.
113. Guyer, AJ, and Richardson, G: Current concepts review: total ankle arthroplasty. *Foot Ankle Int* 29(2):256–264, 2008.
114. Haddad, SL, et al: Intermediate and long-term outcomes of total ankle arthroplasty and ankle arthrodesis. A systematic review of the literature. *J Bone Joint Surg Am* 89(9):1899–1905, 2007.
115. Haji, A, et al: Percutaneous versus open tendo-achilles repair. *Foot Ankle Int* 25(4):215–218, 2004.
116. Hall, EA, et al: Strength-training protocols to improve deficits in participants with chronic ankle instability: a randomized controlled trial. *J Athl Train* 50(1):36–44, 2015.
117. Hall, JPL, et al: The biomechanical differences between barefoot and shod distance running: a systematic review and preliminary meta-analysis. *Sports Med* 43(12):1335–1353, 2013.
118. Hals, TM, Sitler, MR, and Mattacola, CG: Effect of a semi-rigid ankle stabilizer on performance in persons with functional ankle instability. *J Orthop Sports Phys Ther* 30(9):552–556, 2000.
119. Hamilton, WG: Ankle instability repair: The Broström-Gould procedure. In Kitaoka, HB (ed): *Master Techniques in Orthopedic Surgery: The Foot and Ankle,* ed. 2. Philadelphia: Lippincott Williams & Wilkins, 2002.
120. Han, K, Ricard, MD, and Fellingham, GW: Effects of a 4-week exercise program on balance using elastic tubing as a perturbation force for individuals with a history of ankle sprains. *J Orthop Sports Phys Ther* 39(4):246–255, 2009.
121. Hass, CJ, et al: Chronic ankle instability alters central organization of movement. *Am J Sports Med* 38(4):829–834, 2010.
122. Hasselman, CT, Wong, YS, And Conti, SF: Total ankle replacement. In Kitaoka, HB (ed): *Master Techniques in Orthopedic Surgery: The Foot and Ankle,* ed. 2. Philadelphia: Lippincott Williams & Wilkins: p 583, 2002
123. Henricson, A, Nilsson, J-Å, and Carlsson, Å. 10-year survival of total ankle arthroplasties. *Acta Orthop* 82(6):655–659, 2011.
124. Herman, K, et al: The effectiveness of neuromuscular warm-up strategies that require no additional equipment, for preventing lower limb injuries during sports participation: a systematic review. *BMC Med* 10:75, 2012.
125. Hertel, J: Functional anatomy, pathomechanics, and pathophysiology of lateral ankle instability. *J Athl Train* 37(4):364–375, 2002.
126. Hertel, J: Sensorimotor deficits with ankle sprains and chronic ankle instability. *Clin Sports Med* 27(3):353–370, 2008.
127. Hess, GW: Achilles tendon rupture: a review of etiology, population, anatomy, risk factors, and injury prevention. *Foot Ankle Spec* 3(1): 29–32, 2010.
128. Hiller, CE, Kilbreath, SL, and Refshauge, KM: Chronic ankle instability: evolution of the model. *J Athl Train* 46(2):133–141, 2011.
129. Hiller, CE, et al: Intrinsic predictors of lateral ankle sprain in adolescent dancers: a prospective cohort study. *Clin J Sport Med* 18(1):44–48, 2008.

130. Hintermann, B, et al: Conversion of painful ankle arthrodesis to total ankle arthroplasty. *J Bone Joint Surg Am* 91(4):850–858, 2009.
131. Hintermann, B, et al: The HINTEGRA ankle: rationale and short-term results of 122 consecutive ankles. *Clin Orthop Rel Research* 424:57–68, 2004.
132. Hirai, D, Docherty, CL, and Schrader, J: Severity of functional and mechanical ankle instability in an active population. *Foot Ankle Int* 30(11):1071–1077, 2009.
133. Horterer, H, et al: Sports activity in patients with total ankle replacement. *Sports Orthop Traumatol* 31:34–40, 2015.
134. House, C, Reece, A, and Roiz de Sa, D: Shock-absorbing insoles reduce the incidence of lower limb overuse injuries sustained during Royal Marine training. *Mil Med* 178(6):683–689, 2013.
135. Hsu, AR, et al: Intermediate and long-term outcomes of the modified Brostrom-Evans procedure for lateral ankle ligament reconstruction. *Foot Ankle Spec* 9(2):131–139, 2016.
136. Hsu, AR, et al: Clinical outcomes and complications of percutaneous Achilles repair system versus open technique for acute Achilles tendon ruptures. *Foot Ankle Int* 36(11):1279–1286, 2015.
137. Hua, Y, et al: Anatomical reconstruction of the lateral ligaments of the ankle with semitendinosus allograft. *Int Orthop* 36(10):2027–2031, 2012.
138. Hua, Y, et al: Combination of modified Broström procedure with ankle arthroscopy for chronic ankle instability accompanied by intra-articular symptoms. *Arthrosc J Arthrosc Relat Surg* 26(4):524–528, 2010.
139. Huang, J, et al: Rehabilitation regimen after surgical treatment of acute Achilles tendon ruptures: a systematic review with meta-analysis. *Am J Sports Med* 43(4):1008–1016, 2015.
140. Hunt, KJ, et al: Ankle joint contact loads and displacement with progressive syndesmotic injury. *Foot Ankle Int* 36(9):1095–1103, 2015.
141. Hupperets, MDW, Verhagen, EALM, and van Mechelen, W: Effect of unsupervised home based proprioceptive training on recurrences of ankle sprain: randomised controlled trial. *BMJ* 339:b2684, 2009.
142. Hutchinson, ID, et al: How do hindfoot fusions affect ankle biomechanics: A cadaver model. *Clin Orthop* 474(4):1008–1016, 2016.
143. Hyer, CF, and Vancourt, R: Arthroscopic repair of lateral ankle instability by using the thermal-assisted capsular shift procedure: a review of 4 cases. *J Foot Ankle Surg* 43(2):104–109, 2004.
144. Hyland, MR, et al: Randomized controlled trial of calcaneal taping, sham taping, and plantar fascia stretching for the short-term management of plantar heel pain. *J Orthop Sports Phys Ther* 36(6):364–371, 2006.
145. Ishikawa, S: Arthroscopy of the foot and ankle. In Canale ST & Beaty JH (ed)*Campbell's Operative Orthopaedics,* ed. 12. Philadelphia, PA, Elsevier/Mosby; 2013, pp 2379–2392.
146. Jaakkola, JI, and Mann, RA: A review of rheumatoid arthritis affecting the foot and ankle. *Foot Ankle Int* 25(12):866–874, 2004.
147. Janssen, KW, van Mechelen, W, and Verhagen, EALM: Bracing superior to neuromuscular training for the prevention of self-reported recurrent ankle sprains: a three-arm randomised controlled trial. *Br J Sports Med* 48(16):1235–1239, 2014.
148. Jiang, N, et al: Operative versus nonoperative treatment for acute Achilles tendon rupture: a meta-analysis based on current evidence. *Int Orthop* 36(4):765–773, 2012.
149. Johnson, P, et al: New regimen for eccentric calf-muscle training in patients with chronic insertional Achilles tendinopathy: results of a pilot study. *Br J Sports Med* 42:746–749, 2008.
150. Jones, C, et al: Understanding the postoperative course and rehabilitation protocol for total ankle arthroplasty. *Foot Ankle Spec* 8(3):203–208, 2015.
151. Jones, MH, and Amendola, AS: Acute treatment of inversion ankle sprains: immobilization versus functional treatment. *Clin Orthop* 455:169–172, 2007.
152. Jones, MP, Khan, RJK, and Smith, RLC: Surgical interventions for treating acute Achilles tendon rupture: key findings from a recent Cochrane Review. *J Bone Jt Surg Am* 94(12):e88, 2012.
153. Jung, D-Y, et al: Effect of medial arch support on displacement of the myotendinous junction of the gastrocnemius during standing wall stretching. *J Orthop Sports Phys Ther* 39(12):867–874, 2009.
154. Kaminski, TW, et al: National Athletic Trainers' Association position statement: Conservative management and prevention of ankle sprains in athletes. *J Athl Train* 48(4):528–545, 2013.
155. Kangas, J, et al: Achilles tendon elongation after rupture repair: a randomized comparison of 2 postoperative regimens. *Am J Sports Med* 35(1):59–64, 2007.
156. Kangas, J, et al: Early functional treatment versus early immobilization in tension of the musculotendinous unit after Achilles rupture repair: a prospective, randomized, clinical study. *J Trauma* 54(6):1171–1181, 2003.
157. Kauranen, KJ, and Leppilahti, JI: Motor performance of the foot after Achilles rupture repair. *Int J Sports Med* 22(2):154–158, 2001.
158. Kavlak, Y, et al: Outcome of orthoses intervention in the rheumatoid foot. *Foot Ankle Int* 24:494–499, 2003.
159. Kemler, E, et al: A systematic review on the treatment of acute ankle sprain: brace versus other functional treatment types. *Sports Med Auckl NZ* 41(3):185–197, 2011.
160. Kerkhoffs, GMMJ, et al: Surgical versus conservative treatment for acute injuries of the lateral ligament complex of the ankle in adults. *Cochrane Database Syst Rev* (2):CD000380, 2007.
161. Kerkhoffs, GMMJ, et al: Functional treatment after surgical repair of acute Achilles tendon rupture: wrap vs walking cast. *Arch Orthop Trauma Surg* 122(2):102–105, 2002.
162. Khan, RJ, and Carey Smith, RL: Surgical interventions for treating acute Achilles tendon ruptures. *Cochrane Database Syst Rev* (9):CD003674, 2010.
163. Khan, RJK, et al: Treatment of acute Achilles tendon ruptures. A meta-analysis of randomized, controlled trials. *J Bone Joint Surg Am* 87(10): 2202–2210, 2005.
164. Khawaji, B, and Soames, R: The anterior talofibular ligament: a detailed morphological study. *Foot* 25(3):141–147, 2015.
165. Kile, TA: Ankle arthrodesis. In Morrey, BF (ed): *Reconstructive Surgery of the Joints,* ed. 2. New York: Churchill Livingstone, 1996, p 1771.
166. Kim, ES, et al: Arthroscopic anterior talofibular ligament repair for chronic ankle instability with a suture anchor technique. *Orthopedics* 34(4):273, 2011.
167. Kitaoka, HB: Complications of replacement arthroplasty of the ankle. In Morrey, BF (ed): *Joint Replacement Arthroplasty*, ed. 3. Philadelphia: Churchill Livingstone, 2003, pp 1133–1150.
168. Kitaoka, HB: Subtalar arthrodesis In Kitaoka, HB (ed): *Master Techniques in Orthopedic Surgery: The Foot and Ankle*, ed. 2. Philadelphia: Lippincott Williams & Wilkins, 2013, pp 315–324.
169. Kjaer, M, et al: Metabolic activity and collagen turnover in human tendon in response to physical activity. *J Musculoskelet Neuronal Interact* 5(1):41–52, 2005.
170. Knecht, SI, et al: The Agility total ankle arthroplasty. Seven to sixteen-year follow-up. *J Bone Joint Surg Am* 86–A(6):1161–1171, 2004.
171. Knupp, M, et al: Chronic ankle instability (medial and lateral). *Clin Sports Med* 34(4):679–688, 2015.
172. Kofoed, H, and Lundberg-Jensen, A: Ankle arthroplasty in patients younger and older than 50 years: a prospective series with long-term follow-up. *Foot Ankle Int* 20(8):501–506, 1999.
173. Kofoed, H, and Sorensen, TS: Ankle arthroplasty for rheumatoid arthritis and osteoarthritis: prospective long-term study of cemented replacements. *J Bone Joint Surg Br* 80(2):328–332, 1998.
174. Kofotolis, N, and Kellis, E: Ankle sprain injuries: a 2-year prospective cohort study in female Greek professional basketball players. *J Athl Train* 42(3):388–394, 2007.
175. Kofotolis, ND, Kellis, E, and Vlachopoulos, SP: Ankle sprain injuries and risk factors in amateur soccer players during a 2-year period. *Am J Sports Med* 35(3):458–466, 2007.
176. Krause, FG, et al: Impact of complications in total ankle replacement and ankle arthrodesis analyzed with a validated outcome measurement. *J Bone Joint Surg Am* 93(9):830–839, 2011.

177. Krips, R, et al: Sports activity level after surgical treatment for chronic anterolateral ankle instability. A multicenter study. *Am J Sports Med* 30(1):13–19, 2002.
178. Kulig, K, et al: Nonsurgical management of posterior tibial tendon dysfunction with orthoses and resistive exercise: a randomized controlled trial. *Phys Ther* 89(1):26–37, 2009.
179. Kwon, DG, et al: Arthroplasty versus arthrodesis for end-stage ankle arthritis: decision analysis using Markov model. *Int Orthop* 35(11): 1647–1653, 2011.
180. Labek, G, et al: Revision rates after total ankle arthroplasty in sample-based clinical studies and national registries. *Foot Ankle Int* 32(8): 740–745, 2011.
181. Labek, G, et al: Impact of implant developers on published outcome and reproducibility of cohort-based clinical studies in arthroplasty. *J Bone Joint Surg Am* 93(3):55–61, 2011.
182. Labek, G, et al: Outcome after total ankle arthroplasty-results and findings from worldwide arthroplasty registers. *Int Orthop* 37(9): 1677–1682, 2013.
183. Lamm, BM, and Wynes, J: Immediate weightbearing after Lapidus arthrodesis with external fixation. *J Foot Ankle Surg* 53(5):577–583, 2014.
184. Lantto, I, et al: Early functional treatment versus cast immobilization in tension after Achilles rupture repair: results of a prospective randomized trial with 10 or more years of follow-up. *Am J Sports Med* 43(9):2302–2309, 2015.
185. Lantto, I, et al: A prospective randomized trial comparing surgical and nonsurgical treatments of acute Achilles tendon ruptures. *Am J Sports Med* 44(9):2406–2414, 2016.
186. Lardenoye, S, et al: The effect of taping versus semi-rigid bracing on patient outcome and satisfaction in ankle sprains: a prospective, randomized controlled trial. *BMC Musculoskelet Disord* 13:81, 2012.
187. Lee, KT, et al: Long-term results after modified Brostrom procedure without calcaneofibular ligament reconstruction. *Foot Ankle Int* 32(2):153–157, 2011.
188. Leppänen, M, et al: Interventions to prevent sports related injuries: a systematic review and meta-analysis of randomised controlled trials. *Sports Med* 44(4):473–486, 2014.
189. Lieberman, DE, et al: Foot strike patterns and collision forces in habitually barefoot versus shod runners. *Nature* 463(7280):531–535, 2010.
190. Lieberman, DE: What we can learn about running from barefoot running: an evolutionary medical perspective. *Exerc Sport Sci Rev* 40(2):63–72, 2012.
191. Lim, J, Dalal, R, and Waseen, M: Percutaneous vs. open repair of the ruptured Achilles tendon—a prospective randomized controlled study. *Foot Ankle Int* 22:559–568, 2001.
192. Linens, SW, et al: Postural-stability tests that identify individuals with chronic ankle instability. *J Athl Train* 49(1):15–23, 2014.
193. Longo, UG, et al: Acute Achilles tendon rupture in athletes. *Foot Ankle Clin* 18(2):319–38, 2013.
194. Lorenz, DS, and Pontillo, M: Is there evidence to support a forefoot strike pattern in barefoot runners? A review. *Sports Health Multidiscip Approach* 4(6):480–484, 2012.
195. Loudon, JK, Reiman, MP, and Sylvain, J: The efficacy of manual joint mobilisation/manipulation in treatment of lateral ankle sprains: a systematic review. *Br J Sports Med* 48(5):365–370, 2014.
196. Lui, TH: A minimally invasive "overwrapping" technique for repairing neglected ruptures of the Achilles tendon. *J Foot Ankle Surg* 53(6): 806–809, 2014.
197. Macaulay, AA, van Valkenburg, SM, and DiGiovanni, CW: Sport and activity restrictions following total ankle replacement: a survey of orthopaedic foot and ankle specialists. *Foot Ankle Surg* 21(4):260–265, 2015.
198. Maffulli, N, et al: Isolated anterior talofibular ligament Broström repair for chronic lateral ankle instability: 9-year follow-up. *Am J Sports Med* 41(4):858–64, 2013.
199. Maffulli, N, et al: Less-invasive semitendinosus tendon graft augmentation for the reconstruction of chronic tears of the Achilles tendon. *Am J Sports Med* 41(4):865–871, 2013.
200. Maffulli, N, et al: Achilles tendon ruptures in elite athletes. *Foot Ankle Int* 32(1):9–15, 2011.
201. Maffulli, N, et al: Minimally invasive surgery for Achilles tendon pathologies. *Open Access J Sports Med* 1:95–103, 2010.
202. Maffulli, N, et al: Less-invasive reconstruction of chronic Achilles tendon ruptures using a peroneus brevis tendon transfer. *Am J Sports Med* 38(11):2304–2312, 2010.
203. Maffulli, N, et al: Early weightbearing and ankle mobilization after open repair of acute midsubstance tears of the Achilles tendon. *Am J Sports Med* 31(5):692–700, 2003.
204. Maffulli, N, et al: No adverse effect of early weight bearing following open repair of acute tears of the Achilles tendon. *J Sports Med Phys Fitness* 43(3):367–379, 2003.
205. Magee, D: *Orthopedic Physical Assessment*. St. Louis, MO, Elsevier Health Sciences, 2014.
206. Mahieu, NN, et al: Intrinsic risk factors for the development of Achilles tendon overuse injury: a prospective study. *Am J Sports Med* 34(2): 226–235, 2006.
207. Mai, HT, et al: The NFL orthopaedic surgery outcomes database (NO-SOD): The effect of common orthopaedic procedures on football careers. *Am J Sports Med* 44(9):2255–2262, 2016.
208. Man, IOW, Morrissey, MC, and Cywinski, JK: Effect of neuromuscular electrical stimulation on ankle swelling in the early period after ankle sprain. *Phys Ther* 87(1):53–65, 2007.
209. Mann, RA, DeOrio, JK, and Mann, JA: Total ankle arthroplasty. In Kitaoka, HB (ed). *Master Techniques in Orthopedic Surgery: The Foot and Ankle*, ed. 3. Philadelphia: Lippincott Williams & Wilkins, 2013, pp 551–568.
210. Marie, I, et al: Tendinous disorders attributed to statins: a study on ninety-six spontaneous reports in the period 1990-2005 and review of the literature. *Arthritis Rheum* 59(3):367–372, 2008.
211. Martin, RL, and Kivlan, B: The ankle and foot complex. In Levangie, PK, and Norkin, CC (eds): *Joint Structure and Function*, ed. 5. Philadelphia: F.A. Davis, 2011, pp. 440–481.
212. Martin, RL, et al: Ankle stability and movement coordination impairments: ankle ligament sprains. *J Orthop Sports Phys Ther* 43(9):A1–40, 2013.
213. Martin, RL, et al: Heel pain-plantar fasciitis: revision 2014. *J Orthop Sports Phys Ther* 44(11):A1–33, 2014.
214. Martin, RL, Stewart, GW, and Conti, SF: Posttraumatic ankle arthritis: an update on conservative and surgical management. *J Orthop Sports Phys Ther* 37(5):253–259, 2007.
215. Matheny, LM, et al: Activity level and function after lateral ankle ligament repair versus reconstruction. *Am J Sports Med* 44(5): 1301–1308, 2016.
216. Matsui, K, et al: Minimally invasive surgical treatment for chronic ankle instability: a systematic review. *Knee Surg Sports Traumatol Arthrosc* 24(4):1040–1048, 2016.
217. Matsui, K, et al: Early recovery after arthroscopic repair compared to open repair of the anterior talofibular ligament for lateral instability of the ankle. *Arch Orthop Trauma Surg* 136(1):93–100, 2016.
218. McClinton, SM, Cleland, JA, and Flynn, TW: Predictors of response to physical therapy intervention for plantar heel pain. *Foot Ankle Int* 36(4):408–416, 2015.
219. McCullough, KA, Shaw, CM, and Anderson, RB: mini-open repair of Achilles rupture in the national football league. *J Surg Orthop Adv* 23(4):179–183, 2014.
220. McGovern, RP, and Martin, RL: Managing ankle ligament sprains and tears: current opinion. *Open Access J Sports Med* 7:33–42, 2016.
221. McGuine, TA, Brooks, A, and Hetzel, S: The effect of lace-up ankle braces on injury rates in high school basketball players. *Am J Sports Med* 39(9):1840–1848, 2011.
222. McGuine, TA, et al: The effect of lace-up ankle braces on injury rates in high school football players. *Am J Sports Med* 40(1):49–57, 2012.
223. McGuine, TA, and Keene, JS: The effect of a balance training program on the risk of ankle sprains in high school athletes. *Am J Sports Med* 34(7):1103–1111, 2006.

224. McKeon, PO, and Hertel, J: Systematic review of postural control and lateral ankle instability, part II: is balance training clinically effective? *J Athl Train* 43(3):305–315, 2008.
225. McKeon, PO, and Hertel, J: Systematic review of postural control and lateral ankle instability, part I: can deficits be detected with instrumented testing. *J Athl Train* 43(3):293–304, 2008.
226. McPoil, TG, et al: Heel pain—plantar fasciitis: clinical practice guidelines linked to the international classification of function, disability, and health from the orthopaedic section of the American Physical Therapy Association. *J Orthop Sports Phys Ther* 38(4):A1–A18, 2008.
227. Mendel, FC, et al: Effect of high-voltage pulsed current on recovery after grades I and II lateral ankle sprains. *J Sport Rehabil* 19(4):399–410, 2010.
228. Metz, R, et al: Effect of complications after minimally invasive surgical repair of acute Achilles tendon ruptures: report on 211 cases. *Am J Sports Med* 39(4):820–824, 2011.
229. Metz, R, et al: Acute Achilles tendon rupture: minimally invasive surgery versus nonoperative treatment with immediate full weightbearing—a randomized controlled trial. *Am J Sports Med* 36(9):1688–1694, 2008.
230. Metzl, JA, Ahmad, CS, and Levine, WN: The ruptured Achilles tendon: operative and non-operative treatment options. *Curr Rev Musculoskelet Med* 1(2):161–164, 2008.
231. Michelson, J: Triple arthrodesis of the Hindfoot. In Kitaoka, HB (ed): *Master Techniques in Orthopedic Surgery: The Foot and Ankle,* ed. 3. Philadelphia: Lippincott Williams & Wilkins, 2013, pp 343–360.
232. Michelson, J, and Amis, JA: Talus-calcaneus-cuboid (triple) arthrodesis. In Kitaoka, HB (ed): *Master Techniques in Orthopedic Surgery: The Foot and Ankle,* ed. 3. Philadelphia: Lippincott Williams & Wilkins, 2013, pp 343–360.
233. Michener, LA, and Kulig, K: Not all tendons are created equal: Implications for differing treatment approaches. *J Orthop Sports Phys Ther* 45(11):829–832, 2015.
234. Mickel, TJ, et al: Prophylactic bracing versus taping for the prevention of ankle sprains in high school athletes: a prospective, randomized trial. *J Foot Ankle Surg* 45(6):360–365, 2006.
235. Miyamoto, W, et al: Accelerated versus traditional rehabilitation after anterior talofibular Ligament reconstruction for chronic lateral instability of the ankle in athletes. *Am J Sports Med* 42(6):1441–1447, 2014.
236. Mohammadi, F: Comparison of 3 preventive methods to reduce the recurrence of ankle inversion sprains in male soccer players. *Am J Sports Med* 35(6):922–926, 2007.
237. Moller, M, et al: Acute rupture of tendon Achilles. A prospective randomised study of comparison between surgical and non-surgical treatment. *J Bone Joint Surg Br* 83(6):843–848, 2001.
238. Molloy, A, and Wood, EV: Complications of the treatment of Achilles tendon rupture. *Foot Ankle Clin* 14(4):745–759, 2009.
239. Mulier, T, et al: The management of chronic Achilles tendon ruptures: gastrocnemius turn down flap with or without flexor hallucis longus transfer. *Foot Ankle Surg.* 9(3):151–156, 2003.
240. Mullen, S, et al: Barefoot running: The effects of an 8-week barefoot training program. *Orthop J Sports Med* 2(3):1–5, 2014.
241. Mulligan, BR: *Manual Therapy "NAGS", "SNAGS", "MWM's": etc,* ed. 4. Wellington: Plane View Press, 1999.
242. Murphy, GA: Ankle arthrodesis. In Canale ST and Beaty JH (ed)*Campbell's Operative Orthopaedics,* ed. 12. Philadelphia, PA, Elsevier/Mosby; 2013: pp 503–529.
243. Murphy, GA: Total ankle arthroplasty. In Canale ST & Beaty JH (eds) *Campbell's Operative Orthopaedics,* ed. 12. Philadelphia, PA, Elsevier/ Mosby; 2013: pp 486–502.
244. Muscarella, V, Sadri, S, and Pusateri, J: Indications and considerations of foot and ankle arthrodesis. *Clin Podiatr Med Surg* 29(1):1–9, 2012.
245. Myerson, MS, and Mroczek, K: Perioperative complications of total ankle arthroplasty. *Foot Ankle Int* 24(1):17–21, 2003.
246. Naal, FD, et al: Habitual physical activity and sports participation after total ankle arthroplasty. *Am J Sports Med* 237(1):95–102, 2009.
247. Neville, CG, and Houck, JR: Choosing among 3 ankle-foot orthoses for a patient with stage II posterior tibial tendon dysfunction. *J Orthop Sports Phys Ther* 39(11):816–824, 2009.
248. Nielsen, KK, Linde, F, and Jensen, NC: The outcome of arthroscopic and open surgery ankle arthrodesis: A comparative retrospective study on 107 patients. *Foot Ankle Surg* 14(3):153–157, 2008.
249. Nilsson-Helander, K, et al: Acute Achilles tendon rupture: a randomized, controlled study comparing surgical and nonsurgical treatments using validated outcome measures. *Am J Sports Med* 38(11):2186–2193, 2010.
250. Noelle, S, et al: Total ankle arthroplasty factors: age, obesity, and complications. *Int Orthop* 37:1789–1794, 2013.
251. Nunley, JA, et al: Intermediate to long-term outcomes of the STAR Total Ankle Replacement: the patient perspective. *J Bone Joint Surg Am* 94(1):43–48, 2012.
252. Oatis, CA: Biomechanics of the foot and ankle under static conditions. *Phys Ther* 68(12):1815–1821, 1988.
253. Olmsted, LC, et al: Prophylactic ankle taping and bracing: A numbers-needed-to-treat and cost-benefit analysis. *J Athl Train* 39(1):95–100, 2004.
254. Olney, SJ, and Eng, J: Gait. In Levangie, PK, and Norkin, CC (eds): *Joint Structure and Function,* ed. 5. Philadelphia: F.A. Davis, 2011, pp 528–571, 2011.
255. Olsson, N, et al: Ability to perform a single heel-rise is significantly related to patient-reported outcome after Achilles tendon rupture. *Scand J Med Sci Sports* 24(1):152–158, 2014.
256. Olsson, N, et al: Major functional deficits persist 2 years after acute Achilles tendon rupture. *Knee Surg Sports Traumatol Arthrosc* 19(8): 1385–1393, 2011.
257. Olsson, N, et al: Predictors of clinical outcome after acute Achilles tendon ruptures. *Am J Sports Med* 42(6):1448–1455, 2014.
258. Olsson, N, et al: Stable surgical repair with accelerated rehabilitation versus nonsurgical treatment for acute Achilles tendon ruptures: a randomized controlled study. *Am J Sports Med* 41(12):2867–2876, 2013.
259. Palmieri-Smith, RM, Hopkins, JT, and Brown, TN: Peroneal activation deficits in persons with functional ankle instability. *Am J Sports Med* 37(5):982–988, 2009.
260. Panikkar, K, et al: A comparison of open and arthroscopic ankle fusion. *Foot Ankle Surg* 9(3):169–172, 2003.
261. Papadopoulos, ES, Nikolopoulos, CS, and Athanasopoulos, S: The effect of different skin-ankle brace application pressures with and without shoes on single-limb balance, electromyographic activation onset and peroneal reaction time of lower limb muscles. *Foot* 18(4):228–236, 2008.
262. Parekh, SG, et al: Epidemiology and outcomes of Achilles tendon ruptures in the National Football League. *Foot Ankle Spec* 2(6):283–286, 2009.
263. Patton, D, Kiewiet, N, and Brage, M: Infected total ankle arthroplasty: risk factors and treatment options. *Foot Ankle Int* 36(6):626–634, 2015.
264. Pearce, CJ, et al: Rehabilitation after anatomical ankle ligament repair or reconstruction. *Knee Surg Sports Traumatol Arthrosc Off J ESSKA* 24(4):1130–1139, 2016.
265. Pedersen, E, et al: Outcome of total ankle arthroplasty in patients with rheumatoid arthritis and noninflammatory arthritis. A multicenter cohort study comparing clinical outcome and safety. *J Bone Joint Surg Am* 96(21):1768–1775, 2014.
266. Pereira, H, et al: Arthroscopic repair of ankle instability with all-soft knotless anchors. *Arthrosc Tech* 5(1):e99–e107, 2016.
267. Perry, J, and Burnfield, J. *Gait Analysis: Normal and Pathological Function,* ed. 2. Thorofare, NJ, Slack, 2010.
268. Petersen, W, et al: Treatment of acute ankle ligament injuries: a systematic review. *Arch Orthop Trauma Surg* 133(8):1129–1141, 2013.
269. Peterson, KS, et al: Surgical considerations for the neglected or chronic Achilles tendon rupture: a combined technique for reconstruction. *J Foot Ankle Surg* 53(5):664–671, 2014.
270. Petrera, M, et al: Short- to medium-term outcomes after a modified Broström repair for lateral ankle instability with immediate postoperative weightbearing. *Am J Sports Med* 42(7):1542–1548, 2014.
271. Pihlajamäki, H, et al: Surgical versus functional treatment for acute ruptures of the lateral ligament complex of the ankle in young men: a randomized controlled trial. *J Bone Joint Surg Am* 92(14):2367–2374, 2010.

272. Prisk, VR, et al: Lateral ligament repair and reconstruction restore neither contact mechanics of the ankle joint nor motion patterns of the hindfoot. *J Bone Joint Surg Am* 92(14):2375–2386, 2010.
273. Pugely, AJ, et al: Trends in the use of total ankle replacement and ankle arthrodesis in the United States Medicare population. *Foot Ankle Int* 35(3):207–215, 2014.
274. Rahnama, L, et al: Attentional demands and postural control in athletes with and without functional ankle instability. *J Orthop Sports Phys Ther* 40(3):180–187, 2010.
275. Raikin, SM, Garras, DN, and Krapchev, PV: Achilles tendon injuries in a United States population. *Foot Ankle Int* 34(4):475–480, 2013.
276. Raikin, SM, et al: Trends in treatment of advanced ankle arthropathy by total ankle replacement or ankle fusion. *Foot Ankle Int* 35(3): 216–224, 2014.
277. Rao, S, et al: Shoe inserts alter plantar loading and function in patients with midfoot arthritis. *J Orthop Sports Phys Ther* 39(7):522–531, 2009.
278. Rasmussen, O, Tovberg-Jensen, I, and Hedeboe, J: An analysis of the function of the posterior talofibular ligament. *Int Orthop* 7:41–48, 1983.
279. Rettig, AC, et al: Potential risk of rerupture in primary Achilles tendon repair in athletes younger than 30 years of age. *Am J Sports Med* 33(1):119–23, 2005.
280. Richardson, D: Arthritis of the foot. In Canale ST and Beaty JH (eds) *Campbell's Operative Orthopaedics,* ed. 12. Philadelphia, PA, Elsevier/Mosby; 2013, pp 4027–4056.
281. Richardson, D: Sports injuries of the ankle. In Canale ST and Beaty JH (eds) *Campbell's Operative Orthopaedics,* ed. 12. Philadelphia: Elsevier/Mosby; 2013, pp 4213–4253.
282. Riva, D, et al: Proprioceptive training and injury prevention in a professional men's basketball team: A six-year prospective study. *J Strength Cond Res* 30(2):461–475, 2016.
283. Rodrigues-Pinto, R, et al: Total ankle replacement in patients under the age of 50. Should the indications be revised? *Foot Ankle Surg* 19(4): 229–233, 2013.
284. Roemer, FW, et al: Ligamentous injuries and the risk of associated tissue damage in acute ankle sprains in athletes: A cross-sectional MRI study. *Am J Sports Med* 42(7):1549–1557, 2014.
285. Romeo, G, et al: Recreational sports activities after calcaneal fractures and subsequent subtalar joint arthrodesis. *J Foot Ankle Surg* 54(6): 1057–1061, 2015.
286. Rosenbaum, D, et al: First ray resection arthroplasty versus arthrodesis in the treatment of the rheumatoid foot. *Foot Ankle Int* 32(6):589–594, 2011.
287. Rotem-Lehrer, N, and Laufer, Y: Effect of focus of attention on transfer of a postural control task following an ankle sprain. *J Orthop Sports Phys Ther* 37(9):564–569, 2007.
288. Rouhani, H, et al: Multi-segment foot kinematics after total ankle replacement and ankle arthrodesis during relatively long-distance gait. *Gait Posture* 36(3):561–566, 2012.
289. Roussignol, X: Arthroscopic tibiotalar and subtalar joint arthrodesis. *Orthop Traumatol Surg Res* 102(1):S195–S203, 2016.
290. Saltzman, CL, et al: Surgeon training and complications in total ankle arthroplasty. *Foot Ankle Int* 24(6):514–518, 2003.
291. Saltzman, CL, et al: Prospective controlled trial of STAR total ankle replacement versus ankle fusion: initial results. *Foot Ankle Int* 30(7): 579–596, 2009.
292. Saltzman, CL, et al: Total ankle replacement revisited. *J Orthop Sports Phys Ther* 30(2):56–67, 2000.
293. Sammarco, GJ, and Hockenbury, RT: Biomechanics of the foot and ankle. In Nordin, M, and Frankel, VH (eds): *Basic Biomechanics of the Musculoskeletal System,* ed. 3. Philadelphia: Lippincott Williams & Wilkins, 2001, p 222.
294. Sammarco, V: Ankle arthrodesis with onlay graft. In Kitaoka, HB (ed): *Master Techniques in Orthopedic Surgery: The Foot and Ankle,* ed. 3. Philadelphia: Lippincott Williams & Wilkins, 2013, pp 583–596.
295. Santos, MJ, and Liu, W: Possible factors related to functional ankle instability. *J Orthop Sports Phys Ther* 38(3):150–157, 2008.
296. Schenck, RC, and Coughlin, MJ: Lateral ankle instability and revision surgery alternatives in the athlete. *Foot Ankle Clin* 14(2):205–214, 2009.
297. Schiftan, GS, Ross, LA, and Hahne, AJ: The effectiveness of proprioceptive training in preventing ankle sprains in sporting populations: a systematic review and meta-analysis. *J Sci Med Sport* 18(3):238–244, 2015.
298. Schilders, E, et al: Clinical tip: Achilles tendon repair with accelerated rehabilitation program. *Foot Ankle Int* 26(5):412–415, 2005.
299. Schipper, ON, et al: Effect of obesity on total ankle arthroplasty outcomes. *Foot Ankle Int* 37(1):1–7, 2016.
300. Schipper, ON, et al: Effect of diabetes mellitus on perioperative complications and hospital outcomes after ankle arthrodesis and total ankle arthroplasty. *Foot Ankle Int* 36(3):258–267, 2015.
301. Schmidt, R, et al: Reconstruction of the lateral ligaments: do the anatomical procedures restore physiologic ankle kinematics? *Foot Ankle Int* 25(1):31–36, 2004.
302. Schuberth, JM, Patel, S, and Zarutsky, E: Perioperative complications of the Agility total ankle replacement in 50 initial, consecutive cases. *J Foot Ankle Surg* 45(3):139–146, 2006.
303. Schuh, R, et al: Total ankle arthroplasty versus ankle arthrodesis. Comparison of sports, recreational activities and functional outcome. *Int Orthop* 36(6):1207–1214, 2012.
304. Self, BP, Harris, S, and Greenwald, RM: Ankle biomechanics during impact landings on uneven surfaces. *Foot Ankle Int* 21(2):138–144, 2000.
305. Sekiya, H, et al: Arthroscopic-assisted tibiotalocalcaneal arthrodesis using an intramedullary nail with fins: a case report. *J Foot Ankle Surg* 45(4):266–270, 2006.
306. Sharma, J, et al: Biomechanical and lifestyle risk factors for medial tibia stress syndrome in army recruits: a prospective study. *Gait Posture* 33(3):361–365, 2011.
307. Shi, K, et al: Hydroxyapatite augmentation for bone atrophy in total ankle replacement in rheumatoid arthritis. *J Foot Ankle Surg* 45(5): 316–321, 2006.
308. Shrader, JA: Nonsurgical management of the foot and ankle affected by rheumatoid arthritis. *J Orthop Sports Phys Ther* 29(12):703–717, 1999.
309. Silbernagel, KG, and Crossley, KM: A proposed return-to-sport program for patients with midportion Achilles tendinopathy: Rationale and implementation. *J Orthop Sports Phys Ther* 45(11):876–886, 2015.
310. Silbernagel, KG, et al: Evaluation of lower leg function in patients with Achilles tendinopathy. *Knee Surg Sports Traumatol Arthrosc* 14(11): 1207–1217, 2006.
311. Silbernagel, KG, et al: A new measurement of heel-rise endurance with the ability to detect functional deficits in patients with Achilles tendon rupture. *Knee Surg Sports Traumatol Arthrosc* 18(2):258–264, 2010.
312. Silbernagel, KG, Steele, R, and Manal, K: Deficits in heel-rise height and Achilles tendon elongation occur in patients recovering from an Achilles tendon rupture. *Am J Sports Med* 40(7):1564–1571, 2012.
313. Singer, S, et al: Ankle arthroplasty and ankle arthrodesis: gait analysis compared with normal controls. *J Bone Joint Surg Am* 95(24):e191 (1–10), 2013.
314. Sirveaux, F, et al: Increasing shoe instep improves gait dynamics in patients with a tibiotalar arthrodesis. *Clin Orthop* 442:204–209, 2006.
315. Smith, RW: Ankle arthrodesis. In Kitaoka, HB (ed): *Master Techniques in Orthopedic Surgery: The Foot and Ankle,* ed. 2. Philadelphia: Lippincott Williams & Wilkins, 2013, pp. 533–549.
316. Snyder, AR, et al: The influence of high-voltage electrical stimulation on edema formation after acute injury: a systematic review. *J Sport Rehabil* 19(4):436–451, 2010.
317. Solan, MC, Carne, A, and Davies, MS: Gastrocnemius shortening and heel pain. *Foot Ankle Clin* 19(4):719–738, 2014.
318. SooHoo, NF, Zingmond, DS, and Ko, CY: Comparison of reoperation rates following ankle arthrodesis and total ankle arthroplasty. *J Bone Joint Surg Am* 89(10):2143–2149, 2007.
319. Soroceanu, A, et al: Surgical versus nonsurgical treatment of acute Achilles tendon rupture: a meta-analysis of randomized trials. *J Bone Joint Surg Am* 94(23):2136–2143, 2012.

320. Southerland, CC: Arthroscopic reconstruction of the unstable ankle. In Nyska, M, and Mann, G (eds): *The Unstable Ankle*. Champaign, IL: Human Kinetics, 2002, pp 238–249.
321. Spirt, AA, Assal, M, and Hansen, ST: Complications and failure after total ankle arthroplasty. *J Bone Joint Surg Am* 86–A(6):1172–1178, 2004.
322. Squadrone, R, and Gallozzi, C: Biomechanical and physiological comparison of barefoot and two shod conditions in experienced barefoot runners. *J Sports Med Phys Fitness* 49(1):6–13, 2009.
323. Stavrou, M, et al: Review article: treatment for Achilles tendon ruptures in athletes. *J Orthop Surg* 21(2):232–235, 2013.
324. Steffen, K, et al: Self-reported injury history and lower limb function as risk factors for injuries in female youth soccer. *Am J Sports Med* 36(4):700–708, 2008.
325. Stegeman, M, et al: Outcome after operative fusion of the tarsal joints: A systematic review. *J Foot Ankle Surg* 54(4):636–645, 2015.
326. Stephenson, K, Saltzman, CL, and Brotzman, SB: Foot and ankle injuries. In Brotzman, SB, and Wilk, KE: *Clinical Orthopedic Rehabilitation*, ed. 2. Philadelphia: CV Mosby, 2003, pp 371–441.
327. Stockton, B, and Boyles, RE: Osteochondral lesion of the talus. *J Orthop Sports Phys Ther* 40(4):238–238, 2010.
328. Stone, JW: Arthroscopic ankle arthrodesis. In Kitaoka, HB (ed): *Master Techniques in Orthopedic Surgery: The Foot and Ankle*, ed. 3. Philadelphia: Lippincott Williams & Wilkins, 2013, pp 569–582.
329. Subotnick, SI: Return to sport after delayed surgical reconstruction for ankle instability. In Nyska, M, and Mann, G (eds): *The Unstable Ankle*. Champaign, IL: Human Kinetics, 2002, pp 201–205.
330. Suchak, AA, et al: The influence of early weight-bearing compared with non-weight-bearing after surgical repair of the Achilles tendon. *J Bone Joint Surg Am* 90(9):1876–1883, 2008.
331. Suckel, A, et al: Talonavicular arthrodesis or triple arthrodesis: peak pressure in the adjacent joints measured in 8 cadaver specimens. *Acta Orthop* 78(5):592–597, 2007.
332. Sugimoto, K, et al: Reconstruction of the lateral ankle ligaments with bone-patellar tendon graft in patients with chronic ankle instability: a preliminary report. *Am J Sports Med* 30(3):340–346, 2002.
333. Sugimoto, K, et al: Chondral injuries of the ankle with recurrent lateral instability: an arthroscopic study. *J Bone Joint Surg Am* 91(1):99–106, 2009.
334. Sung, W, Weil, L, and Weil, LS: Retrospective comparative study of operative repair of hammertoe deformity. *Foot Ankle Spec* 7(3): 185–192, 2014.
335. Svantesson, U, et al: Muscle fatigue in a standing heel-rise test. *Scand J Rehabil Med* 30(2):67–72, 1998.
336. Takao, M, et al: Ankle arthroscopic reconstruction of lateral ligaments (ankle anti-ROLL). *Arthrosc Tech* 4(5):e595–e600, 2015.
337. Takao, M, et al: Arthroscopic anterior talofibular ligament repair for lateral instability of the ankle. *Knee Surg Sports Traumatol Arthrosc* 24(4):1003–1006, 2016.
338. Takao, M, et al: Anatomical reconstruction of the lateral ligaments of the ankle with a gracilis autograft: a new technique using an interference fit anchoring system. *Am J Sports Med* 33(6):814–823, 2005.
339. Takao, M, et al: Arthroscopic drilling for chondral, subchondral, and combined chondral-subchondral lesions of the talar dome. *Arthrosc J Arthrosc Relat Surg* 19(5):524–530, 2003.
340. Tenenbaum, S, Coleman, SC, and Brodsky, JW: Improvement in gait following combined ankle and subtalar arthrodesis. *J Bone Joint Surg Am* 96(22):1863–1869, 2014.
341. Terrell, RD, et al: Comparison of practice patterns in total ankle replacement and ankle fusion in the United States. *Foot Ankle Int* 34(11): 1486–1492, 2013.
342. Terrier, R, et al: Impaired control of weight bearing ankle inversion in subjects with chronic ankle instability. *Clin Biomech* Bristol Avon 29(4):439–443, 2014.
343. Thelen, S, et al: The influence of talonavicular versus double arthrodesis on load dependent motion of the midtarsal joint. *Arch Orthop Trauma Surg* 130(1):47–53, 2010.
344. Thevendran, G, Younger, A, and Pinney, S: Current concepts review: risk factors for nonunions in foot and ankle arthrodeses. *Foot Ankle Int* 33(11):1031–1040, 2012.
345. Thomas, JL, et al: The diagnosis and treatment of heel pain: a clinical practice guideline-revision 2010. *J Foot Ankle Surg* 49(3):S1–S19, 2010.
346. Thomas, RH, and Daniels, TR: Ankle arthritis. *J Bone Joint Surg Am* 85–A(5):923–936, 2003.
347. Thomas, R, Daniels, TR, and Parker, K: Gait analysis and functional outcomes following ankle arthrodesis for isolated ankle arthritis. *J Bone Joint Surg* 88A:526–535, 2006.
348. Townshend, D, et al: Arthroscopic versus open ankle arthrodesis: a multicenter comparative case series. *J Bone Joint Surg Am* 95(2):98–102, 2013.
349. Turner, NSI, and Campbell, DCI: Prosthetic intervention of the great toe. In Morrey, BF (ed): *Joint Replacement Arthroplasty*, ed. 3. Philadelphia: Churchill Livingstone, 2003, pp 1121–1132.
350. Tweed, JL, Campbell, JA, and Avil, SJ: Biomechanical risk factors in the development of medial tibial stress syndrome in distance runners. *J Am Podiatr Med Assoc* 98(6):436–444, 2008.
351. Tyler, TF, et al: Risk factors for noncontact ankle sprains in high school football players: the role of previous ankle sprains and body mass index. *Am J Sports Med* 34(3):471–475, 2006.
352. Uquillas, CA, et al: Everything Achilles: knowledge update and current concepts in management: AAOS exhibit selection. *J Bone Joint Surg Am* 97(14):1187–1195, 2015.
353. Valderrabano, V, et al: Kinematic changes after fusion and total replacement of the ankle: part 1: range of motion. *Foot Ankle Int* 24(12): 881–887, 2003.
354. Valderrabano, V, et al: Sports and recreation activity of ankle arthritis patients before and after total ankle replacement. *Am J Sports Med* 34(6):993–999, 2006.
355. Valderrabano, V, et al: Mobile- and fixed-bearing total ankle prostheses: is there really a difference? *Foot Ankle Clin* 17(4):565–585, 2012.
356. Valovich McLeod, TC: The effectiveness of balance training programs on reducing the incidence of ankle sprains in adolescent athletes. *J Sport Rehabil* 17(3):316–323, 2008.
357. van den Bekerom, MPJ, et al: The anatomy in relation to injury of the lateral collateral ligaments of the ankle: a current concepts review. *Clin Anat* 21(7):619–626, 2008.
358. van den Bekerom, et al: What is the evidence for rest, ice, compression, and elevation therapy in the treatment of ankle sprains in adults? *J Athl Train* 47(4):435–443, 2012.
359. van der Eng, DM, et al: Rerupture rate after early weightbearing in operative versus conservative treatment of Achilles tendon ruptures: a meta-analysis. *J Foot Ankle Surg* 52(5):622–628, 2013.
360. van Heiningen, J, Vliet Vlieland, TPM, and van der Heide, HJL: The mid-term outcome of total ankle arthroplasty and ankle fusion in rheumatoid arthritis: a systematic review. *BMC Musculoskelet Disord* 14:306, 2013.
361. Vega, J, et al: All-inside arthroscopic lateral collateral ligament repair for ankle instability with a knotless suture anchor technique. *Foot Ankle Int* 34(12):1701–1709, 2013.
362. Verhagen, E, et al: The effect of a proprioceptive balance board training program for the prevention of ankle sprains: a prospective controlled trial. *Am J Sports Med* 32(6):1385–1393, 2004.
363. Verhagen, EALM: What does therapeutic ultrasound add to recovery from acute ankle sprain? A review. *Clin J Sport Med* 23(1):84–85, 2013.
364. Verhagen, RAW, et al: Systematic review of treatment strategies for osteochondral defects of the talar dome. *Foot Ankle Clin* 8(2):233–242, 2003.
365. Vertullo, CJ, and Nunley, JA: Participation in sports after arthrodesis of the foot or ankle. *Foot Ankle Int* 23(7):625–628, 2002.
366. Vicenzino, B, et al: Initial changes in posterior talar glide and dorsiflexion of the ankle after mobilization with movement in individuals with recurrent ankle sprain. *J Orthop Sports Phys Ther* 36(7):464–471, 2006.

367. Villarreal, AD, Andersen, CR, and Panchbhavi, VK: A survey on management of chronic Achilles tendon ruptures. *Am J Orthop* 41(3): 126–131, 2012.
368. Wang, Y, et al: Effects of ankle arthrodesis on biomechanical performance of the entire foot. *PLoS ONE* 10(7): e0134340, 2015.
369. Wapner, KL: Delayed repair of the Achilles tendon. In Kitaoka, HB (ed): *Master Techniques in Orthopedic Surgery: The Foot and Ankle,* ed. 2. Philadelphia: Lippincott Williams & Wilkins, 2002, pp 323–335.
370. Waterman, BR, et al: The epidemiology of ankle sprains in the United States. *J Bone Jt Surg Am* 92(13):2279–2284, 2010.
371. Werner, BC, et al: Obesity is associated with increased complications after operative management of end-stage ankle arthritis. *Foot Ankle Int* 36(8):863–870, 2015.
372. White, WJ, McCollum, GA, and Calder, JDF: Return to sport following acute lateral ligament repair of the ankle in professional athletes. *Knee Surg Sports Traumatol Arthrosc* 24(4):1124–1129, 2016.
373. Whitting, JW, et al: Dorsiflexion capacity affects Achilles tendon loading during drop landings. *Med Sci Sports Exerc* 43(4):706–713, 2011.
374. Wikstrom, EA, et al: Bilateral balance impairments after lateral ankle trauma: a systematic review and meta-analysis. *Gait Posture* 31(4): 407–414, 2010.
375. Wilkins, R, and Bisson, LJ: Operative versus nonoperative management of acute Achilles tendon ruptures: a quantitative systematic review of randomized controlled trials. *Am J Sports Med* 40(9):2154–2160, 2012.
376. Willems, TM, et al: Gait-related risk factors for exercise-related lower-leg pain during shod running. *Med Sci Sports Exerc* 39(2):330–339, 2007.
377. Willits, K, et al: Operative versus nonoperative treatment of acute Achilles tendon ruptures: a multicenter randomized trial using accelerated functional rehabilitation. *J Bone Joint Surg Am* 92(17): 2767–2775, 2010.
378. Wong, J, Barrass, V, and Maffulli, N: Quantitative review of operative and nonoperative management of Achilles tendon ruptures. *Am J Sports Med* 30(4):565–575, 2002.
379. Yasui, Y, et al: Open versus arthroscopic ankle arthrodesis: a comparison of subsequent procedures in a large database. *J Foot Ankle Surg* 55(4):777–781, 2016.
380. Yotsumoto, T, Miyamoto, W, and Uchio, Y: Novel approach to repair of acute Achilles tendon rupture: early recovery without postoperative fixation or orthosis. *Am J Sports Med* 38(2):287–292, 2010.
381. Young, B, et al: A combined treatment approach emphasizing impairment-based manual physical therapy for plantar heel pain: a case series. *J Orthop Sports Phys Ther* 34(11):725–733, 2004.
382. Zhang, H, et al: Surgical versus conservative intervention for acute Achilles tendon rupture: A PRISMA-compliant systematic review of overlapping meta-analyses. *Medicine* 94(45):e1951, 2015.
383. Zhao, H, et al: A systematic review of outcome and failure rate of uncemented Scandinavian total ankle replacement. *Int Orthop* 35(12): 1751–1758, 2011.
384. Ziai, P, et al: The role of the medial ligaments in lateral stabilization of the ankle joint: an in vitro study. *Knee Surg Sports Traumatol Arthrosc* 23(7):1900–1906, 2015.
385. Zwipp, H, et al: High union rates and function scores at midterm followup with ankle arthrodesis using a four screw technique. *Clin Orthop* 468(4):958–968, 2010.

CHAPTER

23

Advanced Functional Training

LYNN COLBY, PT, MS ■ CAROLYN KISNER, PT, MS
■ JOHN BORSTAD, PT, PHD

Functional training involves developing and progressing exercise programs that enable patients to regain their pre-injury level of function. For individuals wishing to return to high-level work, leisure, recreational, or athletic activities, rehabilitation must progress sufficiently to meet the anticipated demands of those activities. For the therapist, it requires a continuous process of decision-making that involves:

- A thorough knowledge of human anatomy, physiology, biomechanics, and function.
- An understanding of tissue healing, especially the effect of time on healing and the response of tissues to imposed stresses.
- An understanding of neuromuscular responses to various forms of exercise.
- The ability to examine and evaluate the structural and functional impairments that restrict activity and full functional participation within the context of personal and societal expectations.
- Knowledge of diagnoses, surgical and therapeutic exercise interventions, special precautions, and each patient's potential for achieving the projected outcomes.

Functional training can begin in the early phases of rehabilitation with specific muscle activation and training techniques designed to develop a balance in the strength and timing of contractions among synergists and antagonists. Because proximal stability is critical for coordinated functioning of the extremities, exercises to develop stability and balance are also incorporated into the early phases of the rehabilitation.

As muscle strength, endurance, and control of the involved region(s) improve, greater emphasis is placed on strengthening muscle groups in functional patterns, using both weight-bearing and nonweight-bearing exercises. Care is taken to ensure that the activity of stronger muscles does not dominate the weaker, impaired muscles during the execution of these functional patterns. As function improves, the exercises can become more activity specific.

Functional motor skills encompass an array of movements completed using multiple postures, at varying speeds, and over many repetitions or durations of time. The cornerstone of a functionally relevant therapeutic exercise program is the inclusion of task-specific movements that are superimposed on sufficient stability, balance, and muscle function to meet the necessary, expected, and desired functional demands in a patient's life.

The purpose of this chapter is to describe a variety of advanced functional training exercises that involve the total body and may be appropriate for the final phase of rehabilitation. The chapter is divided into two sections. The first section focuses on advanced exercises for stability and balance and the second on advanced exercises for strength and power. Exercises selected for this phase of rehabilitation are based on the patient's desired outcome and emphasize the motor skills needed to achieve that outcome.

CLINICAL TIP

For all exercises, always stay within the healing constraints of the impaired tissues. Be aware of the likely tissue stresses imposed by the position, motion, intensity, and speed of each exercise. Initially, emphasize correct joint and body alignment with proper movement velocity during the exercise. Then, as the intensity of an exercise can be progressed, decrease the repetitions (or time) until the patient is able to perform the activity safely and effectively.

Exercises for Stability and Balance

Guidelines Revisited

Stability describes the ability to maintain or adequately return a body or system to a state of equilibrium when external forces impart a perturbation to that body or system. The concept that proximal stability is a requisite for controlled distal mobility and safe and effective function can be applied not only to general postural stability, but also to individual joints.

Joint stability. Stability of each joint in the body is necessary for effective function. Examples of joint stability include the ability to maintain scapular position and glenohumeral joint alignment so the humeral muscles can safely coordinate movement of the upper extremity[4] (see Chapter 17). Other examples include coordinated segmental and global stability of the spine for postural alignment and safe body mechanics (see Chapters 14 and 16) and stability of the hips, knees, and ankles for control during functional weight-bearing activities (see Chapters 20 through 22). Because specific exercises for joint stability are described in detail in the respective chapters, the reader is referred to those chapters for study before progressing to the advanced exercises described in this chapter.

Postural stability and balance. For an individual to be able to execute functional activities, balance—or postural stability—is necessary to maintain the position of the body in equilibrium within the environment. These concepts are described in detail in Chapter 8. In addition, stability and balance exercises in upright postures that are appropriate early in a rehabilitation program are described in each of the lower extremity chapters. Parameters for progressing balance exercises are summarized in Table 23.1.

TABLE 23.1 Parameters for Progressing Balance Exercises

Parameters	Progression
Upright posture	
	▪ Sitting→kneeling→standing
Base of support	
	▪ Sitting: feet on floor→feet off floor ▪ Standing: wide→narrow base ▪ Standing: Double leg stance→tandem stance→single-leg stance
Support surface	
	▪ Stationary, firm, or flat surface→moving, soft, uneven surface (ball, wobble board, slide board, sand, gravel, grass) ▪ Wide surface→narrow (balance beam, half foam roll)
Superimposed movements	
	▪ Head, trunk, extremity movements ▪ Small→large-range extremity movements ▪ Unresisted→resisted (free weights, elastic resistance)
Perturbations	
	▪ Anticipated→unanticipated ▪ Low magnitude→high magnitude ▪ Slow speed→high speed
Environment	
	▪ Surroundings nonmoving (closed)→moving (open)
Functional tasks	
	▪ Simple→complex tasks ▪ Single→multiple tasks

CLINICAL TIP

As patients progress through advanced rehabilitative exercises, remind them frequently to maintain the spine in a neutral position and to activate the trunk muscles in order to stabilize the spine against imposed forces. If at any time the patient shows signs of insufficient trunk stability (such as lack of control of spinal posture or increased painful symptoms), review and implement the spinal stabilization exercises as described in Chapter 16.

Advanced Stabilization and Balance Exercises

Sitting

When the individual is able to sit on a firm, stable surface and maintain balance while reaching in all directions under various loads, progress training by having them perform the same tasks while sitting on an unstable surface. Surface suggestions include a foam cushion, rocker board, BOSU®, or large gym ball.

Sitting and Reaching

Have the patient balance on an unstable surface and reach in various directions, first with one extremity, then with both. Add resistance to the motions as the patient is able (Fig. 23.1).

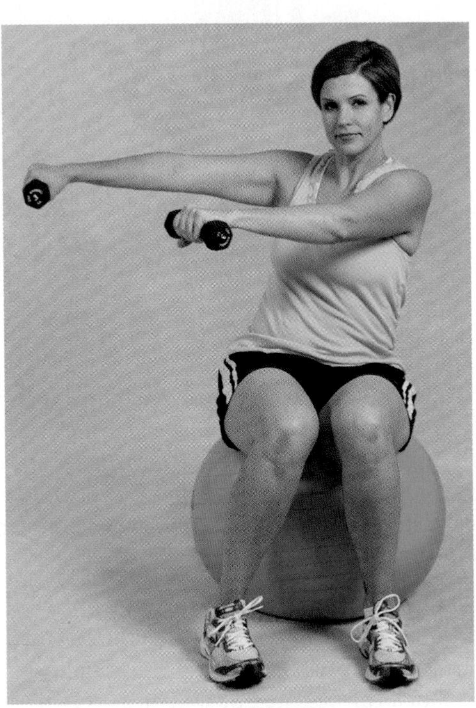

FIGURE 23.1 Resisted reaching movements while maintaining sitting balance on an unstable surface.

Sitting With External Perturbations

While the patient maintains sitting balance on an unstable surface:

- Move the surface in various directions, first slowly, then more quickly.
- Pull on a length of elastic resistance held by the patient. Alter the speed and direction of pull.
- Toss a ball to the patient, requiring him or her to reach out in various directions and return the toss (Fig. 23.2).

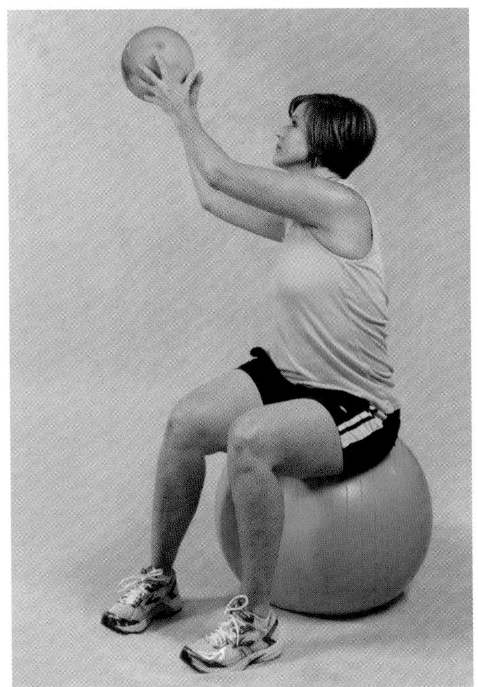

FIGURE 23.2 Maintaining sitting balance while catching and returning a ball.

- Increase the challenge by integrating a plyometric component into the balance activity, such as catching and tossing a weighted ball.
- Manually push on the patient's trunk while they perform reaching activities. Vary the amount, point of application, timing, and direction of manual force used.

NOTE: Refer to the next section of this chapter for examples of plyometric exercises that also improve a patient's balance.

Kneeling

Kneeling activities can be performed in the *half-kneeling* (balancing on one knee with the other extremity forward and foot planted on the floor) or *high-kneeling* (tall-kneeling on both knees) positions. The level of challenge can be adjusted or progressed by having the patient reach in various directions under loaded and unloaded conditions, kneel on stable or unstable surfaces, and respond to perturbations.

Kneeling on a Stable Surface

- In the half-kneeling position, loop an exercise band under the forward foot and have the patient perform diagonal upper extremity patterns against the resistance (Fig. 23.3 A).
- While in a half-kneeling or high-kneeling position, have the patient reach and lift a weighted object from the floor with one or both hands, and then move the weighted object upward and outward in various patterns of motion and return (Fig. 23.3 B).
- While in a half-kneeling or high-kneeling position, toss a ball and have the patient catch and then return it. Progress this activity by gradually tossing the ball away from the trunk in multiple directions and with varying velocities.

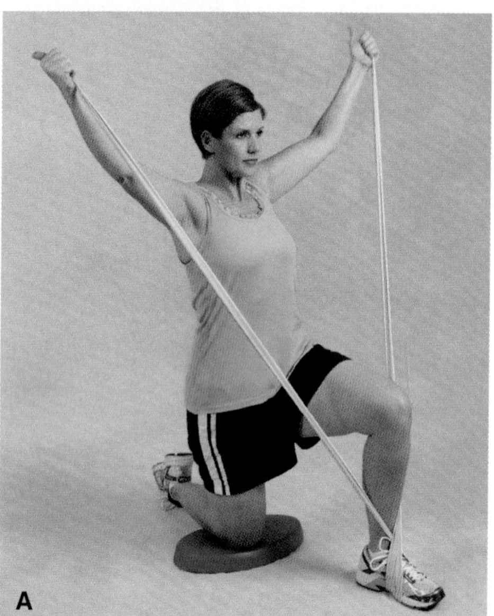

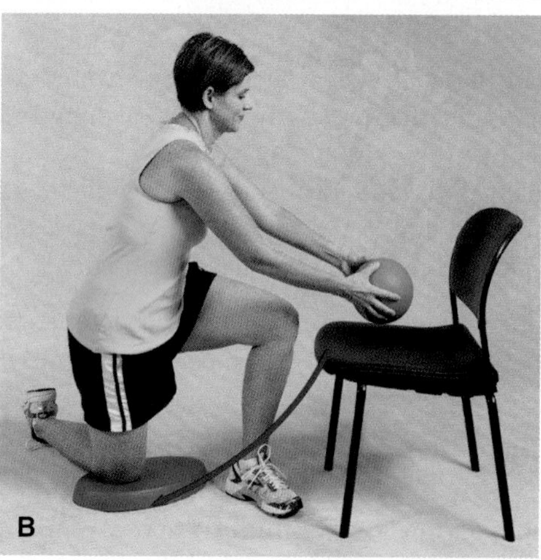

FIGURE 23.3 Balancing in half-kneeling position **(A)** while performing diagonal patterns against elastic resistance; and **(B)** while moving a weighted object from a chair to the floor.

Kneeling on an Unstable Surface

- Have the patient kneel on a foam roller, balance board, BOSU®, or partially deflated large therapy ball and perform arm motions in various directions; progress the activity by having the patient move the arms against resistance.
- While kneeling on an unstable surface, have the patient catch and return a ball. Progress by using a weighted ball (Fig. 23.4) or adjusting the location and speed of the toss.

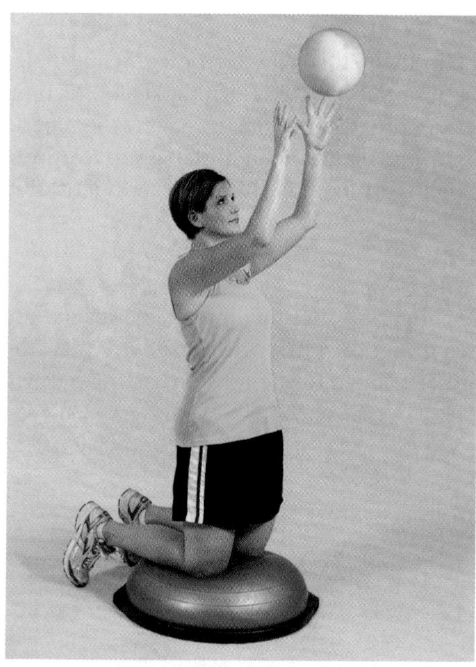

FIGURE 23.4 Balancing in high-kneeling position on a BOSU® while catching and tossing a ball.

Bilateral Stance

Once the individual can stand upright and maintain balance while reaching in all directions and while managing imposed loads (free weights, pulley system, or elastic resistance), the patient is ready to progress to exercises that provide a greater challenge to stability and balance, first in bilateral stance and progressing to unilateral stance.

Bilateral Stance on a Stable Surface VIDEO 23.1

- Begin with the patient standing with both feet on the floor, shoulder width apart, or in a stride position.
  - Toss a ball (unweighted or weighted) that requires the patient to reach outward, upward, or downward to catch and return it. When indicated, remind the patient to maintain a neutral spine, to contract the abdominals when reaching upward to stabilize the spine, or to rotate

at the hips rather than the spine when reaching outward or downward.
    - Perform various arm motions against elastic resistance, with free weights, or while shaking a BodyBlade®.
- Progress to balancing in *tandem stance*. Have the patient stand on a stable, narrow surface, such as a line on the floor or a balance beam. Apply quick alternating manual resistance against the patient's pelvis (Fig. 23.5), or apply quick pulling motions to elastic resistance held by the patient. Vary the timing, direction, amount, and point of application of the forces used to adjust or progress this activity.

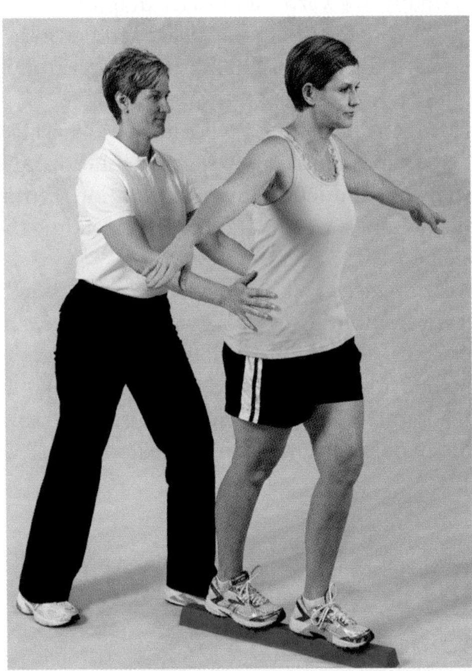

FIGURE 23.5 Balancing in tandem stance on a balance beam with quick alternating resistance applied against the pelvis.

- Progress to *tandem walking* on a narrow but stable surface. Manual perturbations to the pelvis and trunk can be added to further challenge the patient.

Bilateral Stance on an Unstable Surface

VIDEO 23.2

- While on a balance board or BOSU®, have patient rock the platform forward and backward and side-to-side while attempting to control the motion and maintain balance. Instruct the patient to prevent the edges of the platform from hitting the floor.
- Have the patient stand on a foam half-roller (curved side down), a balance board, or BOSU®; add the following perturbations as the patient is able.
    - Apply quick alternating resistance against the patient's pelvis.
    - Have the patient perform various arm motions against elastic resistance, with free weights (Fig. 23.6), or while shaking a BodyBlade®.
    - Toss a ball (unweighted or weighted) back and forth to the patient (Fig. 23.7).
    - Have the patient perform partial squats (Fig. 23.8).

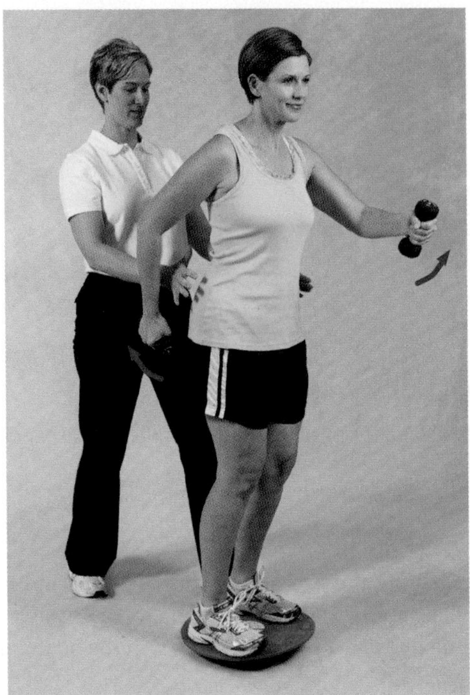

FIGURE 23.6 Balancing in bilateral stance on a balance board while performing arm movements.

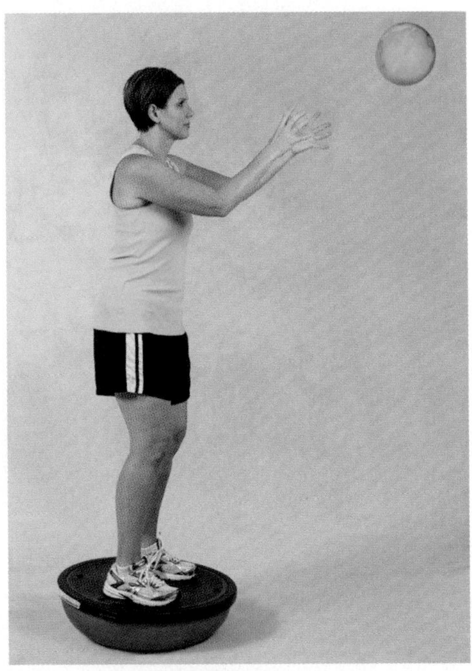

FIGURE 23.7 Balancing in bilateral stance on a BOSU® while catching and tossing a ball.

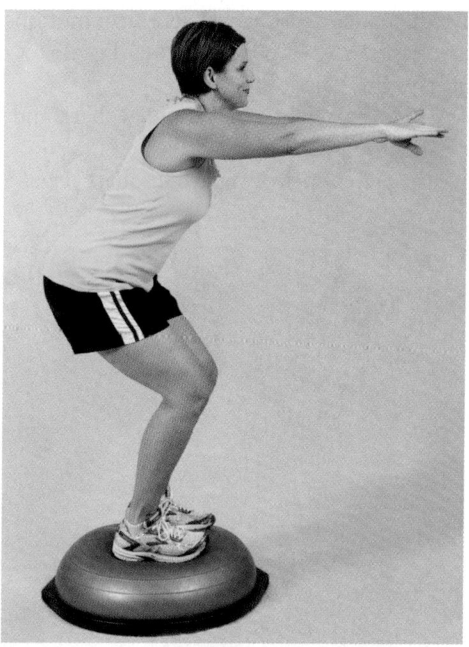

FIGURE 23.8 Balancing on an unstable surface while performing partial squats.

Unilateral Stance

Begin by having the patient practice standing in unilateral stance on a stable surface, progressing to an unstable surface and adding perturbations as described in the bilateral stance exercises.

Unilateral Stance on a Stable Surface

VIDEO 23.3

- Have the patient perform upper extremity diagonal patterns, unilaterally or bilaterally, using free weights or elastic bands (tubing) while balancing on one lower extremity (Fig. 23.9). When using elastic resistance, change the angle of pull to vary the challenge and balance response.
- Have the patient, while balancing on one lower extremity, practice various lower extremity patterns that replicate functional activities. The following are suggestions:
  - Place a star pattern (such as four intersecting lines) on the floor. Have the patient place one foot on the center of the pattern and then touch the opposite foot on each of the lines of the pattern: directly forward, diagonally forward, sideways, diagonally backward (Fig. 23.10 A), straight backward, and crossed behind (Fig. 23.10 B). Then switch feet and repeat the pattern on the opposite side.
  - Perform an alternating PNF pattern, such as D_1 flexion (flexion, adduction, and external rotation)/extension (extension, abduction, internal rotation) with one leg while holding a weight and flexing/extending the opposite elbow (Fig. 23.11).
  - Have the patient walk sideways, then progress to braiding or carioca motions using forward and backward crossover steps. This requires alternating balance reactions from one lower extremity to the other.
  - Bend or rotate to one side while performing a partial squat to lift an object from a chair or the floor (Fig. 23.12).

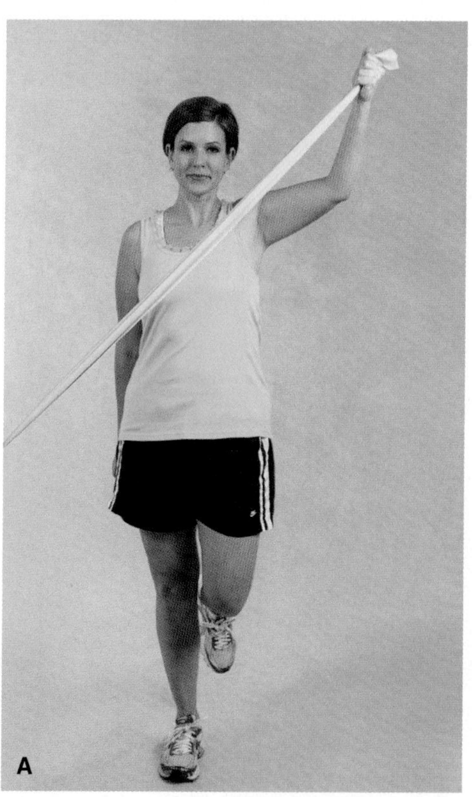

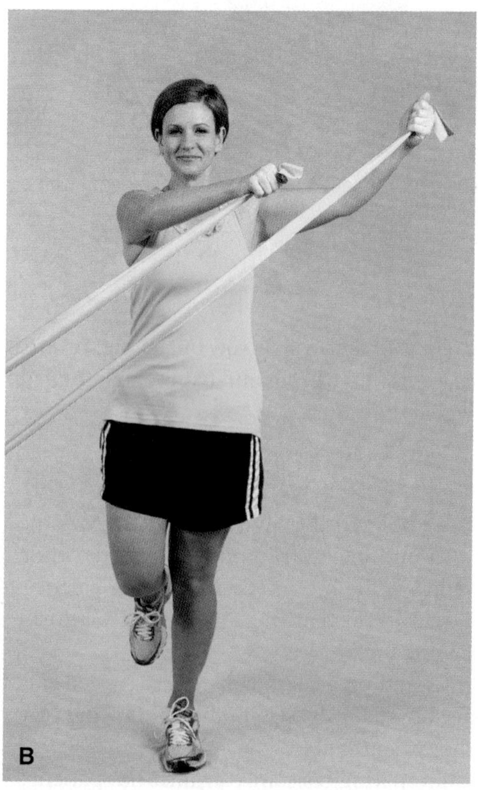

FIGURE 23.9 Balancing in unilateral stance while performing upper extremity diagonal patterns against elastic resistance: **(A)** unilaterally; and **(B)** bilaterally.

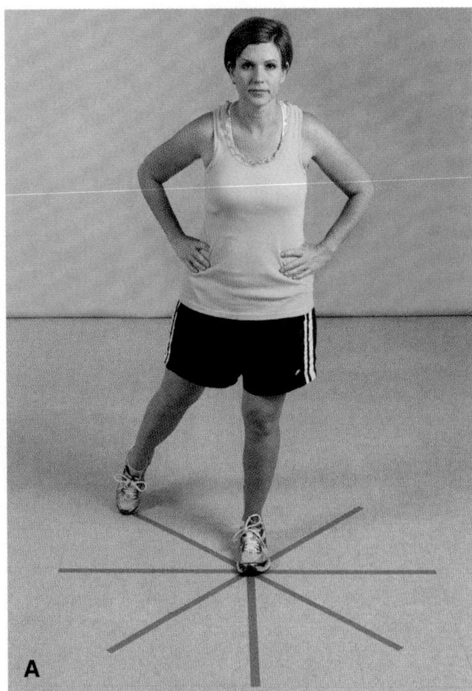

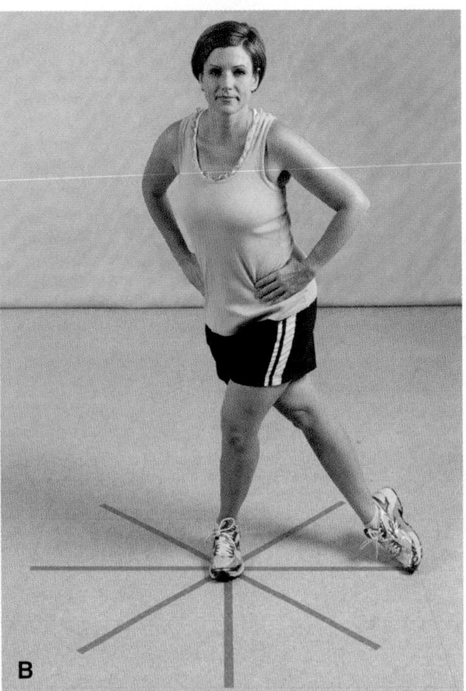

FIGURE 23.10 Maintaining balance while touching one foot on each of the lines of a star pattern on the floor and returning to the center; **(A)** diagonally backward and **(B)** crossed behind stationary leg.

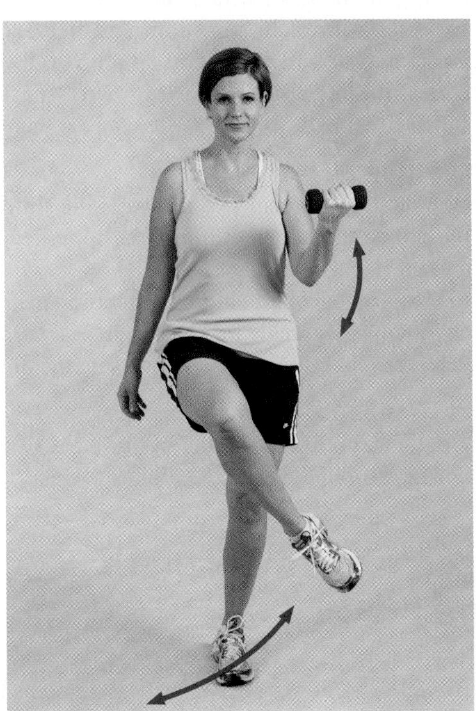

FIGURE 23.11 Balancing in unilateral stance while performing a diagonal pattern with one lower extremity. Upper extremity motions add additional challenges to balance.

- Reach outward with arms while bending forward and extending one leg as in a "skater" position (Fig. 23.13 A). Increase the challenge by picking up a weight from the floor or by alternately moving the arms in a windmill manner (without or with weights in each hand) (Fig. 23.13 B).

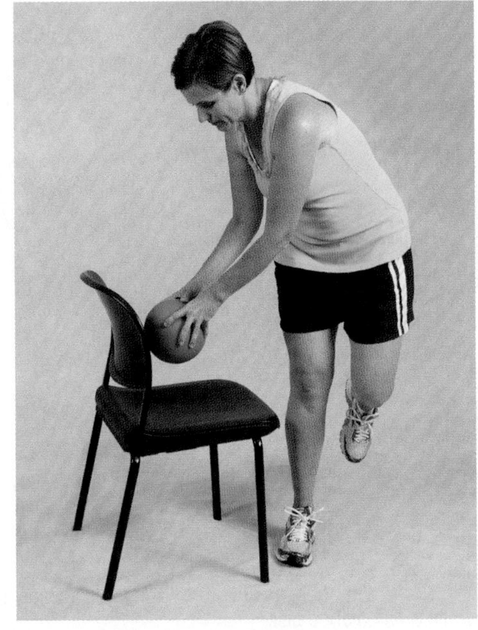

FIGURE 23.12 Partial squatting in unilateral stance, leaning to one side and picking up an object.

Unilateral Stance on an Unstable Surface

- Have the patient stand on the round and then flat side of a BOSU® or on a balance board or disc, and apply resistance against the patient's trunk or to upper extremity movements using elastic resistance (Fig. 23.14).
- While balancing on an unstable surface, have the patient swing one leg forward and backward, first slowly, then with increasing speeds.

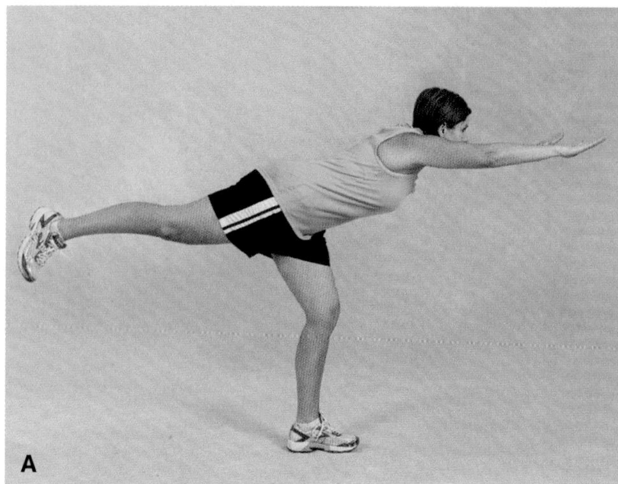

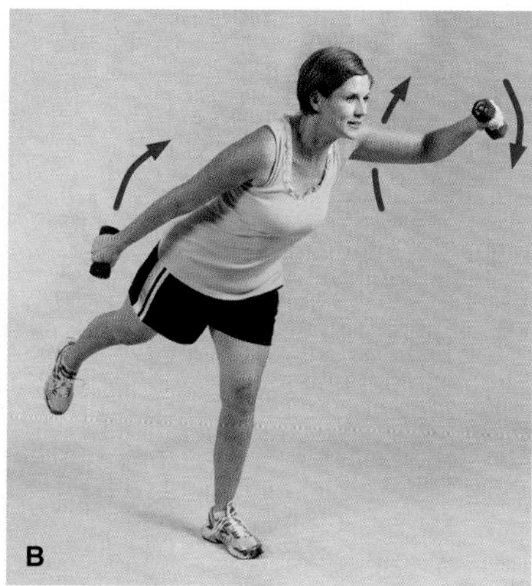

FIGURE 23.13 Maintaining balance in unilateral stance: **(A)** while bending forward at the hips and reaching out with both arms; and **(B)** while performing a windmill motion using handheld weights.

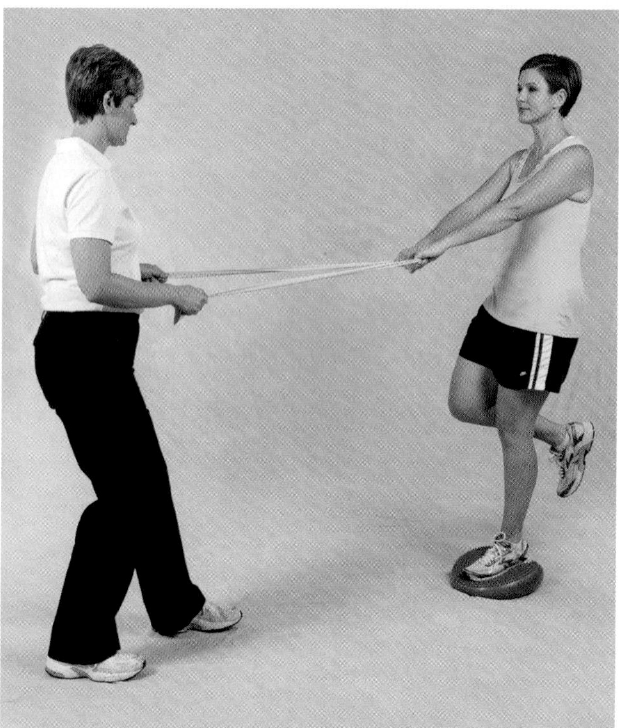

FIGURE 23.14 Perturbations in unilateral stance using elastic resistance while on a balance disc.

Moving and Planting Activities VIDEO 23.4

Movement followed by planting the foot (or feet) not only requires coordinated movements to stop the body's progression in one direction, but also a rapid balance response to keep from falling. These activities also prepare the individual for skills that involve rapid reversals of direction and agility drills.

Jump and "Freeze"

- Have the patient jump down from a platform or low step and hold the end position (Fig. 23.15 A). Progress to jumping up onto the platform.
- When the patient has learned one-legged balance and demonstrates control in the jump-and-freeze exercise, progress to having him or her hop up onto or down from a step and holding the end position with that one leg (Fig. 23.15 B).

Side Shuffle and "Freeze"

- Have the patient perform two to three side shuffles and hold the end position, then shuffle in the opposite direction and "freeze" (Fig. 23.16).
- Vary the pattern to include shuffling in multiple directions, such as moving diagonally forward then backward or in a curved pattern, freezing and then reversing the direction.

Run and "Freeze"

Have the patient run forward, sideways, and backwards and "freeze" when you call out "freeze" or blow a whistle.

Exercises for Strength and Power

Muscle strength and power are two critical elements for successful performance of many high-demand functional tasks and activities, such as moving heavy objects in the workplace and home or meeting the demands required for many sports. Muscle endurance also is necessary when functional or recreational tasks must be repeated or sustained over time. When designing functional rehabilitation programs for patients, recognize that some functional activities may involve slow, controlled, or repetitive movements, while other activities may require bursts of movement or quick changes of direction.

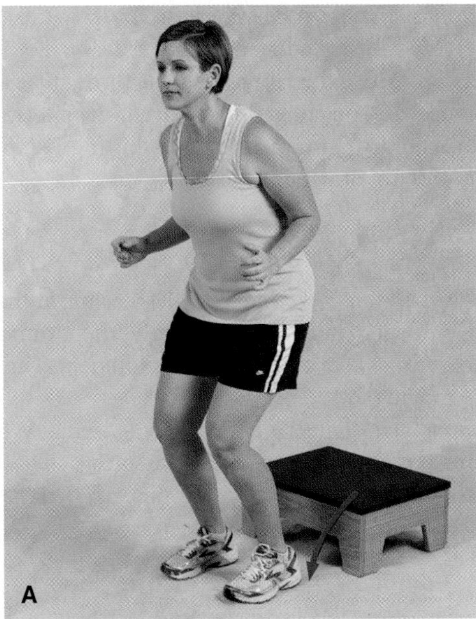

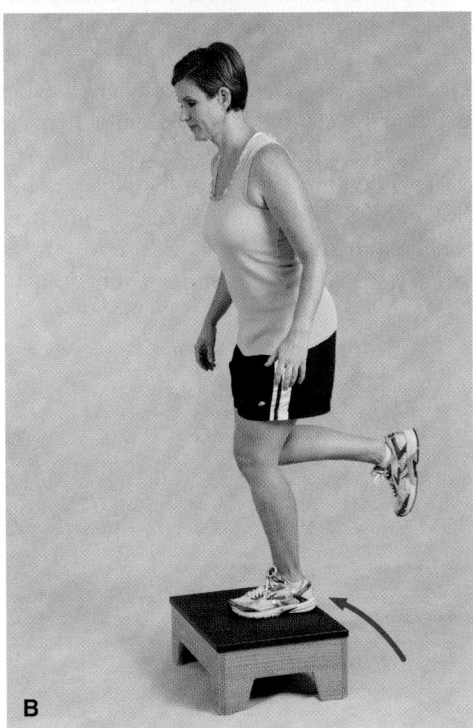

FIGURE 23.15 Jump and freeze sequence and progression: **(A)** jumping down from a step and holding the end position and **(B)** hopping up onto a step and holding the end position.

In many cases, functional activities involve some combination of these movement and force requirements and the patient should be involved in defining their specific circumstances. Once these functional activities are defined, an effective exercise program can be developed that addresses the specific areas of muscle performance associated with each patient's physically demanding activities.

The remainder of this chapter focuses on exercises designed to improve muscle strength and/or power output—specifically,

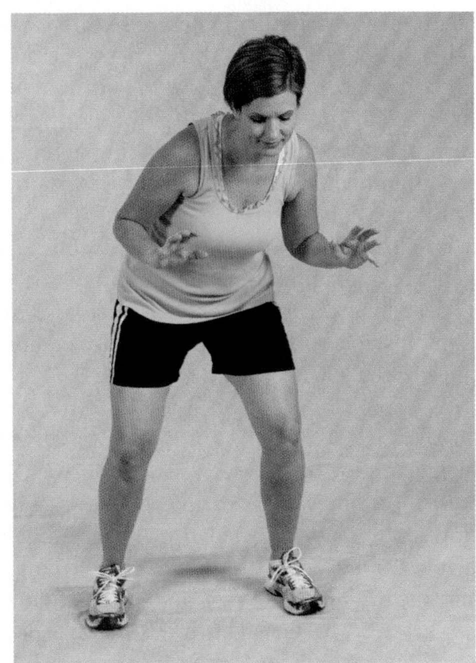

FIGURE 23.16 Side shuffle and freeze.

advanced strengthening exercises for the upper and lower extremities, and plyometric exercises, which involve high force movements performed at rapid speeds. All of the exercises described are built on the foundational constructs of dynamic stability of proximal body regions (shoulder girdle, trunk, pelvic girdle) and balance. Somewhat paradoxically, a program of advanced strengthening exercises and plyometric training also imposes significant demands on a patient's balance and dynamic stability, which improves these areas of physical function.[10]

CLINICAL TIP

When teaching a patient a program of advanced strengthening and plyometric exercises, always emphasize the patient's use of proper exercise technique before increasing the resistance imposed, the number repetitions and sets of an exercise, or the number of exercises in a treatment session.

Advanced Strengthening Exercises

As discussed in Chapter 6, progressive resistance is a necessary element of exercises designed to develop muscle strength, while increasing the duration of exercise (repetitions or time) is necessary to develop muscle endurance. The strengthening exercises in this section use functionally based and total body movement patterns against the resistance of body weight or external loads. They are implemented during the advanced phase of rehabilitation in preparation for the patients return to high-demand tasks and activities.

Many advanced strengthening exercises are carried out using weight machines designed to target specific muscle groups or by using a variety of set-ups with weight-pulley systems and isokinetic equipment. However, the exercises in this section can be performed using simple but versatile resistance equipment, such as handheld weights or elastic bands or tubing. Other exercises suggest using equipment typically employed for cardiopulmonary training, such as a treadmill or stepping machine. Furthermore, some of the exercises described can be progressed by performing the exercises on unstable surfaces such as balance equipment to impose greater challenges.

Advanced Strengthening: Upper Extremities

The following upper extremity exercises, performed in either weight-bearing or nonweight-bearing positions, are designed to develop strength of selected upper extremity muscle groups. However, advanced upper extremity strengthening also requires activation of the trunk and lower extremity musculature. Therefore, be sure that the patient has developed sufficient scapular, shoulder girdle, and trunk stability plus sufficient balance in upright positions before progressing to these exercises.

Exercises With a BodyBlade®

- *Patient position and procedure:* While sitting or standing, have the patient hold and shake the blade with one or both hands in a variety of shoulder positions with the elbow(s) extended or flexed (Fig. 23.17 A and B). Vary the speed, direction, and size of oscillations used by the patient to alter the perturbations generated by the blade.
- *Progression:* Move the vibrating blade through a variety of anatomical and diagonal upper extremity patterns. Incorporate trunk rotation and weight shifting on the lower extremities for a total body exercise.

Upper Extremity Weight-Bearing Exercises Using Selected Equipment

- *Hand-walking on a treadmill:* While kneeling at the end of the treadmill, have the patient "walk" with his or her hands while bearing weight through the shoulders. The surface can be moving forward or backward.
- *"Climbing" with hands on a stepping machine:* While in a kneeling position and with each hand on a step of the unit, have the patient alternately push on each pedal to target scapular stabilizers and elbow extensors.

Pushing/Pulling and Lifting/Lowering Exercises

The following exercises involve various pushing and pulling or lifting and lowering motions. They are useful for developing upper extremity strength for functional tasks that require concentric and eccentric control of shoulder, elbow, and forearm musculature in combined movement patterns for moving objects of varying sizes and weights from one place to another. Depending on the size of the object to be moved, an exercise may be performed bilaterally or unilaterally. It is important to remind the patient to use proper body mechanics by maintaining a neutral spine and contracting the trunk

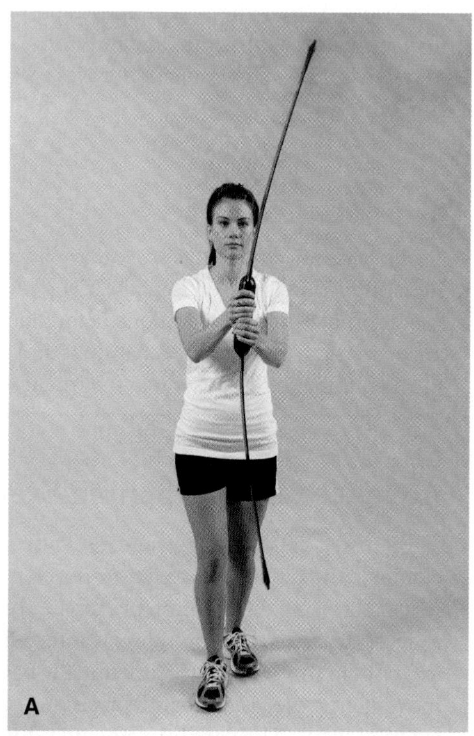

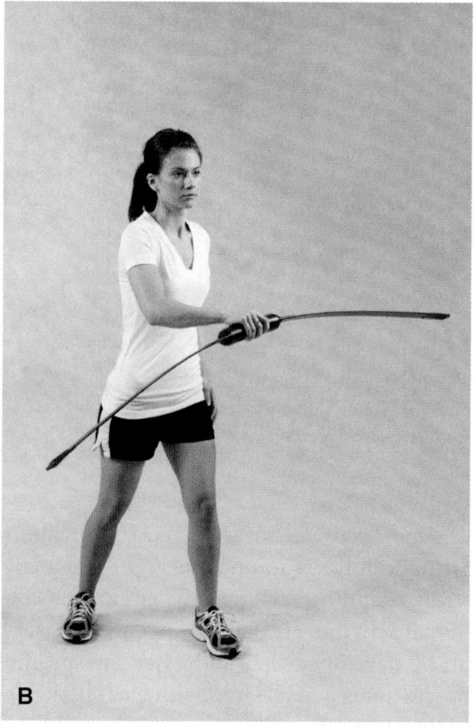

FIGURE 23.17 Exercises with a BodyBlade®: **(A)** bilateral isometric strengthening of shoulder rotators with additional activation of trunk stabilizers; and **(B)** unilateral isometric strengthening of elbow flexors/extensors.

stabilizing muscles during the task and by maintaining a stable base of support during each of these exercises.

- *Pushing or pulling motions*
  - Perform pushing and pulling motions against the resistance of an elastic band by moving the upper extremities in forward, backward, upward, and downward directions.
  - Using an upper extremity ergometer, perform pushing or pulling motions, "pedaling" against resistance in a forward or backward direction. Adjust the direction, speed, and arc of motion to replicate various functional tasks.
  - Reposition a heavy crate on a level surface by pulling (Fig. 23.18) or pushing (see Fig. 18.21) it from one place to another.

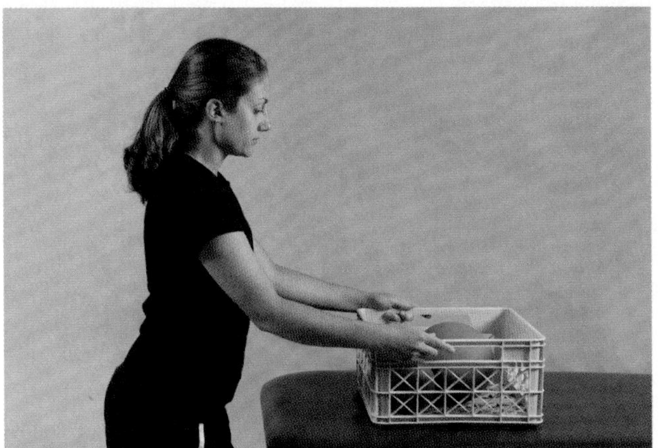

FIGURE 23.18 Strengthening shoulder and elbow musculature by pulling (sliding) a heavy object from one position to another.

- *Lifting or lowering motions*
  - Lift a weighted crate from the surface of a table, hold it close to the body, and lower it to a different position on the table.
  - Lift and lower a heavy object to and/or from high and low surfaces (Fig. 23.19).

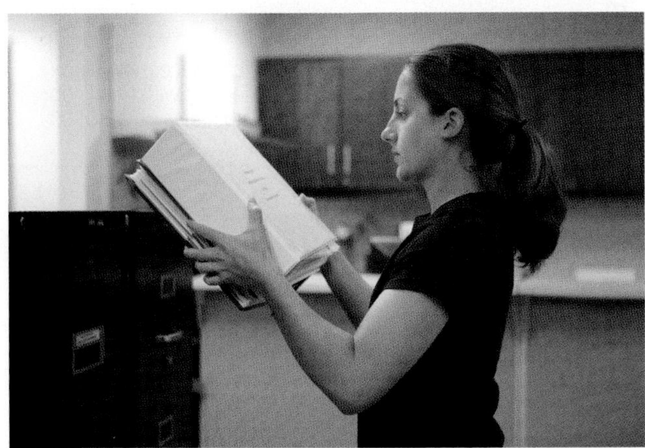

FIGURE 23.19 Strengthening shoulder and elbow musculature by lifting or lowering a heavy object to and from a high surface.

Seated Push-Ups on Unstable Surfaces

VIDEO 23.5

- *Patient position and procedure:* While in a long-sitting position on the floor with heels placed on a firm foam roller or BOSU®, have the patient lift the hips from the floor by performing a seated push-up (Fig. 23.20 A).
- *Patient position and procedure:* Have the patient sit on a firm foam roller, the flat side of a BOSU®, or a balance board with legs on the floor and hands on the unstable surface at either side of the hips and lift the hips upward by performing a seated push-up (Fig. 23.20 B). Progress by increasing the time spent with the hips lifted or by raising one leg off the support surface.

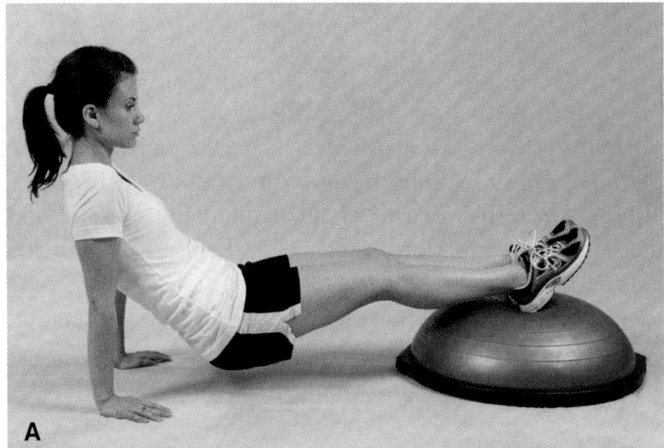

A

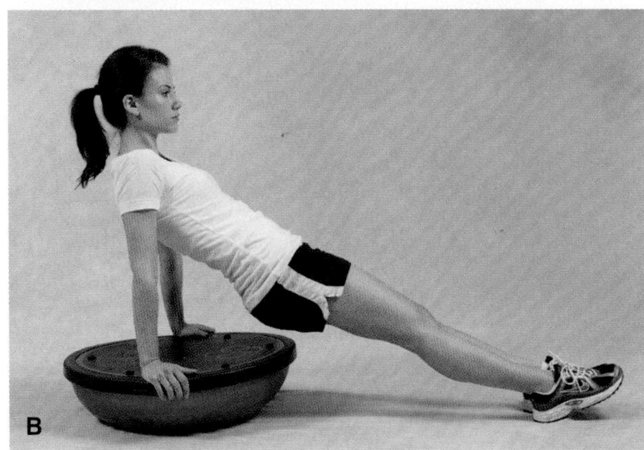

B

FIGURE 23.20 Seated push-ups in a long-sitting position **(A)** with lower legs on an unstable (soft) surface; and **(B)** with hands on an unstable surface.

Prone Push-Ups in a Head-Down Position

Patient position and procedure: Once the patient can perform a prone push-up with hands and feet on the floor, progress to a prone push-up in a head-down position on an incline board, over a therapy ball, or on the floor with feet elevated on a platform to shift greater body weight to the upper extremities (Fig. 23.21).

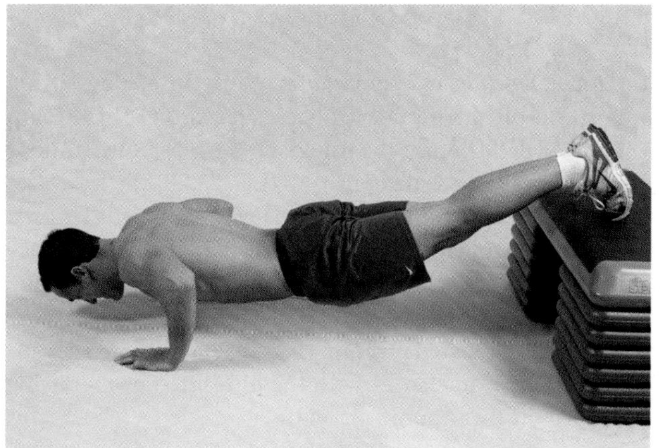

FIGURE 23.21 Prone push-ups in a head-down position.

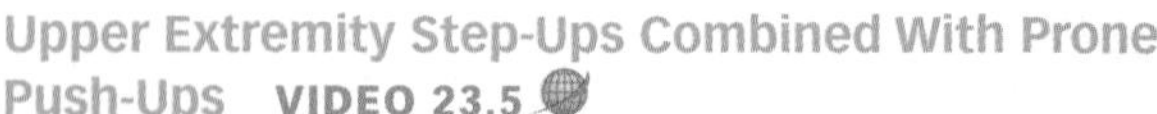

Upper Extremity Step-Ups Combined With Prone Push-Ups VIDEO 23.5

Patient position and procedure: Have the patient perform a prone push-up with both hands on the floor. While maintaining the push-up position, move one hand up onto and then off of a low platform (Fig. 23.22). Repeat the sequence, gradually increasing the number of repetitions. This exercise increases the weight-bearing force on the extremity that remains on the floor.

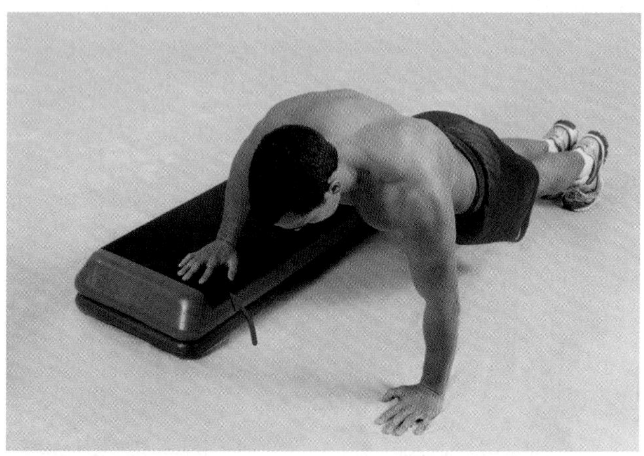

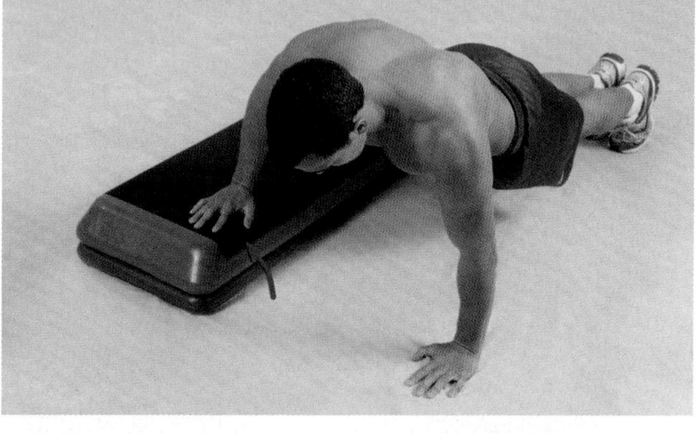

FIGURE 23.22 Upper extremity step-up with the right upper extremity following a prone push-up.

Prone Push-Ups on Unstable Surfaces

- *Patient position and procedure:* Have the patient perform a series of push-ups with hands on the floor and knees on a foam roller (Fig. 23.23 A).
- *Patient position and procedure:* Have the patient perform a series of push-ups with hands on a foam roller or small ball and knees or feet on the floor (Fig. 23.23 B).
- *Patient position and procedure:* Have the patient perform a series of push-ups with hands on a balance board, BOSU®, or small ball and knees on a foam roller (Fig. 23.23 C).

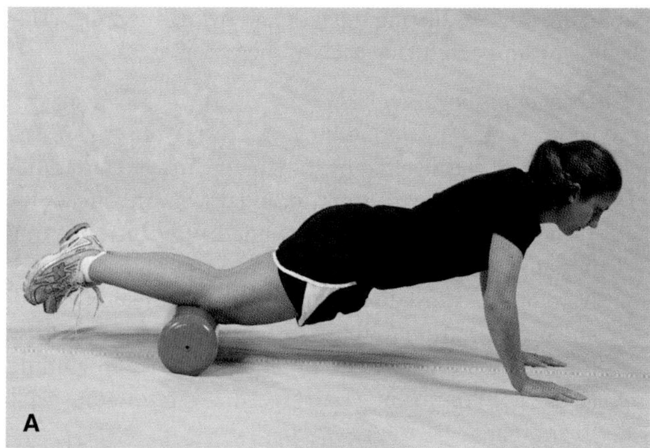

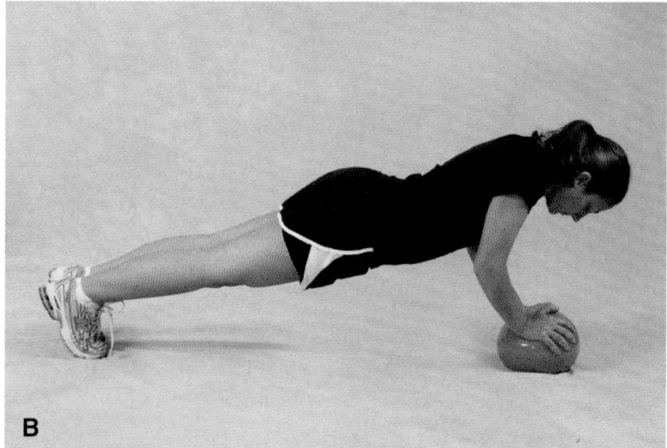

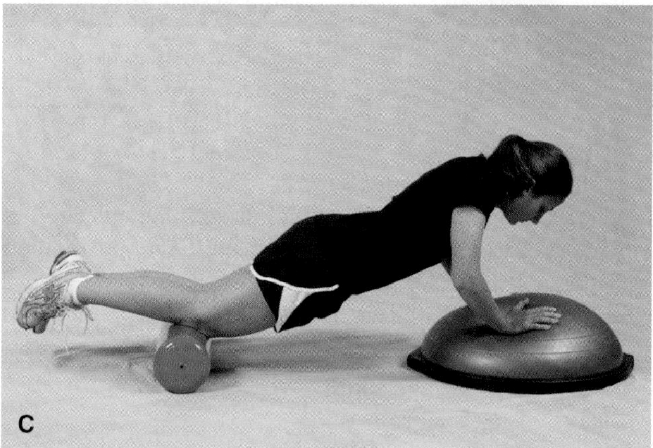

FIGURE 23.23 Prone push-ups on unstable surfaces: **(A)** with hands on the floor and knees on a foam roller; **(B)** with hands on a small ball and feet on the floor; and **(C)** with hands on a BOSU® and knees on a foam roller.

Ball "Walk-Out" VIDEO 23.5

- *Patient position and procedure:* In a prone position with hands on the floor and lower extremities on a large therapy ball, have the patient "walk" forward and then backward on the hands while keeping the lower extremities in contact with the ball (Fig. 23.24). To increase the challenge, perform prone push-ups between the forward and backward "walking" phases.

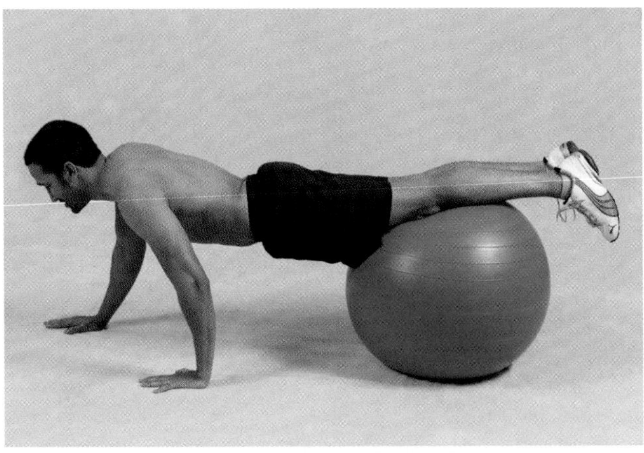

FIGURE 23.24 Ball "walk-out" on hands with lower extremities rolling on a large therapy ball.

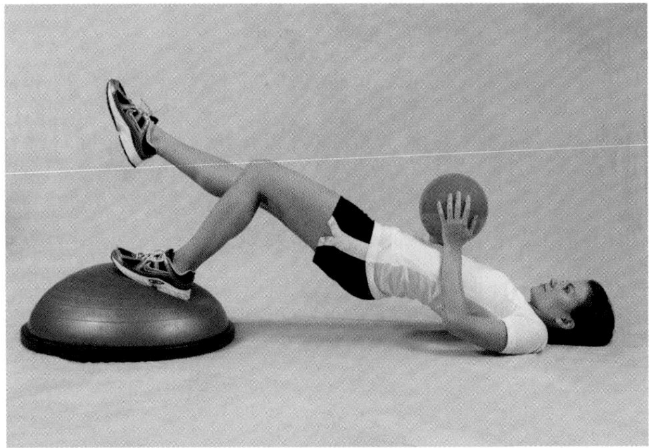

FIGURE 23.25 Unilateral supine pelvic bridge on an unstable surface while holding a weighted ball in both hands for additional resistance.

Plantar-Grade "Walking"

Plantar-grade walking with weight on hands and feet (also referred to as "bear-walking") places considerable weight through the upper extremities and can be used to develop strength of the musculature that stabilizes the scapulothoracic and glenohumeral joints.

- *Patient position and procedure:* Have the patient assume the plantar-grade position on hands and feet and "walk" forward bearing weight through all four limbs.
- *Progression:* Perform plantar-grade "walking" against the resistance of an elastic cord harnessed around the pelvis and fixed to the wall or to a heavy piece of equipment.

Advanced Strengthening: Lower Extremities

VIDEO 23.6

The following exercises, some of which are progressions of exercises described in Chapters 20 through 22, are performed in functional movement patterns against progressive resistance and are implemented to develop increased lower extremity strength. Many of these exercises also improve dynamic stability of the trunk and balance.

Unilateral Supine Pelvic Bridges

Patient position and procedure: With one foot planted on the floor and the other extremity off the floor in either hip/knee flexion or hip flexion and knee extension, have the patient lift and lower the pelvis first against body weight and then while holding a weighted ball in both hands. Increase the challenge by planting the weight-bearing foot on an unstable surface, such as a BOSU® or small balance disk (Fig. 23.25).

Supine Pelvic Bridges on an Elevated Surface

- *Patient position and procedure:* While on the floor in a long-sitting position with both feet on a chair, platform, or a large therapy ball and hands on the floor, have the patient extend the hips, lifting them from the floor (Fig. 23.26).
- *Progression:* Lift the hips from the floor with just one foot placed on the chair or platform and the other leg flexed toward the chest.

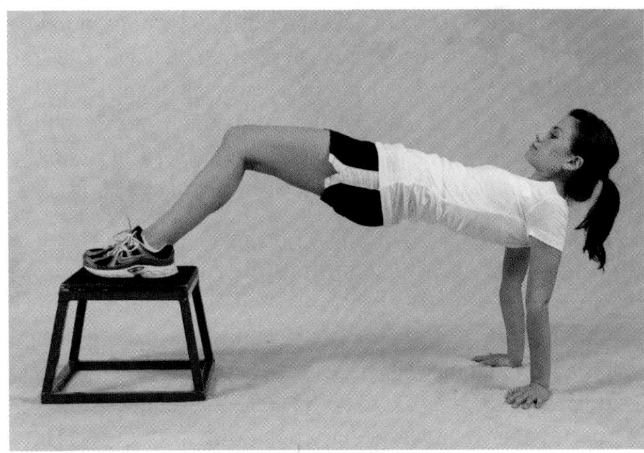

FIGURE 23.26 Supine pelvic bridge with the lower extremities elevated on a platform or chair and hands on the floor.

Supine Hamstring Curls on a Ball **VIDEO 23.6** 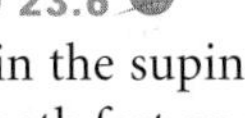

- *Patient position and procedure:* While lying in the supine position on the floor, have the patient place both feet on a large therapy ball and roll it toward the hips by flexing the knees (Fig. 23.27). In addition to strengthening the hamstrings, this exercise also challenges the trunk stabilizers.
- *Progression:* Have the patient perform the exercise unilaterally by lifting one foot off the ball and rolling the ball toward the hips with just one foot on the ball.

Hamstrings or Quadriceps Strengthening: Kneeling

- *Patient position and procedure:* Have the patient begin in a high-kneeling position on a padded surface for comfort.
- *To strengthen the hamstrings:* While manually stabilizing the patient's lower legs, have the patient lean *forward* from the vertical position as far as possible (Fig. 23.28 A), keeping the trunk erect and maintaining balance, and then return to the upright position by flexing the knees. In addition to strengthening the hamstrings eccentrically and concentrically in a closed-chain position, this exercise provides a significant challenge to the patient's balance.

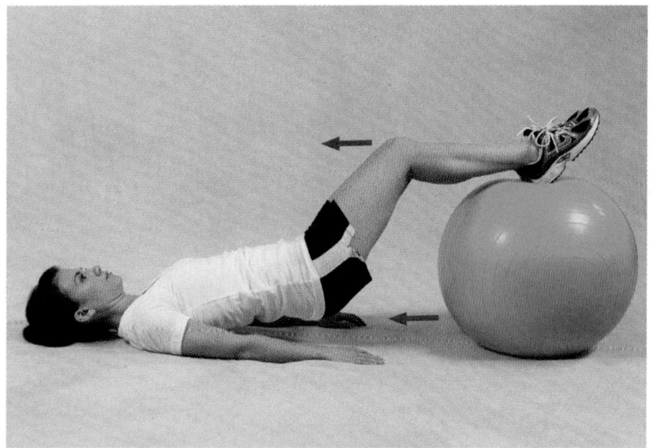

FIGURE 23.27 Supine hamstring curls on a ball.

- *To strengthen the quadriceps:* Have the patient lean *backward* as far as possible from the upright position without touching the buttocks to the heels and then return to the high-kneeling position. As the patient leans backward, the quadriceps contract eccentrically to control movement at the knees and then concentrically as the patient returns to the vertical position.
- *Progression:* Add a weight held close to the chest for additional resistance (Fig. 23.28 B).

Unilateral Wall Slides: Standing

- *Patient position and procedure:* While in unilateral stance with the back against a wall and weight-bearing foot several feet away from the wall, have the patient slide down the wall until the knee is flexed to 90° (Fig. 23.29), making sure the knee avoids valgus and stays posterior to the toes. Hold the position, and then return to a standing position. This exercise strengthens the hip and knee extensors eccentrically and concentrically.
- *Progression:* Hold weights in both hands for additional resistance. Gradually increase the number of repetitions and/or the duration that the 90° position is held. Increase the challenge by placing a large therapy ball behind the back for these exercises.

Deep Squats

- *Patient position and procedure:* In bilateral stance with feet a comfortable distance apart, have the patient perform a deep squat by flexing the hips and knees (Fig. 23.30). Keep body weight distributed posteriorly through the heels, and be sure to keep the lower legs as vertical as possible to the floor so that the knees do not move anterior to the toes. Hold the deep squat position, and then return to the standing position. Have the patient hold both arms out in front of the body for balance or place one hand lightly on a countertop, if necessary.
- *Progression:* Perform repeated deep squats while holding weights or by combining squats with resisted upper extremity motions. This activity is beneficial for developing body mechanics in individuals who do heavy lifting in the work setting.

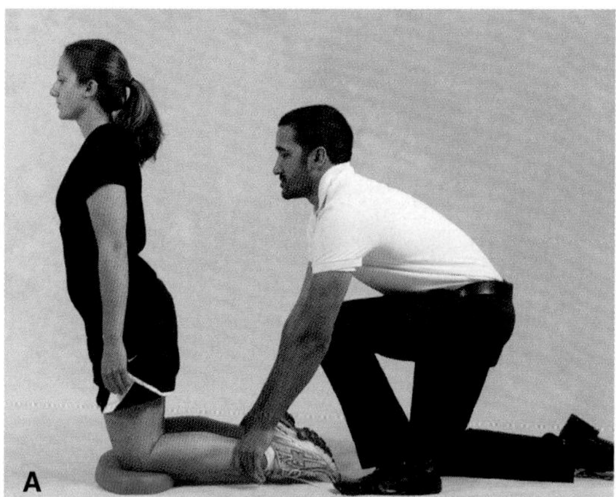

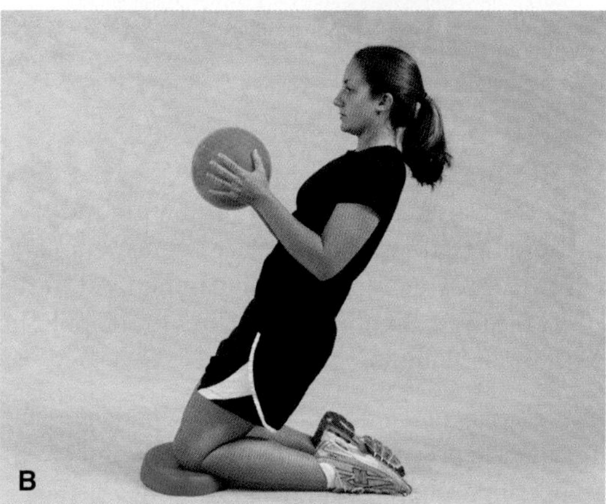

FIGURE 23.28 (A) Strengthening the hamstrings against the resistance of body weight by leaning forward from a high-kneeling position; **(B)** strengthening the quadriceps by leaning backward from the high-kneeling position while holding a weighted ball for additional resistance.

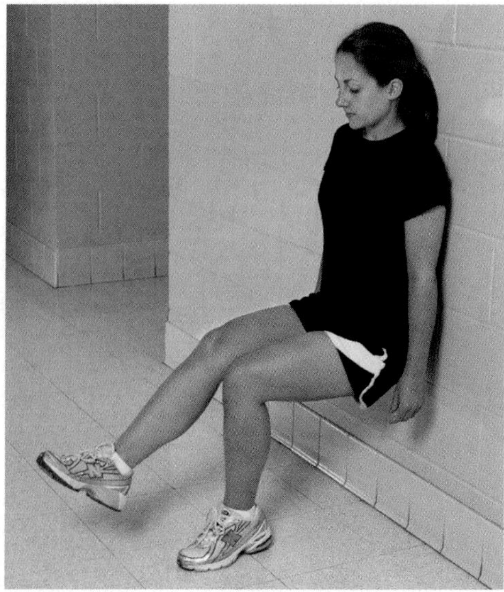

FIGURE 23.29 Unilateral wall slides in standing with a midrange hold.

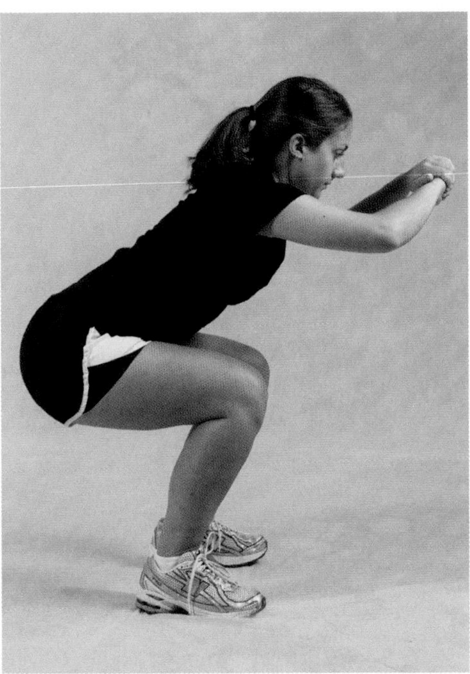

FIGURE 23.30 Deep squats with an end-range hold, while trying to keep the knees posterior to the toes.

Variations of Lunges **VIDEO 23.6**

- *Deep forward lunge:* While maintaining the trunk in an erect position, have the patient place one foot forward and perform a deep lunge, flexing the forward knee to a 90° position but keeping the lower leg vertical and the knee posterior to the toes (Fig. 23.31 A); then return to the standing position. Place one hand lightly on a stable surface (wall, countertop) for balance, if necessary.
  - As balance improves, have the patient perform deep forward lunges while holding a weighted ball away from the chest and performing trunk rotation.
  - Place the forward foot on an unstable surface, such as a balance disk, while performing the forward lunge exercise.

FOCUS ON EVIDENCE

Although the forward lunge exercise typically is performed with the trunk erect, there is evidence demonstrating that changing the position of the trunk and upper extremities alters the recruitment of muscle groups in the lead lower extremity during the lunge. Farrokhi and colleagues[9] conducted a motion analysis and electromyographic (EMG) study of the lead lower extremity during variations of the forward lunge exercise with ten healthy adults (five men, five women) as subjects. The investigators found that there was a small but statistically significant increase in hip extensor muscle (gluteus maximus and biceps femoris) recruitment of the lead leg when forward lunges were performed with the

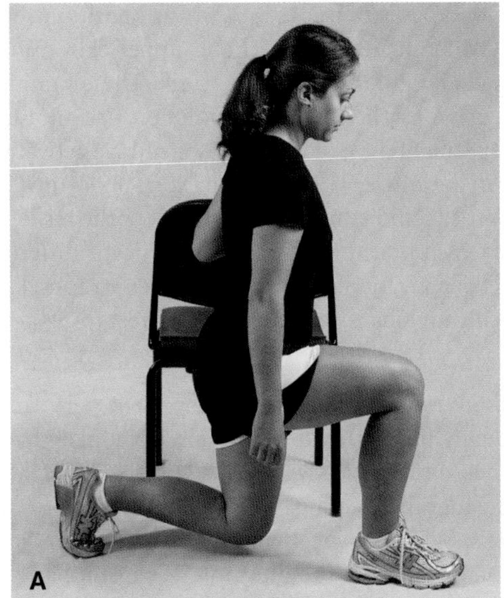

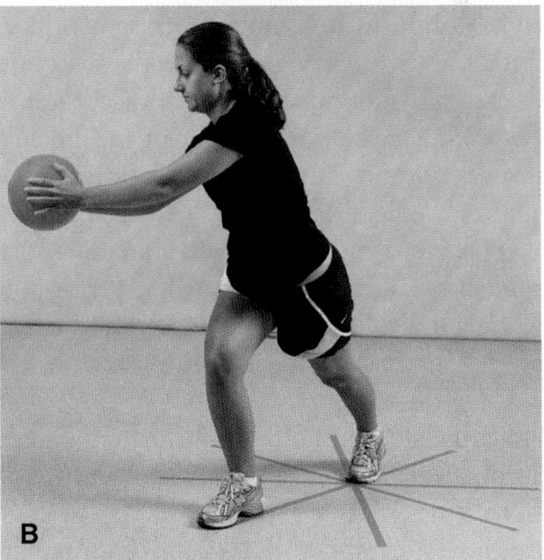

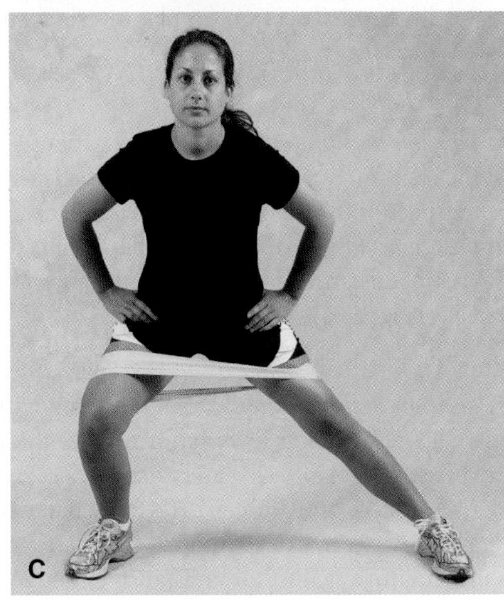

FIGURE 23.31 **(A)** Deep forward lunge while lightly touching a stable surface for balance; **(B)** multidirectional lunges on a star pattern on the floor; and **(C)** deep lateral lunge against elastic resistance.

trunk and upper extremities in a forward position compared with when the trunk was erect and upper extremities were positioned along the sides of the trunk. These findings confirmed a previously held clinical assumption. In contrast, despite clinical speculation that knee extensor muscle activation may increase in the lead leg if forward lunges are performed with the arms overhead and trunk in full extension, the results of this study revealed that there were no significant differences in the levels of activation of hip or knee extensor muscle groups compared with lunges performed in the erect trunk position.

- *Multidirectional lunges:* Have the patient perform lunges diagonally forward, out to the side, diagonally backward, and then directly backward. This sequence is facilitated by placing four intersecting lines on the floor (in a star pattern or like spokes of a wheel) and having the patient keep one foot planted where the lines intersect. The patient steps out onto each line (Fig. 23.31 B) and returns to the upright position. Motion in the same direction can be repeated multiple times before progressing to the next line, or the patient can step out onto each line in succession.
- *Lunges against added resistance:* Increase the difficulty of the exercise by performing lunges against elastic resistance looped around the lower legs (Fig. 23.31 C) or holding weights or a weighted ball, wearing a weight belt, or holding a barbell on the shoulders. Controlling weights while performing lunges is beneficial for developing strength for individuals returning to work settings that require heavy lifting.
- *Lunge-walking:* Perform a series of lunges in various directions to move across the floor or to pick up objects of decreasing height (e.g., 16 to 4 in.) from various places on the floor.
- *Lunge-jumps:* Refer to the description and figure (see Fig. 23.63) in the next section on plyometric training.

Sitting Down and Standing Up From a Chair Against Elastic Resistance

- *Patient position and procedure:* Have the patient sit down against the resistance of an elastic band looped around the posterior aspect of the pelvis (Fig. 23.32 A).
- *Patient position and procedure:* Have the patient stand up against elastic resistance looped around the anterior aspect of the pelvis (Fig. 23.32 B).

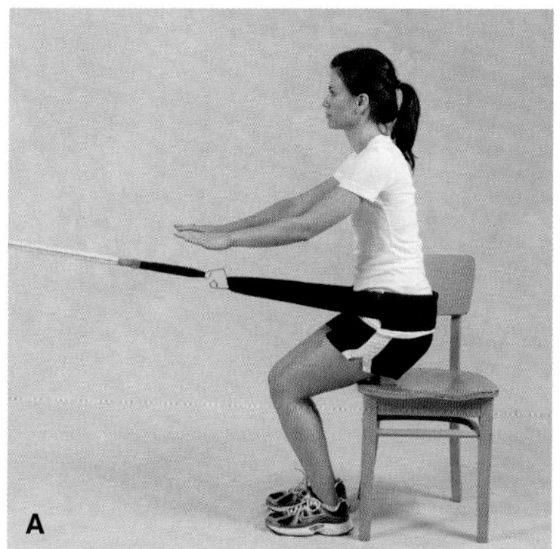

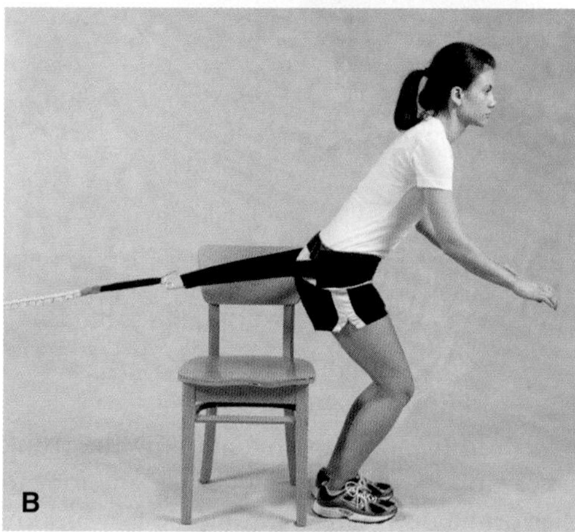

FIGURE 23.32 **(A)** Sitting down; and **(B)** standing up against elastic resistance.

Bilateral or Unilateral Heel-Lowering Over a Step

- *Patient position and procedure:* While standing with heels over the edge of a step or low platform, have the patient perform bilateral heel lowering and raising. Place one hand *lightly* on a railing or a stable surface for balance. Heel lowering imposes eccentric loading of the gastrocnemius-soleus musculature against the resistance of body weight.
- *Progression:* Perform the same exercise while wearing a weight belt or vest or holding weights (Fig. 23.33), then progress to unilateral stance.

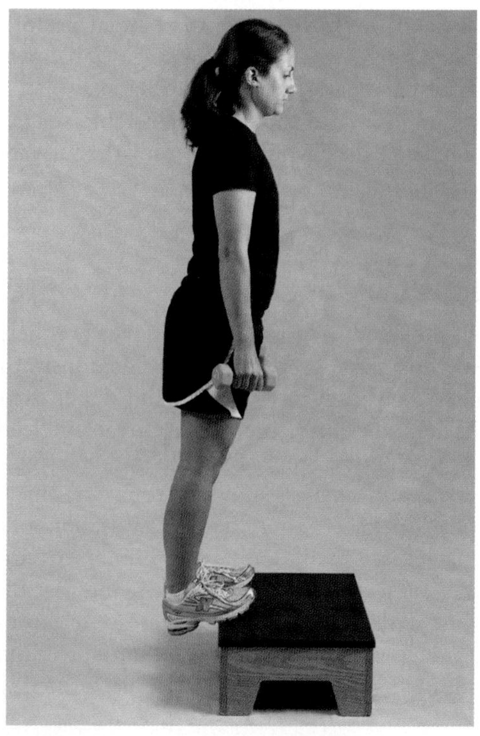

FIGURE 23.33 Heel-lowering over a step while holding weights for additional resistance.

Band Walking

- *Patient position and procedure:* Have the patient walk forward (Fig. 23.34 A), sideward (Fig. 23.34 B), and backward against elastic resistance looped around the pelvis.

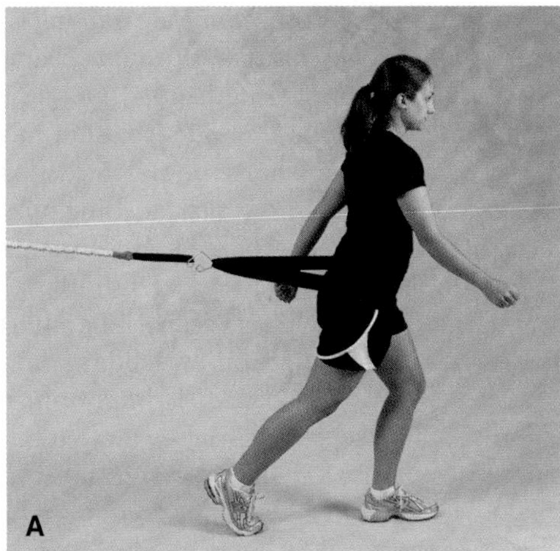

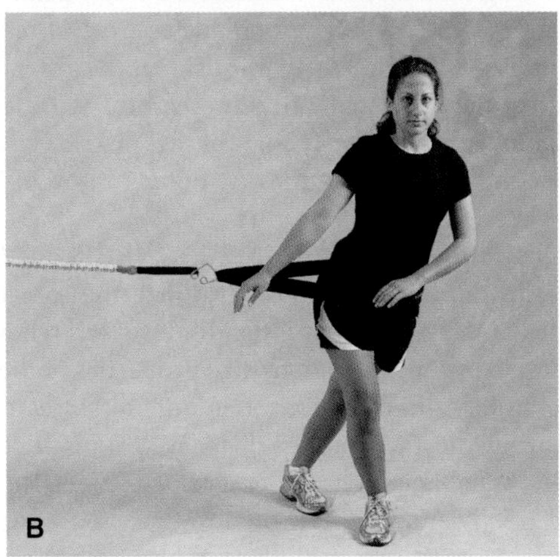

FIGURE 23.34 Band walking: **(A)** in a forward direction; and **(B)** in a sideward direction against elastic resistance looped around the pelvis.

- *Patient position and procedure:* Have the patient walk forward against elastic resistance looped around the thighs for closed-chain strengthening of the external rotators (Fig. 23.35).

Pulling or Pushing a Heavy Object

- *Patient position and procedure:* With the arms positioned in a stable and comfortable position, have the patient use primarily lower extremity strength to pull (Fig. 23.36) or push a heavy object, such as a weighted sled or cart, across the floor. Select positions for pulling or pushing similar to the anticipated work-related tasks or sport activity. Be certain the patient uses proper body mechanics.
- *Progression:* Gradually increase the amount of weight moved from one place to another.

Resisted Running Start and Resisted Running

Patient position and procedure: While wearing a harness placed around the trunk and pelvis, have the patient move from the starting position typically assumed prior to a sprint and then run forward against the resistance of a heavy-grade elastic cord that is attached to the harness and affixed to the wall or a stationary surface (Fig. 23.37). As an alternative, the patient can perform backward running against resistance.

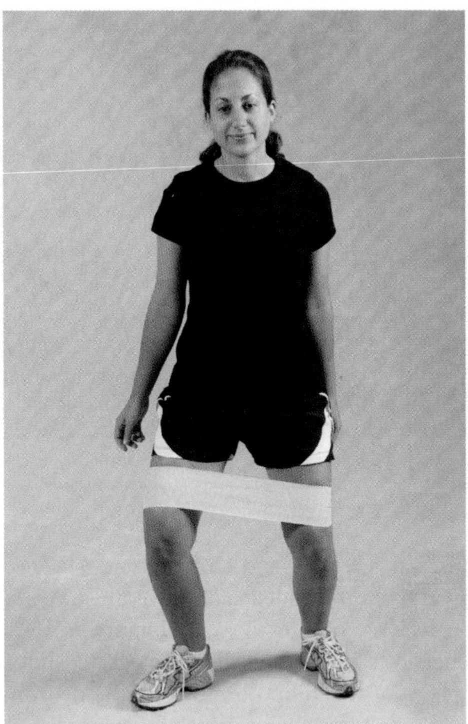

FIGURE 23.35 Band walking in a forward direction against elastic resistance looped around the thighs for closed-chain strengthening of the hip external rotators.

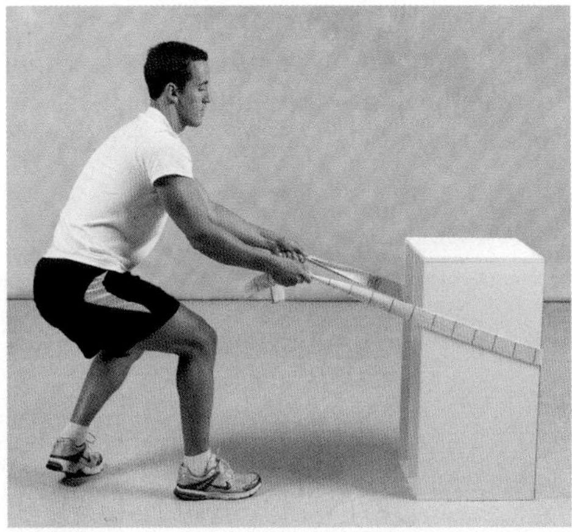

FIGURE 23.36 Pulling increasingly heavy objects across the floor.

Plyometric Training: Stretch-Shortening Drills

Most pieces of equipment used for resistance training, such as free weights, weight machines, or weight-pulley systems, are designed for developing advanced levels of strength by providing resistance during slow, controlled movements. However, functional movements during high-demand occupational or sport-related activities often require reactive bursts of force or power that are not developed concurrently during most strength-building exercises. A program of high-intensity, high-velocity exercises, known as *plyometric training*, not only improves muscle strength, but also develops power output, quick

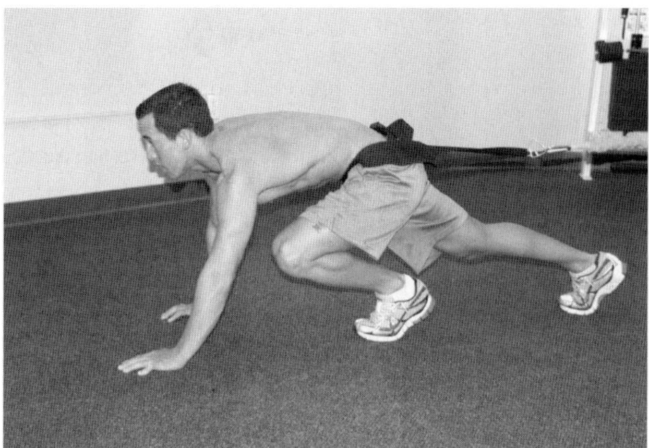

FIGURE 23.37 Resisted running start.

neuromuscular reactions, and coordination.[5,6,13] This form of exercise is also recommended to improve athletic performance and reduce the risk of musculoskeletal injury.[5,6,8,11,19]

Plyometric training typically is integrated into the advanced phase of rehabilitation to train the neuromuscular system to react quickly in preparation for rapid starting and stopping movements or quick changes of direction. This form of training is appropriate only for carefully selected patients who wish to return to high-demand functional activities and sports.

Definitions and Characteristics

Plyometric training,[5,13,16] also called *stretch-shortening drills*[19] or stretch-strengthening drills,[17] employs high-velocity eccentric to concentric muscle loading, reflexive reactions, and functional movement patterns. Plyometric training is defined as a system of high-velocity resistance training characterized by a rapid, resisted, eccentric (lengthening) muscle contraction, followed immediately by a rapid reversal of movement using a resisted concentric (shortening) contraction of the same muscle.[13,18,19] The rapid eccentric loading phase is the stretch cycle, and the concentric phase is the shortening cycle. The period of time between the stretch and shortening cycles is known as the amortization phase. During the amortization phase, the muscle reverses its action, switching from deceleration to acceleration of the load. It is important that the amortization phase be kept very brief by a rapid reversal of movements to capitalize on the increased tension in the muscle.[6]

Body weight or external forms of loading, such as elastic bands or a weighted ball, are possible sources of resistance. An example of a stretch-shortening drill for the lower extremities against the resistance of body weight is represented in Figure 23.38. Additional examples of plyometric training for the upper and lower extremities are noted in Box 23.1.

Neurological and Biomechanical Influences

Plyometric training is thought to utilize the series-elastic properties of connective tissues and the stretch reflex of the neuromuscular unit. The spring-like properties of the series-elastic components of muscle-tendon units create elastic energy during the initial stretch phase as the muscle contracts eccentrically and lengthens under tension. This elastic energy is stored briefly and then returned to the system during the concentric contraction that follows. The storage and release of this elastic energy augments the force production of the concentric muscle contraction.[1,5,13,16]

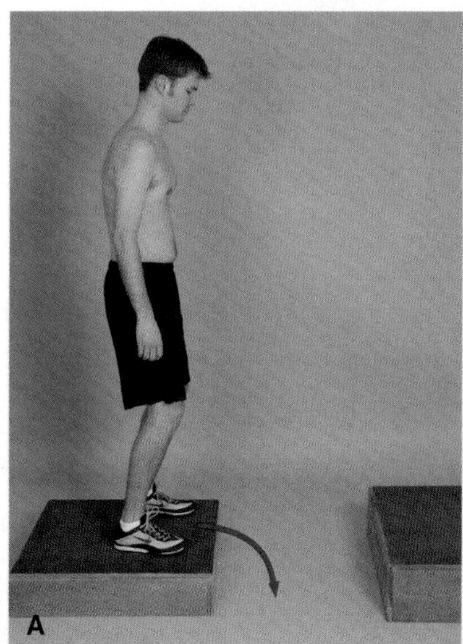

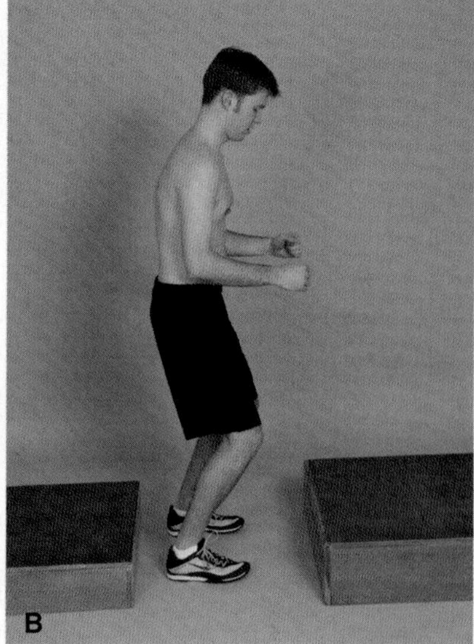

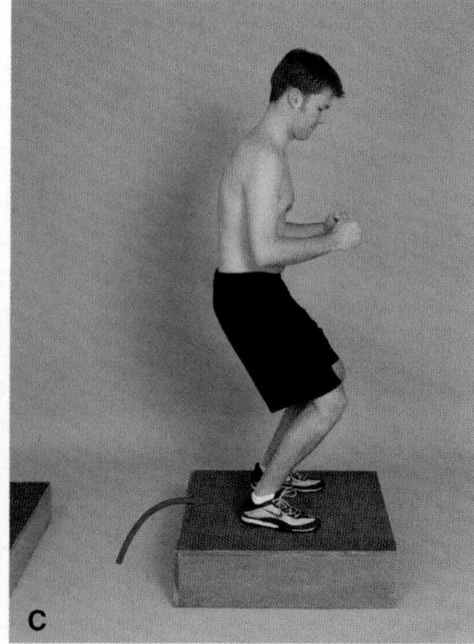

FIGURE 23.38 Plyometric lower extremity sequence against the resistance of body weight: **(A)** patient stands on a low platform; **(B)** jumps off the platform to the floor, controlling the impact with a loaded, lengthening contraction of the hip and knee extensors and plantar flexors—the stretch phase; and **(C)** then without delay jumps forward onto the next platform using a concentric contraction of the same muscle groups—the shortening phase.

BOX 23.1 Plyometric Activities for the Upper and Lower Extremities

Upper Extremities
- Catching and throwing a weighted ball with a partner or against a wall, bilaterally then unilaterally
- Stretch-shortening drills with elastic tubing using anatomical and diagonal motions
- Swinging a weighted object (ball, golf club, bat)
- Dribbling a ball on the floor or against a wall
- Push-offs from a wall or countertop while standing
- Drop push-ups from a low platform to the floor and back onto the platform
- Clap push-ups

Lower Extremities
- Repetitive jumping on the floor: in place; forward/backward; side-to-side; diagonally to four corners; jump with rotation; zigzag jumping; later, jump on foam
- Vertical jumps and reaches and proper landing
- Multiple jumps across a floor (bounding)
- Box jumps: initially off and freeze, then off and back on box, increasing speed and height
- Side-to-side jumps (box to floor to box)
- Jumping over objects on the floor
- Hopping activities: in place, across a surface, and over objects on the floor
- Depth jumps (advanced): jumping from a box, squatting to absorb the shock, and then jumping and reaching as high as possible

The stretch-shortening cycle is thought to stimulate the proprioceptors of muscles, tendons, ligaments, and joints; increase the excitability of the neuromuscular receptors; and improve the reactivity of the neuromuscular system. Therefore, the term *reactive neuromuscular training* also has been used to describe this exercise approach. More specifically, the loaded, eccentric contraction is thought to prepare the contractile elements of the muscle for the concentric contraction by stimulation and activation of the monosynaptic stretch reflex.[5,7,16] Muscle spindles, the receptors that lie in parallel with muscle fibers, sense the length of a muscle and the velocity of stretch applied to a muscle and transmit this information to the CNS via afferent pathways. Efferent signals are returned to the muscle from the CNS, which reflexively facilitates activation of a shortening contraction.[3,12] Based on this mechanism, the more rapid the eccentric muscle contraction, the more likely it is that the stretch reflex will be activated and the concentric contraction enhanced.

It is suggested that the ability to capture the stored elastic energy and activate neural facilitation depends on the velocity and magnitude of the stretch and the transition time between the stretch and shortening phases (the amortization phase).[4,13] A decrease in the duration of the amortization phase theoretically increases the force output during the shortening cycle.[1,5,16,18]

Effects of Plyometric Training

The evidence supporting the effectiveness of plyometric training for developing muscle strength and power is substantial.[13] There is also evidence indicating that plyometric training is associated with an increase in a muscle's ability to resist stretch, which may enhance the muscle's dynamic restraint capabilities.[1] In addition, there is promising evidence to suggest that plyometric training may enhance physical performance[2,11] and decrease the incidence of lower extremity injury.[14,15]

FOCUS ON EVIDENCE

The results of a recent systematic review and meta-analysis of the literature support the conclusions of many previous studies that plyometric training is an effective method to improve muscle strength and power. Greatest gains in strength have been shown to occur when plyometric training was combined with progressive weight training. The review also indicated that plyometric training is beneficial for individuals with moderately low as well as high fitness levels prior to the start of training.[13]

Studies also have investigated the impact of plyometric training on performance of selected upper and lower extremity activities. Carter and colleagues[2] carried out a prospective study of the effect of a plyometric program on throwing velocity in a group of intercollegiate baseball players. Following pre-testing of throwing velocity and isokinetic strength of the shoulder rotators, participants were randomly assigned to either the plyometric training group (n = 13) or the control group (n = 11). Both groups participated in an off-season strength and conditioning program that included exercises with elastic resistance for the shoulder rotators, but only the experimental group performed a program of six plyometric exercises with a weighted ball for the upper extremities twice weekly for 8 weeks. At the conclusion of the program, the throwing velocity of the plyometric group increased significantly compared with the control group, but there continued to be no significant differences in shoulder strength between groups. The investigators concluded that a combined program of strengthening exercises and plyometric training is superior for improving throwing velocity than strengthening exercises alone.

In a prospective study by Hewett,[11] two groups of high school-aged female athletes were monitored during a season of participation in one of three sports (soccer, volleyball, and basketball). One group (n = 366) participated in a 6-week preseason training program, whereas the other group (n = 463) did not. The preseason training focused on jumping and landing techniques. At the end of the sport season, there was a significantly higher incidence (3.6 times higher) of knee injury in the untrained group than in the trained group. The investigators concluded that preseason plyometric training may reduce the risk of knee injury in female athletes, possibly owing to increased dynamic knee stability.

Application and Progression of Plyometric Exercises

Plyometric training is appropriate only in the advanced phases of rehabilitation for carefully selected, active individuals who must achieve a high level of physical performance during specific, high-demand activities.

CONTRAINDICATIONS: Plyometric activities should not be implemented in the presence of inflammation, pain, or significant joint instability.[4,6]

Preparation for plyometrics. Prior to initiating plyometric training, the patient should have an adequate base of muscle strength and endurance, as well as flexibility in the muscles to be exercised.[6] Criteria that should be met to begin plyometric training usually include an 80% to 85% level of strength of the involved muscle groups (compared to the contralateral extremity) and 90% to 95% *pain-free* ROM of the moving joints.[5] Sufficient strength and stability of proximal regions of the body (trunk and limb) for balance and postural control are also necessary. For example, scapulothoracic stability with the absence of scapular winging is necessary before engaging in a progression of advanced push-ups.

Specificity of training. A plyometric exercise should be designed with specific functional activities in mind and should include movement patterns that replicate the desired activity.

Progression and parameters. When planning and implementing a plyometric training program, exercises should be sequenced from easy to difficult and progressed gradually. Box 23.2 summarizes a sequence of sample activities for upper extremity plyometric training.[2,5,16,18,19] Programs should also be individually designed to meet each patient's needs and goals. Note that prior to initiating each session of plyometric activities, a series of warm-up exercises should be performed to reduce the risk of injury to the contracting muscle groups.

The following parameters should be considered when progressing a plyometric program:

- ***Speed.*** Exercises should be performed rapidly but safely. The rate of stretch of the contracting muscle is more important than the amount of stretch.[13,16] Emphasis should be placed on decreasing the amortization phase when transitioning from the eccentric to the concentric contraction. This trains the muscle to generate tension in the shortest time possible. If a jumping activity is performed, for example, progression of the plyometric activity should center on reducing the time on the ground between each jump.
- ***Intensity.*** Resistance should be increased gradually so as not to slow down the activity. Methods for increasing external resistance include using a weight belt or vest, heavier weighted balls, or heavier grade elastic resistance; progressing from double-leg to single-leg activities; and increasing the height of platforms for jumping and hopping activities. Intensity also may be increased by progressing from simple to complex movements.

BOX 23.2 Sample Plyometric Sequence for the Upper Extremities

Warm-Up Activities

- Trunk exercises holding lightweight ball: rotation, side-bending, and chopping motions
- Upper extremity exercises in anatomical and diagonal planes of motion with light-grade elastic tubing
- Prone push-ups

For each of the following plyometric activities, perform a quick reversal between the eccentric and concentric phases.

- Bilateral throwing motions with a weighted ball to and from an exercise partner: bilateral chest press, bilateral overhead throw, and bilateral side throw
- ER/IR against elastic tubing (first with the arm positioned slightly away from the side of the trunk in some shoulder abduction and then in the 90/90 position of shoulder and elbow)
- Diagonal patterns against elastic resistance
- Unilateral catching/throwing motions with a weighted ball: side throws→overhead throws→baseball throws

Additional Exercises

- Trunk exercises holding weighted ball: abdominal curl-ups, back extension, sit-up and bilateral throw, and long sitting throws
- Push-offs from a wall or countertop while in a standing position
- Clap push-ups
- Drop push-ups: prone push-ups from platform to floor and back to platform

- ***Repetitions, frequency, and duration.*** The number of repetitions of an activity should be increased as long as proper exercise technique is maintained by the patient. The number of plyometric exercises in a single session also is increased gradually, working up to perhaps six different activities.[2] The optimal frequency of plyometric sessions is two sessions per week, which allows a 48- to 72-hour recovery period between sessions.[5,13,16] Maximum training benefits typically occur within an 8- to 10-week duration.[13]

Precautions. Because of the emphasis on eccentric loading and rapid reversal to concentric muscle contractions, the potential for tissue damage is increased with plyometric activities. As with other forms of high-intensity resistance training, special precautions must be followed to ensure patient safety.[5,6,16] These precautions are listed in Box 23.3.

Plyometric Exercises: Upper Extremities

Plyometric exercises for the upper extremities can be performed in a variety of nonweight-bearing and weight-bearing positions, using motions and resistance that target a muscle group or using combined movement patterns that involve multiple muscle groups throughout the entire upper extremity.[2,4,6,8,19] Many combined patterns used in plyometric

BOX 23.3 Precautions for Plyometric Training

- If high-stress, shock-absorbing activities are not permissible, do not incorporate plyometric training into a patient's rehabilitation program.
- If a decision is made to include plyometric activities in a rehabilitation program for children or elderly patients, select only beginning-level stretch-shortening drills against light resistance. Do not include high-impact, heavy-load activities—such as drop jumps or weighted jumps—that could place excessive stress on joints.
- Be sure the patient has adequate flexibility and strength before initiating plyometric exercises.
- Wear shoes that provide support for lower extremity plyometrics.
- Always warm-up prior to plyometric training with a series of active, dynamic trunk and extremity exercises.
- During jumping activities, emphasize learning techniques for a safe landing before progressing to rebounding.
- Progress repetitions of an exercise before increasing the level of resistance used or the height or length of jumps.
- For high-level athletes who progress to high-intensity plyometric drills, increase the rest intervals between sets and decrease the frequency of drills as the intensity of the drills increases.
- Allow adequate time for recovery with 48 to 72 hours between sessions of plyometric activities.
- Stop an exercise if a patient can no longer perform the plyometric activity with good form and landing technique because of fatigue.

activities incorporate trunk stability and balance into the movement sequence and often simulate desired functional motor skills that occur during work or recreational activities.

A variety of plyometric exercises for the upper extremities that could be incorporated into the final phase of rehabilitation as a component of advanced functional training are presented in this section.

Bilateral Diagonal Upper Extremity Movements

Patient position and procedure: While standing and holding a weighted ball with both hands, have the patient perform diagonal patterns (D_1 or D_2) with a quick transition from the flexion to extension patterns. Incorporate trunk rotation into the movement patterns. These exercises also develop dynamic stability of the trunk rotators and lower extremities.

Bilateral Chest Press and Throw: Supine

Patient position and procedure: Supine with both hands reaching toward the ceiling. Have the patient catch a weighted ball dropped from above by the therapist (Fig. 23.39), control and lower it to the chest (eccentric phase), and then quickly throw it vertically back to the therapist. As the ball moves toward the chest, shoulder flexors and elbow extensors are loaded eccentrically.

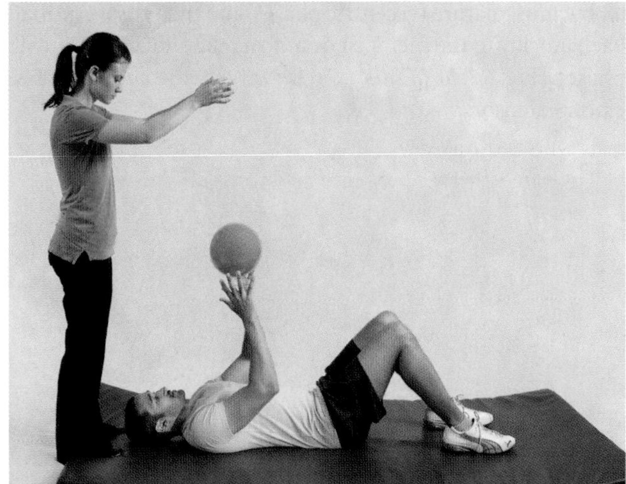

FIGURE 23.39 Bilateral chest press and throw—supine.

Bilateral Chest Press and Throw: Standing

Patient position and procedure: While standing and with feet placed in a stride position for balance, have the patient catch a weighted ball with both hands, bringing it to the chest (eccentric phase) (Fig. 23.40), and then throw it back to the therapist or onto a rebounder (concentric phase).

Bilateral Overhead Catch and Throw

Patient position and procedure: While standing and with feet placed in a stride position for balance, have the patient use both hands to catch a weighted ball thrown over the head, controlling the momentum of the ball with shoulder and

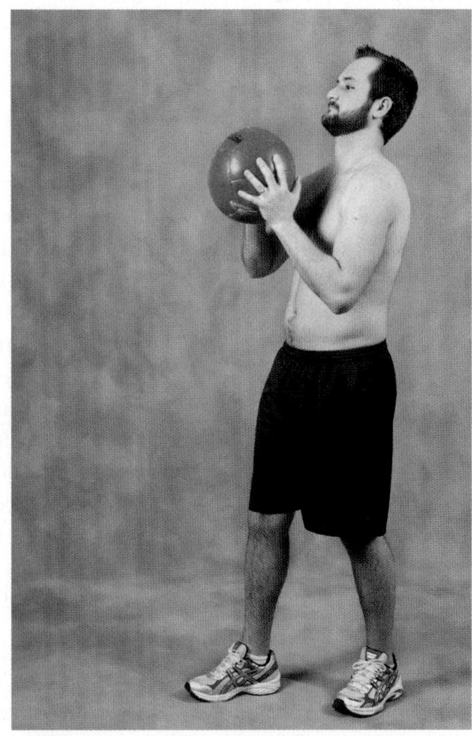

FIGURE 23.40 Bilateral chest press and throw—standing.

elbow musculature (eccentric phase), and then throw the ball back quickly to the therapist or onto a rebounder (concentric phase) (Fig. 23.41). This exercise targets the shoulder and elbow extensors.

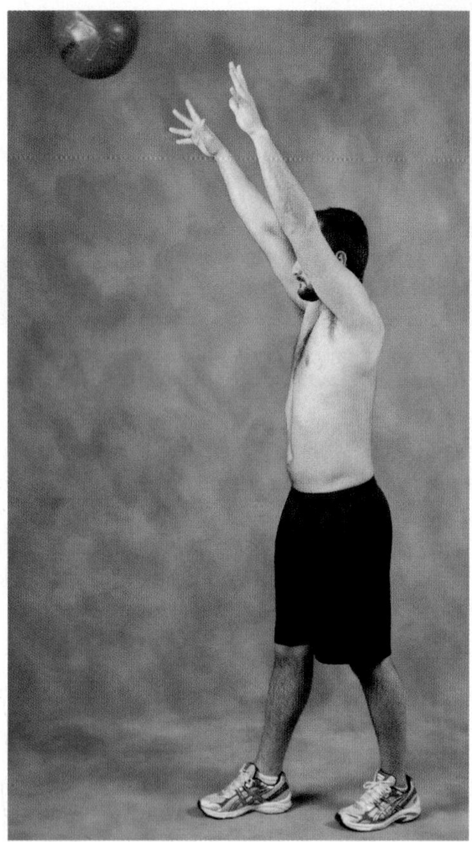

FIGURE 23.41 Bilateral overhead catch and throw.

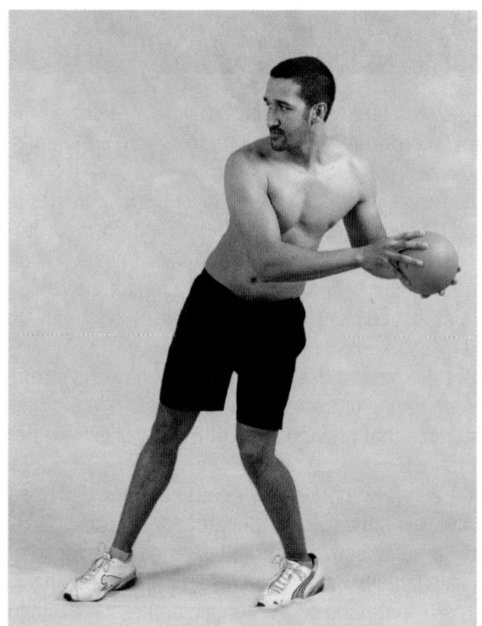

FIGURE 23.42 Bilateral side throw and catch using horizontal abduction and adduction of the shoulders and trunk rotation.

Bilateral Horizontal Side Throw and Catch

VIDEO 23.7

Patient position and procedure: While standing with one side of the body about 10 feet away from a rebounder, have the patient hold a weighted ball in both hands with arms positioned across the chest and then throw the ball toward the rebounder by rotating the trunk and moving the arms across the chest in the transverse plane. The patient then catches the ball as it bounces back from the rebounder, controlling the momentum of the ball by allowing the arms to move back across the chest and rotating the trunk (eccentric phase). The patient then throws the ball back to the rebounder by reversing the movements of the arms and trunk (concentric phase) (Fig. 23.42). This exercise targets the horizontal abductors and adductors of the shoulder and trunk rotators. If a rebounder is not available, the exercise can be performed with a therapist or exercise partner.

Hand-To-Hand Overhead Catch and Throw

Patient position and procedure: While standing or kneeling with both upper extremities elevated to about 120° (aligned just anterior to the frontal plane of the trunk), elbows extended, and forearms supinated (palms facing upward), have the patient throw a bean bag or weighted ball over the head with one upper extremity and catch it with the opposite hand, controlling the weight of the ball with that shoulder (eccentric phase). Then throw the ball back to the other hand by abducting the shoulder (concentric phase). Repeat the sequence as if juggling the ball overhead (Fig. 23.43). This exercises targets the shoulder abductors.

Unilateral Plyometric Shoulder Exercises Using Elastic Resistance

Plyometric activities using elastic resistance can be set up to target individual or multiple muscle groups depending on the patient's position, the line of pull of the elastic, and which joints are moving during the exercise. (Refer to Chapter 6 to review the principles of use of elastic resistance products.) Set-ups for the shoulder rotators are described here.

- *Patient position and procedure:* To target the external rotators of the shoulder, have the patient stand facing a wall or doorframe and grasp one end of a length of elastic tubing or band attached to the wall at eye level. Begin with the shoulder and elbow in the 90/90 position (shoulder abducted 90° and in full external rotation and the elbow flexed 90°) (Fig. 23.44). Have the patient release the externally rotated position, controlling movement into internal rotation (eccentric phase), and then quickly reverse the motion by moving the shoulder into external rotation (concentric phase). The elastic should remain taut throughout the exercise.
- *Patient position and procedure:* To target the internal rotators of the shoulder, have the patient stand facing away from the doorframe or wall to which the elastic resistance is

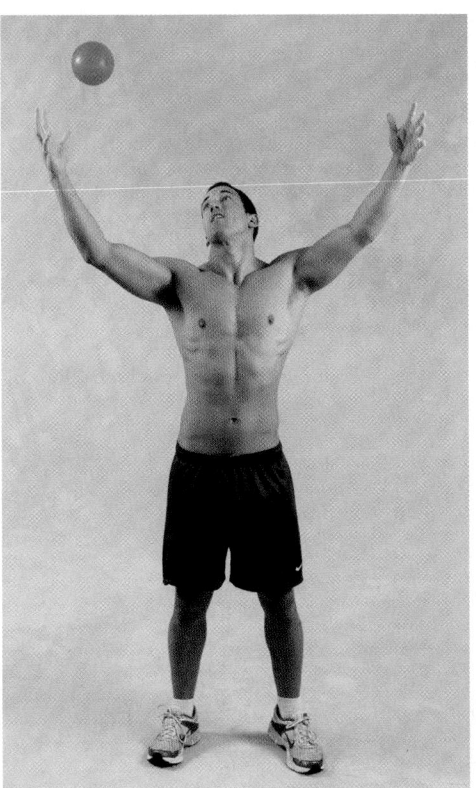

FIGURE 23.43 Hand-to-hand overhead catch and throw.

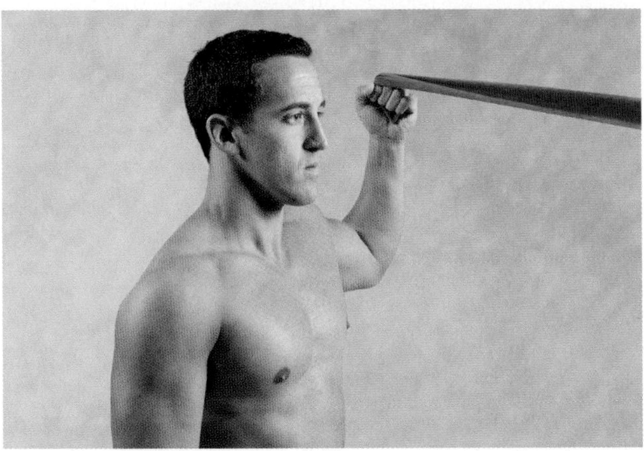

FIGURE 23.44 Unilateral plyometric exercise for the shoulder external rotators using elastic resistance.

attached. Begin with tension on the elastic while the shoulder is in 90° abduction and full internal rotation, and control movement of the shoulder into external rotation (eccentric phase), then quickly return to internal rotation (concentric phase).

Bounce a Weighted Ball: Prone-Lying

Patient position and procedure: While lying prone on a table with the scapula retracted and the upper arm supported on the table, position the shoulder in 90° abduction and external rotation and the elbow in 90° flexion. Have the patient bounce a weighted ball on the floor by internally rotating the shoulder; catch it, moving the shoulder back into external rotation under control (eccentric phase); and quickly bounce it again by internally rotating the shoulder (concentric phase) (Fig. 23.45). This exercise targets the shoulder internal rotators.

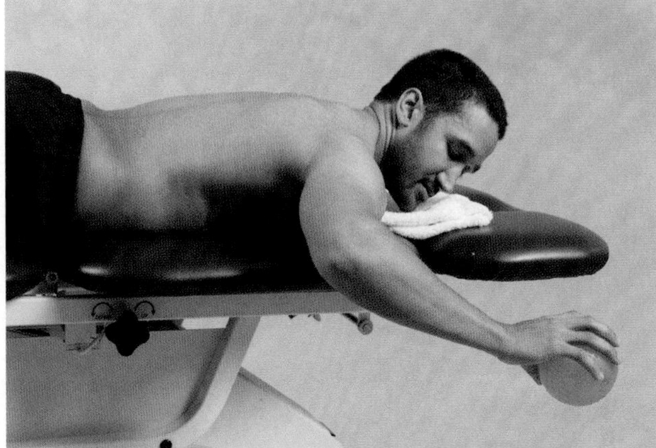

FIGURE 23.45 Unilateral plyometric exercise for the shoulder internal rotators—bounce a weighted ball in the prone-lying position.

Unilateral Side Catch and Throw

These exercises target the internal rotators of shoulder.

- *Patient position and procedure:* While standing in the stride position and with the shoulder positioned in some degree of abduction (upper arm slightly away from the trunk), have the patient face the therapist, catch a weighted ball thrown to one side by the therapist, allowing the shoulder to externally rotate to control the momentum of the ball (eccentric phase) (Fig. 23.46 A), and return the ball using primarily shoulder internal rotation (concentric phase). If a rebounder is available, the patient can perform the exercise independently.
- *Patient position and procedure:* While standing in the stride position and with the shoulder abducted and externally rotated and the elbow flexed, have the patient catch and throw a weighted ball using shoulder rotation (a simulated baseball throw) (Fig. 23.46 B). Incorporate trunk rotation in the backward and forward motion of the shoulder. **VIDEO 23.7**

Unilateral Reverse Catch and Throw

This exercise primarily targets the external rotators of the shoulder in the end-range.

Patient position and procedure: Have the patient assume a half-kneeling position, facing away from the therapist, with the involved shoulder abducted 90° and externally rotated, the elbow flexed to 90°, and the forearm pronated (palm facing therapist). Instruct the patient to look at the hand and catch a soft, lightweight object (ball or bean bag) thrown toward the hand by the therapist; control the momentum of the object by allowing the shoulder to move into internal rotation;

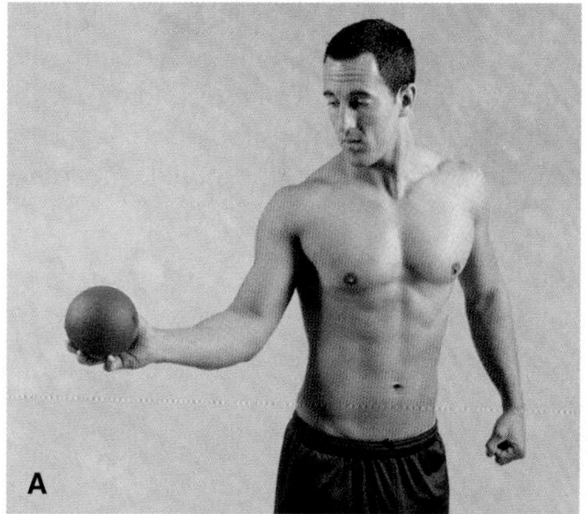

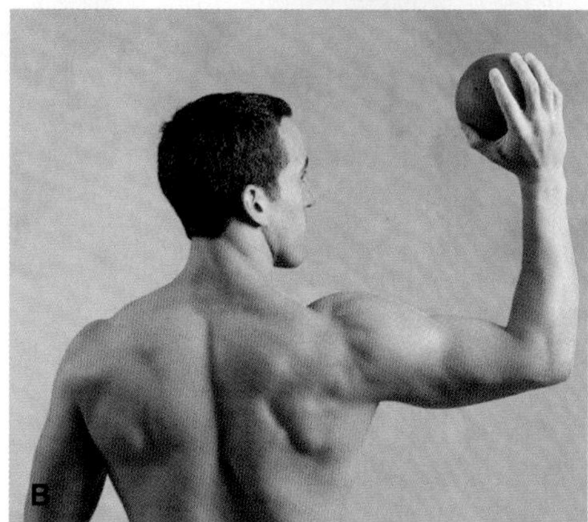

FIGURE 23.46 Unilateral plyometric exercise for the shoulder internal rotators: **(A)** side catch and throw; and **(B)** a simulated baseball throw with the shoulder abducted to 90° and elbow flexed.

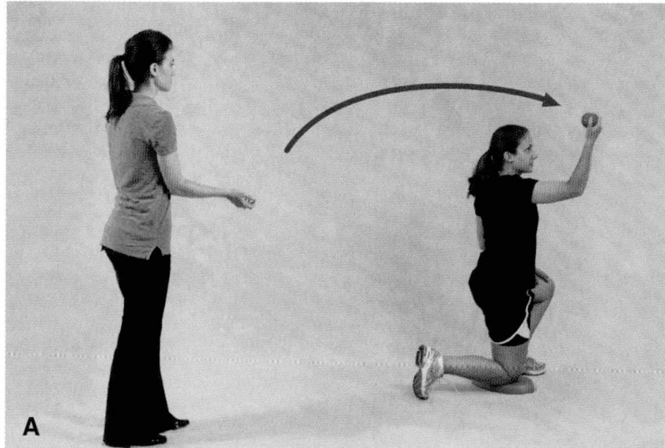

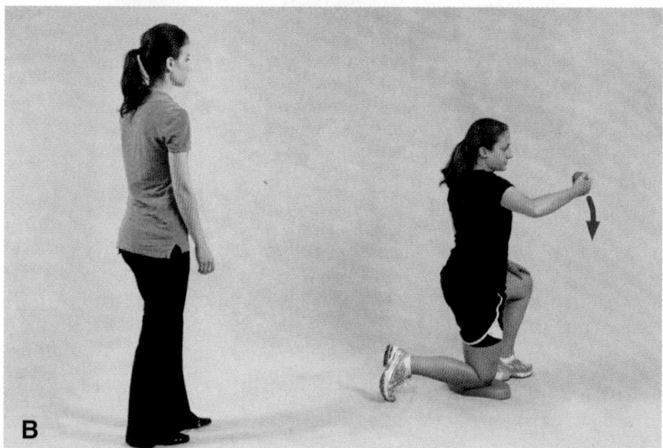

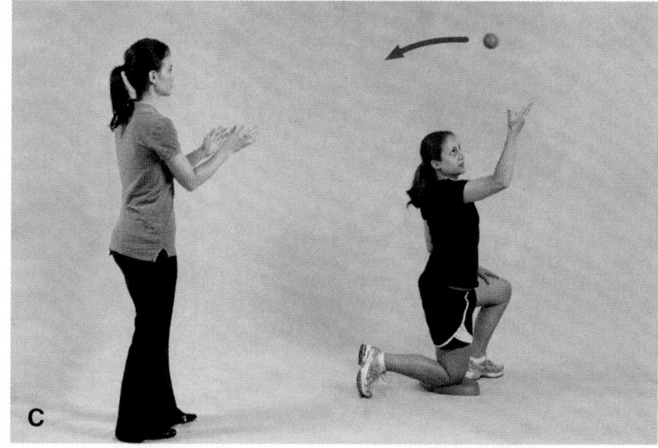

FIGURE 23.47 Unilateral plyometric exercise for the shoulder external rotators—reverse catch and throw: The patient **(A)** catches a soft, lightweight object with the shoulder abducted and externally rotated and the elbow flexed; **(B)** allows the shoulder to internally rotate with control; and **(C)** externally rotates the shoulder to throw the object back to the therapist.

and then quickly throw the object back to the therapist by externally rotating the shoulder (Fig. 23.47 A, B, and C).

Throw and Catch With Elbow Action

- *Patient position and procedure:* While in a standing position and with the arm positioned along the side of the trunk, have the patient throw a weighted ball into the air with one hand, using primarily elbow flexion; catch it, allowing the elbow to extend with control (eccentric phase); and then quickly throw it into the air again (concentric phase) (Fig. 23.48). This exercise targets the elbow flexors.
- *Patient position and procedure:* While standing and with one or both arms positioned overhead, have the patient catch a weighted ball and return it to the therapist or to a rebounder using primarily elbow action. This exercise targets the elbow extensors and can be done bilaterally or unilaterally.

Unilateral Throw and Catch With Wrist Action

Patient position and procedure: While seated, have the patient stabilize the elbow on the thigh in about 90° flexion, and with the forearm supinated, toss a weighted ball or bean bag into the air using primarily wrist flexion; catch it, allowing the wrist to extend under control (eccentric phases); and then quickly toss it into the air again (concentric phase) (Fig. 23.49). This exercise targets the wrist flexors.

Simulated Sport Activities

- Dribble a weighted ball or basketball against a wall (Fig. 23.50) or on the floor using either elbow or wrist actions. This activity targets either the elbow extensors or wrist flexors.
- Bounce a tennis ball or racquetball into the air or onto the floor (forearm supinated or pronated, respectively) with a short-handled racquet, progressing to a long-handled racquet. These activities emphasize the wrist flexors. In

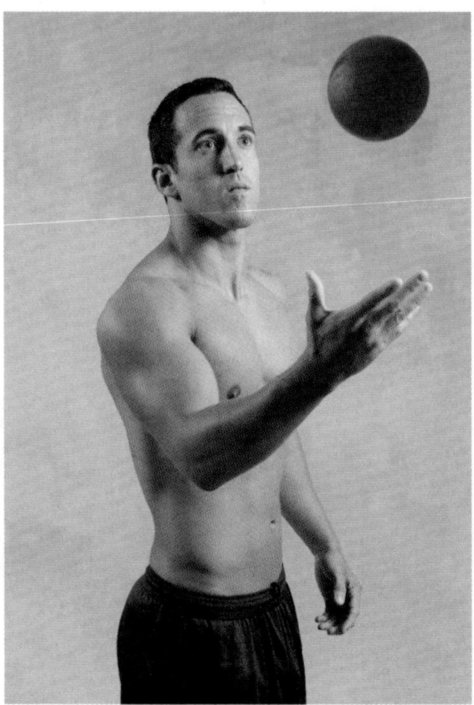

FIGURE 23.48 Unilateral plyometric exercise targeting the elbow flexors.

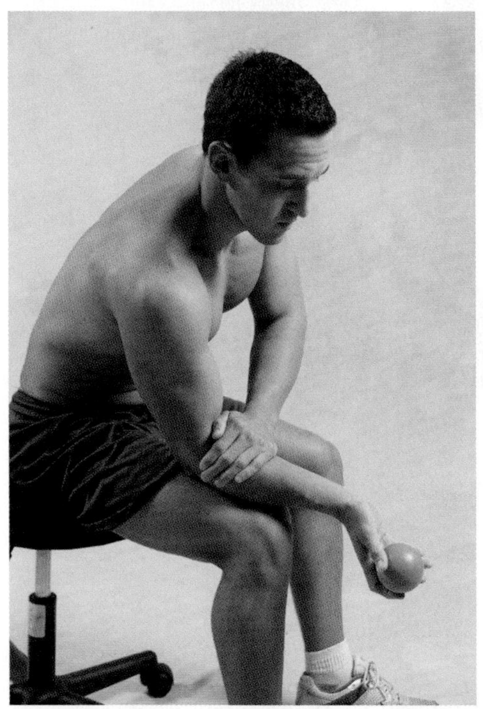

FIGURE 23.49 Unilateral plyometric exercise targeting the wrist flexors.

contrast, bouncing a ball into the air with the forearm pronated emphasizes the wrist extensors (Fig. 23.51).

- Swing a weighted golf club (Fig. 23.52) or baseball bat. The backward motion followed by a rapid reversal forward provides the plyometric stimulus.

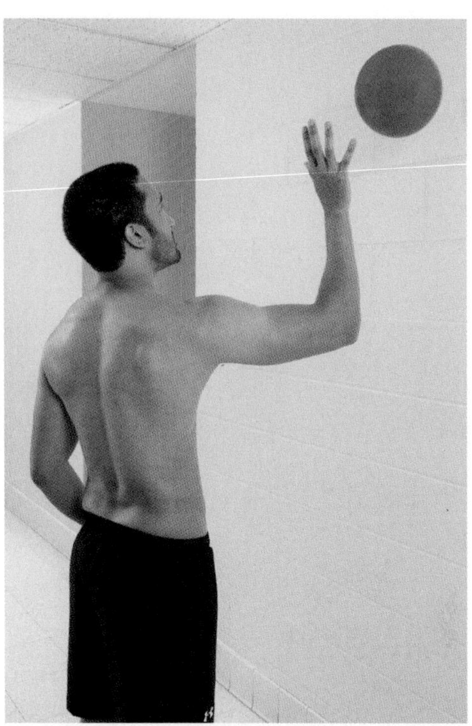

FIGURE 23.50 Dribble a ball against the wall to target the wrist flexors.

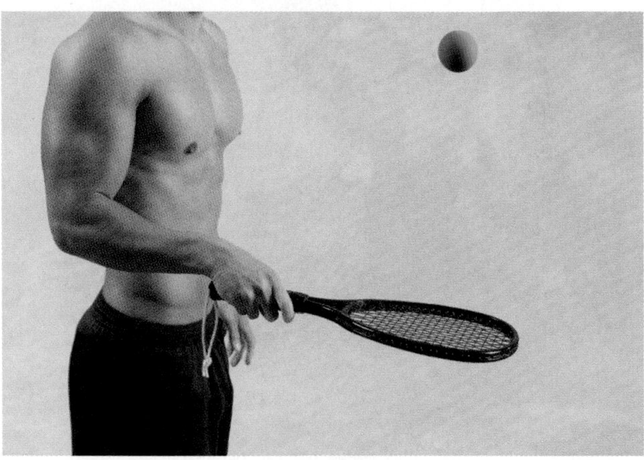

FIGURE 23.51 Using a short-handled racquet, bounce a ball into the air with the forearm pronated to target the wrist extensors.

Upper Extremity Weight-Bearing Movements on a Slide Board

Use of a slide board, such as a ProFitterTM, provides an unstable, moving surface for performing shoulder exercises that require quick changes of direction combined with weight bearing through the upper extremities.

- *Patient position and procedure:* Have the patient place both hands on a spring-loaded slide board while kneeling along one side of the equipment. Shift the arms side-to-side from the shoulders (Fig. 23.53), gradually increasing the speed of the shoulder movements and changes of direction.

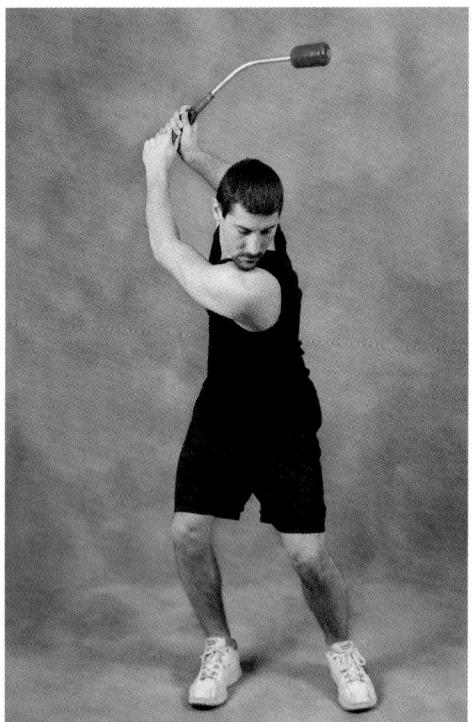

FIGURE 23.52 Practice a golf swing using a weighted club.

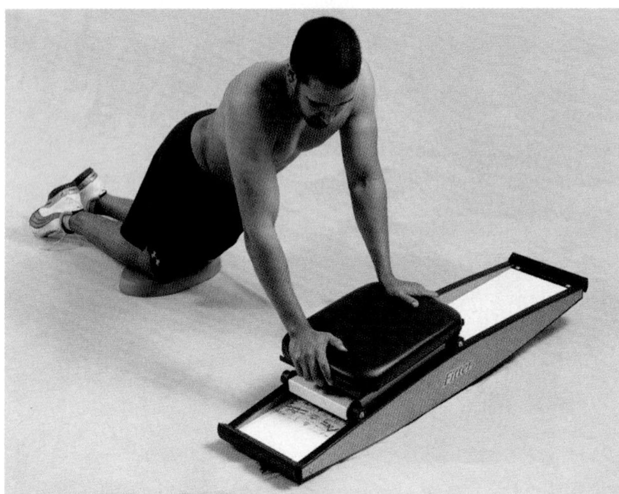

FIGURE 23.53 Bilateral plyometric exercise while bearing weight through the upper extremities—side-to-side movements with quick changes of direction on a ProFitter®.

- *Patient position and procedure:* Have the patient kneel at one end of the slide board and move the arms forward and backward from the shoulders.
- *Progression:* Perform the same movements while kneeling and bearing weight on one hand.

Push-Offs From a Wall

- *Patient position and procedure:* While the patient is standing several feet away from a wall (or countertop), gently push the patient directly forward toward the wall. Instruct the patient to catch himself/herself with equal weight on both hands, allowing the elbows to flex under control (eccentric phase) as the trunk moves toward the wall (Fig. 23.54 A). Then have the patient quickly push away from the wall with both hands (concentric phase) (Fig. 23.54 B), catch the patient as he/she falls backward, and then push the patient forward again to repeat the sequence.

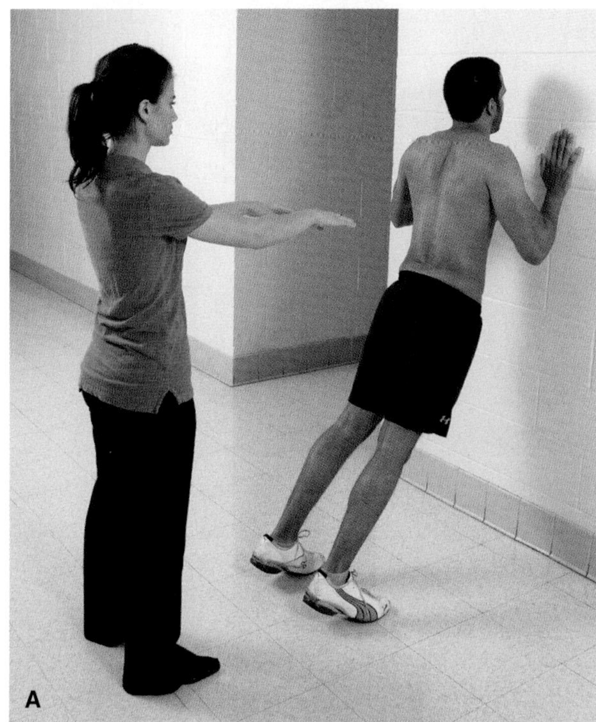

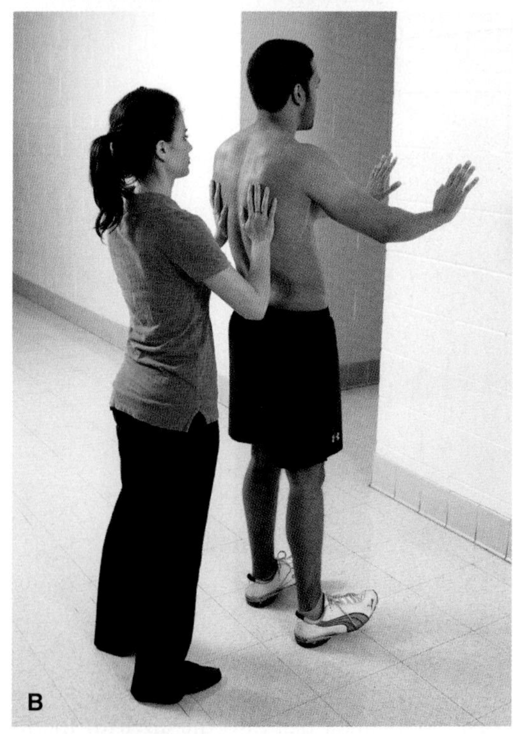

FIGURE 23.54 Repeated push-offs from a wall: **(A)** falling directly forward toward the wall and catching self with both hands; and **(B)** pushing away from the wall to the upright position.

- *Alternative activity:* Have the patient perform the sequence independently by falling forward to the wall and quickly pushing away.
- *Progression:* Have the patient use one hand to catch self and push away from the wall.

Side-to-Side Push-Offs From a Waist-Level Surface VIDEO 23.8

Patient position and procedure: While standing and maintaining both feet approximately 3 feet away from a waist-height, stable surface (countertop, heavy table), have the patient fall forward and slightly to the right of midline and catch self with hands on the edge of the countertop or table; push off and shift arms and trunk to the left; catch self with both hands; and push off again, moving arms and trunk back to the right, past midline (Fig. 23.55). This exercise alternately places greater weight on the right and then the left upper extremity.

Variations of Prone Push-Ups VIDEO 23.8

- *Clap push-ups*: While on the floor, have the patient perform a forceful prone push-up from knees or feet; clap hands together; catch self with both hands, allowing elbows to flex (eccentric phase); and quickly perform another push-up (concentric phase).
- *Drop push-ups*: Have the patient perform a prone push-up from knees or feet with hands on platforms positioned shoulder width apart. Drop both hands and the chest to the floor, controlling the descent of the trunk (eccentric phase); quickly perform another push-up (concentric phase); and return both hands to the platforms (Fig. 23.56 A, B, and C).

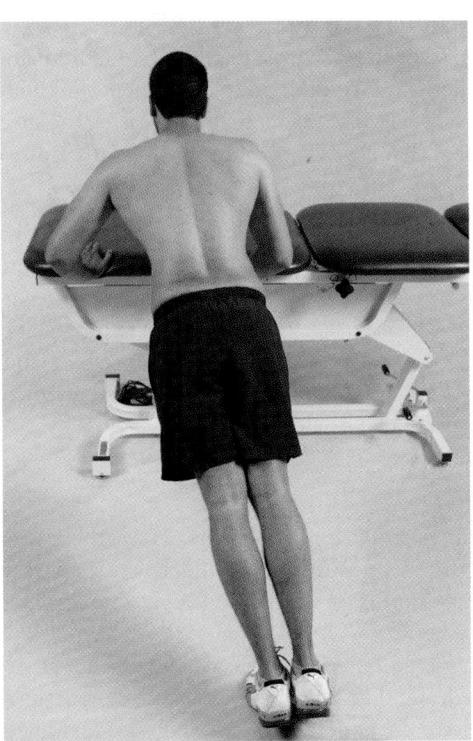

FIGURE 23.55 Alternating side-to-side push-offs to and from a stable, waist-high surface.

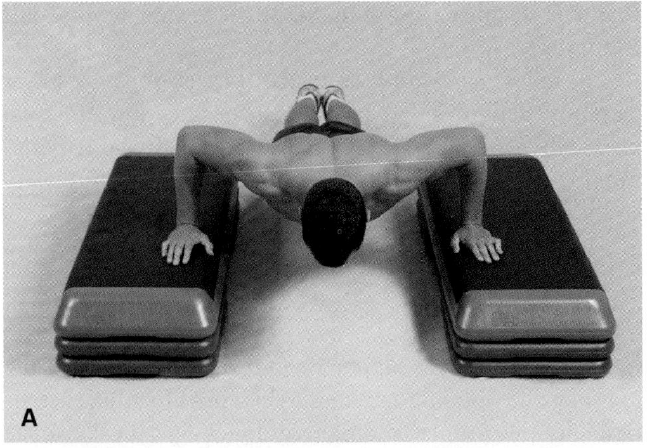

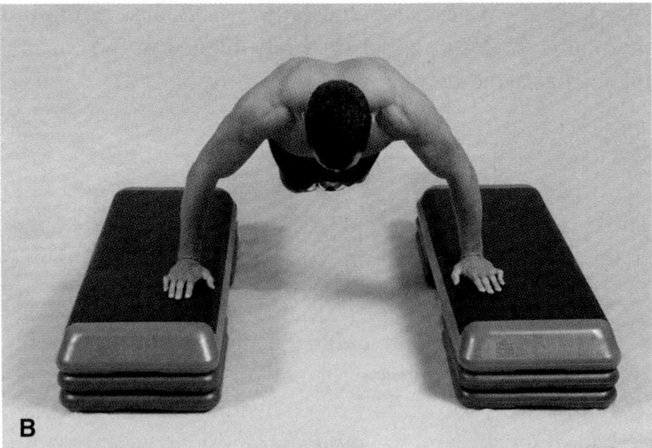

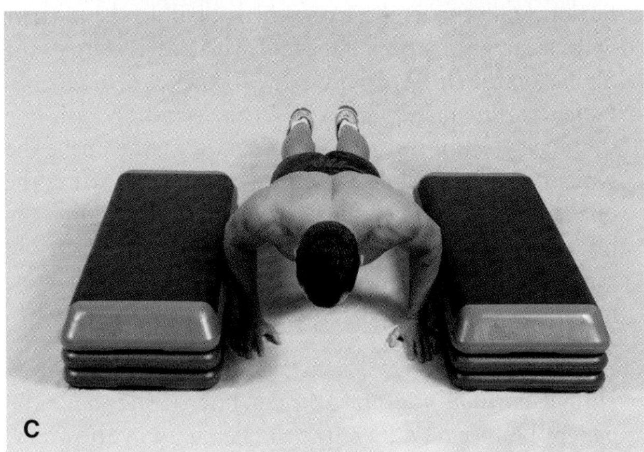

FIGURE 23.56 Drop push-ups in the prone position: **(A)** Starting position; **(B)** prone push-up; and **(C)** drop hands to floor, allowing elbows to flex. Push up from the floor and quickly return hands to platforms as in *(A)*.

Plyometric Exercises: Lower Extremities

Most plyometric exercises for the lower extremities are performed while standing and require eccentric and concentric control of the hip and knee extensors and ankle plantarflexors against body weight.[6] These exercises require postural stability and balance because of the quick changes of direction involved. Plyometric activities can be progressed by adding an external load (a weighted belt, vest, or backpack) to augment body weight or by first performing the exercises in bilateral stance (jumping) and then in unilateral stance (hopping).

The following plyometric exercises are examples of lower extremity activities that can be incorporated into the final phase of rehabilitation in preparation for functional activities ranging from community ambulation to high-intensity sports.

CLINICAL TIP

Have the patient wear supportive footwear when performing jumping and hopping activities. When teaching these activities, reinforce proper landing techniques. Specifically, make sure the patient flexes the knee(s) for shock absorption but maintains the lower leg(s) vertically aligned in the coronal plane, thus avoiding valgus collapse at the knee(s).

Kicking a Ball

These exercises involve rapid eccentric and concentric open-chain contractions of hip musculature. Be sure the patient is wearing shoes during kicking activities.

- *Patient position and procedure:* While standing and facing an exercise partner, have the patient swing one lower extremity backward into hip extension (eccentric phase), then quickly swing the same extremity forward into hip flexion (concentric phase) and kick a ball to the partner with the anterior aspect of the foot. This activity targets the hip flexors and knee extensors.
- *Patient position and procedure:* While standing with one shoulder positioned toward an exercise partner, have the patient stand on the leg closer to the partner, swing the opposite hip into abduction, and then quickly adduct the hip to kick the ball back to the partner using the medial aspect of the foot (as in a soccer kick). This exercise targets the hip adductors.

Sit-to-Stand From a Ball

- *Patient position and procedure:* While sitting, have the patient bounce on a therapy ball (stabilized by the therapist), come to a partial standing position, and then sit back down on the ball and quickly come to a partial standing position again (Fig. 23.57). Progress the exercise by eventually coming to a full standing position. This activity requires contraction of the hip and knee extensors against the resistance of body weight. To be effective, rapid reversals must occur between the lowering (eccentric) and standing-up (concentric) phases.

Bilateral Heel Raises on a Mini-Trampoline

Patient position and procedure: In bilateral stance, have the patient bounce on a mini-trampoline by performing repeated heel raising and lowering. This activity targets the gastrocnemius-soleus muscle groups.

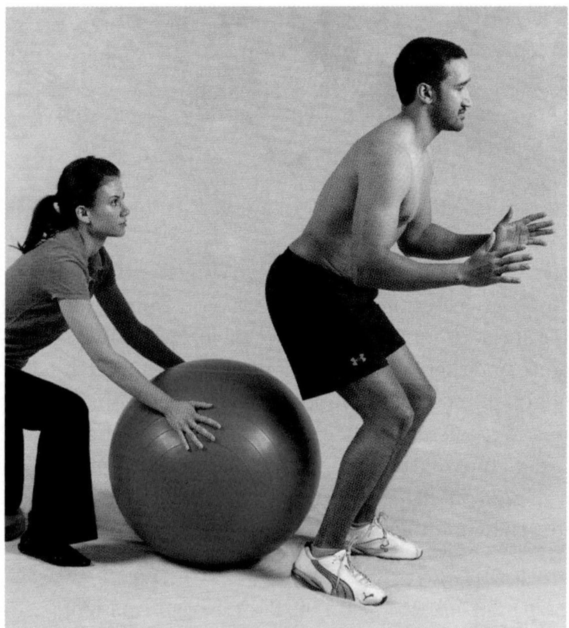

FIGURE 23.57 Moving from sit-to-stand by bouncing on a ball.

Side-to-Side Shuffle

Patient position and procedure: Have the patient take several quick side steps to the right and then back to the left, and repeat. This exercise requires rapid contractions of the hip abductors and adductors against body weight during each change of direction.

Side-to-Side Movements on a Slide Board

Patient position and procedure: While standing on a slide board, such as a Pro-Fitter®, have the patient shift body weight side-to-side (Fig. 23.58), gradually increasing the speed of the directional changes as skill and coordination improve.

Squat Jumps VIDEO 23.9

Patient position and procedure: Have the patient move quickly from a standing position into a squat position (eccentric phase) (Fig. 23.59 A), quickly transition to a vertical jump (concentric phase) (Fig. 23.59 B), return to the squat position, and then perform another vertical jump. When landing and moving into the squat position, be sure the patient keeps the lower legs aligned as close to vertical as possible to prevent valgus collapse.

Bounding

- *Patient position and procedure:* Have the patient start with the feet positioned shoulder width apart and take multiple jumps forward in a straight line across the floor (Fig. 23.60).
- *Progressions:* Increase the speed at which the activity is performed, and then increase the distance of each jump. When able, have the patient perform single-leg forward hopping across the floor.

Four-Quadrant Jumps or Hops VIDEO 23.9

- *Patient position and procedure:* Using two lines on the floor intersecting at right angles as a guide, have the patient jump forward, backward, side-to-side, and diagonally from one quadrant to another, using quick directional changes (Fig. 23.61).

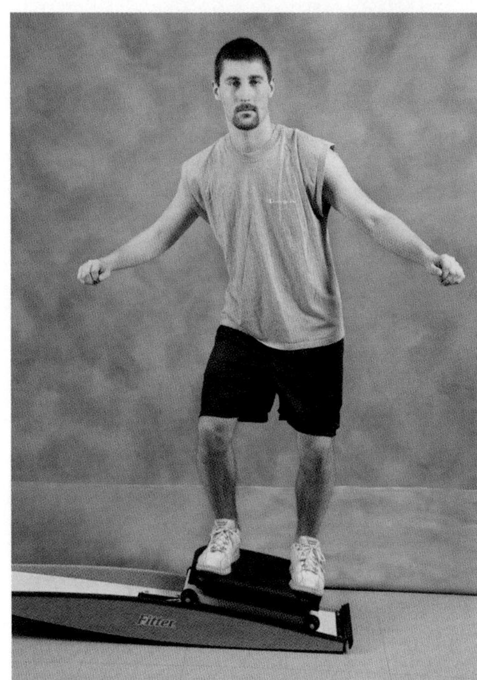

FIGURE 23.58 Side-to-side movements on a Pro-Fitter®.

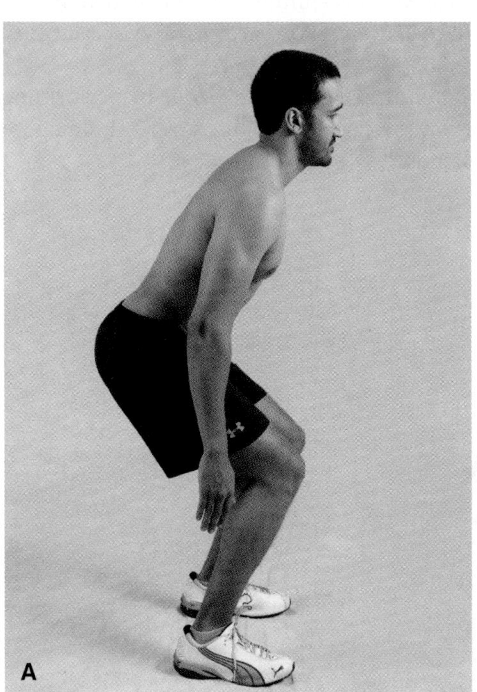

FIGURE 23.59 Squat jumps: **(A)** from a squat position, perform a

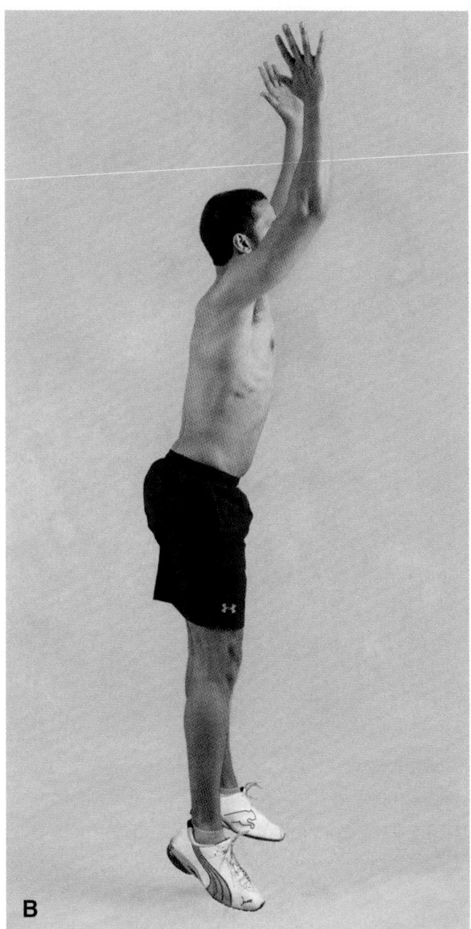

FIGURE 23.59 **(B)** vertical jump.

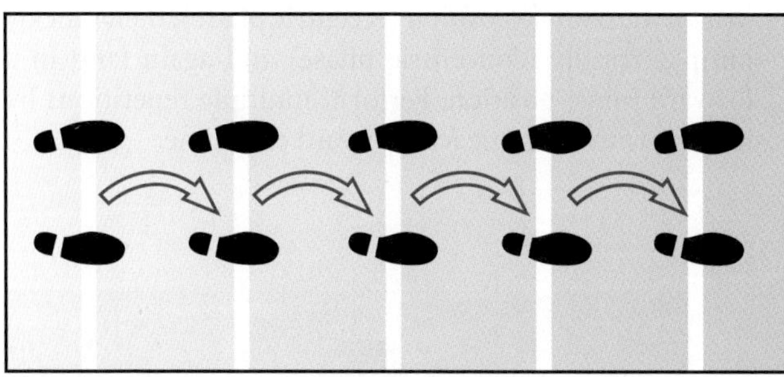

FIGURE 23.60 Bounding: a series of forward jumps across a floor.

Tuck Jumps

- *Patient position and procedure:* Have the patient begin in standing position, quickly lower the body into a squat position (eccentric phase), perform a tuck jump as high as possible, bringing the knees toward the chest (Fig. 23.62), and then land in proper alignment and return to the squat position to initiate the next tuck jump.
- *Progression:* Perform a series of side-to-side tuck jumps over a barrier.

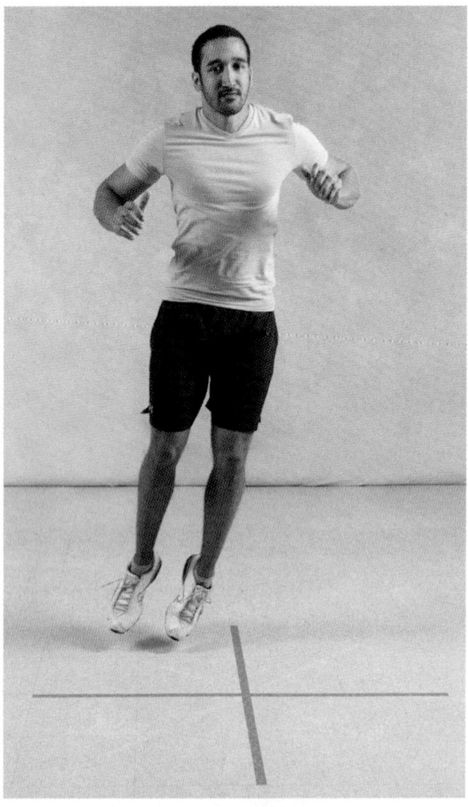

FIGURE 23.61 Four-quadrant jumping or hopping.

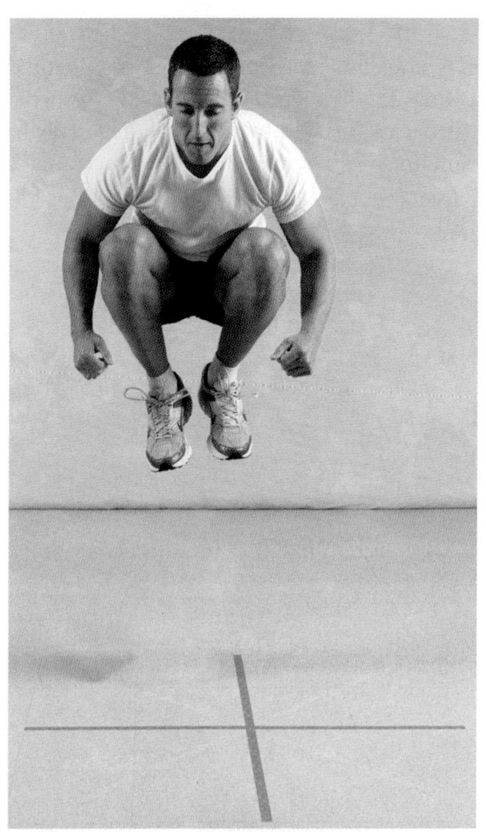

FIGURE 23.62 Tuck jump.

Lunge Jumps VIDEO 23.9

- *Patient position and procedure:* Have the patient begin in a symmetrical standing position, jump vertically, and land in a forward lunge position (eccentric phase); then quickly jump vertically (concentric phase) and again land in a forward lunge position. Perform multiple repetitions by landing with the same foot forward each time.
- *Alternative activity—Scissor-lunge jumps:* Perform a sequence of lunge-jumps, alternately bringing the right and then left foot forward, as in a scissoring motion (Fig. 23.63 A, B, and C).
- *Progression:* Increase the challenge by performing lunge-jumps while wearing a weighted vest or holding weights in both hands.

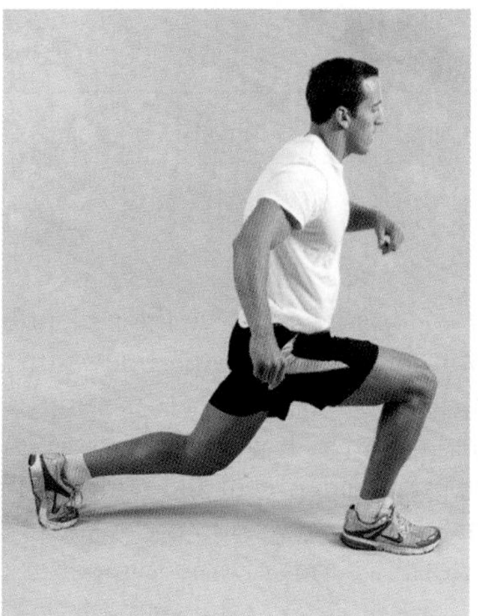

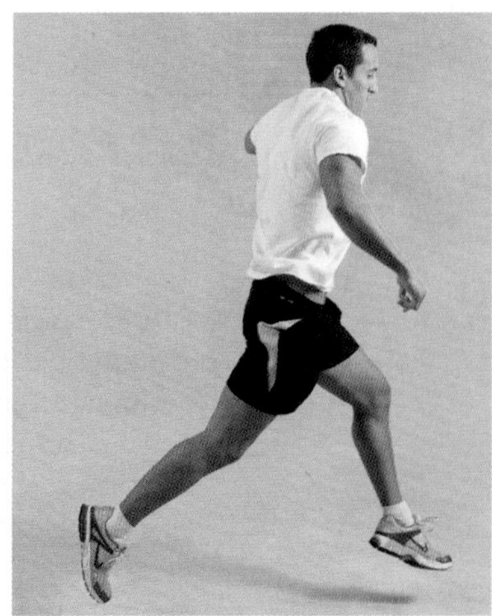

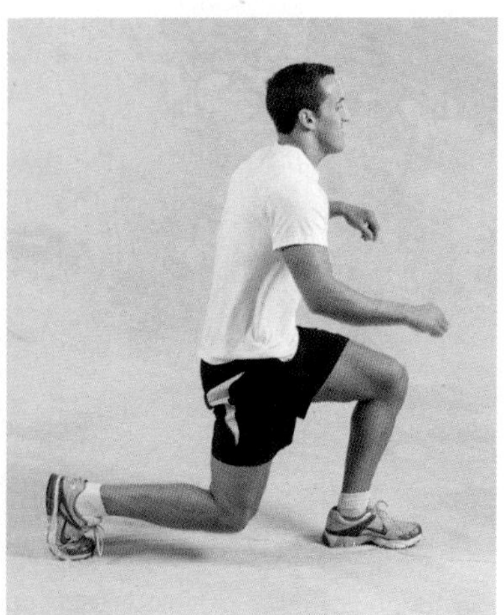

FIGURE 23.63 (A), (B), and **(C)** Lunge-jumps: alternately landing with right, then left lower extremity forward.

Zigzag Forward Jumping or Hopping

Patient position and procedure: Have the patient jump or hop across the floor in a zigzag pattern marked on the floor (Fig. 23.64). Progress by increasing the speed of jumping or hopping and the distance between jumps or hops.

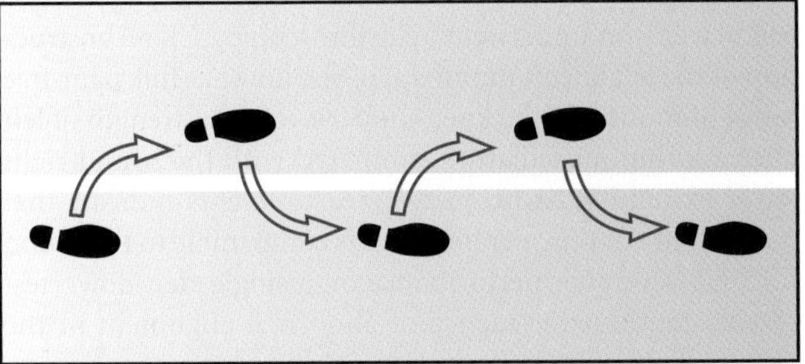

FIGURE 23.64 Zigzag forward hopping.

Hopping Over Objects VIDEO 23.9

Patient position and procedure: Have the patient hop over objects of various sizes placed on the floor like an obstacle course (Fig. 23.65).

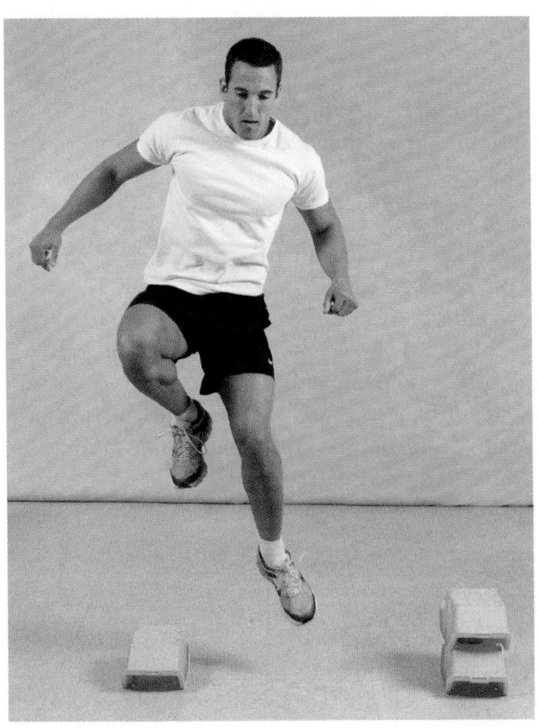

FIGURE 23.65 Lateral hopping over objects of varying sizes set up in an obstacle course on the floor.

Single Platform Jumping or Hopping

Patient position and procedure: Have the patient jump and progress to hopping onto and off of a single, low platform in forward (Fig. 23.66), backward, and lateral directions, being certain to use proper landing technique. To progress, first increase the speed and repetitions of the jumping or hopping activity, then increase the height of the platform.

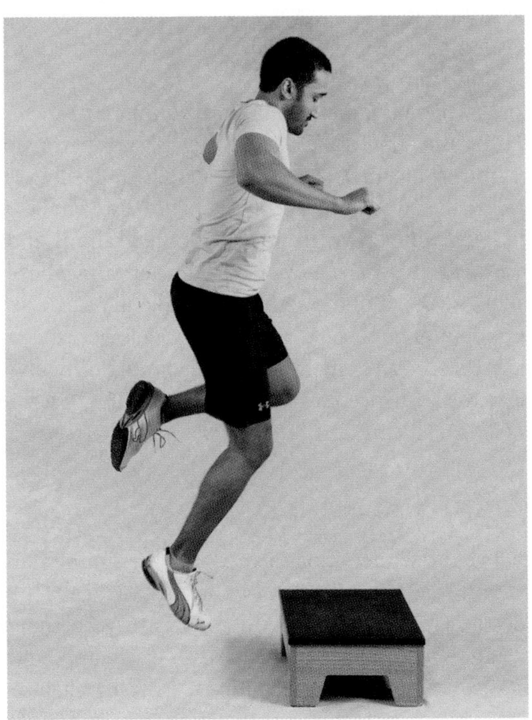

FIGURE 23.66 Hopping onto and off of a single platform using proper landing technique.

Multiple Platform Jumping or Hopping

Patient position and procedure: Have the patient jump (or hop) in a forward direction off of a platform to the floor and then jump forward again onto another platform (see Fig. 23.38 A, B, and C). Progress by performing the sequence more rapidly or by increasing the height of the platforms.

Independent Learning Activities

Critical Thinking Questions

1. Review the principles of balance training described in Chapter 8. Describe how each of the advanced balance activities presented in this chapter (Chapter 23) can be used to enhance the static, dynamic, anticipatory, or reactive aspects of balance.
2. Develop a sequence of balance activities in the standing position from least to most difficult, using progressively more challenging movements and equipment.
3. Identify the benefits, as well as the risks, of performing a program of plyometric exercises (stretch-shortening drills).
4. Analyze the plyometric training activities listed in Box 23.1, and determine in which muscle groups training-induced gains in strength and power would occur and what functional tasks each of the activities could enhance.
5. Develop a plyometric sequence for the lower extremities and trunk progressing from simple to more difficult (similar to the sequence for the upper extremities described in Box 23.3).

Laboratory Activities

1. Practice the sequence of balance activities in the standing position that you developed to answer Critical Thinking Question #2. Take turns with a laboratory partner role-playing the therapist and the patient. If you are the therapist, use proper safety precautions, critically analyze how your patient performs each balance task, and give your patient feedback to facilitate learning correct alignment and technique.
2. Perform and analyze a variety of plyometric exercises for the upper or lower extremities, and identify which muscle groups are loaded eccentrically or concentrically during the two phases of each activity.
   - Catch and throw a weighted ball with both hands (or one hand) while in the supine, prone, and upright positions.
   - While kneeling and with hands placed on a slide board and elbows extended, move the arms forward and backward or side-to-side.
   - While standing a few feet from a wall, fall forward, catching yourself with both hands, and then push off the wall to return to a standing position.
   - In the prone position, perform bilateral drop push-ups to and from two low platforms.
   - While standing on a mini-trampoline, bounce your heels off and on the surface using only ankle motion.
   - Jump off of and back onto a low platform—forward, backward, and side-to-side.

Case Studies

Case Study #1

You have been following a 21-year-old female college volleyball player who underwent an arthroscopic ACL reconstruction of the left knee 4 months ago. She now has full, pain-free range of motion of the knee and 80% to 85% strength of left knee and hip musculature compared with the sound right lower extremity. Arthrometer measurements indicate that A-P stability of the operated knee is comparable to the sound side. However, her performance on a single step-down test reveals continued evidence of abnormal alignment of the operated lower extremity (excessive hip adduction, and internal rotation, knee valgus, and foot pronation). She has been given approval by her surgeon to return to intercollegiate play by 6 months postoperatively following completion of an advanced training program individualized to her needs and goals.

- Develop an 8-week training program of advanced strengthening, balance, and plyometric drills for this patient. Identify specific exercises that would be included in each training session and how the exercises will be progressed over the 8-week period.
- In addition to exercises to enhance stability, control, and strength of the lower extremity, identify exercises that should be included to improve her upper extremity function.

Case Study #2

You have been working with a 35-year-old "weekend warrior" who was diagnosed with chronic tennis elbow. His symptoms are now under control, and he wants to return to competitive play at the local tennis club. Develop a training program of advanced strengthening and plyometric drills for this individual. Identify each exercise and its progression in terms of repetitions, resistance, control, and precautions. Include both upper and lower extremity drills and progressions that include total body-coordinated effort.

Additional Case Studies

For additional study, review the following case studies from previous chapters and modify your exercise interventions to include advanced drills based on the information you studied in this chapter.

1. Case study #4 in Chapter 17
2. Case studies #2 and #3 in Chapter 20
3. Case studies #2, #3, and #4 Chapter 22

REFERENCES

1. Benn, C, et al: The effects of serial stretch loading on stretch work and stretch-shorten cycle performance in the knee musculature. *J Orthop Sports Phys Ther* 27(6):412–422, 1998.
2. Carter, AB, et al: Effects of high volume upper extremity plyometric training on throwing velocity and functional strength ratios of the shoulder rotators in collegiate baseball players. *J Strength Cond Res* 21(1): 208–215, 2007.
3. Chleboun, G: Muscle structure and function. In Levangie, PK, and Norkin, CC (eds): *Joint Structure and Function: A Comprehensive Analysis,* ed. 5. Philadelphia: F.A. Davis, 2011, pp 109–137.
4. Cools, AMJ, et al: Rehabilitation of scapular dyskinesis: from the office worker to the elite overhead athlete. *Br J Sports Med* 48(8):482–489, 2013.
5. Chu, DA, and Cordier, DJ: Plyometrics in rehabilitation. In Ellenbecker, TS (ed): *Knee Ligament Rehabilitation.* New York: Churchill Livingstone, 2000, p 321.
6. Davies, G, Riemann, BL, and Manske, R: Current concepts of plyometric exercise. *International J Sports Phys Ther* 10(6):760–786, 2015.
7. Drury, DG: The role of eccentric exercise in strengthening muscle. *Orthop Phys Ther Clin North Am* 9:515, 2000.
8. Ellenbecker, TS, Pieczynski, TE, and Davies, GJ: Rehabilitation of the elbow following sports injury. *Clin Sports Med* 29:33–60, 2010.
9. Farrokhi, S, et al: Trunk position influences the kinematics, kinetics, and muscle activity of the lead lower extremity during the forward lunge exercise. *J Orthop Sports Phys Ther* 38(7):403–409, 2008.
10. Filipa, A, et al: Neuromuscular training improves performance on the star excursion balance test in young female athletes. *J Orthop Sports Phys Ther* 40(9):551–558, 2010.
11. Hewett, TE: The effect of neuromuscular training on the incidence of knee injury in female athletes: a prospective study. *Am J Sports Med* 27(6):699–706, 1999.
12. McArdle, WD, Katch, FL, and Katch, VL: *Exercise Physiology: Nutrition, Energy, and Human Performance,* ed. 7. Philadelphia: Wolters Kluwer/ Lippincott Williams & Wilkins, 2009.
13. Săez-Săez de Villarreal, E, Requena, B, and Newton, RU: Does plyometric training improve strength performance? A meta-analysis. *J Sci Med Sport* 13:513–522, 2010.
14. Silvers, HJ, and Mandelbaum, BR: Preseason conditioning to prevent soccer injuries in young women. *Clin J Sports Med* 11(3):206, 2001.
15. Stanton, P, and Purdam, C: Hamstring injuries in sprinting: the role of eccentric exercise. *J Orthop Sports Phys Ther* 10(9):343–349, 1989.
16. Voight, M, and Tippett, S: Plyometric exercise in rehabilitation. In Prentice, WE, and Voight, ML (eds): *Techniques in Musculoskeletal Rehabilitation.* New York: McGraw-Hill, 2001, pp 167–178.
17. Voight, ML: Stretch strengthening: an introduction to plyometrics. *Orthop Phys Ther Clin North Am* 1:243–252, 1992.
18. Voight, ML, and Draovitch, P: Plyometrics. In Albert, M (ed): *Eccentric Muscle Training in Sports and Orthopedics,* ed. 2. New York: Churchill Livingstone, 1995, p 149.
19. Wilk, KE, et al: Stretch-shortening drills for the upper extremities: theory and clinical application. *J Orthop Sports Phys Ther* 17: 225–239, 1993.

CHAPTER 24

Exercise for the Older Adult

BARBARA BILLEK-SAWHNEY, PT, EDD, DPT, GCS
RAJIV SAWHNEY, PT, DPT, MS, OCS

The "graying of America" and "graying of the world" are realistic descriptors of the population trend in the United States and many parts of the world. The graying of the population is a universal, developmental gift of 20th century science and technology. With the introduction of antibiotics, insulin, vaccinations, modern surgical techniques, and other medical advancements, adults are living longer.

The life expectancy in North America, most of Europe, and Australia is an average of 75 years of age.[201] In the US, life expectancy at birth for the total population is 78.8 years, 76.4 for men and 81.2 for women.[47] Thirteen percent to 14% of the 318 million citizens of the US (approximately one out of eight) are over 65 years of age.

This is in comparison to 20% of the German and Italian populations and only 3% of the population in Uganda. The age structure of the world has also changed; between 1970 and 2014, the world's population of individuals over 65 years of age or older increased from 5% to 7%. Thus, in the profession of physical therapy, most clinicians can anticipate working with the older adult in some capacity.

"Aging leads to a decline in strength and an associated loss of independence."[65] The importance of this specialty chapter is succinctly stated in the above quote! Physical therapists are able to appropriately adapt interventions to meet the needs of the older adult and enable them to optimize their functional potential. Throughout this chapter, the value of exercise and physical activity for older adults will be addressed.

Definitions and Descriptions Applied to Older Adults

Definitions: Quantitative and Qualitative

Who are older adults? The answer is quite variable when considering roles that change as one ages. Historically, the standard has been 65 years of age based on Medicare eligibility. With the increase in life expectancy, coupled with a 117% increase in the percentage of adults over 65 years of age employed in the workforce,[52] one could question if this continues to define the "older adult." But, 65 years of age is still being used as the "specified age" for categorizing an individual as an "older adult."

The presentation of an older adult is quite variable.[175] A 75-year-old individual may be an athlete, may be working full or part time, or may be a sedentary individual with multiple medical problems having difficulty performing basic activities of daily living (ADLs). Clinicians may document, "patient appears younger than chronological age" or "patient appears older than chronological age." In reality, there is great variability in the older adult population which is reflected in the three case scenarios described in Box 24.1.

As illustrated in Box 24.1, the older adult population can be subdivided into young-old, mid-old, and old-old. However, these stages are overgeneralizations and may not reflect all older adults.

- The *young-old* are those 65 to 74 years of age and generally includes recently retired people who enjoy the results of their employment. The young-old may be busy caring for their parents and assisting with babysitting and transporting their grandchildren in their leisure time. Or, this individual may continue to work because of interest in their work, financial needs, social interaction, or some combination of above. Lou, in Case 1, is in the group of young-old.
- The *mid-old* are 75 to 84 years of age. Generally, the mid-old are experiencing more age-related changes and may work toward simplifying their lives; many may rest during the day. Mary Jane, in Case 2, is an example of mid-old.
- The *old-old* are over 85 years of age and typically have significant decline in physical functioning. They may reflect on the meaning of their lives, their relationships, and contributions to society.[180, 243] As noted in Case 3, Juan has just entered the old-old stage at age 85.

Example of Progression of Aging

When Juan was in the young-old stage he was busy caring for his mother and mother-in-law, was actively engaged in helping to care for his grandchildren, and maintained a small business as a part-time endeavor. In the mid-old stage he began to have more complaints of hip pain due to osteoarthritis (OA). As his grandchildren aged and parents died and he no longer maintained his business, he was less engaged and subsequently, less active. During this stage he continued to do yard work and car maintenance but became very sedentary. In his current old-old stage, he is experiencing more medical problems and numerous issues related to inactivity; he spends extended periods of time isolated and reflective.

BOX 24.1 Three Case Scenarios of Older Adults

Case 1: YOUNG-OLD:
Lou is a 72-year-old male who works out regularly at the local YMCA. He is also a part-time employee in the fitness center at the same facility. His past medical history is unremarkable, and he describes himself as a long time exercise advocate. He has run two to four marathons a year for more than 10 years and also participates in sprint triathlons. Lou recently ran a marathon and reports that this marathon seemed much longer than 26 miles and that it was his worst time ever. He complains of left knee pain. On inspection, Lou is healthy appearing and looks much younger than his chronological age; he has tortuous veins in both legs below the knees.

Case 2: MID-OLD:
Mary Jane is an 82-year-old female who has a long-standing history of cardiac disease, multiple myocardial infarctions, coronary artery bypass grafting (20 and 35 years ago), hypertension, Raynaud's phenomenon, and arterial insufficiency, as well as a history of uterine cancer and a radical hysterectomy 40 years ago. She has long-standing low back, cervical, hip, and shoulder pain attributed to osteoarthritis. Mary Jane reports she takes 13 medications each day. She demonstrates a pronounced kyphosis and forward head posture. She reports she is 5′2″ and weighs 89 pounds, but appears to be approximately 4′9″ in height. Mary Jane reports that the doctor did not say she has osteoporosis. The therapist believes it is likely due to Mary Jane's vertical height loss of 5″. She admits to having occasional falls but no real injuries. She describes days of dizziness where she has difficulty getting out of bed. Her children report an increase in confusion, but that it appears to be episodic. They believe their mother is having mini-strokes. The strokes have not been diagnosed. Mary Jane is independent in IADLs and manages the finances for rental properties. She enjoys cooking, working in her yard, spending time with family, and participating in church events. She denies participating in regular exercise but reports she is able to walk three to four blocks, go up and down flights of steps several times/day, and perform arm exercises with the elastic band she was given when she attended outpatient physical therapy 4 months ago.

Case 3: OLD-OLD:
Juan is an 86-year-old male who is a retired steel mill worker and who resides with his wife. He is being seen by a home health physical therapist following an episode of internal bleeding, a 3-day acute hospitalization, and two blood transfusions. Currently his primary complaint is shortness of breath. Prior to this illness, he was independent in ADLs, including yard work and car maintenance, driving, visiting a fraternal organization, and attending his grandchildren's activities. His past medical history includes osteoarthritis bilaterally in hips, hands, and knees (including left total hip arthroplasty 10 years ago), as well as T2DM, asbestosis, obesity, obstructive sleep apnea (he does not use a continuous positive airway pressure [CPAP] machine), and diminished hearing. He gets up at approximately 11:00 a.m. each day and takes a nap at 2:00 p.m. Although not diagnosed, he has characteristics of sarcopenic obesity. At his peak, Juan was 5′8″ and 225 pounds. His hospital record reveals he is 198 pounds, and he appears to be 5′5″ in height.

Healthy People 2020

The *Healthy People 2020* vision for an older adult is to "increase the proportion of older adults with reduced physical or cognitive function who engage in light, moderate, or vigorous leisure-time physical activities."[111] It is reported that 29.3% of the older adult population experience moderate to severe functional limitations. In addition, approximately one in three "older adults with reduced physical or cognitive function engaged in light, moderate, or vigorous leisure-time physical activities in 2008." [111] Males are more engaged in physical activities than females, and Caucasians are 10% more involved in physical activities than other racial groups.

Complexity of Diagnoses in the Older Population

The medical model of a one-to-one ratio of symptoms to diagnosis is atypical in the older adult population seeking medical care or physical therapy services. More characteristic of older adults is the presence of multiple medical problems or a chronic disease, which may cause a myriad of problems. In the prior paragraph, the incidence of functional limitations was described. Those functional limitations may be due to various factors and may reflect the presence of multiple medical problems. Approximately 92% of older adults are reported to have at least one chronic condition, while 77% of older adults have a minimum of two chronic conditions.[170]

The case of Mary Jane (see Case 2 in Box 24.1) exemplifies this concept of multiple medical problems. Mary Jane had a radical hysterectomy at age 37 secondary to cancer and subsequently experienced early menopause. Severe coronary artery disease, myocardial infarction, and coronary artery bypass grafting were other medical problems she experienced. In the absence of hormone replacement or other preventative intervention, Mary Jane appears to have osteoporosis based on her height loss and flexed posture, although she has not had clinical testing to confirm the diagnosis. Mary Jane takes 13 medications each day. Adverse drug reactions from her cardiac medications and polypharmacy may result in orthostatic hypotension and her complaints of dizziness. The polypharmacy and cardiac medications are a risk factor for falls.

Chronic conditions, injuries, and new medical problems may each impact the quality of life in older adults. Type II diabetes mellitus (T2DM), OA, congestive heart failure, and dementia are chronic conditions that many older adults experience.[170] For example, Juan (see Case 3 in Box 24.1) had end-stage OA of the hip during the stage of young-old. Consequently, he restricted his walking due to pain. This restricted mobility impacted strength, functional mobility, and balance. Now his sedentary behavior further impacts his quality of life including the development of T2DM. This cascading effect is cyclical resulting in even greater problems.[87,128]

Health Trends in the Aging Population

Fair or poor health is the descriptor that almost 25% (23.1%) of the older adult population in the US use to describe their health.[169] A snapshot view of the "older person's health" and incidence of diagnoses can be found in ONLINE Table 24.1 available on the FA Davis web site.

The incidence of diseases varies slightly from the mortality incidence. For example, heart disease and cancer account for approximately half of all deaths in the US, while arthritis is the most common disability.[44,47,115,169,186] The 15 leading causes of death among individuals 65 years of age and older in the US in 2013 were heart disease, cancer, stroke, chronic lower respiratory disease (such as emphysema), accidents (such as falls), cerebrovascular accident, Alzheimer's disease, diabetes, influenza and pneumonia, kidney disease, suicide, septicemia, chronic liver disease, hypertension, Parkinson's disease, and pneumonitis.[245]

Wellness Aging Model Related to Illness, Injury, and Immobility

As people age, loss of strength, loss of muscle mass, and senescence occur. This results in impaired function and greater dependence in the performance of functional activities.[27,36,54,70,92,128,206,208,213,216] These functional impairments can be quantified, with 14% of older adults requiring assistance with ADLs and 35% having difficulty with functional activities necessary for independence.[65] Sehl and Yates[216] extrapolated information from 54,274 subjects into a linear model on various systems of the body and described a loss rate of every system of the body. This loss rate is up to 3% per year beginning at age 30 and continuing up to the age of 70. When individuals are physically active, they typically function more independently than people who have disease or pathology. Illness, chronic disease, injury, and immobility each impact age-related changes. Kauffman[128] refers to the concept of age-related declines in function as "linear senescence," while Brown[36] refers to this concept as the "compression of infirmity." These concepts are collectively depicted in the Wellness Aging Model Related to Illness, Injury, and Immobility (WAMI-3) illustrated in Figure 24.1.

In this model, age is depicted on the X-axis while impairments of structure and function, such as muscular and bone strength, longevity, mental well-being, fall risk, and functional mobility, are depicted on the Y-axis. This right skewed curvilinear shape demonstrates the need for physical activity and exercise as one ages. Individuals who are physically active may have a rightward shift in function while disease, injury, and inactivity result in a leftward shift in function. Billek-Sawhney and Wells[22] applied this relationship to individuals undergoing cancer treatment. Disease specific factors such as cancer related fatigue and nausea were plotted on the Y-axis and the effect of cancer treatments over time on the X-axis. With physical activity and exercise improvement was seen in strength, energy

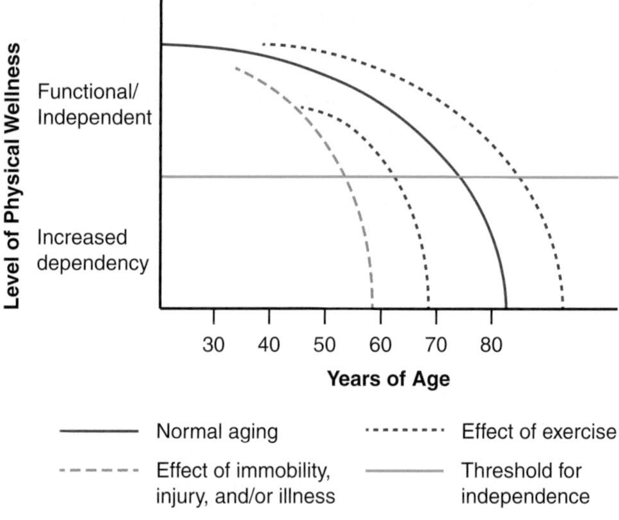

FIGURE 24.1 Wellness Aging Model related to Illness, Injury, and Immobility (WAMI-3) demonstrating the effects of immobility, illness, and/or injury on wellness and aging. Age is depicted on the x-axis; impairments of structure and function, including but not limited to strength, power, bone density, fall risk, and functional mobility, are depicted on the y-axis. Wellness, physical activity, and exercise will result in a rightward shift to decrease the slope of the curve.

level, mental well-being and functional status. This model can be applied to a multitude of medical diagnoses, immobility, and physical inactivity and serves as the basis for the importance of remaining active as one ages. The WAMI-3 is a modification and compilation from numerous diagrams and exemplifies the concept that physical activity and exercise add life to years.[22,36,67,128,168] Wellness, physical activity, and exercise will result in a rightward shift to decrease the slope of decline.

FOCUS ON EVIDENCE

In a study of almost 900 older adults, a slower rate of decline in mobility was reported to be associated with a greater rate of physical activity.[38] Each additional hour of physical activity was associated with about a 3% decrease in the rate of mobility decline when measured on an 8-foot walk and 360° turn. It was concluded that both physical activity and leg strength predict decline in mobility in older adults.

Aging: Primary and Secondary

Primary aging is a universal, developmental process from the passage of time. This differs from secondary aging in the older adult resulting from disease, disuse, the environment, and other factors.[180,233] An example of secondary aging is an older adult with T2DM who develops cardiac disease and peripheral neuropathies.

Effects of Aging or Senescence on the Body Systems

Senescence (*senescere* in Latin, meaning "to grow old") occurs with a decrease in physiological effectiveness of the various systems at an average of 2% per year starting at 30 years of age.[155,216] Through the aging processes, there is a degradation of function of the vital organs. As we age, every cell, tissue, organ, and system of the body changes. Most visible is the graying of the hair, the flexed posture, muscle mass loss, and the wrinkles on the face. Similar aging processes are masked but still occurring beneath the skin.

Immune dysregulation, described as *immunosenescence*, is the age related deterioration of the immune system causing cancer, infection, and autoimmune disease. The changes in the immune system are evident with the increased prevalence of cancer in the older adult. The decreased effectiveness at the cellular and tissue level results in increased susceptibility to infection and impaired surveillance or monitoring of one's condition for the presentation of an illness.[101] In addition, the initial presentation of illness may differ. For example, the presentation of a urinary tract infection in an older adult may be an altered mental status rather than the usual signs of fever or infection.

The impact of exercise and physical activity on aging can be illustrated by looking at results of stress testing. The maximum oxygen consumption, better known as VO_{2MAX}, is described in Chapter 7. The calculation of VO_{2max} is typically done with stress testing. Viewing the formula and seeing the components of the formula change in response to aging, immobility, and exercise/physical activity, as summarized in Table 24.1, enhances the reader's understanding of the importance of the WAMI-3. The reader is referred to several sources for detailed information on stress testing and calculating VO_{2max} using the Fick Equation.[18,161,164,249]

Cellular and Organ Changes

Cellular changes occur with aging and may include atrophy, hypertrophy, hyperplasia, dysplasia, and neoplasia. In older adults, atrophy of muscles and the brain may occur, hypertrophy can occur at the heart and kidneys, hyperplasia may occur of the prostate, dysplasia in the cervix, and neoplasia in squamous cell carcinomas. These changes are also reflected in the maximal oxygen consumption at the heart, vascular system, and muscular level.

Senescence at the cellular level results in lipofuscin, a fatty brown pigment and other fatty substances, which build up in tissue. The accumulation of lipofuscin is a hallmark of aging and is not degradable.[235] Connective tissue becomes stiffer. Therapists recognize these changes in the musculoskeletal system, but it also occurs in organs, blood vessels, and airways, making them more rigid. The changes occurring in the membranes of tissues in the lungs impact the transport of oxygen and nutrients to tissues and negatively affect the removal of carbon dioxide and other wastes. These changes or losses occur gradually and are not noticeable unless coupled with

TABLE 24.1 Maximal Oxygen Consumption and the Impact of Aging, Illness, Injury, Immobility, and Exercise on Physical Activity

	Maximal Oxygen Consumption (VO2max)		Cardiac Output (CO or Q)				Arteriovenous Oxygen Difference (a-vO2)	Comments
	VO2max	=	HR	x	SV	x	(a-vO2)	CO = HR xS V
Aging	↓		RHR- no change MHR- ↓		↓		↓	With aging declines are seen in the effectiveness of each component.
Illness	↓		RHR- ↑or↓ MHR- ↓		↓		↓	With illness various factors can be impacted; for example, heart muscle weakness from a myocardial infarction decreases SV.
Immobility	↓		RHR- ↑ MHR- ↓		↓		↓	Similar to aging, immobility impacts each component negatively.
With exercise/ physical training	↑		RHR- ↓ MHR- ↑		↑		↑	Greater capillary density. Enhanced ability to extract oxygen. Increase in number and size of mitochondria.

disease, at which time a causal chain type of effect may occur leading to a cascade of medical issues.

Organ Reserve Changes

Generally, there is a reserve associated with the function of organs. Cardiac reserve exemplifies this concept. At age 20, the heart "is capable of pumping about 10 times the amount of blood that is actually needed to keep the body alive. After age 30, an average of 1% of this reserve is lost each year."[156] Organ reserve losses have the greatest impact on the heart, lungs, and kidneys.[75] The amount of loss varies among organs in the same individual and between individuals. This concept can be applied to the case of Mary Jane described in Box 24.1; Mary Jane has severe cardiac disease but does not appear to have age-related losses in her respiratory system.

System Changes

The endocrine (hormone production), immune, integumentary, musculoskeletal, reproductive, urinary, cardiopulmonary, vascular, sensory, and central nervous systems are each impacted by the aging process, and their function can be viewed as the solid line in the WAMI-3 (see Fig. 24.1). Many, although not all, systems of the body demonstrate a rightward shift from exercise. For example, the musculoskeletal system demonstrates a rightward shift with exercise, but conversely, the integumentary system with the thinning, graying, and loss of hair does not appear to respond to exercise and activity.[86] In response to aging, changes in the systems of the body not only impact the function of the organs, but can also impact the body's ability to function. Age-related changes in the musculoskeletal system impact strength; posture; gait; coordination; speed of movement; and, consequentially, an individual's ability to function. The age-related changes to the musculoskeletal system are highlighted in ONLINE Table 24.2.

Neuromuscular and Musculoskeletal System Changes

Normal aging results in muscle mass loss beginning in the fourth decade of life but escalates with advancing age. Over the age of 40 muscle mass loss/year is 0.5%, over the age of 50 it increases to 1% to 2%, and over the age of 60 loss/year is 3%.[131,210,258,274] In older adults who are sedentary, this rate of decline is increased. This is coupled by changes in the quality of the muscle tissue. The rate of decrease in strength and power are greater in sedentary individuals as compared to those who are physically active, resulting in a leftward shift in senescence (see Fig. 24.1).[210] Older adults 70 years of age and older, when compared to younger adults, demonstrate a 50% decrease in strength and a 75% decrease in power.[31,112] The loss of muscle mass and strength occurs as a result of many factors, including a reduction in both size and number of muscle fibers, a selective reduction in Type II fibers, a decrease in neural activation, and an increase in antagonistic co-activation (Fig. 24.2).[110,213,229] When a muscle fiber loses it innervation, motor units will

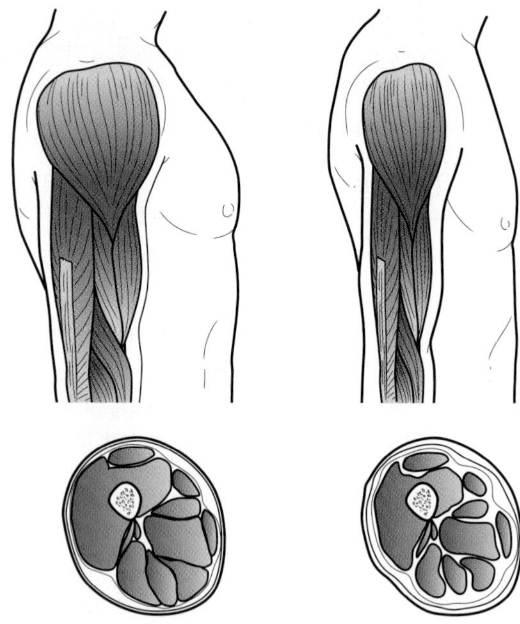

FIGURE 24.2 Age-related changes in muscle mass in the arm showing a lateral view and the related cross-sectional area.

die and compound the loss of muscle fibers. By 60 years of age, there is approximately a 50% loss of the motor units innervating individual muscle fibers because of the death of the alpha-motorneurons at the spinal cord.[213] The disease of sarcopenia, which is associated with aging and the loss of muscle mass, will be discussed in the section on sarcopenia later in this chapter.

Muscle weakness affects gait and activities such as ascending and descending stairs. Gait disorders are commonly associated with aging; 35% of adults over 70 years of age have an abnormal gait. Decreases in gait speed and stride length commonly occur.[39,152] Walking, the most prevalent physical activity, has a greater energy cost in older adults than younger adults. Wert and colleagues[261] stress the need for the physical therapist to assess gait and to specifically evaluate older adult patients for the absence of hip extension, for wider step width, and for slower gait speed. These gait deviations result in a loss of efficiency. Similar losses in efficiency with greater effort required also occur with ADLs in older adults.[125] Thus, older adults are less energy efficient and expend more energy when walking and performing ADLs than younger individuals.

Changes in the musculoskeletal system, such as osteoporosis, osteopenia, and OA, with accompanying pain, stiffness, and deformity, affect balance and the number of falls experienced by older adults.[119] Neuromuscular changes result in mobility loss and impaired function. Coupled together, these changes affect the independence and quality of the older adult's life.[229]

Sensory Changes

Sensory changes associated with aging profoundly impact older adult patients at a functional level resulting in quality of life issues. For example, when considering loss of vision, the older adult may have difficulty reading his or her prescribed home exercise program or completing the necessary patient registration and/or outcomes questionnaires. With aging, the amount of peripheral vision (known as peripheral visual field) has decreases. This, combined with loss of rotation in the cervical spine, may affect driving safety. Wearing bifocals to address the presbyopia affects walking and use of stairs and curbs, thus putting the older adult at risk for falls.[51] In addition, use of bifocals, coupled with changes in position sense and muscular weakness, affects balance and risk of falls. (See Chapter 8 for a discussion on balance exercise programs to address fall risk in the elderly.)

Effects of Decreased Activity

Immobility

Historically, bed rest was prescribed for a multitude of medical problems from back pain to myocardial infarction. Immobility negatively impacts every system of the body and results in a leftward shift on the WAMI-3 (see Fig. 24.1). There are various medical complications associated with prolonged immobility, including orthostatic hypotension, increased heart rate, decreased cardiac reserve, atelectasis, pneumonia, deep venous thrombosis, pulmonary emboli, urinary retention, constipation, muscle atrophy (leading to generalized weakness), contractures, soft tissue changes, metabolic inflexibility (including insulin resistance), osteoporosis, impaired sensory perception, skin breakdown, and psychological manifestations such as depression.[62,71,103,223] The need for early mobilization of patients is now commonly practiced; where it is not, it should become a standard of practice.

Similar to the effects of aging, each organ system is impacted negatively by immobilization. For example, when considering cardiac function, the stroke volume decreases approximately 12% following the first 30 days of inactivity, and the maximal heart rate is also decreased. Subsequently, maximal oxygen uptake is decreased, and total blood volume and hemoglobin concentration are also decreased, making a less efficient cardiovascular (CV) system and less reserve.[14,103,128,231,264] These concepts are highlighted in the impact on maximal oxygen consumption in Table 24.1.

Muscle disuse results in atrophy and loss of muscle strength at the rate of approximately 12% a week or 1% to 1.5% per day from bed rest.[124] Loss of strength in the legs occurs twice as fast as in the arms, with the quadriceps and back extensors showing the greatest loss. As much as 50% strength loss can occur with 3 weeks of bed rest, while the recovery of strength is only 10% per week.[23,56,138,182] In muscles that are larger and better trained, there is quicker recovery of strength.[124] The loss of strength and muscle atrophy impacts much more than just strength and power; muscle fatigue due to reduced oxidative capacity in extracting oxygen, metabolic activity, protein breakdown and loss, increased concentrations of cortisol, and glucose metabolism and function are also affected.[23,124]

Hypokinesis

Hypokinesia is defined as an "abnormally diminished muscular function or mobility."[166] This sedentary behavior in older adults is manifested in minimal energy expenditure and inactivity. Juan in Case 3 (see Box 24.1) illustrates the concept of hypokinesis. Juan is recumbent or sits for extended periods of time and is inactive. At the age of 85, he sleeps in a recliner or in his bed until 11:00 a.m. each morning, and then after eating breakfast, he goes back to bed for a nap. He is upright and watching television until dinner at 5:00 p.m. The only time Juan leaves home is for medical appointments and occasionally to go to a fraternal organization. Generally, he is back to sleep before 10:00 p.m.

 **FOCUS ON EVIDENCE**

A systematic review by Harvey and colleagues[107] on the prevalence of sedentary behaviors in older adults reports that the majority of older adults are sedentary, that approximately 60% of older adults report sitting >4 hours/day, and one study described 67% of the older population as sedentary >8.5 hours/day.

Sedentary Behavior

The lack of physical activity, or sedentary behavior, is now recognized as a modifiable risk factor for a multitude of illnesses. Sedentary behavior is described as spending a great deal of time in a recumbent or sitting position and low energy expenditure behavior (<1.5 METS during waking hours). As a reference, the performance of basic ADLs, such as grooming, eating, toileting, bathing, and dressing, has a metabolic equivalent level of 1.0 to 2.5 METS. Instrumental ADLs, including light housekeeping, doing laundry, washing dishes, setting the table, or making a bed, increase the energy required to 1.5 to 4.0 METS. The American Heart Association reports the risk of CV disease is directly related to sedentary behavior. Adults who watch >4 hours of television/day have a 46% increased risk of death from any cause and 80% increased risk of death from CV disease. In addition, those who are physically active and maintain a healthy weight live approximately 7 years longer than inactive adults who are obese.[10] (See Chapter 7 for additional information on energy expenditure and training for patients with chronic illness.)

Loss Of Functional Mobility

The WAMI-3 (see Fig. 24.1) visually depicts the decreases in functional mobility, musculoskeletal strength and power, bone strength, CV and pulmonary function, but it fails to describe how these changes impact an individual's ability to participate in daily activities in the home and community. The association between the recommended strength training guidelines of twice a week and functional limitations has been described by the National Health Interview Survey of 6,763 older adults.[48] Almost 51% of the older adult population reported functional limitations with stooping, bending, or kneeling. The older adults who performed strength training twice a week reported having less difficulty with the nine functional activities investigated. The nine activities included:

1. Walking 0.25 miles, approximately 3 city blocks
2. Ascending 10 steps without resting
3. Standing for approximately 2 hours
4. Sitting for 2 hours
5. Stooping, bending, or kneeling
6. Reaching overhead
7. Grasping or handling small objects with fingers
8. Lifting and carrying 10 pounds ("like a full grocery bag")
9. Pushing or pulling large objects ("like a living room chair")

The report found that older adults with functional limitations were the least likely to perform strength training. Kraschnewski and colleagues[135] report that older adults with functional impairments believe they are too weak to perform strengthening activities. This belief impacts self-efficacy and requires a paradigm shift. As physical therapists, we can be instrumental in making this shift through education, mentoring, and guiding the older adult in strengthening interventions.

The WAMI-3 can also apply to the loss of functional activities such as ambulation. The walking ability of older adults changes with the aging process. This is exemplified in the US, where 17.3% of adults aged 55 to 64 years and 56.1% of individuals over age 85 report difficulty walking 0.25 miles (402 m).[214] Ambulation is directly impacted as one ages but may be improved through strength training.[81,93,135,164,178,233] Sayers[213] describes a curvilinear relationship between the strength of muscle and the ability to perform functional activities.

When individuals gain strength, there is an improvement in the performance of function to a specific point at which further strength improvements result only in minimal changes of function. When applying this concept to Cases 1 and 3 in Box 24.1, if the ages of both Lou and Juan are hypothetically reset at age 75, Lou will be stronger than Juan at baseline. Then, even if they have the same strength gains, Lou's functional improvements will be less than Juan's due to a higher baseline level.

Benefits of Physical Activity and Exercise

There are a multitude of benefits to being physically active, especially in older adults. The primary benefits include (1) slowing physiological changes of aging; (2) optimizing body composition; (3) supporting psychological and cognitive health; (4) managing chronic disease; (5) decreasing the risk of developing chronic diseases; (6) minimizing risk of physical disability; and (7) increasing lifespan.[195] The phrase "adding life to years" is used by multiple sources[272] to address the need for healthy aging and is also a benefit of physical therapy rehabilitation. This concept can be further stated that "adding life to years" requires physical activity and resistance training.

The Choosing Wisely Initiative

It is not unusual to observe older patients performing exercise programs that do not provide enough resistance to develop strength to improve function. To merely sit and perform leg kicks or marches with a 1- or 2-lb weight for 3 sets of 10 repetitions may be underdosed and nonspecific and should lead the therapist to question the purpose of the exercises.

In 2014, the "Choosing Wisely" initiative between the American Physical Therapy Association (APTA) and the American Board of Internal Medicine Foundation addressed underdosed strength training programs in older adults. In one of its five recommendations, the APTA stresses the importance of developing an exercise program that matches frequency, intensity, and duration of exercise to the older adult's abilities and goals. Box 24.2 cites the statement and provides an explanation. It is critical when developing a strengthening program that the patient's needs are fully assessed and appropriate interventions are prescribed that improve function.

Justification for Exercise and Physical Activity

With resistance training, muscular strength, power, and endurance can improve in the older adult and deter the effects of aging and improve mobility. Improving strength and mobility has been shown to improve balance and reduce the incidence of falls and resulting fractures.[117,120,137,145,220,221,238] Activities of daily living can be performed with less effort, and thus functional independence can be maintained for a longer period of time.[195] Despite this, only about 21% of all older adults and less than 10% of older adults greater than 85 years of age regularly perform physical activities.[195] The importance of power is well documented as being more strongly related to performance of ADLs than strength alone.

Interestingly, there is strong evidence that physical activity reduces the risk of premature death. There is a dose response associated with this concept. Therefore, the risk of premature death declines with greater time and frequency (minutes/week) of physical activity. These benefits are described in Box 24.3.

Progressive resistance strength training can increase muscle mass, strength, power, functional mobility, and the performance of ADLs.[117, 206] High intensity or power training results in even greater strength adaptations compared to low and moderate intensity training. Power training enhances functional tasks like sit to stand and climbing stairs[229] and minimizes functional limitations and disabilities.[203] Functionally, the ability to perform sit-to-stand, ambulate without an assistive device, and alter the ability for an older adult to increase their self-selected gait speed have been shown to improve with high intensity progressive resistance training.[206] The benefits of physical activity increase as the intensity, frequency, and duration of exercising increases.[21]

It should be noted that skeletal muscles have secondary roles that include metabolism, glycogen storage, body temperature regulation, joint stabilization, and endocrine function. Thus, the importance of increasing muscle mass or minimizing its loss with aging must be considered as a secondary benefit to resistance training.[238] This is critical when considering pharmacokinetics and aging. Most simplistically, pharmacokinetics is drug absorption, distribution, metabolism, and secretion.[204] With aging, the sensitivity to drugs may be impacted.[154]

The decline in bone density that generally occurs with increased age can be lessened with exercise. There is a lower risk of hip fracture in physically active older adults, especially women. Individuals who perform 120 to 300 minutes of moderate intensity physical activity each week have a reduced risk of hip fracture. Both physical activity and exercise are beneficial and require voluntary movements resulting in calorie expenditure. Physical activities incorporate any movements like household cleaning, stair climbing, gardening, and shopping at stores. Exercise, a form of physical activity, is planned, structured, and repetitive in nature; it includes weight training, exercise classes, and aerobics.[171]

BOX 24.2 APTA Choosing Wisely Statement on Strength Training Programs in Older Adults

"Don't prescribe under-dosed strength training programs for older adults. Instead, match the frequency, intensity and duration of exercise to the individual's abilities and goals."[8,11]

"Improved strength in older adults is associated with improved health, quality of life and functional capacity, and with a reduced risk of falls. Older adults are often prescribed low dose exercise and physical activity that are physiologically inadequate to increase gains in muscle strength. Failure to establish accurate baseline levels of strength limits the adequacy of the strength training dosage and progression, and thus limits the benefits of the training. A carefully developed and individualized strength training program may have significant health benefits for older adults."[8,11]

FOCUS ON EVIDENCE

A meta-study looking at 160 trials on the benefits of exercise on the CV system found that not all people experience the same benefits from exercise. They reported that exercise has multiple beneficial effects and significantly improves CV fitness and biomarkers, such as lipid profiles, and also that in individuals less than 50 years of age; men; and individuals with T2DM, hypertension, dyslipidemia, or metabolic syndrome the benefits to exercise are greater.[144]

The long-term impact of a 1-year strength-training program in older adults was studied by Kennis and colleagues.[131] After 1-year of training, muscular performance improved for those in the exercise group. Seven years after cessation of the

BOX 24.3 Benefits of Physical Activity and Exercise in the Older Adult (Reprinted with permission from the Office of Disease Prevention and Health Promotion[185])

Strong Evidence
- Lower risk of early death
- Lower risk of coronary heart disease
- Lower risk of stroke
- Lower risk of high blood pressure
- Lower risk of adverse blood lipid profile
- Lower risk of type II diabetes mellitus
- Lower risk of metabolic syndrome
- Lower risk of colon cancer
- Lower risk of breast cancer
- Prevention of weight gain
- Weight loss, particularly when combined with reduced calorie intake
- Improved cardiorespiratory and muscular fitness
- Prevention of falls
- Reduced depression
- Better cognitive function (for older adults)

Moderate to Strong Evidence
- Better functional health (for older adults)
- Reduced abdominal obesity

Moderate Evidence
- Lower risk of hip fracture
- Lower risk of lung cancer
- Lower risk of endometrial cancer
- Weight maintenance after weight loss
- Increased bone density
- Improved sleep quality

Other Benefits
- Enhanced immune function through aerobic training. Aerobic, not resistance, training has been shown to impact chronic inflammation and thereby impact the immune system.[101] This strengthens the argument to employ a multidimensional program in conjunction with a resistance training program.
- Improved spatial awareness, visual, and physical reactions. Fregala et al[86] found that spatial awareness and visual and physical reactions are each improved with resistance training. This benefit may be related to the decreased risk of falls, accident avoidance, and improved cognitive function. The potential cognitive benefits of resistance exercise may enhance the quality of life in older adults.
- Increased joint ROM. This is believed to be due to the actual performance of movement rather than the strengthening exercises.[206]
- Less symptomatic intermittent claudication.[190]
- Decreased fall risk.[17,68,137,145,187,206,226]

exercise intervention, age-related declines were less for the exercise participants than for nonparticipants.

Detraining was studied by Harris et al.[106] Following cessation of a training program, there were significant decreases in strength at weeks 6 and 20 postexercise, but strength was significantly greater than prior to the start of the training program.

Physical therapists play a unique role in enhancing the quality of life of older adults by addressing impairments through exercise, health promotion, and disease prevention. There is a plethora of evidence supporting the positive benefits of exercise and activity in aging adults.[86,91,101,104,131,149,153,190,196,197,206,226,233,238,257,259] The rightward shift in Figure 24.1 provides a visible display of the benefits of exercise.

Considerations Prior to Implementation of Exercise

Examination and evaluation of the older adult are critical prior to establishing exercise interventions and must take into consideration the normal aging of the body systems as well as the complexity of diagnoses as described in the previous section of this chapter. The reader is referred to several physical therapy texts cited in the reference list that describe examination procedures.[151,60,100,209] ONLINE Table 24.3 available on the FA Davis web site summarizes inspection, interview, tests and measures, and patient management considerations for the older adult. Key items to emphasize when examining the older adult are described in this section.

Examination of the Aging Adult: Highlights

Medications

During the interview it is critical to not only review the medications, but also to count the number of medications that a patient is taking. Polypharmacy is defined as the use of ≥ three or four medications and is a fall risk factor in older adults. In addition, when the medications include diuretics, antiarrhythmics, and psychotropics, the risk of falls is increased.[105,139,140,242,276] The pharmacokinetics of drugs and how the drugs are removed from the body occur at a slower rate in older adults, and lower doses may be necessary. Unfortunately, the side effects of medications may result in a multitude of secondary symptoms. The role of the physical therapist and pharmacotherapy is variable by practice setting and beyond the scope of this chapter. The patient's ability to take their medications as prescribed, follow the prescribed regimen, and continue blood testing when taking medications are each critical issues for the older adult. For example, Mary Jane (see Box 24.1) defers taking her diuretics when leaving her house to minimize her frequency of urination.

This may result in greater fatigue and uncompensated heart failure.

The 2016 PAR-Q+

The Physical Activity Readiness Questionnaire (PAR-Q) was developed in 1978 and revised in 2002. The PAR-Q has been used worldwide as a preparticipation health screening tool to determine if an individual is healthy enough to participate in exercise and physical activity. Unfortunately, both of these self-report forms are outdated and were designed for individuals aged 15 to 69.[35,195,239] When used on older adults, there are numerous false-positive responses, leading to a large portion of older adults being required to have medical clearance prior to engaging in physical activity and exercise.[41,42,122,212,237,254,255,256] The PAR-Q+ was introduced in 2011 and is frequently revised. The 4-page 2016 PAR-Q+ is available online on the FA Davis web site and is also available at http://eparmedx.com/?page_id=79. The 2016 PAR-Q+ begins with seven screening questions. If the questions are answered negatively, the patient is cleared to participate in exercise. If any of the items are positive, there are follow-up questions. The 2016 PAR-Q+ differs from prior forms by reducing the barrier of seeing a physician for medical clearance before participating in physical activity. "The risks of being physically inactive far outweigh the small, transient risks seen after acute exercise in both asymptomatic and symptomatic populations across the lifespan."[35] The 2016 PAR-Q+ is recommended for preparticipation screening for outpatient physical therapy as a component of the physical therapy examination process.

As physical therapists, use of the 2016 PAR-Q+ does not eliminate applying clinical expertise employed as exercise professionals but builds upon basic examination skills. Ongoing monitoring is a critical component of physical therapy. Obtaining vital signs at resting, immediate post activity, and recovery, plus perceived exertion (see page 968 on the Borg scale) help determine if interventions are at the appropriate level or if they need to be adjusted in intensity.

Global Health Initiative and the Physical Activity Vital Signs

The concept of "Exercise is Medicine"®[7] is a global health initiative developed in 2007 by the American College of Sports Medicine (ACSM) to elevate physical activity.[7,108,135,146] The focus of EIM is based on the premise that physical activity is integral for the prevention and treatment of disease.[7] This initiative is also important for older adults.

To assess the level of physical activity, the ACSM advocates employing the Physical Activity Vital Signs (PAVS). The PAVS was first introduced in 2010, demonstrated validity,[58] and can be quickly performed in less than a minute.[7] Two questions comprise the PAVS, which query the average number of days and minutes an individual performs physical activity. The questions are:

1. "How many days a week do you engage in moderate to strenuous exercise (like a brisk walk)?"
2. "On average, how many minutes per day do you exercise at this level?"

The PAVS has been found to have a positive impact on metabolic outcomes.[97] In addition, body mass index and obesity are related to the PAVS; the higher the activity level the lower the body mass index and obesity.[98]

Fracture Risk Assessment Index and Balance

Perry and Downey[193] stress the need for physical therapists to incorporate routine screening of older adults using the World Health Organizations Fracture Risk Assessment Tool[269] (FRAX®) and screening for fall risk. The FRAX® tool is available online and is available in multiple languages. This tool looks at country, bone mineral density, age, gender, and clinical risk factors to calculate the 10-year probability of a fracture. The clinical risk factors include low body mass index, prior fragility fracture, parental history of a hip fracture, use of glucocorticoids, current smoking, alcohol intake of ≥ three units/day, rheumatoid arthritis, or other secondary causes of osteoporosis.[163,269] Falls are the causal factor for approximately 90% of all appendicular fractures. Thus, it is critical to assess fall risk and perform appropriate interventions coupled with strengthening exercises.[184] Refer to Chapter 8 for an in-depth discussion of balance assessment and interventions.

Objective Measures to Assess Strength, Power, Fall Risk, and Functional Mobility in the Older Adult

To assess strength, power, fall risk, and functional mobility in older adults, various tests and measures can be used. Some commonly performed tests for the older adult to assess strength and power are handgrip strength, five-time sit-to-stand test (FTSTS), 30-second sit-to-stand (30s-STS), and the time to ascend stairs.[72,220,252] When working with the older adult, the use of a standardized test with a temporal component may provide greater insight into the power, balance, endurance, reserve, morbidity, and mortality. Table 24.2 highlights several measures that may be used when examining the older adult. The temporal component to a test provides insight into the individual's power. The specifics and written guidelines for the tests and measures described in Table 24.2 can be found at several Internet sites, including but not limited to the ones identified in Box 24.4.

Power. It is imperative for physical therapists to use tests and measures to assess power because power is lost quicker than strength with aging. Power is directly related to an individual's ability to maintain independence and the risk of falls. The greater a person's power, the more independent and lower the fall risk.[220,238] Because of the explosive nature and time factor in most of the tests listed in Table 24.2, they provide an objective measure of power. Of the various tests described in Table 24.2, grip strength is only slightly associated with power. This test is valuable as it is a predictor of mobility. In addition, the 6-minute walk test (6MWT) looks at the maximum distance a person can cover in 6-minutes and thus how CV pulmonary considerations and muscular endurance impact performance. The energy pathways used for each of these tests can be found in Chapter 7. For example, the 30s-STS is anaerobic and uses

TABLE 24.2 Tests for Older Adults[2,14,88,114,183,192,228,234]

Test	Description	Interpretation
Stair Climb Power Test	Test not standardized. Functionally based measure of leg strength, power, and functional performance in older adults. Patients are timed on their ascent of stairs. A handrail can be used for safety but not to assist the ascent.	This test, although sensitive, has great variability and lacks norms. Recommended to compare pre- and post-interventions, keeping all factors the same; i.e., number of steps, use of railing, up and down or ascent only, reciprocal or non-reciprocal pattern, and directions.[183] Stair climbing is an item of the Dynamic Gait Index, and Functional Gait Assessment scoring is not temporal but is on the impairment scale.
Gait Speed Self-Selected AND Fast-Paced	A straight path is used of 10 m or 20 m in length, individuals are timed for the middle 5 m or 10 m to eliminate acceleration and deceleration time. Comparing the self-selected to fast-paced gait speed provides input on a person's gait reserve.	Normal walking speed is 1.2 to 1.4 m/s; speeds of ≤0.4 m/s are classified as household ambulators, speeds of 0.4 to 0.8 m/s are classified as limited community ambulators, and those walking at speeds of 0.8 m/s to 1.2 m/s are classified as community ambulators.
Timed Up and Go (TUG)	From sitting in a standard chair, individuals are timed as they rise from sitting, walk 3 m (10'), turn, walk back to chair, and sit.	Older adults who take ≥12 s are at high risk for falling.
30-Second Sit to Stand	From sitting in a standard chair, the number of repetitions an individual performs of sit to stand are counted in 30 s.	An older adult scoring ≤14.5 repetitions is at increased risk of falling.
Five Time Sit to Stand	From sitting in a standard chair, individuals are timed for the repeated performance of five repetitions from sit to stand.	A cutoff score of <15 s is predictive of fallers in older adults.
Grip strength	From sitting in a standard chair with back, pelvis, and knees close to 90°, shoulder adducted and neutrally rotated, elbow flexed at 90°, forearm neutral, wrist held between 0°-15° of ulnar deviation; forearm is not supported by examiner or armrest; dynamometer is presented vertically and in line with the forearm; the maximum grip is the mean of three trials.	In women, 20 kg was identified as a predictor for decreased mobility (sensitivity = 0.67, specificity = 0.73). In normal-weight men, it is 33 kg; in overweight men, it is 39 kg; in obese men, it is 40 kg.
6-Minute Walk Test (6MWT)[14]	A submaximal walking test measuring the maximal distance an individual can walk in 6 minutes. Walkway recommended is 30 m (100 ft), instructed to walk pathway for 6 minutes continually. Permitted to rest as needed. The distance walked in 6 minutes is measured. Gathering data on the level of perceived exertion and vitals enhances interpretation.	This test was originally developed for chronic respiratory disease and has since been modified in length and applied to different populations (geriatrics, pulmonary disease, stroke, Parkinson's, osteoarthritis).[114] The minimal detectable age in geriatrics is 58.21 m (190.98 ft).[192] For the community-dwelling elderly without assistive devices, the mean distances by age and gender are as follows:[228] Years / Males / Females 60–69 / 572 m / 538 m 70–79 / 527 m / 471 m 80–89 / 417 m / 392 m

BOX 24.4 Websites Where Standardized Tests and Measures Can Be Found

American Physical Therapy Association, and the Neurology Section Outcome Measures Recommendations: http://www.neuropt.org/professional-resources/neurology-section-outcome-measures-recommendations
Assessments, Stroke Engine: http://www.strokengine.ca/assess/
Australian Lung Foundation, Pulmonary Rehabilitation Toolkit: http://www.pulmonaryrehab.com.au/index.asp?page=2
Centers for Disease Control STEADI Older Adult Fall Prevention: http://www.cdc.gov/steadi/[51]
Geriatric Examination Tool Kit by the Academy of Geriatric Physical Therapy: http://geriatrictoolkit.missouri.edu/SoG-Joint-Report-2013-GCode-Tests.pdf
Osteoarthritis Research Society International recommended performance-based tests: http://oarsi.org/sites/default/files/docs/2013/manual.pdf
Outcome Measures in Stroke Rehabilitation, Chapter 21, Evidence-Based Review of Stroke Rehabilitation: http://ebrsr.com/evidence-review/21-outcome-measures
Rehabilitation Measures Database: http://www.rehabmeasures.org/default.aspx

ATP-PC and lactic acid while the 6MWT is aerobic and uses oxidative phosphorylation.[162]

Gait, falls, balance, endurance. Gait or walking speed is a commonly performed test that can predict future health status, functional decline, risk of falling, and fear of falling. The progression or regression of walking speed is linked to changes in the quality of life.[88]

- The Timed Up and Go (TUG) can assess fall risk and shed insight into power, gait, and balance status of an individual.[51,160,199,219,262]
- The 30s-STS is used to assess lower body strength, power, muscular endurance, and balance.[51,126,165,273] Another option to assess STS is the FTSTS test, which assesses strength, power, and balance.[26,37,66] Assessing STS for 30 seconds allows greater insight about the patient's muscular endurance.[263]

Grip Strength. Grip strength, similar to gait speed, is reported to predict mortality, disability, and time spent in a hospital and can be considered a vital sign.[24,25] Negative health outcomes can be predicted from a weaker hand grip value.[24,25,69,136,158,188,241]

Exercise Prescription for the Older Adult

Multidimensional Program

A balanced exercise program of aerobic, flexibility, balance, and resistance exercises should be a part of healthy living (Fig. 24.3) and is essential for the older adult.[43,129,164] The principles of developing exercises for each of these parameters are described in Part II of this textbook, with guidelines for each region of the body in Part IV. The effects of aging on the body systems and special concerns that these have in older adults are presented earlier in this chapter. Also, the importance of a detailed examination for the older

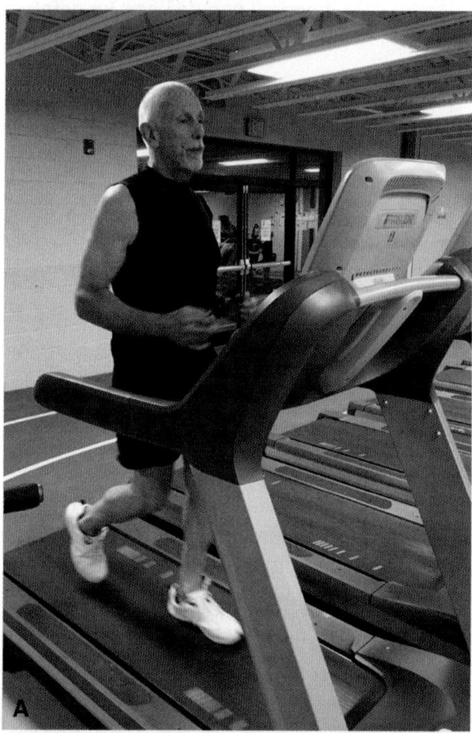

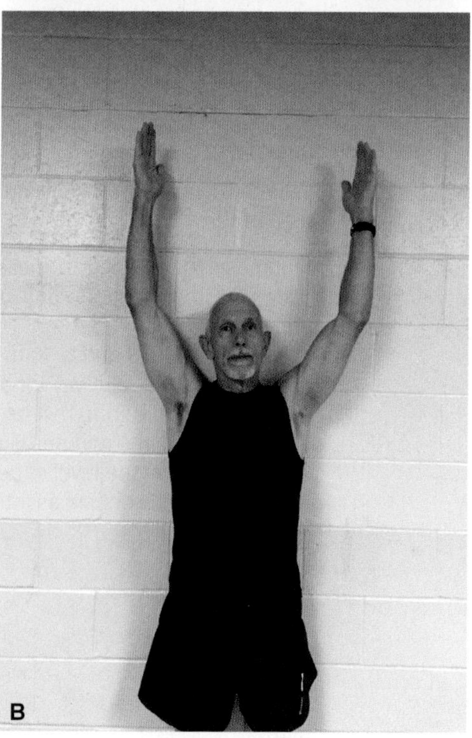

FIGURE 24.3 A balanced exercise program includes **(A)** aerobic, **(B)** flexibility,

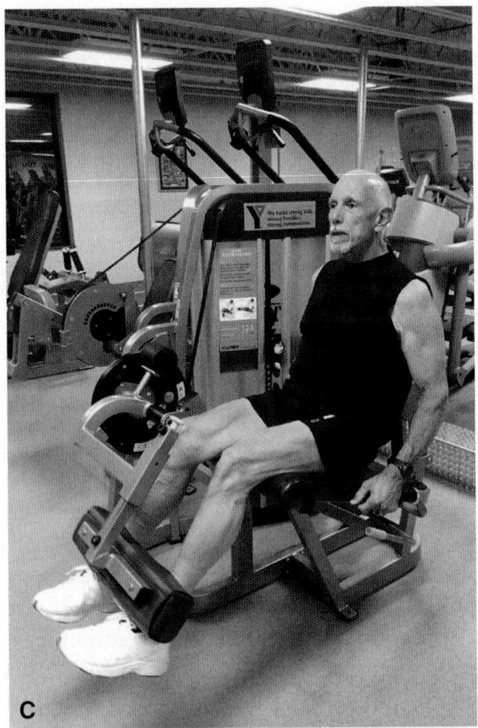

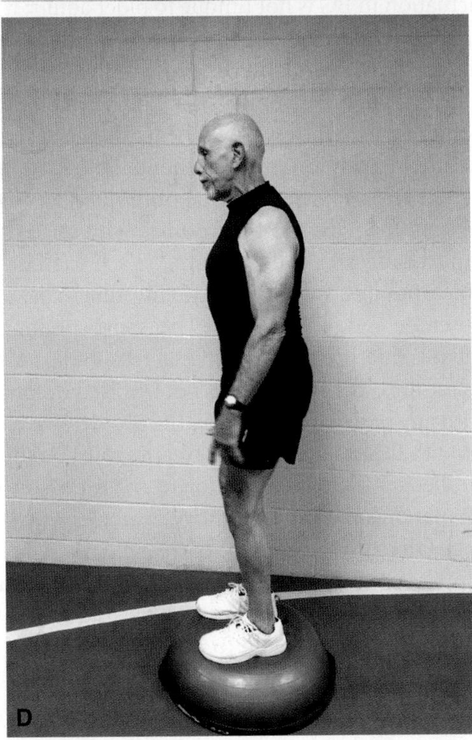

FIGURE 24.3—cont'd (C) resistance, and (D) balance exercises.

patient in order to identify the structural and functional impairments and related comorbidities is emphasized in order to develop a safe exercise program. The key point is, the exercise program should challenge the patient at his or her current level and then must be progressed so functional goals can be attained while monitoring the older adult for safety at all times.

Aerobic Exercise for the Older Adult

Principles of aerobic exercise are described in Chapter 7, including specific guidelines for patients with coronary disease, the deconditioned individual, and patients with chronic diseases, as well as for the older adult in general.

Guidelines Revisited

When providing instructions for aerobic exercises with the older adult, it is important to remember:

- Maximum heart rate is age related and decreases with age (220 minus age is a general guideline).
- Stroke volume decreases with age, resulting in decreased cardiac output.
- Arteriovenous oxygen difference decreases as a result of decreased lean body mass and low oxygen-carrying capacity.
- Maximum oxygen uptake decreases so that aerobic capacity decreases about 10% per decade in sedentary men.
- Blood pressure increases because of increased peripheral vascular resistance.
- Respiratory rate increases and maximum voluntary ventilation decreases with age.

Recommendations

Recommendations for aerobic training are to participate in 150 minutes of moderate-intensity aerobic activity (brisk walking) or 75 minutes of vigorous-intensity aerobic activity (jogging or running) every week or an equivalent mix of moderate and vigorous intensity aerobic activity, Bouts of activity may be as short as 10 minutes at a time, just so the total time is obtained per week.[197]

Talk test. The talk test is a simple concept that can be employed when working with patients. The concept of being able to maintain a conversation or talk while performing an activity is thought to correlate with moderate-intensity aerobic exercise, while only being able to say a few words without taking a breath or having difficulty maintaining a conversation correlates with vigorous intensity. The talk test has been demonstrated to be a gauge of aerobic exercise intensity.[50,84,194,207,268]

Flexibility Exercises for the Older Adult

Principles of stretching and flexibility exercises are presented in detail in Chapter 4.

Guidelines Revisited

When providing instructions for mobility exercises with the older adult, it is important to remember:

- A low-intensity, long-duration stretch is the safest and most effective form of stretch.
- With age, there is a decrease in the maximum tensile strength and the rate of adaptation to tissue stress is

slower resulting in increased tendency for tears with stretching.

- With co-morbidities such as nutritional deficiencies, hormonal imbalances, and dialysis, connective tissue may become injured at lower levels of tissue stress.

Recommendations

For long-lasting effects of flexibility and stretching, it is critical to use any newly gained range of motion (ROM). Encourage the older adult to include daily activities that require reaching overhead, out to the side, and behind the back, as well as moving their trunk, neck, and lower extremity joints through as much ROM as possible.

Balance Training for the Older Adult

Chapter 8 provides background material and principles of exercises for impaired balance and includes an extensive section on evidence-based balance exercise programs for fall prevention in the elderly. Later in this chapter (see the section on Common Disorders in Older Adults and Exercise Recommendations), there is a discussion on the risk of falls in the older adult with a detailed discussion on the importance of balance training as well as strengthening exercises and task-specific exercises to reduce the risk.

Guidelines Revisited

When providing instructions for balance exercises with the older adult, it is important to remember:

- Be sure the person has good sitting balance before proceeding to standing activities
- Have safety measures in place such as a secure surface where the individual can grab with one or two hands if necessary
- Challenge the person at a level where they are safe. Consider:
  - Base of support (standing double leg, tandem stance, single leg stance)
  - Support surface (stationary, flat, moving, soft, wobble board)
  - Superimposed movements (head, trunk, extremity, small to large range)
  - Perturbations (anticipated, magnitude, speed)
  - Surroundings (nonmoving, moving)
- Incorporate functional tasks when ready
  - Sit to stand using hands on arm rests, progress to no use of hands
  - Rising up on toes; progress to toe walking
  - Rocking back onto heels; progress to heel walking
  - Walk, then turn around
  - Side walking, backward walking
  - Reaching overhead, behind, to each side, toward the floor

Recommendations

Exercise classes such as tai chi or other group balance exercise programs may provide a fun environment while teaching movement patterns that require balance. Encourage each individual to perform balance activities independently at home at least 15 to 20 minutes per day and progress to more challenging activities as able.

Resistance Exercise for the Older Adult

Principles of resistance exercise and general procedures for developing resistance programs are described in detail in Chapter 6. Resistance exercises are often neglected as a person ages, yet research has documented the value of strength training for maintaining functional independence as well as recovery from various pathologic conditions.[101,104,117,137,185,187,190,206] High intensity progressive resistance exercise has been demonstrated to be safe in older adults up to 96 years of age.[206] Although the principles of resistance exercise training for younger adults also apply to older adults,[233] the exercises may need to be modified due to medical conditions such as osteoporosis, progressions may be slower because of degenerative changes, greater attention to safety and injury prevention may be necessary due to cognitive as well as physical changes, and sessions may be delayed due to fluctuations in blood glucose (BG) levels. This fluctuation in BG is not unique to older adults; it is mentioned here due to diabetes being one of the most common causes of death in older adults and one of the most common chronic diseases in older adults (see ONLINE Table 24.1).

Although nonspecific exercise is better than no exercise, it is essential for older adults to receive an individualized examination of their specific needs and be prescribed a program to meet those needs. This must be coupled with ongoing monitoring and changes in the program.[17] Each exercise session should incorporate a warm-up, flexibility, functional or sport-specific exercise, and cool-down.[196] The "sport-specific exercise" component is interpreted as functional retraining and balance exercises for the older adult who is not involved in sports.

As with any patient, when initiating progressive resistance exercises with the older adult, the exercise must be supervised and modified so the patient performs the exercise correctly. Too often patients use compensatory strategies when exercising or may fail to do the exercise correctly. Thus, when introducing a patient to resistance exercises, initially use a lower weight to enhance learning the correct technique.[206] This also enables the connective tissue to adapt to the training with gradual increases in the number of repetitions and resistance to achieve overload.[195,197]

Safety and Special Precautions

Although resistance training has been shown to be safe in older adults, ongoing exercise supervision is necessary to assess for overtraining weakness, exacerbation of a musculoskeletal complaint, or exercising above the patient's level of the CV, pulmonary, or musculoskeletal capabilities. Use subthreshold intensities if symptoms increase with exercise. When performing resistance exercises, normal breathing is advocated,[164,195] and work only within the pain-free ranges.[195]

Guidelines Revisited and Recommendations

Exercise and Equipment Choices

Based on the results of the examination, determine what muscles and patterns of movement need to be strengthened to achieve the established goals. Determine safe positions and appropriate equipment that will match the capability of the patient at his or her current level, provide a challenge to progress, and address the specificity of training principle in order to meet the needs of the patient. For example, a patient who is seen in a home care setting may do well with functionally based resistance exercises such as those illustrated in Figure 24.4.

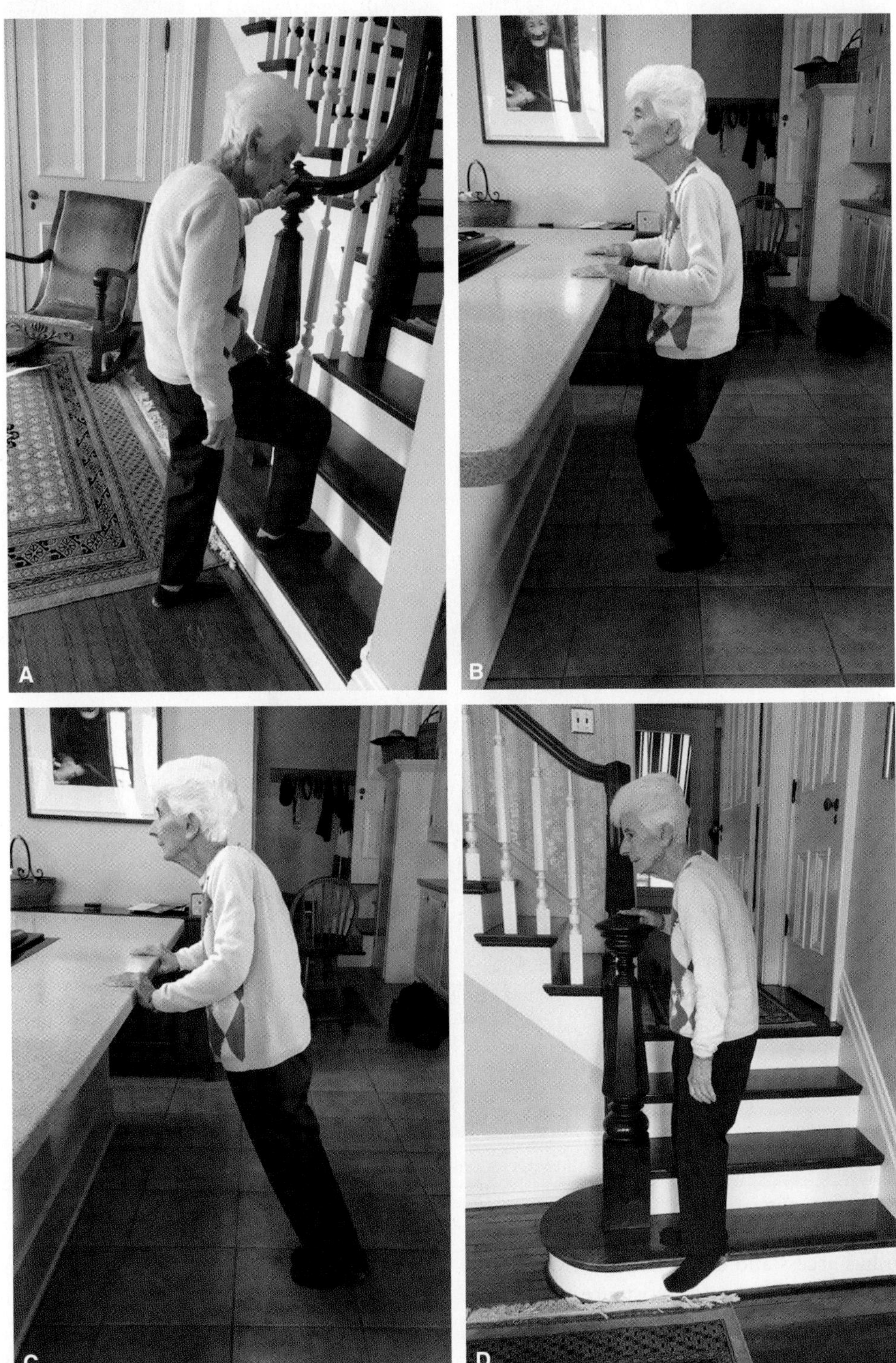

FIGURE 24.4 An example of a program that can be done in the home-care setting. **(A)** Ambulation and stairs, **(B)** mini-squats, **(C)** modified push-ups and/or planks, **(D)** lateral step-ups,

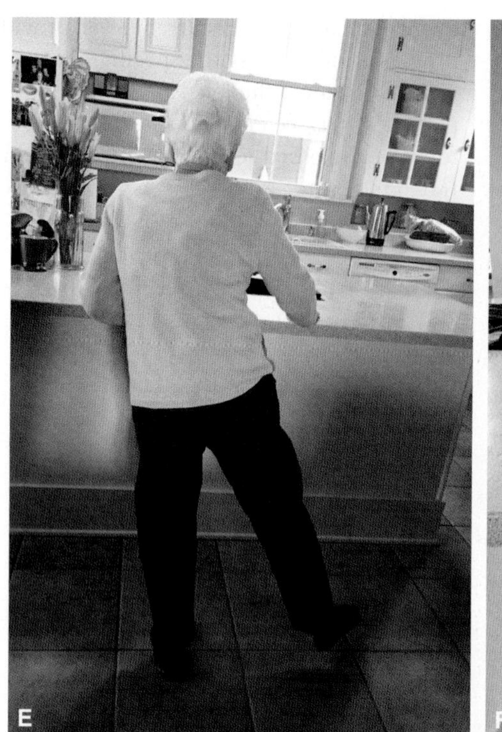

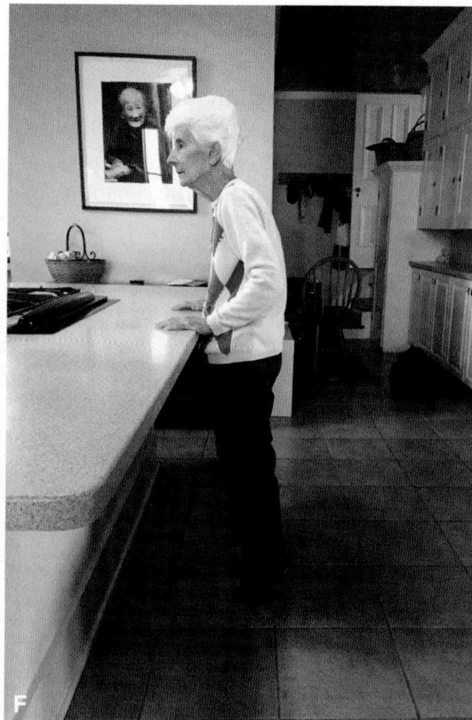

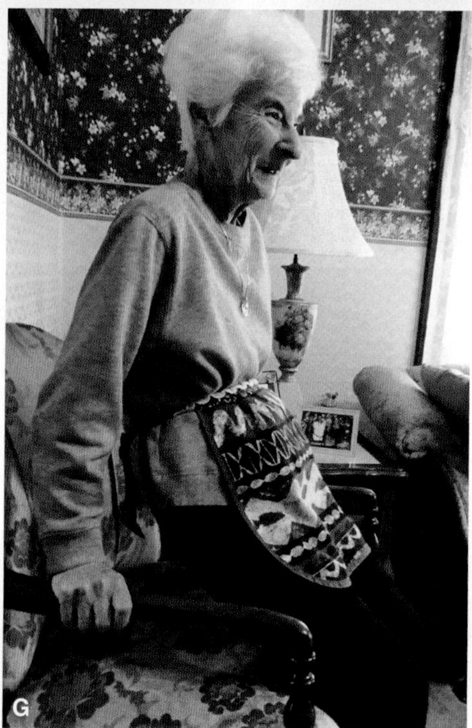

FIGURE 24.4—cont'd **(E)** hip abduction, **(F)** heel rises, and **(G)** repeated sitting push-ups/sit to stand.

A patient who has access and enjoys using a fitness facility may prefer machines that provide resistance, while another patient may prefer free weights. The use of elastic resistance bands has also been found to be effective and valuable for strength and power training in older adults and can easily be adapted for use in the clinic, gym, or home setting (Fig. 24.5).[89,110,148,157,238] Some forms of resistance may meet several goals. For example, patients may wear a weighted vest for strengthening purposes and/or to increase body weight with the benefit of enhancing bone density. (The use of a weighted vest will be discussed in the osteoporosis section.) A secondary benefit to using weight training machines is improvement in balance. This is due to the need for multiple transfers and transitional movements to get on and off of the exercise equipment. If a person does 3 sets of 10 different exercises on 8 machines, that individual will perform many transfers.

Table 24.3 provides suggestions of exercises that can be used to include 8 to 10 muscle groups in a resistance training program for the older adult. Many of the exercises are illustrated in the spine and extremity chapters (see Chapters 16 through 23).

Exercise and Equipment Choices: Modifications

When working with an older adult patient, the presence of comorbidities such as shoulder OA, rotator cuff injury, osteopenia,

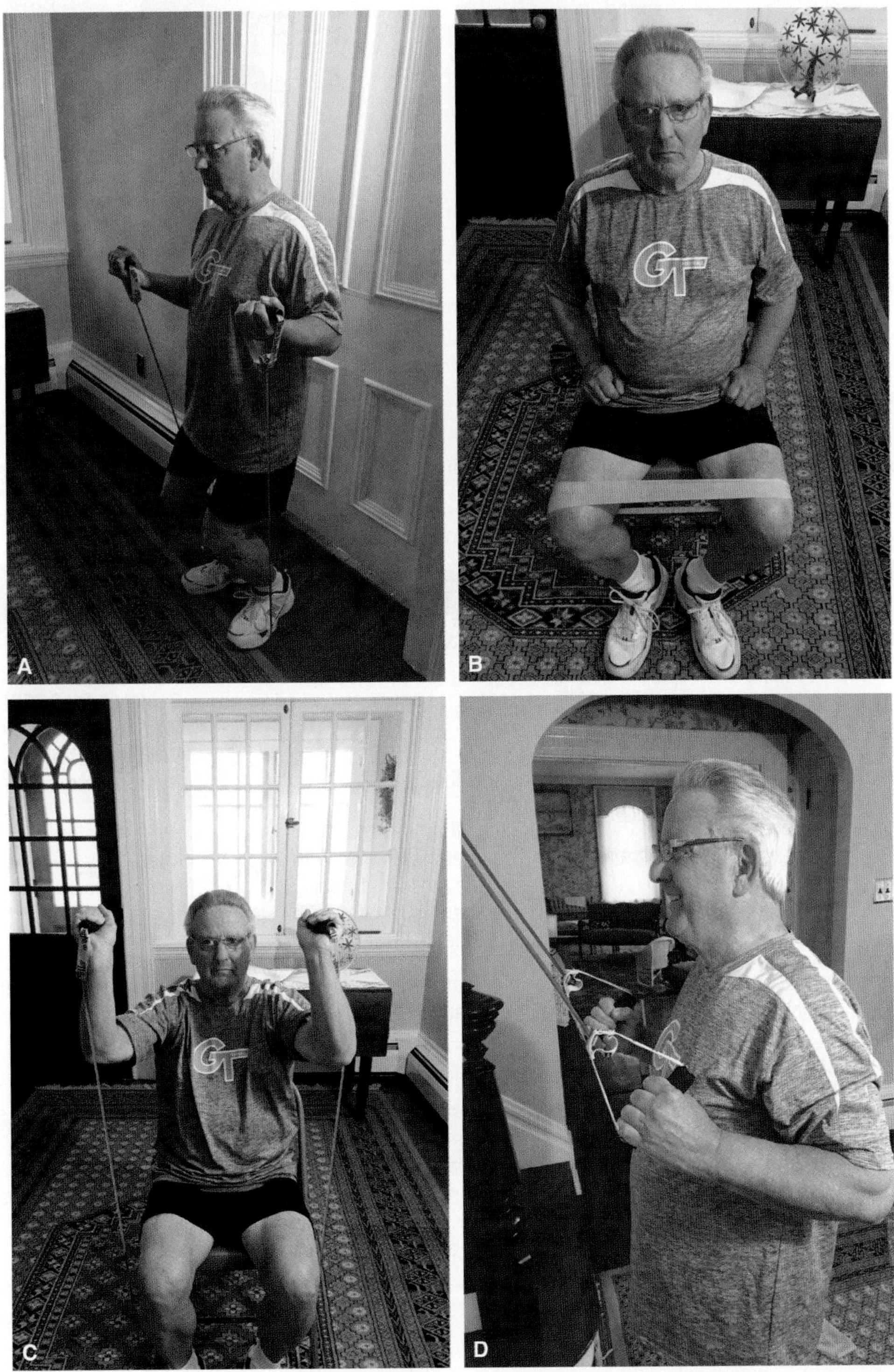

FIGURE 24.5 Examples of exercises that can be done using elastic resistance bands in the home setting. **(A)** Mini-squats/leg press, **(B)** hip abduction with lateral rotation, **(C)** shoulder presses, **(D)** lat pull-downs,

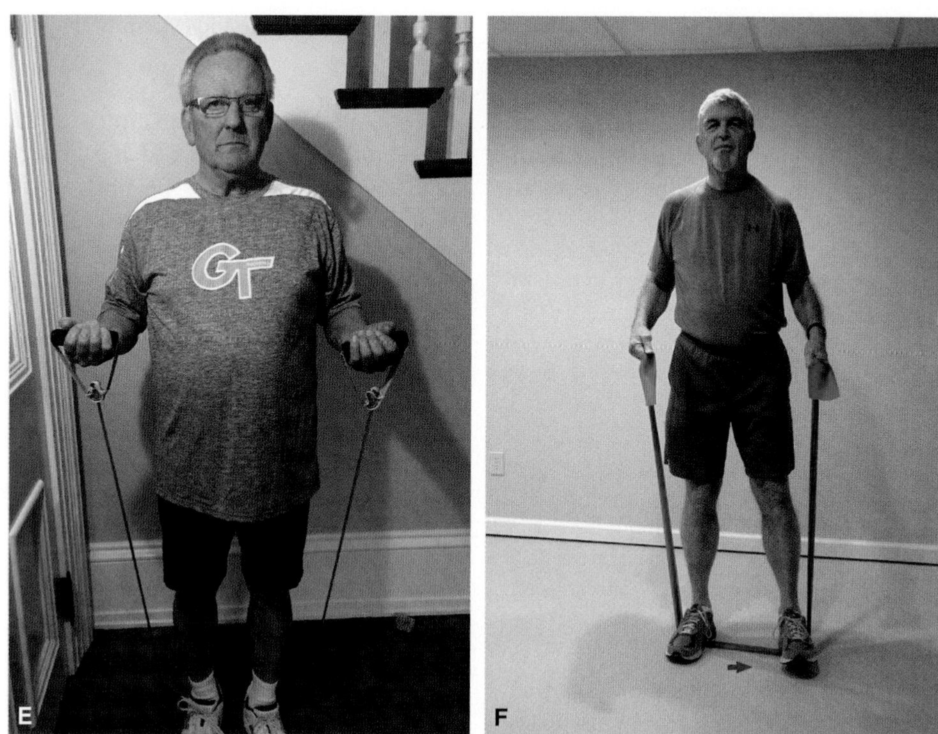

FIGURE 24.5—cont'd (E) biceps curl, and **(F)** weight-bearing hip abduction with the patient walking sideways (or performing repeated hip abduction).

TABLE 24.3 Resistance Training of Key Muscle Groups for Older Adults Using Machines, Weight Bearing, and Dynamic Constant External Resistance

Muscle Group	Machine	Weight Bearing	Dynamic Constant External Resistance (DCER) Using Free Weights, Resistance Bands, Weighted Balls, Cable System, etc.
Hip Extensors	Leg press Hip extension machine	Bridging (hamstring recruitment is greater with less knee flexion; gluteal recruitment is greater with more knee flexion)	Hip extension Knee curls Hip extension with knee flexion
Knee Extensors	Knee extension machine	Mini-squats Wall squats Steps Lunges	Knee extension with long and short arc quads Straight leg raise
Hip Abductors	Hip abduction machine	Standing hip abductions, works the limb abducting and isometrically the weight-bearing limb Elastic resistance around distal thighs or ankles and monster walk	Supine, prone, and side-lying hip abductions Clam shells Standing/cable, elastic band hip abductions

Continued

TABLE 24.3 Resistance Training of Key Muscle Groups for Older Adults Using Machines, Weight Bearing, and Dynamic Constant External Resistance—cont'd

Muscle Group	Machine	Weight Bearing	Dynamic Constant External Resistance (DCER) Using Free Weights, Resistance Bands, Weighted Balls, Cable System, etc.
Hip External Rotators		Monster walks with elastic resistance around knees Diagonal hip abduction/ external rotation with elastic resistance around ankles to emphasize gluteus medius	Sitting or side-lying clam shells with elastic resistance around knees
Ankle Plantar Flexors	Leg press	Heel rises	Heel rises holding weights; long sitting with elastic resistance under foot
Trunk Flexors	Straight and rotational abdominal machine **CONTRAINDICATION:** Trunk flexion with potential or actual diagnosis of osteopenia/osteoporosis. Alternative is stabilization exercises.	Plank Side plank Ball roll out using a large gym ball Modify exercises if painful, shoulders may need to be in less flexion	Curl-up/crunches Stabilization exercise progression beginning supine, progressing to sitting and standing with resistance **CONTRAINDICATION:** Trunk flexion (curl-ups and crunches) with osteopenia/osteoporosis
Trunk Extensors	Trunk extension machine **CAUTION:** arthritis or stenosis may cause neurologic symptoms	Bridging	Stabilization exercise progression beginning in quadruped, progressing to sitting and standing with resistance
Scapular Retractors, Shoulder Extensors	Pull down machine, rowing	Corner press-out (with back to corner)	Y and T positions with weight in prone or over a large gym ball; sitting using elastic resistance/ cable system
Shoulder External Rotators	Cable system		Side-lying or sitting shoulder external rotation
Shoulder Abductors	Lateral raise machine	Quadruped moving diagonally or straight plane Moving a ball on the wall	Lateral raises Shoulder flexion Shoulder extension
Elbow Flexors	Biceps curl machine	Pull-ups and assisted pull-ups; using an assist may enable successful performance of pull-ups; seated pull-ups	Curls
Elbow Extensors	Elbow extension machine	Push-ups with a plus Wall push-ups with a plus Dips	Elbow extension

or a loss in ROM, result in a need to modify exercises to the patient's ability (Fig. 24.6). The exercises should not be painful or exacerbate a potential problem. For example, rather than performing trunk curls or crunches, which cause vertebral body compression, have the patient with osteoporosis do partial range on a large gym ball or BOSU(tm) to a neutral spine position avoiding full range into trunk flexion.

Exercise modifications that challenge the individual can also be adapted for those who have the loss of independent ambulation (Fig. 24.7). The patient's constraints dictate the selection of the interventions. For example, if a patient has limited space, performing exercises at their kitchen counter may provide a stable surface for closed chain and balance exercises (see Fig. 24.4 B, C, E and F and Fig 24.9 later in the chapter).

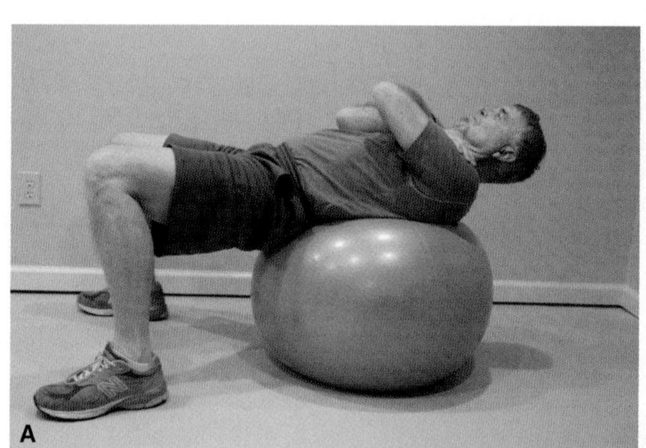

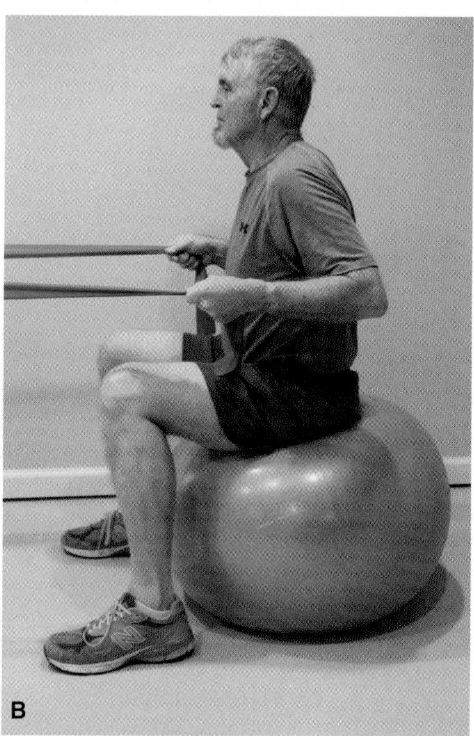

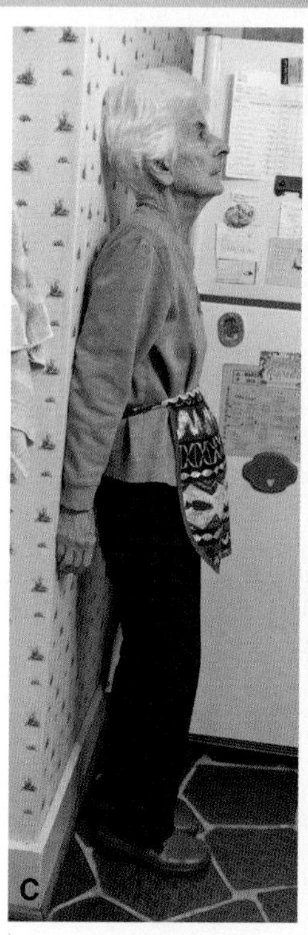

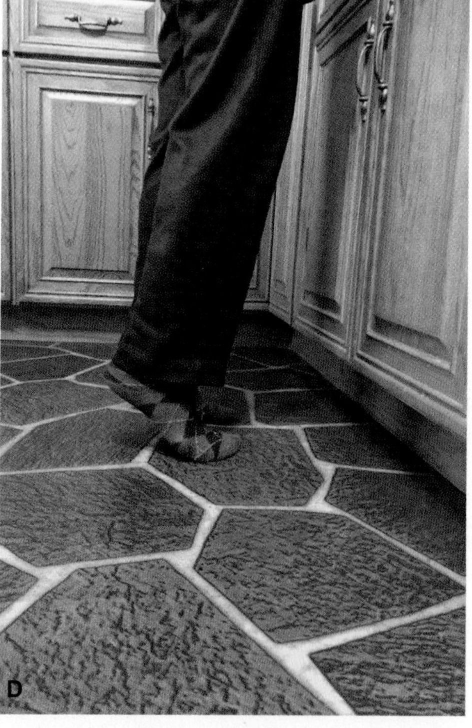

FIGURE 24.6 Examples of exercise modifications to meet the needs of older adults. **(A)** Abdominal strengthening without going into trunk flexion using a large gym ball through partial range, **(B)** sitting balance combined with strengthening extensor postural muscles, **(C)** posture training using a wall for tactile cues, and **(D)** weight-bearing plantar flexion with support.

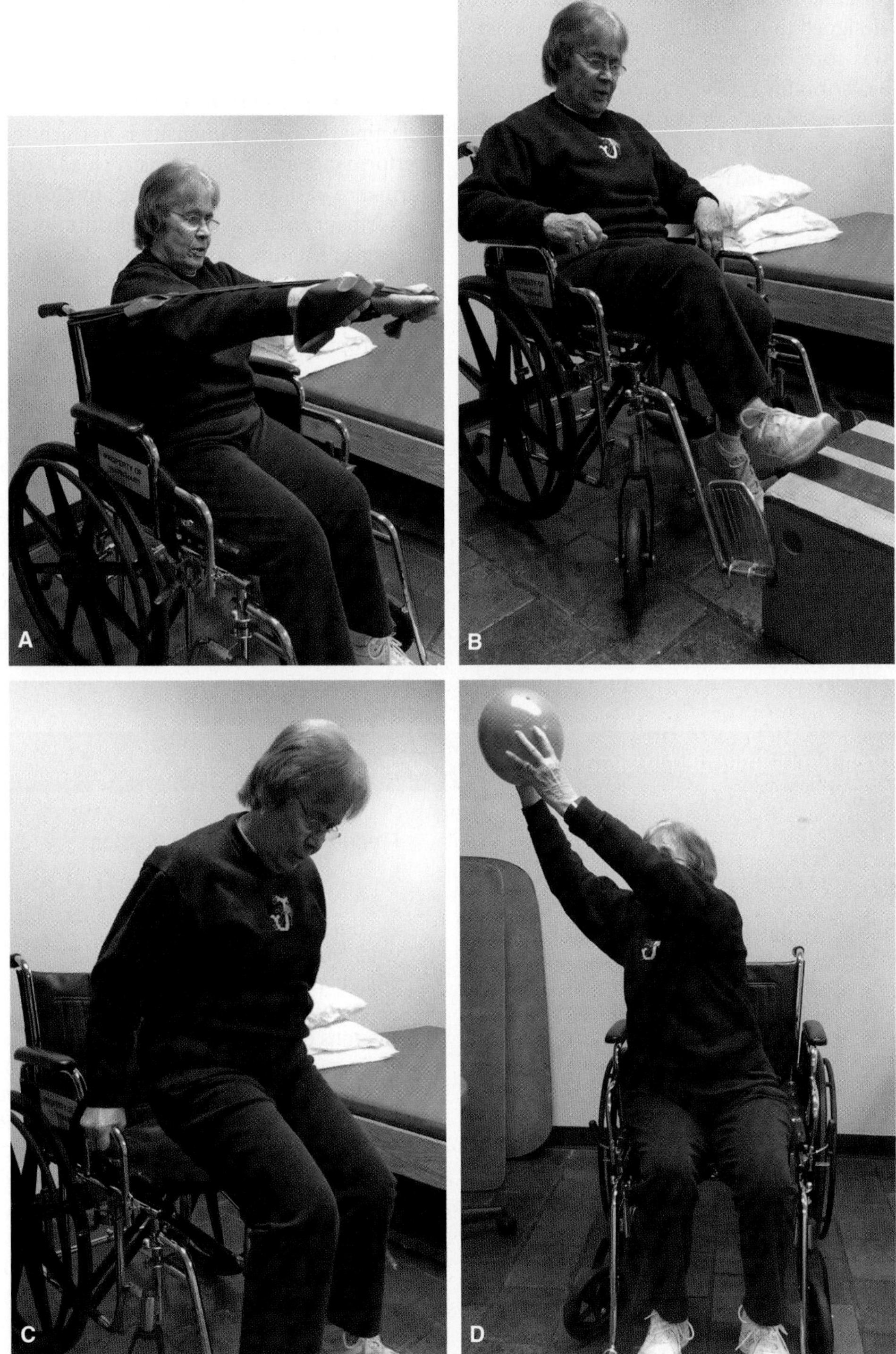

FIGURE 24.7 An example exercises that have been modified to meet the needs of an older adult in a wheelchair. **(A)** Scapular protraction with resisted band, **(B)** seated step ups (raise height as patient improves), **(C)** sitting push-up with feet on the floor, and **(D)** seated diagonal patterns with ball (can use weighted ball).

Intensity of Exercise

Intensity is based on load, repetitions, and sets as described in Chapter 6. Avers and Brown[16] report that when exercise or activities are performed below the 60% 1 RM, slight improvements of 5% to 10% may occur on strength tests but that recruitment of motor units and motor learning rather than actual strength changes in the muscle may be the reason. The initial rapid strength gains achieved following the start of resistance training is attributed to neural adaptations and motor learning. Patients are often discharged from therapy before the 12 weeks necessary to achieve actual strength gains.[210] Thus, it is essential for therapists and assistants to educate the patients on the need to continue exercising following discharge by participating in community based programs or by exercising independently.

Borg scale. The original Borg 6 to 20 scale (see Box 25.4 in Chapter 25) was designed to match the heart rate response; i.e., a score of 9 was correlated with very light effort and a heart rate of 90 beats/minute.[30] The 6 to 20 scale was considered difficult to understand, so the revised 0 to 10 scale was developed (see Box 6.6 in Chapter 6). Although subjective measures of exercise intensity, both Borg scales provide valuable insight into the intensity of exercise. To determine 60% of a 1-RM intensity, various strategies may be employed. Avers and Brown[16] report the 60% threshold is when an individual can perform 15 repetitions with a rating of perceived exertion (RPE) of 12 to 13 on the original Borg scale or a 3 to 4 on the modified Borg scale. This is described as work or effort of "fairly light" to "moderately hard." When using either Borg scale to measure intensity, it is critical to take the time to explain the scale including the values at each end of the scale. The patient is advised to rate their total amount of exertion and fatigue combining all sensations including physical stress, effort, and fatigue and to avoid focusing on one aspect such as leg pain. The therapist should confirm the patient's self-report or level of exertion by repeating the number back to the patient. The use of either of Borg's RPE scales is especially helpful when heart-rate measurements are difficult or when a patient is on medications that impact heart rate responses to physical activity.[29,195,248]

Determining amount of resistance. Another approach to selecting the correct intensity is to teach the correct exercise performance at a lower intensity (load) and observe the performance of the exercise, noting any change in the quality of performance, such as muscle substitutions or inability to go through the entire range. (Refer to Box 6.2 in Chapter 6 for specific signs of muscle fatigue.) If the individual is able to complete 8 repetitions correctly but less than 15, the intensity is appropriate. If unable to complete 8 repetitions or shows signs of muscle fatigue, the weight should be decreased. If 15 repetitions is too easy, the weight should be increased.

Various strengthening protocol intensities are recommended for the older adult. Table 24.4 highlights several of these for comparison.

Sets

Research by Ribeiro and colleagues[210] demonstrated that performing 3 sets of resistance training is more effective for strengthening muscles than performing 1 set of exercises in

TABLE 24.4 Three Recommended Resistance Training Protocols for Older Adults

Intensity	Sets	Repetitions per Set (reps/set)	Frequency	Progression	Power
Recommendations from Avers and Brown.[16]					
60% of 1 RM is the minimal exercise load necessary	1 set for untrained individuals, (more sets if possible, although risk of injury increases with multiple sets)	Set reps at desired intensity	2-3 times/ week;24 to 48 hours of rest between sessions of same muscle group	Increase load 2%-10% once able to perform 12 to 15 reps	Initiate power once 2 sets of an exercise are performed with good form and no pain at an initial load 20% of 1 RM. Gradually increase toward 60% of 1 RM.
Recommendations from Haskell et al[108] and Nelson et al.[179]					
Moderate to high intensity (on modified Borg 3 = moderate and 5 = strong or heavy)	1 set if goal is to increase strength; 2-3 sets are more effective	8-12 reps	≥2-times/ week	Gradual increases in the amount of weight or the days/ week	Not addressed
Recommendations from Symons & Swank.[233]					
50%-80% 1 RM	2 to 3 sets	10-15 reps	2-3 days/week	Not specified	Must include higher velocity resistance exercise incorporated into training

older women following 12 weeks of training. Thus, when advocating continuation of progressive resistance exercise training after a patient is discharged from physical therapy, if the goal is to continue to increase muscle strength, three sets are recommended.[210] Ratamess and colleagues[205] recommended a 1- to 2-minute rest between moderate velocity sets but an increase to 3 to 5 minutes of rest for high-velocity training. In lieu of a patient or client sitting on a piece of equipment for that rest period to expire, it is recommended that the person employ *active recovery* and work a different muscle group. For example, to apply active recovery to Lou, described in Case 1 in Box 24.1, he would perform his strengthening exercises by doing one set on the leg press machine, then one set on the hamstring curl machine, then one set on the rowing machine, and then one set of dips. After completing the first set of all four exercises, he would repeat the circuit for a second set and then a third set. The cycling through of different muscle groups provides the needed rest or recovery.

Frequency of Exercise

Twenty-four to 48 hours are recommended between resistance training sessions for the same muscle groups for safe adaptation when working at an intensity of 60%.[129] In various practice settings, such as acute care, subacute rehabilitation, and skilled care, patients may be seen once or twice daily 5 to 7 days/week. In these circumstances, focusing on different muscle groups or varying activities such as task-specific skills, posture, balance, endurance, strengthening, and stretching should be alternated between sessions in order to allow tissues to safely adapt.[16] Incorporating other dimensions of rehabilitation, such as neuromuscular re-education and balance exercises, is invaluable when considering the potential need for functional interventions. The need to employ a multidimensional exercise program, as described in the next section, is recommended.[129, 157] A minimum frequency of performing a strengthening exercise to impact bone and muscle is two sessions/week.[129]

Speed of Exercise—Power

With aging there is a preferential loss of power attributed to the loss of type II muscle fibers and a decrease in velocity of contraction.[112,208,213] Power training should not be implemented with the older adult until a base has been established; i.e., the ability to perform three sets of each exercise prior to adding a power component to the training.

To address power, the rapid movement of light resistance is described as most practical and widely acceptable.[208] Patients should perform the concentric phase of each repetition as rapidly as possible, with the combined eccentric-concentric cycle being approximately 2 to 3 seconds.[110,167,208,232] (Table 24.5 provides guidelines for power training with older adults.[112]) Similar to the guidelines for resistance training, a 48-hour recovery is recommended between power training. Mizko and colleagues[167] found power training to be more efficacious than strength training to improve function in community dwelling older adults (mean age 72.5 +/- 6.3 years).

TABLE 24.5 Guidelines for Incorporating Power Into Resistance Training for Older Adults[112]

Set 1	8 repetitions	45% 1 RM
Set 2	8 repetitions	60% 1 RM
Set 3	≥8 repetitions	75% 1 RM

The concentric portion of each repetition should be performed as rapidly as possible. The eccentric portions should be controlled over approximately 3 seconds.

Progression

When progressing an exercise program, the same guidelines follow as for other populations but with continual monitoring for safety and the potential onset of injury or overwork weakness. It is essential to start at lower intensity and progress slowly.

Functional Training for the Older Adult

Functional training is most often geared toward attaining independence or improving basic activities such as steps, raising up and lowering self in a chair, reaching items overhead or on the floor, or simply walking. Efficiency, time to perform a task, effort, and the quality of the task may be incorporated in the interventions. The tests described in Table 24.2 will help to guide the therapist in designing appropriate interventions to enhance function. Thus, if the problem is sit to stand, then the patient needs to work on the task of sit to stand. If, initially, the muscles are too weak to perform the function without substitution, then focusing on the specific weak muscles also becomes part of the exercise intervention.

Common Disorders in Older Adults and Exercise Recommendations

With the "graying of America" and the life expectancy increasing, many diseases that affect older adults have become more prevalent. In this section, several common problems seen in older adults provide a background prior to discussing exercise interventions. One's medical diagnosis does not define the physical therapy treatment plan, although knowledge of the medical condition alerts the therapist to special considerations, precautions, and/or contraindications to interventions. The medical diagnosis should be used in conjunction with the clinical examination to determine the structural and functional impairments and to establish realistic goals for improving participation in functional activities. Numerous chronic conditions, as listed in ONLINE Table 24.1, and multiple other illness and injuries may threaten the older adults' independence. This section addresses common conditions and diagnoses seen in older adults, including falls, osteoporosis, sarcopenia, OA, obesity, cancer, T2DM, and incontinence. Each of these will be briefly described with cross references to other chapters within this text where additional information is presented.

Falls in Older Adults

Background

As people age there is an increased incidence in the number of falls. One out of every three older adults falls each year, with 20% of those falls resulting in serious injuries.[17,51,90,109,116] This incidence is even greater in the institutionalized elderly. Over the past decade, the number of deaths directly attributed to the injuries from falls has increased and is anticipated to increase with the aging of the Baby Boomer generation.

Fall Risk Assessment

All older adult patients should be screened for fall risk.[17,51] Each patient should be asked:

1. Have you fallen in the past year?
   - If yes—how many times did you fall?
   - If yes—were you injured when you fell?
2. Do you feel unsteady when standing or walking?
3. Do you have a fear of falling?

The above three questions are from the CDC's Stopping Elderly Accidents, Deaths, and Injuries (STEADI) initiative.[51] Screening items 1 and 2 are also recommended by Avin and colleagues in the Clinical Guidance Statement from the Academy of Geriatric Physical Therapy on the management of falls in community-dwelling older adults.[17] The need to perform a multifactorial fall risk assessment is not necessary for all patients 65 and older but is essential when screening indicates a prior fall in the past 12 months, difficulty with walking or balance, or a fear of falling.[17]

CLINICAL TIP

The STEADI Older Adult Fall Prevention[51] website from the CDC is valuable for all therapists and assistants working with older adults: http://www.cdc.gov/steadi/index.html. The STEADI initiative provides a comprehensive tool kit with educational information for health-care providers and older adult patients. Instructional videos and a webinar are also available. An Algorithm for Fall Risk Assessment and Interventions developed by the STEADI initiative is shown in Figure 24.8 to provide guidance for screening, examination, and interventions useful for physical therapists working with the older individual at risk for falling.[51]

Importance of Exercise to Reduce Fall Risks

A multidimensional program that includes resistance exercises, balance exercises, task specific training (gait, sit to stand, rising from the floor), correction of both environmental hazards, and selection of proper footwear should be included in patient interventions.[17.145-227] The Academy of Geriatric Physical Therapy of the APTA list these five specific recommendations based on strong level 1 evidence.[17]

Nonspecific exercise, low-intensity exercise, and generic group exercise programs may not meet the needs of older adults and reduce fall risk.[17] It is critical to recognize the need for long-term adherence: a dosage of at least 50 hours of challenging exercise (e.g. 2 hours/week for at least 6 months) is needed.[17] Improvements do not occur spontaneously and require more time than is generally approved by insurance companies; therefore, education on the importance of continuing the prescribed exercise program is critical.

Resistance Training

Improvements in balance and a decrease in falls occur from strength training in older adults.[137,145] The causes of falls are multifactorial with weakness of the legs being an intrinsic risk factor. Strengthening the muscles of the trunk and lower extremities with resistance exercises and power training is related to reducing falls.[68,137,187] Strength training has been found to benefit postural control and to decrease variability of reactions during stabilization training.[68] In addition, strengthening the trunk muscles has been shown to improve performance of ADLs in older adults by contributing to efficiency in use of upper and lower extremities and improved balance. A systematic review by Grenacher and colleagues[96] supports the use of core strengthening and Pilates exercises either as an adjunct with or alternative to traditional balance and/or resistance training programs for older adults.

Tai Chi

Tai chi is a mind and body practice that arose centuries ago from Asia. It incorporates postures, gentle movements, mental focus, breathing, and relaxation and has proven to be beneficial in decreasing fall risk.[130,148,173] When the movements are performed quickly, tai chi is considered a form of self-defense. Tai chi also benefits heart disease, cancer, and other chronic diseases such as Parkinson's, OA, and fibromyalgia. It has been reported to improve pain, sleep, and anxiety.[173] When performing tai chi, strength, self-awareness, deep breathing, static and dynamic balance, ROM, endurance, positioning and postural awareness, weight bearing, and relaxation are incorporated into the various movements performed.[130,148,173]

Balance Training

The ability to maintain balance requires complex integration of the somatosensory, visual, and vestibular systems—all of which are affected with aging. Impairments involving balance are described in detail in Chapter 8, with a description of risk assessment (see Tables 8.2 and 8.3) and interventions (see Boxes 8.4 and 8.5, Table 8.4, and related figures in Chapter 8). Similar to progressing resistance exercises, progress balance interventions that safely challenge the patient (Fig. 24.9).

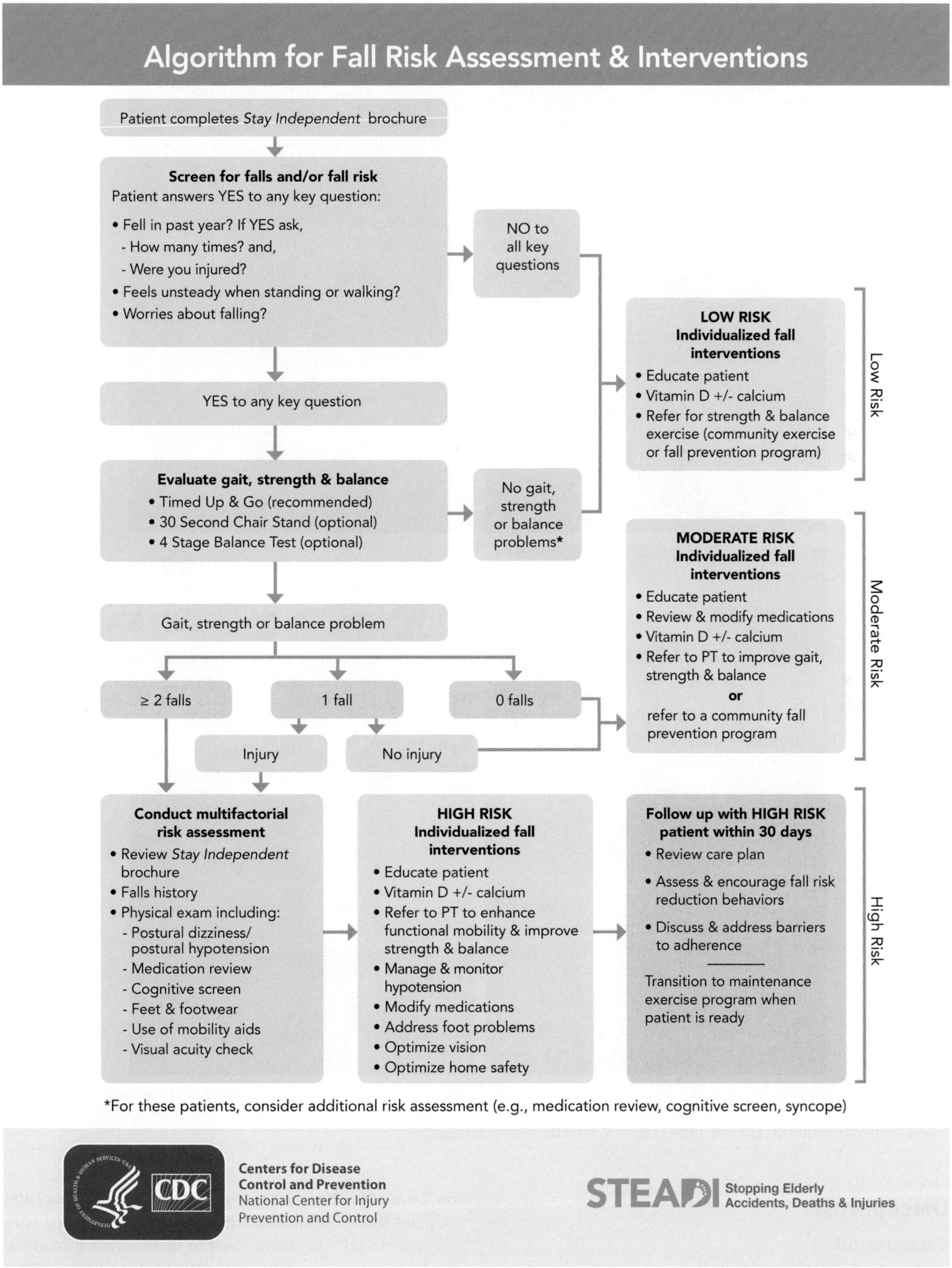

Algorithm for Fall Risk Assessment & Interventions

Patient completes *Stay Independent* brochure

Screen for falls and/or fall risk
Patient answers YES to any key question:

- Fell in past year? If YES ask,
  - How many times? and,
  - Were you injured?
- Feels unsteady when standing or walking?
- Worries about falling?

NO to all key questions → LOW RISK

YES to any key question

Evaluate gait, strength & balance

- Timed Up & Go (recommended)
- 30 Second Chair Stand (optional)
- 4 Stage Balance Test (optional)

No gait, strength or balance problems* → LOW RISK

Gait, strength or balance problem

≥ 2 falls → Conduct multifactorial risk assessment

1 fall → Injury → Conduct multifactorial risk assessment; No injury → MODERATE RISK

0 falls → MODERATE RISK

LOW RISK
Individualized fall interventions

- Educate patient
- Vitamin D +/- calcium
- Refer for strength & balance exercise (community exercise or fall prevention program)

Low Risk

MODERATE RISK
Individualized fall interventions

- Educate patient
- Review & modify medications
- Vitamin D +/- calcium
- Refer to PT to improve gait, strength & balance

or

refer to a community fall prevention program

Moderate Risk

Conduct multifactorial risk assessment

- Review *Stay Independent* brochure
- Falls history
- Physical exam including:
  - Postural dizziness/ postural hypotension
  - Medication review
  - Cognitive screen
  - Feet & footwear
  - Use of mobility aids
  - Visual acuity check

HIGH RISK
Individualized fall interventions

- Educate patient
- Vitamin D +/- calcium
- Refer to PT to enhance functional mobility & improve strength & balance
- Manage & monitor hypotension
- Modify medications
- Address foot problems
- Optimize vision
- Optimize home safety

Follow up with HIGH RISK patient within 30 days

- Review care plan
- Assess & encourage fall risk reduction behaviors
- Discuss & address barriers to adherence

Transition to maintenance exercise program when patient is ready

High Risk

*For these patients, consider additional risk assessment (e.g., medication review, cognitive screen, syncope)

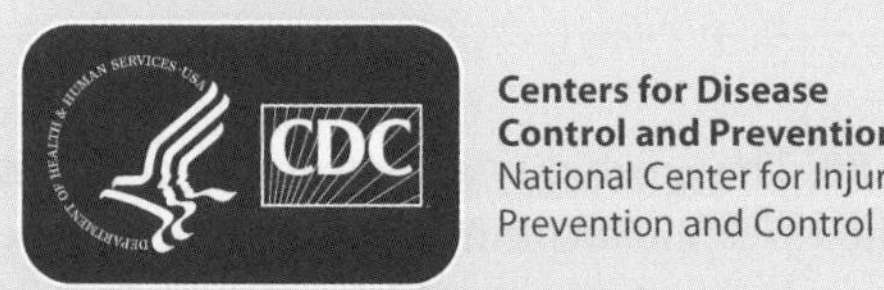

Centers for Disease Control and Prevention
National Center for Injury Prevention and Control

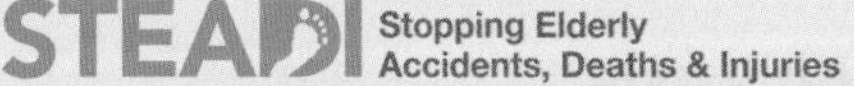

FIGURE 24.8 Algorithm for Fall Risk Assessment and Interventions from STEADI[51] *(Reproduced with permission from the Centers for Disease Control and Prevention: http://www.cdc.gov/steadi/)*

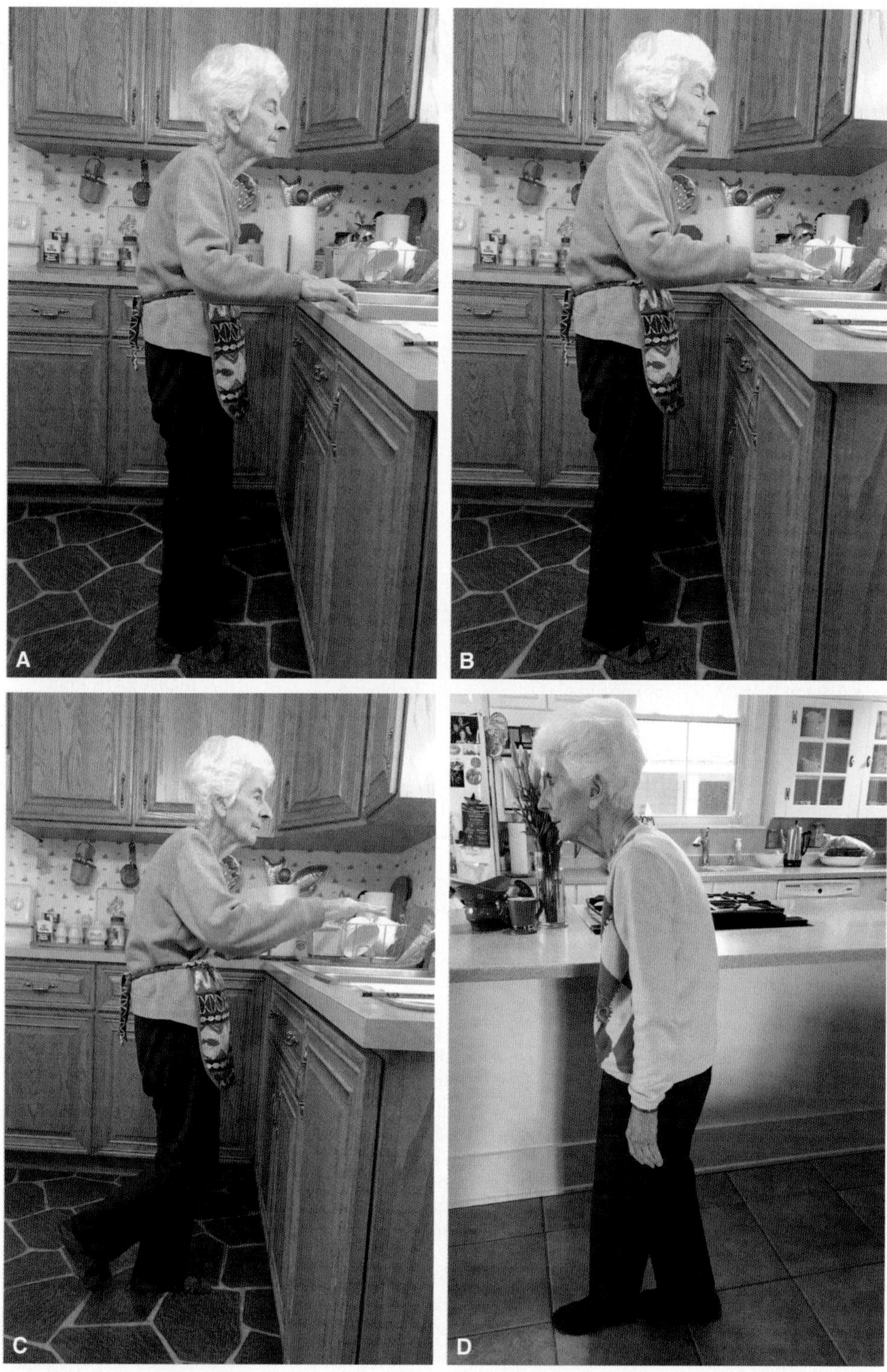

FIGURE 24.9 An example of balance exercise progression in the home setting by modifyingthe amount of support through the hands. **(A)** Both hands using light tactile cues, with eyes closed for greater challenge; **(B)** both hands hovering above the support surface, with eyes closed for greater challenge; **(C)** one-legged standing; and **(D)** tandem Romberg.

Osteoporosis

Background

Osteoporosis is considered to be the most common bony disorder resulting in risk of fractures. Peak bone mass is attained by the third decade of a woman's life with approximately 30% loss by age 80. The morbidity and mortality of hip fractures is one of the three most common fractures associated with osteoporosis. Hip fractures result in up to a 25% increase in mortality within 1 year following the fracture, with another 25% of patients requiring long-term care and the remaining 50% not attaining their pre-hip fracture status.[184] (Refer to

Chapter 6 and Box 6.13 for a discussion of pathological fractures and precautions, and to Chapter 11 for a detailed description of osteoporosis and recommendations for exercise interventions.)

Considerations for Interventions

Strength training, weight-bearing exercises, and postural extension exercises are hallmark interventions for older adults for primary, secondary, and tertiary prevention associated with osteoporosis or osteopenia. Generally this is coupled with a well-balanced diet, adequate calcium and vitamin D, smoking cessation, minimal alcohol consumption, fall prevention strategies, and possible pharmacological interventions.[184,265] Box 24.5 summarizes considerations and recommendations when working with the older adult with or at risk for osteoporosis. (See also Box 6.13 in Chapter 6 for precautions that should be taken with resistance exercise.)

Importance of Exercise in Managing Osteoporosis

Postural Training

The employment of spinal extension and postural exercises is critical when considering the incidence of compression fractures in individuals with or at risk of osteoporosis. Schultz and colleagues[215] found that with the trunk at 30° of flexion, the compression load on the third lumbar vertebra is 1,800 N with the arms at the chest and 2,610 N when holding 2 kg (4.4 lb) of weight in each hand. This is significantly greater than the 300 to 1,200 N of force necessary to fracture an osteoporotic vertebra.[77]

Resistance Training and Weight-Bearing Exercises

Muscle contractions and mechanical loading of the spine and extremities utilizing resistance training and weight-bearing exercises stimulate osteoblastic activity for improving bone density and reducing fracture risk.[27,118,200] Weight-bearing and endurance activities (three to five times/week) and resistance exercise (two to three times/week) are recommended for bone health.[134] A systematic review on the effectiveness of resistance exercise for older adults with decreased bone density concluded that resistance training was beneficial on the self-reported physical function and ADLs.[265]

Weight-bearing exercises such as walking, jogging, and stair climbing also have the benefit of improving cardiopulmonary fitness. These interventions for primary, secondary, and tertiary osteoporosis are summarized in Table 24.6.

Weighted Vests

Another less commonly used option but one that shows positive results is the use of a weighted vest in the management of osteoporosis (Fig. 24.10).[110,218,224,267] Weighted vests are also used for power training, walking, and other activities. Weighted vests increase resistance and body weight while exercising, walking, and performing ADLs. Increasing an individual's weight via the vest serves as a stimulus for increasing bone density while the wearer is physically active.

Recommended guidelines for use of weighted vests. It is essential that the vest is adjustable, that the majority of the weight be on the pelvis, and that there are no areas causing pain. Similar to the use of orthotics, when initiating the use

BOX 24.5 Considerations and Recommendations for Management of Patients With Osteoporosis

Considerations

- Height loss of >1.5" (3.8 cm) increases the likelihood of a vertebral fracture being present[184]
- At high risk for fragility fractures
- When trunk is in flexion, there is greater compressive loads on the vertebra
- Only 20% of individuals with osteoporotic compression fractures receive treatment

Recommendations

- Screen all patients for fall risk.
- Utilize the FRAX to screen all patients for fracture risk.[193,269]
- Educate on risks and importance of exercise.
- Have the patient:
  - Perform weight-bearing, strengthening exercises and resistance exercise that emphasize postural extension two to three times/week.
  - Perform endurance, weight-bearing activities three to five times/week.
  - Perform core and abdominal strengthening in a nonflexed position.
  - Employ good body mechanics with spine in neutral.
- Make appropriate referrals for bone density screening and nutritional consult.

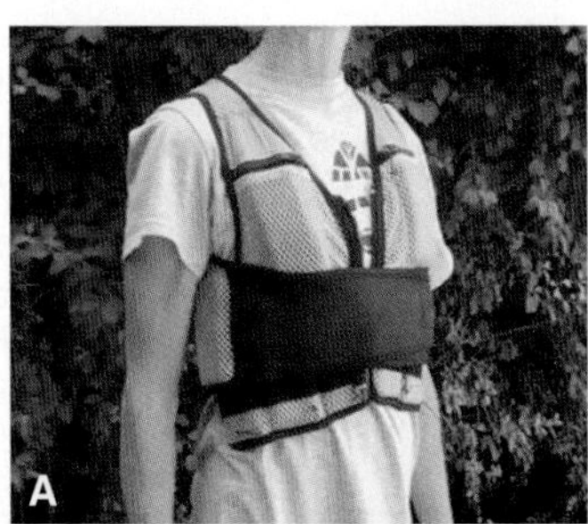

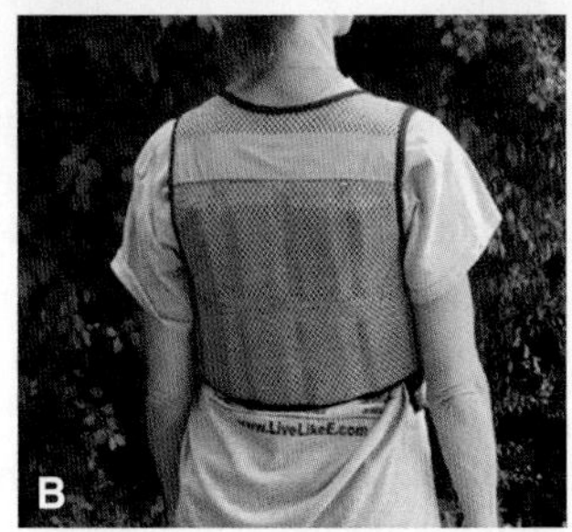

FIGURE 24.10 **(A)** Anterior and **(B)** posterior images of a weighted vest used in the management of osteoporosis and/or to increase body weight for resistance exercises.

TABLE 24.6 Management of Primary, Secondary, and Tertiary Osteoporosis

	Description	Clinical Examples	Interview, Tests, and Measures	Interventions
Primary	Prevention of osteoporosis or osteopenia in someone susceptible to the problem or disease through strategies to promote general health	56-year-old female being seen for DeQuervain's of her hand. Family history of osteoporosis; cessation of menses 2-years ago. On inspection, patient is thin but muscular in nature.	Have you experienced height loss? Have you had any fractures as an adult? Have you taken steroids? Do you smoke or have alcohol regularly? Ask if willing to look at total patient, consider measuring height, objective posture measurement like tragus to wall; employ the FRAX.	Focus on education, postural and weight-bearing exercises, resistance training, body mechanics, and nutrition.
Secondary	Early diagnosis of osteoporosis or osteopenia made through screening; early diagnosis enables initiation of intervention	60-year-old female with a diagnosis of osteoporosis. She is referred to PT for spinal stenosis and disc herniation at C4-5, C5-6, and C6-7, neck pain, and radicular symptoms. She is being managed conservatively and has begun taking calcium and osteoporosis medications to increase bone density prior to surgical interventions and fusion of the spine.	Assess for myelopthic changes, bowel and bladder involvement, loss of balance, weakness of legs, and hyperreflexia. Query regarding the Physical Activity Vital Signs (PAVS); what type of exercise is performed by the patient and willingness to modify or make changes. Assess deep tendon reflexes, Babinski Hoffman's, and clonus.	Interventions are same as primary prevention interventions but emphasize progressive ambulation and weight-bearing exercises.
Tertiary	Clinical diagnosis of osteoporosis and presence of fragility fractures, interventions designed to limit the degree of disability, promote recovery of function, and minimize the disease progression	75-year-old female who is being seen 10-weeks post fragility fracture of the femoral neck secondary to a fall while walking on level surface. Patient has a history of 2 spinal compression fractures and a height loss of 3". Patient is being seen through home health care (recently returned home from skilled care). She is ambulating with a standard cane, weight bearing as tolerated.	Ask if patient experiences pain at rest or with activity. Ask about current level of function and prior level of function. Does the patient have a fear of falling or any self-restriction of activities? Use objective measures such as gait speed, TUG, 30s-STS, grip, and posture.	Focus on function. Progressively challenge the patient as the status improves. Employ task-specific training and weight-bearing exercises.

of weighted vests, start slowly and progress gradually. Shaw and Stone[218] used a beginning vest weight of 5% of body weight with a 1% to 2% increase until 10% of body weight was achieved. This was followed by a more gradual 0.5% to 1% increase in weight every 2 weeks until 20% of body weight was attained. It is recommended that the vest be worn 3 days/week for resistance power exercises such as jumping or for several hours daily while being active.[85,218,224,267] A website selling the vests advocates 1 hour/day, 5 days/week, with a maximum vest weight of 16 pounds.[85] Because there is a paucity of clinically based evidence related to usage, the authors of this chapter recommend monitoring patients for their ability to maintain good posture and the absence of pain with a gradual, monitored increase in vest weight until attaining a desired weight. Similarly, the time spent wearing the vest is to start low and gradually progress usage. The use of the weighted vest for low-weight individuals should be used as long as the individual is ambulatory and able to tolerate it. If necessary or in response to medical changes, the amount of weight should be adjusted appropriately. Guidelines for their use in pediatric physical therapy and sensory processing disorders are not applicable for the older adult.

It is known that a body mass index (BMI) <21 kg/m2 is a risk factor for low bone mass density. For those with a low BMI, by determining a weight for a BMI >21 kg/m2, a goal for a reasonable maximum load with the vest can be attained.

PRECAUTION: Some patients may not tolerate the weighted vest due to clinical fragility, pain, or weakness.[224,267]

FOCUS ON EVIDENCE

A 6-month study with 1-year follow-up of 42 individuals with osteopenia consisting of a progressive exercise and education program was designed to establish the feasibility and adherence to the intervention, identify any adverse events, and document changes in lower extremity function. The resistance portion of the program included use of weight vests to increase resistance during the group exercise sessions, which were conducted two times/week under supervision of a therapist and 1 time/week at home. Data for 31 participants that were available at the 1-year follow-up showed that the program was feasible, had sufficient progression of training, and had high adherence with no adverse events. There were significant improvements in femoral trochanter bone mineral density, as well as quadriceps strength and dynamic balance, with overall improvement in lower extremity function.[102]

Sarcopenia/Frailty

Background

The etymology of *sarcopenia* has a Greek origin from *sarx* (flesh) and *penia* (poverty).[240] It is more than the age-associated loss of muscle mass. Sarcopenia causes a cascade of responses leading to frailty impacting balance, gait, and function.[63] This disease is a progressive 3% to 8% loss of lean muscle mass each decade beginning with the third decade, and it is believed to affect 30% of adults greater than 60 years old and 50% of older adults greater than 80 years (see Fig. 24.2).[70,73,117,155,203,22,230,240] The importance of regular resistance exercise coupled with protein intake is necessary in order to minimize the loss of muscle mass. Marcell[155] reports, "the only agreed-upon intervention ... (for sarcopenia) was regular physical exercise, stressing weight-training for elderly men and women."

Sarcopenic obesity. An individual who has both sarcopenia and obesity is described as having sarcopenic obesity (Fig. 24.11). The concept of sarcopenic obesity is when skeletal muscle mass is deficient relative to fat tissue.[63] This diagnosis is based on a measure of fat mass and skeletal muscle mass of the thigh using dual-energy X-ray absorptiometry (DXA) or magnetic resonance imaging (MRI). It is estimated that 4% to 12% of individuals over 60 years of age have sarcopenic obesity. This disease is managed with loss of fat, increased protein intake, and performance of resistance training.[63,70]

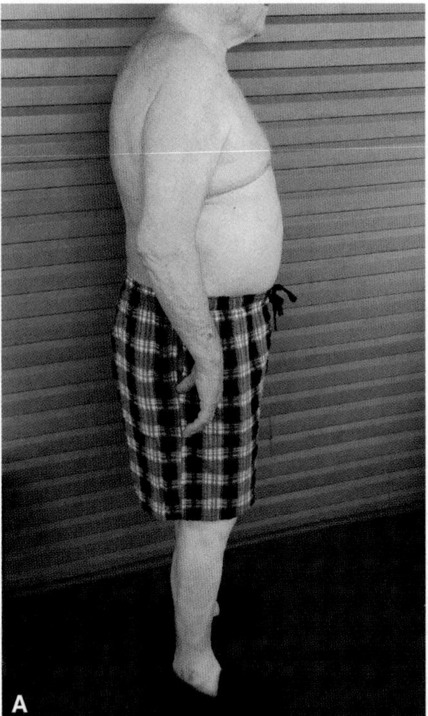

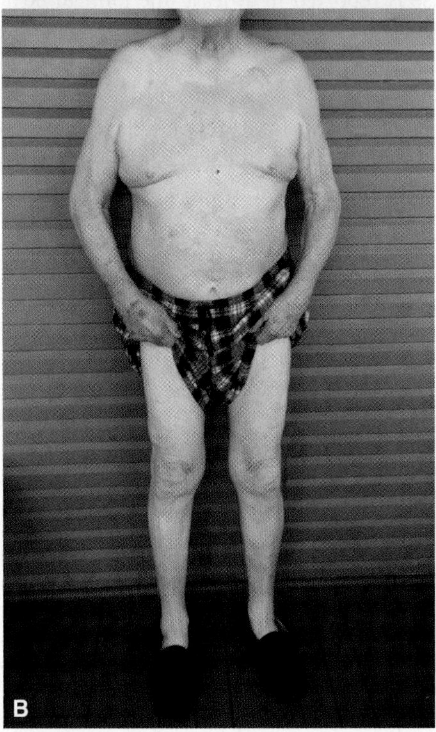

FIGURE 24.11 An older individual with sarcopenic obesity; **(A)** side view showing posture and **(B)** front view showing atrophy in legs greater than arms.

Considerations for Interventions

When working with the frail elderly population, it is critical to consider the risk of a fatigue fracture, the potential for loss of balance and falls, the nutrition of the patient, and whether the demands of an exercise program exceeds nutritional intake.

(Refer to Chapter 6 and Box 6.13 for a discussion of pathological fractures and precautions and to Chapter 8 for information on balance and falls.)

Importance of Exercise in Managing Sarcopenia

The multifactorial nature of sarcopenia has many facets partially attributed to inactivity and atrophy of fast-twitch (type II) muscle fibers that are recruited during high-intensity, anaerobic exercise. Physical inactivity coupled with motor unit remodeling, decreased hormone levels, and decreased protein synthesis may contribute to sarcopenia. Fortunately, with resistance exercise, sarcopenia may be partially reversed or progression of the loss slowed.[53,63,70,117,155,189,203,220,229,230,240]

Osteoarthritis

Background

Osteoarthritis is a common chronic disease affecting 30% to 50% of adults over age 65.[147] Among older adults, OA is the most common form of arthritis, with the greatest incidence in the knees followed by the hips.[159] This wear and tear degenerative disease is reported in at least one joint in 80% of older adults. Involvement of the hands occurs frequently, but the involvement of the knees and hips is reported to be more disabling. (Refer to Chapter 11 for a detailed description of OA and management guidelines for treatment. Also refer to Chapters 15 and 17 through 22 for specific guidelines for the treatment of OA in the spine and each of the extremity joints.)

Considerations for Interventions

When initially greeting an older adult patient, the therapist may take note of the patient's hands and the presence of Heberden or Bouchard nodes at the distal interphalangeal and proximal interphalangeal joints, respectively. The patient may also have genu varum, genu valgum, calcaneal valgum, or other deformities associated with OA.

Patients with OA must learn to value the importance of exercise; how to self-manage during painful exacerbations; and how to work on strengthening, stretching, balance, and aerobics during less painful times. Integrating the knowledge of biomechanics with observations of the patient performing exercises is critical in guiding the patient in correct exercise performance. For the patient to attain the ability to self-manage their disease, the patient must be aware of the impact of alignment and what to expect when performing exercises rather than adopting the adage "no pain, no gain."

When working with patients with OA:

- Avoid vigorous, repetitive movements on unstable joints.
- Be cautious if there is pain in the hands impacting grip when working with free weights or elastic bands.
- Observe the alignment, performance, and response to exercise and modify when indicated.
- Modify the program when a patient has increased pain, fatigue, weakness, or joint swelling to decrease stress on the joint.
- Avoid stretching, strengthening, and aerobic exercise that exacerbate symptoms during acute joint flare-ups, but continue to do ROM to the involved joint(s) and balance activities if symptoms allow.
- Emphasize moving all joints through their full ROMs at least one time each day to prevent loss in ROM.

Weight loss or maintenance of ideal weight may decrease compressive forces but must be considered in relationship to worsening the osteoporosis risk of fracture.

Importance of Exercise in Managing OA

Despite having OA, older adults should strive to be physically active by exercising to minimize their risk of developing other chronic diseases and lower their body weight. In addition, the lack of activity can further compound the problem of OA and subsequently contribute to falls, osteoporosis, and sarcopenia. Unfortunately, many patients with OA who are experiencing pain refrain from exercise and physical activity. Mat and colleagues[159] reported that OA of the knee is a risk factor for falls in older adults and that strength training, tai chi, and aerobic exercises improve balance and reduce fall risk in older adults. The benefits of regular exercise for individuals with OA are many. Exercise has been shown to reduce pain while enhancing physical function, quality of life, and mental health in individuals with OA.[197] For example, the performance of 130 to 150 minutes/week of moderate-intensity, low-impact aerobics helps to manage pain, improve the ability to perform daily activities, improve the quality of life, decrease the level of fatigue, and improve ROM. This is complimented by better weight control and less metabolic abnormalities.[141]

Aquatic physical therapy is highlighted in Chapter 9 of this book. The benefits of a 12-week aquatic program in people with hip and knee OA has been demonstrated for pain reduction. In addition, it may improve self-reports of disability and improve quality of life.[19,113]

Obesity

Background

The obesity epidemic that plagues the US is becoming a global problem. The US no longer leads the world in the incidence of obesity.[225] For all age groups, including older adults, the obesity epidemic is increasing.[251] From 1980 to 2013, the estimated number of overweight or obese individuals worldwide increased to 36.9% in men and 38% in women.[181] More than 33% of people over 65 years of age in the US are obese; the incidence is greatest for the young old and least for the old-old.[80] The co-morbidity of obesity may compound other problems that impact older adults. Excessive abdominal adiposity is associated with increased risk of morbidity and mortality.[270]

Changes in Body Composition

As people age, there are changes in the body composition with a decrease in the fat-free mass, an increase in fat mass, and height loss from vertebral body compression and scoliosis. Abdominal adiposity, which is assessed by measuring the circumference of the waist, provides the clinician with insight into an individual's health status.[61,123,174,176,177,198,253,271] According to the National Institutes of Health, "Although waist circumference and BMI are interrelated, waist circumference provides an independent prediction of risk over and above that of BMI."[176] The American Heart Association, National Heart, Lung, and Blood Institute establishes >88 cm (35") for women and >102 cm (40") for men as the criteria for abdominal adiposity. The International Diabetes Federation[236] uses different cut-points for individuals of different ethnic groups with cut-points as low as >80 cm (31.5") for women and >90 cm (35.5") for men. In individuals of very short or very tall stature, waist circumference should be less than half of their height. For example, if a female patient is 1.44 m (4'9") in height, their waist circumference should be <72 cm (28.5"). This is more appropriate than using the cut-point of >88 cm (35").

In addition to measuring waist circumference, neck circumference may shed light into the potential of obstructive sleep apnea. A neck circumference ≥16" (40.6 cm) in women and ≥17" (43.2 cm) in men plus being overweight or obese are both risk factors for obstructive sleep apnea (OSA).[4] The prevalence of OSA increases between middle and older age. Neck size correlates with adiposity in non-athletic patients. When a large neck is noted on the inspection, the patient should be asked if they snore when sleeping, if sleep is interrupted, if they feel fatigued or unrefreshed in the morning, or if they feel irritable or forgetful.

Impact on the Metabolic System

Individuals with visceral adiposity have increased risk of metabolic abnormalities, including decreased glucose tolerance, reduced insulin sensitivity, and abnormal lipid profiles, which increased the risk for T2DM and CV disease.[123,132] Other health risks associated with being overweight and obese include OA, sleep apnea, and hypertension.[123]

Impact on the Respiratory System

The impact of obesity on the respiratory system is underappreciated.[275] Weight gain and increased body mass index are directly related with decreased lung volumes characteristic of restrictive lung dysfunction. Abdominal adiposity directly impacts diaphragmatic excursion, decreased inspiratory volume, and an increased work in breathing. Obesity hypoventilation syndrome may occur with clinical obesity when the body mass index is >30 kg/m2. Secondary problems impairing respiration, such as hypercapnia, may occur in obese patients. When evaluating and treating an older adult with obesity, these comorbidities will have an effect on any exercise program and may require modification to maintain safe parameters.

Considerations for Interventions

Health-care providers in a multitude of settings assess obesity through various measures, including BMI, waist-hip ratio, or simple waist circumference. To determine BMI, use a table, smartphone app, or a person's weight in kilograms divided by height in meters squared. The formula for BMI is:

$$BMI = weight\ (kg)\ /\ [height\ (m)]^2$$
$$(in\ pounds\ and\ inches,\ BMI = weight\ (lb)\ /\ [height\ (in)]2 \times 703)$$

In athletes and individuals who are muscular, BMI may overestimate body fat, and in older persons, BMI may underestimate body fat.[45,49,174] The WHO reports that it is unclear which measurement is most indicative of CV disease risk, while other references recommend use of waist to hip ratio due to the direct relationship of CV risk with central adiposity.[40,59,198,253]

Because of the relationship of obesity with restrictive lung dysfunction, it is critical to observe the older adult during any physical activity. Is breathing labored, noted by the use of accessory muscles of respiration? Does phonation decrease? Can the patient talk without shortness of breath at rest or with activity (talk test)? Does the patient limit their speech to take a breath (phonation)? If a patient has shortness of breath at rest, dyspnea on exertion, or a pulmonary problem such as emphysema, it may be appropriate to determine the patient's oxygen saturation. Does it decrease then with activity initiation and quickly return to baseline with activity cessation? What is the respiratory rate? Is the patient on supplemental oxygen? If not, is it necessary? Should it be titrated to a higher flow rate when performing exercise? Are sitting activities preferred over being recumbent due to orthopnea?

Looking at the whole patient is paramount. An obese patient who complains of knee pain must be counseled on the impact of obesity and the benefits of healthy eating and physical activity. To increase activity while decreasing the impact of ground reaction forces on the weight-bearing joints, utilize a pool for their exercise program (see Chapter 9) or have the patient exercise while sitting on a chair, mat, or large exercise ball. It is well established that patients who receive counseling will lose weight and exercise more than patients who do not receive counseling.[246] When working with overweight and obese patients, it is critical to avoid stigmatizing and stereotyping them.[202,217] Box 24.6 highlights key points when discussing weight loss with your patient.

Importance of Exercise in Managing Obesity

Incorporating physical activity is essential for a successful weight loss program and in maintaining weight loss.[74,121,132] Weight loss through diet may result in loss of fat-free mass and lean body mass, while exercise combined with calorie restriction may prevent the loss of muscle. With the loss of muscle mass associated with aging, it is critical to optimize lean body mass by addressing obesity through a program that increases energy expenditure and decreases energy intake.[49,74,32,251]

Cancer

Background

Cancer falls behind heart disease as the second most common cause of death in the US. Aging is the greatest risk factor for developing cancer; it is referred to as a disease of the elderly,

BOX 24.6 Considerations for Discussing Weight Loss[202,217,246]

- During the examination, address the patient's main physical therapy need first.
- If indicated, measure abdominal circumference at the midpoint between lower margin of last palpable rib and top of iliac crest in the standing position with a stretch resistant tape. Record "obesity" as a precaution.
- Perform secondary tests and measures as indicated including vital signs at rest, immediately post activity, and recovery.
- Explain findings to the patient in a nonjudgmental manner. For example, "Your body weight or waist size may increase your risk for health problems. Can we talk about my concerns?" Open discussion about weight respectfully using terms such as weight and unhealthy body weight. What is the patient's readiness to change?
- Employ the "teach back" method to ensure patient understands implications of obesity on their health status. The "teach back" method is when the patient (or family member) is asked to explain in their own words what was taught by the therapist to check for understanding.[1, 3]
- Provide valuable resources, including possible referrals to dietitians, specialty clinics, and support groups.
- Document patient education.

with the median age for occurrence of all types of cancer being 68 years.[78] The lifetime probability of developing cancer is one in two for males and one in three for females. The likelihood of dying from cancer is one in four for males and one in five for females. It is estimated that nutrition, inactivity, and excess weight may account for 25% to 33% of cancers in high-income countries like the US.[21]

Considerations for Interventions

Years after treatment has ended, the cancer survivor remains at risk for recurrence of the primary cancer, development of metastases, and/or development of new cancers, Metastasis may occur at any time; primary tumors may metastasize to secondary tumors in bone, lymph nodes, lung, liver, and brain. Cancers of the breast, lung, and prostate are more likely to metastasize to bone. The development of bone pain in a cancer survivor should be considered suspicious and a red flag. Initially the bone pain may cycle and increase with activity and then become continuous (ACS, bone metastasis). The pain may change and become aching or sharp in nature; skeletal pain should be considered as potential metastasis until proven otherwise.[5,22] When the spine is involved, spinal cord compression may occur.[5]

If there is metastasis to the bone, the patient is at risk for pathological fracture.[5,22] For example, an 80-year-old female patient who was cancer-free for 10 years presented with an acute spiral fracture of the humerus from lifting a toaster. Originally, this patient was screened for abuse and later found to have stage IV cancer with metastasis to the bone, lungs, and liver from her primary site of breast cancer. Thus, it is critical to regularly screen patients despite a remote history of cancer. Because of the increased risk of pathologic fracture, modify the intensity as well as application site of resistance when designing strengthening programs.

A therapist working with a patient undergoing cancer treatment or a cancer survivor must consider the patient's laboratory values. However this information may not be readily accessible for therapists practicing in a free-standing practice setting. Consequently, it is essential to screen the patient for changes in health status. For example, increased fatigue when performing an exercise program may be indicative of a low hemoglobin level. Electronic medical records may allow access to important information such as platelets, white blood cell count, neutrophils, International Normalized Ratio (INR), red blood cell count, hemoglobin, and hematocrit. The reader is referred to Billek-Sawhney and Wells[22] for in-depth information on laboratory values of specific importance in the patient with cancer.

Hospitals may have specific criteria for when to hold therapy or proceed based on laboratory values. It is critical to consider in the goals for physical therapy. In hospitals, nursing homes, and home health therapy, ensuring the patient is safe to access the bathroom and perform ADLs is essential. This differs greatly from the performance of aerobic or resistance exercise for wellness. For example, a patient with a hemoglobin of 8.1 g/dL could be evaluated for their ability to walk around their home or room to perform basic ADLs but not for performance of resistance exercises.

When the neutrophils, a type of white blood cell, become critically low the patient is described as being neutropenic. This means that the patient is at high risk for bacterial infections. Therapists always need to adhere to infection control through proper hand washing and cleaning of equipment, as well as the wearing of a mask when experiencing cold-like symptoms. In addition, when working with patients at increased risk of infection, consider the benefit of treating them in a private treatment room or an area where there is less exposure to bacteria and other contaminants, or have them wear a mask to minimize risk of an airborne infection.

Importance of Exercise With Cancer

The adoption of a physically active lifestyle (150 minutes of moderate-intensity aerobic activity each week) has been shown to be beneficial in preventing cancer, during cancer treatment, and during survivorship. This has been well documented for many forms of cancer.[6] The relationship between exercise and physical activity and maintaining an ideal body weight is related to a lower risk of colon, breast, lung, and prostate cancer. Regular physical activity has preventive benefits for cancer survivors and can reduce the risk of new chronic disease. In survivors with breast or colon cancer, the likelihood of recurrence or premature death is lessened in those who exercise.[197]

The deleterious effects of cancer and the treatments for it can be lessened through physical activity and exercise.[22,222] Rehabilitation may reduce the adverse effects of pain, fatigue, strength loss, decreased CV capacity, lymphedema, depression, anxiety, osteoporosis or osteopenia, nausea, and numerous other side effects of treatment. Cancer-related fatigue is the most common complaint during cancer treatments. It affects 70% to 100% of individuals during and after cancer treatment and has been shown to be responsive to exercise. The benefits of exercise have been demonstrated with aerobic exercise and resistance exercise. Silver and Gilchrist[222] report a 40% to 50% lower fatigue level in cancer survivors who exercise.

CLINICAL TIP

According to Curtis and colleagues,[64] normally with exercise there is an increase in heart rate that quickly returns to baseline. When this recovery is slowed in patients (i.e., the patients' recovery is <22 beats/min at 2 minutes following exercise when measured in supine), it is considered an abnormal hemodynamic response; the physician should be notified and an ECG recommended.

Type 2 Diabetes Mellitus

Background

The incidence of T2DM is estimated to be 9.3% of the US population and is now in epidemic proportions. This percentage increases to 25.9% of individuals 65 years or older. Ninety percent to 95% of the cases of diabetes mellitus are T2DM.[57]

Considerations for Interventions

Exercise Risks in T2DM

Considering the risk of coronary artery disease and other comorbidities of T2DM, it may be necessary for patients to have medical clearance prior to participating in an exercise program.[164,195] Uncontrolled metabolic disease, including T2DM, is considered a relative contraindication and a relative risk factor to exercise participation. The position statement by ACSM and the ADA state "exercise stress testing is advised primarily for sedentary individuals with diabetes who want to undertake activity more intense than brisk walking."[57] Brisk walking, at 3 miles per hour or faster, falls into the category of moderate intensity exercise. The recommended RPE level of 12 to 13, or "somewhat hard," on the original Borg RPE scale (see Box 25.4 in Chapter 25), is the corresponding description.[9]

Medical Monitoring

Electrocardiogram (ECG) stress testing is recommended for individuals who are:[12,57]

- Older than age 40 with or without CV disease risk factors not including T2DM
- Older than age 30 with one of the following: T2DM for more than 10 years, hypertension, cigarette smoking, dyslipidemia, retinopathy, or nephropathy
- Has known or suspected CAD, cerebrovascular disease, and/or peripheral neuropathy
- Has autonomic neuropathy
- Has advanced nephropathy with concomitant renal failure

In many PT practice settings, patients are commonly seen who have a known diagnosis of T2DM, are hypertensive, have CAD, neuropathy, nephropathy, retinopathy, and smoke. These characteristics may be commonly reported in the patient with T2DM following an amputation. Thus, if ECG results and/or testing has not been done or is not available, it is critical to initiate patients at a low-level exercise program and monitor responses.

Hypoglycemia and Insulin

Hypoglycemia is reported as the "most serious problem" for people with diabetes.[195] The risk of hypoglycemia (low BG level) is less common in individuals with T2DM who do not take insulin or insulin-releasing medications, also known as secretagogues. Those individuals who do use insulin or secretagogues should supplement their exercise with carbohydrates to prevent hypoglycemia. Exercise should not be initiated if the BG is too low or too high. Exercise guidelines based on BG levels are described in Table 24.7. If these guidelines are impractical in some practice settings, the recommendation of using 100 to 300 mg/dL is employed for exercise.[12,191]

PRECAUTIONS: When working with individuals with T2DM who use insulin:[191,244]

- Avoid exercise when insulin is peaking.
- Advise the patient to exercise the same time each day.
- Consider the timing of the last meal, regularly assess the blood sugar level; if it is low, have the patient eat and delay exercise; if it is high, be cautious and carefully monitor the patient when exercising.
- Use caution when exercising the muscles where the insulin was just injected to avoid speeding up the pharmacodynamics.
- Maintain hydration.
- Recognize that hypoglycemia may occur for up to 48 hours post exercise.
- Assess feet for absence of protective sensation.

With the advent of insulin pumps, also known as continuous subcutaneous insulin infusion (CSII), individuals with diabetes have continuous subcutaneous insulin delivery to attain a tighter glucose control and less BG excursions. The safety guidelines for insulin pumps are commonly provided by the pump manufacturer.[33,99,142] In general, with exercise the amount of insulin from the pump should be less due to the exercise-induced BG drop. This can be programmed into the pump by the patient. Thus, it is recommended that patients check their blood sugar level before, during, or after exercise, especially when new to exercise or having recently received an insulin pump. The above guidelines should be employed and, in general, if exercise is greater than 30 minutes additional carbohydrates are suggested. In addition, the amount of insulin may need to be decreased after exercise. Caution should be used to avoid friction from exercise around the infusion site.[15]

TABLE 24.7 Exercise Guidelines Based on Blood Glucose Levels (Modified from Partridge et al[191] with permission)

Blood Glucose Level	What To Do	Comments
<70 mg/dL	Exercise should not be initiated	Immediately provide carbohydrates (fruit juice, hard candy, glucose table or gel) and recheck blood glucose; seek emergent medical attention if symptoms worsen
70–100 mg/dL	Snack	15 g carbohydrate every hour of mild-moderately intense activity; 25-50 g with moderate or greater intensity; hydrate
100–300 mg/dL	Proceed with exercise program	Strenuous activity or activity of long duration (1-2 hr) requires increased carbohydrate intake; hydrate well
>300 mg/dL and on oral medications	Trial of activity 10-15 min and recheck	If blood glucose rises, stop activity; if blood glucose drops, continue checking every 10-15 min
>300 mg/DL and on insulin	Check for ketosis (urine dipstick or glucometer that measures ketosis)	If (+) ketones, avoid activity; if (-) ketones, participate with close blood glucose monitoring every 10-15 min

Other Complications

The presence of underlying microvascular complications such as retinopathy, nephropathy, and peripheral and/or autonomic neuropathy provides the clinician with insight into the severity of T2DM and the patient's ability to exercise. In these individuals caution must be employed to avoid high-intensity exercises due to the risk of potentially worsening the microvascular complications.[57,95,191] In addition, it is critical to perform a comprehensive foot examination and assess shoe wear due to the potential of insensitive feet, Charcot joint, neuropathy, and/or neuropathic ulcers.

Importance of Exercise in Managing T2DM

The management of T2DM is described as a three-pronged approach that includes exercise, diet, and medication.[57,91,191] These three prongs should be grounded on a solid base of patient education. Education is critical for self-management in regard to exercise, diet, and pharmacotherapy. It is essential to realize that improvements can be made in the systemic insulin action through exercise. Moderate aerobic exercise improves blood sugar levels and insulin action. Furthermore, combining aerobic and resistance exercise is more effective than either intervention alone.[57] A 12-week resistance exercise program was found to improve muscle strength and function in older adults who were either healthy, prediabetic, or diagnosed with T2DM. Regular exercise and physical activity for individuals with T2DM can reduce the risk of other diseases and help improve body weight. There are greater benefits with increased time and greater intensity of exercise.[197]

Urinary Incontinence

Background

Urinary incontinence affects from 26% to 46% of older adults.[32,94,266] It is associated with advancing age, impaired cognition, and decreased mobility. In men it may follow treatment of prostate cancer, and in women it may occur after menopause due to the decrease in estrogen levels. Despite this, it is not considered a normal occurrence of primary aging. In stress urinary incontinence (SUI), the muscles that help with micturition may become weak from loss of muscle mass and disuse so that urine may escape with little pressure. Depending on the resource, there are four to five types of incontinence; Box 24.7 highlights the most common forms.[32,94,247,266] SUI occurs when coughing, laughing, sneezing, jogging, or jumping cause pressure on the bladder that is not stopped by muscular contraction. Urge, overactive bladder, functional incontinence, or overflow incontinence may occur in isolation or in combination with each other.

BOX 24.7 Common Forms of Urinary Incontinence

Stress Urinary Incontinence
- Most common form of incontinence
- Weak pelvic floor muscles that allow urine to escape when exercising, sneezing, lifting, or even laughing

Urge Urinary Incontinence (aka Overactive Bladder)
- The bladder muscles contract and pass urine before the bladder is full causing a need to urinate, described as "key in the door" syndrome in which leakage begins prior to accessing the toilet

Mixed Incontinence
- When the patient experiences both SUI and urge incontinence

Functional Incontinence (aka Insensible Urinary Incontinence)
- The person may be unaware of the need to go to the toilet (insensible) or may not get to the toilet in time due to functional mobility limitations (functional)

Considerations for Interventions

In addition to medication and/or surgery, the management of SUI may include referral to physical therapy for the pelvic floor exercises, as well as lifestyle, and behavioral changes.[32,94,266] The basics of this specialty area of practice are valuable for all physical therapists and assistants working with older adults in every practice setting. Pelvic floor musculature exercises can be taught in various ways to increase strength and develop bladder control.[82] Within 3 to 6 weeks of daily muscular strengthening exercise, bladder control may improve. Similar to traditional strengthening, changes may occur initially from neural adaptations but may take as long as 3 months, and overexercising may result in overwork weakness. If improvements are not noted, the patient should be referred to a physical therapist who specializes in treatment of the pelvic floor.

Importance of Exercise in Managing Incontinence

Pelvic floor exercises are an effective approach of conservative management of incontinence.[76] These exercises are described in Chapter 25. The treatment of pelvic organ prolapse, painful intercourse, and other pelvic floor issues are beyond the scope of this text. For additional information the reader is referred to the APTA's Section on Women's Health.[28,34]

Summary

Contrary to the ageism stereotype that an older adult cannot learn new things, the older adult, most assuredly, can learn. "Because it may take older adults more time to encode, store, and retrieve information, the rate at which new information is learned can be slower, and older adults have a greater need for repetition of new information."[13] This may be the case with exercise. Changes associated with aging can be combatted with exercise and physical activity but require a long-term commitment. Physical activity through exercise is a viable option to pharmacological interventions for both disease prevention and management of disease.[129,164]

There are many stereotypes associated with aging, one being that once you are "old" you cannot get stronger! That is a myth that must change through patient education, appropriate interventions, and role modeling. It is critical to become the change agent and create this paradigm shift away from underdosed strengthening, flexibility, endurance, and balance activities to examining the patient's status, prescribing appropriate interventions, and modifying and adjusting the patient's exercise program as the patient's status changes. Physical therapists must look at the total patient and incorporate wellness and walk the talk! A summary of practice considerations to promote physical activity in the older adult are presented in Box 24.8.

BOX 24.8 Physical Therapy Practice Considerations to Promote Physical Activity in the Older Adult

"Walk the Talk"

- Encourage older adults and role model a paradigm shift from being sedentary to becoming active after retirement.
- Be visible and excited with exercise and physical activity ideas.
- Create an environment for patient socialization.
- Encourage adherence to a routine.
- Demonstrate an interest in patients' activity level.
- Encourage other members of your department or clinic in the process.
- Promote physical activity by having flyers on display, sponsoring programs, and being visible in the community.
- Assess and promote physical activity with EVERY patient.
- Prescribe the appropriate level of physical activity after determining readiness to change.
- Provide the appropriate exercise prescription that addresses the patient's level and allows for continued improvement, and modify the interventions as the patient's status changes.
- Ensure that the interventions meet the interests and abilities of the older adult.
- Serve as a resource following discharge from physical therapy.
- Consider having an onsite wellness program for patients at a nominal cost.
- Provide a resource list of local community programs and professionals that can be recommended to patients.
- Develop a network for exercise referrals.
- Be available to the patients and referral sources for consultation, guidance, and collaboration.

Independent Learning Activities

Critical Thinking and Discussion

1. Review the subpopulations of older, young-old, mid-old, and old-old adults. In small groups, discuss various older adults that you know who are in each subpopulation in each of these categories that reflect healthy aging and non-healthy aging. Describe their physical presentation and functional mobility.
2. Reflect on the "Choosing Wisely" initiative between the APTA and the American Board of Internal Medicine Foundation and underdosed strength training programs in older adults. How does this compare to your observations and practice as a student or therapist? What could be done to change the following interventions to "dose-appropriate" strengthening? Change the following three exercises to be dose appropriate: (a) full arc knee extension, leg kicks with a 2-lb weight, (b) rowing with elastic resistance band while in a sitting position against back support, and (c) performing standing mini-squats with a walker.
3. Apply the WAMI-3 to the following scenarios to explain to a patient the need to participate in resistance exercise: (a) a patient with knee OA who has pain and difficulty descending stairs, (b) a patient with peripheral vascular insufficiency, and (c) a patient who had a femoral neck fracture and open reduction with internal fixation.
4. Differentiate the primary and secondary aging process for the patients in Box 24.1.
5. Develop an in-service instructional presentation that addresses changes with aging and the importance of physical activity and resistance exercise.
6. How does a lifestyle of sedentary behavior negatively impact older adults? How is this reflected on the WAMI-3 Model?
7. Why is it critical to perform standardized tests when examining older adult patients? What tests would be most appropriate to perform in a home health setting where there is not a clear path to assess gait? What tests would be most appropriate for the older adult patient being seen in an inpatient physical therapy setting?
8. An older adult patient with a new diagnosis of osteoporosis is being seen bedside in an acute care hospital following a spinal compression fracture of T10; the patient does not want to participate in physical therapy. Discuss strategies that can be used to educate and motivate the patient to address the benefits of therapy and deleterious effects of immobility.
9. A 78-year-old male patient is being seen in an acute care hospital secondary to sepsis following a pacemaker replacement. He is able to ambulate at 0.3 m/s. Document the assessment or professional interpretation of this test to qualify him for skilled physical therapy in a nursing home following acute discharge.
10. Similar to Question 9, this patient performs the FTSTS but requires the use of his hands to perform five repetitions in 25 seconds. Document the test results and the professional interpretation of the performance on the test.
11. Why is it essential to include power exercises in a strength training program of older adults?
12. A 68-year-old female patient who is obese experiences an increase in her OA hip pain following the initiation of a resistance training program. What may have caused this pain? What should be done to address the pain?
13. What techniques can be employed to initiate the conversation of weight loss with older adult patients?
14. What questions should be incorporated into the patient interview of a 65-year-old patient with T1DM or T2DM to ensure the patient can tolerate resistance exercise? What strategies can be employed to ensure that the patient continues resistance training after discharge from physical therapy?
15. You observe that your new 72-year-old female patient uses accessory muscles when breathing and has decreased phonation, a blue tinge to lips, and clubbing of the digits. What special precautions will you need to employ when working with this patient?

Laboratory Practice

1. Develop and perform a comprehensive/multidimensional program of exercises for each of the patients in Box 24.1.
2. Develop and perform interventions for primary, secondary, and tertiary osteoporosis for the patients in Table 24.6.
3. A 91-year-old female who lives independently at home is interested in "getting stronger." Her past medical history includes a transient ischemic attack, osteoporosis, myocardial infarction, breast cancer, and pelvic sling surgery for incontinence. She has a history of three falls in the past year. She has a wheeled walker that she is willing to use outside her home. Develop a comprehensive program—including education—that can be done using the following: the counter at her kitchen sink, the flight of steps to her second floor with one railing, and a standard kitchen chair with arm rests. Explain how "getting stronger" includes balance and aerobic capacity.
4. A 65-year-old male travels frequently for his work. He would like to use elastic resistance bands and/or his own body weight for strengthening. Develop a comprehensive program working 8 to 10 major muscle groups including his core.
5. Perform each of the tests and measures described in this chapter, including TUG, gait speed, 30s-STS, FTSTS, and the tragus-to-wall measure.

Case Studies

1. Using Case Study 1 described in Box 24.1, answer the following questions:
   a. On examination of Lou for his left knee pain, it is apparent that he has restricted ankle dorsiflexion with tightness of his gastrocnemius tighter than his soleus muscle. What specific stretches are recommended for Lou? What specific instructions should be given to Lou? Develop written instructions.
   b. Lou demonstrates hip internal rotation and increased knee pain on reciprocal stair descent. Demonstrate and perform specific interventions that can be performed without equipment.
   c. Address the above muscle weakness problem again, but employ weight lifting equipment.
2. Using Case Study 2 described in Box 24.1 the following is observed as you walk Mary Jane back to the examining room:
   a. Mary Jane appears to be frail and has a very kyphotic posture, causing her to be bent and look down toward the floor. While ambulating toward the examination room, you note she has an effective gait speed but has two episodes where she demonstrates a deviation in her path. From this brief introduction, what critical questions should you ask this patient? What tests should you perform to further assess balance?
   b. What measurements should be taken as a result of the observation of flexed posture? Are there any red flags that warrant safety precautions and possible referral for bone density testing? If so, what are they?
   c. Mary Jane frequently has episodes of dizziness that may be caused by her cardiac medications. Also, her prescription for beta blockers may blunt her heart rate response to exercise. What precautions will be necessary while she exercises?
   d. Based on Mary Jane's vertical height loss, document the assessment and the need to rule out osteoporosis and propose appropriate recommendations.
3. Using Case Study 3 described in Box 24.1, answer the following questions:
   a. How have the neuromuscular and musculoskeletal complaints affected Juan's functional independence and ability to participate in social activities outside his home?
   b. Juan is not willing to attend outpatient physical therapy and states he will perform only three exercises. What exercises would you recommend that he perform and why those three exercises?
   c. Write "1" objective and measurable goal for Juan related to educating him on the importance of physical activity and exercise that meets documentation guidelines for reimbursement.
   d. What specific tests and measures would best measure the decline in Juan's functional mobility?
   e. Document Juan's performance on the 30s-STS test, the interpretation of these findings, and an appropriate goal. When performing STS, Juan requires use of his arms. He is only able to perform four repetitions.

REFERENCES

1. Agency for Healthcare Research and Quality: *Health Literacy Universal Precautions Toolkit,* ed. 2. Available at http://www.ahrq.gov/sites/default/files/ publications/files/healthlittoolkit2_3.pdf. Accessed March 2, 2016.
2. Almeida, GJ, et al: Interrater reliability and validity of the stair ascend/descent test in subjects with total knee arthroplasty. *Arch Phys Med Rehabil* 91(6):932–938, 2010.
3. Always Use Teach-back! Training tool kit–45 minute interactive module. Available at http://www.teachbacktraining.org. Accessed July 12, 2016.
4. American Academy of Sleep Medicine: Obstructive sleep apnea, 2008. Available at http://www.aasmnet.org/resources/factsheets/sleepapnea.pdf. Accessed March 2, 2016.
5. American Cancer Society: Bone metastasis, 2016. Available at http://www.cancer.org/treatment/understandingyourdiagnosis/bonemetastasis/bone-metastasis-what-is-bone-mets. Accessed June 2, 2016.
6. American Cancer Society: Cancer facts and figures 2014. Available at http://www.cancer.org/acs/groups/content/@research/documents/document/acspc-041777.pdf. Accessed June 26, 2016.
7. American College of Sports Medicine: Exercise is medicine, *Healthcare Providers' Action Guide.* Available at http://exerciseismedicine.org/assets/page_documents/Complete%20HCP%20Action%20Guide.pdf. Accessed March 2, 2016.
8. American Family Physician: Choosing wisely. Available at http://www.aafp.org/afp/recommendations/viewRecommendation.htm?recommendationId=210 , Accessed April 11, 2016.
9. American Heart Association: Moderate to vigorous – what is your level of intensity? Available at http://www.heart.org/HEARTORG/GettingHealthy/PhysicalActivity/FitnessBasics/Moderate-to-Vigorous—-What-is-your-level-of-intensity_UCM_463775_Article.jsp. Accessed March 2, 2016.
10. American Heart Association: Physical activity improves quality of life, 2015. Available at http://www.heart.org/HEARTORG/GettingHealthy/PhysicalActivity/FitnessBasics/Physical-activity-improves-quality-of-life_UCM_307977_Article.jsp. Accessed 7/21/2015.
11. American Physical Therapy Association: Five things physical therapists and patients should question, http://www.choosingwisely.org/societies/american-physical-therapy-association/. Accessed April 11, 2016.
12. American Physical Therapy Association: Physical fitness and type II diabetes based on best available practice. *Supplement to PT Magazine.* October 2007. Available at www.apta.org/pfsp. Accessed March 2, 2016.
13. American Psychological Association: Older adults' health & age related changes, 1998. Available at http://www.apa.org/pi/aging/resources/guides/older-adults.pdf. Accessed July 7, 2015.
14. American Thoracic Society: ATS statement: guidelines for the six-minute walk test. *Am J Repir Crit Care Med* 166:111–117, 2002.
15. Anima Corporation: Physical activity, ANM-14-4309A, 2015. Available at http://www.animas.com/sites/default/files/pdf/Physical%20%20Activity.pdf. Accessed June 27, 2016.
16. Avers, D, and Brown, M: White paper: Strength training for the older adult. *J Geri Phys Ther* 32(4):148–158, 2009.
17. Avin, KG, et al: Management of falls in community dwelling older adults: clinical guidance statement from the Academy of Geriatric Physical Therapy of the American Physical Therapy Association. *Phys Ther* 95(6):815–834, 2015.
18. Bacon, AP, et al: VO2max trainability and high intensity interval training in humans: a meta-analysis. *Public Lib of Sci* 16(8):e73182, 1–7, 2013.
19. Bartels, E, et al: Aquatic exercise for people with osteoarthritis in the knee or hip. *Cochrane Reviews.* March 23, 2016.
20. Bassey, EJ, et al: Leg extensor power and functional performance in very old men and women. *Clin Sci* 82:321–327, 1992.

21. Berger, NA, et al: Cancer in the elderly. *Trans Am Clin Climatol Assoc* 117:147–156, 2006.
22. Billek-Sawhney, B, and Wells, CL: Oncology implications for exercise and rehabilitation. *J Acute Care Phys Ther*, 18(4):12–19, Winter 2010.
23. Bloomfield, SA: Changes in musculoskeletal structure and function with prolonged bed rest. *Med Sci Sport Ex* 29(2):197–206, 1997.
24. Bohannon, RW: Grip strength predicts outcomes: letters to the editor. *Age Ageing* 3:320–323, 2006.
25. Bohannon, RW.: Hand-grip dynamometry predicts future outcomes in aging adults. *J Geriatr Phys Ther* 31:3–10, 2008.
26. Bohannon, RW: Reference values for the five-repetition sit-to-stand test: a descriptive meta-analysis of data from elders. *Percept Mot Skills* 103(1):215–222, 2006.
27. Bonaiuti, D, et al: Exercise for preventing and treating osteoporosis in postmenopausal women. *Cochrane Reviews.* April 22, 2002.
28. Borello-France DF, et al: Pelvic-floor muscle function in women with pelvic organ prolapse. *Phys Ther* 87(4):399–407, 2007.
29. Borg, GA: *Borg's Rating of Perceived Exertion and Pain Scales.* Champaign, IL: Human Kinetics, 1998.
30. Borg, GA: Psychophysical bases of perceived exertion. *Med Sci Sports Exerc* 14:377–381, 1982.
31. Bosco, C, and Komi, PV: Influence of aging on the mechanical behavior or leg extensor muscles. *Eur J Appl Physiol Occup Physiol* 45:209–212, 1980.
32. Boyle, E: *Incontinence Management of the Geriatric Patient.* UPMC Geriatric Residency Program, Capstone Project, Pittsburgh, PA, November 2015.
33. Boyle, ME, et al: Guidelines for application of continuous subcutaneous insulin infusion (insulin pump) therapy in the perioperative period. *J Diab Sci Tech* 6(1):184–190, 2012.
34. Braekken, IH, et al: Can pelvic floor muscle training reverse pelvic organ prolapse and reduce prolapse symptoms. An assessor-blinded, randomized, controlled trial. *Am J Obstet Gyn* 203(2):170.e1–170.e7, 2010.
35. Bredin, SS, et al: PAR-Q+ and ePARmed-X+: New risk stratification and physical activity clearance strategy for physicians and patients alike. *Can Fam Phys* 59:273–277, 2013.
36. Brown, MB: Strength training and aging. *Top Geriatr Rehabil* 15(3):1–5, 2000.
37. Buatois, S, et al. Five times sit to stand test is a predictor of recurrent falls in healthy community-living subjects aged 65 and older. *J Am Geriatr Soc* 56(8):1575–1577, 2008.
38. Buchman, AS, et al: Physical activity and leg strength predict decline in mobility performance in older adults. *J Am Geriatr Soc* 55:1618–1623, 2007.
39. Camicioli, R, and Rosana, C: Understanding gait in aging (part 1). International Parkinson and Movement Disorder Society. Available at http://www.movementdisorders.org/MDS/News/Online-Web-Edition/Archived-Editions/Series-on-Gait—-Part-1.htm. Accessed October 12, 2015.
40. Cancer Council Victoria: Be a healthy weight. Available at http://www.cutyourcancerrisk.org.au/how-to-cut-cancer-risk/maintain-weight#.V21CvUuIz8s. Accessed June 20, 2016.
41. Cardinal, BJ, and Cardinal, MK: Screening efficiency of the revised physical activity readiness questionnaire in older adults. *J Aging Phys Activity* 3:299–308, 1995.
42. Cardinal, BJ, Esters, J, and Cardinal, MK: Evaluation of the revised physical activity readiness questionnaire in older adults. *Med and Science in Sports and Exer* 28:468–472, 1996.
43. Carvalho, J, et al: Isokinetic strength benefits after 24 weeks of multicomponent exercise training and combined training in older adults. *Aging Clin Exp Res* 22(1):63–69, 2010.
44. Centers for Disease Control and Prevention: Chronic disease prevention and health promotion, chronic disease overview, February 23, 2016. Available at http://www.cdc.gov/chronicdisease/overview/index.htm. Accessed June 16, 2016.
45. Centers for Disease Control and Prevention: Healthy weight, about adult BMI, 2014. Available at http://www.cdc.gov/healthyweight/assessing/bmi/adult_bmi/index.html. Accessed June 25, 2016.
46. Centers for Disease Control and Prevention: Important facts about falling. Available at http://www.cdc.gov/homeandrecreationalsafety/falls/adultfalls.html. Accessed March 2, 2016.
47. Centers for Disease Control and Prevention, National Center for Health Statistics: Deaths and mortality. Available at http://www.cdc.gov/nchs/fastats/deaths.htm. Accessed June 27, 2016.
48. Centers for Disease Control and Prevention: National Health Interview Survey, 2014. Available at http://www.cdc.gov/nchs/nhis.htm. Accessed April 12, 2016.
49. Centers for Disease Control and Prevention: Physical activity for a healthy weight, 2015. Available at http://www.cdc.gov/healthyweight/physical_activity/. Accessed March 11, 2016.
50. Centers for Disease Control and Prevention: Physical activity: measuring physical activity intensity. Available at http://www.cdc.gov/physicalactivity/basics/measuring/index.html. Accessed June 29, 2016.
51. Centers for Disease Control and Prevention: STEADI older adult fall prevention: prevention. Available at http://www.cdc.gov/steadi/. Accessed June 27, 2016.
52. Centers for Disease Control and Prevention: The National Institute for Occupational Safety and Health: Productive aging, and work. Available at http://www.cdc.gov/niosh/topics/productiveaging/dataandstatistics.html. Accessed June 27, 2016.
53. Chien, MY, Kuo, HK, and Wu, YT: Sarcopenia, cardiopulmonary fitness, and physical disability in community-dwelling elderly people. *Am Phys Ther Assn* 20(9):1277–1287, 2010.
54. Chmelo, EA, et al: Heterogeneity of physical function responses to exercise training in older adults. *J Am Geriatr Soc* 63:462–469, 2015.
55. Chodzko-Zajko, WJ, et al: ACSM, position. Stand, exercise and physical activity for older adults. *Med Sci Sports Ex* 41(7):1510–1530, 2009.
56. Choi, JY, Tasota, FJ, and Hoffman, LA: Mobility interventions to improve outcomes in patients undergoing mechanical ventilation: a review of the literature. *Biol Res Nurs* 10:21–33, 2008.
57. Colberg, SR, et al: Exercise and type 2 diabetes: American College of Sports Medicine and the American Diabetes Association: joint position statement. *Med & Sci in Sports & Exer* 42(12):2282–2303, 2010.
58. Coleman, KJ, et al: Initial validation of an exercise "vital sign" in electronic medical records. *Med Sci Sports Exerc* 44(11):2071–2076, 2012.
59. Collins N. Waist to height ratio 'more accurate than BMI.' *The Telegraph.* May 13, 2013. Available at http://www.telegraph.co.uk/news/health/news/10054519/Waist-to-height-ratio-more-accurate-than-BMI.html. Accessed June 23, 2016.
60. Cook, CE, and Hegedus, EJ: *Orthopedic Physical Examination Tests, An Evidence-Based Approach,* ed. 2. London: Pearson, 2013.
61. Cornier, MA, et al: Assessing adiposity: a scientific statement from the American Heart Association. *Circulation* 124:1996–2019, 2011.
62. Creutzfeldt, CJ, and Hough, CL: Get out of bed: immobility in the neurologic ICU. *Crit Care Med* 43(4):926–927, 2015.
63. Cruz-Jentoft, AJ, et al: Sarcopenia: European consensus on definition and diagnosis. *Age Ageing* 39(4):412–423, 2010.
64. Curtis, JM, et al: Prevalence and predictors of abnormal cardiovascular responses to exercise testing among individuals with type 2 diabetes the look AHEAD (action for health in diabetes) study. *Diabetes Care* 33(4):901–907, 2010.
65. Daly, M, et al: Upper extremity muscle volumes and functional strength after resistance training in older adults. *J Aging Phys Act* 21:186–207, 2013.
66. Deems-Dluhy, S, et al: Vestibular EDGE task force of the Neurology Section of the APTA: rehab measures: five times sit to stand test. Available at http://www.rehabmeasures.org/Lists/RehabMeasures/DispForm.aspx?ID=1015. Accessed July 12, 2016.
67. Dempsey, JA, and Seals, DR: Aging, exercise and cardiopulmonary function. In Lamb DR, Gisolfi, CV, and Nadel, E (eds): *Exercise in Older Adults. Perspectives in Exercise Science and Sports Medicines.* Carmel, IN: Cooper Publishing Group, 1995, pp 237–298.
68. DeSousa, PD, et al. Resistance strength training's effects on late components of postural responses in the elderly. *J Aging and Phys Activity* 21:208–331, 2013.

69. Desrossiers, J, et al: Normative data for grip strength of elderly men and women. *Am J Occup Ther.* 49(7):637–644, 1995.
70. Deutz, NEP, et al: Protein intake and exercise for optimal muscle function with gaining: recommendations from the ESPEN expert group. *Clin Nutri* 33:929–936, 2014.
71. Dittmer, DK, Teasell, R: Complications of immobilization and bed rest. Part 1: musculoskeletal and cardiovascular complications. *Can Fam Phys* 39:1428–1432, 1435–1437, 1993.
72. Dobson, F, et al: Osteoarthritis Research Society International, University of Melbourne. Recommended performance-based tests to assess physical function in people diagnosed with hip or knee osteoarthritis. Available at https://www.oarsi.org/sites/default/files/docs/2013/manual.pdf. Accessed June 27, 2016.
73. Doherty, TJ: Invited review: aging and sarcopenia. *J App Physiology.* 95(4):1717–1727, 2003.
74. Donnelly, JE, et al: American College of Sports Medicine position stand. Appropriate physical activity intervention strategies for weight loss and prevention of weight regain for adults. *Med Sci Sports Ex* 41(2):459–471, 2009.
75. Dugdale, DC, Zieve, D, and Black, B: Aging changes in organs-tissue-cells. US National Library of Medicine. Available at http://www.nlm.nih.gov/medlineplus/ency/article/004012.htm. Accessed July 7, 2015.
76. Dumoulin, C, and Hay-Smith, J: Pelvic floor muscle training versus no treatment, or inactive control treatments, for urinary incontinence in women. *Cochrane Database Syst Rev* 20(1):CD005654, 2010.
77. Edmondston, SJ, et al: Ex vivo estimation of thoracolumbar vertebral body compressive strength: the relative contributions of bone densitometry and vertebral morphometry. *Osteoporosis Int.* 7:42–148, 1997.
78. Ersler, WB: Cancer: a disease of the elderly. Available at http://www.oncologypractice.com/jso/journal/articles/0104s205.pdf. Accessed July 1, 2015.
79. Evans, WJ: Exercise strategies should be designed to increase muscle power. *J Geron: Bio Sci* 55A:M309–M310, 2000.
80. Falkhouri, THI, et al: Prevalence of obesity among older adults in the United States, 2007-2010. CDC, National Center for Health Statistics, NCHS Data Brief No. 106, September 2012. Available at http://www.cdc.gov/nchs/data/databriefs/db106.htm. Accessed June 6, 2016.
81. Fiatarone, MA, et al: Exercise training and nutritional supplementation for physical frailty in very elderly people. *N Engl J Med* 33:1769–1775, 1994.
82. Fine, P, et al: Teaching and practicing of pelvic floor muscle exercises in primiparous women during pregnancy and the postpartum period. *Am J Obstet Gyn* 197(1):107.e1–107e5, 2007.
83. Foldvari, M, et al: Association of muscle power with functional status in community-dwelling elderly women. *J Geron: Bio Sci* 55A:M192–M199, 2000.
84. Foster, C, et al: The talk test as a marker of exercise training intensity. *J Cardiopul Rehab Prev* 28(1):24–30, 2008.
85. Free, P: Weight vest for osteoporosis. Available at http://weightvest 4osteoporosis.com/. Accessed June 28, 2016.
86. Fregala, MS, et al: Resistance exercise may improve spatial awareness and visual reaction in older adults. *J Strength Cond Res* 28(8):2079–2087, 2014.
87. Fried, LP, et al: Diagnosis of illness presentation in the elderly. *J Am Geriatr Soc* 39:117–123, 1991.
88. Fritz, S, and Lusardi, M: White paper: walking speed: the sixth vital sign. *J Geri PT* 32(2):2–5, 2009.
89. Frontera, WR: Aging muscle. *Crit Rev Phys Rehabil Med* 18(1):63–93, 2006.
90. Fuller, GF: Falls in the elderly. *Am Fam Physician* 61(7):2159–2168, 2000.
91. Geirsdottir, OF, et al: Effect of 12-week resistance exercise program on body composition, muscle strength, physical function, and glucose metabolism in healthy, insulin-resistant, and diabetic elderly Icelanders. *J of Gerontol A Biol Sci Med Sci* 67(11):1259–1265, 2012.
92. Geirsdottir, OF, et al: Muscular strength and physical function in elderly adults 6-18 months after a 12-week resistance exercise program. *Scand J Pulbic Health* 43:76–82, 2015.
93. Gennuso KP, et al: Resistance training congruent with minimal guidelines improves functions in older adults: a pilot study. *J Phys Act Health* 10:769–776, 2013.
94. Ghaderi, F, and Oskouei, AE: Physiotherapy for women with stress urinary incontinence: a review article. *J Phys Ther Sci* 26(9):1493–1499, 2014.
95. Goodman, CC, and Fuller, KS: *Pathology: Implications for the Physical Therapist,* ed. 4. St. Louis: Saunders Elsevier, 2015.
96. Granacher, U, et al: The importance of trunk muscle strength for balance, functional performance, and fall prevention in seniors: a systematic review. *Sports Med* 43:627–641, 2013.
97. Grant, RW, et al: Exercise as a vital sign: a quasi-experimental analysis of a health system intervention to collect patient-reported exercise levels. *J Gen Intern Med* 29(2):341–348, 2014.
98. Greenwood, JL, Joy, EA, and Stanford, JB: The physical activity vital sign: a primary care tool to guide counseling for obesity. *J Phys Act Health* 7(5)571–576, 2010.
99. Grunberger, G, et al: AACE consensus statement. Statement by the American Association of Clinical Endocrinologists Consensus Panel on Insulin Pump Management. *B Endocrine Practice,* 16(5):September/October, 2010.
100. Gulick, D: *Ortho Notes Clinical Examination Pocket Guide.* Philadelphia, PA: F.A. Davis, 2013.
101. Haaland, DA, et al: Is regular exercise a friend or foe of the gaining immune system? A systematic review. *Clin J Sport Med* 18(6):539–548, 2008.
102. Hakestad, K, et al: Exercises including weight vests and a patient education program for women with osteopenia: a feasibility study of the OsteoACTIVE rehabilitation program. *J Orthop Sports Phys Ther* 45(2):97–105, 2015.
103. Hamburg, NM, et al: Physical inactivity rapidly induces insulin resistance and microvascular dysfunction in healthy volunteers. *Arterioscler Thromb Vasc Biol* 27: 2650–2656, 2007.
104. Hamer, M, et al: Physical activity and mortality risk in patients with cardiovascular disease: possible protective mechanisms? *Med and Sci in Sports & Exer* 44(1):84–88, 2012.
105. Hammond, T, and Wilson, A: Polypharmacy and falls in the elderly: A literature review. *Nurs Midwifery Stud* 2(2):171–175, 2013.
106. Harris, C, et al: Detraining in the older adult: effects of prior training intensity on strength retention. *J Strength and Conditioning Res* 2(3):813–818, 2007.
107. Harvey, JA, Chastin, SFM, and Skelton, DA: Prevalence of sedentary behavior in older adults: A systematic review. *Int J Environ Res Public Health* 10(12):6645–6661, 2013.
108. Haskell, WL, et al: Physical activity and public health. Updated recommendation for adults from the American College of Sports Medicine and the American Heart Association. *Circ* 116:1081–1093, 2007.
109. Hausdorff, JM, Rios, DA, and Edelber, HK: Gait variability and fall risk in community-living older adults: a 1-year prospective study. *Arch Phys Med Rehab,* 82:1050–1056, 2001.
110. Hazell, T, Kenno, K, and Jakobi, J: Functional benefit of power training for older adults. *J Aging Phys Act* 15:349–359, 2007.
111. *Healthy People 2020.* Available at https://www.healthypeople.gov/2020/topics-objectives/topic/older-adults. Accessed June 11, 2015.
112. Henwood, TR, Rick, S, and Taafe, DR: Strength versus muscle power-specific resistance training in community-dwelling older adults. *J Geron Med Sci* 63A(1):83–91, 2008.
113. Hinman, RS, Heywood, SE, and Day, AR: Aquatic physical therapy for hip and knee osteoarthritis: Results of a single-blind randomized controlled trial. *Phys Ther* 87(1):32–43, 2007.
114. Hoder, J, and Edge, PD: Rehab measures: 6 minute walk test. Task Force of the Neurology Section of the APTA. Available at http://www.rehabmeasures.org/Lists/RehabMeasures/PrintView.aspx?ID=895. Accessed February 29, 2016.
115. Hootman. JM, et al: Prevalence and most common causes of disability among adults—United States, 2005. *MMWR* 58(16):421–426, 2009.

116. Hornbrook, MC, et al: Preventing falls among community dwelling older persons: results from a randomized trial. *Gerontologist* 34:16–23, 1994.
117. Hunter, GR, McCarthy, JP, and Bamman, MM: Effects of resistance training on older adults. *Sports Med* 34:329–349, 2004.
118. Huntoon, EA, Schmidt, CK, and Sinaki, M: Significantly fewer refractures after vertebroplasty in patients who engage in back-extensor-strengthening exercises. *May Clin Proc* 83(1):54–57, 2008.
119. Hurd, R, Zieve, D, and Oglivie, I: Aging changes in the bones-muscles-joints. *US National Library of Medicine, MedlinePlus.* Available at https://medlineplus.gov/ency/article/004015.htm. Accessed July 12, 2016.
120. Ivey, FM, et al: Effects of age, gender, and myostatin genotype on the hypertrophic response to heavy resistance strength training. *J Gerontol A Biol Sci Med Sci* 55(11):M641–M648, 2000.
121. Jakicic, JM, et al: American College of Sports Medicine position stand. Appropriate intervention strategies for weight loss and prevention of weight gain for adults. *Med Sci in Sports and Exer* 33(12)2145–2156, 2001.
122. Jamnik, VK, Giedhill, N, and Shephard, RR: Revised clearance for participation in physical activity: Greater screening responsibility for qualified university-educated fitness professionals. *J Appl Physiol Nutri Metab* 32:1191–1197, 2007.
123. Jensen, MD, et al: 2013 AHA/ACC/TOS guideline for the management of overweight and obesity in adults, a report of the American College of Cardiology/American Heart Association Task Force on Practice Guidelines and The Obesity Society. *Circ* 129 (suppl 2):S102–S138, 2014.
124. Jiricka, MK: Activity tolerance and fatigue pathophysiology: concepts of altered health states. In Porth, CM (ed): *Essentials of Pathophysiology: Concepts of Altered Health States.* Philadelphia: Lippincott Williams & Wilkins, 2008.
125. John, EB, Liu, W, and Gregory, RW: Biomechanics of muscular effort: Age-related changes. *Med Sci in Sports & Ex* 41(2):418–425, 2009.
126. Jones, CJ, Rikli, RE, and Beam, W: A 30-s chair stand test as a measure of lower body strength in community-residing older adults. *Res Q Exerc Sport* 70:113–119, 1999.
127. Judge, JO: Gait disorders in the elderly, professional version. *Merck Manual, Professional Version*, 2013. Available at http://www.merckmanuals.com/professional/geriatrics/gait-disorders-in-the-elderly/gait-disorders-in-the-elderly. Accessed July 7, 2015.
128. Kauffman, TL: Wholeness of the individual. In Kauffman, TL, et al (eds): *A Comprehensive Guide to Geriatric Rehabilitation.* Philadelphia: Elsevier, 2014, pp 3–6.
129. Kemmler, W, and von Stengel, S. Exercise frequency, health risk factors, and disease of the elderly. *Arch Phys Med Rehab* 94:2046–2053, 2013.
130. Kendrick, D, et al: Exercise for reducing fear of falling in older people living in the community. *Cochrane Database Syst Rev* 2014(11):CD009848.
131. Kennis, E, et al: Long-term impact of strength training on muscle strength characteristics in older adults. *Arch Phys Med Rehabil* 94:2054–2060, 2013.
132. Klein, S, et al: Weight management through lifestyle modification for the prevention and management of type 2 diabetes: rationale and strength, ADA Statement. *Am J Clin Nutr* 80(2):257-263, 2004.
133. Knight, J, Nigam, Y, and Jones, A. Effects of bedrest 1: cardiovascular, respiratory and haematological systems. *Nurs Times* 105(21):16–20, 2009.
134. Kohrt, WM, et al: American College of Sports Medicine Position Stand physical activity and bone health. *Med Sci Sports Ex* 36(11):1985-1996, 2004.
135. Kraschnewski, JL, et al: Is exercise used as medicine? Association of meeting strength training guidelines and functional limitations among older US adults. *Prev Med* 66:1–5, 2014.
136. Lamb, M: Rehab measures: hand-held dynamometer/grip strength. Available at http://www.rehabmeasures.org/Lists/RehabMeasures/DispForm.aspx?ID=1185. Accessed August 26, 2015.
137. Lee, IH, and Park, SY: Balance improvement by strength training for the elderly. *J Phys Ther Sci* 25:1591–1593, 2013.
138. Lehman, CA: Phenomena of concern to the clinical nurse specialist. In Foster, JB, and Prevost, SE (eds): *Advanced Nursing of Adults in Acute Care.* Philadelphia: F.A. Davis, 2012, p 36.
139. Leipzig, RM, Cumming, RG, and Tinetti, ME: Drugs and falls in older people: a systematic review and meta-analysis: I. Psychotropic drugs. *J Am Geriatri Soc* 47(1):30–39, 1999.
140. Leipzig, RM, Cumming, RG, and Tinetti, ME: Drugs and falls in older people: a systematic review and meta-analysis: II. Cardiac and analgesic drugs. *J Am Geriatri Soc* 47(1):40–50, 1999.
141. Leong, DJ, and Sun, HB: Osteoarthritis – why exercise? *J Exerc Sports Orthop* 1(1):4, 2014.
142. Leonhardi, BJ, et al: Use of continuous subcutaneous insulin infusion (insulin pump) therapy in the hospital: a review of one institution's experience. *J Diabetes Sci Technol* 2(6):948–962, 2008.
143. Li, F, et al: Tai chi and fall reductions in older adults: a randomized controlled trial. *J Gerontol A Biol Sci Med Sci* 2005(60):187–194.
144. Lin, X, et al: Effects of exercise training on cardiorespiratory fitness and biomarkers of cardiometabolic health: a systematic review and meta_analysis of randomized controlled trials. Available at http://jaha.ahajournals.org/citmgr?gca=ahaoa%3B4%2F7%2Fe002014. Accessed July 8, 2015.
145. Liu-Ambrose, T, et al: Both resistance and agility training reduce fall risk in 75-85 year old women with low bone mass: a six-month randomized controlled trial. *J Am Geriatr Soc* 52(5):657–665, 2004.
146. Lobelo, F, Stoutenberg, M, and Hutber, A: The Exercise Is Medicine Global Health Initiative: a 2014 update. *Br J Sports Med.* 48(22):1627–1633, 2013.
147. Loesser, RF: Age-related changes in the musculoskeletal system and the development of osteoarthritis. *Clin Geriatr Med* 26(3):371–386, 2010.
148. Lubans, DR, et al: Pilot randomized controlled trial: Elastic-resistance-training and lifestyle-activity interventions for sedentary older adults. *J Aging Phys Act* 21:20–32, 2013.
149. Lucotti, P, et al: Aerobic and resistance training effects compared to aerobic training alone in obese type 2 diabetic patients on diet treatment. *Diabetes Res Clin Prac* 94(3):395–403, 2011.
150. Macfarlane, DJ, et al: Validity and normative data for thirty-second chair stand test in elderly community-dwelling Hong Kong Chinese. *Am J Hum Biol* 18(3):418–421, 2006.
151. Magee, DJ: *Orthopedic Physical Assessment,* ed. 6. Missouri: Saunders, Elsevier, 2013.
152. Maki, BE: Gait changes in older adults: predictors of falls or indicators of fear? *JABS* 45(3):313–320, 1997.
153. Mancia, G, et al: 2007 Guidelines for management of arterial hypertension: the Task Force for the Management of Arterial Hypertension of the European Society of Hypertension (ESH) and the European Society of Cardiology (ESC). *J Hypertens* 25(6):1105–1187, 2007.
154. Mangoni, AA, and Jackson, SH: Age-related changes in pharmacokinetics and pharmacodynamics: basic principles and practical applications. *Br J Clin Pharm* 57:6–14, 2004.
155. Marcell, TJ: Sarcopenia: Causes, consequences, and preventions. *J Gerontol A Biol Sci* 58A(10):911–916, 2003.
156. Martin, LJ, Zieve, D, and Ogilvie, I: Aging changes in organs – tissue – cells. *Medline Plus.* Available at https://www.nlm.nih.gov/medlineplus/ency/article/004012.htm. Accessed June 29, 2016.
157. Martins, WR, et al: Elastic resistance training to increase muscle strength in elderly: a systematic review with meta-analysis. *Arch Geron Geri* 57:8–15, 2013.
158. Massy-Westropp, NM, et al: Hand grip strength: age and gender stratified normative data in a population-based study. *BMC Res Notes* 4:127, 2011.
159. Mat, S, et al: Systematic review of physical therapies for improving balance and reducing falls risk in osteoarthritis of the knee: a systematic review. *Age Ageing* 44:16–24, 2015.
160. Mathias S, Nayak US, and Isaacs B: Balance in elderly patients: the "get-up and go" test. *Arch Phys Med Rehab* 67(6):387, 1986.
161. McArdle, WD, Katch, FI, and Katch, VL: *Essentials of Exercise Physiology,* ed. 4. Philadelphia: Lippincott Williams & Wilkins, 2011.

162. McArdle, WD, Katch, FI, and Katch, VL: *Exercise Physiology, Nutrition, Energy, and Human Performance*, ed. 8. Philadelphia: Lippincott Williams & Wilkins, 2014.
163. McCloskey, E, and the International Osteoporosis Foundation (2009): FRAX. Identifying people at high risk of fracture. Available at http://www.iofbonehealth.org/sites/default/files/PDFs/WOD%20Reports/FRAX_report_09.pdf. Accessed February 29, 2016.
164. McDermott, AY, and Mernitz, H: Exercise and older patients: prescribing guidelines. *Am Acad Fam Phys* 74(3):437–444, 2006.
165. Macfarlane, DJ, et al: Validity and normative data for thirty-second chair stand test in elderly community-dwelling Hong Kong Chinese. *Am J Hum Biol* 18(3):418–421, 2006.
166. Merriam-Webster Medical Dictionary: Hypokinesia. Available at http://www.merriam-webster.com/medical/hypokinesia. Accessed July 7, 2015.
167. Miszko, TA, et al: Effect of strength and power training on physical function in community-dwelling older adults. *J Geron: Bio Sci* 58A:171–175, 2003.
168. Mithal, A, et al: Impact of nutrition on muscle mass, strength, and performance in older adults. *Osteoporos Int* 24(5):1555–1566, 2013.
169. National Center for Health Statistics: Health, United States, 2014. US DHHS, CDC, DHHS Publication No. 2015-1232. Available at http://www.cdc.gov/nchs/data/hus/hus14.pdf#001. Accessed July 12, 2016.
170. National Council on Aging: Healthy aging facts, 2016. Available at https://www.ncoa.org/resources/fact-sheet-healthy-aging/. Accessed June 27, 2016.
171. National Institute on Aging: Health and aging, exercise and physical activity: your everyday guide from the National Institute on Aging (2015). Available at https://www.nia.nih.gov/health/publication/exercise-physical-activity/introduction. Accessed July 8, 2015.
172. National Institute of Health: Aging changes in the bones-muscles-joints, 2014. Available at https://www.nlm.nih.gov/medlineplus/ency/article/004015.htm. Accessed April 12, 2016.
173. National Institute of Health, National Center for Complementary and Integrative Health: Tai chi and qi gong: in depth. Available at https://nccih.nih.gov/health/taichi/introduction.htm. Accessed June 27, 2016.
174. National Institute of Health, National Heart, Lung, and Blood Institute: Aim for a healthy weight. Assessing your weight and health risk. Available at http://www.nhlbi.nih.gov/health/educational/lose_wt/risk.htm. Accessed July 12, 2016.
175. National Institute of Health, National Institute on Aging, Global Health and Aging: Changing role of the family. Available at https://www.nia.nih.gov/research/publication/global-health-and-aging/changing-role-family. Accessed June 27, 2016.
176. National Institute of Health: Obesity guidelines. Available at http://www.nhlbi.nih.gov/health-pro/guidelines/current/obesity-guidelines/e_textbook/txgd/4142.htm. Accessed March 2, 2016.
177. National Institute of Health: Clinical guidelines of the identification, evaluation, and treatment of overweight and obesity in adults, the evidence report. Publication, No. 98-4083. Available at http://www.nhlbi.nih.gov/files/docs/guidelines/ob_gdlns.pdf. Accessed May 4, 2016.
178. Nelson, ME, et al: Effects of high-intensity strength training on multiple risk factors for osteoporotic fractures: a randomized controlled trial. *JAMA* 272:1909–1914, 1994.
179. Nelson, ME, et al: Physical activity and public health in older adults. *Circulation* 116: 1094–1105, 2007.
180. Newson, P: Presentation of illness in the elderly patient. *Nurs Resident Care* 9(5):218–221, 2007.
181. Ng, M, et al: Global, regional, and national prevalence of overweight and obesity in children and adults during 1980-2013: a systematic analysis for the Global Burden of Disease Study 2013. *Lancet* 384(9945):766–781, 2014.
182. Nigam, Y, Night, J, and Jones, A. Effects of bedrest 3: musculoskeletal and immune systems, skin and self-perception. *Nurse Times* 105(23):18–22, 2009.
183. Nigthingale, EJ, Pourkazemi, F, and Hiller, CE: Systematic review of timed stair tests. *JRRD* 51(3):335–350, 2014.
184. North American Menopause Society: Position statement: management of osteoporosis in postmenopausal women: 2010. *Menopause* 17(1):25–54, 2010.
185. Office of Disease Prevention and Health Promotion: Physical activity guidelines, Ch 2: physical activity has many benefits. Available at http://health.gov/paguidelines/guidelines/chapter2.aspx. Accessed April 12, 2016.
186. Older Americans 2012: Key indicators of well-being. Available at http://www.agingstats.gov/main_site/data/2012_documents/docs/entirechartbook.pdf. Accessed March 12, 2016.
187. Orr, R, Raymond, J, and Singh, MA: Efficacy of progressive resistance training on balance performance in older adults. A systematic review of randomized controlled trials. *Sports Med* 38(4):317–343, 2008.
188. Osterrieder, K, and Schultheis, S: Are decreased gait speed and grip strength reliable indicators for predicting loss of function in elderly patients? *GeriNotes* 21(5):16–20, 2014.
189. Paddon-Jones, D, and Rasmussen, BB: Dietary protein recommendations and the prevention of sarcopenia: protein, amino acid metabolism and therapy. *Curr Opin Clin Nutr Metab Care* 12(1):86–90, 2009.
190. Parmenter, BJ, et al: High-intensity progressive resistance training improves flat-ground walking in older adults with symptomatic peripheral arterial disease. *J Am Geriatr Soc* 61:1964–1970, 2013.
191. Partridge, T, Billek-Sawhney, B, and Partridge, J: Type II diabetes mellitus: exercise prescription and application for physical therapy. *GeriTopics* 19(1):12–20, 2011.
192. Perera, S, et al: Meaningful change and responsiveness in common physical performance measures in older adults. *J Am Geri Soc* 54(5):743–749, 2006.
193. Perry, SB, and Downey, PA: Fracture risk and preventions: a multidimensional approach. *Phys Ther* 92(1):164–178, 2012.
194. Persinger, R, et al: Consistency of the talk test for exercise prescription. *Med Sci Sports Ex* 36(9):1632–1636, 2004.
195. Pescatello, LS, et al: *American College of Sports Medicine. ACSM's Guidelines for Exercise Testing and Prescription*, ed. 9. Philadelphia: Lippincott Williams, & Wilkins, 2014.
196. Pescatello, LS, et al. American College of Sports Medicine position stand. Exercise and hypertension. *Med Sci Sports Exerc* 36(3):533–553, 2004.
197. Physical Activity Guidelines for Americans: Health.gov, chapter 5. Available at http://health.gov/paguidelines/guidelines/chapter5.aspx. Accessed August 23, 2015.
198. Pischon, T, Nothlings, U, and Boeing, H. Obesity and cancer. *Proc Nutri Soci* 67(2):1280145, 2008.
199. Podsiadlo, D, and Richardson, S: The timed "up & go": a test of basic functional mobility for frail elderly persons. *J Am Geriatr Soc* 39(2):142–148, 1991.
200. Polidoulis, I, Beyene, J, and Cheung, AM: The effect of exercise on pQCT parameters of bone structure and strength in postmenopausal women—a systematic review and meta-analysis of randomized controlled trials. *Osteoporos Inter* 23(1):39–51, 2012.
201. Population Reference Bureau: 2014 world population data sheet. Available at http://www.prb.org/pdf14/2014-world-population-data-sheet_eng.pdf. Accessed June 11, 2015.
202. Puhl, R, and Heuer, C: The stigma of obesity: a review and update. *Obesity* 17:941–964, 2009.
203. Puthoff, ML, and Nielsen, DH: Relationships among impairments in lower-extremity strength and power, functional limitations and disability in older adults. *Phys Ther* 87(10):1334–1347, 2007.
204. Ratain, MJ, and Plunkett, WK: Principles of pharmacodynamics. In Kufe, DW, et al (eds): *Holland-Frei Cancer Medicine,* ed. 6. Hamilton, ON: BC Decker, 2003.
205. Ratamess, NA, et al: Progression models in resistance training for healthy adults. *Med Sci Sports Ex*41(3):687–708, 2009.
206. Raymond, MJ, et al: Systematic review of high-intensity progressive resistance strength training of the lower limb compared with other intensities of strength training in older adults. *Arch Phys Med Rehabil* 94:1458–1972, 2013.

207. Reed, JL, and Pipe, Al: The talk test: a useful tool for prescribing and monitoring exercise intensity. *Curr Opin Cardiol* 29(5):475–480, 2014.
208. Reid, K, et al: Comparative effects of light or heavy resistance power training for improving lower extremity power and physical performance in mobility-limited older adults. *J Gero Series A: Bio Sci Med Sci* 70(3):374–380, 2015.
209. Reiman, MP: *Orthopedic Clinical Examination With Web Resource.* Champaign, IL: Human Kinetics, 2016.
210. Ribeiro, AS, et al: Resistance training in older women: comparison of singles vs multiple sets on muscle strength and body composition. *Isokinetics and Exer Sci* 23:53–60, 2015.
211. Rice, CL: Muscle function at the motor unit level: consequences of aging. *Top Geriatr Rehabil* 15(3):70–82, 2000.
212. Riebe, D, et al: Updating ACSM's recommendations for exercise preparticipation health screening. *Med Sci Sports Ex* 47(11):2473–2479, 2015.
213. Sayers, S: High-speed power training: a novel approach to resistance training in older men and women. A brief review and pilot study. *J Strength Cond Res* 21(2):518, 2007.
214. Schoenborn, CA, and Heyman, KM: Health characteristics of adults aged 55 years and over: US, 2004-2007. National Health Statistic Report 1-31. Available at http://www.cdc.gov/nchs/data/nhsr/nhsr016.pdf. Accessed August 12, 2015.
215. Schultz, A, et al: Loads in the lumbar spine—validation of a biomechanical analysis by measurements of intradiscal pressures and myoelectric signals. *J Bone Joint Surg [Am]* 64:713–720, 1982.
216. Sehl, ME, and Yates, FE: Kinetics of human aging. Rates of senescence between ages 30 and 70 years in healthy people. *J Gerontol A Biol Sci Med Sci* 56(5):B198–B208, 2011.
217. Setchell, J, et al: Physical therapists' ways of talking about overweight and obesity: Clinical implications. *Phys Ther* 96(6):865–875, 2016.
218. Shaw, JM, and Snow, CM: Weighted vest exercise improves indices of fall risk in older women. *J Geron Med Sci* 53(1):M53–M58, 1998.
219. Shumway-Cook, A, Brauer, S, and Woolacott, M. Predicting the probability for falls in community-dwelling older adults using the Timed Up & Go Test. *Phys Ther* 80(9):896–903, 2000.
220. Signorile, JF: Targeting muscular strength, power, and endurance. *ACSMs Health Fit J* 17(5):24–32, 2013.
221. Sillanpää, E, et al: Combined strength and endurance training improves health-related quality of life in healthy middle-aged and older adults. *Int J Sports Med* 33:981–986, 2012.
222. Silver, JK, and Gilchrist, LS: Cancer rehabilitation with a focus on evidence-based outpatient physical and occupational therapy interventions. *AJPMR* 90(suppl):S5–S15, 2011.
223. Singh, NA, Clements, KM, and Singh, MAF: The efficacy of exercise as a long-term antidepressant in elderly subjects: a randomized, controlled trial. *J Gerontol: Med Sci* 56A(8):M497–M504, 2001.
224. Snow, CM, et al: Long-term exercise using weighted vests prevents hip bone loss in postmenopausal women. *J Geron Med Sci* 55A(9): M489–M491, 2000.
225. Social Progress Index: Obesity data table, 2015. Available at http://www.socialprogressimperative.org/data/spi#data_table/countries/idr28/dim1,dim2,com7,idr28,dim3. Accessed April 11, 2016.
226. Sousa, N, and Mendes, R: Comparison of effects of resistance and multicomponent training on falls prevention in institutionalized elderly women. *JAGS* 63(2):396–397, 2015.
227. Sousa, N, et al: The long-term effects of aerobic training versus combined training on physical fitness and cardiovascular diseases risk factors in overweight elderly men with high blood pressures. *Br J Sports Med* 47e3:9, 2013.
228. Steffen, TM, et al: Age- and gender-related test performance in community-dwelling elderly people: six-minute walk test, Berg Balance Scale, Timed Up & Go Test, and gait speeds. *Phys Ther* 82(2):128–137, 2002.
229. Steib, S, Schoene, D, and Pfeifer, K: Dose-response relationship of resistance training in older adults: a meta-analysis. *Med Sci Sports Ex* 42(5):902–914, 2010.
230. Stewart, VH, Saunders, DH, and Greig, CA: Responsiveness of muscle size and strength to physical training in very elderly people: a systematic review. *Scan J Med Sci Sports* 24:e1–e10, 2014.
231. Stuempfle, K, and Drury, DG: The physiological consequences of bed rest. *J Exercise Physiol Online* 10(3):32–41, 2007.
232. Suzuki, T, Bean, JF, and Fielding, RA: Muscle power of the ankle flexors predicts functional performance in community-dwelling older women. *J Am Geriatr Soc* 49(9):1161–1167, 2001.
233. Symons, TB, and Swank, AM: Exercise testing and training strategies for healthy and frail elderly. *ACSM's Health & Fitness Journal* 19(2):32–35, 2015.
234. Tan, FYH, et al: Reliability of the stair-climb test (SCT) of cardiorespiratory fitness. *Adv Exerc Sports Physiol* 10(3):77–83, 2004.
235. Terman, A, and Brunk, UT: Lipofuscin. *J Biochem Cell Biol* 36(8): 1400–1404, 2004.
236. The International Diabetes Federation: The IDF consensus worldwide definition of the metabolic syndrome. Available at http://www.idf.org/webdata/docs/MetSyndrome_FINAL.pdf. Accessed July 13, 2016.
237. The New PAR-Q+ and ePARmed-X+: Official website. Available at http://eparmedx.com/. Accessed July 12, 2016.
238. Thiebaud, RS, Funk, MD, and Abe, T: Home-based resistance training for older adults: a systematic review. *Geriatrics & Gerontology Intl* 14:750–757, 2014.
239. Thomas, S, Reading, J, and Shephard, RJ: Revision of the Physical Activity Readiness Questionnaire (PAR-Q). *Can J Spt Sci* 17(4):338–345, 1992.
240. Thompson, DR: Sarcopenia. *Clin Geriatr Med* 26:331–346, 2010.
241. Tieland, M, et al: Handgrip strength does not represent an appropriate measure to evaluate changes in muscle strength during an exercise intervention program in frail older people. *Int J Sport Nutrition and Ex Metab* 25:27–36, 2015.
242. Tinetti, ME: Preventing falls in elderly persons. *N Engl J Med* 348:42–49, 2003.
243. Transgenerational.org: The demographics of aging. Available at http://transgenerational.org/aging/demographics.htm. Accessed June 17, 2015.
244. US Department of Health and Human Services, Health Resources and Services Administration: Lower extremity amputation prevention, 2012. Available at http://www.hrsa.gov/hansensdisease/leap/. Accessed April 11, 2016.
245. US Department of Health and Human Service, National Vital Statistics Reports: Department of Health and Human Services deaths data for 2013. Available at http://www.cdc.gov/nchs/data/nvsr/nvsr64/nvsr64_02.pdf. Accessed June 27, 2016.
246. US Department of Health and Human Services: Talking with patients about weight loss: tips for primary care providers. NIH publication 05-5634. Available at http://www.niddk.nih.gov/health-information/health-topics/weight-control/talking-with-patients-about-weight-loss-tips-for-primary-care/Documents/TalkingWPAWL.pdf. Accessed April 11, 2016.
247. US Department of Health and Human Services: Urinary incontinence in women. NIH publication 08-4132. Available at http://kidney.niddk.nih.gov/KUDiseases/pubs/uiwomen/UI-Women_508.pdf. Accessed July 12, 2016.
248. Uttter, AC, Kang, J, and Robertson, RJ: ACSM current comment perceived exertion. *ACSM*, 2000. Available at https://www.acsm.org/docs/current-comments/perceivedexertion.pdf. Accessed April 11, 2016.
249. Valentour, J: The Fick Equation by the American Council on Exercise. Available at https://www.acefitness.org/blog/1545/the-fick-equation. Accessed March 22, 2016.
250. Vella, C, and Kravitz L: Sarcopenia: the mystery of muscle loss. *IDEA Personal Trainer* 13(4):30–35, 2002.
251. Villareal, DT, et al: Obesity in older adults: technical review and position statement of the American Society for Nutrition and NAASO, The Obesity Society. *Am J Clin Nutr* 2(5):923–934, 2005. Available at http://ajcn.nutrition.org/content/82/5/923.long. Accessed May 24, 2017.
252. Wanderley, FAC, et al: Aerobic versus resistance training effects on health-related quality of life body composition, and function of older adults. *J Ap Geron* 34(3):143–165, 2015.

253. Wang, Y, et al: Comparison of abdominal adiposity and overall obesity in predicting risk of type 2 diabetes among men. *Am J Clin Nutr* 81, 555–563, 2005.
254. Warburton, DER, et al: Evidence-based risk assessment and recommendations for physical activity clearance; consensus document 2011. *APNM* 36(S1):S266–s298, 2011.
255. Warburton, DER, et al: The ePARmed-X+ physician clearance follow-up. *Health Fitness J Canada* 7(2):35–38, 2014.
256. Warburton, DER, et al: The Physical Activity Readiness Questionnaire for Everyone (PAR-Q+) and Electronic Physical Activity Readiness Medical Examination (ePARmed-X+). *Health Fitness J Canada* 4(2):3–23, 2011.
257. Warburton, DER, Nicol, CW, and Bredin, SSD: Health benefits of physical activity: the Evidence. *CMAJ* 174(6):801–809, 2006.
258. Waters, DL, et al: Advantages of dietary, exercise-related, and therapeutic interventions to prevent and treat sarcopenia in adult patients: an update. *Clin Interventions Aging* 5:259–270, 2010.
259. Wen, CP, et al: Minimum amount of physical activity for reduced mortality and extended life expectancy: a prospective cohort study. *Lancet* 378(9798):1244–1253, 2011.
261. Wert, DM, et al: Gait biomechanics, spatial and temporal characteristics, and the energy cost of walking in older adults with impaired mobility. *Phys Ther* 90:977–985, 2010.
262. Whitney, JC, Lord, SR, and Close, JC: Streamlining assessment and intervention in a falls clinic using the Timed Up and Go Test and Physiological Profile assessments. *Age Ageing* 34(6):567–571, 2005.
263. Whitney, SL, et al: Clinical measurement of sit-to-stand performance in people with balance disorders: validity of data for the five-times-sit-to-stand test. *Phys Ther* 85(10):1034–1045, 2005.
264. Wick, JY: Bedrest: implications for the aging population. *Pharm Times,* 2011. Available at http://www.pharmacytimes.com/publications/issue/2011/January2011/FeatureBedrest-0111. Accessed April 12, 2016.
265. Wilhelm, M, et al: Effect of resistance exercises on function in older adults with osteoporosis or osteopenia: a systematic review. *Physiother Canada* 64(4):386–394, 2012. Available at https://www.ncbi.nlm.nih.gov/pmc/articles/PMC3484910/. Accessed May 24, 2017.
266. Wilson, L, et al: Annual direct cost of urinary incontinence. *Obstet Gynecol* 98:398–406, 2001.
267. Winters-Stone, KM, and Snow, CM: Site-specific response of bone to exercise in premenopausal women. *Bone* Dec;39(6):1203–1209, 2006.
268. Woltmann, ML, et al: Evident that the talk test can be used to regulate exercise intensity. *J Strength Cond Res* 29(5):1248–1254, 2015.
269. World Health Organization: FRAX WHO Fracture Risk Assessment Tool. Available at http://www.shef.ac.uk/FRAX/. Accessed June 4, 2016.
270. World Health Organization: Obesity and overweight, fact sheet no. 311. Available at http://www.who.int/mediacentre/factsheets/fs311/en/. Accessed May 4, 2016.
271. World Health Organization: Waist circumference and waist-hip ratio, report of a WHO expert consultation, 2008. Available at http://whqlibdoc.who.int/publications/2011/9789241501491_eng.pdf. Accessed March 2, 2016.
272. World Health Organization: World Health Day 2012: adding life to years. Available at http://www.wpro.who.int/mediacentre/releases/2012/20120404/en/. Accessed November 21, 2015.
273. Wright, AA, et al: A comparison of 3 methodological approaches to defining major clinically important improvement of 4 performance measures in patients with hip osteoarthritis. *J Orthop Sports Phys Ther* 41(5):319–327, 2011.
274. Zacker, RJ: Health related implications and management of sarcopenia. *J Am Acad Phys Assistants* 19(10):24–29, 2006.
275. Zammit, C, et al: Obesity and respiratory disease. *Int J Gen Med* 2010. Available at http://www.ncbi.nlm.nih.gov/pmc/articles/PMC2990395/pdf/ijgm-3-335.pdf. Accessed March 2, 2016.
276. Ziere, G, et al: Polypharmacy and falls in the middle age and elderly population. *Br J Clin Pharmacol* 61(2):218–223, 2006.

CHAPTER 25

Women's Health: Obstetrics and Pelvic Floor

BARBARA SETTLES HUGE, PT ■ CAROLYN KISNER, PT, MS

Throughout a woman's life cycle, specific gender differences need to be recognized for their relevance to rehabilitation. Recent research has shown repeatedly that women have specific and distinct physiological processes that extend beyond the obvious considerations of anatomy and hormones, including differences in symptoms of heart attacks and in metabolism of medications.[77] Clearly, the pregnant or postpartum patient presents a unique gender-based clinical challenge for the physical therapist. Although pregnancy is a time of tremendous musculoskeletal, physiological, and emotional change, it is nonetheless a state of wellness. Pregnant women are typically well motivated, willing to learn, and highly responsive to treatment suggestions. For many women, the therapist is able to assess and monitor the physical changes with the primary focus on maintaining wellness. The ability to educate women about the role of exercise and health promotion during this key life transition provides a significant professional opportunity and responsibility.

In cases of musculoskeletal impairment related to pregnancy, the therapist is able to examine and treat the patient by incorporating knowledge of injury and tissue healing with knowledge of the changes during pregnancy. By considering a broader, lifespan perspective, all female patients can benefit from education regarding the role of the pelvic floor muscles in musculoskeletal health, specifically in trunk stabilization. Evidence is growing regarding prevention of pelvic floor impairments; when women receive individualized interventions, improvement is seen in pelvic floor awareness and activation and in symptom reduction.[17,53,86,87] Specialized treatment of pelvic floor dysfunction is critical to quality of life (QOL) for women experiencing incontinence, pelvic organ prolapse (POP), and a variety of pelvic pain syndromes. As a natural progression of expertise in pelvic floor interventions, physical therapists are also treating males with urinary incontinence and other pelvic floor impairments. Although all physical therapists can easily incorporate activation of the pelvic floor muscles as a key component of trunk stabilization and training in body mechanics, true proficiency can come only with further training and mentoring. Advanced study of pelvic floor anatomy, evaluation, and treatment is highly recommended for therapists who wish to specialize in this area. Clinical Specialization in Women's Health (WCS), available through the American Physical Therapy Association since 2010, is another option for postgraduate training.

This chapter provides readers with basic information about the systemic changes of pregnancy as a foundation for the development of safe and effective exercise programs. In addition, a review of pelvic floor anatomy, function, and dysfunction serves as an introduction to the treatment of pelvic floor disorders. The chapter emphasizes modification of general exercises to meet the needs of the obstetric patient and provides information to assist in the development of an exercise program for an uncomplicated pregnancy. Cesarean delivery, high-risk pregnancy, and the special needs of patients with these conditions are also discussed.

Overview of Pregnancy, Labor, and Related Conditions

Characteristics of Pregnancy and Labor

Pregnancy

Pregnancy, which spans 40 weeks from conception to delivery, is divided into three trimesters, with characteristic changes during each.[78,102]

First Trimester Changes

During the first trimester (weeks 0 through 12), the following occur:

- Implantation of the fertilized ovum in the uterus occurs 7 to 10 days after fertilization.
- The mother is very fatigued, urinates more frequently, and may experience nausea and/or vomiting ("morning" sickness).
- Breast size may increase.
- There is a relatively small weight gain of 0 to 1,455 g (0 to 3 lb is normal).
- Emotional changes may occur.
- By the end of the 12th week, the fetus is 6- to 7-cm long and weighs approximately 20 g (2 oz). The fetus now can kick, turn its head, and swallow and has a beating heart, but these movements are not yet felt by the mother.

Second Trimester Changes

During the second trimester (weeks 13 through 26), the following occur:

- The pregnancy becomes visible to others.
- The mother begins to feel movement at around 20 weeks.
- Most women now feel very good. Nausea and fatigue have usually disappeared.
- By the end of the second trimester, the fetus is 19 to 23 cm (14 in.) in length and weighs approximately 600 g (1 to 2 lb).
- The fetus now has eyebrows, eyelashes, and fingernails.

Third Trimester Changes

During the third trimester (weeks 27 through 40), the following occur:

- The uterus is now very large and has regular contractions, although these may be felt only occasionally.
- Common complaints during the third trimester are frequent urination, back pain, leg edema and fatigue, round ligament pain, shortness of breath, and constipation.
- By the time of birth, the baby will be 33- to 39-cm long (16 to 19 in.) and will weigh approximately 3,400 g (7 lb, although a range of 5 to 10 lb is normal).

NOTE: Although pregnancy typically lasts 40 weeks, the range of 38 to 42 weeks is considered full term.

Labor

Labor is divided into three stages, each containing specific events.[22,78] While the exact mechanism that initiates labor is not known, continued study reveals the complexity of the hormonal triggers from both the maternal and fetal circulation.[95] Regular and strong involuntary contractions of the smooth muscles of the uterus are the primary symptom of labor. True labor produces palpable changes in the cervix, which are known as effacement and dilation (Fig. 25.1).

- ***Effacement*** is the shortening or thinning of the cervix from a thickness of 5 cm (2 in.) before onset of labor to the thickness of a piece of paper.
- ***Dilation*** is the opening of the cervix from the diameter of a fingertip to approximately 10 cm (4 in.).

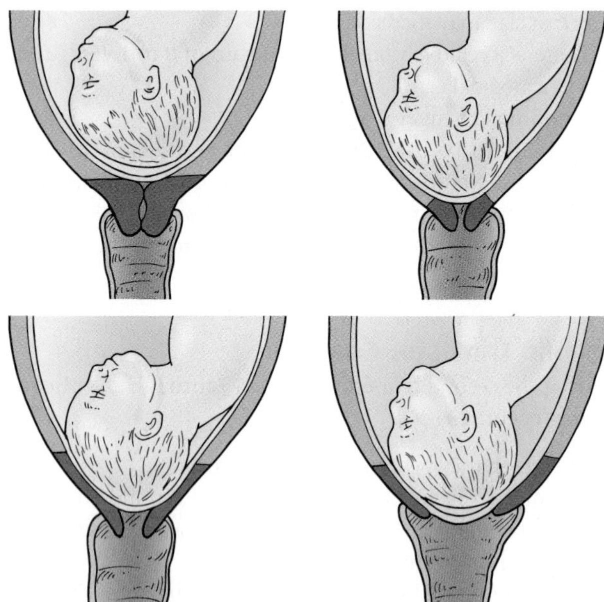

FIGURE 25.1 Effacement and dilation of the cervix. *(Adapted from Ward, S, and Hisley, S: Maternal-Child Nursing Care. Philadelphia: F.A. Davis, 2009, with permission.)*

Labor: Stage 1

Some women experience initial cervical dilation and effacement before they are in true labor. However, by the end of this stage, the cervix is fully dilated, and there is no doubt that a baby is about to be delivered. Stage 1 of labor is divided into three major phases.

Cervical dilation phase. The cervix dilates from 0 to 3 cm (0 to 1 in.) and will almost completely efface. Uterine contractions occur from the top down, causing the cervix to open and pushing the fetus downward.

Middle phase. The cervix dilates from 4 to 7 cm (1 to 3 in.). Contractions are stronger and more regular.

Transition phase. The cervix dilates from 8 to 10 cm (3 to 4 in.), and dilation is complete. Uterine contractions are very strong and close together.

Labor: Stage 2

Stage 2 involves "pushing" and expulsion of the fetus. Intra-abdominal pressure is the primary force expelling the fetus; it is produced by voluntary contraction of the abdominal muscles and diaphragm. Relaxation and stretching of the pelvic floor during stage 2 are also necessary for successful vaginal delivery. Uterine contractions may last as long as 90 seconds during this stage.

Fetal descent. Position changes (cardinal movements) by the fetus allow it to pass through the pelvis and be born (Fig. 25.2).[78] The position changes are described as:

- ***Engagement.*** The greatest transverse diameter of the fetal head passes through the pelvic inlet (the superior opening of the minor pelvis).
- ***Descent.*** Continued downward progression of the fetus occurs.
- ***Flexion.*** The fetal chin is brought closer to its thorax; this occurs when the descending head meets resistance from the walls and floor of the pelvis and the cervix.
- ***Internal rotation.*** The fetus turns its occiput toward the mother's symphysis pubis when the fetal head reaches the level of the ischial spines.
- ***Extension.*** The flexed fetal head reaches the introitus; the fetus extends its head, bringing the base of the occiput in direct contact with the inferior margin of the maternal symphysis pubis; this phase ends when the fetal head is delivered.
- ***External rotation.*** The fetus rotates its occiput toward the mother's sacrum to allow the fetal shoulders to pass through the pelvis.

Expulsion The fetal anterior shoulder passes under the symphysis pubis, and the rest of the body follows.

Labor: Stage 3

Placental stage (expulsion of the placenta). After delivery, the uterus continues to contract and shrink, causing the placenta to detach and be expelled.

- As the uterus decreases in size, the placenta detaches from the uterine wall, blood vessels are constricted, and bleeding slows. This can occur 5 to 30 minutes after the baby is delivered.
- A hematoma forms over the uterine placental site to prevent further significant blood loss; mild bleeding persists for 3 to 6 weeks after delivery.

Uterine involution. The uterus continues to contract and decrease in size for 3 to 6 weeks after delivery; the uterus always remains slightly enlarged over its prepregnant size.

Anatomical and Physiological Changes of Pregnancy

Considerable changes occur in the woman's body as the pregnancy progresses.[7,22,67,78,]

Weight Gain During Pregnancy

Current recommendations for weight gain during a singleton pregnancy are an average of 25 to 35 lb[71,78] with a distribution as shown in Box 25.1.

Changes in Organ Systems

Uterus and Related Connective Tissue

Uterus. The uterus increases from a prepregnant size of 5 by 10 cm (2 by 4 in.) to 25 by 36 cm (10 by 14 in.). It increases five to six times in size, 3,000 to 4,000 times in capacity, and 20 times in weight by the end of pregnancy. By the end of pregnancy, each muscle cell in the uterus has increased approximately 10 times over its prepregnancy

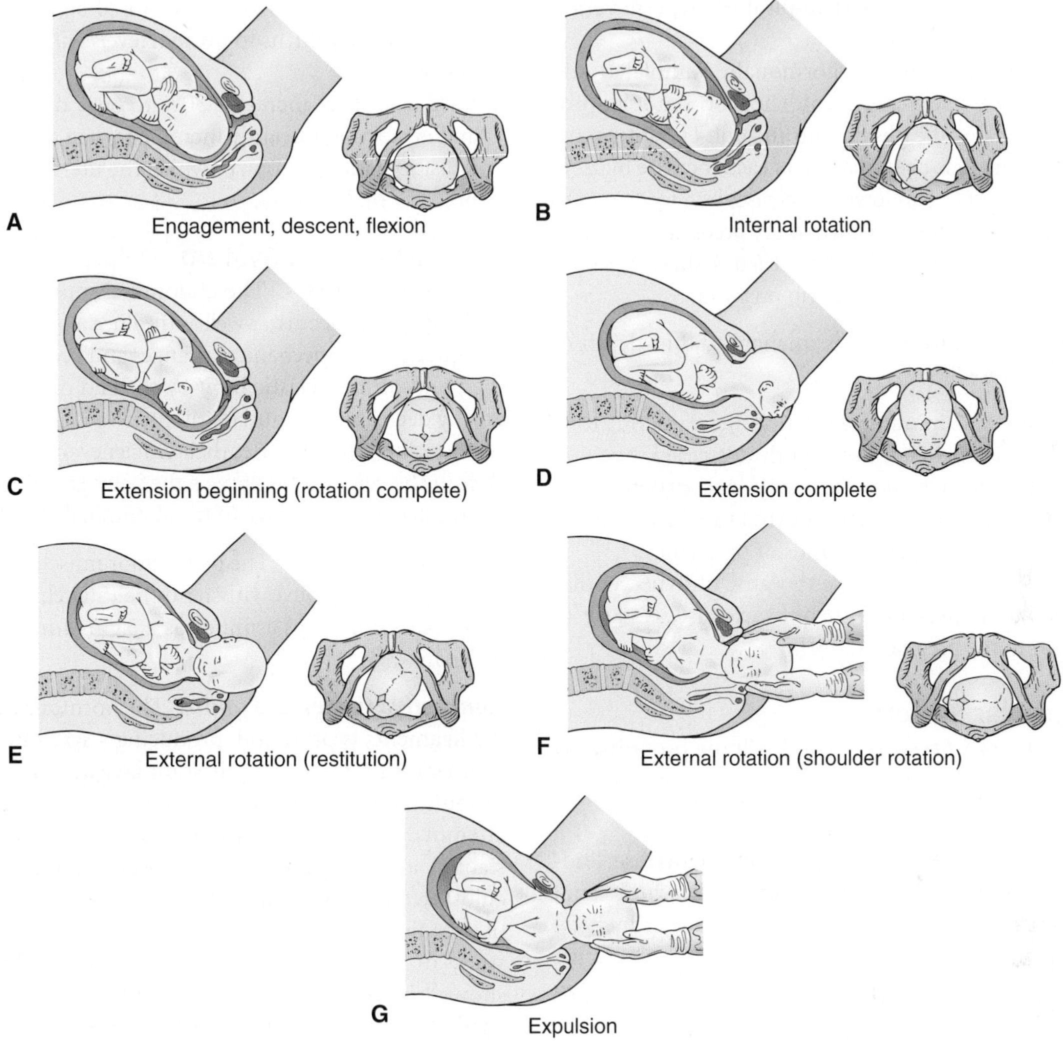

FIGURE 25.2 Principal movements in the mechanism of labor and delivery, left occiput anterior position. *(From Ward, S, and Hisley, S:* Maternal-Child Nursing Care. *Philadelphia: F.A. Davis, 2009, with permission.)*

BOX 25.1 Total Weight Gain (Ranges) for Single Fetus

■ Baby	3.36–3.88 kg	(7–8 lb)
■ Placenta	0.48–0.72 kg	(2–3 lb)
■ Amniotic fluid	0.72–0.97 kg	(2–3 lb)
■ Uterus and breasts	2.42–2.66 kg	(4–8 lb)
■ Blood and fluid	1.94–3.99 kg	(4 lb)
■ Fat stores	0.48–2.91 kg	(5–9 lb)
■ Total:	9.70–14.55 kg	(25–35 lb)

length.[125] Once the uterus expands upward and leaves the pelvis, it becomes an abdominal rather than a pelvic organ.

Connective tissues. Ligaments connected to the pelvic organs are more fibroelastic than ligaments supporting joint structures. The fascial tissues, which surround and enclose the organs in a continuous sheet, also include a significant amount of smooth muscle fibers.[38] The round and broad ligaments, as well as the cardinal-uterosacral complex, all provide suspensory support for the uterus.

Urinary System

Kidneys. The kidneys increase in length by 1 cm (0.5 in.).

Ureters. The ureters enter the bladder at a perpendicular angle because of uterine enlargement. This may result in a reflux of urine out of the bladder and back into the ureter; therefore, during pregnancy, there is an increased chance of developing urinary tract infections because of urinary stasis.

Pulmonary System

Hormonal influences. Hormone changes affect pulmonary secretions and rib cage position.

- Edema and tissue congestion of the upper respiratory tract begin early in pregnancy because of hormonal changes.

Hormonally stimulated upper respiratory hypersecretion also occurs.

- Changes in rib position are hormonally stimulated and occur prior to uterine enlargement. The subcostal angle progressively increases; the ribs flare up and out. The anteroposterior and transverse chest diameters each increase by 2 cm (1 in.). Total chest circumference increases by 5 to 7 cm (2 to 3 in.) and does not always return to the prepregnant state.
- The diaphragm is elevated by 4 cm (1.5 in.); this is a passive change caused by the change in rib position.

Respiration. Respiration rate is unchanged, but depth of respiration increases.[78]

- Tidal volume and minute ventilation increase, but total lung capacity is unchanged or slightly decreased.[78,125]
- There is a 15% to 20% increase in oxygen consumption; a natural state of hyperventilation exists throughout pregnancy to meet the oxygen demands of pregnancy.[78, 125]
- The work of breathing increases because of hyperventilation; dyspnea is present with mild exercise as early as 20 weeks into the pregnancy. [78,125]

Cardiovascular System

Blood volume and pressure. Blood volume progressively increases 35% to 50% (1.5 to 2 L) throughout pregnancy and returns to normal by 6 to 8 weeks after delivery.

- Plasma increase is greater than red blood cell increase, leading to the "physiologic anemia" of pregnancy, which is not a true anemia but is representative of the greater increase of plasma volume. The increase in plasma volume occurs as a result of hormonal stimulation to meet the oxygen demands of pregnancy.
- Venous pressure in the lower extremities increases during standing as a result of increased uterine size and increased venous distensibility.
- Pressure in the inferior vena cava rises in late pregnancy, especially in the supine position, because of compression by the uterus just below the diaphragm. In some women, the decline in venous return and resulting decrease in cardiac output may lead to symptomatic supine hypotensive syndrome. The aorta is partially occluded in the supine position.
- Blood pressure decreases early in the first trimester. There is a slight decrease of systolic pressure and a greater decrease of diastolic pressure. Blood pressure reaches its lowest level approximately midway through pregnancy and then rises gradually from midpregnancy to reach the prepregnant level approximately 6 weeks after delivery. Although cardiac output increases, blood pressure decreases because of venous distensibility.

Heart. Heart size increases, and the heart is elevated because of the movement of the diaphragm.

- Heart rhythm disturbances are more common during pregnancy.
- Heart rate usually increases 10 to 20 beats per minute by full term and returns to normal levels within 6 weeks after delivery.
- Cardiac output increases 30% to 60% during pregnancy and is most significantly increased when a woman is in the left side-lying position, in which the uterus places the least pressure on the aorta.

Musculoskeletal System

Abdominal muscles. The abdominal muscles, particularly both sides of the rectus, as well as the linea alba, are all subjected to significant biomechanical changes and become stretched to the point of their elastic limit by the end of pregnancy. This greatly decreases the muscles' ability to generate a strong contraction and thus decreases their efficiency of contraction. The shift in the center of gravity as the baby grows also decreases the mechanical advantage of the abdominal muscles.[68,125]

Pelvic floor muscles. The pelvic floor muscles, in their antigravity position, must withstand the total change in weight; the pelvic floor drops as much as 2.5 cm (1 in.) as a result of pregnancy.[120]

Connective tissues and joints. The hormonal influence on the ligaments is profound, producing a systemic decrease in ligamentous tensile strength. Joint laxity has been measured in multiple joints during pregnancy and postpartum, with attempts to correlate hormonal levels with changes in joint stability and also to determine the connection between musculoskeletal impairments related to childbearing with levels of estradiol, progesterone, relaxin, and cortisol. A longitudinal study of 35 pregnant women that measured wrist laxity showed increases in each of the above serum levels with significant correlation found only between cortisol levels and increased laxity. The authors propose that individual differences in hormonal receptors could account for the mixed findings over many years of studies. Better understanding of these hormonal influences is pertinent as it relates to persistent pelvic pain or risk of POP.[84]

- Clinically, it appears that these physiological changes lead to increased vulnerability to injury in weight-bearing joints of the back, pelvis, and lower extremities during pregnancy.

Thermoregulatory System

Metabolic rate. During pregnancy, basal metabolic rate and heat production increase.[4]

- An additional intake of 300 calories per day is needed to meet the basic metabolic needs of pregnancy.
- In pregnant women, normal fasting blood glucose levels are lower than in nonpregnant women.[4]

Changes in Posture and Balance

Center of Gravity

The center of gravity shifts upward and forward because of the enlargement of the uterus and breasts. This requires postural compensations to maintain balance and stability (Fig. 25.3).[7,67,125]

- The *lumbar and cervical lordoses* increase to compensate for the shift in the center of gravity.
- The *shoulder girdle and upper back* become rounded with scapular protraction and upper extremity internal rotation because of breast enlargement; this postural tendency persists in the postpartum period due to infant care demands. Tightness of the pectoralis muscles and weakness of the scapular stabilizers may be preexisting to or induced by the pregnancy postural changes.
- The *suboccipital muscles* respond in an effort to maintain appropriate eye level (optical righting reflex) and to moderate forward head posture along with the change in shoulder alignment.
- A tendency toward genu recurvatum will shift weight toward the heels in an attempt to counteract the anterior pull of the growing fetus.
- Changes in posture do not automatically correct after childbirth, and the pregnant posture may become habitual. In addition, many childcare activities contribute to persistent postural faults and asymmetry.

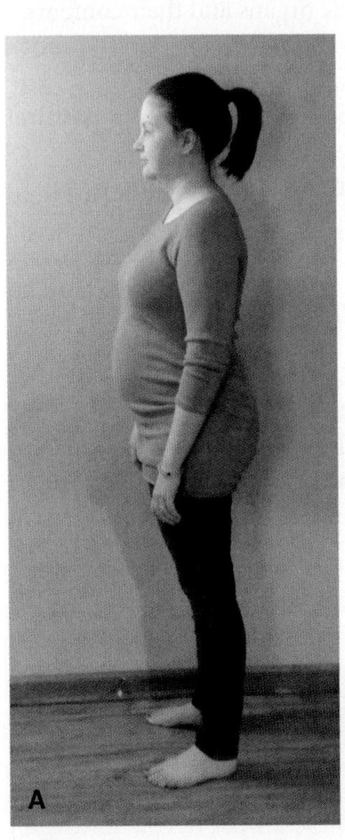

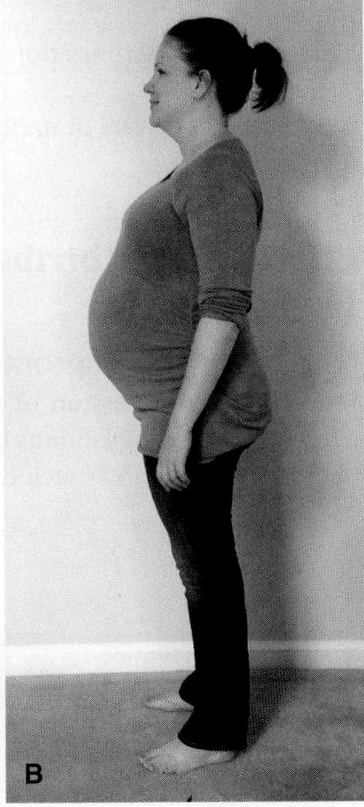

FIGURE 25.3 Change in posture as pregnancy progresses: **(A)** 23 weeks, **(B)** 34 weeks.

Balance

With the increased weight and redistribution of body mass, there are compensations to maintain balance.[7,125]

- The pregnant woman usually walks with a wider base of support and increased external rotation at the hips.
- This change in stance, along with growth of the baby, makes some activities such as walking, stooping, stair climbing, lifting, reaching, and other activities of daily living (ADLs) progressively more challenging.
- Activities requiring fine balance and rapid changes in direction, such as aerobic dancing and bicycle riding, may become difficult to do, especially during the third trimester, so added caution is necessary in order to avoid falling.[4]

Overview of Pelvic Floor Anatomy, Function, and Dysfunction

Treatment of pelvic floor impairments has become more visible and available in the physical therapy community over the past 15 to 20 years. As a result, both male and female clients with pelvic floor dysfunction are now seeking, and being referred for, rehabilitation in larger numbers. Advanced and in-depth study of anatomy, including internal pelvic floor muscle assessment, physiology, evaluation, and treatment, continues to be highly recommended for therapists who specialize in this area. Physicians and consumers, particularly with the increase of social media use, are also more aware of the need for expert practitioners when seeking treatment for pelvic floor dysfunction. As an example, a closed Facebook support group for women experiencing POP attracted over 3,000 members in less than 4 years (from 2011 to 2015), representing all 50 states in the United States and 38 countries, with ages ranging from teens to mid-80s.[101]

Pelvic Floor Musculature

The pelvic floor musculature is composed of multiple elements in a funnel-shaped orientation, with boney attachments to the pubic bone and the coccyx. Laterally, the tissues blend into a fascial layer overlying the obturator internus. The prime mover of the pelvic floor is the levator ani. The levator ani, in combination with the coccygeus, forms the pelvic diaphragm. The most superficial muscles of the pelvic floor include the superficial transverse perineal muscles, the ischiocavernosus, the bulbocavernosus (called bulbospongiosus in men), and the external anal sphincter. Both the right and left sides of the pelvic floor complex contribute fibers to the perineal body located superficially between the vagina/scrotum and external anal sphincter (Fig. 25.4). The structure and action of the muscles of each layer are summarized in Table 25.1. The combined action of these muscles creates a superior force toward the heart and a puckering or drawstring motion around the sphincters.[112]

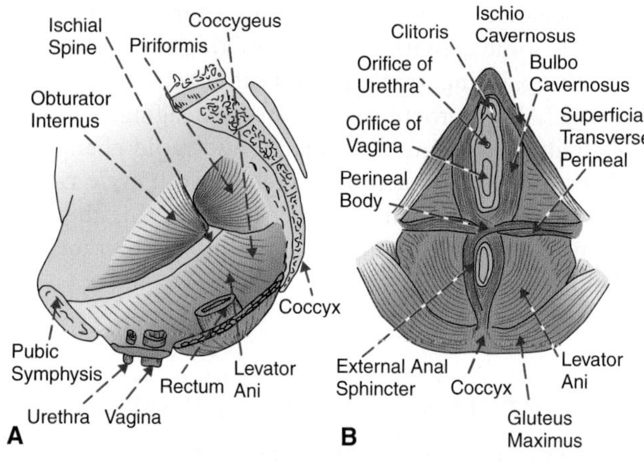

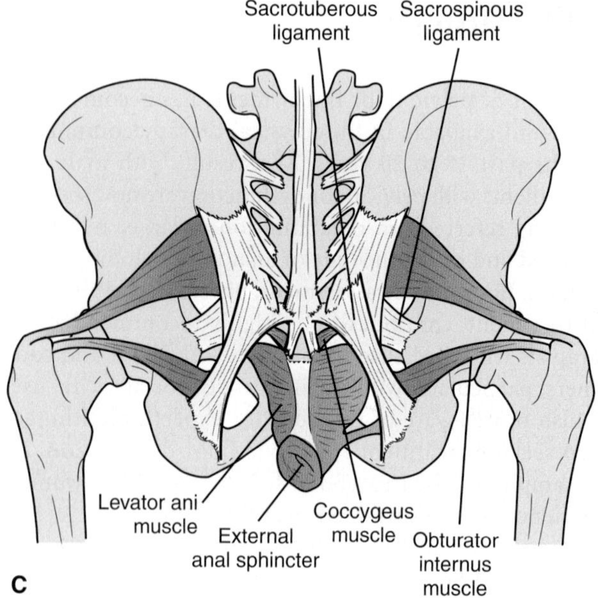

FIGURE 25.4 Pelvic floor muscles. **(A)** Sagittal section—note sling/hammock orientation; **(B)** viewed from below—note figure-eight orientation of the muscles around the orifice of the urethra/vagina and the anal sphincter; and **(C)** posterior view—note the funnel shape of the pelvic muscles.

Female Pelvic Floor

The female pelvic floor allows for passage of the urethra, vagina, and rectum. This automatically results in less intrinsic stability and pelvic organ support when compared to the male anatomy. The urogenital hiatus is the opening through which the urethra and vagina pass; measurement of this opening is being used as an objective measure in research design.[119]

Innervation

Recent cadaveric studies have uncovered many variations in configuration of the nerves to the pelvic floor complex.[11,59,124] The nerve supply to the perineal tissues includes the pudendal nerve (with its three terminal branches, the dorsal, perineal and rectal), the levator ani nerve, and direct branches from the sacral nerve roots, with conflicting findings as to sacral levels. These dual and variable innervations provide a safeguard in particular against damage during labor and vaginal delivery, which would be more likely with a single-nerve arrangement.

Function

The pelvic floor musculature has the following essential roles:

- Provide support for the pelvic organs and their contents
- Withstand increases in intra-abdominal pressure —"shock absorber"
- Contribute to stabilization of the spine/pelvis for postural stability[109]
- Sphincteric closure of urethra, vagina, and anus
- Sexual response

Effect of Childbirth on the Pelvic Floor

Neurological Compromise

Stretch and compression of the pudendal and levator ani nerves occur during labor as the baby's head travels through the birth canal. This stretch can be 20% to 35% of the total

TABLE 25.1 Female and Male Pelvic Floor Anatomy: From Superficial to Deep

Muscle Layer	Structure	Action
Superficial (outlet: primarily sexual function)		
	Ischiocavernosus	Maintains erection of clitoris or penis
	Bulbocavernosus in females; bulbospongiosus in males	Vaginal "sphincter" closure, erection of clitoris or penis, empties urethra in males
	Superficial transverse perineal	Fixes perineal body
	External anal sphincter	Closure of anus

Continued

TABLE 25.1 Female and Male Pelvic Floor Anatomy: From Superficial to Deep—cont'd

Muscle Layer	Structure	Action
Perineal membrane (formerly urogenital diaphragm)		
	Deep transverse perineal	Compression of urethra and ventral wall of vagina
	Compressor urethrae Urethrovaginal sphincter	Support of the perineal body and introitus
Pelvic diaphragm (primary muscular support)		
	Levator ani ■ Pubococcygeus ■ Puborectalis ■ Iliococcygeus	Prime mover of the pelvic floor, puborectalis aids in closure of the rectum
	Coccygeus (Ischiococcygeus)	Flexes coccyx

length of the nerve structures and has been found to be more significant in the posterior portion of the perineum.[80,114] This compromise to the nerve tissue is most intense during pushing (the second stage of labor), through the completion of vaginal delivery.

Muscular Impairment

Extreme stretching of all pelvic floor tissues is inherent in the process of labor and vaginal delivery. Recent computerized simulations of the biomechanics of childbirth are adding to the understanding of these impairments.[80] Muscle and/or ligamentous injury during labor and delivery diminishes the maximal closure pressure of the pelvic floor complex, which makes the entire system more vulnerable to increased intra-abdominal pressure and changes force transmission to the distal vagina, possibly contributing to prolapse of the bladder, urethra, vagina, uterus, small intestine, and rectum.[9]

The pelvic floor musculature may also be torn or incised during the birth process. Additional soft tissue lacerations can occur as a result of forceps use, necessitating suturing throughout the musculature and into the vaginal vault.

Episiotomy

An episiotomy is an incision made in the perineal body (see Fig. 25.4B). It is automatically considered a second-degree laceration according to the following classification of perineal lacerations.[78]

- First degree—only skin
- Second degree—includes underlying superficial muscle layer
- Third degree—extends to anal sphincter
- Fourth degree—tears through the sphincter and into the rectum, possibly into the deeper muscular layer of the pelvic floor (see Fig. 25.4 A)

Although episiotomy is common, occurring in 33% to 54% of vaginal deliveries, there is no strong medical evidence supporting its use. In fact, outcomes with episiotomy are worse in some cases, including pain with intercourse and extension into the external and internal anal sphincter or rectum. Pelvic floor dysfunctions such as incontinence and organ prolapse need further study relative to history of episiotomy.[76] Anal sphincter defects were linked with fecal incontinence in the postpartum period as far as 6 months after delivery in a study done by the Pelvic Floor Disorders Network.[20] Long-term follow up (beyond 1 year postpartum) is very limited.

Differences in recovery of pelvic floor strength in women with and without episiotomy have been documented with continued lack of consensus as to benefit of this procedure.[76] There is consistent agreement in the literature that episiotomy is closely associated with forceps-assisted delivery; additionally, if epidural anesthesia, forceps, and episiotomy are all utilized during labor and delivery, the risk of anal sphincter tear is even greater.[1,20,47,64,74] Pregnant women have many questions about labor in general and episiotomy in particular; the clinician is able to provide education and support for the patient as she explores birthing options with her physician.

FOCUS ON EVIDENCE

A randomized, controlled trial of 459 Canadian women during their first pregnancy found a significant protective effect against third- and fourth-degree tears (extensions following episiotomy) in women who participated in "strenuous" exercise three or more times per week. The researchers defined "strenuous" exercise as bicycling, jogging, tennis, skiing, and weight training, as opposed to "nonstrenuous" exercise such as walking, swimming, prenatal classes, and yoga. Data were collected regarding type, frequency, and duration of exercise for a 12-month period including prepregnancy and postpartum time frames. In the "strenuous" exercise group, 200 of the women did *not* have third- or fourth-degree tears compared with only 25 women who did experience this tearing. In addition, this study helped dispel the theory that serious exercisers may have overdeveloped perineal musculature; these women were not at increased risk for episiotomy when compared to casual exercisers.[74]

Classification of Pelvic Floor Dysfunction

This is a very broad category that encompasses bladder, bowel, and sexual symptoms in males and females in a variety of combinations. Some patients present with pelvic floor disuse atrophy, weakness, or nerve damage; others will have overactive pelvic floor musculature. Pelvic pain is another far-reaching, nonspecific diagnosis; many of these patients will be seen by multiple doctors prior to musculo-skeletal etiology being considered.

Pelvic Organ Prolapse

A prolapse is a supportive impairment that results in vaginal protrusion. It refers to the descent of any of the pelvic viscera out of their normal alignment because of muscular, fascial, and/or ligamentous deficits and because of increased abdominal pressure (Fig. 25.5). A prolapse often worsens over time and with subsequent pregnancies. Other contributing factors include chronic increases in intra-abdominal pressure (such as constipation or increased BMI), menopause, and possibly significant lifting or exertion.[96]

- A cross-sectional study found stage I prolapse in 33% of the subjects and stage II descent in 62.9%. The sample included 270 women with a mean age of 68.3 years and median parity of three vaginal births.[96] In another study, over 1,900 U.S. women were assessed for symptomatic prolapse and other pelvic floor dysfunctions with findings of prevalence in up to 49.7% of the sample correlated with increased age, increased parity, and increased weight.[98] This is critically important information for all clinicians prescribing trunk stabilization programs for female patients regardless of diagnosis.

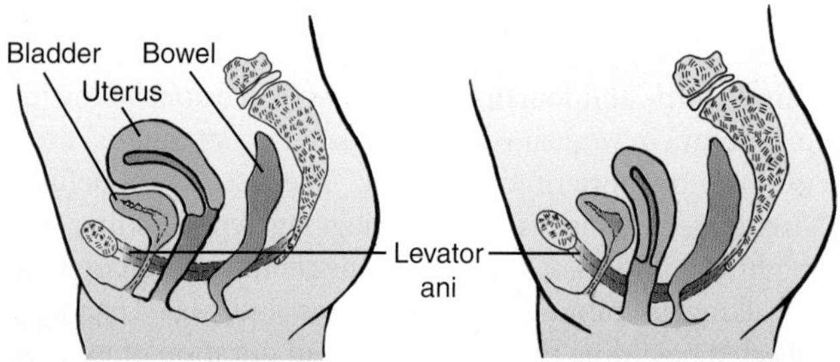

FIGURE 25.5 **(A)** Good pelvic floor support with a firm base, organs in normal position. **(B)** Inadequate support, pelvic organs descend.

- From a biomechanical aspect, activation of the pelvic floor is necessary in coordination with deep segmental muscle activation of the multifidus and transversus abdominis (see Chapters 13 and 15) to prevent excessive downward forces during all daily activities.

 **FOCUS ON EVIDENCE**

Creating an "ideal" program to achieve motor learning of the pelvic floor is complicated by differing study results. A landmark study done by Dr. Bump showed that brief verbal instruction alone was not effective in teaching correct pelvic floor contraction technique in 50% of women and, in fact, caused increased downward pressures to the bladder in 25% of their sample rather than producing an appropriate superiorly directed force.[26] Other studies have confirmed repeatedly that skilled individualized intervention is needed as many women perform pelvic floor contractions incorrectly.[15] Studies in normal individuals promote the use of a transverse abdominus contraction as a way to facilitate a synergistic contraction of the pelvic floor.[109,110] However, coordinated recruitment of the trunk muscles and the pelvic floor cannot be assumed across the board in a standard rehabilitation setting. Ideally, co-contraction of the pelvic floor with the deep segmental muscles would be confirmed internally prior to prescribing more challenging positions and activities.

- As prolapse progresses, functional changes occur as a result of perineal pressure and heaviness, including low back pain, abdominal pressure or pain, and difficulties with bladder and bowel elimination.[23] These symptoms can interfere with exercise; recreation; household responsibilities, including yard work; and occasionally the ability to work outside the home.[96]

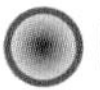 **FOCUS ON EVIDENCE**

A 2011 Cochran review highlighted rigorous trials to support pelvic floor muscle exercise in the treatment of prolapse with specific recommendations for longer follow-up and varied combinations of interventions.[61]

Urinary or Fecal Incontinence

Involuntary loss of bladder or bowel contents, frequently a result of both neuromuscular and musculoskeletal impairments, may occur in combination with prolapse. A conservative estimate of people affected with urinary or fecal incontinence is 25 million in the United States alone.[90] Women are twice as likely to have these symptoms as men.[43] In a recent prevalence study of noninstitutionalized persons over the age of 65, over 25% of men and 50% of women reported urinary incontinence.[58] These patients often have significant social discomfort, anxiety regarding leakage, and hygiene concerns. Significant financial implications exist for both the individual and the larger society. In a systematic review, analysis of costs for women in the United States, including both conservative and surgical interventions, totaled over $12 billion per year.[32] Types of incontinence are summarized in Box 25.2.

FOCUS ON EVIDENCE

Multiple studies have shown statistically significant improvement in urinary leakage as a result of a program of pelvic floor strengthening.[46,81,87,88,108,122] Decrease in postprostatectomy leakage in men has also been documented after pelvic floor exercise, at times in combination with biofeedback.[57,81,125]

Functional improvements (decreased urinary incontinence and improved pelvic floor strength) have been noted in late pregnancy and from 3 to 12 months postpartum in a number of studies.[87,88,108]

There is strong evidence in support of skilled intervention for pelvic floor dysfunction. The inclusion of physical therapists in the first line of treatment allows integration of exercise physiology and progressive strengthening principles to treatment protocols along with proper instruction and close follow-up.[15] Bø[16] summarized current findings in support of pelvic floor rehabilitation in the treatment of stress urinary incontinence:

- Strength training of the pelvic floor (using principles of exercise physiology) improves structural support of the organs and connective tissue in addition to facilitating more effective recruitment of motor units and more consistent, proficient contractions.
- Counterbracing with the pelvic floor musculature, done intentionally and habitually prior to increases in intra-abdominal pressure, becomes a form of behavioral modification with "trigger" activities such as lifting and coughing.

BOX 25.2 Types of Lower Urinary Tract Impairments[1]

- **Stress urinary incontinence**: loss of urine with increased abdominal pressure (exertion, cough, sneeze) may present in isolation or combined with urge incontinence
- **Urgency**: sudden desire to void, hard to ignore, may be called overactive bladder
- **Urge urinary incontinence**: loss of urine associated with a strong sense of urgency
- **Detrusor overactivity**: bladder contractions during filling phase, seen on urodynamics
- **Retention incontinence**: hypotonic or acontractile bladder leads to dribbling of urine or interrupted flow (previously called Overflow)
- **Functional incontinence**: related to other impairments such as arthritis, Parkinson's, dementia, medications

Pain and Overactivity of the Pelvic Floor and Surrounding Musculature

Pain and overactivity may be related to delayed healing of perineal lacerations, trauma to the soft tissues and/or the pelvic girdle joints during delivery, pelvic obliquity, multiple gynecologic/visceral diagnoses, cauda equina involvement, and scar tissue restrictions, as well as high incidence clinically of protective muscle spasm, guarding, and anxiety regarding movement in general. Central sensitization and pain education are key factors in treatment planning.[29]

- One study described "nonmenstrual" pelvic pain as being most commonly caused by endometriosis, adhesions, interstitial cystitis, or irritable bowel syndrome, occurring in as much as 20% of women aged 15 to 50.[18] In another study with a total sample of 581 women (aged 18 to 45), the following prevalence was found: pelvic pain, 39%; dyspareunia (pain with intercourse), 46%; and dysmenorrhea, 90%.[68]
- Functional impairments may include pain with ADLs, decreased sitting tolerance, dyspareunia, and difficulty with elimination of bladder and bowel contents. In patients with pelvic pain impairments, often referred to as chronic pelvic pain (CPP), persistent tightness of the lumbar paraspinals and hip flexors is typically present.[10]
- Because of the breadth of this topic, treatment recommendations are conflicting. Attention is being given to the correlation of pelvic pain with a history of sexual abuse, which highlights the need for multidisciplinary assessment in order to address all potential causative factors. Sexual abuse continues to be underreported, yet recent studies cite rates of 20% to 25% of women who report childhood sexual trauma.[69,102,105]

Risk Factors for Dysfunction in the Female Population

Childbirth

Childbirth is clearly the most significant risk factor for female pelvic floor impairments. The process of labor, particularly with vaginal delivery and current medical management, can produce significant trauma to the structures of the pelvic floor.

- A longitudinal cohort study with follow-up 15 years after delivery (n = 55) showed that stress incontinence during the first pregnancy doubled the risk of reoccurrence 15 years later.[41] With respect to risk of future POP, in a cohort study of over 17,000 women, those with one delivery were four times more likely, and those with two children were over eight times more likely to have a subsequent hospital admission for POP. However, this study did not distinguish mode of delivery.[82]
- Other potential obstetric risk factors include mothers older than 30 years of age, multiple deliveries, prolonged second stage (over 1-2 hours) of labor, forced pushing, use of forceps, vacuum extraction or oxytocin, third- or fourth-degree perineal tears, and birth weight greater than 8 lb.[56,68,75,97,116,123]

Other Causes

Women who have never been pregnant may also present with pelvic floor dysfunction. Excessive straining because of chronic constipation, smoking, chronic cough, obesity, and hysterectomy can contribute to these impairments in any woman.[5,13,43,,123] More recent studies are uncovering a connection between high impact exercise and urinary leakage, even in young athletes.[40] The role of estrogen in the development of incontinence is still unclear, with some studies citing estrogen depletion as a risk factor,[43] and others finding a connection between incontinence and oral estrogen-replacement therapy.[66,123] High caffeine intake has been cited as a specific risk factor for urge incontinence,[25,66] and reduction of caffeine, combined with dietary modifications and pelvic floor exercises, has led to improved continence.[25]

Considerations for Treatment of Pelvic Floor Dysfunction in the Male Population

As physical therapists become more knowledgeable and proficient in female pelvic floor impairments, it may be an "easy" and natural transition to add services for male (and possibly pediatric clients). Continued training for therapists is imperative and available. Teaching of pelvic floor awareness and correct exercise technique is similar as for women in terms of explaining the anatomy and function of the musculature. However, men can see movement of the base of the penis and scrotum, which gives them more immediate feedback regarding accurate identification of the pelvic floor muscles. The primary contributing factor for pelvic floor dysfunction in men is prostate enlargement or prostate cancer treatment; otherwise, many of the same topics of discussion apply (i.e., increases in intra-abdominal pressure, caffeine) when educating these clients. Evidence is growing for this population as well in terms of optimal rehabilitation approaches.[57,85,91,106,122]

Interventions for Pelvic Floor Impairments

Management of both women and men with pelvic floor impairments involves a comprehensive approach. Management guidelines for pelvic floor impairments are summarized in Box 25.3. Exercises for the pelvic floor are described in the exercise section of this chapter.

BOX 25.3 MANAGEMENT GUIDELINES—
Pelvic Floor Impairments

Potential Impairments of Structure and Function, Activity Limitations, and Participation Restrictions

Pelvic floor muscle weakness, soft tissue disruption
Lack of sphincter control resulting in urinary or fecal incontinence
Organ prolapse
Poor proprioceptive awareness and disuse atrophy of the pelvic floor muscles
Lack of knowledge of pelvic floor muscle function
Over activity of pelvic floor muscles along with pain and/or voiding dysfunction
Limited participation in work, social, and community activities related to:
- frequent urges/poor sphincter control/pain and discomfort
- potential skin breakdown, hygiene concerns

Plan of Care	Interventions
1. Educate the patient	1. Explain the anatomy and function of the pelvic floor. Explain intervention approach for specific impairments. Increase awareness of risk factors for pelvic floor impairments (weight gain, constipation, etc.). Educate regarding skin care as needed.
2. Coordinate intervention with other professionals	2. Consult with physician regarding medications, further diagnostic testing. Consult with dietitian regarding diet. Refer for internal pelvic floor musculoskeletal assessment as needed.
3. Develop self-management strategies	3. Increase awareness of bladder irritants, impact of bowel function on bladder symptoms, and recommended fluid/fiber intake. Use voiding diary to record baseline information and monitor improvements in leakage and urgency.

BOX 25.3 MANAGEMENT GUIDELINES—
Pelvic Floor Impairments—cont'd

Plan of Care	Interventions
	Use exercise log. Teach urge suppression techniques. Incorporate pain management and self-care strategies.
4. Screen for unresolved postpartum impairments	4. Assess strength/integrity of abdominal wall, postural asymmetries, history of other musculoskeletal issues.
5. Develop awareness and control of the pelvic floor musculature for life-long daily functional use	5. Increase implementation of pelvic floor activation and relaxation as appropriate for retention of motor patterns and integration with ADLs.

Patient Education

Teach the patient about pelvic floor anatomy and function. Place emphasis on appreciating all three dimensions of the muscle complex: the sling/hammock fibers, the figure-eight orientation of the musculature, and the "funnel" configuration extending inferiorly to the outlet (see Fig. 25.4). Use visual aids to help the patient visualize the fibers that run anterior-posterior as well as superior-inferior (to create a "lifting" motion toward the heart), as well as the circumferential fibers (which produce a drawstring or "pucker" effect). Verbal cues that seem to be effective include "tighten your muscles as if to hold back gas and urine" along with visualizing the lift and pucker motions. Be specific with gender differences, mentioning the image of tightening around the vaginal opening and movement of the penis and scrotum as appropriate.

Provide individual instruction in exercise performance. Detailed, individual exercise instruction is linked to significant proprioceptive improvement and meets the criteria for skilled care. Successful strengthening is unlikely without this individualized educational component along with later confirmation of correct exercise performance.[15]

Teach bladder and bowel management. Regardless of primary symptoms, it is important to educate all clients on behavioral management specifically concerning bladder irritants and fiber intake. Most clients are motivated to apply tools that will improve continence; however, cutting back on caffeinated beverages and improving fiber intake can be very challenging. Help the patient develop a routine for keeping track of and then modifying the daily habits that affect the impairments. Suggestions include:

- **Voiding diary**. Have the client record all voids, any time there is an "accident," and cause of leakage if known (cough, sneeze). Also have the patient record amount/frequency/type of all fluids, and food intake if monitoring fiber. If protective garments are used, record type and number per day. Many sample diaries can be found on the Internet.
- **Exercise log**. Have the patient record, or check off, when pelvic floor exercises are performed as well as any general fitness exercises.
- **Urge suppression techniques**. With urge incontinence have the patient practice techniques to calm the sudden strong urge to urinate or leak urine.[43] Suggestions include:
  - Remaining calm (panic makes the urge worse)
  - Use pelvic floor contractions[27,113]
  - Standing still or sitting down until the urge disappears—usually 1 minute
  - Thinking of something else as a distraction
  - Trying not to rush to the toilet
  - Continue with normal activity or visit the toilet after the urge disappears. To help retrain the bladder, try a 5-minute delay then calmly walking to the bathroom.

Review the diary and exercise log periodically with the patient to note progress and provide additional education as needed.

Neuromuscular Re-education

Facilitate pelvic floor muscular activation. Neuromuscular re-education is essential because many women have significant disuse atrophy and proprioceptive deficits of the pelvic floor muscles. Internal techniques of assessment and treatment may be indicated for optimal patient outcomes. For example, manual stretch facilitation (a proprioceptive neuromuscular facilitation technique) to the levator ani at the vaginal or anal orifice can be an effective treatment option for clinicians with appropriate training.

Initially, emphasize correct identification of the pelvic floor musculature, with the goal of the patient learning isolated contractions of the pelvic floor. Many patients exhibit excessive accessory muscle recruitment (such as the gluteals, hip adductors, and abdominals) or the tendency to breath hold during attempts to recruit the pelvic floor muscles. Monitor for these substitutions during early treatment sessions to eliminate their use. Palpate the pelvic floor muscles at the perineal body over thin layers of fabric to verify correct activation, and then teach this palpation technique to the patient for use at home to assist in the re-education process. Once the patient learns to isolate and improve coordination of the pelvic floor contractions progress the instruction to integration of pelvic floor activity with ADLs, lumbar stabilization, and other functional strengthening exercises.

Biofeedback

Use biofeedback with instrumentation. The definition of biofeedback is "the technique of using monitoring devices to furnish information regarding ... bodily function ... in an attempt to gain some voluntary control over that function" (www.thefreedictionary.com). This can be accomplished by a creative physical therapist in a number of ways. There are multiple types of instruments that can be used to provide sensory feedback as the pelvic floor muscles contract around the device. Some are pressurized objects that allow for isotonic strengthening. Traditional surface electromyography (SEMG) sensors are solid and provide isometric resistance to the muscular contraction. SEMG can also be applied through peri-anal sensors for patients who are not candidates for internal assessment or treatment. SEMG provides immediate visual and/or auditory feedback regarding pelvic floor activity, which improves patient comprehension, appropriate recruitment patterns, and proprioceptive awareness. It is particularly invaluable for pelvic floor re-education and retention of motor learning pathways owing to generalized lack of knowledge of the muscles' existence, let alone their function and importance. Motor learning, which is facilitated through the "real-time" capabilities of the equipment, is greatly enhanced when compared to exercise without this intervention.

Combine biofeedback with exercises. Specific exercises to address pelvic floor impairments are listed in the exercise section of the chapter. The use of exercise and biofeedback, including SEMG for treatment of pelvic floor dysfunction in both male and female populations, has been studied with mixed results.[27,43,57,103,106,126]The need for further research is great.

Manual Treatment and Modalities

Manual treatment and modalities, including intravaginal and intrarectal techniques, also play a role in the treatment of all pelvic floor disorders. Advanced training is necessary for true expertise with internal techniques.

FOCUS ON EVIDENCE

FitzGerald[48] analyzed improvement in pelvic pain and urinary urgency and frequency comparing specific pelvic floor myofascial release techniques to "global therapeutic massage." A significantly higher proportion of the 81 women in the study improved with the direct physical therapy interventions versus massage ($p = 0.0012$).

Pregnancy-Induced Pathology

The combined influence of hormones, weight gain, and postural changes of pregnancy contributes to a variety of impairments (in addition to pelvic floor dysfunction that was described in the previous section) that can be addressed with physical therapy.

Diastasis Recti

Diastasis rectus abdominis (DRA) is separation of the rectus abdominis muscles in the midline at the linea alba. Elizabeth Noble was the first physical therapist to describe rehabilitation for this condition.[93] The etiology of this separation is unknown; however, the continuity and integrity of the abdominal musculature are disrupted (Fig. 25.6). Any separation larger than two finger widths is considered significant.[19,28,93] Currently other methods of assessment and treatment are being explored (for example, rehabilitative ultrasound or calipers versus manual palpation to measure separation) in order to determine best practice.[73]

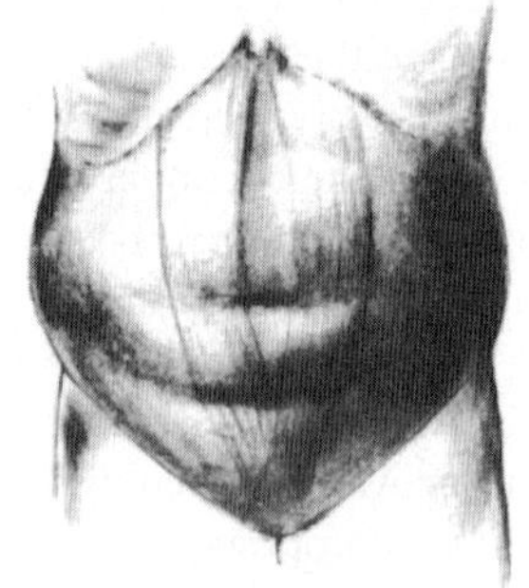
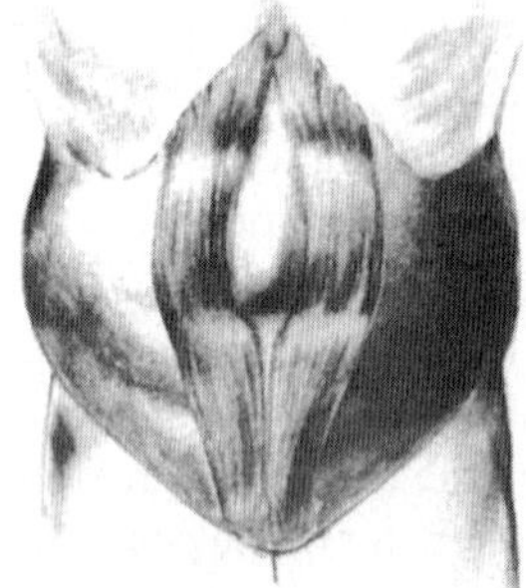

FIGURE 25.6 Diagrammatic representations of diastasis recti. *(From Boissonnault, JS, and Kotarinos, RK: Diastasis recti. In Wilder, E [ed]:* Obstetric and Gynecologic Physical Therapy, Vol. 20, *ed. 1. New York: Churchill Livingstone, 1988, p 91, with permission.)*

Incidence

This condition is frequently seen in the childbearing woman, although it is not exclusive to this population. In one study, Boissonnault and Blaschak[19] tested 89 women for separation of the rectus abdominis muscles. The sample included one group of women who were not pregnant, one group for each trimester of pregnancy, and two postpartum groups. The incidence in this study ranged from none in the nonpregnant and first trimester women, to 27% in the second trimester, to a high of 66% in the third trimester. Also of interest is that 36% of the women between 5 weeks and 3 months postpartum continued to display a separation. A study by Bursch[28] found a significant diastasis in 62.5% of postpartum women tested within 92 hours of delivery. In a population of 547 women seen in a urogynecology practice, 52% of the primarily menopausal women had persistent diastasis recti; 66% of those with DRA also had various combinations of stress or fecal incontinence and POP.[118]

- Diastasis recti may occur in pregnancy as a result of hormonal effects on the connective tissue and the biomechanical changes of pregnancy; it may also develop during labor, especially with excessive breath holding during the second stage.[120] It causes no discomfort.
- It can occur above, below, or at the level of the umbilicus but appears to be less common below the umbilicus.
- It appears to be less common in women with good abdominal tone before pregnancy.[19]
- Clinically, a diastasis may be found in women well past their childbearing years[118] (Fig. 25.7 A) and also in men (Fig. 25.7 B). Routine assessment for this condition is highly recommended in all clients and can easily be done in conjunction with abdominal strength testing.

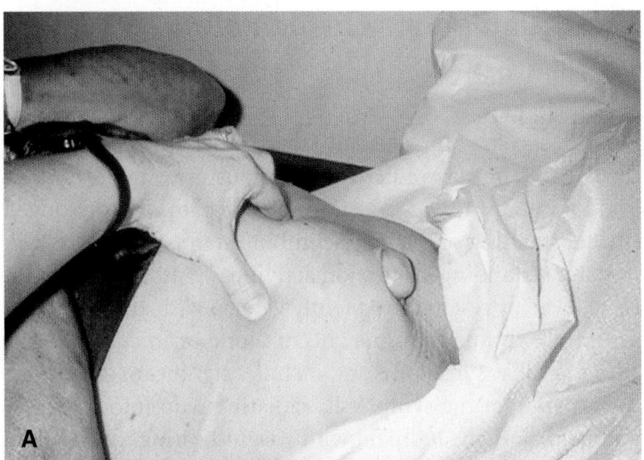

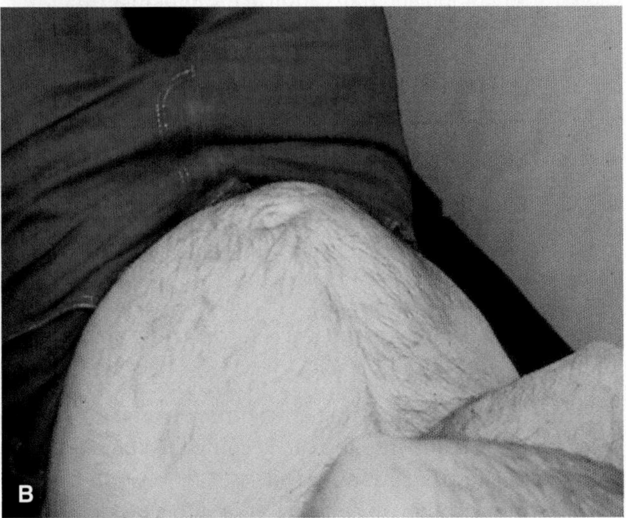

FIGURE 25.7 **(A)** Diastasis recti abdominus (DRA) of an 82-year-old woman who currently has urinary incontinence and emphysema. The DRA began with earlier pregnancies and is now exacerbated with coughing. Note the umbilical hernia. **(B)** DRA in a 54-year-old male truck driver with low back pain and significant deconditioning.

Significance

The condition of diastasis recti may produce musculoskeletal complaints, such as low back pain, possibly as a result of decreased ability of the abdominal musculature and thoracolumbar fascia to stabilize the pelvis and lumbar spine.

Activity limitations. Activity limitations can also occur, such as inability to perform independent supine-to-sitting transitions because of extreme loss of the mechanical alignment and function of the rectus muscle. Again, this finding is not exclusive to women in the childbearing years.

Decreased fetal protection. In severe separations, the remaining midline layers of abdominal wall tissue are skin, fascia, subcutaneous fat, and peritoneum.[19,28,120] The lack of muscular support provides less protection for the fetus.

Potential for herniation. Severe cases of diastasis recti may progress to herniation of the abdominal viscera through the separation at the linea alba. This degree of separation requires surgical repair. Rehabilitation following this type of repair may include components of C-section rehabilitation, with specific precautions and input from the referring surgeon. There may be a need for very slow progression depending on the severity of the diastasis and type of repair.

Examination for Diastasis Recti

Test all patients for the presence of diastasis recti before prescribing any abdominal exercises. Repeat this test throughout pregnancy and rehabilitation, and make appropriate modifications to existing exercises. This is a very quick assessment to incorporate with other trunk testing procedures.

Instruct female patients to perform a self-test on or after the third postpartum day for optimal accuracy. Until 3 days after delivery, the abdominal musculature has inadequate tone for valid test results.[93,120]

Patient position and procedure: Hook-lying. Have the patient slowly raise his/her head and shoulders off the floor, reaching hands toward the knees, until the spines of the scapulae leave the floor. Place the fingers of one hand horizontally across the midline of the abdomen at the umbilicus (Fig. 25.8); also test above and below the umbilicus. If a

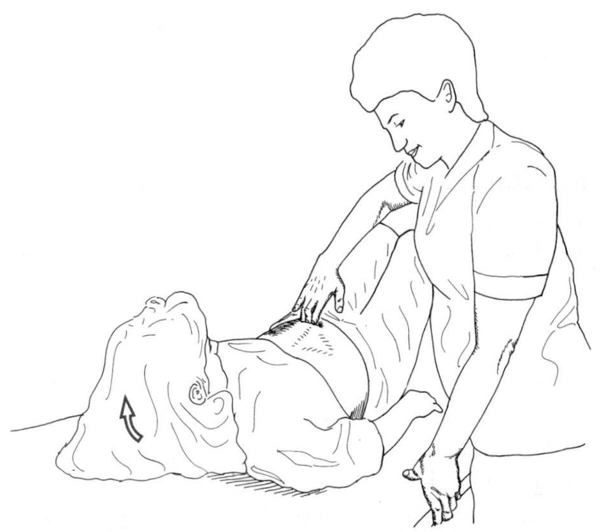

FIGURE 25.8 Diastasis recti test.

separation exists, the fingers will sink into the gap between the rectus muscles, or a visible bulge between the rectus bellies may be appreciated. Document the number of fingers that can be placed between the muscle bellies and identify if the separation is above, below, or at the level of the umbilicus.[93]

Intervention for Diastasis Recti

Teach the patient to perform the corrective exercise for diastasis recti (see Fig. 25.11 and accompanying text later in this chapter) until the separation is decreased to 2 cm or less prior to resuming more strenuous abdominal strengthening that increases intra-abdominal pressure.[93,120] Transverse abdominis exercises may be incorporated with the caution against breath holding. Once correction has been obtained, strengthening of the obliques and more advanced abdominal work can be resumed.[67]

Posture-Related Back Pain

Back pain commonly occurs because of the postural changes of pregnancy, increased ligamentous laxity, hormonal influences, and decreased abdominal muscle function.[5,7,39,67,93,100,,108,125]

Incidence

Back pain is reported by 50% to 80% of pregnant women at some point during pregnancy.[51,92] This condition contributes to lost work days, decreased functional ability, and QOL scores. In addition, symptoms may continue in the postpartum period, with prevalence in as many as 68% of women, for as long as 12 months after delivery.[92,99] Women who are physically fit generally have less back pain during pregnancy.[103]

Characteristics

The symptoms of low back pain usually worsen with muscle fatigue from static postures or as the day progresses; symptoms are usually relieved with rest or change of position.

Interventions

Low back pain symptoms can be treated effectively with many traditional low back exercises, proper body mechanics, posture instructions, and improvement in work techniques, along with superficial modality application.[93,120] The use of deep heating agents, electrical stimulation, and traction is generally contraindicated during pregnancy.

FOCUS ON EVIDENCE

Garshasbi and Faghih Zadeh[51] studied more than 200 primigravid women (pregnant for the first time) in a prospective randomized study on the effect of exercise and the intensity of low back pain during pregnancy. Subjects were excluded if they had a history of exercise before pregnancy or history of orthopedic conditions. The exercise group was in a supervised exercise program for 3 hr/wk for 12 weeks in the second and early third trimesters; the control group was women who were homemakers and had no significant change in activity level. The groups were statistically equal in maternal and neonatal weight gain, as well as length of pregnancy. The exercise group experienced significant decrease in intensity of low back pain by the end of the study, whereas intensity was increased in the control group. The study did not describe the nature of the symptoms or differentiate between postural pain and sacroiliac pain. Interestingly, there was no significant difference in the change in lordosis between the two groups.

A 2007 Cochrane review found pregnancy specific exercises—including "water gymnastics"—to provide relief of back or pelvic pain more than typical prenatal care alone, although the effect was small due to potential bias in the studies.[104] In 2015 this subject was revisited with a larger number of studies in the review. Moderate- to low-quality evidence documented that land exercise for low back pain reduces functional disability and sick days more than standard prenatal care. There are continued questions due to heterogeneity in study design and small numbers of subjects.[79]

Sacroiliac/Pelvic Girdle Pain

Characteristics

Sacroiliac pain is localized to the posterior pelvis and is described as stabbing deep into the buttocks distal and lateral to L5/S1. Pain may radiate into the posterior thigh or knee but not into the foot. Symptoms include pain with prolonged sitting, standing or walking, climbing stairs, turning in bed, unilateral standing, or torsion activities. Symptoms may not be relieved by rest and frequently worsen with activity. Pubic symphysis dysfunction may occur alone or in combination with sacroiliac symptoms and includes significant tenderness to palpation at the symphysis, radiating pain into the groin and medial thigh, and pain with weight bearing. In addition, excessive separation and translation at the joint may occur.[39,120] One study reported a four times greater incidence of posterior pelvic pain than low back pain in pregnant women.[100]

Interventions

Treat pelvic girdle and sacroiliac symptoms via modification or elimination of activities that may further aggravate sensitive tissue, stabilization exercises, and the use of belts and corsets to provide external support to the pelvis.

Activity modification. Help the patient adapt her daily activities to minimize asymmetrical forces acting on the trunk and pelvis. For example, teach:

- getting into a car by sitting down first, then pivoting both legs and the trunk into the car, keeping the knees together
- log rolling for transitions in bed
- side-lying symmetry by placing a pillow between the knees and under the abdomen
- modifying sexual positions to avoid full range of hip abduction
- avoiding single-leg weight bearing, excessive abduction, and sitting on very soft surfaces
- avoiding climbing more than one step at a time, swinging one leg out of bed at a time when getting up, or crossing the legs when sitting[39,120]

Exercise modification. Modify exercises so as not to aggravate the condition. Avoid exercises that require single-leg weight bearing and excessive hip abduction or hyperextension. Teach the patient to activate the pelvic floor and transverse abdominals when transitioning from one position to another and with any lifting in order to stabilize the trunk and pelvis.

FOCUS ON EVIDENCE

A randomized, clinical trial with 2-year follow-up looked at long-term effects of physical therapy for pelvic girdle pain in the postpartum period.[121] Each group had 20 weeks of treatment, with the control group focusing on modalities, manual therapy, and general exercises. In addition, the second group had specific focus on trunk/hip stabilizing exercises, with particular attention to the transverse abdominals. All participants received individual instruction from an experienced physical therapist. Outcome measures included the Oswestry Disability Questionnaire, pain scales, and a health-related QOL tool that measured eight subscales. At 1 year postpartum, the group with specific stabilizing exercises showed significantly better scores on all measures of those three tools, except for the social functioning subscale of the QOL tool. The same measurements were collected at 2 years' post-delivery, and the benefit for the stabilization group persisted, with significant differences in functional status and morning and evening pain. The specific exercise group had scores on QOL comparable to those of a representative group of the general population.

External stabilization. Use of external stabilization such as belts or corsets designed for use during pregnancy helps reduce posterior pelvic pain, especially when walking.

 **FOCUS ON EVIDENCE**

Ostgaard and colleagues[100] found that the use of nonelastic external stabilization designed for use during pregnancy helped reduce posterior pelvic pain in 82% of women. This was a large, randomized, controlled study (n = 407). More recent studies have validated the use of external stabilization for pelvic girdle pain (n = 118)[92] but found no effect with a support belt in cases of pubic symphysis pain (n = 87).[39]

The ***Clinical Practice Guidelines (CPGs) for Pelvic Girdle Pain in the Antepartum Population*** recommend using support belts for the antepartum patient with pelvic girdle pain and also state there is need for further research to clarify initial application, duration, and specific patient classifications because of conflicting evidence.[37]

Varicose Veins

Varicosities are aggravated in pregnancy by the increased uterine weight, venous stasis in the legs, and increased venous distensibility.

Characteristics

Varicosities can present in the first trimester and are more prevalent with repeated pregnancies. They can occur in the lower extremities, the rectum (hemorrhoids), or vulva. Symptoms usually include heaviness or aching discomfort, especially with dependent leg positions; intensity may become severe as the pregnancy progresses. In addition, pregnant women are more susceptible to deep vein thrombosis.[120]

Interventions

Exercise modification. If there is discomfort, modify exercises so that minimal dependent positioning of the legs occurs.

External support. Encourage the patient to wear elastic support stockings to provide an external pressure gradient against the distended veins, to perform lower extremity exercises, and to elevate the lower extremities as often as possible. Vulvar varicosities may benefit from use of external support to provide counter-pressure and support to the tissues.[93]

Joint Laxity

Significance

All joint structures are at increased risk of injury during pregnancy and during the immediate postpartum period.[84] The tensile quality of the ligamentous support is decreased, and therefore injury can occur if women are not educated regarding joint protection. There is much controversy regarding the impact of postpartum hormone levels; however, elevated levels have been found 3 to 5 months after delivery.[120] This elevation may persist even longer if the woman is nursing. Many patients are aware of persistent symptoms in conjunction with the menstrual cycle, and this correlation is certainly seen clinically.

Interventions

Exercise modification. Teach the woman safe exercises to perform during the childbearing year, including modification of exercises to decrease excessive joint stress (see exercises described in the management section of this chapter).

Aerobic exercise. Suggest non-weight bearing or less stressful aerobic activities such as swimming, walking, or stationary biking, particularly for women who were relatively sedentary before pregnancy. Other activities that may be initiated in pregnancy include modified yoga or Pilates and strength training.[4]

Nerve Compression Syndromes

Causes

Impairments from conditions such as thoracic outlet syndrome (TOS) or carpal tunnel syndrome (CTS) may be caused by one or more of the following in pregnancy: postural changes in the neck and upper quarter, fluid retention, hormonal changes, or circulatory compromise. Overall, women are three times as likely as men to experience CTS. Occurrence in pregnancy can be as high as 41%.[103] (See Chapter 13 for a discussion of CTS and TOS and Chapter 14 for a discussion of posture.)

Nerve compression syndromes (for example, of the lateral femoral cutaneous nerve) may also occur in the lower extremities because of the weight of the fetus, fluid retention, hormonal changes, or circulatory compromise.

Interventions

Typical protocols include postural correction exercises, manual techniques, ergonomic assessment, and modalities (see Chapter 13 for management of nerve compression syndromes). A static wrist orthosis may be used in the treatment of CTS. Carpal tunnel surgery in the pregnant population is rare because symptoms generally resolve soon after delivery; a longer course of the problem has been noted in women who breastfeed.[120]

Exercise Interventions for Pelvic Floor Impairments, Pregnancy, Labor, and Related Conditions

Exercise for the Pelvic Floor

Pelvic floor muscle training is a valuable modality regardless of a patient's presentation or cause of symptoms.[13,16,26,31,45,47,49,50,66,67,87,88,93,103,108,120,125] Although this chapter is geared toward women's health, men with pelvic floor impairments may benefit from exercise interventions and are therefore included in this material. Many men and women are unfamiliar with the presence of the pelvic floor muscles and are even less aware of their function and role in daily activities. For women, symptoms are often linked with the childbearing years owing to the stress of pregnancy, labor, and delivery on the pelvic floor. For men, bladder and/or bowel impairments or sexual dysfunction may co-exist with prostate enlargement, cancer, surgery, or cancer related treatment.[57,85,91,106,122] The management guidelines outlined in Box 25.3 and exercises presented in this section are therefore used when treating the range of impairments described in this chapter in both female and male clients.

Pelvic Floor Awareness and Training

Begin pelvic floor exercises with an empty bladder. Gravity-assisted positioning (hips higher than the heart, such as supported bridge or elbows/knees position) may be indicated initially for some clients with extreme weakness and proprioceptive deficits. Explore various positions to maximize patient awareness and motor learning with progression into more challenging activities/positions as functional application becomes feasible.

Contract-Relax

Instruct the client to tighten the pelvic floor as if attempting to stop urine flow or hold back gas. Hold for 3 to 5 seconds, and relax for at least the same length of time. Repeat as many as 10 times (if performed with proper technique). As pelvic floor muscle fibers fatigue, substitution with the gluteals, abdominals, or hip adductors may occur. To maximize proprioception and motor learning, it is important initially to emphasize identification and isolation of the pelvic floor and avoid the substitute muscle actions.[115] In addition, watch for Valsalva's maneuver; if necessary, have the client count out loud to encourage normal breathing patterns.

Quick Contractions

Have the client perform quick, repeated contractions of the pelvic floor muscles while maintaining a normal breathing rate and keeping accessory muscles relaxed. Try for 15 to 20 repetitions per set. This type II fiber response is important to develop in order to withstand pressure from above, especially with coughing or sneezing.

"Elevator" Exercise

Instruct the client to imagine riding in an elevator. As the elevator goes up from one floor to the next, she contracts the pelvic floor muscles a little "higher." As strength and awareness improve, add more "floors" to the sequence of the contraction. Another way to increase difficulty is to ask for relaxation of the muscles gradually, as if the elevator were descending one floor at a time. This component requires an eccentric contraction and is very challenging.

Pelvic Floor Relaxation

- Instruct the client to contract the pelvic floor as in the strengthening exercise, then allow total voluntary release and relaxation of the pelvic floor. Emphasize use of the "elevator" imagery, with particular attention to taking the elevator to the "basement."
- Pelvic floor relaxation is closely linked with effective breathing and relaxation of the facial muscles. Emphasize slow, deep breath and allow the pelvic floor to completely relax and soften. For a woman, relaxation of the pelvic floor is extremely important during stage 2 of labor and vaginal delivery.[50,93,120]
- Chronic inability to relax the pelvic floor muscles may lead to impairments such as pelvic floor overactivity, pain with intercourse (dyspareunia), or voiding dysfunction. (Please refer to the earlier information on pelvic pain syndromes.) If the patient presents with these symptoms, only prescribe submaximal, quick contractions in order not to increase tension; in addition, increase the rest time between pelvic floor contractions and sets. Use of surface EMG for downtraining, and muscle reeducation is invaluable with these impairments for increasing awareness of holding patterns, pain inhibition, and resting levels.

CLINICAL TIP

For optimal outcomes, pelvic floor contractions should be incorporated into routine ADLs, particularly activities that are "triggers" for leakage due to increased intra-abdominal pressure; used for stabilization prior to coughing or sneezing; and continued for life-long health benefits.[16,66] From a neurophysiology standpoint, voluntary pelvic floor contractions create reflex inhibition through Bradley's Loop 3, which inhibits internal urethral sphincter relaxation and relaxes the detrusor muscle, leading to less urinary urgency and improved voiding intervals.[113]

Related Exercises for Pelvic Floor Stabilization

Hip Rotation[72]

Patient position: To recruit greater pelvic floor muscle activity, instruct the patient to sit tall (avoid slouching), with feet on the floor.[111]

- Have the client first perform active internal and external rotation by moving each leg outward and inward
- *For resisted hip external rotation,* place a resistance band around the distal thighs and instruct the client to roll their knees out against the band (the feet remain on the floor with heels touching and toes pointed outward to form a V), and hold the contraction for 5 seconds (Fig. 25.9 A).
- *For resisted hip internal rotation,* place an inflatable ball (approximately 9") between the knees and instruct the client to squeeze the ball by rolling their knees inward (the feet remain on the floor with the toes touching and heels sliding apart), and hold the contraction for 5 seconds (Fig. 25.9 B).

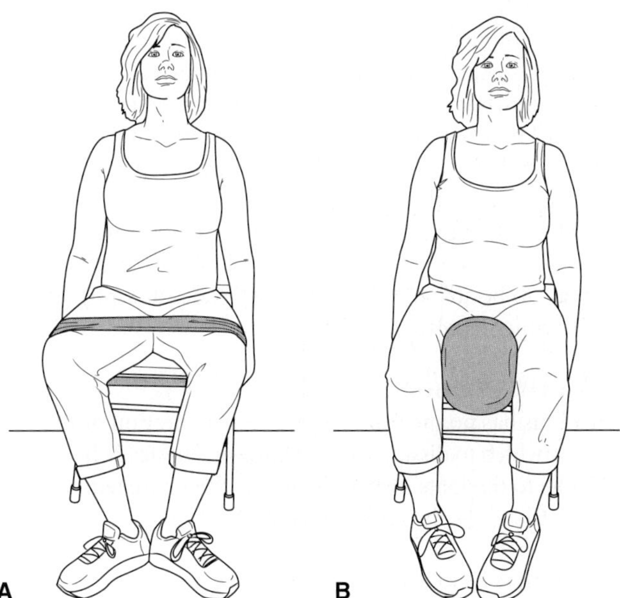

FIGURE 25.9 Hip rotation exercises to recruit pelvic floor muscle activity. **(A)** Resisted external rotation using a resistance band (note feet remain on floor in V position with heels touching), and **(B)** resisted internal rotation squeezing a ball between the knees (feet remain on floor and heels slide outward).

Stabilization Exercises

Ideally, pelvic floor muscles contract in synchrony with the deep segmental muscles of the spine (multifidus and transverses abdominis); stabilization exercises may be helpful to facilitate contraction of the pelvic floor as a component of pelvic floor motor learning.[14,109,110] These exercises are described in Chapter 16. When used during pregnancy, specific precautions are identified later in this chapter.

Aerobic Exercise During Pregnancy

Many women who have been doing aerobic exercises choose to continue exercising during pregnancy to maintain their cardiopulmonary fitness. Maternal[4,8,33,35,70,125] and fetal[4,33,31,36,50,70,117,125] responses have been well studied; therefore, this information is used to guide both the therapist and the patient in determining necessary modifications to an existing exercise program. The physiological effects of aerobic exercise to both the mother as well as fetus are described, followed by recommendations for fitness exercise.

Maternal Response to Aerobic Exercise

Blood Flow

Aerobic exercise does not reduce blood flow to the brain and heart. It does, however, cause a redistribution of blood flow away from the internal organs (and possibly the uterus) and toward the working muscles. This raises two concerns: that the reduction in blood flow may decrease the oxygen and nutrient availability to the fetus and that uterine contractions and preterm labor may be stimulated.[33] Stroke volume and cardiac output both increase with steady-state exercise. This, coupled with increased blood volume and reduction in systemic vascular resistance during pregnancy, may help offset the effects of the vascular shunting.

Respiratory Rate

The maternal respiration rate appears to adapt to mild exercise but does not increase proportionately with moderate and severe exercise when compared with a nonpregnant state. The pregnant woman reaches a maximum exercise capacity at a lower work level than a nonpregnant woman because of the increased oxygen requirements of exercise.

Hematocrit Level

The maternal hematocrit level during pregnancy is lowered; however, it rises as many as 10 percentage points within

15 minutes of beginning vigorous exercise. This condition continues for as many as 4 weeks postpartum. As a result, cardiac reserve is decreased during exercise.

Inferior Vena Cava Compression

Compression of the inferior vena cava by the uterus can occur after the fourth month of pregnancy, with relative obstruction of venous return. This leads to decreased cardiac output and orthostatic hypotension. It occurs most often in supine or static standing positions, and therefore prolonged time in these positions should be avoided.[4]

Energy Needs

Hypoglycemia occurs more readily during pregnancy; therefore, adequate carbohydrate intake is important for the pregnant woman who exercises.[31] A caloric intake of an additional 500 calories per day is suggested to support the energy needs of pregnancy and exercise, dependent on the intensity and duration of the exercise. In comparison, a sedentary pregnant woman requires a 300 calorie per day increase.[6]

Core Temperature

Vigorous physical activity and dehydration through perspiration lead to increased core temperature in anyone who exercises. Concern has been expressed over this occurring in the pregnant woman because of the relationship of elevated core temperature to neural tube defects of the fetus. Studies report that during pregnancy the core temperature of physically fit women actually decreases during exercise. These women appeared to be more efficient in regulating their core temperature, and thus the thermal stress on the embryo and fetus is reduced.[31,35]

Uterine Contractions

Norepinephrine and epinephrine levels increase with exercise. Norepinephrine increases the strength and frequency of uterine contractions. This may pose a problem for the woman at risk of premature labor, although the association is small.[4]

Responses of Healthy Women

Regular physical activity is beneficial for most pregnant women in terms of both physical and psychological wellness, and it also aids in weight management. Moderate-intensity aerobic activities are generally recommended in healthy pregnancy and the postpartum period for at least 150 min/wk.[4] Additionally, studies have shown that healthy women who continue to run throughout pregnancy deliver an average of 5 to 7 days sooner compared with controls.[33,34] Clapp[33-35] found that exercise, including weight bearing (even with ballistic motions such as during aerobic dancing), can be performed in midpregnancy and late pregnancy without risk of preterm labor or premature rupture of the membranes. Women who wish to continue strenuous or competitive exercise or participate in specific athletic training require close supervision by a specialist during pregnancy.[4,117]

Fetal Response to Maternal Aerobic Exercise

No human research has conclusively proven a detrimental fetal response to mild- or moderate-intensity maternal exercise. Recent studies suggest that even vigorous exercise does not have the detrimental effects on the fetus that once were feared, and therefore restrictions on exercise because of concerns for the effects on the embryo and fetus have been lessened. In fact, fit women who maintained their volume of exercise after 20 weeks' gestation delivered babies with lower fat mass than those who decreased exercise intensity midway through the pregnancy.[33-35] Given the epidemic of obesity in the United States, the need for future research to define further the connections between fetal nutrition and adult disease is imperative.[36]

Blood Flow

A 50% or greater reduction of uterine blood flow is necessary before fetal well-being is affected (based on animal research). No studies have documented such decreases in pregnant women who exercise, even vigorously. It is suggested that the cardiovascular adaptations in exercising women offset any redistribution of blood to muscles during exercise.[33]

Fetal Heart Rate

Brief submaximal maternal exercise (as much as 70% maternal aerobic power) does not adversely affect fetal heart rate (FHR).[4] The FHR usually increases 10 to 30 beats/minute at the onset of maternal exercise. After mild to moderate maternal exercise, the FHR usually returns to normal levels within 15 minutes, but in some cases of strenuous maternal exercise, the FHR may remain elevated as long as 30 min. Fetal bradycardia (indicating fetal asphyxia) during maternal exercise has been reported in the literature with the return to pre-exercise FHR levels within 3 minutes after maternal exercise, followed by a brief period of fetal tachycardia.[50] The healthy fetus appears to be able to tolerate brief episodes of asphyxia with no detrimental results.

Heat Dissipation

The fetus has no mechanism such as perspiration or respiration by which to dissipate heat. However, physically fit women are able to dissipate heat and regulate their core temperature more efficiently, thus reducing risk.[33]

Newborn Status

Newborn children of women who continue endurance exercises into the third trimester of pregnancy are reported to have an average decrease in birth weight of 310 g. There is no change in head circumference or heel-crown length. Further study of these children (as old as 5 years of age) has shown slightly better neurodevelopmental status in addition to higher percentage of lean body mass.[35]

Recommendations for Aerobic Training

NOTE: These recommendations are for pregnant women with no maternal or fetal risk factors.*

- It is strongly recommended that all women participate in mild to moderate exercise, for both strength and cardiopulmonary benefits, for at least 15- to 30-minutes most days of the week. Individualized programs based on prepregnancy fitness levels are preferable.[4,117]
- Currently, there are no data in humans suggesting that pregnant women need to decrease their intensity of exercise or lower their target heart rates, but because of decreased oxygen supply, it is advisable to modify exercise intensity according to their tolerance.
  - Conventional (age-based) target heart rate zones may be too aggressive for the average pregnant patient.
  - Use of the Borg scale of perceived exertion (Box 25.4) is more appropriate in this population, with exertion between 12 and 14 suggested during uncomplicated pregnancy.[4,21,117]
  - When fatigued, a woman should stop exercising, and she should never exercise to exhaustion.
- Activities to avoid include contact sports, anything with a high risk of abdominal trauma or falling, "hot" yoga or "hot" Pilates, high-altitude activities (greater than 6,000 ft), and scuba diving. The fetus is at increased risk of decompression sickness during scuba diving.[4, 117]
- Nonweight-bearing aerobic exercises, such as stationary cycling, swimming, or water aerobics, will minimize the risk of injury throughout pregnancy and the postpartum period.
- If the woman cannot safely maintain balance because of the shifting and increasing weight, have her modify exercises that could result in falling and injuring herself or the fetus. An example would be the need to modify or eliminate racquet sports as pregnancy progresses.[4]
- Adequate caloric intake for nutrition, adequate fluid intake, and appropriate clothing for heat dissipation are critical.
- Resumption of prepregnancy exercise routines during the postpartum period should be gradual. However, initiation of pelvic floor exercises immediately postpartum may reduce or possibly prevent symptoms and duration of incontinence.[4,86-88]
- Physiological and morphological changes of pregnancy continue for a minimum of 4 to 6 weeks postpartum—longer if the woman is breastfeeding. Encourage continued joint protection.

*4,7,8,21,33-36,44,51,67,70,87,88,93,103,108,114,117,120,125

BOX 25.4 Borg Rating Scale for Perceived Exertion (RPE)[21]

6—Very, very light
7
8
9—Very light
10
11—Fairly light
12
13—Moderately hard
14
15—Hard
16
17—Very hard
18
19—Very, very hard
20—Exhaustion

- Breastfeeding women can be reassured that moderate exercise does not impair quantity or quality of breast milk or infant growth.
  - Rate of weight loss in the postpartum period is variable in women who are lactating; an additional 500 calories/day are needed to support production of breast milk.[67]
  - Water intake continues to be important; 12 or more glasses per day are recommended.
  - There may be a short-term increase in lactic acid secreted in breast milk after high-intensity exercise; if the baby appears to eat less after an exercise session, this can easily be remedied by nursing before exercise. In addition, feeding the baby prior to exercise will reduce discomfort from any breast engorgement.[4,67,117]

ABSOLUTE CONTRAINDICATIONS TO AEROBIC EXERCISE DURING PREGNANCY:

- Hemodynamically significant heart disease
- Restrictive lung disease
- Incompetent cervix: early dilation of the cervix before full term, or cerclage
- Vaginal bleeding, especially second or third trimester
- Placenta previa after 26 weeks gestation: placenta is located on the uterus in a position in which it may detach before the baby is delivered
- Multiple gestation with risk of premature labor[4,67,94]
- Preeclampsia or pregnancy-induced hypertension
- Rupture of membranes: loss of amniotic fluid before the onset of labor
- Premature labor: labor beginning before the 37th week of pregnancy
- Maternal type 1 diabetes
- Severe anemia

NOTE: See also precautions and relative contraindications to exercise in general in the following section.

Exercise for the Uncomplicated Pregnancy and Postpartum

Exercise classes during pregnancy and after childbirth are designed to minimize impairments and help the woman maintain or regain function while she is preparing for the arrival of the baby and then caring for the infant.* The potential structural and functional impairments and the management guidelines related to uncomplicated pregnancies are summarized in Box 25.5, and a suggested sequence for teaching an exercise class is listed in Box 25.6.[7,8,120,125]

*4,7,8,44,51,52,67,70,87,88,92,93,100,103,104,108,114,117,120,121,125

Guidelines and techniques for exercise class instruction are included in this section.[4,7,8,67,93,117,120,125] In addition, interventions for women receiving individualized care for specific impairments are noted throughout this section. Interventions for special situations such as cesarean childbirth and high-risk pregnancy are described in the following sections.

Guidelines for Managing the Pregnant Woman

Suggest that your patients discuss with their physicians any guidelines or restrictions to exercise before engaging in an exercise program, either in a class or on a one-to-one basis. As always, follow your state practice act for physical therapy regarding referral, evaluation, and treatment.

BOX 25.5 MANAGEMENT GUIDELINES—Pregnancy and Postpartum

Potential Impairments of Structure and Function

Musculoskeletal pain and muscle imbalances from faulty postures
Poor body mechanics related to lack of knowledge, changing body size, and physical demands of child care
Lower extremity edema and discomfort from altered circulation and varicose veins
Pelvic floor impairments, including:
- Urinary or fecal incontinence
- Organ prolapse
- Overactivity
- Poor episiotomy healing
- Poor proprioceptive awareness and disuse atrophy
- Pain throughout the pelvic girdle/trunk

Abdominal muscle stretch, trauma, and diastasis recti
Potential decrease in cardiovascular fitness
Lack of knowledge of body changes and safe exercises to use during and after pregnancy
Changing body image
Lack of physical preparation (strength, endurance, relaxation) necessary for labor and delivery
Lack of knowledge of appropriate positioning for optimal comfort in labor and delivery
Lack of adequate postpartum rehabilitation
Anxiety regarding childbirth due to history of abuse

Plan of Care	Interventions
1. Develop awareness and control of posture during and after pregnancy.	1. Stretch, train, and strengthen postural muscles. Posture awareness.
2. Learn safe body mechanics.	2. Body mechanics in sitting, standing, lifting, and lying, as well as transitions from one position to another. Body mechanics with baby equipment and childcare activities. Position options for labor and delivery.
3. Develop upper extremity strength for the demands of infant care.	3. Resistive exercises to appropriate muscles.

BOX 25.5 MANAGEMENT GUIDELINES— Pregnancy and Postpartum—cont'd

Plan of Care	Interventions
4. Promote increased body awareness and a positive body image.	4. Body awareness and proprioception activities. Reinforce posture.
5. Prepare the lower extremities for the demands of increased weight bearing and circulatory compromise.	5. Elastic support stockings. Safe stretching exercises. Toning and resistive exercises to appropriate muscles.
6. Develop awareness and control of the pelvic floor musculature.	6. Isolate pelvic floor muscle contraction and relaxation. Muscle control and integration with ADLs.
7. Maintain abdominal function and prevent or correct diastasis recti.	7. Monitor diastasis recti. Diastasis recti exercises. Safe abdominal-strengthening exercises with diastasis recti protection/correction.
8. Promote or maintain safe cardiovascular fitness.	8. Safe progression of aerobic exercises.
9. Teach about the changes of pregnancy and birth.	9. Patient/family instruction. Refer to other disciplines as indicated.
10. Develop relaxation skills.	10. Relaxation and breathing techniques
11. Prevent impairments associated with pregnancy.	11. Education about potential problems of pregnancy, prevention techniques, and appropriate exercises.
12. Prepare physically for labor, delivery, and postpartum activities.	12. Strengthen muscles needed in labor and delivery, and train responses. Comfort measures and relaxation techniques for labor and delivery.
13. Provide education on safe postpartum exercise progression.	13. Postpartum exercise instruction.
14. Develop awareness of treatment options for pelvic floor dysfunction.	14. Comprehensive approach for prolapse, incontinence, or overactivity.

BOX 25.6 Suggested Sequence for Exercises Classes

1. General rhythmic activities to "warm-up"
2. Gentle selective stretching for postural alignment and for perineum and adductor flexibility
3. Aerobic activity for cardiovascular conditioning (duration/intensity may need to be individualized)
4. Postural exercises; upper/lower extremity strengthening and individualized abdominal exercises
5. Cool-down activities
6. Pelvic floor exercises
7. Relaxation techniques
8. Labor and delivery techniques/positions
9. Educational information
10. Postpartum exercise instruction (e.g., when to begin exercises, how to safely progress, precautions) because the patient may not be attending a postpartum class. Include education regarding body mechanics relative to childcare.

Examination. Individually examine each woman before participation to screen for preexisting musculoskeletal problems, posture, and fitness level.

Education. Educate your patients that increased uterine cramping *may* occur with moderate activity; this is acceptable as long as the cramping stops when the activity is completed. Teach your patient all exercise guidelines and precautions so that exercises may be carried out safely at home. Include the following:

- Do not exceed 5 minutes of supine positioning at any one time after the first trimester of pregnancy to avoid vena cava compression by the uterus. Educate your patients that compression of the vena cava also occurs with motionless standing. For supine exercise, place a small wedge or rolled towel under the right hip to lessen the effects of uterine compression on abdominal vessels and to improve cardiac output. The wedge turns the patient slightly toward the left (Fig. 25.10).[8] This modification is also helpful during physical therapy evaluation and treatment when the patient is positioned supine.

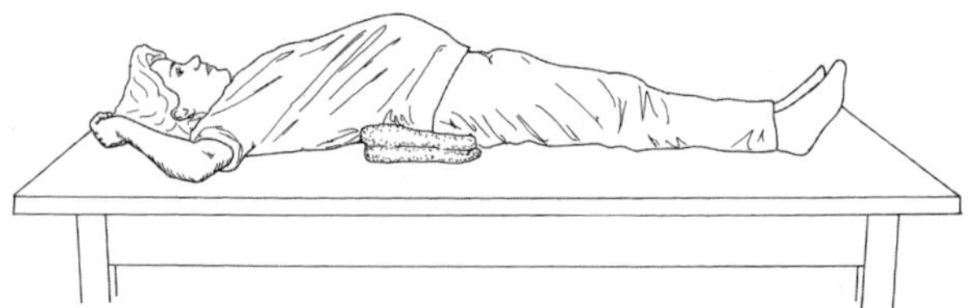

FIGURE 25.10 To prevent inferior vena cava compression when the patient is lying supine, a folded towel can be placed under the right side of the pelvis so the patient is tipped slightly to the left.

- To avoid the effects of orthostatic hypotension, instruct the woman to always rise slowly when moving from lying down or sitting to standing positions.
- Discourage breath holding and avoid activities that tend to elicit Valsalva's maneuver because this may lead to undesirable downward forces on the uterus and pelvic floor. In addition, breath holding causes stress to the cardiovascular system in terms of cardiac output, blood pressure, and heart rate.
- Break frequently for fluid replenishment. The risk of dehydration during exercise is increased in pregnancy. Avoid exercising in high temperature or humidity. Increase water intake in proportion to time spent exercising and as environmental temperature increases.
- Encourage complete bladder emptying before exercise. A full bladder places increased stress on an already vulnerable pelvic floor.
- Include appropriate warm-up and cool-down activities.
- Modify or discontinue any exercise that causes pain.
- Limit activities in which single-leg weight bearing is required, such as standing leg kicks. In addition to possible loss of balance, these activities can promote sacroiliac or pubic symphysis discomfort.

Stretching/flexibility. Choose stretching exercises that are specific to a single muscle or muscle group; do not involve several groups at once. Asymmetrical stretching or stretching multiple muscle groups can promote joint instability.

- Avoid ballistic movements.
- Do not allow any joint to be taken beyond its normal physiological range.
- Use caution with hamstring and adductor stretches. Overstretching of these muscle groups can increase pelvic instability or hypermobility.

CLINICAL TIP

Consider use of muscle energy techniques using light resistance for a client with pelvic instability and one whose pelvic boney landmarks are out of alignment. (See Chapter 15 for description of techniques.)

Muscle performance and aerobic fitness. In addition to pelvic floor training and aerobic exercising that have already been presented in this chapter, specific areas to emphasize and selected exercise techniques for the woman during pregnancy and to prepare for labor and delivery are described in the following sections.

FOCUS ON EVIDENCE

The ***CPGs*** from the Section on Women's Health and the Orthopaedic Sections of the American Physical Therapy Association recommend the use of exercise in the antepartum population with pelvic girdle pain. The guidelines also recommend exercise for pelvic girdle and low back pain but are not conclusive as to type due to conflicting evidence in varied populations and variety of exercise interventions.[37]

Precautions and Contraindications to Exercise during Pregnancy

There are some circumstances in which exercise is contraindicated or requires very specific restrictions and precautions.[4,6,7,24,37,52,54,30,67,93,94,103,114,117,120,125] Discussion of interventions for patients with high-risk pregnancy are described later in this chapter.

PRECAUTIONS: Observe participants closely for signs of overexertion or complications. The following signs are reasons to *discontinue exercise* and *contact a physician*.[4,117]

- Vaginal bleeding
- Persistent pain, especially in the chest, pelvic girdle, or low back
- Leakage of amniotic fluid

- Regular painful uterine contractions that persist beyond the exercise session
- Decreased fetal movements
- Persistent shortness of breath, especially before exertion
- Irregular heartbeat
- Tachycardia
- Headache
- Dizziness/faintness
- Swelling/pain in the calf (rule out phlebitis)
- Difficulty in walking or maintaining balance

CLINICAL TIP

Keep in mind when developing intervention programs, whether providing advice to a class or providing individual therapy, that most physical agents are *contraindicated* in pregnancy. Superficial heat or ice may be beneficial to relieve pain/spasm and improve circulation.

- Electric stimulation may be added postpartum to modulate pain and to stimulate muscle contractions, respectively.
- Ultrasound may be helpful in cases of poor episiotomy healing and persistent painful scar tissue, including reports of dyspareunia.[65]

RELATIVE CONTRAINDICATIONS: The woman with one or more of the following conditions may participate in an exercise program under close observation by a physician and a therapist as long as no further complications arise.[4,6,8,24,67,93] Exercises often require modification.[4,117] Discuss with referring practitioner.

- Poorly controlled type 1 diabetes, hypertension, seizure disorder or hyperthyroidism
- History of extremely sedentary lifestyle
- Musculoskeletal complaints and/or pain presenting with orthopedic limitations
- Overheating
- Extreme morbid obesity or extreme underweight (BMI below 12) or eating disorder
- Diastasis recti
- Heavy smoker
- Unevaluated maternal cardiac arrhythmia
- Chronic bronchitis
- Intrauterine growth retardation in current pregnancy

NOTE: Refer to the absolute contraindications to aerobic exercise identified in the aerobic section.

Critical Areas of Emphasis and Selected Exercise Techniques

Pelvic Floor Exercises

Pelvic floor exercises were described earlier in this section since they are useful for treating multiple conditions. It is worth emphasizing here the importance of including pelvic floor exercises when managing the pregnant woman.

Posture Exercises

The growing fetus places added stress on postural muscles as the center of gravity shifts forward and upward and the spine shifts to compensate and maintain stability. In addition, after delivery, activities involving holding and caring for the baby stress postural muscles. Muscles that require emphasis are listed in Box 25.7 with reference to respective chapters where the exercises are described. Adaptations of specific exercises for the pregnant woman are described in this section.

Use caution when implementing flexibility and stretching exercises. Remember that connective tissues and supporting joint structures are more vulnerable during pregnancy and the immediate postpartum period because of hormonal changes. Resistance exercises are performed at a low intensity.

Corrective Exercises for Diastasis Recti

Always check for diastasis recti before initiating abdominal exercises. Use only the corrective exercises (head lift or head lift with pelvic tilt) until the separation is 2 cm (two finger widths) or less.[93]

Head Lift

Patient position and procedure: Hook-lying with hands crossed over midline at the level of the diastasis for support. Have the client exhale and lift only the head off the floor while at the same time, using her hands to gently approximate the rectus muscles toward midline (Fig. 25.11), then lower the head slowly and relax. This exercise emphasizes the rectus abdominis muscle and minimizes the obliques. If a client cannot successfully reach across her abdomen, use a sheet

BOX 25.7 Selected Stretching and Resistance Exercises During Pregnancy

Stretching (With Caution)

- Upper neck extensors and scalenes (Chapter 16)
- Scapular protractors, shoulder internal rotators, and levator scapulae (Chapter 17)
- Low back extensors (Chapter 16)
- Hip flexors, adductors, and hamstrings (Chapter 20) CAUTION: women with pelvic instabilities should not overstretch these muscles
- Ankle plantarflexors (Chapter 22)

Strengthening (Low Intensity With Modifications Described in This Chapter)

- Upper neck flexors and lower neck and upper thoracic extensors (Chapter 16)
- Scapular retractors and depressors (Chapter 17)
- Shoulder external rotators (Chapter 17)
- Trunk stabilizers with precautions if diastasis recti present (Chapter 16)
- Hip extensors (Chapter 20)
- Knee extensors (Chapter 21)
- Ankle dorsiflexors (Chapter 22)

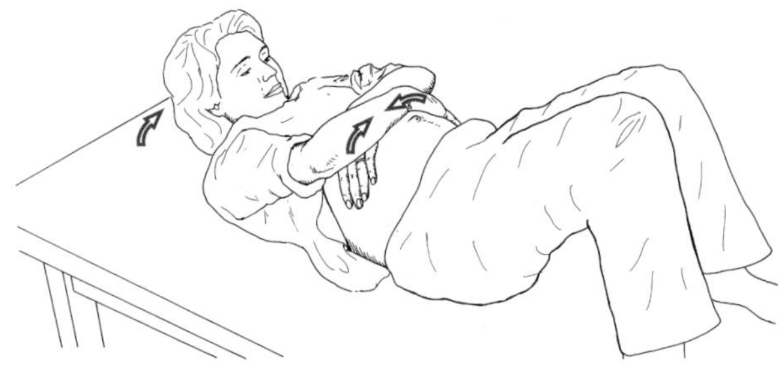

FIGURE 25.11 Corrective exercise for diastasis recti. The patient gently approximates the rectus muscle toward the midline by pulling with the crossed arms.

wrapped around the trunk at the level of the separation to provide support and approximation.[93]

Head Lift With Pelvic Tilt

Patient position and procedure: Hook-lying. The arms are crossed over the diastasis for support as described in the "head lift" exercise. Have the patient slowly lift only the head off the floor while approximating the rectus muscles and performing a posterior pelvic tilt, then slowly lower the head and relax. Perform all abdominal contractions with an exhalation to minimize intra-abdominal pressure.

Stabilization Exercises

Exercises for activating the abdominal and low back muscles and developing control of their stabilizing function in the lumbar spine and pelvis are described in Chapter 16 (see Table 16.4 and Figs. 16.47 and 16.48 [Level 3 A–C]; see also Table 16.5 and Fig. 16.49 A–D). Initiate and progress the exercises at the intensity that the woman is able to safely control. Emphasize slow, controlled breathing while developing the stabilizing function of the muscles. As pregnancy progresses, the abdominals will undergo extreme overstretching, and the pelvic floor complex will be progressively challenged by increased weight. These biomechanical changes make it even more challenging to teach pelvic floor activation in pregnancy without confirmation of internal assessment. As a result, core exercise prescription in particular must be adapted to meet the needs of each individual, and periodic reassessment must be done (approximately every 4 weeks during pregnancy).

PRECAUTIONS:

- Because the trunk muscles are contracting isometrically in many of the stabilization exercises, there is a tendency to hold the breath; this is detrimental to the blood pressure and heart rate. Caution the woman to maintain a relaxed breathing pattern and exhale during the exertion phase of each exercise.
- If diastasis recti is present, adapt the stabilization exercises to protect the linea alba as described in the Corrective Exercises for Diastasis Recti section. Any progression of postpartum abdominal strengthening exercises should be postponed until the diastasis has been corrected to two finger widths or less.
- Keep in mind the 5-minute time limit for supine positioning when prescribing abdominal exercises after 13 weeks' gestation.

FOCUS ON EVIDENCE

An evidence based review of studies dealing with low-back pain and pelvic girdle pain reported statistical significance for the relief of pain and improved function during advancing pregnancy utilizing stability ball exercises and progressive core stabilization exercises.[12]

Dynamic Trunk Exercises

Pelvic Motion Training

These exercises are helpful in cases of posture-related back pain; they are beneficial for improving proprioceptive awareness, as well as lumbar, pelvic, and hip mobility.

Pelvic tilt exercises. Begin in quadruped (on hands and knees). Instruct the patient to perform a posterior pelvic tilt. While the patient keeps her back straight, have her isometrically tighten (imagine drawing in) the lower abdominals and hold, then release and perform an anterior tilt through very small range.

- For additional exercise, while holding the abdominals in and the back straight, have the woman laterally flex the trunk to the right (side-bend to the right), looking at the right hip, then reverse to the left.
- Have the woman practice pelvic tilt exercises in a variety of positions, including side-lying and standing.

Pelvic clock.[44] With the woman hook-lying, ask her to visualize the face of a clock on her lower abdomen. The umbilicus is 12 o'clock and the pubic symphysis is 6 o'clock. The patient's legs may move slightly while performing this exercise.

- Have her begin with gentle movements back and forth between 12 and 6 o'clock (the basic pelvic tilt exercise).
- Then ask her to move back and forth between 3 o'clock (weight shifted to left hip) and 9 o'clock (weight shifted to the right hip).
- Then move slowly and smoothly (in a clockwise manner) from 12 to 3 to 6 to 9 and then back to 12 o'clock. With repetition, the movement can become somewhat faster.

Eventually, these will become automatic, rhythmical movements and will not require such concentration on each number of the clock. Continue relaxed breathing throughout the exercise, and do not force any part of the movement. If the patient has difficulty with the motion, make the clock "smaller" until coordination improves.

Pelvic clock progressions. Use the visual imagery of cutting the face of the clock in half so that there is a right side and a left side or a top half and a bottom half. Have the woman move her pelvis through the arc on the one side and back through the middle of the clock, and then move the pelvis through the opposite side and back through the middle. Initially, the woman may notice asymmetry when comparing the halves; this will improve with time.

- Once the patient understands and is able to perform the clockwise pattern, have her do counterclockwise motions with all of the activities mentioned previously, and then progress the exercises to the sitting position.

Trunk Curls

- Curl-ups and curl-downs are classic abdominal exercises but should not be used during pregnancy. If a woman chooses to continue with trunk curls, they should only be used in the early stages of pregnancy *if tolerated and if no diastasis recti is present.* Have a pregnant patient protect the linea alba with crossed hands (see Fig. 25.11) while performing trunk curls.
- This precaution should also be followed when performing diagonal curls (carried out to emphasize the oblique muscles). Have the woman lift one shoulder toward the outside of the opposite knee as she curls up and down while protecting the linea alba with crossed hands.

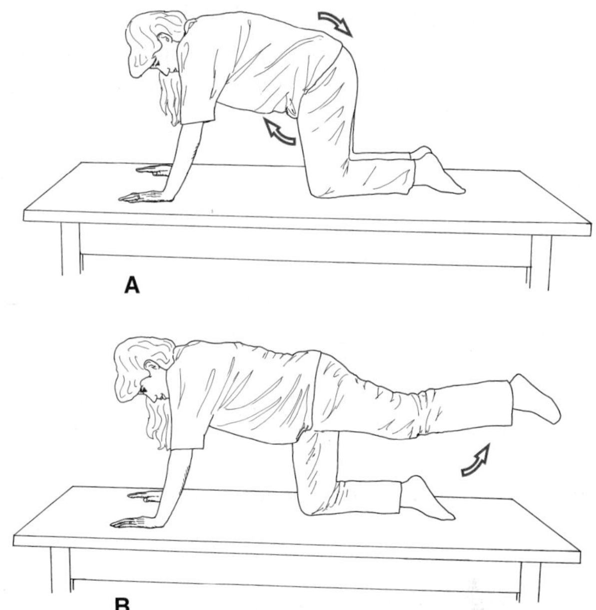

FIGURE 25.12 All-fours leg-raising. **(A)** Patient assumes quadruped position with posterior pelvic tilt. **(B)** Leg is raised only until it is in line with the trunk.

Modified Upper and Lower Extremity Strengthening

As the abdomen enlarges, it becomes impossible to comfortably assume the prone position. Exercises that are usually performed in the prone position must be modified.

Standing Push-Ups

Patient position and procedure: Standing, facing a wall, feet pointing straight forward, shoulder width apart, and approximately an arm-length away from the wall. The palms are placed on the wall at shoulder height. Have the woman slowly bend the elbows, bringing her upper body close to the wall, maintaining a stable trunk and pelvic position, and keeping the heels on the floor. Her elbows should be shoulder height. She then slowly pushes with her arms, bringing the body back to the original position.

Supine Bridging

Patient position and procedure: Supine in the hook-lying position. Have the woman perform a posterior pelvic tilt and then lift her pelvis off the floor. She can do repetitive bridges or hold the bridge position and alternately flex and extend her upper extremities to emphasize the stabilization function of the hip extensors and trunk musculature (see Fig. 20.28).

Quadruped Hip Extension

Patient position and procedure: On hands and knees (hands may be in fists or palms may be open and flat). Instruct the woman to first perform a posterior pelvic tilt and then slowly lift one leg, extending the hip to a level no higher than the pelvis while maintaining the posterior pelvic tilt (Fig. 25.12). She then slowly lowers the leg and repeats with the opposite side. The knee may remain flexed or extended during the exercise. Monitor this exercise, and discontinue if there is stress on the sacroiliac joints or ligaments. If the woman cannot stabilize the pelvis while lifting the leg, have her just slide one leg posteriorly along the floor and return (see Fig. 16.50 A).

Modified Squatting

Wall slides and supported squatting exercises are used to strengthen the hip and knee extensors for good body mechanics and to help stretch the perineal area for flexibility during the delivery process. In addition, if the woman wishes to use squatting for labor and delivery, the muscles must be strengthened and endurance trained in advance.

- *Patient position and procedure:* Standing with back against a wall and her feet shoulder width apart. Have the woman slide her back down the wall as her hips and knees flex only as far as is comfortable, then slide back up (see Fig. 20.29).
- *Patient position and procedure:* Standing with feet shoulder width apart or wider, facing a counter, chair, or wall on which the woman can rest her hands and/or forearms for support. Have the woman slowly squat as far as is comfortable, keeping knees apart and over the feet and keeping the back straight. To protect her feet, she should wear shoes with good arch support. A woman with knee problems should perform only partial range of the squat. For optimal success with squatting during stage 2 of labor (pushing), increase the duration of the squat gradually to 60 to 90 seconds as tolerated.

Scapular Retraction

When scapular retraction exercises become difficult in the prone position, the woman should continue strengthening in the sitting or standing position (see Figs. 17.46 and 17.47.)

Perineum and Adductor Flexibility

In addition to modified squatting previously described, these flexibility exercises prepare the legs and pelvis for childbirth.[7,93,120] Discontinue if any irritation or pain occurs at the pubic symphysis.

Self-Stretching

- *Patient position and procedure:* Supine or side-lying. Instruct the woman to abduct the hips and pull the knees toward the sides of her chest and hold the position for as long as is comfortable (at least to the count of 10).
- *Patient position and procedure:* Sitting on a short stool with the hips abducted as far as comfortable and feet flat on the floor. Have her flex forward slightly at the hips (keeping the lumbar spine in neutral), or have her gently press her knees outward with her hands for an additional stretch.

Relaxation and Breathing Exercises for Use During Labor

Developing the ability to relax requires awareness of stress and muscle tension. Techniques of conscious relaxation allow the individual to manage and respond to a variety of imposed stresses by being mentally alert to the task at hand while relaxing tense muscles that are superfluous to the activity (see Chapter 4). This is particularly important during labor and delivery when there are times that the woman should relax and allow the physiologic processes to occur without excessive tension in unrelated muscles.[93] Additional relaxation techniques for managing stress are described in Chapter 14. The following guidelines are most effective for the pregnant woman if consistently practiced in preparation for labor and delivery.

Visual Imagery

Use instrumental music and verbal guidance. Instruct the woman to concentrate on a relaxing image such as the beach, mountains, or a favorite vacation spot. Suggest that she focus on the same image throughout the pregnancy so that the image can be called up to the conscious level when recognizing the need to relax during labor. These techniques have been found to be helpful in various pain conditions as well as for anxiety.[89]

Muscle Setting

- Have the woman lie in a comfortable position.
- Have her begin with the lower body. Instruct her to gently contract and then relax first the muscles in the feet, then legs, thighs, pelvic floor, and buttocks.
- Next, progress to the upper extremities and trunk, then to the neck and facial muscles.
- Reinforce the importance of remaining awake and aware of the contrasting sensations of the muscles. Emphasize "softening" of the muscles as the session continues.
- Add deep, slow, relaxed breathing to the routine.

Selective Tension

Progress the training by emphasizing awareness of muscles contracting in one part of the body while remaining relaxed in other parts. For example, while she is tensing the fist and upper extremity, the feet and legs should be limp. Reinforce the comparison between the two sensations and the ability to control both tension and relaxation.

CLINICAL TIP

While practicing *selective tension*, have your client work with a partner who gently shakes the extremity that is "relaxed" to make sure there is no tension in it.

Breathing

- Slow, deep breathing (with relaxation of the upper thorax) is the most efficient method for exchange of air to use with relaxation techniques and for controlled breathing during labor.
- Teach the woman to relax the abdomen during inspiration so that it feels as though the abdominal cavity is "filling up" and the ribs are expanding laterally. During exhalation, the abdominal cavity becomes smaller; active contraction of the abdominal muscles is not necessary with relaxed breathing.
- To prevent hyperventilation, emphasize a slow rate of breathing. Caution the woman to decrease the intensity of the breathing if she experiences dizziness or feels tingling in the lips and fingers.

Relaxation and Breathing During Labor

First Stage

As labor progresses, the contractions of the uterus become stronger, longer, and closer together. Relaxation during the contractions becomes more difficult. Provide the woman with suggested techniques to assist in relaxation.[93]

- Ensure the woman has emotional support from the father, family member, or special friend to provide encouragement and assist with overall comfort.
- Seek comfortable positions including walking, hands and knees, lying on pillows, or lying or sitting on a Swiss ball (Fig. 25.13); include gentle repeated rhythmical motions such as pelvic rocking.
- Breathe slowly with each contraction; use visual imagery, such as muscles softening like butter, and attempt to relax. Some women find it helpful to focus their attention on a specific visual object. Other suggestions include singing, talking, or moaning during each contraction to prevent breath holding and encourage slow breathing.
- During transition (near the end of the first stage), there is often an urge to push. Teach the woman to use quick blowing techniques, using the cheeks, not the abdominal muscles, to overcome the desire to push until the appropriate time.

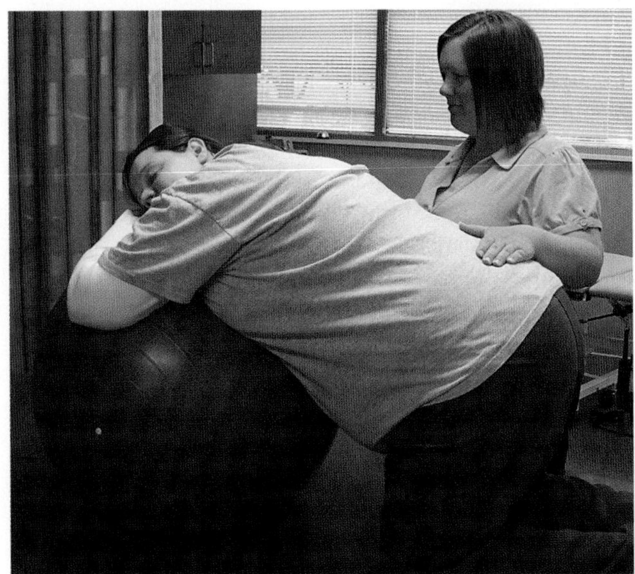

FIGURE 25.13 The use of a stability ball in labor can provide relief of back pain and the comfort of rhythmical, relaxing movements. The labor coach can massage the back and/or hip muscles and apply heat or ice if desired.

- Massage or apply pressure to any areas of pain or discomfort, such as the low back. Using the hands may help distract the focus from the contractions.
- Apply heat or cold for local symptoms; wipe the face with a wet washcloth.

Second Stage

Once dilation of the cervix has occurred, the woman may become more active in the birth process by assisting in pushing the baby down the birth canal.[93] Teach her the following techniques:

- While bearing down, take in a breath, contract the abdominal wall, and slowly breathe out. This will cause increased pressure within the abdomen along with relaxation of the pelvic floor.

PRECAUTION: Tell the woman that if she holds her breath, there will be increased tension and resistance in the pelvic floor. In addition, exertion with a closed glottis, known as Valsalva's maneuver, has adverse effects on the cardiovascular system.

- For maximum efficiency, maintain relaxation in the extremities, especially the legs and perineum. Keeping the face and jaw relaxed assists with this.
- Between contractions, perform total body relaxation.
- As the baby is delivered, just "let go," and breathe with light pants or groans to relax the pelvic floor as it stretches.

Unsafe Postures and Exercises During Pregnancy

Bilateral straight-leg raising. This exercise typically places more stress on the abdominal muscles and low back than they can tolerate. It can cause back injury or diastasis recti and therefore should not be attempted.

"Fire hydrant" exercise. This exercise is performed on hands and knees, and one hip is abducted and externally rotated at a time (the "image" of a dog at a fire hydrant). If the leg is elevated too high, the sacroiliac joint and lumbar vertebrae can be stressed. It should be avoided by any woman who has preexisting sacroiliac joint symptoms or women in whom symptoms develop.

All-fours (quadruped) hip extension. This exercise can be performed safely only as explained earlier in this chapter (see Fig. 25.12). It becomes unsafe and can cause low back pain when the leg is elevated beyond the physiologic range of hip extension, causing the pelvis to tilt anteriorly and the lumbar spine to hyperextend.

Unilateral weight-bearing activities. Weight bearing on one leg (which includes slouched standing with the majority of weight shifted to one leg and the pelvis tilted down on the opposite side) during pregnancy can cause sacroiliac joint irritation and should be avoided by women with preexisting sacroiliac joint symptoms. Unilateral weight bearing also can cause balance problems because of the increasing body weight and shifting of the center of gravity. This posture becomes a significant problem postpartum when the woman carries her growing child on one hip. Any asymmetries become accentuated, and painful compensations may develop.

Exercise Critical to the Postpartum Period

After an uncomplicated vaginal delivery, exercise can be started as soon as the woman feels able to exercise and has been cleared by her physician or midwife.[4,6,67,87,88,93,51,108,117]

Pelvic floor strengthening. Exercises should be resumed as soon after the birth as possible. These exercises increase circulation and aid healing of lacerations or episiotomy. Combining pelvic floor contractions with feeding or changing the baby may help them become integrated into the daily routine. When treating a postpartum client in the clinic, emphasize the life-long need for pelvic floor exercise, especially when lifting or with significant exertion, to allow the pelvic floor muscles to provide additional "shock absorption" and trunk support.

Diastasis recti correction. The testing procedure for diastasis recti was described earlier in this chapter. The mother should be taught this test and encouraged to perform it on the third postpartum day. Corrective exercises (see Fig. 25.11) should continue until the separation is two finger widths or less. At that time, more vigorous abdominal exercise can be resumed.

Aerobic and strengthening exercises. As soon as the woman feels able, resume cardiopulmonary exercise and light resistance training with gradually increasing intensity. It is suggested that a physical examination, including assessment of pelvic floor integrity be conducted before the onset of vigorous exercise or sport-specific training.

PRECAUTIONS: Because the woman may not be seen for exercise instruction after the delivery, inform her of the following precautions:

- If bleeding increases or turns bright red, exercise should be postponed. Tell her to rest more and allow a longer recovery time.
- Joint laxity may be present for some time after delivery, especially if breastfeeding. Precautions should be taken to protect the joints as described previously.[7,120,125] Adequate warm-up and cool-down time is important.

Cesarean Childbirth

A *cesarean section* (C-section) is the delivery of a baby through an incision in the abdominal wall and uterus rather than through the pelvis and vagina.[3,52, 54,60, 67] General, spinal, or epidural anesthesia may be used.

Significance to Physical Therapists

Surgical Risks

C-section delivery is now at an all-time high and is the most commonly performed surgical procedure in the world. In 2013, C-sections in the United States reached a record high rate of 32.7%.[62] This number has fluctuated in the past 3 to 4 decades, in part depending on the type of hospital and the population it served. Since the early 1990s, the American College of Obstetricians and Gynecologists (ACOG) has discouraged repeat C-sections as routine practice, and the *Healthy People 2010* goal was to reduce the primary rate to 15%, with a target rate for repeat cesareans at 63%.[127] The Vaginal Birth After Cesarean (VBAC) movement was a factor in reducing C-sections from 1990 to 1996; however, since then, the rates have continued to climb. The medical community is continuing to discuss the short- and long-term benefits and harms to both mother and baby of a trial of labor following a previous C-section. Pregnant clients will have many questions regarding this evidence. Al-Zirqi and colleagues[2] identified specific risk factors for uterine rupture with a VBAC and determined that absolute risk was low (5/1,000 births; n= 18,794). However, the use of prostaglandin induction significantly increased the odds for rupture when compared to spontaneous labor.

Recently, the perceived "convenience" of a C-section is becoming a factor, leading to increases in not only repeat, but also elective, C-sections. In reality, there is conflicting evidence that cesarean delivery may aid in prevention of future pelvic floor dysfunction.[9,55,60,116] These risks and benefits will continue to be discussed as long-term maternal and fetal outcomes are detailed in the literature. Because these statistics continue to fluctuate and more changes will be inevitable as our health-care system evolves, physical therapists must stay informed in order to address these issues with all pregnant patients so each patient will know the risks and benefits when making their own decision.[2,9,54,60,74,83,116,120,123]

Interventions

Pelvic floor rehabilitation. Women who have had a cesarean delivery may still require pelvic floor rehabilitation. Many women experience a lengthy labor, including prolonged second stage (pushing), before a C-section is deemed necessary. Therefore, the pelvic floor musculature and the pudendal and levator ani nerves may still be compromised. Also, pregnancy itself creates significant strain on the pelvic floor musculature and other soft tissues.

Postsurgical rehabilitation. Postpartum intervention for the woman who has had a cesarean delivery is similar to that of the woman who has had a vaginal delivery. However, a C-section is a major abdominal surgery with all the risks and complications of such surgeries, and therefore the woman may also require general postsurgical rehabilitation.[54,60,120] Impairments and management guidelines are summarized in Box 25.8.

BOX 25.8 MANAGEMENT GUIDELINES—**Postcesarean Section**

Potential Impairments of Structure and Function

Risk of pulmonary, gastrointestinal, or vascular complications

Postsurgical pain and discomfort

Development of adhesions at incision site

Faulty posture

Pelvic floor dysfunction
- Urinary or fecal incontinence
- Organ prolapse
- Overactivity
- Poor proprioceptive awareness and disuse atrophy
- Pain throughout the pelvic girdle/trunk

Abdominal weakness, diastasis recti

General functional restrictions of post delivery

BOX 25.8 MANAGEMENT GUIDELINES—Postcesarean Section—cont'd

Plan of Care	Interventions
1. Improve pulmonary function and decrease the risk of pneumonia	1. Breathing instruction, coughing, and/or huffing
2. Decrease incisional pain with coughing, movement, or breastfeeding	2. Postoperative TENS; support incision with pillow when coughing or breastfeeding Incisional support with pillow or hands with movement education regarding incisional care and risk of injury
3. Prevent postsurgical vascular or gastrointestinal complications	3. Active leg exercises Early ambulation Teach abdominal massage to stimulate peristalsis[63]
4. Enhance incisional circulation and healing; prevent adhesion formation.	4. Gentle abdominal exercise with incisional support Scar mobilization and friction massage
5. Decrease postsurgical discomfort from flatulence, itching, or catheter	5. Positioning instruction, massage, and supportive exercises
6. Correct posture	6. Posture instruction, particularly regarding childcare
7. Prevent injury and reduce low back pain	7. Instruction in incisional splinting and positioning for ADLs Body mechanics instruction
8. Prevent pelvic floor dysfunction	8. Pelvic floor exercises Education regarding risk factors and types of pelvic floor dysfunction
9. Develop abdominal strength	9. Abdominal exercise progression, including corrective exercises for diastasis recti

Emotional support. All childbirth preparation classes do not adequately educate and prepare couples for the experience of a cesarean delivery. As a result, the woman with an unplanned C-section frequently feels as if her body has failed her, causing her to have more conflicting emotions than a woman who has experienced a "normal" vaginal delivery.

Suggested Activities for the Patient Following a Cesarean Section

Exercises

- Instruct the woman during her pregnancy in all appropriate exercises, with indicated precautions.
- Instruct the woman to begin preventive exercises as soon as possible during the recovery period.[52,67,93,94]
  - Ankle pumping, active lower extremity range of motion (ROM), and walking are used to promote circulation and prevent venous stasis.
  - Pelvic floor exercises are used to regain strength, function, and control of the muscles of the perineum.
  - Deep breathing and coughing or huffing are used to prevent pulmonary complications (see instructions that follow).
- Progress abdominal exercises slowly. Check for diastasis recti, and protect the area of the incision to improve comfort. Initiate nonstressful muscle-setting techniques and progress as tolerated, based on the degree of separation.[52,67,93,94,120]
- Teach posture correction as necessary. Retrain postural awareness and help realign posture with indicated therapeutic exercise. Develop control of the shoulder girdle muscles as they respond to the increased stress of caring for the new baby.
- Reinforce the value of deep diaphragmatic breathing techniques for pulmonary ventilation, especially when exercising, and relaxed breathing techniques to relieve stress and promote relaxation.
- Inform the woman that she should wait at least 6 to 8 weeks before resuming vigorous exercise. Emphasize the importance of progressing at a safe and controlled pace and not expecting to begin at her prepregnancy level.

Coughing or Huffing

Coughing is difficult following a C-section because of incisional pain. An alternative is huffing.[93] A huff is an outward breath caused by the upper abdominals contracting up and in against the diaphragm to push air out of the lungs. The abdominals are pulled up and in, rather than pushed out, causing decreased pressure in the abdominal cavity and less strain on the incision. Huffing must be done quickly to generate sufficient force to expel mucus. Instruct the patient to support the incision with a pillow or the hands and say "ha" forcefully and repetitively while contracting the abdominal muscles.

Interventions to Relieve Intestinal Gas Pains

Abdominal massage or kneading. Have the patient lie supine or on the left side. This is very effective and typically done with either long or circular strokes. Begin on the right side at the ascending colon, stroking upward, then stroke across the transverse colon from right to left and down the descending colon, then finish with an "S" stroke along the sigmoid colon. This can also be particularly beneficial in stimulating peristalsis and improving constipation in general.[63]

Pelvic tilting and/or bridging. These can be done in conjunction with massage.

Bridge and twist. Have the patient maintain a position of bridging while twisting her hips to the right and left.

Scar Mobilization

Cross-friction massage should be initiated around the incision site as soon as sufficient healing has occurred. This will minimize adhesions that may contribute to postural problems and back pain.

High-Risk Pregnancy

A *high-risk pregnancy* is one that is complicated by disease or problems that put the mother or fetus at risk for illness or death before, during, or after delivery. Conditions may be preexisting, induced by pregnancy, or caused by an abnormal physiologic reaction during pregnancy.[54,67] The goal of medical intervention is to prevent preterm delivery. Historically bed rest has been used, as well as restriction of activity and medications when appropriate. Recent guidelines from ACOG are advising against routine bed rest, however. "Although frequently prescribed, bed rest is only rarely indicated and, in most cases, allowing ambulation should be considered. Patients prescribed prolonged bed rest or restricted physical activity are at risk of venous thromboembolism, bone demineralization, and deconditioning."[4] Prolonged bed rest can impact not just the musculoskeletal system, but also pulmonary, cardiovascular, and metabolic functions. Although these women may initially be seen in the home or as inpatients, the deconditioning present continues to create functional restrictions for the postpartum client in terms of strength and endurance, making this scenario ideal for further physical therapy intervention. Here again, as with pelvic floor dysfunction, advanced education for the therapist and specialized care is required for successful outcomes.[7,54,67,103,108,120]

High-Risk Conditions

Premature onset of labor. If cervical dilation, effacement, and/or uterine contractions begin before 37 weeks' gestation, this is considered preterm labor. Clearly, the health of the baby is of primary concern if these signs are present. The mechanism for this condition is still unclear.[67]

Preterm rupture of membranes. If the amniotic sac breaks and amniotic fluid is lost before onset of labor, it can be dangerous to the fetus if fetal development is complete. Labor may begin spontaneously after the membranes rupture. The chance for fetal infection also increases when the protection of the amniotic sac is lost. Leakage of amniotic fluid is an indication for immediate medical attention.

Incompetent cervix. An incompetent cervix is the painless dilation of the cervix that occurs in the second trimester (after 16 weeks' gestation) or early in the third trimester of pregnancy. Intervention may include cerclage (stitches in the cervix to keep it closed). If the dilation continues, it may lead to premature membrane rupture and delivery of a fetus too small to survive.

Placenta previa. The placenta attaches too low on the uterus, near the cervix. As the cervix dilates, the placenta begins to separate from the uterus and may present before the fetus, thus endangering fetal life. The primary symptom is intermittent, recurrent, or painless bleeding that increases in intensity.

Pregnancy-related hypertension or preeclampsia. Characterized by hypertension, protein in the urine, and severe fluid retention, preeclampsia can progress to maternal convulsions, coma, and death if it becomes severe (eclampsia). It usually occurs in the third trimester and disappears after birth. The cause is not understood.

Multiple gestation. More than one fetus develops. Complications of multiple gestations include premature onset of labor and birth, increased incidence of perinatal mortality, lower-birth-weight infants, and increased incidence of maternal complications (e.g., hypertension).

Diabetes. Diabetes can be present before pregnancy or may occur as a result of the physiological stress of pregnancy. Gestational diabetes mellitus (GDM), which presents or is first recognized in pregnancy, affects 7% of pregnant women and usually disappears after pregnancy; however, as many as 50% of these women may develop type 2 diabetes within 10 years.[30] Inactivity and excessive weight gain in pregnancy has been found to be an independent risk factor for GDM.[4]

Unlike many of the previously discussed high-risk conditions, women with gestational diabetes may be appropriate candidates for more traditional physical therapy interventions.[4] Supervised, individualized exercise programs are excellent options. Parameters for exercise in pregnancy for women with gestational diabetes were published by the American Diabetes Association in 2006.[6] They support aerobic exercise with limited duration and at 50% maximum aerobic capacity; alternatively, the Borg scale may be used with a range of 11 to 13 rate of perceived exertion (RPE) as maximal activity level (see Box 25.4). With appropriate monitoring of fetal/uterine activity, maternal heart rate, and blood glucose levels, exercise duration of 15 to 30 minutes appears to be safe.[67] Instruct patients to monitor for any postexercise uterine activity; contractions need to be fewer than one every 15 minutes.[6,67]

Exercise may actually prevent gestational diabetes in obese pregnant women.[4] In particular, recumbent bicycling or arm ergometer exercises stabilize and lower glucose levels.[103]

 **FOCUS ON EVIDENCE**

In a randomized study of overweight women with gestational diabetes (n=32), the control group was treated with diet alone, while the remaining women also participated in circuit resistance training. The diet-plus-exercise group was able to postpone the use of insulin therapy until later in the pregnancy ($p < 0.05$) and was also prescribed less insulin overall ($p < 0.05$) than the diet-alone group.[24] A recent systematic review assessed both prevention and management of gestational diabetes with inconclusive results, possibly linked to compliance issues. There is some evidence that physical activity in pregnancy contributes to glycemic control and reduced use of insulin in these women.[107]

Management Guidelines and Precautions for High-Risk Pregnancies

Establish an individually designed exercise program for each woman with a high-risk pregnancy based on diagnosis, limitations, physical therapy examination, evaluation, and consultation with the physician. Activities must address patient needs but should not further complicate the condition.[7,120] Management guidelines for the woman who is confined to bed because of her high-risk status are summarized in Box 25.9.

BOX 25.9 MANAGEMENT GUIDELINES— High-Risk Pregnancy

Potential Impairments of Structure and Function, and Activity Limitations

Primary activity limitations are inability to be out of bed and move about and prolonged static positioning, contributing to the following impairments:

- Joint stiffness and muscle aches
- Muscle weakness and disuse atrophy
- Vascular complications including risk of thrombosis and decreased uterine blood flow
- Decreased proprioception in distal body parts
- Constipation caused by lack of exercise
- Postural changes
- Boredom

Emotional stress; patient may be at risk of losing the baby

Guilt from the belief that some activity caused the problem or that the patient did not take good enough care of herself

Anxiety about her home situation, older children, finances, or the impending birth

Plan of Care	Interventions
1. Decrease stiffness	1. Positioning instructions; assess for supports Facilitation of joint motion in available range
2. Maintain muscle length and bulk	2. Stretching and strengthening exercises within limits imposed by the physician
3. Maximize circulation; prevent deep-vein thrombosis	3. Ankle pumping; ROM
4. Improve proprioception	4. Movement activities for as many body parts as possible
5. Improve posture within available limits	5. Posture instruction, modified as necessary based on allowed activity level Bed mobility and transfer techniques if able (avoid Valsalva's maneuver)

Continued

BOX 25.9 MANAGEMENT GUIDELINES—High-Risk Pregnancy—cont'd

Plan of Care	Interventions
6. Relieve boredom	6. Vary activities and positioning for exercises; encourage interaction with others on bed rest (http://www.sidelines.org)
7. Enhance relaxation	7. Relaxation techniques/stress management
8. Prepare for delivery	8. Childbirth education, breathing training, and exercises to assist and prepare for labor
9. Enhance postpartum recovery	9. Exercise instruction and home program for postpartum period Body mechanics instruction, particularly related to childcare

Develop good rapport with the patient and instill trust. Closely monitor the patient during all activities; re-evaluate after each treatment, and note any changes. It is also important to teach the patient self-monitoring techniques so that she will be alert to adverse reactions and respond appropriately.

- Prolonged static positioning is a primary concern. The position of choice for the high-risk patient is left side-lying, which is optimal for reducing pressure on the inferior vena cava and for maximizing cardiac output, thereby enhancing maternal and fetal circulation.
- Some exercises, especially abdominal exercises, may stimulate uterine contractions. If this occurs, modify or discontinue them.
- Monitor and report any uterine contractions, bleeding, or amniotic fluid loss.
- Do not allow use of Valsalva's maneuver. Avoid any activities that increase intra-abdominal pressure. Body mechanics and postural instruction may stimulate abdominal contractions, so be sure the patient does not strain and closely monitor for adverse symptoms.
- Keep the exercises simple. Have the patient do them slowly, smoothly, and with minimal exertion.
- Many high-risk pregnancies result in cesarean deliveries, so educate the woman about cesarean delivery rehabilitation.
- Incorporate maximum muscle efficiency into each movement.
- Teach the patient self-monitoring techniques.

Exercise Suggestions With High-Risk Pregnancies

Exercise suggestions are adaptations of interventions that have already been described that should be considered for the bed-bound patient with a high-risk pregnancy.[7,103,120] Exercises to include are summarized in Box 25.10.

Positioning

- Left side-lying to prevent vena cava compression, enhance cardiac output, and decrease lower extremity edema
- Pillows between the knees and under the abdomen when side-lying
- Supine positioning for short periods, with a wedge placed under the right hip to decrease inferior vena cava compression (see Fig. 25.10)
- Modified prone positioning (side-lying, partially rolled toward prone, with pillow under abdomen) to decrease low back discomfort and pressure

BOX 25.10 Bed Exercises for High-Risk Pregnancy

- Patient supine (with wedge under the right hip), semireclined, or side-lying
- Cervical active ROM and chin tucks
- Backward shoulder circles (scapular retraction); reach to ceiling (protraction)
- Unilateral upper extremity diagonal patterns
- Shoulder, elbow flexion/extension; arm circles in side-lying
- Forearm pronation/supination; wrist flexion/extension, hand open/close
- Pelvic tilts
- Abdominal exercises (per physician consultation)
- Pelvic floor exercises (per physician consultation)
- Quad and gluteal isometric sets
- Unilateral hip abduction and adduction, internal/external rotation
- Unilateral hip and knee flexion/extension in side-lying
- Ankle pumping, ankle circles, ankle "alphabet"
- Toe flexion/extension

ROM

- Active ROM of all joints
- Motions should be slow, nonstressful, and through the full range if possible
- Teach in a gravity-neutral position if antigravity ROM is too much exertion
- Individualize the number of repetitions and frequency to the woman's condition

Ambulation/Standing

Historically, getting out of bed has been contraindicated with high-risk pregnancies; this will likely continue to evolve in varied health-care settings.[4] In the past, women would be upright only for using the bathroom or to shower. When allowed:

- Encourage good posture in ambulation
- Tip-toe or heel walking to emphasize calf muscles
- Gentle, partial-range squatting to emphasize hip and thigh muscles

Relaxation Techniques, Bed Mobility, and Transfer Activities

- Relaxation as in the uncomplicated pregnancy
- Moving up, down, and side-to-side in bed
- Log rolling: incorporate neck and upper and lower extremities to aid movement
- Supine-to-sitting: use log-roll technique, assisted by arms

Preparation for Labor

- Relaxation techniques
- Substitutions for squatting: supine, sitting, or side-lying, bringing flexed knees toward chest (hips will have to be abducted)
- Pelvic floor relaxation
- Breathing exercises: minimize forced abdominal exhalations

Postpartum Exercise Instruction

Instructions are the same as previously described in the uncomplicated pregnancy section.

Independent Learning Activities

Critical Thinking and Discussion

1. Describe three normal changes of pregnancy that will affect exercise tolerance.
2. Explain the clinical significance of diastasis recti, the testing procedure, and the corrective exercise.
3. Differentiate between postural and sacroiliac back pain in the pregnant patient.
4. Name five risk factors for pelvic floor dysfunction.
5. What exercise guidelines are most helpful for a woman who has not exercised prior to becoming pregnant?
6. Discuss optimal positioning for an uncomplicated labor and delivery in terms of biomechanics, gravity, and energy conservation.
7. Vaginal delivery places great stretch and compression on which nerves?

Laboratory Practice

1. Practice giving instructions to a lab partner on how to perform the following exercises. Observe that they are being done correctly. Reverse the experience and provide feedback.
   - Diastasis recti exercises
   - Pelvic clock exercises
   - Breathing and relaxation for the different stages of labor and delivery
2. Practice giving instructions, and get verbal feedback as to the success of instructions for the pelvic floor awareness training and strengthening exercises.
3. Observe an exercise class for pregnant women. Critique the effectiveness and inclusiveness of the instruction.

Case Studies

Case Study 1

Ms. V is a 32-year-old pregnant woman referred with a diagnosis of "low back pain" that became severe at 24 weeks' gestation. She reports (L) lumbar/thoracic, (R) anterior rib/pectoral, and cervical symptoms, which are worsening as the pregnancy progresses. Before her pregnancy, she wore a custom-made bra (32-MM), which is now much too small and provides inadequate support. Wearing this bra greatly increases her cervical and upper trapezius symptoms. Wearing a sports bra or standing more than 10 to 15 minutes causes increased low back symptoms. Pain is severely limiting her daily activities both at home and in the community. She has difficulty climbing stairs, grocery shopping, doing laundry, and other household chores. She is wakened at night by pain and also reports numbness in her lower extremities at night. She is a single mother of a 6-year-old son. Pertinent medical history includes a weight gain of 100 lb with her previous pregnancy, C-section delivery, and removal of fibrocystic breast tissue three times. She has no systemic medical conditions or medications other than prenatal vitamins. Current weight: 238 lb, height: 5′4″.

Clinical Findings

Postural assessment reveals marked forward head/shoulders with internal rotation at both shoulder joints, significant lordosis (cervical and lumbar), recurvatum bilaterally, decreased longitudinal arches, and increased base of support with excessive external rotation (ER) at both hips. All dynamic movements are pain inhibited: frequent weight shift and asymmetrical transitions, antalgic gait pattern with increased ER of hips. Lumbar extension and (L) cervical rotation most limited by pain and spasm.

Diastasis recti of 9 cm noted above umbilicus; abdominal strength 3–/5. Pelvic landmarks difficult to assess due to adipose tissue; leg lengths appear equal. Slight tenderness over pubic symphysis with palpation.

- Identify the impairments and functional limitations.
- Identify goals that deal with impairments and functional limitations.
- Develop a treatment plan to meet the goals; identify specific interventions and parameters, number of times she will be seen, and any follow-up or referrals that you believe will be necessary.

Case Study 2

Mrs. W is a 71-year-old woman with an 11-year history of urinary incontinence and urgency. She experiences frequent, large-volume accidents, using 8 to 10 large incontinence pads and 8 panty liners per day for garment protection. Voiding frequency is 13 to 16 times every 24 hours. She also reports constipation and straining for evacuation, which improves with increased fiber intake. Caffeine intake is two servings per day. Mrs. W is a nonsmoker. She is much less active with social and community activities as a result of this problem. Urodynamic testing revealed diminished bladder capacity at 150 cc and confirmed the diagnosis of detrusor instability.

Pertinent medical history includes nine pregnancies and seven live births (G9, P7) with one breech presentation. LBP and "sciatic nerve problems" of long standing were reported with lumbar fusion done when she was 44 and 48 years of age. Other surgical history includes rectocele/cystocele repair when she was 36 and partial hysterectomy when she was 37. Hypertension and asthma are both well controlled with medication.

Clinical Findings

Pelvic floor muscle assessment reveals poor sensory awareness, decreased resting tone, and an MMT of 2/5. Patient able to hold a contraction 4 seconds and repeat 10 "quick flicks" in 10 seconds. Accessory recruitment of the abdominals noted. Pressure perineometry confirms muscle weakness with 6.35 cm of water pressure generated. Levator ani contraction is enhanced with stretch facilitation to the pelvic floor (R > L).

Abdominal strength is 3/5. Diastasis recti noted above the umbilicus of 4.5 cm. Diaphragmatic breathing pattern present; no Valsalva's with exertion. All dynamic movements of the trunk are mildly restricted because of lumbar fusion.

The patient underwent physical therapy treatments approximately 18 months ago and is independent with her low back program. (Because of insurance limitations of 10 visits, the patient requested primary attention to pelvic floor dysfunction and incontinence.)

- Identify the impairments and functional limitations.
- Identify goals that deal with the impairments and functional limitations.
- Design a treatment plan to meet the goals; identify specific interventions and parameters, number of times she will be seen, and any follow-up or referrals that you believe will be necessary.

WEB RESOURCES

http://www.womenshealthapta.org (Section on Women's Health, APTA)
http://www.pfdn.rti.org (Pelvic Floor Disorders Network)
http://www.nafc.org (National Association for Continence)
http://www.pelvicpain.org (International Pelvic Pain Society)
http://www.sidelines.org (High-risk pregnancy support)
http://sis.nlm.nih.gov/outreach/whrhome.html (Women's health resources)
http://www.healthywomen.org
www.ustoo.org (International Prostate Cancer Education & Support)

REFERENCES

1. Abrams, P et al: The standardization of terminology of lower urinary tract function: report from the standardization sub-committee of the International Continence Society. *Neurouol Urodyn*21:167–178, 2002.
2. Allen, RE, and Hanson, RW: Episiotomy in low-risk vaginal deliveries. *J Am Board Fam Pract* 18:8–12, 2005.
3. Al-Zirqi, I, et al: Uterine rupture after previous caesarean section. *BJOG* 117(7):809–820, 2010.
4. American College of Obstetricians and Gynecologists: Physical activity and exercise during pregnancy and the postpartum period. Committee Opinion No. 650. *Obstet Gynecol* 126:e135–e142. 2015.
5. American College of Obstetrics and Gynecology: Nutrition During Pregnancy. Available at http://www.acog.org/publications/patient_education/bp001.cfm#pregnancy. Accessed July 29, 2010.
6. American Diabetes Association: Standards of medical care in diabetes, 2006 position statement. *Diabetes Care* 29:S4–S42, 2006.
7. American Physical Therapy Associatio: *Perinatal Exercise Guidelines: Section on Obstetrics and Gynecology.* Alexandria, VA, 1986.
8. Artal, R, and Wiswell, R: *Exercise in Pregnancy.* Baltimore: Williams & Wilkins, 1986.
9. Ashton-Miller, J, and DeLancey, J: On the biomechanics of vaginal birth and common sequelae. *Annu Rev Biomed Eng* 11:163–176, 2009.
10. Baker, PK: Musculoskeletal problems.. In Steege, J, et al (eds): *Chronic Pelvic Pain: An Integrated Approach.* Philadelphia: WB Saunders, 215–240, 1998.
11. Barber, MD, et al: Innervation of the female levator ani muscles. *Am J Obstet Gynecol* 187(1):64–71, 2002.
12. Belegolovsky, I, et al: The effectiveness of exercise in treatment of pregnancy-related lumbar and pelvic girdle pain: a meta-analysis and evidence-based review. *J Women's Health Phys Ther* 39(2):53–64, 2015.
13. Benson, JT (ed): *Female Pelvic Floor Disorders: Investigation and Management.* New York: WW Norton, 1992.
14. Bø, K, et al: Constriction of the levator hiatus during instruction of pelvic floor or transversus abdominis contraction: a 4D ultrasound study. *Intl Urogyn J* 20(1):27–32, 2009.
15. Bø, K, et al: Lower urinary tract symptoms and pelvic floor muscle exercise adherence after 15 years, part 1. *Ob & Gyn*105(5):999–1005, 2005.
16. Bø, K: Pelvic floor muscle training is effective in treatment of stress urinary incontinence, but how does it work? *Int Urogynecol J Pelvic Floor Dysfunct* 15:76–84, 2004.
17. Bø, K, et al: Transabdominal ultrasound measurement of pelvic floor muscle activity when activated directly or via a transversus abdominis muscle contraction. *Neurourol Urodynam* 22:582–588, 2003.
18. Boardman, R, and Jackson, B: Below the belt: approach to chronic pelvic pain. *Can Fam Physician* 52(12):1556–1562, 2006.

19. Boissonnault, J, and Blaschak, M: Incidence of diastasis recti abdominis during the childbearing years. *Phys Ther* 68:1082–1086, 1988.
20. Borello-France, D, et al: Fecal and urinary incontinence in primiparous women: the Childbirth and Pelvic Symptoms (CAPS) Study. *Obstet Gynecol* 108:863–872, 2006.
21. Borg, G: Psychophysical bases of perceived exertion. *Med Sci Sports Exerc* 14:377–381, 1982.
22. Boston Women's Health Book Collective: *The New Our Bodies, Ourselves,* ed. 35. New York: Simon & Schuster, 2005.
23. Bradley, CS, et al: Bowel symptoms in women planning surgery for pelvic organ prolapse. *Am J Obstet Gynecol* 195(6):1814–1819, 2006.
24. Brankston, GN, et al: Resistance exercise decreases the need for insulin in overweight women with gestational diabetes mellitus. *Am J Obstet Gynecol* 190(1):188–193, 2004.
25. Bryant, CM, et al: A randomized trial of the effects of caffeine upon frequency, urgency and urge incontinence. *Neurourol Urodyn* 19:501–502, 2000.
26. Bump, R, et al: Assessment of Kegel pelvic muscle exercise performance after brief verbal instruction. *Am J Obstet Gynecol* 165:322–329, 1991.
27. Burgio, KL, et al: Behavioral versus drug treatment for urge urinary incontinence in older women. *JAMA* 280(23):1995–2000, 1998.
28. Bursch, S: Interrater reliability of diastasis recti abdominis measurement. *Phys Ther* 67(7):1077–1079, 1987.
29. Butler, DS, and Moseley, GL, Sunyata: *Explain Pain.* Adelaide: Noigroup Publications, 2003.
30. Centers for Disease Control and Prevention: Check Your Knowledge: Diabetes and Pregnancy. Available at http://www.cdc.gov/Features/DiabetesPregnancy. Accessed July 24, 2010.
31. Chiarelli, P, and O'Keefe, D: Physiotherapy for the pelvic floor. *Austral J Physiother* 27(4):103–108, 1981.
32. Chong, EC, et al: The financial burden of stress urinary incontinence among women in the United States. *Curr Urol Rep* 12(5):358–362, 2011.
33. Clapp, JF: A clinical approach to exercise during pregnancy. *Clin Sports Med* 13(2):443–458, 1994.
34. Clapp, JF: Exercise and fetal health. *J Dev Physiol* 15(1):9–14, 1991.
35. Clapp, JF: Exercise during pregnancy: a clinical update. *Clin Sports Med* 19(2):273–286, 2000.
36. Clapp, JF, et al: Continuing regular exercise during pregnancy: effect of exercise volume on fetoplacental growth. *Am J Obstet Gynecol* 186: 142–147, 2002.
37. Clinton, S, et al: Pelvic girdle pain in the antepartum population: physical therapy clinical practice guidelines linked to the International Classification of Functioning, Disability, and Health from the section on women's health and the orthopaedic section of the American Physical Therapy Association. *J Women's Health Phys Ther* 41(2):102–125, 2017.
38. DeLancey, JOL, and Richardson, AC: Anatomy of genital support. In Benson, JT (ed): *Female Pelvic Floor Disorders: Investigation and Management.* New York: WW Norton, 19–26, 1992.
39. Depledge, J, et al: Management of symphysis pubis dysfunction during pregnancy using exercise and pelvic support belts. *Phys Ther* 85: 1290–1300, 2005.
40. Dockter, M, et al: Prevalence of urinary incontinence: a comparative study of collegiate female athletes and non-athletic controls. *J Women's Health Phys Ther* 31(1):12–17, 2007.
41. Dolan, L, et al: Stress incontinence and pelvic floor neurophysiology 15 years after the first delivery. *BJOG* 110(12):1107–1114, 2003.
42. Dorey, G, et al: Developing a pelvic floor muscle training regimen for use in a trial intervention. *Physiother* 95:199–208, 2009.
43. Fantl, JA, et al: *Urinary Incontinence in Adults: Acute and Chronic Management.* Clinical Practice Guideline No. 2, AHCPR Publication No. 96–0682. Rockville, MD: U.S. Department of HHS, Public Health Service, 1996.
44. Feldenkrais, M: *Awareness Through Movement: Health Exercises for Personal Growth,* ed. 1. New York: Harper & Row, 1972.
45. Figuers, C, et al: "A Comparison of Pelvic Floor Muscle Activity and Urinary Incontinence Between Weight_Bearing Female Athletes and Female Non_Athletes." *J Women's Health Phys Ther* 31(1):24–25, 2007.
46. Fisher, K, and Riolo, L: What is the evidence regarding specific methods of pelvic floor exercise for a patient with urinary stress incontinence and mild anterior wall prolapse? *Phys Ther* 84(8):744–753, 2004.
47. FitzGerald, MP, et al: Risk factors for anal sphincter tear during vaginal delivery. *Obstet Gynecol* 109:29–34, 2007.
48. FitzGerald, M, et al: Randomized multicenter clinical trial of myofascial physical therapy in women with interstitial cystitis/painful bladder syndrome and pelvic floor tenderness. *J Urology* 187:2113–2118, 2012.
49. Frahm, J: Strengthening the pelvic floor. *Clin Man Phys Ther* 5(3): 30–33, 1985.
50. Freyder, SC: Exercising while pregnant. *J Orthop Sports Phys Ther* 10: 358–365, 1989.
51. Garshasbi, A, and Faghih Zadeh, S: The effect of exercise on the intensity of low back pain in pregnant women. *Int J Gynaecol Obstet* 88(3): 271–275, 2005.
52. Gent, D, and Gottlieb, K: Cesarean rehabilitation. *Clin Man Phys Ther* 5:14, 1985.
53. Giarenis, I, and Robinson, D: Prevention and management of pelvic organ prolapse. *F1000Prime Reports* 6:77, 2014.
54. Gilbert, E, and Harman, J: *High-Risk Pregnancy and Delivery,* ed. 1. St. Louis: CV Mosby, 1986.
55. Glazener, C, et al: Childbirth and prolapse: long-term associations with the symptoms and objective measurement of pelvic organ prolapse. *Brit J Gynecol* 120:161–168, 2013.
56. 5Goldberg, R: Effects of pregnancy and childbirth on the pelvic floor. In Culligan, P, and Goldberg, R (eds): *Urogynecology in Primary Care.* London: Springer Science and Business Media, 2007, pp 21–33.
57. Goode, PS, et al: Behavioral therapy with or without biofeedback and pelvic floor electrical stimulation for persistent post-prostatectomy incontinence: a randomized controlled trial. *J Am Med Assn* 305(2):151–159, 2011.
58. Gorina Y, et al: Prevalence of incontinence among older Americans. National Center for Health Statistics. *Vital Health Stat* 3(36), p 5, 2014.
59. Grigorescu, BA, et al: Innervation of the levator ani muscles: description of the nerve branches to the pubococcygeus, iliococcygeus, and puborectalis muscles. *Int Urogynecol J Pelvic Floor Dysfunct* 19(1):107–116, 2008.
60. Guise, JM, et al: *Vaginal Birth After Cesarean: New Insights. Evidence Report/Technology Assessment No. 191.* AHRQ Publication No.10-E001. Rockville, MD: Agency for Healthcare Research and Quality, 2010.
61. Hagen, S, and Stark, D: Conservative prevention and management of pelvic organ prolapse in women. *Cochrane Database Syst Rev* 12:CD003882, 2011.
62. Hamilton, B, et.al.: Births: Preliminary data for 2013. National vital statistics reports; vol 63 no 2. Hyattsville, MD: National Center for Health Statistics, 2014. Available at http://www.cdc.gov/nchs/fastats/delivery.htm. (2013 figures) Accessed July 3, 2015.
63. Harrington, K, and Haskvitz, E: Managing a patient's constipation with physical therapy. *Phys Ther Nov* 86:1511–1519, 2006.
64. Hartmann, K, et al: Outcomes of routine episiotomy. *JAMA* 293: 2141–2148, 2005.
65. Hay-Smith, J: Therapeutic ultrasound for postpartum perineal pain and dyspareunia. *Cochrane Database Syst Rev* 3:CD000495. 1998.
66. Holroyd-Leduc, J, and Straus, S: Management of urinary incontinence in women. *JAMA* 291:986–995, 2004.
67. Irion, J, and Irion, G (eds): *Women's Health in Physical Therapy.* Baltimore: Lippincott Williams & Wilkins, 2010.
68. Jamieson, D, and Steege, J: The prevalence of dysmenorrhea, dyspareunia, pelvic pain, and irritable bowel syndrome in primary care practices. *Obstet Gynecol* 87(1):55–58, 1996.
69. Jarrell, J, et al: Consensus guidelines for the management of chronic pelvic pain. *J Obstet Gynaecol Can* 27(8):781–826, 2005.
70. Jarski, RW, and Trippett, DL: The risks and benefits of exercise during pregnancy. *J Fam Pract* 30(2):185–189, 1990.
71. Johnson, T: Gain Weight Safely During Your Pregnancy. Available at http://www.webmd.com/baby/guide/healthy-weight-gain#1 Accessed May 24, 2017.
72. Jordre, B, and Schweinle, W: Comparing resisted hip rotation with pelvic floor muscle training in women with stress urinary incontinence: a pilot study. *J Women's Health Phys Ther* 38(2):81–89, 2014.
73. Keeler, J, et al: Diastasis recti abdominis: a survey of women's health specialists for current physical therapy clinical practice for postpartum women. *J Women's Health Phys Ther* 36(3):131–142, 2012.

74. Klein, M, et al: Determinants of vaginal-perineal integrity and pelvic floor functioning in childbirth. *Am J Obstet Gynecol* 176(2):403–410, 1997.
75. Laine, K, et al: Prevalence and risk factors for anal incontinence after obstetric anal sphincter rupture. *Acta Obst Gynecol Scand* 90(4):319–324, 2011.
76. Lappen, J, and Gossett, D: Changes in episiotomy practice: evidence-based medicine in action. *Expert Rev of Obstet Gynecol* 5(3):301–309, 2010.
77. Legato, M: *Eve's Rib: The Groundbreaking Guide to Women's Health.* New York: Three Rivers Press, 2002.
78. Leveno, K, et al: *Williams Manual of Obstetrics,* ed. 21. McGraw-Hill Companies, New York, New York 2003.
79. Liddle, SD, and Pennick, V: Interventions for preventing and treating low-back and pelvic pain during pregnancy. *Cochrane Database Syst Rev* 9:CD001139, 2015.
80. Lien, K, et al: Pudendal nerve stretch during vaginal birth: a 3D computer simulation. *Am J Obstetrics and Gynecol* 192:1669–1676, 2005.
81. MacDonald, R, et al: Pelvic floor muscle training to improve urinary incontinence after radical prostatectomy: a systematic review of effectiveness. *BJU International* 100:76–81, 2007.
82. Mantl, J, et al: Epidemiology of genital prolapse: observations from the Oxford Family Planning Association Study. *BJOG* 104:579–585, 1997.
83. Markel Feldt, C: Applying the Guide to Physical Therapist Practice to women's health physical therapy: part II. *J Women's Health Phys Ther* 24:1, 2000.
84. Marnach, M, et al: Characterization of the relationship between joint laxity and maternal hormones in pregnancy. *Ob & Gyn* 101(2):331–335, 2003.
85. Mayo Clinic: Men's health: Kegel exercises for men can help improve bladder control and possibly improve sexual performance. Available at http://www.mayoclinic.org/kegel-exercises-for-men/ART-20045074?p=1. Accessed July 31, 2015.
86. Mørkved, S, and Bø, K: Effect of pelvic floor muscle training during pregnancy and after childbirth on prevention and treatment of urinary incontinence: a systematic review. *Br J Sports Med* 48(4):299–310, 2014.
87. Morkved, S, and Bø, K: Effect of postpartum pelvic floor muscle training in prevention and treatment of urinary incontinence: a one-year follow up. *BJOG* 107(8):1022–1028, 2002.
88. Morkved, S, et al: Pelvic floor muscle training during pregnancy to prevent urinary incontinence: a single-blind randomized controlled trial. *Obstet Gynecol* 101(2):313–319, 2003.
89. Naparstek, B: *Staying Well With Guided Imagery.* New York, New York, Grand Central Publishing, 2008.
90. National Association for Continence. Conditions overview. Available at http://www.nafc.org/conditions/. Accessed November 22, 2015.
91. Newman, DK, et al: An evidence-based strategy for the conservative management of the male patient with incontinence. *Curr Opin Urol* 24(6):553–559, 2014.
92. Nilsson-Wikmar, L, et al: Effect of three different physical therapy treatments on pain and activity in pregnant women with pelvic girdle pain: a randomized clinical trial with 3, 6, and 12 months follow-up postpartum. *Spine* 30(8):850–856, 2005.
93. Noble, E: *Essential Exercises for the Childbearing Year,* ed. 4. Harwich: New Life Images, Boston, 1995.
94. Noble, E: *Having Twins,* ed. 3. Boston: Houghton Mifflin, 2003.
95. Norwitz, E, and Robinson, J: Scientific review of *The Control of Labor. Fetal Monitoring, Pregnancy and Birth.* Available at http://www.obgyn.net/fetal-monitoring/scientific-review-control-labor#sthash.qzboYgLe.dpuf. Accessed September 23, 2015.
96. Nygaard, I, et al: Pelvic organ prolapse in older women: prevalence and risk factors. *Obstet Gynecol* 104(3):489–497, 2004.
97. Nygaard, I, et al: Physical activity in women planning sacrocolpopexy. *Int Urogyn J* 18:33–37, 2007.
98. Nygaard, I, et al: Prevalence of symptomatic pelvic floor disorders in US women. *JAMA* 300(11):1311–1316, 2008.
99. Olsson, C, and Nilsson-Wikmar, L: Health-related quality of life and physical ability among pregnant women with and without back pain in late pregnancy. *Acta Obstet Gynecol Scand* 83(4):351–357, 2004.
100. Ostgaard, HC, et al: Reduction of back and posterior pelvic pain in pregnancy. *Spine* 19(8):894–900, 1994.
101. Palm, S: Personal correspondence with founder of Association for Pelvic Organ Prolapse Support and closed group on Facebook. November 9, 2015.
102. Paras, ML, et al: Sexual abuse and lifetime diagnosis of somatic disorders: a systematic review and meta-analysis. *JAMA* 302(5):550–561, 2009.
103. Pauls, J: *Therapeutic Approaches to Women's Health: A Program of Exercise and Education.* Gaithersburg, MD: Aspen, 1995.
104. Pennick, VE, and Young, G: Interventions for preventing and treating pelvic and back pain in pregnancy. *Cochrane Database Syst Rev* 18(2): CD001139, 2007.
105. Peters, AA, et al: A randomized clinical trial to compare two different approaches in women with chronic pelvic pain. *Obstet Gynecol* 77(5): 740–744, 1999.
106. Ribeiro, LHS, et al: Long-term effect of early postoperative pelvic floor biofeedback on continence in men undergoing radical prostatectomy: a prospective, randomized, controlled trial. *J Urol*184(3):1034–1039, 2010.
107. Ruchat, SM, and Mottola, M: The important role of physical activity in the prevention and management of gestational diabetes mellitus. *Diabetes/Metab Res Rev*29(5):334–346, 2013.
108. Sampselle, C, et al: Effect of pelvic muscle exercise on transient incontinence during pregnancy and after birth. *Obstet Gynecol* 91(3):406–412, 1998.
109. Sapsford, RR, et al: Co-activation of the abdominal and pelvic floor muscles during voluntary exercises. *Neuro Urodynam* 20:31–42, 2001.
110. Sapsford, R: Rehabilitation of pelvic floor muscles utilizing trunk stabilization. *Man Ther* 9(1):3–12, 2004.
111. Sapsford, RR, et al: Pelvic floor muscle activity in different sitting postures in continent and incontinent women. *Arch Phys Med Rehabil* 89(9):1741–1747, 2008.
112. Santiesteban, A: Electromyographic and dynamometric characteristics of female pelvic floor musculature. *Phys Ther* 68(3):344–351, 1988.
113. Shafik, A: A study of the continence mechanism of the external urethral sphincter with identification of the voluntary urinary inhibition reflex. *J of Urology* 162(6):1967–1971, 1999.
114. Shrock, P, Simkin, P, and Shearer, M: Teaching prenatal exercise: part II—exercises to think twice about. *Birth Fam J* 8(3):167–175, 1981.
115. Shumway-Cook, A, and Woollcott, MH: *MOTOR Control: Translating Research Into Clinical Practice.* Philadelphia: Lippincott Williams & Wilkins, 2007.
116. Snooks, SJ, et al: Risk factors in childbirth causing damage to the pelvic floor innervation. *Int J Colorect Dis* 1(1):20–24, 1986.
117. Society of Obstetricians and Gynaecologists of Canada and the Canadian Society for Exercise Physiology: Exercise in pregnancy and the postpartum period. Joint guidelines. *J Obstet Gynaecol Can* 25(6):516–522, 2003.
118. Spitznagle, T, et al: Prevalence of diastasis recti abdominis in an urogynecological population. *Int Urogyn J Pelvic Floor Dysfunct* 18(3): 321–328, 2007.
119. Staer-Jensen, J, et al: Postpartum recovery of levator hiatus and bladder neck mobility in relation to pregnancy. *Obstet Gynecol* 125(3):531–539, 2015.
120. Stephenson, R, and O'Connor, L: *Obstetric and Gynecologic Care in Physical Therapy,* ed. 2. Thorofare, NJ: Charles B. Slack, 2000.
121. Stuge, B, et al: The efficacy of a treatment program focusing on specific stabilizing exercises for pelvic girdle pain after pregnancy—a two-year follow-up of a randomized, clinical trial. *Spine* (29)10:E197–E203, 2004.
122. Tienforti, D, et al: Efficacy of an assisted low-intensity programme of perioperative pelvic floor muscle training in improving the recovery of continence after radical prostatectomy: a randomized controlled trial. *BJU International* 110:1004–1010, 2012.
123. Thom, D, et al: Evaluation of parturition and other reproductive variables as risk factors for urinary incontinence in later life. *Obstet Gynecol* 90:983–989, 1997.
124. Wallner, C, et al: Innervation of the pelvic floor muscles: a reappraisal for the levator ani nerve. *Obstet Gynecol* 108(3 pt, 1):529–534, 2006.
125. Wilder, E (ed): *Obstetric and Gynecologic Physical Therapy: Clinics in Physical Therapy, Vol. 20,* ed. 1. New York: Churchill Livingstone, 1988.
126. Wilder, E (ed): *The Gynecological Manual,* ed. 2. Alexandria, VA: APTA, Section on Women's Health, 2000.
127. Wright, D: Maternal, Infant, and Child Health Progress Review. Available at http://www.healthypeople.gov/Data/2010prog/focus16/2007Focus16.pdf. Accessed Sept 20, 2010.

CHAPTER

26

Management of Lymphatic Disorders

KAREN L. HOCK, PT, MS, CLT-LANA ■ LYNN ALLEN COLBY, PT, MS

Impairments of the lymphatic system can lead to lymphatic insufficiencies that can result in significant physical impairments and subsequent loss of function of either the upper or lower extremities. Disturbances in structure or function can lead to accumulation of lymphatic fluids in the tissue of the body that affect the physiological health of the tissue, impair joint mobility, and impact daily functioning. Lymphatic dysfunction can be a result of a congenital or hereditary abnormality or can be caused by trauma, infection, or treatment for a cancer.

To contribute to the effective management of patients with lymphatic disorders, a therapist must possess a sound understanding of the underlying pathologies and the clinical manifestations of many types of lymphatic disorders, as well as the interplay between the lymphatic and venous systems. A therapist must also be aware of the use, effectiveness, and limitations of therapeutic exercise in the comprehensive management and rehabilitation of patients with lymphatic insufficiencies.

Disorders of the Lymphatic System

Structure and Function of the Lymphatic System

The primary function of the lymphatic system is to collect and transport fluid from the interstitial spaces back to the venous circulation (Fig. 26.1).[36,57,62,69,86,133.135] This is accomplished with a series of lymph vessels and lymph nodes.[36,69,135] The lymphatic system also has a role in the body's immune function.[36,69,86,133,135] When the lymphatic system is compromised either by impairment of lymphatic structures or by an overload of lymphatic fluid, the result is swelling in the tissue spaces. Edema is a natural consequence of trauma to and subsequent healing of soft tissues. If the lymphatic system is compromised and does not function efficiently, lymphedema develops and impedes wound healing.

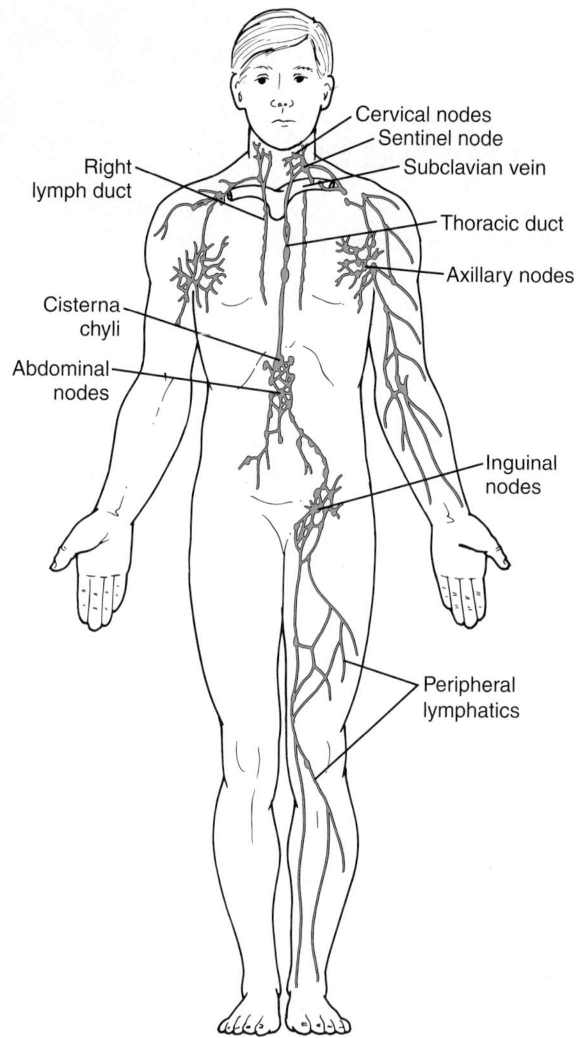

FIGURE 26.1 Major vessels of the lymphatic system.

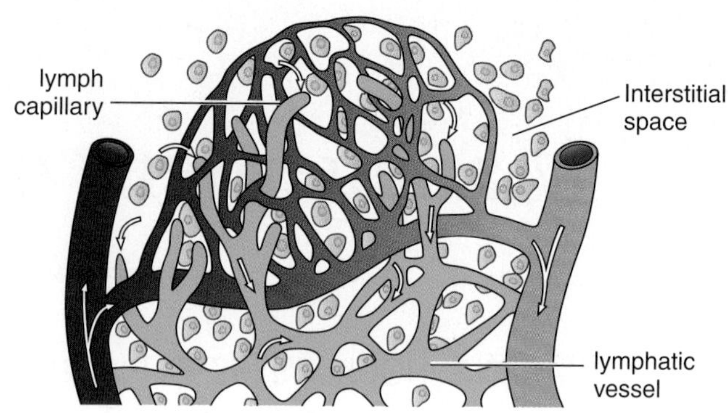

FIGURE 26.2 Lymph capillary and larger lymph vessel.

Lymphedema is an excessive and persistent accumulation of extravascular and extracellular fluid and proteins in tissue spaces.[12,22,32,57,69.74,135] It occurs when lymph volume exceeds the capacity of the lymph transport system, and it is associated with a disturbance of the water and protein balance across the capillary membrane. An increased concentration of proteins draws larger amounts of water into interstitial spaces, leading to lymphedema.[32,51,69,135] The accumulation of the extracellular fluid and protein causes a proliferation of adipose tissue in the affected area.[14,15,86] Furthermore, many disorders of the cardiopulmonary system can cause the load on lymphatic vessels to exceed their transport capacity and subsequently cause lymphedema.[51,74,107]

Anatomy of the Lymphatic System

The lymphatic system is an open system.[36,69,70,135] The lymphatic capillaries are situated close to the blood capillaries and are responsible for pulling the fluid into the lymphatic circulation (Fig. 26.2).[36,57,70.133.135] Once inside the lymphatic vessels, the fluid is transported from lymph nodes to lymphatic trunks.[36,69,70,133,135] The end result is the collection of the lymphatic fluid at the venous angles. In total, the body has 600 to 700 lymph nodes with the largest grouping found in the head and neck, around the intestines, and in the axilla and groin.[36,135]

Physiology of the Lymphatic System

The main components of lymphatic fluid are water and protein found in the extracellular spaces.[32,36,51,69,70] In a normal state, the lymphatic system transports this fluid back to the venous circulation. The amount of fluid transported is the lymphatic load, and the amount of fluid the lymphatic system can transport is the transport capacity.[36,69,135] When the balance in the interstitium is disrupted, whether by an increased lymphatic load or a decreased transport capacity, lymphedema can develop.[32,36,51,135] Lymphatic load is increased when the venous system is unable to transport the required amount of fluid, which can occur in a patient with a venous insufficiency.[69] Transport capacity is affected when the structures of the lymphatic system are impaired, for example, following surgery to remove lymph nodes in a patient with cancer.

Types of Lymphedema

Lymphedema can be classified as primary, meaning there is an inherent problem with the structures of the lymphatic system, or secondary, meaning there is an injury to lymphatic structures.[36,51,69,135] This injury may be in the form of surgery, radiation, trauma, or infection. Lymphedema can also be caused by a combination of lymphatic-venous dysfunction commonly seen in patients with chronic venous insufficiency. Remember, lymphedema is not a disease but rather a symptom of a malfunctioning lymphatic system.

Primary Lymphedema

Primary lymphedema, although uncommon, is the result of insufficient development (dysplasia) and congenital malformation of the lymphatic system.[50,69]

Primary lymphedema can be divided according to the age of presentation:[36,51,69]

- *Congenital*: presents at birth and is sometimes known as Milroy's disease
- *Praecox (early)*: develops prior to 35 years of age
- *Tarda*: develops after 35 years of age

Primary lymphedema typically affects more females than males and presents more often in the extremities, more so in the lower than upper extremities. However, it can be seen in other areas of the body as well.[36,51,70,135] If not managed properly, this type of lymphedema can progress over time and present with skin changes (hyperkeratosis) and increased skin folds and skin creases.[36,51,62,124,128]

Secondary Lymphedema

Most of the patients seen by health-care practitioners for management of lymphedema have secondary lymphedema.[101] By far, the most common causes of secondary lymphedema are related to the comprehensive management of cancers of the breast, pelvis, and abdomen.[4,11,12,44,50,51,101,102] Secondary lymphedema is classified by the cause of the injury to the lymphatic structures including the following:

- Surgery
- Inflammation and infection
- Obstruction or fibrosis
- Combined venous-lymphatic dysfunction (chronic venous insufficiency)

Surgical Dissection of Lymph Nodes

Lymph nodes and vessels often are surgically removed (lymphadenectomy) as an aspect of treatment of a primary malignancy or metastatic disease. For example, lymph node sampling is performed in most types of breast cancer surgeries to determine the extent and progression of breast cancer.[13,19,44,59] Likewise, pelvic or inguinal lymph node excision often is necessary for the treatment of pelvic or abdominal cancers.[4,101,102]

Infection and Inflammation

Inflammation of the lymph vessels (*lymphangitis*) or lymph nodes (*lymphadenitis*) and enlargement of lymph nodes (*lymphadenopathy*) can occur as the result of a systemic infection or local trauma. Any of these conditions can cause disruption of lymph circulation.[50,51,69,135]

Obstruction or Fibrosis

Trauma, surgery, and neoplasms can block or impair the lymphatic circulation.[51,69,123] Radiation therapy associated with treatment of malignant tumors also can cause fibrosis of vessels.[4,13]

Combined Venous-Lymphatic Dysfunction

Although not a primary disorder of the lymphatic system, chronic venous insufficiency and varicose veins are associated with venous stasis and accumulation of edema in the extremities.[45,50,65,135] Dependent, peripheral edema, occurring with long periods of standing or sitting, is a common manifestation of chronic venous dysfunction. Edema decreases if the limb is elevated. Patients often report dull aching or tiredness in the affected extremity.[27,33,45,50,65,96,135] If the insufficiency is associated with varicose veins, venous distention (bulging) also is notable. When edema persists, the skin becomes less supple over time and takes on a brownish pigmentation.

With time, a continued increase in the lymphatic work load imposed by the venous system causes a combined venous-lymphatic dysfunction. The lymphatic system begins to lose efficiency with the increased workload imposed over time, and a mixed edema results.[135] A venous-lymphatic dysfunction has a mixture of low protein edema from the venous system and a high protein edema from the lymphatic system. This combined dysfunction is termed *phlebolymphedema*.[18,35]

Several characteristics distinguish the venous component from lymphedema in phlebolymphedema. Skin changes, typically hyperpigmentation, are present in chronic venous insufficiency. Clinical findings typical of the lymphedema component include pitting swelling in the dorsal aspect of the foot with swelling in the toes.[18,35]

Clinical Manifestations of Lymphatic Disorders

Lymphedema

Location. When lymphedema develops, it is most often apparent in the distal extremities, particularly over the dorsum of the foot or hand.[32,51] The term *dependent edema* describes the accumulation of fluids in the peripheral aspects of the limbs, particularly when the distal segments are lower than the heart. In contrast, lymphedema can manifest more centrally, for example, in the axilla, groin, or even the trunk.[32,50,69,135] Thorough assessment of the entire limb and regional area is important to define the extent of swelling.

Severity. The severity of lymphedema may be described quantitatively or qualitatively. Lymphedema is described by the severity of changes that occur in skin and subcutaneous tissues. The three categories—pitting, brawny, and weeping edema—are described in Box 26.1. Although all three types reflect a significant degree of lymphedema, they are listed in order of severity, from least severe to most severe.[19,22,50,111]

CLINICAL TIP

When skin is interrupted in a patient with lymphedema, it is common to note a seeping of clear, yellow-tinged fluid that is slightly thicker than vascular fluid in consistency. This increased viscosity comes from the high level of protein contained in the fluid transported by the lymphatic system. If the fluid is leaking out of the pores without interruption of the skin, this signals a severe nature to the condition.

Another common way to define the severity of lymphedema is through staging. Staging refers to the physical

BOX 26.1 Severity of Lymphedema

- **Pitting edema.** Pressure on the edematous tissues with the fingertips causes an indentation of the skin that persists for several seconds after the pressure is removed. This reflects significant but short-duration edema with little or no fibrotic changes in skin or subcutaneous tissues.
- **Brawny edema.** Pressure on the edematous areas feels hard with palpation. This reflects a more severe form of interstitial swelling with progressive, fibrotic changes in subcutaneous tissues.
- **Weeping edema.** This represents the most severe and long-duration form of lymphedema. Fluids leak from cuts or sores; wound healing is significantly impaired. Lymphedema of this severity occurs almost exclusively in the lower extremities.

condition of the limb only.[62] The stages are described in Box 26.2.[36,62,70,135] Stage 0 or the latency stage might present with the greatest possibility for reducing the onset of worsening lymphedema. This is especially true in the patient with secondary lymphedema from cancer surgery.

Increased Size of the Limb

As the volume of interstitial fluid in the limb increases, so does the size of the limb (weight and girth).[17,51,65,135] Increased volume, in turn, causes tautness of the skin and susceptibility to skin breakdown.[19,69]

BOX 26.2 Stages of Lymphedema

Stage 0—Latency Stage
- No outward swelling noted
- Essentially asymptomatic with occasional reports of heaviness in the extremity
- Despite reduced transport capacity, the body is still able to accommodate the lymphatic load

Stage I—Reversible Stage
- Elevation reduces swelling
- No tissue fibrosis
- Swelling is soft or pitting

Stage II—Spontaneously Irreversible
- Fibrosis of tissue; brawny, hard swelling
- Swelling is no longer pitting
- Positive Stemmer sign
- Frequent infections may occur

Stage III—Lymphostatic Elephantiasis
- Positive Stemmer sign
- Significant increase in limb volume
- Typical skin changes noted (hyperkeratosis, papillomas, deep skin folds)
- Bacterial and fungal infections of the skin and nails more common

Descriptors, such as mild, moderate, and severe, sometimes are based on how much larger the size of the edematous limb is compared to the non-involved limb.[74] However, there are no standard definitions associated with size and severity.

Sensory Disturbances

Paresthesia (tingling, itching, or numbness) or occasionally a mild, aching pain may be felt, particularly in the fingers or toes. In many instances the condition is painless, and the patient perceives only a sense of heaviness of the limb. Fine finger coordination also may be impaired as the result of the sensory disturbances.[19,51,93,111]

Stiffness and Limited Range of Motion

Range of motion (ROM) decreases in the fingers and wrist or toes and ankle or even in the more proximal joints, leading to decreased functional mobility of the involved segments.[19,82]

Decreased Resistance to Infection

Wound healing is delayed, and frequent infections (e.g., cellulitis) may occur.[51,64,65,135] Cellulitis is a common health condition in patients with lymphedema.[86] Early recognition and treatment of cellulitis has shown to be important in reducing further tissue damage.[30,129]

Examination and Evaluation of Lymphatic Function

A patient's history, a systems review, and specific tests and measures provide information to determine impairments and functional limitations that can arise from lymphatic disorders and the presence of lymphedema. Key components in the examination process that are particularly relevant when lymphatic dysfunction is suspected or lymphedema is present are summarized in this section.[20,33,82,114,135] Other tests and measurements, such as vital signs, ROM, strength, posture, and sensory, functional, and cardiopulmonary testing, are also appropriate.

History and Systems Review

Note any history of infection, trauma, surgery, or radiation therapy. If a patient has a history of cancer and received chemotherapy, a review of the treatment and duration of the chemotherapy treatment is also important. The onset and duration of lymphedema, delayed wound healing, or previous treatment of lymphedema are pertinent pieces of information. Identify the occupation or daily activities of the patient, and determine if long periods of standing or sitting are required. Specific questioning to determine a pattern to the swelling can also aid in treatment planning.

Examination of Skin Integrity

Visual inspection and palpation of the skin provide information about the integrity of the skin. The location of the edema should be noted. When the limb is in a dependent position, palpate the skin to determine the type and severity of lymphedema and changes in skin and subcutaneous tissues. Describe the thickness and density of the tissue in each area of the limb. Areas of pitting, brawny, or weeping edema should be noted.

CLINICAL TIP

When palpating the skin over lymph nodes, note any tenderness of the nodes (cervical, supraclavicular, or inguinal). Tenderness may or may not indicate ongoing infection or serious disease.[46] Evidence of warm, enlarged, tender, painless, or adherent nodes should be reported to the physician.

The presence of wounds or scars and the color and appearance of the skin, which is often shiny and red in the edematous limb, should be noted. Document any papillomas, hyperkeratosis, or darkening of the skin, especially in the lower extremities. Photographic documentation is convenient in the clinical or home setting and provides visual evidence of changes in skin integrity. If a wound or scar is identified, its size should be noted, as should scar mobility or the presence of inflammation or infection in a wound.

A positive Stemmer sign, an indication of stage II or III lymphedema, may be identified during palpation (Fig. 26.3). It is considered positive if the skin on the dorsal surface of the fingers or toes cannot be pinched or is difficult to pinch compared with the uninvolved limb.[36,70,100,125,135] A positive Stemmer sign can be indicative of a worsening condition.

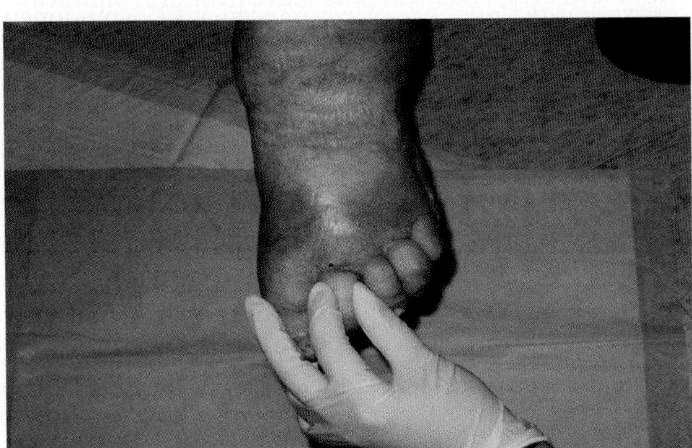

FIGURE 26.3 Stemmer sign: Objective test for lymphedema in the extremities. *(From Hetrick, H: Lymphedema complicating healing. In McCulloch, JM, and Kloth, LC (eds):* Wound Healing: Evidence-Based Management, *ed. 4. Philadelphia: F.A. Davis, 2010, p 283, with permission.)*

Girth Measurements

Circumferential measurements of the involved limb should be taken and compared with the non-involved limb if the problem is unilateral.[17,93] Identify specific intervals or landmarks at which measurements are taken so measurements during subsequent examinations are reliable. Use of circumferential measurements at anatomical landmarks has been shown to be a valid and reliable method of calculating limb volume.[2,113]

Volumetric Measurements

An alternative method of measuring limb size is to immerse the limb in a tank of water to a predetermined anatomical landmark and measure the volume of water displaced.[17,113] Although this method also has been shown to be valid and reliable, for routine clinical use, it is more cumbersome and less practical than girth measurements.[2,113]

Perometer Measurements

A perometer calculates limb volume through the use of infrared light and opto-electric sensors. The perometer scans the limb without direct contact on the skin, making this an efficient form of volumetric measurement.[3] However, the cost and size of the perometer make this technology unrealistic for most clinical facilities.

Bioimpedance Measurements

Bioimpedance measurements involve the use of a low-level, alternating electrical current to measure the resistance to the flow through the extracellular fluid in the upper extremities.[31,99,122] The higher the resistance to flow, the more extracellular fluid present. Testing is fairly easy to perform, requiring only placement of skin electrodes.

For any bioimpedance value to be meaningful, initial testing must take place prior to surgery.[38,78,108] Testing can then be performed at set intervals throughout the treatment continuum. This affords the opportunity for intervention at an earlier stage in the development of lymphedema. Other factors that affect volume in the body can theoretically affect the bioimpedance reading; therefore, this must be considered.[31,78,99,100,122] Bioimpedance is gaining acceptance in clinical practice as an effective method of detecting early, perhaps subclinical, lymphedema.[38,63,108]

Lymphedema Risk Reduction

If a patient is at risk of developing lymphedema secondary to infection, inflammation, obstruction, surgical removal of lymphatic structures, chronic venous insufficiency, or an increased body mass index (BMI), reducing the risk of lymphedema should be the priority of patient management. In some situations, such as after removal of lymph nodes or vessels, risk-reducing measures may be needed for a lifetime. Even when a patient takes every measure to reduce the risk of edema, it still may develop at some time, particularly after trauma to or surgical removal of lymph vessels. Box 26.3 summarizes precautions and measures to reduce the risk of lymphedema.* The education of patients in the importance of risk reduction has been shown to be effective in lowering lymphedema symptoms.[39,40,49,78]

*3,13,19,52,55,58,70,82,92,98,111,116,123

BOX 26.3 Precautions, Risk Reduction, and Self-Management of Lymphedema

Reducing the Risk of Lymphedema

- Keep moving. Standing or sitting for long periods of time can cause pooling of fluid in the legs. Sit with both feet on the floor instead of legs crossed.
- When traveling long distances by car, stop periodically, and walk around or support an involved upper extremity on the car's window ledge or seat back.
- Elevate involved limb(s), and perform repetitive pumping exercises frequently during the day.
- Be cautious about performing vigorous, repetitive activities with the involved limb.
- Monitor the weight used with exercise. Increase weight slowly, and assess for feelings of heaviness, throbbing, or aching in the limb.
- Carry heavy loads, such as a heavy backpack or shoulder bag, over your uninvolved shoulder.
- If you have lymphedema, wear compressive garments while exercising.
- Wear clothing and jewelry that does not leave a mark or imprint on your skin when removed.
- Monitor diet to maintain an ideal weight and minimize sodium intake.
- If possible, have blood pressures, needle sticks, and blood draws performed in the uninvolved upper extremity or lower extremity.

Skin Care

- Keep the skin clean and supple; use moisturizers and sunscreen, but avoid perfumed lotions.
- Immediately attend to a skin abrasion or cut, an insect bite, a blister, or a burn.
- Protect hands and feet; wear socks or hose, properly fitting shoes, rubber gloves, oven mitts, etc.
- Use protective gloves when in contact with harsh detergents and chemicals.
- Use caution when cutting nails. Push back cuticles instead of trimming.
- Use an electric razor when shaving legs or underarms. If the underarm area is numb, use your eyes to ensure that good skin integrity was maintained.
- Avoid hot baths, whirlpools, and saunas that elevate the body's core temperature.
- Seek immediate medical care if infection is suspected. An infection may present with warmth, redness, tenderness, or rash on the skin. A fever may or may not be present.
- Consult your physician immediately if a new onset of swelling is noted that does not resolve in 1 to 2 days.

Management of Lymphedema

Background and Rationale

Comprehensive management of lymphedema involves a combination of appropriate medical management and direct therapeutic intervention by a therapist combined with self-management by the patient. Treatment also includes appropriate pharmacological management for infection control and prevention or removal of excessive fluid and proteins.[12,50,69]

Because there is no cure for lymphedema, the main goal of treatment is to minimize the lymphedema as much as possible or return the lymphedema to a latency stage. In addition, the health of the tissue is important. Other goals include reducing risk of infection and softening of fibrotic tissue.[36,135]

The overall objective of management, when lymphedema has developed, is to improve drainage of obstructed areas and, theoretically, to channel fluids into more centrally located lymph structures that carry the fluid to the venous system. In order to affect the reduction of lymphatic and/or venous edema, the following should be considered.

- Interstitial pressure is increased by external forces. These external forces can be from manual lymphatic drainage (MLD) or compression therapy. An increased interstitial pressure causes an increased uptake of fluid. There is an increase of lymph production as more fluid enters the lymphatic system as well as an increase in the resorption of fluid by the venous system.[36,78,135]
- Elevation can assist fluid return in stage I lymphedema or in venous edema. If elevation produces a reduction, then a mild compression therapy (i.e., compression garment) may be indicated.[32,62,69,70,123]
- Dynamic pressure changes within the body can assist lymphatic flow. Pressure changes can be in the form of diaphragmatic breathing or with muscle contractions. Breathing changes intrathoracic pressure and causes an increased uptake of lymph fluid in lymphatic trunks and ducts. Active muscle contractions change pressure in a localized area, enhancing the movement of lymph within lymph vessels. A muscle contraction combined with external forces from a bandage or compression garment can be even more effective in the movement of fluid.[36,70,104,135]

Comprehensive Regimens and Components

A comprehensive approach to the management of lymphedema is referred to in the literature by a variety of terms, including complex lymphedema therapy, complete or complex decongestive therapy (CDT), or decongestive lymphatic therapy.* Treatment typically is divided into two phases. Phase I is the intensive treatment phase, and phase II is the maintenance phase. The goal of phase I treatment is reduction, whereas the goal of phase II treatment is long-term management.[19,62,70,135] Therapist-directed care is replaced by patient-directed care as treatment moves from phase I to phase II. Box 26.4 summarizes the components of these programs.

Manual lymphatic drainage. MLD involves slow, very light repetitive stroking and circular massage movements done in a specific sequence with the involved extremity.[78,9,23,24,29,67,113,134,135] Proximal congestion in the trunk, groin, buttock, or axilla is cleared first to make room for fluid from the more distal areas. The direction of the

*8,9,23,24,29,60,73,75,76,103,112,134,135

BOX 26.4 Components of a Decongestive Lymphatic Therapy Program

Phase I
- Manual lymphatic drainage (MLD)
- Multiple layer compression bandaging
- Skin and nail care
- Exercise

Phase II
- Self-MLD by the patient
- Compression therapy
  - Compression garment during the day
  - Multiple layer bandaging in the evening/night
- Skin and nail care
- Exercise

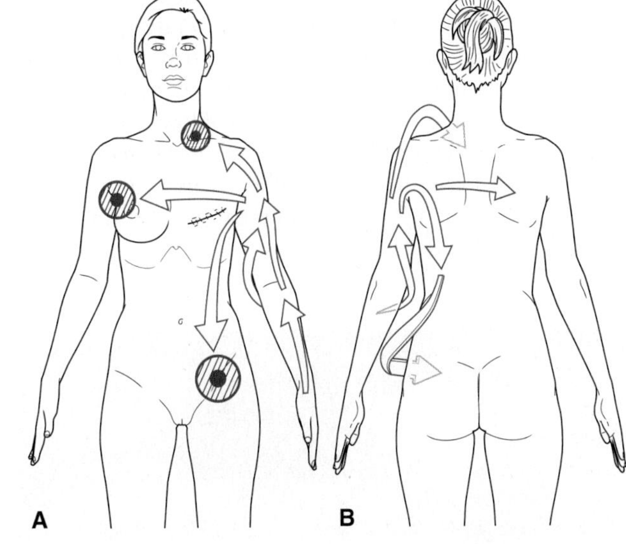

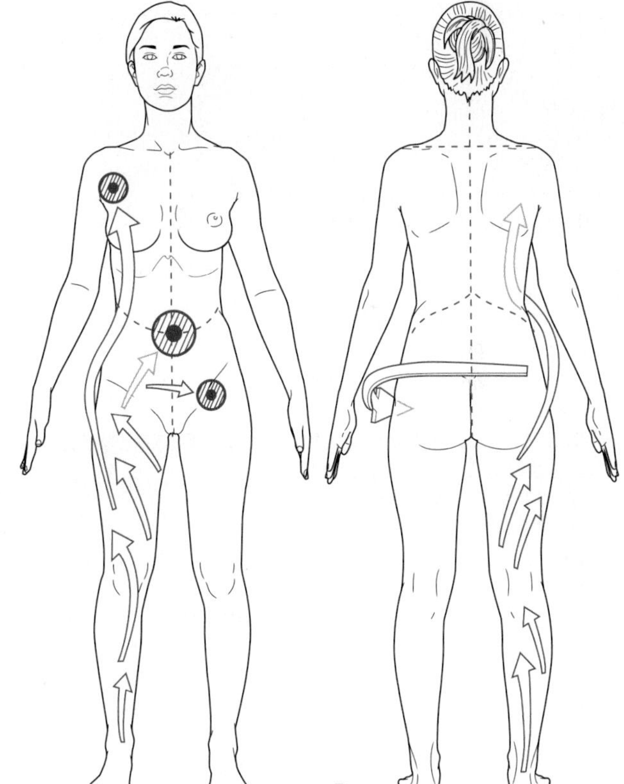

FIGURE 26.4 Application of manual lymphatic drainage sequences for **(A & B)** upper extremity and **(C & D)** lower extremity lymphatic pathways.

massage is toward specific lymph nodes and usually involves distal-to-proximal stroking. Fluid in the involved extremity is then cleared, first in the proximal portion and then in the distal portion of the limb. Because MLD is extremely labor and time intensive, methods of self-massage are taught to a patient as soon as possible in a treatment program. The manual technique involved in lymphatic drainage is positively correlated to the results seen in tissue decongestion.[36,135] The specific techniques of MLD include several principles:[36,135]

- Hand position should match the anatomical shape and size of the area being treated.
- The pressure applied in each stroke should maximize the elasticity available in the superficial tissue. Too much pressure can cause vasodilation.
- Each stroke has a working phase and a resting phase. The purpose of the working phase is to move fluid into the lymphatic system, with the directional stretch facilitating the lymphatic angions.[30,107] The resting phase elicits a pressure change in the tissue and allows the lymph fluid to fill the lymphatic collectors.
- Repetition of the strokes is needed to help reduce the high viscosity of the lymphatic fluid.
- MLD sequences direct lymphatic fluid from an area of congestion, across lymphatic water sheds to an area of no tissue congestion.

Application of these principles for upper and lower extremity clearance of lymphedema is depicted in Figure 26.4.[135]

Exercise. Active ROM, stretching, and low-intensity resistance exercises are integrated with manual drainage techniques.[6,12,19,23,25,26,73,80,84,85,91,135] Exercises are performed while wearing a compressive garment or bandages and in a specific sequence to facilitate lymphatic flow. A low-intensity cardiovascular/pulmonary endurance activity, such as bicycling, often follows ROM and strengthening exercises. Specific exercises and a suggested sequence for the upper and lower extremities, compiled from several sources, are described and illustrated in the last section of this chapter.

Compression therapy. The type of compression used depends on the phase of treatment. During phase I of treatment, only low-stretch bandages are used, which provide a low resting pressure on a limb but a high working pressure.[36,135] High-stretch sports bandages, such as Ace™ wraps, are not recommended for treating lymphedema.[9,12,19,123] Given that a low-stretch bandage has a low resting pressure, the bandage can be worn during the day and at night. During the active reduction phase of treatment, it is recommended that compression be applied in the form of low-stretch bandaging at all times except for bathing.[36,105,135] Under the low-stretch bandage, nonwoven padding is used and can be combined with foam pads to aid in the softening and reduction of fibrotic tissue (Fig. 26.5).

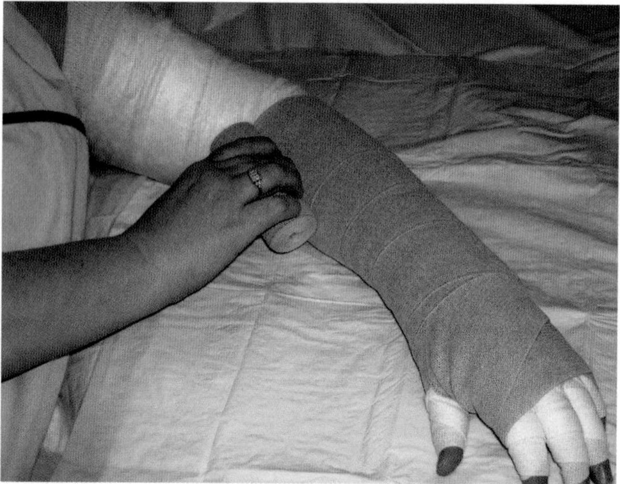

FIGURE 26.5 Upper extremity multilayer bandaging with padding from the upper arm to the hand.

As a patient moves from phase I to a maintenance phase of treatment, compression is transitioned from low-stretch bandaging at all times to a compression garment during the day. A compression garment has a high resting pressure and low working pressure.[36,135] Therefore, the use of a garment is not recommended during long periods of inactivity (night rest). The garment should be viewed as a method to maintain limb size during the day, giving a patient a more cosmetic appearance and ease of wearing clothing. During phase II, it is still recommended that a patient wear the low-stretch bandages at night.[19,105] In summary, the bandages are used for continued limb reduction, and a garment keeps the size of the extremity stable.

Compression garments are made in specific compression categories or classes (Table 26.1).[19,105,135] Patients can most often be fit with a premade garment, but custom garments are available. For patients with lymphedema of the trunk, genital area, or face, custom garments can be fabricated.

FOCUS ON EVIDENCE

Forner-Cordero and coinvestigators[37] conducted a study to identify the factors that best predicted response to CDT. A prospective multicenter, controlled cohort study was undertaken with 171 patients with breast cancer–related lymphedema. Following statistical analysis, compliance with bandaging was one of the most predictive indicators of response to CDT. The length of time from the development of the lymphedema to treatment did not predict response to treatment in this study.

TABLE 26.1 Garment Compression Classification

Class of Compression	mm Hg	Indications
Class 1		
	20–30 mm Hg	■ Mild lymphedema ■ Typically used for UE, not LE ■ Patient with fragile skin or the elderly
Class 2		
	30–40 mm Hg	■ Most commonly used for stage II UE lymphedema ■ Minimum compression for LE lymphedema
Class 3		
	40–50 mm Hg	■ Rarely used for UE lymphedema ■ Typically for stage II LE lymphedema ■ For patients with LE lymphedema involved in high-intensity, repetitive activities
Class 4		
	50–60 mm Hg	■ Rarely used ■ Only for LE lymphedema ■ Only available as custom-made garments

LE, Lower extremity; *UE*, upper extremity

However, there was an inverse correlation between severity of lymphedema and response to CDT.

Another form of compression therapy is a pneumatic compression pump.[79,132] The use of compression pumps, however, has been controversial over the years. Studies have shown that a compression pump can be a positive adjuvant therapy to CDT but should not be the sole therapeutic modality in the treatment of lymphedema.[77,82,112] The main criticism of pump compression is the pumping of fluid in a distal to proximal sequence, which is opposite of the principles of MLD. There is also the potential to cause swelling in adjoining areas of the body, mainly the genital area, for a patient with lower extremity edema.[10] When used correctly, a pneumatic compression pump can be a positive therapeutic intervention, especially in severe or refractory cases. More advanced pumps are now available that follow the sequence of MLD more closely, treating the trunk first and then the extremity in a proximal-to-distal sequence. Recommendations for pressure and timing settings to effectively elicit lymph flow with an intermittent pneumatic compression device have been reported in the literature.[132]

Skin care and hygiene. Lymphedema predisposes the patient to skin breakdown, infection, and delayed wound healing. Meticulous attention to skin care and protection of the edematous limb are essential elements of self-management of lymphedema.[12,24,82,123]

Surgical Intervention for Lymphedema

A surgical procedure, such as a lymphovenous bypass or a vascularized lymph node transfer, may be chosen for management of lymphedema depending on the availability of intact lymphatic channels and the extent of fibrosis in the tissue. The purpose of these surgical interventions is to facilitate restoration of the physiological balance in the tissue by eliminating the excess of protein and other cellular components in the extracellular space.[62,110] With a lymphovenous bypass, lymphatic channels are identified along the length of the limb and are anastomosed with a venule of corresponding size.[27,28,62,110] In a lymph node transfer a lymph node from a distant site along with vasculature is transplanted in the affected limb.[62,110] Liposuction is another surgical option that has been shown to be effective in long-term follow-up studies.[14,15,86] Liposuction reduces the overall girth of a limb by removing the proliferation of adipose tissue.[14,15,62]

A growing body of evidence has become available in the literature to support the benefits and efficacy of selected surgical interventions.[7,14,15,27,28] The results of these studies have shown that the majority of patients following surgical intervention report subjective, symptomatic improvement. However, improvements identified by objective testing have been reported in a lesser percentage of patients.[27,28,95] Irrespective of the surgical approach taken, patients must continue with many of the presurgical interventions for lymphedema management, including daily compression therapy.

Online Resources

A valuable resource for patients and health-care professionals is the National Lymphedema Network (www.lymphnet.org). This nonprofit organization provides education and guidance about lymphedema. Other resources include the National Comprehensive Cancer Network (www.nccn.org), the Peninsula Medical, Inc., website (www.lymphedema.org), and Lymph Notes (www.lymphnotes.com).

Breast Cancer–Related Lymphatic Dysfunction

Background

Breast cancer–related dysfunction of the lymphatic system and subsequent lymphedema of the upper extremity is a somewhat common and potentially serious complication of the treatment for breast cancer. The incidence of lymphedema following surgical intervention for breast cancer varies widely in the literature.* Much of the variation is related to how lymphedema is diagnosed and defined. Some studies quantify lymphedema in the upper extremity only, whereas other studies define breast cancer–related lymphedema as including the remaining breast or chest wall and trunk. Other factors contributing to the variation in incidence of lymphedema reported are the use of sentinel lymph node biopsy versus axillary dissection. The time of onset of lymphedema also varies widely in the literature, with onset varying from 6 months to 3 years in the majority of patients who develop persistent swelling.[53,55,94,116]

Current treatment for breast cancer involves a multimodality approach. Surgery, chemotherapy or hormonal therapy, and radiation may be employed. The type of surgery performed, the extent of axillary nodes removed, and the use of radiation all affect the incidence of lymphedema in a patient with breast cancer.

Axillary dissection and removal of lymph nodes interrupt and slow the circulation of lymph, which in turn can lead to lymphedema.[6,13,19,34] Radiation therapy can cause fibrosis of tissues in the area of the axilla, which obstructs the lymphatic vessels and contributes to pooling of lymph in the arm and hand.[6,13,19,34] The extent of the axillary dissection and exposure to radiation is associated with the degree of risk for lymphedema to develop. In addition, shoulder motion can become impaired as the result of incisional pain, delayed wound healing, skin ulcerations (associated with radiation therapy), and postoperative weakness of the muscles of the shoulder girdle.[19,82]

A comprehensive approach to postoperative management that emphasizes patient education and includes therapeutic exercise and other direct interventions to reduce the risk of or to treat lymphedema and other impairments or limitations of function are key to successful outcomes.[4,12,19,43,82,98]

*2,42,54,71,81,94,106,117

As with most cancers, the diagnosis of breast cancer and the ensuing treatments have an enormous emotional impact on patients and their families.[15,90] The advent of breast cancer–related lymphedema not only has an impact on a breast cancer survivor's physical function, but also is known to have a significantly adverse effect on health-related quality of life, making prevention—and if it develops, aggressive treatment—of lymphedema a high priority for management.[72,94,102]

Surgical Procedures

Surgical treatment of breast cancer falls into two broad categories—mastectomy and breast-conserving surgery—both of which are coupled with either sentinel lymph node biopsy and/or axillary lymph node dissection. Differences in surgical procedures are related to the extent of removal of breast tissue and surrounding or underlying soft tissues.[1,8,56] A course of radiation therapy routinely follows surgery to decrease the risk of regional recurrence of the disease in patients who undergo breast-conserving surgeries. Chemotherapy also may be initiated preoperatively or postoperatively to reduce the risk of systemic spread of the disease.

Mastectomy

Mastectomy involves removing the entire breast. In addition, a mastectomy may involve removing the fascia over the chest muscle. With late-stage, invasive disease, a radical mastectomy in which the pectoralis muscles also are excised may be required, leading to significant muscle weakness and impaired shoulder function.

Breast-Conserving Surgery

Options for resecting the tumor and preserving a portion of the breast include lumpectomy, which involves excision of the mass and a margin of healthy surrounding breast tissue, or segmental mastectomy (also known as quadrectomy), which is excision of the affected quadrant of the breast. Rather than mastectomy, these procedures are being used increasingly in combination with adjuvant therapy for patients with stage I or II tumors.[1,56]

There are now multiple randomized clinical trials that show that the 10- to 20-year survival rate for patients with stage I or II disease who underwent breast-conserving surgery combined with radiation therapy is equivalent to that achieved by patients who underwent mastectomy alone or mastectomy with adjuvant therapy.[1]

Patients who undergo breast-conserving procedures without removal of lymph nodes are still at risk for developing postoperative lymphedema and impaired shoulder mobility because of potential complications from radiation therapy and biopsy of at least one lymph node.[19,82]

Evaluation of Lymph Node Involvement

In the past, axillary lymph node dissection was a standard part of mastectomy and breast-conserving surgery.[1,56] A minimum of a level I and, most often, a level II axillary dissection was performed. Currently, the sentinel lymph node biopsy is used to determine disease presence in the axilla, therefore sparing removal of uninvolved lymph nodes when possible.

Sentinel lymph node biopsy is used with patients who present with no clinically evident disease in the axilla.[119] With a radiosensitive substance, the specific lymph nodes that a tumor first drains into are identified and removed.[135] If clear, research has shown that an axillary dissection is not required and risk of disease in further lymph nodes is low.[16] If the sentinel lymph nodes show signs of disease, then axillary lymph nodes are removed. More extensive dissection for metastatic or regional bulky disease removes the nodes under the pectoralis minor muscle or around the clavicle.

Breast Reconstruction Options

Depending on breast cancer presentation and staging at the time of diagnosis, a woman may have a choice of breast conservation or mastectomy. If a mastectomy is chosen, then reconstruction (immediate versus delayed) may be considered. A patient's body type, breast size, and tumor size become factors in the determination of which procedures are viable options. Immediate reconstruction is done at the time of the definitive breast cancer surgery so that an additional surgery is not required. However, an immediate reconstruction increases surgical time and length of stay in the hospital. Delayed reconstruction requires an additional surgery at some point following the completion of breast cancer treatment but gives a woman additional time to consider reconstructive options.[68,97]

Implications for physical therapy management during postoperative rehabilitation depend on the reconstructive approach performed (Table 26.2).[115] Alloplastic procedures, using expanders and implants, construct a "breast pocket" under the pectoralis muscle on the chest wall, whereas autologous procedures involve use of a women's own tissue to reconstruct the breast. These procedures can include tissue only or muscle as well.[68,97]

Radiation Therapy

Radiation therapy is rarely used as the sole treatment intervention for breast cancer. Most often radiation is employed following breast-conserving surgery as an adjuvant treatment modality.[71] Radiation delivered to the whole breast is standard following breast-conserving therapy. The parameters of the radiation field include the tissue from the clavicle to 2 cm below the inframammary line and from the midsternum to the mid-axillary line laterally.[90] Radiation typically is delivered over a course of 5 to 6 weeks with effects not felt until 2 to 3 weeks into treatment. In patients who undergo mastectomy, depending on the disease presentation, radiation may be offered. The radiation field usually includes the surgical scar, chest wall, and sometimes the regional lymphatics.

Radiation causes changes in most types of soft tissue and can be categorized as having acute or chronic effects.[71] Acute

TABLE 26.2 Implications for Rehabilitation Following Breast Reconstruction Surgery

Procedure	Implications for Rehabilitation
Alloplastic	
■ Tissue expander/ implant	■ Pectoralis muscle tightness ■ Impaired shoulder girdle alignment ■ Decreased shoulder range of motion
Autologous	
■ TRAM Flap* (transverse rectus abdominis muscle)	■ Impaired trunk posture ■ Core muscle weakness, especially if unilateral
■ LD Flap* (latissimus dorsi)	■ Rotator cuff insufficiency ■ Impaired shoulder girdle alignment
■ DIEP Flap* (deep inferior epigastric perforator)	■ Impaired trunk posture

*Flap integrity and perfusion are of primary importance.

effects of radiation include acute dermatitis or skin burn. Chronic or late effects of radiation involve tissue fibrosis that can restrict ROM and changes to lymphatic vessel function.[120] It is important to note that the chronic effects of radiation can extend for many years following the end of the radiation therapy.[121]

Impairments and Complications Related to Breast Cancer Treatment

The following impairments and complications may occur in association with treatment of breast cancer. Many of these problems are interrelated and must be considered jointly when a comprehensive postoperative rehabilitation program is developed for the patient.*

Postoperative Pain

Incisional pain. A transverse incision across the chest wall is made to remove the breast tissue and underlying fascia on the chest musculature. The incision extends into the axilla for lymph node dissection. Postoperatively, the sutured skin over the breast area may feel tight along the incision. Movement of the arm pulls on the incision and is uncomfortable for the patient. Healing of the incision may be delayed as the result of radiation therapy. Delayed wound healing, in turn, prolongs pain in the area of the incision.

Posterior cervical and shoulder girdle pain. Pain and muscle spasm may occur in the neck and shoulder region as a result of muscle guarding. The levator scapulae, teres major and minor, and infraspinatus often are tender to palpation and can restrict active shoulder motion. Decreased use of the involved upper extremity after surgery due to pain sets the stage for the patient to develop a chronic frozen shoulder and increases the likelihood of lymphedema in the hand and arm.

Postoperative Vascular and Pulmonary Complications

Decreased activity and extended time in bed increase venous stasis and the risk of a deep vein thrombosis (DVT). Risk of pulmonary complications, such as pneumonia, also is higher because of the patient's reduced activity level. Incisional pain may make the patient reluctant to cough or breathe deeply, both of which are necessary postoperatively to keep the airways clear of fluid accumulation.

Lymphedema

As noted previously, patients who undergo any level of lymph node dissection or whose treatment regimen includes radiation therapy remain at risk throughout life for developing ipsilateral upper extremity lymphedema.[6,19,82,135] Lymphedema can occur almost immediately after lymph node dissection, during the course of radiation therapy, or many months or even years after treatment has been completed. It is typically evident in the hand and arm but occasionally develops in the anterior chest wall, remaining breast, or back area.[6,13,19,82,93,135] In turn, lymphedema leads to impaired upper extremity function, poor cosmesis, and emotional distress.[19,41,93,111]

FOCUS ON EVIDENCE

Fu et al[40] conducted a study involving two groups of breast cancer survivors. One group received breast cancer–related lymphedema education during their treatment for breast cancer. The other group received no lymphedema-specific education. Information was collected from both groups to identify physical symptoms and overall knowledge related to lymphedema following treatment. In both groups, the mean number of physical symptoms reported was three. However, fewer women in the intervention group than in the control group reported physical symptoms such as swelling, heaviness, limited shoulder movement, seroma formation, or breast swelling. As a result of this study, the authors recommended the active engagement of breast cancer survivors in education regarding ways to reduce the risk of lymphedema.

Chest Wall Adhesions

Restrictive scarring of underlying tissues on the chest wall can develop as the result of surgery, radiation fibrosis, or wound infection. Chest wall adhesions can lead to increased risk of postoperative pulmonary complications, restricted mobility

*5,11,13,19,41,43,47,48,59,82,93,127,130,135

of the shoulder, postural asymmetry and dysfunction, and discomfort in the neck, shoulder girdle, and upper back.

Decreased Shoulder Mobility

It is well documented that patients may experience temporary and sometimes long-term loss of shoulder mobility after surgery or radiation therapy for treatment of breast cancer.[6,48,59,72,82,98,109,126,127,130] Factors contributing to impaired shoulder mobility after surgery are listed in Box 26.5.

One of these factors, lymphatic cording, or axillary web syndrome (AWS), is a fairly new term for a condition that is quite common in patients treated for breast cancer. The incidence among breast cancer survivors ranges from 28% to 36%.[118,120] However, the incidence varies in the literature, and onset can be as soon as one week following surgery to years later.[87,120,131] AWS is thought to be caused by the interruption of the lymphatics in the axilla following a sentinel lymph node biopsy or axillary dissection, with resulting thrombosis of lymphatic channels.[54,72] Visually, AWS can be described as a web of skin covering "cords" that are more visible with shoulder abduction (Fig. 26.6).[66,87] These cords can extend from the axilla distally to the antecubital space and into the forearm. Lymphatic cording can be painful and limit movement of the entire upper extremity.[19,66] Patients often present with complaints of pain that extends down the arm, even into the hand. Cording can also be seen in the lateral trunk.[120] Numbness or tingling may also be reported. Treatment for AWS typically includes gentle stretching and soft tissue release of the lymphatic cord, as well as MLD.[66,120] AWS may resolve if left untreated, but more research is needed to clarify long-term outcomes.[131]

BOX 26.5 Factors Contributing to Impaired Shoulder Mobility After Breast Cancer Surgery

- Incisional pain immediately after surgery or associated with delayed wound healing
- Muscle guarding and tenderness of the shoulder and posterior cervical musculature
- Need for protected shoulder ROM until the surgical drain is removed
- Fibrosis of soft tissues in the axillary region due to adjuvant radiation therapy
- Adherence of scar tissue to the chest wall, causing adhesions
- Temporary or permanent weakness of the muscles of the shoulder girdle
- Rounded shoulders and kyphotic or scoliotic trunk posture associated with age or incisional pain
- A feeling of heaviness of the upper extremity due to lymphedema
- Decreased use of the hand and arm for functional activities
- Axillary web syndrome

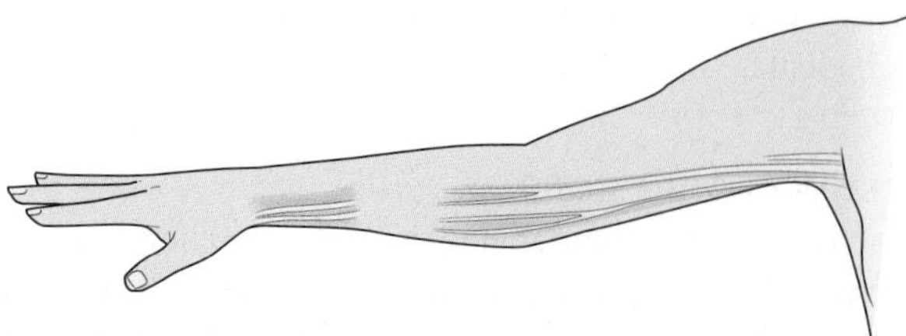

FIGURE 26.6 Axillary web syndrome.

 **FOCUS ON EVIDENCE**

Verbelen and coinvestigators[118] conducted a systematic review of the literature to identify the shoulder impairments found in patients following sentinel lymph node biopsy. The shoulder and arm impairments identified included loss of mobility and strength, pain, AWS, and sensory disorders. The highest incidence of restricted range of motion occurred at 1 month following surgery, with shoulder abduction and forward flexion being most limited. Shoulder abduction and internal rotation remained restricted in approximately 40% of patients at 2 years.

Weakness of the Involved Upper Extremity

Shoulder weakness. If the long thoracic nerve is traumatized during axillary dissection and removal of lymph nodes, this results in weakness of the serratus anterior and compromised stability of the scapula, limiting active flexion and abduction of the arm. Faulty shoulder mechanics and use of substitute motions with the upper trapezius and levator scapulae during overhead reaching can cause subacromial impingement and shoulder pain. Shoulder impingement, in turn, can be a precursor to a frozen shoulder. If the pectoralis muscles were disturbed, which occurs with a radical mastectomy for advanced disease, weakness is evident in horizontal adduction.

Decreased grip strength. Grip strength is often diminished as the result of lymphedema and secondary stiffness of the fingers.

Postural Malalignment

The patient may sit or stand with rounded shoulders and kyphosis because of pain, skin tightness, or psychological reasons. An increase in thoracic kyphosis associated with aging is commonly seen in the older patient.[47] This contributes to faulty shoulder mechanics and eventually restricts active use of the involved upper extremity. Asymmetry of the trunk and abnormal scapular alignment may occur as the result of a subtle lateral weight shift, particularly in a large-breasted woman.

Fatigue and Decreased Endurance

Patients undergoing radiation therapy or chemotherapy often experience debilitating fatigue.[1,44,72] Fatigue has been reported by more than 60% of patients undergoing cancer treatment.[21,88]

Many cancer survivors experience fatigue for months, even years, after treatment has been completed.[83] Anemia may develop as a result of chemotherapy. Nutritional intake and subsequent energy stores may be diminished, particularly if a patient is experiencing nausea for several days after a cycle of chemotherapy.

Fatigue is also associated with depression. As a result, exercise tolerance and endurance during functional activities are markedly reduced. Multiple studies support the initiation of an exercise program as one of the most effective methods to combat fatigue related to cancer treatment.[21,88,89] The findings of a recent systematic review and meta-analysis by Meneses-Echavez[83] demonstrated that supervised aerobic exercise is the most beneficial form of exercise.

Psychological Considerations

A patient undergoing treatment for breast cancer experiences a wide range of emotional and social issues.[111] The needs and concerns of both the patient and the family must be considered. The patient and family members must cope with the potentially life-threatening nature of the disease and a difficult treatment regimen. It is common for a patient to feel anxiety, agitation, anger, depression, a sense of loss, and significant mood swings during treatment of and recovery from breast cancer.

In addition to the obvious physical disfigurement and altered body image associated with mastectomy, medications such as immunosuppressants and corticosteroids can affect the emotional state of a patient. Psychological manifestations affect physical well-being and can contribute to general fatigue, the patient's perception of functional disability, and motivation during treatment.

Guidelines for Management Following Breast Cancer Surgery

Guidelines for postoperative management for the patient who has undergone a mastectomy or breast-conserving surgery and who may currently be receiving adjuvant therapy are outlined in Box 26.6. The guidelines identify therapeutic interventions for common impairments during the early postoperative period and those that could develop at a later time.

NOTE: The guidelines outlined in Box 26.6 also can be modified to prevent or manage problems that can develop in the trunk and lower extremities after surgery for abdominal or pelvic cancers and accompanying inguinal lymph node dissection.

Special Considerations

Patient education. The length of an in-hospital stay following surgery for breast cancer is short. Ideally, intervention by the therapist is initiated preoperatively with an emphasis on patient education for reducing the risk of postoperative complications and impairments, including pulmonary complications, thromboemboli, lymphedema, and loss of shoulder mobility. Recommendations for reducing the risk of

BOX 26.6 MANAGEMENT GUIDELINES—
After Surgery for Breast Cancer

Potential Postoperative Structural and Functional Impairments

- Pulmonary and circulatory complications
- Lymphedema
- Restricted mobility of the upper extremity
- Postural malalignment
- Weakness and decreased functional use of the upper extremity
- Fatigue and decreased endurance for functional activities
- Emotional and social adjustments

Plan of Care	Interventions
1. Prepare the patient for postoperative self-management	1. Interdisciplinary patient education involving all aspects of potential impairments and functional limitations Self-management activities and preparation for participation in a home program as indicated per surgical protocol
2. Prevent postoperative pulmonary complications and thromboemboli	2. Pre- or postoperative instruction in deep breathing, emphasizing maximal inspirations and effective coughing Active ankle exercises (calf-pumping exercises)

Continued

BOX 26.6 MANAGEMENT GUIDELINES—
After Surgery for Breast Cancer—cont'd

Plan of Care	Intervention
3. Minimize postoperative swelling	3. Elevation of the involved upper extremity on pillows (about 30°) while the patient is in bed or sitting in a chair Squeeze a ball on the operative side to produce a pumping action in the muscles Early ROM exercises **PRECAUTION:** Avoid static, dependent positioning of the arm
4. Identify and treat early signs of lymphedema should it develop	4. Manual lymphatic drainage massage Daily regimen of exercises to include flexibility and strengthening exercises Compression therapy (low-stretch compression bandaging and/or compression garments) Adherence to lymphedema risk-reducing behaviors (see Box 26.3)
5. Prevent postural deformities	5. Posture-awareness training; encourage the patient to assume an erect posture when sitting or standing to minimize a rounded shoulder posture Posture exercises with an emphasis on scapular retraction exercises
6. Prevent muscle tension and guarding in cervical musculature	6. Active ROM of the cervical spine to promote relaxation Shoulder shrugging and shoulder circle exercises Gentle massage to cervical musculature
7. Prevent restricted mobility of the upper extremity	7. Shoulder motion performed within protected ROM, usually no more than 90° of elevation of the arm until after removal of drains No repetitive motion until drains removed
8. Regain strength and functional use of the involved extremity	8. Initiate resistance exercise following full postoperative healing. Consider exercise parameters if patient is at risk for lymphedema or has lingering weakness in the involved extremity
9. Improve exercise tolerance and sense of well-being; reduce fatigue	9. Graded, low-intensity aerobic exercise such as walking or cycling
10. Provide information about resources for patient and family support and ongoing patient education	10. Resources: American Cancer Society for family support and ongoing patient education (www.cancer.org); National Breast Cancer Coalition (www.nobreastcancer.org); National Lymphedema Network (www.lymphnet.org)

PRECAUTIONS: Observe the incision and sutures carefully during exercises. Avoid any undue tension on the incision or blanching of the scar during shoulder ROM. Avoid exercises with the involved arm in a dependent position. Progress graded exercise program slowly, particularly if the patient is receiving adjuvant therapy. Consider other adjuvant therapies when designing an exercise program.

lymphedema or for self-management if it develops is reviewed with the patient (see Box 26.3). Following surgery, once the drains are removed, an exercise program can then be individualized based on a patient's surgical procedure and anticipated adjuvant treatments.

Exercise. The postoperative exercise program focuses on three main areas: improving shoulder function, regaining an overall level of fitness, and reducing the risk of or managing lymphedema. Early, but protected, assisted or active ROM of the shoulder is the key to restoring shoulder mobility. Postoperative risks that contribute to restricted shoulder mobility were summarized previously (see Box 26.5).[1,19,56,82,85] These risks are highest during the early postoperative period until drains have been removed and the incision has healed.

CLINICAL TIP

Radiation therapy to the axillary and breast areas can delay wound healing beyond the typical 3- to 4-week period.[1,56] Even after initial healing of the incision, the scar has a tendency to contract and can become adherent to underlying tissues, which, in turn, can restrict shoulder motion. Because radiation changes can occur months following treatment, educating the patient to continue with ROM and flexibility exercises should be encouraged. Deep-breathing exercises should also be performed regularly if the chest wall was included in the radiation field.[121]

Although strengthening exercises and aerobic conditioning are important for upper extremity function and total body fitness, considerations should be taken in an exercise program. Programming considerations may include the type of chemotherapy given and the specific side effects of the drugs. For example, some chemotherapy can cause peripheral neuropathy, proximal muscle weakness, and differing fatigue patterns.[61,88] Exercises must be progressed gradually, excessive fatigue must be avoided, and energy conservation must be emphasized. Exercise precautions for a patient undergoing treatment are noted in Box 26.7.[6,19,72,85,88,98]

Early intervention for reducing the risk of lymphedema and upper extremity mobility impairments is often advocated by therapists and suggested in descriptive articles in the literature. However, patients often are not referred for postoperative rehabilitation until after impairments and activity limitations have developed. This may be due to concerns raised in the literature[34] that early postoperative ROM could delay wound healing or that exercises, if performed too vigorously, could initiate or exacerbate lymphedema. In addition, few studies have rigorously investigated the efficacy of specific interventions or rehabilitation protocols.[82,126] A recent review of the literature on exercise and cancer-related lymphedema revealed, however, that exercise neither worsened pre-existing lymphedema nor was associated with a significant increase in the occurrence of lymphedema.[6]

BOX 26.7 Exercise Precautions During Treatment of Breast Cancer

- Exercise only at a moderate level and never to the point that the affected arm aches, throbs, or feels heavy during or after exercise, even if there is no evidence of lymphedema.
- Adjust the timing of exercise during cycles of radiation therapy or chemotherapy. With some chemotherapy medications, a patient can develop cardiac arrhythmia or cardiomyopathy.[61]
- Avoid exercising 1 to 2 hrs before blood is drawn.
- Gradually return to a regular pattern of exercise and recreational activities based on the fitness level prior to diagnosis and specific side effects of treatment.
- Be aware of blood counts, including white blood cell count and hemoglobin and platelet counts when designing exercise programs.

From the information available in the literature, the following recommendations for exercise are made:*

- Integrate ROM, flexibility, and strengthening exercises into a patient's comprehensive plan of care.
- Implement posture-awareness training and exercise early in a postoperative program to prevent postural malalignment and muscle imbalance, especially following mastectomy.
- Include moderate-intensity aerobic conditioning exercises to improve fitness and quality of life and to reduce chemotherapy-related fatigue.
- Progress all forms of exercise gradually, and teach the patients individualized exercise parameters based on specific surgical interventions and adjuvant therapies.

Community and Online Resources

Reach to Recovery is a one-to-one patient education program sponsored by the American Cancer Society (www.cancer.org). Representatives of this program, most of whom are breast cancer survivors, provide emotional support to the patient and family, as well as current information on breast prostheses and reconstructive surgery. The National Lymphedema Network (www.lymphnet.org) and the National Comprehensive Cancer Network (www.nccn.org) are other valuable sources of information for patients at risk for or who have developed lymphedema.

Exercises for the Management of Lymphedema

Background and Rationale

As noted previously in this chapter, exercise is just one aspect of a decongestive lymphatic therapy program. The rationale for including exercise in the comprehensive treatment of

*5,11,12,13, 17,19,41,48,60,76,80,84,85,91,112,126,127,134,135

patients with upper or lower extremity lymphedema is to move and drain lymph fluid to reduce the edema and to improve the functional use of the involved limb or limbs. The principles and rationale upon which exercises for lymphatic drainage are based are summarized in Box 26.8.[6,84,91,135]

The exercises employed in lymph drainage regimens cover a wide spectrum of therapeutic exercise interventions, specifically deep breathing, flexibility, strengthening, and cardiovascular conditioning exercises, combined with a sequence of lymphatic drainage exercises. Exercise regimens have been described in an extensive number of publications.*

No particular combination or sequence of exercises has been shown to be superior to another. Although an older critical review of the literature[75] indicated that the effectiveness of exercise regimens for lymph drainage was based primarily on clinical observations and opinions of experienced practitioners or case reports, there is now an emerging body of evidence documenting the efficacy of specific components of these programs.[6,60,80,82,112]

Components of Exercise Regimens for Management of Lymphedema

Deep Breathing Exercises

Deep breathing is interwoven throughout exercise regimens for the management of lymphedema. It has been suggested that the use of abdominal-diaphragmatic breathing assists in the movement of lymphatic fluid as the diaphragm descends during a deep inspiration and the abdominals contract during a controlled, maximum expiration.[19] Changes in intra-abdominal and intrathoracic pressures create a gentle, continual pumping action that moves fluids in the central lymphatic vessels, which run superiorly in the chest cavity and drain into the venous system in the neck (see Fig. 26.1).

*8,9,19,23-26,58,60,73,75,76,84,85,91,98,102,112,134,135

Flexibility Exercises

Gentle, self-stretching exercises are used to minimize soft tissue and joint hypomobility, particularly in proximal areas of the body that may contribute to static postures and lymph congestion.

Strengthening and Muscular Endurance Exercises

Both isometric and dynamic exercises using self-resistance, elastic resistance, and weights or weight machines are appropriate if done against light resistance (initially 1 to 2 lb) and progressing resistance and repetitions gradually.[91] Regardless of whether lymphedema has developed, it is important to monitor the circumferential size and the skin texture of the involved limb closely to determine whether an appropriate intensity of exercise has been established. Emphasis is placed on improving endurance and strength of central and peripheral muscle groups that enhance an erect posture and minimize fatigue in muscles that contribute to the efficiency of the lymphatic pump mechanism.

Cardiovascular Conditioning Exercises

Activities such as upper extremity ergometry, swimming, cycling, and walking increase circulation and stimulate lymphatic flow.[19,91] Thirty minutes of aerobic endurance exercises complement lymph drainage exercises. Conditioning exercises are done at low intensity (at 40% to 50% of the target heart rate) when lymphedema is present and at higher intensities (as high as an 80% level) when the lymphedema has been reduced and exercise is otherwise safe.[19,84]

BOX 26.8 Exercises for Lymphatic Drainage: Principles and Rationale

- Contraction of muscles pumps fluids by direct compression of the collecting lymphatic vessels.
- Exercise reduces soft tissue and joint hypomobility that can contribute to static positioning and lead to lymphostasis.
- Exercise strengthens and prevents atrophy of muscles of the limbs, which improves the efficiency of the lymphatic pump.
- Exercise increases heart rate and arterial pulsations, which in turn contribute to lymph flow.
- Exercise should be sequenced to clear the central lymphatic reservoirs before the peripheral areas.
- Wearing a compression sleeve or compression bandaging during exercises enhances lymph flow and protein resorption more efficiently than exercising without bandages.

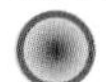 **FOCUS ON EVIDENCE**

In a randomized, controlled study by Schmitz and associates,[104] weight lifting was studied in a group of 141 breast cancer survivors with stable upper extremity lymphedema over a 1-year period. The exercise intervention consisted of progressive weight lifting twice a week and the use of a compression sleeve during exercise. The authors of the investigation hypothesized that controlled resistance training could improve the functional ability of the affected arm to withstand the insults of daily living. Women in the study ranged from 1 to 15 years following diagnosis.

The intervention program included cardiovascular as well as resistance exercise in a controlled and supervised setting. Exercises were advanced gradually. Results of the study demonstrated that a program of weight lifting did not adversely affect lymphedema in the study participants. Additionally, the results showed that when compared with the control group, women in the intervention (weight-lifting) group reported fewer complaints about their affected arm and hand and had increased overall muscle strength and fewer lymphedema exacerbations following completion of the study.

Lymphatic Drainage Exercises

Lymphatic drainage exercises, often referred to as pumping exercises, move fluids through lymphatic channels. Active, repetitive ROM exercises are performed throughout each session. The exercises follow a specific sequence to move lymph away from congested areas.[19,23,25,26,135] It is similar to the sequence of massage applied during manual lymph drainage.[67,91,113] In general, the exercises first focus on proximal areas of the body to clear central collecting vessels and then involve distal muscle groups to begin to move peripheral edema in a centripetal direction to the central lymph vessels. The affected upper or lower extremity or extremities are held in an elevated position during many of the exercises. Static, dependent postures are avoided. Self-massage also is interspersed throughout the exercise sequence to further enhance drainage. These exercises also maintain mobility of the involved limbs.

Guidelines for Lymphatic Drainage Exercises

The patient should follow these guidelines when performing a sequence of lymphatic drainage exercises. These guidelines apply to management of upper or lower extremity lymphedema and reflect the combined opinions of several authors and experts in the field.[19,23-25,84,135]

Preparation for Lymphatic Drainage Exercises

- Set aside approximately 20 to 30 minutes for each exercise session.
- Perform exercises twice daily every day.
- Have needed equipment at hand, such as a foam roll, wedge, or exercise wand.

During Lymphatic Drainage Exercises

- Wear compression bandages or a customized compression garment if the patient has lymphedema.
- Precede lymphatic drainage exercises with diaphragmatic breathing.
- Follow a specified order of exercises.
- Perform active, repetitive movements slowly, about 1 to 2 seconds per repetition.
- Elevate the involved limb above the heart during distal pumping exercises.
- Combine deep-breathing exercises with active movements of the head, neck, trunk, and limbs.
- Initially, perform a low number of repetitions. Increase repetitions gradually to avoid excessive fatigue.
- Do not exercise to the point at which the edematous limb aches.
- Incorporate self-massage into the exercise sequence to further enhance lymph drainage.
- Maintain good posture during exercises.
- When strengthening exercises are added to the lymph drainage sequence, use light resistance and avoid excessive muscle fatigue.

Follow-Up to Lymphatic Drainage Exercises

- Set aside time several times per week for low-intensity aerobic exercise activities, such as walking or bicycling for 30 minutes.
- Carefully check for signs of redness or increased swelling or reports of aching or throbbing in the edematous limb, any of which could indicate that the level of exercise was excessive.

Selected Exercises for Lymphatic Drainage: Upper and Lower Extremity Sequences

The selection and sequences of exercises described in this section and summarized in Box 26.9 are designed to assist in the drainage of upper or lower extremity lymphedema. Many of the individual exercises suggested in lymphedema protocols, such as ROM of the cervical spine and some of the shoulder girdle or upper extremity exercises, are not exclusively used for lymph drainage. They also are used to improve mobility and strength. Several of the exercises highlighted in this section already have been described in previous chapters in this text. Only those exercises or variations of exercises that are somewhat unique or not previously addressed are described or illustrated in this section.

Sequence of Exercises

- Diaphragmatic breathing is performed prior to lymphatic drainage exercises.
- Exercises for lymphatic drainage should follow a particular sequence to assist lymph flow. The central and proximal lymphatic vessels, such as the abdominal, inguinal, and cervical nodes (see Fig. 26.1), are cleared first with trunk, pelvic, hip, and cervical exercises. Then, for the most part, exercises proceed distally from shoulders to fingers or from hips to toes. If lymph nodes have been surgically removed (e.g., with a unilateral axillary node dissection for breast cancer or a bilateral inguinal node dissection for cancers of the abdominal or pelvic organs), lymph must be channeled to the remaining nodes in the body.

NOTE: Because no single sequence of exercises has been shown to be more effective than another, the upper and lower extremity sequences of exercises outlined in this section do not reflect the exercises included in any one specific protocol. Rather, the exercise sequences are based on the recommendations of numerous authors.[19,23-25,60,80,82,84,112,135] Sequences of exercises for upper or lower extremity lymphedema are summarized in the remaining portion of this chapter. Therapists are encouraged to

BOX 26.9 Sequence of Selected Exercises for Management of Upper or Lower Extremity Lymphedema

Exercises Common to Upper and Lower Extremity Regimens

NOTE: Start an upper or lower extremity regimen with these exercises.

- Deep breathing exercises
- Posterior pelvic tilts and partial curl-ups
- Cervical ROM
- Bilateral scapular movements

Upper Extremity Exercises

- Active circumduction with the involved arm elevated while lying supine
- Bilateral active movements of the arms while lying supine or on a foam roll
- Bilateral hand press while lying supine or sitting
- Shoulder stretches (with wand, doorway, or towel) while standing
- Active elbow, forearm, wrist, and finger exercises of the involved arm
- Bilateral horizontal abduction and adduction of the shoulders
- Overhead wall press while standing
- Finger exercises
- Partial curl-ups
- Rest with involved upper extremity elevated

Lower Extremity Exercises

- Alternate knee to chest exercises
- Bilateral knees to chest
- Gluteal setting and posterior pelvic tilts
- Single knee to chest with the involved lower extremity
- External rotation of the hips while lying supine with both legs elevated and resting on a wedge or wall
- Active knee flexion of the involved lower extremity while lying supine
- Active plantarflexion and dorsiflexion and circumduction of the ankles while lying supine with lower extremities elevated
- Active hip and knee flexion with legs externally rotated and elevated against a wall
- Active cycling and scissoring movements with legs elevated
- Bilateral knee to chest exercises, followed by partial curl-ups
- Rest with lower extremities elevated

modify or add other exercises to the sequences in this chapter as they see fit to meet the individual needs of their patients.

Exercises Common to Upper and Lower Extremity Sequences

These initial exercises should be included in programs for unilateral or bilateral upper or lower extremity lymphedema. They are designed to help the patient relax and then to clear the central channels and nodes.

- ***Diaphragmatic breathing***
  - Have the patient assume a comfortable supine position.
  - Place hands lightly on the abdomen.
  - Inhale deeply through the nose, feeling the abdomen rise against the hands; exhale by blowing air out of the mouth, as if blowing through a straw.
  - Perform diaphragmatic breathing periodically throughout the entire sequence and throughout the day. Avoid breath-holding and the Valsalva maneuver.
- ***Posterior pelvic tilts and partial curl-ups.*** Perform these exercises in the supine position with hips and knees flexed.
- ***Unilateral knee-to-chest movements.*** These exercises are designed to target the inguinal nodes and are important even for upper extremity lymphedema.
  - In the supine position, flex one hip and knee and grasp the lower leg. Pull the knee to the chest. Gently press or bounce the thigh against the abdomen and chest about 15 times.
  - Repeat the procedure with the opposite lower extremity.
  - If lymphedema is present in only one lower extremity, initiate the knee-to-chest exercises with the uninvolved lower extremity.
- ***Cervical ROM.*** Perform each motion for a count of five for five repetitions.
  - Rotation
  - Lateral flexion
- ***Scapular exercises.*** Perform each exercise for a count of five for five repetitions.
  - Active elevation and depression (shoulder shrugs)
  - Active shoulder rolls
  - Active scapular retraction and protraction; with arms at sides and elbows flexed, bilaterally retract the scapulae, pointing elbows posteriorly and medially, and then protract the scapulae

CLINICAL TIP

Be sure to shrug the shoulders as high as possible and then actively pull down the shoulders (depress the scapulae) as far as possible.

Exercises Specifically for Upper Extremity Lymphedema Clearance

The following sequence of exercises is performed after the general, total body exercises just described. The exercises, which are performed in a proximal-to-distal sequence, are done specifically for upper extremity lymph clearance.

CLINICAL TIP

Periodically during the exercise sequence, have the patient perform self-massage to the axillary node area of the *uninvolved* side proceeding from the axilla to the chest.

- ***Active circumduction of the arm (Fig. 26.7).*** While lying supine, flex the involved arm to 90° (reach toward the ceiling) and perform active circular movements of the arm about 6 to 12 in. in diameter. Do this clockwise and counterclockwise, five repetitions in each direction.

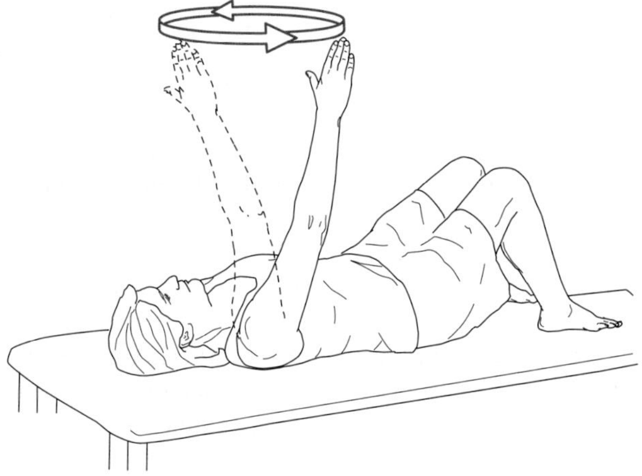

FIGURE 26.7 Active circumduction of the edematous extremity.

PRECAUTION: Avoid pendular motions or circumduction of the edematous upper extremity with the arm in a dependent position.

- ***Exercises on a foam roll (Fig. 26.8).*** While lying supine on a firm foam roll (approximately 6 in. in diameter), perform horizontal abduction and adduction, as well as flexion and extension of the shoulder. These movements target congested axillary nodes and are done unilaterally. For home exercises, if special equipment such as an Ethyfoam® roller is not available, have the patient perform these exercises on a foam pool "noodle." Although the diameter is smaller, a towel or folded sheet can be wrapped around the foam "noodle" to increase the diameter of the roll.

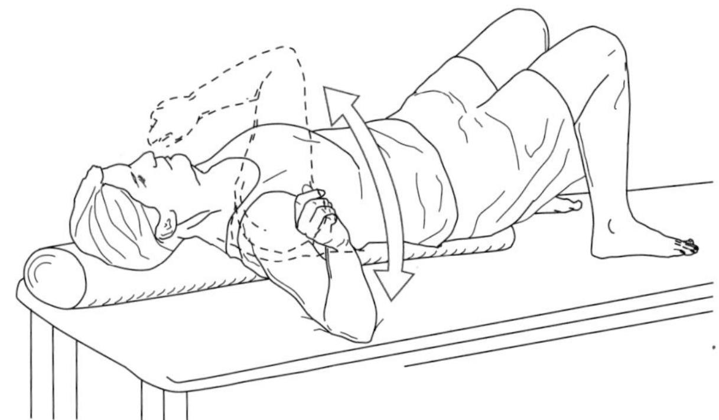

FIGURE 26.8 Active shoulder exercises while lying on a firm, foam roll.

- ***Bilateral hand press.*** With arms elevated to shoulder level or higher and with the elbows flexed, place the palms of the hands together in front of the chest or head. Press the palms together (for an isometric contraction of the pectoralis major muscles) while breathing in for a count of five. Relax, and then repeat as many as five times.
- ***Wand exercise, doorway or corner stretch, and towel stretch.*** Incorporate several exercises to increase shoulder mobility and to decrease congestion and assist lymph flow in the upper extremity. Hold the position of stretch for several seconds with each repetition. These exercises are described and illustrated in Chapter 17.
- ***Unilateral arm exercises with the arm elevated.*** The following exercises are done with the patient seated and the arm supported at shoulder level on a tabletop or countertop or with the patient supine and the arm supported on a wedge or elevated overhead.
  - Shoulder rotation with the elbow extended. Turn the palm up, then down, by rotating the shoulder, not simply pronating and supinating the forearm.
  - Elbow flexion and extension
  - Circumduction of the wrist
  - Hand opening and closing
- ***Bilateral horizontal abduction and horizontal adduction.*** While standing or sitting, place both hands behind the head. Horizontally adduct and abduct the shoulders by bringing the elbows together and then pointing them laterally.
- ***Overhead wall press.*** Face a wall; place one or both palms on the wall with the hands above shoulder level. Gently press the palms into the wall for several seconds without moving the body. Relax, and repeat approximately five times.
- ***Wrist and finger exercises.*** If swelling is present in the wrist and hand, repetitive active finger movements are indicated with the arm elevated.
  - After performing the overhead wall press as just described, keep the heel of the hand on the wall and alternatively move all of the fingers away from and back to the wall (Fig. 26.9).
  - In the same position as just described, alternately press individual fingers into the wall, as if playing a piano, while keeping the heel of the hand in contact with the wall.
  - Place the palms of both hands together with the hands overhead or at least above shoulder level. One finger at a time, press matching fingers together and then pull them away from each other.

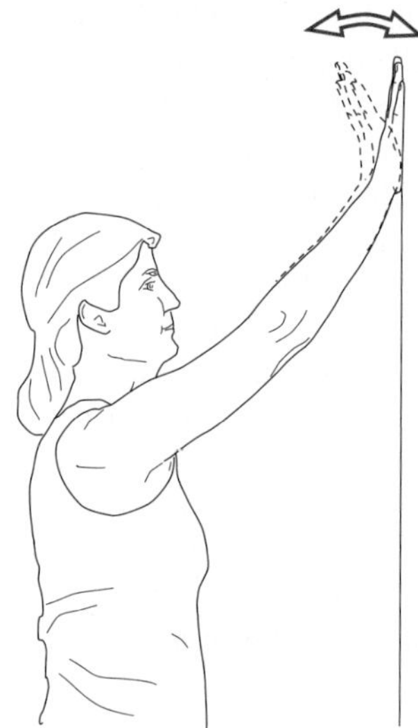

FIGURE 26.9 Overhead wall press.

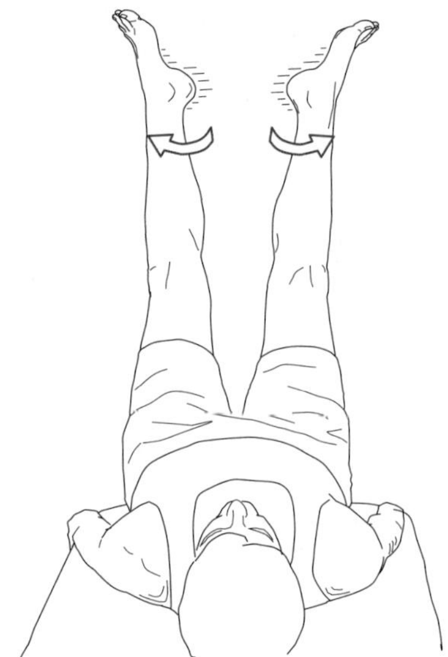

FIGURE 26.10 Repeated outward rotation of the hips with legs elevated and resting on a wall.

- ***Partial curl-ups.*** To complete the exercise sequence, perform additional curl-ups (about five repetitions) with hands sliding on the thighs.
- ***Rest.*** Rest in a supine position with the involved arm elevated on pillows for about 30 minutes after completing the exercise sequence.

Exercises Specifically for Lower Extremity Lymphedema Clearance

NOTE: After completing the general lower body, neck, and shoulder exercises previously described, have the patient perform self-massage first to the axillary lymph nodes on the involved side of the body. Then massage the lower abdominal area superiorly to the waist and then laterally and superiorly to the axillary area of the involved side. This sequence is repeated periodically throughout the lower extremity exercise sequence.

- ***Unilateral knee-to-chest movements.*** In the supine position, repeat this exercise for another 15 repetitions. If lymphedema is present in only one lower extremity, perform repeated knee-to-chest movements with the uninvolved leg first and then the involved leg.
- ***Bilateral knees to chest.*** In the supine position, flex both hips and knees, grasp both thighs, and gently pull them to the abdomen and chest. Repeat 10 to 15 times.
- ***Gluteal setting and posterior pelvic tilts.*** Repeat five times, holding each contraction for several seconds and then slowly releasing.
- ***External rotation of the hips (Fig. 26.10).*** Lie in the supine position with the legs elevated and resting against a wall or on a wedge. Externally rotate the hips, pressing the buttocks together and holding the outwardly rotated position. Repeat several times.
- ***Knee flexion to clear the popliteal area.*** While lying in the supine position and keeping the uninvolved lower extremity extended, flex the involved hip and knee enough to clear the foot from the mat table. Actively flex the knee as far as possible by quickly moving the heel to the buttocks. Repeat approximately 15 times.
- ***Active ankle movements.*** With both legs elevated and propped against a wall, or with just the involved leg propped against a door frame and the uninvolved leg resting on the floor, actively plantarflex the ankle and curl the toes; then dorsiflex the ankle and extend the toes as far as possible for multiple repetitions. Lastly, actively circumduct the foot clockwise and counterclockwise for several repetitions.
- ***Wall slides in external rotation (Fig. 26.11).*** With the feet propped up against the wall, legs externally rotated, and heels touching, slide both feet down the wall as far as possible and then back up the wall for several repetitions.

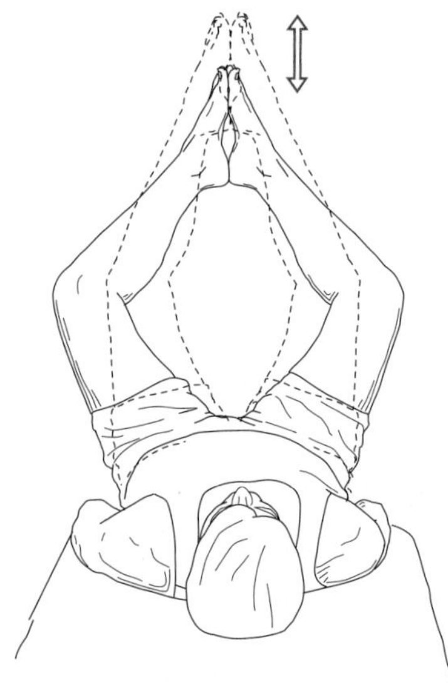

FIGURE 26.11 Sliding feet up and down a wall with hips externally rotated.

- ***Leg movements in the air (Fig. 26.12).*** With both hips flexed and the back flat on the floor and both feet pointed to the ceiling, alternately move the legs, simulating cycling, walking, and scissoring motions.

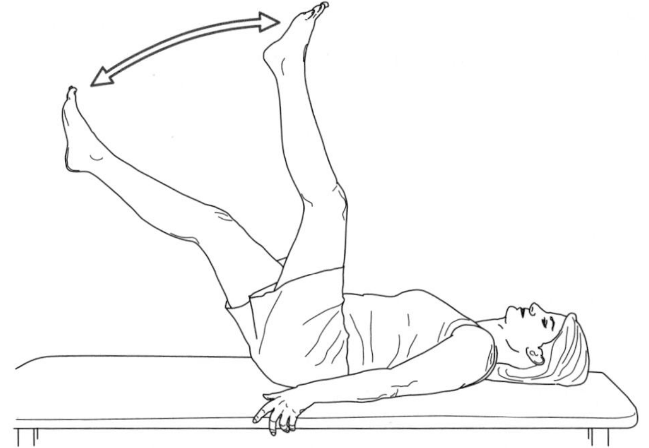

FIGURE 26.12 Repetitive walking movements.

- ***Hip adduction across the midline (Fig. 26.13).*** Lie in the supine position with the uninvolved leg extended. Flex the hip and knee of the involved leg. Grasp the lateral aspect of the knee with the contralateral hand; pull the involved knee repeatedly across the midline in a rocking motion.

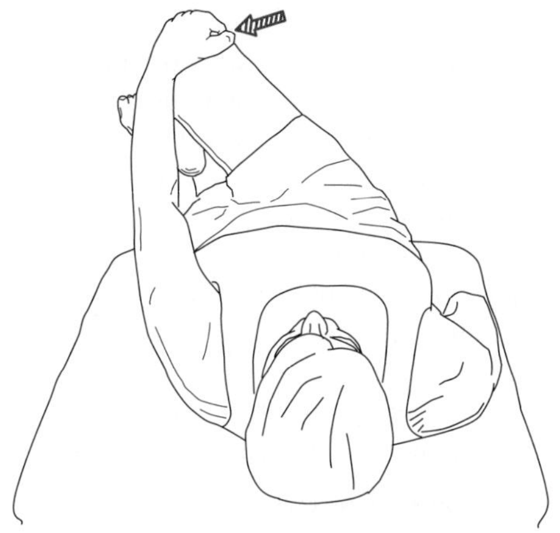

FIGURE 26.13 Hip adduction across the midline to clear inguinal nodes.

NOTE: If lymphedema is bilateral, repeat this exercise with the other lower extremity.

- ***Bilateral knee to chest.*** Repeat bilateral gentle, bouncing movements of the legs previously described.
- ***Partial curl-ups.*** To complete the exercise sequence, perform additional partial curl-ups, about five repetitions.
- ***Rest.*** With feet elevated and legs propped up against the wall, rest in this position for several minutes after completing exercises. Then rest the legs partially elevated on a wedge, and remain in this position for another 30 minutes.

Independent Learning Activities

Critical Thinking and Discussion

1. You have been asked to participate in a patient education program at your community's cancer society for patients who have undergone treatment for breast cancer. Your responsibility in this program is to help breast cancer survivors reduce the risk of physical impairments and functional limitations associated with their surgery and any related adjuvant therapies. Outline the components of such a program, and explain the rationale for the activities you have chosen to include.
2. A patient has developed lymphedema as a result of a right mastectomy 5 years ago. She presents to physical therapy with finger and hand swelling extending proximally to the upper arm. Elevation has not been effective. The tissue is pitting in the hand but hard to palpation in the forearm. Stage this lymphedema and outline a proposed treatment plan describing the pathways that would be used for MLD.
3. Describe the anatomy of the lymphatic system. Explain the terms *transport capacity* and *lymphatic load*.
4. Outline the components of CDT and the relationship between each component. Describe a home management program that corresponds to CDT.

Laboratory Practice

Perform the sequence of exercises and suggested repetitions for the exercise plan you have designed for Case 1, Case 2, and Case 3.

Case Studies

Case 1

Ms. L underwent surgery for metastatic pelvic cancer and lymphadenectomy (lymph node dissection) 3 months ago. She also received a series of radiation therapy treatments as part of her comprehensive oncological management. About 2 weeks ago, she began to notice bilateral swelling in her legs, most notably in her feet and ankles.

She has been referred by her oncologist to the outpatient facility where you work to "evaluate and treat" her for her lymphedema. Describe the examination procedures you would use in your evaluation, and then develop a plan of care, including a program of exercise, to help her manage and reduce her lymphedema and prevent potential complications related to the lymphedema.

Case 2

Mrs. B is a 50-year-old female who recently underwent a lumpectomy and axillary lymph node dissection. She is referred to physical therapy following the removal of her surgical drain. She will be starting chemotherapy shortly, followed by a course of radiation therapy. She reports that prior to her diagnosis and surgery, she was an active individual who enjoyed a variety of recreational activities, including swimming, doubles tennis, and camping, and would like to return to those activities as soon as possible. Design a postoperative exercise program taking into consideration the upcoming chemotherapy and radiation therapy.

Case 3

Ms. H is a 33-year-old female recently diagnosed with stage II breast cancer on her dominant side. Her physician has recommended a mastectomy based on the location and size of the tumor. Ms. H would prefer to conserve her breast but is advised that a lumpectomy would leave her with a less than optimal cosmetic outcome. She is now considering the following options: latissimus dorsi flap, TRAM flap, DIEP flap, or tissue expander with eventual permanent implant. Design a postoperative rehabilitation program for each surgical reconstruction procedure.

REFERENCES

1. Abeloff, MD, et al: Breast. In Abeloff, MD, et al (eds.): *Clinical Oncology,* ed. 2. New York: Churchill Livingstone, 2000, p 2051.
2. Armer, J: The problem of post-breast cancer lymphedema: impact and measurement issues. *Cancer Invest*1:76–83, 2005.
3. Armer, JM, et al: Best-practice guidelines in assessment, risk reduction, management, and surveillance for post-breast cancer lymphedema. *Curr Breast Cancer Rep* 5:134–144, 2013.
4. Bergan, JJ: Effect of cancer therapy on lower extremity lymphedema. *Natl Lymphedema Network Newsletter* 11(1):1999.
5. Bertelli, G, et al: Conservative treatment of postmastectomy lymphedema: a controlled randomized trial. *Am Oncol* 2(8):575–578, 1991.
6. Bicego, D, et al: Exercise for women with or at risk for breast cancer-related lymphedema. *Phys Ther* 86(10):1398–1405, 2006.
7. Boccardo, F, et al: Lymphatic microsurgery to treat lymphedema: techniques and indications for better results. *Ann Plast Surg* Aug;71(2): 191–195, 2013.
8. Boris, M, et al: Lymphedema reduction by noninvasive complex lymphedema therapy. *Oncology* 8(9):95–106, 1994.
9. Boris, M, Weindorf, S, and Lasinski, B: Persistence of lymphedema reduction after noninvasive complex lymphedema therapy. *Oncology* 11(1):99–109, 1997.
10. Boris, M, Weindorf, S, and Lasinski, BB: The risk of genital edema after external pump compression for lower limb lymphedema. *Lymphology* 31(1):15–20, 1998.
11. Brennan, MJ: Lymphedema following the surgical treatment of breast cancer: a review of pathophysiology and treatment. *J Pain Symptom Manage* 7(2):110–116, 1992.
12. Brennan, MJ, DePompodo, RW, and Garden, FH: Focused review: postmastectomy lymphedema. *Arch Phys Med Rehabil* 77(3 Suppl):S74–S80, 1996.
13. Brennan, MJ, and Miller, L: Overview of treatment options in the management of lymphedema. *Cancer* 83(12 Suppl):2821–2827, 1998.
14. Brorson, H, and Freccero, C: Liposuction as a treatment for lymphoedema. *1st Jobst Scientific Symposium*, 2008. Available at http://www.eurolymphology.org/wp-content/uploads/2011/01/5-page-11-25-Brorson-proof-10.pdf. Accessed May 25, 2017.
15. Brorson, H: Liposuction in arm lymphedema treatment. *Scand J Surg* 92:287–295, 2003.
16. Buchholz, TA, Avritscher, R, and Yu, T: Identifying the "sentinel lymph nodes" for arm drainage as a strategy for minimizing the lymphedema risk after breast cancer therapy. *Breast Cancer Res Treat* 116:539–541, 2009.
17. Bunce, IH, et al: Postmastectomy lymphoedema treatment and measurement. *Med J Aust* 161(2):125–128, 1994.
18. Bunke, N, et al: Phlebolymphedema: usually unrecognized, often poorly treated. *Perspect Vasc Surg EndovascTher* 21(2):65–68, 2009.
19. Burt, J, and White, G: *Lymphedema: A Breast Cancer Patient's Guide to Prevention and Healing.* Alameda, CA: Hunter House, 1999.
20. Cameron, MH: *Physical Agents in Rehabilitation: From Research to Practice.* Philadelphia: WB Saunders, 1999.
21. Carroll, JK, et al: Pharmacologic treatment of cancer-related fatigue. *The Oncologist* 12(Suppl 1):43–51, 2007.
22. Casley-Smith, JR: *Exercises for Patients With Lymphedema of the Arm,* ed. 2. Adelaide, Australia: Lymphoedema Association of Australia, 1991.
23. Casley-Smith, JR: *Exercises for Patients With Lymphedema of the Leg,* ed. 2. Adelaide, Australia: Lymphoedema Association of Australia, 1991.
24. Casley-Smith, JR: *Information About Lymphoedema for Patients,* ed. 6. Malvern, Australia: Lymphoedema Association of Australia, 1997.
25. Casley-Smith, JR: Treatment for lymphedema of the arm—The Casley-Smith method. *Cancer* 83(Suppl):2843–2860, 1998.
26. Casley-Smith, JR, and Casley-Smith, JR: Modern treatment of lymphoedema. I. Complex physical therapy: the first 200 Australian limbs. *Aust J Dermatol* 33(2):61–68, 1992.
27. Chang, DW: Lymphaticovenular bypass for lymphedema management in breast cancer patients: a prospective study. *Plast ReconstrSurg* 126(3):752–758, 2010.
28. Chang, DW, Suami, H, and Skoracki, R: A prospective analysis of 100 consecutive lymphovenous bypass cases for treatment of extremity lymphedema. *Plast Reconstr Surg* 132(5):1305–1314, 2013.
29. Connell, M: Complete decongestive therapy. *Innovations Breast Cancer Care* 3:93, 1998.
30. Connor, MP, and Gamelli, R: Challenges of cellulitis in a lymphedematous extremity: a case report. *Cases J* 22(2):9377, 2009.
31. Czerniec, SA, et al: Assessment of breast cancer-related arm lymphedema: comparison of physical measurement methods and self-report. *Cancer Invest*28:54–62, 2010.
32. Daroczy, J: Pathology of lymphedema. *Clin Dermatol* 13(5):433–444, 1995.
33. Eisenhardt, JR: Evaluation and physical treatment of the patient with peripheral vascular disorders. In Irwin, S, and Tecklin, JS (eds): *Cardiopulmonary Physical Therapy,* ed. 3. St. Louis: Mosby Year Book, 1995, pp 215–233.
34. Erickson, V, et al: Arm edema in breast cancer patients. *J Natl Cancer Inst* 93:96–111, 2001.
35. Farrow, W: Phlebolymphedema-a common underdiagnosed and undertreated problem in the wound care clinic. *J Am Col Certif Wound Spec*2(1):14–23, 2010.
36. Földi, M, Földi, E, and Kubik, S: *Textbook of Lymphology.* Müchen: Urban & Fischer/Elsevier, 2003.
37. Forner-Cordero, I, et al: Predictive factors of response to decongestive therapy in patients with breast cancer-related lymphedema. *Ann Surg Oncol* 17:744–751, 2010.
38. Fu, MR, et al: L-DEX Ration in detecting breast cancer-related lymphedema: reliability, sensitivity, and specificity. *Lymphology* 46:85–96, 2013.
39. Fu, MR, et al: Proactive approach to lymphedema risk reduction: a prospective study. *Ann Surg Oncol* 21:3481–3489, 2014.

40. Fu, MR, et al: The effect of providing information about lymphedema on the cognitive and symptom outcomes of breast cancer survivors. *Ann Surg Oncol* 17:1847–1853, 2010.
41. Ganz, PA: The quality of life after breast cancer: solving the problem of lymphedema. *N Engl J Med* 340(5):383–385, 1999.
42. Golshan, G, Martin, WJ, and Dowlatshahi, K: Sentinel lymph node biopsy lowers the rate of lymphedema when compared with standard axillary lymph node dissection. *AmSurg*69:209–212, 2003.
43. Goodman, CC: The female genital/reproductive system. In Goodman, CC, and Fuller, KS (eds): *Pathology: Implications for Physical Therapists,* ed. 3. St Louis: Saunders Elsevier, 2009, pp 986–1036.
44. Goodman, CC: Oncology. In Goodman, CC, and Fuller, KS (eds): *Pathology: Implications for Physical Therapists,* ed. 3. St. Louis: Saunders Elsevier, 2009, pp 348–391.
45. Goodman, CC, and Smirnova, IV: The cardiovascular system. In Goodman, CC, and Fuller, KS (eds): *Pathology: Implications for Physical Therapists,* ed. 3. St Louis: Saunders Elsevier, 2009, pp 519–641.
46. Goodman, CC, and Snyder, TEK: *Differential Diagnosis for Physical Therapists: Screening for Referral,* ed. 4. St Louis: Saunders-Elsevier, 2007.
47. Gudas, SA: Neoplasms of the breast. In Kauffman, TL (ed): *Geriatric Rehabilitation Manual.* New York: Churchill Livingstone, 1999, p 182.
48. Guttman, H, et al: Achievements of physical therapy in patients after modified radical mastectomy compared with quadrantectomy, axillary dissection, and radiation for carcinoma of the breast. *Arch Surg* 125: 389–391, 1990.
49. Hack, TF, et al: Predictors of arm morbidity following breast cancer surgery. *Psychooncology* 19(11):1205–1212, 2010.
50. Hansen, M: *Pathophysiology: Foundations of Disease and Clinical Intervention.* Philadelphia: WB Saunders, 1998.
51. Harwood, CA, and Mortimer, PS: Causes and clinical manifestations of lymphatic failure. *Clin Dermatol* 13(5):459–471, 1995.
52. Hayes, S, Cornish, B, and Newman, B: Comparison of methods to diagnose lymphoedema among breast cancer survivors: 6-month follow-up. *Breast Cancer Res and Treat* 89:221–226, 2005.
53. Hayes, SC, et al: Lymphedema after breast cancer: incidence, risk factors, and effect on upper body function. *J Clin Onc* 26(21):3536–3542, 2008.
54. Helms, G, et al: Shoulder-arm morbidity in patients with sentinel node biopsy and complete axillary dissection: data from a prospective randomized trial. *Eur J Surg Oncol* 35(7):696–701, 2009.
55. Helyer, LK, et al: Obesity is a risk factor for developing postoperative lymphedema in breast cancer patients. *Breast J* 16(1):48–54, 2010.
56. Henderson, IC: Breast cancer. In Murphy, GP, Lawrence, W, and Lenhard, RE (eds): *Clinical Oncology,* ed. 2. Atlanta: American Cancer Society, 1995, p 198.
57. Hetrick, H: Lymphedema complicating healing. In McCulloch, JM, and Kloth, LC (eds): *Wound Healing: Evidence-Based Management,* ed. 4. Philadelphia: F.A. Davis, 2010, pp 279–291.
58. Hewitson, JW: Management of lower extremity lymphedema. *National Lymphedema Network Newsletter* 9(3):1, 1997.
59. Hladiuk, M, et al: Arm function after axillary dissection for breast cancer: a pilot study to provide parameter estimates. *J Surg Oncol* 50(1):47–52, 1992.
60. Holtgrefe, KM: Twice-weekly completed decongestive physical therapy in the management of secondary lymphedema of the lower extremities. *Phys Ther* 86(8):1128–1136, 2006.
61. Iltis, M: Cancer chemotherapy toxicity guidelines for the physical therapist. *Rehabil Oncol* 4(3):1986.
62. International Society of Lymphology: 2013 consensus document of the diagnosis and treatment of peripheral lymphedema. *Lymphology* 46:1–11, 2013.
63. Iyigun, ZE, et al: Bioelectrical impedance for detecting and monitoring lymphedema in patients with breast cancer. Preliminary results of the Florence Nightingale Breast Study Group. *Lymphat ResBiol* 13(1):40–45, March 2015.
64. Keeley, VL: Lymphoedema and cellulitis: chicken or egg? *Br J Dermatol* 158(6):1175–1176, 2008.
65. Kelly, DG: Vascular, lymphatic, and integumentary disorders. In O'Sullivan, SB, Schmitz, TJ, and Fulk, GD (eds): *Physical Rehabilitation,* ed. 6. Philadelphia: F.A. Davis, 2014, pp 577–633.
66. Kepics, J: Treatment of axillary web syndrome: a case report using manual techniques. *Dr. Vodder School International.* Available at www.vodderschool.com/treatment_of_axillary_web_syndrome. Accessed May 25, 2017.
67. Kurtz, I: *Textbook of Dr. Vodder's Manual Lymphatic Drainage, Vol 2. Therapy,* ed. 2. Heidelberg: Karl F. Haug, 1989.
68. Lamp, S, and Lester, J: Reconstruction of the breast following mastectomy. *Semin Oncol Nurs*31(2):134–145, 2015.
69. Lasinski, B: The lymphatic system. In Goodman, CC, and Fuller, KS (eds): *Pathology: Implications for Physical Therapists,* ed. 3. St Louis: Saunders Elsevier, 2009, pp 642–677.
70. Lawenda, BD, Mondry, TE, and Johnstone, PA: Lymphedema: a primer on the identification and management of a chronic condition in oncologic treatment. *CA Cancer J Clin* 59(1):8–24, 2009.
71. Lawenda, BD, and Mondry, TE: The effects of radiation therapy on the lymphatic system: acute and latent effects. *Natl Lymphedema Netw Newslett* 20(3):1–5, 2008.
72. Lemieux, J, Bordeleau, LJ, and Goodwin, PJ: Medical, psychosocial, and health-related quality of life issues in breast cancer survivors. In Ganz, P (ed): *Cancer Survivorship.* New York: Springer Science+Business Media, LLC, 2007, pp 122–144.
73. Lerner, R: What's new in lymphedema therapy in America? *Int J Angiol* 7(3):191–196, 1998.
74. Logan, V: Incidence and prevalence of lymphedema: a literature review. *J Clin Nurs* 4(4):213–219, 1995.
75. Mason, M: The treatment of lymphoedema by complex physical therapy. *Aust J Physiother* 39:41–45, 1993.
76. Matthews, K, and Smith, J: Effectiveness of modified complex physical therapy for lymphoedema treatment. *Aust J Physiother* 42(4):323–328, 1996.
77. Mayrovitz, HN: Interface pressures produced by two different types of lymphedema therapy devices. *Phys Ther* 87(10):1379–1388, 2007.
78. Mayrovitz, HN: The standard of care for lymphedema: current concepts and physiological considerations. *Lymphat Res Biol* 7(2):101–108, 2009.
79. McGarvey, CL: Pneumatic compression devices for lymphedema. *Rehabil Oncol* 10:16–17, 1992.
80. McKenzie, DC, and Kalda, AL: Effect of upper extremity exercise on secondary lymphedema in breast cancer patients: a pilot study. *J Clin Oncol* 21:463–466, 2003.
81. McLaughlin, SA, et al: Prevalence of lymphedema in women with breast cancer 5 years after sentinel lymph node biopsy or axillary dissection: objective measurements. *J Clin Oncol* 26(32):5213–5219, 2008.
82. Megens, A, and Harris, S: Physical therapist management of lymphedema following treatment for breast cancer: a critical review of its effectiveness. *Phys Ther* 78(12):1302–1311, 1998.
83. Meneses-Echavez, JF: Effects of supervised exercise on cancer related fatigue in breast cancer survivors: A systematic review and meta-analysis. *BMC Cancer* 21(Feb):77, 2015.
84. Miller, LT: Exercise in the management of breast cancer-related lymphedema. *Innovations Breast Cancer Care* 3(4):101–106, 1998.
85. Miller, LT: The enigma of exercise: participation in an exercise program after breast cancer surgery. *Natl Lymphedema Netw Newslett* 8(4): 1996.
86. Mortimer, PS, et al: New developments in clinical aspects of lymphatic disease. *JClin Invest*124(3):915–921, 2014.
87. Moskovitz, AH, et al: Axillary web syndrome after axillary dissection. *Am J Surg* 181(5):434–439, 2001.
88. Mustian, KM, et al: Integrative nonpharmacologic behavioral interventions for the management of cancer related fatigue. *The Oncologist* 12(Suppl 1):52–67, 2007.
89. National Comprehensive Cancer Network: *NCCN Practice Guidelines in Oncology: Cancer-Related Fatigue,* V.2., 2007. Available at www.nccn.org. Accessed May 25, 2017.
90. National Comprehensive Cancer Network: *NCCN Practice Guidelines in Oncology: Invasive Breast Cancer—Principles of Radiation Therapy,* V.2, 2010. Available at www.nccn.org. Accessed March 23, 2010.

91. National Lymphedema Network: Position statement: exercise. Nov 2013. Available at www.lymphnet.org. Accessed May 25, 2017.
92. National Lymphedema Network: Position statement: lymphedema risk reduction practices. May 2012. Available at www.lymphnet.org. Accessed January 8, 2010.
93. Norman, SA, et al: Development and validation of a telephone questionnaire to characterize lymphedema in women treated for breast cancer. *Phys Ther* 81(6):1192–1205, 2001.
94. Paskett, ED, et al: The epidemiology of arm and hand swelling in premenopausal breast cancer survivors. *Cancer Epidemiol Biomarkers Prev* 16(4):775–782, 2007.
95. Patel, KM, et al: A prospective evaluation of lymphedema-specific quality-of-life outcomes following vascularized lymph node transfer. *Ann Surg Oncol* 22(7):2424–2430, July 2015.
96. Peters, K, et al: Lower leg subcutaneous blood flow during walking and passive dependency in chronic venous insufficiency. *Br J Dermatol* 124(2):177–180, 1991.
97. Piper, M, et al. Oncoplastic breast surgery: current strategies. *Gland Surgery* 4(2):154–163, 2015.
98. Price, J, and Purtell, J: Teaming up to prevent and treat lymphedema. *Am J Nurs* 7(9):23, 1997.
99. Ridner, SH, et al: Bioelectric impedance for detecting upper limb lymphedema in nonlaboratory settings. *Lymphat Res Biol* 7(1):11–15, 2009.
100. Rockson, SG: The unique biology of lymphatic edema. *LymphatRes Biol* 7(2):97–100, 2009.
101. Rockson, SG: Secondary lymphedema of the lower extremities. *Natl Lymphedema Network Newsletter* 10(3):1–3, 1998.
102. Rockson, SG, et al: Diagnosis and management of lymphedema. *Cancer* 83(Suppl):2882–2885, 1998.
103. Ross, C: Complex physical therapy: a treatment note. *NZ J Physiother* 22(3):19–21, 1994.
104. Schmitz, KH, et al: Weight lifting in women with breast-cancer-related lymphedema. *N Engl J Med* 361(7):664–673, 2009.
105. Schuchhardt, C, Pritschow, H, and Weissleder, H: Therapy concepts. In Weissleder, H, and Schuchhardt, C (eds): *Lymphedema Diagnosis and Therapy.* Koln, Germany: Viavital, 2001, pp 336–362.
106. Sener, SF, et al: Lymphedema after sentinel lymphadenectomy for breast carcinoma. *Cancer* 92(4):748–752, 2001.
107. Simonian, SJ, et al: Differential diagnosis of lymphedema. In Tretbar, LL, Morgan, CL, Lee, BB, Simonian, SJ, and Blandeau, B (eds): *Lymphedema: Diagnosis and Treatment.* London: Springer, 2008, pp 12–20.
108. Soran, A, et al: The importance of detection of subclinical lymphedema for the prevention of breast cancer-related clinical lymphedema after axillary lymph node dissection: A prospective observational study. *Lymph Res and Biol* 12(4): 289–294, 2014.
109. Springer, BA, et al: Pre-operative assessment enables early diagnosis and recovery of shoulder function in patients with breast cancer. *Breast Cancer Res Treat* 120(1):135–147, 2010.
110. Suami, H, and Chang, DW: Overview of surgical treatments for breast cancer-related lymphedema. *PlastReconstr Surg* 126(6):1853–1863, 2010.
111. Swirsky, J, and Nannery, DS: *Coping with Lymphedema.* Garden City Park, NY: Avery Publishing, 1998.
112. Szuba, A, Achalu, R, and Rockson, SG: Decongestive lymphatic therapy for patients with breast carcinoma-associated lymphedema: a randomized, prospective study of a role for adjunctive intermittent pneumatic compression. *Cancer* 95:2260–2267, 2002.
113. Tappan, FM, and Benjamin, PJ: *Tappan's Handbook of Healing Massage.* Stamford, CT: Appleton & Lange, 1998.
114. Taylor, R, et al: Reliability and validity of arm volume measurements for assessment of lymphedema. *Phys Ther* 86(2):205–214, 2006.
115. Teixeira, L, and Sandrin, F: The role of physiotherapy in the plastic surgery patients after oncological breast surgery. *Gland Surgery* 3(1): 43–47, 2014.
116. Togawa, K: Risk factors for self-reported arm lymphedema among female breast cancer survivors: a prospective cohort study. *Breast Cancer Res*16:414, 201.
117. Tsai, RJ, et al: The risk of developing arm lymphedema among breast cancer survivors: a meta-analysis of treatment factors. *Ann Surg Oncol* 16(7):1959–1972, 2009.
118. Verbelen, H, et al: Shoulder and arm morbidity in sentinel node-negative breast cancer patients: a systematic review. *Breast Cancer Res Treatment* 144:21–31, 2014.
119. Voutsadakis, IA, and Spadafora, S: Axillary lymph node management in breast cancer with positive sentinel lymph node biopsy. *World JClin Oncol* 6(1):1–6, 2015.
120. Walrath, J, et al: Axillary web syndrome: a complication of breast cancer: what the orthopaedic physical therapist needs to know. *Orthopaedic Practice* 27(2):94–103, 2015.
121. Walton, J: The effects of radiotherapy: their relationship to rehabilitation.*Rehabil Oncol*5(1&2):1987.
122. Ward, LC, Czerniec, S, and Kilbreath, SL: Operational equivalence of bioimpedance indices and perometry for the assessment of unilateral arm lymphedema. *Lymphat Res Biol* 7(2):81–85, 2009.
123. Weiss, JM: Treatment of leg edema and wounds in patients with severe musculoskeletal injuries. *Phys Ther* 78(10):1104–1013, 1998.
124. Weissleder, H, and Schuchhardt, C: Primary lymphedema. In Weissleder, H, and Schuchhardt, C (eds.): *Lymphedema Diagnosis and Therapy.* Koln, Germany: Viavital, 2001, pp 98–113.
125. Weissleder, H: Examination methods. In Weissleder, H, and Schuchhardt, C (eds): *Lymphedema Diagnosis and Therapy.* Koln, Germany: Viavital, 2001, pp 49–90.
126. Wingate, L: Efficacy of physical therapy for patients who have undergone mastectomies. *Phys Ther* 65(6):896–900, 1985.
127. Wingate, L, et al: Rehabilitation of the mastectomy patient: a randomized, blind, prospective study. *Arch Phys Med Rehabil* 70:21–24, 1989.
128. Wittlinger, H, and Wittlinger, G (eds.): *Textbook of Dr. Vodder's Manuel Lymphatic Drainage,* ed. 5. Brussels: Haug International, English version (translated by Harris, R), 1992.
129. Woo, PCY, et al: Cellulitis complicating lymphedema. *Eur J Clin Microbiol Infect Dis* 19(4):294–297, 2000.
130. Woods, EN: Reaching out to patients with breast cancer. *Clin Manage Phys Ther* 12:58–63, 1992.
131. Yeung, WM, et al: A systematic review of axillary web syndrome (AWS). *J Cancer Surviv* 9(4):576–598, 2015. .
132. Zaleska, M, et al: Pressures and timing of intermittent pneumatic compression devices for efficient tissue fluid and lymph flow in limbs with lymphedema. *Lymphat Res Biol*11(4):227–232, 2013.
133. Zawieja, DC: Proceedings of a mini-symposium: Lymphedema—an overview of the biology, diagnosis, and treatment of the disease (contractile physiology of lymphatics). *Lymphat Res Biol* 7(2):87, 2009.
134. Zuther, JE: Treatment of lymphedema with complete decongestive physiotherapy. *Natl Lymphedema Netw Newslett* 2(2):1999.
135. Zuther, JE, and Norton, S: *Lymphedema Management: A Comprehensive Guide for Practitioners,* ed. 3. New York: Thieme, 2013.

Index

Note: Page numbers followed by f indicate figures; t, tables.

B

D

F

G

H

I

J

K

L

N

O

P

Q

R

S

T

U

V

W

Y

Z